DIAGNOSTIC PATHOLOGY

Neoplastic Dermatopathology

SECOND EDITION

CASSARINO | DADRAS

LINDBERG · KO · BILLINGS · AUERBACH

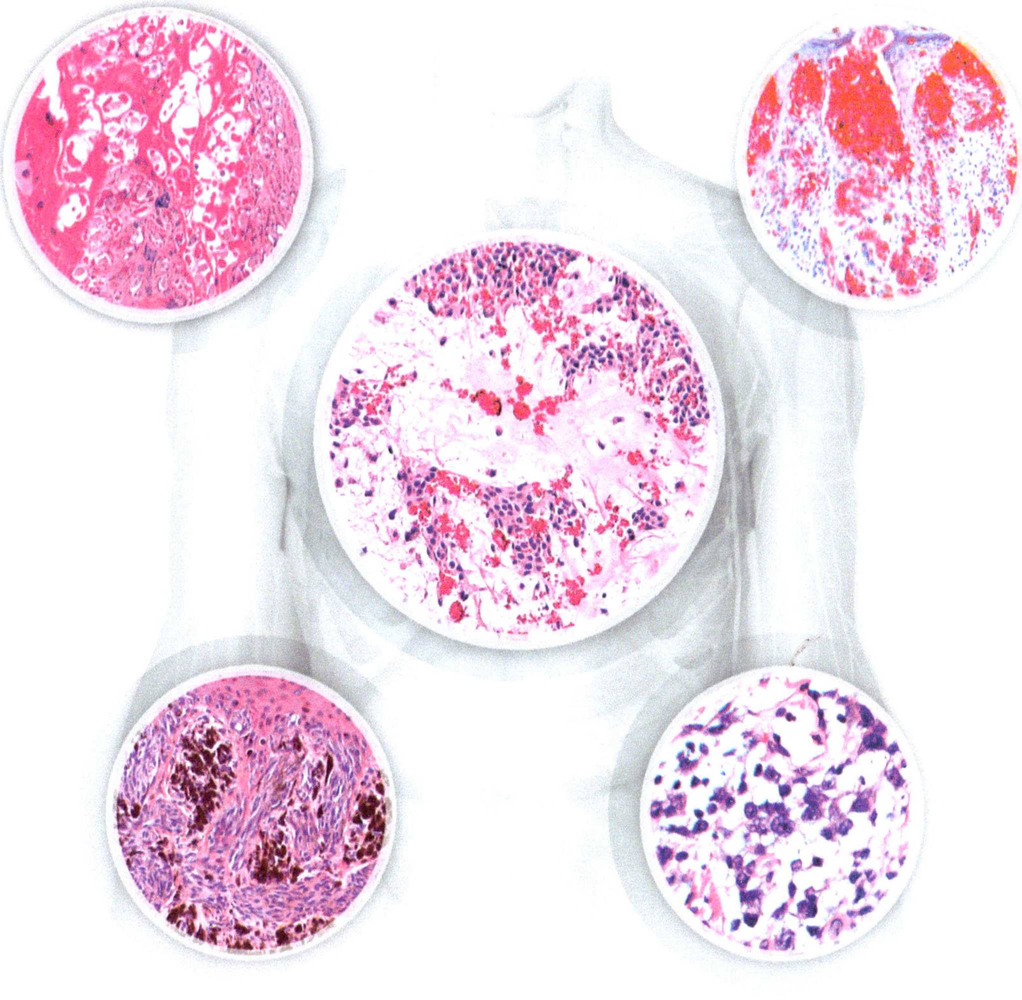

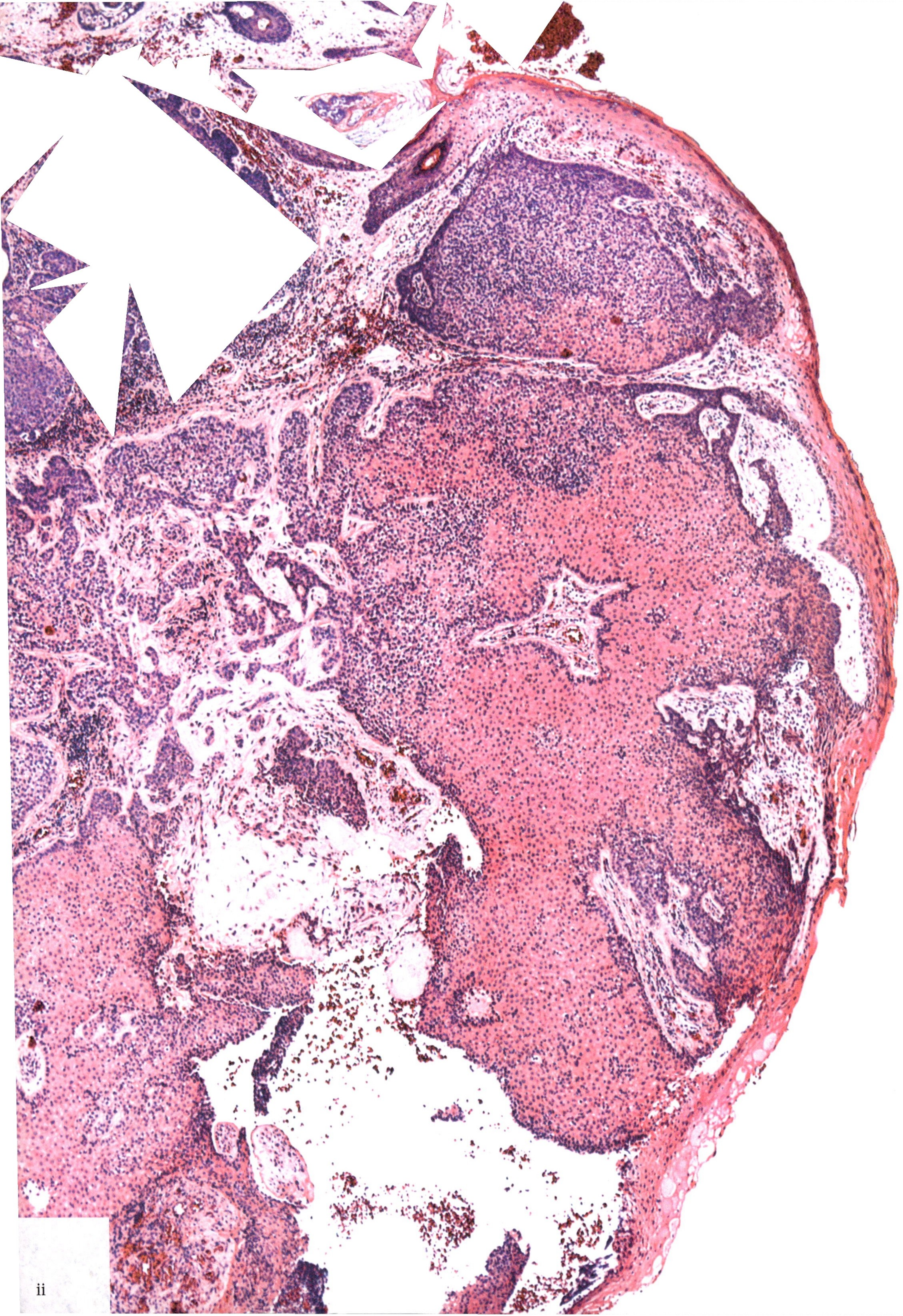
ii

DIAGNOSTIC PATHOLOGY

Neoplastic Dermatopathology

SECOND EDITION

David S. Cassarino, MD, PhD

Consultant Dermatopathologist and Staff Pathologist
Southern California Permanente Medical Group
Los Angeles, California
Clinical Professor
Department of Dermatology
University of California, Irvine
Irvine, California

Soheil Sam Dadras, MD, PhD

Associate Professor of Dermatology
Departments of Dermatology,
Pathology, and Genetics and Genomic Sciences
UConn Health
Farmington, Connecticut

Matthew R. Lindberg, MD
Assistant Professor
Department of Pathology
University of Arkansas for Medical Sciences
Little Rock, Arkansas

Christine J. Ko, MD
Professor of Dermatology and Pathology
Yale University
New Haven, Connecticut

Steven D. Billings, MD
Co-Director, Dermatopathology Section
Department of Pathology
Cleveland Clinic
Cleveland, Ohio

Aaron Auerbach, MD, MPH
Staff Pathologist
Department of Hematopathology
The Joint Pathology Center
Bethesda, Maryland

ELSEVIER

1600 John F. Kennedy Blvd.
Ste 1800
Philadelphia, PA 19103-2899

DIAGNOSTIC PATHOLOGY: NEOPLASTIC DERMATOPATHOLOGY, SECOND EDITION ISBN: 978-0-323-44310-4

Notices

Knowledge and best practice in this field are constantly changing. As new research and experience broaden our understanding, changes in research methods, professional practices, or medical treatment may become necessary.

Practitioners and researchers must always rely on their own experience and knowledge in evaluating and using any information, methods, compounds, or experiments described herein. In using such information or methods they should be mindful of their own safety and the safety of others, including parties for whom they have a professional responsibility.

With respect to any drug or pharmaceutical products identified, readers are advised to check the most current information provided (i) on procedures featured or (ii) by the manufacturer of each product to be administered, to verify the recommended dose or formula, the method and duration of administration, and contraindications. It is the responsibility of practitioners, relying on their own experience and knowledge of their patients, to make diagnoses, to determine dosages and the best treatment for each individual patient, and to take all appropriate safety precautions.

To the fullest extent of the law, neither the Publisher nor the authors, contributors, or editors, assume any liability for any injury and/or damage to persons or property as a matter of products liability, negligence or otherwise, or from any use or operation of any methods, products, instructions, or ideas contained in the material herein.

The opinions and assertions herein are the private views of the authors and are not to be construed as official or as reflecting the views of the Department of the Army or the Department of Defense.

Publisher Cataloging-in-Publication Data

Names: Cassarino, David. | Dadras, Soheil Sam.
Title: Diagnostic pathology. Neoplastic dermatopathology / [edited by] David Cassarino and Soheil Sam Dadras.
Other titles: Neoplastic dermatopathology.
Description: Second edition. | Salt Lake City, UT : Elsevier, Inc., [2016] | Includes bibliographical references and index.
Identifiers: ISBN 978-0-323-44310-4
Subjects: LCSH: Skin--Tumors--Diagnosis--Handbooks, manuals, etc. | MESH: Skin Neoplasms--pathology--Atlases. | Skin Neoplasms--diagnosis--Atlases.
Classification: LCC RC280.S5 D53 2016 | NLM WR 17 | DDC 616.99'477--dc23

International Standard Book Number: 978-0-323-44310-4

Cover Designer: Tom M. Olson, BA

Printed in the United States of America by King Printing Co., Inc.

Last digit is the print number: 9 8 7 6 5 4 3

Dedications

To my beautiful wife, Lulit, and my exasperating and inspiring children, Carmella, Marcus, and Azarius.

DSC

I am indebted to my parents, Mercedeh and Mojtaba, for having sacrificed much so I could seek higher education. I am grateful to my wife, Hanan, for putting up with my working long hours.

SSD

To my wife, Rani, for her love and support.

MRL

To Peter, Dylan, and Owen.

CJK

I would like to thank my family for their continued support and my residents and fellows who teach me so much.

SDB

In loving memory of Romeo. With inspiration from Suzann, Ann, Donald, Shayna-Jahna, Ben and Zachary, Hal and Laurie.

AA

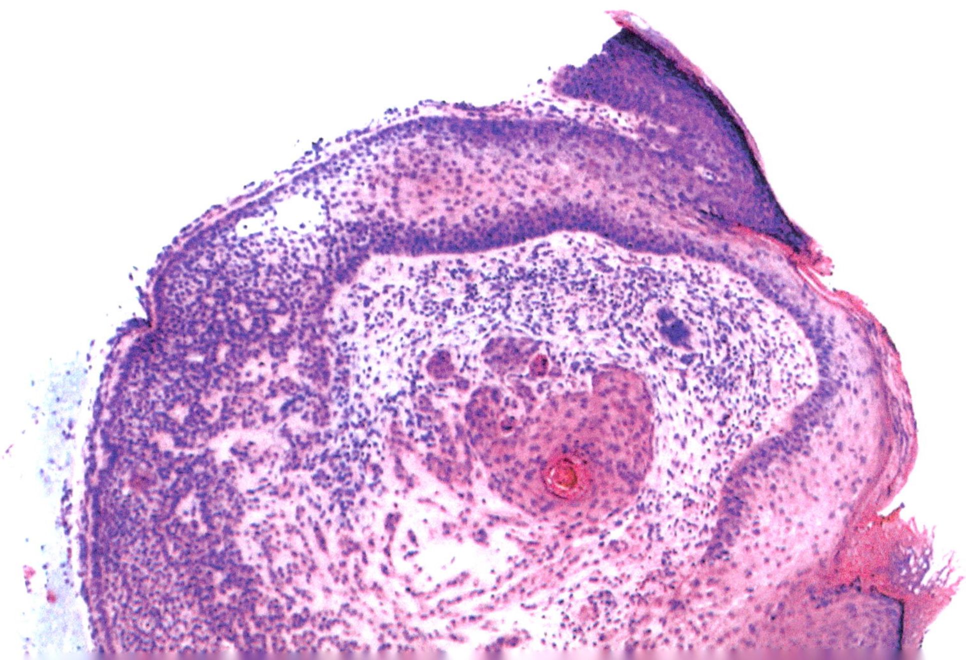

Contributing Authors

Elsa F. Velazquez, MD
Director of Dermatopathology
Miraca Life Sciences
Assistant Professor of Dermatology
Director of the Dermatopathology Fellowship Program
Tufts University School of Medicine
Boston, Massachusetts

Elizabeth A. Montgomery, MD
Professor of Pathology and Oncology
and Orthopedic Surgery
Johns Hopkins University Medical Institutions
Baltimore, Maryland

Hyemin Pomerantz, MD
Resident Physician
Department of Dermatology
Hofstra Northwell School of Medicine
Manhasset, New York

Jeremy C. Wallentine, MD
Staff Pathologist
Intermountain Healthcare and
Utah Pathology Services, Inc.
Intermountain Medical Center
Salt Lake City, Utah

Lester D. R. Thompson, MD
Consultant Pathologist
Southern California Permanente Medical Group
Woodland Hills, California

Senait W. Dyson, MD
Dermatopathologist
Dyson Dermatology, PLLC
Tucson, Arizona

Jerad M. Gardner, MD
Assistant Professor of Pathology and Dermatology
Program Director, Dermatopathology Fellowship
University of Arkansas for Medical Sciences
Little Rock, Arkansas

Cyril Fisher, MD, DSc, FRCPath
Consultant Histopathologist
Royal Marsden NHS Foundation Trust
Professor of Tumour Pathology
Institute of Cancer Research
University of London
London, United Kingdom

Jessica M. Comstock, MD
Assistant Professor
University of Utah Department of Pathology
Division of Pediatric Pathology
Primary Children's Hospital
Salt Lake City, Utah

Sa A. Wang, MD
Associate Professor
Department of Hematopathology
The University of Texas MD Anderson Cancer Center
Houston, Texas

Amitabh Srivastava, MD
Associate Professor of Pathology
Harvard Medical School
Associate Director, Surgical Pathology
Director, Surgical Pathology Fellowship Program
Brigham and Women's Hospital
Boston, Massachusetts

Artur Zembowicz, MD, PhD
Professor of Anatomic and Clinical Pathology
Tufts Medical School
Senior Staff
Lahey Clinic
Burlington, Massachusetts
Medical Director
Dermatopathology Consultations, LLC
Needham, Massachusetts

David Lucas, MD
Professor of Pathology
Department of Pathology
University of Michigan Medical School
Ann Arbor, Michigan

Thomas Mentzel, MD
Dermatopathology Bodensee
Associated Professor, Department of Pathology
University of Freiburg, Germany
Friedrichshafen, Germany

Susan Müller, DMD, MS
Atlanta Oral Pathology
Professor Emeritus
Department of Otolaryngology,
Head and Neck Surgery
Emory University School of Medicine
Atlanta, Georgia

Khin Thway, MD, FRCPath
Consultant Histopathologist
Sarcoma Unit
Royal Marsden Hospital
London, United Kingdom

Francisco Vega, MD, PhD
Professor of Pathology
Professor of Medicine
Director of Hematopathology
Department of Pathology and Laboratory Medicine
University of Miami/Sylvester
Comprehensive Cancer Center
Miami, Florida

Cary Chisholm, MD
Dermatopathologist
Central Texas Pathology Laboratory
Waco, Texas

Brenda L. Nelson, DDS, MS
Consulting Pathologist
Naval Medical Center, San Diego
San Diego, California

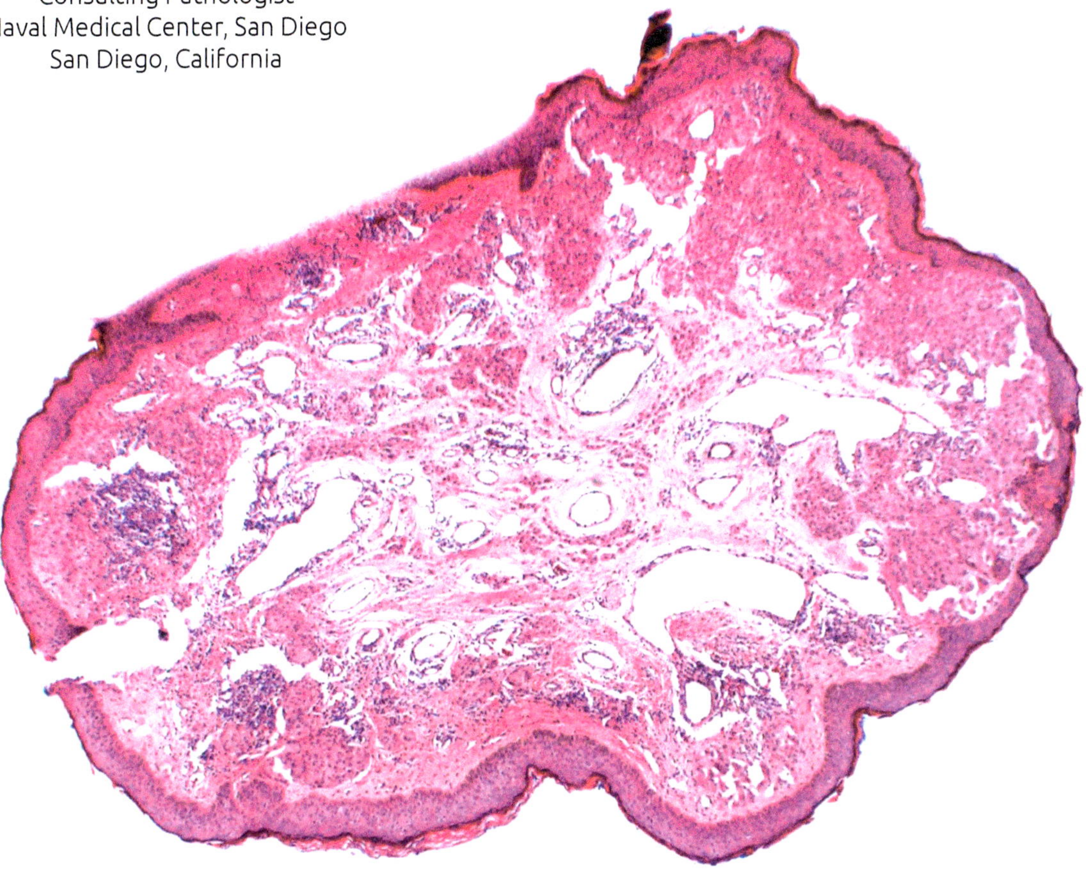

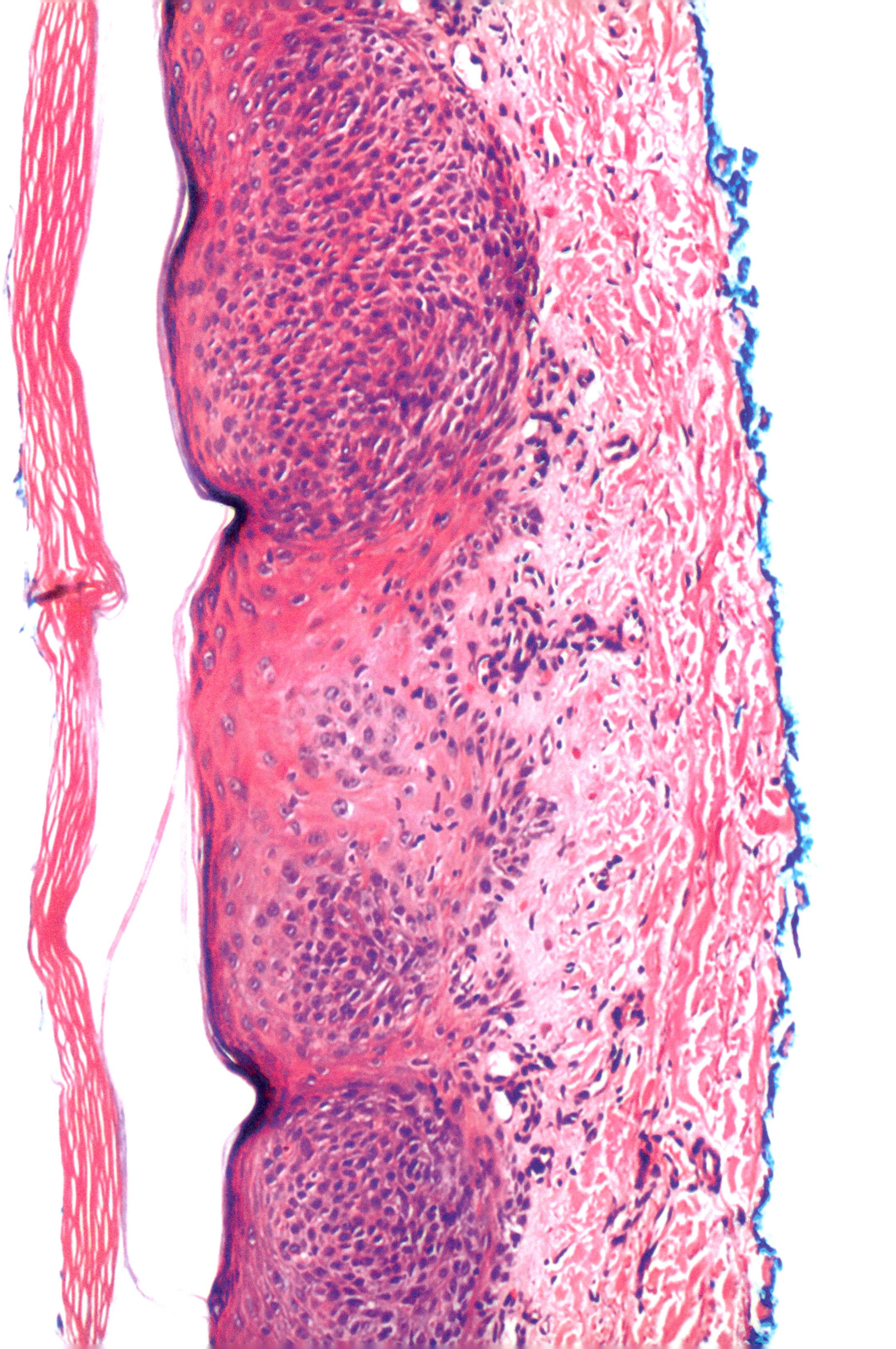

Preface

Cutaneous neoplasms include a wide array of benign and malignant proliferations showing diverse etiology and differentiation. Many unusual and rare tumors unique to the skin have been described, and many proliferations more commonly seen in other organ systems, especially soft tissue and lymphatic tumors, can also involve the skin either primarily or secondarily. Many of these entities can be difficult to precisely classify, as they may show overlapping features with other tumors in the differential and can prove challenging for general pathologists, dermatologists, and even dermatopathologists in some cases. This second edition of *Diagnostic Pathology: Neoplastic Dermatopathology* is designed as a concise, practical, and richly illustrated reference covering the broad array of cutaneous neoplasms and their differential diagnoses to allow for accurate interpretation and diagnosis.

Although there are many dermatopathology textbooks currently available, they are mostly traditional textbooks written in a paragraph-based format, with relatively few clinical and histologic photographs. In contrast, this book is lavishly illustrated and written in a detailed yet concise bulleted format, which facilitates the reader's ability to quickly find relevant information. Each chapter includes critical information such as definitions, etiology/pathogenesis, epidemiology, clinical presentation, prognosis and treatment, histologic findings, ancillary techniques including immunohistochemistry and molecular pathology, differential diagnosis, and pathologic interpretation pearls. In addition, current CAP-approved staging protocols for tumors, including melanoma and squamous cell carcinoma, are also included for reference. Moreover, the carefully annotated histological images focus on the histopathological features, making them readily recognizable.

As in other subspecialities of pathology, there is a rapidly growing body of knowledge in dermatopathology, including new diagnostic immunohistochemical, molecular, and genetic techniques, making it difficult for any textbook to remain fully up to date. To that end, this book includes Expert Consult, an ebook that provides users access to relevant topics, fully searchable text, and a complete listing of antibodies.

We hope that *Diagnostic Pathology: Neoplastic Dermatopathology*, Second Edition will be a useful and valuable reference for in-training and practicing pathologists, dermatologists, and dermatopathologists.

David S. Cassarino, MD, PhD
Consultant Dermatopathologist and Staff Pathologist
Southern California Permanente Medical Group
Los Angeles, California
Clinical Professor
Department of Dermatology
University of California, Irvine
Irvine, California

Soheil Sam Dadras, MD, PhD
Associate Professor of Dermatology
Departments of Dermatology, Pathology, and Genetics and Genomic Sciences
UConn Health Center
Farmington, Connecticut

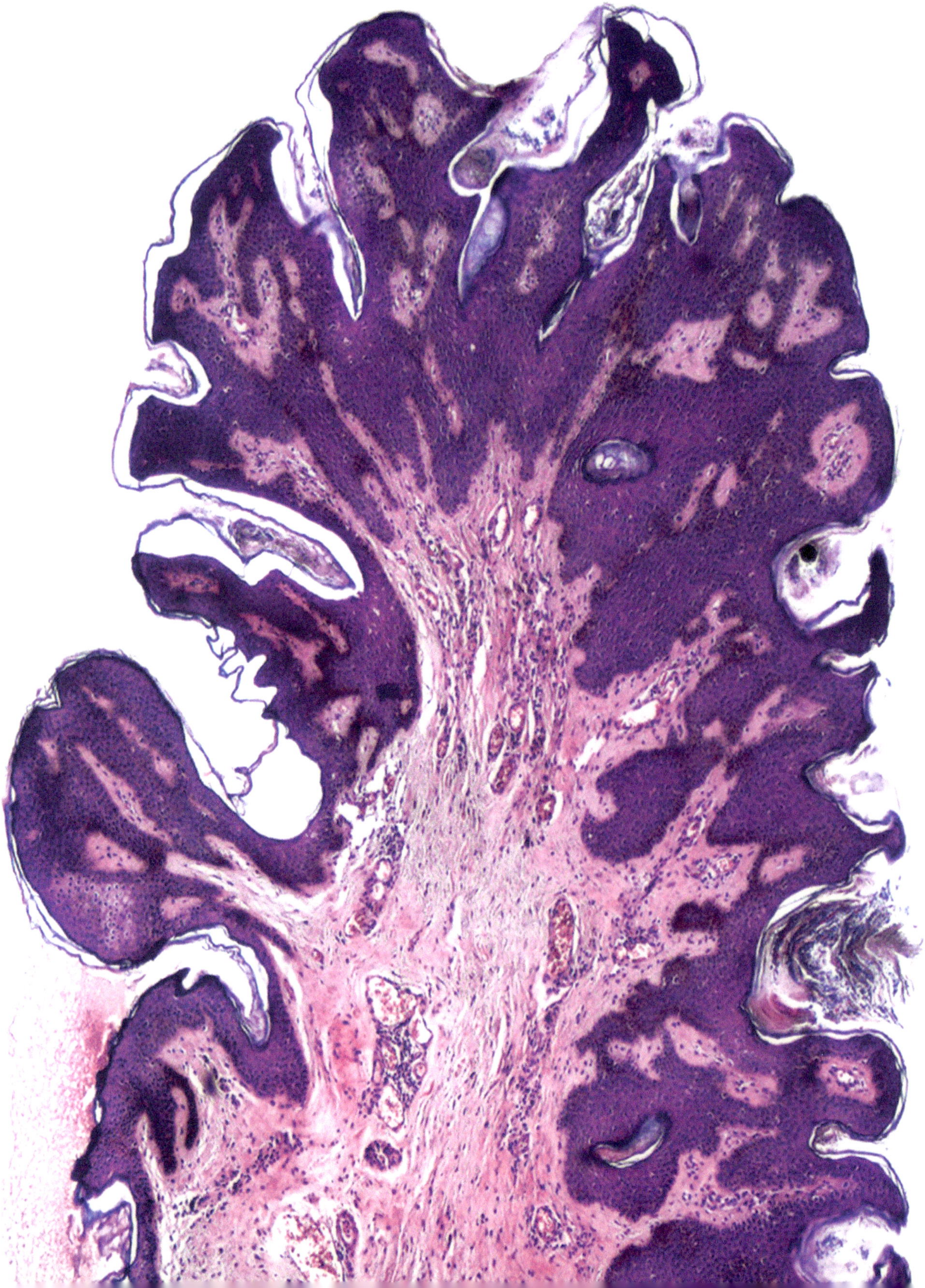

Acknowledgments

Text Editors

Arthur Gelsinger, MA
Nina I. Bennett, BA
Tricia L. Cannon, BA
Lisa A. Gervais, BS
Karen E. Concannon, MA, PhD
Matt W. Hoecherl, BS

Image Editors

Jeffrey J. Marmorstone, BS
Lisa A. M. Steadman, BS

Illustrations

Laura C. Sesto, MA
Lane R. Bennion, MS
Richard Coombs, MS

Art Direction and Design

Tom M. Olson, BA
Laura C. Sesto, MA

Lead Editor

Terry W. Ferrell, MS

Production Coordinators

Angela M. G. Terry, BA
Rebecca L. Hutchinson, BA
Emily Fassett, BA

ELSEVIER

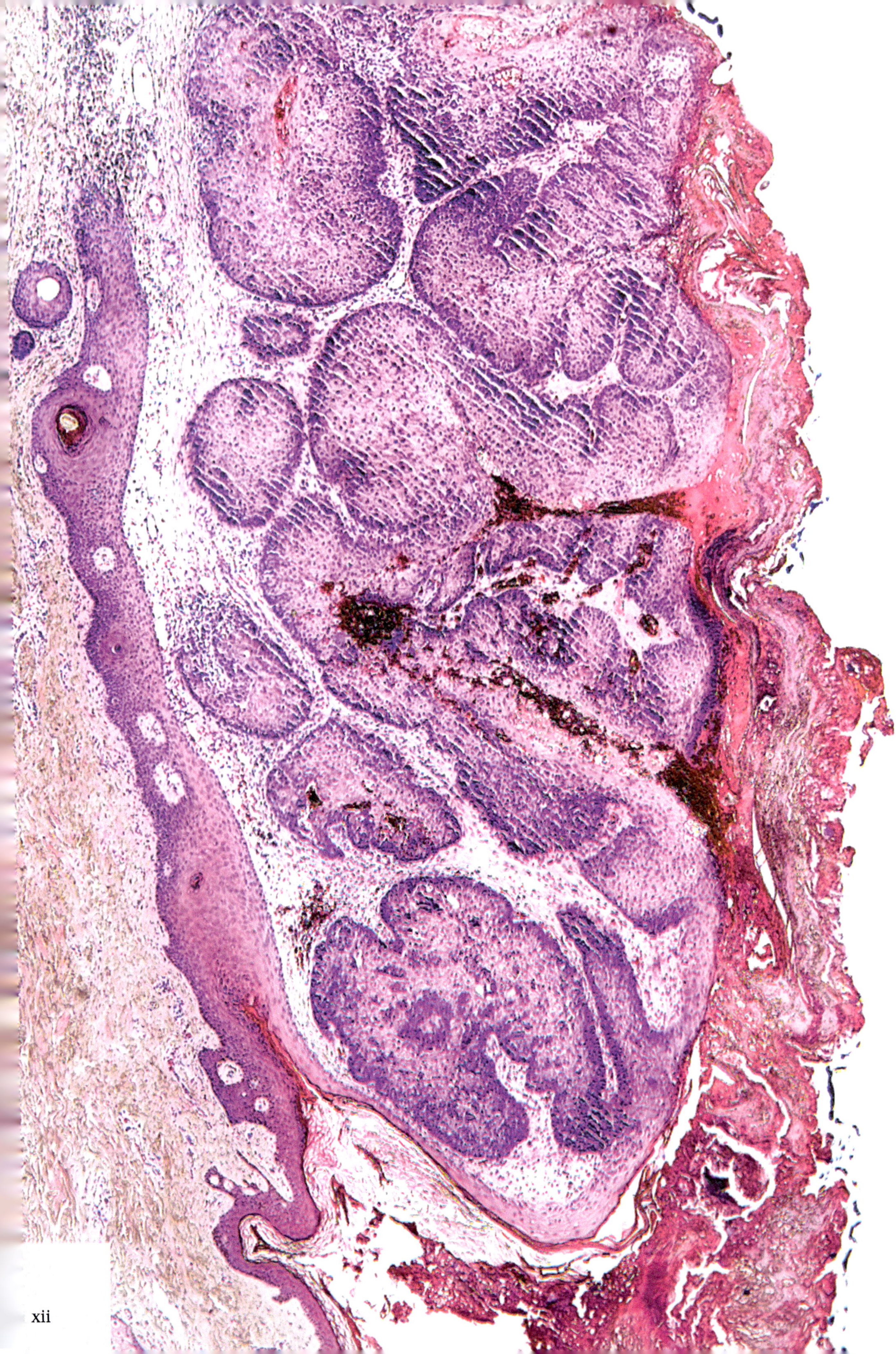

Sections

TABLE OF CONTENTS

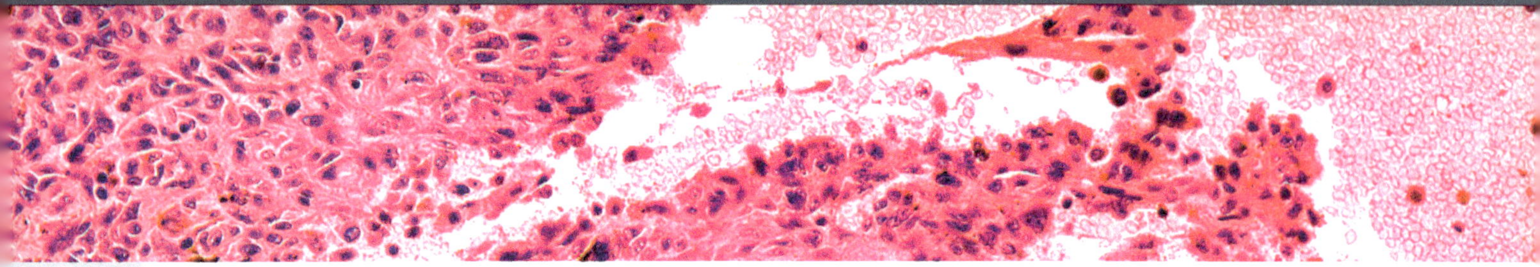

Part I: Nonmelanocytic Tumors of Skin

SECTION 1: EPITHELIAL CYSTS

SECTION 2: EPIDERMAL TUMORS

BENIGN EPIDERMAL TUMORS AND PROLIFERATIVE LESIONS

PREMALIGNANT AND MALIGNANT EPIDERMAL TUMORS

TABLE OF CONTENTS

TABLE OF CONTENTS

TABLE OF CONTENTS

TABLE OF CONTENTS

TABLE OF CONTENTS

DIAGNOSTIC PATHOLOGY

Neoplastic Dermatopathology

SECOND EDITION

CASSARINO | DADRAS

LINDBERG • KO • BILLINGS • AUERBACH

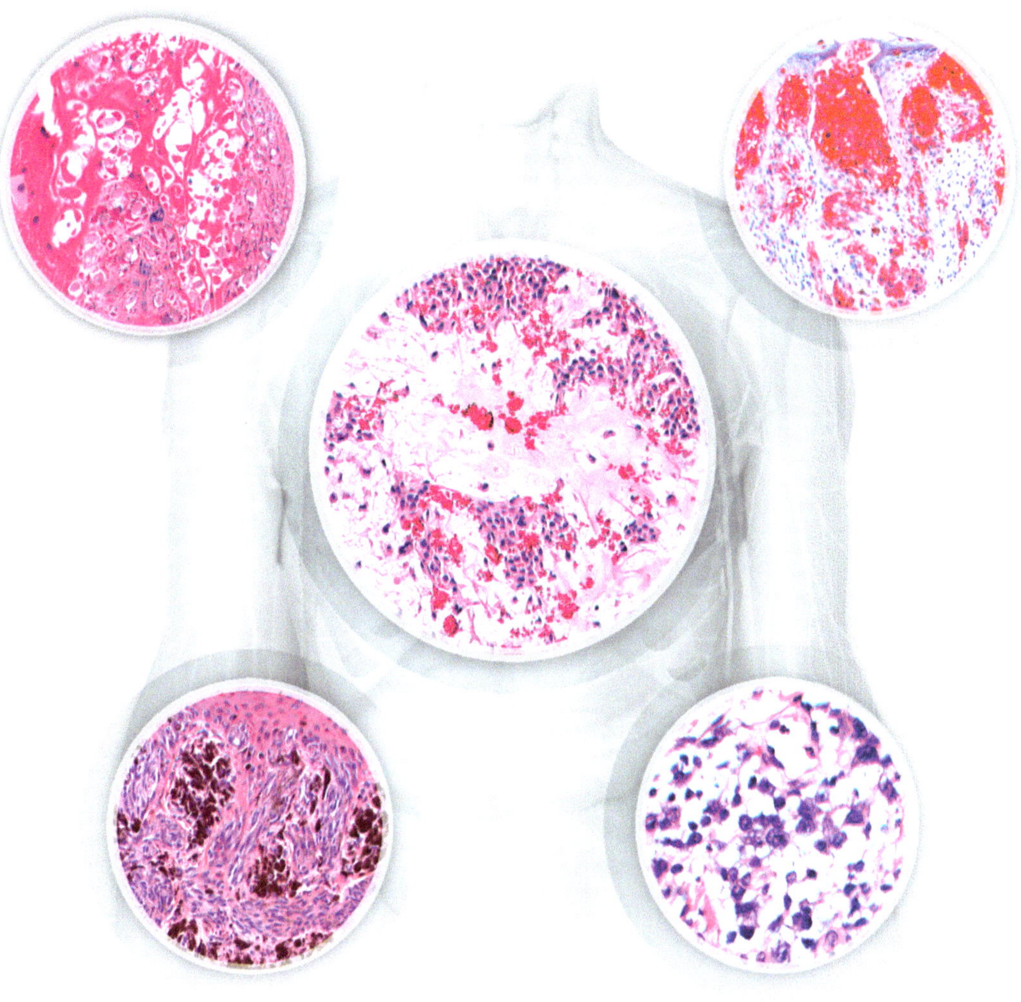

PART I
SECTION 1
Epithelial Cysts

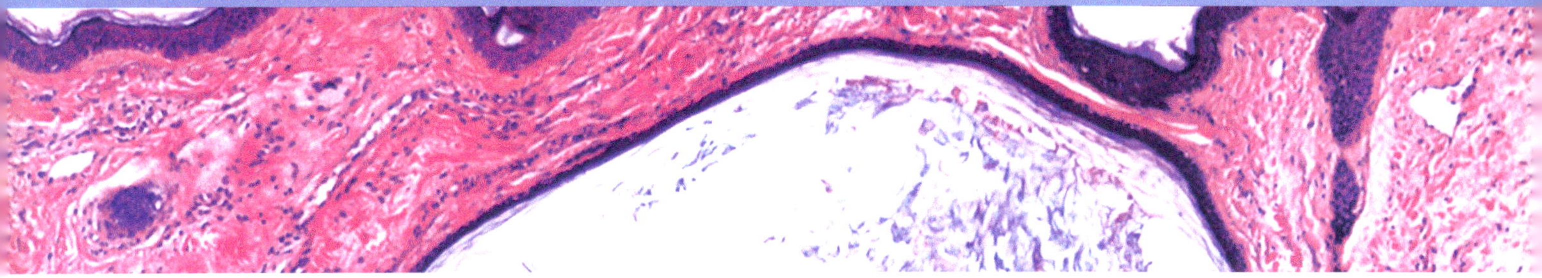

Epidermoid/Epidermal Inclusion Cyst

KEY FACTS

ETIOLOGY/PATHOGENESIS

- Infundibular cyst variant
  - Secondary to damage to pilosebaceous unit
- Implantation (inclusion) cyst variant
  - Secondary to penetrating trauma

CLINICAL ISSUES

- Very common lesions
- Usually affecting face, neck, and trunk
- Other locations: Labia majora, scrotum
- Multiple lesions should raise suspicion for Gardner syndrome
- Multiple lesions may be seen in organ transplant patients taking cyclosporin A and other immunosuppressants

MICROSCOPIC

- Unilocular cyst
- Lined by squamous epithelium with granular layer
- Contains laminated (basket weave) keratin
- May rupture and become inflamed
  - Keratin granuloma
  - Old ruptured lesions may be totally replaced by fibrosis and granulomatous inflammation
    - Cyst epithelium may disappear
    - Presence of keratin material may help to make diagnosis
  - Scrotal calcinosis my represent late stage of ruptured epidermoid cyst
- Hybrid cysts show mixed features of epidermoid and pilar cysts (rare)
  - Pilomatrixoma-like features should raise suspicion for Gardner syndrome

TOP DIFFERENTIAL DIAGNOSES

- Tricholemmal (pilar) cyst
- Vellus hair cyst
- Dermoid cyst
- HPV-related epidermoid cyst

Epidermoid Cyst

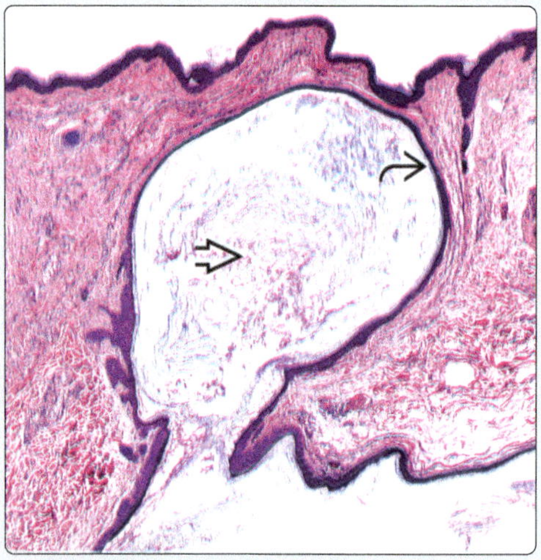

Epidermoid Cyst Lining

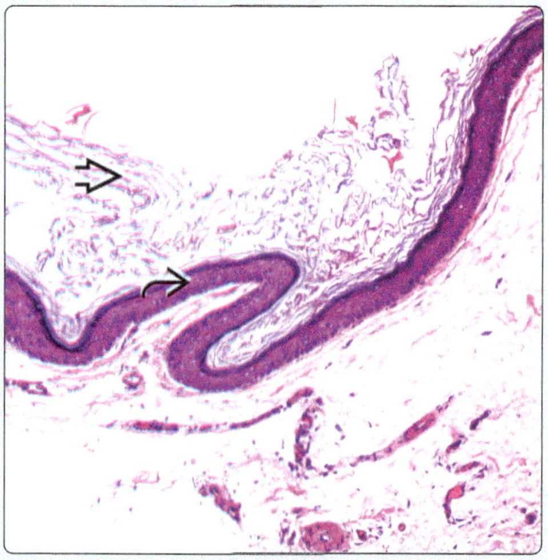

(Left) *A solitary epidermoid cyst is appreciated in the dermis. Note the thin squamous epithelium ↷ and abundant keratin contents ⇒. The punctum is not represented in this section.* **(Right)** *High magnification shows that the contents of the epidermoid cyst consist of laminated orthokeratotic material ⇒. The cyst lining is composed of a bland-appearing squamous epithelium ↷, similar to the epidermis.*

Ruptured Epidermoid Cyst

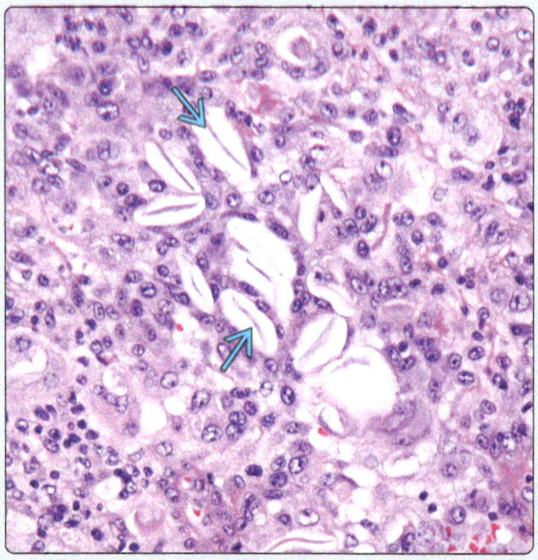

Hybrid Epidermoid and Pilomatrical Cyst

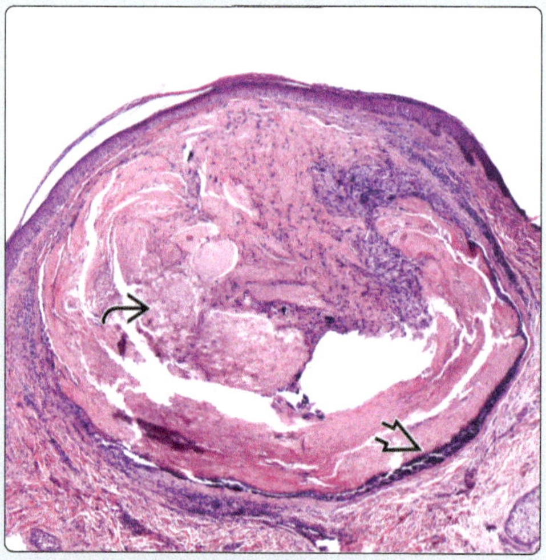

(Left) *Even when the epithelium is not identified, the presence of a foreign body giant cell reaction to keratin material → is characteristic of a ruptured epidermoid cyst.* **(Right)** *Hybrid cyst with combined epidermoid and pilomatrical features may be associated with Gardner syndrome. Basaloid/matrical cells in the wall ⇒ and ghost cells ↷ admixed with the keratin contents are characteristic of these cysts.*

TERMINOLOGY

Abbreviations

- Epidermoid/epidermal inclusion cyst (EIC)

Synonyms

- Infundibular cyst

Definitions

- Unilocular cysts lined by epidermis-like epithelium

ETIOLOGY/PATHOGENESIS

Etiology

- Damage to pilosebaceous unit
  - Infundibular cyst variant
    - Cystically dilated follicular infundibulum
    - Usually shows connection to surface (punctum)
  - Implantation (inclusion) cyst variant
    - Secondary to trauma (e.g., surgery, sewing needle)
    - No connection to epidermis
- Cyclosporin treatment in transplant recipients
- Multiple lesions may be associated with Gardner (familial adenomatosis polyposis, *APC* gene mutation) syndrome

CLINICAL ISSUES

Epidemiology

- Incidence
  - Very common
- Age
  - Young and middle-aged adults
- Sex
  - Both genders equally affected

Site

- Preferentially face, neck, and trunk
- Scrotum and labia majora are also common

Presentation

- Dome-shaped lesions with smooth surface
  - May show dark dot-like punctum on surface
- A few millimeters to a few centimeters in diameter

Prognosis

- Can rupture and become inflamed &/or infected
- Benign lesions with excellent prognosis
- Malignant transformation is exceptional

MACROSCOPIC

General Features

- Cut sections show dermal &/or subcutaneous unilocular cystic structure
  - Thin, white, smooth wall and cheesy contents

MICROSCOPIC

Histologic Features

- Unilocular cyst
- Lined by squamous epithelium with granular layer
- Contains laminated (basket weave) keratin
- Ruptured lesions are surrounded by acute/suppurative and granulomatous inflammation with giant cells
  - In older ruptured lesions, epithelial lining may disappear
    - Fibrosis and foreign body giant cell reaction with variable amounts of keratin material (keratin granuloma)
    - Most common cause of granulomatous inflammation in dermis and subcutis is ruptured epidermoid cyst
- Hybrid cysts show mixed features of epidermoid and pilar cysts (rare)
  - Pilomatrixoma-like features (presence of basaloid cells and ghost cells) should raise suspicion for Gardner syndrome
- EIC may coexist with melanocytic nevi (common)
  - May explain increase in size of mole
- Exceptionally, malignant tumors may arise in association with epidermoid cysts
  - Squamous cell carcinoma (in situ and invasive)
  - Basal cell carcinoma
  - Paget disease and neuroendocrine carcinoma

DIFFERENTIAL DIAGNOSIS

Tricholemmal (Pilar) Cyst

- Absence of granular layer
- Eosinophilic compact (not laminated) keratin

Vellus Hair Cyst

- Thin squamous epithelium with granular layer
- Laminated keratin contents with numerous small hair shafts

Dermoid Cyst

- Stratified squamous epithelium with granular layer and laminated keratin contents
- Associated hair follicles and sebaceous glands

Verrucous Cyst

- Epidermoid cyst variant associated with HPV (koilocytosis may be present)
- Papillomatous acanthotic epithelium with prominent hypergranulosis (enlarged keratohyalin granules)

DIAGNOSTIC CHECKLIST

Pathologic Interpretation Pearls

- In older ruptured epidermoid cysts, wall may disappear
  - Residual keratin material admixed with granulomatous inflammation is clue to diagnosis

SELECTED REFERENCES

1. Solanki A et al: Scrotal calcinosis: pathogenetic link with epidermal cyst. BMJ Case Rep. 2015
2. Urabe K et al: Pilomatricoma-like changes in the epidermoid cysts of Gardner syndrome with an APC gene mutation. J Dermatol. 31(3):255-7, 2004
3. Schoendorff C et al: Multiple epidermoid cysts in a renal transplant recipient taking cyclosporine A. Cutis. 50(1):36-8, 1992
4. Perse RM et al: Trabecular (Merkel cell) carcinoma arising in the wall of an epidermal cyst. Am J Dermatopathol. 9(5):423-7, 1987
5. McGavran MH et al: Keratinous cysts of the skin. Identification and differentiation of pilar cysts from epidermal cysts. Arch Dermatol. 94(4):499-508, 1966

Pilar (Tricholemmal) Cyst

KEY FACTS

TERMINOLOGY

- Trichilemmal cyst
- Isthmus-catagen cyst

CLINICAL ISSUES

- 90% of pilar cysts present on scalp
- 2nd most common type of cutaneous cyst
- Most common in adults

MICROSCOPIC

- Circumscribed simple cyst
- Filled with dense eosinophilic keratin
- Stratified squamous epithelium
- Abrupt keratinization from large polygonal keratinocytes
- Granular layer generally absent
- Rupture with associated granulomatous response common

TOP DIFFERENTIAL DIAGNOSES

- Proliferating pilar cyst
  - Architecturally more complex
  - Multiloculated
  - Squamous eddies
  - Mitotic activity
- Malignant proliferating pilar cyst/tumor
  - Infiltrative growth
  - Cytologic atypia and mitotic activity
- Epidermoid cyst
  - Well-developed granular layer
  - Epidermal keratinization
- Hybrid cyst
  - Has distinct features of both epidermoid and pilar cyst

DIAGNOSTIC CHECKLIST

- Abrupt tricholemmal keratinization is key diagnostic feature
- Simple unilocular cyst

Pilar Cyst Involving Scalp

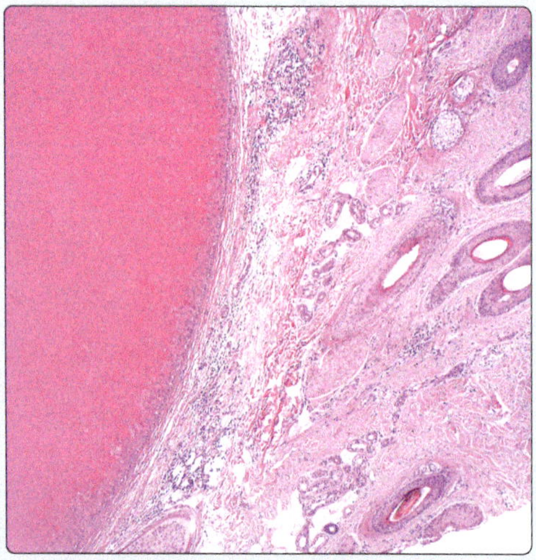

Well-Circumscribed Simple Cyst

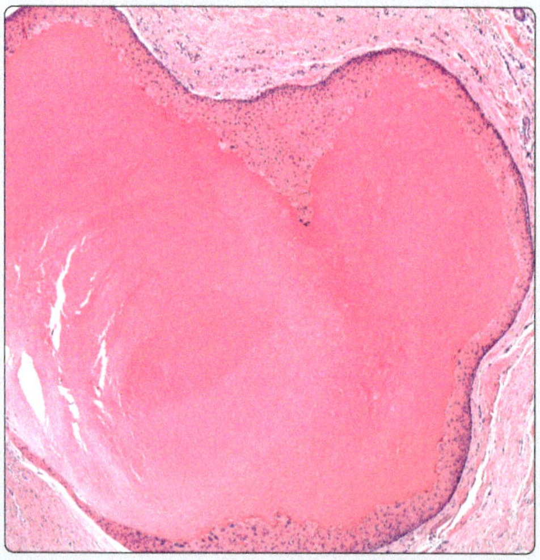

(Left) *The scalp is the most common location for pilar cysts, though they can rarely occur almost anywhere.* **(Right)** *Pilar cysts are well-circumscribed simple cysts involving the dermis &/or subcutis. No granular layer is seen, even at low magnification.*

High-Power Image of Pilar Cyst

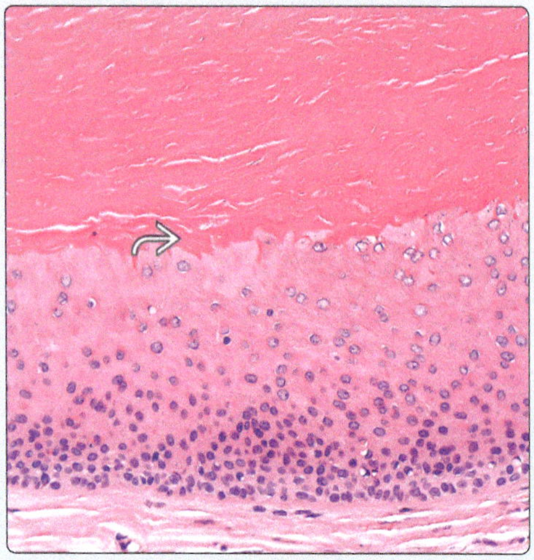

Ruptured Pilar Cyst

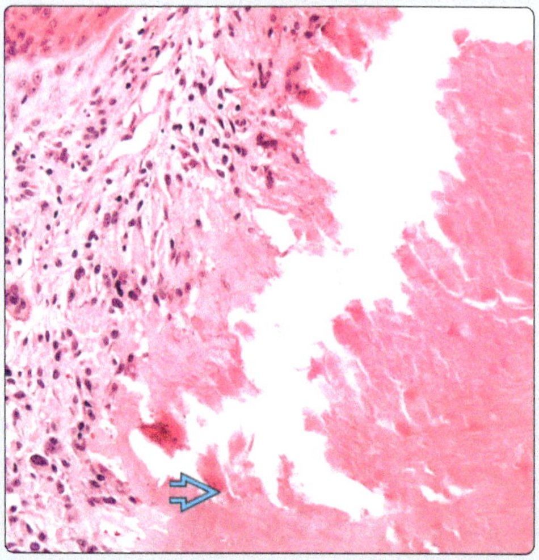

(Left) *The epithelium at the interface with the keratin is composed of large polygonal keratinocytes with abundant eosinophilic cytoplasm. There is abrupt keratinization ➔ without a granular layer, but scattered keratohyaline granules may be seen.* **(Right)** *Pilar cysts often rupture, resulting in granulomatous inflammation. Recognition of cyst remnants ➾ help make the diagnosis.*

TERMINOLOGY

Synonyms

- Pilar cyst
- Trichilemmal cyst
- Isthmus-catagen cyst

Definitions

- Benign unilocular cyst lined by squamous epithelium lacking granular layer and containing abundant dense keratin material

CLINICAL ISSUES

Epidemiology

- Incidence
    - 2nd most common type of cutaneous cyst
- Age
    - Most common in adults
- Sex
    - More common in women than men

Site

- 90% of pilar cysts present on scalp

Presentation

- Usually present as asymptomatic lesion on scalp as dermal or subcutaneous nodule
- Multiple lesions common
- Autosomal dominant inheritance common in multiple lesion

Treatment

- Surgical approaches
    - Simple excision

Prognosis

- Benign lesions
- Proliferating pilar (tricholemmal) cysts or malignant pilar (tricholemmal) cysts may rarely arise in pilar cysts

MACROSCOPIC

General Features

- Dermal or subcutaneous cystic structure

Sections to Be Submitted

- Representative sections appropriate

Size

- Wide range, can be < 0.5 cm to several cm in size

MICROSCOPIC

Histologic Features

- Circumscribed simple cyst located in dermis &/or subcutaneous tissue
- Filled with dense laminated eosinophilic keratin
- Stratified squamous epithelium lining cyst
- Abrupt keratinization from large polygonal keratinocytes
    - So-called tricholemmal keratinization
- Granular layer generally absent
    - Occasionally, cells with a few keratohyaline granules may be seen
- Calcification in up to 25% of cases
- Rupture with associated granulomatous response common
- Rarely have associated sebaceous or apocrine glands

DIFFERENTIAL DIAGNOSIS

Proliferating Pilar Cyst/Tumor

- Multiloculated cystic neoplasm
- Nodules of proliferating squamous cells
- Squamous eddies
- Mitotic activity present, especially in peripheral cells
- At least focal abrupt tricholemmal keratinization present

Malignant Proliferating Pilar Cyst/Tumor

- Similar to proliferating pilar tumor but with at least focal areas of
    - Infiltrative growth
    - Cytologic atypia
    - Mitotic activity ± atypical mitotic figures

Epidermoid Cyst/Epidermal Inclusion Cyst

- Unilocular cyst
- Squamous epithelial lining
- Intact granular layer
- Epidermal keratinization with loose layers of keratin, not dense eosinophilic tricholemmal keratinization as in pilar cyst

Hybrid Cyst

- Combination of epidermoid cyst and pilar cyst
- Upper portion has features of epidermoid cyst
- Lower portion resembles pilar cyst

DIAGNOSTIC CHECKLIST

Pathologic Interpretation Pearls

- Abrupt tricholemmal keratinization is key feature
    - If there is both trichilemmal keratinization and epidermal keratinization, consider hybrid cyst
- Simple unilocular cyst
    - If architectural complexity present, consider proliferating pilar cyst or malignant proliferating pilar cyst
- Rupture is common
    - Granulomatous inflammation can partially obscure histologic features

SELECTED REFERENCES

1. Eskander A et al: Squamous cell carcinoma arising in a proliferating pilar (trichilemmal) cyst with nodal and distant metastases. J Otolaryngol Head Neck Surg. 39(5):E63-7, 2010
2. Karaman E et al: Giant trichilemmal cyst at the neck region. J Craniofac Surg. 20(3):961-2, 2009
3. Anolik R et al: Proliferating trichilemmal cyst with focal calcification. Dermatol Online J. 14(10):25, 2008
4. Berk DR et al: Milia: a review and classification. J Am Acad Dermatol. 59(6):1050-63, 2008
5. González-Vela MC et al: Proliferating trichilemmal cyst associated with an epidermal nevus. J Dermatol. 35(1):52-4, 2008
6. Takeda H et al: Hybrid cyst: case reports and review of 15 cases in Japan. J Eur Acad Dermatol Venereol. 17(1):83-6, 2003
7. Vandeweyer E et al: Cutaneous cysts: a plea for systematic analysis. Acta Chir Belg. 103(5):507-10, 2003
8. Leppard BJ et al: The natural history of trichilemmal cysts. Br J Dermatol. 94(4):379-90, 1976

Proliferating Pilar (Tricholemmal) Cyst/Tumor

KEY FACTS

TERMINOLOGY

- Proliferating pilar tumor (PPT), proliferating pilar cyst (PPC), proliferating trichilemmal cyst/tumor
  - Multicystic squamous neoplasm composed of mature keratinocytes lining keratin-filled spaces

CLINICAL ISSUES

- Typically occur on scalp (90% of cases) in older adults
- Much more common in female than male patients
- Most cases of PPT behave in benign fashion, but malignant PPTs are aggressive tumors that have high rate of metastasis

MACROSCOPIC

- Large tumors, 6 cm or greater in most cases

MICROSCOPIC

- Cystic spaces are irregularly formed and anastomosing
- Cysts show keratinization without granular layer
- Large, multicystic, dermal-based tumor with squamous lining and spaces containing dense keratin
- Peripheral palisading of basilar layer is typically present, and there may be thickened basement membrane
- Occasional mitotic figures are present, but no high-grade atypia or increased mitotic activity should be present

TOP DIFFERENTIAL DIAGNOSES

- Pilar/tricholemmal cyst
  - Unicystic structure lined by mature squamous cells
- Proliferating epidermoid cyst
  - Shows overlapping features with PPT but has granular layer and laminated keratin
- Malignant PPT (squamous cell carcinoma arising in PPT)
  - Larger than benign PPTs, clinically often present as rapidly enlarging nodular mass lesion
  - Show greater cytologic atypia and mitotic activity, infiltrative features

Low Magnification of PPT

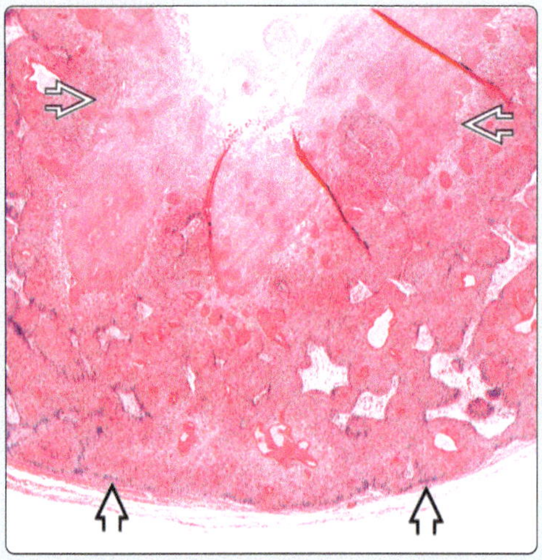

High Magnification of PPT

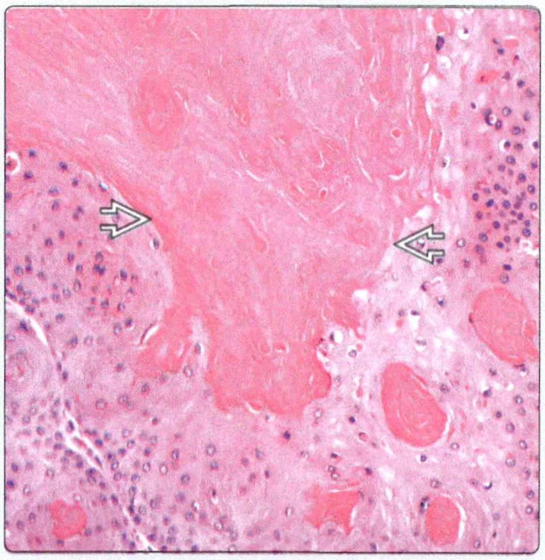

(Left) *Scanning magnification of proliferating pilar tumor (PPT) shows a smooth-bordered ⇨, circumscribed tumor composed of thickened cords of squamous cells surrounding a large cystic cavity ➡ containing abundant keratin material.* **(Right)** *High-magnification examination of a benign PPT shows bland squamous keratinocytes with abundant eosinophilic cytoplasm surrounding keratin-filled spaces. Note the lack of an intervening granular layer ➡.*

PPT With Bland Cytologic Features

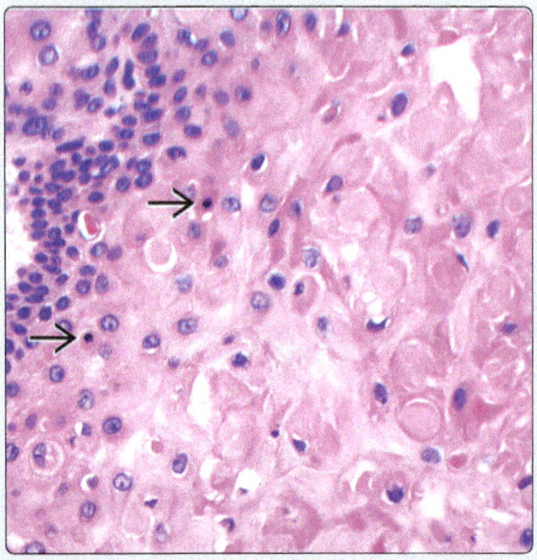

PPT With Keratinization

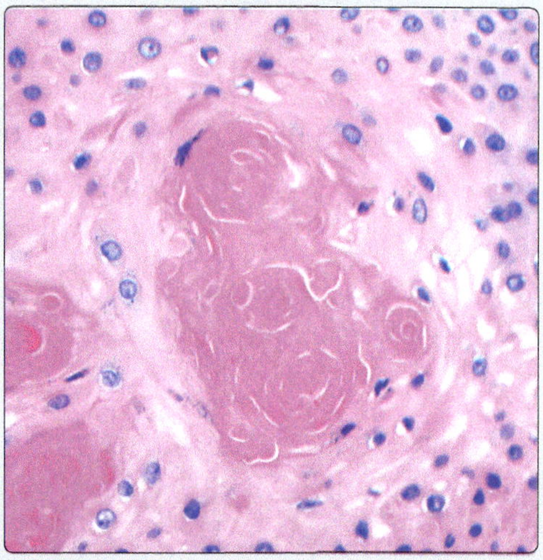

(Left) *High-magnification examination shows the bland cytologic features of the squamous cells, which show uniform nuclei, small nucleoli, and abundant amounts of dense eosinophilic cytoplasm. Scattered dyskeratotic keratinocytes are present →.* **(Right)** *High-magnification examination shows several small foci of dense keratin material surrounded by bland-appearing squamous cells.*

TERMINOLOGY

Abbreviations

- Proliferating pilar tumor (PPT)
- Proliferating pilar cyst (PPC)

Synonyms

- Proliferating trichilemmal cyst/tumor

Definitions

- Multicystic squamous neoplasm composed of mature keratinocytes lining keratin-filled spaces

ETIOLOGY/PATHOGENESIS

Unknown

- Postulated that most cases arise in preexisting pilar (tricholemmal) cyst; may be related to chronic inflammation or trauma

CLINICAL ISSUES

Epidemiology

- Incidence
  - Uncommon tumors
- Age
  - Typically occur in older adults
- Sex
  - Much more common in female than male patients

Site

- Typically occur on scalp (90%); also may occur on face, trunk, and extremities

Treatment

- Surgical approaches
  - Complete surgical excision is recommended in order to prevent recurrence and malignant transformation

Prognosis

- PPTs behave in benign fashion, but malignant PPTs are aggressive tumors that have high rate of metastasis

MACROSCOPIC

General Features

- Often multicystic dermal-based tumors that may involve subcutis

Size

- Large tumors, most are 6 cm or greater in diameter

MICROSCOPIC

Histologic Features

- Large, multicystic, dermal-based tumor with squamous lining and spaces containing dense keratin
  - Typically symmetric and well-circumscribed at low-power examination
  - Cystic spaces are irregularly formed and anastomosing
    - Cysts are filled with abundant, dense, eosinophilic keratin (similar to pilar/tricholemmal cysts)
    - Cells lining cyst show keratinization without granular layer (tricholemmal/pilar-type keratinization), unlike proliferating epidermoid cyst (PEC), which shows granular layer
  - Squamous eddies may be seen in cyst lining
  - Peripheral palisading of basilar layer is typically present, and there may be thickened basement membrane
  - Squamous epithelial cells show mild enlargement and nuclear hyperchromasia
  - Occasional mitotic figures are present, but no high-grade atypia or increased mitotic activity should be present
- Focal epidermal connections may be present in minority (about 25%) of cases

DIFFERENTIAL DIAGNOSIS

Pilar/Tricholemmal Cyst

- Unicystic structure lined by mature squamous cells that keratinize without granular layer
- Cyst contains abundant, dense, laminated keratin and may show focal calcifications
- May be found in association with PPT, as most PPTs likely arise in preexisting pilar cysts

Proliferating Epidermoid Cyst

- Shows overlapping features with PPT but exhibits granular layer and loose tiers of laminated keratin (similar to epidermoid/epidermal inclusion cysts)
- Hybrid lesions that show features of both PPT and PEC may be encountered

Malignant PPT (Squamous Cell Carcinoma Arising in PPT)

- Tumors are usually larger than benign PPTs and clinically often present as rapidly enlarging nodular mass lesion, may be ulcerated or bleeding
- May arise in PPT but shows greater cytologic atypia and mitotic activity, with infiltrative features
  - Typically resembles conventional squamous cell carcinoma, but may also show features of spindle cell/sarcomatoid carcinoma in some cases
- Malignant PPTs are aggressive carcinomas, with high incidence of local recurrence and metastasis (up to 30% reported)

SELECTED REFERENCES

1. Cassarino DS et al: Cutaneous squamous cell carcinoma: a comprehensive clinicopathologic classification–part two. J Cutan Pathol. 33(4):261-79, 2006
2. Ye J et al: Proliferating pilar tumors: a clinicopathologic study of 76 cases with a proposal for definition of benign and malignant variants. Am J Clin Pathol. 122(4):566-74, 2004
3. Haas N et al: Carcinoma arising in a proliferating trichilemmal cyst expresses fetal and trichilemmal hair phenotype. Am J Dermatopathol. 24(4):340-4, 2002
4. Mathis ED et al: Malignant proliferating trichilemmal tumor. Am J Clin Oncol. 24(4):351-3, 2001
5. Sau P et al: Proliferating epithelial cysts. Clinicopathological analysis of 96 cases. J Cutan Pathol. 22(5):394-406, 1995
6. Rutty GN et al: Malignant change in trichilemmal cysts: a study of cell proliferation and DNA content. Histopathology. 21(5):465-8, 1992
7. Mehregan AH et al: Malignant proliferating trichilemmal tumors–report of three cases. J Dermatol Surg Oncol. 13(12):1339-42, 1987
8. Amaral AL et al: Proliferating pilar (trichilemmal) cyst. Report of two cases, one with carcinomatous transformation and one with distant metastases. Arch Pathol Lab Med. 108(10):808-10, 1984
9. Jones EW: Proliferating epidermoid cysts. Arch Dermatol. 94(1):11-9, 1966

(Left) *Scanning magnification view of a PPT shows a smooth-bordered tumor composed of thickened cords of squamous keratinocytes surrounding a large cystic cavity that contains abundant keratin material.* **(Right)** *High-magnification examination of a PPT shows bland squamous keratinocytes with abundant eosinophilic cytoplasm surrounding multiple keratin-filled spaces that lack an intervening granular layer.*

Low Magnification of PPT

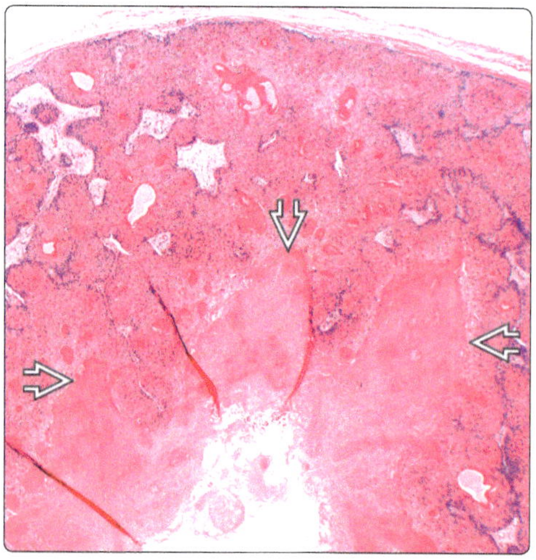

High Magnification of PPT

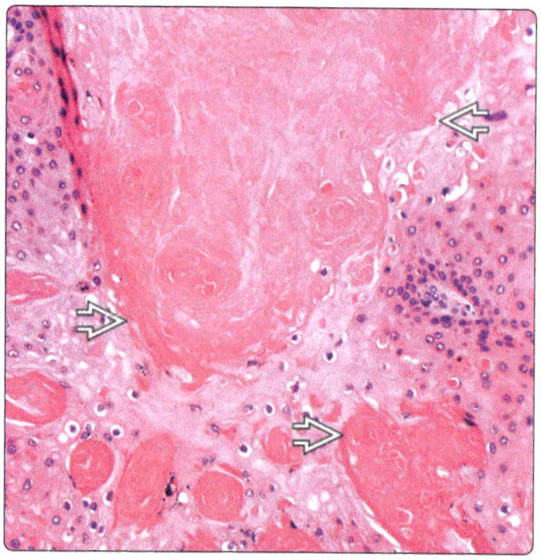

(Left) *PPT with clear cell features shows a circumscribed cystic space lined by thickened cords of pale to clear-staining squamous cells surrounding a central cystic cavity with dense keratin and focal calcifications.* **(Right)** *Higher magnification of the tumor shows a cellular area composed of enlarged but bland-appearing squamoid cells with abundant pale eosinophilic to clear-staining cytoplasm.*

PPT With Clear Cell Features

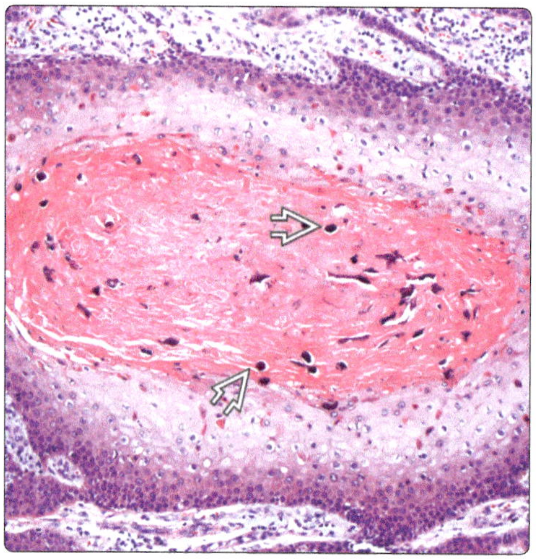

PPT With Clear Cell Features

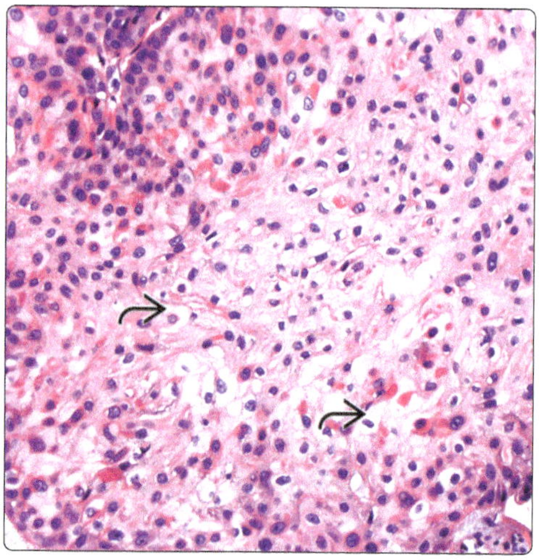

(Left) *High magnification shows the pale to clear-staining squamous cells with abundant cytoplasm and small round nuclei lacking significant atypia.* **(Right)** *Scanning magnification shows a proliferating cystic neoplasm with combined features of a proliferating epidermoid cyst (showing a granular layer and loose, laminated keratin) and a proliferating pilar cyst (lacking a granular layer and showing dense eosinophilic keratin).*

High Magnification of PPT With Clear Cell Features

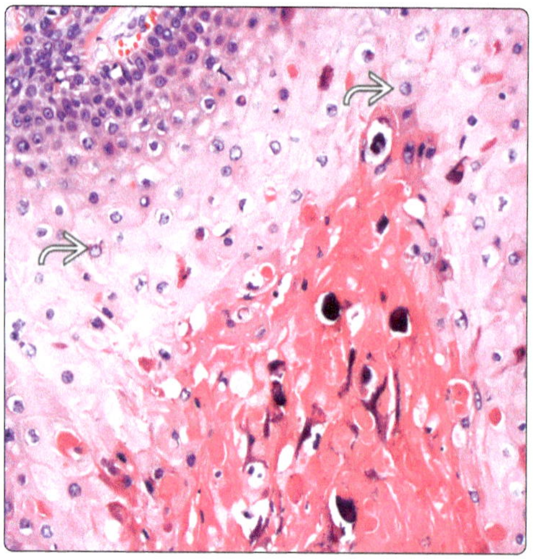

Combined PPT/Proliferating Pilar Cyst and Proliferating Epidermoid Cyst

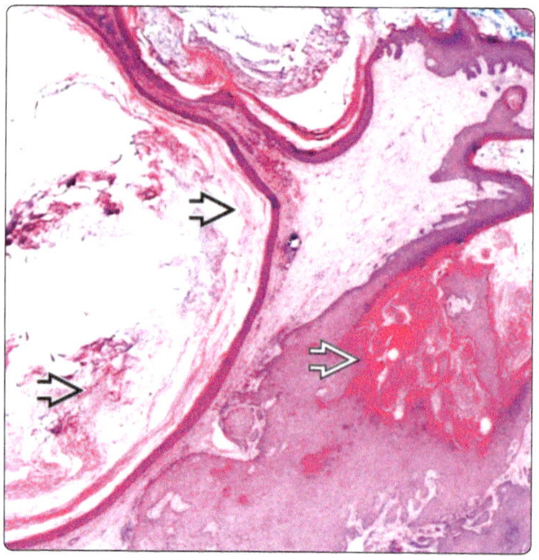

Differential Diagnosis: Malignant PPT

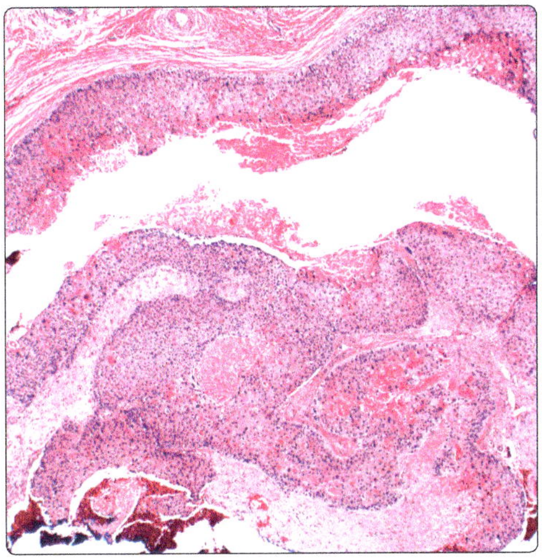

Malignant PPT at Low Magnification

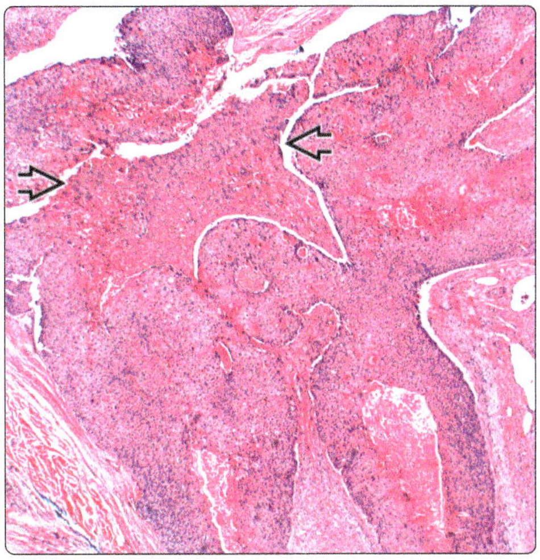

(Left) *Low-magnification view of a malignant PPT shows cystic spaces lined by enlarged, atypical squamous cells.* **(Right)** *Malignant PPT composed of irregular, anastomosing cords of enlarged, atypical squamous cells with areas of keratinization and necrotic cellular debris ⇨ is seen.*

Malignant PPT at High Magnification With Marked Cytologic Atypia

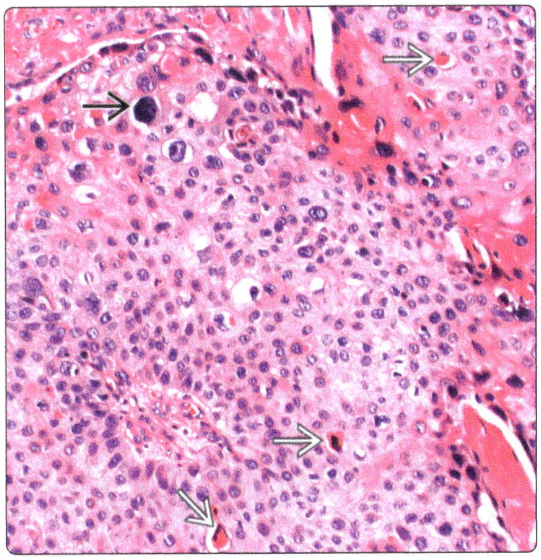

Malignant PPT with Multiple Mitotic Figures

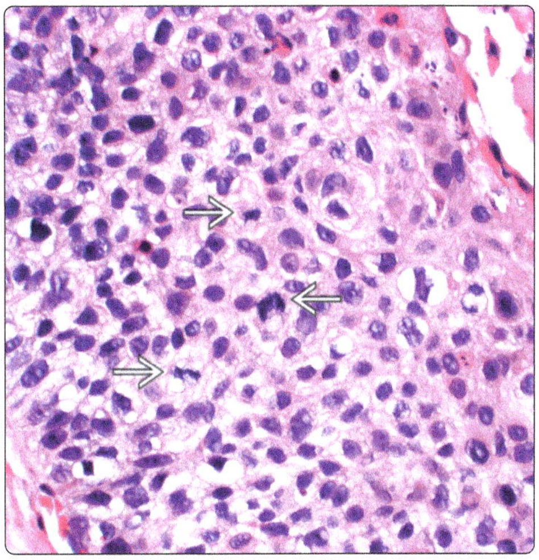

(Left) *High-magnification view of a malignant PPT demonstrates nuclear pleomorphism with marked nuclear enlargement ⇨ and atypia, along with scattered mitotic figures and dyskeratotic cells ➡.* **(Right)** *High magnification of a malignant PPT shows nuclear hyperchromasia, irregular nuclear borders, and multiple mitotic figures ➡ in a single high-power field.*

Infiltrative Malignant PPT

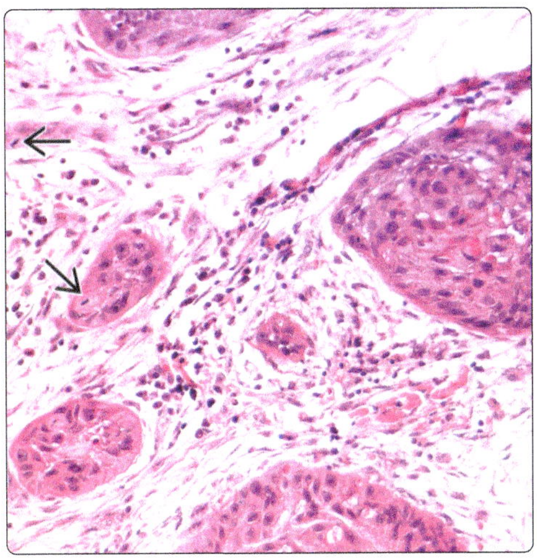

p63 Immunohistochemistry in Malignant PPT

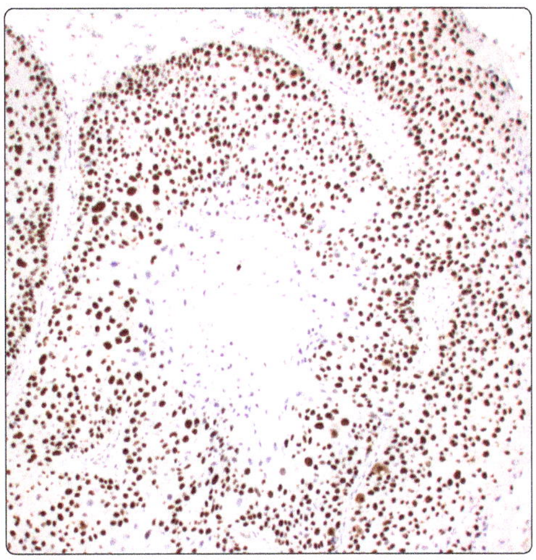

(Left) *Another example of a malignant PPT shows infiltrating small islands of atypical squamous cells in an inflamed, edematous stroma. Scattered mitotic figures are present ⇨.* **(Right)** *Immunohistochemical stain for p63 in a malignant PPT shows strong and diffuse nuclear staining; p63 is not a specific marker for PPT, but it is positive in most adnexal tumors, and thus favors a primary cutaneous carcinoma over a metastatic tumor to the skin.*

KEY FACTS

TERMINOLOGY

- Epidermoid cysts associated with human papillomavirus (HPV) infection

ETIOLOGY/PATHOGENESIS

- HPV-related cysts
  - Verrucous cysts
    - Associated with HPV-20 and -34
  - Epidermoid cyst of palm and sole
    - Associated with HPV-60 and -57

CLINICAL ISSUES

- Rare lesions that present in adults
- Verrucous cysts
  - Face, neck, and trunk
- Epidermoid cyst of palm and sole
  - Palms and soles
- May rupture and become inflamed or infected

MICROSCOPIC

- Verrucous epidermal cyst
  - Papillary and acanthotic squamous epithelium
  - Hyper- and orthokeratosis, with focal parakeratosis
  - Hypergranulosis
  - Keratohyalin granules and koilocytic change
- Epidermoid cyst of palm and sole
  - Epidermal-like lining
  - Eosinophilic intracytoplasmic inclusions
  - Vacuolated cells

TOP DIFFERENTIAL DIAGNOSES

- Epidermoid (epidermal inclusion) cyst
  - Presence of granular layer
  - No viral cytopathic changes
- Trichilemmal (pilar) cyst
  - Squamous epithelium without granular layer
  - No viral cytopathic changes

(Left) *This verrucous epidermal cyst shows an acanthotic and papillated ➲ cystic epithelial structure in the dermis. The lumen contains keratin and degenerating inflammatory cells.* **(Right)** *Higher magnification shows the acanthotic and papillomatous squamous-lining epithelium with foci of koilocytosis ➡.*

Human Papillomavirus-Related Epidermal Cyst

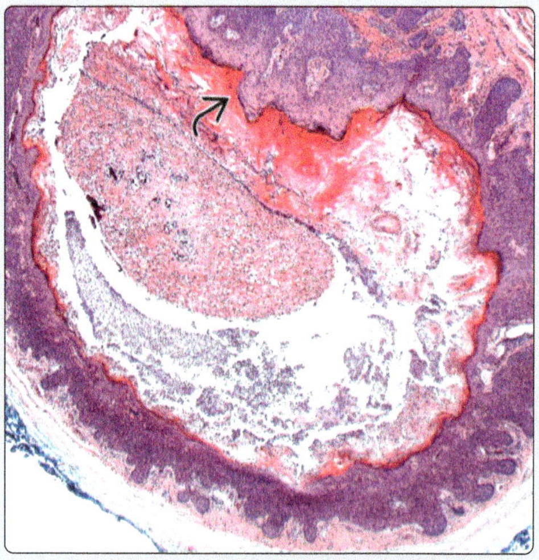

Human Papillomavirus-Related Epidermal Cyst at Higher Magnification

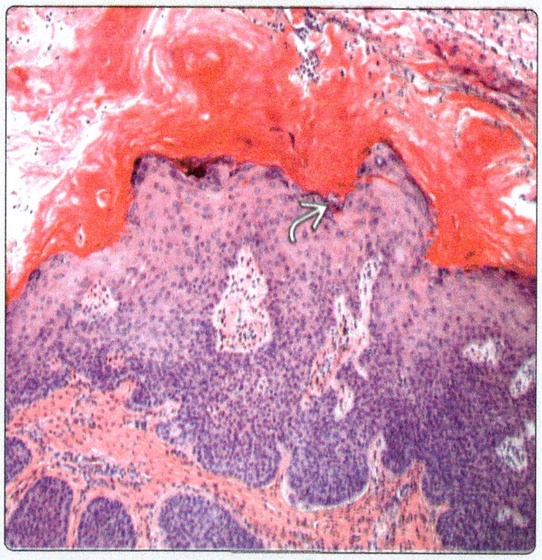

(Left) *The acanthotic squamous epithelium of a verrucous cyst shows areas of koilocytosis and prominent squamous whorls ➡, similar to an irritated seborrheic keratosis.* **(Right)** *High magnification shows the acanthotic epithelium of a human papillomavirus (HPV)-related verrucous epidermal cyst showing prominent keratohyaline granules ⇨ and koilocytosis ➲.*

Human Papillomavirus-Related Epidermal Cyst With Acanthotic Lining

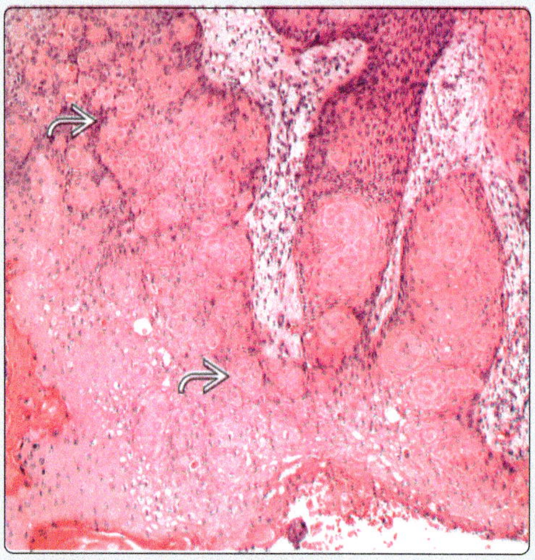

High Magnification of Human Papillomavirus-Related Epidermal Cyst

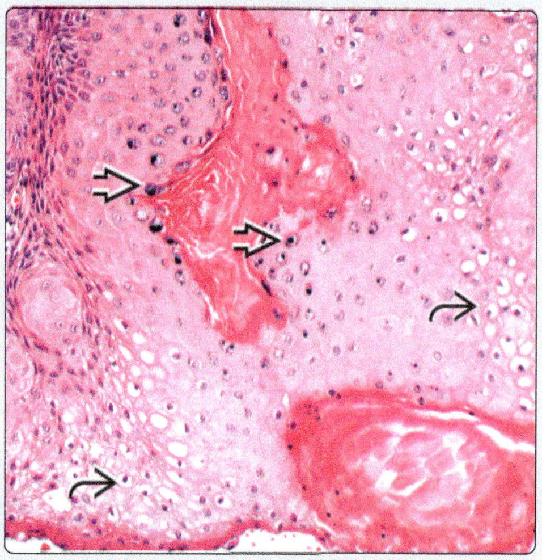

TERMINOLOGY

Synonyms

- Verrucous cyst, epidermoid cyst of palm and sole

Definitions

- Epidermoid cysts associated with human papillomavirus (HPV) infection

ETIOLOGY/PATHOGENESIS

Infectious Agents

- HPV
  - Verrucous cysts have been reported to be associated with HPV-20 and -34 (epidermodysplasia verruciformis strains)
  - Epidermoid cyst of palm and sole mainly associated with HPV-60 and -57
    - Traumatic implantation of HPV-infected epidermis (or perhaps eccrine ducts) into dermis

CLINICAL ISSUES

Epidemiology

- Incidence
  - Rare
- Age
  - Adults
- Sex
  - Both genders equally affected
- Ethnicity
  - HPV-related cysts of soles and palms mainly affect Japanese

Site

- Verrucous cysts
  - Face, neck, trunk
- Cysts of palms and soles
  - Palms and soles

Presentation

- Dome-shaped lesion

Prognosis

- Cosmetic problems
- May rupture and become inflamed or infected
- Benign lesions with excellent prognosis

MACROSCOPIC

General Features

- Dome-shaped lesion sometimes showing dark punctum on surface
- Cut sections show dermal &/or subcutaneous unilocular round cyst
  - Thin to slightly papillary white wall and cheesy yellowish contents

MICROSCOPIC

Histologic Features

- Verrucous cysts
  - Papillary and acanthotic squamous epithelium with hypergranulosis and hyperkeratosis (focal parakeratosis)
    - Keratohyalin granules and koilocytic changes
  - Part of cyst shows classical features of epidermoid cyst or, less often, pilar cyst
  - May or may not show connection to overlying epidermis
- Epidermoid cyst of palm and sole
  - Epidermis-like lining as in classical epidermoid cyst
    - Eosinophilic intracytoplasmic inclusions in wall
    - Vacuolated cells in keratin contents
  - Electron microscopy
    - Viral inclusions
- Less well-characterized variant of HPV-related cyst with molluscum-like inclusions has also been described
  - Usually affects big toe and is associated with HPV-1

Cytologic Features

- Verrucous cyst
  - Prominent keratohyalin granules and koilocytosis
- Epidermoid cyst of sole
  - Intracytoplasmic eosinophilic inclusions

ANCILLARY TESTS

Immunohistochemistry

- May confirm presence of HPV

DIFFERENTIAL DIAGNOSIS

Epidermoid (Epidermal Inclusion) Cyst

- Epidermis-like smooth lining without papillary surface
- Presence of granular layer
- Abundant laminated keratin
- No viral cytopathic changes

Tricholemmal (Pilar) Cyst

- Squamous epithelium without granular layer
- Compact (tricholemmal) keratinization
- Absence of viral cytopathic changes

Molluscum contagiosum

- Large characteristic inclusions

DIAGNOSTIC CHECKLIST

Pathologic Interpretation Pearls

- Papillary surface with hypergranulosis and koilocytic changes in verrucous cysts
- Intracytoplasmic eosinophilic inclusions in HPV-related cysts of soles and palms

SELECTED REFERENCES

1. Sato Y et al: Human papillomavirus-associated plantar epidermoid cysts: MR and US imaging appearance. Skeletal Radiol. 43(2):257-61, 2014
2. Pusiol T et al: Squamous cell carcinoma arising in epidermal and human papillomavirus associated cysts: report of three cases. Pathologica. 102(3):88-92, 2010
3. Kohno M et al: Human papillomavirus 1 induced epidermoid cystic structure mimicking molluscum bodies. J Eur Acad Dermatol Venereol. 22(10):1242-4, 2008
4. Misago N et al: Verrucous trichilemmal cyst containing human papillomavirus. Clin Exp Dermatol. 30(1):38-9, 2005
5. Egawa K et al: Human papillomavirus 57 identified in a plantar epidermoid cyst. Br J Dermatol. 138(3):510-4, 1998
6. Reis MD et al: Verrucous cyst. Eur J Dermatol. 8(3):186-8, 1998
7. Kato N et al: Two cases of plantar epidermal cyst associated with human papillomavirus. Clin Exp Dermatol. 17(4):252-6, 1992

Vellus Hair Cyst

KEY FACTS

TERMINOLOGY

- Vellus hair cyst (VHC)
- Eruptive vellus hair cyst (EVHC)
- Similar histology to epidermoid cysts, but with addition of multiple intraluminal vellus hairs

ETIOLOGY/PATHOGENESIS

- Can present concomitantly with steatocystoma multiplex (SM) and milial cysts
- Some consider VHC and SM to be variation of same entity

CLINICAL ISSUES

- Uncommon lesions
- Typically occur in children and young adults
- Present as small, discrete, asymptomatic follicular papules; often on chest
- Usually multiple (up to a few hundred lesions)
- Treatment not necessary but may be done for cosmetic purposes
    - Mechanical dermabrasion, retinoids, needle evacuation, simple excision, or laser therapy

MICROSCOPIC

- Dermal cyst lined by bland stratified squamous epithelium with granular layer
- Intraluminal laminated keratin debris and numerous vellus hair shafts
- Small hair follicles/pilosebaceous units may be seen attached to cyst wall

TOP DIFFERENTIAL DIAGNOSES

- Epidermoid (epidermal inclusion, follicular infundibular) cyst
    - Lacks intraluminal vellus hairs
- Milial cyst
- Steatocystoma
- Trichofolliculoma

Clinical Photograph of Eruptive Vellus Hair Cysts

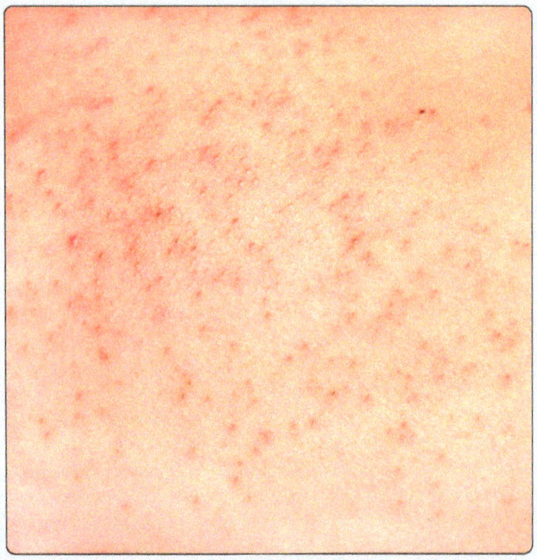

Vellus Hair Cyst

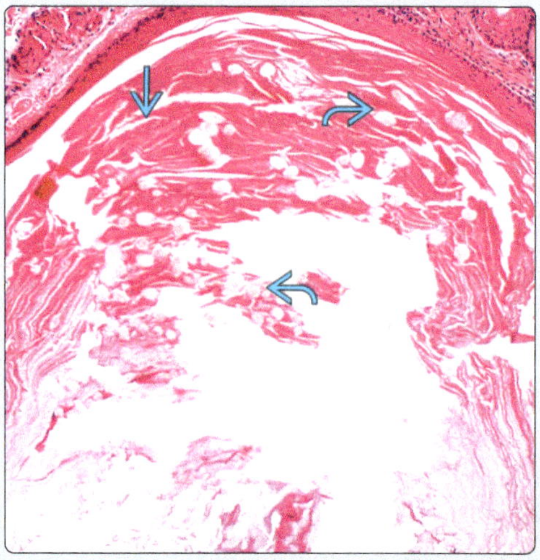

(Left) *Multiple, slightly brownish, small follicular papules are seen on the chest. This is a classic presentation of eruptive vellus hair cysts. (Courtesy J. Wu, MD.)* **(Right)** *Low magnification shows a cyst lined by a keratinizing squamous epithelium. The cyst contents include laminated keratin → and numerous transversely sectioned hair shafts →.*

Vellus Hair Cyst With Pilosebaceous Unit

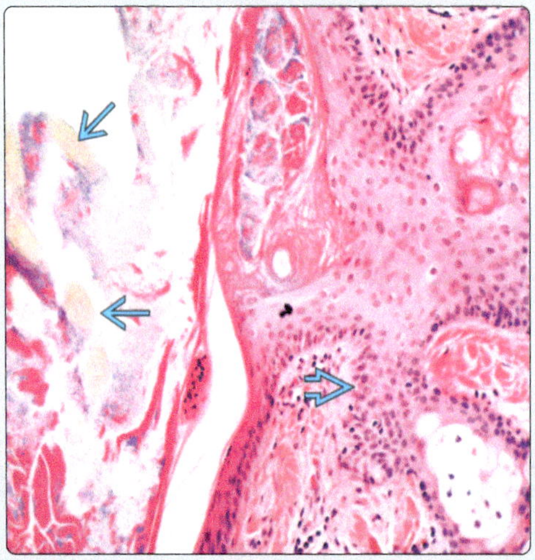

Ruptured Vellus Hair Cyst

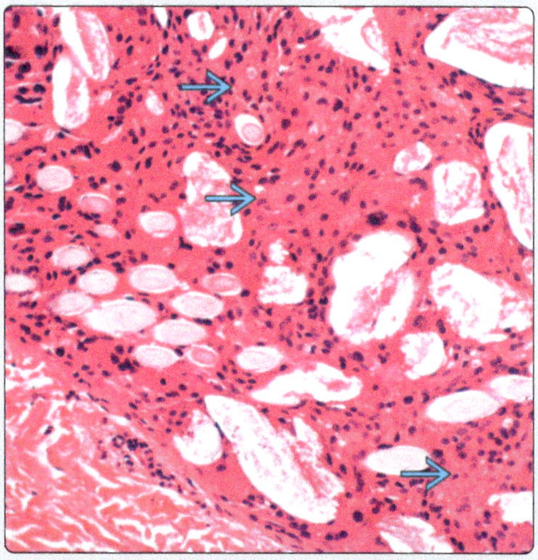

(Left) *Some cysts may show a pilosebaceous unit attached to the cyst wall →. Fragments of hair shafts are also present within the cystic space →.* **(Right)** *Ruptured vellus hair cysts are often accompanied by an exuberant foreign body granulomatous response → as is illustrated here, with many hair shafts surrounded by inflammation.*

TERMINOLOGY

Abbreviations

- Vellus hair cyst (VHC)

Synonyms

- Eruptive vellus hair cyst (EVHC)

Definitions

- Similar histology to epidermoid (follicular, infundibular type) cyst with addition of intraluminal vellus hairs

ETIOLOGY/PATHOGENESIS

Genetics

- Rare cases reported to be autosomal dominant
  - Rarely associated with the following diseases
    - Ectodermal dysplasia (anhidrotic and hidrotic)
    - Lowe syndrome (oculocerebrorenal syndrome)
    - Pachyonychia congenita

Associations

- Can present concomitantly with steatocystoma multiplex (SM) and milial cysts
  - Some consider VHC and SM to be variation of same entity
    - Considered to arise from 1 pilosebaceous duct
    - Designation as multiple pilosebaceous cysts, which has been used to define both of these entities
  - Cytokeratin (CK) studies, however, have suggested that VHC and SM are distinct entities
    - Vellus hair cysts express CK17
    - Steatocystoma multiplex expresses CK10 and CK17

CLINICAL ISSUES

Epidemiology

- Incidence
  - Uncommon
- Age
  - Children and young adults
- Sex
  - No gender predilection
- Ethnicity
  - No race predilection

Site

- Commonly on chest
- Upper extremities and other sites can be affected

Presentation

- Small (1-4 mm), discrete, asymptomatic papules
  - Skin-colored, erythematous, yellowish, brown, or bluish-gray
  - Occasional central umbilication
- Usually multiple (up to a few hundred lesions)

Treatment

- Not necessary
  - If cosmetically bothersome: Mechanical dermabrasion, retinoids, needle evacuation, simple excision, or laser treatment are some options
  - May spontaneously resolve

Prognosis

- Excellent, no malignant potential

MACROSCOPIC

General Features

- Usually small, skin-colored papule

MICROSCOPIC

Histologic Features

- Dermal cyst lined by bland stratified squamous epithelium with granular layer
- Intraluminal laminated keratin and numerous transversely and obliquely sectioned vellus hair shafts
  - Hair shafts are doubly refractile with polarized light
- Small hair follicles/pilosebaceous units may be seen attached to cyst wall
- Cyst can rupture and show surrounding granulomatous inflammation

Cytologic Features

- Bland squamous cells with uniform nuclei, small nucleoli, and eosinophilic cytoplasm

DIFFERENTIAL DIAGNOSIS

Epidermoid (Epidermal Inclusion, Follicular Infundibular) Cyst

- Typically larger in size
- Lacks intraluminal vellus hairs

Milial Cyst

- Small follicular cyst that lacks intraluminal vellus hairs

Steatocystoma

- Corrugated, eosinophilic cuticle lines inside of cyst wall
- Cyst lacks keratin and granular layer in cyst wall
- Associated sebaceous glands and small follicles usually present

Trichofolliculoma

- Usually solitary lesion
- Multiple primitive hair follicles open into larger follicle

DIAGNOSTIC CHECKLIST

Pathologic Interpretation Pearls

- Small epidermoid (follicular infundibular) cyst with intraluminal vellus hairs

SELECTED REFERENCES

1. Pauline G et al: Eruptive vellus hair cysts: an original case occurring in twins. Int J Dermatol. 54(6):e209-12, 2015
2. Shi G et al: Clinicopathological features and expression of four keratins (K10, K14, K17 and K19) in six cases of eruptive vellus hair cysts. Clin Exp Dermatol. 39(4):496-9, 2014
3. Patrizi A et al: Persistent milia, steatocystoma multiplex and eruptive vellus hair cysts: variable expression of multiple pilosebaceous cysts within an affected family. Dermatology. 196(4):392-6, 1998
4. Kiene P et al: Eruptive vellus hair cysts and steatocystoma multiplex. variants of one entity? Br J Dermatol. 134(2):365-7, 1996
5. Sexton M et al: Eruptive vellus hair cysts. A follicular cyst of the sebaceous duct (sometimes). Am J Dermatopathol. 11(4):364-8, 1989

KEY FACTS

TERMINOLOGY

- Benign cyst derived from sebaceous duct that may present as multiple lesions (steatocystoma multiplex) or as single lesion (simplex)

CLINICAL ISSUES

- Steatocystoma multiplex usually presents in adolescents, simplex in adults
- May occur at any site, but trunk most common location overall
- Steatocystoma multiplex: Multiple translucent flesh-colored to yellow dome-shaped papules or nodules
- Steatocystoma simplex: Solitary translucent flesh-colored to yellow dome-shaped papule or nodule

MICROSCOPIC

- Thin-walled multiloculated cyst located in dermis
- Undulating, eosinophilic cuticle forms inner lining of cyst
- Sebaceous lobules usually identified within cyst wall
- Lacks granular layer

TOP DIFFERENTIAL DIAGNOSES

- Vellus hair cyst
  - Has granular layer, rather than eosinophilic cuticle of steatocystoma
  - Lacks associated sebaceous glands
- Dermoid cyst
  - Occurs in younger patients
  - Has granular layer, rather than eosinophilic cuticle of steatocystoma
- Epidermoid cyst/epidermal inclusion cyst
  - Has granular layer
  - Lacks sebaceous glands in cyst wall
- Pilar cyst
  - Exhibits abrupt trichilemmal keratinization
  - Lack sebaceous glands

Steatocystoma With Multiple Thin-Walled Cystic Spaces

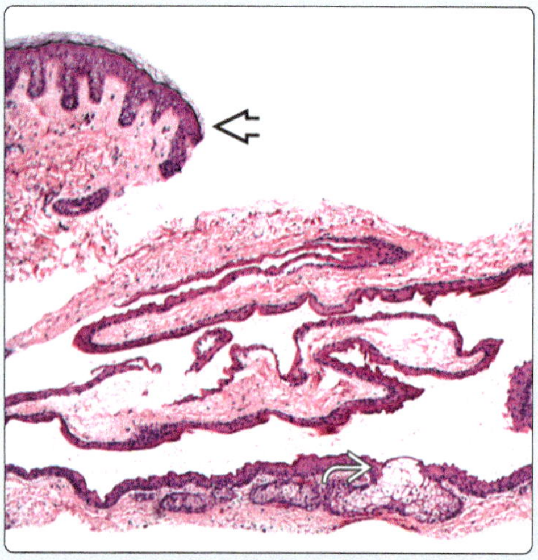

Typical Steatocystoma With Sebaceous Glands

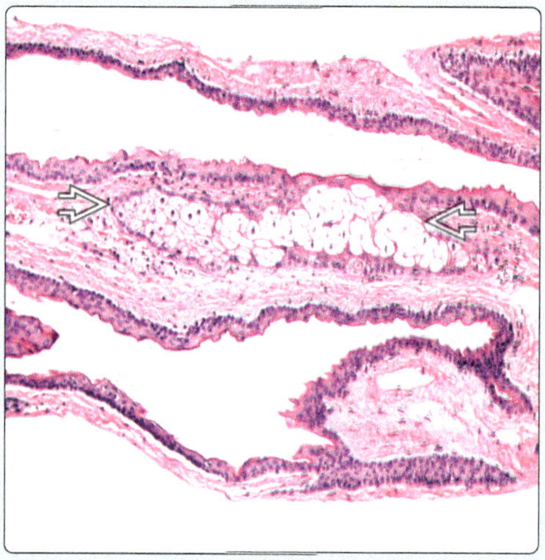

(Left) *Steatocystomas present as thin-walled dermal cysts. Note the normal epidermis in the upper left corner and sebaceous glands in the cyst wall.* **(Right)** *The cyst is lined by a thin squamous epithelial lining that has an eosinophilic cuticle and is associated with sebaceous glands.*

High Magnification of Lining of Steatocystoma

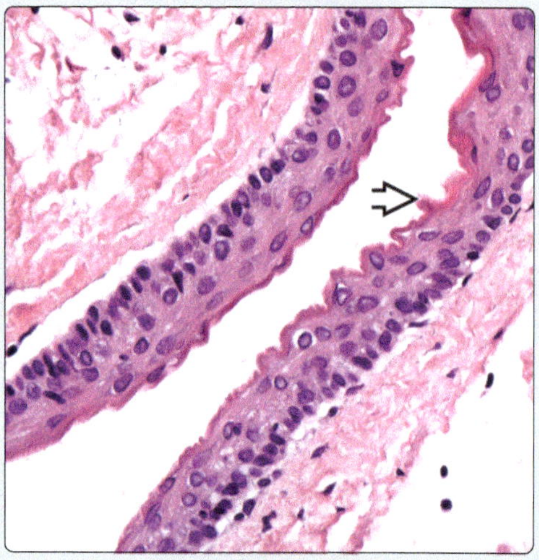

High Magnification of Steatocystoma With Vellus Hair Shaft

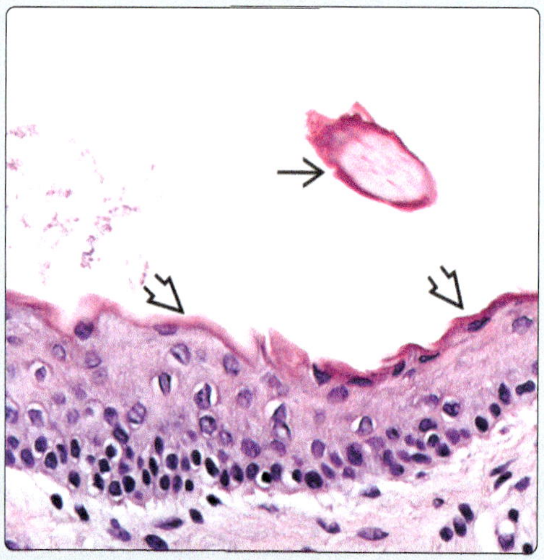

(Left) *The key diagnostic feature is the eosinophilic cuticle lining the cyst wall. It has an undulating crenulated appearance.* **(Right)** *The eosinophilic cuticle with its undulating, crenulated appearance is a key diagnostic feature. This cyst also has a fragment of a vellus hair shaft, a feature sometimes seen in steatocystomas.*

TERMINOLOGY

Definitions

- Benign cyst derived from sebaceous duct that may present as multiple lesions (steatocystoma multiplex) or as single lesion (steatocystoma simplex)

CLINICAL ISSUES

Epidemiology

- Incidence
  - Uncommon
- Age
  - Steatocystoma multiplex usually presents in adolescents
  - Steatocystoma simplex usually presents in adults

Site

- May occur at any site, but trunk is most common location for steatocystoma multiplex
  - Axillae and groin commonly affected in female patients
- Steatocystoma simplex most common on face, neck, chest, and axillae

Presentation

- Steatocystoma multiplex
  - Autosomal dominant inheritance or sporadic
  - Multiple translucent flesh-colored to yellow dome-shaped papules or nodules
- Steatocystoma simplex
  - Sporadic; no mode of inheritance
  - Solitary translucent flesh-colored to yellow dome-shaped papule or nodule

Treatment

- For steatocystoma multiplex, no treatment is necessary, as lesions are often too numerous to excise
- Excision is option for specific bothersome lesions or lesions that have ruptured, resulting in inflammatory response
- Simple excision can be offered for solitary lesions of steatocystoma simplex

Prognosis

- Benign lesions with no malignant potential

MACROSCOPIC

General Features

- Dermal-based cystic lesion; sectioning often releases dark, oily fluid

Size

- Usually between 3 mm and 3 cm

MICROSCOPIC

Histologic Features

- Thin-walled multiloculated cyst located in dermis
- Stratified squamous epithelial lining
  - Undulating, densely eosinophilic cuticle forms inner lining of cyst wall
  - Absent granular layer
- Sebaceous lobules usually identified within cyst wall
- Associated primitive follicle and vellus hairs may also be seen
- Cystic space is usually empty except for occasional presence of vellus hairs

DIFFERENTIAL DIAGNOSIS

Vellus Hair Cyst

- Dermal cyst lined by bland squamous epithelium
- Contains numerous vellus hairs
- Lining epithelium has granular layer, unlike steatocystoma
- Rare hybrid cysts may show combined features of vellus hair cyst and steatocystoma

Dermoid Cyst

- Presents at birth or in infancy
- Head and neck location, most common around eyes
- Cyst lined by stratified squamous epithelium with granular layer
- Sebaceous lobules and follicular structures often present in wall of cyst
- Multiple hair shafts often present

Epidermoid Cyst/Epidermal Inclusion Cyst

- Simple cyst lined by squamous epithelium
- Shows prominent granular layer and contains loose keratin
- Lacks follicular structures and vellus hairs

Pilar (Tricholemmal) Cyst

- Simple cyst lined by squamous epithelium
- Solitary or multiple
- Lacks granular layer and contains dense laminated keratin, often with calcifications

Cutaneous Keratocyst

- Usually associated with Gorlin-Goltz syndrome (nevoid basal cell carcinoma syndrome), but rare cases are sporadic
- Shows identical epithelial lining, with eosinophilic cuticle, as in steatocystoma
- Lacks associated sebaceous glands, vellus hairs, and primitive hair follicles

DIAGNOSTIC CHECKLIST

Pathologic Interpretation Pearls

- Undulating, eosinophilic cuticle is key microscopic feature
- Sebaceous glands in or closely associated with cyst wall should prompt consideration of steatocystoma
  - Sebaceous glands sometimes sparse or even absent

SELECTED REFERENCES

1. Marzano AV et al: Familial syringoma: report of two cases with a published work review and the unique association with steatocystoma multiplex. J Dermatol. 36(3):154-8, 2009
2. Cassarino DS et al: Cutaneous keratocyst arising independently of the nevoid basal cell carcinoma syndrome. Am J Dermatopathol. 27(2):177-8, 2005
3. Cambiaghi S et al: Steatocystoma multiplex and leuconychia in a child with Alagille syndrome. Br J Dermatol. 138(1):150-4, 1998
4. Covello SP et al: Keratin 17 mutations cause either steatocystoma multiplex or pachyonychia congenita type 2. Br J Dermatol. 139(3):475-80, 1998
5. Requena L et al: A facial variant of steatocystoma multiplex. Cutis. 51(6):449-52, 1993
6. Olsen DB et al: Steatocystoma simplex in the oral cavity: a previously undescribed condition. Oral Surg Oral Med Oral Pathol. 66(5):605-7, 1988
7. Leppard B et al: Gardner's syndrome and steatocystoma multiplex. Two unusual genetically determined conditions occurring in same patient. J Med Genet. 13(5):407-11, 1976

Cutaneous Keratocyst

KEY FACTS

TERMINOLOGY

- Nevoid basal cell carcinoma syndrome (NBCCS) cutaneous cyst/Gorlin-Goltz syndrome-associated cutaneous cysts
- Rare cutaneous cysts showing features identical to oral keratocysts

ETIOLOGY/PATHOGENESIS

- Most cases are associated with NBCCS/Gorlin-Goltz syndrome
  - Gorlin-Goltz syndrome: Multiple cutaneous basal cell carcinomas, odontogenic keratocysts of jaw, palmar and plantar pits, rare medulloblastomas, and skeletal abnormalities
- Rare cases not associated with NBCCS also reported

CLINICAL ISSUES

- Extremely rare lesions
- Typically occur on head and neck region but can occur at other sites
- Dermal cysts, usually multiple lesions, but may be single

MICROSCOPIC

- Dermal-based cystic proliferation lined by 2-5 cell layers of bland squamous cells
- Typically shows corrugated eosinophilic lining (cuticle) and parakeratosis on luminal surface
- No evidence of follicular or sebaceous differentiation (unlike steatocystoma)

TOP DIFFERENTIAL DIAGNOSES

- Steatocystoma
- Epidermoid (epidermal inclusion) cyst
- Pilar (tricholemmal) cyst
- Vellus hair cyst
- Hidrocystoma

DIAGNOSTIC CHECKLIST

- Bland squamous-lined cyst, which typically shows prominent corrugated eosinophilic lining (cuticle)

Scanning Magnification of Cutaneous Keratocyst

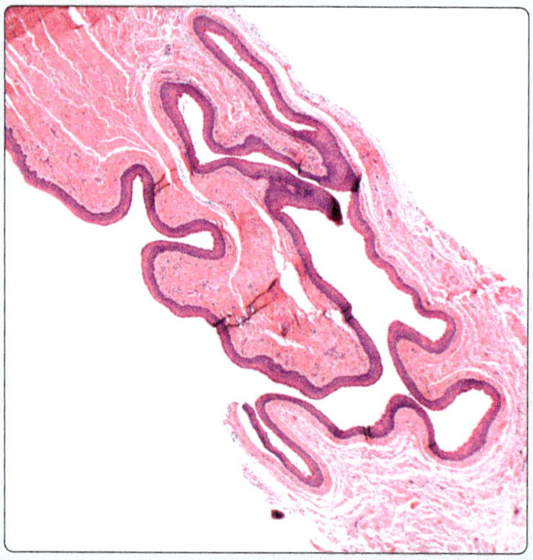

Intermediate Magnification of Cutaneous Keratocyst

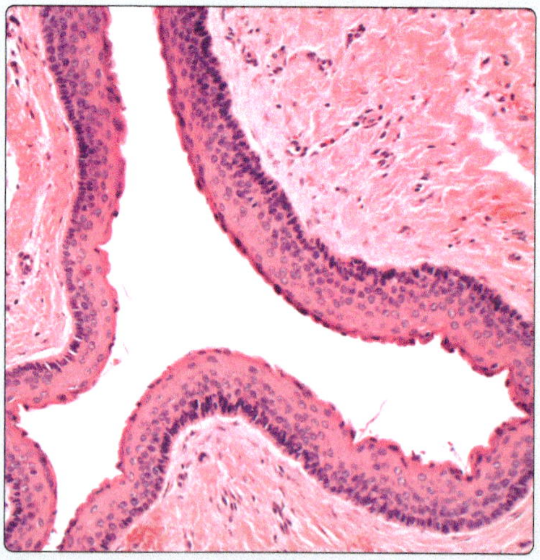

(Left) *Scanning magnification view of a cutaneous keratocyst shows an undulating squamous epithelium lining the irregularly shaped cystic spaces. There are no associated sebaceous glands, unlike steatocystoma.* **(Right)** *The cyst shows a bland, multilayered squamous lining surrounding an irregularly shaped cystic space.*

High Magnification of Dense Eosinophilic Cuticle of Keratocyst

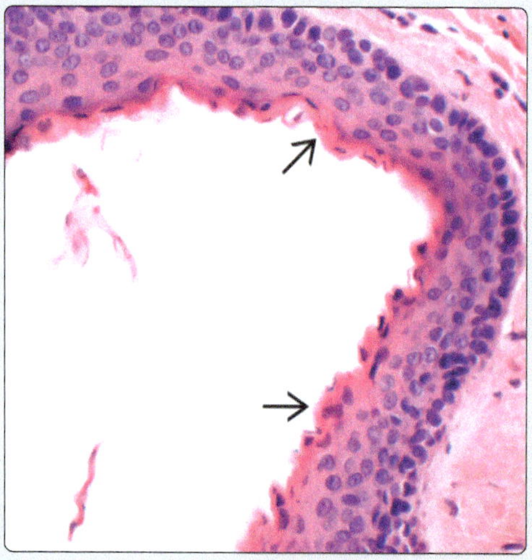

Dense Eosinophilic Cuticle of Keratocyst

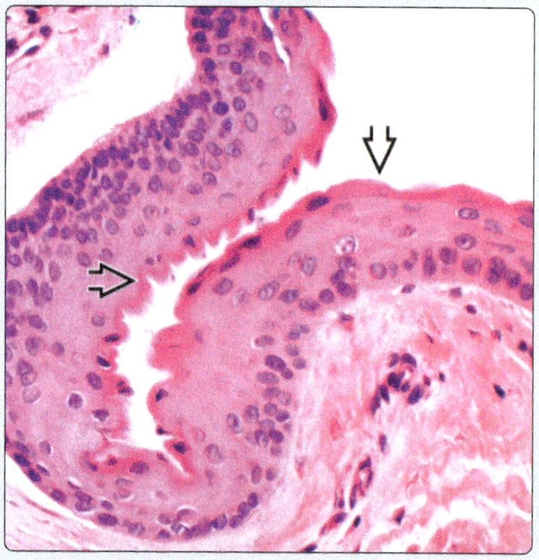

(Left) *High-magnification view of the lining of the cyst shows a bland, multilayered squamous epithelium with a dense eosinophilic cuticle ➡ and parakeratosis lining the cystic space.* **(Right)** *Another high magnification of a cutaneous keratocyst shows a bland squamous epithelium with a dense eosinophilic, jagged-appearing cuticle ⇨ lining the cystic space.*

TERMINOLOGY

Synonyms

- Nevoid basal cell carcinoma syndrome (NBCCS)/Gorlin-Goltz syndrome-associated cutaneous cyst

Definitions

- Rare cutaneous cyst showing features identical to oral keratocysts, often associated with NBCCS

ETIOLOGY/PATHOGENESIS

Genetic

- Most cases are associated with NBCCS (Gorlin-Goltz syndrome: Multiple cutaneous basal cell carcinomas, odontogenic keratocysts of jaw, palmar and plantar pits, rare medulloblastomas, and skeletal abnormalities)
  - Mutations for NBCCS in *PTCH1* gene on chromosome 9q22.3-q31, which encodes receptor for the Sonic Hedgehog signaling pathway
- Rare cases not associated with NBCCS also reported

CLINICAL ISSUES

Epidemiology

- Incidence
  - Extremely rare lesions
- Age
  - Typically occur in older adults

Site

- Variable, but typically on head and neck region

Presentation

- Dermal cyst; usually multiple lesions but may be single

Treatment

- Surgical approaches
  - Incision and drainage
  - Not necessary, but complete conservative excision may be performed to prevent recurrence

Prognosis

- Excellent; no malignant potential, but diagnosis should prompt clinical examination for other tumors (e.g., basal cell carcinomas, odontogenic keratocysts, medulloblastomas), as well as genetic studies for NBCCS

MACROSCOPIC

General Features

- Dark, oily fluid contents seen on gross sectioning

Size

- Typically small cystic lesion

MICROSCOPIC

Histologic Features

- Dermal-based cystic proliferation lined by 2-5 cell layers of bland-appearing squamous cells
  - Typically shows corrugated eosinophilic lining (cuticle) and parakeratosis on luminal surface, lacking granular layer, very similar to steatocystoma
- Clear proteinaceous cystic contents
- No evidence of follicular or sebaceous differentiation (unlike steatocystoma)

Cytologic Features

- Bland squamous cells with abundant eosinophilic cytoplasm

DIFFERENTIAL DIAGNOSIS

Steatocystoma

- Often multiple (steatocystoma multiplex)
- Similar cyst lining, lacking granular layer, but connections to sebaceous glands or primitive follicles, by definition, should be present (especially if multiple deeper level sections examined)

Epidermoid (Epidermal Inclusion) Cyst

- Keratinizing squamous lining with granular layer and lacking eosinophilic cuticle
- Usually shows abundant laminated keratin contents; may show hair fragments
- Often rupture and are associated with mixed acute and granulomatous inflammatory infiltrate

Pilar (Tricholemmal) Cyst

- Keratinizing squamous lining without granular layer and lacking eosinophilic cuticle
- Abundant dense hyalinized keratin contents, often with calcifications

Vellus Hair Cyst

- Large cystic follicular structure demonstrating numerous intraluminal miniaturized hairs
- Lacks classic eosinophilic corrugated lining of keratocyst and steatocystoma

Hidrocystoma

- Thin (1-2 cell layers thick) cyst lining composed of cuboidal epithelial cells, often with apocrine features
- Lacks corrugated lining of keratocyst

DIAGNOSTIC CHECKLIST

Pathologic Interpretation Pearls

- Bland squamous-lined cyst, which typically shows prominent corrugated eosinophilic lining (cuticle)

SELECTED REFERENCES

1. Makhija M: Cutaneous keratocyst and steatocystoma unified as sebaceous duct cyst, a hamartoma resembling the sebaceous duct. Am J Dermatopathol. 37(11):871-3, 2015
2. Tirado M et al: Histologic and immunohistochemical characteristics of cutaneous cysts in Goltz-Gorlin syndrome: clues for differentiation of nonsyndromic cysts. Am J Dermatopathol. 36(11):892-8, 2014
3. Fernandez-Flores A: Cutaneous keratocyst: a renaming as isthmic-anagenic cyst proposal. Am J Dermatopathol. 30(1):87-9, 2008
4. Peñaranda JM et al: Cutaneous keratocyst not associated to gorlin syndrome: an incidental finding in a healthy male. Am J Dermatopathol. 29(6):584-5, 2007
5. Cassarino DS et al: Cutaneous keratocyst arising independently of the nevoid basal cell carcinoma syndrome. Am J Dermatopathol. 27(2):177-8, 2005
6. Manfredi M et al: Nevoid basal cell carcinoma syndrome: a review of the literature. Int J Oral Maxillofac Surg. 33(2):117-24, 2004
7. Hamel AF et al: The cutaneous keratocyst: a rare hallmark of the nevoid basal cell carcinoma syndrome. Int J Surg Pathol. 11(1):36, 2003
8. Barr RJ et al: Cutaneous keratocysts of nevoid basal cell carcinoma syndrome. J Am Acad Dermatol. 14(4):572-6, 1986
9. Gorlin RJ et al: Multiple nevoid basal-cell epithelioma, jaw cysts and bifid rib. A syndrome. N Engl J Med. 262:908-12, 1960

Milial Cysts

KEY FACTS

TERMINOLOGY
- Small epidermoid/infundibular cyst

CLINICAL ISSUES
- Very common lesions
- Can occur at any age
- No gender predilection
- Primary milial cysts
  - Occur spontaneously and typically seen on face
  - Rarely on mucosa (Epstein pearls) and palate (Bohn nodules)
- Secondary milial cysts
  - Occur at sites of trauma (i.e., after surgery, dermabrasion, burns, laser resurfacing)
  - Sites of subepidermal blistering diseases such as bullous pemphigoid and porphyria cutanea tarda
- Eruptive milia
  - Very rare
  - May be idiopathic or familial, autosomal dominant inheritance
- Milia en plaque
  - Very rare
  - Multiple milia on erythematous and edematous plaque

MICROSCOPIC
- Dermal-based, small cystic structures
- Lined by squamous epithelium with granular layer, similar to epidermal inclusion cyst
- Abundant intraluminal laminated keratin debris

TOP DIFFERENTIAL DIAGNOSES
- Epidermoid (epidermal inclusion, follicular infundibular) cyst
  - Larger cysts
- Vellus hair cyst
  - Contain multiple vellus hair shafts
- Steatocystoma

Low Magnification of Milial Cysts

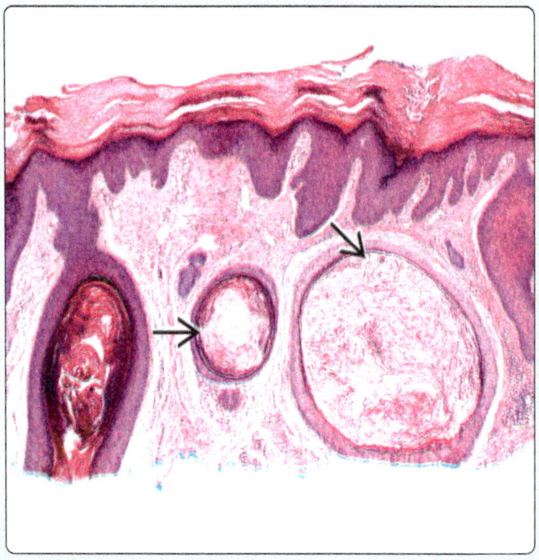

Keratin Debris Within Milia

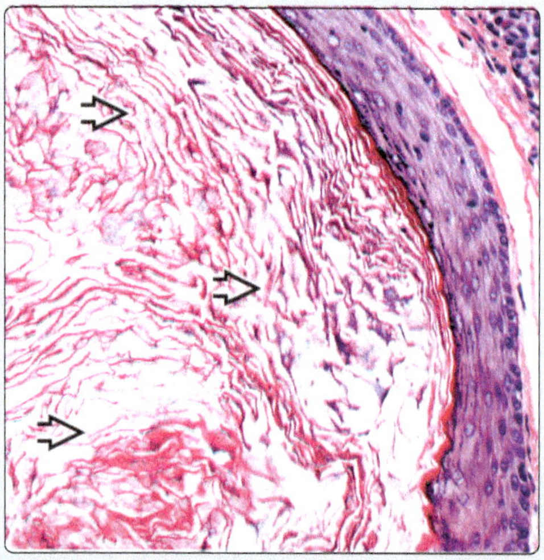

(Left) *Low magnification shows multiple small dermal cysts, which appear essentially identical to miniature epidermoid/follicular, infundibular-type cysts.* **(Right)** *The cyst contains abundant loose keratin flakes; granular layer is easily identified.*

Milial Cyst With Stromal Calcifications

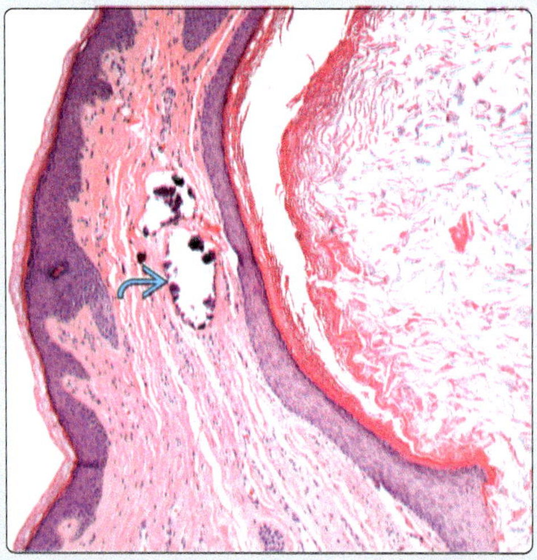

Milial Cyst With Rupture and Incidental Syringoma

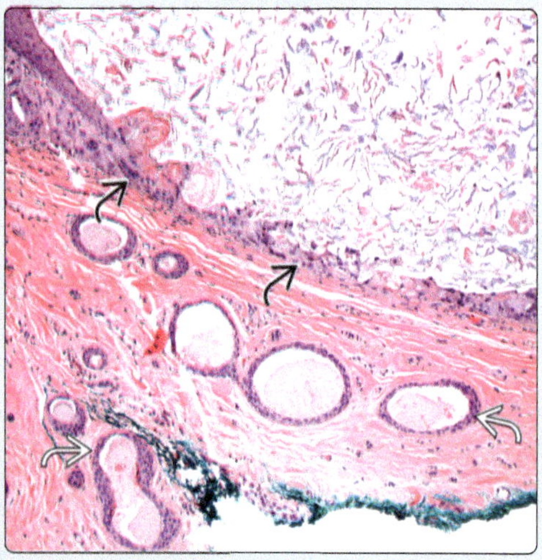

(Left) *This image shows a milial cyst with adjacent stromal calcifications and mild fibrosis, changes likely due to previous rupture of the cyst.* **(Right)** *This milial cyst shows evidence of rupture, with associated granulomatous inflammation partially replacing its wall. There was also a small incidental syringoma in this biopsy.*

TERMINOLOGY

Synonyms

- Milial

Definitions

- Basically small epidermal inclusion/epidermoid (follicular, infundibular-type) cysts

CLINICAL ISSUES

Epidemiology

- Incidence
  - Very common
- Age
  - Any age
    - Newborns, children, and adults
- Sex
  - No gender predilection
- Ethnicity
  - No race predilection

Site

- Primary milial cysts
  - Face
- Secondary milial cysts
  - Any site

Presentation

- Primary milial cysts
  - Occur spontaneously
  - Typically seen on face
    - Rarely on mucosa (Epstein pearls) and palate (Bohn nodules)
  - Common in newborns
- Secondary milial cysts
  - Sites of trauma
    - After surgery, dermabrasion, burns, laser resurfacing
  - Sites of subepidermal blistering diseases such as
    - Bullous pemphigoid
    - Porphyria cutanea tarda
    - Epidermolysis bullosa
    - Bullous lichen planus
- Eruptive milial are very rare
  - Idiopathic
  - Familial, autosomal dominant inheritance
  - Rarely associated with genodermatoses, including
    - Basaloid follicular hamartoma syndrome
    - Bazex syndrome
    - Rombo syndrome
    - Gardner syndrome
    - Orofaciodigital syndrome
- Milial en plaque
  - Very rare
  - Multiple milia on erythematous and edematous plaque
  - Head and neck

Treatment

- Not necessary
  - If cosmetically bothersome: Needle evacuation, mechanical dermabrasion, retinoids, and laser treatment are some options

Prognosis

- Excellent, no malignant potential

MACROSCOPIC

General Features

- Small, skin-colored to whitish, firm papules

Size

- 1-2 mm

MICROSCOPIC

Histologic Features

- Dermal-based, small cystic structures
  - Often multiple
- Lined by stratified squamous epithelium with granular layer
  - Appear similar to epidermal inclusion/epidermoid cysts
- Abundant intraluminal laminated keratin debris

Cytologic Features

- Bland squamous cells with small uniform nuclei and eosinophilic cytoplasm
- No mitoses

DIFFERENTIAL DIAGNOSIS

Epidermoid (Epidermal Inclusion, Follicular Infundibular) Cyst

- Larger; otherwise shows same histology, with abundant intraluminal keratin and granular layer

Vellus Hair Cyst

- Larger, similar to epidermoid cysts
- Shows numerous intraluminal vellus hairs

Steatocystoma

- Shows eosinophilic corrugated lining
- Lacks intraluminal keratin
- Typically has attached sebaceous glands and often vellus follicles

DIAGNOSTIC CHECKLIST

Pathologic Interpretation Pearls

- Small cyst with squamous epithelium and keratin cyst content

SELECTED REFERENCES

1. Hallaji Z et al: Bilateral retro-auricular milia en plaque: a case report and review of the literature. Dermatol Online J. 16(1):12, 2010
2. Leong T et al: Pronounced secondary milia precipitated by a superficial traumatic abrasion in a 4-year-old boy. J Pediatr. 156(5):854, 2010
3. Pozo J et al: Variants of milia successfully treated with CO(2) laser vaporization. J Cosmet Laser Ther. 12(4):191-4, 2010
4. Berk DR et al: Milia: a review and classification. J Am Acad Dermatol. 59(6):1050-63, 2008
5. Dogra S et al: Milia en plaque. J Eur Acad Dermatol Venereol. 19(2):263-4, 2005
6. Langley RG et al: Multiple eruptive milia: report of a case, review of the literature, and a classification. J Am Acad Dermatol. 37(2 Pt 2):353-6, 1997
7. Wolfe SF et al: Eruptive milia. Cutis. 60(4):183-4, 1997
8. Inman P: Milia following bullous dermatitis. Br J Dermatol. 81(2):132-3, 1969

Hidrocystoma (Apocrine and Eccrine)

KEY FACTS

TERMINOLOGY

- Cystic, dome-shaped, translucent papules with bluish hue commonly found on eyelids
- Synonyms include
  - Cystadenoma (apocrine and eccrine)
  - Papillary apocrine gland cyst
  - Sudoriferous cyst

ETIOLOGY/PATHOGENESIS

- Most hidrocystomas are now considered to be of apocrine origin

CLINICAL ISSUES

- Relatively common lesions
- Predominately occur on face, especially in periorbital region
- Occur in adults, no particular age group
- Slightly more common in female than male patients
- Appear as translucent to bluish, dome-shaped papule
- Treatment not necessary in most cases

MICROSCOPIC

- Dermal unilocular or multilocular cyst
- Often no cyst contents, appears empty
- Cystic spaces lined by 1-2 layers of cuboidal or columnar epithelium
- Papillary projection into cyst cavity: Decapitation secretion typically present
- Secretory cells occasionally contain pigment granules
- PAS-positive, diastase-resistant granules are also seen in secretory cells
- Beneath secretory cells are elongated myoepithelial cells

TOP DIFFERENTIAL DIAGNOSES

- Apocrine (papillary) cystadenoma
- Median raphe cysts
- Cutaneous ciliated cyst

Low Magnification of Apocrine Hidrocystoma

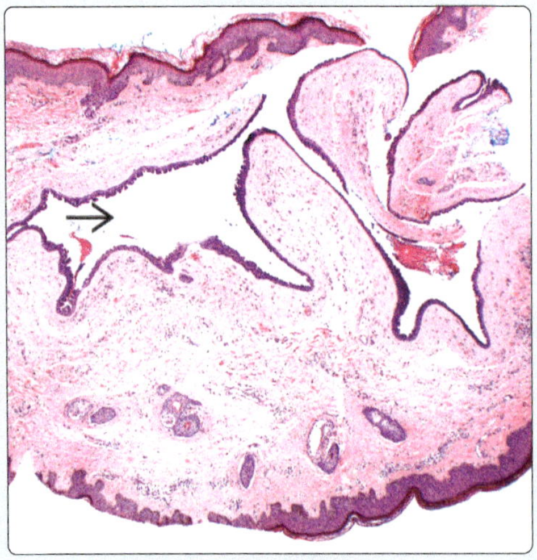

Higher Magnification of Apocrine Hidrocystoma

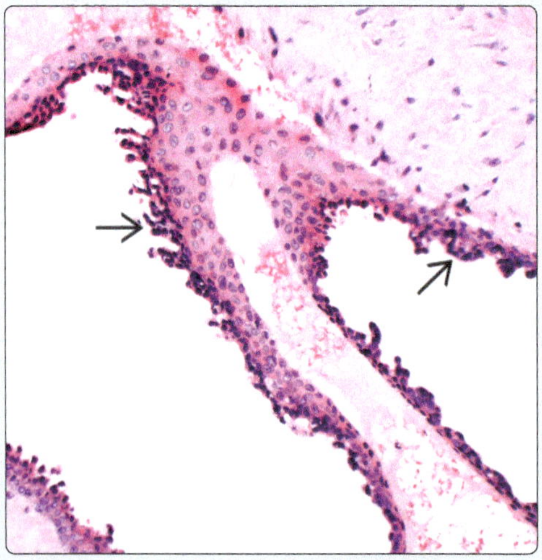

(Left) *Hidrocystoma on low magnification shows characteristic thin-walled, dermal-based, clear cystic spaces →.* **(Right)** *Higher magnification of an apocrine hidrocystoma shows a thin layer of bland-appearing apocrine epithelium → lining the cystic lumina.*

Papillary Hidrocystoma

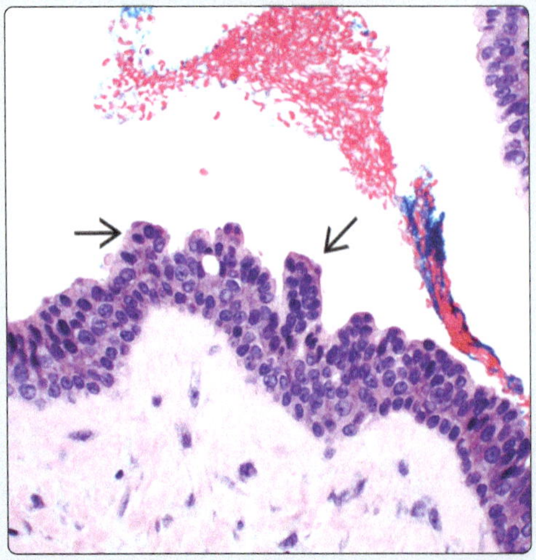

Papillary Hidrocystoma (Cystadenoma)

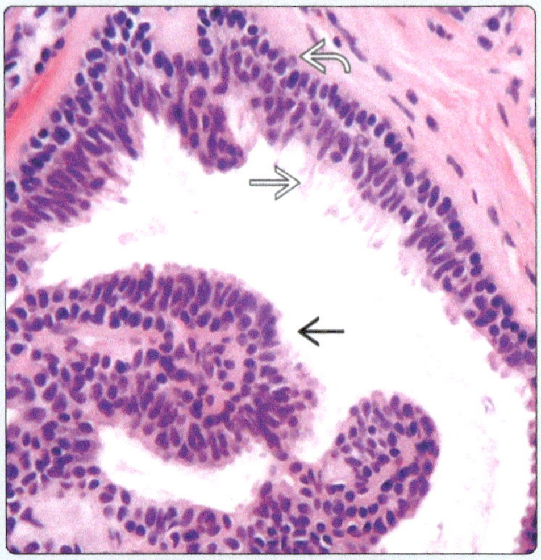

(Left) *Hyperplastic epithelial lining with small, thin papillary projections → can be seen in some cases.* **(Right)** *More cellular lesions are considered cystadenomas. Two or more layers of cuboidal-columnar epithelium → line the cyst. An outer layer of myoepithelial cells ↩ is present. Prominent decapitation secretion ⇨ (indicative of apocrine differentiation) is seen.*

TERMINOLOGY

Synonyms

- Cystadenoma (apocrine and eccrine)
- Apocrine gland cyst

Definitions

- Cystic, dome-shaped, translucent papules with bluish hue commonly found on eyelids

ETIOLOGY/PATHOGENESIS

Eccrine vs. Apocrine Hidrocystomas

- Most hidrocystomas are now considered to be of apocrine origin
- Apocrine hidrocystoma
  - Usually multiloculate
  - Cytoplasmic projections into cyst cavity: Decapitation secretion present
- Eccrine hidrocystoma
  - Usually unilocular
  - No decapitation secretion

CLINICAL ISSUES

Epidemiology

- Incidence
  - Relatively common
- Age
  - Adults, no particular age group
- Sex
  - Female slightly more than male patients

Site

- Commonly on face
  - Predominately in periorbital region

Presentation

- Translucent to bluish, dome-shaped papule
- Solitary or multiple

Treatment

- Not necessary
  - If cosmetically bothersome, needle evacuation or simple excision are some options

Prognosis

- Excellent, no malignant potential

MACROSCOPIC

General Features

- During sectioning, clear, brownish, or blackish fluid is released, and cyst collapses

Size

- Commonly 1-15 mm

MICROSCOPIC

Histologic Features

- Dermal-based unilocular or multilocular cyst
- Often, no cyst contents: Appears empty
  - Cyst contents often leak during incision or during sectioning of tissue
- Cystic spaces lined by 1-2 layers of cuboidal or columnar epithelium
  - Secretory cells have abundant eosinophilic cytoplasm and basally located nucleus
  - Foci of hyperplasia and papillomatous areas of secretory cells
    - Occasionally with papillary projections into cyst space
    - Cytoplasmic projections consistent with decapitation secretion
    - If prominent hyperplasia and connective tissue core are present, considered to be cystadenoma
  - PAS(+), diastase-resistant granules are seen in secretory cells
- Secretory cells occasionally contain pigment granules
  - Cause brownish-blue color of cystic fluid
  - This pigment is neither melanin nor hemosiderin
- Beneath secretory cells are elongated myoepithelial cells

Cytologic Features

- Secretory cells are bland cuboidal or columnar epithelium

DIFFERENTIAL DIAGNOSIS

Apocrine (Papillary) Cystadenoma

- Some consider this entity to be type of apocrine hidrocystoma
- Studies, however, have shown this to be proliferative tumor and not simple cyst like most hidrocystomas
  - Papillary projections with fibrous core
  - Increased mitotic rate within secretory cells
    - Increased Ki-67 staining

Median Raphe Cysts

- Located on ventral penis, scrotum, or perineum
- Cyst is lined by pseudostratified columnar epithelium
  - Occasional mucin-containing cells present
  - Rarely, ciliated cells present

Cutaneous Ciliated Cyst

- Lower extremities of women
- Cyst is lined by ciliated cuboidal to columnar epithelium
  - Foci of pseudostratified epithelium common

DIAGNOSTIC CHECKLIST

Pathologic Interpretation Pearls

- Dermal, empty unilocular or multilocular cyst
- Cyst lined by 1-2 layers of cuboidal or columnar epithelium

SELECTED REFERENCES

1. Jakobiec FA et al: A reappraisal of eyelid eccrine and apocrine hidrocystomas: microanatomic and immunohistochemical studies of 40 lesions. Am J Ophthalmol. 151(2):358-74, 2011
2. Verma SB: Multiple apocrine hidrocystomas: a confusing clinical diagnosis. An Bras Dermatol. 85(2):260-3, 2010
3. Sugiyama A et al: Apocrine cystadenoma and apocrine hidrocystoma: examination of 21 cases with emphasis on nomenclature according to proliferative features. J Cutan Pathol. 34(12):912-7, 2007
4. Simón RS et al: Does eccrine hidrocystoma exist? J Cutan Pathol. 25(3):182-4, 1998
5. Macmillan A et al: Hidrocystoma. Br J Dermatol. 88(2):201-2, 1973

KEY FACTS

TERMINOLOGY

- Solitary, dome-shaped, skin-colored to translucent papule
- Synonyms
  - Digital myxoid cyst
  - Digital synovial cyst
  - Periungual ganglions

ETIOLOGY/PATHOGENESIS

- Unclear etiology
- Most view digital mucous cyst and digital myxoid cyst to be synonymous

CLINICAL ISSUES

- Relatively common lesions
- Mostly occur in adults
- Slight female predilection
- Most commonly present on dorsum of fingers
- Excellent prognosis, no malignant potential
- Treatment not necessary in most cases
  - Only for symptoms such as pain, or if cosmetically bothersome

MICROSCOPIC

- Subepidermal cystic space or clefts with collection of mucin and stellate fibroblasts
- No epithelial lining present
- Overlying epidermis is often thinned
- Surrounding collagen is often compressed
- Often show increased numbers of small blood vessels
- Mucin is positive with colloidal iron and Alcian blue stains

TOP DIFFERENTIAL DIAGNOSES

- Ganglion cyst
- Focal mucinosis
- Cutaneous myxoma (superficial angiomyxoma)

Low Magnification of Digital Mucus Cyst

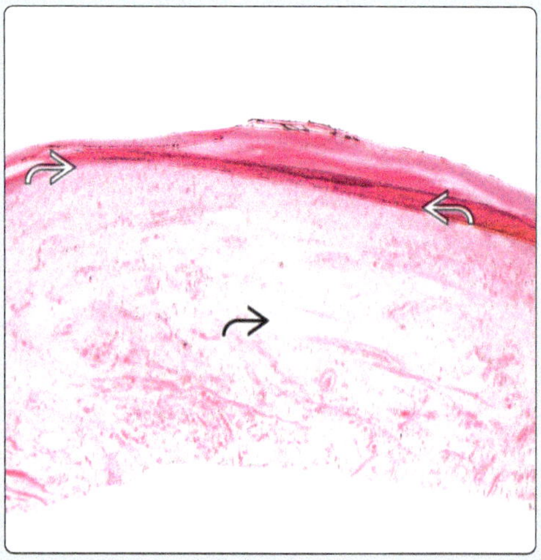

Higher Magnification of Digital Mucus Cyst

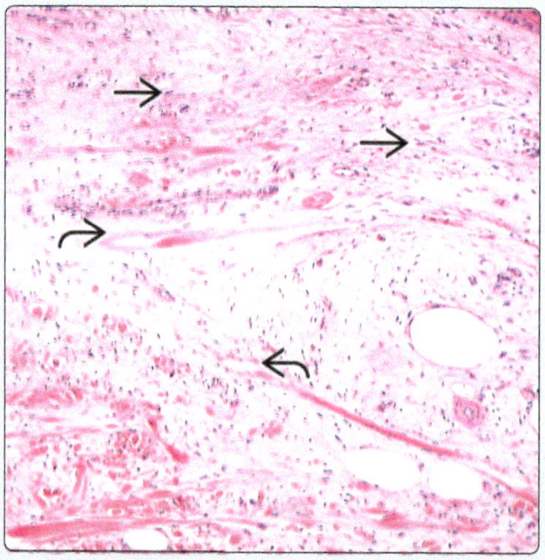

(Left) *Earlier lesions show pools of mucin infiltrating between collagen bundles. Prominent effacement of the overlying epidermal rete ridges is present.* **(Right)** *Within the mucinous matrix, an increased number of small vessels and stromal fibroblasts are seen.*

Digital Mucous Cyst With Grenz Zone

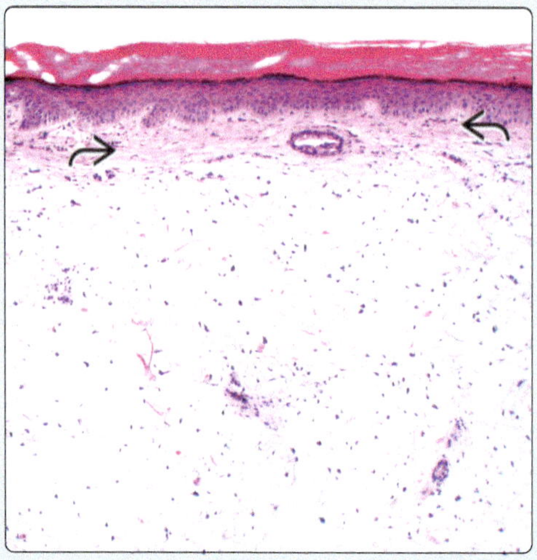

Deep Dermal Involvement

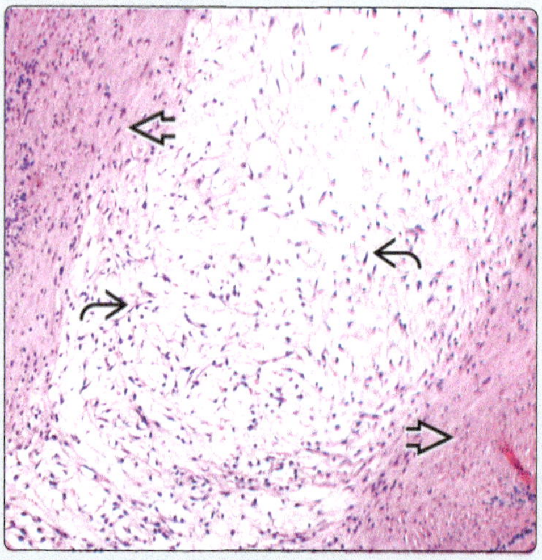

(Left) *Digital mucous cyst at low magnification shows that the epidermis is separated from the mucinous deposits by a thin grenz zone.* **(Right)** *Deep dermal area involved by digital mucous cyst shows a central collection of prominent mucinous material with increased numbers of small, spindle-shaped fibroblasts surrounded by compressed stroma.*

TERMINOLOGY

Abbreviations

- Digital mucous cyst (DMC)

Synonyms

- Digital myxoid cyst
- Digital synovial cyst
- Nail cysts
- Periungual ganglions
- Myxomatous cutaneous cysts

Definitions

- Solitary, dome-shaped, skin-colored to translucent papule

ETIOLOGY/PATHOGENESIS

Unclear Etiology

- There are 2 views as to possible etiology
  - Lesions near proximal nail may be due to local synthesis of mucin by fibroblasts
    - Identical to focal mucinosis of skin and are termed DMC
  - Lesions on distal interphalangeal joint may be due to herniation of joint lining
    - Identical to ganglion and are termed myxoid cyst
- Most view DMC and digital myxoid cyst to be synonymous

CLINICAL ISSUES

Epidemiology

- Incidence
  - Relatively common
- Age
  - Adults
- Sex
  - Slight female predilection
- Ethnicity
  - No ethnic predilection

Site

- Dorsum of fingers
  - Occasionally dorsum of toes

Presentation

- Solitary papule
- Dorsum of fingers, typically at base of nail
- Can cause deformity of involved nail

Treatment

- Not necessary
  - Most cases are asymptomatic
- For symptoms such as pain or if cosmetically bothersome
  - Steroid injection
  - Electrocautery
  - Chemical cautery
  - Lesions tend to recur and often require multiple treatments

Prognosis

- Excellent, no malignant potential

MACROSCOPIC

General Features

- Gelatinous fluid contents released during gross sectioning

Size

- Commonly 3-7 mm

MICROSCOPIC

Histologic Features

- Subepidermal cystic space or clefts with collection of mucin and stellate fibroblasts
  - Overlying acral skin with stratum lucidum is diagnostic clue
- No epithelial lining present
- Overlying epidermis is often thinned
- Surrounding collagen is often compressed
- Usually show increased numbers of small blood vessels
- Mucin is strongly positive with colloidal iron and Alcian blue stains

Cytologic Features

- Bland-appearing, small stromal fibroblasts

DIFFERENTIAL DIAGNOSIS

Ganglion Cyst

- DMC may be considered superficial variant of ganglion cyst
  - Ganglion cysts are larger and more deeply located; usually located around wrists

Focal Mucinosis

- Histologically identical findings
- Location distinguishes from DMC (not on fingers)

Cutaneous Myxoma (Superficial Angiomyxoma)

- Solitary or multiple (associated with Carney complex)
- Prominent myxoid stroma with increased numbers of fibroblasts
- Differs from DMC by increased vascularity

DIAGNOSTIC CHECKLIST

Clinically Relevant Pathologic Features

- Cystic space with mucin on finger is characteristic for DMC

Pathologic Interpretation Pearls

- Subepidermal collection of mucin with stellate fibroblasts
- No epithelial lining and overlying thin acral skin with stratum lucidum

SELECTED REFERENCES

1. Salerni G et al: Dermatoscopic pattern of digital mucous cyst: report of three cases. Dermatol Pract Concept. 4(4):65-7, 2014
2. Li K et al: Digital mucous cysts. J Cutan Med Surg. 14(5):199-206, 2010
3. Misago N et al: Digital superficial angiomyxoma. Clin Exp Dermatol. 32(5):536-8, 2007
4. Lawrence C: Skin excision and osteophyte removal is not required in the surgical treatment of digital myxoid cysts. Arch Dermatol. 141(12):1560-4, 2005
5. Sonnex TS: Digital myxoid cysts: a review. Cutis. 37(2):89-94, 1986

Bronchogenic Cyst

KEY FACTS

TERMINOLOGY

- Rare congenital malformation of ventral foregut

CLINICAL ISSUES

- Pediatric population; rare in adults
- Midline superficial presternal or suprasternal is most common neck location
  - Less commonly: Lateral, thyroid, or subcutaneous
- M:F = 4:1
- Presents with airway compression, dysphagia, or infection, or may be asymptomatic
- Complete surgical excision is treatment of choice
- Excellent long-term clinical prognosis

IMAGING

- Best study: Contrast-enhanced MR T1WI or T2WI to show well-defined, solitary, smooth-bordered mass

MACROSCOPIC

- Grossly tubular, altered by infection
- Cut sections show clear serous to mucoid material

MICROSCOPIC

- Cyst lined by respiratory-type epithelium
- Cyst wall with mucoserous glands, hyaline cartilage, and smooth muscle

TOP DIFFERENTIAL DIAGNOSES

- Teratoma
- Dermoid cyst
- Branchial cleft cyst
- Thyroglossal duct cyst
- Cystic hygroma (lymphangioma)

Cyst Wall With Cartilage and Glands

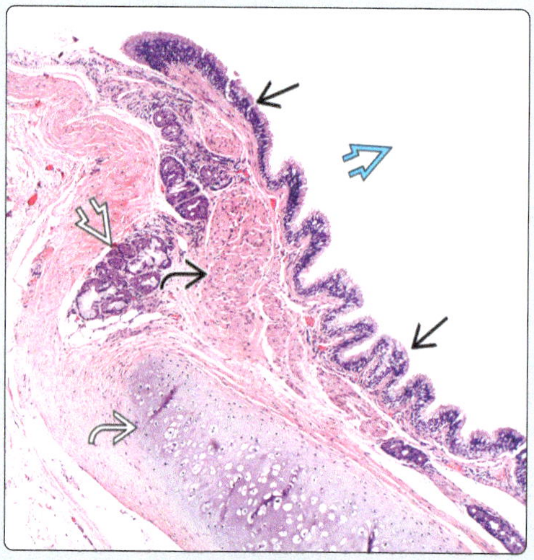

Ciliated Respiratory Epithelium

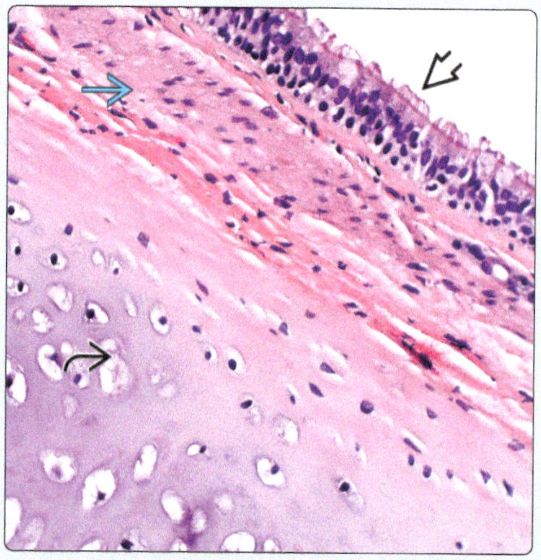

(Left) *This hematoxylin and eosin shows all the major features of a bronchogenic cyst: A cyst space lined by respiratory-type epithelium with a fibrous connective tissue wall that contains mucoserous glands, hyaline cartilage and smooth muscle. Multiple step sections may be needed to identify the different components.* **(Right)** *High-power image shows ciliated respiratory-type epithelium overlying a band of smooth muscle closely associated with cartilage.*

Wall Contents

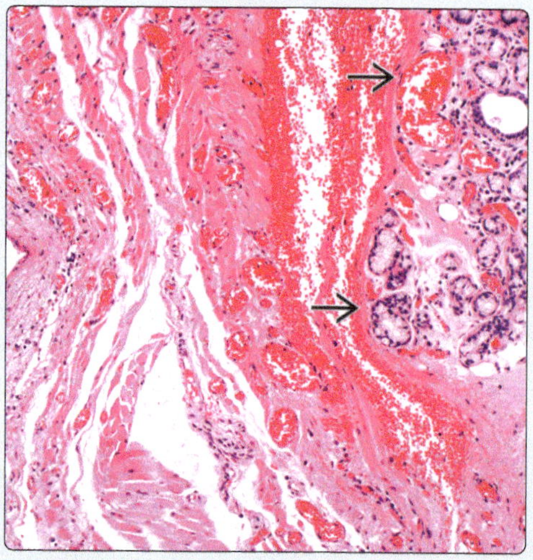

Highlighting of Smooth Muscle

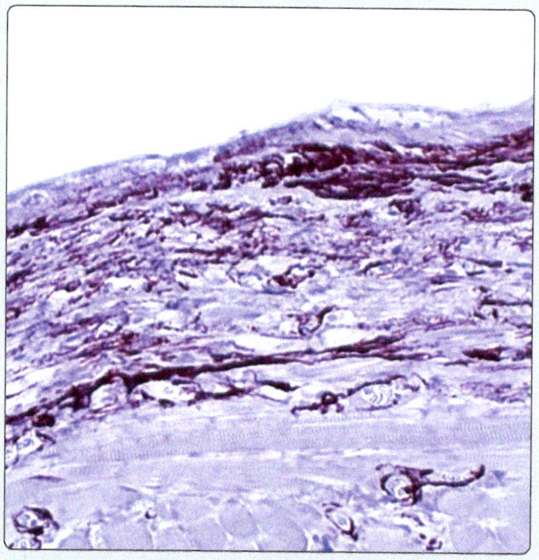

(Left) *Hematoxylin and eosin shows the fibrous wall of a bronchogenic cyst. Seromucinous glands are found throughout the wall and may contribute to the mucoid material found within the cyst.* **(Right)** *Smooth muscle, highlighted with smooth muscle actin, is characteristic within the wall of a bronchogenic cyst. Other cysts in the differential diagnosis, such as branchial cleft cysts and thyroglossal duct cysts, lack smooth muscle.*

TERMINOLOGY

Synonyms

- Bronchial cyst

Definitions

- Rare congenital malformation of ventral foregut
  - Enteric cyst, neurenteric cysts are part of same family

ETIOLOGY/PATHOGENESIS

Embryogenesis

- Derived from small buds of diverticula that separate from foregut during formation of tracheobronchial tree
- Usually between 26th-40th day of gestation

CLINICAL ISSUES

Epidemiology

- Incidence
  - Rare
- Age
  - Pediatric population; rare in adults
- Sex
  - M:F = 4:1

Site

- **Cervical**
  - Midline superficial presternal or suprasternal is most common location
  - Less commonly: Lateral, thyroid, or subcutaneous
- **Noncervical**
  - Mediastinum
  - Around hilum

Presentation

- Compression of airway: Respiratory distress, cough, dyspnea
- Dysphagia
- Infection may be uncommon
  - Drainage associated with sinus tract
  - Fever
- Asymptomatic presentation is uncommon

Endoscopic Findings

- May show compression of laryngotracheal axis

Treatment

- Options, risks, complications
  - Drainage and infection are possible complications
- Surgical approaches
  - Complete surgical excision is treatment of choice
    - Neck exploration and selective dissection via transcervical approach
    - Great vessels and recurrent laryngeal nerve are at risk
    - If sinus tract is present, it should be removed with cyst
  - Drainage and ablation
    - Indicated for only high-risk adults

Prognosis

- Excellent long-term clinical prognosis
- Recurrence develops if incompletely excised
- Rare cases of carcinoma arising from bronchogenic cyst

IMAGING

Radiographic Findings

- Best study: Contrast-enhanced T1WI or T2WI MR to show homogeneously increased signal
- Well-defined, solitary, smooth-bordered mass

MACROSCOPIC

General Features

- Grossly tubular, altered by infection
- Cut sections show clear serous to mucoid material

MICROSCOPIC

Histologic Features

- Cyst lined by respiratory-type epithelium
  - Ciliated
  - Pseudostratified
  - Columnar
  - Epithelium may be altered by infection: Stratified squamous
- Cyst wall contains
  - Mucoserous glands
  - Hyaline cartilage
  - Haphazard smooth muscle
  - Scant lymphoid tissue

ANCILLARY TESTS

Cytology

- Normal ciliated columnar cells
- Serous or mucinous material

DIFFERENTIAL DIAGNOSIS

Teratoma

- Tissues from sites other than respiratory tract

Dermoid Cyst

- Hair and skin appendages
- Squamous epithelium

Branchial Cleft Cyst

- Lymphoid tissue arranged in germinal centers
- Typically has stratified squamous epithelium
- Lacks smooth muscle and cartilage
- Clinically, usually found laterally

Thyroglossal Duct Cyst

- Usually has thyroid follicles
- Lacks smooth muscle and cartilage

Cystic Hygroma (Lymphangioma)

- Variably sized lymphatic vessels

SELECTED REFERENCES

1. Mattingly JK et al: Cervical bronchogenic cysts: case report and review of the literature. Am J Otolaryngol. 35(5):655-7, 2014
2. Crespo Del Hierro J et al: Cervical bronchogenic cysts. Acta Otorrinolaringol Esp. 64(5):379-81, 2013
3. Moz U et al: Bronchogenic cysts of the neck: a rare localization and review of the literature. Acta Otorhinolaryngol Ital. 29(1):36-40, 2009
4. Newkirk KA et al: Bronchogenic cysts of the neck in adults. Ann Otol Rhinol Laryngol. 113(9):691-5, 2004

Branchial Cleft Cyst

KEY FACTS

TERMINOLOGY

- Branchial cleft cyst (BCC) refers to congenital developmental lateral cervical cyst derived from remnants of 2nd branchial apparatus

ETIOLOGY/PATHOGENESIS

- Failure of obliteration of cervical sinus results in 2nd branchial cleft remnant (cyst, sinus, or fistula)

CLINICAL ISSUES

- BCC: ~ 20% of all congenital cervical cysts
- Bimodal presentation (< 5 years; 20-40 years)
- Waxing and waning, painless, compressible, cervical swelling
  - Enlarges after upper respiratory tract infection
- Along anterior border of sternocleidomastoid muscle
- Initial work-up of suspected branchial cleft anomaly (in order)
  - Intravenous or oral antibiotics (if infected), FNA, endoscopy &/or radiographic studies, surgery
- Complete surgical excision yields low recurrence risk

MICROSCOPIC

- Cyst lined by various types of epithelium (90% stratified squamous)
  - Basement membrane often beneath epithelium
- Lymphoid aggregates in cyst wall
- Lumen is filled with keratinaceous debris in many cases

ANCILLARY TESTS

- p16 may show focal, strong staining of superficial squamous epithelium and interdigitating cells

TOP DIFFERENTIAL DIAGNOSES

- Metastatic cystic squamous cell carcinoma, bronchiogenic cyst, cervical thymic cyst, metastatic cystic thyroid papillary carcinoma, thyroglossal duct cyst, dermoid cyst, laryngocele

CT of 2nd Branchial Cleft Cyst

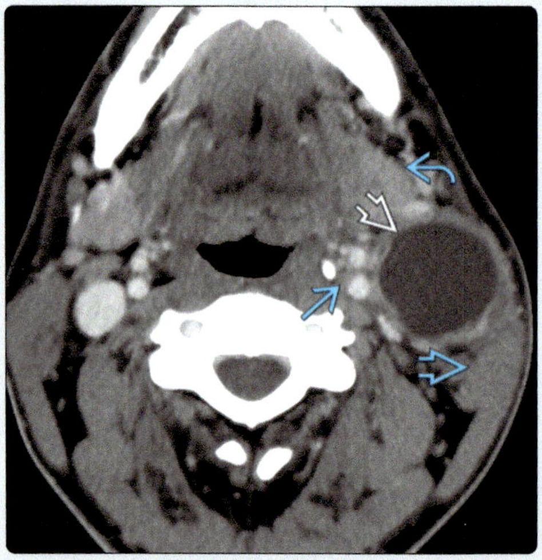

Gross Photo of Branchial Cleft Cyst

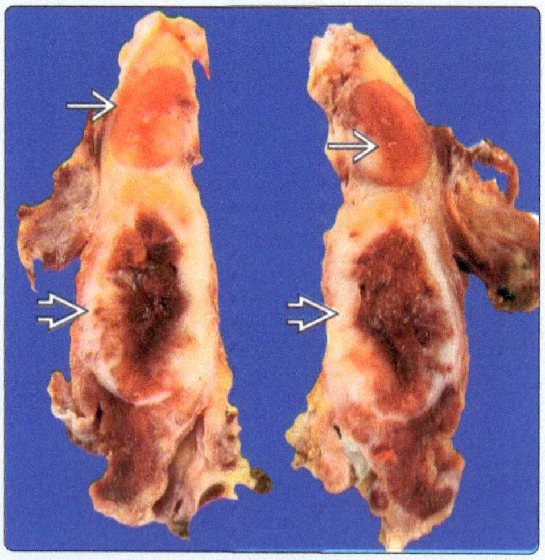

(Left) *Axial contrast-enhanced CT reveals a 2nd branchial cleft cyst (BCC) located posterior to the submandibular gland, lateral to the carotid space, and anterior to the sternomastoid muscle. Capsule thickening suggests inflammation.* **(Right)** *The resection specimen includes a benign lymph node, separate from the cyst immediately below. Note the thick, fibrous connective tissue wall surrounding the cyst, filled with hemorrhagic and keratinaceous material.*

Keratinaceous Debris in Branchial Cleft Cyst

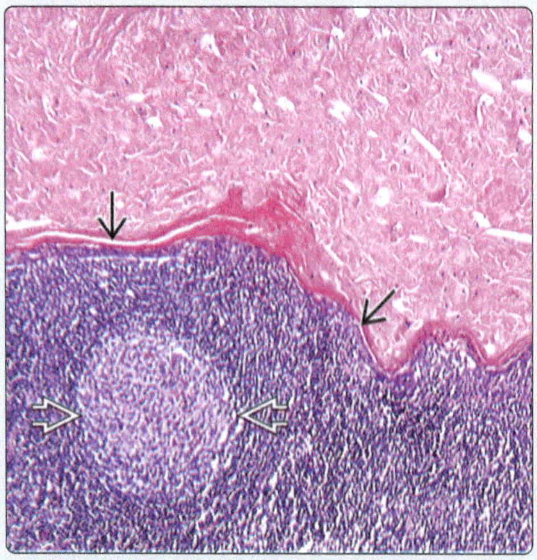

Metaplastic Squamous-Lined Cyst

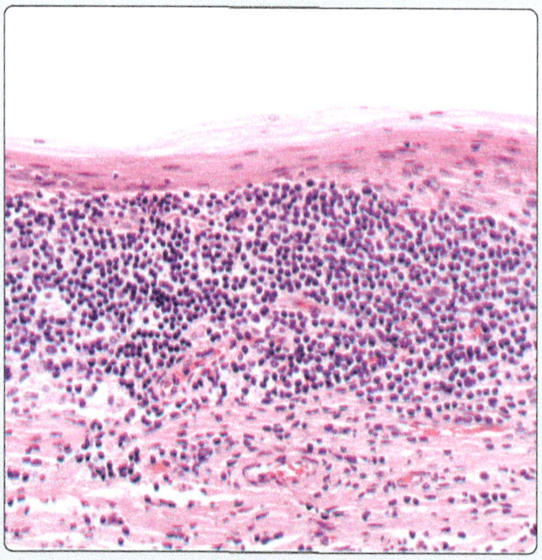

(Left) *The lumen of this BCC is filled with keratinaceous debris. There is a thin, squamous epithelium without any atypia. There is a germinal center within the associated lymphoid tissue.* **(Right)** *The cyst is lined by metaplastic squamous epithelium subtended by a very thin basement membrane between the epithelium and lymphoid tissue. Metaplasia is usually seen in patients who have had previous infection.*

TERMINOLOGY

Abbreviations

- Branchial cleft cyst (BCC)

Synonyms

- Lateral neck cyst
- Cervical lymphoepithelial cyst

Definitions

- By convention, BCC refers to congenital developmental lateral cervical cyst derived from remnants of 2nd branchial apparatus
  - ~ 80-90% of all branchial anomalies arise from 2nd branchial apparatus
  - Encompasses branchial cyst, sinus, or fistula

ETIOLOGY/PATHOGENESIS

Branchial Apparatus

- Precursor of many head and neck structures
- 2nd branchial arch overgrows 2nd, 3rd, and 4th clefts, forming "cervical sinus"
- Embryogenesis usually complete by 6-7 weeks of gestation
- Failure of obliteration of cervical sinus results in 2nd branchial cleft remnant (cyst, sinus, or fistula)
  - Sinus is respiratory epithelium lined, but squamous metaplasia and lymphoid hyperplasia develop as consequence of immunologic stimulation during infection
- 2nd branchial cleft fistula extends from skin anterior to sternocleidomastoid muscle (SCM), through carotid artery bifurcation to terminate in tonsillar fossa
- 3rd and 4th BCCs are very uncommon (< 5%)
  - Recurrent neck abscess or acute suppurative thyroiditis
  - Vast majority on left side (90-95%)
- Some authors posit cystic transformation of cervical lymph nodes (specifically in adults)

CLINICAL ISSUES

Epidemiology

- Incidence
  - Uncommon
    - Still, BCC are 1 of most commonly encountered congenital anomalies in pediatric otolaryngic practice
    - Thyroglossal duct cysts are most common
  - BCC accounts for ~ 20% of all congenital cervical cysts
    - Cysts > > sinuses (3:1)
  - ~ 80-90% of all branchial cleft anomalies are 2nd BCCs
  - 4th branchial cleft anomalies are rare and involve larynx (neonatal stridor and recurrent deep neck infection)
- Age
  - Bimodal presentation
    - < 5 years old (24%)
    - 20-40 years old (75%)
    - ~ 1% in > 50 years
- Sex
  - Equal gender distribution

Site

- Lateral neck near mandibular angle
- Along anterior border of SCM
  - Anywhere from hyoid bone to suprasternal notch
- Curiously, left-sided predominance for 4th branchial anomalies (> 90%)

Presentation

- Painless cervical swelling
  - Along anterior border of SCM
  - Often present for long duration
  - May be painful (if infected)
- Waxing and waning lesion
  - Frequently enlarges in concert with upper respiratory tract infection
  - Patients present during phase of recent enlargement
  - May lie dormant (clinically silent) for years
- Compressible, fluctuant
- Mucoid or pus-like secretions from sinus tract skin opening (when opening is present)
  - Patients present with external fistulae ± internal opening
- Clinically, some lesions may mimic parotid mass or odontogenic infection
- Bilateral lesions are usually identified in syndromic or familial association
- Clinically, 1st or 4th BCC more likely to have incision and drainage procedures, resulting in recurrence
- **Important**: Must consider metastatic cystic squamous cell carcinoma (SCC) in adults

Endoscopic Findings

- Advocated as part of initial assessment of neck cyst
  - Assess internal opening or draining sinus/fistula

Natural History

- Repeated infections and inflammation

Treatment

- Options, risks, complications
  - Initial work-up of suspected branchial cleft anomaly (in order)
    - Intravenous or oral antibiotics (if infected)
    - Fine-needle aspiration
    - Endoscopy (concurrent with surgery in some cases)
    - Radiographic studies
    - Surgery in nonresolving cases
  - Avoid repeated incision and drainage, as it yields high recurrence rate
  - Noninfected lesions are more easily removed than infected lesions
  - Entire fistula tract must be removed to prevent recurrence
  - Complications include possible wound infection and cranial nerve paresis
- Surgical approaches
  - Combined simultaneous endoscopic identification of sinus tract with lateral external cervical dissection
    - Cauterization of fistula used by some practitioners
    - Endoscopic placement of catheter into sinus lumen before surgical exploration
  - Complete surgical excision
    - May be difficult in recurrent cases due to scarring
    - Excision performed during quiescent phase (no active infection; 6-8 weeks after antibiotics)

- May need to include thyroid lobectomy to decrease recurrences
  - Must dissect around cyst bed to exclude fistula
    - If superomedial tract: Usually ends in faucial tonsil
    - If inferior tract: Travels down carotid space, exiting in supraclavicular area skin

Prognosis

- Lesions are benign without malignant potential
- Recurrence rate is variable
  - < 3% if not infected before surgery
  - ~ 20% if infected or previously incised/drained or incompletely removed

IMAGING

Radiographic Findings

- Combination of radiographic studies and endoscopy greatly improve surgical management and outcome
- Contrast CT (or MR) will easily suggest this diagnosis and differentiate it from solid mass
- Well-circumscribed nonenhancing low-density cystic mass with smooth cavity and thin wall (unless infected)
  - If infected, wall is thicker and enhances (cellulitis)
- Cystic, ovoid to rounded mucoid density mass in characteristic location is diagnostic
- Location
  - Posterolateral to submandibular gland
  - Lateral to carotid space
  - Anteromedial to SCM
  - Most are at or immediately caudal to mandibular angle
- Focal rim of cyst extending to carotid bifurcation
  - Notch sign is pathognomonic for 2nd BCC

MACROSCOPIC

General Features

- Unilocular, containing clear to grumous material

Size

- Wide range, up to 10 cm

MICROSCOPIC

Histologic Features

- Usually unilocular cyst
- Cyst lined by various types of epithelium
  - Stratified squamous (90%)
  - Respiratory epithelium (~ 8%)
    - Considered native lining in uninflamed cyst
  - Transitions or both (2%)
- Lumen is filled with keratinaceous debris in many cases
- Lymphoid aggregates usually subtend epithelial lining
  - Basement membrane frequently seen between epithelium and lymphoid elements
- Reactive germinal centers commonly present (~ 80%)
- Lymph node architecture is not present
  - No subcapsular sinus, medullary region, or interfollicular zone
- Acute and chronic inflammation frequently present
- Foreign body giant cell reaction within wall of cyst
- Fibrosis is frequently seen
  - Not heavy, thick "capsule" formation seen in metastatic cystic SCC
- Salivary gland tissue may be detected in wall
- Adnexa and cartilage are not seen in this type of BCC
  - Only seen in 1st BCCs/sinuses
- Absence of dysplasia, pleomorphism, increased mitoses, and carcinoma

ANCILLARY TESTS

Cytology

- Fine-needle aspiration is recommended in evaluation of all neck cysts
  - Usually of residual cyst post antibiotic therapy
- Thick, yellow, pus-like material is aspirated
- Smears are generally cellular
- Composed of anucleate squames and mature squamous epithelium
  - Columnar respiratory type cells are less common
- Amorphous debris often associated with macrophages
- Lymphoid infiltrate, including plasma cells
- Acute inflammatory cells if infected

Immunohistochemistry

- Variety of keratins are positive, depending on type of lining
  - Pseudostratified respiratory, transitional, stratified keratinizing, or nonkeratinizing squamous epithelium
- p16 negative in BCC while positive in metastatic SCC of oropharyngeal origin
- Isolated cells are strongly positive with p16, usually in epithelial cells surrounded by lymphocytes (interdigitating cells)
- p16 may show focal, strong staining of superficial squamous epithelium and interdigitating cells
- Glucose transporter 1 (GLUT1) negative in BCC but positive in metastatic cystic SCC

DIFFERENTIAL DIAGNOSIS

Metastatic Cystic Squamous Cell Carcinoma

- Jugulodigastric lymph node most commonly affected
- Unilocular cyst
- Very thick and well-developed capsule
- Subcapsular sinus, medullary zone, and interfollicular zones usually identified
- Ribbon-like distribution of atypical epithelium
- Lack of maturation, cellular enlargement, mitoses
- Pleomorphism is often limited and subtle, although can be profound in some cases
- Primary usually identified in
  - Tonsil and base of tongue: Frequently p16 positive
  - Nasopharynx: Frequently EBER positive
- Primary branchiogenic carcinoma **does not** exist

Bronchogenic Cyst

- Identified in subcutaneous tissue of supraclavicular region
- Radiographic appearance is different from BCC: Low in neck
- Cyst is lined by respiratory mucosa
- Cyst wall containing smooth muscle and bronchial glands

Cervical Thymic Cyst

- Often develop in children
- Affecting lateral cervical region
  - Angle of mandible to sternum, although usually lower neck
- Thymic tissue is present in cyst wall
  - Hassall corpuscles (squamous eddies)
  - Calcifications
  - Lymphoid elements

Metastatic Cystic Thyroid Papillary Carcinoma

- Lymph node architecture is easily identified
- May be unilocular lesion, with only serum or clear fluid in lumen
- Lining shows characteristic features of thyroid papillary carcinoma
  - Large cuboidal to columnar cells
  - Cellular crowding and overlapping
  - Cells have high nuclear:cytoplasmic ratio
  - Nuclear features of papillary carcinoma
    - Nuclear grooves, nuclear contour irregularities, nuclear folds
    - Nuclear enlargement, oval and elongated nuclei with overlapping
    - Intranuclear cytoplasmic inclusions
    - Nuclear chromatin clearing with condensation along nuclear membranes
  - Papillary architecture is frequently absent
  - **Positive**: Thyroglobulin, TTF-1, pax-8

Lymphangioma

- Generally clinical consideration
- Usually involves posterior cervical space
- Endothelial-lined spaces with serum, lymphocytes, and smooth muscle wall

Thyroglossal Duct Cyst

- Midline location or just off midline
- Cyst lined by squamous or respiratory epithelium that is associated with thyroid tissue
  - Thyroid tissue is often quite limited in extent
- Hyoid bone involved

Dermoid Cyst

- Sequestration of ectodermal tissue only
- Floor of mouth is most common location
- Squamous lining without lymphoid elements
- **No** other components
  - Muscle, nerve, or cartilage

Laryngocele

- Midline lesion, seldom confused with BCC
- Clinically classified into internal, external, and mixed types
- Lacks lymphoid stroma

SELECTED REFERENCES

1. Gaddikeri S et al: Congenital cystic neck masses: embryology and imaging appearances, with clinicopathological correlation. Curr Probl Diagn Radiol. 43(2):55-67, 2014
2. Zaifullah S et al: Diagnosis and treatment of branchial cleft anomalies in UKMMC: a 10-year retrospective study. Eur Arch Otorhinolaryngol. 270(4):1501-6, 2013
3. Goins MR et al: Pediatric neck masses. Oral Maxillofac Surg Clin North Am. 24(3):457-68, 2012
4. Guldfred LA et al: Branchial cleft anomalies: accuracy of pre-operative diagnosis, clinical presentation and management. J Laryngol Otol. 126(6):598-604, 2012
5. Slater J et al: Role of fine needle aspiration cytology in the preoperative investigation of branchial cysts. ANZ J Surg. 82(1-2):42-5, 2012
6. Veivers D et al: Lateral cervical cysts: an Australian perspective. ANZ J Surg. 82(11):799-802, 2012
7. Nicoucar K et al: Management of congenital fourth branchial arch anomalies: a review and analysis of published cases. J Pediatr Surg. 44(7):1432-9, 2009
8. Ozolek JA: Selective pathologies of the head and neck in children: a developmental perspective. Adv Anat Pathol. 16(5):332-58, 2009
9. Pai RK et al: p16(INK4A) immunohistochemical staining may be helpful in distinguishing branchial cleft cysts from cystic squamous cell carcinomas originating in the oropharynx. Cancer. 117(2):108-19, 2009
10. Doshi J et al: Branchial cyst side predilection: fact or fiction? Ann Otol Rhinol Laryngol. 116(2):112-4, 2007
11. Kadhim AL et al: Pearls and pitfalls in the management of branchial cyst. J Laryngol Otol. 118(12):946-50, 2004
12. Thompson LD: Branchial cleft cyst. Ear Nose Throat J. 83(11):740, 2004
13. Weiner MF et al: Diagnostic value of GLUT-1 immunoreactivity to distinguish benign from malignant cystic squamous lesions of the head and neck in fine-needle aspiration biopsy material. Diagn Cytopathol. 31(5):294-9, 2004
14. Glosser JW et al: Branchial cleft or cervical lymphoepithelial cysts: etiology and management. J Am Dent Assoc. 134(1):81-6, 2003
15. Prasad KK et al: Cervical thymic cyst: report of a case and review of the literature. Indian J Pathol Microbiol. 44(4):483-5, 2001
16. Koeller KK et al: Congenital cystic masses of the neck: radiologic-pathologic correlation. Radiographics. 19(1):121-46; quiz 152-3, 1999
17. Edmonds JL et al: Third branchial anomalies. Avoiding recurrences. Arch Otolaryngol Head Neck Surg. 123(4):438-41, 1997
18. Regauer S et al: Lateral neck cysts–the branchial theory revisited. A critical review and clinicopathological study of 97 cases with special emphasis on cytokeratin expression. APMIS. 105(8):623-30, 1997
19. Thompson LD: Diagnostically challenging lesions in head and neck pathology. Eur Arch Otorhinolaryngol. 254(8):357-66, 1997
20. Choi SS et al: Branchial anomalies: a review of 52 cases. Laryngoscope. 105(9 Pt 1):909-13, 1995
21. Clevens RA et al: Familial bilateral branchial cleft cysts. Ear Nose Throat J. 74(6):419-21, 1995
22. Blackwell KE et al: Functional neck dissection for treatment of recurrent branchial remnants. Arch Otolaryngol Head Neck Surg. 120(4):417-21, 1994
23. Golledge J et al: The aetiology of lateral cervical (branchial) cysts: past and present theories. J Laryngol Otol. 108(8):653-9, 1994
24. Todd NW: Common congenital anomalies of the neck. Embryology and surgical anatomy. Surg Clin North Am. 73(4):599-610, 1993
25. Rosenfeld RM et al: Fourth branchial pouch sinus: diagnosis and treatment. Otolaryngol Head Neck Surg. 105(1):44-50, 1991
26. Takimoto T et al: Branchial cleft (pouch) anomalies: a review of 42 cases. Auris Nasus Larynx. 18(1):87-92, 1991
27. Godin MS et al: Fourth branchial pouch sinus: principles of diagnosis and management. Laryngoscope. 100(2 Pt 1):174-8, 1990
28. Kenealy JF et al: Branchial cleft anomalies: a five-year retrospective review. Trans Pa Acad Ophthalmol Otolaryngol. 42:1022-5, 1990
29. Doi O et al: Branchial remnants: a review of 58 cases. J Pediatr Surg. 23(9):789-92, 1988
30. Harnsberger HR et al: Branchial cleft anomalies and their mimics: computed tomographic evaluation. Radiology. 152(3):739-48, 1984

Branchial Cleft Cyst

(**Left**) *The failure of a branchial apparatus cleft (c) or pouch (p) to involute or fuse during embryologic development results in the development of 2nd, 3rd, and 4th branchial cleft anomalies.* (**Right**) *CT shows a low-attenuation nonenhancing right BCC anterolateral to the carotid sheath, anteromedial to the sternocleidomastoid muscle (SCM), and posterolateral to the submandibular gland. This is characteristic of a noninflamed BCC.*

Branchial Apparatus Development Graphic

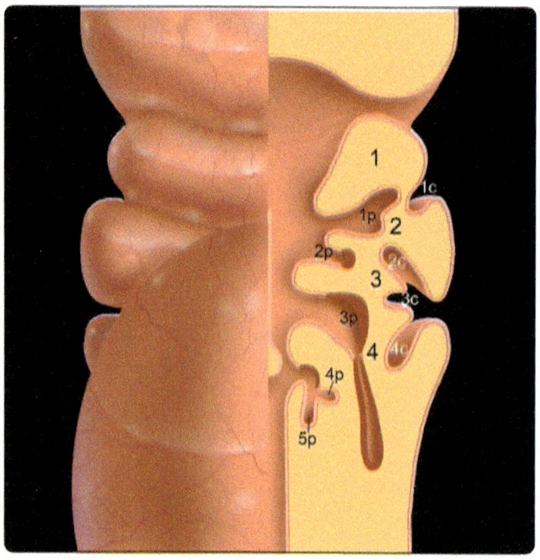

CT of Nonenhancing Branchial Cleft Cyst

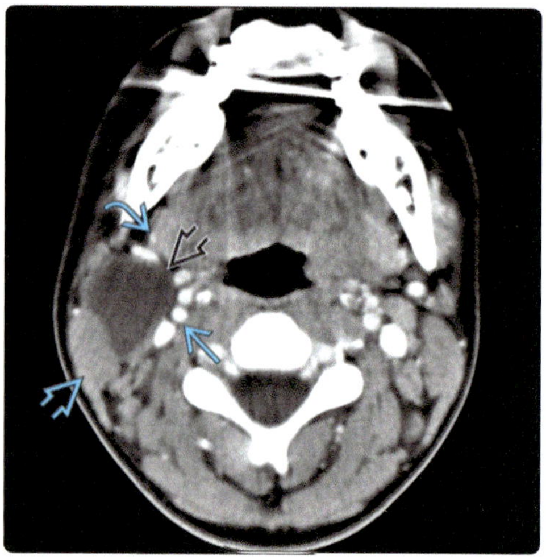

(**Left**) *A 2nd BCC/sinus/fistula can develop anywhere along the normal development of the branchial pouches and arches. The opening in the tonsil may be associated with a tract along the anterior border of the SCM, which extends to a supraclavicular skin opening.* (**Right**) *Plain film image from a lipiodol fistulogram demonstrates the presence of a complete fistulous tract extending from the tonsillar fossa in the oropharynx to the right supraclavicular fossa skin opening.*

Graphic of Branchial Apparatus Tract

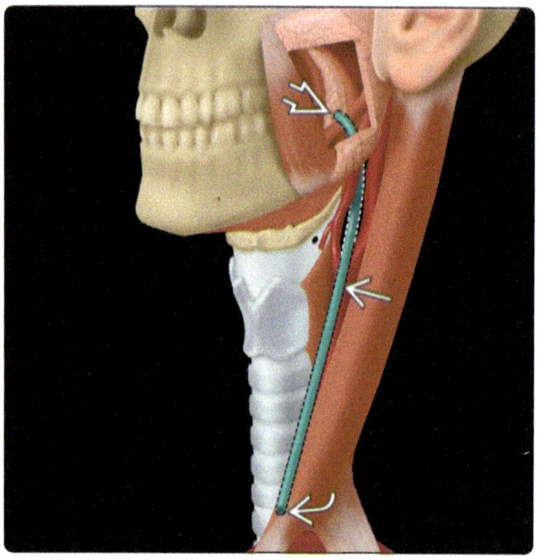

Fistulogram of Branchial Cleft Cyst Tract

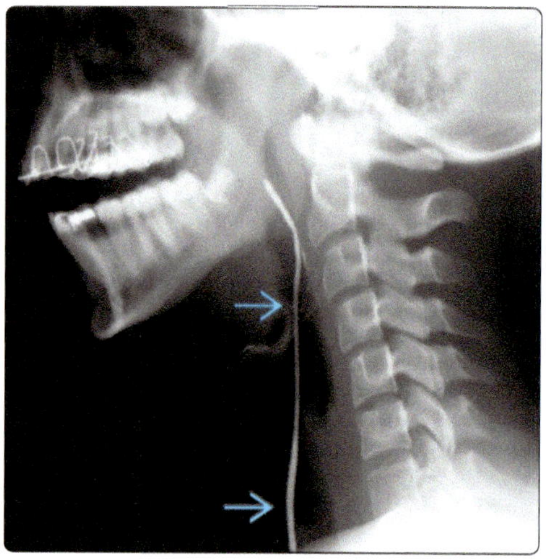

(**Left**) *This clinical photograph shows a compressible lateral neck mass in a young adult man, quite characteristic for a 2nd BCC. The patient came to clinical attention after an upper respiratory tract viral infection.* (**Right**) *The cyst has been retracted out of the operative field, highlighting the intimate association with the muscles, veins, arteries, and nerves of the neck.*

Mass in Lateral Neck of Young Man

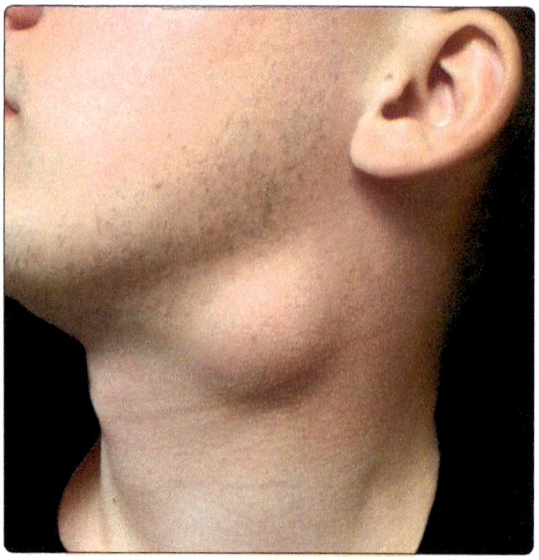

Intraoperative Photograph of Branchial Cleft Cyst

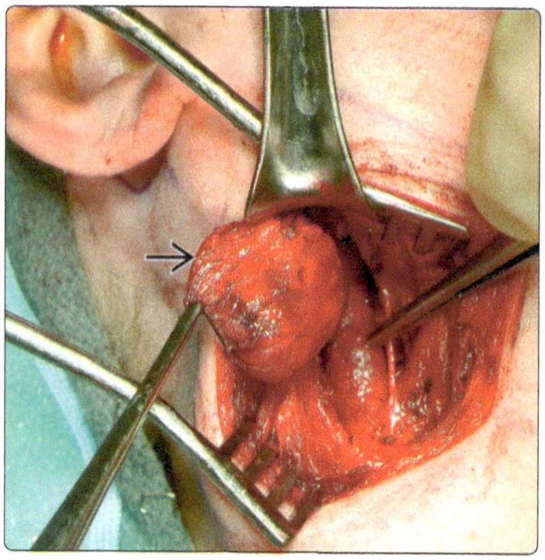

Unilocular Cyst With Mature Squamous Lining

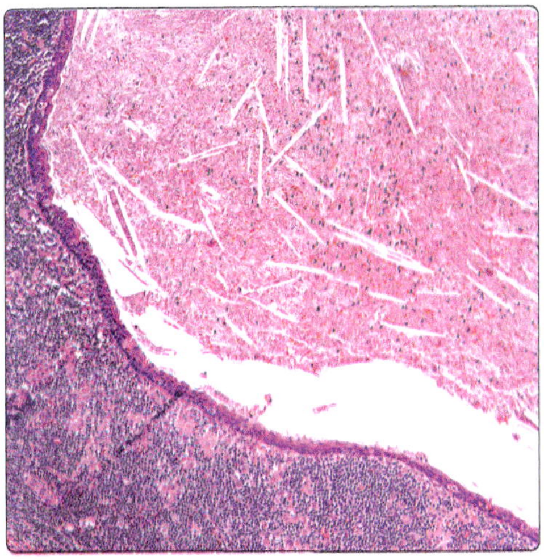

Cyst Lined by Metaplastic Squamous Cells

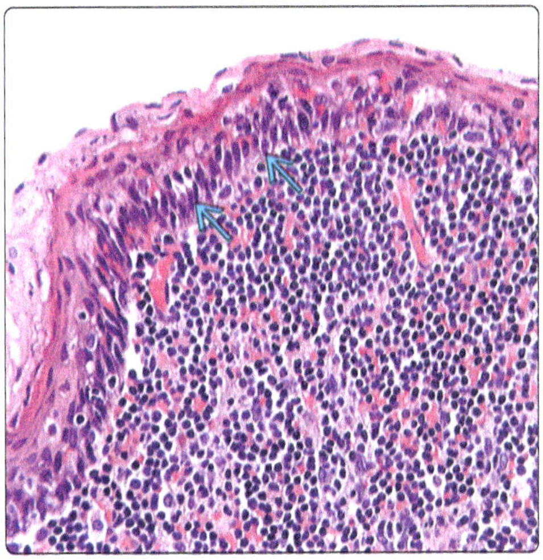

(Left) *As seen here, there is a very thin, mature squamous epithelium lining the unilocular cyst. There is keratinaceous debris with cholesterol clefts. The stroma contains lymphoid elements.* **(Right)** *The cyst is lined by metaplastic squamous epithelium, although a residuum of columnar epithelium is still present ➔. There is a very thin basement membrane between the epithelium and lymphoid tissue.*

Mature Squamous Epithelium

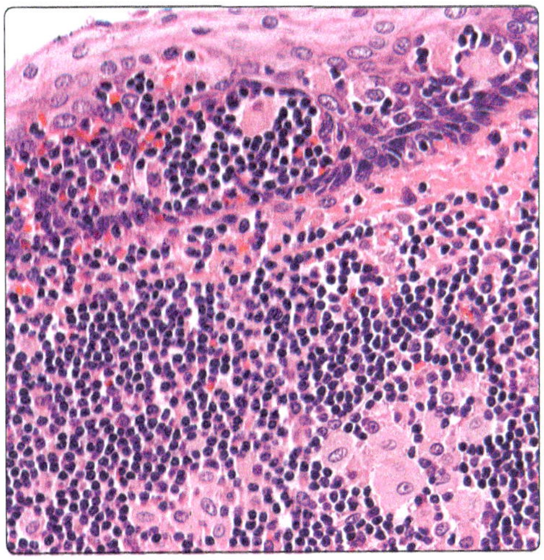

Anucleated Squames With Debris

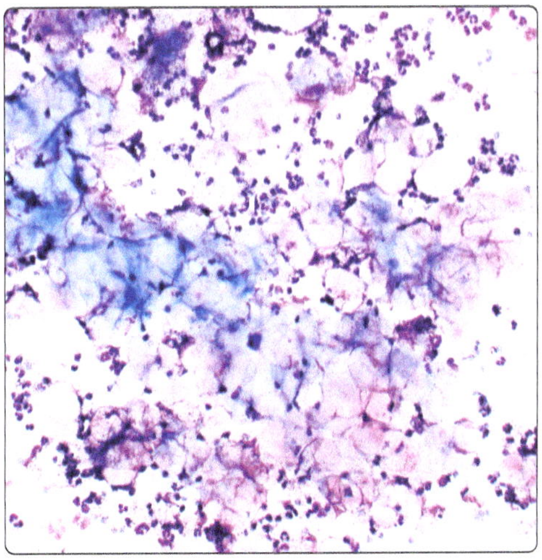

(Left) *The squamous epithelium seen here is mature and lacks cytologic atypia. A well-developed basement membrane is seen, separating the epithelium from the stroma. Histiocytes are also present within the lymphoid background.* **(Right)** *Numerous acute inflammatory cells are seen in direct association with the anucleated squamous cells. Keratin debris like this is quite characteristic of a BCC. There are no cytologic atypia and no irregular cell shapes.*

Neutrophils With Anucleated Squames

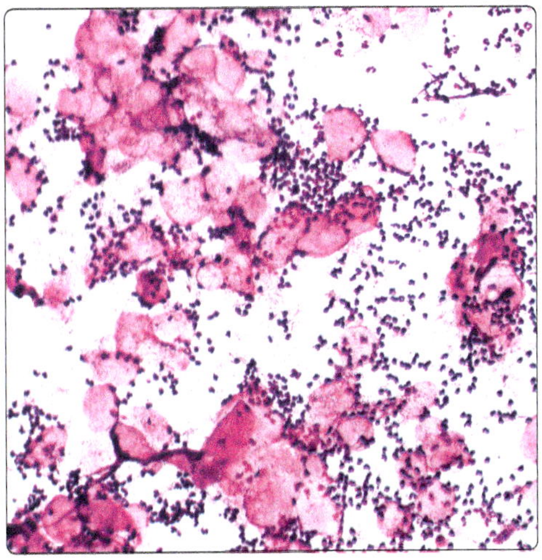

p16 Focal Reaction in Interdigitating Cells

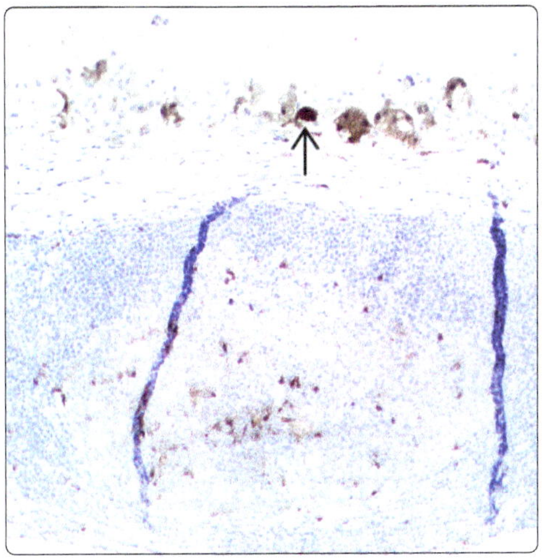

(Left) *There are many neutrophils intimately associated with squamous and anucleated squames in this smear from a BCC. There are no pleomorphism, no irregular shapes, and no mitotic figures. Necrosis is absent, although debris is present.* **(Right)** *Focal, strong positive reaction with p16 of selected epithelial cells ➔ within the cyst lining of a BCC is shown. This type of limited reaction is common in inflamed or infected BCC.*

KEY FACTS

TERMINOLOGY

- Older terms
  - Parameatal cyst, paraurethral cyst, genitoperineal cyst, mucoid cyst
- Midline developmental cyst found at any point from external urethral meatus to anus

ETIOLOGY/PATHOGENESIS

- Defective embryological closure of median raphe
  - Abnormal closure of urogenital swellings
- Anomalous separation of columnar epithelium from urethra

CLINICAL ISSUES

- Solitary cyst
- Typically < 1 cm in size
- May be located at any point between meatus urethralis and anus
  - Most frequent location is ventral glans

MICROSCOPIC

- Located in dermis/lamina propria
- Most frequently lined by
  - Pseudostratified columnar epithelium (similar to urethral epithelium)
- Other less frequent lining (focal to extensive)
  - Mucinous
  - Squamous
    - Keratinizing
    - Nonkeratinizing
  - Apocrine
  - Ciliated

TOP DIFFERENTIAL DIAGNOSES

- Epidermoid inclusion cyst
- Dermoid cyst
- Steatocystoma
- Apocrine hidrocystoma/cystadenoma

Median Raphe Cyst

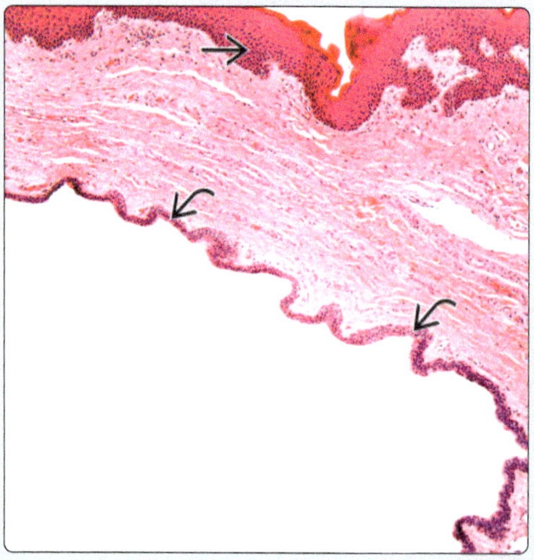

Medium Raphe Cyst With Squamous Epithelium

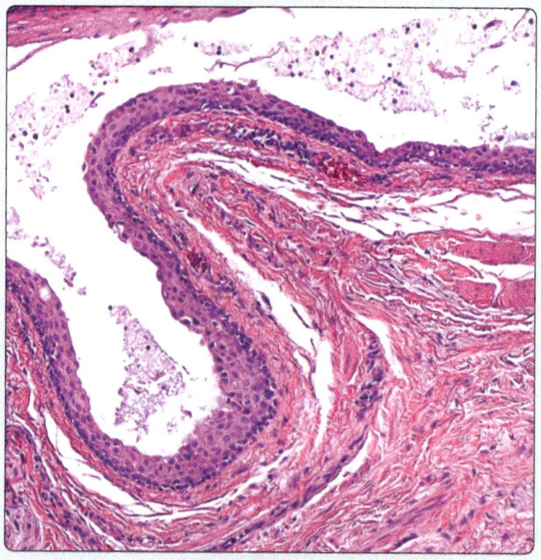

(Left) *This median raphe cyst ⮳ is located in the dermis without connection with the overlying surface epidermis ➔.* **(Right)** *A minority of medium raphe cysts are lined by squamous epithelium, as shown in this picture. Note the lack of keratinization or a granular layer.*

Medium Raphe Cyst With Columnar Epithelium

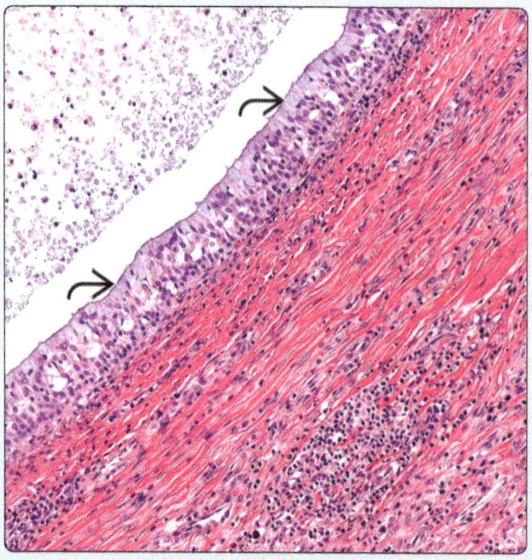

Medium Raphe Cyst: Immunohistochemistry for Cytokeratins

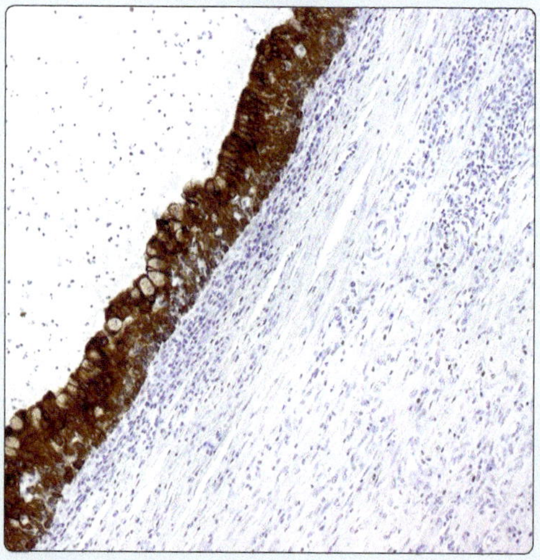

(Left) *This median raphe cyst is lined by pseudostratified columnar epithelium with mucin-containing cells on the surface ⮳. This type of epithelium is seen in the majority of these lesions.* **(Right)** *The multilayered epithelium is positive for cytokeratin AE1/AE3.*

TERMINOLOGY

Definitions

- Midline developmental cyst found from external urethral meatus to anus
- Older terms include: Parameatal cyst, paraurethral cyst, genitoperineal cyst, mucoid cyst, urethroid cyst, and hydrocystoma/apocrine cystadenoma

ETIOLOGY/PATHOGENESIS

Developmental Anomaly

- Thought to arise from defective embryological closure of median raphe
- Some may result from anomalous budding and separation of columnar epithelium from urethra

CLINICAL ISSUES

Epidemiology

- Incidence
  - Rare, but account for majority of penile cystic lesions reported in literature
- Age
  - Congenital cyst that becomes apparent in young adults
- Sex
  - Male patients

Presentation

- Solitary cyst
  - Less frequently multiple
  - Multiple lesions in linear arrangement have been described
- Usually located on ventral aspect of penis
  - But may occur at any point between meatus urethralis and anus
  - Predilection for glans
- Usually present as papule/nodule
  - Polypoid lesions are rare
- Usually measure < 1 cm
- Spontaneous regression is rare
- Median raphe canal is probably closely related to median raphe cyst
  - Presents as elongated canal in ventral portion of penis

Treatment

- Surgical approaches
  - Simple excision

Prognosis

- Excellent
- Malignant transformation is anecdotal

MACROSCOPIC

General Features

- Solitary cyst
- Clear contents
  - Turbid when mucous cells are prominent
- Asymptomatic

Size

- A few millimeters

Sections to Be Submitted

- Specimen usually consists of entire cyst

MICROSCOPIC

Histologic Features

- Lined by pseudostratified columnar epithelium
  - 1-4 cells in thickness (may be flattened on the surface)
- May contain mucin-secreting columnar cells (goblet cells)
- Other types of lining (from focal to extensive)
  - Mucin-secreting columnar cells (goblet cells)
    - Often admixed with the pseudostratified columnar epithelium
  - Squamous (keratinizing or not)
  - Ciliated
  - Apocrine
- Epithelium may be pigmented
  - Melanocytes may be admixed with epithelial cells

ANCILLARY TESTS

Immunohistochemistry

- Epithelial lining positive for AE1/AE3, CAM5.2, CK13, CK7, p63 and GATA-3
  - CK7 stains upper portion of epithelium
  - p63 stains lower portion of epithelium
- Negative for CK20 and human milk fat globule 1

DIFFERENTIAL DIAGNOSIS

Epidermoid/Epidermal Inclusion Cyst

- Lacks pseudostratified columnar/mucous lining

Dermoid Cyst

- Squamous lining with associated adnexal structures (hair follicles and sebaceous glands)

Apocrine Hidrocystoma/Cystadenoma

- Usually only lined by 2-cell layer, with inner apocrine cells and outer myoepithelial cells
- Apocrine cells are positive for GCDFP1

Steatocystoma

- Thick eosinophilic-staining hyaline cuticle lining surface
- Attached sebaceous glands

DIAGNOSTIC CHECKLIST

Pathologic Interpretation Pearls

- No connection to overlying epidermis
- Lined by pseudostratified columnar epithelium

SELECTED REFERENCES

1. Lezcano C et al: Clinicopathological features and histogenesis of penile cysts. Semin Diagn Pathol. 32(3):245-8, 2015
2. LaCarrubba F et al: Canal versus cysts of the penile median raphe: advancing diagnostic methods using videodermatoscopy. Pediatr Dermatol. 27(6):667-9, 2010
3. Colmenero I et al: [Pigmented cyst of the median raphe of the scrotum in a boy.] Actas Dermosifiliogr. 100(7):633-4, 2009
4. Krauel L et al: Median raphe cysts of the perineum in children. Urology. 71(5):830-1, 2008
5. Barua JM et al: Squamous cell carcinoma arising in a para-urethral cyst. Br J Urol. 80(1):158-9, 1997

Cutaneous Ciliated Cyst

KEY FACTS

TERMINOLOGY

- Most likely 2 different entities
  - Cutaneous müllerian cyst
  - Eccrine cutaneous ciliated cyst

ETIOLOGY/PATHOGENESIS

- Müllerian (paramesonephric) heterotopia
- Metaplasia of sweat gland epithelium

CLINICAL ISSUES

- Cutaneous müllerian cyst: Typically affects limbs of young female patients
- Eccrine cutaneous ciliated cyst: Affects men and women, more variable locations

MICROSCOPIC

- Ciliated pseudostratified cuboidal or columnar epithelium
  - May show apocrine, squamous, and mucinous foci
- Unilocular in most cases (rarely multilocular)

TOP DIFFERENTIAL DIAGNOSES

- Bronchogenic cyst
  - Precordial location
  - Pseudostratified ciliated cuboidal/columnar epithelium
  - Adjacent tissue may show lymphoid follicles
- Branchial cleft cyst
  - Near jaw angle
  - Stratified squamous epithelium
  - Adjacent tissue shows prominent lymphoid follicles
- Thyroglossal cyst
  - Midline neck (moves with swallowing)
  - Pseudostratified cuboidal/columnar (often ciliated) epithelium
  - Adjacent tissue often shows thyroid follicles
- Thymic cyst
  - Anterior neck
  - Squamous or ciliated cuboidal/columnar
  - Adjacent tissue shows thymic remnants

Cutaneous Ciliated Cyst

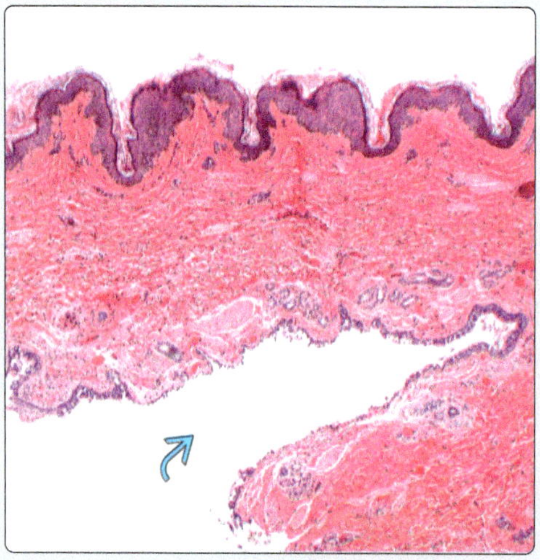

Cutaneous Ciliated Cyst Lining at Higher Magnification

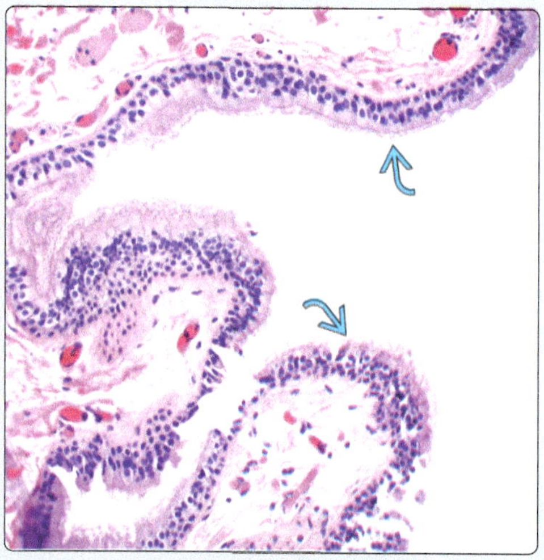

(Left) *Cutaneous ciliated cyst ↷ presents as a unilocular cavity within the dermis. Occasionally, they may be located in the subcutis.* **(Right)** *The cyst is lined by a pseudostratified and ciliated columnar epithelium. Note the cilia on the surface ↷ and lack of a granular layer of keratin.*

Cutaneous Ciliated Cyst Wall

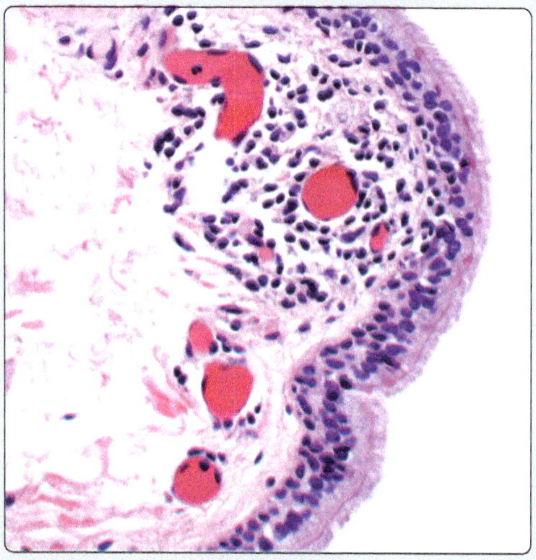

Cutaneous Ciliated Cyst at High Magnification

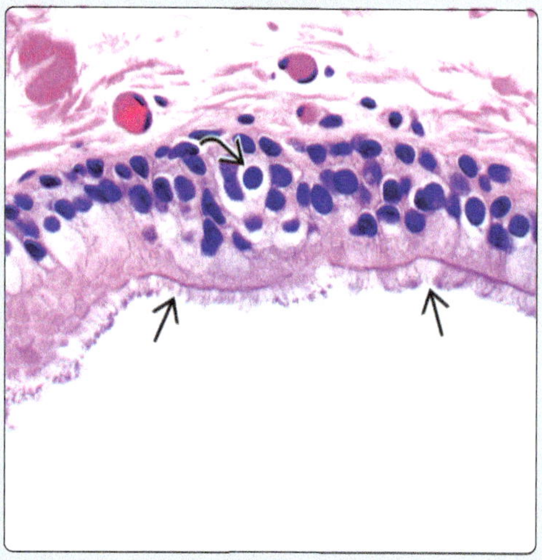

(Left) *The fibroconnective tissue underlying the cyst wall shows small, dilated blood vessels with a mild lymphoid infiltrate. Smooth muscle bundles are usually absent.* **(Right)** *High magnification shows a cutaneous ciliated cyst. The epithelial lining is pseudostratified columnar with a prominent ciliated surface ➙. There are intercalated dark nuclei ↷, similar to the epithelium of the fallopian tube.*

TERMINOLOGY

Definitions

- Solitary cutaneous cyst with ciliated epithelium
- Probably 2 different origin/entities
  - Cutaneous müllerian cyst
  - Eccrine cutaneous ciliated cyst

ETIOLOGY/PATHOGENESIS

Developmental Anomaly

- Müllerian (paramesonephric) heterotopia
  - Migration abnormality during fetal development

Metaplasia of Preexisting Cyst

- Sweat gland cyst (eccrine cutaneous ciliated cyst)

CLINICAL ISSUES

Epidemiology

- Incidence
  - Very rare
- Age
  - Müllerian ciliated cyst: Women in 2nd-4th decades
  - Eccrine cutaneous ciliated cyst: Men and women in 2nd-6th decades
- Sex
  - Müllerian ciliated cyst: Female predilection
  - Eccrine cutaneous ciliated cyst: Men and women

Site

- Müllerian ciliated cyst: Lower extremities
  - Thigh > buttock > calf > foot
  - Cases reported in unusual locations may represent eccrine cutaneous ciliated cyst
- Eccrine cutaneous ciliated cyst
  - More variable locations: Scalp, cheek, trunk, extremities

Presentation

- Cutaneous müllerian cyst: Solitary cyst affecting limbs of female patients shortly after menarche
  - Become clinically symptomatic during high estrogen states such as puberty and pregnancy
- Eccrine cutaneous ciliated cyst: More variable presentation

Treatment

- Surgical excision is curative

Prognosis

- Excellent

MACROSCOPIC

General Features

- Solitary cyst in deep dermis &/or subcutis

Size

- Up to several centimeters

MICROSCOPIC

Histologic Features

- Unilocular in most cases (rarely multilocular)
- Intraluminal papillae may be seen
- Pseudostratified cuboidal or columnar epithelium with ciliated surface
  - Similar to epithelium of fallopian tubes (intercalated dark cells may be present)
  - Squamous metaplasia is common
  - Mucin-secreting cells and apocrine cells are rare
- Fibrovascular stroma without smooth muscle bundles
  - Variable degree of inflammation

ANCILLARY TESTS

Immunohistochemistry

- Cutaneous müllerian cyst
  - Positive: CAM5.2, CK7, EMA, ER, PR, WT1, pax-8
  - Negative: CEA, GCDFP-15, CK20, p63
- Eccrine cutaneous ciliated cyst
  - Positive: CAM5.2, CK7, CEA, EMA, GCDFP-15, S100, p63
  - Negative: CK20, ER, PR, WT1, pax-8

DIFFERENTIAL DIAGNOSIS

Bronchogenic Cyst

- Presents on neck, usually midline in male patients
- Ciliated epithelium occasionally surrounded by lymphoid tissue

Branchial Cleft Cyst

- Presents on neck, usually lateral
- Stratified squamous epithelium surrounded by prominent lymphoid follicles
  - Occasionally cuboidal/columnar ciliated epithelium

Thyroglossal Duct Cyst

- Ciliated epithelium surrounded by thyroid tissue

Thymic Cyst

- Squamous or ciliated epithelium surrounded by thymic remnants

Mature Cystic Teratoma

- Stratified squamous epithelium-associated hair follicles and sebaceous glands
- Adjacent tissue often contains smooth muscle bundles

DIAGNOSTIC CHECKLIST

Pathologic Interpretation Pearls

- Cutaneous müllerian cyst has epithelial lining similar to that of fallopian tubes
- ER, PR, WT1, pax-8 positivity in cutaneous ciliated cysts of limb of young female patients supports müllerian origin

SELECTED REFERENCES

1. Joehlin-Price AS et al: PAX-8 expression in cutaneous ciliated cysts: evidence for Müllerian origin. Am J Dermatopathol. 36(2):167-70, 2014
2. Oh JS et al: Müllerian-type, cutaneous ciliated cyst in the gluteal cleft mimicking a pilonidal cyst. Pediatr Surg Int. 30(5):545-8, 2014
3. Reserva JL et al: Cutaneous ciliated cyst of the scalp: a case report of a cutaneous ciliated eccrine cyst and a brief review of the literature. Am J Dermatopathol. 36(8):679-82, 2014
4. Rodrigo-Nicolás B et al: Müllerian and eccrine cutaneous ciliated cysts: two different entities? The contribution of WT-1 and PAX8 to diagnosis. J Cutan Pathol. 40(6):608-10, 2013
5. Hung T et al: Cutaneous ciliated cyst on the finger: a cutaneous mullerian cyst. Am J Dermatopathol. 34(3):335-8, 2012
6. Farmer ER et al: Cutaneous ciliated cysts. Arch Dermatol. 114(1):70-3, 1978

PART I
SECTION 2
Epidermal Tumors

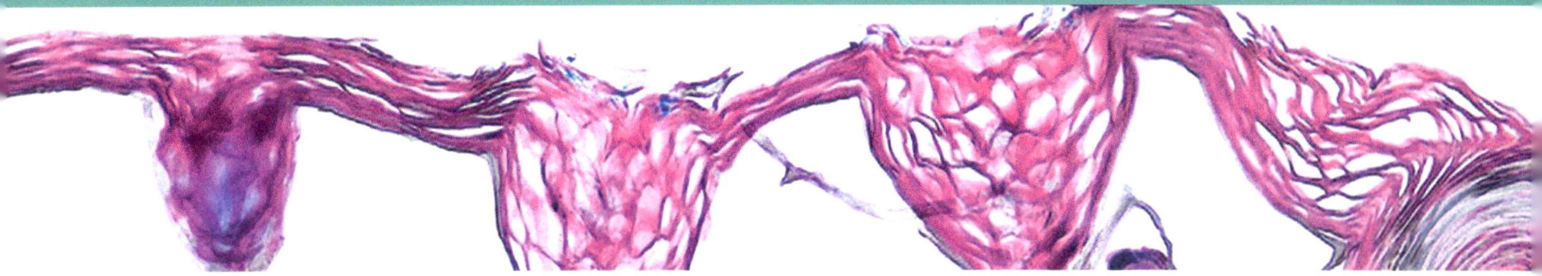

Benign Epidermal Tumors and Proliferative Lesions

Premalignant and Malignant Epidermal Tumors

Epidermal Nevus

KEY FACTS

TERMINOLOGY

- Developmental malformation of epidermis with keratinocytic hyperplasia

CLASSIFICATION

- Nevus verrucosus
  - Localized, wart-like variants, solitary or multiple
- Nevus unius lateris
  - Long, linear lesions on unilateral extremities
- Ichthyosis hystrix
  - Large, bilateral lesions on trunk

ETIOLOGY/PATHOGENESIS

- Epidermal nevus syndrome includes neurological, ocular, and skeletal abnormalities

CLINICAL ISSUES

- Common sites include neck, trunk, and extremities
- May present together with nevus sebaceus, woolly hair nevus, and nevus comedonicus
- Small lesion can be excised, larger lesions can be treated by laser or cryotherapy

MICROSCOPIC

- At least 10 different patterns, > 1 pattern can coexist in single lesion
- Common pattern includes hyperkeratosis with papillomatosis and acanthosis
- Inflammatory linear verrucous epidermal nevus is considered subtype of epidermal nevus

TOP DIFFERENTIAL DIAGNOSES

- Seborrheic keratosis
- Acanthosis nigricans
- Confluent and reticulated papillomatosis of Gougerot and Carteaud
- Organoid nevus (nevus sebaceous)

Hyperpigmented Epidermal Nevus

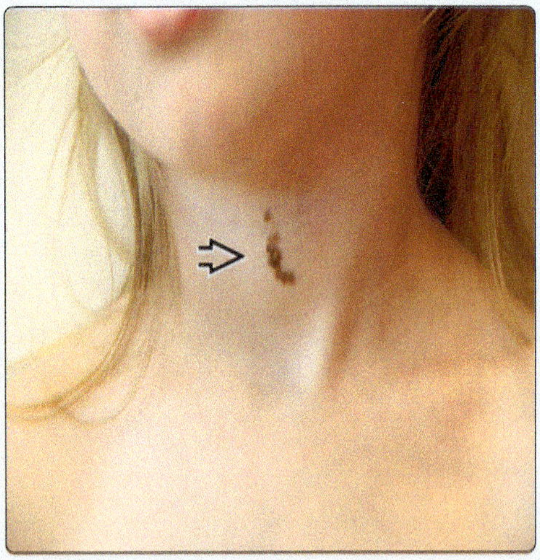

Classic Histology of Epidermal Nevus

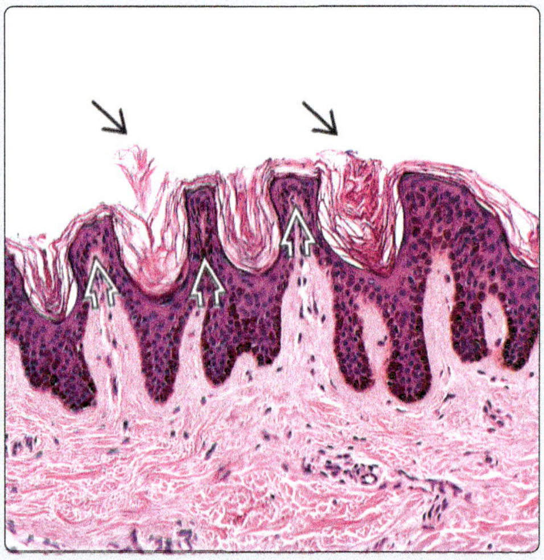

(Left) *An example of an epidermal nevus exhibits hyperpigmented, curvilinear, mammillated plaque ⇨ on the anterior, midline neck of a girl. (Courtesy J. Finch, MD.)* **(Right)** *Epidermal nevus shows orthokeratotic hyperkeratosis ⇨ overlying epidermal papillomatosis ➡. Note hyperpigmentation in the basal keratinocytes. (Courtesy C. Cockerell, MD.)*

Hypopigmented Epidermal Nevus

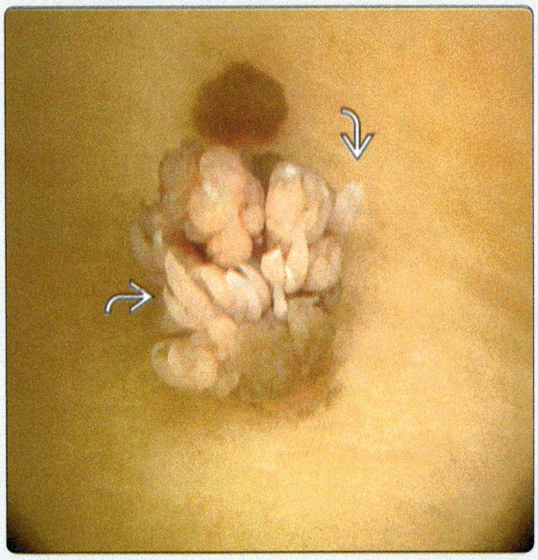

Histology Resembles Seborrheic Keratosis

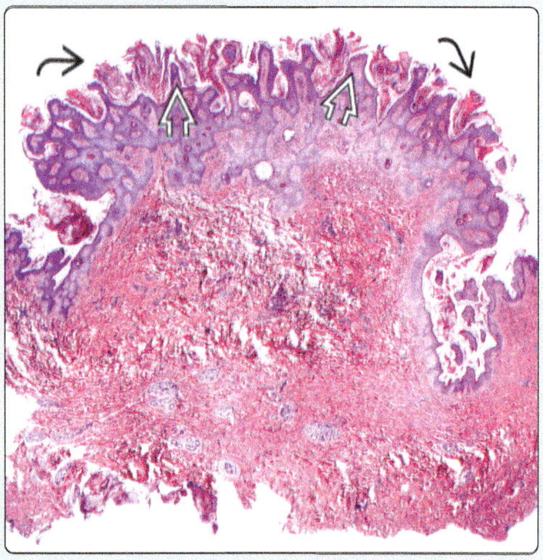

(Left) *In this example of epidermal nevus in another child, a cauliflower-like, hypopigmented, and exophytic tumor clinically resembles a wart. Note the finger-like projections ➡. (Courtesy J. Finch, MD.)* **(Right)** *Under low magnification, prominent orthokeratotic hyperkeratosis ⇨ (scale without nucleated cells) and papillomatosis ➡ (church spire-like acanthosis) are constant features of epidermal nevus.*

TERMINOLOGY

Synonyms

- Nevus verrucosus: Localized, wart-like variants, solitary or multiple
- Nevus unius lateris: Long, linear lesions on unilateral extremities
- Ichthyosis hystrix: Large, bilateral lesions on trunk

Definitions

- Developmental malformation of epidermis with hyperplasia of keratinocytes

ETIOLOGY/PATHOGENESIS

Epidermal Nevus Syndrome

- Epidermal nevi (usually extensive) with
  - Neurological abnormalities (epilepsy, mental retardation)
  - Ocular abnormalities (cataracts)
  - Skeletal anomalies (kyphoscoliosis, limb hypertrophy)
- Various systemic cancers at young age

Other Associations

- Polyostotic fibrous dysplasia
- Proteus syndrome
- Phakomatosis pigmentokeratotica

CLINICAL ISSUES

Epidemiology

- Age
  - Usually present at birth; develops during early childhood or can be seen in adulthood

Site

- Neck, trunk, extremities

Presentation

- May present together with nevus sebaceus, woolly hair nevus, and nevus comedonicus
- Associated with number of diseases and syndromes; look for other clinical findings

Treatment

- Small lesion can be excised; larger lesions can be treated by laser or cryotherapy

Prognosis

- Very rarely, benign tumors can arise within epidermal nevi
  - Basal cell carcinoma, squamous cell carcinoma, and keratoacanthoma
  - Adnexal tumors like eccrine syringofibroadenoma or syringocystadenoma papilliferum

MACROSCOPIC

General Features

- Single or multiple with scaly discoloration
- Warty plaque
- May be linear or zosteriform

MICROSCOPIC

Histologic Features

- At least 10 different patterns
  - > 1 pattern can exist in single nevus
- Common patterns
  - Broad papillomatosis and acanthosis with overlying hyperkeratosis
  - Thickened granular layer
  - Increased basal melanin pigment
- Less common patterns resemble
  - Acrokeratosis verruciformis
  - Epidermolytic hyperkeratosis
  - Seborrheic keratosis: Elongated rete ridges with flat bottoms

Inflammatory Linear Verrucous Epidermal Nevus

- Subtype of epidermal nevus
- Pruritic linear eruption on lower extremities
- May resemble linear psoriasis

Nevus Comedonicus

- Distinct entity, though sometimes grouped as a histologic pattern of epidermal nevus
- Grouped or linear comedonal papules
- Dilated keratin-filled invaginations of epidermis

DIFFERENTIAL DIAGNOSIS

Seborrheic Keratosis

- Clinically distinctive, well-demarcated "stuck-on" lesions occurring in older patients
  - Avoid misdiagnosing seborrheic keratosis in children
- Pseudohorn cysts are more common
- Epidermal nevi show rete ridges with flat bottoms

Acanthosis Nigricans

- Symmetric, velvety-appearing plaques in axillae and neck region
- Mild epidermal acanthosis with hyperkeratosis and papillomatosis

Confluent and Reticulated Papillomatosis of Gougerot and Carteaud

- Clinical appearance more diffuse and reticulated
- Undulating papillomatosis with mild acanthosis

Organoid Nevus (Nevus Sebaceous)

- Prominent sebaceous hyperplasia attached to overlying papillomatosis
- Loss or hypoplasia of hair follicles
- Could have ectatic apocrine glands

SELECTED REFERENCES

1. Happle R: The group of epidermal nevus syndromes Part I. Well defined phenotypes. J Am Acad Dermatol. 63(1):1-22; quiz 23-4, 2010
2. Happle R: The group of epidermal nevus syndromes Part II. Less well defined phenotypes. J Am Acad Dermatol. 63(1):25-30; quiz 31-2, 2010
3. Cabanillas M et al: Epidermal nevus syndrome associated with polyostotic fibrous dysplasia, CNS lipoma, and aplasia cutis. Dermatol Online J. 15(10):7, 2009

(Left) *Grouped, skin-colored papules coalesce to form a zosteriform plaque to the flank of an infant in this example of epidermal nevus. (Courtesy J. Finch, MD.)* **(Right)** *An example of epidermal nevus on the chin of an African American child shows a hyperpigmented to black plaque. Note the area of unaffected skin ➡ can be a clue. (Courtesy J. Finch, MD.)*

Can Present as Zosteriform Plaque

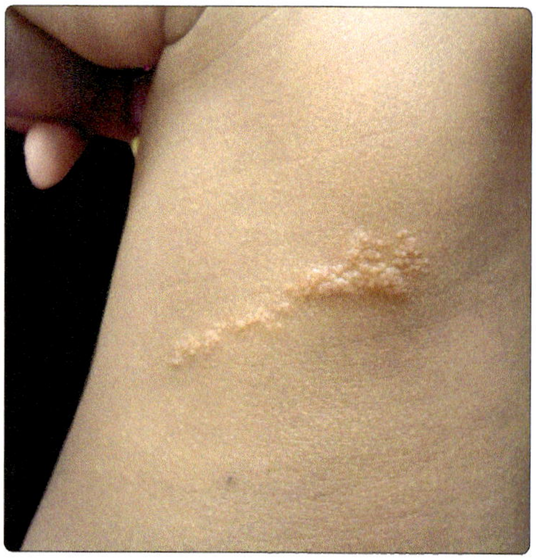

Hyperpigmented Papule With Linear Tale

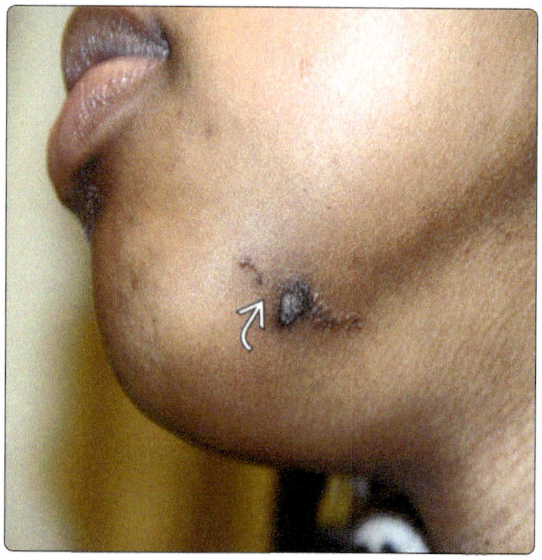

(Left) *Coalescing red-brown, flat papules on the trunk of an older adult can clinically mimic herpes zoster. (Courtesy J. Finch, MD.)* **(Right)** *Epidermal nevus can also present as a wart, as in this child, showing broad bands of flat-top hypopigmented plaque on the dorsal forearm and extensor wrist. (Courtesy University of Utah Department of Dermatology.)*

Can Mimic Herpes Zoster in Adults

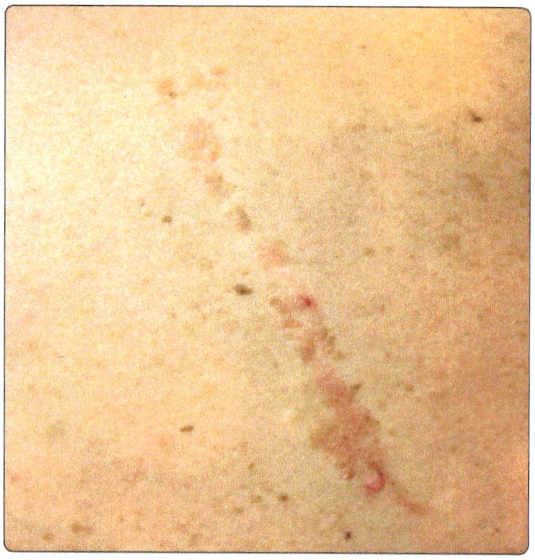

Flat Top Hypopigmented Plaque

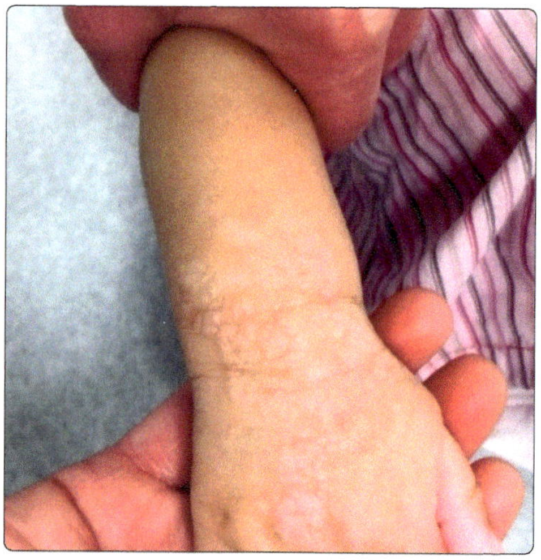

(Left) *Confluent and reticulated papillomatosis can histologically resemble epidermal nevus. However, the acanthosis ➡ is present in the valley between papillomatous projections ➡ in the former. (Courtesy G. Fraga, MD.)* **(Right)** *Low magnification shows a common type of epidermal nevus with prominent hyperkeratosis ➡, papillomatosis ➡, and acanthosis ➡.*

CARP Resembles Epidermal Nevus

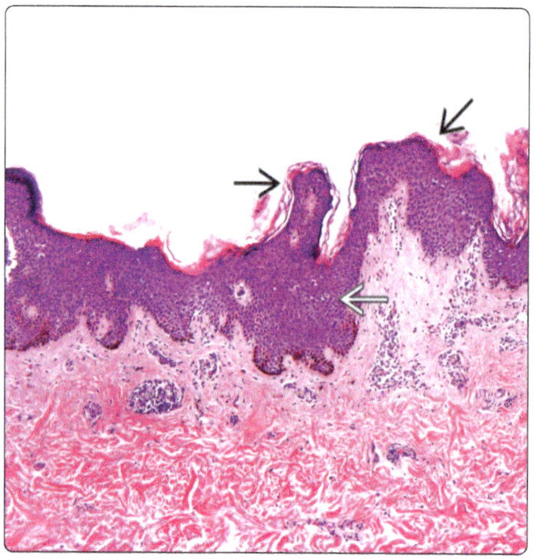

Classic Histology With Stalk

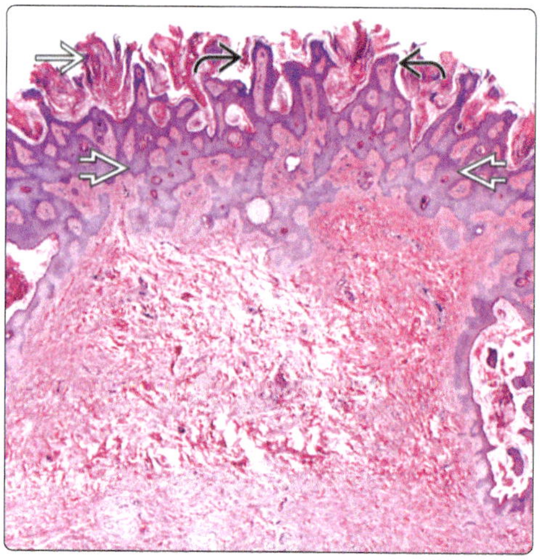

Exophytic Epidermal Tumor

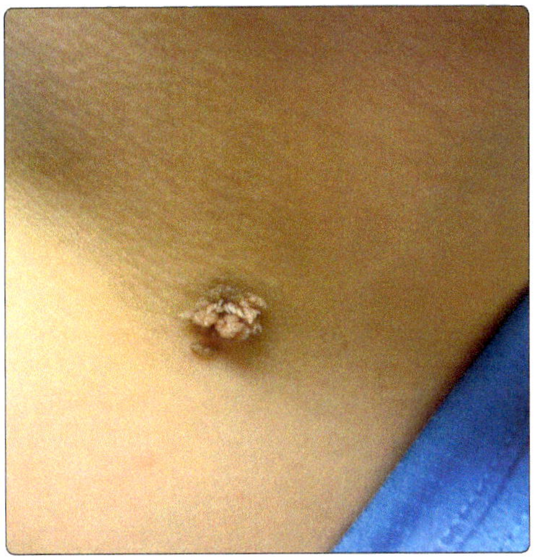

Resembles CARP or Seborrheic Keratosis

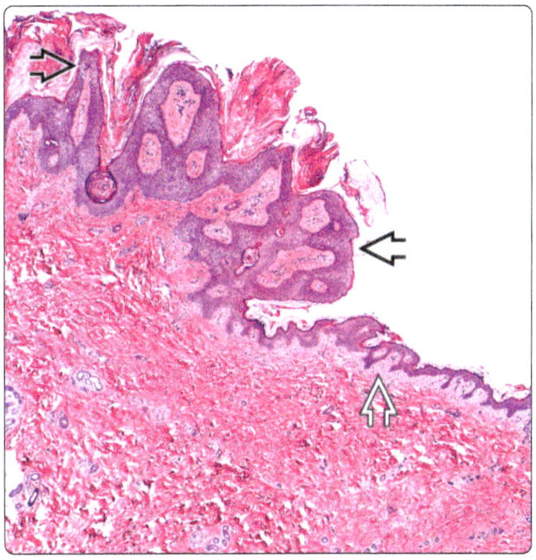

(Left) *Grouping of warty papules can mimic a verruca vulgaris. (Courtesy J. Finch.)* **(Right)** *Epidermal nevus ➯ is sharply demarcated from the adjacent normal epidermis ➯. There is marked acanthosis and papillomatosis.*

Hyperpigmented Variant

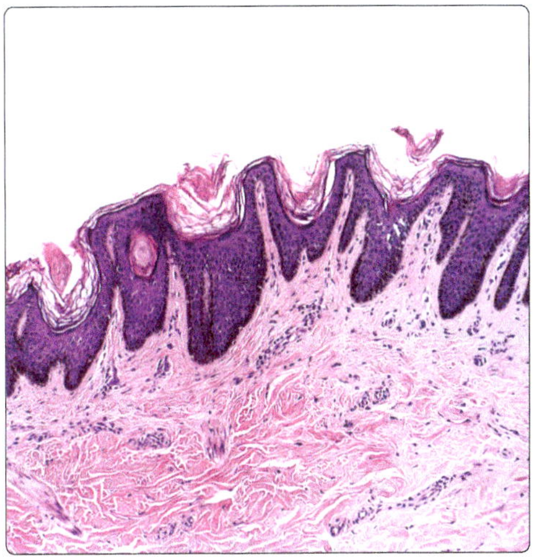

Low-Power View of Epidermal Nevus

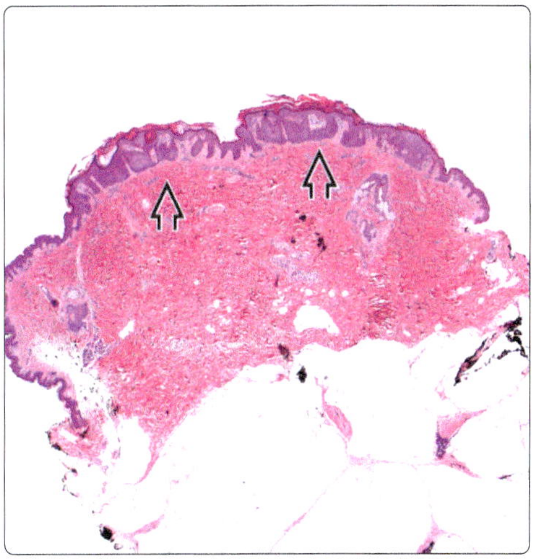

(Left) *Increased melanin content resembles a pigmented seborrheic keratosis.* **(Right)** *The broad epidermal plaque ➯ is shown at low magnification. The epidermis shows acanthosis and hyperpigmentation.*

Inflamed Epidermal Nevus

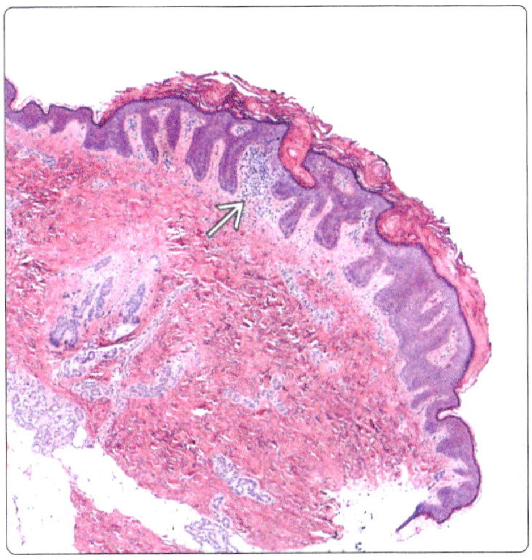

Epidermal Nevus With Normal Adnexae

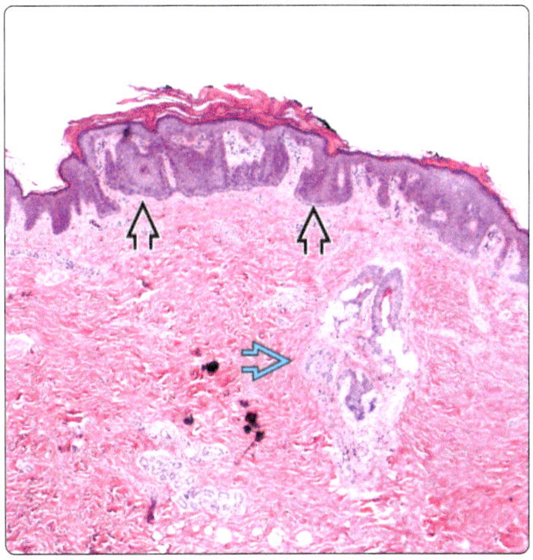

(Left) *The same epidermal nevus shows focal inflammation in the dermis ➯, an uncommon feature. The abrupt demarcation from normal epidermis is again seen.* **(Right)** *The same epidermal nevus shows acanthosis with broad, flat bottoms ➯ and hyperkeratosis. The underlying dermis has normal adnexal structures ➯, unlike a sebaceous nevus.*

Seborrheic Keratosis (and Variants)

KEY FACTS

TERMINOLOGY

- Seborrheic keratosis (SK)
- Benign epidermal proliferation

CLINICAL ISSUES

- Very common in middle-aged to elderly patients
- Usually affecting face, chest, and back

MACROSCOPIC

- Sharply delineated plaques with greasy appearance
- Verruciform or flat surface with keratotic plugs
- Flesh-colored to brown-black

MICROSCOPIC

- Exophytic/endophytic acanthotic lesion
- Composed of basaloid and squamoid cells
- Ortho-hyperkeratosis
- Often hyperpigmented
- Variable degree of inflammation
- Variants of SK include
  - Acanthotic
  - Papillomatous (hyperkeratotic)
  - Adenoid (reticulated)
  - Clonal (irritated SK variant)
  - Inverted follicular keratosis (likely irritated SK variant)
  - Lichenoid SK
  - Desmoplastic
  - Adamantinoid
  - SK with pseudorosettes

TOP DIFFERENTIAL DIAGNOSES

- Verruca vulgaris
- Hypertrophic actinic keratosis
- Squamous cell carcinoma in situ
- Epidermal nevus
- Acanthosis nigricans
- Confluent and reticulated papillomatosis (CARP)
- Hidroacanthoma simplex

Seborrheic Keratosis

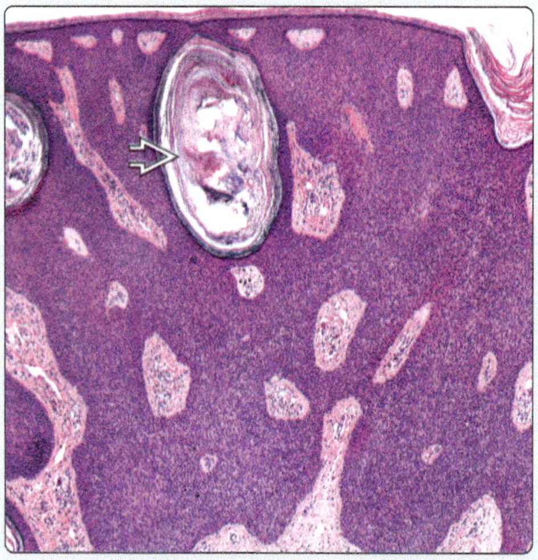

Acanthotic and Pigmented Seborrheic Keratosis

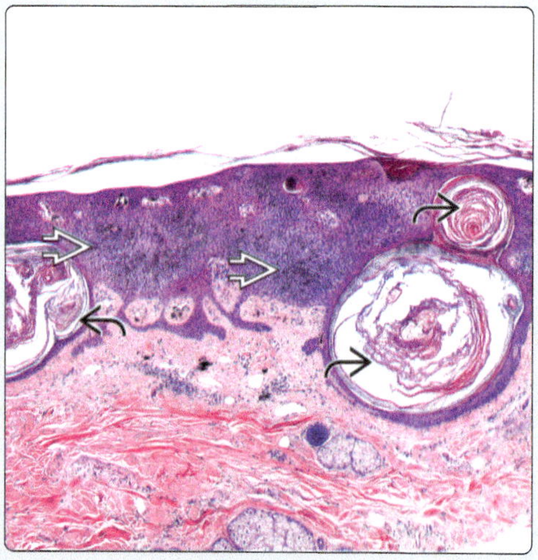

(Left) *Seborrheic keratosis (SK), acanthotic/endophytic variant shows smooth, rounded surface and thickened epithelium. The lesion is predominantly composed of basaloid cells with prominent horn cysts.* **(Right)** *Acanthotic and pigmented SK is characterized by a flat surface and marked acanthosis and prominent horn cysts. Note the presence of abundant melanin within the basaloid keratinocytes.*

Acanthotic Seborrheic Keratosis

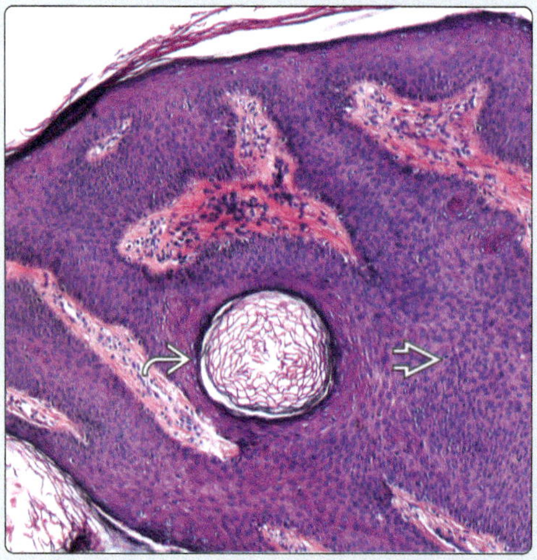

Adenoid Seborrheic Keratosis

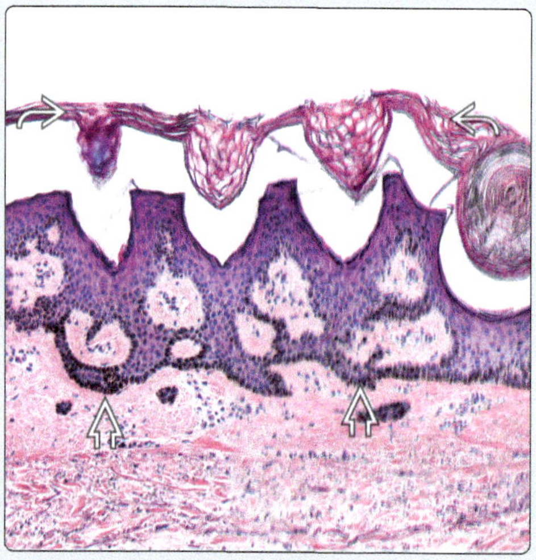

(Left) *Acanthotic variant of SK is characterized by broad columns of bland and uniform basaloid cells showing intervening horn cysts and areas with early clonal features.* **(Right)** *Adenoid seborrheic keratosis composed of narrow and hyperpigmented trabeculae is shown. This variant of SK may evolve from a solar lentigo. Note the basket weave, orthokeratotic surface.*

TERMINOLOGY

Abbreviations

- Seborrheic keratosis (SK)

Definitions

- Benign epidermal proliferation

ETIOLOGY/PATHOGENESIS

Benign Epidermal Tumor

- Monoclonal
  - Likely neoplasm rather than hyperplasia

CLINICAL ISSUES

Epidemiology

- Incidence
  - Very common
- Age
  - Middle-aged and elderly
    - Affecting ~ 20% of elderly population

Site

- Most common on face, chest, and back
  - May be found anywhere except palms and soles

Presentation

- Sharply delineated plaques with greasy appearance
- Solitary or multiple
- Verruciform or flat surface
  - Surface shows characteristic keratotic plugs
- Soft and friable
- Round or oval
- From flesh-colored to brown-black
  - Darkly pigmented lesions may be clinically mistaken for melanoma
- Often appearing as "stuck-on" skin surface
- Inverted follicular keratosis variant presents as warty papulonodule
- Multiple inverted follicular keratoses in Cowden syndrome
- Leser-Trélat sign
  - Sudden onset of multiple seborrheic keratoses
    - Usually associated with internal malignancies (most commonly gastric adenocarcinoma)

Prognosis

- Excellent
- SKs are benign tumors
  - Very rarely, squamous cell carcinoma (SCC) in situ or invasive SCC can arise in SK

MACROSCOPIC

General Features

- Exophytic tumors
  - Verruciform/warty or smooth surface

Size

- A few mm to a few cm in diameter

Sections to Be Submitted

- As lesions are small, they tend to be almost entirely sampled in most biopsies

MICROSCOPIC

Histologic Features

- Symmetric, sharply defined tumors
- Exophytic, endophytic, or combination of both
- Overlying orthohyperkeratosis ("starry sky") often present
  - Heavily inflamed, irritated, or infarcted SK may show foci of parakeratosis
- Composed of bland-appearing basaloid and squamoid cells (variable amounts of each)
- Keratin-filled invaginations and small pseudocysts (pseudohorn cysts) are characteristic
- Nests of keratinocytes (squamous eddies) may be seen in irritated lesions
  - Apparently related to acrotrichia
- Frequently hyperpigmented
  - Melanocytes may be increased in number and size
    - Melanoacanthomas are SKs with marked melanocytic proliferation and pigmentation
- Tricholemmal differentiation (glycogen-rich) may be focally present
- Sebaceous differentiation is uncommon
- Acantholysis &/or dyskeratosis occasionally seen
- Many different variants of SK have been described
  - **Acanthotic SK**
    - Smooth, rounded and orthohyperkeratotic surface
    - Acanthotic and often pigmented
    - Basaloid cells predominate over squamoid cells
    - Horn cysts tend to be prominent
  - **Papillomatous (verrucous) SK**
    - Acanthosis and papillomatosis
    - Overlying orthohyperkeratosis may be prominent
    - Squamoid cells predominate over basaloid cells
    - Prominent horn cysts
  - **Adenoid (reticulated) SK**
    - Orthohyperkeratosis
    - Flat or papillomatous surface
    - Thin, proliferating strands emanating from epidermis
      - Often pigmented
    - Basaloid cells predominate over squamoid cells
    - Horn cysts are absent or sparse
  - **Clonal SK (type of irritated SK)**
    - Borst-Jadassohn phenomenon: Oval to round aggregates of monotonous intraepidermal keratinocytes
    - CK10(-) nested pattern in clonal SK may be helpful to distinguish it from pagetoid SCCIS
  - **Inverted follicular keratosis (type of irritated SK)**
    - Endophytic growth pattern
      - Often involving follicles
    - Prominent squamous eddies
  - **Inflammatory SK**
    - Any variant of SK may be inflamed
  - **Lichenoid SK**
    - Prominent lymphoid infiltrate with variable melanophages

 - Apoptotic cells (Civatte bodies)
 - May evolve to lichenoid keratosis (lichen planus-like keratosis)
 - **Desmoplastic SK**
 - Bulk of lesion is typical SK
 - Irregular cords and strands of squamous cells surrounded by desmoplastic stroma at base
 - May mimic invasive SCC
 - **Adamantinoid SK**
 - Very unusual variant
 - Small basaloid keratinocytes with spindled cytoplasm
 - Intercellular mucin
 - **SK with pseudorosettes**
 - Very rare
 - Basaloid cells arranged around central small spaces
- Malignant transformation is exceptional
 - Rare cases of SCC in situ and invasive SCC arising in SK have been described
- Collision of SK with benign and malignant neoplasms may also rarely occur (e.g., SCC, BCC, nevi, or melanoma)

DIFFERENTIAL DIAGNOSIS

Verruca Vulgaris

- Hypergranulosis and usually dense compact hyperkeratosis with tiers of parakeratosis (not "starry sky" of SK)
- Koilocytosis typically present
- Intracorneal hemorrhage
- "Toeing in" of epidermis at peripheral edges

Hypertrophic Actinic Keratosis

- Alternating foci of ortho- and parakeratosis
- Atypical keratinocytes present underneath parakeratotic foci

Stucco Keratosis

- Multiple tiny lesions affecting extremities of elderly patients
- Microscopically indistinguishable from early SK (may be considered an SK variant)
- Acanthosis with church spire appearance

Condyloma Acuminatum

- SK-like lesions in genital areas usually represent old condyloma acuminatums
- May show horn pseudocysts and basaloid cells

Epidermal Nevus

- Often present at birth or appear during childhood
- Microscopically may be indistinguishable from SK

Acanthosis Nigricans

- Associated with diabetes, obesity, internal malignancies, and other systemic conditions
- Symmetrical, pigmented plaques in flexural areas
- Histologically may be indistinguishable from SK
- Mild acanthosis with papillomatosis and hyperkeratosis
- Horn cysts are not present

Confluent and Reticulated Papillomatosis

- Histologically may be indistinguishable from early SK
- Mild acanthosis with papillomatosis and hyperkeratosis
- Horn cysts are not present

Arsenical and Tar Keratosis

- Mild acanthosis with papillomatosis and hyperkeratosis
- Histologically may be indistinguishable from early seborrheic keratosis

Clear Cell Acanthoma

- Psoriasiform hyperplasia and parakeratosis containing neutrophils
- Sharp demarcation from adjacent epidermis
- Lesional keratinocytes have abundant pale cytoplasm

Poroma and Hidroacanthoma Simplex

- Nests of basaloid adnexal cells attached to (poroma) or in epidermis (hidroacanthoma simplex)
- Cells are usually smaller than basaloid cells of SK
- Poromatous cells often contain glycogen
- Scattered ductal structures may be present

Squamous Cell Carcinoma In Situ

- Full-thickness keratinocytic atypia
- Mitoses including in upper levels of the epidermis
- Confluent parakeratosis

Dermatofibroma (Overlying Epidermal Changes)

- Surface of dermatofibromas may show SK-like features, with acanthosis and basilar hyperpigmentation

DIAGNOSTIC CHECKLIST

Pathologic Interpretation Pearls

- In superficial biopsies, presence of orthokeratosis with appearance of "starry sky" is a hint to underlying SK
- Inflamed SKs may show reactive keratinocytic atypia
 - Entire infarcted papillae are often seen on top of atypical foci
- Many different variants of SK have been described
 - Overlapping features are common
- SK-like lesions in genital areas often represent condyloma acuminata

SELECTED REFERENCES

1. Wu YH et al: Seborrheic keratosis with bowenoid transformation: the immunohistochemical features and its association with human papillomavirus infection. Am J Dermatopathol. 37(6):462-8, 2015
2. Böer-Auer A et al: Cytokeratin 10-negative nested pattern enables sure distinction of clonal seborrheic keratosis from pagetoid Bowen's disease. J Cutan Pathol. 39(2):225-33, 2012
3. Battistella M et al: From hidroacanthoma simplex to poroid hidradenoma: clinicopathologic and immunohistochemic study of poroid neoplasms and reappraisal of their histogenesis. Am J Dermatopathol. 32(5):459-68, 2010
4. Choi HJ et al: Squamous eddies in irritated seborrheic keratosis. Am J Dermatopathol. 2007 Feb;29(1):28-31. Erratum in: Am J Dermatopathol. 29(2):229, 2007
5. Requena L et al: Seborrheic keratosis with pseudorosettes and adamantinoid seborrheic keratosis: two new histopathologic variants. J Cutan Pathol. 33 Suppl 2:42-5, 2006
6. King R et al: Desmoplastic seborrheic keratosis. Am J Dermatopathol. 25(3):210-4, 2003

Papillomatous Seborrheic Keratosis

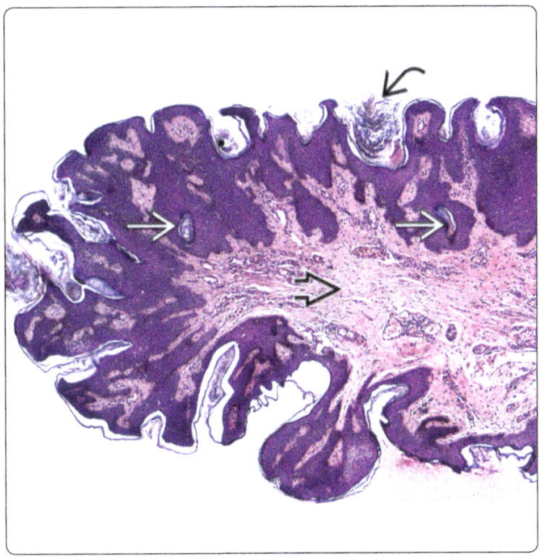

Prominent Pseudohorn Cysts

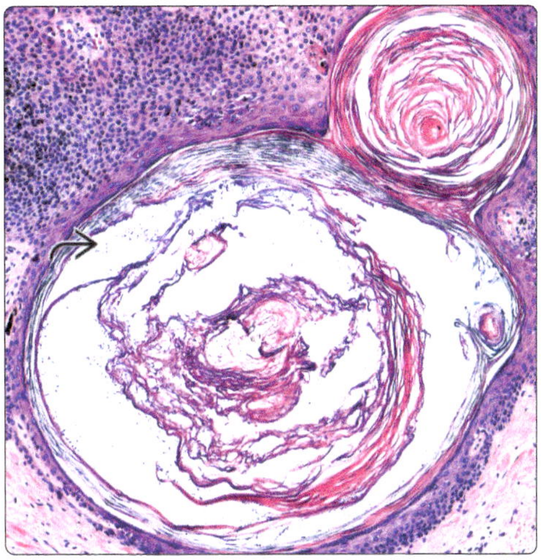

(Left) *Papillomatous SK shows hyperkeratosis ⇗, papillomatosis, acanthosis, and horn cysts ➡. This lesion is from the axilla, where SKs can share some features with acrochordons. Note the prominent stromal core ⇨ without adnexal structures.* **(Right)** *Horn cysts may be absent or numerous, tiny to large. Note the large horn cyst ⇗ in this SK. These horn cysts may rupture and be associated with a dermal granulomatous foreign body giant cell reaction in some cases.*

Clonal Seborrheic Keratosis

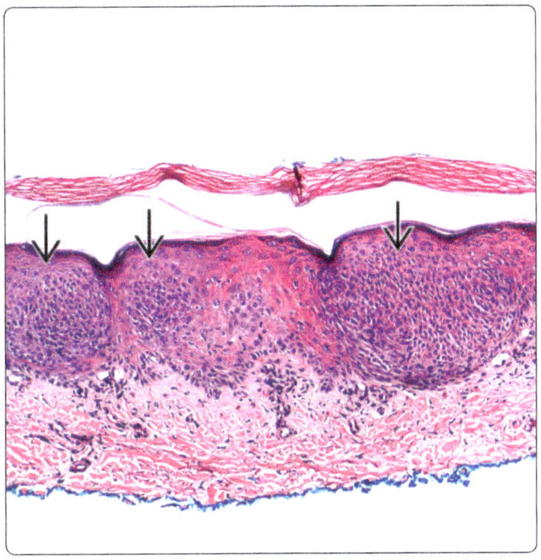

Clonal Seborrheic Keratosis at Higher Magnification

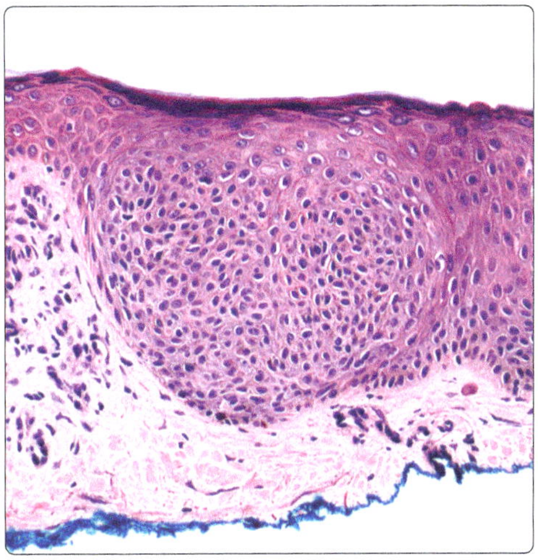

(Left) *Clonal SK with round to oval, intraepidermal aggregates of keratinocytes shows the so-called Borst-Jadassohn phenomenon ⇨.* **(Right)** *Nests of bland-appearing neoplastic keratinocytes surrounded by normal epidermis are characteristic of clonal SK. Borst-Jadassohn phenomenon (epithelioma) likely refers more to a histopathological pattern rather than a distinct entity, as clonal SKs and hidroacanthoma simplex also show this pattern.*

Early/Macular Seborrheic Keratosis

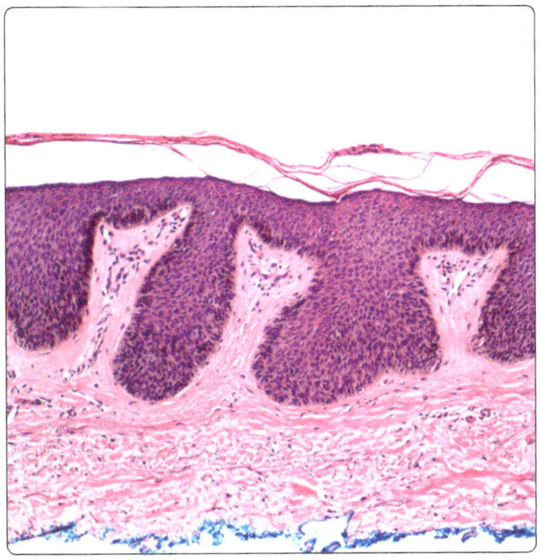

Early Seborrheic Keratosis

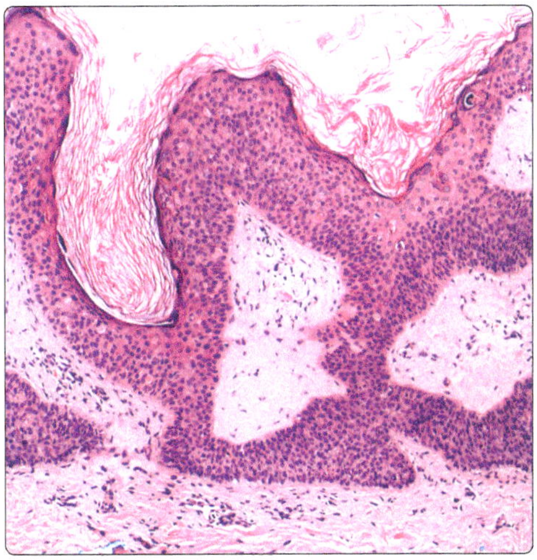

(Left) *Horn cysts are absent or sparse in macular (early) SK. Because of their flat surface, these lesions may clinically mimic lentigo or dysplastic nevi.* **(Right)** *This early SK is characterized by orthokeratosis, mild papillomatosis, mild acanthosis, and predominance of basaloid cells. Horn cysts are not present in this area. The lesion has mixed features of a hyperkeratotic (papillomatous) and adenoid (reticulated) SK.*

(Left) *This example of irritated/traumatized SK with inverted follicular keratosis features shows prominent acanthosis and multiple foci of intraepidermal clefting present. Note the dense overlying serum crust with degenerating neutrophils present.* **(Right)** *Note the conspicuous squamous eddies in this irritated SK with features of an inverted follicular keratosis. Squamoid cells predominate over basaloid cells.*

Irritated SK With Acantholytic Features

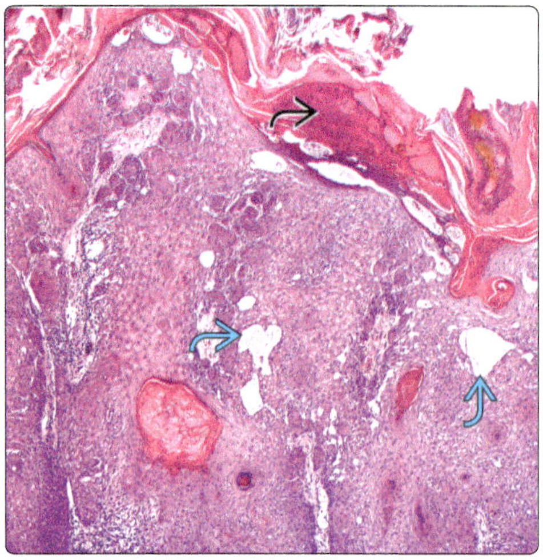

Irritated Seborrheic Keratosis

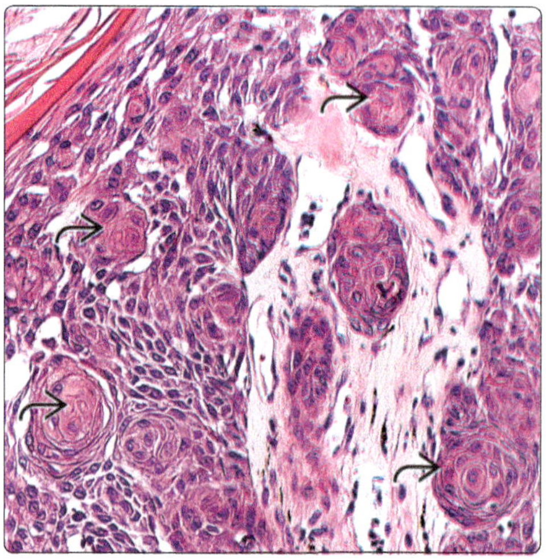

(Left) *Partially infarcted SK shows entire papillae with their epithelium and stromal cores infarcted. The viable portion may show a variable degree of reactive keratinocytic atypia.* **(Right)** *Partially infarcted SK shows reactive atypia and prominent squamous eddies. The atypical keratinocytes are enlarged and show nuclear atypia and a few mitoses. However, markedly pleomorphic nuclei, mitoses in the upper epithelium, and atypical mitoses are usually not seen.*

Infarcted Seborrheic Keratosis

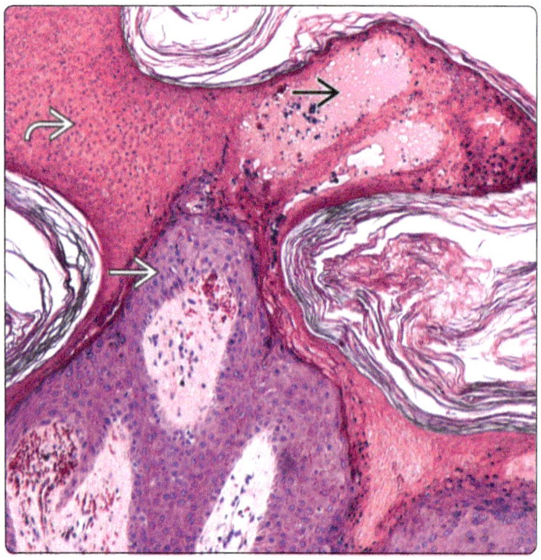

Infarcted Seborrheic Keratosis

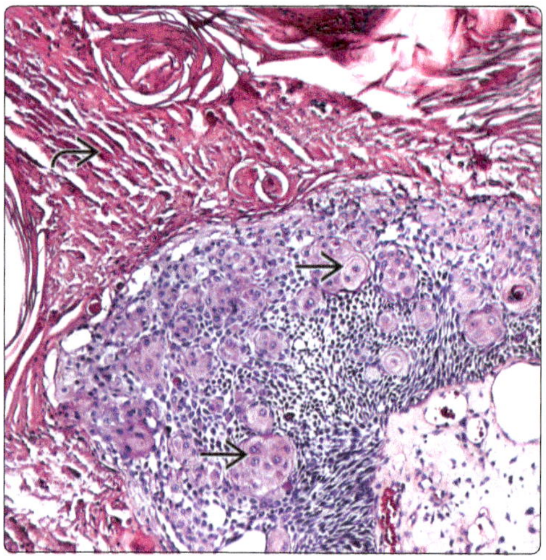

(Left) *Characteristic keratin layer of a SK is seen here. Unless the lesion is irritated, inflamed or infarcted, the keratin layer is orthokeratotic. Some authors describe this pattern as "van Gogh sky" or "starry sky" for the resemblance with his paintings.* **(Right)** *Stromal amyloid deposition is occasionally seen in SKs. Note the homogeneous eosinophilic and globular dermal deposits. This is keratin-derived amyloid (the same as in macular and lichen amyloidosis) and has no clinical significance.*

Orthokeratotic Keratin Layer Overlying Seborrheic Keratosis

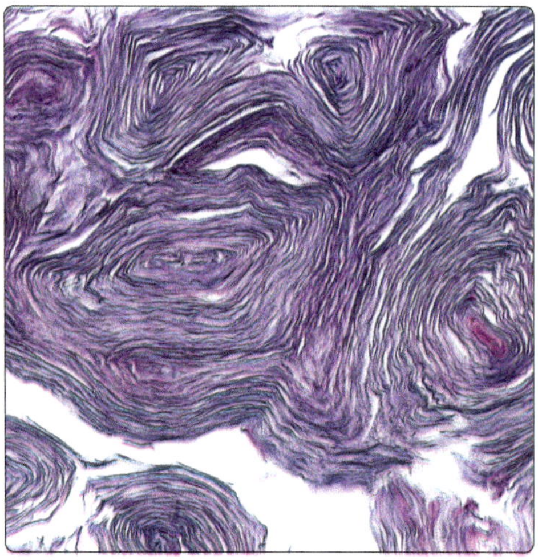

Seborrheic Keratosis With Amyloid

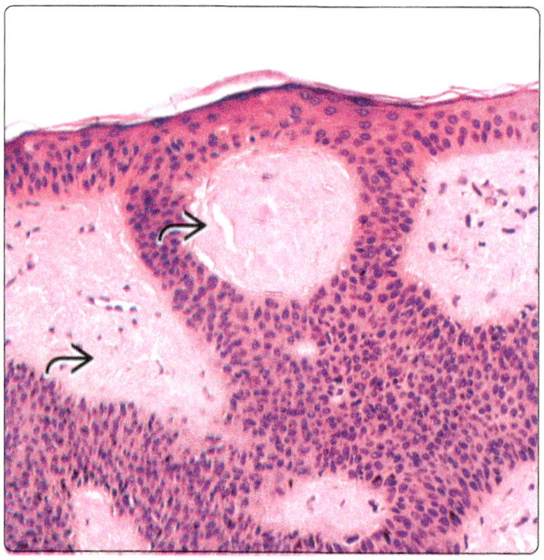

Irritated and Acantholytic SK

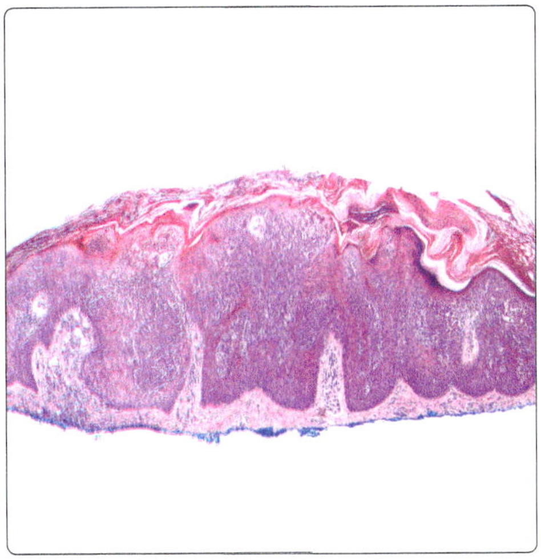

Acantholytic SK at Higher Magnification

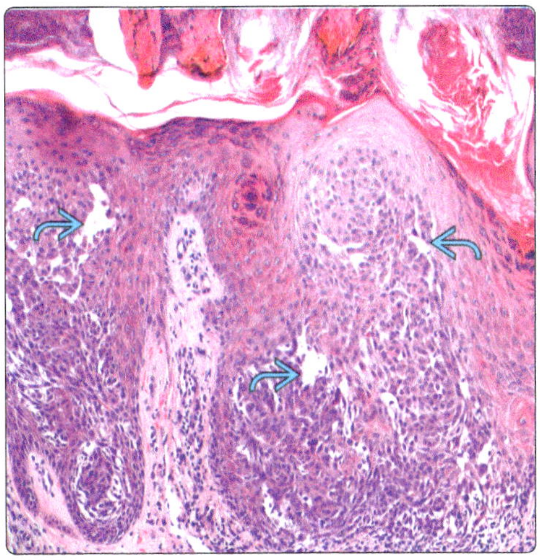

(Left) *Low magnification of an irritated SK shows prominent acanthosis and foci of acantholysis. Pseudohorn cysts are not present in this field, and the low-power differential could include an acantholytic squamous cell carcinoma in situ.* **(Right)** *Higher magnification of this irritated SK shows whorls of bland keratinocytes and acantholysis, with multiple areas of intraepidermal clefting present.*

Differential Diagnosis: Acantholytic SCC In Situ

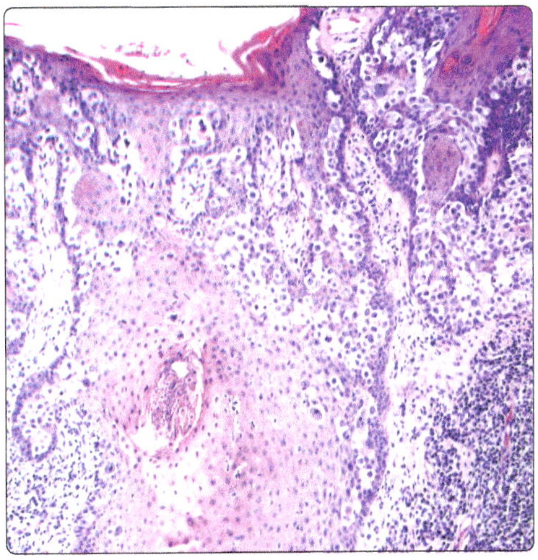

Differential Diagnosis: Pigmented Poroma

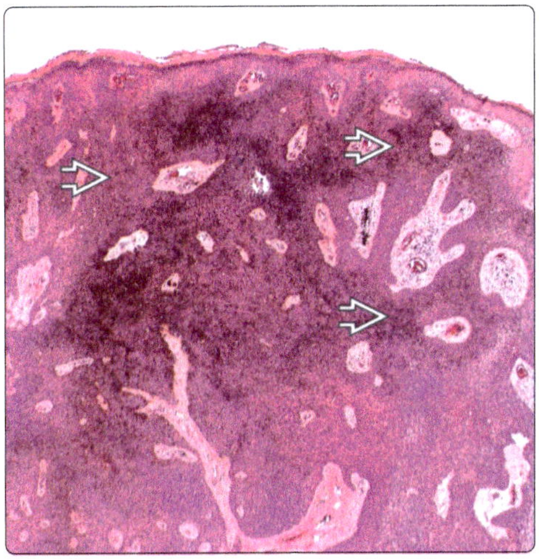

(Left) *Acantholytic SCC in situ at low magnification can simulate an irritated and acantholytic SK. However, cytologic atypia and mitoses are easily identified at higher magnification.* **(Right)** *Pigmented poroma is a relatively common variant that can mimic a pigmented acanthotic SK. However, besides the heavy pigmentation, it shows features typical of poroma, being composed of basaloid to squamoid cells forming multiple thickened, anastomosing connections between tumor cords.*

Differential Diagnosis: Verruca

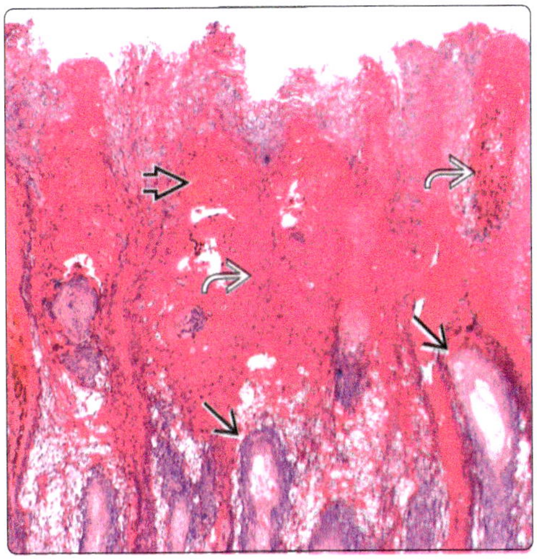

Differential Diagnosis: Verruca Vulgaris

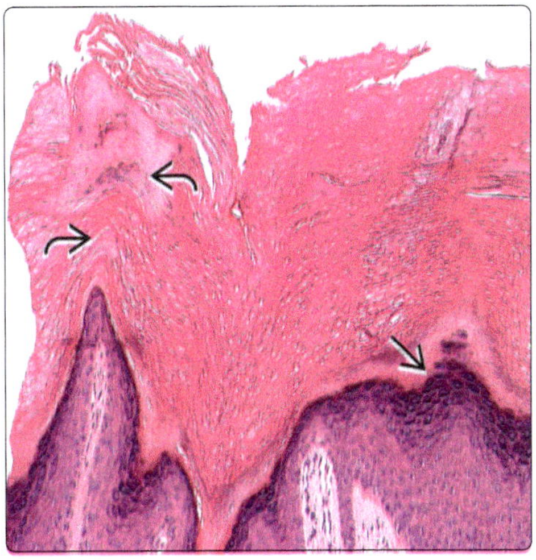

(Left) *Warts often enter the differential diagnosis with papillomatous SKs but typically show more dense hyperkeratosis and parakeratosis. This palmoplantar wart (myrmecia) shows marked papillomatosis with thick overlying hyperkeratosis, parakeratosis, and intracorneal hemorrhage.* **(Right)** *Low magnification of the surface of a verruca vulgaris shows epidermal papillomatosis with hypergranulosis and overlying dense hyperkeratosis and tiers of parakeratosis.*

Pseudoepitheliomatous Hyperplasia

KEY FACTS

TERMINOLOGY

- Pseudoepitheliomatous hyperplasia (PEH): Florid proliferation of epidermis that mimics squamous cell carcinoma
- Pseudocarcinomatous hyperplasia

ETIOLOGY/PATHOGENESIS

- Reaction pattern overlying particular tumors such as
  - Granular cell tumor
  - Lymphoma
- Reaction pattern in certain inflammatory conditions such as
  - Lichen planus
  - Lupus erythematosus
- Reaction pattern overlying certain infections
  - Particularly deep fungal
- Reaction pattern overlying tattoos
  - Particularly red pigment

CLINICAL ISSUES

- Variable presentation, depending upon underlying condition
- Excellent prognosis, no malignant potential

MICROSCOPIC

- Hyperplasia of epidermis
- Base of hyperplastic epidermis may show broad rete or jagged borders
- May seem to predominantly involve hair follicles and other adnexal structures
- Varying depth (but never into subcutis)
- Squamous eddies may be prominent
- Minimal keratinocyte atypia

TOP DIFFERENTIAL DIAGNOSES

- Squamous cell carcinoma
- Keratoacanthoma
- Hypertrophic lupus erythematosus

(Left) *Pseudoepitheliomatous hyperplasia (PEH) associated with a tattoo shows irregular downgrowth of the epidermis with bulbous rete →. Black tattoo pigment and inflammation are present in the dermis.* **(Right)** *Higher magnification of PEH associated with a tattoo shows prominent epidermal hyperplasia above black tattoo pigment → deposits in the dermis.*

PEH

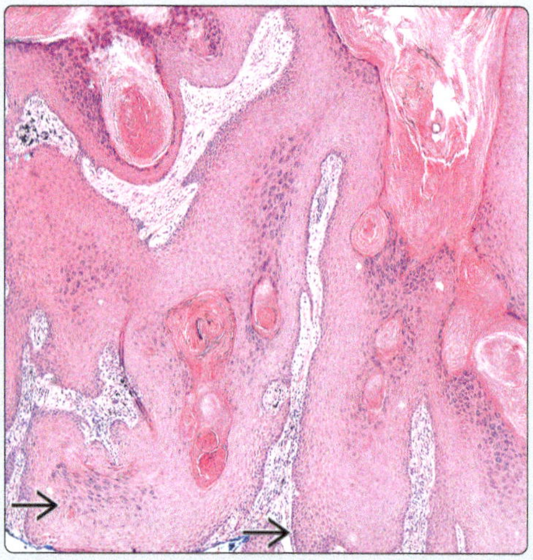

PEH Associated With Tattoo

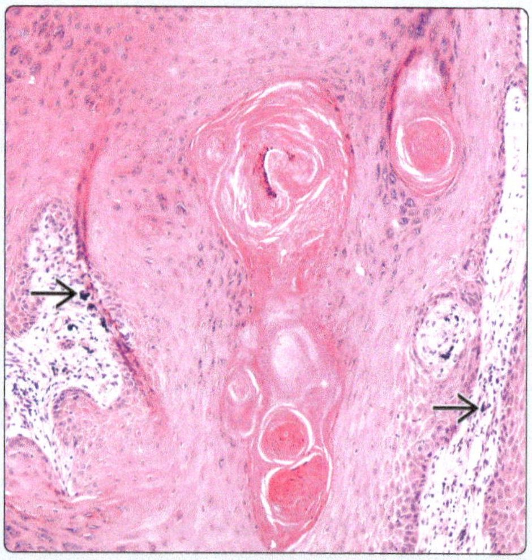

(Left) *In this example of PEH → associated with a primary cutaneous anaplastic large cell lymphoma (ALCL), the epithelium is obscured by atypical lymphocytes → and eosinophils.* **(Right)** *Cytologic atypia is absent in PEH. There is parakeratosis →, but a true squamous pearl is not evident.*

PEH Associated With ALCL

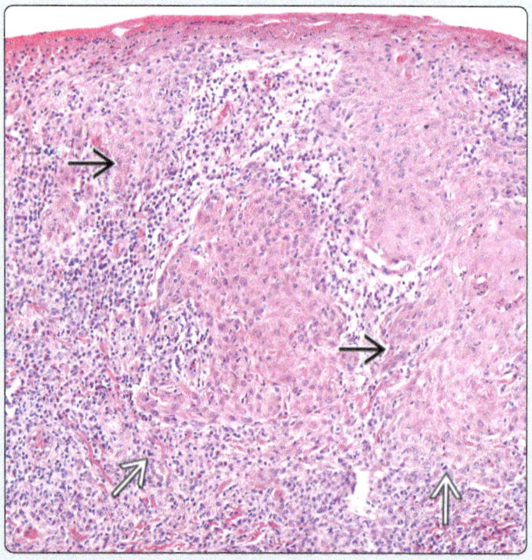

PEH at High Magnification

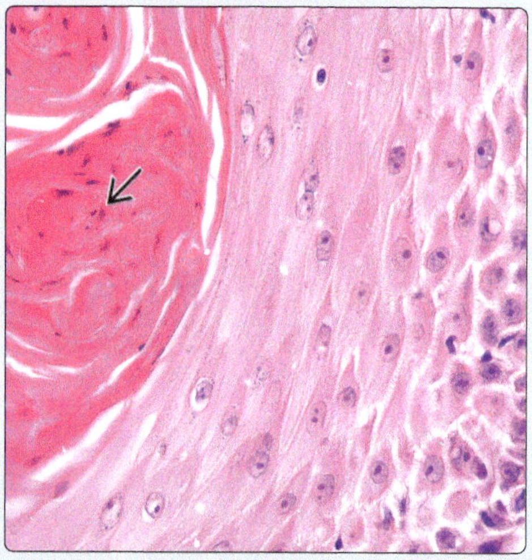

TERMINOLOGY

Abbreviations

- Pseudoepitheliomatous hyperplasia (PEH)

Synonyms

- Pseudocarcinomatous hyperplasia

Definitions

- Florid proliferation of epidermis that mimics squamous cell carcinoma
- Reaction pattern that may be secondary to chronic irritation/trauma

ETIOLOGY/PATHOGENESIS

Associated or Underlying Conditions

- Tumors
  - e.g., granular cell tumor
- Inflammatory conditions
  - e.g., lupus erythematosus, lichen sclerosus
- Infections
  - Particularly deep fungal
  - Also consider syphilis, mycobacteria
- Tattoos

CLINICAL ISSUES

Presentation

- Variable, depending upon underlying condition

Prognosis

- Excellent, no malignant potential

MICROSCOPIC

Histologic Features

- Hyperplasia of epidermis
- Base of hyperplastic epidermis may show broad rete or jagged borders
- Varying depth (but never into subcutis)
- May seem to predominantly involve hair follicles and other adnexal structures
- Squamous eddies may be prominent
- Associated inflammation may be granulomatous
- Should prompt evaluation for underlying/associated process, including
  - Tumors
    - e.g., granular cell tumor, malignant melanoma, Spitz nevus, lymphoma
  - Infections
    - e.g., deep fungal, granuloma inguinale, syphilis, acid-fast bacilli
  - Inflammatory conditions
    - e.g., lupus erythematosus, lichen sclerosus
  - Tattoos
  - Prurigo nodularis/lichen simplex chronicus
    - May show areas of PEH

Cytologic Features

- Minimal keratinocyte atypia
- Cells are polygonal with central, round nuclei, small nucleoli, and intercellular bridges
- Individually necrotic cells are rare

DIFFERENTIAL DIAGNOSIS

Squamous Cell Carcinoma

- Well-differentiated squamous cell carcinoma (SCC) generally shows squamous cell carcinoma features not commonly seen in PEH, including
  - Infiltrative areas
  - Cytologic atypia, atypical mitoses
  - Squamous pearls

Keratoacanthoma

- Crateriform architecture with central keratin
- Keratinocytes with glassy pink cytoplasm
- Elastic fiber trapping, dermal fibrosis, and eosinophilic/neutrophilic abscesses may be present
- Clinically should have history of rapid growth and should spontaneously resolve

Hypertrophic Lupus Erythematosus

- Adjacent features compatible with lupus should be present
  - Interface changes
  - Basement membrane thickening
  - Follicular plugging
  - Perivascular and periadnexal lymphocytic infiltrate

Hypertrophic Lichen Planus

- Hyperplasia of epidermis
- Lichenoid lymphocytic infiltrate concentrated at tips of elongated rete
- Clinically often on lower legs; pruritic

Pyodermatitis Vegetans

- Vegetating plaque with pustules
- May be associated with inflammatory bowel disease
- Florid epithelial hyperplasia with eosinophilic/neutrophilic abscesses
- Direct immunofluorescence negative
- Clinicopathologic correlation important

Pemphigus Vegetans

- Florid epithelial hyperplasia with eosinophilic abscesses
- Direct immunofluorescence positive for intercellular IgG &/or C3

Halogenoderma (Iododerma, Bromoderma)

- Florid hyperplasia of epidermis secondary to ingestion of halogens

DIAGNOSTIC CHECKLIST

Pathologic Interpretation Pearls

- Special stains for infectious organisms often performed
- Special immunohistochemical stains are not routinely performed

SELECTED REFERENCES

1. McFaddin C et al: Desmoplastic trichoepithelioma with pseudocarcinomatous hyperplasia: a report of three cases. J Cutan Pathol. 42(2):102-7, 2015
2. Chakrabarti S et al: Pseudoepitheliomatous hyperplasia: a clinical entity mistaken for squamous cell carcinoma. J Cutan Aesthet Surg. 7(4):232-4, 2014

KEY FACTS

TERMINOLOGY

- Warty dyskeratoma (WD)

CLINICAL ISSUES

- Solitary (very rarely multiple)
- Umbilicated papule or nodule
- Often on head or neck
- Rarely mucosa

MICROSCOPIC

- Cup-shaped lesion
- Sometimes associated with hair follicles
- Hyperkeratosis and parakeratosis
- Suprabasilar acantholysis with villi at base
- Mixed inflammatory infiltrate in dermis
- Corp ronds
  - Round to slightly oval nucleus with pink cytoplasm
- Grains
  - Raisinoid nuclei with pink cytoplasm
- Minimal to no cytologic atypia

TOP DIFFERENTIAL DIAGNOSES

- Darier disease
  - Histologically similar
  - Clinically different
    - Multiple lesions in seborrheic distribution
- Acantholytic dyskeratotic acanthoma
  - Similar to WD
    - Both have acantholysis and dyskeratosis
    - Both are usually clinically solitary lesions
  - Unlike WD
    - Not cup-shaped or associated with hair follicles
    - Flat-based lesion
- Acantholytic squamous cell carcinoma
  - Infiltrative
  - Cytologic atypia
  - Atypical mitoses

Warty Dyskeratoma: Low-Power Architecture

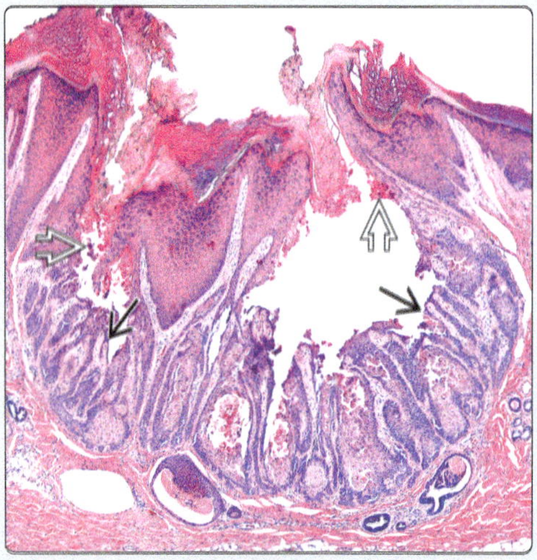

Warty Dyskeratoma: Acantholytic Dyskeratosis

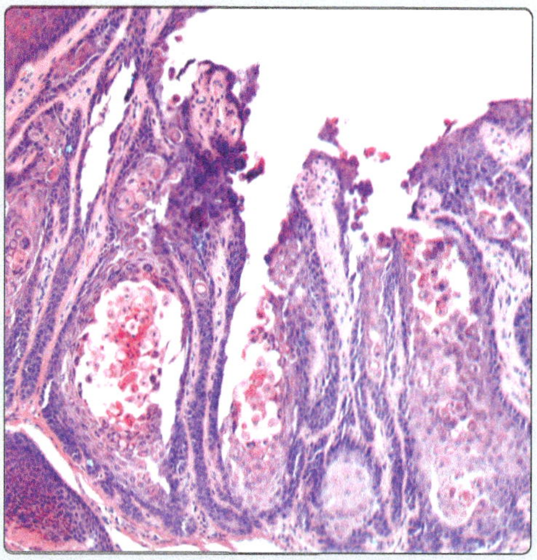

(Left) *This is a low-power view of a warty dyskeratoma, a cup-shaped lesion. There is hyperkeratosis and parakeratosis above central acantholytic dyskeratosis ➡ with villi at the base ➡.* **(Right)** *Acantholysis and dyskeratosis within the hyperplastic epithelial cup are seen here.*

Acantholytic Dyskeratosis: Prominent Grains

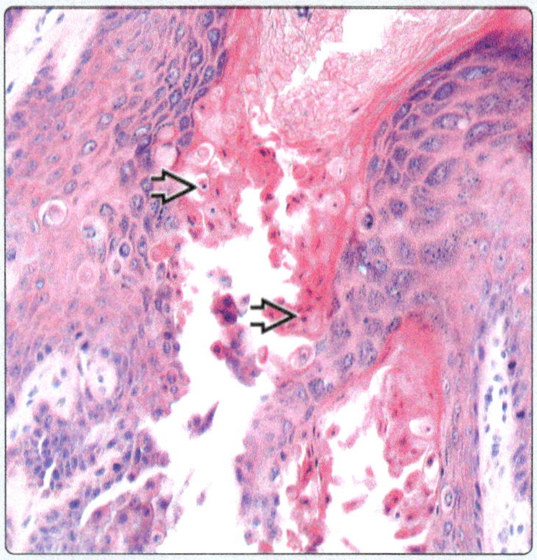

Acantholytic Dyskeratosis: Prominent Corp Ronds

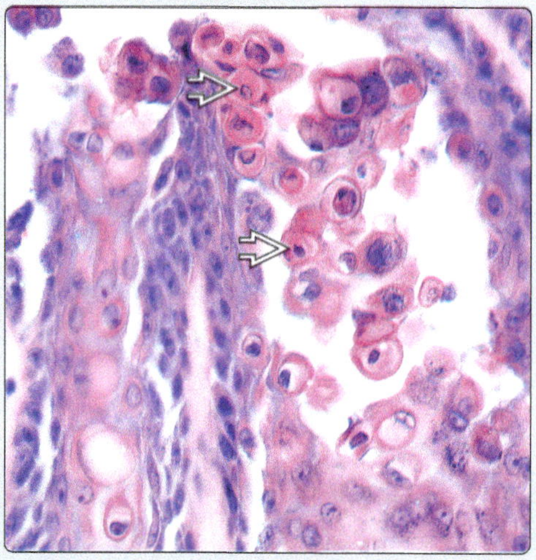

(Left) *Higher magnification shows numerous grains ➡ below hyperkeratosis.* **(Right)** *A high-power view shows the central acantholytic dyskeratosis in a warty dyskeratoma. There are corp ronds (central round to slightly oval shrunken nuclei with surrounding pink cytoplasm) ➡.*

TERMINOLOGY

Abbreviations

- Warty dyskeratoma (WD)

Definitions

- Cup-shaped epidermal proliferation
- Acantholysis is present
- Dyskeratosis (corp ronds and grains) is present

ETIOLOGY/PATHOGENESIS

Pathophysiology

- Germline mutations in *ATP2A2* not described (as are seen in Darier disease)
- Human papilloma virus infection has not been associated with WD

CLINICAL ISSUES

Epidemiology

- Age
  - Middle-aged to older patients

Site

- Often on head or neck, may be in genital area
- Mucosal lesions uncommon but described

Presentation

- Solitary, very rarely multiple, umbilicated papule or nodule

Treatment

- Biopsy/excision generally curative

Prognosis

- Benign, no malignant potential

MICROSCOPIC

Histologic Features

- Cup-shaped lesion
- Occasionally cystic or nodular
- May be associated with hair follicles in some cases
- Hyperkeratosis and parakeratosis
- Suprabasilar acantholysis
- Corp ronds and grains
- Villi at base
- Mixed inflammatory infiltrate in dermis

Cytologic Features

- Corp ronds (dyskeratotic cells with round to slightly oval nucleus with eosinophilic cytoplasm)
- Grains (raisinoid nuclei with dense eosinophilic cytoplasm)
- Minimal to no cytologic atypia

DIFFERENTIAL DIAGNOSIS

Darier Disease

- Autosomal dominant genetic disorder
- Mutations in *ATP2A2* gene
- Multiple hyperkeratotic, greasy papules
- Seborrheic (face, scalp, chest, upper back) distribution
- Histology similar to WD, but it lacks cup shape
  - Acantholysis and dyskeratosis beneath hyperkeratosis
  - Clinicopathologic correlation necessary

Grover Disease

- Multiple slightly eroded papules, may be pruritic
- Affects chest and upper back of middle-aged to older males
- Histology may be similar to WD
  - More commonly, acantholysis and dyskeratosis limited to a few rete, without prominent overlying hyperkeratosis
- Multiple patterns of acantholysis may be present
  - WD-like, full-thickness acantholysis (Hailey-Hailey-like), suprabasilar acantholysis (pemphigus vulgaris-like), subcorneal acantholysis

Acantholytic Acanthoma

- Solitary lesion
- Often on trunk of middle-aged to older individuals
- Unlike WD, dyskeratosis is not present

Acantholytic Dyskeratotic Acanthoma

- Solitary lesion
- Often on trunk of middle-aged to older individuals
- Like WD, acantholysis and dyskeratosis present
- Unlike WD, overall architecture is flat
  - Not associated with hair follicles

Acantholytic Actinic Keratosis

- Generally not cup-shaped
- Typically spares hair follicles
- Cytologic atypia present in basal layer with acantholysis
- Corp ronds and grains not prominent

Acantholytic Squamous Cell Carcinoma

- Endophytic lesion
- Infiltrative growth pattern
- Acantholysis present
- Corp ronds and grains not prominent
- Cytologic atypia and mitoses usually easily identified

Acantholytic Dermatosis of Genital (Vulvocrural) Area

- Multiple papules and plaques in genital area
- Lesions with similar histology absent on other areas of body
- More common in women
- Histology may be WD-like or show acantholysis without dyskeratosis

DIAGNOSTIC CHECKLIST

Pathologic Interpretation Pearls

- Cup-shaped lesion with hyperkeratosis
- Acantholytic dyskeratosis (corp ronds and grains)

SELECTED REFERENCES

1. Lora V et al: Warty Dyskeratoma as a Cutaneous Horn of the Mons Pubis. Am J Dermatopathol. 37(10):802-4, 2015
2. Phelps PO et al: Warty Dyskeratoma of the Eyelid. Ophthalmology. 122(7):1282, 2015
3. Ugras N et al: Multiple warty dyskeratomas: case report. Iran J Public Health. 43(8):1145-7, 2014
4. Kaddu S et al: Warty dyskeratoma--"follicular dyskeratoma": analysis of clinicopathologic features of a distinctive follicular adnexal neoplasm. J Am Acad Dermatol. 47(3):423-8, 2002
5. Brownstein MH: The benign acanthomas. J Cutan Pathol. 12(3-4):172-88, 1985

Acantholytic and Acantholytic Dyskeratotic Acanthoma

KEY FACTS

TERMINOLOGY

- Benign lesions with flat, plaque-like architecture and acantholysis
- **Acantholytic acanthoma**
- **Acantholytic dyskeratotic acanthoma**

CLINICAL ISSUES

- Generally a solitary papule
- Often on trunk
- Often submitted to "rule out basal cell carcinoma"

MICROSCOPIC

- Flat, plaque-like architecture
- Minimal to no cytologic atypia
- Acantholytic acanthoma
  - Acantholysis without dyskeratosis
- Acantholytic dyskeratotic acanthoma
  - Acantholysis with dyskeratosis
  - Corp ronds and grains

TOP DIFFERENTIAL DIAGNOSES

- Warty dyskeratoma
- Grover disease
- Hailey-Hailey disease
- Darier disease
- Pemphigus vulgaris
- Pemphigus foliaceus
- Acantholytic actinic keratosis
- Acantholytic squamous cell carcinoma
- Acantholytic dermatosis of genital (vulvocrural) area

DIAGNOSTIC CHECKLIST

- Acantholytic and acantholytic dyskeratotic acanthoma
  - Flat, plaque-like architecture
    - Not cup shaped
    - Not associated with hair follicles
  - Rounding up of keratinocytes (acantholysis)
  - Minimal to no cytologic atypia

Acantholytic Acanthoma

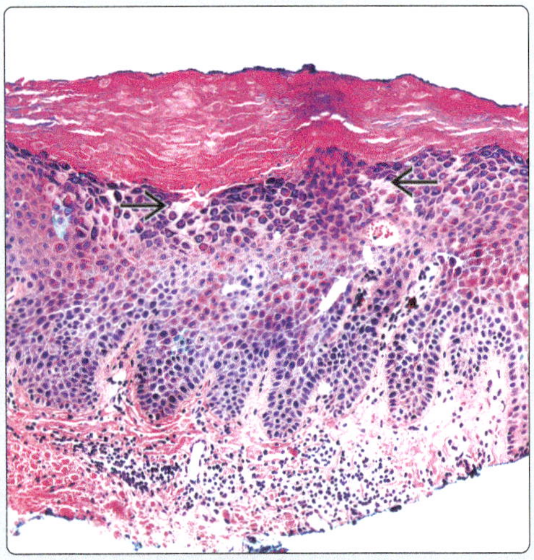

Acantholytic Dyskeratotic Acanthoma

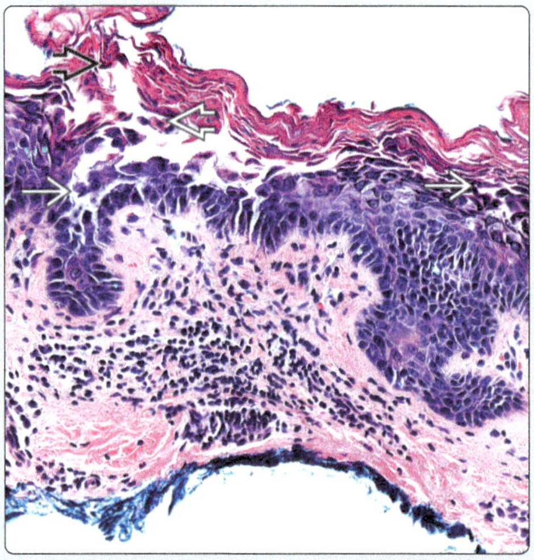

(Left) *An acantholytic acanthoma is a solitary keratosis characterized by acantholysis (dyscohesion of keratinocytes) ⇨, which is full thickness in this example. There is a lack of dyskeratosis (corp ronds and grains).* **(Right)** *An acantholytic dyskeratotic acanthoma is a solitary keratosis with acantholysis ➡ and dyskeratosis (corp ronds ➡ and grains ⇨). The overall architecture is flat and plaque-like.*

Acantholytic Acanthoma

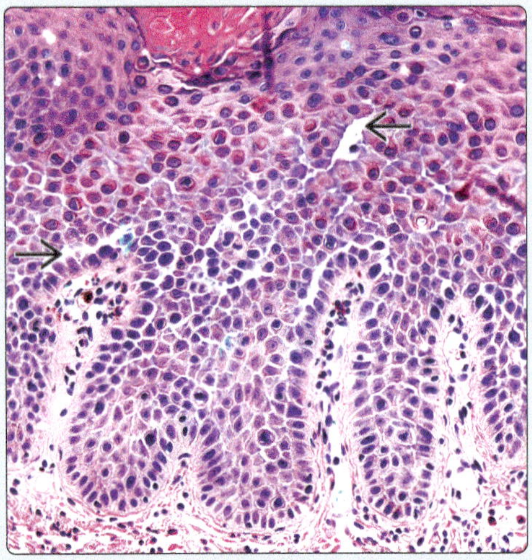

Acantholytic Acanthoma

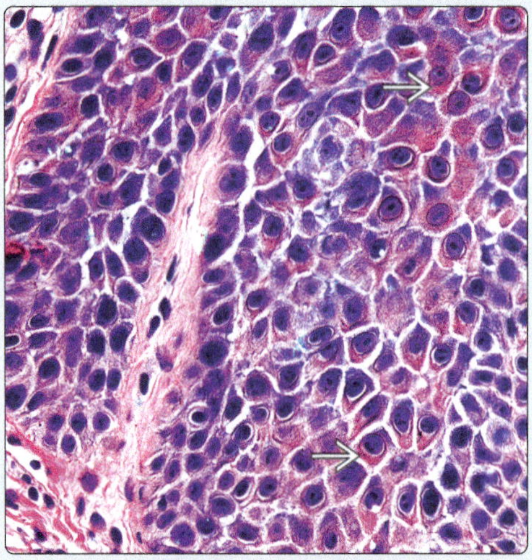

(Left) *Intermediate-magnification view of an acantholytic acanthoma shows dyscohesion of keratinocytes (acantholysis) ⇨. Dyskeratosis is not prominent.* **(Right)** *High-magnification view of an acantholytic acanthoma reveals acantholytic cells that lack cytologic atypia and have pink cytoplasm ➡ due to clumped tonofilaments.*

TERMINOLOGY

Synonyms

- Some consider these 2 entities synonymous
- Criterion used to separate them is presence or absence of dyskeratosis (corp ronds and grains)

Definitions

- Benign lesions with flat, plaque-like architecture and acantholysis
- **Acantholytic acanthoma**
  - Absent dyskeratosis (corp ronds and grains)
- **Acantholytic dyskeratotic acanthoma**
  - Dyskeratosis present

CLINICAL ISSUES

Presentation

- Generally solitary papule
- Often on trunk
- Often submitted to "rule out basal cell carcinoma"

Prognosis

- Benign, no malignant potential

MICROSCOPIC

Histologic Features

- Acantholytic and acantholytic dyskeratotic acanthoma
  - Flat, plaque-like architecture
- Acantholytic acanthoma
  - Acantholysis without dyskeratosis
  - Acantholysis may be suprabasilar or full thickness
- Acantholytic dyskeratotic acanthoma
  - Acantholysis with dyskeratosis (corp ronds and grains)
  - Acantholysis may be suprabasilar or subcorneal

Cytologic Features

- Acantholytic and acantholytic dyskeratotic acanthoma
  - Minimal to no cytologic atypia
  - Rounding up of keratinocytes (acantholysis)
- Acantholytic dyskeratotic acanthoma
  - Corp ronds (round to minimally oval nuclei with surrounding pink cytoplasm) present

DIFFERENTIAL DIAGNOSIS

Warty Dyskeratoma

- Often on head and neck
- Hyperkeratosis over cup-shaped lesion
- Dyskeratosis present

Grover Disease

- Multiple slightly eroded papules
- Affects chest and upper back
- Typically in middle-aged to older men
- 4 patterns of acantholysis can be present
  - Darier like (acantholysis and dyskeratosis)
  - Full-thickness acantholysis
  - Suprabasilar acantholysis
  - Subcorneal acantholysis

Hailey-Hailey Disease

- Eroded, macerated, erythematous plaques in intertriginous areas
- Histology shows full-thickness acantholysis
  - Often likened to dilapidated brick wall
- Generally lacks dyskeratosis

Darier Disease

- Autosomal dominant genetic disorder
- Multiple hyperkeratotic, greasy papules
- Seborrheic (face, scalp, chest, upper back) distribution
- Acantholysis and dyskeratosis beneath hyperkeratosis

Pemphigus Vulgaris and Foliaceus

- Multiple flaccid blisters and erosions generally present
- Pemphigus vulgaris: Suprabasilar acantholysis, lacks dyskeratosis, involves adnexal structures
- Pemphigus foliaceus: Subcorneal acantholysis
- Direct immunofluorescence shows intercellular staining with IgG and C3

Acantholytic Actinic Keratosis

- Cytologic atypia present in basal layer with acantholysis
- Dyskeratosis not prominent

Acantholytic Squamous Cell Carcinoma

- Endophytic and infiltrative growth pattern
- Acantholysis of atypical keratinocytes
- Atypical mitoses present

Acantholytic Dermatosis of Genital (Vulvocrural) Area

- Multiple papules and plaques in genital area
- Lesions with similar histology absent on other areas of body
- Can be difficult to distinguish from Hailey-Hailey disease (benign familial pemphigus)

DIAGNOSTIC CHECKLIST

Pathologic Interpretation Pearls

- Acantholytic and acantholytic dyskeratotic acanthoma
  - Flat, plaque-like architecture
  - Rounding up of keratinocytes (acantholysis)
- Acantholytic dyskeratotic acanthoma
  - Acantholysis
  - Corp ronds (round to minimally oval nuclei with surrounding pink cytoplasm) present
  - Grains (raisinoid, shrunken nuclei with pink cytoplasm) present

SELECTED REFERENCES

1. Goldenberg A et al: Acantholytic dyskeratotic acanthoma: case report and review of the literature. Dermatol Pract Concept. 4(3):25-30, 2014
2. Pernet C et al: Genitoperineal papular acantholytic dyskeratosis is allelic to Hailey-Hailey disease. Br J Dermatol. 167(1):210-2, 2012
3. Fernández-Figueras MT et al: Grover disease: a reappraisal of histopathological diagnostic criteria in 120 cases. Am J Dermatopathol. 32(6):541-9, 2010
4. Ko CJ et al: Acantholytic dyskeratotic acanthoma: a variant of a benign keratosis. J Cutan Pathol. 35(3):298-301, 2008
5. Cooper PH: Acantholytic dermatosis localized to the vulvocrural area. J Cutan Pathol. 16(2):81-4, 1989

Verruca Vulgaris (and Variants)

KEY FACTS

TERMINOLOGY

- Verruca vulgaris (VV)
- Common warts
- Palmoplantar warts (myrmecia)
- Flat warts (verruca plana)

ETIOLOGY/PATHOGENESIS

- Causal relationship with numerous human papillomavirus (HPV) types
- Numerous HPV types implicated, including HPV-1, 2, 3, 4, 7, 10, 27, 29, and 57

CLINICAL ISSUES

- Common sites include fingers & hands (VV), palms & soles (palmoplantar warts), face & dorsal hands (flat warts)

MICROSCOPIC

- Exophytic/endophytic papillomatous proliferation with hypergranulosis, dense overlying hyperkeratosis, and tiers of parakeratosis
- Intracorneal hemorrhage typically present
- Periphery often shows pointing inward of basilar epidermis
- Superficial keratinocytes show perinuclear halos and prominent keratohyaline granules
  - Palmoplantar warts show especially prominent keratohyaline inclusions
- Lesions may be irritated and inflamed, often associated with reactive atypia

TOP DIFFERENTIAL DIAGNOSES

- Verrucous keratosis
- Seborrheic keratosis
- Lichen simplex chronicus
- Hypertrophic lichen planus
- Verrucous carcinoma
- Epidermodysplasia verruciformis

Clinical Photograph of Verrucae

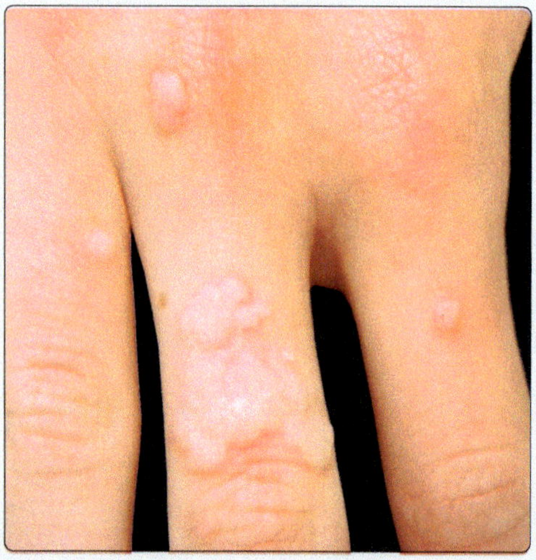

Verruca Vulgaris

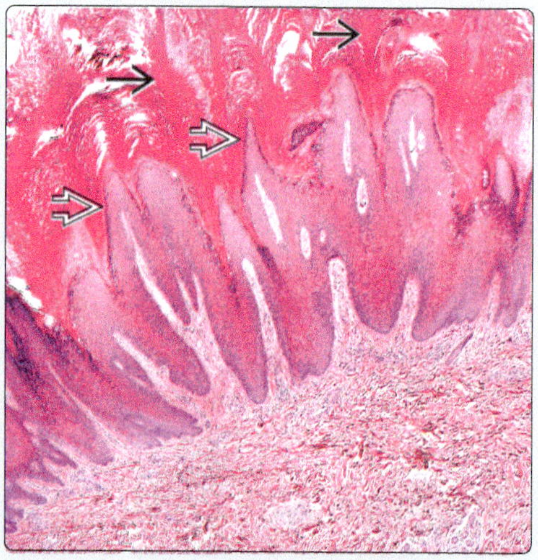

(Left) *Clinical photograph shows multiple verrucae on the dorsal hand and fingers. (Courtesy J. Wu, MD.)* **(Right)** *This verruca vulgaris (VV) shows dense hyperkeratosis →, parakeratosis, acanthosis, and marked papillomatosis ⇨. Most lesions show few or no dermal changes.*

Palmoplantar Wart With Prominent Papillomatosis

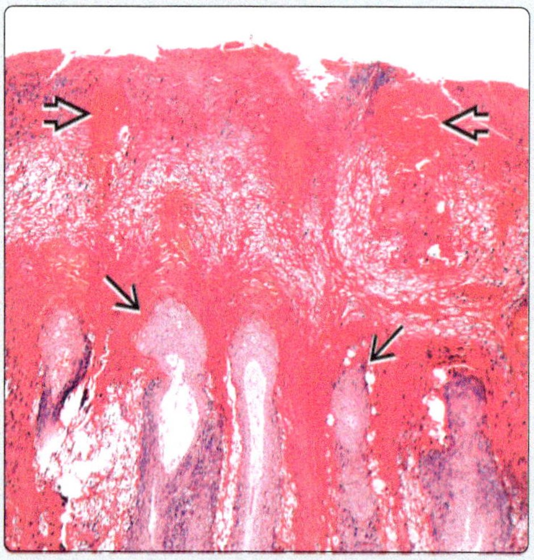

Palmoplantar Wart With Prominent Keratohyaline Granules

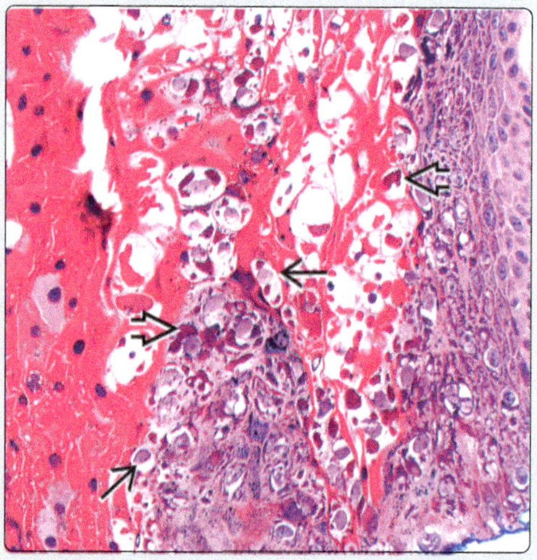

(Left) *Scanning magnification of a palmoplantar wart (myrmecia) shows prominent papillomatosis → with thick overlying hyperkeratosis and parakeratosis with areas of hemorrhage ⇨.* **(Right)** *Palmoplantar warts (myrmecia) often show especially prominent koilocytes with perinuclear halos → and large, dense keratohyaline inclusions ⇨.*

TERMINOLOGY

Abbreviations

- Verruca vulgaris (VV)

Synonyms

- **Variants**
  - Palmoplantar warts (myrmecia)
  - Flat warts (verruca plana)

Definitions

- Human papillomavirus (HPV)-related benign epidermal proliferation

ETIOLOGY/PATHOGENESIS

Infectious Agents

- Causal relationship established with numerous HPV types, including HPV-1, 2, 3, 4, 7, 10, 27, 29, and 57

CLINICAL ISSUES

Epidemiology

- Incidence
  - Very common lesions
- Age
  - Common in children and young adults, but can occur at any age

Site

- Common sites include fingers and dorsal hands (VV), palms and soles (palmoplantar warts), face and dorsal hands (flat warts)

Presentation

- Small papular to plaque-like lesions

Natural History

- Grow rapidly, then stabilize

Treatment

- Drugs
  - Topical therapy with podophyllin or other antiviral medications

Prognosis

- Excellent, unless immunosuppressed

MACROSCOPIC

General Features

- Often exophytic-appearing scaly (hyperkeratotic) lesion

MICROSCOPIC

Histologic Features

- Exophytic and endophytic papillomatous epidermal proliferation
  - Epidermal acanthosis with hypergranulosis, dense overlying hyperkeratosis, and tiers of parakeratosis (church spires)
    - Flat warts show acanthosis and hyperkeratosis but lack significant papillomatosis and parakeratosis
  - Intracorneal hemorrhage typically present
  - Periphery of lesion shows pointing (toeing) inward of basilar epidermis
  - Superficial keratinocytes may show perinuclear halos and prominent keratohyaline granules
    - Palmoplantar warts (myrmecia) show especially prominent keratohyaline inclusions, which appear basophilic
- Lesions may be irritated and inflamed, often associated with reactive atypia
  - Mitotic figures often present within basilar layer, especially in irritated/inflamed lesions, but are not present in upper levels of epidermis
- Dermal papillae often show dilated capillaries

DIFFERENTIAL DIAGNOSIS

Verrucous Keratosis

- Epidermal proliferation with acanthosis and irregular papillomatosis, but lacks diagnostic features of VV
- Often used for partial/nondiagnostic biopsies, in which lesion cannot be definitively classified

Seborrheic Keratosis

- Verrucous seborrheic keratosis (SK) shows epidermal hyperplasia with papillomatous projections
- Intraepidermal pseudohorn cysts filled with keratin whorls

Lichen Simplex Chronicus

- Irregular epidermal hyperplasia with hypergranulosis and overlying hyperkeratosis
- Lacks tiers of parakeratosis and toeing in of peripheral epidermis

Hypertrophic Lichen Planus

- Shows irregular epidermal acanthosis, often with sawtooth pattern
- Superficial dermis shows dense, band-like, chronic inflammatory infiltrate

Verrucous Carcinoma

- Papillomatous proliferation demonstrating prominent elongated, bulbous rete ridges extending deeply into dermis
- Bland cytologic features with large squamous keratinocytes showing abundant dense eosinophilic cytoplasm

Epidermodysplasia Verruciformis

- May be inherited (genodermatosis) or related to immunosuppression (i.e., AIDS)
- Histologic features are similar to verruca plana, but cells show basophilic cytoplasm and prominent keratohyaline granules

SELECTED REFERENCES

1. Smola S: Human papillomaviruses and skin cancer. Adv Exp Med Biol. 810:192-207, 2014
2. Bruggink SC et al: Natural course of cutaneous warts among primary schoolchildren: a prospective cohort study. Ann Fam Med. 11(5):437-41, 2013
3. Antonsson A: Review: antibodies to cutaneous human papillomaviruses. J Med Virol. 84(5):814-22, 2012
4. Barcelos AC et al: Comparative analysis of the expression of cytokeratins (1, 10, 14, 16, 4), involucrin, filaggrin and e-cadherin in plane warts and epidermodysplasia verruciformis plane wart-type lesions. J Cutan Pathol. 36(6):647-54, 2009

(Left) *This VV shows acanthosis and papillomatosis, typical of verruca. Note the inward turning (toeing in) of the elongated rete ridges at the edge of the lesion →, also a characteristic finding.* **(Right)** *Another example of VV shows marked papillomatosis with overlying hyperkeratosis and tiers of parakeratosis →. The superficial dermis underlying this VV shows prominent telangiectasia, a finding commonly seen in verrucae.*

Verruca Vulgaris With Toeing In of Peripheral Rete Ridges

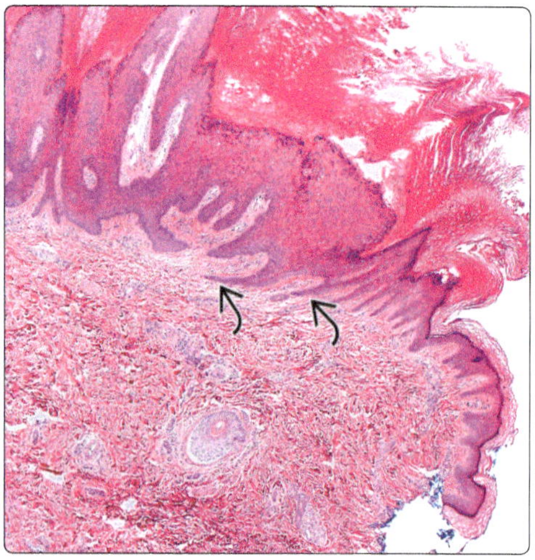

Higher Magnification of Verruca Vulgaris

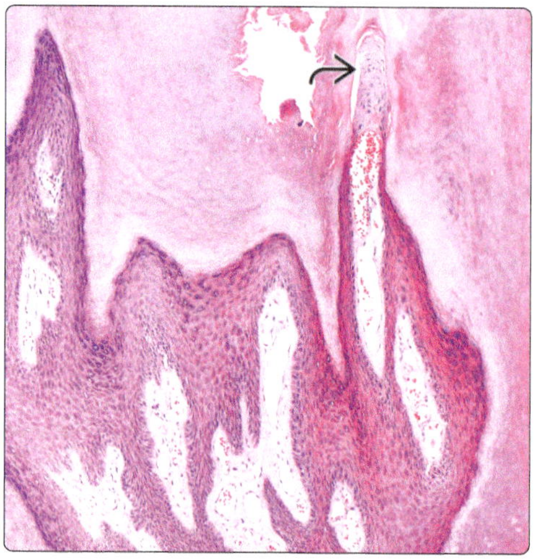

(Left) *Low magnification of a flat wart demonstrates mild epidermal acanthosis and dense overlying hyperkeratosis and parakeratosis. This lesion was treated (with liquid nitrogen) prior to biopsy, and it shows foci of intracorneal hemorrhage → and superficial necrosis →, consistent with treatment effects.* **(Right)** *High magnification of a flat wart shows hypergranulosis, dense hyperkeratosis, and scattered superficial koilocytic cells → with perinuclear halos.*

Verruca Plana (Flat Wart)

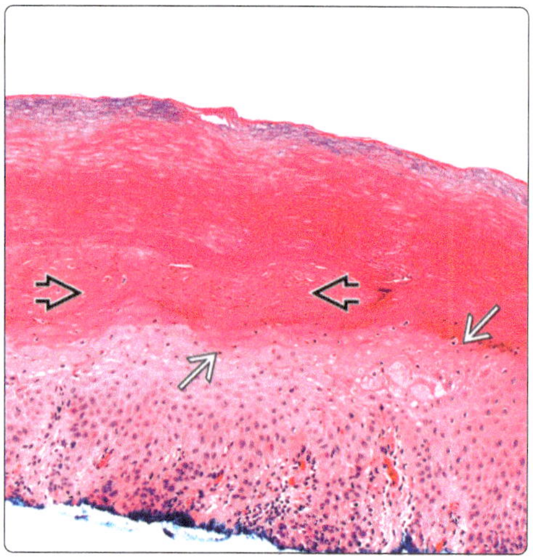

Verruca Plana at High Magnification

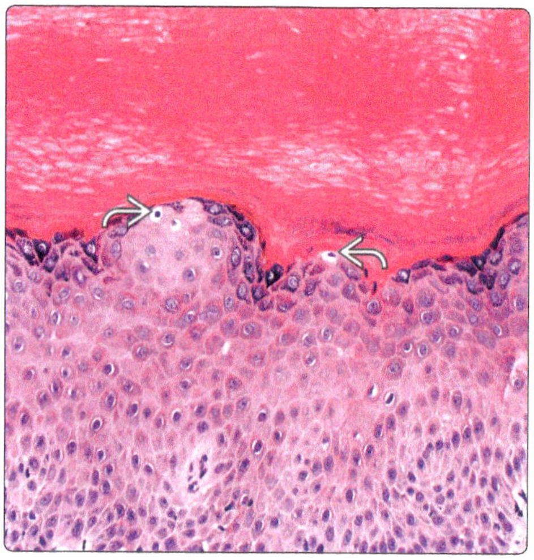

(Left) *This verruca vulgaris shows epidermal acanthosis and papillomatosis with dense overlying hyperkeratosis, tiers of parakeratosis →, and areas of serum crusting →, with collections of neutrophils and focal acute hemorrhage →.* **(Right)** *Palmoplantar wart at high magnification shows especially prominent koilocytes with perinuclear halos → and large, dense keratohyaline inclusions →.*

Superficial Portion of Irritated Verruca Vulgaris

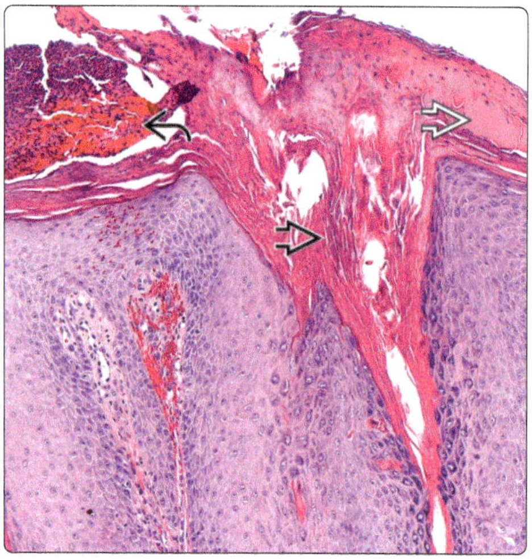

Palmoplantar Wart With Prominent Keratohyaline Granules

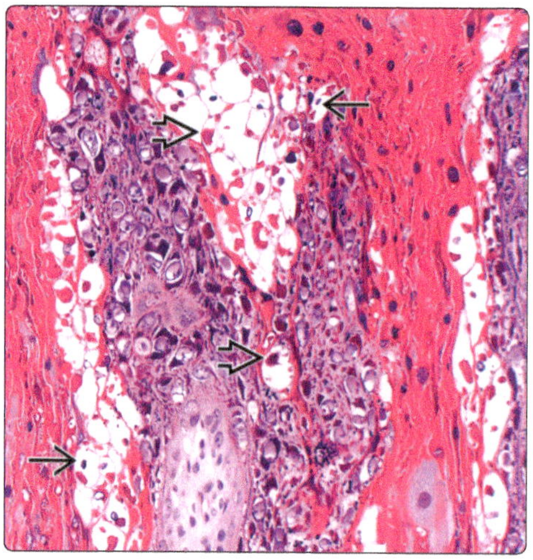

Differential Diagnosis: SCC In Situ Arising in Verruca Vulgaris

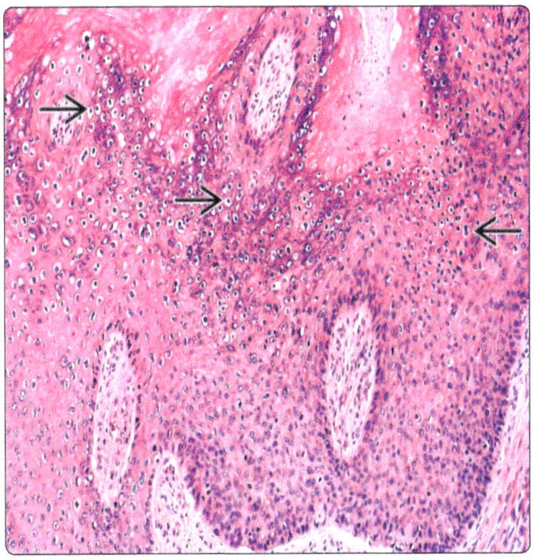

Differential Diagnosis: Squamous Cell Carcinoma In Situ

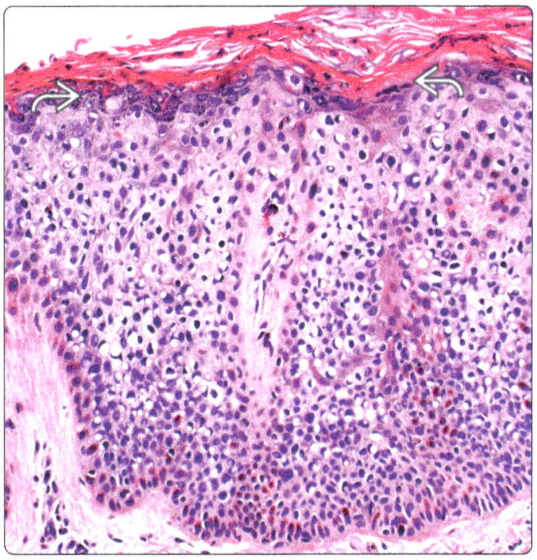

(Left) *A rare example of squamous cell carcinoma in situ (Bowen disease) arising in association with a VV is shown. Note the numerous superficial koilocytes.* **(Right)** *This is an example of a clear cell squamous cell carcinoma in situ, which shows epidermal acanthosis, slight papillomatosis, and focally prominent hypergranulosis. However, the epidermis is filled with atypical pale to clear-staining keratinocytes.*

Differential Diagnosis: Verrucous Carcinoma

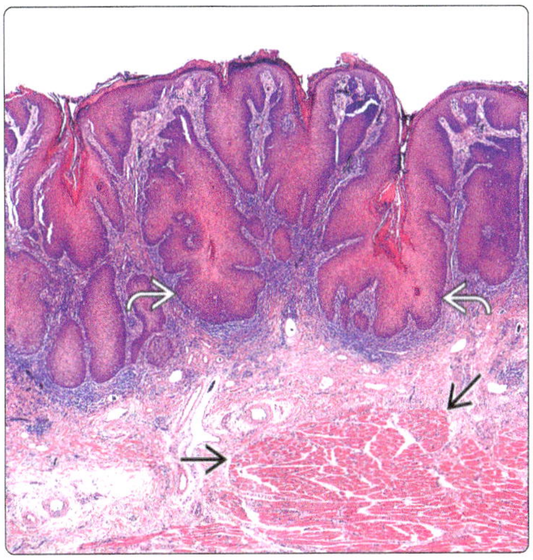

Differential Diagnosis: Verrucous Carcinoma

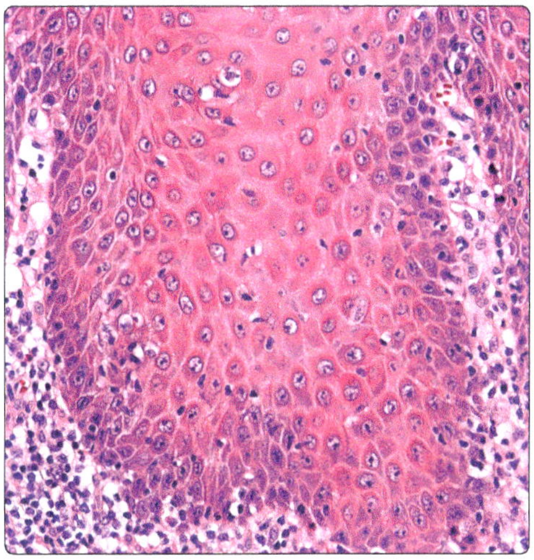

(Left) *Verrucous carcinoma shows prominent endophytic downgrowths with bulbous rete ridges surrounded by chronic inflammation. Note the deep pushing invasion approaching bundles of skeletal muscle.* **(Right)** *High magnification of a verrucous carcinoma shows the bland cytologic features of the squamous cells. The cells are enlarged and show abundant dense, eosinophilic cytoplasm, but there is minimal cytologic atypia.*

Differential Diagnosis: Epidermodysplasia Verruciformis

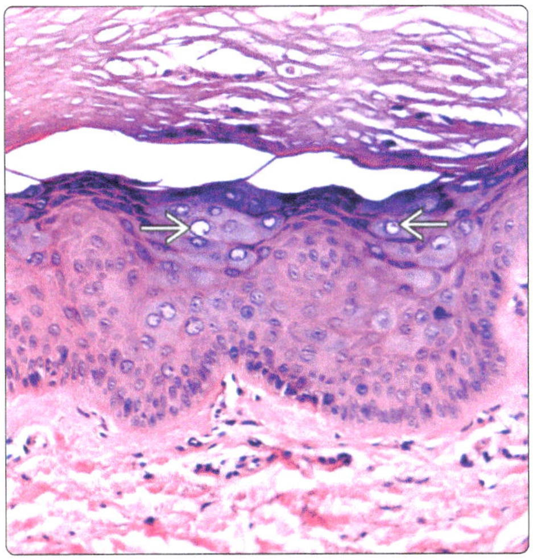

Differential Diagnosis: Hypertrophic Lichen Planus

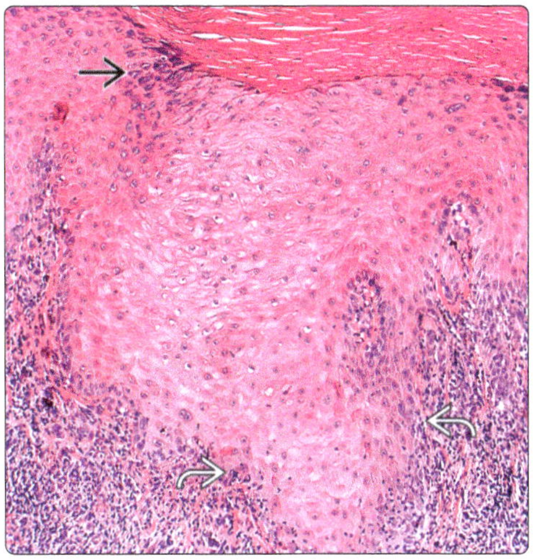

(Left) *This example of epidermodysplasia verruciformis shows mild epidermal acanthosis and a proliferation of enlarged, bluish gray-staining keratinocytes with nuclear clearing.* **(Right)** *High magnification of hypertrophic lichen planus shows epidermal acanthosis with hypergranulosis. The superficial dermis shows a dense lymphoid infiltrate with scattered exocytosis into the basilar epithelium.*

Condyloma Acuminatum (Genital Wart)

KEY FACTS

ETIOLOGY/PATHOGENESIS

- HPV-related lesion
- Low-risk HPV serotypes (6, 11) predominate

CLINICAL ISSUES

- Very common STD
- Preferentially affecting anogenital region
- Lesions tend to recur

MACROSCOPIC

- From flat to exophytic, cauliflower-like lesions
- Measuring from a few mm to several cm
- Giant condylomas are large lesions measuring > 5 cm

MICROSCOPIC

- Acanthosis with variable papillomatosis and prominent fibrovascular cores
- Broad and sharply defined lower border
- Conspicuous koilocytosis
  - Irregular wrinkled nuclei
  - Bi- and multinucleation
  - Perinuclear vacuolization
- Old lesions may mimic seborrheic keratoses

ANCILLARY TESTS

- Immunostain for p16 is negative (there is no overexpression)
- In situ hybridization and PCR usually show presence of low-risk HPV (HPV 6 to 11)

TOP DIFFERENTIAL DIAGNOSES

- Verrucous carcinoma
- Warty carcinoma
- Papillomatosis of glans corona (pearly penile papules)
- Bowenoid papulosis
- Squamous cell carcinoma in situ or warty/basaloid penile intraepithelial neoplasia

Low-Power View of Condyloma Acuminatum

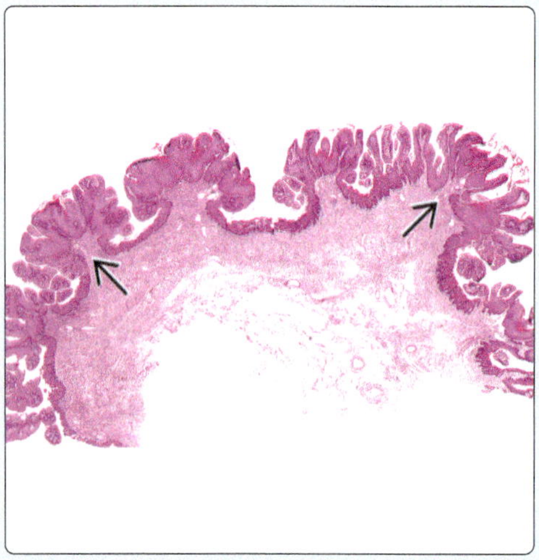

Prominent Koilocytosis in Condyloma Acuminatum

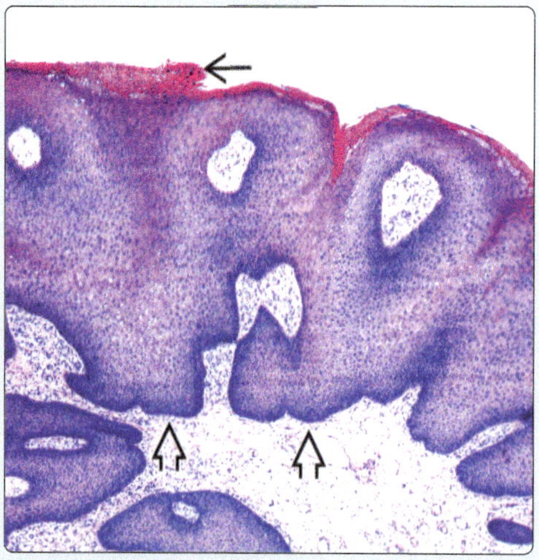

(Left) *Condyloma acuminatum shows an exophytic papillomatous growth, regular and broad tumor base, and easily recognizable fibrovascular cores* →. **(Right)** *Condyloma acuminatum is characterized by marked acanthosis, slight (as in this example) to marked papillomatosis, and a sharply demarcated, bulbous base* ⇒. *Note the focal parakeratosis* →.

Higher Power View of Koilocytic Change

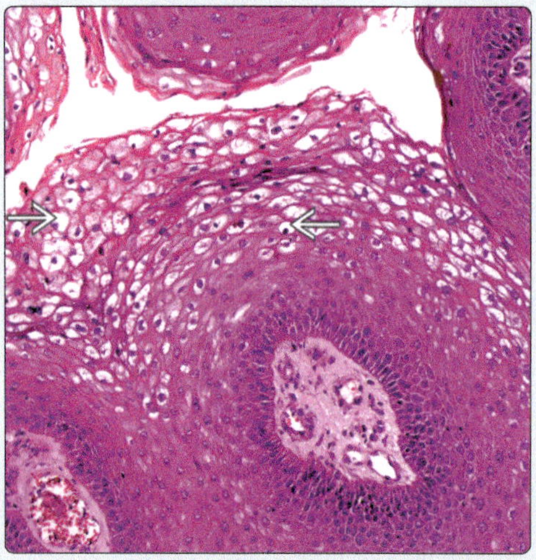

Binucleated Koilocytes in Condyloma Acuminatum

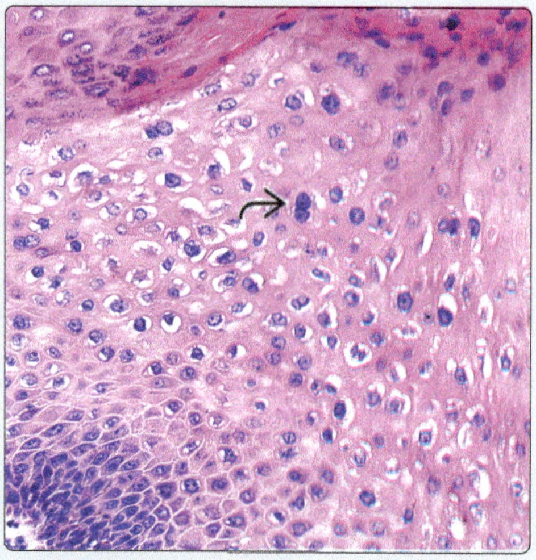

(Left) *Condyloma acuminatum is characterized by koilocytic change (nuclear wrinkling, a perinuclear halo* ➡*, and often bi- and multinucleated nuclei). Koilocytosis tend to be confined to upper levels of the epithelium in contrast with warty carcinoma, where koilocytic change extends to deep infiltrative foci.* **(Right)** *Koilocytes have eosinophilic cytoplasm and are characterized by clear perinuclear halos and wrinkled and hyperchromatic nuclei. Binucleation is common* ↪.

TERMINOLOGY

Synonyms

- Genital wart

Definitions

- Exophytic and verruciform benign epithelial lesions

ETIOLOGY/PATHOGENESIS

Infectious Agents

- Caused by HPV
  - Low-risk serotypes 6 and 11 (90% of cases)
  - Other serotypes include 16, 18, 30-32, 42-44, 51-55
  - > 1 serotype may be found in lesion

CLINICAL ISSUES

Epidemiology

- Incidence
  - Very common STD
  - Penile lesions are more common in uncircumcised men than in circumcised ones
  - Topical treatment of vulvar dermatosis with corticosteroids and tacrolimus may reactivate old/latent lesions
  - Penile subclinical lesions appear to be more frequent in sexual partners of women with cervical intraepithelial neoplasia
- Age
  - Most frequent in young adults
    - 2nd and 3rd decades of life
  - Uncommon in children
    - Such cases should raise suspicion of sexual abuse
    - HPV has been detected in young girls with lichen sclerosus without history of sexual abuse
    - Spontaneous regression is common in children
      - ~ 50% of cases
- Sex
  - Affect both sexes

Site

- Predilection for anogenital area
  - Males: Glans, prepuce, shaft
    - May extend to meatus
  - Females: Labia minora, interlabial sulcus, area around introitus
    - May extend into introitus
  - Both sexes: Perianal and more rarely oral cavity
  - Other less frequent locations: Abdomen, breast (nipple/areola)

Presentation

- Soft fleshy verruciform plaques
- Filiform lesions
- Lesion in coronal sulcus and vulva may be bulkier and macerated
- Flat (nearly macular lesions) may occur
- Tiny inconspicuous lesions may be difficult to detect
- Immunocompromised patients may show extensive lesions

Natural History

- Usually sexually transmitted
  - Spreads rapidly
- Variable incubation period
  - Usually 2-3 months
- Condylomas tend to recur
  - In ~ 30% of cases
  - May be due to persistence of HPV DNA in dermis &/or hair follicles

Treatment

- For small tumors: Cryosurgery, electrofulguration, laser ablation, and topical treatments
- For medium-sized and large tumors: Surgical excision

Prognosis

- Benign lesions
  - High recurrence rate (~ 30%)
- Malignant transformation is rare in condyloma acuminatum
  - More frequent in larger lesions (giant condyloma)
- Patients with condyloma often have other sexually transmitted diseases
- HPV vaccine holds promise for future

MACROSCOPIC

General Features

- Size ranges from few mm to several cm

MICROSCOPIC

Histologic Features

- Arborescent acanthotic papillae with prominent fibrovascular cores
  - Some lesions may be flat
- Variable parakeratosis and orthokeratosis
- Koilocytosis
  - Best seen in upper portion of epithelium of papillae and upper portion of declivities
  - Koilocytes exhibit perinuclear vacuolization
  - Wrinkled and hyperchromatic nuclei
  - Frequent bi- and multinucleation
- Sharply defined base that is broad and flat
- Condylomata may show horn pseudocysts
- Old condylomata may show little to no koilocytosis
  - Old condylomata may look very similar to seborrheic keratoses
  - Seborrheic keratosis-like lesions in genital areas are very often associated with HPV
- Condylomata treated with resin of podophyllin
  - May show pallor of upper epithelium
  - Nuclear enlargement
  - Increased numbers of mitotic figures (not atypical)
  - Scattered necrotic keratinocytes
  - Differential diagnosis includes carcinoma in situ and bowenoid papulosis
    - History of treatment is important
  - Changes disappear after week

ANCILLARY TESTS

Immunohistochemistry

- p16 immunostain is usually negative (no overexpression)
- Ki-67(+) only in basilar portions of lesion

In Situ Hybridization

- Association with low-risk HPV
  - Most frequently 6-11

PCR

- Association with low-risk HPV
  - Most frequently 6-11

DIFFERENTIAL DIAGNOSIS

Verrucous Carcinoma

- HPV unrelated in most cases
- No koilocytosis
- Acanthotic papillae with thin fibrovascular cores
- Prominent keratin valleys between papillae
- Minimal cytologic atypia
- Broad and pushing tumor base

Giant Condyloma

- Condyloma measuring > 5 cm in size
- More prominent endophytic pattern of growth
- May harbor foci of squamous cell carcinoma (SCC)
  - Malignant foci tend to be located in deep portions
  - Keratinizing SCC of usual type
    - Most commonly associated subtype
  - Generous sampling of giant condylomata is recommended
- Recommend avoiding term Buschke-Löwenstein tumor
  - Confusing term that has been used for different lesions in literature
    - (e.g., condylomas, verrucous carcinomas, papillary SCC)

Warty Carcinoma

- Affects older patients
- Associated with high-risk HPV
- Atypical koilocytosis
  - Nuclear pleomorphism
  - Numerous mitoses
    - Atypical mitosis may be seen
- Koilocytic change is seen throughout tumor
  - Including deep infiltrative aggregates
- Tumor base is variable
  - Jagged and irregular (more frequent)
  - Bulbous and well defined (mimicking base of condylomas)
    - High-power view to highlight cytological features is important when patten of growth mimics condyloma
- p16 overexpression is common in warty carcinoma
  - Condylomas are negative with p16

Papillary Carcinoma, Not Otherwise Specified

- HPV unrelated in most cases
- No koilocytosis
- Complex papillae with branching fibrovascular cores
- Cytologic atypia ranges from mild to moderate
- Jagged and irregular tumor base

Papillomatosis of Glans Corona (Pearly Penile Papules)

- Very common
  - ~ 1/3 of normal males
- Uniform small lesions
- Usually arranged in 2-3 rows on dorsal aspect of glans corona
- Histologically correspond to small fibroepithelial papillomas
  - HPV unrelated
  - No koilocytosis

Bowenoid Papulosis

- Full-thickness atypia of squamous epithelium
- Identical to warty and basaloid penile intraepithelial neoplasia (PeIN)
- Condylomata after treatment with podophyllin may mimic bowenoid papulosis

Warty/Basaloid Penile Intraepithelial Neoplasia or Squamous Cell Carcinoma In Situ

- Full-thickness epithelial replacement by atypical cells with numerous mitoses
  - Basaloid cells predominate in basaloid PeIN
  - Atypical koilocytes are prominent in warty PeIN
  - Mixed lesions with basaloid and warty features are very common
- Condylomata after treatment with podophyllin may mimic warty/basaloid PeIN
  - Treated condylomas may show increased in mitotic figures
    - Atypical mitosis should not be seen in treated condylomata
    - History of treatment is important to make distinction

DIAGNOSTIC CHECKLIST

Pathologic Interpretation Pearls

- Condylomata treated with podophyllin may show degenerative changes including nuclear enlargement and metaphase arrest
  - May mimic squamous cell carcinoma In situ

SELECTED REFERENCES

1. Arroyo LS et al: Distribution of genital human papillomavirus genotypes in benign clinical manifestations among men from Northern Spain. BMC Public Health. 16(1):81, 2016
2. Shimizu A et al: Keratotic condyloma acuminatum. J Dermatol. ePub, 2016
3. Sturegård E et al: Human papillomavirus typing in reporting of condyloma. Sex Transm Dis. 40(2):123-9, 2013
4. Nordenvall C et al: Cancer risk among patients with condylomata acuminata. Int J Cancer. 119(4):888-93, 2006
5. Buechner SA: Common skin disorders of the penis. BJU Int. 90(5):498-506, 2002
6. Li J et al: "Seborrheic keratoses" that contain human papillomavirus are condylomata acuminata. Am J Dermatopathol. 16(4):398-405; discussion 406-8, 1994

Condyloma Acuminatum (Genital Wart)

Papillomatosis and Branching Fibrovascular Cores

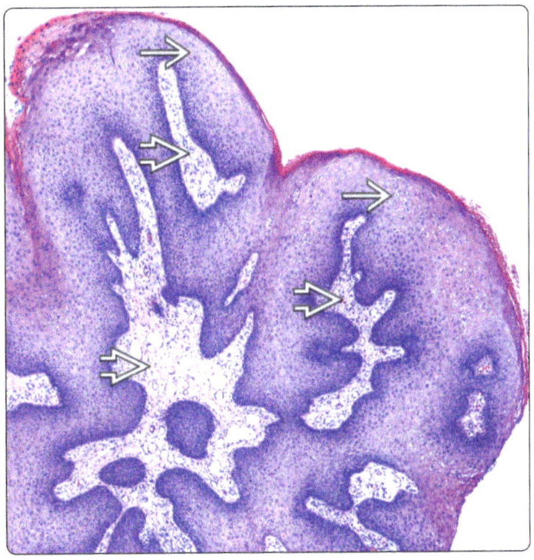

Koilocytic Change

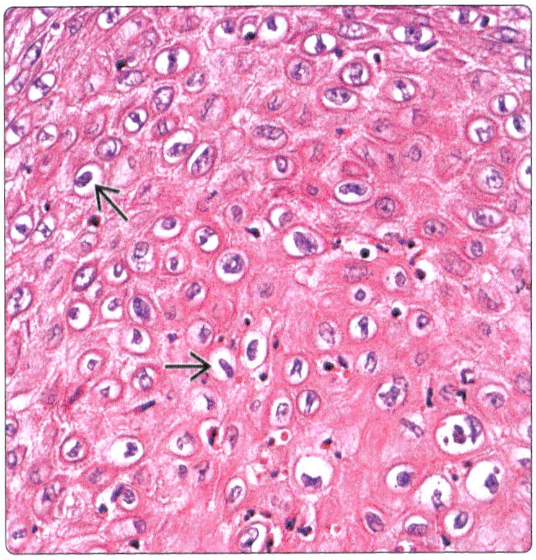

(Left) *Condyloma acuminatum is characterized by papillomatosis with acanthotic epithelium and prominent fibrovascular cores.* *Koilocytes are usually prominent in the upper portion of the epithelium.* **(Right)** *Koilocytes are characterized by clear perinuclear halos and wrinkled and hyperchromatic nuclei. Cytoplasm is eosinophilic, cellular borders are distinctive, and binucleation is common.*

Parakeratosis Overlying Koilocytes

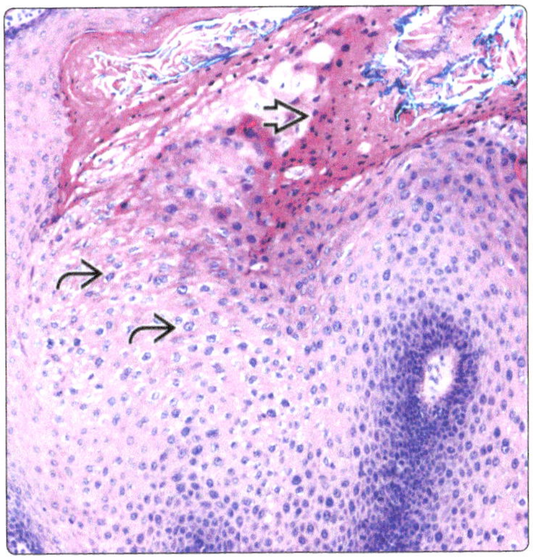

Seborrheic Keratosis-Like Condyloma

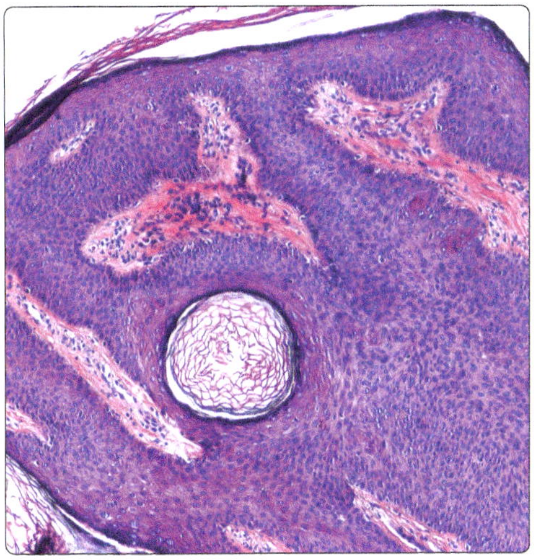

(Left) *High magnification shows koilocytes with perinuclear vacuolization and wrinkled nuclei seen in the upper portions of the acanthotic papilla. There is also parakeratosis with large nuclei.* **(Right)** *Koilocytosis may be less evident in older condylomata. Furthermore, such lesions may show horn pseudocysts, mimicking a seborrheic keratosis. However, most of these lesions are positive for HPV by in situ hybridization or immunohistochemistry.*

HPV In Situ Hybridization

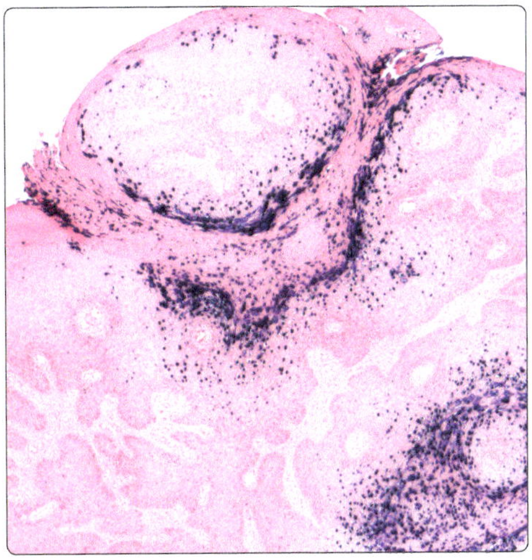

HPV In Situ Hybridization

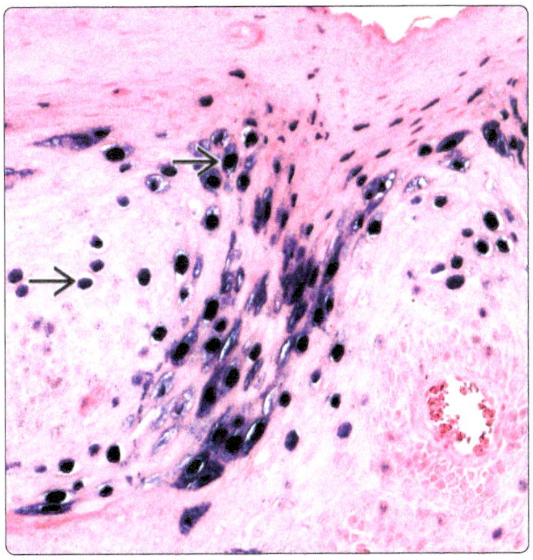

(Left) *In situ hybridization shows strongly positive nuclear staining for low-risk HPV-6.* **(Right)** *HPV-6 is the most frequent genotype associated with condyloma acuminatum as supported by in situ hybridization in this case. Dark blue nuclear staining indicates a positive result.*

KEY FACTS

ETIOLOGY/PATHOGENESIS

- Chronic rubbing/scratching induces discrete papules/nodules

CLINICAL ISSUES

- Generally on extremities but sometimes on trunk or posterior scalp

MICROSCOPIC

- Hyperkeratosis
- Focal parakeratosis
- Hypergranulosis
- Acanthosis and sometimes pseudoepitheliomatous hyperplasia
- Vertical streaking of collagen fibers in papillary dermis
- Minimal keratinocyte atypia

TOP DIFFERENTIAL DIAGNOSES

- Squamous cell carcinoma
  - Dermal infiltration
  - Greater cytologic atypia
  - Mitoses present
- Keratoacanthoma
  - Crateriform pattern
  - History of rapid growth
- Lichen simplex chronicus
  - On continuum with prurigo nodularis
  - Clinically presents as flat plaque rather than nodule
- Pseudoepitheliomatous hyperplasia
  - Secondary to infection
    - Deep fungal
    - Atypical mycobacterial
  - Associated with other tumors
    - Granular cell tumor
    - Lymphomas
  - Overlying a tattoo

Low-Power View of Prurigo Nodularis

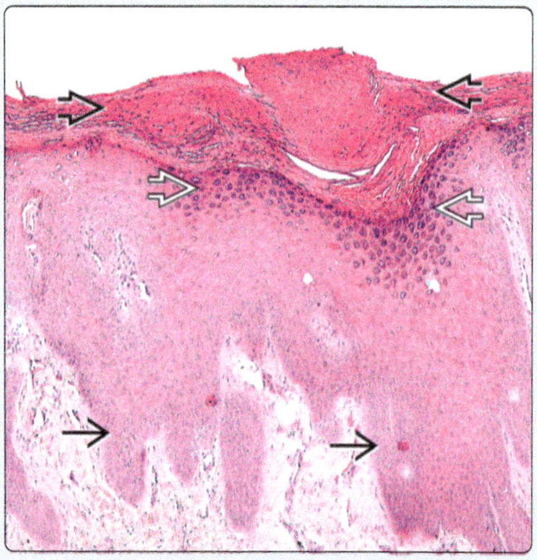

Higher Magnification of PN

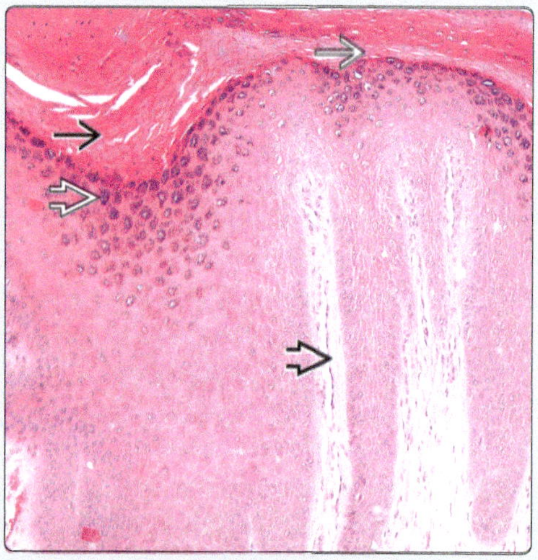

(Left) *Low-power view of PN shows prominent hyperkeratosis, parakeratosis, and hypergranulosis overlying irregular acanthosis with vertical streaking of collagen in the papillary dermis.* **(Right)** *Prurigo nodularis shows hyperkeratosis, a stratum lucidum, hypergranulosis, and vertical streaking of collagen bundles in the dermis.*

High Magnification of PR With Hypergranulosis

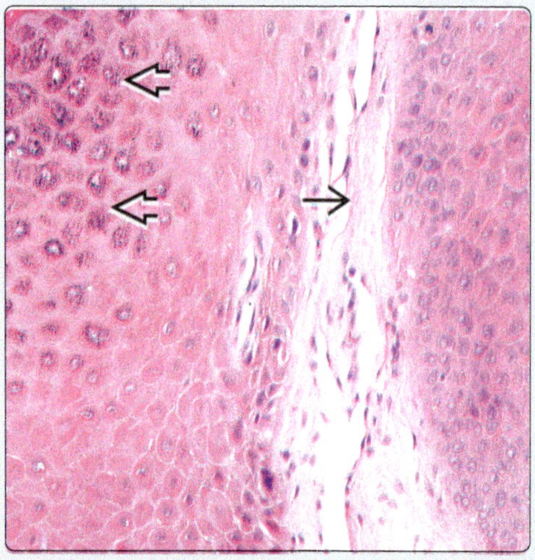

High Magnification of PN

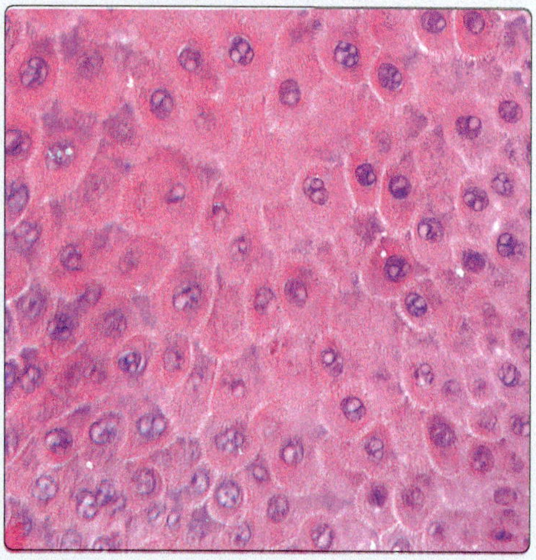

(Left) *High magnification of prurigo nodularis shows hypergranulosis. There is vertical streaking of collagen bundles present in the papillary dermis, a finding seen in both prurigo nodularis and lichen simplex chronicus.* **(Right)** *High magnification shows a lack of cytologic atypia in the keratinocytes.*

TERMINOLOGY

Abbreviations

- Prurigo nodularis (PN)

Definitions

- Pruritic nodules
- Generally on extensor surfaces of extremities
- Secondary to chronic rubbing/scratching

ETIOLOGY/PATHOGENESIS

Pathophysiology

- Chronic rubbing/scratching induces discrete papules/nodules
- True cause of pruritus leading to chronic rubbing/scratching often unknown
- Papillary dermal nerves increased in number compared to normal skin
- Conditions sometimes present that cause pruritus include
  - Atopic dermatitis
  - Diabetes mellitus
  - Renal failure
  - Liver failure
  - Psychiatric disorders
  - Internal malignancy
  - HIV infection

CLINICAL ISSUES

Presentation

- Most commonly seen in middle-aged to elderly individuals
- Generally on extremities but sometimes on trunk or posterior scalp
- Discrete papules or nodules
  - Often slightly scaly
  - Sometimes hyperpigmented
  - May be crusted or show other signs of trauma

Laboratory Tests

- Depending on history, consider ordering
  - CBC
  - Liver function tests
  - Renal function tests

Treatment

- Prevent rubbing/scratching
  - Occlusion may be key
- Topical therapies to reduce pruritus may be helpful
  - Corticosteroids, calcineurin inhibitors, capsaicin, menthol, pramoxine, other antipruritics
- Intralesional corticosteroids
- In some cases, UV light treatments or oral treatments (corticosteroids, antihistamines, anxiolytics, gabapentin, thalidomide) or IM methotrexate may be necessary

Prognosis

- Resolution with elimination of chronic rubbing/scratching

MICROSCOPIC

Histologic Features

- Hyperkeratosis with stratum lucidum, focal parakeratosis
- Acanthosis and sometimes pseudoepitheliomatous hyperplasia
- Cup-shaped, exo-/endophytic or more plaque-like with overlap with lichen simplex chronicus
- Vertical streaking of collagen fibers in papillary dermis
- Perivascular lymphocytes, histiocytes, and sometimes neutrophils &/or eosinophils
- Thickened dermal nerve fibers sometimes present

Cytologic Features

- Minimal keratinocyte atypia
- Cells are polygonal with central round nuclei, small nucleoli, and intercellular bridges
- Individually necrotic cells rare

DIFFERENTIAL DIAGNOSIS

Squamous Cell Carcinoma

- Infiltrative areas with cytologic atypia, atypical mitoses, squamous pearls
- May be difficult to exclude underlying squamous cell carcinoma with certainty in superficial shave biopsy specimens

Keratoacanthoma

- Crateriform architecture with central keratin
- Keratinocytes with abundant glassy pink cytoplasm
- Elastic fiber trapping, dermal fibrosis, and eosinophilic/neutrophilic abscesses may be present
- Clinically, keratoacanthoma typically has history of rapid growth and spontaneously resolves

Lichen Simplex Chronicus

- On histologic continuum with prurigo nodularis
- Clinically flat plaque rather than papule or nodule (clinical correlation necessary)

Deep Fungal Infection

- Histologic features of pseudoepitheliomatous hyperplasia
- Granulomatous inflammation and abscesses often present
- Special stains should highlight fungal organisms

Atypical Mycobacterial Infection

- Histologic features of pseudoepitheliomatous hyperplasia
- Special stains should highlight acid-fast bacteria
- Culture may be necessary

Pemphigoid Nodularis

- Clinically similar with pruritic papules and nodules
- Presence of bullous lesions a helpful clue
- Histologic findings similar to PN
- Direct immunofluorescence positive for linear IgG &/or C3 at dermoepidermal junction

SELECTED REFERENCES

1. Spring P et al: Prurigo nodularis: retrospective study of 13 cases managed with methotrexate. Clin Exp Dermatol. 39(4):468-73, 2014
2. Haas S et al: Low density of sympathetic nerve fibers relative to substance P-positive nerve fibers in lesional skin of chronic pruritus and prurigo nodularis. J Dermatol Sci. 58(3):193-7, 2010
3. Weigelt N et al: Prurigo nodularis: systematic analysis of 58 histological criteria in 136 patients. J Cutan Pathol. 37(5):578-86, 2010
4. Powell AM et al: Pemphigoid nodularis (non-bullous): a clinicopathological study of five cases. Br J Dermatol. 147(2):343-9, 2002

KEY FACTS

TERMINOLOGY

- Proliferation of enlarged and mildly atypical keratinocytes in sun-damaged skin without diagnostic features of actinic keratosis
- Variously considered to be related to solar lentigo, seborrheic keratosis, or actinic keratosis

ETIOLOGY/PATHOGENESIS

- Most cases associated with UV radiation
- HPV types have been detected in some studies

CLINICAL ISSUES

- Typically occur in older adults (mean: 75 yr)
- Usually present in head and neck region or extremities
- Excellent prognosis, very low malignant potential

MICROSCOPIC

- Epidermal acanthosis with proliferation of enlarged keratinocytes with proportionately enlarged nuclei
- Overlying hypergranulosis and hyperkeratosis usually present
- Mitotic figures rare
- May show background of solar lentigo changes (basilar pigmentation and elongated rete ridges) in some cases

TOP DIFFERENTIAL DIAGNOSES

- Actinic keratosis
  - Proliferation of atypical keratinocytes typically confined to basilar 1/3 of epidermis
  - Overlying parakeratosis and basilar budding usually seen
- Solar lentigo (lentigo senilis)
  - Elongated, hyperpigmented rete ridges
  - Lacks keratinocyte atypia/pleomorphism
- Seborrheic keratosis
  - More prominent epidermal acanthosis with pseudohorn cysts

Large Cell Acanthoma

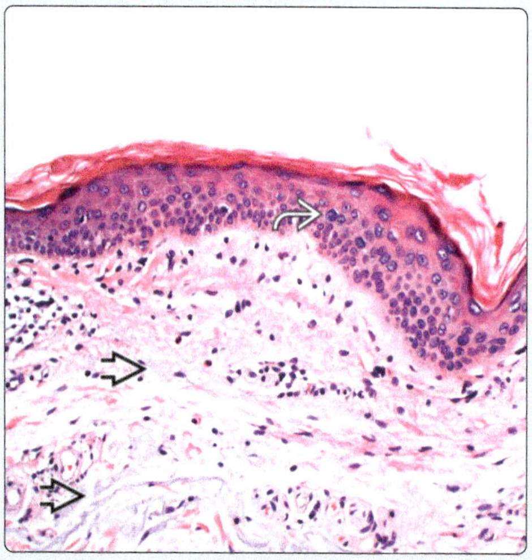

Large Cell Acanthoma at High Magnification

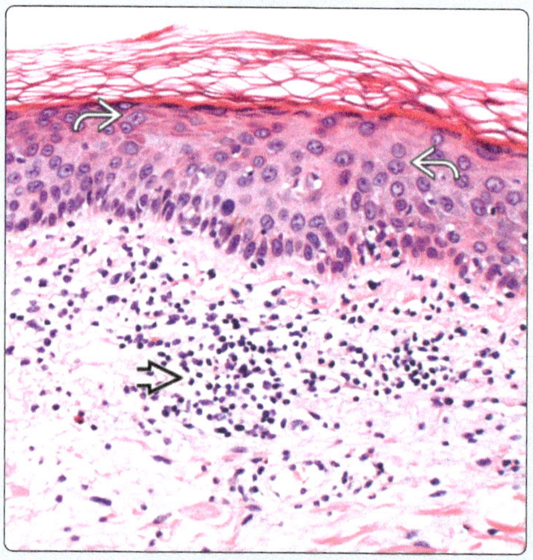

(Left) *LCA shows an intraepidermal proliferation of enlarged keratinocytes ➡ in a disorganized pattern. There is no basilar budding or overlying parakeratosis typical of an actinic keratosis. Note the prominent solar elastosis ⇨ in dermis.* **(Right)** *Higher power of LCA shows enlarged keratinocytes ➡ involving the mid to upper layers of epidermis with overlying basket-weave orthokeratosis. The dermis shows solar elastosis and mild chronic inflammatory infiltrate ⇨.*

Large Cell Acanthoma at Low Magnification

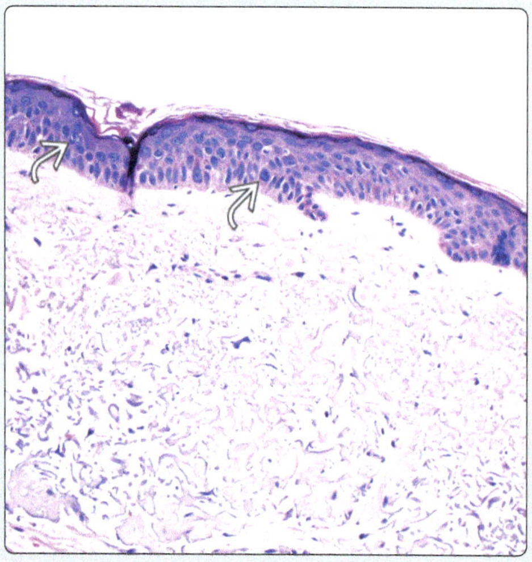

Large Cell Acanthoma at High Magnification

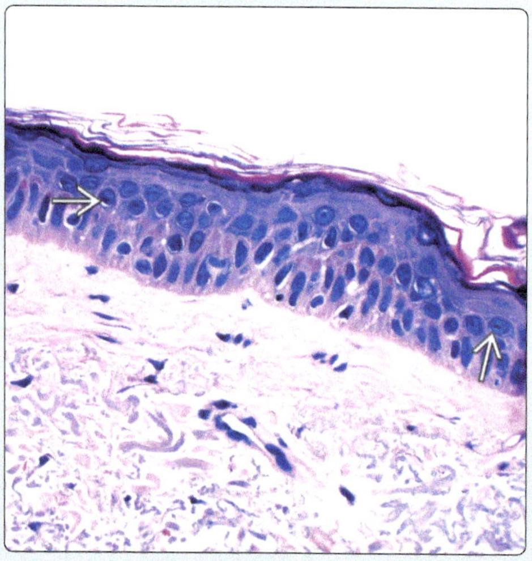

(Left) *Another example of LCA shows an intraepidermal proliferation of enlarged squamous cells ➡. There is a lack of basilar budding or overlying parakeratosis typical of actinic keratosis.* **(Right)** *The cells show nuclear enlargement, hyperchromasia, and focally prominent nucleoli ➡, but no mitotic figures are identified.*

TERMINOLOGY

Abbreviations

- Large cell acanthoma (LCA)

Definitions

- Proliferation of enlarged and mildly atypical keratinocytes in sun-damaged skin without diagnostic features of actinic keratosis (AK)
  - Has been variously considered to be related to or variant of solar lentigo, seborrheic keratosis (stucco keratosis) (SK), or AK

ETIOLOGY/PATHOGENESIS

Environmental Exposure

- Most cases associated with UV radiation (chronic solar damage)

Infectious Agents

- HPV types have been detected in some studies

CLINICAL ISSUES

Epidemiology

- Incidence
  - Uncommon lesions but may be underreported
- Age
  - Typically occur in older adults (mean: 75 yr)
- Sex
  - ~ equal distribution or slight female predominance

Site

- Usually head and neck region or extremities

Presentation

- Hyperkeratotic patch, usually well-demarcated lesion

Natural History

- Most cases do not regress, but only rare cases are associated with squamous cell carcinoma in situ (Bowen disease)

Treatment

- Surgical approaches
  - Not necessary in most cases, given benign behavior of majority of these lesions

Prognosis

- Excellent, very low malignant potential

MACROSCOPIC

Size

- Small lesions, usually < 1 cm in greatest dimension

MICROSCOPIC

Histologic Features

- Epidermal acanthosis and intraepidermal proliferation of enlarged keratinocytes with proportionately enlarged nuclei
  - Cells show abundant eosinophilic cytoplasm and hyperchromatic-staining nuclei
- Overlying hypergranulosis and hyperkeratosis usually present
- Lesion is typically sharply demarcated from adjacent normal epidermis
- May show mild basilar pigmentation and elongated rete ridges in some cases, suggesting derivation from, or association with, solar lentigo
- Mitotic figures rare

Cytologic Features

- Enlarged, mildly atypical squamous keratinocytes with large nuclei and small to focally prominent nucleoli

ANCILLARY TESTS

Immunohistochemistry

- Increased expression of nuclear proliferative markers including Ki-67 and PCNA

Genetic Testing

- Cells are mostly aneuploid

DIFFERENTIAL DIAGNOSIS

Actinic Keratosis

- Proliferation of atypical keratinocytes typically confined to basilar 1/3 of epidermis
- Overlying parakeratosis very common
- Basilar budding of atypical cells usually present
- Mitotic figures often easily identified (as opposed to rare in LCA)

Solar Lentigo (Lentigo Senilis)

- Elongated, hyperpigmented rete ridges
  - May also be seen in some case of LCA, suggesting association with, or derivation from, solar lentigo
- Background of severe solar elastosis
- Lacks degree of cellular and nuclear enlargement of LCA

Seborrheic Keratosis

- Classically shows prominent epidermal acanthosis with pseudohorn cysts
  - Degree of acanthosis is greater than that in LCA in most cases
  - Pseudohorn cysts lacking in LCA
- Stucco keratosis variant of seborrheic keratosis shows milder acanthosis with papillomatosis and lacks pseudohorn cysts
- Lacks degree of enlargement of lesional cells seen in LCA

SELECTED REFERENCES

1. Fraga GR et al: Large cell acanthoma: a variant of solar lentigo with cellular hypertrophy. J Cutan Pathol. 41(9):733-9, 2014
2. Patsatsi A et al: Large cell acanthoma: a debate throughout the decades. Dermatol Pract Concept. 4(1):43-5, 2014
3. Garrido-Ríos AA et al: Human papillomavirus detection in multiple large-cell acanthomas. J Eur Acad Dermatol Venereol. 23(4):454-5, 2009
4. Mehregan DR et al: Large cell acanthoma. Int J Dermatol. 42(1):36-9, 2003
5. Argenyi ZB et al: Large-cell acanthoma of the skin. A study by image analysis cytometry and immunohistochemistry. Am J Dermatopathol. 16(2):140-4, 1994
6. Sánchez Yus E et al: Large-cell acanthoma is a distinctive condition. Am J Dermatopathol. 14(2):140-7; discussion 148, 1992
7. Rahbari H et al: Large cell acanthoma. One of the actinic keratoses. Arch Dermatol. 114(1):49-52, 1978

Clear Cell Acanthoma

KEY FACTS

CLINICAL ISSUES

- Epidemiology
  - Common in middle-aged women
- Site
  - Generally on lower legs
- Morphology
  - Solitary lesion, rarely multiple
  - Pink-red, shiny papule or plaque

MICROSCOPIC

- Acanthosis of pale or clear cells
  - Sharply demarcated from adjacent, normal epidermis
- Often overlying parakeratosis, sometimes with neutrophils
- Pale or clear cells
  - Glycogen filled, PAS(+)
- Minimal to no cytologic atypia

TOP DIFFERENTIAL DIAGNOSES

- Psoriasis
  - Similar parakeratosis but often with neutrophils
  - Acanthosis with hypogranulosis
  - Prominent vessels in papillary dermis
  - Increased suprabasilar mitoses
- Psoriasiform keratosis
  - Similar findings to psoriasis
  - Solitary lesion
- Tricholemmoma
  - Pale or clear cells in lobular configuration
  - Peripheral palisading and thickened basement membrane
- Clear cell Bowen disease
  - Cytologic atypia, mitoses, &/or full-thickness disorder
- Dermatophyte infection
  - Keratinocytes generally not pale or clear
  - Hyphae in stratum corneum
- Verruciform xanthoma

Clear Cell Acanthoma at Low Magnification

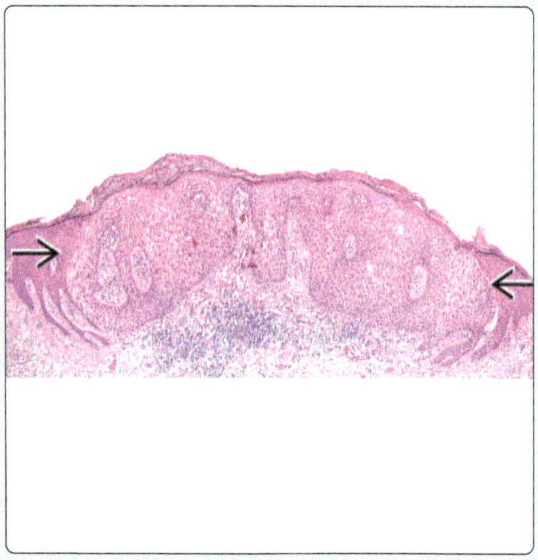

Clear Cell Acanthoma at Higher Magnification

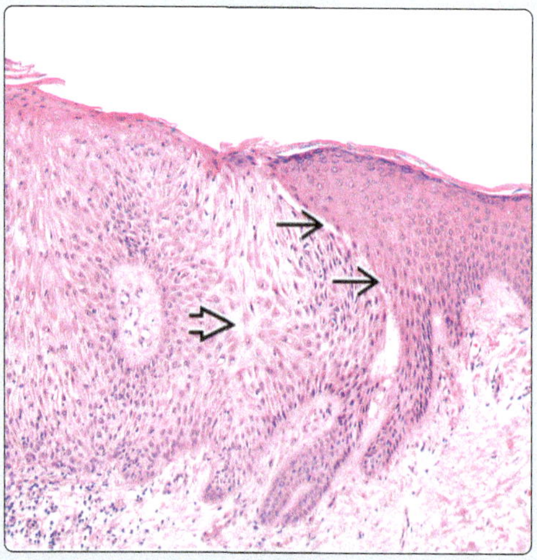

(Left) *Clear cell acanthoma at low-power magnification shows clear/pale cells in an acanthotic epidermis. The lesion is sharply demarcated from the surrounding epidermis →.* **(Right)** *In this intermediate-power magnification of clear cell acanthoma, there are clear/pale cells ⇨ with overlying parakeratosis. The lesion is sharply demarcated from the adjacent normal epidermis →.*

Border of Clear Cell Acanthoma

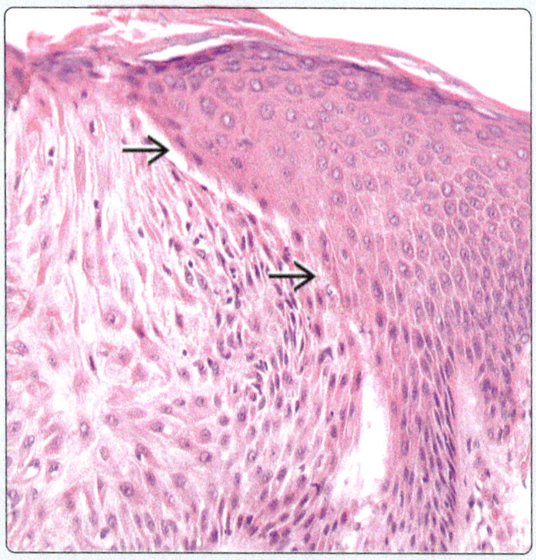

PAS Stain in Clear Cell Acanthoma

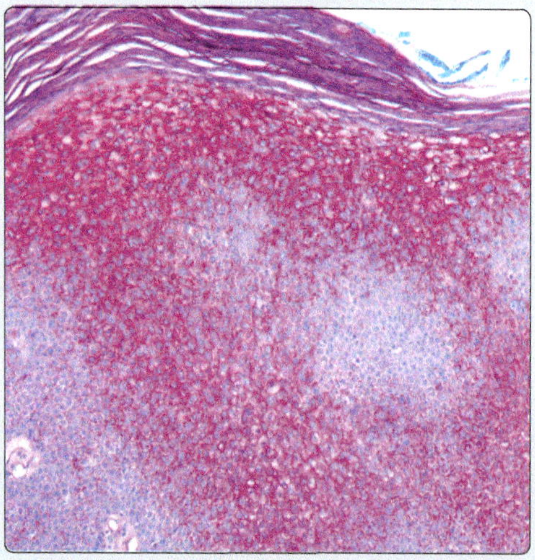

(Left) *Pale/clear cells are sharply demarcated from the normal, surrounding epidermis →. There is a lack of cytologic atypia. Mitoses are not increased.* **(Right)** *The lesional cells of CCA contain glycogen and are bright pink/purple with the periodic acid-Schiff (PAS) stain.*

TERMINOLOGY

Abbreviations

- Clear cell acanthoma (CCA)

Synonyms

- Degos acanthoma, pale cell acanthoma

Definitions

- Benign epidermal tumor, generally on lower legs of women
- Epidermal acanthosis with pale or clear cells, often with overlying parakeratosis
- Pale or clear cells sharply demarcated from adjacent, normal epidermis

ETIOLOGY/PATHOGENESIS

Pathogenesis

- Some consider this reactive proliferation of epidermis rather than true neoplasm

CLINICAL ISSUES

Epidemiology

- Sex
  - More common in middle-aged women

Site

- Generally on lower legs

Presentation

- Solitary, pink-red, shiny papule or plaque
- White scale may be seen at periphery

Treatment

- Biopsy is generally curative

Prognosis

- Benign, no malignant potential

MACROSCOPIC

Dermatoscopy

- Characteristic dot-like vessels in linear arrangements

MICROSCOPIC

Histologic Features

- Epidermal acanthosis with proliferation of pale or clear cells
- Often overlying parakeratosis, sometimes with neutrophils
- Pale or clear cells sharply demarcated from adjacent, normal epidermis
- Pale or clear cells stain bright pink/purple with periodic-acid Schiff (PAS), with diastase sensitivity

DIFFERENTIAL DIAGNOSIS

Psoriasis

- Varying clinical presentations
  - Commonly multiple plaques with silvery scale favoring elbows/knees/scalp/lower back
- Regular acanthosis with hypogranulosis
- Confluent parakeratosis with collections of neutrophils
- Unlike CCA
  - Not composed of pale or clear cells that are sharply demarcated from adjacent epidermis
  - Increased basilar and suprabasilar mitoses
  - Thinning of suprapapillary plates
  - Dilated vessels in papillary dermis

Psoriasiform Keratosis

- Solitary papule
- Patients without history of psoriasis
- Hyperkeratosis and parakeratosis with neutrophils overlying acanthosis

Tricholemmoma

- 2 main clinical presentations
  - Solitary papule on sun-damaged skin
  - Multiple, slightly verrucous papules on central face associated with Cowden syndrome
- Hyperkeratosis and parakeratosis
- Sometimes papillomatous
- Hyperplastic epidermis composed of clear or pale cells with
  - Peripheral palisaded basal layer
  - Thickened basement membrane

Clear Cell Bowen Disease

- Confluent parakeratosis
- Regular or irregular acanthosis
- Atypical keratinocytes and atypical mitoses in full thickness of epidermis
- Keratinocytes are clear or pale

Dermatophyte Infection

- Like CCA, may have confluent parakeratosis with neutrophils
- Unlike CCA, dermatophyte infection is characterized by
  - Epidermis not composed of pale/clear cells that are sharply demarcated from adjacent epidermis
  - Special stains (e.g., PAS) that highlight fungal hyphae in stratum corneum

Verruciform Xanthoma

- Like CCA, may have confluent parakeratosis with neutrophils
- Unlike CCA, verruciform xanthoma shows
  - Often polypoid architecture
  - Papillary dermis containing foamy cells

DIAGNOSTIC CHECKLIST

Pathologic Interpretation Pearls

- Acanthosis of pale or clear cells with overlying parakeratosis, sharply demarcated from adjacent, normal epidermis

SELECTED REFERENCES

1. Tiodorovic-Zivkovic D et al: Dermoscopy of clear cell acanthoma. J Am Acad Dermatol. 72(1 Suppl):S47-9, 2015
2. Miyake T et al: Histopathological correlation to the dermoscopic feature of "string of pearls" in clear cell acanthoma. Eur J Dermatol. 24(4):498-9, 2014
3. Saeki H et al: Pigmented clear cell acanthoma of the finger simulating pigmented nevus. Int J Dermatol. 53(12):e579-81, 2014
4. Zedek DC et al: Clear-cell acanthoma versus acanthosis: a psoriasiform reaction pattern lacking tricholemmal differentiation. Am J Dermatopathol. 29(4):378-84, 2007

Clear Cell Papulosis

KEY FACTS

TERMINOLOGY

- Multiple, hypopigmented to white, flat-topped papules and macules
- Generally on lower trunk/suprapubic area
- Almost always in young children, especially Asian

MICROSCOPIC

- Clear to pale cells with abundant cytoplasm
- Cells concentrated in basal layers of epidermis
- Cells single or in clusters, positive for CK7
- Nuclear atypia and pleomorphism absent

TOP DIFFERENTIAL DIAGNOSES

- Clear cells of Toker
  - Clinical history differs; incidental finding in nipple/areola, breast, and vulva
  - Histologic findings similar to clear cell papulosis
    - Clear to pale cells with abundant cytoplasm in epidermis
  - Unlike clear cell papulosis, clear/pale cells often scattered into upper portions of epidermis
- Pagetoid dyskeratosis
  - Clinical history differs; incidental finding
  - Clusters of pale cells in spinous layer
- Paget disease
  - Clinical history: Generally affects unilateral nipple/areola in older adults
  - Clear to pale cells with abundant cytoplasm scattered at all levels in epidermis
  - Nuclear atypia present
- Extramammary Paget disease
  - Clinical history: Presents as erythematous patch or plaque, usually in groin/perineal area
  - Clear to pale cells with abundant cytoplasm scattered at all levels in epidermis
  - Nuclear atypia present

Clinical Photograph of Clear Cell Papulosis

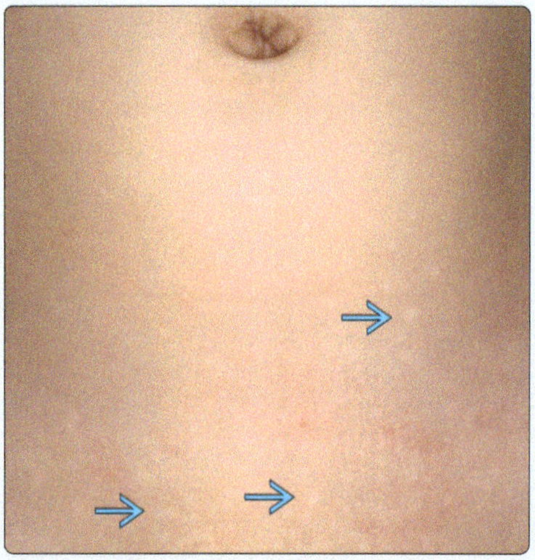

Clinical Photograph of Clear Cell Papulosis

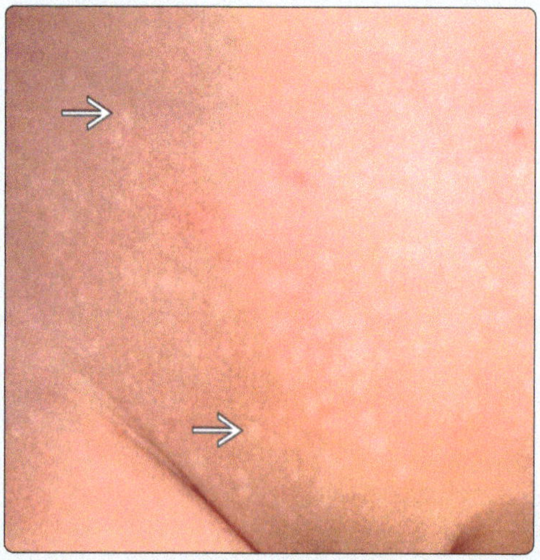

(Left) *There are hypopigmented macules → on the lower abdomen of this child.* **(Right)** *Hypopigmented macules and flat-topped papules → are visible on the lower abdomen/suprapubic area. (Courtesy R. Hui, MD.)*

Clear Cell Papulosis

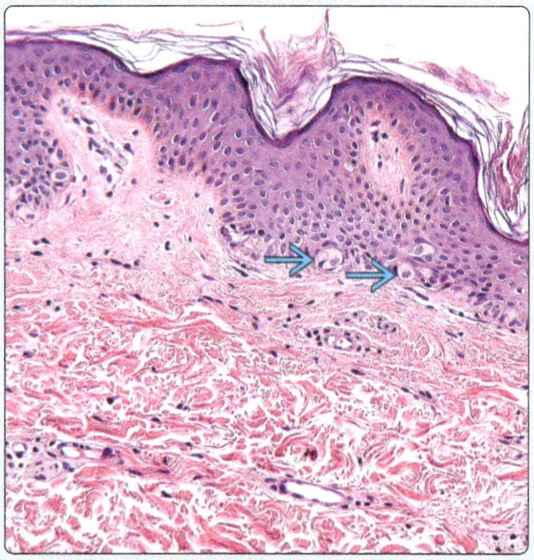

Clear Cell Papulosis

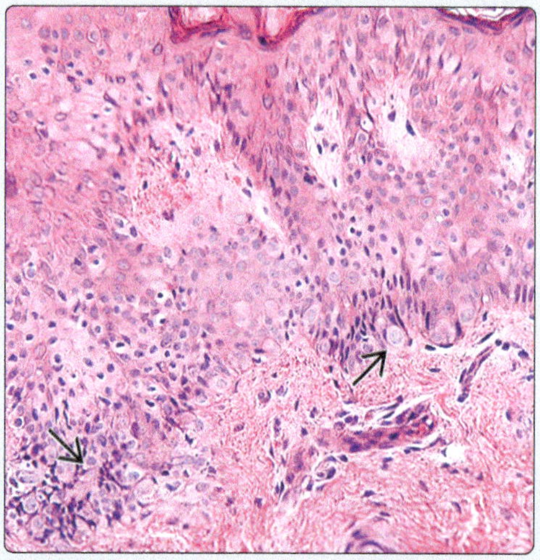

(Left) *There are clear cells →, without significant atypia, in the basal layer of the epidermis.* **(Right)** *Clear/pale cells → are seen with abundant cytoplasm in the basal and suprabasal layers of a hyperkeratotic and acanthotic epidermis. (Courtesy R. Hui, MD.)*

TERMINOLOGY

Definitions

- Rare disorder of multiple, hypopigmented to white, flat-topped papules and macules
- Generally on lower trunk
- Almost always in young children, often of Asian descent
- Histopathology characteristic, with clear/pale cells in basal layer of acanthotic epidermis

ETIOLOGY/PATHOGENESIS

Pathogenesis

- Clear cells may be normal component of epidermis along "milk lines," type of glandular epithelial cell
- Others postulate that clear cells are derived from eccrine secretory gland
  - Based on staining of clear cells with IKH-4, carcinoembryonic antigen, and CAM5.2
- Genetic component is postulated, as siblings may be affected

CLINICAL ISSUES

Epidemiology

- Age
  - Young children: Mean = 1.7 yr
  - Exceptionally reported in adults
- Sex
  - Slight female predominance
- Ethnicity
  - Often in patients of Asian descent

Site

- Generally on lower trunk/suprapubic area
- Also reported on chest, axillae, inguinal area, lower back/buttocks, and extremities
- Sometimes described as affecting trunk along "milk lines," which run from anterior axillae to upper medial thighs

Presentation

- Multiple, often symmetric, hypopigmented to white, flat-topped papules and macules; asymptomatic
- 1-10 mm in diameter
- Number of skin lesions ranges from 2 to > 100; average of 10-20

Natural History

- Lesions increase in number, become stable, and then regress with age

Treatment

- Treatment is not necessary, as many patients develop spontaneous regression

Prognosis

- Benign condition without malignant potential

MICROSCOPIC

Histologic Features

- Clear to pale cells, singly or in clusters, with abundant cytoplasm concentrated in basal layers of epidermis
- Cells occasionally in suprabasal layers
- Epidermis acanthotic and hyperkeratotic
- Decreased basal layer melanin pigmentation
- Clear to pale cells stain with
  - PAS
  - Mucin stains (variable)
  - Cytokeratin stains (including CK7)
  - CEA
  - EMA
  - GCDFP-15
- Clear to pale cells reportedly negative with HER2

Cytologic Features

- Clear to pale cells with abundant cytoplasm
- Nuclei are round to oval and sometimes slightly indented, inconspicuous nucleoli

DIFFERENTIAL DIAGNOSIS

Clear Cells of Toker

- Clinical history differs: Incidental finding in nipple/areola, breast, and vulva
- Histologic findings similar to clear cell papulosis
  - Clear to pale cells with abundant cytoplasm in epidermis
- Unlike clear cell papulosis, clear/pale cells often scattered into upper portions of epidermis

Pagetoid Dyskeratosis

- No clinical history; incidental finding
- Clusters of pale cells in spinous layer

Paget Disease

- Clinical history is distinctive: Generally affects unilateral nipple/areola in older adults
- Clear to pale cells with abundant cytoplasm scattered at all levels in epidermis
- Nuclear atypia present

Extramammary Paget Disease

- Clinical history differs, with extramammary Paget disease presenting as erythematous patch or plaque, usually in groin/perineal area
- Clear to pale cells with abundant cytoplasm scattered at all levels in epidermis
- Nuclear atypia present

DIAGNOSTIC CHECKLIST

Pathologic Interpretation Pearls

- Clear to pale cells with abundant cytoplasm concentrated in basal layer of epidermis
- Clear cells single or in groups
- No nuclear atypia

SELECTED REFERENCES

1. Hashemi P et al: Multicentric primary extramammary Paget disease: a Toker cell disorder? Cutis. 94(1):35-8, 2014
2. Wysong A et al: Clear-cell papulosis: a rare entity that may be misconstrued pathologically as normal skin. Pediatr Dermatol. 29(2):195-8, 2012
3. Tseng FW et al: Long-term follow-up study of clear cell papulosis. J Am Acad Dermatol. 63(2):266-73, 2010
4. Yu Y et al: Clear cell papulosis: a connection of clear cells to toker cells or paget disease. Arch Dermatol. 145(9):1066-8, 2009
5. Farley-Loftus R et al: Clear cell papulosis. Dermatol Online J. 14(10):19, 2008
6. Kim YC et al: Clear cell papulosis: an immunohistochemical study to determine histogenesis. J Cutan Pathol. 29(1):11-4, 2002

Toker Cell Hyperplasia

KEY FACTS

TERMINOLOGY

- Increase in number of Toker cells in epidermis
- Absence of underlying ductal carcinoma
- Mimics Paget disease of nipple

CLINICAL ISSUES

- Very rare, incidental finding; nipple normal clinically/grossly

MICROSCOPIC

- Round to slightly oval nuclei
- Abundant cytoplasm that is slightly pale to clear
- No pleomorphism
- CK7 positive; negative with CD138 and p53

TOP DIFFERENTIAL DIAGNOSES

- Paget disease of nipple
  - Clinical history differs
    - Generally affects unilateral nipple/areola in older adults
  - Clear to pale cells with abundant cytoplasm scattered at all levels in epidermis
  - Nuclear atypia present
    - Hyperchromatic nuclei
    - Prominent eosinophilic cytoplasm
  - Variable mitotic activity
- Pagetoid dyskeratosis
  - Clusters of somewhat pale or clear keratinocytes
    - Slightly shrunken nuclei
    - Perinuclear halo
  - Possibly related to trauma
  - Cells do not mark with CK7
- Clear cell papulosis
  - Clinical presentation differs
    - Child with multiple hypopigmented, white to flesh-colored papules on lower abdomen/groin area
  - Scattered, benign-appearing cells in basal layer of acanthotic epidermis
  - Cells stain with CK7

Toker Cell Hyperplasia

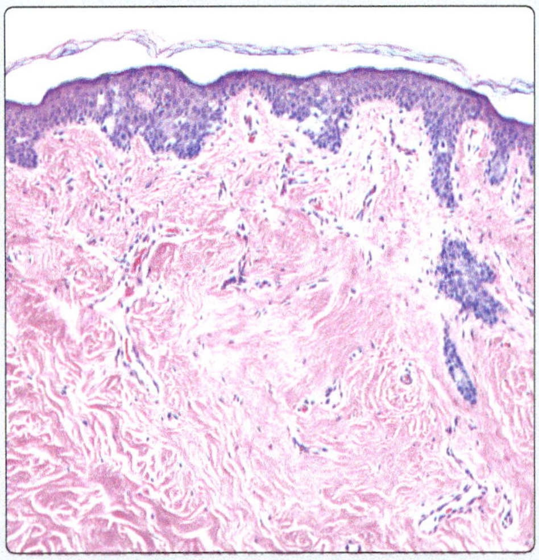

Toker Cell Hyperplasia at Higher Magnification

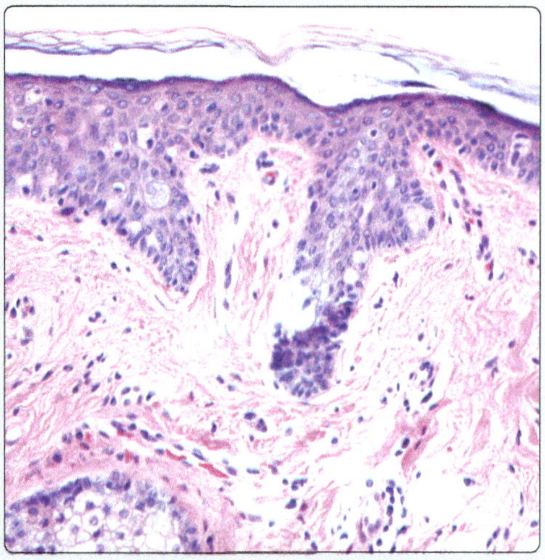

(Left) *Toker cell hyperplasia is a rare histopathologic finding. Toker cells, a normal component of the nipple epithelium, are increased in number and may mimic Paget disease of the nipple.* **(Right)** *At this magnification, the scattered, hyperplastic Toker cells in the epidermis mimic Paget disease of the nipple.*

Toker Cell Hyperplasia at High Magnification

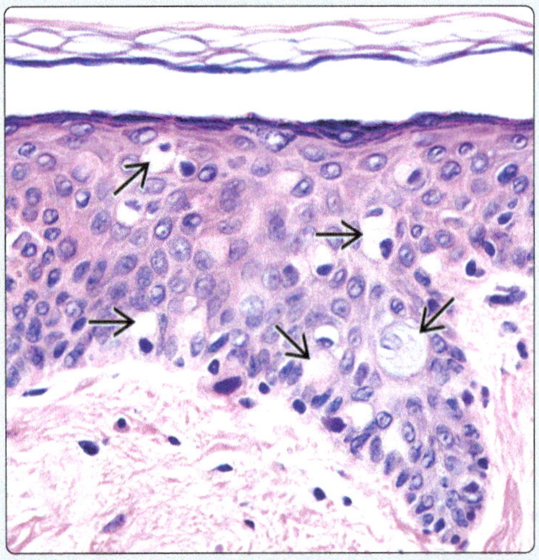

Toker Cell Hyperplasia: CK7 Immunohistochemistry

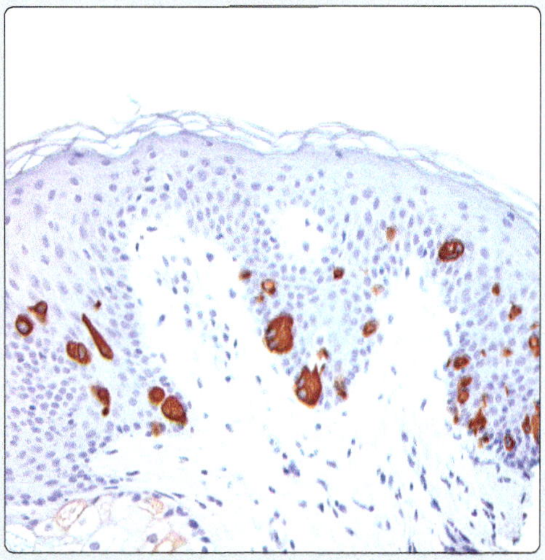

(Left) *This is a high-magnification view of Toker cell hyperplasia. Toker cells ➡ have bland nuclei with expanded, pale to clear-staining cytoplasm. They are in the basal and suprabasal layers of the epidermis.* **(Right)** *In Toker cell hyperplasia, Toker cells are evident by light microscopy, and they are also highlighted by CK7 staining. The bland cells are scattered in the basal and suprabasal layers.*

TERMINOLOGY

Definitions

- Increase in number of Toker cells in epidermis
- Absence of underlying ductal carcinoma
- Mimics Paget disease of nipple
- Awareness important to avoid overdiagnosis of Paget disease

CLINICAL ISSUES

Epidemiology

- Incidence
  - Toker cells present by light microscopy in ~ 10% of normal nipples
  - Toker cells also described in
    - Vulva
    - Accessory nipples
    - Along milk line of epidermis
    - Overlying nipple duct adenoma/florid papillomatosis of nipple
  - Toker cell hyperplasia
    - Rare
    - Described in 2 cases out of 340 in Toker's original series
    - Increase in number of Toker cells, mimicking Paget disease of nipple
    - Absence of underlying ductal carcinoma
    - Clinically normal nipple

Presentation

- Incidental finding, normal nipple grossly/clinically

Treatment

- Excision with clear margins has been recommended

Prognosis

- Hyperplasia that mimics Paget disease is rare; in reported cases, excision with negative margins seems to portend excellent prognosis

MICROSCOPIC

Histologic Features

- Slightly enlarged cells in epidermis
- Cells lack atypia and pleomorphism
- Cells concentrated in basal and suprabasal layers
- Often arranged in single units, but occasionally clustered
- Mitoses should not be present
- Inflammation absent
- Immunohistochemical findings
  - Positive with CK7, EMA, CAM5.2
  - Negative with CK20, GCDFP-15, 34bE12, S100, HER2, CD138, and p53

Cytologic Features

- Round to slightly oval nuclei
- Cytoplasm abundant and slightly pale to clear
- No pleomorphism

DIFFERENTIAL DIAGNOSIS

Paget Disease of the Nipple

- Clinical history differs
  - Generally affects unilateral nipple/areola in older adults
- Clear to pale cells with abundant cytoplasm scattered at all levels in epidermis
- Nuclear atypia present, variable mitotic activity

Extramammary Paget Disease

- Clinical history differs
  - Erythematous patch or plaque, usually in groin/perineal area
- Clear to pale cells with abundant cytoplasm scattered at all levels in epidermis
- Nuclear atypia present
- Variable mitotic activity

Pagetoid Dyskeratosis

- Clusters of somewhat pale or clear keratinocytes
  - Slightly shrunken nuclei
  - Perinuclear halo
- Possibly related to trauma
- Cells do not mark with CK7

Clear Cell Papulosis

- Clinical presentation differs
  - Child with multiple hypopigmented, white to flesh-colored papules on lower abdomen/groin area
- Scattered, benign-appearing cells in basal layer of acanthotic epidermis
- Cells stain with CK7

DIAGNOSTIC CHECKLIST

Pathologic Interpretation Pearls

- Slightly enlarged cells in basal and suprabasal epidermis
  - Lack atypia and pleomorphism
  - Predominately single units
  - Occasionally clustered
  - CK7 positive, EMA positive
  - Negative with CD138, p53
- Degree of hyperplasia mimics Paget disease, but cells are not atypical and mitoses are absent

SELECTED REFERENCES

1. Val-Bernal JF et al: The nipple-areola complex epidermis: a prospective systematic study in adult autopsies. Am J Dermatopathol. 32(8):787-93, 2010
2. Di Tommaso L et al: Toker cells of the breast. Morphological and immunohistochemical characterization of 40 cases. Hum Pathol. 39(9):1295-300, 2008
3. Garijo MF et al: Pagetoid dyskeratosis of the nipple epidermis: an incidental finding mimicking Paget's disease of the nipple. APMIS. 116(2):139-46, 2008
4. Willman JH et al: Vulvar clear cells of Toker: precursors of extramammary Paget's disease. Am J Dermatopathol. 27(3):185-8, 2005
5. Willman JH et al: Clear cells of Toker in accessory nipples. J Cutan Pathol. 30(4):256-60, 2003
6. Lundquist K et al: Intraepidermal cytokeratin 7 expression is not restricted to Paget cells but is also seen in Toker cells and Merkel cells. Am J Surg Pathol. 23(2):212-9, 1999
7. Decaussin M et al: Paget's disease versus Toker cell hyperplasia in a supernumerary nipple. Virchows Arch. 432(3):289-91, 1998
8. Toker C: Clear cells of the nipple epidermis. Cancer. 25(3):601-10, 1970

Actinic Keratosis

KEY FACTS

TERMINOLOGY

- Actinic keratosis (AK)
- Solar keratosis
- Atypical intraepidermal proliferation of keratinocytes typically confined to basilar portion of epidermis

ETIOLOGY/PATHOGENESIS

- Ultraviolet light (primarily UVB) induces mutations in DNA (p53 most common)

CLINICAL ISSUES

- Very common lesions, estimated to affect up to 10-40% of adult Caucasians; higher incidence in areas with heavy sun exposure (i.e., Australia)
- Mostly occurs in Caucasians, much less common in other races
- Excellent in vast majority of cases, as only ~ 2-3% progress to invasive SCC

MICROSCOPIC

- Basilar budding of atypical cells
- Cells show nuclear enlargement, hyperchromasia, and prominent nucleoli
- Overlying parakeratosis present
- Lesional cells usually do not involve follicles (as opposed to Bowen disease)
- Histologic subtypes include hypertrophic, atrophic, pigmented, lichenoid, and bowenoid AK

TOP DIFFERENTIAL DIAGNOSES

- Squamous cell carcinoma (SCC)
- Bowen disease (SCC in situ)
- Basal cell carcinoma (BCC), superficial-multicentric and basosquamous types
- Melanoma in situ (lentigo maligna type)
- Discoid lupus erythematosus
- Lichen planus (LP) and LP-like keratosis [benign lichenoid keratosis (BLK)]

Clinical Photograph of Actinic Keratosis

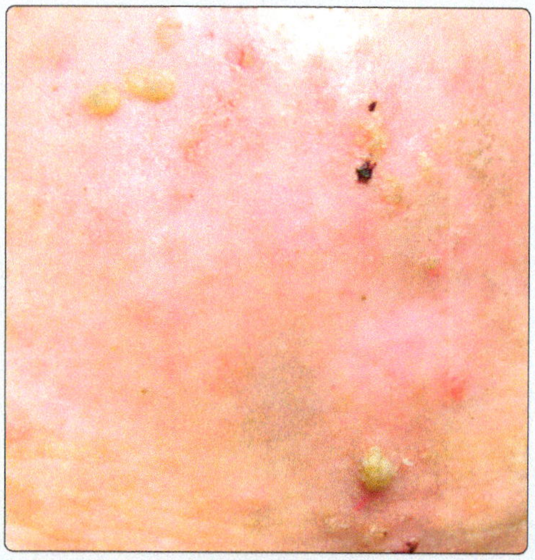

Bowenoid Actinic Keratosis

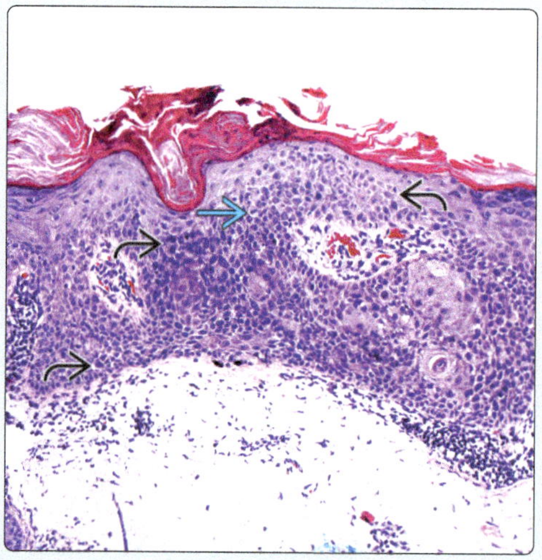

(Left) *Clinical photograph of the scalp of an elderly patient shows multiple actinic keratoses (AKs) with prominent crusting. (Courtesy J. Wu, MD.)* **(Right)** *Bowenoid AK shows basilar to midepidermal involvement by atypical cells, with a mitotic figure. Overlying hyperkeratosis and parakeratosis are also present.*

Classic Actinic Keratosis With Overlying Parakeratosis

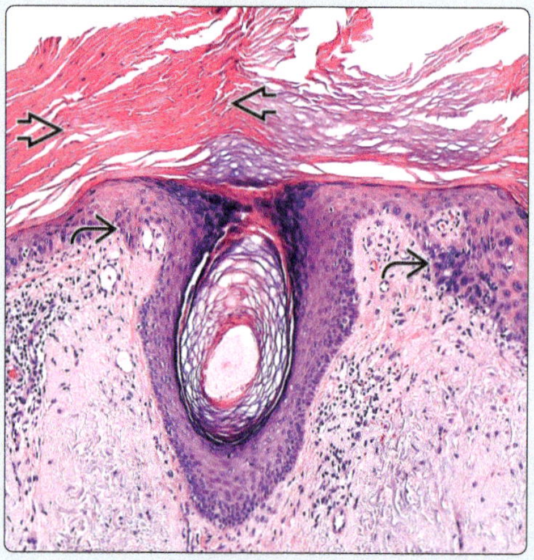

Actinic Keratosis at High Magnification

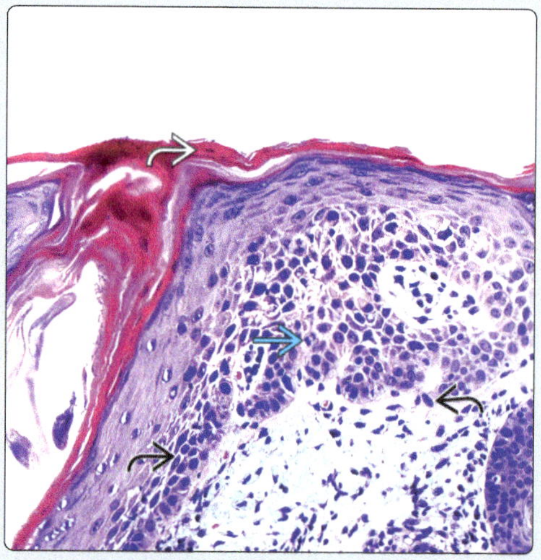

(Left) *Low-magnification view of an AK shows basilar keratinocytic budding and atypia, with sparing of a central hair follicle. Areas of prominent overlying parakeratosis are also present.* **(Right)** *Another AK involving the superficial portion of a hair follicle shows basilar keratinocytic budding and atypia, with a mitotic figure. Parakeratosis is also present within and overlying the follicle.*

TERMINOLOGY

Abbreviations

- Actinic keratosis (AK)

Synonyms

- Solar keratosis
- Often considered precancer or form of early squamous cell carcinoma (SCC) in situ

Definitions

- Atypical intraepidermal proliferation of keratinocytes typically confined to basilar portion of epidermis, with very low risk for progression to invasive SCC

ETIOLOGY/PATHOGENESIS

Solar Damage

- Ultraviolet light (primarily UVB) induces mutations in DNA, which leads to abnormal proliferation of intraepidermal keratinocytes
- *TP53* mutations are most common genetic alteration identified

CLINICAL ISSUES

Epidemiology

- Incidence
    - Very common lesions, estimated to affect up to 10-40% of adult Caucasians; higher incidence in areas with heavy sun exposure (i.e., Australia)
- Age
    - Older adults typically affected
- Sex
    - Males more common than females
- Ethnicity
    - Mostly occurs in Caucasians; much less common in other races

Site

- Sun-exposed sites, especially face, head and neck, dorsal hands, and forearms

Presentation

- Scaly papules and plaques, often multiple

Natural History

- Minority of cases progress to invasive SCC

Treatment

- Options, risks, complications
    - Controversial whether treatment is necessary in all cases, but most clinicians opt for treatment to avoid potential development of SCC
- Surgical approaches
    - Conservative excision of lesions is not necessary in most cases (unless there is clinical suspicion for invasive SCC) but is curative
- Drugs
    - Topical therapy with drugs such as 5-fluorouracil, diclofenac, or imiquimod may be used
    - Liquid nitrogen (cryotherapy) frequently used
    - Photodynamic therapy is also emerging treatment that may be useful for extensive AK

Prognosis

- Excellent in vast majority of cases, as only ~ 2-3% progress to invasive SCC
- Most invasive SCCs arising in AK are low grade, but aggressive cases may also occur

MACROSCOPIC

Size

- Usually small (< 1 cm) papules, but larger lesions may occur

MICROSCOPIC

Histologic Features

- Intraepidermal proliferation of atypical keratinocytes, typically confined to basilar 1/3 of epithelium
    - Basilar budding of atypical cells
    - Cells show nuclear enlargement, hyperchromasia, and prominent nucleoli
    - Abundant eosinophilic-staining cytoplasm
    - Increased numbers of mitotic figures usually present
- Overlying parakeratosis present in vast majority of cases; hypogranulosis may also be present
- Lesional cells usually do not involve follicles (as opposed to Bowen disease) and adnexal ducts
    - Leads to alternating red and blue tiers of parakeratosis (overlying AK) and hyper/orthokeratosis (overlying follicles and eccrine ducts)
- Histologic subtypes
    - **Hypertrophic AK**
        - Shows epidermal hyperplasia, often psoriasiform, with prominent overlying hyperkeratosis and parakeratosis
        - Dermal fibrosis and vertical collagen bundles often present, suggesting lichen simplex chronicus changes (due to chronic excoriation) superimposed on AK
    - **Atrophic AK**
        - Shows thinning of epidermis and flattening of rete ridges, and may involve superficial portions of adnexal structures
        - Dense hyperkeratosis usually is present; parakeratosis is more focal than usual
    - **Acantholytic AK**
        - Shows dyscohesive atypical basilar cells and clefts between AK and overlying benign keratinocytes
        - Dyskeratotic cells often present
    - **Pigmented AK**
        - Shows basilar hyperpigmentation
        - Melanophages often present in dermis
        - May be confused with melanoma in situ in some cases
        - Immunohistochemistry for melanocytic markers and cytokeratins can be used to distinguish these lesions
    - **Lichenoid AK**
        - Has dense, band-like inflammatory infiltrate present in superficial dermis
        - Shows mild basal-vacuolar alteration and scattered dyskeratotic keratinocytes
    - **Bowenoid AK**
        - Involves greater proportion of epidermis (up to 1/2 or 2/3 thickness)
        - Does not show full-thickness involvement, which should be diagnosed as SCC in situ (Bowen disease)

- Proliferative AK (controversial variant)
  - Closely related to hypertrophic AK, but nests and finger-like projections of atypical keratinocytes extend into upper dermis
  - Involvement of follicular epithelium frequently present
  - Many dermatopathologists would consider these lesions to be superficially invasive SCC

Cytologic Features

- Enlarged squamous cells with irregular, hyperchromatic-staining nuclei, enlarged nucleoli
- Abundant dense, eosinophilic-staining cytoplasm

ANCILLARY TESTS

Immunohistochemistry

- Not necessary, except in very few special situations
  - **AK vs. superficial or basosquamous-type basal cell carcinoma (BCC)**
    - BER-EP4 positive in BCC; negative in AK
    - Bcl-2 often strongly positive in BCC; weak or negative in AK
  - **Pigmented AK vs. melanoma in situ**
    - Cytokeratins (including CK-PAN and high molecular weight CKs) and melanocytic markers (HMB-45, SOX10, or MITF1)
    - MART-1/Melan-A least useful in this situation, as it often shows staining of pigmented keratinocytes

DIFFERENTIAL DIAGNOSIS

Squamous Cell Carcinoma

- Vast majority of cases of invasive SCC arise in associated AK (over 90%)
- Invasive cells extend through basement membrane into (at least) superficial dermis
- Cannot be excluded with certainty in cases where AK involves base of biopsy
  - Should be diagnosed as at least AK; underlying SCC cannot be excluded, given involvement of base of biopsy

Bowen Disease (Squamous Cell Carcinoma In Situ)

- Involves full thickness of epidermis, with atypical cells extending into granular cell layer
- Usually spares basilar layer, producing so-called eyeliner sign
- Involves hair follicles and adnexal structures as opposed to AK, which typically spares them

Basal Cell Carcinoma, Basosquamous and Superficial-Multicentric Types

- Proliferation of superficial basaloid cells with peripheral palisading
- May be difficult to distinguish in some cases of very small, superficial shave biopsies, where lesional cells are transected at base of biopsy
  - Especially if ulceration and inflammation present (may be associated with/induce squamoid features in BCC)
- Often see at least focal tumor-stromal retraction artifact and superficial surrounding mucinous stroma

Melanoma In Situ (Lentigo Maligna Type)

- May be difficult to separate from pigmented AK in some cases
- Cells are typically more spindle-shaped with angulated, hyperchromatic-staining nuclei; show lentiginous pattern ± nesting
- Lacks overlying parakeratosis (unless irritated)
- Immunohistochemistry for cytokeratins (including CK-PAN and high molecular weight CKs) and melanocytic markers (HMB-45, SOX10, &/or MiTF1) allows for distinction in most cases

Discoid Lupus Erythematosus

- Atrophic lichenoid AK may occasionally be difficult to separate from lupus, as both show atrophy of epidermis
- Reactive atypia may be present in basilar keratinocytes
- Interface changes with exocytosis of lymphocytes into basilar epidermis, basal vacuolization, and dyskeratotic cells should be present
- Additional findings may include follicular plugging, basement membrane thickening, dermal mucin, and periadnexal inflammation

Lichen Planus and Lichen Planus-Like Keratosis/Benign Lichenoid Keratosis

- Lichenoid AK may mimic lichen planus (LP) or benign lichenoid keratosis (BLK) in some cases, especially at low magnification
- Basal vacuolization and dyskeratotic cells typical of LP and BLK, though also present in lichenoid AK
- Cytologic atypia and budding of keratinocytes are main diagnostic features for lichenoid AK

SELECTED REFERENCES

1. Philipp-Dormston WG: Field cancerization: from molecular basis to selective field-directed management of actinic keratosis. Curr Probl Dermatol. 46:115-21, 2015
2. Stockfleth E et al: New topical treatment options for actinic keratosis: a systematic review. Acta Derm Venereol. ePub, 2015
3. Zalaudek I et al: Dermoscopy of actinic keratosis, intraepidermal carcinoma and squamous cell carcinoma. Curr Probl Dermatol. 46:70-6, 2015
4. Fenske NA et al: Actinic keratoses: past, present and future. J Drugs Dermatol. 9(5 Suppl ODAC Conf Pt 1):s45-9, 2010
5. Ferrándiz C: Update on actinic keratosis in clinical trial experience with imiquimod. Br J Dermatol. 157 Suppl 2:32-3, 2007
6. Roewert-Huber J et al: Pathology and pathobiology of actinic (solar) keratosis - an update. Br J Dermatol. 157 Suppl 2:18-20, 2007
7. Cassarino DS et al: Cutaneous squamous cell carcinoma: a comprehensive clinicopathologic classification. Part one. J Cutan Pathol. 33(3):191-206, 2006
8. Gold MH et al: Current treatments of actinic keratosis. J Drugs Dermatol. 5(2 Suppl):17-25, 2006
9. Wheeland RG: The pitfalls of treating all actinic keratoses as squamous cell carcinomas. Semin Cutan Med Surg. 24(3):152-4, 2005
10. Anwar J et al: The development of actinic keratosis into invasive squamous cell carcinoma: evidence and evolving classification schemes. Clin Dermatol. 22(3):189-96, 2004
11. Epstein E: Quantifying actinic keratosis: assessing the evidence. Am J Clin Dermatol. 5(3):141-4, 2004
12. Oppel T et al: Actinic keratosis: the key event in the evolution from photoaged skin to squamous cell carcinoma. Therapy based on pathogenetic and clinical aspects. Skin Pharmacol Physiol. 17(2):67-76, 2004
13. Tran H et al: Summary of actinic keratosis studies with imiquimod 5% cream. Br J Dermatol. 149 Suppl 66:37-9, 2003
14. Ortonne JP: From actinic keratosis to squamous cell carcinoma. Br J Dermatol. 146 Suppl 61:20-3, 2002
15. Salasche SJ: Epidemiology of actinic keratoses and squamous cell carcinoma. J Am Acad Dermatol. 42(1 Pt 2):4-7, 2000
16. Tope WD et al: Ber-EP4-positive phenotype differentiates actinic keratosis from superficial basal cell carcinoma. Dermatol Surg. 26(5):415-8, 2000

Hypertropic Actinic Keratosis

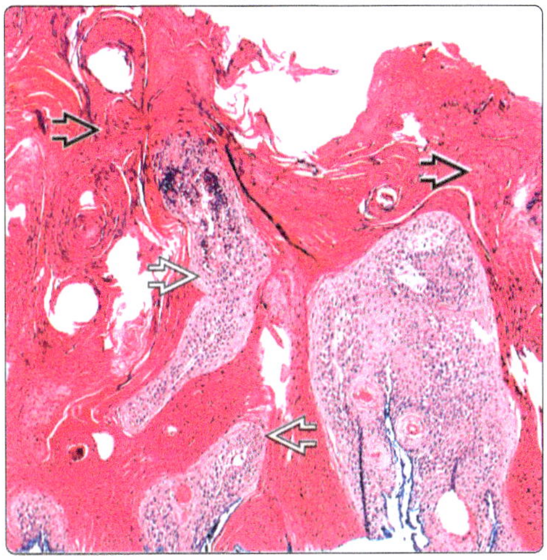

Acantholytic Actinic Keratosis

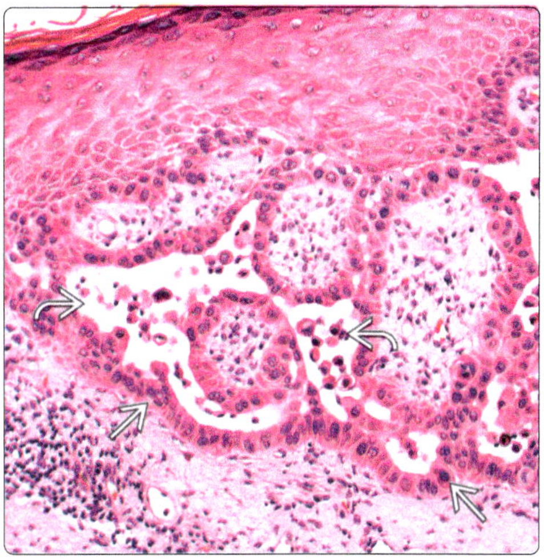

(Left) *Scanning magnification view of a hypertropic AK shows prominent dense hyperkeratosis and parakeratosis , with epidermal acanthosis with papillomatosis .* **(Right)** *This is an example of an acantholytic AK demonstrating prominent suprabasilar acantholysis overlying a layer of atypical basilar keratinocytes .*

Bowenoid Actinic Keratosis

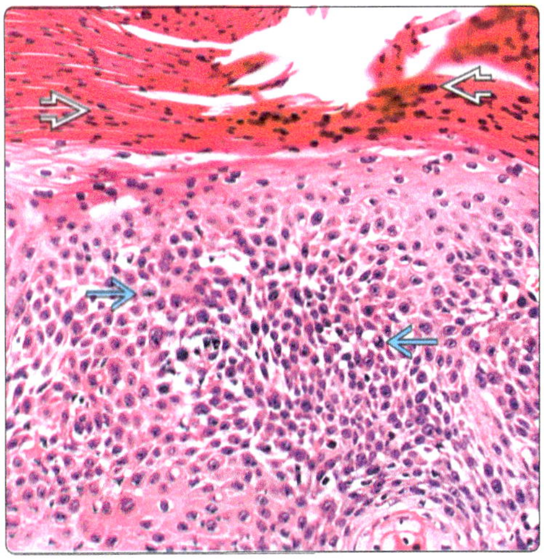

Bowenoid Actinic Keratosis

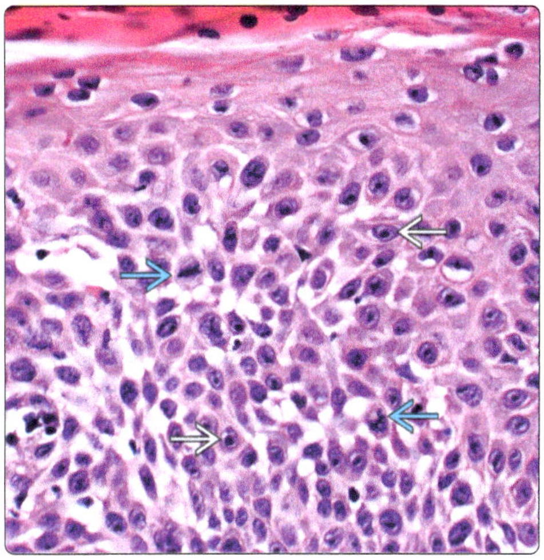

(Left) *Bowenoid AK demonstrates prominent parakeratosis overlying a proliferation of atypical keratinocytes involving the basilar 2/3 of the epidermis. Multiple suprabasilar mitotic figures are easily identified .* **(Right)** *High magnification of a bowenoid AK shows markedly enlarged and atypical-appearing keratinocytes with hyperchromatic nuclei, prominent nucleoli , and dense eosinophilic-staining cytoplasm. Mitotic figures are scattered throughout the lesion.*

Immunohistochemistry for p53 in Bowenoid Actinic Keratosis

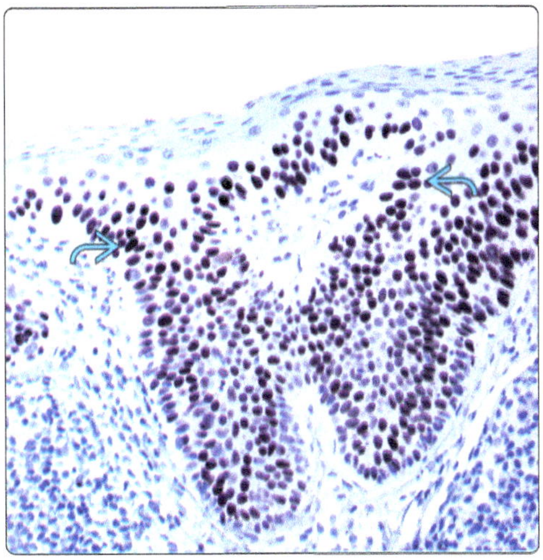

Immunohistochemistry for Ki-67 in Actinic Keratosis

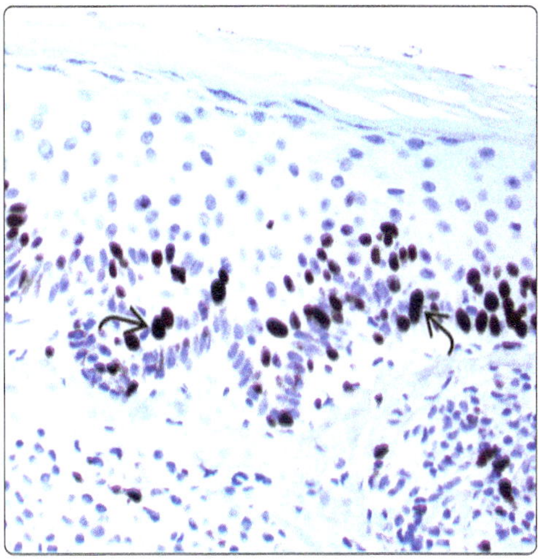

(Left) *Immunohistochemistry for p53 in a bowenoid AK shows strong nuclear staining in the atypical keratinocytes, which involve the lower 1/2-2/3 of the epidermis.* **(Right)** *Immunohistochemistry for Ki-67 highlights an elevated basilar proliferative rate in AK. Note the enlarged, atypical nuclei staining .*

Actinic Cheilitis

KEY FACTS

TERMINOLOGY

- Actinic cheilitis (AC)
- Actinic keratosis (AK) of lip

ETIOLOGY/PATHOGENESIS

- Chronic sun exposure, especially UVB rays

CLINICAL ISSUES

- Excellent prognosis in most cases, low risk of developing SCCis and invasive SCC
- Conservative excision may be performed to prevent development of SCC but is not necessary in most cases

MICROSCOPIC

- Mucosa may be hyperplastic or atrophic-appearing
- Often show overlying parakeratosis alternating with orthokeratosis
- Basilar keratinocytic atypia with budding
- Increased mitotic activity typically present in basilar layers
- May involve 1/2-2/3 of mucosal thickness (Bowenoid features) in some cases
- Prominent solar elastosis, variable telangiectasia, and mild to moderately dense inflammatory infiltrate

TOP DIFFERENTIAL DIAGNOSES

- Squamous cell carcinoma in situ (Bowen disease)
  - Full-thickness keratinocytic atypia, often with prominent suprabasilar mitoses and apoptotic figures
- Squamous cell carcinoma (SCC)
  - Invasive islands of atypical keratinocytes involving stroma
- Actinic cheilitis prurigo
  - Most common in Native Americans, usually presents in summer months after sun exposure
- Contact cheilitis
  - Similar to contact dermatitis, with spongiosis and eosinophils
- Plasma cell cheilitis

Clinical Photograph of Actinic Cheilitis

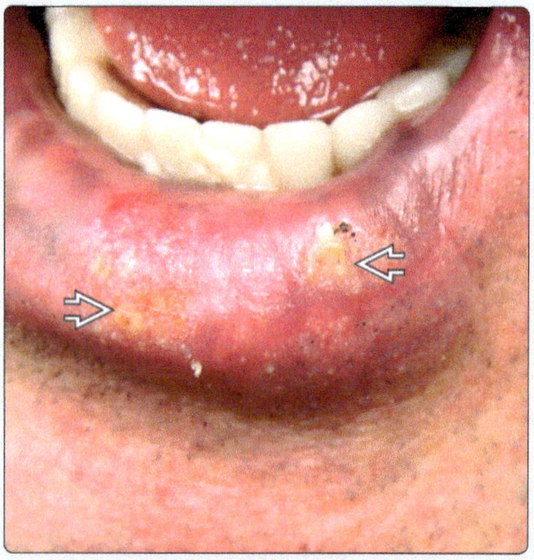

Actinic Cheilitis Histologic Findings

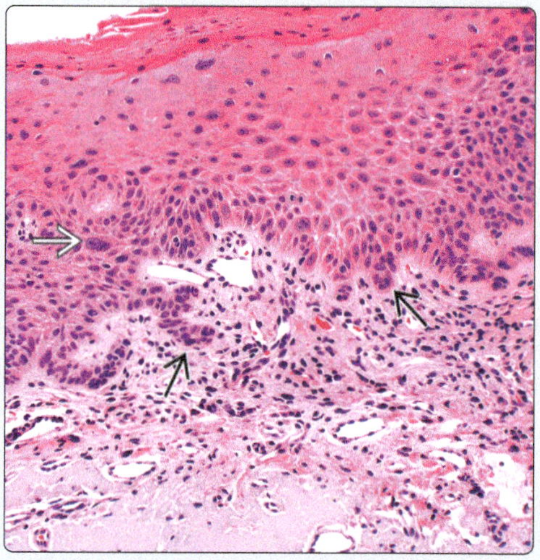

(Left) *This clinical photograph shows actinic cheilitis (AC) diffusely involving the lower lip with associated crusting ➡. (Courtesy J. Wu, MD.)* **(Right)** *Histologic section of AC shows mucosal acanthosis with overlying parakeratosis. There is irregular budding ➡ and basilar atypia, with many of the cells showing enlarged, hyperchromatic-staining nuclei ➡.*

AC With Prominent Acanthosis

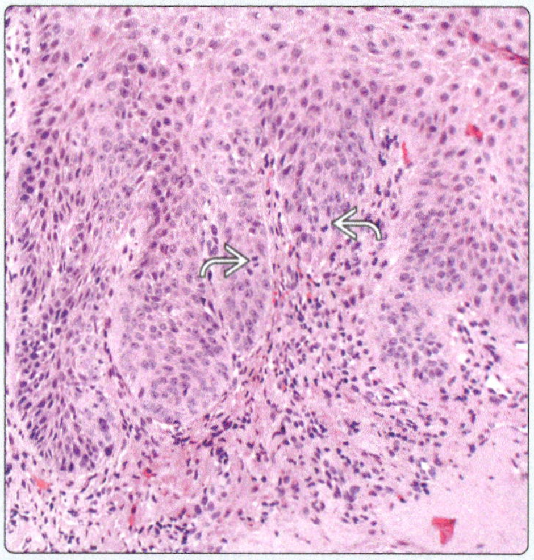

Increased Ki-67 Staining in AC

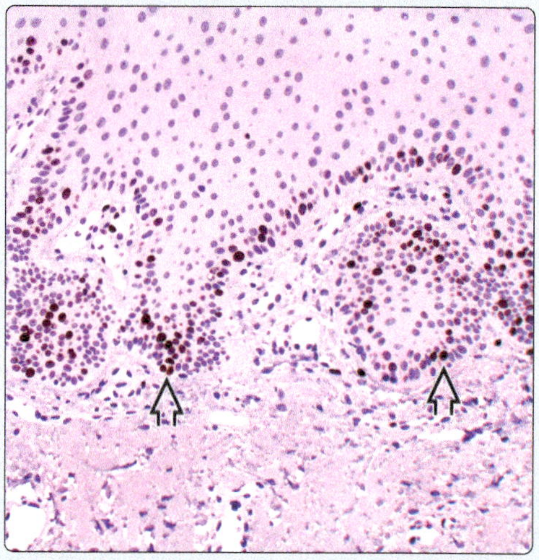

(Left) *AC with prominent mucosal acanthosis and elongation of the rete ridges is shown. Atypical keratinocytes involve the lower 1/3 of the epithelium, and scattered mitotic figures are easily identified ➡.* **(Right)** *Immunohistochemistry for Ki-67 shows increased proliferative activity with strong nuclear staining in numerous basilar keratinocytes ➡.*

TERMINOLOGY

Abbreviations

- Actinic cheilitis (AC)

Synonyms

- Actinic keratosis (AK) of lip
- Solar cheilosis
- Cheilosis exfoliativa

Definitions

- Proliferation of atypical keratinocytes involving basilar layers of mucosal epithelium
- Minority of cases may transform into squamous cell carcinoma in situ (SCCis) or invasive squamous cell carcinoma (SCC)

ETIOLOGY/PATHOGENESIS

Environmental Exposure

- Chronic sun exposure, especially UVB rays
- Smoking and chronic irritation are also risk factors

Infectious Agents

- Herpes virus infection and syphilis implicated in rare cases

CLINICAL ISSUES

Epidemiology

- Age
  - Occurs in older adults with longstanding solar damage
- Sex
  - Much more common in males than females
- Ethnicity
  - Most commonly occurs in Caucasians

Site

- Most often presents on lower lip in vermilion zone

Presentation

- Dry, whitish gray, scaly plaques with erythema
  - Recurrent crusting and healing may occur
- Erosions and ulcerations may be present
- Large areas of lip may be involved

Treatment

- Surgical approaches
  - Conservative excision may be performed to prevent development of SCC, but is not necessary in most cases
- Drugs
  - Similar to AKs, often treated with liquid nitrogen (cryotherapy), imiquimod, diclofenac, or 5-fluorouracil

Prognosis

- Excellent in most cases, low risk of developing SCCis and invasive SCC

MICROSCOPIC

Histologic Features

- Mucosa may be hyperplastic or atrophic
- Often show overlying parakeratosis alternating with orthokeratosis
- Basilar keratinocytic atypia with budding, similar to AK
  - May involve 1/2-2/3 of mucosal thickness (Bowenoid features) in some cases
- Increased mitotic activity typically present in basilar layers
- Submucosal tissue shows prominent solar elastosis, variable telangiectasia, and mild to moderately dense inflammatory infiltrate
  - Intense inflammatory infiltrate should raise the possibility of adjacent invasive SCC

Cytologic Features

- Cells show mild to moderate atypia, with nuclear enlargement, hyperchromasia, and enlarged nucleoli

DIFFERENTIAL DIAGNOSIS

Squamous Cell Carcinoma In Situ (Bowen Disease)

- Full-thickness keratinocytic atypia (dysplasia), often with prominent suprabasilar mitoses and apoptotic figures
- May develop in some cases of actinic cheilitis

Squamous Cell Carcinoma

- Invasive islands of atypical keratinocytes involving submucosal stroma
- Often associated with ulceration and dense inflammatory infiltrate
- May arise in preexisting actinic cheilitis
  - Prolonged ulceration should raise possibility of development of SCC

Actinic Cheilitis Prurigo

- Most common in Native Americans, usually presents in summer months after sun exposure
- Epithelial spongiosis with superficial and deep perivascular lymphocytic infiltrate
- May show mucosal acanthosis and parakeratosis, but it lacks significant cytologic atypia

Contact Cheilitis

- Similar to contact dermatitis on cutaneous surfaces
- Spongiosis and intraepithelial lymphocytes present; eosinophils often present in stroma
- Lacks significant cytologic atypia of basilar keratinocytes

Plasma Cell Cheilitis

- Prominent plasmacytic infiltrate in submucosal stroma
- Lacks significant overlying epithelial atypia

SELECTED REFERENCES

1. Yazdani Abyaneh MA et al: Photodynamic therapy for actinic cheilitis: a systematic review. Dermatol Surg. 41(2):189-98, 2015
2. de Santana Sarmento DJ et al: Actinic cheilitis: clinicopathologic profile and association with degree of dysplasia. Int J Dermatol. 53(4):466-72, 2014
3. Poulopoulos AK et al: Expression of matrix metalloproteinases 9 and 12 in actinic cheilitis. World J Exp Med. 3(3):43-9, 2013
4. Castiñeiras I et al: Actinic cheilitis: evolution to squamous cell carcinoma after carbon dioxide laser vaporization. A study of 43 cases. J Dermatolog Treat. 21(1):49-53, 2010
5. Cavalcante AS et al: Actinic cheilitis: clinical and histological features. J Oral Maxillofac Surg. 66(3):498-503, 2008
6. Ulrich C et al: Management of actinic cheilitis using diclofenac 3% gel: a report of six cases. Br J Dermatol. 156 Suppl 3:43-6, 2007
7. Picascia DD et al: Actinic cheilitis: a review of the etiology, differential diagnosis, and treatment. J Am Acad Dermatol. 17(2 Pt 1):255-64, 1987

Squamous Cell Carcinoma In Situ (Bowen Disease)

KEY FACTS

TERMINOLOGY

- Squamous cell carcinoma in situ (SCCis)
- Synonyms: Bowen disease, squamous intraepithelial neoplasia
- Full-thickness intraepidermal atypia of squamous keratinocytes often with numerous mitotic figures and apoptotic cells

ETIOLOGY/PATHOGENESIS

- Chronic UV radiation strongly implicated in SCCis
- Some cases of SCCis are related to HPV infection, particularly in anogenital sites

CLINICAL ISSUES

- Small risk for invasive squamous cell carcinoma
- Most common on head and neck region, other sun-exposed sites
- Complete surgical excision is standard and definitive therapy
- Mohs surgery often performed for facial lesions to minimize amount of tissue taken
- Topical therapy with immunomodulators, including imiquimod or 5-fluorouracil, may be used
- Excellent in most cases

MICROSCOPIC

- Cells are usually markedly enlarged and atypical-appearing, with nuclear hyperchromasia and enlarged nucleoli
- Basilar keratinocytes are often spared, leading to so-called eyeliner sign
- Overlying parakeratosis is usually diffusely present, without skip areas over adnexal structures
- Numerous intraepidermal mitotic figures and apoptotic figures typically present

TOP DIFFERENTIAL DIAGNOSES

- Actinic keratosis
- Invasive squamous cell carcinoma
- Paget disease and other pagetoid in situ carcinomas

Clinical Photograph of SCCis on Forearm

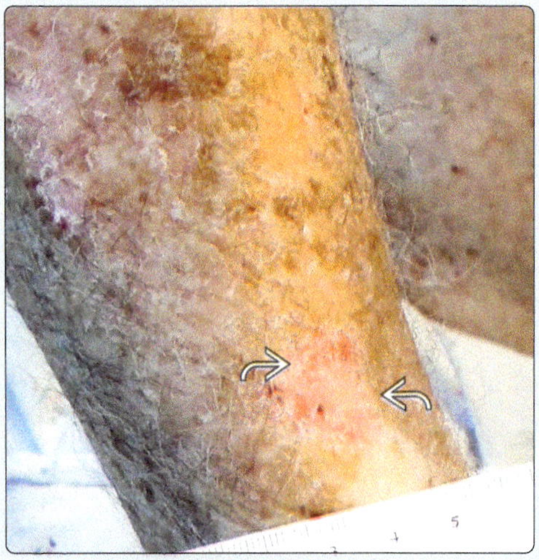

SCCis (Bowen Disease)

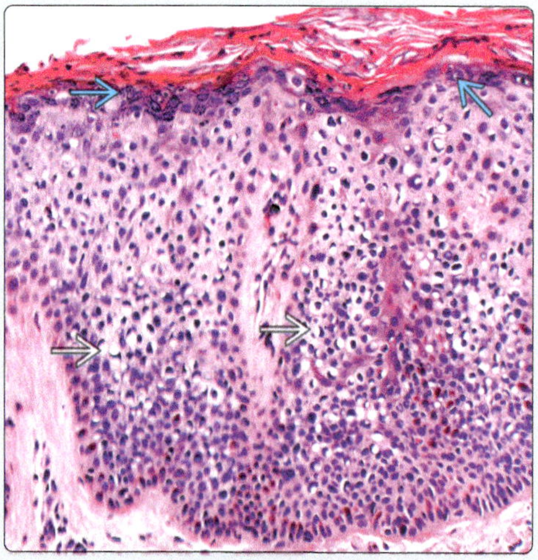

(Left) *This is an example of squamous cell carcinoma in situ (SCCis)/Bowen disease presenting as an erythematous plaque on the forearm of an elderly male patient who had a history of multiple skin cancers.* **(Right)** *Bowen disease (SCCis) is characterized by a proliferation of atypical intraepidermal keratinocytes filling the entire epidermis, including the granular layer. Many of the cells show cytoplasmic clearing.*

SCCis at High Magnification

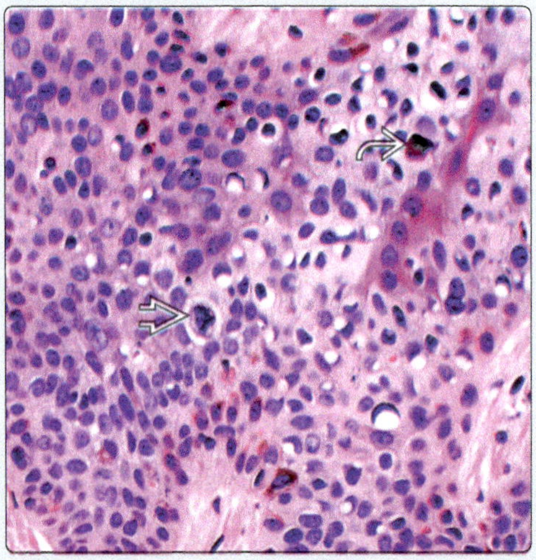

Verrucoid SCCis

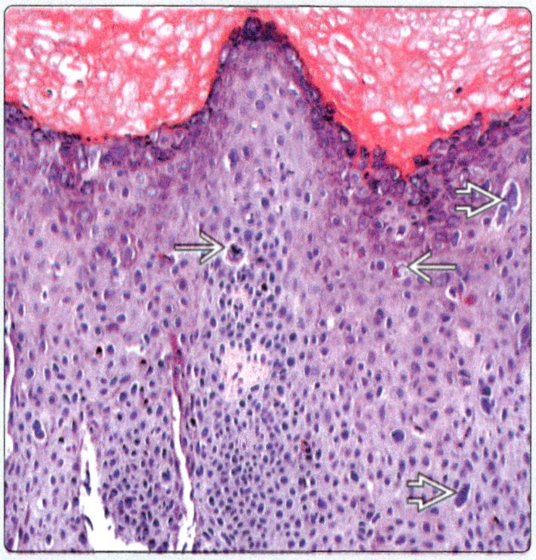

(Left) *High magnification of Bowen disease shows prominent cytologic atypia, an atypical mitotic figure in the midepidermis, and apoptotic cells.* **(Right)** *Verrucoid SCCis shows hypergranulosis, mild papillomatosis, and superficial koilocytic-appearing cells, suggesting an HPV etiology. Note the scattered mitotic figures and enlarged, bizarre-appearing, hyperchromatic-staining nuclei.*

TERMINOLOGY

Abbreviations

- Squamous cell carcinoma in situ (SCCis)

Synonyms

- Bowen disease

Definitions

- Full-thickness intraepidermal atypia of squamous keratinocytes, often with numerous mitotic figures and apoptotic cells

ETIOLOGY/PATHOGENESIS

Sun Exposure

- Chronic UV radiation strongly implicated in SCCis

Immunosuppression

- Increased risk of developing SCCis in immunosuppressed patients, especially organ transplant recipients

CLINICAL ISSUES

Site

- Most common on head and neck region, other sun-exposed sites

Presentation

- Scaly patch or plaque lesion

Treatment

- Surgical approaches
  - Complete surgical excision is standard and definitive therapy
  - Mohs surgery often performed for facial lesions to minimize amount of tissue taken
  - Electrodesiccation and curettage may also be used
- Drugs
  - Topical therapy with immunomodulators, including imiquimod or 5-fluorouracil, may be used
    - Patients with extensive lesions or poor surgical candidates

Prognosis

- Excellent in most cases
- Small risk for invasive squamous cell carcinoma

MACROSCOPIC

General Features

- Broad, superficial lesion with epidermal thickening and overlying scale

MICROSCOPIC

Histologic Features

- Atypical intraepidermal proliferation of squamous cells extending into upper levels of epidermis
  - Basilar keratinocytes are often spared, leading to so-called eyeliner sign
- Overlying parakeratosis often diffusely present, without skip areas over adnexal structures
- Follicular epithelial involvement is typically seen
- Cells are usually markedly enlarged and atypical-appearing, with nuclear hyperchromasia and enlarged nucleoli
- Numerous intraepidermal mitotic figures and apoptotic bodies typically present

Cytologic Features

- Enlarged cells with dense eosinophilic-staining cytoplasm, enlarged hyperchromatic-staining nuclei, and prominent nucleoli

DIFFERENTIAL DIAGNOSIS

Actinic Keratosis

- Defined as atypical proliferation of basilar keratinocytes not involving full epidermal thickness
  - However, bowenoid actinic keratosis can be difficult and somewhat subjective to separate from SCCis, as it can involve 1/2-2/3 of epidermal thickness
- Typically spares adnexal structures, while SCCis involves them

Invasive Squamous Cell Carcinoma

- Shows infiltrative nests, cords, &/or single cells in dermis
- May only be focally/superficially invasive in some cases and can be easily overlooked on scanning magnification
- Superficial biopsies in which SCCis is transected at base of biopsy cannot be definitively evaluated for invasion
  - Such cases should be signed out as at least in situ, with comment stating that underlying invasive carcinoma cannot be excluded with certainty

Paget Disease and Other Pagetoid In Situ Carcinomas

- In differential diagnosis with pagetoid Bowen disease
- Cells are epithelioid-appearing and show abundant amphophilic to clear or foamy-appearing cytoplasm
- Immunohistochemistry typically shows strong positivity for CK7, CEA, EMA, and GCDFP-15; ER/PR positive in many cases, especially mammary Paget
- Other pagetoid carcinomas including pagetoid sebaceous carcinoma (EMA, CK7, and androgen R+) and Merkel cell carcinoma (CK20, synaptophysin, chromogranin positive) may be in the differential

SELECTED REFERENCES

1. Övermark M et al: A Retrospective Study of Treatment of Squamous Cell Carcinoma In situ. Acta Derm Venereol. ePub, 2015
2. Dallaglio K et al: Expression of nuclear survivin in normal skin and squamous cell carcinoma: a possible role in tumour invasion. Br J Cancer. 110(1):199-207, 2014
3. Aung PP et al: Apoptosis and in situ and invasive squamous cell carcinoma in sun-exposed sites. Am J Dermatopathol. 35(8):797-803, 2013
4. Chuang GS et al: Incidence of invasive squamous cell carcinomas in biopsy-proven squamous cell carcinomas in situ sent for Mohs micrographic surgery. Dermatol Surg. 38(9):1456-60, 2012
5. Nakanishi G et al: Human papillomavirus genome integration in multifocal vulvar Bowen's disease and squamous cell carcinoma. Clin Exp Dermatol. 34(8):e965-7, 2009
6. Hama N et al: Detection of mucosal human papilloma virus DNA in bowenoid papulosis, Bowen's disease and squamous cell carcinoma of the skin. J Dermatol. 33(5):331-7, 2006
7. Campbell C et al: p53 mutations are common and early events that precede tumor invasion in squamous cell neoplasia of the skin. J Invest Dermatol. 100(6):746-8, 1993

(Left) *Low magnification of a clear cell SCCis shows epidermal acanthosis with expansion of the epidermis by atypical keratinocytes, many of which show pale to clear cytoplasm. Note the focal overlying parakeratosis.* **(Right)** *Clear cell SCCis shows a proliferation of pale to clear-staining atypical keratinocytes filling the epidermis. Numerous mitotic figures are easily identified. Scattered intraepidermal pigmented cells and focal papillary dermal pigment incontinence are seen.*

Clear Cell SCCis at Low Magnification

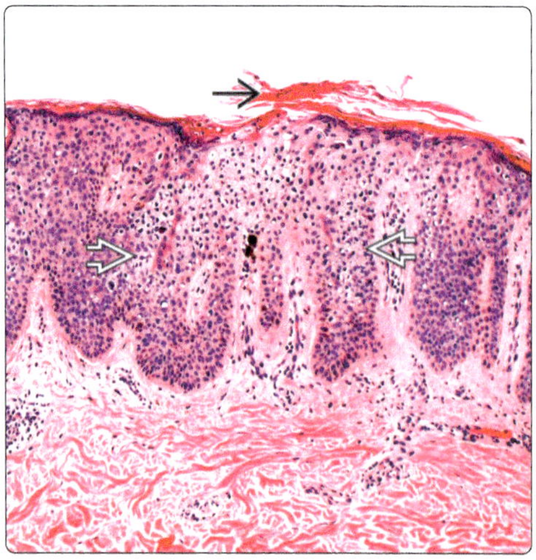

Clear Cell SCCis at High Magnification

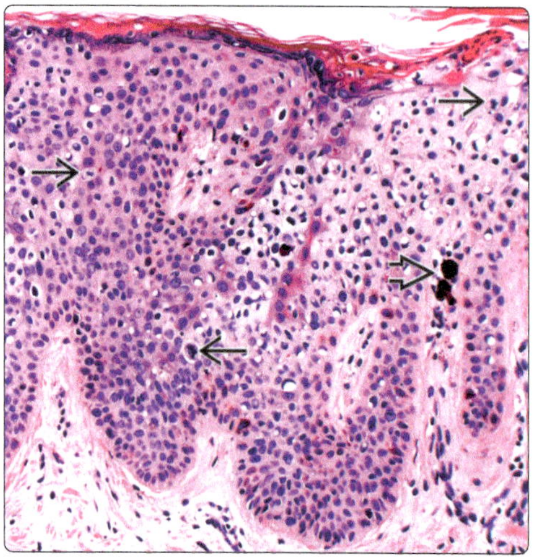

(Left) *Pagetoid clear cell SCCis shows upward spread of clusters of atypical squamous cells with abundant clear cytoplasm extending into the granular layer, with overlying parakeratosis. Note the preserved basilar layer of benign keratinocytes.* **(Right)** *High magnification of a pagetoid clear cell SCCis shows a disordered proliferation of cells with prominent cytologic atypia, including nuclear hyperchromasia and enlarged nucleoli, as well as multiple mitotic figures in the mid to upper epidermis.*

Pagetoid Clear Cell SCCis (Bowen Disease)

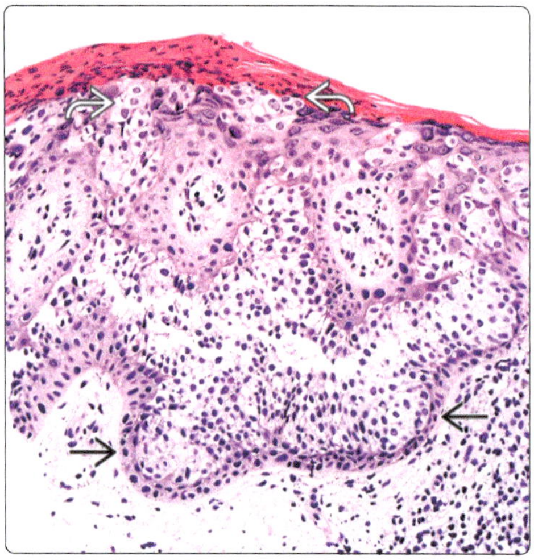

Pagetoid Clear Cell SCCis at High Magnification

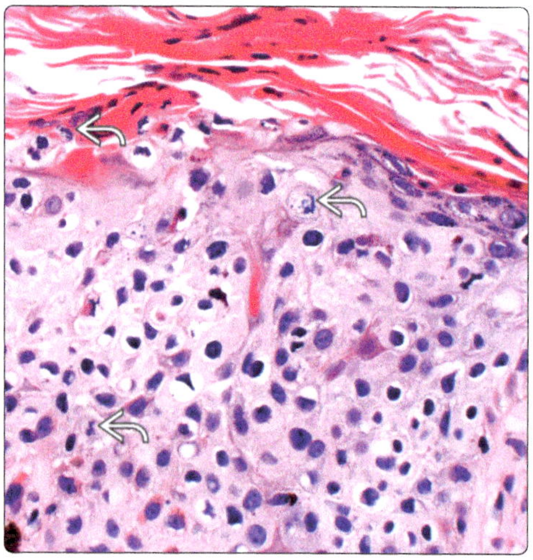

(Left) *Acantholytic SCCis shows clefting and spaces around many of the atypical intraepidermal keratinocytes. There is also florid involvement of a hair follicle.* **(Right)** *Higher Magnification of acantholytic SCCis involving the superficial portion of a follicle is shown. Note the markedly atypical cells with large nucleoli.*

Acantholytic SCCis Involving Hair Follicle

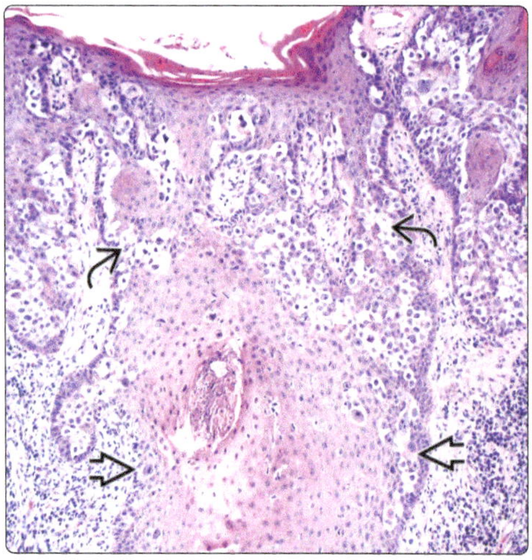

Acantholytic SCCis Involving Hair Follicle

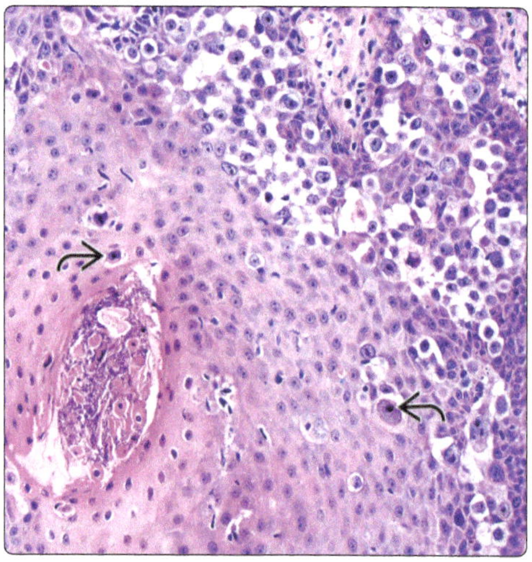

Differential Diagnosis: Actinic Keratosis

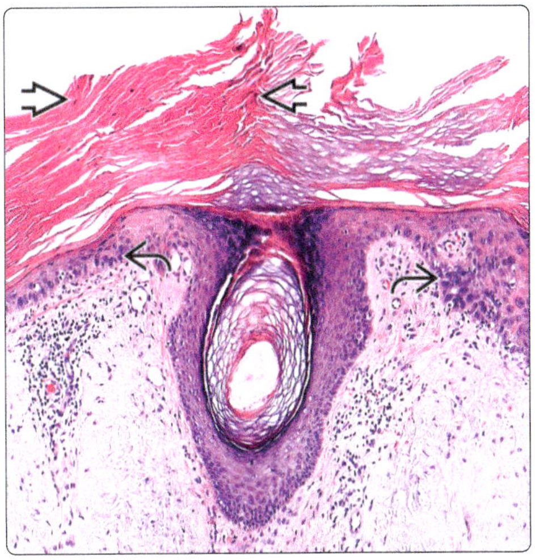

Differential Diagnosis: Bowenoid Actinic Keratosis

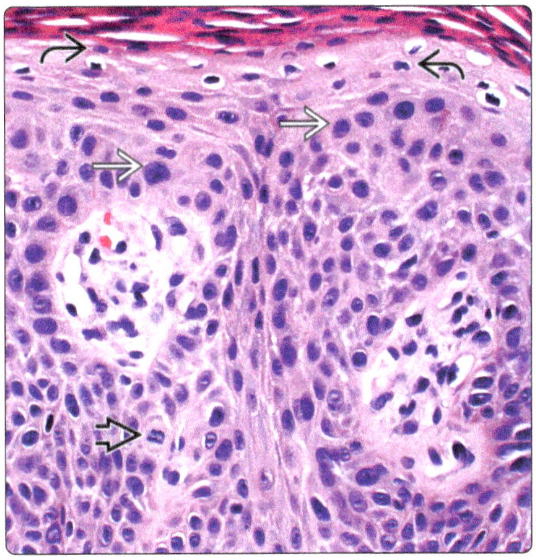

(Left) *Actinic keratosis classically shows basilar keratinocytic atypia surrounding, but sparing, a hair follicle (which are typically involved in Bowen disease). There is prominent overlying hyperkeratosis and parakeratosis .* **(Right)** *Bowenoid actinic keratosis shows atypical keratinocytes involving the lower and midlevels of the epidermis, but sparing the upper levels, which show smaller, more bland-appearing keratinocytes . Basilar mitotic figures are identified .*

Differential Diagnosis: Extramammary Paget Disease

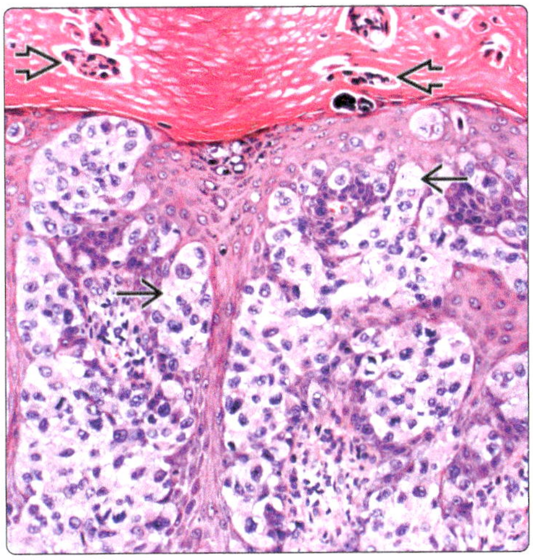

Differential Diagnosis: Pagetoid Sebaceous Carcinoma

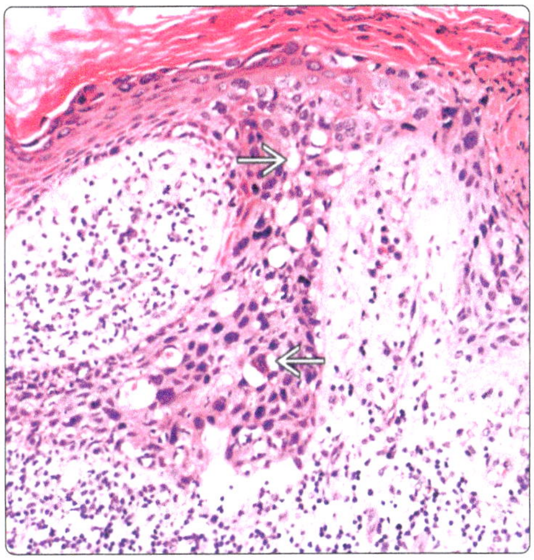

(Left) *Extramammary Paget disease shows prominent intraepidermal nests of epithelioid cells with abundant eosinophilic to vacuolated cytoplasm. Numerous pagetoid single cells and nests extend into the stratum corneum .* **(Right)** *This pagetoid sebaceous carcinoma in situ shows an intraepidermal proliferation of clear cells with cytoplasmic vacuoles and nuclear hyperchromasia. IHC for markers including EMA, CK7, and androgen receptor are useful in confirming the diagnosis.*

Differential Diagnosis: Verrucous Carcinoma

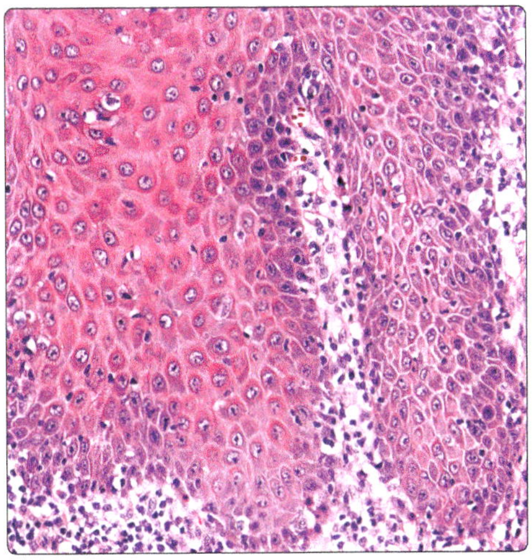

Differential Diagnosis: Pagetoid Merkel Cell Carcinoma

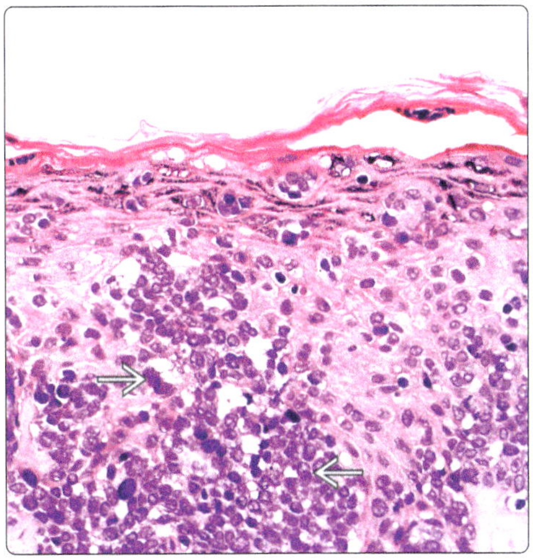

(Left) *Verrucous carcinoma shows expansion of the epidermis by enlarged squamous keratinocytes with minimal cytologic atypia. Cells typically show dense eosinophilic cytoplasm and vesicular chromatin.* **(Right)** *Pagetoid Merkel cell carcinoma shows a proliferation of atypical cells with hyperchromatic to vesicular nuclei with focal molding . Merkel cell carcinoma may show pagetoid spread in up to 15-20% of cases. IHC for CK20 and neuroendocrine markers can confirm the diagnosis.*

Bowenoid Papulosis

KEY FACTS

TERMINOLOGY

- Bowenoid papulosis (BP)

ETIOLOGY/PATHOGENESIS

- Most often related to HPV-16

CLINICAL ISSUES

- Often multifocal
- Benign-looking papules and macules with flat surface
  - May show verruciform surface
  - Rare linear presentation has been described
- Affect labia majora in females
- Usually affect skin of shaft in males
- Lesions affecting young healthy patients usually regress spontaneously
- Risk of progression to invasive disease is related to
  - Older age
  - Immunosuppression

MICROSCOPIC

- Proliferation of atypical basaloid and koilocytic cells arranged as
  - Scattered single units or patches
  - Involving full thickness of epithelium
- Granular layer may be preserved
- Ortho- or parakeratosis
- Most cases are indistinguishable from SCCis

TOP DIFFERENTIAL DIAGNOSES

- Vulvar and penile intraepithelial neoplasia (VIN and PeIN)
  - Despite benign appearance, BP may be identical to VIN and PeIN histologically
  - Clinical correlation is crucial to make distinction
- Treated condyloma
  - Pallor of epithelium, nuclear enlargement, necrotic keratinocytes
  - Increase number of mitotic figures (metaphase arrest)
  - No atypical mitosis

Early Lesion of Bowenoid Papulosis

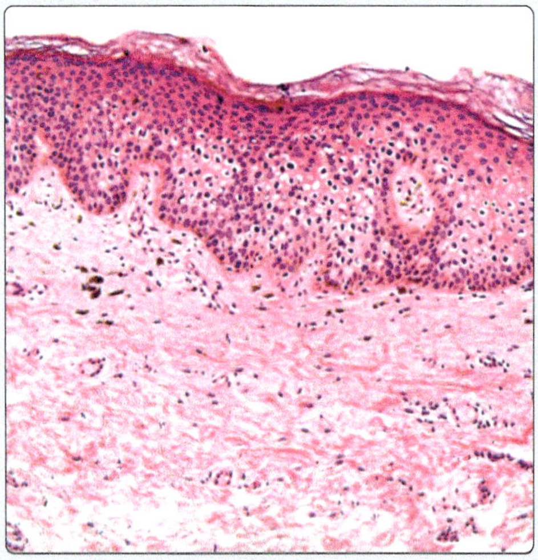

Bowenoid Papulosis With Basilar Hyperpigmentation

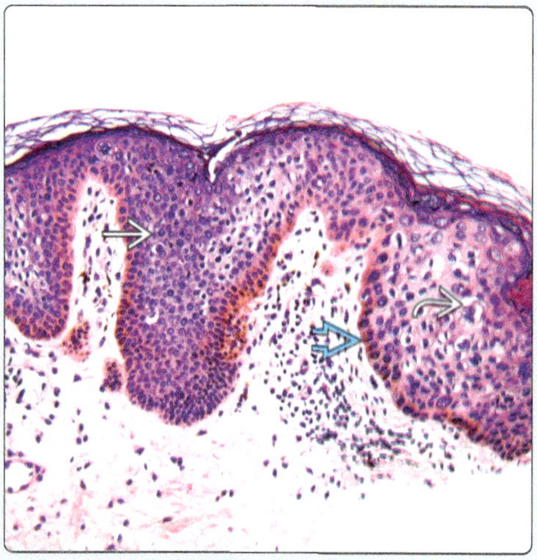

(Left) *At low-power examination of an early lesion, the changes may be subtle, and the condition may be difficult to distinguish from a flat condyloma.* **(Right)** *Patchy foci of full-thickness keratinocytic atypia are usually seen in bowenoid papulosis. Atypical cells vary from small basaloid to larger and more pleomorphic with koilocytic-like changes. Note the hyperpigmentation of the basal layer.*

Bowenoid Papulosis at Higher Magnification

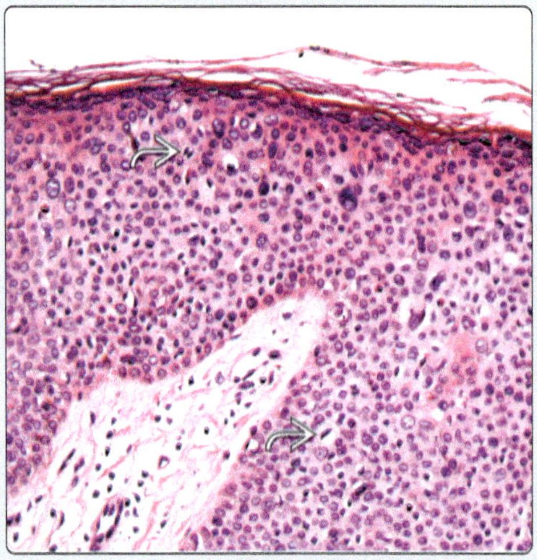

Bowenoid Papulosis at High Magnification

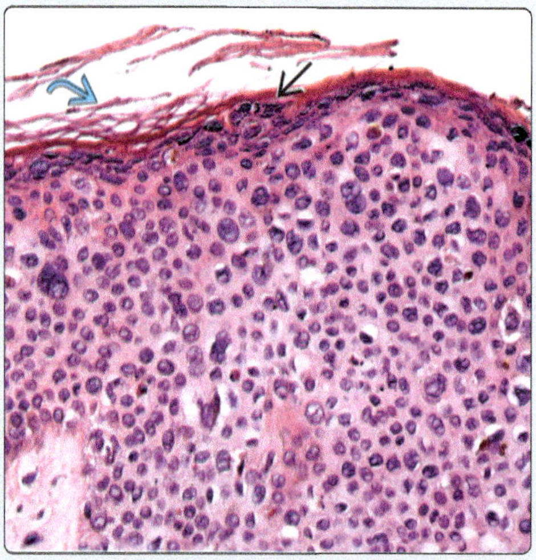

(Left) *Bowenoid papulosis shows atypical keratinocytes throughout the full thickness of the epithelium. There are several mitoses and koilocytic change.* **(Right)** *Higher power view shows atypical basaloid and koilocytic cells replacing the epidermis. Despite the atypical features, the granular layer is preserved, and there is overlying orthokeratosis.*

TERMINOLOGY

Abbreviations

- Bowenoid papulosis (BP)

Synonyms

- Multicentric pigmented Bowen disease

Definitions

- Multifocal HPV-related, papular, preneoplastic condition affecting anogenital region in sexually active young adults

ETIOLOGY/PATHOGENESIS

Etiology

- Related to high-risk types of HPV, especially type 16
  - Other types of HPV (18, 31, 32, 33, 34, 35, 39, 42, 48, 51, 52, 53, and 54) have also been implicated
- Usually transmitted via sexual contact

Pathogenesis

- Oncogenic HPV elaborate proteins that interfere with normal cellular homeostasis

CLINICAL ISSUES

Epidemiology

- Incidence
  - Unknown and probably underestimated
  - Immunosuppression, including HIV infection, greatly increases risk for bowenoid papulosis
- Age
  - 20-40 yr

Presentation

- Solitary or, more often, multiple soft papules and macules with flat surface
  - Surface may be verruciform
- Small (0.2-1 cm in diameter); red, brown, or flesh colored
- In males
  - Affects skin of shaft, epithelium of glans, coronal sulcus, foreskin, or perianal area
- In females
  - Labia majora is most frequent site
  - Spread to other vulvar areas is common; perianal lesions may occur
  - Lesions tend to be bilateral and hyperpigmented
- Extraanogenital lesions are exceptional
- Usually asymptomatic
  - May be pruritic or painful
- Lesions in immunosuppressed patients tend to be more widespread

Treatment

- Usually may be treated with locally destructive modalities
  - Important to remember that BP may be multifocal and has malignant potential; therefore, clinical follow-up is advised

Prognosis

- Most BP lesions run benign course with spontaneous regression occurring within several months
- Some lesions (especially in older or immunocompromised patients) last longer or never regress at all
- Minority of lesions evolve to invasive squamous cell carcinoma (SCC)
- Females with BP and female partners of men with BP have increased risk of cervical intraepithelial neoplasia

MICROSCOPIC

Histologic Features

- Proliferation of atypical cells with high nuclear:cytoplasmic ratio (basaloid cells) that may be scattered throughout epidermis
- Koilocytic-like changes are also seen in most cases
- Range of atypia from scattered atypical cells to low-grade dysplasia to full-thickness atypia of squamous epithelium
- Morphological features are indistinguishable from HPV-related vulvar and penile intraepithelial neoplasia (VIN and PeIN)
- Variable increased pigmentation of basal layer
- Overlying ortho- or parakeratosis
- Granular layer may be preserved

DIFFERENTIAL DIAGNOSIS

Squamous Cell Carcinoma In Situ (HPV-Related VIN and PeIN)

- Histopathological features may be identical to those of SCCIS
- Clinical correlation is crucial to make distinction

Treated Flat Condyloma (After Podophyllin Application)

- Pallor of epithelium, nuclear enlargement, necrotic keratinocytes
- Increase in number of mitotic figures (metaphase arrest)
- Atypical mitoses should not be seen

DIAGNOSTIC CHECKLIST

Pathologic Interpretation Pearls

- Histologically, most cases are indistinguishable from SCCis
  - Presence of only scattered atypical cells or more patchy pattern of full-thickness squamous dysplasia may suggest BP
- Clinical correlation is needed to make this distinction

SELECTED REFERENCES

1. Lee HJ et al: A case of isolated bowenoid papulosis of the nipple. Ann Dermatol. 26(3):381-4, 2014
2. Feng J et al: Spontaneous regression of bowenoid papulosis. Dermatol Online J. 19(5):18185, 2013
3. Zhou L et al: Expression of cyclin D1 and cyclin E significantly associates with human papillomavirus subtypes in Bowenoid papulosis. Acta Histochem. 115(4):339-43, 2013
4. Kumei A et al: Multiple linear bowenoid papulosis without surrounding papules. J Dermatol. 39(10):862-3, 2012
5. Shim WH et al: Bowenoid papulosis of the vulva and subsequent periungual Bowen's disease Induced by the same mucosal HPVs. Ann Dermatol. 23(4):493-6, 2011
6. Liu H et al: Expression of p16 and hTERT protein is associated with the presence of high-risk human papillomavirus in Bowenoid papulosis. J Cutan Pathol. 33(8):551-8, 2006
7. Obalek S et al: Bowenoid papulosis of the male and female genitalia: risk of cervical neoplasia. J Am Acad Dermatol. 14(3):433-44, 1986

Penile and Vulvar Intraepithelial Neoplasia

KEY FACTS

TERMINOLOGY

- Recommended terminology for HPV-associated squamous lesions of anogenital tract is low-grade squamous intraepithelial lesion (LSIL) and high-grade squamous intraepithelial lesion (HSIL/SCCIS)
- Differentiated VIN/PeIN is considered high-grade lesion

MICROSCOPIC

- Differentiated (simplex) PeIN and VIN (HPV-unrelated)
  - Elongated and anastomosing rete ridges
  - Atypical basal cells with hyperchromatic-staining nuclei
  - Subtle abnormal maturation (large, eosinophilic keratinocytes)
  - Whorling and keratin pearl formation
  - Usually associated with LS&A
  - Preferential association with HPV-unrelated variants of invasive SCC (i.e., keratinizing SCC)
- Basaloid, warty, and mixed (warty/basaloid) PeIN and VIN (a.k.a. usual VIN, HPV-related)
  - Basaloid VIN/PeIN: Basaloid cells replace most to full thickness of epithelium
  - Warty VIN/PeIN: Pleomorphic cells with koilocytic changes replace most to full thickness of epithelium
  - Warty-basaloid VIN/PeIN: Pleomorphic cells with koilocytic changes seen on upper epithelium and basaloid cells replace lower epithelium
  - Basaloid, warty, and mixed (warty/basaloid) PeIN and VIN is usually seen adjacent to HPV-related variants of invasive SCC (basaloid and warty types)

ANCILLARY TESTS

- p16 diffuse (block) positivity is seen in HPV-related PeIN and VIN
- Differentiated PeIN and VIN are negative (or show non-block patchy positivity) with p16

TOP DIFFERENTIAL DIAGNOSES

- Squamous hyperplasia/lichen simplex chronicus
- Condyloma acuminatum

Differentiated (Simplex) PeIN

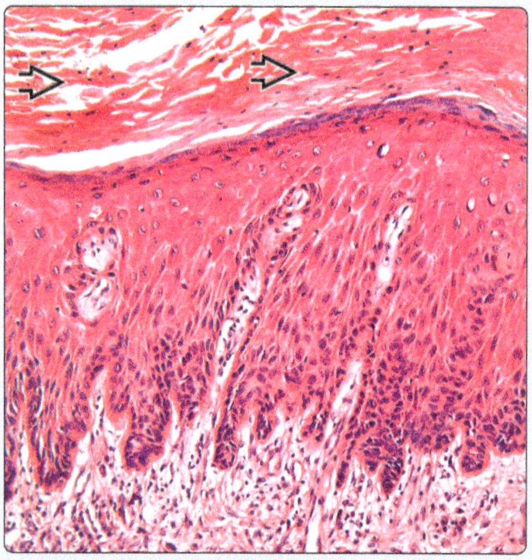

Keratin Pearls in Differentiated VIN and PeIN

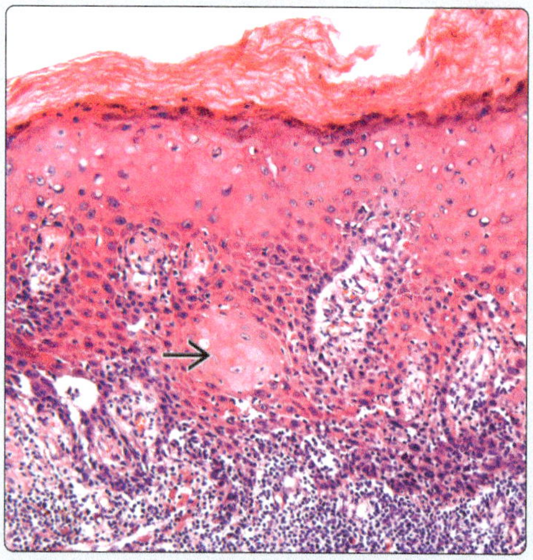

(Left) *Acanthotic epithelium with subtle abnormal maturation and hyperchromatic-staining atypical basilar cells are features of differentiated penile intraepithelial neoplasia/vulvar intraepithelial neoplasia (PeIN/VIN). Prominent parakeratosis is seen on the surface* ⇨. **(Right)** *Enlarged keratinocytes with abundant eosinophilic cytoplasm throughout most of the epithelium are seen in differentiated PeIN/VIN. Characteristic keratin pearl formation is present* ⇨.

Warty PeIN and VIN (HSIL, Warty Type)

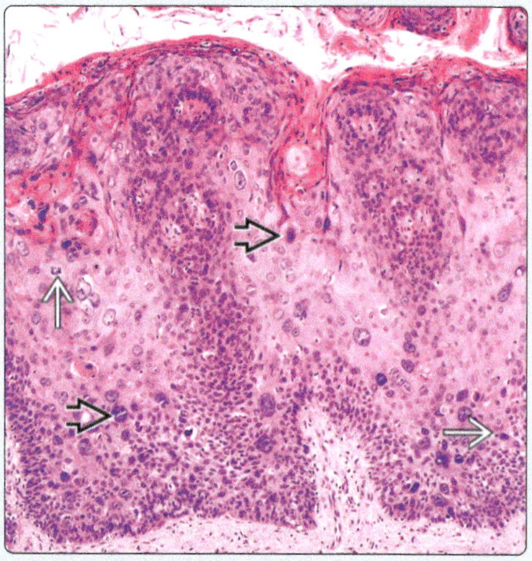

HSIL (Basaloid Type)

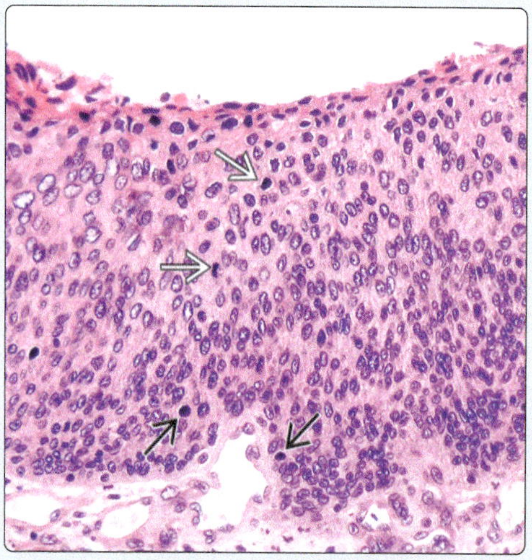

(Left) *Warty PeIN and VIN show pleomorphic and hyperchromatic-staining nuclei* ⇨, *bi- and multinucleation, and multiple mitoses* ➡ *throughout the epithelium.* **(Right)** *The epithelium is completely replaced by atypical cells with basaloid features. Numerous mitoses* ➡ *and apoptotic bodies* ⇨ *are seen. The diagnosis of carcinoma in situ is easily achieved in high-grade basaloid PeIN and VIN.*

TERMINOLOGY

Abbreviations

- Penile intraepithelial neoplasia (PeIN)
- Vulvar intraepithelial neoplasia (VIN)
- Lower anogenital squamous terminology (LAST)
  - Low-grade squamous intraepithelial lesion (LSIL), vulvar and penile
  - High-grade squamous intraepithelial lesion (HSIL), vulvar and penile

Synonyms

- Erythroplasia of Queyrat, Bowen disease, squamous cell carcinoma in situ (SCCIS)

Definitions

- VIN and PeIN are considered intraepithelial (in situ) precursor lesions of invasive SCC
- LAST (2012) recommends 2-tiered nomenclature system for HPV-related precursor lesions (applicable to entire anogenital region)
  - LSIL (includes some flat and atypical condyloma, VIN 1 and PeIN 1, low-grade dysplasia)
  - HSIL (includes VIN 2-3, PeIN 2-3, moderate and severe dysplasia, SCCIS)
  - Recommended terminology for HPV-associated squamous lesions of anogenital tract is LSIL and HSIL, which may be further classified by applicable -IN subcategorization
    - e.g., HSIL, PeIN 3, warty-basaloid
    - e.g., HSIL, VIN 3, usual type
- HPV-unrelated precursor lesions
  - Differentiated/simplex VIN
  - Differentiated/simplex PeIN

ETIOLOGY/PATHOGENESIS

Pathogenesis

- Bimodal pathway of tumor progression in vulvar and penile SCC (HPV-related and HPV-unrelated)
  - Basaloid, warty, and mixed (warty/basaloid) VIN and PeIN, a.k.a. "usual type" VIN/PeIN are HPV-related (especially HPV-16)
    - Warty PeIN has been recently shown to demonstrate heterogeneous pattern of HPV genotypes
  - Differentiated (simplex) VIN and PeIN are **not** HPV-related
    - May be related to lichen sclerosus et atrophicus (LS&A)
    - May be associated with *P53* mutations

CLINICAL ISSUES

Epidemiology

- Incidence
  - Real incidence is unknown
  - 2/3 associated with invasive SCC
- Age
  - 5th and 6th decades
    - About 1/2 of patients with VIN are < 40 years old

Presentation

- Differentiated PeIN and VIN
  - Older patients
  - Usually arises in setting of chronic scarring, inflammatory dermatosis, especially lichen sclerosus et atrophicus (LS&A)
- Warty, basaloid, and mixed PeIN and VIN (a.k.a. VIN of "usual type" in vulvar pathology)
  - Younger patients
  - May have history of condyloma
  - May be multicentric
    - Important to screen entire anogenital region
  - Immunocompromised patients tend to have HPV-related variants of VIN/PeIN

Treatment

- Surgery, locally destructive treatments

Prognosis

- Most studies are retrospective and real prognosis remains unknown

MACROSCOPIC

General Features

- VIN and PeIN have heterogeneous gross appearance
- Solitary or multifocal
- Flat to slightly elevated, hyperkeratotic or even condylomatous lesions
- Pearly white, moist, erythematous, dark brown/black macules, papules, or plaques

MICROSCOPIC

Histologic Features

- **Differentiated (simplex) PeIN and VIN**
  - Considered high-grade lesion (SCCIS)
  - Thickened epithelium
  - Elongated and anastomosing rete ridges
  - Atypical basal cells with hyperchromatic nuclei
  - Subtle abnormal maturation (enlarged keratinocytes with abundant eosinophilic cytoplasm)
  - Whorling and keratin pearl formation (usually in deep rete ridges)
  - Prominent intercellular bridges (spongiosis and sometimes acantholysis)
  - Parakeratosis is frequent
  - Absence of koilocytosis
    - Differentiated PeIN/VIN is unrelated to HPV
  - Often see associated LS&A
- **Penile and vulvar SIL/PeIN and VIN (warty, basaloid, and mixed variants, a.k.a "usual VIN")**
  - Squamous epithelium is replaced by different percentages of 2 types of cells
    - Basaloid (blue) cells
    - Pleomorphic (pink/koilocytic) cells with perinuclear halo and frequent bi-/multinucleation
  - Most lesions are high grade (HSIL): PeIN 2-3 and VIN 2-3 (atypical cells replacing > 2/3 of squamous epithelium)
    - Atypical/dysplastic cells may extend down epithelium of hair follicles
  - Low-grade lesions (LSIL/PeIN/VIN 1) with atypical cells involving lower portion of epithelium are rare
  - **Warty PeIN/VIN**

- Undulating/spiky surface with atypical parakeratosis
- Pleomorphic cells with koilocytic changes (multinucleation, irregular nuclear contours, perinuclear halos) replace epithelium
- Mitoses tend to be numerous

- **Basaloid PeIN/VIN**
  - Epithelium replaced by monotonous population of small immature cells with high nuclear:cytoplasmic ratios
  - Apoptosis and mitotic figures are numerous
- **Mixed PeIN/VIN (warty-basaloid)**
  - Lower part of epithelium is replaced by basaloid cells
  - Upper portion of epithelium shows features of warty PeIN/VIN
  - Surface often slightly undulated/papillary
  - Mitoses and apoptoses are prominent
- **Other less well-characterized variants of PeIN and VIN**
  - Pleomorphic, spindle cell, clear cel, pagetoid etc.

ANCILLARY TESTS

Immunohistochemistry

- HPV-related PeIN and VIN
  - p16 is typically positive
    - Strong and diffuse (block) positive p16 results support diagnosis of HPV-related PeIN and VIN
    - p16 recommended for use as adjudication tool for cases in which there is disagreement in diagnosis, with caveat that differential diagnosis includes precancerous lesion (-IN2 or -IN3)
  - Ki-67 tends to show basal and suprabasal to diffuse positivity
  - p53 is variable and in general not helpful
- Differentiated PeIN and VIN
  - p16 is negative (or shows only focal/patchy positivity)
  - Ki-67 tends to show basal and suprabasal to diffuse positivity
  - p53
    - Basal and suprabasal to diffuse positivity
      - Typically seen in association with missense mutation
    - Negative/absent (p53-null)
      - Associated with nonsense mutations or deletions, with undetectable p53 protein in tumor cells

DIFFERENTIAL DIAGNOSIS

Squamous Hyperplasia/Lichen Simplex Chronicus

- Reactive condition that may be confused with differentiated VIN/PeIN
- Basilar atypia and abnormal maturation are not seen
- Frequently seen associated with chronic inflammatory conditions, LS&A and adjacent to SCC

Condyloma Acuminatum

- Koilocytosis confined to upper epithelium
- Absence of nuclear atypia and pleomorphism
- Mitoses are scant and confined to lower epithelium
- Associated with low-risk HPV (usually 6 and 11)
- Usually p16(-)

Bowenoid Papulosis

- Represents clinical subset of vulvar and penile HSIL in which multiple small, red-brown papules occur in genital area of young patients (20-40 years)
  - Indistinguishable from warty, basaloid, and mixed PeIN/VIN on histology alone
  - Clinical correlation is essential for diagnosis

DIAGNOSTIC CHECKLIST

Pathologic Interpretation Pearls

- Differentiated PeIN: At low power, atypia seems to be present only in lower levels of epidermis
  - At higher power, it is more clear that there is subtle but abnormal maturation in all levels of epithelium
- Warty, basaloid, and mixed PeIN are HPV-related, and p16 may be useful morphologic surrogate
- Precursor squamous lesions affecting anogenital tract sites are morphologically identical in both sexes; without clinical information, anatomical site and gender would be impossible to determine with certainty

SELECTED REFERENCES

1. Bornstein J et al: The 2015 international society for the study of vulvovaginal disease (ISSVD) terminology of vulvar squamous intraepithelial lesions. Obstet Gynecol. 127(2):264-8, 2016
2. Hoang LN et al: Squamous precursor lesions of the vulva: current classification and diagnostic challenges. Pathology. ePub, 2016
3. Saglam O et al: No viral association found in a set of differentiated vulvar intraepithelial neoplasia cases by human papillomavirus and pan-viral microarray testing. PLoS One. 10(4):e0125292, 2015
4. Singh N et al: Expanding the morphologic spectrum of differentiated VIN (dVIN) through detailed mapping of cases with p53 loss. Am J Surg Pathol. 39(1):52-60, 2015
5. Darragh TM et al: The Lower Anogenital Squamous Terminology Standardization project for HPV-associated lesions: background and consensus recommendations from the College of American Pathologists and the American Society for Colposcopy and Cervical Pathology. Int J Gynecol Pathol. 32(1):76-115, 2013
6. de Sanjosé S et al: Worldwide human papillomavirus genotype attribution in over 2000 cases of intraepithelial and invasive lesions of the vulva. Eur J Cancer. 49(16):3450-61, 2013
7. Chaux A et al: Distribution and characterization of subtypes of penile intraepithelial neoplasia and their association with invasive carcinomas: a pathological study of 139 lesions in 121 patients. Hum Pathol. 43(7):1020-7, 2012
8. Darragh TM et al: The Lower Anogenital Squamous Terminology Standardization Project for HPV-Associated Lesions: Background and Consensus Recommendations from the College of American Pathologists and the American Society for Colposcopy and Cervical Pathology. Arch Pathol Lab Med. 136(10):1266-97, 2012
9. Velazquez EF et al: Histologic classification of penile intraepithelial neoplasia. Semin Diagn Pathol. 29(2):96-102, 2012
10. Chaux A et al: Distinctive association of p16INK4a overexpression with penile intraepithelial neoplasia depicting warty and/or basaloid features: a study of 141 cases evaluating a new nomenclature. Am J Surg Pathol. 34(3):385-92, 2010

Clinical Photograph of VIN Adjacent to Invasive SCC

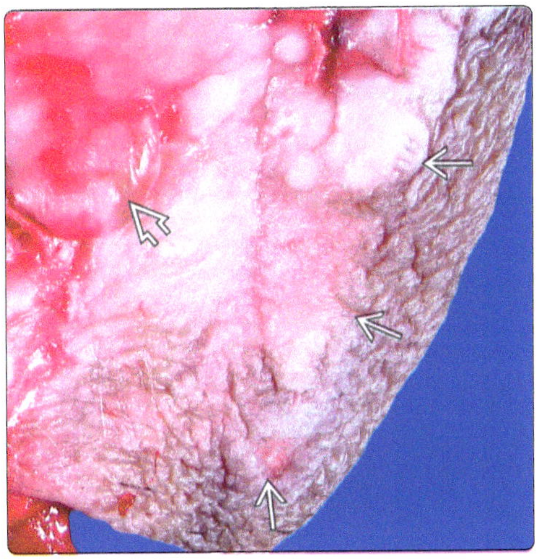

Elongated Rete Ridges in Differentiated Lesions

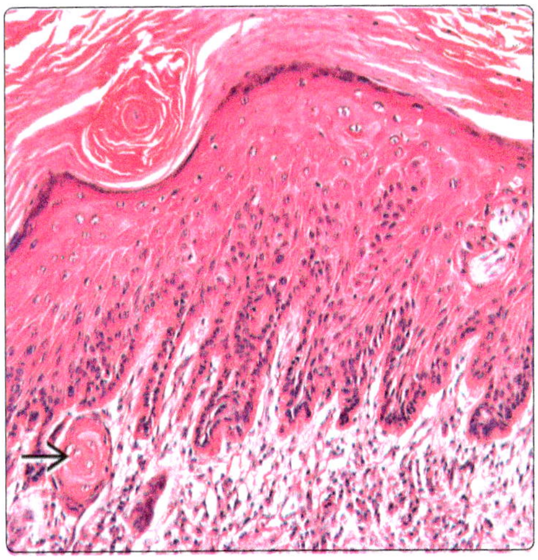

(Left) *Vulvar intraepithelial neoplasia may appear as a raised, thickened, white plaque . This lesion is associated with an invasive component that is exophytic. (Courtesy T. Quinn, MD.)* **(Right)** *Characteristic features of PeIN and VIN include elongated rete ridges and atypical basilar cells. Abnormal maturation, spongiosis, keratin pearl formation , and parakeratosis are also appreciated.*

Differentiated PeIN and LS

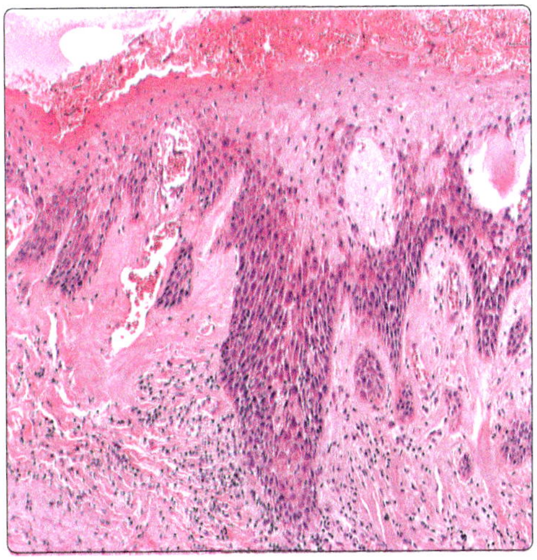

Confluent Parakeratosis in Differentiated Precursor Lesions

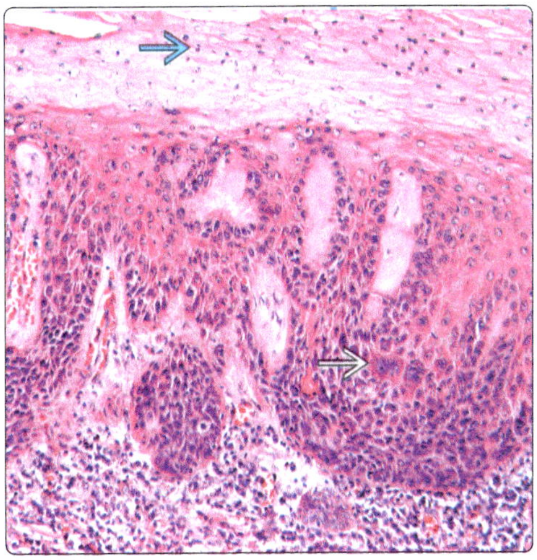

(Left) *There is a markedly thickened epithelium with atypical basal and parabasal cells in this example of differentiated PeIN arising in a background of lichen sclerosus.* **(Right)** *Differentiated VIN/PeIN shows parakeratosis and atypical basilar cells. A few cells showing more frankly atypical nuclei are seen in this example. There is also a thickened basement membrane and hyalinization of the upper lamina propria corresponding to associated lichen sclerosus.*

Hyperplastic Epithelium Adjacent to SCCIS

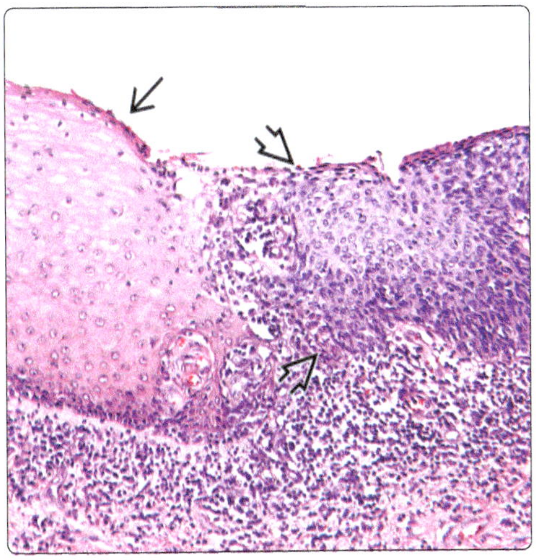

Staining for p16: En-Block Positivity Characteristic of HSIL

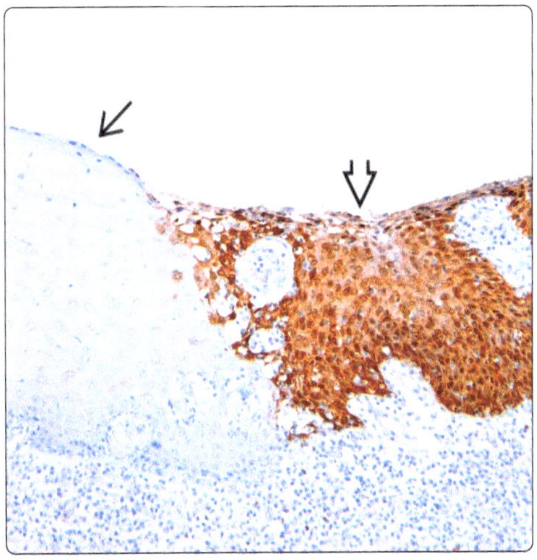

(Left) *This picture illustrates a sharp demarcation between the atypical epithelium of basaloid PeIN (SCCIS) on the right and adjacent hyperplastic squamous epithelium without atypia on the left.* **(Right)** *Immunohistochemistry with p16 (surrogate marker for oncogenic HPV) is strongly positive in the area of basaloid PeIN . The adjacent hyperplastic epithelium is negative .*

Epidermodysplasia Verruciformis

KEY FACTS

TERMINOLOGY

- Epidermodysplasia verruciformis (EDV)
- HPV-related intraepidermal proliferation of enlarged, often bluish-gray staining keratinocytes

ETIOLOGY/PATHOGENESIS

- Subtypes implicated include HPV-3, 5, 8, 9, 10, 12
- Majority of cases are familial (genodermatosis)
  - Inherited mutations in *EVER1/TMC6* or *EVER2/TMC8* lead to susceptibility to HPV infection
  - Increased risk for development of in situ and invasive SCC

CLINICAL ISSUES

- As most cases are benign, aggressive treatment not usually indicated
- Topical antivirals (similar to those used for verrucae) may be used
- Liquid nitrogen (cryotherapy) is usually effective
- Radiotherapy should be avoided (increased risk for malignancy)

MICROSCOPIC

- Epidermal acanthosis with proliferation of enlarged cells with abundant bluish-gray staining cytoplasm
- Perinuclear halos usually prominent
- High-grade atypia usually not present
- Mitotic figures are rare

TOP DIFFERENTIAL DIAGNOSES

- Verruca plana
  - Clinically shows overlapping features with EDV
- Actinic keratosis
  - Basilar keratinocytes show budding, nuclear enlargement, and atypia
- Bowen disease/squamous cell carcinoma in situ
- EDV acanthoma

Epidermodysplasia Verruciformis

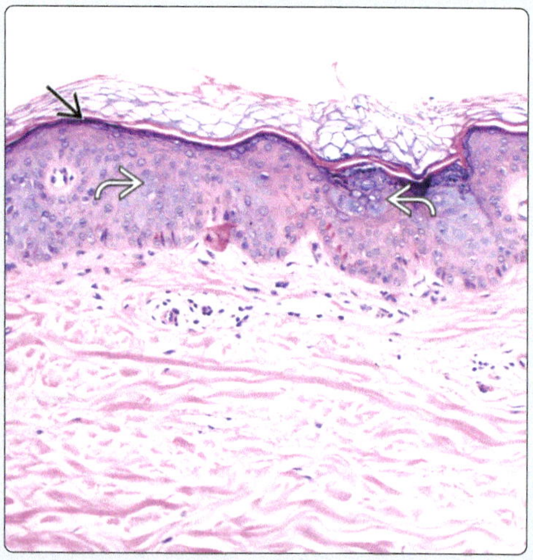

Hypergranulosis, Hyperkeratosis, and Parakeratosis in EDV

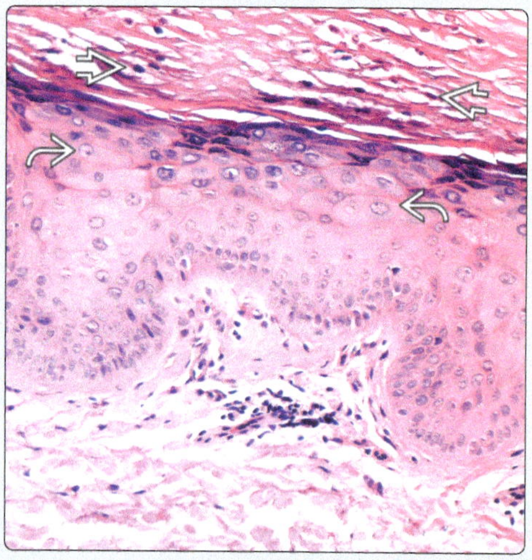

(Left) *Epidermodysplasia verruciformis (EDV) is characterized by irregular epidermal acanthosis associated with an intraepidermal proliferation of enlarged, bluish-gray staining keratinocytes ➡. Note the overlying hypergranulosis ➡.* **(Right)** *Higher magnification of EDV shows a proliferation of enlarged bluish-gray keratinocytes ➡ involving the mid to upper layers of the epidermis. Note the dense overlying hyperkeratosis and parakeratosis ➡.*

Nuclear Clearing in EDV

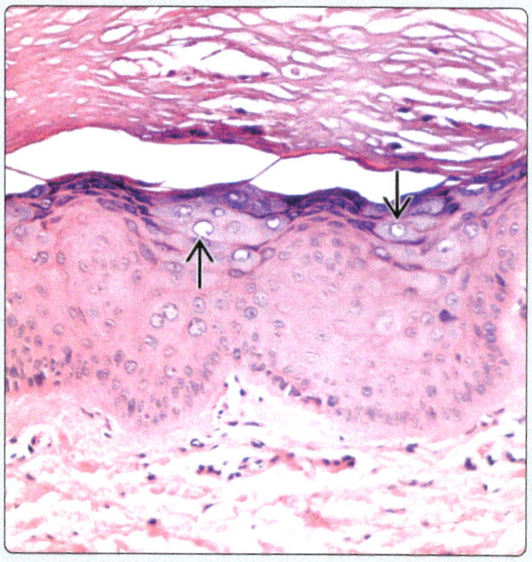

Prominently Bluish/Gray Keratinocytes in EDV

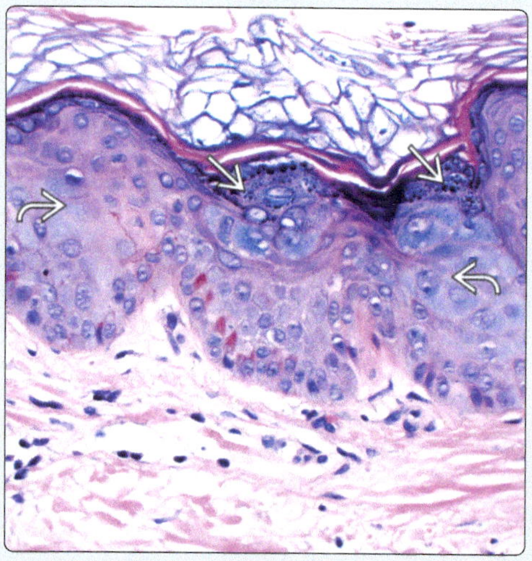

(Left) *Some of the superficial HPV-infected keratinocytes show prominent nuclear clearing ➡.* **(Right)** *High magnification of another example of EDV shows a proliferation of enlarged, bluish-gray staining keratinocytes ➡, some with prominent keratohyaline granules ➡.*

TERMINOLOGY

Abbreviations

- Epidermodysplasia verruciformis (EDV)

Definitions

- HPV-related intraepidermal proliferation of enlarged, often bluish-gray staining keratinocytes

ETIOLOGY/PATHOGENESIS

Environmental Exposure

- HPV infection is established as etiologic agent
- Subtypes implicated include HPV-3, 5, 8, 9, 10, 12

Genetic Condition

- Majority of cases are familial (genodermatosis)
- Inherited mutations in *EVER1/TMC6* or *EVER2/TMC8* lead to susceptibility to infections with HPV
  - Increased risk for development of in situ and invasive squamous cell carcinoma (SCC)

CLINICAL ISSUES

Presentation

- Scaly papules or plaques

Treatment

- Options, risks, complications
  - As most cases are benign, aggressive treatment not usually indicated
  - Radiotherapy reported to increase risk for malignant transformation and should be avoided
- Surgical approaches
  - Excision may be considered in patients considered at higher risk for SCC
- Drugs
  - Topical antivirals [similar to those used for verruca vulgaris (VV)] may be used
  - Liquid nitrogen (cryotherapy) is usually effective

Prognosis

- Risk for malignant transformation increased in genetic forms
- Up to 25-50% of patients may eventually develop in situ or invasive SCC

MICROSCOPIC

Histologic Features

- Epidermal acanthosis with expansion of epidermis by enlarged, mildly atypical-appearing cells
- Cells typically show abundant bluish-gray staining cytoplasm
- Nuclei can be hyperchromatic or cleared out with small nucleoli
  - Perinuclear halos usually prominent
- Mitotic figures are rare
- High-grade atypia usually not present
  - If full-thickness frank atypia present, should be diagnosed as SCCis (Bowen disease), which can arise in EDV

Cytologic Features

- Enlarged squamous cells with abundant bluish-gray cytoplasm
- Nuclear clearing may be seen in some of the cells

Predominant Pattern/Injury Type

- Epithelial proliferation of atypical enlarged squamous cells

DIFFERENTIAL DIAGNOSIS

Verruca Plana

- Clinically shows overlapping features with EDV
- Histologically shows epidermal acanthosis with hypergranulosis and overlying orthokeratosis or hyperkeratosis
- Superficial koilocytic cells with nuclear hyperchromasia and prominent perinuclear halos
- Lacks prominent bluish-gray staining cells of EDV

Actinic Keratosis

- Basilar keratinocytes show nuclear enlargement and atypia
- Basilar budding and overlying parakeratosis usually present
- Mitotic figures usually easily identified
- No bluish-gray staining cells as in EDV

Bowen Disease/Squamous Cell Carcinoma In Situ

- Full-thickness epidermal atypia with enlarged squamous cells
- Numerous mitotic figures usually present
- No bluish-gray staining cells as in EDV

EDV Acanthoma

- Rarely, histologic changes typical of EDV can be seen as single lesion
- May be only finding or may be associated with another benign lesion, including nevus, seborrheic keratosis, or acantholytic acanthoma
- If patient has only 1 lesion, it may be referred to as EDV acanthoma

DIAGNOSTIC CHECKLIST

Pathologic Interpretation Pearls

- Intraepidermal proliferation of enlarged, often bluish-gray staining keratinocytes with perinuclear halos

SELECTED REFERENCES

1. Kim T et al: Development of aggressive squamous cell carcinoma in epidermodysplasia verruciformis associated with human papillomavirus type 22b. Dermatology. 220(4):326-8, 2010
2. Dell'Oste V et al: High beta-HPV DNA loads and strong seroreactivity are present in epidermodysplasia verruciformis. J Invest Dermatol. 129(4):1026-34, 2009
3. Rogers HD et al: Acquired epidermodysplasia verruciformis. J Am Acad Dermatol. 60(2):315-20, 2009
4. Mitsuishi T et al: Epidermodysplasia verruciformis with keratoacanthoma, Bowen's disease and squamous cell carcinoma: isolation of high-risk types of HPV 5 and unknown type of human papillomavirus. J Eur Acad Dermatol Venereol. 22(9):1126-7, 2008
5. Ko CJ et al: Changes of epidermodysplasia verruciformis in benign skin lesions: the EV acanthoma. J Cutan Pathol. 34(1):44-8, 2007
6. Cassarino DS et al: Cutaneous squamous cell carcinoma: a comprehensive clinicopathologic classification. Part one. J Cutan Pathol. 33(3):191-206, 2006
7. Orth G: Genetics of epidermodysplasia verruciformis: Insights into host defense against papillomaviruses. Semin Immunol. 18(6):362-74, 2006

KEY FACTS

ETIOLOGY/PATHOGENESIS

- HPV-unrelated squamous cell carcinoma (SCC)

CLINICAL ISSUES

- Rare tumor
- Affects oral cavity, anogenital area, feet
  - Other locations are less frequent
- Usually solitary
  - Multicentric tumors can occur
- Some cases may be associated with viral warts (plantar lesions)
- Verrucous carcinoma (VC) may arise in setting of longstanding lichen sclerosus (genital tumors)

MACROSCOPIC

- Exophytic papillary tumor
- Broad and pushing base
- Deep burrowing pattern is hallmark of carcinoma cuniculatum (VC variant)

MICROSCOPIC

- Acanthotic papillae
- Slender fibrovascular cores
- Prominent (orange) keratin craters between papillae
- Lack of koilocytosis
- Extremely well differentiated
- Epithelium of papillae and keratin predominate over fibrovascular core
- Pushing, club-shaped base
- Higher grade areas &/or infiltrative borders are not features of pure VC
  - Raises possibility of hybrid (mixed) VC

TOP DIFFERENTIAL DIAGNOSES

- Carcinoma cuniculatum (VC variant)
- Mixed/hybrid VC with foci of SCC of usual type
- Condyloma acuminatum/giant condyloma
- Warty (condylomatous) SCC
- Papillary carcinoma (SCC variant)

Multicentric Verrucous Carcinoma

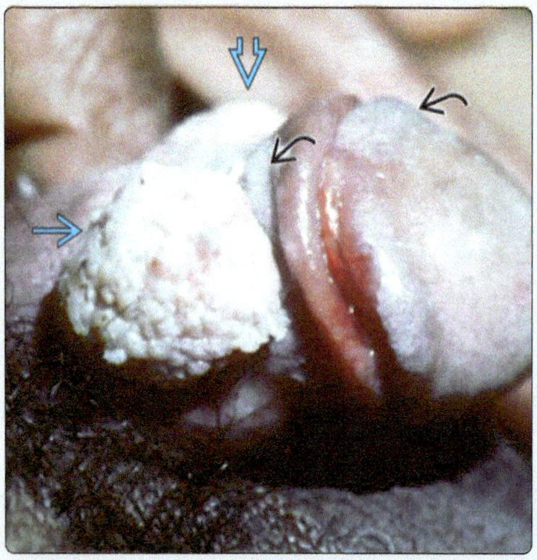

Partial Penectomy Cut Section

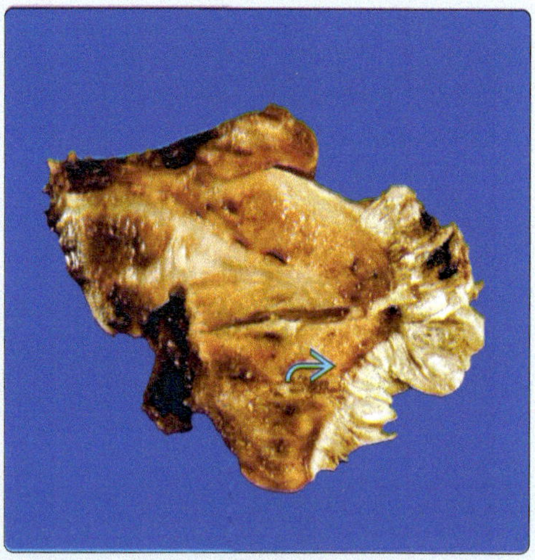

(Left) *Clinical image shows 2 separate verrucous carcinomas (VCs) (one on the right ➔ and the other on the left ⇨) affecting the foreskin of a patient with chronic lichen sclerosus (LS) ➔.* **(Right)** *Cut section of a partial penectomy specimen shows a verruciform tumor with sharp bulbous base ➔ confined to the lamina propria. Note the papillomatous and spiky surface.*

Verrucous Carcinoma and Lichen Sclerosus

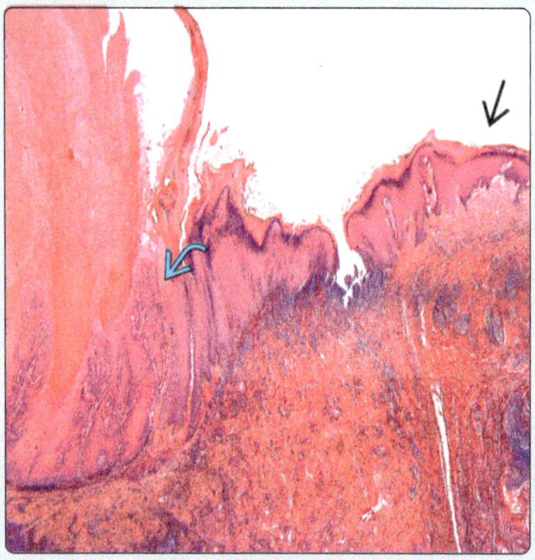

Verrucous Carcinoma

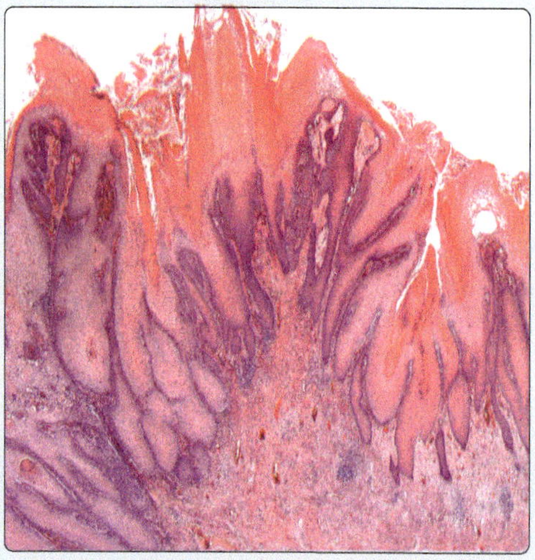

(Left) *Histologic section illustrates a VC ➔ confined to the lamina propria arising in a background of LS ➔.* **(Right)** *Well-differentiated tumor with a well-defined stromal-tumor interface shows papillomatosis, acanthosis, and hyperkeratosis.*

TERMINOLOGY

Abbreviations

- Verrucous carcinoma (VC)
- Squamous cell carcinoma (SCC)

Synonyms

- Buschke-Loewenstein tumor
  - Confusing term that has been used in reference to different papillary/verrucous squamous lesions, including VC
  - We recommend abandoning this term
- Ackerman tumor (oral florid papillomatosis)
  - Older term

Definitions

- Usually human papillomavirus (HPV)-unrelated variant of SCC with papillary surface and bulbous deep borders
- Very well differentiated

ETIOLOGY/PATHOGENESIS

Unknown Pathogenesis

- Most VC are unrelated to HPV
- p53 may play role in its pathogenesis
- Cutaneous lesions may be related to scarring and chronic inflammation
- Anogenital cases may be associated with
  - Phimosis
  - Lichen sclerosus (LS)
  - Lichen simplex chronicus
- Oral VC (Ackerman tumor) may be related to tobacco chewing
- Cutaneous (particularly plantar) lesions may arise within preexisting warts
- Rare cases of anogenital and cutaneous VCs may be associated with low- or high-risk HPV

CLINICAL ISSUES

Epidemiology

- Incidence
  - Rare
- Age
  - 6th-7th decade

Site

- Originally described by Lauren Ackerman in oral cavity
- May also affect anogenital area and skin (sole of foot, finger, nail bed, scalp, wrist, buttocks, etc.)
  - Penile tumors are more frequent on foreskin

Presentation

- Exophytic white-gray neoplasm
- Unicentric tumors are more frequent than multicentric ones
- Anogenital lesions often arise in background of longstanding LS

Treatment

- Surgical

Prognosis

- Pure VCs have excellent prognosis
  - Tumors may recur but almost never metastasize
- Hybrid/mixed VCs have worse prognosis than pure VC
  - Behavior relates to least differentiated component
- There are sporadic reports of sarcomatoid/anaplastic transformation after radiation therapy

MACROSCOPIC

General Features

- Exophytic white-gray neoplasms with papillary, sometimes spiky surface
- Cut sections reveal broad base between tumor and stroma
- Tumors may invade deep dermis and deeper structures
- Irregular jagged borders or foci of necrosis are not features of pure VC

Size

- 1-5 cm in diameter

MICROSCOPIC

Histologic Features

- Extremely well-differentiated squamous neoplasm
- Thick acanthotic papillae
- Slender fibrovascular cores
- Papillae are separated by prominent keratin craters
- Pilling up of orange keratin among acanthotic papillae
- Orthokeratosis
- Parakeratosis may be seen
- Granular layer may be present or absent
- Absence of koilocytosis
- Pushing, club-shaped deep borders
- Adjacent epithelium often shows
  - Verrucous squamous hyperplasia
  - Differentiated vulvar or penile intraepithelial neoplasia
  - Vulvar acanthosis with altered differentiation
  - LS (genital)

Predominant Pattern/Injury Type

- Papillary

Predominant Cell/Compartment Type

- Epithelial, squamous

ANCILLARY TESTS

Immunohistochemistry

- p53 positive (suprabasal extension)
- p16 negative (there is no overexpression)

In Situ Hybridization

- Usually negative for HPV

PCR

- Usually negative for HPV

DIFFERENTIAL DIAGNOSIS

Carcinoma Cuniculatum

- Anogenital, oral, sole of foot
- HPV-unrelated variant of SCC

- Hallmark of lesion is deep burrowing pattern of growth
- Papillary/verrucous surface
- Most tumors correspond to mixed/hybrid VCs
  - Part of tumor has classical features of VC
  - Focal higher grade areas and jagged borders

Mixed (Hybrid) Verrucous Carcinoma

- Tumors showing classical areas of VC associated with other foci that are less differentiated and more infiltrative
- Prognosis is related to less differentiated component

Giant Condyloma

- Large condyloma (measuring > 5 cm)
- Rounded, arborescent papillae
- Koilocytosis on surface
- Usually associated with HPV-6 or -11
- May harbor smaller foci of SCC

Warty (Condylomatous) Carcinoma

- SCC variant usually associated with HPV-16
- Vulvar, penile, or anal locations
- Higher histological grade than VC
- Papillary surface
- Usually infiltrative deep borders
- Prominent koilocytosis throughout neoplasm
- Common in immunosuppressed patients
- Less favorable prognosis than VC

Warty-Basaloid Carcinoma

- Vulvar, penile, or anal locations
- Closely related to warty carcinoma (WC)
- Surface is papillary and shows features of WC
- Deep portion of lesion shows features of basaloid carcinoma
- Most frequently associated with HPV-16
- Prognosis is worse than pure WC

Papillary Carcinoma (SCC Variant)

- HPV-unrelated variant of SCC
- Most commonly affecting genital area
- Well to moderately differentiated SCC
- Papillary surface
- Infiltrative borders
- Less favorable prognosis than VC

Verruca Vulgaris

- Acanthosis, papillomatosis, hypergranulosis, and koilocytosis
- Well-defined deep boundaries

Pseudoepitheliomatous Hyperplasia

- Surface is less papillary
- Downgrowths are more uneven and jagged

DIAGNOSTIC CHECKLIST

Pathologic Interpretation Pearls

- Acanthotic papillae with thin fibrovascular cores
- Piling up of keratin between papillae (keratin craters) is characteristic
  - Keratin is usually orange in color
- Epithelium and keratin predominate over fibrovascular cores
- Club-shaped pushing base
- In partial biopsy, recommended diagnosis is well-differentiated SCC, with verrucous features
  - Acknowledges possibility of unsampled moderately or poorly differentiated invasive conventional carcinoma in definitive excision
  - VCs with foci of moderately or poorly differentiated SCC are considered hybrid/mixed VC
- Carcinoma cuniculatum is variant of VC (usually hybrid VC) with classical burrowing pattern of growth

SELECTED REFERENCES

1. Liu G et al: Verrucous carcinoma of the vulva: a 20 year retrospective study and literature review. J Low Genit Tract Dis. 20(1):114-8, 2016
2. Arisi M et al: Carcinoma cuniculatum of the foot invading the bone mimicking a pseudo-epitheliomatous reaction to an acute osteomyelitis. Dermatol Ther (Heidelb). ePub, 2015
3. Mannweiler S et al: Two major pathways of penile carcinogenesis: HPV-induced penile cancers overexpress p16ink4a, HPV-negative cancers associated with dermatoses express p53, but lack p16ink4a overexpression. J Am Acad Dermatol. 69(1):73-81, 2013
4. Patel KR et al: Verrucous carcinomas of the head and neck, including those with associated squamous cell carcinoma, lack transcriptionally active high-risk human papillomavirus. Hum Pathol. 44(11):2385-92, 2013
5. Chaux A et al: Distribution and characterization of subtypes of penile intraepithelial neoplasia and their association with invasive carcinomas: a pathological study of 139 lesions in 121 patients. Hum Pathol. 43(7):1020-7, 2012
6. del Pino M et al: Comprehensive analysis of human papillomavirus prevalence and the potential role of low-risk types in verrucous carcinoma. Mod Pathol. 25(10):1354-63, 2012
7. Chaux A et al: Papillary squamous cell carcinoma, not otherwise specified (NOS) of the penis: clinicopathologic features, differential diagnosis, and outcome of 35 cases. Am J Surg Pathol. 34(2):223-30, 2010
8. Arduino PG et al: Verrucous oral carcinoma: clinical findings and treatment outcomes in 74 patients in Northwest Italy. Minerva Stomatol. 57(7-8):335-9, 339-41, 2008
9. Velazquez EF et al: Penile squamous cell carcinoma: anatomic, pathologic and viral studies in Paraguay (1993-2007). Anal Quant Cytol Histol. 29(4):185-98, 2007
10. Nascimento AF et al: Vulvar acanthosis with altered differentiation: a precursor to verrucous carcinoma? Am J Surg Pathol. 28(5):638-43, 2004
11. Velazquez EF et al: Limitations in the interpretation of biopsies in patients with penile squamous cell carcinoma. Int J Surg Pathol. 12(2):139-46, 2004
12. Kato N et al: Penile hybrid verrucous-squamous carcinoma associated with a superficial inguinal lymph node metastasis. Am J Dermatopathol. 22(4):339-43, 2000
13. McKee PH et al: Carcinoma (epithelioma) cuniculatum: a clinico-pathological study of nineteen cases and review of the literature. Histopathology. 5(4):425-36, 1981
14. Wilkinson JD et al: A case of carcinoma cuniculatum with coexistant viral plantar wart. Clin Exp Dermatol. 6(6):619-23, 1981

Valleys Filled With Orange Keratin

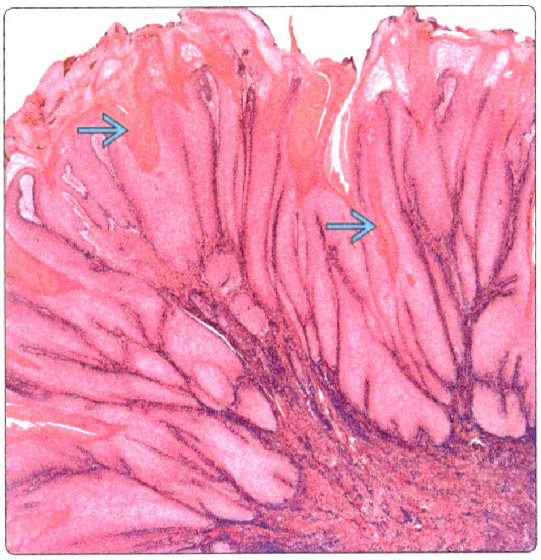

Bulbous Deep Borders in Verrucous Carcinoma

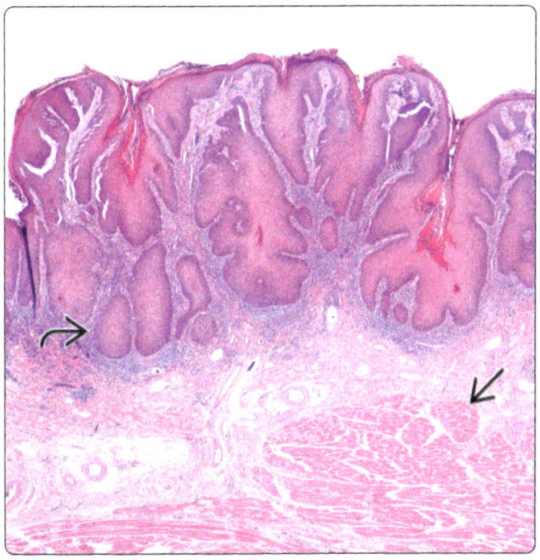

(Left) *Low-power view of a VC illustrates the thick acanthotic papillae, thin fibrovascular cores, and the classic piling up of orange keratin → between papillae.* **(Right)** *VC shows endophytic bulbous downgrowths ↷ surrounded by chronic inflammation. Note blunt-type "pushing invasion" approaching bundles of skeletal muscle ↙.*

Club-Shaped Deep Borders

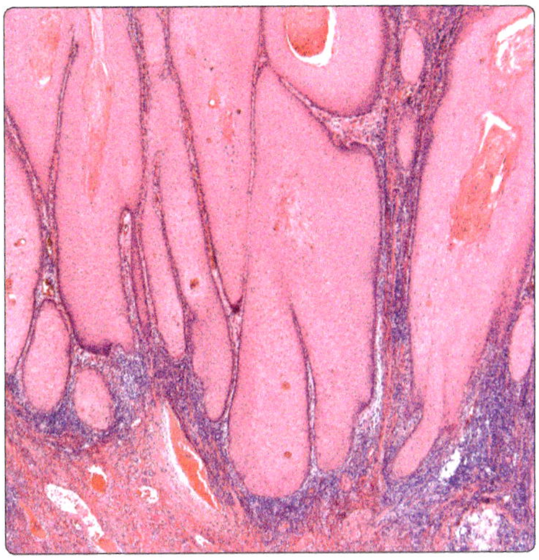

Verrucous Carcinoma is Well-Differentiated Tumor

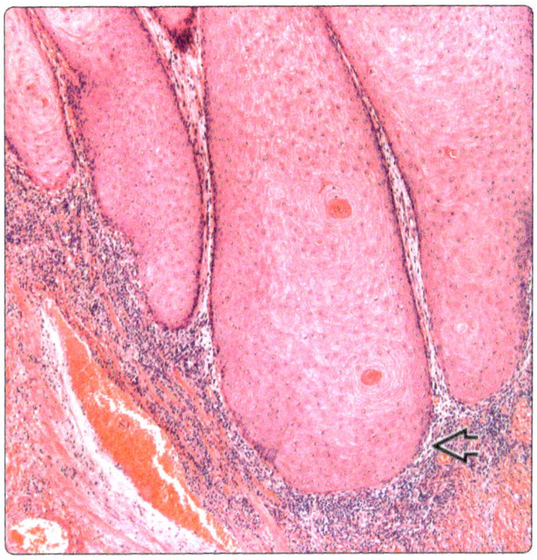

(Left) *Pushing, bulbous, and club-shaped deep borders are characteristic of VC. Note the high degree of differentiation, including at the base of the lesion.* **(Right)** *Pure VC is extremely well differentiated, including its deep portion. The bulbous ⇨ base is a key differentiating feature from pseudoepitheliomatous hyperplasia, which has narrow elongated rete ridges. The degree of differentiation and lack of koilocytosis help to differentiate VC from warty carcinoma.*

Abundant Keratin Material in Verrucous Carcinoma

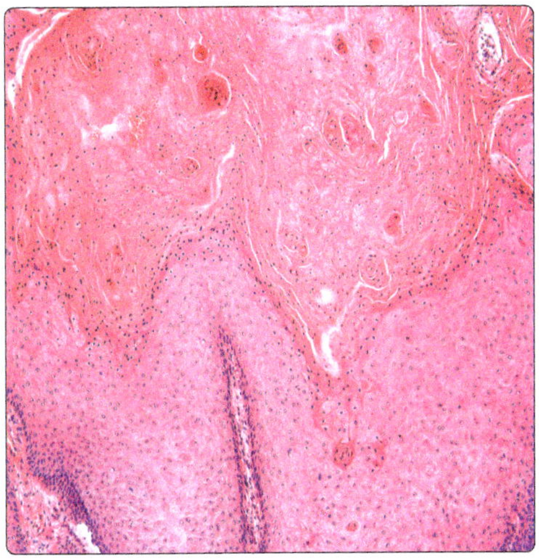

p16 in Verrucous Carcinoma

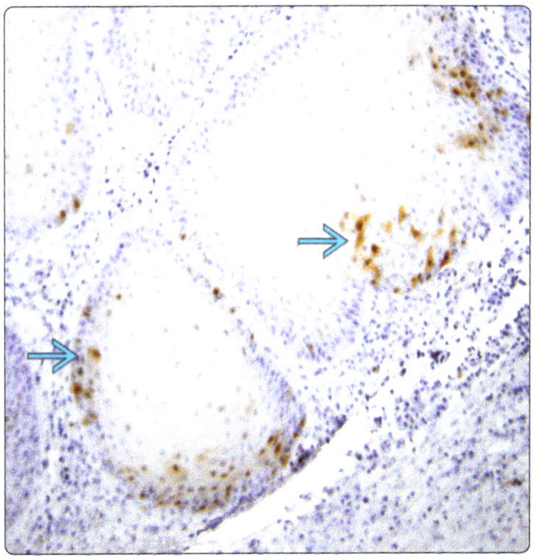

(Left) *Abundant keratin-filled craters are usually seen in VC. In a superficial biopsy specimen in which the entire lesion cannot be examined, the diagnosis of VC can be challenging. Clinical correlation and recommendation for additional sampling may be necessary.* **(Right)** *p16 immunostain may be totally negative or may show patchy staining →. Diffuse positivity (p16 overexpression) is not seen in VC. Such lack of p16 overexpression may be helpful to distinguish VC from warty carcinoma.*

(Left) *Abundant orange keratin and bulbous bases are typical of VC. The acanthotic epithelium and abundant keratin are much more prominent than the thin fibrovascular cores.* **(Right)** *Hybrid/mixed VCs show areas of classical VC associated with less differentiated foci. The less differentiated and infiltrative foci usually show features of keratinizing squamous cell carcinoma of the usual type. In this case, the less-differentiated areas show sarcomatoid features.*

Acanthotic Epithelium and Thin Fibrovascular Cores

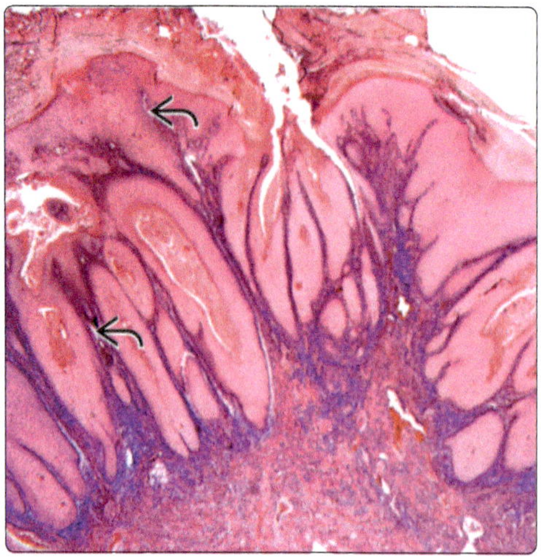

Hybrid (Mixed) Verrucous Carcinoma

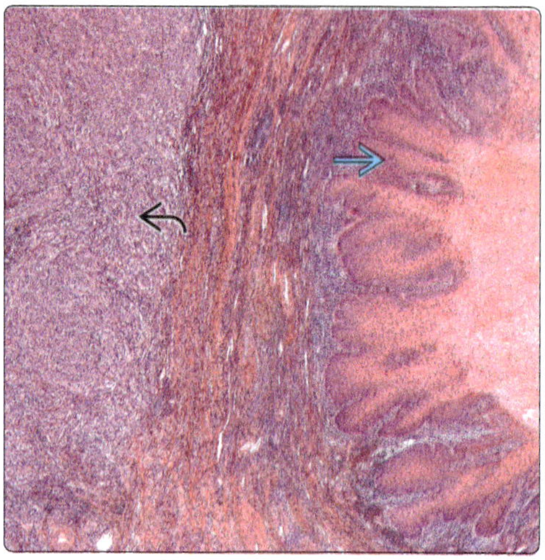

(Left) *VC often arises in a background of longstanding LS. This picture illustrates LS with hyperplastic epithelium. The VC is not included in this picture.* **(Right)** *Differentiated penile intraepithelial neoplasia in the penis and differentiated vulvar intraepithelial neoplasia in the vulva (often associated with LS) are believed to represent a precursor lesion of VC.*

Lichen Sclerosus and Verrucous Carcinoma

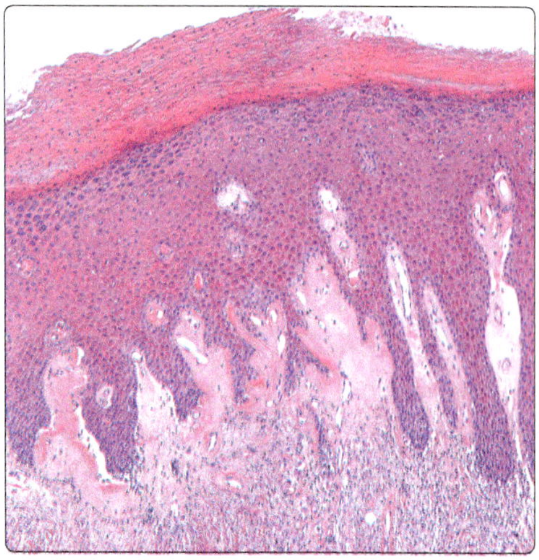

Differentiated Penile Intraepithelial Neoplasia

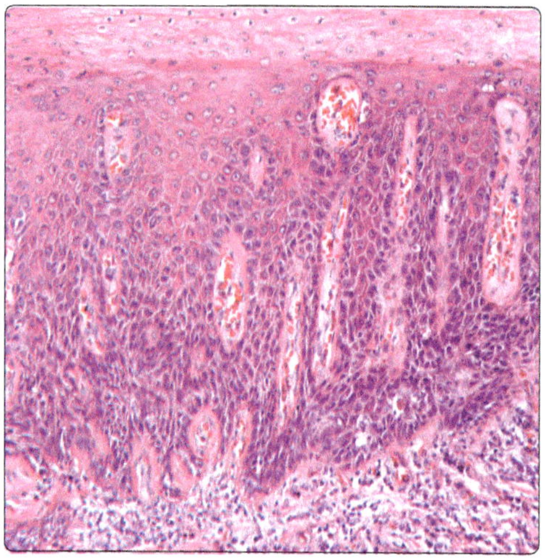

(Left) *Cut section of a penectomy specimen with a carcinoma cuniculatum shows the burrowing pattern, which is the hallmark of this tumor. A deep penetrating burrow is seen growing along the tunica albuginea and invading the corpus cavernosum.* **(Right)** *H&E shows microscopic features of a carcinoma cuniculatum. Most authors consider this tumor to be a variant of VC with hybrid foci. Note the tumoral burrows containing abundant keratin.*

Burrowing Pattern in Carcinoma Cuniculatum

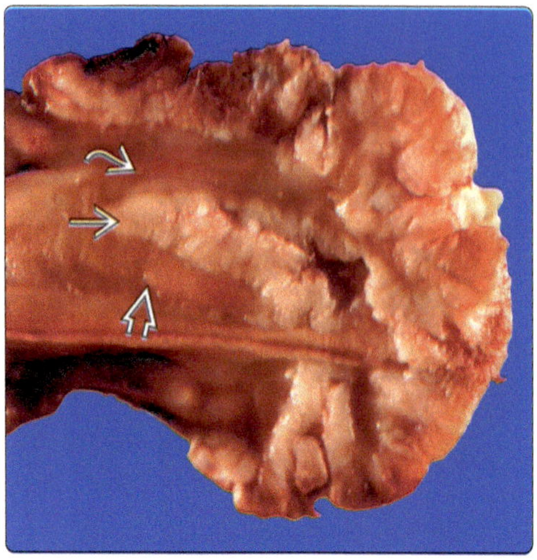

Carcinoma Cuniculatum

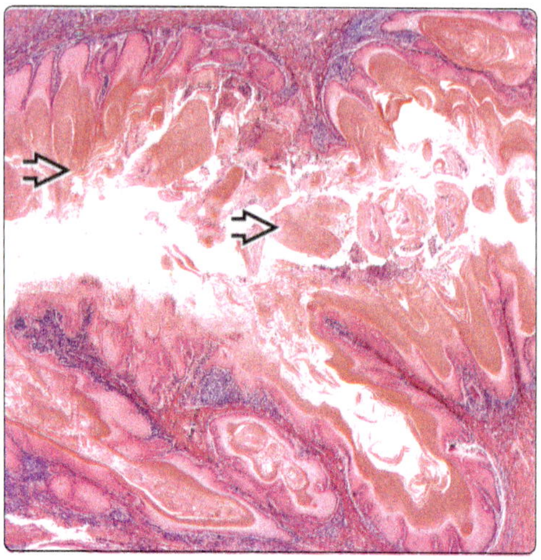

Verrucous Carcinoma Graphic

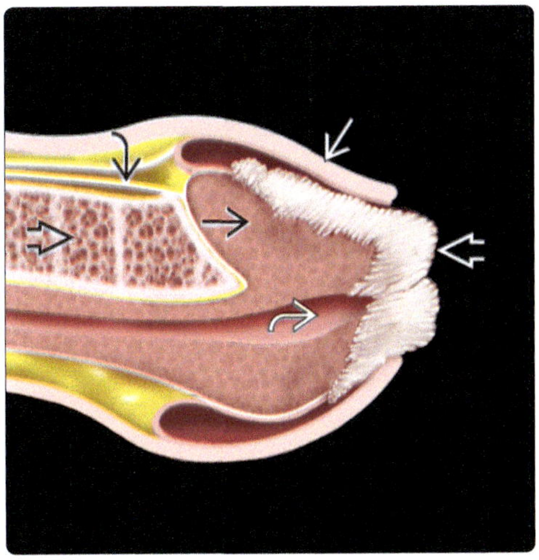

Verrucous Carcinoma

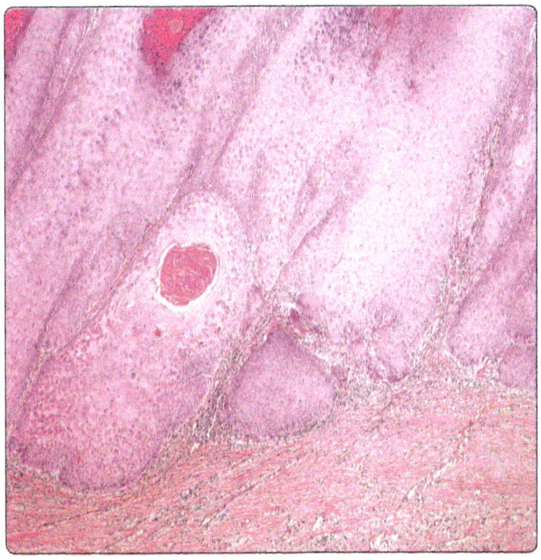

(Left) *Graphic of a VC (white) highlights the papillary, spiky surface and well-demarcated base. Note the VC ⇨, corpus spongiosum ⇨, foreskin ➡, albuginea ↪, corpus cavernosum ⇨, and urethra ↪.* **(Right)** *Well-differentiated tumor with a well-defined stromal-tumor interface shows that there is papillomatosis, acanthosis, and hyperkeratosis.*

Bland Cytology

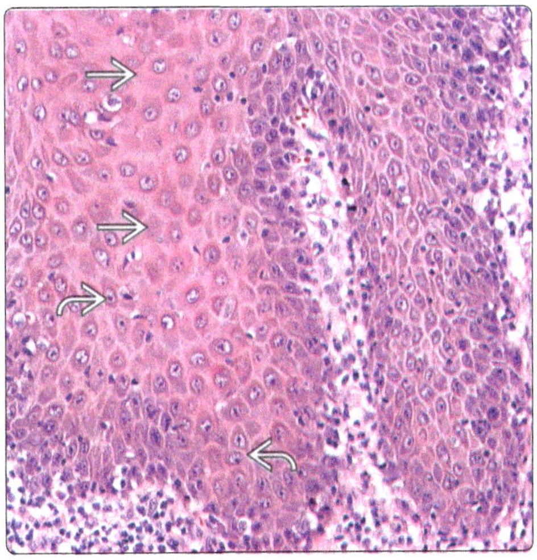

Papillary Carcinoma

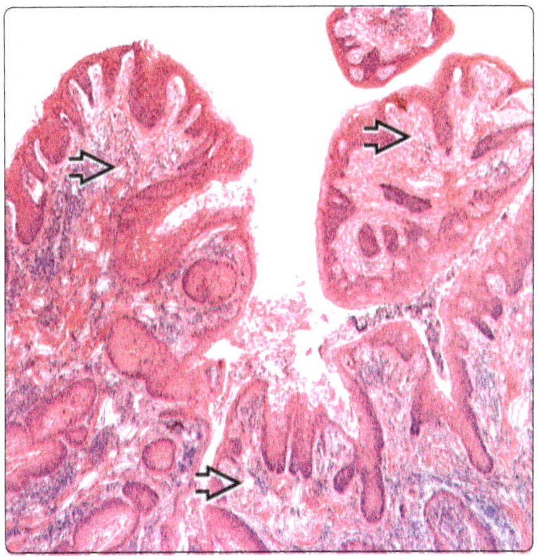

(Left) *High magnification of VC shows enlarged, bland-appearing squamous cells with abundant, dense eosinophilic to amphophilic-staining cytoplasm ➡ and nuclei with vesicular chromatin and small to mildly enlarged nucleoli ↪.* **(Right)** *Papillary carcinoma, not otherwise specified, shows arborescent papillae. Fibrovascular cores ⇨ are more prominent than in VC. Papillary carcinoma is less well differentiated than VC and shows infiltrative deep borders. It is distinguished from warty carcinoma by the lack of koilocytic changes.*

Craters of Keratin

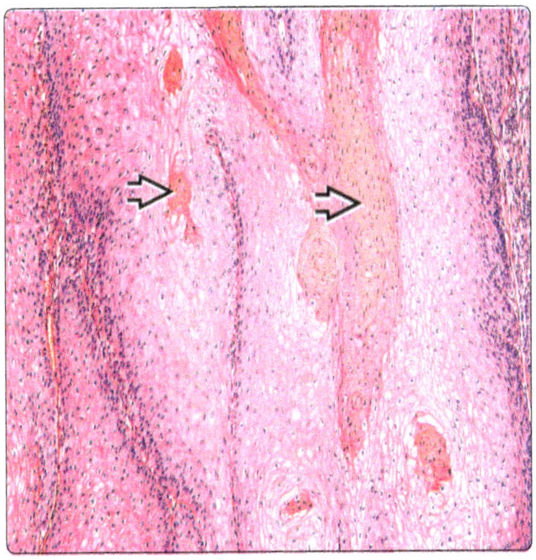

Hybrid (Mixed) Verrucous Carcinoma

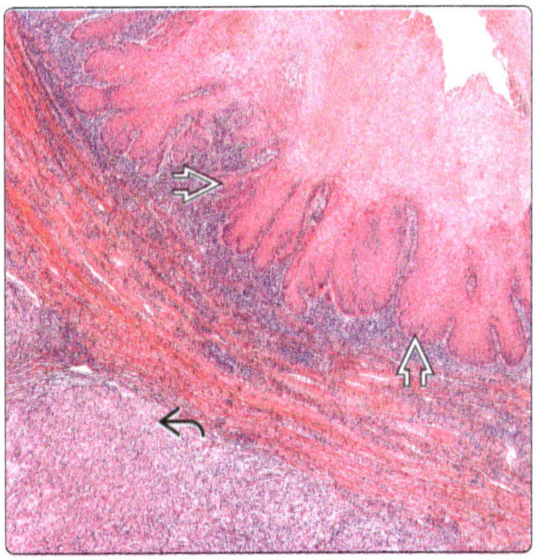

(Left) *High magnification of VC shows a very well-differentiated squamous tumor with craters containing abundant (orange-staining) keratin material ⇨ with parakeratosis.* **(Right)** *Hybrid (mixed) VC shows areas of classic VC ➡ associated with less differentiated areas ↪. These tumors have worse prognosis than pure VC.*

Squamous Cell Carcinoma (and Variants)

KEY FACTS

TERMINOLOGY

- Squamous cell carcinoma (SCC)
  - Malignant epithelial tumor of squamous keratinocytes

ETIOLOGY/PATHOGENESIS

- Most cases are related to UV radiation
- Previous radiation therapy implicated in some cases; usually associated with more aggressive SCC

CLINICAL ISSUES

- Often arises in sun-damaged skin of elderly patients (usually head and neck)
  - Vast majority of cases associated with preexisting actinic keratosis (AK)
- Complete surgical excision is optimal and definitive therapy
- Prognosis usually good in superficial and well-differentiated cases
- Worse prognosis with poorly differentiated, deeply invasive, or aggressive subtypes

MICROSCOPIC

- Proliferation of invasive atypical keratinocytes, often with areas of keratinization (keratin pearls) and squamous eddies
- Cells are present in nests, sheets, and cords
- Cytologically, cells show abundant eosinophilic cytoplasm and large nucleus with vesicular chromatin and prominent nucleoli
- Degree of differentiation is variable, ranging from well to moderately to poorly differentiated
- Multiple variants of differing malignant potential described

TOP DIFFERENTIAL DIAGNOSES

- Basal cell carcinoma
- Atypical fibroxanthoma
- Poorly differentiated carcinoma (Including metastatic)
- Pseudoepitheliomatous hyperplasia
- Keratoacanthoma

Clinical Photograph of Squamous Cell Carcinoma

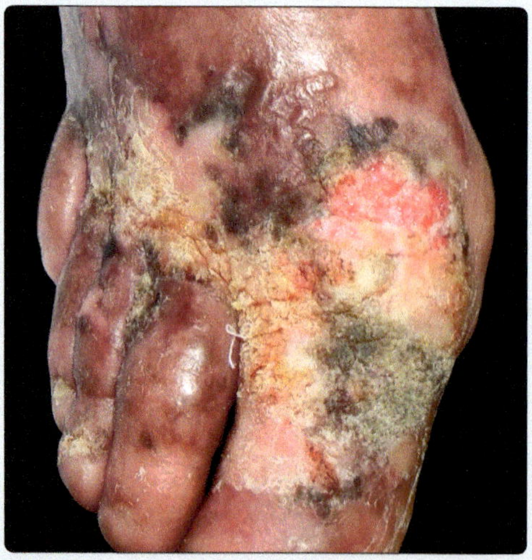

Invasive, Well-Differentiated Squamous Cell Carcinoma

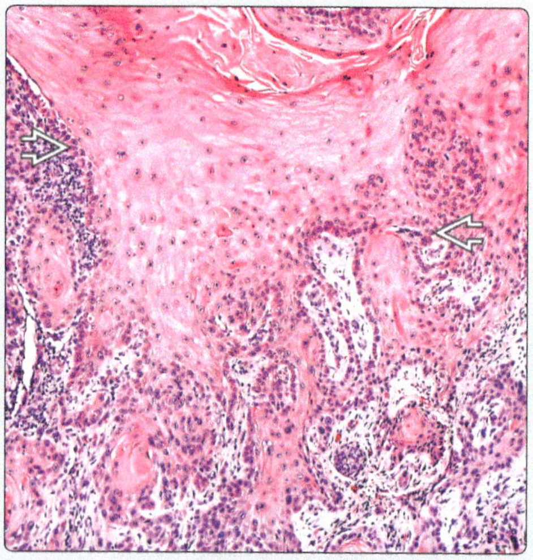

(Left) *Clinical photograph shows an extensive squamous cell carcinoma (SCC) arising on the distal foot in a patient with a history of previous burn injury. (Courtesy S. Yashar, MD.)* **(Right)** *Invasive, well-differentiated SCC is seen arising in association with an actinic keratosis ➡.*

Invasive, Well-Differentiated Squamous Cell Carcinoma on Ear

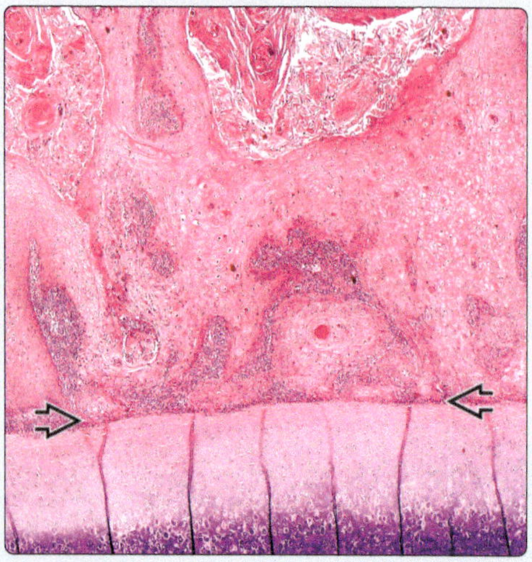

Moderately Differentiated Invasive Squamous Cell Carcinoma

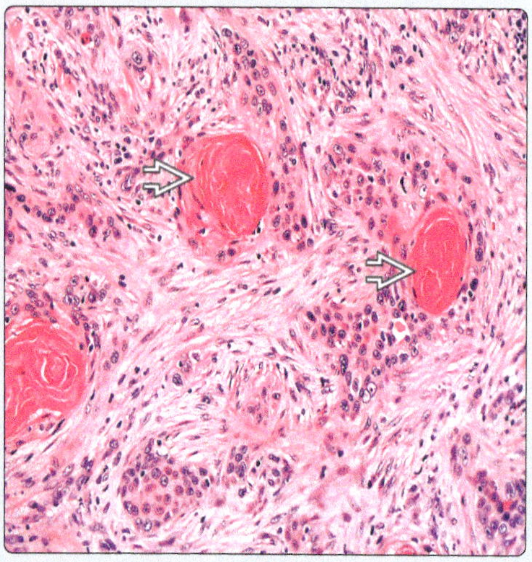

(Left) *Invasive, well-differentiated SCC of the ear invading up to ➡ (but not into) the auricular cartilage is shown.* **(Right)** *Moderately differentiated invasive SCC shows prominent keratin pearls ➡ and a sclerotic stroma with scattered inflammatory cells.*

TERMINOLOGY

Abbreviations

- Squamous cell carcinoma (SCC)

Synonyms

- Sarcomatoid carcinoma (spindle cell carcinoma/carcinosarcoma/metaplastic carcinoma)
- Acantholytic (adenoid/pseudoglandular) SCC
- Verrucous carcinoma: Well-differentiated variant
- Keratoacanthoma (KA): Very well-differentiated variant, regresses spontaneously

Definitions

- Malignant tumor of squamous keratinocytes

ETIOLOGY/PATHOGENESIS

Environmental Exposure

- Most cases are related to UV radiation
- Some cases are likely related to chronic inflammation (i.e., SCC arising in burns, lupus, lichen planus)
- Previous radiation therapy is implicated in some cases; usually associated with more aggressive SCC
- Chronic wounds and burn scars also can be associated with high-risk SCC
- Human papillomavirus is associated with some cases
  - Especially verrucous carcinoma (low grade) and SCC in immunosuppressed patients (high grade)

CLINICAL ISSUES

Epidemiology

- Age
  - Usually in elderly, especially solar-related lesions
  - However, can present in wide age range (34-95 years)
    - Rare cases in children (should prompt genetic studies)
- Sex
  - Slightly more common in males, overall

Presentation

- Slow-growing papular, nodular, or plaque lesion
- Often arises in sun-damaged skin (head and neck tumors)
  - Vast majority of cases associated with preexisting actinic keratosis (AK)
- May be ulcerated or bleeding
- Ear canal and middle ear tumors may present with pain, hearing loss, and discharge

Treatment

- Surgical approaches
  - Complete surgical excision is optimal and definitive therapy
    - Mohs surgery has been shown to be highly effective for most tumors
- Drugs
  - If patients are not surgical candidates, topical chemotherapeutics or immunomodulators may be used
- Radiation
  - May be used for very advanced cases where surgical therapy is not curative

Prognosis

- Usually excellent in most cases
- Worse prognosis with poorly differentiated, deeply invasive, or rare aggressive subtypes
- Site of tumor important for prognosis
  - Lip and ear tumors more aggressive, regardless of degree of differentiation

MACROSCOPIC

General Features

- Papular to nodular or plaque-like lesion; can be exophytic
  - May be ulcerated or hemorrhagic

Size

- Variable; can be small or large lesions

MICROSCOPIC

Histologic Features

- Proliferation of atypical keratinocytes invading into dermis
  - Cells are present in nests, sheets, and infiltrative cords
  - Often show areas of keratinization (keratin pearls) and squamous eddies
  - Attachments to overlying epidermis in most cases
  - Associated AK is very common; less likely, may be associated with SCC in situ (Bowen disease)
  - Cytologically, cells show abundant eosinophilic cytoplasm and large nucleus with vesicular chromatin and prominent nucleoli
  - Intercellular bridges (desmosomes) should be present on high-power examination
  - Presence of dyskeratotic cells (apoptotic keratinocytes) is reliable sign of squamous differentiation
  - If no definite squamous differentiation is present, immunohistochemistry should be used to confirm diagnosis
- Degree of differentiation is variable, ranging from well to moderately to poorly differentiated
  - Amount of keratinization typically decreases and cytologic atypia increases with higher grades
  - Mitotic figures are usually numerous, and atypical forms are found, especially in moderately to poorly differentiated cases
- Multiple variants of differing malignant potential described
  - Low-risk variants include well-differentiated SCC arising in AK, KA, verrucous carcinoma, and tricholemmal (variant of clear cell) carcinoma
  - Intermediate-risk variants include acantholytic (adenoid/pseudoglandular) and lymphoepithelioma-like carcinoma of the skin
  - High-risk variants include spindle cell/sarcomatoid, basaloid, adenosquamous, and desmoplastic
    - Also, radiation, burn scar, and immunosuppression-related SCCs
  - Rare variants of uncertain malignant potential include clear cell SCC, signet ring cell SCC, follicular SCC, papillary SCC, pigmented SCC, and SCC arising from adnexal ducts or cysts

Predominant Pattern/Injury Type

- Epithelioid/squamoid

Predominant Cell/Compartment Type

- Squamous cell

ANCILLARY TESTS

Immunohistochemistry

- Not necessary in well-/moderately differentiated cases but may be needed in poorly differentiated and spindle cell cases
- Cytokeratins are most important markers, especially high molecular weight cytokeratins (HMWCKs)
  - HMWCKs are most sensitive markers for poorly differentiated and spindle cell/sarcomatoid SCC
    - Pankeratin can be lost in poorly differentiated and spindle cell tumors
  - p63 is also very sensitive marker and can be used in addition to HMWCK to confirm diagnosis
- Vimentin is very nonspecific and may be positive in spindle cell/sarcomatoid cases
- Negative staining for other markers, including
  - S100, SOX10, MART-1/Melan-A, and HMB-45 (melanoma)
  - CD10, CD68, and CD99 [atypical fibroxanthoma (AFX)]
  - Actin-sm and desmin (leiomyosarcoma)
  - BER-EP4, androgen receptor (AR), and D2-40 [basal cell carcinoma (BCC) and sebaceous carcinoma]

DIFFERENTIAL DIAGNOSIS

Basal Cell Carcinoma

- Cells are typically smaller, more hyperchromatic, and show peripheral palisading, mucinous stroma, and retraction artifact
- Cytokeratins do not distinguish basal cell carcinoma (BCC) from SCC, but BER-EP4 and AR are almost always positive in BCC; negative in SCC

Atypical Fibroxanthoma

- Usually large, nodular lesion in heavily sun-damaged skin (typically head and neck)
- Immunohistochemistry is essential in excluding poorly differentiated SCC
  - SCC is typically positive for HMWCKs and p63; atypical fibroxanthoma is negative for these markers and often CD10(+) and CD99(+)

Poorly Differentiated Carcinoma (Including Metastatic)

- Clinical history and imaging studies are paramount, as immunohistochemistry may not be able to distinguish some cases from primary SCC
- Adenocarcinomas may show varying degree of ductal/glandular differentiation
  - If present, ductal spaces can be highlighted with markers such as EMA and CEA

Pseudoepitheliomatous Hyperplasia

- Can mimic SCC, especially SCC in situ, but does not show infiltrative features or high-grade cytologic atypia
- Mitotic figures can be numerous but should be in basilar keratinocytes and not atypical

Keratoacanthoma

- Essentially, well-differentiated variant of SCC that spontaneously regresses in most cases
- Typically composed of large, crateriform (cup-like) lesion filled with abundant keratin debris
- Cells are enlarged, with abundant glassy-appearing/hyalinized cytoplasm
- Most cases regress, but giant KA and subungual KA can be aggressive; some may metastasize in immunosuppressed patients

DIAGNOSTIC CHECKLIST

Clinically Relevant Pathologic Features

- Degree of differentiation
- Depth of invasion
  - Deeply invasive tumors have much higher rates of recurrence and metastasis
- Perineural invasion
  - Tumors with perineural invasion have high rates of local recurrence and increased risk of metastasis
- Location of tumor important (i.e., facial sites, including lip and mucosal lesions, are more aggressive)

Pathologic Interpretation Pearls

- Invasive proliferation of epithelioid cells, with areas of keratinization (keratin pearls) and squamous eddies
  - Intercellular bridges (desmosomes) and dyskeratotic cells confirm squamous differentiation in poorly differentiated cases
- Adjacent or overlying AK often present in external ear cases

SELECTED REFERENCES

1. Kallini JR et al: Squamous cell carcinoma of the skin: epidemiology, classification, management, and novel trends. Int J Dermatol. 54(2):130-40, 2015
2. Chu MB et al: Evaluation of the definitions of "high-risk" cutaneous squamous cell carcinoma using the american joint committee on cancer staging criteria and national comprehensive cancer network guidelines. J Skin Cancer. 2014:154340, 2014
3. Emmert S et al: Molecular biology of basal and squamous cell carcinomas. Adv Exp Med Biol. 810:234-52, 2014
4. Yang A et al: Primary cutaneous myxoid spindle cell squamous cell carcinoma: a clinicopathologic study and review of the literature. J Cutan Pathol. 37(4):465-74, 2010
5. Garcia-Zuazaga J et al: Cutaneous squamous cell carcinoma. Adv Dermatol. 24:33-57, 2008
6. Ulrich C et al: Skin cancer in organ transplant recipients--where do we stand today? Am J Transplant. 8(11):2192-8, 2008
7. Weinberg AS et al: Metastatic cutaneous squamous cell carcinoma: an update. Dermatol Surg. 33(8):885-99, 2007
8. Cassarino DS et al: Cutaneous squamous cell carcinoma: a comprehensive clinicopathologic classification--part one. J Cutan Pathol. 33(3):191-206, 2006
9. Cassarino DS et al: Cutaneous squamous cell carcinoma: a comprehensive clinicopathologic classification--part two. J Cutan Pathol. 33(4):261-79, 2006
10. Veness MJ et al: High-risk cutaneous squamous cell carcinoma of the head and neck: results from 266 treated patients with metastatic lymph node disease. Cancer. 106(11):2389-96, 2006
11. Leibovitch I et al: Cutaneous squamous cell carcinoma treated with Mohs micrographic surgery in Australia I. Experience over 10 years. J Am Acad Dermatol. 53(2):253-60, 2005
12. Lindelöf B et al: Cutaneous squamous cell carcinoma in organ transplant recipients: a study of the Swedish cohort with regard to tumor site. Arch Dermatol. 141(4):447-51, 2005
13. Rowe DE et al: Prognostic factors for local recurrence, metastasis, and survival rates in squamous cell carcinoma of the skin, ear, and lip. Implications for treatment modality selection. J Am Acad Dermatol. 26(6):976-90, 1992

Acantholytic (Adenoid) Type of Squamous Cell Carcinoma

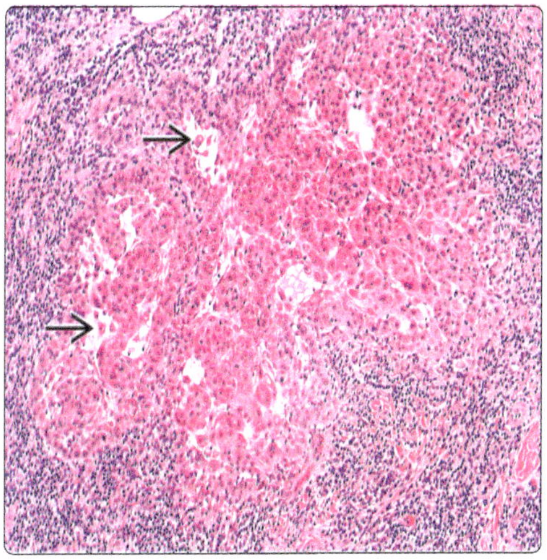

High Magnification of Acantholytic SCC

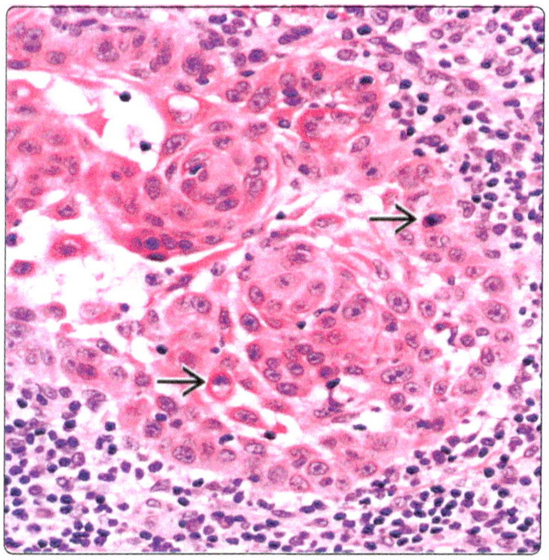

(Left) *Acantholytic (adenoid) type of invasive SCC shows scattered cystic spaces containing dyscohesive squamous cells* ➡*. This variant of SCC may mimic an adenocarcinoma (pseudoglandular SCC) or even an angiosarcoma (pseudovascular SCC).* **(Right)** *High-power view of acantholytic SCC shows large epithelioid cells with dense eosinophilic cytoplasm and scattered dyskeratotic (apoptotic) cells* ➡*. There is an associated heavy inflammatory cell infiltrate.*

Invasive Squamous Cell Carcinoma Arising in Seborrheic Keratosis

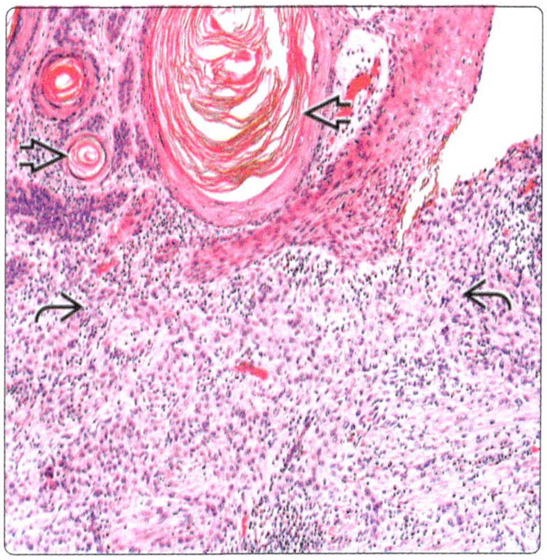

Poorly Differentiated Invasive SCC With Desmoplastic Features

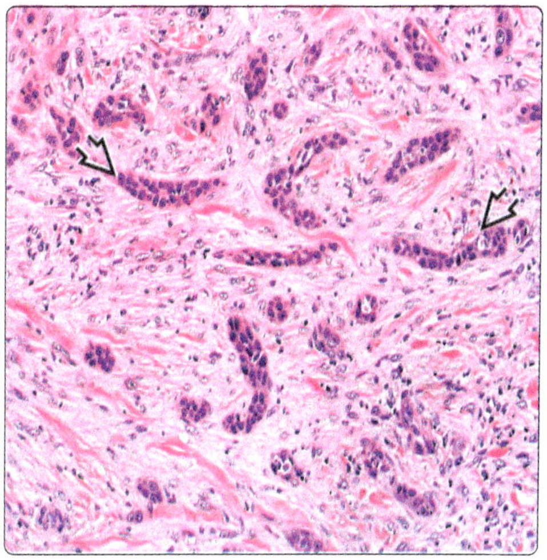

(Left) *A rare invasive SCC arising in association with a seborrheic keratosis shows sheets of moderately to poorly differentiated infiltrating squamous cells* ↗*, with an overlying seborrheic keratosis with pseudohorn cysts present* ⇨*.* **(Right)** *This is an example of a poorly differentiated infiltrating SCC forming cords (mimicking ductal structures)* ⇨*. There is an associated dense desmoplastic stroma.*

Poorly Differentiated Squamous Cell Carcinoma

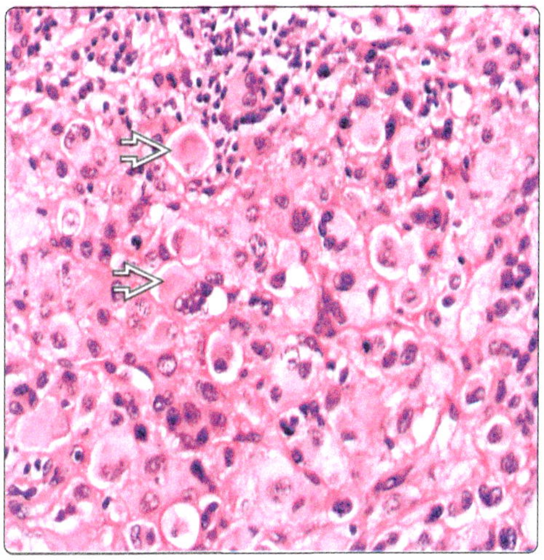

SCC With Lymphoepithelioma-Like Carcinoma Features

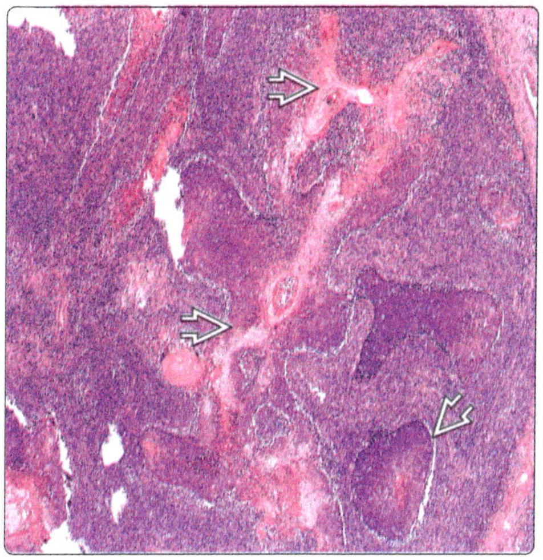

(Left) *High-grade invasive SCC shows a sheet-like proliferation of atypical and pleomorphic epithelioid and multinucleated cells with hyperchromatic nuclei, prominent nucleoli, and abundant glassy-appearing eosinophilic cytoplasm* ➡*.* **(Right)** *Heavily inflamed invasive SCC with moderately differentiated tumor islands* ➡ *composed of basaloid to squamoid cells is surrounded by a sea of inflammatory cells, features suggestive of the lymphoepithelioma-like carcinoma of the skin (LELCS) variant.*

(Left) *Poorly differentiated invasive SCC shows signet ring cell-like features and areas of myxoid stroma ➡ (myxoid SCC).* **(Right)** *Higher power view of poorly differentiated myxoid SCC shows epithelioid to signet ring-like, eosinophilic-staining cells with focal extracellular mucin ➡.*

Poorly Differentiated Squamous Cell Carcinoma With Myxoid Features

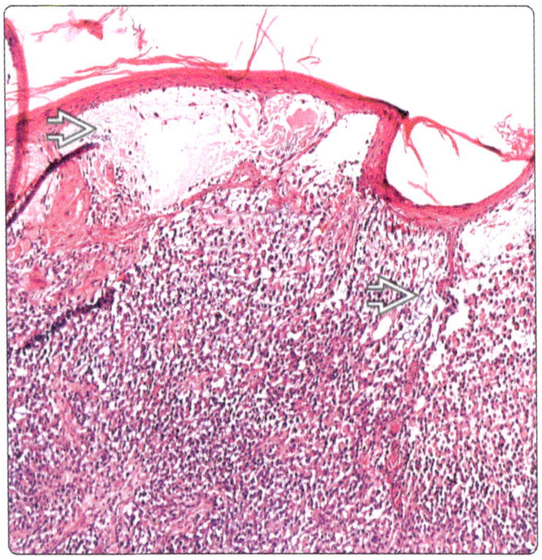

Poorly Differentiated Squamous Cell Carcinoma With Myxoid Features

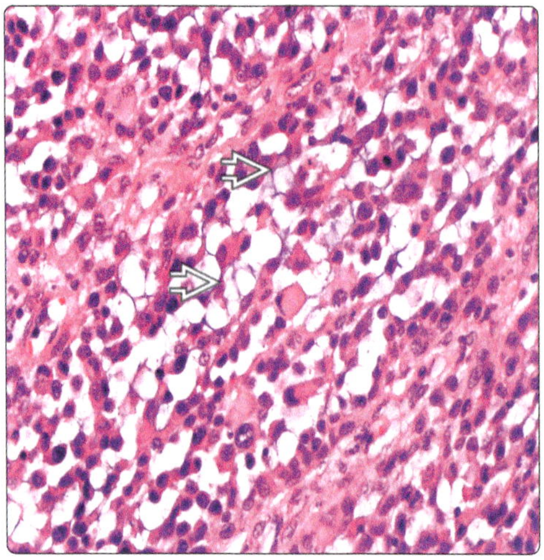

(Left) *Poorly differentiated infiltrating SCC ⇨ associated with a sclerotic (desmoplastic) stroma is shown. This is a high malignant potential variant of SCC.* **(Right)** *SCC in situ (Bowen disease) is seen arising in a longstanding large verruca vulgaris.*

Desmoplastic Squamous Cell Carcinoma

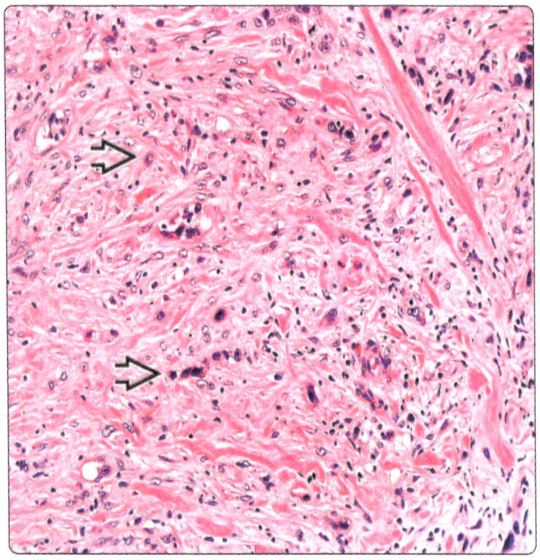

Differential Diagnosis: SCC In Situ (Bowen Disease) Arising in Verruca

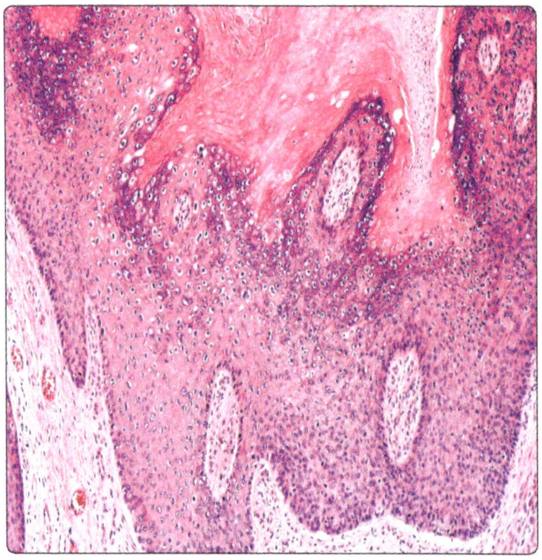

(Left) *Higher power view of the base of the lesion shows tangentially sectioned SCC in situ with smooth borders ⇨ and lack of an infiltrative growth pattern. There is an associated inflammatory cell infiltrate.* **(Right)** *Basosquamous carcinoma [basal cell carcinoma (BCC) with squamous differentiation] can be mistaken for SCC, especially in small, superficial biopsies. Note, however, the areas of peripheral palisading →, typical of BCC.*

Differential Diagnosis: Squamous Cell Carcinoma In Situ Arising in Verruca

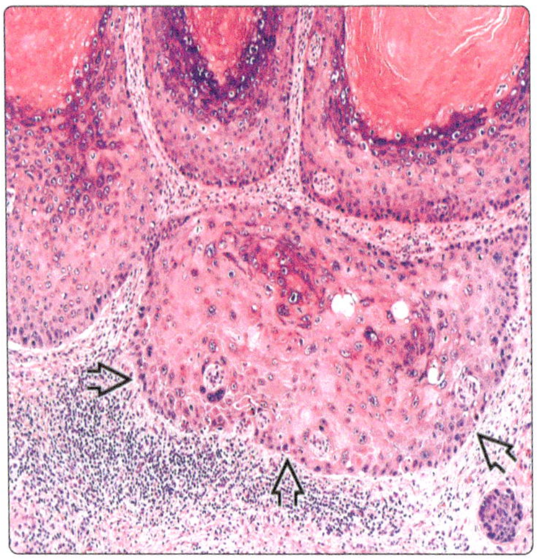

Differential Diagnosis: Basosquamous Carcinoma

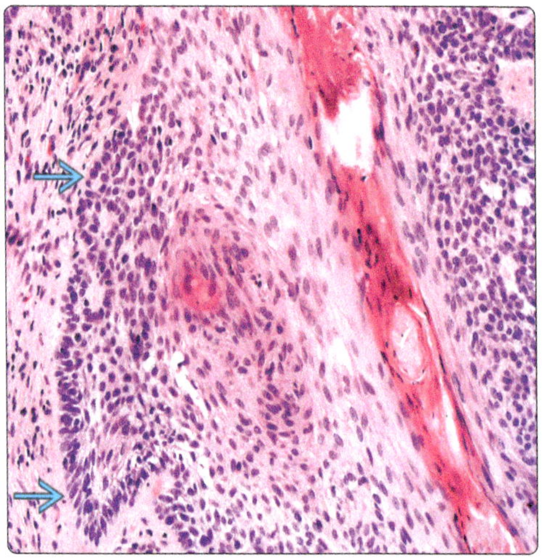

HMWCK Immunohistochemistry in Poorly Differentiated Squamous Cell Carcinoma

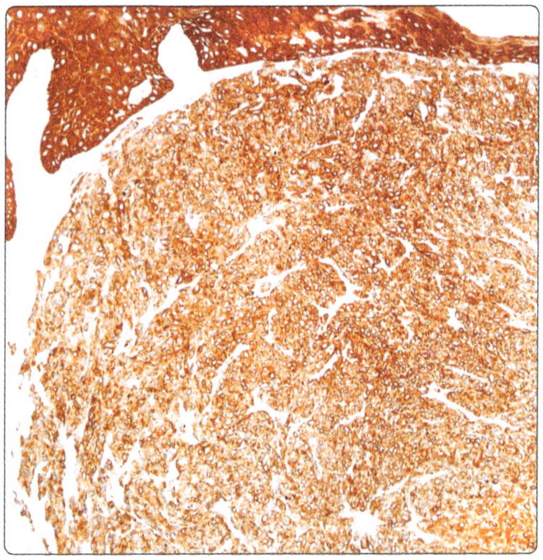

CK-PAN Immunohistochemistry in Poorly Differentiated Squamous Cell Carcinoma

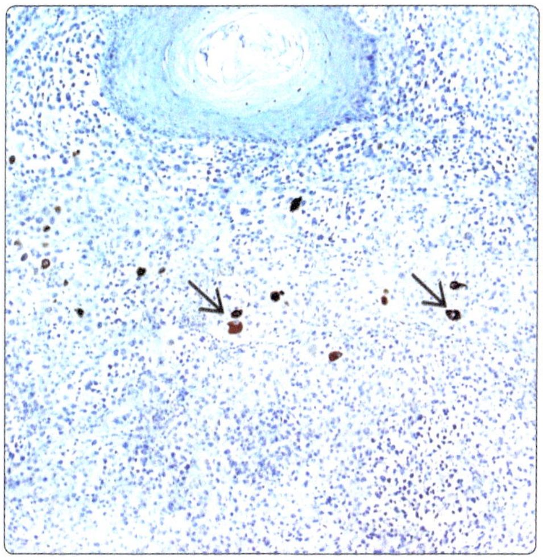

(Left) *CK903 [high molecular weight cytokeratins (HMWCK)] IHC shows strong staining of an invasive, poorly invasive SCC (with strong internal control staining of the overlying epidermis).* **(Right)** *CK-PAN IHC shows only focal staining of a few scattered single cells → in a case of poorly differentiated SCC. CK-PAN is much less sensitive than HMWCKs and p63 in identifying poorly differentiated and sarcomatoid SCC cases.*

CK5/6 in Poorly Differentiated Squamous Cell Carcinoma

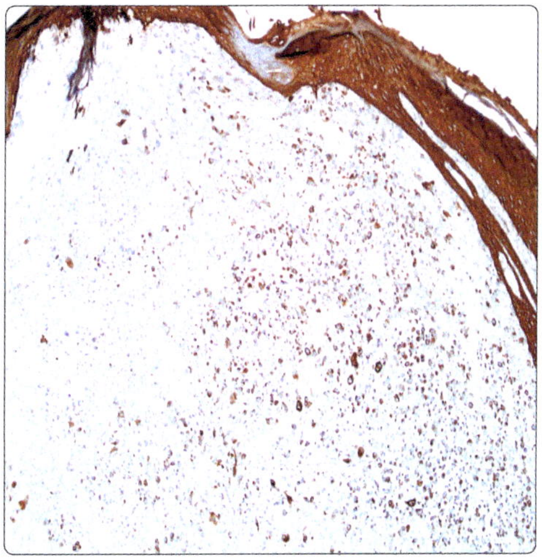

CK5/6 in Poorly Differentiated Squamous Cell Carcinoma

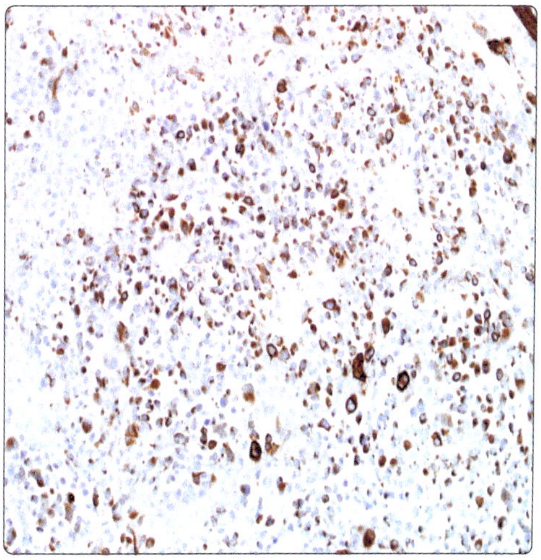

(Left) *CK5/6 (HMWCK) IHC shows strong staining of the epidermis and scattered single cells in a poorly differentiated SCC.* **(Right)** *Higher power view of CK5/6 shows moderate to strong cytoplasmic staining of many of the tumor cells.*

p63 in Lymphoepithelioma-Like Carcinoma SCC

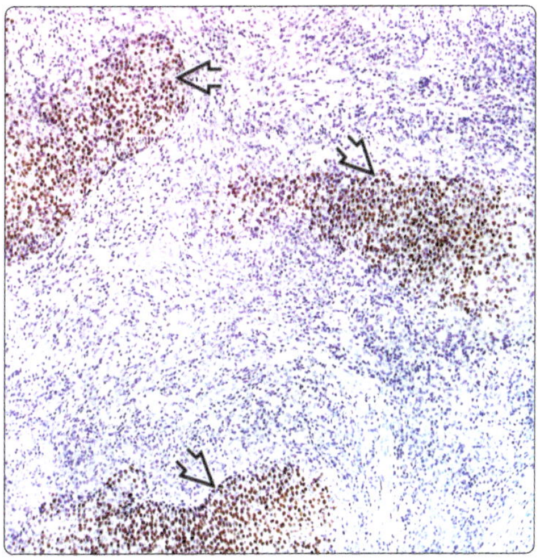

p63 in Poorly Differentiated Squamous Cell Carcinoma

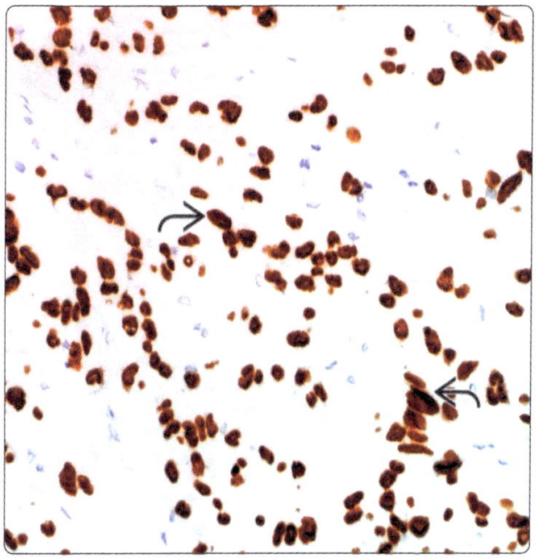

(Left) *IHC stain for p63 in an LELCS shows strong and diffuse nuclear staining in islands of epithelial tumor cells →.* **(Right)** *High-power view of p63 immunohistochemistry shows strong and diffuse nuclear staining of large, irregularly shaped nuclei → in a poorly differentiated infiltrating SCC.*

Keratoacanthoma

KEY FACTS

TERMINOLOGY

- Keratoacanthoma (KA)
- Very well-differentiated form of cutaneous squamous cell carcinoma (SCC), which often spontaneously regresses

ETIOLOGY/PATHOGENESIS

- Similar to other forms of SCC, typically related to chronic solar (UV) damage
- Regression is thought to be due to immune-mediated destruction of squamous cells

CLINICAL ISSUES

- Often dome-shaped with central keratinous plug
- May reach large size, up to 10 cm (giant KA)
- Excellent prognosis; vast majority of cases spontaneously regress
- Head and neck most common, followed by arms, legs

MACROSCOPIC

- Typically large, scaly lesions with central keratinous crater

MICROSCOPIC

- Scanning magnification shows large, nodular, well-differentiated tumor
- Typically appears symmetric with central keratin-filled crater present
- Large squamous cells with abundant, dense eosinophilic-staining cytoplasm and enlarged, hyperchromatic to vesicular-appearing nuclei with prominent nucleoli
- Prominent inflammatory infiltrate, usually with many eosinophils and neutrophils
- Regressing lesions often show epidermal atrophy, dermal fibrosis, and bland cytologic features

TOP DIFFERENTIAL DIAGNOSES

- Conventional well-differentiated SCC
  - Lacks central keratin-filled crater, shows greater cytologic atypia
- Squamous cell carcinoma in situ (SCCis/Bowen disease)
- Verrucous carcinoma

(Left) *Multiple keratoacanthomas can arise in tattoos, most often in the areas of red ink, as in this case.* **(Right)** *Scanning magnification of a keratoacanthoma shows an endophytic-appearing atypical squamous proliferation with prominent, central keratin-filled cavities ➡.*

Clinical Photograph of Multiple Keratoacanthomas Associated With Tattoo

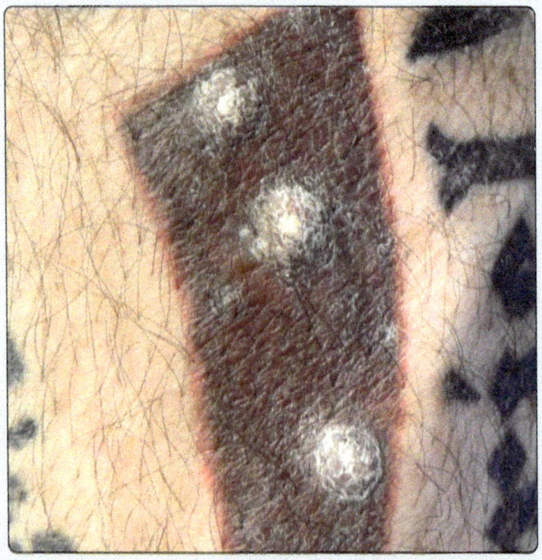

Scanning Magnification of Keratoacanthoma

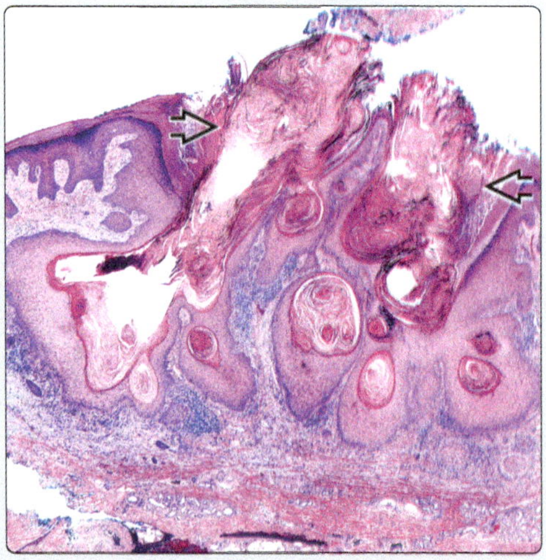

(Left) *Higher magnification of this KA shows enlarged, relatively bland-appearing squamous cells with abundant pale- to eosinophilic-staining cytoplasm. Note the scattered dyskeratotic keratinocytes ➡.* **(Right)** *High magnification shows the relatively bland cytologic features in this lesion, with enlarged pale-staining keratinocytes containing uniform round nuclei and small nucleoli. Note the central collection of dyskeratotic cells ➡.*

Higher Magnification of Keratoacanthoma

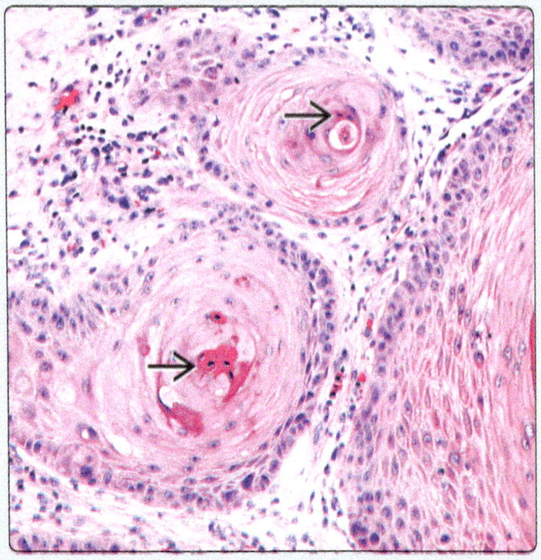

High Magnification of Keratoacanthoma

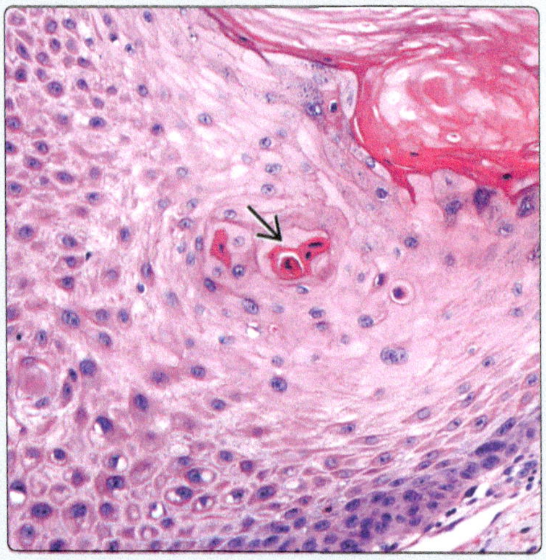

TERMINOLOGY

Abbreviations

- Keratoacanthoma (KA)

Synonyms

- Crateriform ulcer

Definitions

- Very well-differentiated form of cutaneous squamous cell carcinoma (SCC), which often spontaneously regresses

ETIOLOGY/PATHOGENESIS

Environmental Exposure

- Similar to other forms of SCC, typically related to chronic solar (UV) damage
  - Regression is thought to be due to immune-mediated destruction of squamous cells

CLINICAL ISSUES

Epidemiology

- Incidence
  - Relatively common, may represent up to 25% of cases of cutaneous SCC
- Age
  - Older adults, mean is mid 60s
- Sex
  - More common in males
- Ethnicity
  - Most common in Caucasians

Site

- Head and neck most common, followed by arms, legs

Presentation

- Rapidly growing nodular lesion
  - Often dome-shaped with central keratinous plug
  - May reach large size, up to 10 cm (giant keratoacanthoma)

Treatment

- Options, risks, complications
  - Surgical excision is mainstay of treatment, although observation may be acceptable in many cases
- Surgical approaches
  - Complete excision is curative, but likely not necessary in most cases due to spontaneous regression

Prognosis

- Excellent; vast majority of cases spontaneously regress
- Rare case reports of metastatic KA, but most of these are giant or subungual KAs, or in immunosuppressed patients

MACROSCOPIC

General Features

- Typically large, scaly lesions with central keratinous crater

MICROSCOPIC

Histologic Features

- Scanning magnification shows large, nodular, well-differentiated squamous tumor
- Lesion typically appears symmetric with central keratin-filled crater present
- Cells may show infiltrative features at periphery of tumor
  - Perineural and even lymphovascular invasion have been reported in rare cases but do not seem to correlate with increased metastatic potential
- Cells are enlarged, with large nuclei and abundant dense eosinophilic-staining cytoplasm
  - Dyskeratotic cells and mitotic figures usually present, especially in growing lesions
- Prominent inflammatory infiltrate, usually with many eosinophils and neutrophils
- Regressing lesions often show epidermal atrophy and bland cytologic features
  - Dermal fibrosis and chronic inflammation typically present

DIFFERENTIAL DIAGNOSIS

Conventional Squamous Cell Carcinoma

- Well-differentiated SCC may occasionally mimic or arise in KA
- Lacks central keratin-filled crater
- More atypia, mitoses, and infiltrative features
- If lesion appears to be KA, but is only partially sampled, possibility of SCC cannot be excluded

Squamous Cell Carcinoma In Situ (Bowen Disease)

- Not often difficult to distinguish from KA, except in some superficial/partial shave biopsies in which lesion cannot be completely evaluated
- Typically shows prominent cytologic atypia with numerous mitotic figures present throughout full thickness of epidermis

Verrucous Carcinoma

- Shows prominent endophytic and exophytic architecture with deep, bulbous rete ridges
- Lacks central crater of KA
- Cells are large and bland appearing and show similar cytologic features to KA with abundant dense/glassy eosinophilic cytoplasm

SELECTED REFERENCES

1. Ko CJ: Keratoacanthoma: facts and controversies. Clin Dermatol. 28(3):254-61, 2010
2. Weedon DD et al: Squamous cell carcinoma arising in keratoacanthoma: a neglected phenomenon in the elderly. Am J Dermatopathol. 32(5):423-6, 2010
3. Magalhães RF et al: Diagnosis and follow-up of keratoacanthoma-like lesions: clinical-histologic study of 43 cases. J Cutan Med Surg. 12(4):163-73, 2008
4. Cassarino DS et al: Cutaneous squamous cell carcinoma: a comprehensive clinicopathologic classification–part two. J Cutan Pathol. 33(4):261-79, 2006
5. Monroe WM: Keratoacanthoma: a frequent but rarely recognized skin lesion confused with squamous carcinoma. South Med J. 50(7):852-4, 1957

Scanning Magnification of Keratoacanthoma

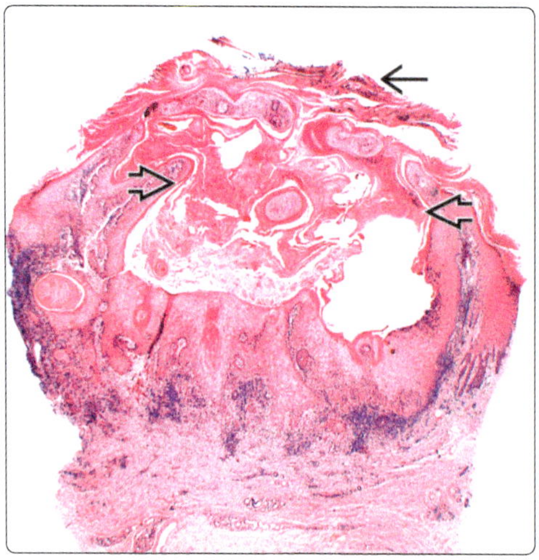

High Magnification of Keratoacanthoma

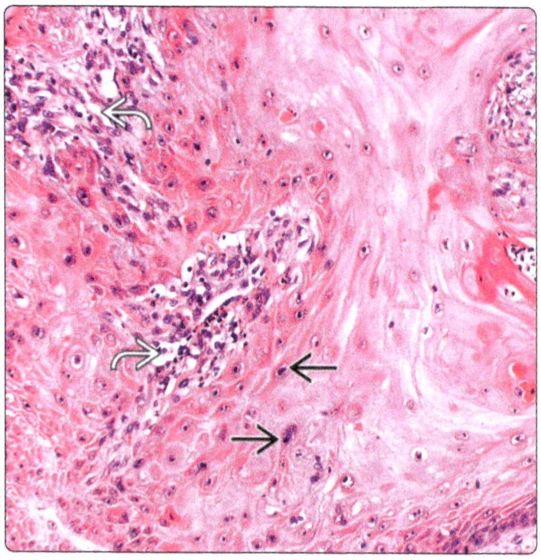

(Left) *Scanning power examination of a relatively small KA shows a symmetric-appearing atypical squamous proliferation with a dilated, central keratin-filled crater and dense overlying parakeratosis.* **(Right)** *High magnification of an area with significant cytologic atypia is characterized by enlarged squamous cells with hyperchromatic nuclei and prominent nucleoli. Note the inflamed papillary dermal stroma.*

Inflammatory Microabscesses in Keratoacanthoma

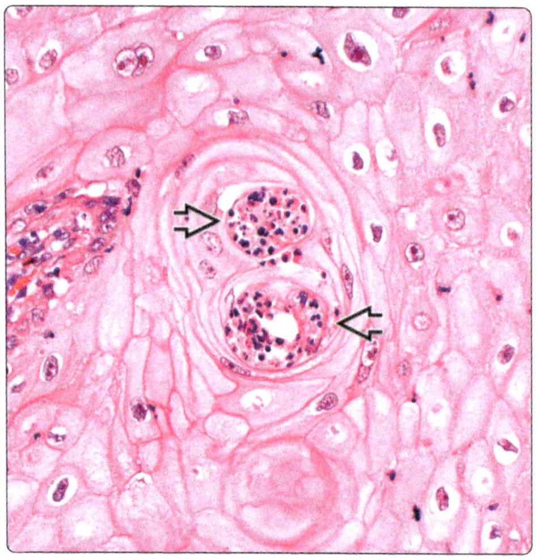

High Magnification of Keratoacanthoma

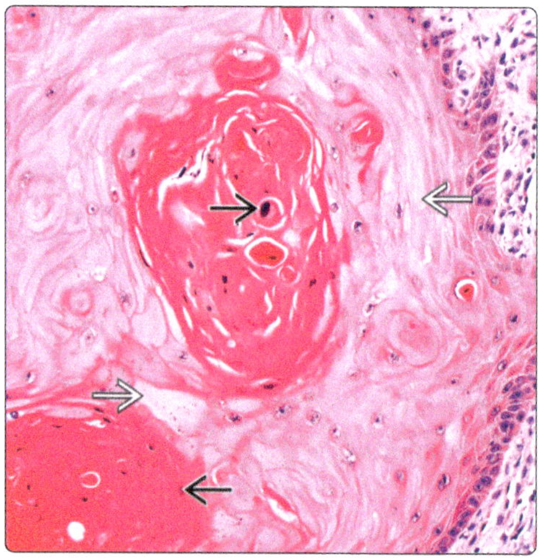

(Left) *Acute inflammation is common in KAs, and intraepithelial microabscesses filled with eosinophils and neutrophils are often seen.* **(Right)** *High magnification shows enlarged keratinocytes with abundant, glassy amphophilic- to eosinophilic-staining cytoplasm. Note the numerous dyskeratotic cells in the foci of keratinization.*

Low Magnification of Endophytic Keratoacanthoma

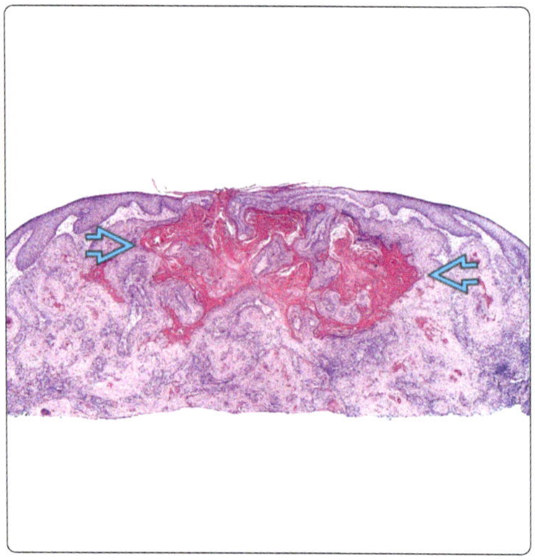

Higher Magnification of Endophytic Keratoacanthoma

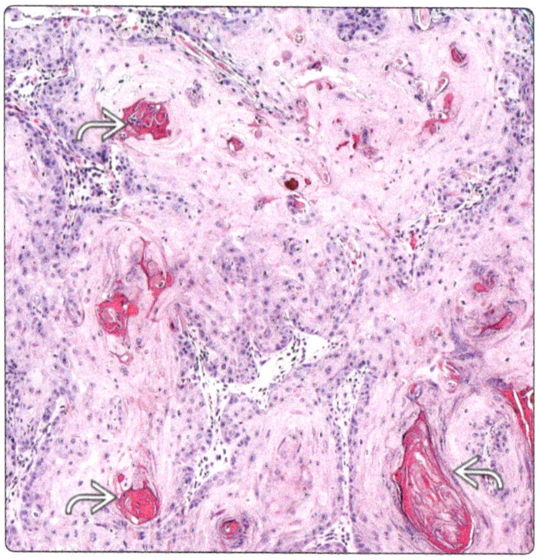

(Left) *This is another example of a KA at low magnification. This case shows an endophytic appearance, with extension of lobules of squamous cells into the dermis. However, a central crateriform area can still be identified.* **(Right)** *Higher magnification of the central area of the endophytic KA shows a proliferation of large, well-differentiated keratinocytes with abundant pale, eosinophilic-staining cytoplasma and multiple foci of keratinization.*

Differential Diagnosis: Squamous Cell Carcinoma

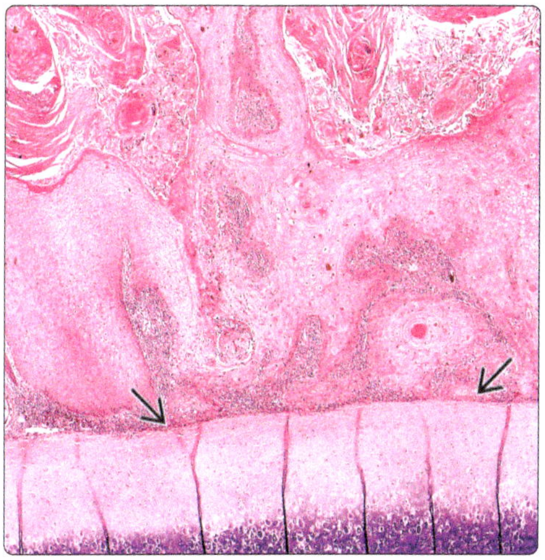

Differential Diagnosis: Squamous Cell Carcinoma

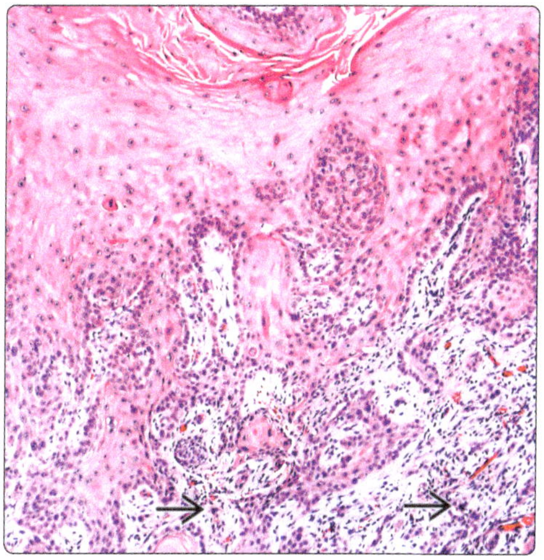

(Left) *This is an example of a well-differentiated SCC with large, glassy-appearing cells mimicking a KA (but lacking the crateriform appearance of KA). This case arose on the ear and invaded deeply to abut the cartilage* ➙. **(Right)** *Higher magnification shows a well-differentiated SCC with some features mimicking a KA, including enlarged squamous cells with abundant glassy-appearing eosinophilic cytoplasm. However, the tumor lacks a central keratin-filled crater, and shows infiltrating single atypical cells in the dermis* ➙.

Differential Diagnosis: Well-Differentiated Squamous Cell Carcinoma

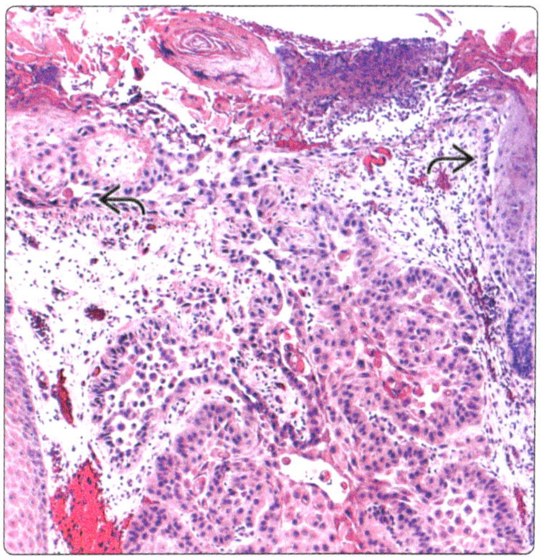

Differential Diagnosis: Moderately Differentiated Squamous Cell Carcinoma

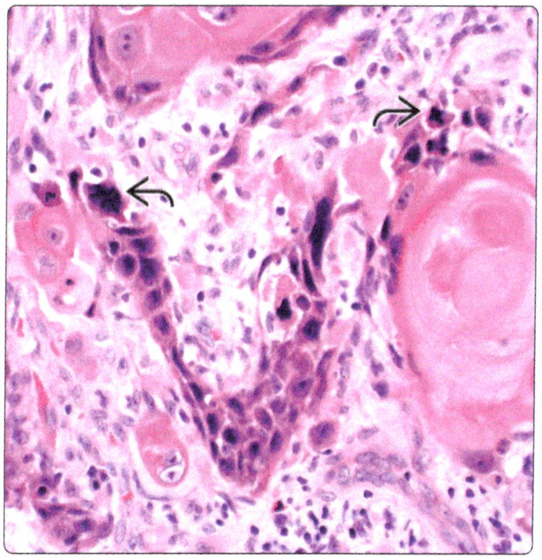

(Left) *KA should be distinguished from cases of conventional SCC, which can be more aggressive. This is an example of an invasive SCC with acantholytic features arising in association with an overlying AK* ➚. **(Right)** *High magnification of an infiltrating, moderately differentiated SCC shows prominent nuclear atypia, pleomorphism, and scattered atypical mitotic figures* ➚. *This degree of atypia should not be seen in KA.*

Differential Diagnosis: Verrucous Carcinoma

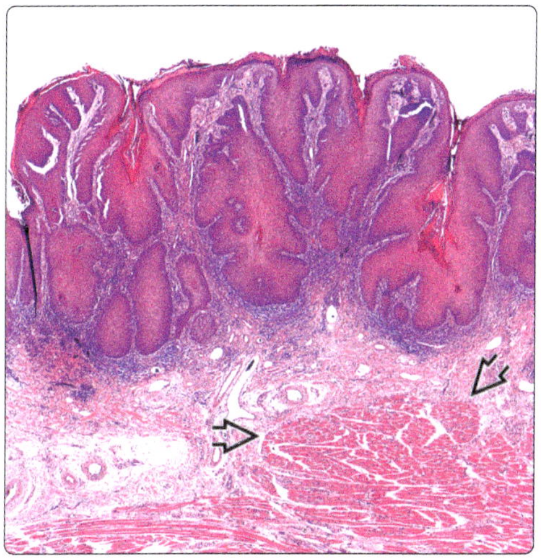

Differential Diagnosis: Verrucous Carcinoma

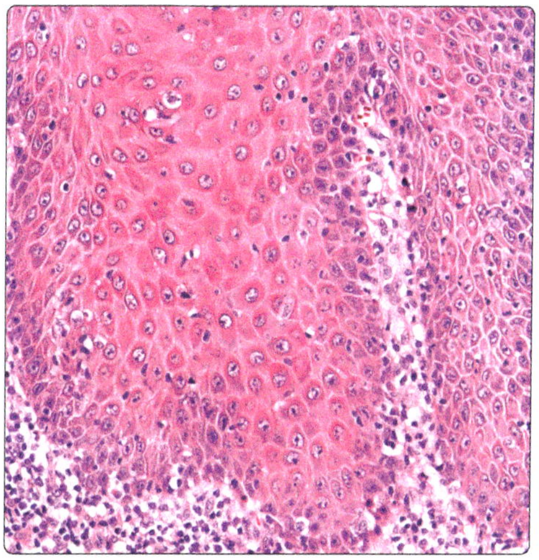

(Left) *Verrucous carcinoma (VC) shows exophytic and endophytic growth patterns with deep pushing invasion. Note underlying skeletal muscle bundles* ➯, *indicating deep extent of invasion.* **(Right)** *High-power examination of VC shows enlarged keratinocytes with dense eosinophilic cytoplasm and nuclei with vesicular chromatin and focally enlarged nucleoli. While the cytologic features can be similar to KA, the architectural features are very different in these tumors.*

Lymphoepithelioma-Like Carcinoma of Skin

KEY FACTS

TERMINOLOGY

- Lymphoepithelioma-like carcinoma of skin (LELCS)
- Poorly differentiated carcinoma with prominent inflammatory infiltrate

ETIOLOGY/PATHOGENESIS

- No relationship with EBV (unlike nasopharyngeal lymphoepitheliomas)

CLINICAL ISSUES

- Extremely rare variant of SCC
- Typically occurs in elderly patients
- Most common in head and neck region
- Complete excision is definitive treatment, similar to invasive SCC
- Low risk of metastasis, but several cases of metastatic disease have been reported

MICROSCOPIC

- Dense dermal infiltrate of predominantly lymphoid cells associated with scattered large epithelioid cells
- Epithelioid cells may form nests or clusters, although they may be difficult to identify due to heavy lymphoid infiltrate
- Focal overlying SCC in situ may be identified in some cases
- Rare cases may represent poorly differentiated adnexal carcinoma

ANCILLARY TESTS

- Epithelioid cells are positive for CKs, especially high molecular weight CKs (CK5-CK6, CK903) and p63
- Lymphoid markers, especially T-cell markers, will highlight dense background lymphoid infiltrate

TOP DIFFERENTIAL DIAGNOSES

- Lymphoma
- Poorly differentiated inflamed carcinoma
- Regressing melanoma with heavy inflammation

Lymphoepithelioma-Like Carcinoma of the Skin

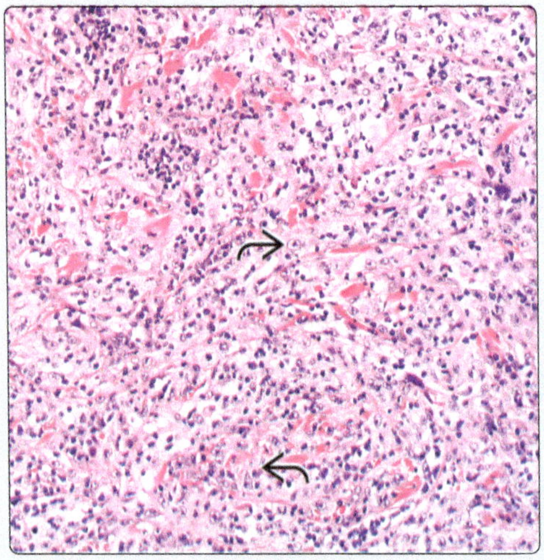

Low Magnification of LELCS

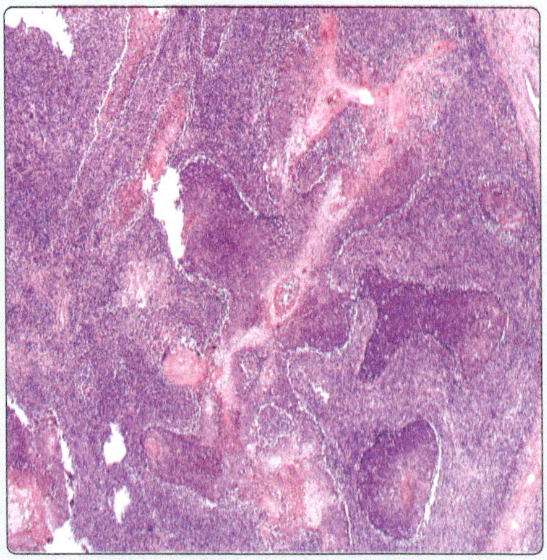

***(Left)** High magnification of lymphoepithelioma-like carcinoma of the skin (LELCS) shows a prominent lymphohistiocytic infiltrate obscuring a background of large, undifferentiated epithelioid-appearing cells →. **(Right)** This is an example of LELCS at low magnification showing large, irregular epithelial islands surrounded by a very dense inflammatory infiltrate.*

High Magnification of LELCS

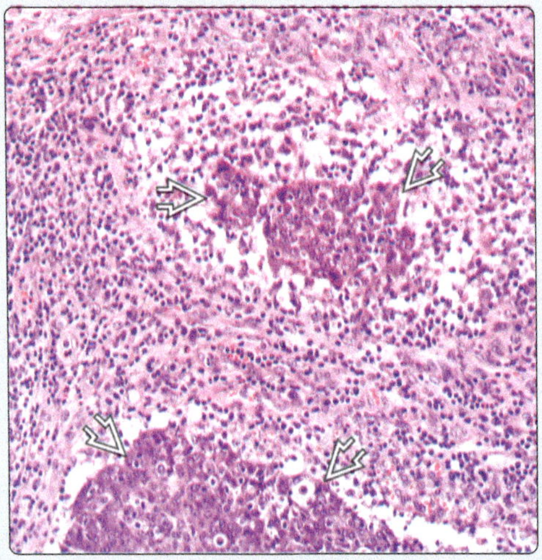

Immunohistochemistry for p63 in LELCS

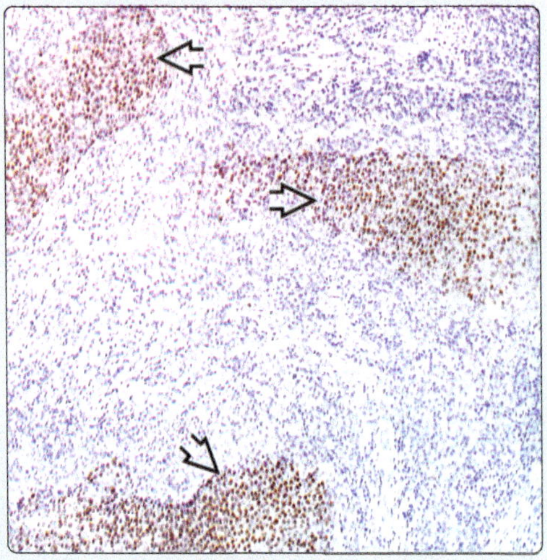

***(Left)** LELCS at high magnification shows islands of atypical basaloid-appearing epithelial cells → surrounded by a dense mixed acute and chronic inflammatory infiltrate. **(Right)** Immunohistochemical stain for p63 shows diffuse nuclear staining → of the epithelial cells, which are in islands surrounded by inflammatory cells.*

TERMINOLOGY

Abbreviations

- Lymphoepithelioma-like carcinoma of skin (LELCS)

Definitions

- Poorly differentiated carcinoma, most likely variant of squamous cell carcinoma (SCC), with prominent inflammatory infiltrate mimicking lymphoepithelioma-like carcinoma of nasopharynx

ETIOLOGY/PATHOGENESIS

Unknown

- No proven relationship with Epstein-Barr virus (EBV), unlike nasopharyngeal lymphoepitheliomas

CLINICAL ISSUES

Epidemiology

- Incidence
  - Extremely rare variant of SCC; < 70 cases reported to date
- Age
  - Typically occurs in elderly patients
- Sex
  - M > F

Site

- Most common in head and neck region

Presentation

- Nodular erythematous lesion

Treatment

- Surgical approaches
  - Complete excision is definitive treatment, similar to invasive SCC

Prognosis

- Low risk of metastasis, but several cases of metastatic disease have been reported
- Currently classified as variant of SCC with intermediate malignant potential

MICROSCOPIC

Histologic Features

- Dermal infiltrate of predominantly lymphoid cells associated with enlarged, atypical epithelioid cells
- Epithelioid cells may form small nests or clusters
  - Tumor cells may be difficult to discern due to heavy lymphoid infiltrate
  - On high-magnification examination, epithelioid cells show enlarged nuclei with vesicular chromatin and prominent nucleoli
- Focal overlying SCC in situ may be identified
- Rare cases may represent poorly differentiated adnexal carcinoma

ANCILLARY TESTS

Immunohistochemistry

- Epithelioid cells are positive for cytokeratins, especially high molecular weight cytokeratins (CK5-CK6, CK903), and p63
- EMA also positive in most cases
- Lymphoid markers, especially T-cell markers, will highlight dense background lymphoid infiltrate

DIFFERENTIAL DIAGNOSIS

Lymphoma

- Atypical lymphocytes lacking epithelial component
- Positive for B- or T-cell markers; negative for cytokeratins and EMA

Poorly Differentiated Inflamed Carcinoma

- Look for areas of well-differentiated carcinoma or overlying carcinoma in situ
- Typically lacks zonation pattern of LELCS
- Immunohistochemistry will be similar to LELCS
- If metastatic tumor, p63 and CK5-CK6 are typically negative; additional organ-specific markers, such as TTF-1, CDX-2, or PSA, may be positive

Regressing Melanoma With Heavy Inflammation

- May be difficult to recognize if only a few residual melanocytes are present
- Overlying melanoma in situ often present
- Immunohistochemistry should show positivity for melanocytic markers including S100, SOX10, Melan-A, HMB-45

DIAGNOSTIC CHECKLIST

Clinically Relevant Pathologic Features

- Size of tumor and depth of invasion likely correlate with prognosis

Pathologic Interpretation Pearls

- Dense dermal infiltrate of predominantly lymphoid cells associated with scattered large atypical epithelioid cells
- Epithelioid cells typically show enlarged nuclei with vesicular chromatin and prominent nucleoli
- Cytokeratins and EMA will highlight epithelial cells
- Lymphoid markers show mixed lymphocytic population

SELECTED REFERENCES

1. Wang G et al: Lymphoepithelioma-like carcinoma vs inflamed squamous cell carcinoma of the skin. JAMA Dermatol. 150(12):1367-8, 2014
2. López V et al: Lymphoepitelioma-like carcinoma of the skin: report of three cases. J Cutan Pathol. 38(1):54-8, 2011
3. Welch PQ et al: Lymphoepithelioma-like carcinoma of head and neck skin: a systematic analysis of 11 cases and review of literature. Oral Surg Oral Med Oral Pathol Oral Radiol Endod. 111(1):78-86, 2011
4. Kazakov DV et al: Absence of Epstein-Barr virus, human papillomavirus, and simian virus 40 in patients of central european origin with lymphoepithelioma-like carcinoma of the skin. Am J Dermatopathol. 29(4):365-9, 2007
5. Cassarino DS et al: Cutaneous squamous cell carcinoma: a comprehensive clinicopathologic classification–part two. J Cutan Pathol. 33(4):261-79, 2006
6. Wick MR et al: Lymphoepithelioma-like carcinoma of the skin with adnexal differentiation. J Cutan Pathol. 18(2):93-102, 1991
7. Swanson SA et al: Lymphoepithelioma-like carcinoma of the skin. Mod Pathol. 1(5):359-65, 1988

Basal Cell Carcinoma

KEY FACTS

TERMINOLOGY

- Basal cell carcinoma (BCC)
- Low-grade malignancy of basal keratinocytes

ETIOLOGY/PATHOGENESIS

- Related to sun exposure, radiation, immunosuppression
- Rare cases are associated with genetic syndromes

CLINICAL ISSUES

- Extremely common: Most common cancer in humans
- Most common in head and neck region (up to 80% of cases)
- Prognosis usually excellent, most cases cured by excision

MICROSCOPIC

- Proliferation of nodules, nests, and cords of basaloid cells with peripheral palisading, stromal retraction artifact, and mucinous material
- Numerous mitotic and apoptotic figures typically present
- Cells show enlarged hyperchromatic nuclei with inconspicuous nucleoli and scant amounts of cytoplasm
- **Superficial multicentric type**: Superficial nests attached to epidermis separated by areas of uninvolved epidermis
- **Nodular type**: Large, rounded, predominantly dermal-based nests with prominent peripheral palisading
- **Micronodular type**: Predominantly dermal-based infiltrative proliferation of small nests
- **Infiltrative type**: Small cords and nests, often deeply invasive
- **Desmoplastic/sclerosing/morpheaform type**: Infiltrative strands and nests associated with dense sclerotic stroma

TOP DIFFERENTIAL DIAGNOSES

- Squamous cell carcinoma
- Actinic keratosis (on superficial shave biopsy)
- Follicular neoplasms (trichoepithelioma and trichoblastoma)
- Merkel cell carcinoma

Clinical Photograph of Basal Cell Carcinoma

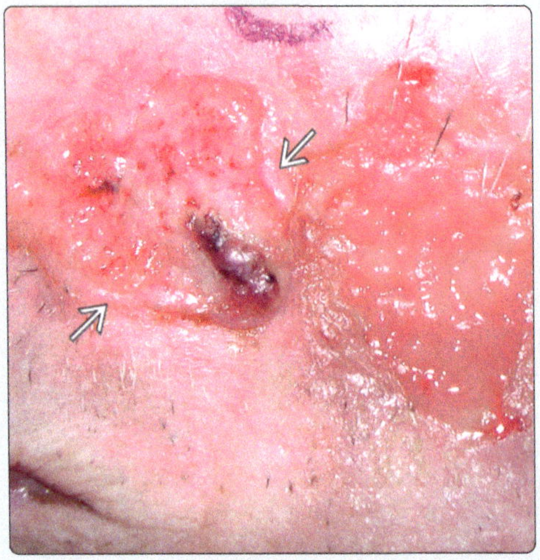

Basal Cell Carcinoma at Low Magnification

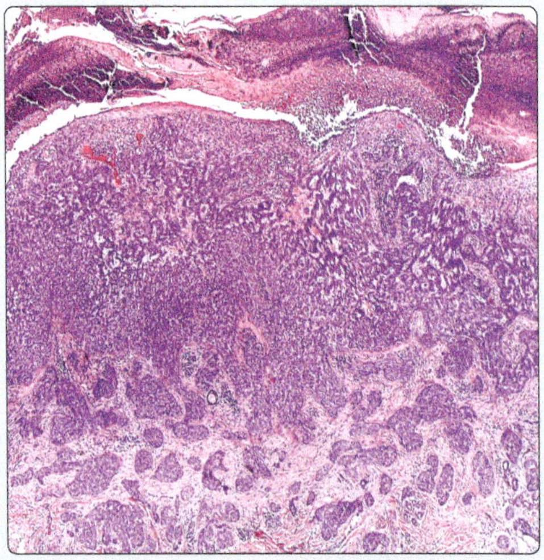

(Left) *Clinical photograph of a large facial basal cell carcinoma (BCC) shows areas of ulceration and granulation-like tissue surrounded by a raised border ⇨. (Courtesy S. Yashar, MD.)* **(Right)** *Low magnification shows a large nodular- and micronodular-type BCC with diffuse overlying ulceration and dense serum crust containing degenerating neutrophils.*

Basal Cell Carcinoma at High Magnification

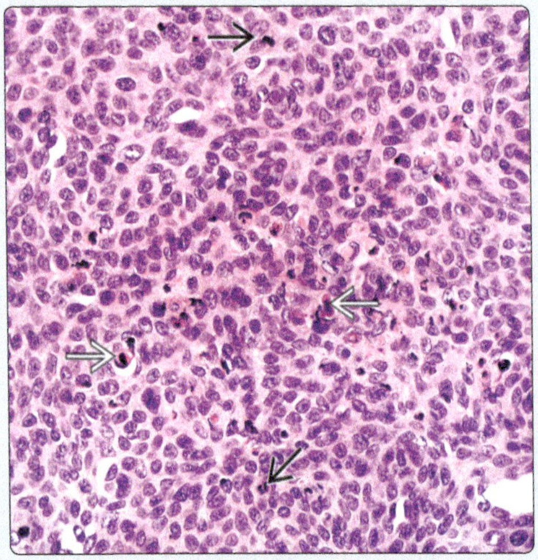

Basal Cell Carcinoma: Micronodular Type

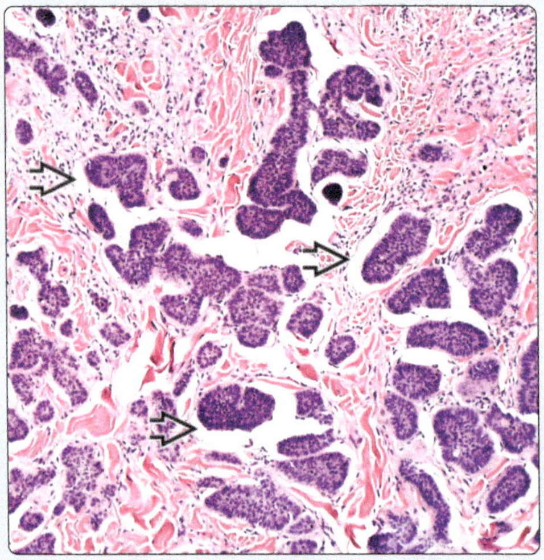

(Left) *High magnification of a nodular BCC shows a sheet-like proliferation of atypical basaloid cells with high nuclear:cytoplasmic ratios and numerous apoptotic ➡ and mitotic figures ⇨.* **(Right)** *Histologic section of a micronodular-type BCC shows a proliferation of small, infiltrative nests of basaloid cells with a prominent retraction artifact ⇨ in a somewhat sclerotic-appearing stroma.*

TERMINOLOGY

Abbreviations

- Basal cell carcinoma (BCC)

Synonyms

- Basal cell epithelioma (BCE)
- Trichoblastic carcinoma (not well accepted and should be discouraged)

Definitions

- Low-grade malignancy of basaloid-appearing keratinocytes

ETIOLOGY/PATHOGENESIS

Multifactorial

- Related to sun exposure (vast majority of cases)
  - Some cases may also be associated with radiation, immunosuppression (organ transplantation), burn scars
    - These cases tend to be more aggressive
- May actually be derived from follicular stem cells (hence, rationale for term trichoblastic carcinoma)

Genetics

- Rare cases are associated with genetic syndromes including nevoid BCC (Gorlin) syndrome, xeroderma pigmentosum, Basex syndrome, Rombo syndrome, and McKusick syndrome
  - Genes implicated include *PTCH1* (Gorlin syndrome), *TP53, SOX9, BMI1, BAX, RMRP*

CLINICAL ISSUES

Epidemiology

- Incidence
  - Extremely common: Most common cancer overall in humans when skin cancers are included
    - Accounts for 70% of primary cutaneous malignancies
- Age
  - Typically older adults; few cases in young adults
    - If in child, should consider genetic syndrome
- Sex
  - Slightly greater incidence in male patients
- Ethnicity
  - Caucasian/light-skinned individuals
  - Rare in individuals with darker skin types

Site

- Most common in head and neck region (up to 80% of cases)
  - ~ 15% occur on trunk and shoulders
  - Very rare cases involve lips, breast, axillae, groin, inguinal region, and genitalia

Presentation

- Typically papular, plaque-like, or nodular lesion
  - Often present as pearly, translucent papule with telangiectasia
  - Larger lesions often ulcerated with bleeding &/or overlying crusting
  - Minority of cases are pigmented, more often in Asians and Africans

Treatment

- Surgical approaches
  - Complete excision or electrodesiccation and curettage
  - Mohs micrographic surgery often used in facial cases

Prognosis

- Usually excellent, cured by local excision
- More aggressive subtypes, including micronodular, infiltrative, desmoplastic, and basosquamous, have higher rate of recurrence and increased (but still very low) risk of metastasis
  - Overall risk of metastasis estimated at 0.05%

MACROSCOPIC

Size

- Variable, small (few mm) to large (several cm)

MICROSCOPIC

Histologic Features

- Tumor is composed of nodules, nests, &/or infiltrative cords
  - Overlying ulceration and serum crusting often present in large tumors
- Proliferation of small basaloid cells with peripheral palisading
- Stromal retraction artifact
  - Between tumor cells and stroma
- Mucinous material often is present in stroma
- Numerous mitotic and apoptotic figures in most cases
- Cells show enlarged, hyperchromatic-staining nuclei with inconspicuous or small nucleoli and scant eosinophilic cytoplasm

Variants

- **Superficial multicentric**: Superficial nests attached to epidermis separated by areas of uninvolved epidermis
- **Nodular**: Large, rounded, predominantly dermal-based nests with prominent peripheral palisading
- **Micronodular**: Predominantly dermal-based infiltrative proliferation of small nests
- **Infiltrative**: Small cords and nests, often deeply invasive
- **Desmoplastic/sclerosing/morpheaform**: Infiltrative strands and nests associated with dense sclerotic stroma
- **Infundibulocystic**: Mature folliculocystic spaces containing keratinous material
- **Basosquamous/metatypical**: Prominent areas of squamous differentiation [may mimic squamous cell carcinoma (SCC)], less peripheral palisading present
- **Fibroepithelioma of Pinkus**: Numerous small, anastomosing cords of basaloid cells attached to epidermis
- Rare variants include adenoid, clear cell, signet ring cell, plasmacytoid/myoepithelial, and BCC with neuroendocrine differentiation

ANCILLARY TESTS

Immunohistochemistry

- Not necessary in most cases except when unusual features present
- BCC vs. trichoepithelioma and trichoblastoma
  - BCC shows greater staining for Bcl-2, p53, and Ki-67
- BCC vs. SCC

- BCC is positive for BER-EP4; SCC is almost always negative
- CK-PAN, high molecular weight cytokeratins, and p63 are not useful, as they are positive in both tumors

DIFFERENTIAL DIAGNOSIS

Squamous Cell Carcinoma

- Most cases are easily separated; however, basosquamous type of BCC shows prominent squamous differentiation
  - Usually, areas of more typical BCC are present, especially at periphery of tumor
  - Overlying actinic keratosis (AK) or Bowen disease often seen in association with SCC
  - BER-EP4 strongly positive in BCC, almost always negative in SCC
- Superficial shave biopsies of ulcerated/inflamed cases may be very difficult or impossible to accurately separate

Actinic Keratosis

- Can be difficult to distinguish on very superficial shave biopsies
  - AK typically shows basilar budding of atypical squamous cells and overlying parakeratosis
  - No mucinous stroma, peripheral palisading, or tumor-stromal retraction artifact should be seen
  - Numerous apoptotic and mitotic figures favor BCC

Follicular Neoplasms (Trichoepithelioma and Trichoblastoma)

- Dermal-based basaloid adnexal neoplasms, may be large and nodular (trichoblastoma)
  - Usually symmetric and well circumscribed at scanning magnification
- Typically lack degree of cytologic atypia, mitoses, and apoptotic figures of BCC
- May show peripheral palisading but mucinous stroma and tumor-stromal retraction artifact typically lacking in benign follicular neoplasms

Merkel Cell Carcinoma

- Nodular to sheet-like proliferation of highly atypical basaloid cells
  - Mucinous stroma and tumor-stromal retraction artifact only rarely identified
  - Peripheral palisading usually absent or only focally present
- Nuclei typically show speckled (salt and pepper) chromatin pattern or nuclear clearing
- Perinuclear dot-like staining with CK20, pancytokeratin, and CAM5.2
- Positive immunoreactivity with neuroendocrine markers

Sebaceous Carcinoma

- Can show prominent areas of basaloid differentiation
- Focal atypical clear/multivacuolated cells with nuclear indentations should be present
- Lacks peripheral palisading, mucinous stroma, or stromal retraction artifact
- Immunohistochemistry may be useful
  - Androgen receptor is positive; also frequently positive in BCC
  - CAM5.2, CD10, and CK7 can be positive or negative; typically negative in BCC
  - EMA often positive in clear cells, although, it is often lost in poorly differentiated cases
  - Strong BER-EP4 and Bcl-2 favor BCC, but they are also positive in some sebaceous carcinomas

DIAGNOSTIC CHECKLIST

Clinically Relevant Pathologic Features

- Aggressive subtypes (micronodular, infiltrative, sclerosing/morpheaform, and basosquamous)
- Deep subcutaneous invasion
- Perineural invasion (< 3% of cases)

Pathologic Interpretation Pearls

- Proliferation of nodules, nests, and cords of small basaloid cells with peripheral palisading, stromal retraction artifact, and mucinous material

SELECTED REFERENCES

1. Gurunluoglu R et al: Nonpersistence of basal cell carcinoma after diagnostic shave biopsy: reconstruction when specimen is negative during surgery. Ann Plast Surg. 74(6):695-8, 2015
2. Webb DV et al: Basal cell carcinoma vs basaloid squamous cell carcinoma of the skin: an immunohistochemical reappraisal. Ann Diagn Pathol. 19(2):70-5, 2015
3. Albert B et al: Interaction of hedgehog and vitamin D signaling pathways in basal cell carcinomas. Adv Exp Med Biol. 810:329-41, 2014
4. Emmert S et al: Molecular biology of basal and squamous cell carcinomas. Adv Exp Med Biol. 810:234-52, 2014
5. Begnini A et al: PTCH1 gene haplotype association with basal cell carcinoma after transplantation. Br J Dermatol. 163(2):364-70, 2010
6. Plaza JA et al: Value of p63 and podoplanin (D2-40) immunoreactivity in the distinction between primary cutaneous tumors and adenocarcinomas metastatic to the skin: a clinicopathologic and immunohistochemical study of 79 cases. J Cutan Pathol. 37(4):403-10, 2010
7. Garcia C et al: Basosquamous carcinoma. J Am Acad Dermatol. 60(1):137-43, 2009
8. Krokowski M et al: Basal cell carcinoma with neuroendocrine differentiation arising in a scar: A case report. Dermatol Online J. 15(10):4, 2009
9. Mosterd K et al: Destructive basal cell carcinoma in a patient with basal cell nevus syndrome and an interstitial deletion of chromosome 9q22. Dermatol Surg. 35(12):2051-3, 2009
10. Cohen PR et al: Basal cell carcinoma with mixed histology: a possible pathogenesis for recurrent skin cancer. Dermatol Surg. 32(4):542-51, 2006
11. Tschen JP et al: Pleomorphic basal cell carcinoma: case reports and review. South Med J. 99(3):296-302, 2006
12. Wadhera A et al: Metastatic basal cell carcinoma: a case report and literature review. How accurate is our incidence data? Dermatol Online J. 12(5):7, 2006
13. Ackerman AB et al: Fibroepithelial tumor of pinkus is trichoblastic (Basal-cell) carcinoma. Am J Dermatopathol. 27(2):155-9, 2005
14. Ting PT et al: Metastatic basal cell carcinoma: report of two cases and literature review. J Cutan Med Surg. 9(1):10-5, 2005
15. Bogdanov-Berezovsky A et al: Risk factors for incomplete excision of basal cell carcinomas. Acta Derm Venereol. 84(1):44-7, 2004
16. Saldanha G et al: Basal cell carcinoma: a dermatopathological and molecular biological update. Br J Dermatol. 148(2):195-202, 2003
17. Kim YC et al: Signet ring cell basal cell carcinoma: a basal cell carcinoma with myoepithelial differentiation. Am J Dermatopathol. 23(6):525-9, 2001
18. Meehan SA et al: Basal cell carcinoma with tumor epithelial and stromal giant cells: a variant of pleomorphic basal cell carcinoma. Am J Dermatopathol. 21(5):473-8, 1999
19. Jones MS et al: The immunohistochemical characteristics of the basosquamous cell carcinoma. Dermatol Surg. 23(3):181-4, 1997
20. Kazantseva IA et al: Immunohistochemical study of primary and recurrent basal cell and metatypical carcinomas of the skin. Am J Dermatopathol. 18(1):35-42, 1996
21. Sina B et al: Fibroepithelioma of Pinkus: eccrine duct spread of basal cell carcinoma. Am J Dermatopathol. 17(6):634-6, 1995
22. Pinkus H: Epithelial and fibroepithelial tumors. Arch Dermatol. 91:24-37, 1965

Pigmented Basal Cell Carcinoma

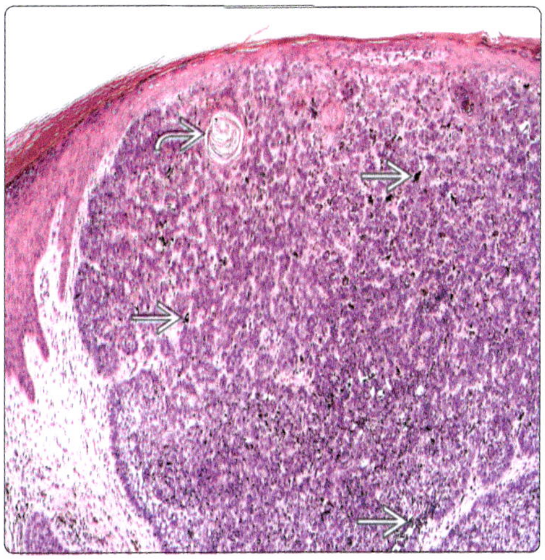

Basal Cell Carcinoma: Clear Cell Type

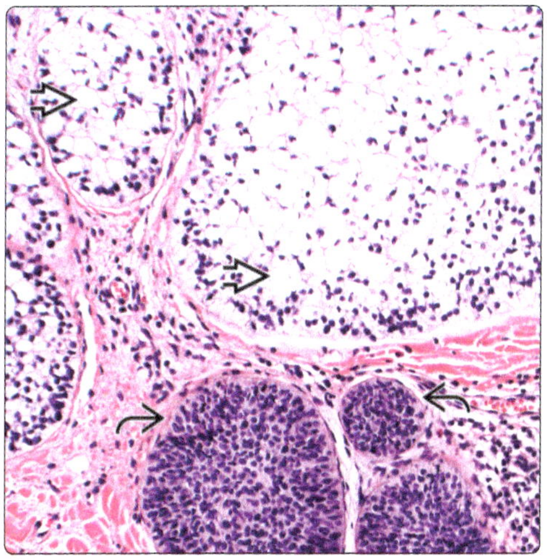

(Left) *Low-power view of a large, pigmented, nodular BCC shows prominent melanin pigmentation throughout the nodule. Note the focal infundibulocystic area.* **(Right)** *Clear cell BCC is composed of large cells with abundant clear cytoplasm and can mimic clear cell squamous cell carcinoma or sebaceous carcinoma in some cases. However, areas of more conventional-appearing BCC are often present, as are seen in the lower portion of this photomicrograph.*

Basal Cell Carcinoma: Basosquamous Type

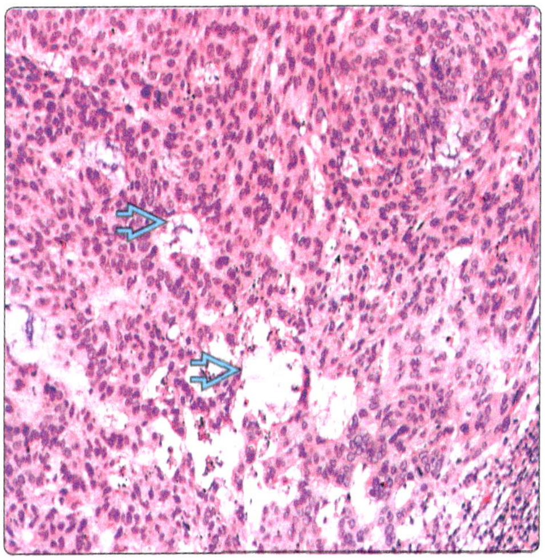

Basal Cell Carcinoma: Fibroepithelioma of Pinkus Type

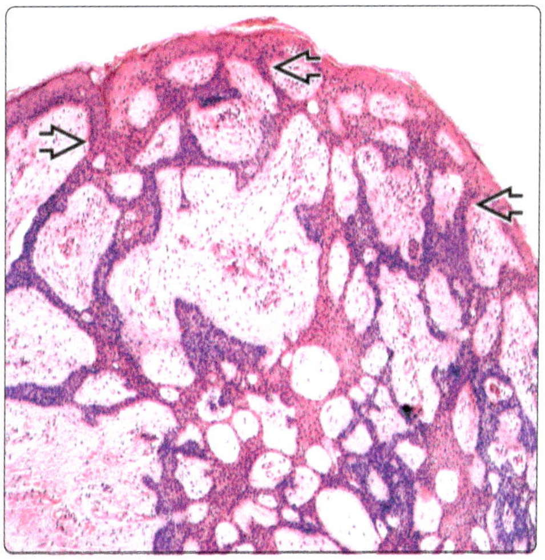

(Left) *Basosquamous-type BCC shows a proliferation of large, squamoid-appearing cells with abundant eosinophilic cytoplasm and focal mucin collections.* **(Right)** *Scanning magnification of a fibroepithelioma of Pinkus-type BCC is characterized by numerous small anastomosing cords of basaloid cells with multiple epidermal connections.*

Basal Cell Carcinoma: Morpheaform (Desmoplastic/Sclerosing) Type

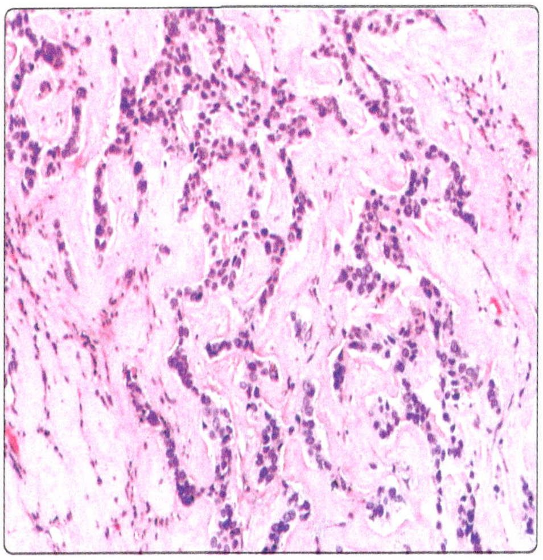

Perineural Invasion in Basal Cell Carcinoma

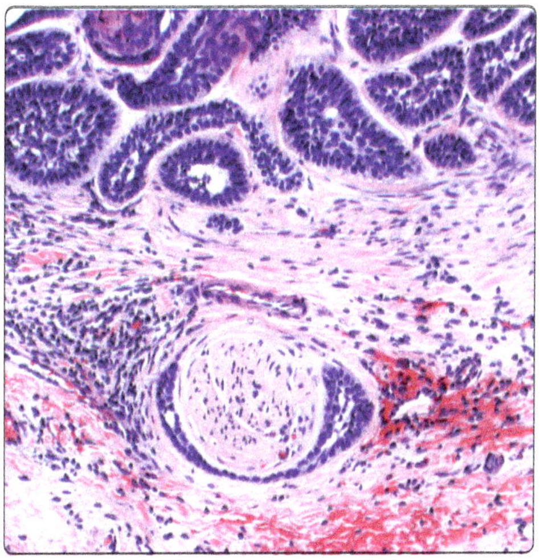

(Left) *Morpheaform (desmoplastic/sclerosing) BCC shows cords of atypical basaloid cells infiltrating a dense, desmoplastic stroma.* **(Right)** *This is an example of perineural invasion in a micronodular-type BCC. Although quite rare, perineural invasion can be seen in larger, more deeply invasive tumors, especially micronodular, infiltrative, and sclerosing/morpheaform types.*

(Left) *Low-power view shows a BCC with adenoid cystic-like features (adenoid BCC) characterized by numerous well-formed cystic spaces containing abundant mucinous material.* **(Right)** *High magnification of a nodular BCC shows a rare markedly enlarged, pleomorphic-appearing tumor cell with a macronucleolus ⇨.*

Basal Cell Carcinoma: Adenoid Type

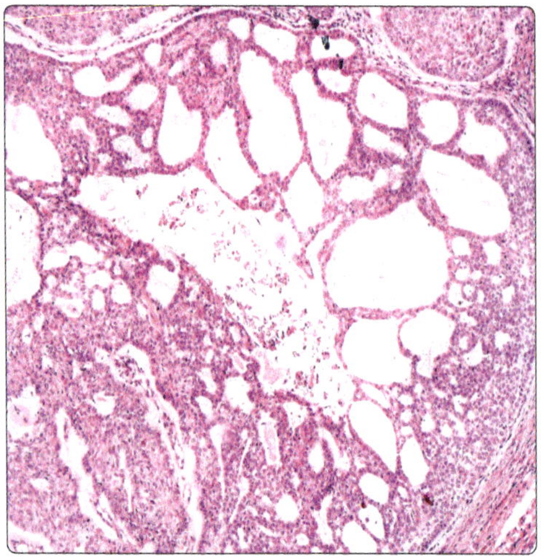

Basal Cell Carcinoma With Pleomorphic Cells

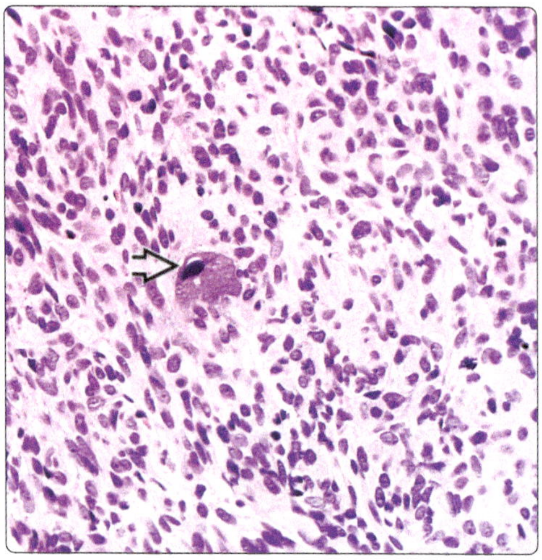

(Left) *High-power magnification of a plasmacytoid BCC shows dense eosinophilic cytoplasmic inclusions ⇨ and displaced nuclei. These cases have been shown to exhibit myoepithelial differentiation.* **(Right)** *Strong and diffuse BER-EP4/CD326 staining is shown in a nodular and infiltrative-type BCC. This marker is typically strongly expressed in BCC, but negative in squamous cell carcinoma (SCC) and many other tumors.*

Basal Cell Carcinoma: Plasmacytoid Type

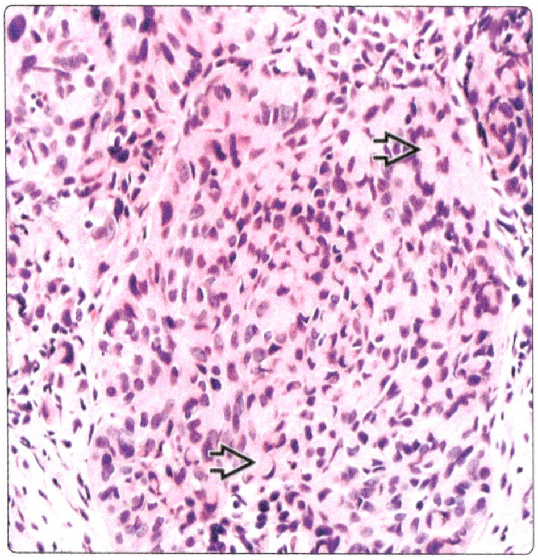

BER-EP4 Immunohistochemical Staining in Basal Cell Carcinoma

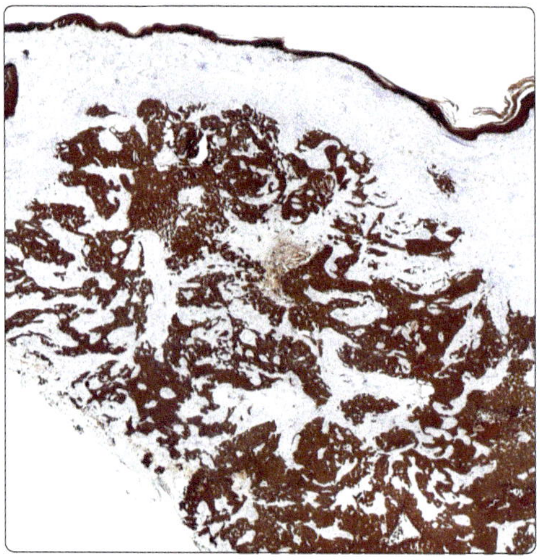

(Left) *Strong and diffuse nuclear Ki-67 immunohistochemical staining is typically seen in BCC.* **(Right)** *Bcl-2 immunohistochemistry in a micronodular BCC shows moderate to strong cytoplasmic staining of the tumor cells.*

Ki-67 Immunohistochemistry in Basal Cell Carcinoma

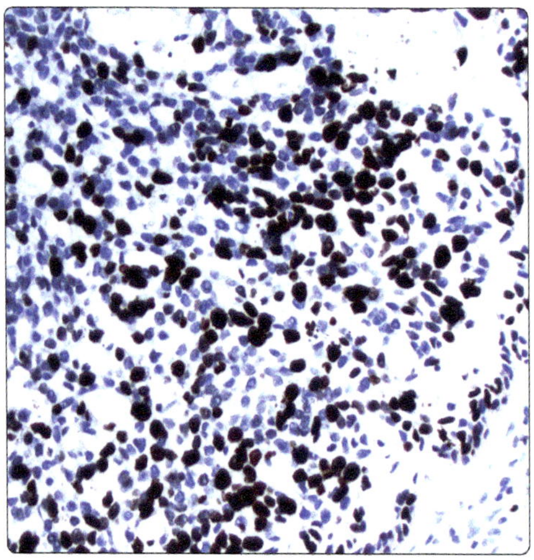

Bcl-2 Staining in Basal Cell Carcinoma

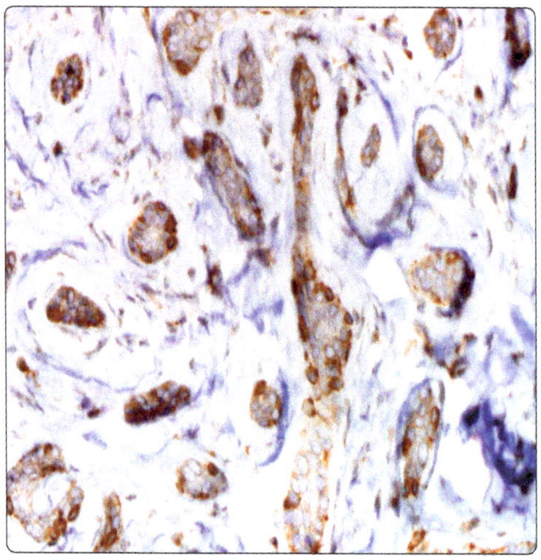

Differential Diagnosis: Squamous Cell Carcinoma

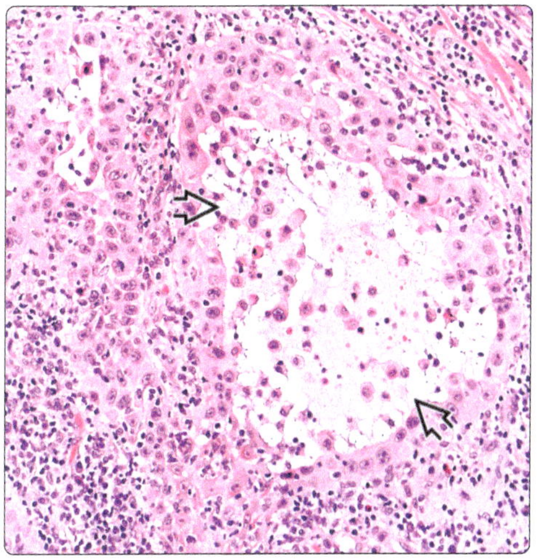

Differential Diagnosis: Infiltrative Squamous Cell Carcinoma

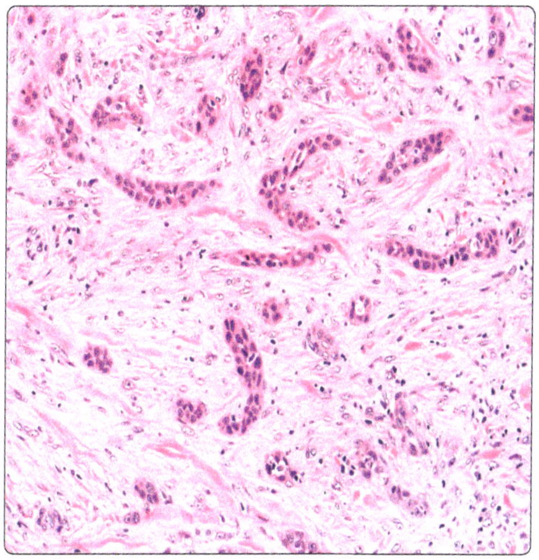

(Left) *SCC can rarely show mucin production, as in this example of acantholytic SCC, but it is typically found within the center of a tumor island, not in the stroma (as in BCC).* **(Right)** *Infiltrative SCC with cord-like structures associated with a desmoplastic stroma can mimic desmoplastic/morpheaform BCC or, less likely, microcystic adnexal carcinoma.*

Differential Diagnosis: Trichoblastoma

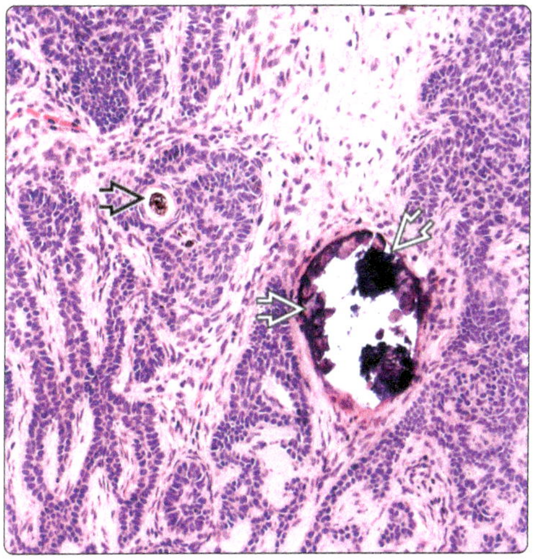

Differential Diagnosis: Trichoblastoma

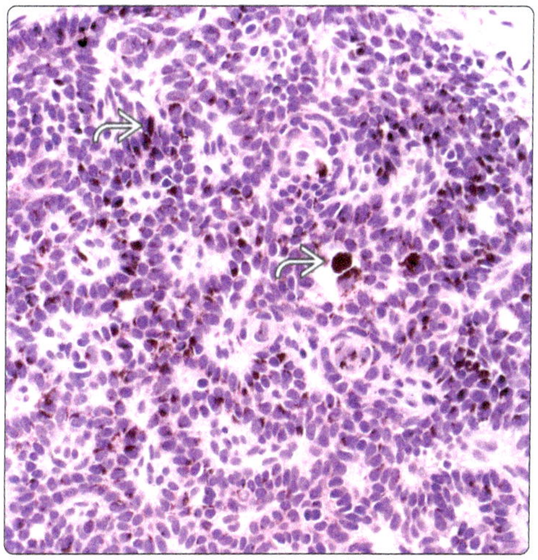

(Left) *Histologic section of a trichoblastoma shows a bland-appearing basaloid tumor in a fibromyxoid stroma lacking a tumor-stromal retraction artifact (as is seen in BCC). There is focal pigmentation and an area of calcification, findings typical of this neoplasm.* **(Right)** *High magnification shows a trichoblastoma with diffuse pigmentation. The lesion is composed of bland-appearing basaloid cells in anastomosing ribbons. Note the bland cytology and lack of mitotic or apoptotic figures.*

Differential Diagnosis: Merkel Cell Carcinoma

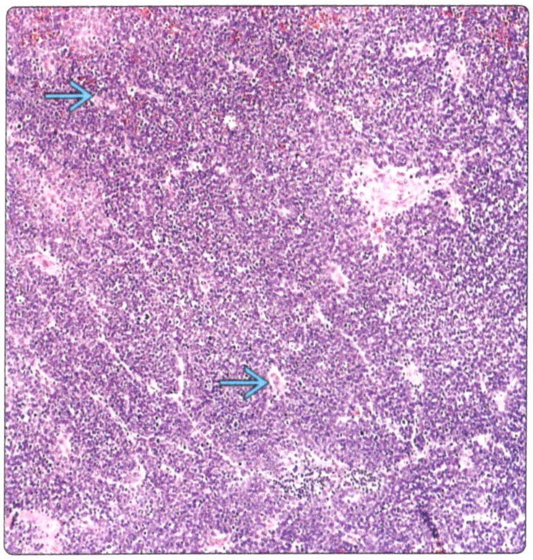

Differential Diagnosis: Merkel Cell Carcinoma

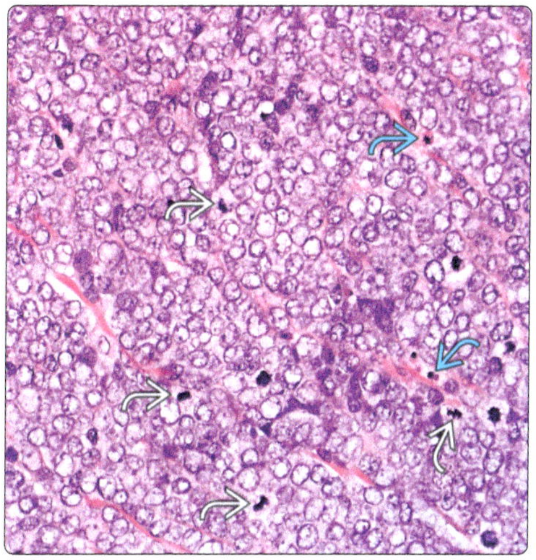

(Left) *Merkel cell carcinoma is typically composed of broad cords and sheet-like collections of highly atypical basaloid cells. There is scant stroma intervening between the neoplastic cells, and no tumor-stromal retraction, peripheral palisading, or mucinous material is present.* **(Right)** *Merkel cell carcinoma at high magnification shows prominent nuclear crowding and atypia, with numerous mitotic and apoptotic figures. Nuclear clearing is also present, a feature not seen in BCC.*

KEY FACTS

TERMINOLOGY

- Extramammary Paget disease (EMPD)

CLINICAL ISSUES

- Erythematous patches or plaques with sharply defined borders
- May clinically mimic chronic eczema

MICROSCOPIC

- Round, large, pale cells in all levels of epidermis arranged as single units or confluent aggregates
  - Sometimes with true glandular formation
- Round vesicular nuclei with prominent nucleoli
- Abundant clear cytoplasm
  - May contain intracytoplasmic melanin
- Absence of intercellular bridges
- Paget cells often extend to adnexal structures
- Flattened basal keratinocytes

ANCILLARY TESTS

- Paget cells are mucin (+)
- Primary EMPD is CK7(+) and CK20(-)
- Secondary EMPD has more variable immunohistochemical profile
  - Secondary EMPD associated with urothelial carcinoma is CK7 and CK20(+)
  - Secondary EMPD associated with anal/rectal carcinoma is CK20(+) and CK7(-)

TOP DIFFERENTIAL DIAGNOSES

- Squamous cell carcinoma in situ
- Melanoma in situ
- Clear cell papulosis
- Benign mucinous metaplasia of penis
- Pagetoid dyskeratosis
- Pagetoid reticulosis
- Melanoma in situ

Clinical Appearance of EMPD

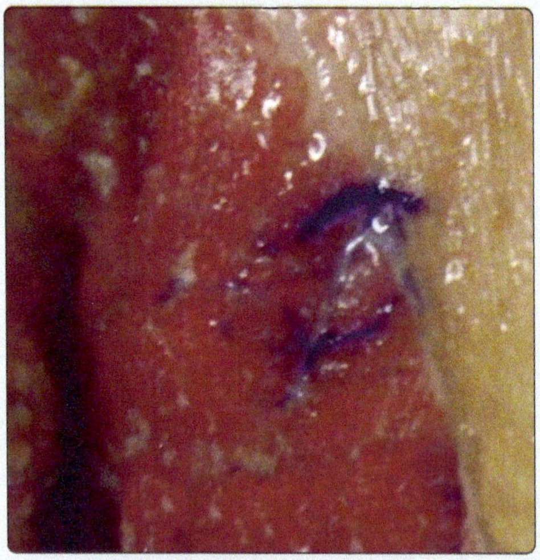

Paget Cells Involving All Levels of Epidermis

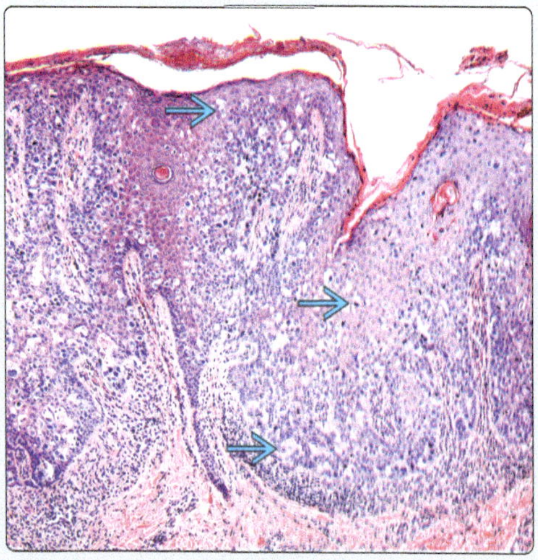

(Left) *This case presented as a large, moist-appearing erythematous patch affecting the groin of an elderly patient.* **(Right)** *Large, pale-staining neoplastic cells ➡ extensively infiltrate all levels of the hyperplastic epidermis in another case of extramammary Paget disease (EMPD). There is a chronic inflammatory infiltrate in the upper dermis.*

Hyperplastic Epidermis With Marked Pagetoid Spread in EMPD

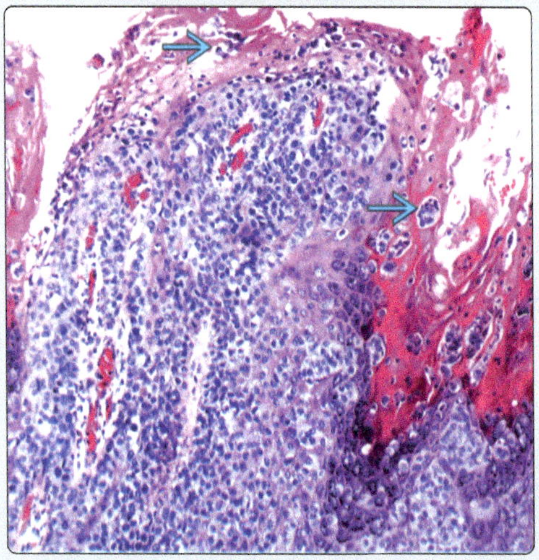

CK7 Expression in EMPD

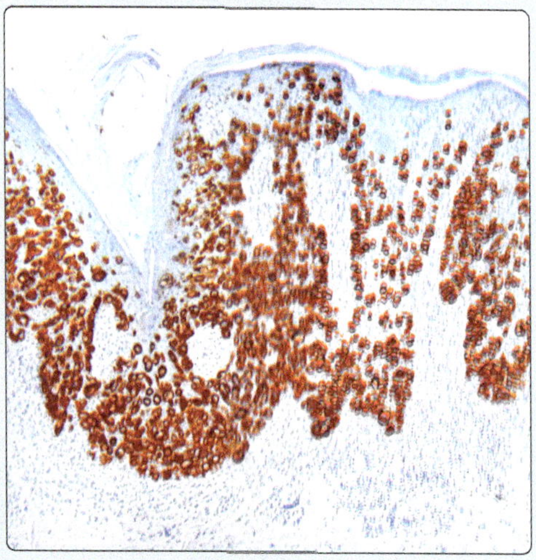

(Left) *The epidermis in this case shows hyperplasia with papillary features. The neoplastic cells are numerous and affect all levels of the epidermis, including the stratum corneum ➡. They are arranged as single units and confluent aggregates.* **(Right)** *CK7 immunohistochemical stain strongly highlights the neoplastic cells throughout the epidermis. The use of CK7 may also assist in defining the margins of the disease.*

TERMINOLOGY

Abbreviations

- Extramammary Paget disease (EMPD)

Definitions

- Adenocarcinoma involving epidermis and commonly extending to epithelium of eccrine glands &/or hair follicles (adenocarcinoma in situ)
- May involve dermis in minority of cases

ETIOLOGY/PATHOGENESIS

Pathogenesis

- Uncertain in most cases
- Cases limited to epidermis are postulated to originate from intraepidermal portion of sweat glands or from intraepidermal stem cells
- Heterogeneous condition; can be classified as primary (cutaneous origin) and secondary (extracutaneous origin)
  - Primary EMPD is rarely associated with underlying sweat gland carcinoma (usually apocrine)
  - Secondary EMPD: Associated with internal carcinoma in 15-29% of cases
    - Genital EMPD is often associated with genitourinary carcinomas and perianal EMPD is more frequently associated with gastrointestinal carcinomas
    - Most frequent in perianal EMPD (underlying rectal carcinoma in 1/3 of cases)

CLINICAL ISSUES

Epidemiology

- Age
  - 6th-8th decades
- Sex
  - F > M

Site

- Skin regions rich in apocrine glands
  - Most common sites: Vulva and perianal region
  - Other sites: Scrotum, perineum, penis, axilla, umbilicus
  - Exceptional sites: Eyelid (accompanying carcinoma of Moll gland), external auditory meatus (associated with ceruminous carcinoma), face, scalp, chest, abdomen, and extremities

Presentation

- Circinate or annular moist erythematous scaly patches or plaques
- Other presentations: Gray-white eczematous patches, hypopigmented or pigmented macules, ulcerated plaques/tumors
- Pruritus is frequent and may precede clinical lesion
- Bleeding, oozing, tenderness, or burning sensation can occur
- EMPD may mimic eczema
- Lesions may be multifocal

Treatment

- Complete surgical excision is treatment of choice for primary EMPD
  - Patients require long-term follow-up because of multifocal nature of condition and high recurrence rate
- Treatment in secondary lesions will depend on associated carcinoma

Prognosis

- Primary EMPD confined to epidermis and epithelium of adnexal structures (in situ carcinoma) has good prognosis when completely excised
- Dermal invasion is associated with worse prognosis; prognosis is related to depth of invasion
  - Invasion of reticular dermis or depth of ≥ 1 mm have been found to indicate higher risk
  - Expression of Ki-67, cyclin-D1, MUC5AC, and loss of E-cadherin, have been shown to increase risk of extracutaneous spread
- Prognosis in secondary Paget disease is related to underlying carcinoma and is usually poor

MACROSCOPIC

General Features

- Erythematous patches or plaques with sharply defined borders

Sections to Be Submitted

- Important to carefully evaluate margins because neoplastic cells may extend beyond clinical borders

Size

- Few millimeters to several centimeters
- Focal or multicentric

MICROSCOPIC

Histologic Features

- Intraepithelial proliferation of large, round, atypical cells (Paget cells)
- Epithelium varies from hyperplastic to atrophic
  - May be eroded or ulcerated
  - Changes similar to syringocystadenoma papilliferum have been described
- Paget cells have abundant pale or vacuolated cytoplasm
  - No intercellular bridges appreciated between them
  - Rare signet cell variant has been described
  - May contain intracytoplasmic melanin
  - Nuclei are large and vesicular
  - Nucleoli prominent
  - Mitoses may be numerous
- Early lesions show only scattered single Paget cells in epidermis
- Advanced lesions show numerous Paget cells that may form confluent aggregates
  - Paget cells compress squamous cells
    - Flattened basal keratinocytes are seen lying between neoplastic cells and underlying dermis
- Neoplastic cells often extend to epithelium of adnexal structures
- Neoplastic cells may form true intraepidermal glandular lumina
- Dermal inflammatory infiltrate is usually present
- Dermal invasion by tumoral cells may rarely occur

Predominant Pattern/Injury Type

- Adenocarcinoma

Predominant Cell/Compartment Type

- Paget cells

ANCILLARY TESTS

Histochemistry

- Mucicarmine
  - Reactivity: Positive
  - Staining pattern: Cytoplasmic

Immunohistochemistry

- Primary EMPD is CEA, low molecular weight cytokeratins (CK7, CAM5.2, AE1/AE3), EMA/MUC1 (+); often GCDFP-15 and AR(+)
- Primary EMPD is CK20, CDX2, and p63 (-)
- Secondary EMPD is usually GCDFP-15, AR, and p63(-)
- Immunohistochemical expression profile of secondary EMPD is related to associated carcinoma
  - Secondary EMPD associated with urothelial carcinoma
    - Usually expresses both CK7 and CK20 and uroplakin-3
    - CEA(-)
  - EMPD secondary to anal/rectal carcinomas
    - Expresses CK20, CEA, and CDX-2
    - Usually CK7 and GCDFP-15 negative
- Primary and secondary EMPD are negative for melanocytic markers, such as S100, MART-1/Melan-A, tyrosinase, and HMB-45

DIFFERENTIAL DIAGNOSIS

Squamous Cell Carcinoma In Situ With Pagetoid Pattern

- Dense eosinophilic-staining cytoplasm and presence of intercellular bridges between neoplastic cells
- HMWCKs (34βE12 and CK5/6) and p63 positive
- May be CK7 and EMA positive
- Mucicarmine and PAS-D (-)
- CEA, GCDFP-15, ER/PR, AR, and CK20 (-)
- Usually CAM5.2(-)

Melanoma In Situ

- Melanoma cells are present in all levels of epidermis, including basal layer
- No flattened keratinocytes seen between melanoma cells and dermis
- Intracytoplasmic melanin in neoplastic cells does not confirm melanoma, as Paget cells can be pigmented
- Dermal invasion is more frequent than in EMPD
- Immunohistochemical expression of melanocytic markers, such as S100, MART-1/Melan-A, and HMB-45

Clear Cell Papulosis (Toker Cell Hyperplasia)

- Young children (more often Asian or Hispanic)
- Small macules or papules affecting lower part of trunk, face
  - Predominantly milk line location
- Clear cells with pagetoid features in lower part of epidermis
- CK7, PAN-CK (AE1/AE3) and CEA (+)
- Usually mucin stains (-)

Benign Mucinous Metaplasia of Penis

- Elderly patients
- Prepuce or glans
- Benign mucin-containing cells in squamous epithelium
- Usually associated with chronic inflammatory conditions

Pagetoid Dyskeratosis

- Reactive process (usually incidental finding)
- Lips, intertriginous and anogenital area, hemorrhoids
- Keratinocytes in upper epidermis show abundant eosinophilic pale cytoplasm
  - Lesional cells are keratinocytes
  - CEA and mucicarmine (-)

Pagetoid Reticulosis

- Rare variant of cutaneous T-cell lymphoma
- Epidermal infiltration by medium- to large-sized T cells with abundant pale cytoplasm
- T cells are CD45 (LCA) and CD3 positive
- T cells may be either CD4 or CD8 positive or (double negative)
- T-cell gene rearrangement can be demonstrated

Merkel Cell Carcinoma

- Rare cases may have prominent epidermotropic component
- Small round blue cells with scant cytoplasm
- Characteristic dot-like pattern with CK20 and PAN-CK (AE1/AE3)
- In minority of cases, may express CK7
- Positive expression of neuroendocrine markers, such as chromogranin and synaptophysin

DIAGNOSTIC CHECKLIST

Clinically Relevant Pathologic Features

- Important to distinguish in situ from invasive lesions
- Important to recognize EMPD associated with underlying sweat gland carcinoma
- Important to rule out associated internal carcinoma

Pathologic Interpretation Pearls

- Flattened basal keratinocytes lying between Paget cells and underlying basement membrane
- Presence of melanin does not rule out Paget disease

SELECTED REFERENCES

1. Konstantinova AM et al: Syringocystadenocarcinoma papilliferum in situ-like changes in extramammary Paget disease: a report of 11 cases. Am J Dermatopathol. ePub, 2016
2. Shu B et al: Primary invasive extramammary Paget disease on penoscrotum: a clinicopathological analysis of 41 cases. Hum Pathol. 47(1):70-7, 2016
3. Terada T: Extramammary Paget disease of signet ring cell carcinoma type: a case report. Am J Dermatopathol. 38(3):249-51, 2016
4. Cohen JM et al: Risk stratification in extramammary Paget disease. Clin Exp Dermatol. 40(5):473-8, 2015
5. Liegl B et al: Mammary and extramammary Paget's disease: an immunohistochemical study of 83 cases. Histopathology. 50(4):439-47, 2007
6. Ohnishi T et al: The use of cytokeratins 7 and 20 in the diagnosis of primary and secondary extramammary Paget's disease. Br J Dermatol. 142(2):243-7, 2000
7. Val-Bernal JF et al: Benign mucinous metaplasia of the penis. a lesion resembling extramammary Paget's disease. J Cutan Pathol. 27(2):76-9, 2000

Pagetoid Epidermal Involvement

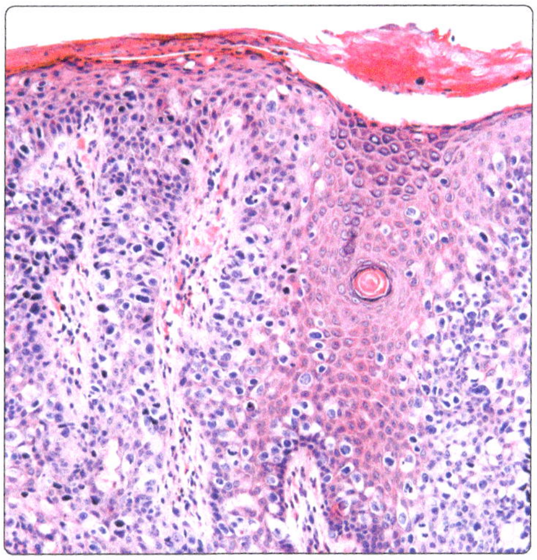

Pale Cytoplasm Characteristic of Paget Cells

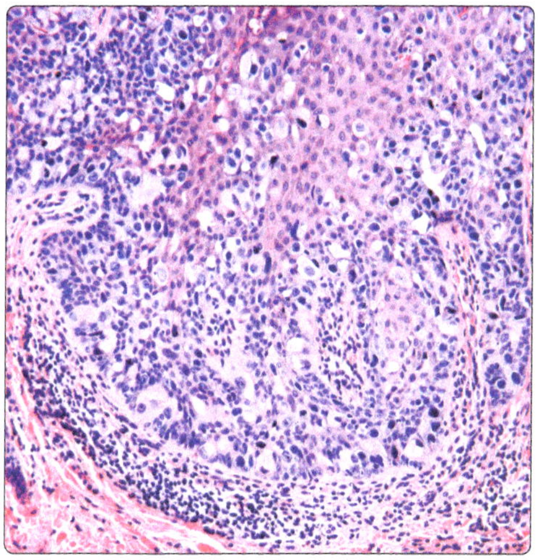

(Left) *Numerous pagetoid cells are present in all levels of the epidermis in this case of extramammary Paget disease. The epidermis is hyperplastic with overlying foci of parakeratosis.* **(Right)** *Paget cells are large, round to oval, and show ample pale to clear-staining cytoplasm on high magnification.*

Flattened Keratinocytes in EMPD

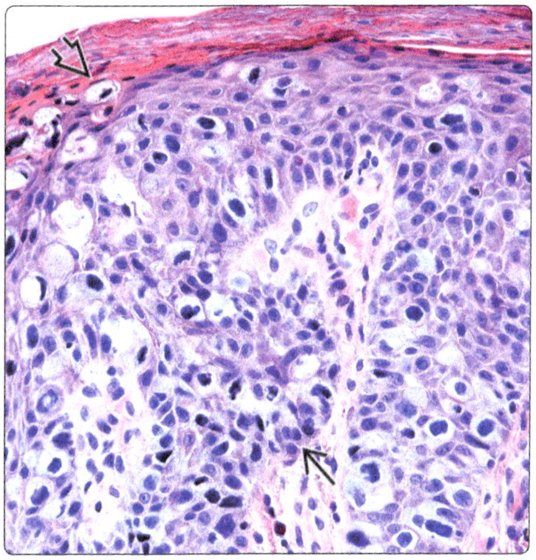

Red Staining With Mucicarmine

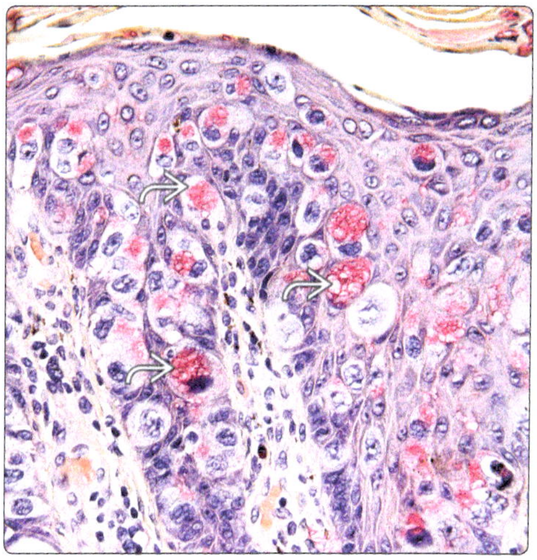

(Left) *Numerous Paget cells ⇒ arranged as single units are seen in all levels of the epidermis, including the cornified layer. Note the flattened basal keratinocytes ⇒.* **(Right)** *A mucicarmine stain shows reddish/pink staining of the cytoplasm ➔ in most cases of EMPD.*

CK20 Expression in Secondary EMPD

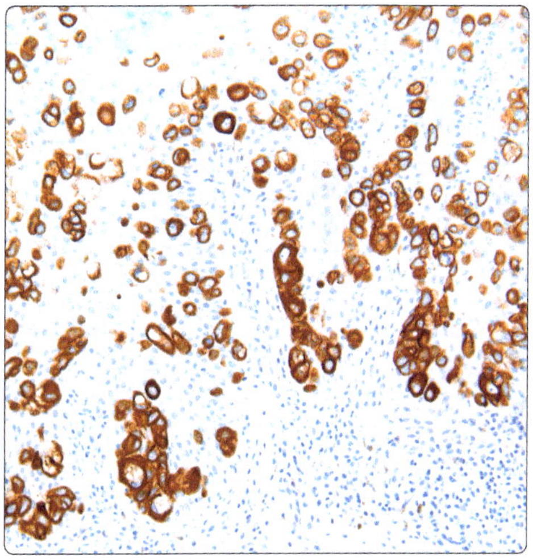

CDX-2 Staining in Secondary EMPD

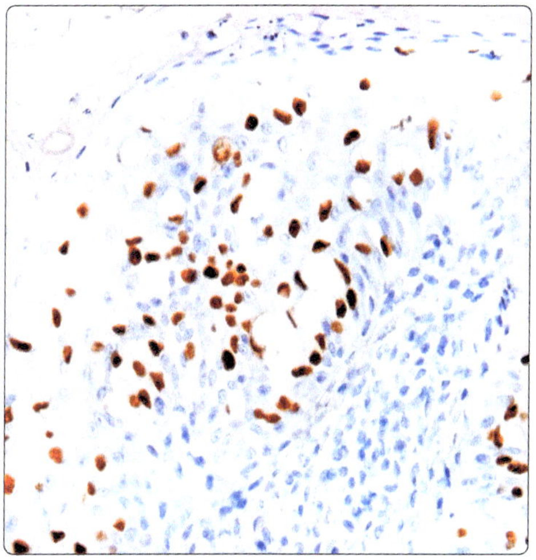

(Left) *Strong CK20 expression by the neoplastic cells is seen in this case of EMPD secondary to underlying rectal/anal carcinoma.* **(Right)** *CDX-2 expression by the Paget cells would be another strong indicator of an associated synchronous or metachronous anal/rectal malignancy in cases of EMPD.*

Squamomelanocytic Tumor

KEY FACTS

TERMINOLOGY

- Admixed histopathologic features of both squamous cell carcinoma and malignant melanoma
- Original descriptions were of dermal-based tumors

CLINICAL ISSUES

- Very rare tumor
- Often elderly patients
- Predilection for head and neck
- Unclear prognosis, as very few cases reported

MICROSCOPIC

- Intermingled populations of cells in dermal nodules
- Predominantly squamoid population
- Smaller melanocytic population (may not be obvious on histologic sections)

TOP DIFFERENTIAL DIAGNOSES

- Squamous cell carcinoma with colonization by melanocytes
  - Predominantly composed of atypical squamous cells, with scattered melanocytes
    - Melanocytes
      - Single, not nested
      - Dendritic shaped
      - Nuclei not atypical
- Pseudoepitheliomatous hyperplasia associated with malignant melanoma
  - Keratinocytes in hyperplastic areas not atypical and connect to epidermal surface
  - Mitoses not prominent
  - Dyskeratosis absent
- Melanocytic matrixoma
  - Dendritic melanocytes intermingled with basaloid epithelial cells with foci of matrical differentiation
- Atypical solid-cystic hidradenoma
  - Lacks population of spindled cells with clear cytoplasm and fine melanin pigment

Squamomelanocytic Tumor

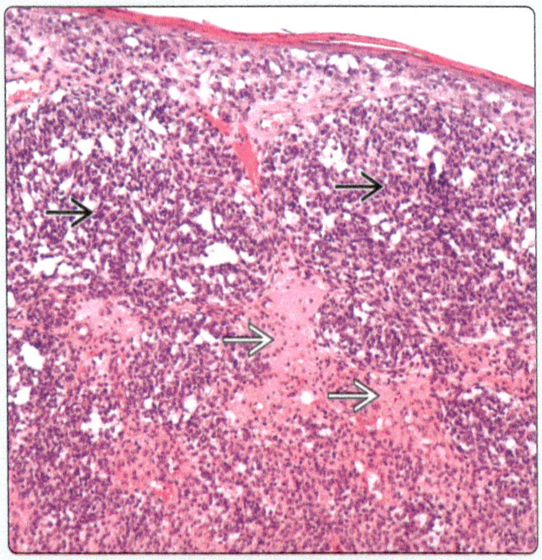

Squamomelanocytic Tumor at High Magnification

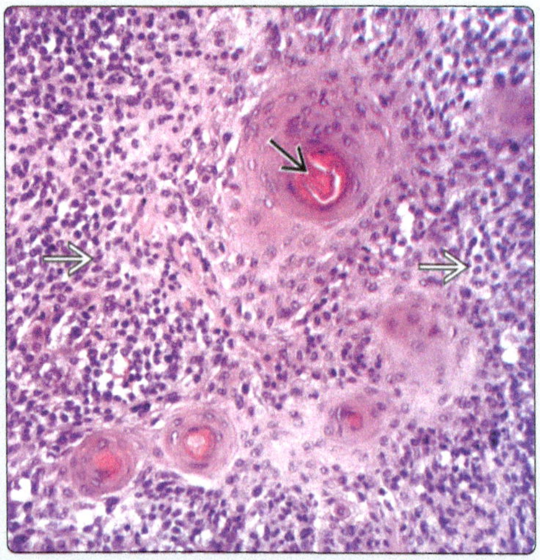

(Left) *Squamomelanocytic tumor is a dermal-based tumor composed of 2 populations of cells: Atypical epithelioid melanocytic cells ⇨ and larger squamoid cells ➡. (Courtesy P. Amerio, MD, PhD.)* **(Right)** *Squamomelanocytic tumor shows squamoid cells with pink cytoplasm in islands, forming keratin pearls ⇨, surrounded by smaller melanocytic cells ➡ with less distinctive cytoplasm. (Courtesy P. Amerio, MD, PhD.)*

Cytokeratin Staining in Squamomelanocytic Tumor

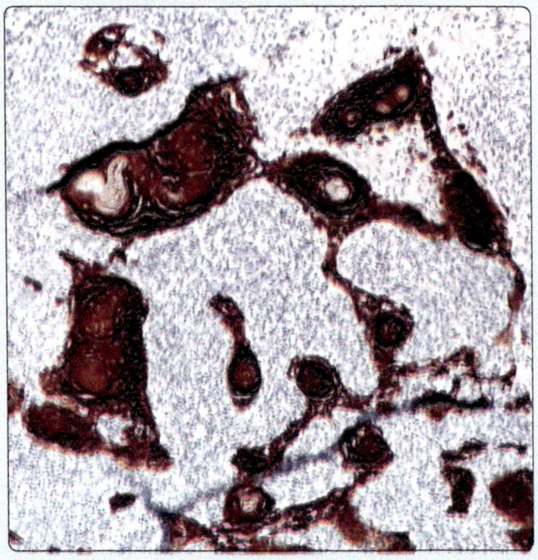

Melan-A Staining in Squamomelanocytic Tumor

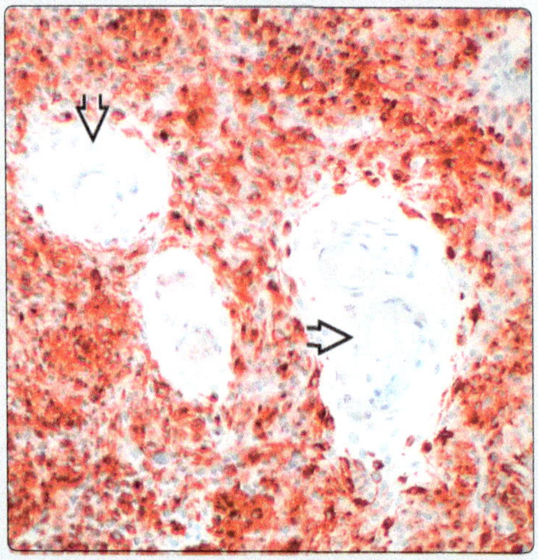

(Left) *Cytokeratin AE1/AE3 strongly highlights the islands of squamoid cells forming keratin. (Courtesy P. Amerio, MD, PhD.)* **(Right)** *Melan-A staining is positive in the melanocytic cells surrounding the negative islands of squamoid cells ⇨. (Courtesy P. Amerio, MD, PhD.)*

TERMINOLOGY

Definitions

- Admixed histopathologic features of both atypical squamoid and melanocytic cells
  - 2 cell types generally within < 1 mm of each other
- Original descriptions were of dermal-based tumors

ETIOLOGY/PATHOGENESIS

Field Cancerization Theory

- Common carcinogen (i.e., ultraviolet light) may lead to proliferation of 2 different cell types

Tumor Collision Theory

- By chance, 2 different cell types have mutations and show clonal proliferation
- Arguing against this theory is presence of identical molecular alterations and immunohistochemical staining patterns in both squamous and melanocytic components of some squamomelanocytic tumors

Tumor Convergent Theory

- Tumors with biphasic differentiation arise from common progenitor cell that undergoes 2 different types of differentiation
- Supporting this theory is presence of identical molecular alterations and immunohistochemical staining patterns in both squamous and melanocytic components of some tumors

CLINICAL ISSUES

Presentation

- Very rare tumor
- Generally elderly patients, often male
- Predilection for head and neck
- Nondescript papule or nodule
  - Blue-black to red or flesh colored

Treatment

- Excision

Prognosis

- Unclear
  - Prognosis may be better than malignant melanoma of same depth
- Local recurrence and widespread metastasis have been reported

MICROSCOPIC

Histologic Features

- Intermingled cell populations in dermal nodules
  - Squamoid cells
    - Pink cytoplasm, hyperchromatic-staining nuclei, atypical mitoses
    - Keratin pearls may be evident
    - Focal ductal differentiation has been described
  - Melanocytes
    - May not be obvious on histologic sections
    - Cells may be highlighted with melanocytic markers such as S100, SOX10, and Melan-A
    - Atypical epithelioid cells in nests may be seen in some cases
  - In some published cases of dermal-based tumors, 3rd population of cells also reported
    - Difficult to appreciate on H&E sections
    - Do not mark with melanocytic or epithelial immunohistochemical stains
- Changes of melanoma in situ often overlie dermal-based tumors

Cytologic Features

- Squamoid cells: Hyperchromatic-staining nuclei, pink cytoplasm, keratin pearls, mitoses
- Melanocytic population
  - May be spindled with clear cytoplasm and fine melanin pigment
  - May be difficult to appreciate; highlighted by melanocytic immunohistochemical stains

ANCILLARY TESTS

Immunohistochemistry

- Squamoid cells stain with cytokeratins, p63
- Melanocytic population stains with S100, SOX10, and other melanocytic markers

DIFFERENTIAL DIAGNOSIS

Squamous Cell Carcinoma With Colonization by Melanocytes

- Melanocytes are not atypical, do not form nests

Pseudoepitheliomatous Hyperplasia Associated With Malignant Melanoma

- Keratinocytes in hyperplastic areas not atypical and connect to epidermal surface

Melanocytic Matrixoma

- Dermal nodule of basaloid and pigmented cells
  - Dendritic melanocytes intermingled with epithelial cells
  - Epithelial cells are small, basaloid (matrical), similar to pilomatrixoma
  - Shadow cells also present

Atypical Solid-Cystic Hidradenoma

- Lacks population of spindled cells with clear cytoplasm and fine melanin pigment

SELECTED REFERENCES

1. Amin SM et al: Combined cutaneous tumors with a melanoma component: A clinical, histologic, and molecular study. J Am Acad Dermatol. 73(3):451-60, 2015
2. Jour G et al: Squamomelanocytic tumor: a case report and further insights into its possible histogenesis. Am J Dermatopathol. 36(6):517-21, 2014
3. Amerio P et al: Metastasizing dermal squamomelanocytic tumour. J Eur Acad Dermatol Venereol. 25(4):489-91, 2011
4. Leonard N et al: Squamomelanocytic tumor: an unusual and distinctive entity of uncertain biological potential. Am J Dermatopathol. 31(5):495-8, 2009
5. Miteva M et al: A rare case of a cutaneous squamomelanocytic tumor: revisiting the histogenesis of combined neoplasms. Am J Dermatopathol. 31(6):599-603, 2009
6. Pool SE et al: Dermal squamo-melanocytic tumor: a unique biphenotypic neoplasm of uncertain biological potential. Hum Pathol. 30(5):525-9, 1999

TERMINOLOGY

Abbreviations

- Primary tumor (pT)
- Regional lymph nodes (pN)
- Metastasis (pM)

Definitions

- **pTX**: Primary tumor cannot be assessed (i.e., primary site unknown, regressed, or partial biopsy)
- **pT0**: No evidence of primary tumor
- **pTis**: Carcinoma in situ
- **pT1**: Tumor 2 cm or less in greatest dimension with fewer than 2 high-risk features
- **pT2**: Tumor greater than 2 cm in greatest dimension ± 1 additional high-risk feature or any size with 2 or more high-risk features
- **pT3**: Tumor with invasion of maxilla, mandible, orbit, or temporal bone
- **pT4**: Tumor with invasion of skeleton (axial or appendicular) or perineural invasion of skull base
- **pNX**: Regional lymph nodes cannot be assessed
- **pN0**: No regional lymph node metastasis
- **pN1**: Metastasis in single ipsilateral lymph node, 3 cm or less in greatest dimension
- **pN2**: Metastasis in 1 or more lymph node, all < 6 cm in greatest dimension
  - pN2a: Metastasis in single ipsilateral lymph node, > 3 cm to < 6 cm in greatest dimension
  - pN2b: Metastasis in multiple ipsilateral lymph nodes, none > 6 cm in greatest dimension
  - pN2c: Metastasis in bilateral or contralateral lymph nodes, none > 6 cm in greatest dimension
- **pN3**: Metastasis in a lymph node, > 6 cm in greatest dimension
- **pMX**: Not applicable or unknown (not necessary to report)
- **pM1**: Distant metastasis
  - Specify site(s), if known

SELECTED REFERENCES

1. Agar NJ et al: Predicting lymph node metastases in cutaneous squamous cell carcinoma: use of a morphological scoring system. N Z Med J. 128(1411):59-67, 2015
2. Brunner M et al: Assessment of the new nodal classification for cutaneous squamous cell carcinoma and its effect on patient stratification. Head Neck. 37(3):336-9, 2015
3. Díaz-Corpas T et al: Squamous cell carcinoma: clinical and pathological features and associated risk factors in an observational study of 118 patients. Actas Dermosifiliogr. 106(10):806-15, 2015
4. Stratigos A et al: Diagnosis and treatment of invasive squamous cell carcinoma of the skin: European consensus-based interdisciplinary guideline. Eur J Cancer. 51(14):1989-2007, 2015
5. Westers-Attema A et al: Correlation between histological findings on punch biopsy specimens and subsequent excision specimens in cutaneous squamous cell carcinoma. Acta Derm Venereol. 95(2):181-5, 2015
6. Ahmed MM et al: Utility of head and neck cutaneous squamous cell carcinoma sentinel node biopsy: a systematic review. Otolaryngol Head Neck Surg. 150(2):180-7, 2014
7. Brougham ND et al: The incidence and risk factors of metastasis for cutaneous squamous cell carcinoma--implications on the T-classification system. J Surg Oncol. 110(7):876-82, 2014
8. Brunner M et al: Comparison of the AJCC N staging system in mucosal and cutaneous squamous head and neck cancer. Laryngoscope. 124(7):1598-602, 2014
9. Chu MB et al: Evaluation of the definitions of "high-risk" cutaneous squamous cell carcinoma using the american joint committee on cancer staging criteria and national comprehensive cancer network guidelines. J Skin Cancer. 2014:154340, 2014
10. Gurney B et al: Management of regional metastatic disease in head and neck cutaneous malignancy. 1. Cutaneous squamous cell carcinoma. Br J Oral Maxillofac Surg. 52(4):294-300, 2014
11. Karia PS et al: Evaluation of American Joint Committee on Cancer, International Union Against Cancer, and Brigham and Women's Hospital tumor staging for cutaneous squamous cell carcinoma. J Clin Oncol. 32(4):327-34, 2014
12. LeBlanc KG Jr et al: Understanding and use of the American Joint Committee on Cancer seventh edition guidelines for cutaneous squamous cell carcinoma: a survey of dermatologic surgeons. Dermatol Surg. 40(5):505-10, 2014
13. Schmitt AR et al: Staging for cutaneous squamous cell carcinoma as a predictor of sentinel lymph node biopsy results: meta-analysis of American Joint Committee on Cancer criteria and a proposed alternative system. JAMA Dermatol. 150(1):19-24, 2014
14. Vasconcelos L et al: Invasive head and neck cutaneous squamous cell carcinoma: clinical and histopathological characteristics, frequency of local recurrence and metastasis. An Bras Dermatol. 89(4):562-8, 2014
15. Jambusaria-Pahlajani A et al: Evaluation of AJCC tumor staging for cutaneous squamous cell carcinoma and a proposed alternative tumor staging system. JAMA Dermatol. 149(4):402-10, 2013
16. Edge SB, et al: AJCC Cancer Staging Manual. 7th Ed. New York, NY: Springer. 301-314, 2010

Clinical Photograph of T1 Squamous Cell Carcinoma on Forehead

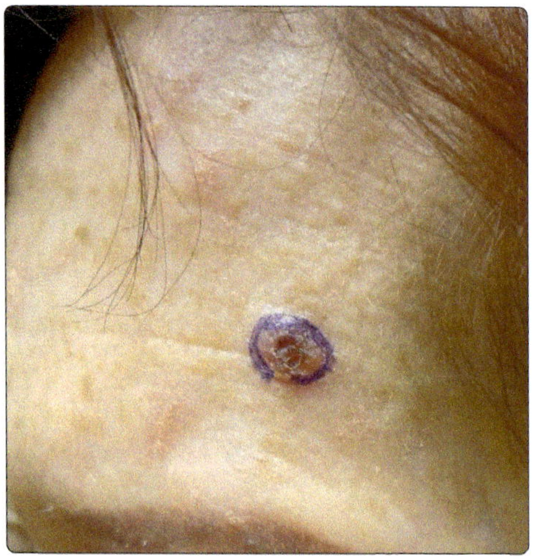

Histologic Section of Invasive, Well- to Moderately Differentiated SCC

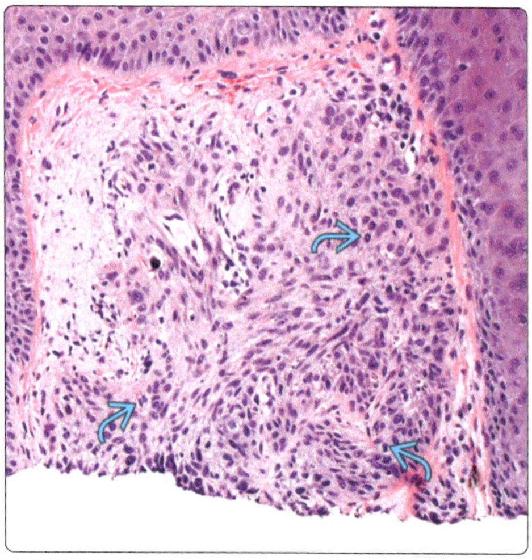

(Left) *This is a small invasive squamous cell carcinoma (SCC) arising on the forehead of an adult female. The tumor is less than 2 cm in greatest dimension and did not have any high-grade features histologically, consistent with a T1 tumor.* **(Right)** *This is an example of a small, superficially invasive, well- to moderately differentiated SCC (T1). Note the enlarged, hyperchromatic staining nuclei with focal spindling and scattered mitoses ➩.*

Squamous Cell Carcinoma In Situ (Tis)

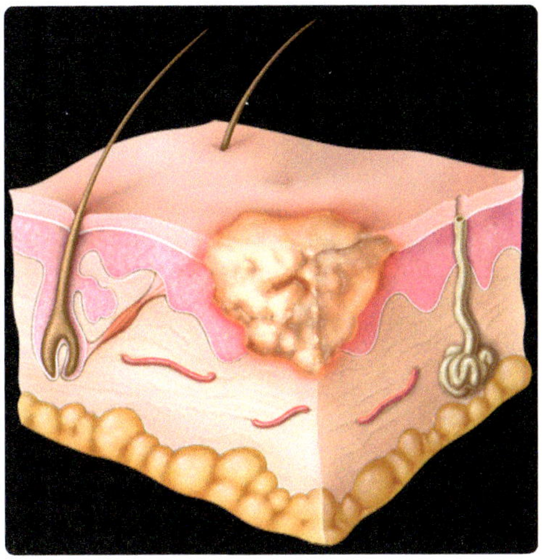

Superficially Invasive Squamous Cell Carcinoma (T1)

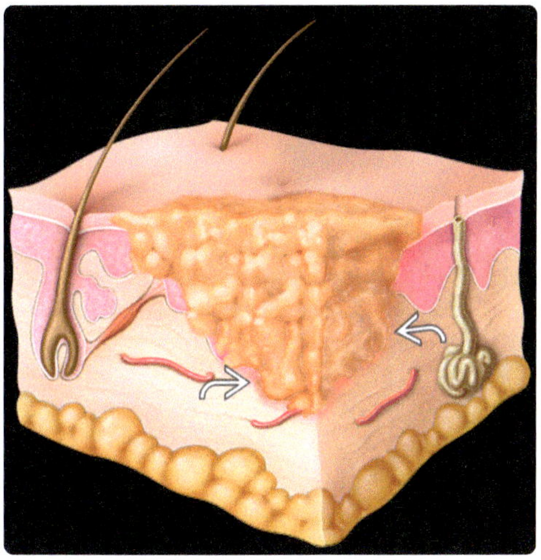

(Left) *Squamous carcinoma in situ (Bowen disease) shows growth limited to the epidermis (Tis).* **(Right)** *Invasive SCC shows superficial invasion into the dermis. This is a tumor ≤ 2 cm in greatest dimension with < 2 high-risk features (T1).*

Deeply Invasive Squamous Cell Carcinoma (T2)

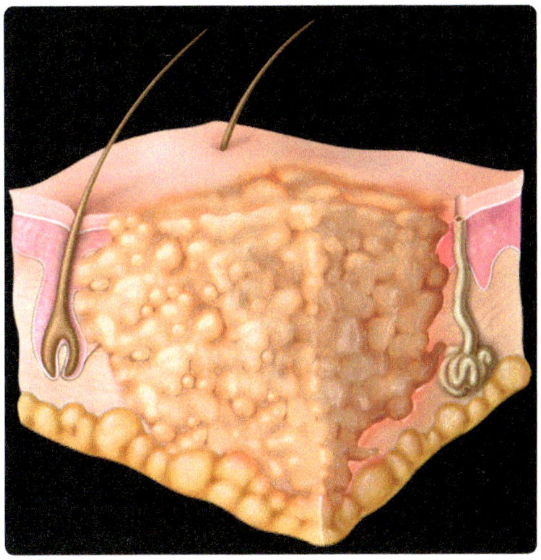

PET/CT of Squamous Cell Carcinoma

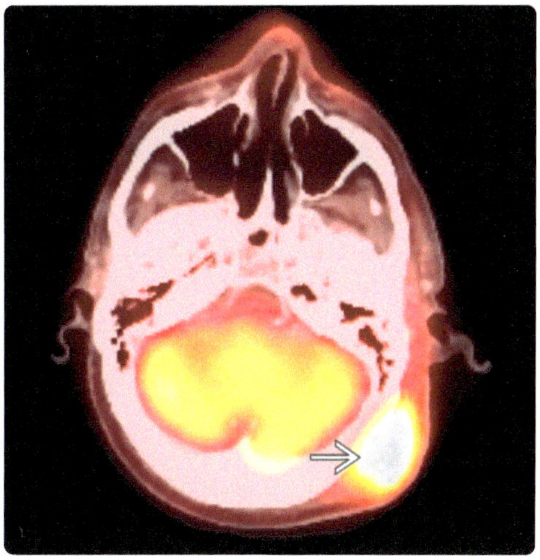

(Left) *A tumor > 2 cm in greatest dimension ± 1 additional high-risk feature or any size with ≥ 2 high-risk features is staged as T2.* **(Right)** *Axial fused PET/CT scan shows an increase in size and metabolic activity of a left scalp mass; excision confirmed an invasive SCC of > 2 cm in greatest dimension (T2).*

PET/CT of Metastatic Squamous Cell Carcinoma

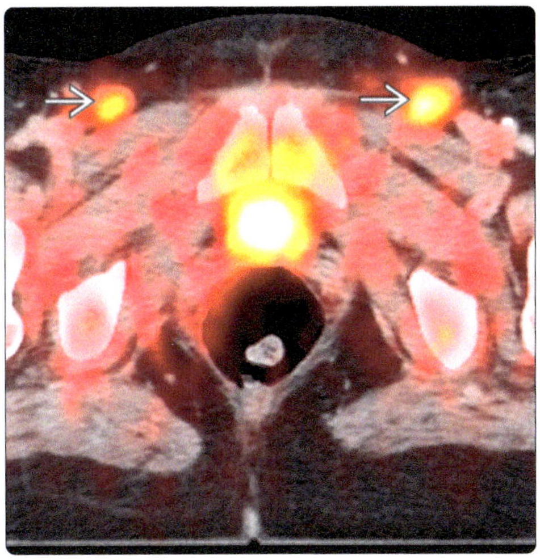

HRCT of Metastatic Squamous Cell Carcinoma

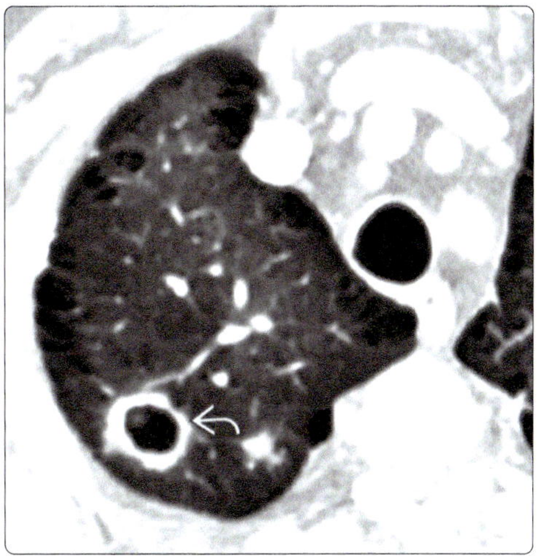

(Left) *Axial fused PET/CT shows bilateral intense inguinal FDG activity, compatible with metastatic nodes (N2c). This is a patient with a known primary anal SCC.* **(Right)** *Axial HRCT of a patient with metastatic SCC shows 2 right upper lobe metastases (M1), 1 of which exhibits cavitation. Note the thick nodular cavity wall, typical of malignancy.*

PART I
SECTION 3

Tumors and Tumor-Like Conditions of the Hair Follicle

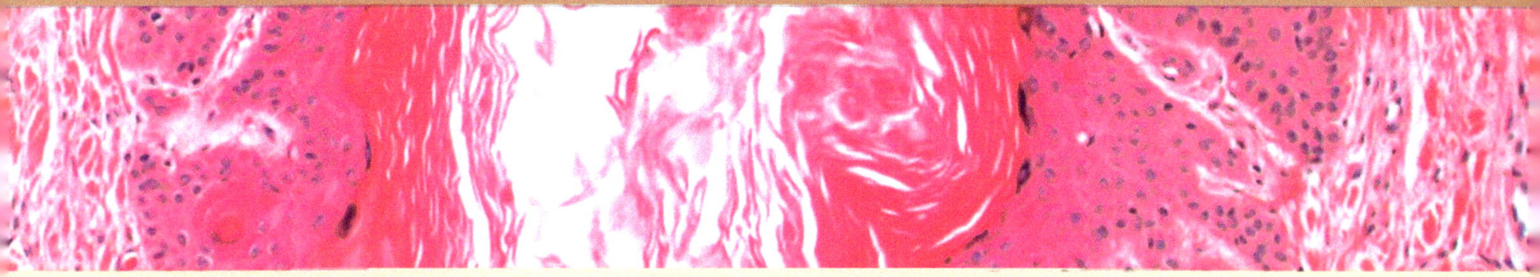

KEY FACTS

TERMINOLOGY

- Nevus sebaceus: Organoid nevus, Jadassohn nevus
- Nevus sebaceus: Hamartoma with abnormalities of epidermis, follicles, sebaceous and apocrine glands
- Basaloid follicular hamartoma: Hamartoma resembling primitive follicles

CLINICAL ISSUES

- Nevus sebaceus
  - Usually presents on scalp in infancy, often at birth
  - Presents as yellowish flat to warty plaque; enlarges during puberty
- Basaloid follicular hamartoma
  - Usually presents in adults

MICROSCOPIC

- Nevus sebaceus
  - Abnormalities of epidermis, follicles, apocrine and sebaceous glands
    - Proliferating sebaceous glands high in dermis; may communicate with epidermal surface
  - Follicles are disorganized with primitive germs
  - Associated tumors arising within nevus sebaceus
    - Trichoblastoma (most common), syringocystadenoma papilliferum, basal cell carcinoma (BCC) (rare)
- Basaloid follicular hamartoma
  - Multifocal islands of basaloid epithelium
  - No retraction artifact; no to rare mitotic activity

TOP DIFFERENTIAL DIAGNOSES

- **DDx of nevus sebaceus**
  - **Epidermal nevus**: Lacks abnormalities of follicles and sweat glands
  - **Sebaceous hyperplasia**: Mature follicles without epidermal changes
- **DDx of basaloid follicular hamartoma**
  - **BCC**: More cytologic atypia, retraction spaces, inflammatory stroma, mitotic activity

(Left) *Nevus sebaceus has an acanthotic epidermis, often with a papillomatous surface →. The follicles have a disorganized appearance →, and there are often associated large sebaceous glands →.* **(Right)** *Basaloid follicular hamartoma is characterized by multifocal islands of basaloid epithelium → resembling primitive follicles that are surrounded by a fibroblastic stroma.*

Nevus Sebaceus

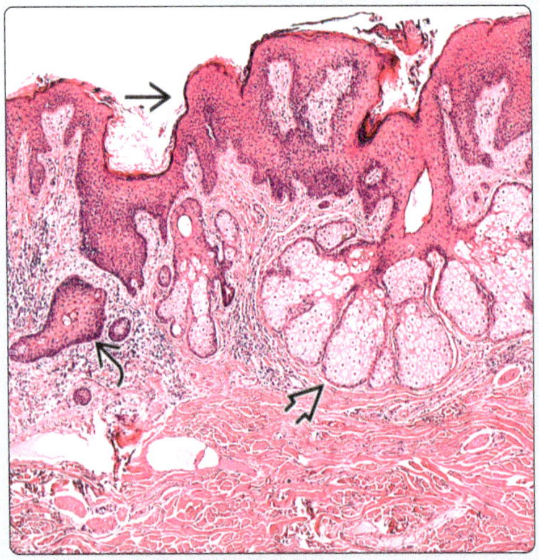

Basaloid Follicular Hamartoma

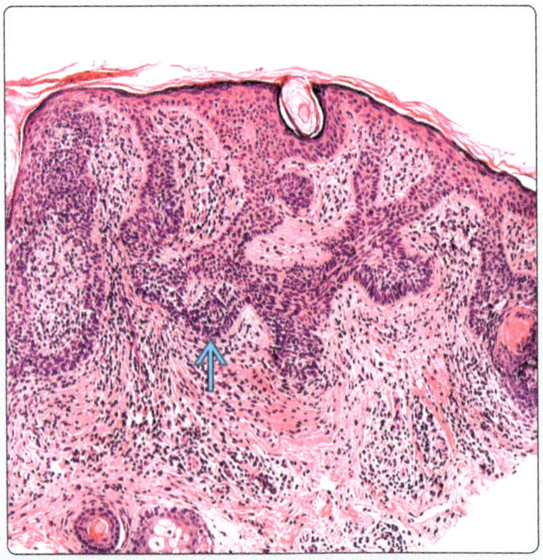

(Left) *This nevus sebaceus demonstrates a papillomatous acanthotic epidermis → overlying disorganized follicles with prominent sebaceous glands →.* **(Right)** *In this nevus sebaceus from a young child, there are disorganized, immature follicles →; sebaceous glands are not prominent in this view but are often hypoplastic before puberty.*

Nevus Sebaceus at Low Magnification

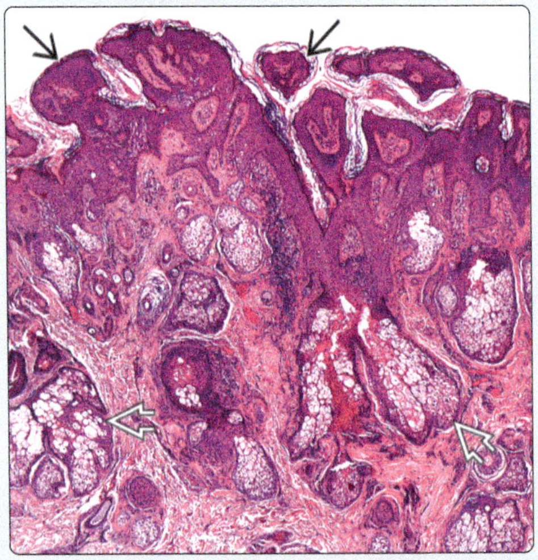

Immature Follicles in Nevus Sebaceus

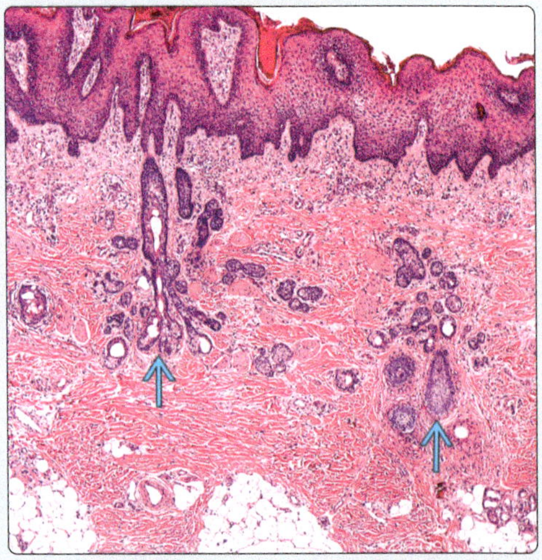

TERMINOLOGY

Synonyms

- Nevus sebaceus: Organoid nevus, Jadassohn nevus

Definitions

- Nevus sebaceus
  - Hamartoma with abnormalities of epidermis, follicles, sebaceous glands, and apocrine glands
- Basaloid follicular hamartoma
  - Hamartoma resembling primitive follicles

ETIOLOGY/PATHOGENESIS

Developmental Anomaly

- Nevus sebaceus
  - Deletion of *PTCH1* (PTCH) gene may play role
- Basaloid follicular hamartoma
  - Possible role for Sonic Hedgehog signaling pathway

CLINICAL ISSUES

Presentation

- Nevus sebaceus
  - Usually presents in infancy, often at birth; often enlarges during puberty
  - Usually involves scalp, less commonly on face, as yellowish flat to warty plaque
- Follicular hamartomas
  - Solitary
    - Elderly patients with flesh-colored papule on face
    - May clinically mimic basal cell carcinoma (BCC)
  - Localized
    - Presents in 3rd-4th decade on head as erythematous to hyperpigmented plaque
  - Linear nevoid
    - Pale brown plaque with follicular papules in linear pattern; may follow dermatome
  - Inherited
    - Autosomal dominant, presents in adulthood
    - Numerous flesh-colored or hyperpigmented papules on head/neck, trunk, and anogenital areas
    - May be associated with alopecia &/or cystic fibrosis

Treatment

- Surgical approaches
  - Excision

Prognosis

- Benign
  - Rarely, BCC can arise in association with nevus sebaceus

MICROSCOPIC

Histologic Features

- **Nevus sebaceus**
  - Acanthosis and papillomatosis of epidermis
    - Similar to changes seen in epidermal nevi
  - Disorganized follicles with primitive germ-like areas
    - Reduction in number of mature follicles
  - Abnormalities of sebaceous glands
    - Disorganized proliferation of sebaceous glands high in dermis
    - May communicate with epidermal surface
    - May not be associated with follicle
    - Sebaceous glands less prominent in young children
  - Abnormalities of sweat glands: Dilated apocrine glands in deep dermis during/after puberty
  - Associated other tumors arising within nevus sebaceus
    - Trichoblastoma (most common), syringocystadenoma papilliferum (next most common), and, rarely, BCC
- **Basaloid follicular hamartoma**
  - Multiple islands of basaloid epithelium affecting most or all pilosebaceous units
    - Islands arranged as anastomosing cords of basaloid epithelium
    - May have squamoid areas and focal horn cysts
    - Epithelium weakly positive for Bcl-2
  - Islands surrounded by loose fibroblastic stroma that is CD34(+)
  - Absence of mature follicular elements (i.e., sebaceous glands)
  - No retraction artifact, no atypia, no to rare mitoses

DIFFERENTIAL DIAGNOSIS

DDx of Nevus Sebaceus

- **Epidermal nevus**
  - Lacks abnormalities of follicles and sebaceous glands
- **Sebaceous hyperplasia**
  - Enlarged sebaceous glands attached to mature follicles or epidermis
  - No overlying epidermal acanthosis or papillomatosis
- **Sebaceous adenoma**
  - Larger nodular sebaceous proliferation, with more prominent layer of immature sebocytes
  - Lacks epidermal changes and primitive follicular structures

DDx of Basaloid Follicular Hamartoma

- **BCC**
  - Retraction artifact, inflammatory mucinous stroma
  - Cytologic atypia and mitoses
  - Immunohistochemistry
    - Epithelium Bcl-2(+); stroma CD34(-)
- **Trichoepithelioma**
  - Areas are indistinguishable from trichoepithelioma
  - Not multifocal like basaloid follicular hamartoma

SELECTED REFERENCES

1. Aslam A et al: Naevus sebaceus: a mosaic RASopathy. Clin Exp Dermatol. 39(1):1-6, 2014
2. Wang E et al: A rare combination of sebaceoma with carcinomatous change (sebaceous carcinoma), trichoblastoma, and poroma arising from a nevus sebaceus. J Cutan Pathol. 40(7):676-82, 2013
3. Mills O et al: Basaloid follicular hamartoma. Arch Pathol Lab Med. 134(8):1215-9, 2010
4. Alessi E et al: Nevus sebaceus. A clinicopathologic study of its evolution. Am J Dermatopathol. 8(1):27-31, 1986
5. Jones EW et al: Naevus sebaceus. A report of 140 cases with special regard to the development of secondary malignant tumours. Br J Dermatol. 82(2):99-117, 1970

(Left) *In this nevus sebaceus, there is prominent papillomatosis ➡, but the enlarged sebaceous glands ➡ lack conspicuous attachment to the epidermis.* **(Right)** *This abnormal sebaceous gland directly communicates with the epidermal surface ➡ and lacks a well-formed associated follicle.*

Nevus Sebaceus With Marked Papillomatosis and Sebaceous Glands

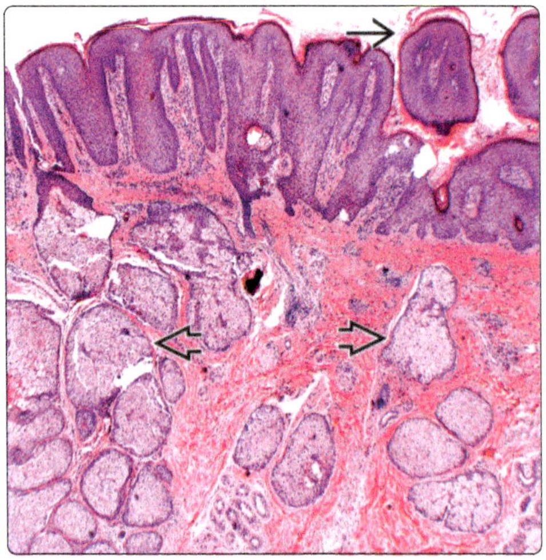

Sebaceous Gland Attached to Epidermis

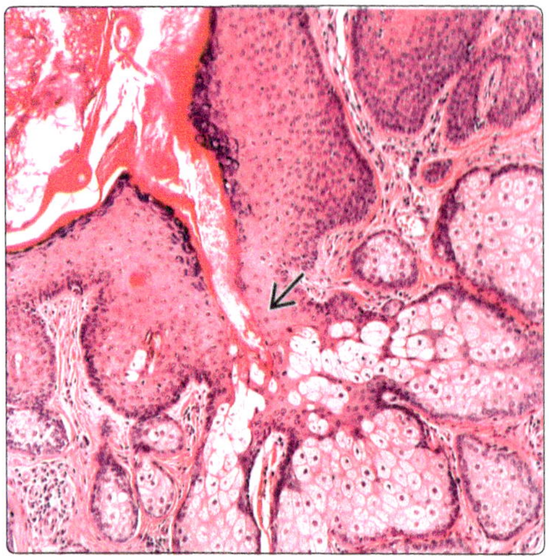

(Left) *In addition to the primitive follicles and enlarged sebaceous glands ➡, there are prominent ectatic apocrine glands ➡ present in some cases.* **(Right)** *High-power image of apocrine glands from nevus sebaceus demonstrates characteristic decapitation secretion ➡.*

Prominent Apocrine Glands

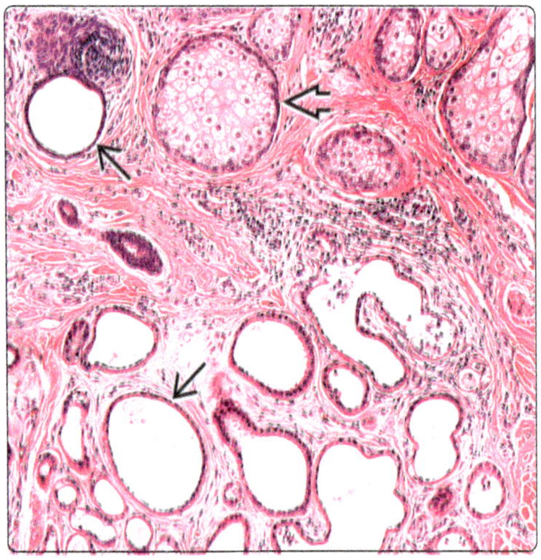

High Magnification of Apocrine Glands

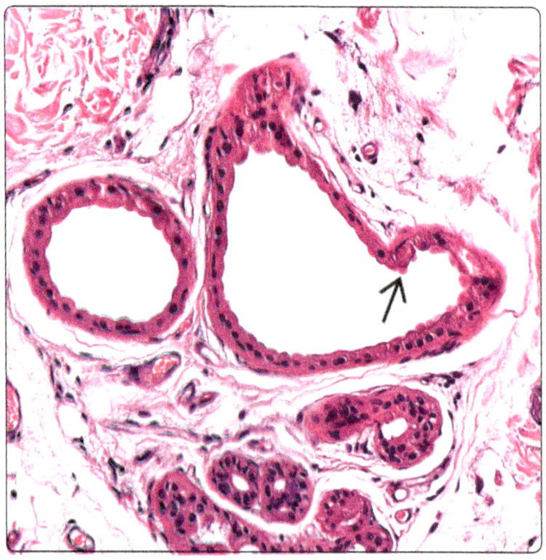

(Left) *Beneath the nevus sebaceus in the upper part of the image, there is a focal area of trichoblastoma ➡ formation. Although there are retraction spaces ➡, there is still a thin rim of stroma mostly surrounding the lobule of trichoblastoma.* **(Right)** *In this nevus sebaceus, there is an associated nodular basal cell carcinoma with prominent peripheral palisading and tumor-stroma retraction spaces ➡. High magnification showed multiple mitoses and apoptotic bodies.*

Nevus Sebaceus With Trichoblastoma

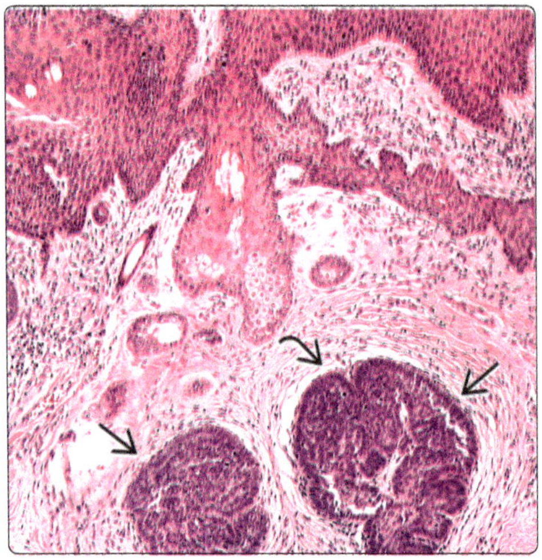

Nevus Sebaceous With Basal Cell Carcinoma

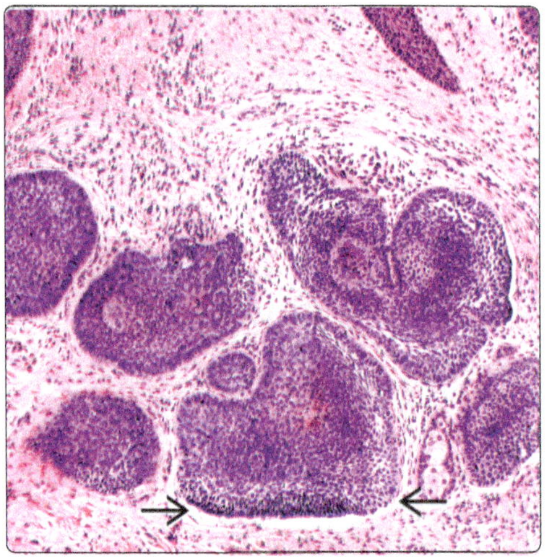

Basaloid Follicular Hamartoma

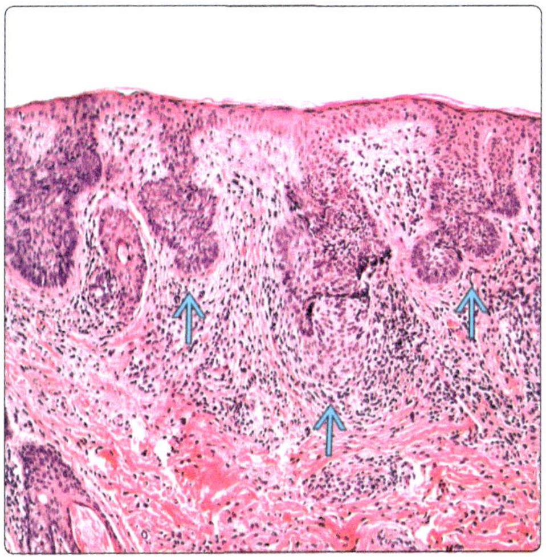

Basaloid Follicular Hamartoma

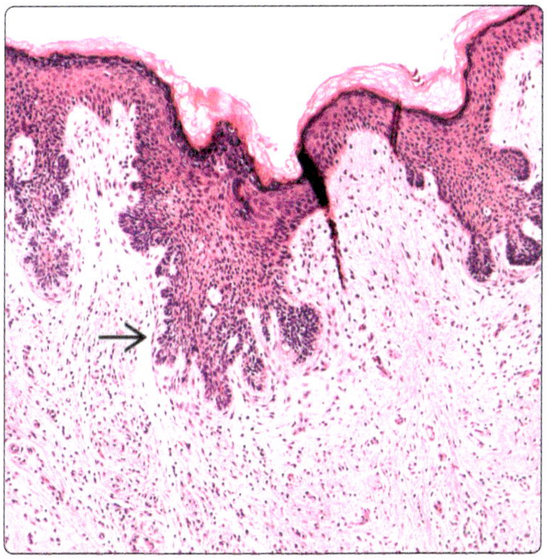

(Left) *Basaloid follicular hamartoma is characterized by a proliferation of basaloid epithelium recapitulating primitive follicles.* **(Right)** *In this early basaloid follicular hamartoma, the primitive follicular structures are not well developed.*

Basaloid Follicular Hamartoma at High Magnification

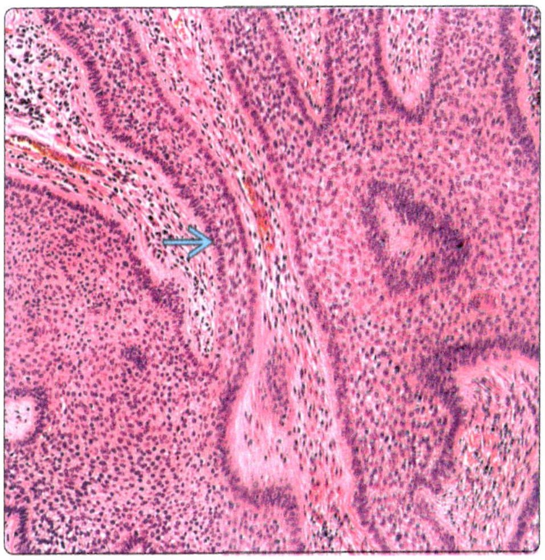

Basaloid Follicular Hamartoma at High Magnification

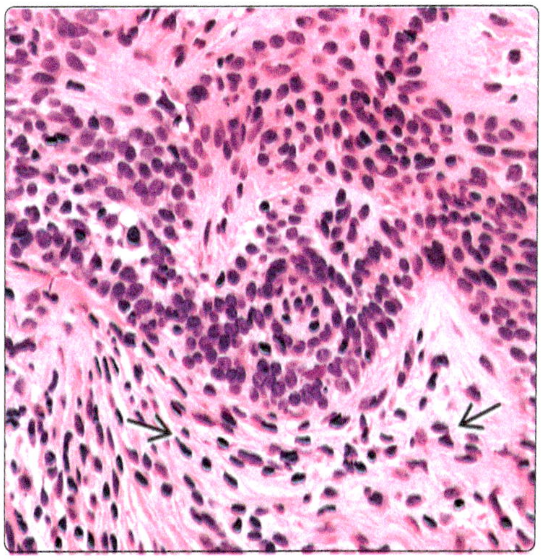

(Left) *This higher power image from a basaloid follicular hamartoma demonstrates anastomosing cords of basaloid epithelium with peripheral palisading. However, there is a conspicuous absence of atypia and mitotic activity.* **(Right)** *The epithelium of basaloid follicular hamartoma is surrounded by a cellular fibroblastic stroma. Note the absence of retraction spaces between the stroma and epithelium, and the lack of mitotic activity.*

Nevus Sebaceus

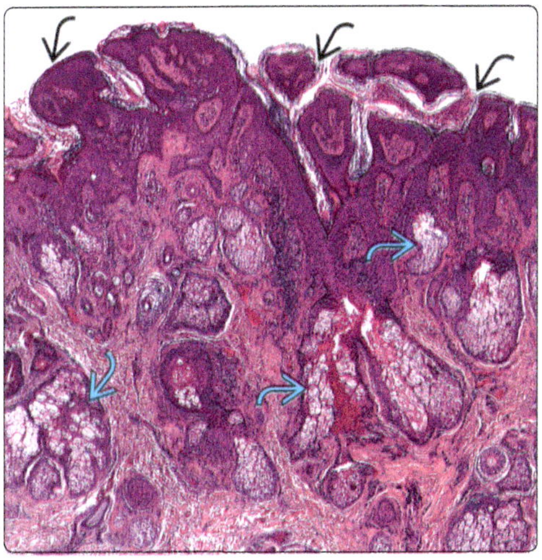

Nevus Sebaceus With Syringocystadenoma Papilliferum

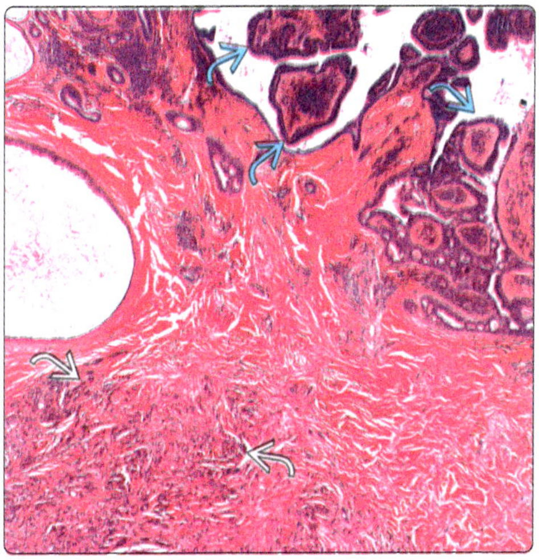

(Left) *Another example of nevus sebaceus shows mammillated papillomatosis with superficially attached sebaceous glands opening to the epidermis. These features are typical of nevus sebaceus.* **(Right)** *Nevus sebaceus can be complicated by development of adnexal tumors, including syringocystadenoma papilliferum. The papillary architecture lined by a 2-cell layer is very characteristic of this tumor. There is also a rare associated apocrine carcinoma in the deeper dermis.*

Trichofolliculoma

KEY FACTS

ETIOLOGY/PATHOGENESIS

- Majority of cases are sporadic

CLINICAL ISSUES

- Benign hamartomatous lesion
- Face is most common location, especially around nose
- No malignant potential
- Usually presents in adults
- Males and females equally affected

MICROSCOPIC

- Folliculocystic tumor that communicates to overlying epidermis
- Cystic space filled with keratinous debris and hair shafts
- Numerous small, primitive follicles radiate around periphery of tumor and communicate with central cystic space
- May have small attached sebaceous glands
- Follicles surrounded by perifollicular stromal sheath
- Focal granulomatous inflammation secondary to rupture may be present

TOP DIFFERENTIAL DIAGNOSES

- Folliculosebaceous cystic hamartoma
  - May also represent later stage/regressing variant of trichofolliculoma, but is typically dermal-based tumor with prominent sebaceous glands
- Dilated pore of Winer
  - Cystically dilated follicle that communicates with overlying epidermis
- Trichoepithelioma
  - Lobules and nests of basaloid epithelium with peripheral palisading
  - Lacks central folliculocystic structure
- Dermoid cyst
  - Cystic lesion lined by bland squamous epithelium with follicular structures and sebaceous glands

Trichofolliculoma

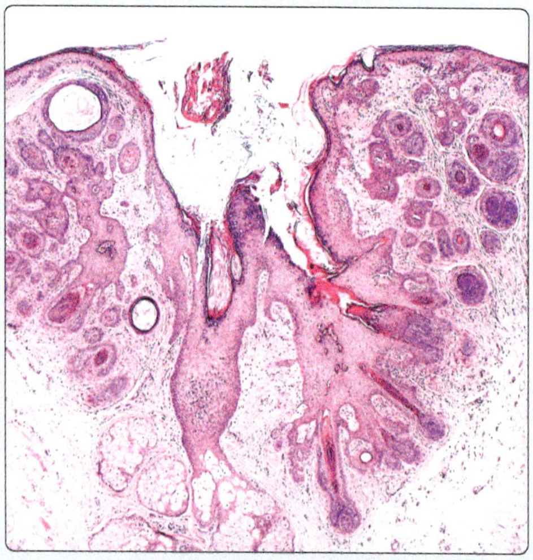

Trichofolliculoma

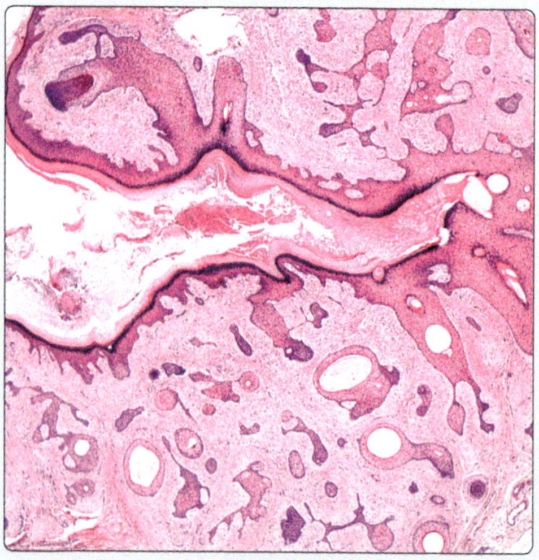

(Left) *Trichofolliculoma is an invaginated cystic tumor lined by keratinizing squamous epithelium that communicates with the overlying epidermis. The central cystic space is usually filled with keratinous debris.* **(Right)** *Trichofolliculoma is characterized by an invaginated cystic lesion lined by mature, keratinizing squamous epithelium that communicates with the overlying epidermis.*

Trichofolliculoma With Radiating Follicular Structures

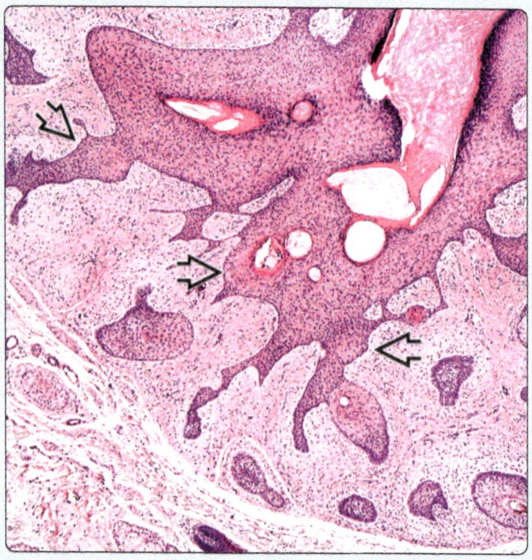

Trichofolliculoma With Primitive Radiating Follicular Structures

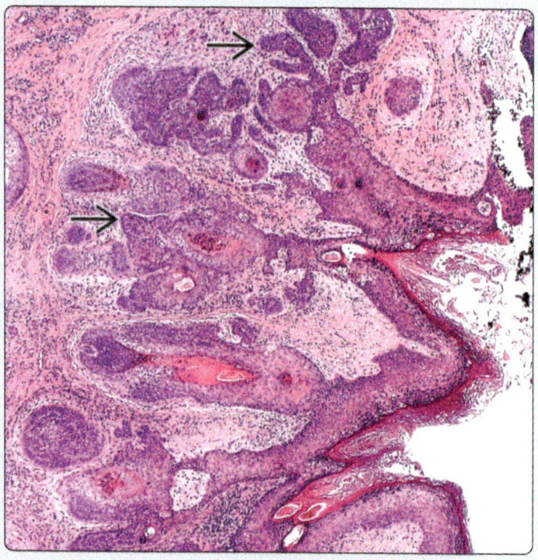

(Left) *Small, branching follicular structures ⇨ radiate out from, and communicate with, the central cystic space.* **(Right)** *Radiating around the central cystic space are numerous primitive follicles that connect with the central cystic space. The follicles often show secondary branching ⇨.*

TERMINOLOGY

Definitions

- Hamartoma with prominent follicular differentiation

ETIOLOGY/PATHOGENESIS

Unknown

- Majority of cases are sporadic

CLINICAL ISSUES

Epidemiology

- Incidence
  - Rare
- Age
  - Usually presents in adults
- Sex
  - Males and females equally affected

Presentation

- Dome-shaped papule with central dilated pore
  - Tuft of white hairs often emerges from opening
- Face is most common location, especially around nose
- Occasionally on scalp, neck, or other locations

Treatment

- Surgical approaches
  - Simple excision is curative

Prognosis

- Benign; no malignant potential

MICROSCOPIC

Histologic Features

- Cystic tumor that communicates to overlying epidermis
  - Cystic space filled with keratinous debris and hair shafts
  - Lined by squamous epithelium with thin granular layer
- Numerous small, primitive follicles radiate around periphery of tumor and communicate with central cystic space
  - Follicles demonstrate some architectural complexity
    - Secondary budding with abortive pilar differentiation
  - May have small attached sebaceous glands
  - Exhibits anagen, catagen, &/or telogen phases of hair cycle
- Follicles surrounded by perifollicular stromal sheath
- Granulomatous inflammation sometimes present

Cytologic Features

- Bland adnexal cells with small nuclei and basophilic- to eosinophilic-staining cytoplasm

Sebaceous Trichofolliculoma (Variant)

- Same architecture as conventional trichofolliculoma
  - Connects to epidermis
  - Central cystic space lined by squamous epithelium
  - Follicles radiating around periphery
- Primary difference: Numerous mature sebaceous lobules

DIFFERENTIAL DIAGNOSIS

Folliculosebaceous Cystic Hamartoma

- May also represent later stage/regressing variant of trichofolliculoma, but is typically dermal-based tumor
- Prominent sebaceous glands
  - More numerous than in conventional trichofolliculoma
- Prominent fibroblastic collagenous stroma surrounding tumor lobules
- Tumor lobules often have distinct clefts

Dilated Pore of Winer

- Cystically dilated follicle that communicates with epidermis
- Irregular epithelial budding radiating out from cyst
- Lacks primitive follicular structures of trichofolliculoma

Trichoepithelioma

- Lobules and nests of basaloid epithelium with peripheral palisading
- Small keratocysts present; often associated with rupture and granulomatous inflammation
- Lacks central cystic space lined by keratinizing squamous epithelium

Dermoid Cyst

- Presents in infants/young children, often on midline face
- Cyst lined by bland squamous epithelium with follicular structures and sebaceous glands
  - Up to 25% of cases also have eccrine &/or apocrine glands
- Lacks communication with overlying epidermis

Panfolliculoma

- Follicular structures do not radiate around central cystic space

DIAGNOSTIC CHECKLIST

Pathologic Interpretation Pearls

- Cystic follicular structure lined by mature squamous epithelium
- Numerous primitive follicular structures radiating from cystic lumen

SELECTED REFERENCES

1. Jégou-Penouil MH et al: [Trichofolliculoma: a retrospective review of 8 cases.] Ann Dermatol Venereol. 142(3):183-8, 2015
2. Bharti JN et al: Trichofolliculoma presenting as lobulated mass: a rare presentation. Int J Trichology. 6(1):19-20, 2014
3. Misago N et al: A revaluation of trichofolliculoma: the histopathological and immunohistochemical features. Am J Dermatopathol. 32(1):35-43, 2010
4. Wu YH: Folliculosebaceous cystic hamartoma or trichofolliculoma? A spectrum of hamartomatous changes inducted by perifollicular stroma in the follicular epithelium. J Cutan Pathol. 35(9):843-8, 2008
5. Kurokawa I et al: Trichofolliculoma: case report with immunohistochemical study of cytokeratins. Br J Dermatol. 148(3):597-8, 2003
6. Schulz T et al: The trichofolliculoma undergoes changes corresponding to the regressing normal hair follicle in its cycle. J Cutan Pathol. 25(7):341-53, 1998
7. Kimura T et al: Folliculosebaceous cystic hamartoma. A distinctive malformation of the skin. Am J Dermatopathol. 13(3):213-20, 1991
8. Gore HC Jr: Trichofolliculoma. Arch Dermatol. 89:385-6, 1964

Trichoadenoma

KEY FACTS

TERMINOLOGY

- Trichoadenoma of Nikolowski

CLINICAL ISSUES

- Solitary papule
- Often on face
- Sometimes on buttock or other sites
- No malignant potential

MICROSCOPIC

- Multiple mature cystic structures in dermis, showing epidermal-type keratinization
- Cysts have granular layer and flaky central keratin
- Interspersed among cystic structures are basaloid tubules and cords
- Fibrotic stroma
- Well circumscribed and not infiltrative
- Verrucous variant (verrucous trichoadenoma) contains vellus hairs
- CK20(+) cells are present in cysts and tubules/cords

TOP DIFFERENTIAL DIAGNOSES

- Trichoepithelioma
  - Basaloid islands, some in grape-like arrangements, with occasional horn cysts
- Trichofolliculoma
  - Central dominant follicle with smaller hair follicles radiating away from central follicle
- Microcystic adnexal carcinoma
  - Cords, tubules, and small clusters of cells with ductal differentiation infiltrate deep into dermis/subcutaneous tissues
- Syringoma
  - Lacks follicular cysts; small cords and tadpoles of cells, with ductal differentiation (eosinophilic cuticle)
- Nevus comedonicus

Low Magnification of Trichoadenoma

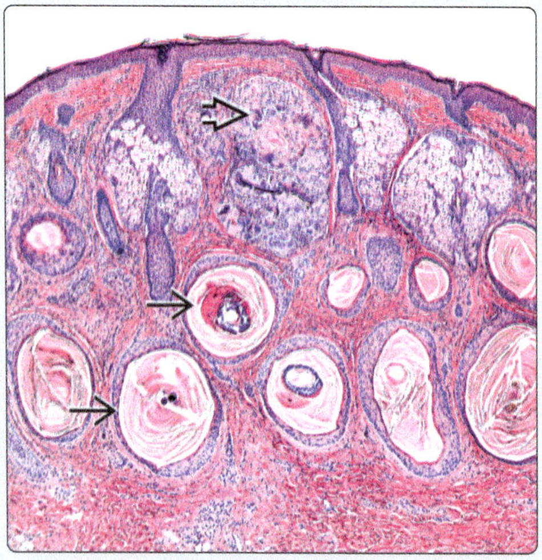

Follicular Cysts in Trichoadenoma

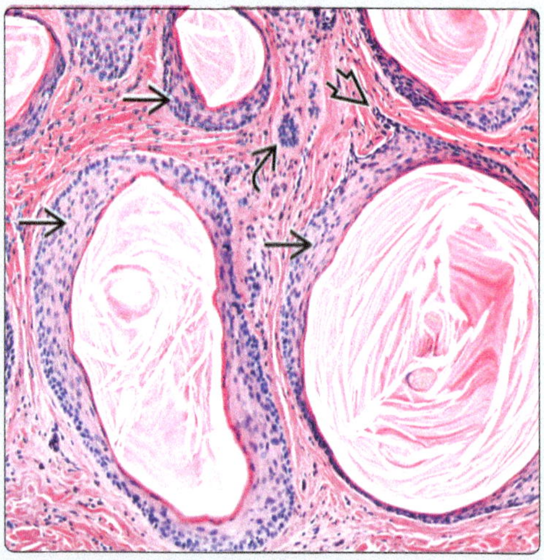

(Left) *Low-magnification view of a trichoadenoma shows a dome-shaped lesion based in the dermis. Note numerous mature horn cysts* →. *There is focal granulomatous inflammation surrounding the keratin debris* ⇨. **(Right)** *In this intermediate-power view of a trichoadenoma, there are numerous horn cysts* → *embedded in a sclerotic stroma. There are a few basaloid buds in the stroma* ↷ *and emanating off the borders of the horn cysts* ⇨.

Higher Magnification of Trichoadenoma

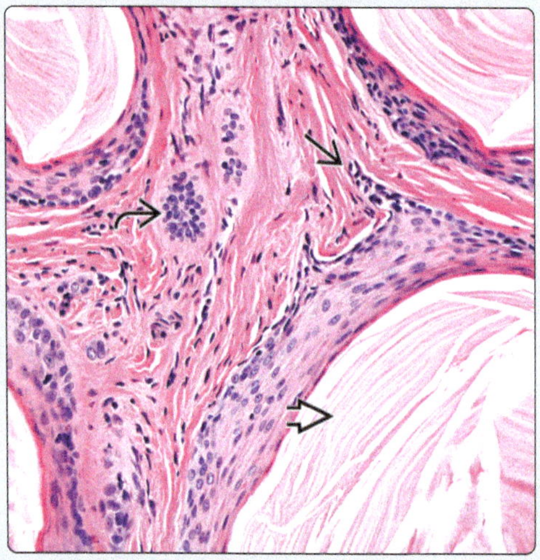

High Magnification of Trichoadenoma

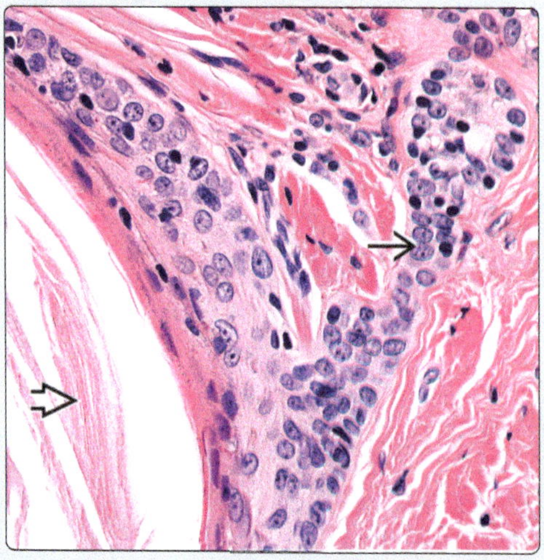

(Left) *High magnification view of a trichoadenoma highlights the sclerotic stroma and the loose keratin debris within the horn cysts* ⇨. *There are basaloid buds arising off of the horn cysts* → *and in the stroma* ↷. **(Right)** *In this high-power view of a trichoadenoma, flaky keratin* ⇨ *is seen within a horn cyst, at the border of which there is a basaloid tubule* →. *The stroma is sclerotic.*

TERMINOLOGY

Synonyms

- Trichoadenoma of Nikolowski

Definitions

- Benign follicular tumor
- Predominance of mature folliculocystic structures in dermis

CLINICAL ISSUES

Site

- Often on face
- Sometimes on buttock or other sites

Presentation

- Solitary papule

Prognosis

- Benign lesions
- No malignant potential

MICROSCOPIC

Histologic Features

- Multiple cystic structures in dermis, showing epidermal-type keratinization and following features
  - Granular layer
  - Flaky central keratin (may see keratin granulomas)
  - CK10(+), suggesting infundibular differentiation
  - No hair follicle formation
- Occasional cysts may show tricholemmal differentiation with
  - Absent granular layer
  - Abrupt keratinization into dense, pink keratin
- Interspersed among cystic structures are basaloid tubules and cords
- CK20(+) cells are present in cysts and tubules/cords
- Fibrovascular stroma
- Well circumscribed
- Verrucous variant (verrucous trichoadenoma) contains vellus hairs

Cytologic Features

- No cytologic atypia

DIFFERENTIAL DIAGNOSIS

Trichoepithelioma

- Basaloid islands, some in grape-like arrangements, with occasional horn cysts
- Papillary mesenchymal bodies present
- Sclerotic stroma

Trichoepithelioma, Desmoplastic

- Occasional horn cysts (but not predominating as in trichoadenoma)
- Basaloid tubules and cords
- Often show calcifications and occasional foreign body giant cell reaction surrounding ruptured cysts
- Sclerotic stroma

Trichofolliculoma

- Central, dominant hair follicle
- Secondary, smaller hair follicles radiating away from central follicle

Panfolliculoma

- May show numerous dermal cystic structures with loose keratin and granular layer
- Also has other islands that show differentiation toward other parts of hair follicle
  - Bulbar
    - May show matrical cells
  - Isthmic
    - May show clear cells or trichohyalin granules

Microcystic Adnexal Carcinoma

- Sometimes has scattered cystic structures in superficial dermis
- Cords, tubules, and small clusters of cells with ductal differentiation infiltrate deep into dermis/subcutaneous tissues
- Cytologic atypia may be minimal
- Often perineural invasion present

Syringoma

- Lacks component of cysts with loose keratin
- Small cords and tadpoles of cells, with ductal differentiation (eosinophilic cuticle)
- Clear cells often present in islands

Nevus Comedonicus

- Multiple cysts in upper dermis with granular cell layer and loose keratin
- Lacks basaloid tubules/cords
- Clinically typically linear lesion, often present from birth

Favre-Racouchot Disease

- Multiple milia (small cysts with granular layer and loose keratin) in background of solar elastosis
- Lacks basaloid tubules/cords
- Clinically numerous open comedones on heavily sun-damaged skin, especially malar area

DIAGNOSTIC CHECKLIST

Pathologic Interpretation Pearls

- Predominance of cystic epithelial islands with rare basaloid tubules/cords in fibrotic stroma
- Well circumscribed and limited to dermis

SELECTED REFERENCES

1. Mahajan SR et al: A rare case of trichoadenoma over the vulva. Indian J Sex Transm Dis. 36(1):83-5, 2015
2. Lever JF et al: Trichoadenoma of an eyelid in an adult mimicking sebaceous cell carcinoma. Ophthal Plast Reconstr Surg. 28(4):e101-2, 2012
3. Shimanovich I et al: Trichoadenoma of Nikolowski is a distinct neoplasm within the spectrum of follicular tumors. J Am Acad Dermatol. 62(2):277-83, 2010
4. Lee WS et al: Congenital trichoadenoma with an unusual clinical manifestation. J Am Acad Dermatol. 57(5):905-6, 2007
5. Kurokawa I et al: Trichoadenoma: cytokeratin expression suggesting differentiation towards the follicular infundibulum and follicular bulge regions. Br J Dermatol. 153(5):1084-6, 2005

Trichoepithelioma

KEY FACTS

TERMINOLOGY

- Trichoepithelioma
- Basaloid follicular proliferation with mixture of primitive follicular structures and mature infundibulocystic keratinizing areas

ETIOLOGY/PATHOGENESIS

- Some cases are inherited as part of genetic syndrome, including Brooke-Spiegler syndrome

CLINICAL ISSUES

- Most commonly occur on the face, but may involve other head and neck sites
- Excellent prognosis, very low recurrence or malignant potential

MICROSCOPIC

- Multiple lobules and nests of basaloid cells, typically confined to superficial dermis
- Scattered areas of infundibulocystic differentiation (keratinizing cysts) are typically present
- Tumor is associated with fibrotic and cellular stroma
- Papillary mesenchymal bodies classically are present
- Calcifications and granulomatous inflammation (reaction to ruptured cysts) often present
- Mucin is almost always absent in stroma
- **Desmoplastic trichoepithelioma**
  - Superficial folliculocystic structures and calcifications
  - Deeper infiltrative-appearing cords and small islands in densely fibrotic stroma

TOP DIFFERENTIAL DIAGNOSES

- Basal cell carcinoma
- Microcystic adnexal carcinoma
- Trichoblastoma
- Trichoadenoma
- Sebaceoma

Clinical Photograph of Multiple Lesions

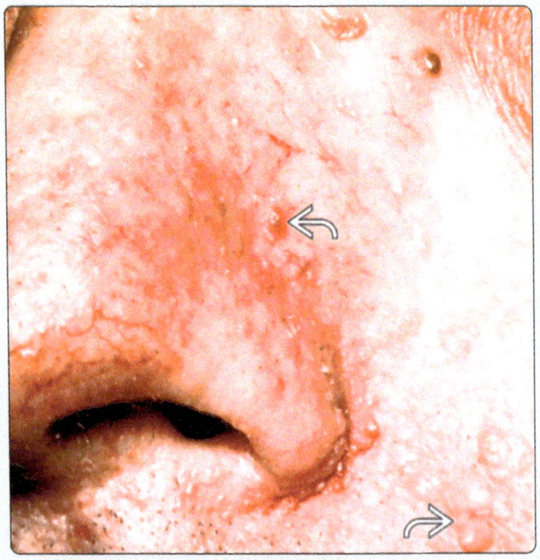

Trichoepithelioma at Low Magnification

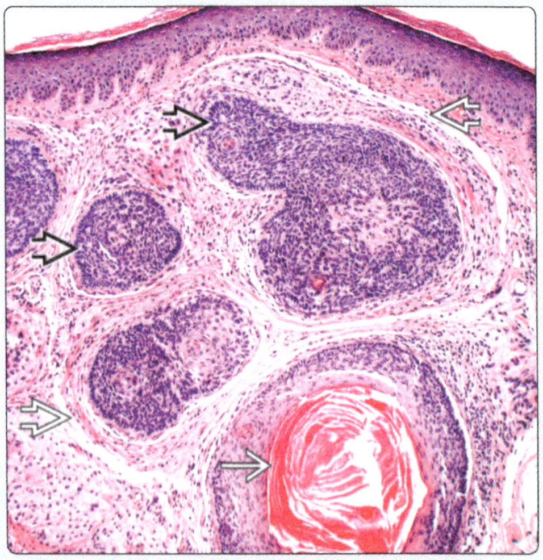

(Left) *Multiple trichoepitheliomas are scattered over the central face and nasolabial area presenting as flesh-colored, 1- to 4-mm papules. (Courtesy B. Hall, MD.)* **(Right)** *Scanning magnification of trichoepithelioma (TE) shows irregular islands of bland basaloid cells with prominent horn cysts and clefts between collagen bundles, rather than the tumor-stromal retraction artifact seen in basal cell carcinoma (BCC).*

Higher Magnification of Papillary Mesenchymal Bodies

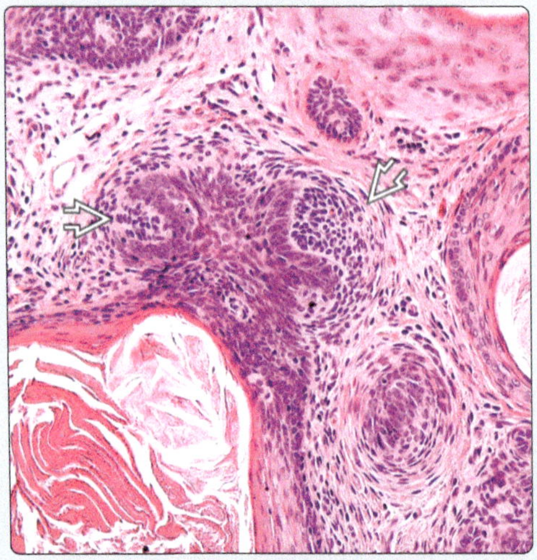

Desmoplastic Trichoepithelioma

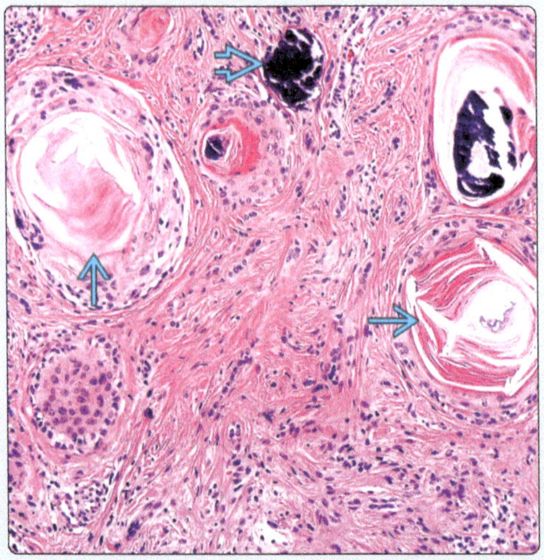

(Left) *High-power view of a TE demonstrates characteristic papillary mesenchymal bodies invaginating into the basaloid cells. (Courtesy A. Bowen, MD.)* **(Right)** *Desmoplastic TE can mimic a morpheaform BCC in some cases. However, the prominent horn cysts and calcifications are more consistent with a TE. (Courtesy G. Fraga, MD.)*

TERMINOLOGY

Abbreviations

- Trichoepithelioma (TE)

Definitions

- Basaloid proliferation with mixture of primitive follicular structures and mature infundibulocystic keratinizing areas

ETIOLOGY/PATHOGENESIS

Genetic

- Some cases are inherited as part of a genetic syndrome, including Brooke-Spiegler, familial TEs, or Rombo syndrome
- Present as multiple lesions, often with cylindromas and spiradenomas (Brooke-Spiegler syndrome)

CLINICAL ISSUES

Epidemiology

- Incidence
  - Relatively common tumors
- Age
  - Usually present in adults
- Sex
  - Slight male predominance

Site

- Most commonly occur on face, but may involve other head and neck sites

Presentation

- Solitary or multiple papules
  - Sporadic cases are typically solitary
  - Inherited cases are usually multiple

Treatment

- Options, risks, complications
  - Surgical excision is curative
  - Should be recommended in partial biopsies in order to exclude basal cell carcinoma (BCC)

Prognosis

- Excellent; very low recurrence or malignant potential
- However, rare cases have been associated with (or progressed to) BCC

MACROSCOPIC

General Features

- Small, superficial dermal-based lesion

MICROSCOPIC

Histologic Features

- Multiple lobules and nests of basaloid cells, typically confined to superficial dermis
- Areas of infundibulocystic differentiation (keratinizing cysts) are present
- Associated fibrotic and cellular stroma
  - Stromal-stromal cleft artifact may be present, but no tumor-stromal clefts (as in BCC)
  - Mucin is almost always absent in the stroma
- Papillary mesenchymal bodies
  - Characterized by invagination of fibroblastic stroma into basaloid nest
- Calcifications and granulomatous inflammation (reaction to ruptured cysts) are often present

Cytologic Features

- Basaloid cells with small, hyperchromatic nuclei, inconspicuous nucleoli, and eosinophilic cytoplasm

Subtype

- **Desmoplastic trichoepithelioma**
  - More common in women
  - Shows superficial folliculocystic structures and calcifications
  - Deeper infiltrative-appearing cords and small islands in densely fibrotic stroma

DIFFERENTIAL DIAGNOSIS

Basal Cell Carcinoma

- Usually shows multiple attachments to overlying epidermis (focal or absent in TE)
- Also shows the following features not seen in TE
  - Prominent peripheral palisading
  - Mucinous stroma
  - Tumor-stroma retraction artifact
  - Numerous mitotic and apoptotic figures
- Immunohistochemistry may be useful in some cases (especially small, partial biopsies)
  - Bcl-2, p53, and Ki-67 all elevated in BCC (low to negative in TE)
  - CK20 highlights Merkel cells in TE (rare or absent in BCC)

Microcystic Adnexal Carcinoma

- Can be difficult, if not impossible, to distinguish from desmoplastic trichoepithelioma in superficial biopsies
- Need to see the base of lesion to evaluate for perineural invasion and deep invasion

Trichoblastoma

- Larger, more nodular tumor that often extends into deep dermis/superficial subcutis
- Histologic features overlap with those of TE, which some dermatopathologists regard as superficial trichoblastoma
  - However, infundibulocystic differentiation more common in TE

SELECTED REFERENCES

1. Kallam AR et al: Basal cell carcinoma developing from trichoepithelioma: review of three cases. J Clin Diagn Res. 10(3):PD17-9, 2016
2. Nuno-Gonzalez A et al: Desmoplastic trichoepithelioma: an infrequent entity not to be missed: report of two cases. Pediatr Dermatol. 32(5):e208-9, 2015
3. Reuven B et al: Multiple trichoepitheliomas associated with a novel heterozygous mutation in the CYLD gene as an adjunct to the histopathological diagnosis. Am J Dermatopathol. 35(4):445-7, 2013
4. Sellheyer K et al: The immunohistochemical differential diagnosis of microcystic adnexal carcinoma, desmoplastic trichoepithelioma and morpheaform basal cell carcinoma using BerEP4 and stem cell markers. J Cutan Pathol. 40(4):363-70, 2013
5. Mamelak AJ et al: Desmoplastic trichoepithelioma. J Am Acad Dermatol. 62(1):102-6, 2010
6. Lum CA et al: Proliferative characterization of basal-cell carcinoma and trichoepithelioma in small biopsy specimens. J Cutan Pathol. 31(8):550-4, 2004

(Left) *Superficial biopsy of a TE shows islands of basaloid cells ➔ with prominent horn cysts ➔ and clefts between collagen bundles ➔, rather than tumor-stromal retraction artifact as in BCC.* **(Right)** *Higher magnification of TE shows basaloid nests with areas of peripheral palisading ➔. Focal intratumoral collections of mucin ➔ can be seen in some cases, but no stromal mucin is present.*

Superficial Dermal Trichoepithelioma

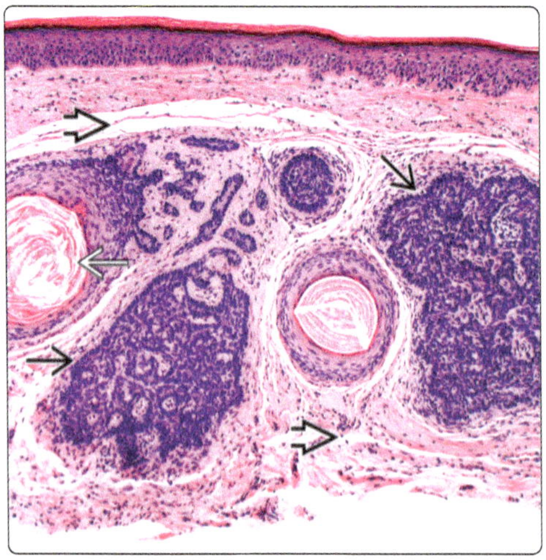

Higher Magnification of Basaloid Nests

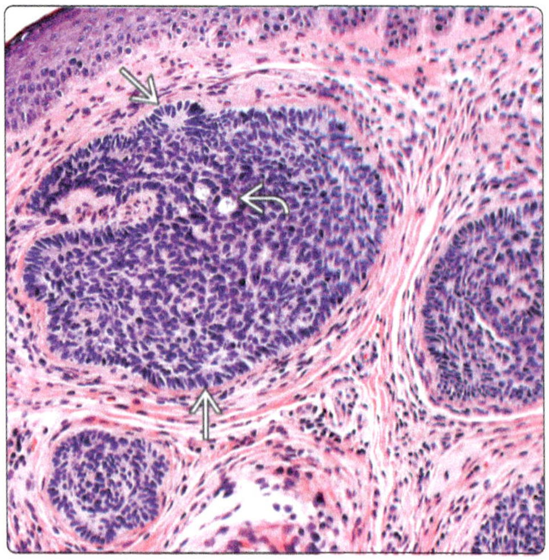

(Left) *TE often shows variably sized nests of more primitive basaloid cells ➔ alternating with areas of more mature-appearing squamous cells ➔ lining follicular cysts. (Courtesy A. Bowen, MD.)* **(Right)** *A deep area of desmoplastic trichoepithelioma shows multiple infiltrative-appearing cords of cells ➔ mimicking a desmoplastic BCC. (Courtesy G. Fraga, MD.)*

Low Magnification of Squamoid Areas

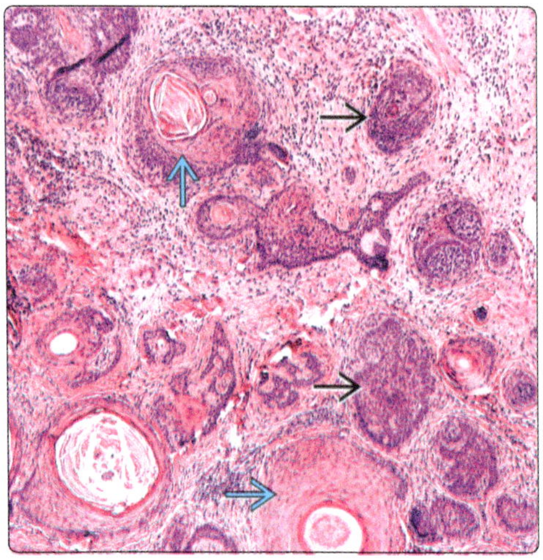

Desmoplastic Trichoepithelioma

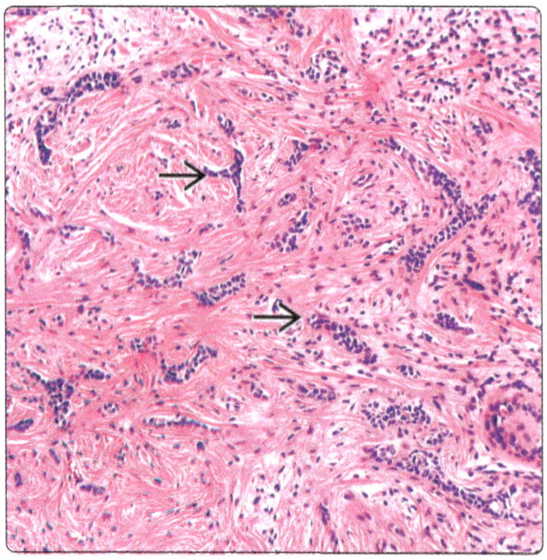

(Left) *CK20 strongly highlights significant numbers of Merkel cells in a TE ➔. These cells are almost always present in benign follicular neoplasms and absent in BCC.* **(Right)** *Other markers that are useful in the differential diagnosis of TE vs. BCC include p53 and Ki-67, both of which are typically low in TE, and significantly elevated in BCC. This is an example of p53 staining, which shows only a few scattered positive nuclei ➔, mostly at the periphery of the tumor.*

CK20 Immunohistochemistry

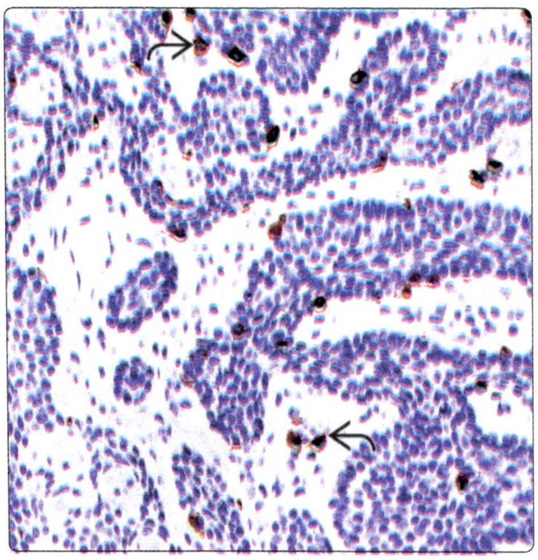

p53 Immunohistochemistry

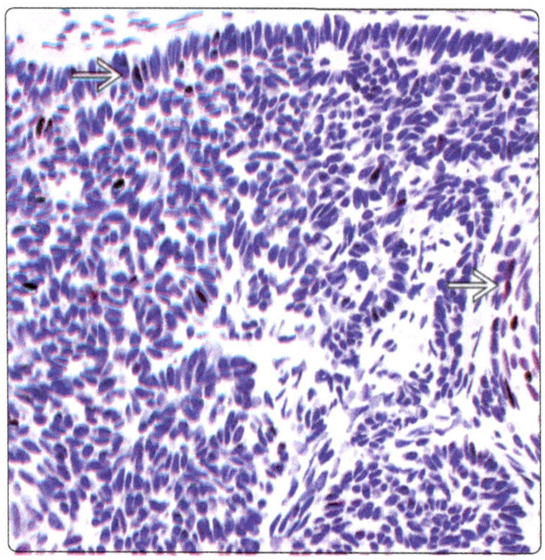

Differential Diagnosis: Trichoblastoma

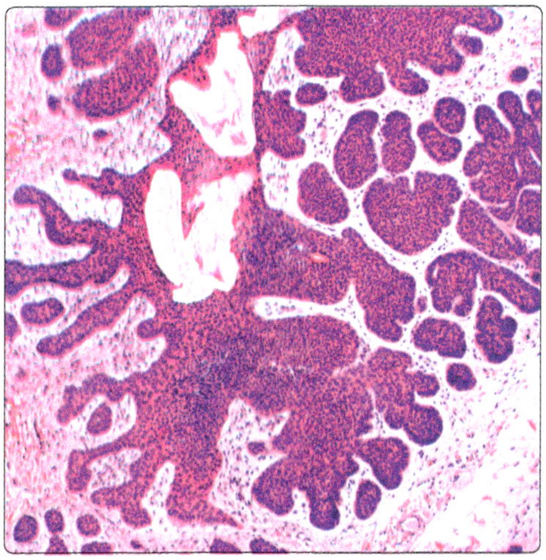

Differential Diagnosis: Sebaceoma

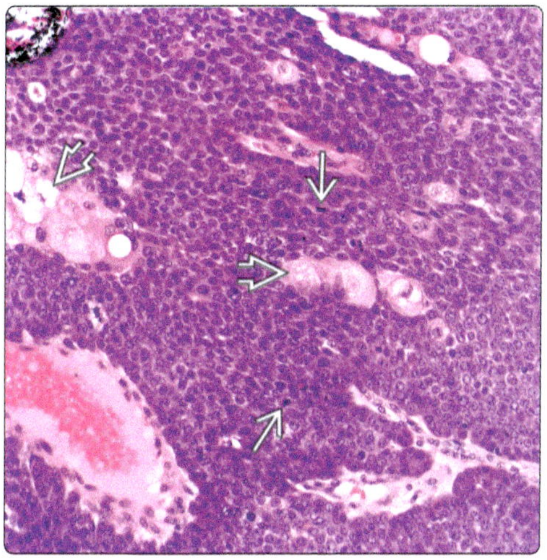

(Left) *Trichoblastoma (TB) is closely related to TE, which may be considered a superficial type of TB. While the histologic findings are similar, TB is typically a larger and deeper nodular lesion, which may even extend into the subcutaneous tissue.* **(Right)** *Sebaceoma shows a predominantly basaloid population of cells with nuclear hyperchromasia surrounding several large clear cells with abundant, multivacuolated cytoplasm. Several mitotic figures are seen, which can be quite numerous in sebaceomas.*

Differential Diagnosis: BCC

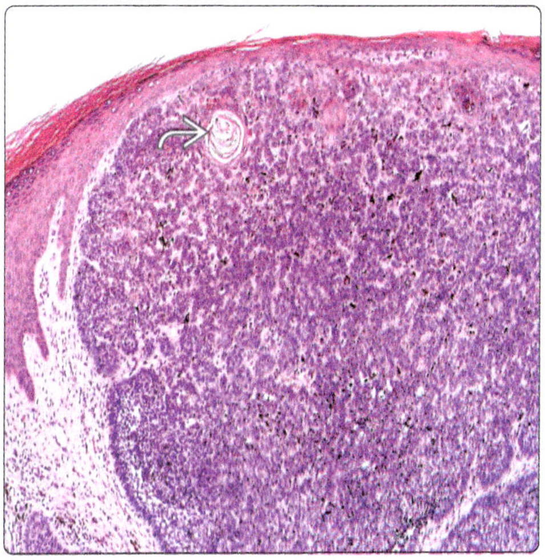

Differential Diagnosis: BCC

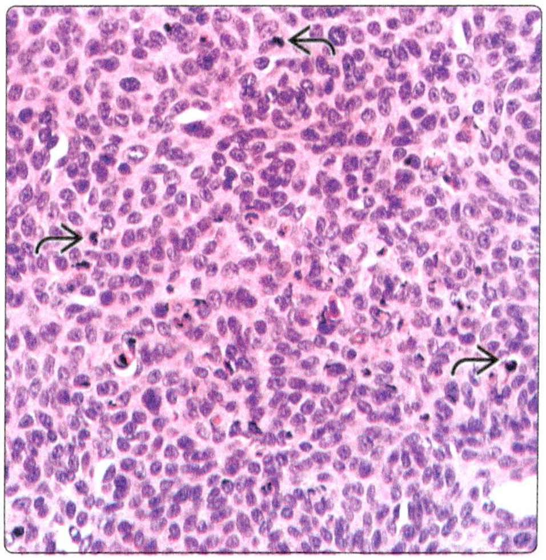

(Left) *This example of BCC shows focal areas of follicular differentiation (i.e., infundibulocystic type BCC); however, the tumor is composed of larger nodules than those seen in TE and shows significant atypia and mitotic activity, consistent with BCC.* **(Right)** *High magnification of a BCC shows numerous mitotic and apoptotic figures, which should be absent or rare in TE.*

Differential Diagnosis: BCC

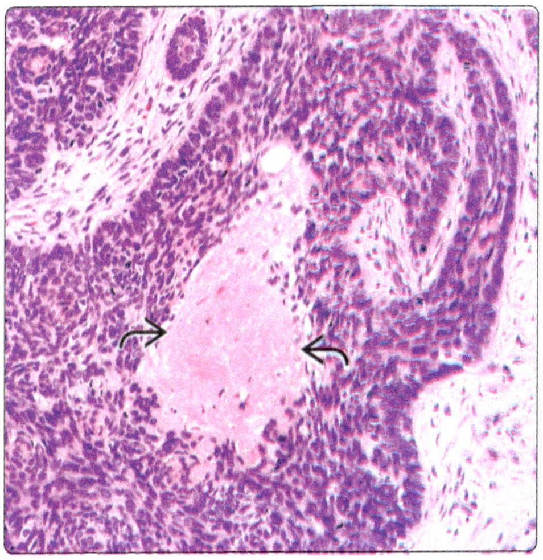

Differential Diagnosis: Merkel Cell Carcinoma

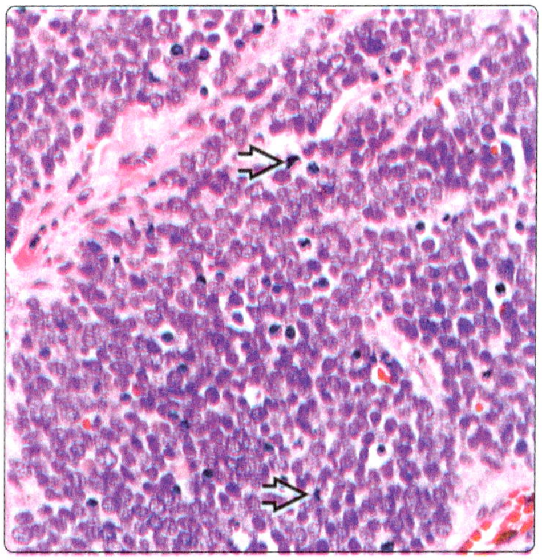

(Left) *This example of BCC showed areas of follicular differentiation (i.e., infundibulocystic type BCC); however, foci comedonecrosis are also identified, consistent with BCC.* **(Right)** *Merkel cell carcinoma can rarely enter the differential diagnosis at low-power examination; however, higher magnification reveals cytologic atypia with numerous apoptotic figures and mitotic figures.*

KEY FACTS

TERMINOLOGY

- Trichoblastoma (TB)
- Synonym: Giant trichoepithelioma
- Benign adnexal tumor showing primitive follicular differentiation

CLINICAL ISSUES

- Head and neck area, especially scalp
  - Can be multiple in some cases
- Rare recurrences and association with, or progression to, malignancy [basal cell carcinoma (BCC)]

MACROSCOPIC

- Nodular lesion involving deep dermis and subcutis
- Large, typically > 1 cm in diameter

MICROSCOPIC

- Large, basaloid-appearing deep dermal-based nodule
  - Composed of irregular lobules and nests of basaloid cells
  - No epidermal connections
- Associated fibrotic stroma with increased numbers of fibroblasts
- Papillary mesenchymal bodies classically present, similar to TE
- Subtypes include trichogerminoma, rippled-pattern trichomatricoma, trichoblastic fibroma, and cutaneous lymphadenoma

TOP DIFFERENTIAL DIAGNOSES

- BCC
  - Usually shows multiple attachments to epidermis, mucinous stroma, and mitotic figures (focal or absent in TB)
- Trichoepithelioma
  - Smaller and more superficial than TB
- Sebaceoma
- Cylindroma
- Spiradenoma

Clinical Photograph of Trichoblastoma on Eyelid

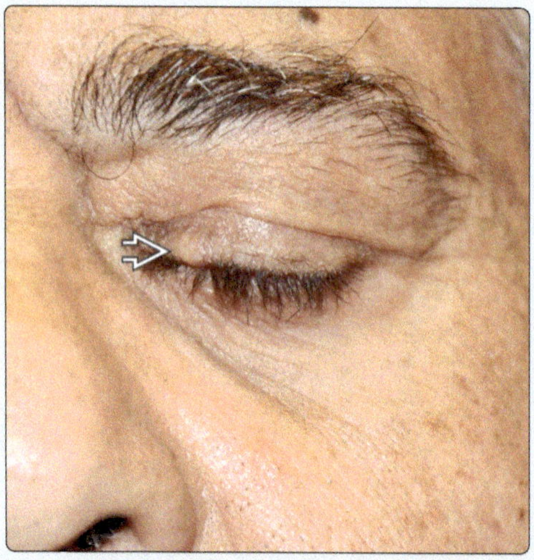

Scanning Magnification of Trichoblastoma

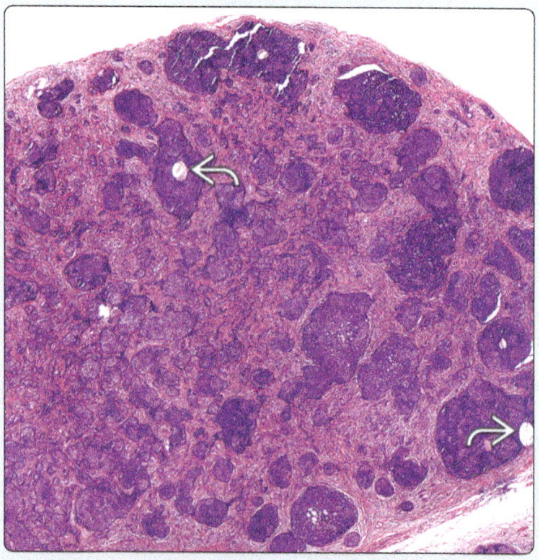

(Left) *Clinical photograph shows a nodular lesion on the eyelid ➡ of a patient with a history of multiple trichoblastomas and trichoepitheliomas (TEs).* **(Right)** *Scanning magnification of a trichoblastoma shows a nodular basaloid proliferation associated with a fibrotic stroma. Note the presence of scattered folliculocystic structures ➡.*

High Magnification of Trichoblastoma

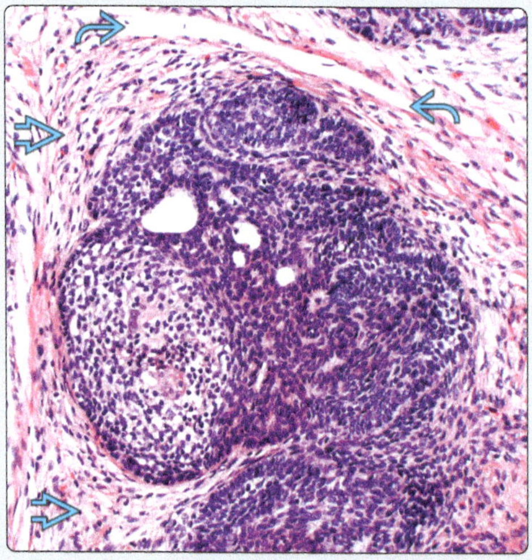

Trichoblastoma With Focal Sebaceous Differentiation

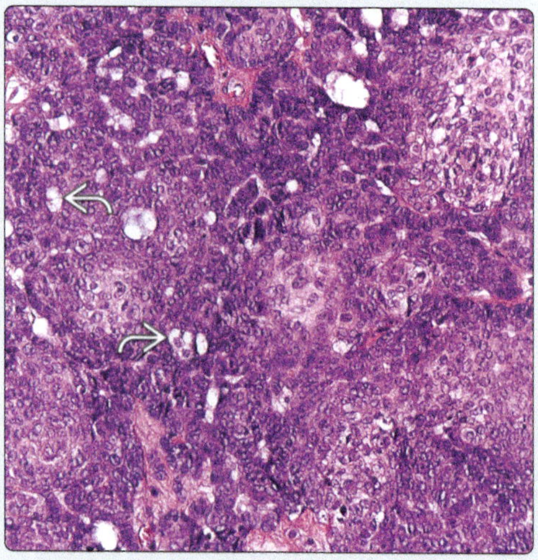

(Left) *High magnification of a trichoblastoma shows a lobular basaloid proliferation associated with a cellular, fibrotic stroma ➡. Note the prominent stromal-stromal retraction artifact ➡.* **(Right)** *Trichoblastoma can show sebaceous differentiation in some cases. Scattered clear cells with multivacuolated cytoplasm are identified ➡.*

TERMINOLOGY

Abbreviations

- Trichoblastoma (TB)

Synonyms

- Giant trichoepithelioma (TE)
- Trichoblastic fibroma
- Cutaneous lymphadenoma

Definitions

- Benign dermal-based adnexal tumor showing primitive follicular differentiation

CLINICAL ISSUES

Epidemiology

- Age
  - Usually occur in adults

Site

- Head and neck area, especially scalp

Presentation

- Dermal nodule/mass lesion
  - Usually single but may rarely be multiple
- Usually asymptomatic

Treatment

- Surgical approaches
  - Complete excision is curative
  - Should be recommended in cases of partial biopsy in order to exclude basal cell carcinoma (BCC)

Prognosis

- Excellent in most cases

MACROSCOPIC

General Features

- Nodular lesion involving deep dermis and subcutis

Size

- Large, typically > 1 cm in diameter

MICROSCOPIC

Histologic Features

- Large, basaloid-appearing deep dermal-based nodule
  - Usually symmetric and shows well-circumscribed borders
  - Composed of irregular lobules and nests of basaloid cells
  - No epidermal connections
- Associated fibrotic stroma with increased numbers of fibroblasts
  - Calcifications and granulomatous inflammation occasionally seen, but less common than in TE
- Papillary mesenchymal bodies classically present, similar to TE
  - Invagination of fibroblastic stroma into primitive follicular structures

Subtypes

- **Cutaneous lymphadenoma**
  - Rare variant with prominent lymphocytic infiltrate and clear cell features
- **Rippled-pattern trichoblastoma**
  - Palisading ribbons of basaloid cells; may resemble Verocay bodies

DIFFERENTIAL DIAGNOSIS

Basal Cell Carcinoma

- BCC usually shows multiple attachments to overlying epidermis (focal or absent in TB)
- BCC also shows following features (lacking in TB)
  - Prominent peripheral palisading
  - Mucinous stroma
  - Tumor-stromal retraction artifact (stromal-stromal retraction seen in TB)
  - Numerous mitotic and apoptotic figures
- Immunohistochemistry may be useful in some cases (particularly small, partial biopsies)
  - Bcl-2, p53, and Ki-67 all elevated in BCC (should be low in TB)
  - CK20 highlights Merkel cells in TB (absent in BCC)

Trichoepithelioma

- Small, papular lesion clinically
- Overlapping histologic features, but TE is smaller, more superficial than TB

Sebaceoma

- More superficial, epidermal- or follicular-based adnexal neoplasm
- Composed of lobules and nests of predominantly basaloid cells with minor population of clear cells
- Scattered mature sebaceous cells with multivacuolated cytoplasm

Cylindroma

- Dermal-based neoplasm composed of basaloid cells with ductal differentiation
- Irregular, jigsaw puzzle pattern of variably shaped lobules and nests
  - Surrounded by hyalinized basement membrane, and nests contain hyalinized globules

Spiradenoma

- Dermal-based nodular basaloid neoplasm with ductal differentiation
- Biphasic cellular population of smaller, darker cells and larger, pale cells
- Numerous lymphocytes typically sprinkled throughout tumor

SELECTED REFERENCES

1. Córdoba A et al: Bcl-2 and CD10 expression in the differential diagnosis of trichoblastoma, basal cell carcinoma, and basal cell carcinoma with follicular differentiation. Int J Dermatol. 48(7):713-7, 2009
2. Graham BS et al: Rippled-pattern sebaceous trichoblastoma. J Cutan Pathol. 27(9):455-9, 2000
3. Jaqueti G et al: Trichoblastoma is the most common neoplasm developed in nevus sebaceus of Jadassohn: a clinicopathologic study of a series of 155 cases. Am J Dermatopathol. 22(2):108-18, 2000
4. Diaz-Cascajo C et al: Cutaneous lymphadenoma. A peculiar variant of nodular trichoblastoma. Am J Dermatopathol. 18(2):186-91, 1996

(Left) *This example of trichoblastoma shows a proliferation of smaller nests and cords of basaloid cells associated with a fibrotic stroma with scattered lymphocytes. Note the small mature folliculocystic structures.* **(Right)** *Pigmented trichoblastoma is a relatively common type that shows occasional cystic spaces and a few cells with melanin pigmentation. Note the adjacent microcalcification.*

Small Cords and Folliculocystic Structures in Trichoblastoma

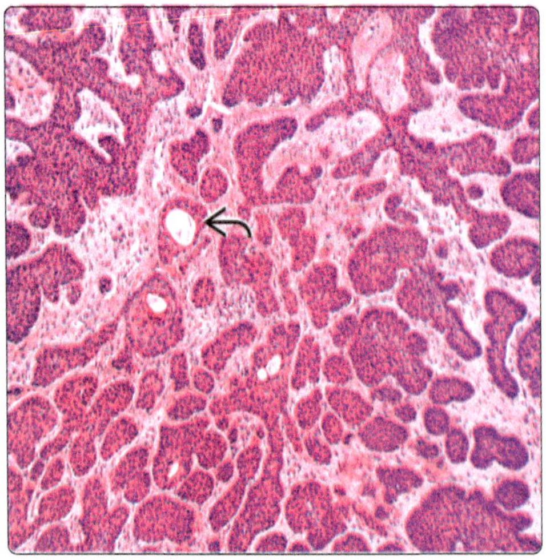

Pigmented Trichoblastoma With Calcifications

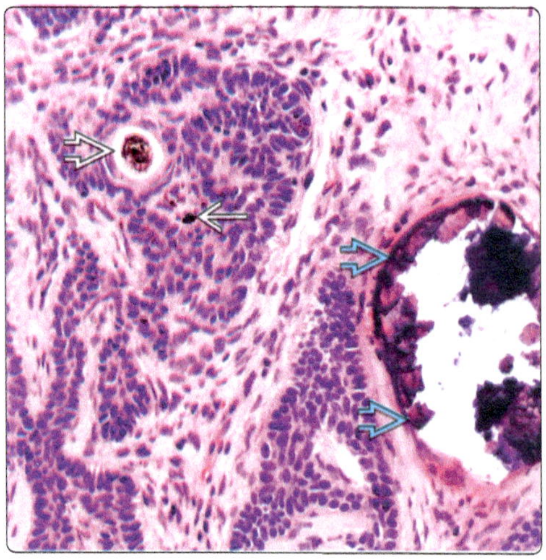

(Left) *High magnification of a folliculocystic structure shows pilar-type keratinization with a central lumen containing dense keratin and a few calcifications.* **(Right)** *High magnification of a papillary mesenchymal body shows invagination of cellular fibroblastic stroma into a peripheral bulb-like area of the tumor.*

High Magnification of Folliculocystic Structure

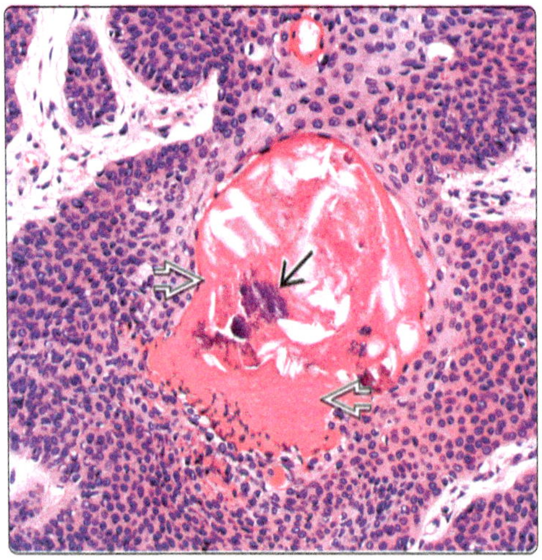

Papillary Mesenchymal Body in Trichoblastoma

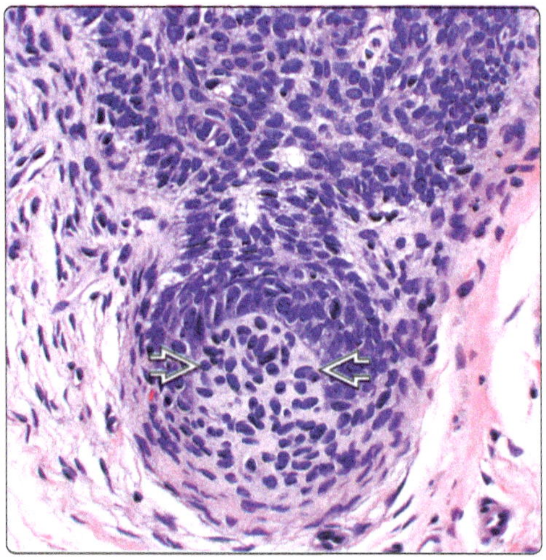

(Left) *Low magnification of a cutaneous lymphadenoma shows a multinodular tumor in the dermis associated with a prominent fibrotic stroma and focal microcalcifications.* **(Right)** *Intermediate-power view of cutaneous lymphadenoma shows small lobules and nests of basaloid cells with peripheral palisading. Note the associated cellular fibrotic stroma with chronic inflammation.*

Trichoblastoma Variant: Cutaneous Lymphadenoma

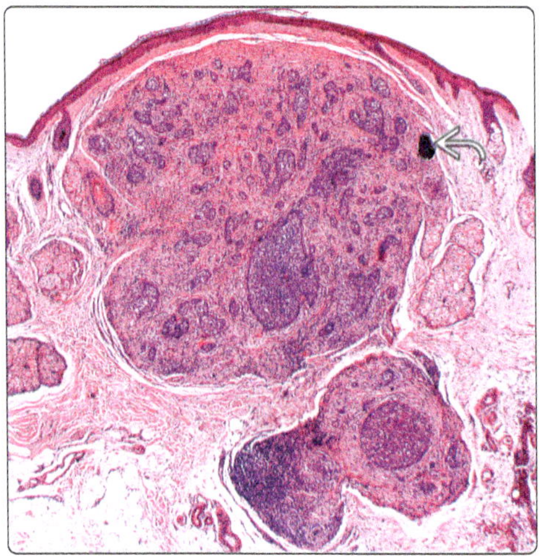

Trichoblastoma Variant: Cutaneous Lymphadenoma

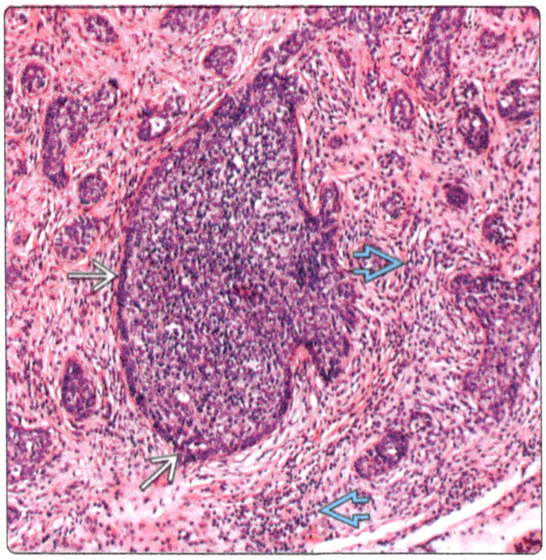

p53 Immunohistochemistry in Trichoblastoma

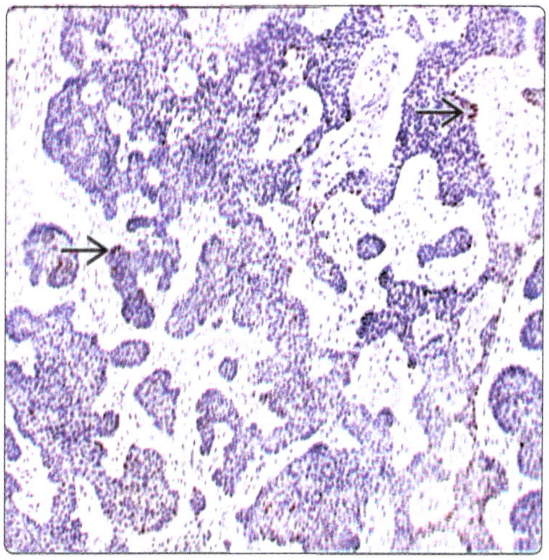

CK20 Immunohistochemistry in Trichoblastoma

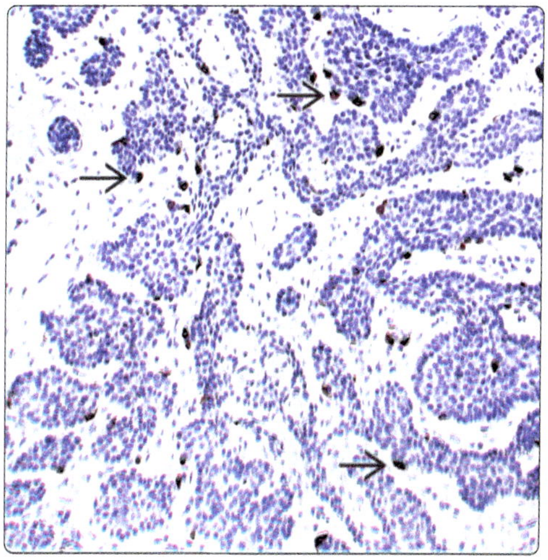

(Left) *Immunohistochemistry for p53 usually shows only focal staining (< 10% of cells staining) in trichoblastoma, usually within scattered peripheral cells ⇨. BCC usually shows much greater labeling with this marker (> 30-40% of cells).* **(Right)** *CK20 highlights Merkel cells ⇨ in TB, which are often quite numerous. Merkel cells are almost always completely absent in BCC, making this a useful marker in their distinction.*

Differential Diagnosis: Trichoepithelioma

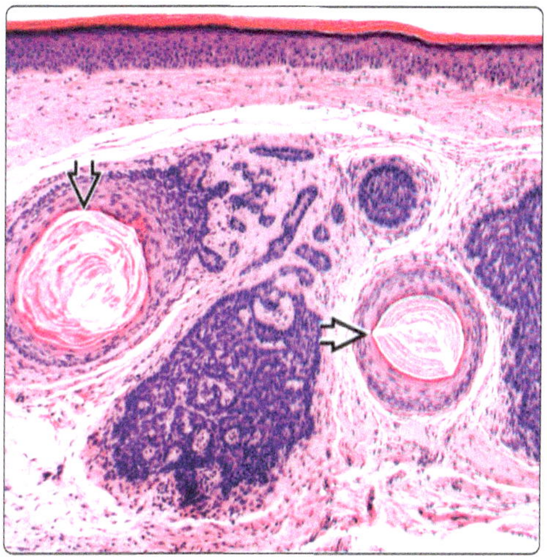

DDx: Cylindroma

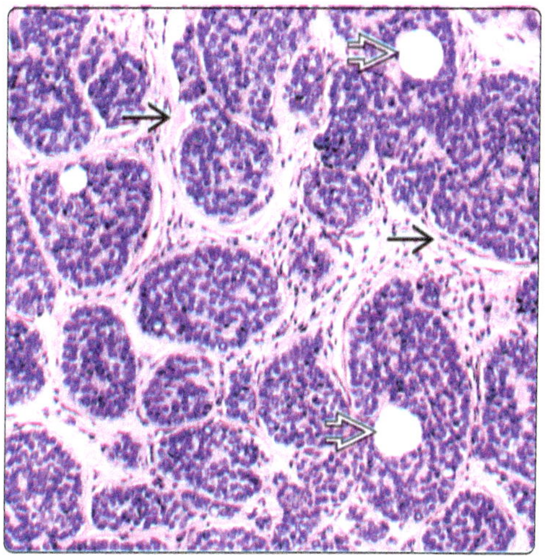

(Left) *TE is a closely related tumor and may even be considered a superficial variant of TB. However, TE is usually smaller and often shows more prominent well-differentiated folliculocystic structures ⇨ than does TB.* **(Right)** *Cylindroma is another nodular, dermal-based basaloid neoplasm. However, cylindroma is composed of irregularly shaped nests of cells surrounded by hyalinized basement membrane ⇨, and ductal structures are easily identified ⇨.*

DDx: Basal Cell Carcinoma

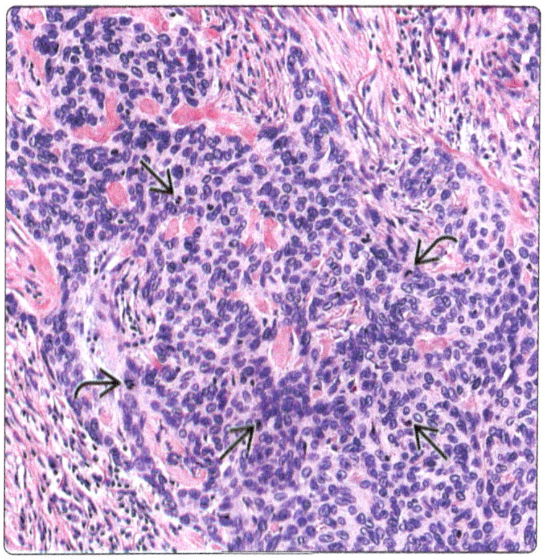

Ki-67 Staining in Basal Cell Carcinoma

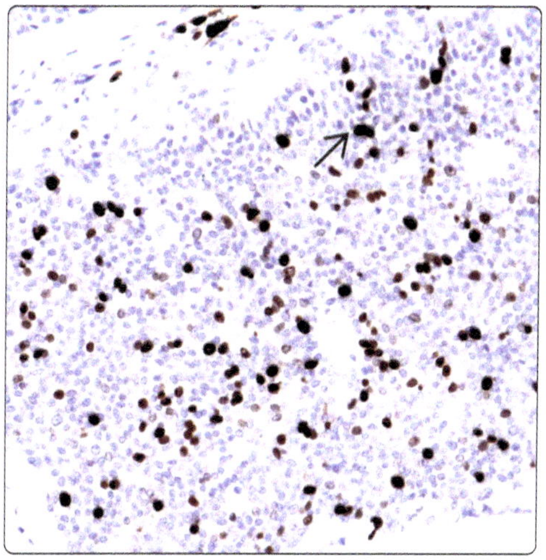

(Left) *Basal cell carcinoma (BCC) may occasionally be difficult to distinguish from TB, especially if classic features, such as mucinous stroma and tumor-stromal retraction artifact, are absent. However, on high-power examination, mitotic ⇨ and apoptotic ⇨ figures are abundant, as opposed to rare in TB.* **(Right)** *Ki-67 stains many more nuclei in this example of BCC, including scattered enlarged, irregular-appearing nuclei ⇨.*

Panfolliculoma

KEY FACTS

TERMINOLOGY

- Benign tumor with differentiation to all segments of hair follicle

CLINICAL ISSUES

- Very rare benign tumors

MICROSCOPIC

- Closely set solid and partially cystic structures with follicular differentiation
- Well circumscribed
- Follicular differentiation includes all components of follicular unit
  - Cystic areas resembling infundibulum with stratified squamous epithelium, granular layer, and basket-weave stratum corneum
  - Areas resembling internal and external root sheath
  - Foci of matrical epithelium
  - Areas resembling hair bulb with papillary mesenchymal bodies

TOP DIFFERENTIAL DIAGNOSES

- Trichoblastoma
  - Less organized
  - Lacks more advanced follicular differentiation
  - Usually composed entirely of basaloid epithelium
- Trichoepithelioma
  - Less organized
  - Also lacks more advanced follicular differentiation
  - Usually composed entirely of basaloid epithelium
- Pilomatrixoma
  - Consists only of matrical epithelium and ghost cells
  - Lacks papillary mesenchymal bodies
- Trichofolliculoma
  - Multiple secondary follicles connecting to large, central, cystically dilated follicular structure
  - Sebaceous glands often present

Low-Power Image of Panfolliculoma

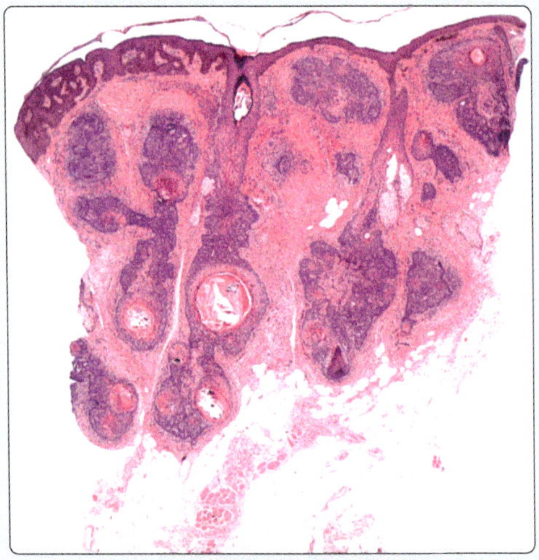

Medium-Power Image of Panfolliculoma Resembling Primitive Follicles

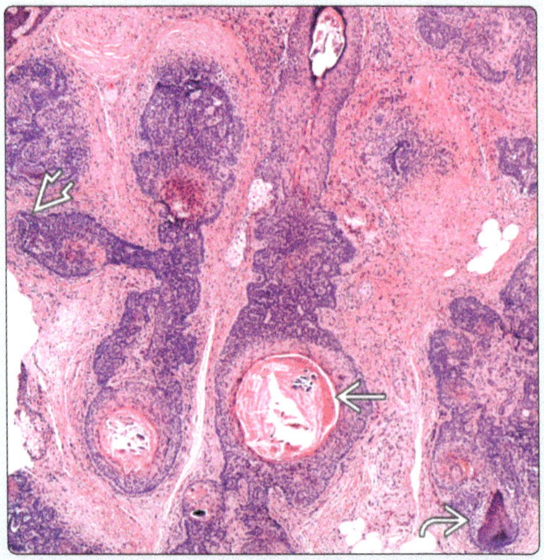

(Left) *Panfolliculoma is characterized by a dermal-based adnexal proliferation recapitulating all levels of the hair follicle.* **(Right)** *Panfolliculoma shows cystic areas lined by stratified squamous epithelium with a granular layer →, basaloid epithelium with papillary mesenchymal bodies →, and inner and outer root sheath →.*

Higher Power Image of Panfolliculoma With Component Resembling Infundibulum

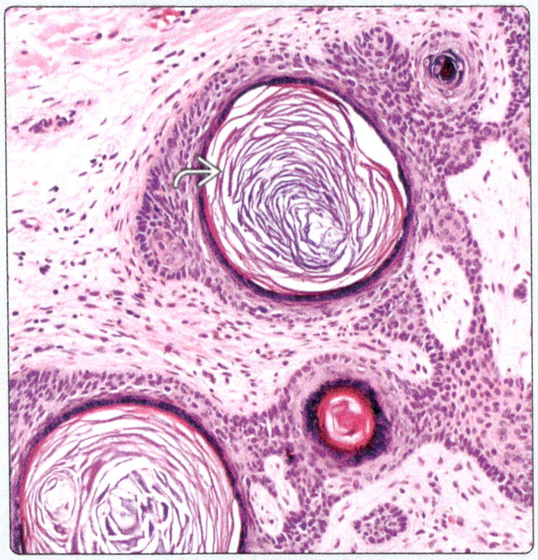

High-Power Image of Panfolliculoma With Hair Bulb Formation

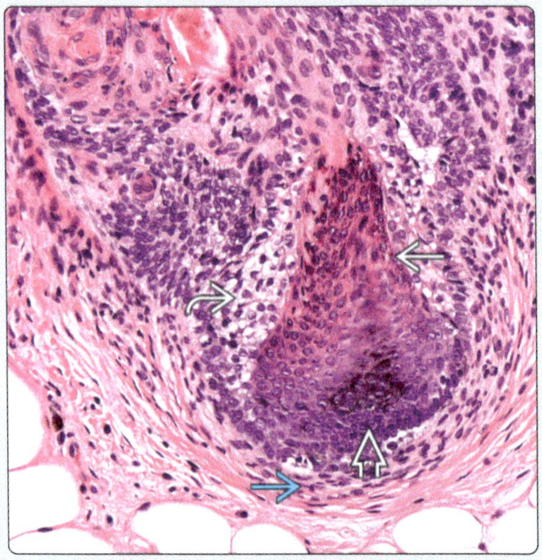

(Left) *The cystic areas are lined by stratified squamous epithelium with a granular layer and filled with abundant laminated keratin →, consistent with infundibular differentiation.* **(Right)** *There is advanced follicular differentiation with external → and internal → root sheath formation, as well as matrical → epithelium. At the base there is a condensation of spindled cells representing a papillary mesenchymal body →.*

TERMINOLOGY

Definitions

- Benign tumor with differentiation that represents all segments of hair follicle

CLINICAL ISSUES

Epidemiology

- Incidence
  - Very rare
- Age
  - Adults
- Sex
  - Men and women affected equally

Site

- Usually involving face or scalp but may occur elsewhere

Presentation

- Mass lesion
  - Slowly growing

Treatment

- Surgical approaches
  - Simple excision is usually curative

Prognosis

- Benign
  - Rare recurrence
  - No malignant transformation

MACROSCOPIC

General Features

- Nodular, dermal-based tumor

Size

- Generally < 3 cm

MICROSCOPIC

Histologic Features

- Well-circumscribed, noninfiltrative, typically dermal-based lesion
- Closely set solid and partially cystic structures with follicular differentiation
- Follicular differentiation represents all components of follicular epithelium
  - Cystic areas resembling infundibulum
    - With stratified squamous epithelium showing granular layer and basket-weave stratum corneum
  - Areas resembling internal and external root sheath, with latter showing clear cell features
  - Areas with matrical epithelium
  - Areas resembling hair bulb with papillary mesenchymal body formation
- Rare intraepidermal cases also described

Cytologic Features

- Small, bland, basaloid, squamoid, and clear cells lacking nuclear irregularities and enlarged nucleoli
- Mitotic figures absent

DIFFERENTIAL DIAGNOSIS

Trichoblastoma

- May have similar low-power appearance
- More primitive follicular neoplasm that typically lacks more advanced follicular differentiation
  - Fewer keratin-filled cysts
  - No external root sheath differentiation with clear cell features
  - Lacks matrical epithelium

Trichoepithelioma

- May have similar low-power appearance, but is usually smaller and more superficial
- Lacks more advanced follicular differentiation
  - No external root sheath differentiation with clear cell features
  - Lacks matrical epithelium
- Often shows calcifications and ruptured cysts with associated granulomatous inflammation

Trichofolliculoma

- Multiple secondary follicles connecting to large, central, cystically dilated follicular structure
  - Panfolliculoma lacks central dilated follicular structure
- Often has sebaceous glands, which are not seen in panfolliculoma
  - Numerous sebaceous glands present in folliculocystic sebaceous hamartoma, which may be considered trichofolliculoma variant

Pilomatrixoma

- Typically occurs in children or young adults
- Consists of basaloid matrical epithelium and shadow (or ghost) cells
- Cystic spaces often present
- Lacks more advanced follicular differentiation
  - No keratin-filled cysts
  - No root sheath differentiation
- Often shows rupture with calcifications and associated granulomatous inflammation

DIAGNOSTIC CHECKLIST

Pathologic Interpretation Pearls

- Closely packed basaloid tumor nodules
- Key feature: All aspects of follicular differentiation present
  - Cystic areas resembling infundibulum
  - Areas with external and internal root sheath differentiation
  - Areas with matrical differentiation
  - Hair bulb formation with papillary mesenchymal bodies

SELECTED REFERENCES

1. Harris A et al: Epidermal panfolliculoma: a report of 2 cases. Am J Dermatopathol. 33(1):e7-10, 2011
2. Tellechea O et al: Trichogerminoma. Am J Dermatopathol. 31(5):480-3, 2009
3. Hoang MP et al: Cystic panfolliculoma. Arch Pathol Lab Med. 130(3):389-92, 2006
4. Ackerman AB et al: Panfolliculoma. In Neoplasms with Follicular Differentiation. London: Lea & Febiger: 461-76, 1993

KEY FACTS

TERMINOLOGY

- Tumor of follicular infundibulum
- Basal cell hamartoma with follicular differentiation
- Bland, superficial, plate-like adnexal proliferation with multiple epidermal attachments

ETIOLOGY/PATHOGENESIS

- May be sporadic (most cases) or part of Cowden syndrome (multiple, often with tricholemmomas)
- Rare cases may be associated with nevus sebaceous (organoid nevus)

CLINICAL ISSUES

- Usually present in elderly adults
- Typically present on face and in head and neck region
- Excellent prognosis; little recurrence potential, and no malignant potential
- Surgical excision is curative

MICROSCOPIC

- Multiple connections between lesion and epidermis
- Tumor is composed of mildly enlarged, bland-appearing squamous keratinocytes
  - Cells show abundant pale to clear-staining cytoplasm
  - Peripheral cells are more basaloid and show palisading
- Multiple small follicular structures typically blend into deeper portions of lesion but do not emerge from surface
- Stroma shows abundant elastic fibers

TOP DIFFERENTIAL DIAGNOSES

- Basal cell carcinoma
- Inverted follicular keratosis
- Tricholemmoma
- Pilar sheath acanthoma

TFI

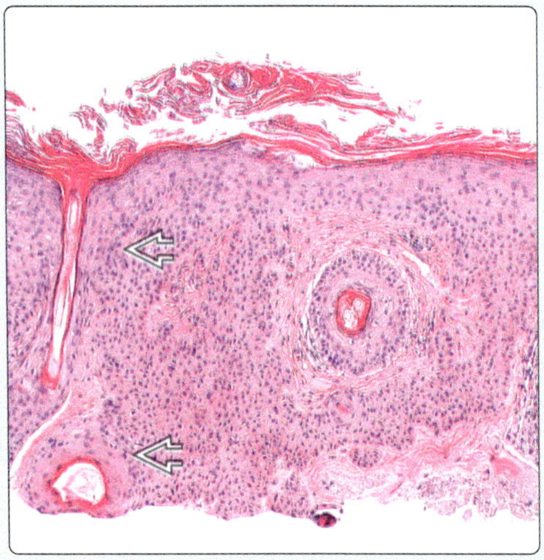

High Magnification of TFI

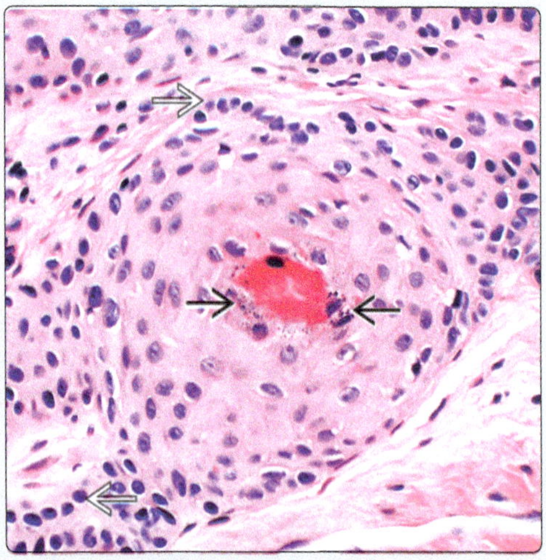

(Left) *Tumor of the follicular infundibulum (TFI) is characterized by a superficial, plate-like distribution parallel to the epidermis. Note the multiple connections to an adjacent follicular structure* ➡. **(Right)** *High magnification of TFI shows a central area of infundibular-type keratinization surrounded by bland squamous cells showing focal cytoplasmic granules* ➡. *Note the focal areas of peripheral palisading* ➡.

TFI With Infundibulocystic Structures

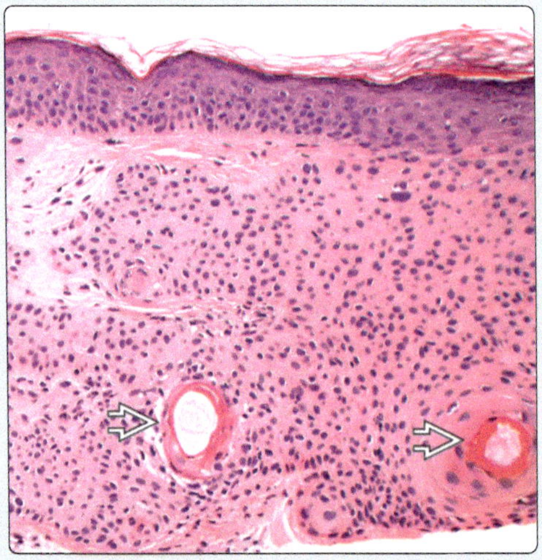

PAS Stain in TFI

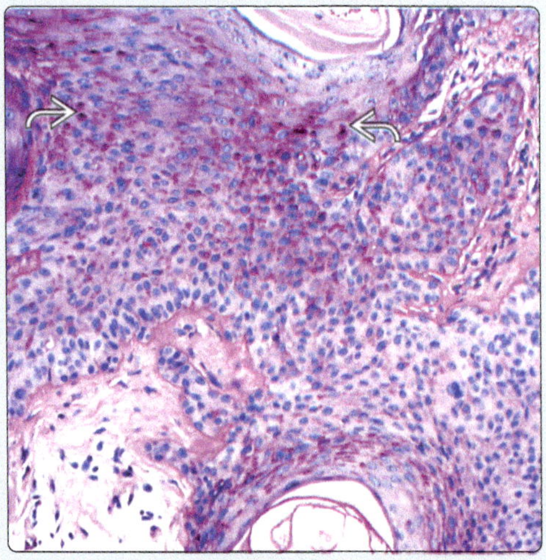

(Left) *Another example of TFI shows a bland proliferation of pale eosinophilic-staining epithelial cells with scattered infundibulocystic structures* ➡. **(Right)** *A PAS stain (without digestion) highlights focally prominent cytoplasmic glycogen collections* ➡.

TERMINOLOGY

Abbreviations

- Tumor of follicular infundibulum (TFI)

Synonyms

- Basal cell hamartoma with follicular differentiation
- Mehregan TFI

Definitions

- Benign proliferation of mature adnexal keratinocytes showing superficial plate-like formation with multiple epidermal attachments

ETIOLOGY/PATHOGENESIS

Unknown

- Most cases are sporadic
- Some cases may be associated with nevus sebaceous (organoid nevus)

Genetic Syndrome

- May represent manifestation of Cowden syndrome
  - Typically multiple lesions, often present with tricholemmomas

CLINICAL ISSUES

Epidemiology

- Incidence
  - Uncommon lesions
- Age
  - Usually present in elderly adults
- Sex
  - More common in women

Site

- Typically present on face and in head and neck region
- May also occur on upper chest

Presentation

- Small, slow-growing papule
  - Smooth or slightly keratotic appearing
  - Rarely may present as multiple lesions (eruptive infundibulomas)

Natural History

- Stable lesions that do not regress

Treatment

- Options, risks, complications
  - Surgical excision is curative but not necessary due to benign nature of lesion

Prognosis

- Excellent; little recurrence potential and no malignant potential

MICROSCOPIC

Histologic Features

- Superficial, plate-like proliferation parallel to epidermis
- Multiple anastomosing connections between lesion and epidermis
- Tumor is composed of mildly enlarged, bland-appearing squamous keratinocytes
  - Cells typically show abundant pale to clear-staining cytoplasm
  - Peripheral cells are more basaloid and show palisading
- Small follicular structures blend into deeper portions of lesion but do not emerge from surface
  - Other evidence of follicular differentiation may include small follicular bulbs, papillary mesenchymal bodies, and occasional hair shafts
- Rarely, ductal structures may be present
- Stroma shows abundant elastic fibers

DIFFERENTIAL DIAGNOSIS

Basal Cell Carcinoma

- TFI may mimic superficial basal cell carcinoma (BCC), as both show peripheral palisading; however
  - Cells are pale- to clear-staining in TFI
  - TFI lacks significant cytologic atypia, mitoses, and apoptotic bodies
- BCC typically lacks plate-like distribution of TFI

Inverted Follicular Keratosis

- Acanthotic, endophytic proliferation of mature squamous keratinocytes
- Squamous eddies and scattered pseudohorn cysts present
- Typically considered variant of irritated seborrheic keratosis

Tricholemmoma

- Lobular proliferation of mature squamoid cells with pale to clear-staining cytoplasm
- Multiple broad connections to epidermis and follicles present
- Lacks plate-like architecture of TFI

Pilar Sheath Acanthoma

- Central dell-like depression
- Composed of thickened epithelium with enlarged, pale-staining keratinocytes
- Lacks superficial, plate-like architecture of TFI

Dilated Pore of Winer

- Central dilated keratin-filled space
- Enlarged comedone-like follicular structure with acanthotic squamous lining
- Lacks superficial, plate-like architecture of TFI

SELECTED REFERENCES

1. Suchonwanit P et al: Eruptive tumors of the follicular infundibulum: an unexpected diagnosis of hypopigmented macules. Dermatol Ther (Heidelb). ePub, 2015
2. Zhu JW et al: Multiple tumors of the follicular infundibulum: a cutaneous reaction pattern? Cutis. 94(6):301-3, 2014
3. Abbas O et al: Tumor of the follicular infundibulum: an epidermal reaction pattern? Am J Dermatopathol. 31(7):626-33, 2009
4. MacGregor JL et al: Basal cell and squamous cell carcinoma occurring within a field of multiple tumors of the follicular infundibulum. Dermatol Surg. 34(11):1567-70, 2008
5. Mahalingam M et al: Tumor of the follicular infundibulum with sebaceous differentiation. J Cutan Pathol. 28(6):314-7, 2001
6. Cribier B et al: Tumor of the follicular infundibulum: a clinicopathologic study. J Am Acad Dermatol. 33(6):979-84, 1995
7. Mehregan AH et al: A tumor of follicular infundibulum. Report of a case. Arch Dermatol. 83:924-7, 1961

Dilated Pore of Winer

KEY FACTS

TERMINOLOGY

- Dilated pore of Winer (DPW)
- Enlarged follicular structure with acanthotic squamous lining and central keratin-filled space

ETIOLOGY/PATHOGENESIS

- May be related to preceding inflammatory cystic acne in some cases
- Solar damage also implicated in cases in elderly patients

CLINICAL ISSUES

- Uncommon, comedone-like lesion lesions
- Head and neck region most common
- May be solitary or multiple
- Excellent prognosis, completely benign (likely nonneoplastic) lesion

MICROSCOPIC

- Enlarged, dilated follicular structure
- Often filled with abundant keratin debris
- Infundibular-type keratinization with granular layer
- Squamous epithelial lining shows acanthosis and finger-like projections
- Small sebaceous glands and vellus hair follicles may be attached to base of lesion
- No infiltrative features, cytologic atypia, or mitotic activity

TOP DIFFERENTIAL DIAGNOSES

- Pilar sheath acanthoma
  - Infundibular structure lined by acanthotic epithelium
  - Fewer finger-like projections than DPW
- Comedone
  - Enlarged, dilated follicular structure, similar to DPW
  - Filled with abundant keratin debris, acute inflammatory cells, and numerous bacterial organisms
- Hair cortex comedo
- Regressing keratoacanthoma

Dilated Pore of Winer

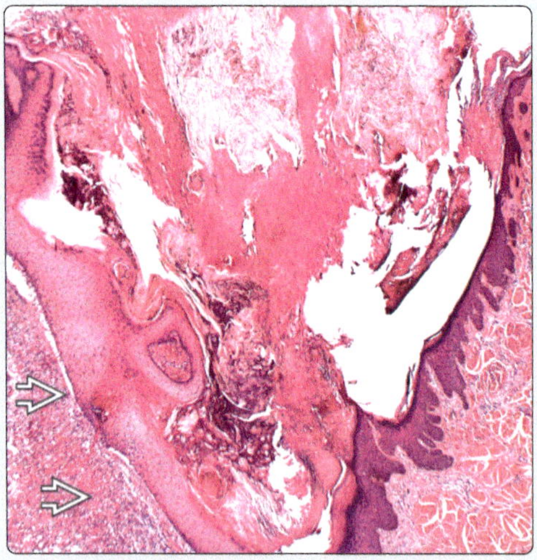

DPW With Acanthotic Lining

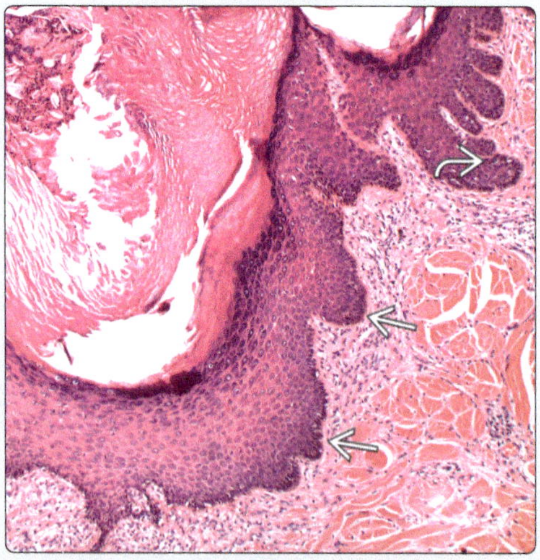

(Left) *Dilated pore of Winer (DPW) at low-power examination shows a follicular structure with a dilated opening filled with keratin debris. This lesion shows focal rupture and associated inflammation →.* **(Right)** *Intermediate magnification of a DPW shows the acanthotic squamous lining epithelium with focal finger-like projections → and mild basilar hyperpigmentation →.*

DPW With Finger-Like Projections

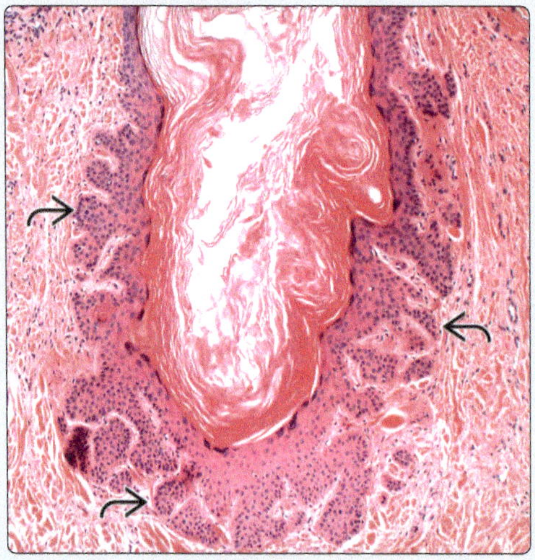

Higher Magnification of Finger-Like Projections

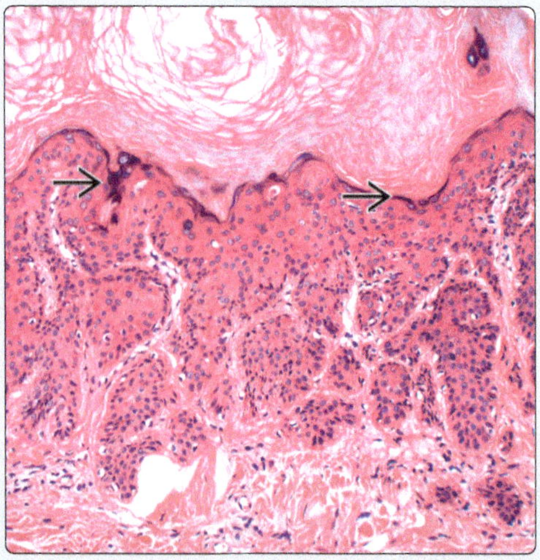

(Left) *A tangentially sectioned area shows a central keratin-filled follicular structure with multiple irregular, radiating finger-like projections →.* **(Right)** *Higher magnification of the finger-like projections surrounding a follicular lumen shows bland squamous epithelial cells forming a granular layer →.*

TERMINOLOGY

Abbreviations

- Dilated pore of Winer (DPW)

Definitions

- Enlarged follicular structure with acanthotic squamous lining and central keratin-filled space

ETIOLOGY/PATHOGENESIS

Unknown

- May be related to preceding inflammatory cystic acne in some cases
- Solar damage also implicated, as most cases occur in elderly

CLINICAL ISSUES

Epidemiology

- Incidence
  - Uncommon lesions
- Age
  - Usually elderly patients

Site

- Head and neck region most common
  - May also occur on trunk

Presentation

- Comedone-like lesion
  - May be solitary or multiple

Treatment

- Options, risks, complications
  - Surgery not necessary, but conservative excision or ablation is curative

Prognosis

- Excellent, completely benign (likely nonneoplastic) lesion

MACROSCOPIC

General Features

- Markedly dilated comedone-like lesion

Size

- Variable; may be up to 2 cm

MICROSCOPIC

Histologic Features

- Enlarged, dilated follicular structure
- May extend into deep dermis
- Often filled with abundant keratin debris
  - Infundibular-type keratinization with granular layer
- Squamous epithelial lining shows acanthosis and finger-like projections into surrounding dermis
  - No infiltrative features present
  - No significant cytologic atypia or mitotic activity present
- Small sebaceous glands and vellus hair follicles may be attached to base of lesion
- Follicular epithelium may show prominent pigmentation in some cases

Cytologic Features

- Bland squamous keratinocytes

DIFFERENTIAL DIAGNOSIS

Pilar Sheath Acanthoma

- Infundibular structure lined by acanthotic epithelium
  - Less dilated and more acanthotic appearing than DPW
  - Fewer finger-like projections than DPW
- Cells show abundant pale- to clear-staining [glycogen-containing, PAS(+), diastase-sensitive] cytoplasm

Comedone

- Enlarged, dilated follicular structure, similar to DPW
- Filled with abundant keratin debris, acute inflammatory cells, and numerous bacterial organisms
- Clinical presentation different from dilated pore of Winer
  - Much more likely to present in adolescents and young adults

Hair Cortex Comedo

- Very rare lesion that is closely related to DPW
- Dilated follicular structure showing central keratinous plug with cornification (similar to cortex of hair shaft)
- Epithelium may show melanin pigmentation
- Stroma may show surrounding granulomatous inflammation

Regressing Keratoacanthoma

- Usually shows irregularly dilated crateriform area
- Epithelium appears more atrophic
- Often lacks significant cytologic atypia or mitotic activity
- Associated with dermal fibrosis and chronic inflammation

DIAGNOSTIC CHECKLIST

Pathologic Interpretation Pearls

- Enlarged, dilated follicular structure filled with keratinous debris
- Squamous epithelial lining shows acanthosis and finger-like projections into surrounding dermis

SELECTED REFERENCES

1. Moreira A et al: Dermoscopy of a dilated pore of Winer. Eur J Dermatol. 20(2):229, 2010
2. Walsh SN et al: Hair cortex comedo: a series of 34 cases. Am J Dermatopathol. 32(8):749-54, 2010
3. Jakobiec FA et al: Winer's dilated pore of the eyelid. Ophthal Plast Reconstr Surg. 25(5):411-3, 2009
4. Carlson-Sweet KL et al: Trichoid basal cell carcinoma found in a dilated pore on the nose. Dermatol Surg. 26(9):874-6, 2000
5. Resnik KS et al: Dilated pore nevus. A histologic variant of nevus comedonicus. Am J Dermatopathol. 15(2):169-71, 1993
6. Hausmann G et al: [The Winer dilated pore.] Med Cutan Ibero Lat Am. 17(1):45-7, 1989
7. Winer LH: The dilated pore, a tricho-epithelioma. J Invest Dermatol. 23(3):181-8, 1954

Pilar Sheath Acanthoma

KEY FACTS

TERMINOLOGY

- Pilar sheath acanthoma
- Mature adnexal proliferation composed of thickened epithelium with enlarged pale-staining keratinocytes

CLINICAL ISSUES

- Rare lesions
- Usually in middle-aged to older adults
- Most often occur on upper lip
- Slow-growing, stable lesion
- Keratotic papule with central pore-like area

MACROSCOPIC

- Superficial keratotic papule

MICROSCOPIC

- Endophytic, lobular proliferation of enlarged, mature squamous cells with prominent acanthosis
- Usually superficial, well circumscribed, and noninfiltrative
- Lobules typically surround follicular structure
- Foci of infundibular-type keratinization
- Cells show abundant pale eosinophilic to clear-staining cytoplasm and small nuclei
- Clear cells contain glycogen, which can be demonstrated by PAS (without diastase digestion)

TOP DIFFERENTIAL DIAGNOSES

- Dilated pore of Winer
- Trichofolliculoma
- Inverted follicular keratosis
- Tumor of follicular infundibulum

DIAGNOSTIC CHECKLIST

- Endophytic proliferation of thickened epithelium with enlarged pale-staining keratinocytes

Pilar Sheath Acanthoma

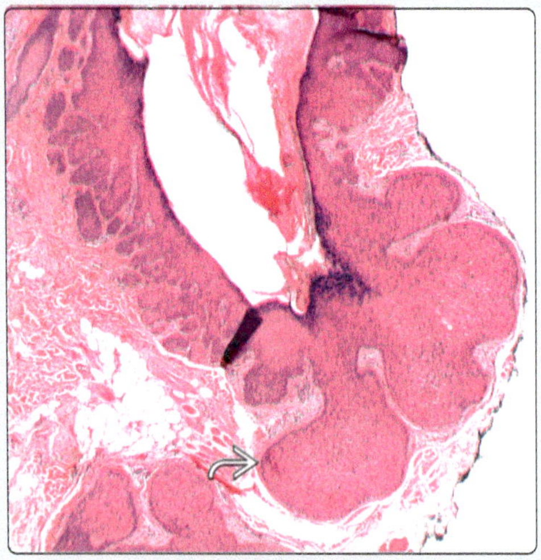

Pilar Sheath Acanthoma at Higher Magnification

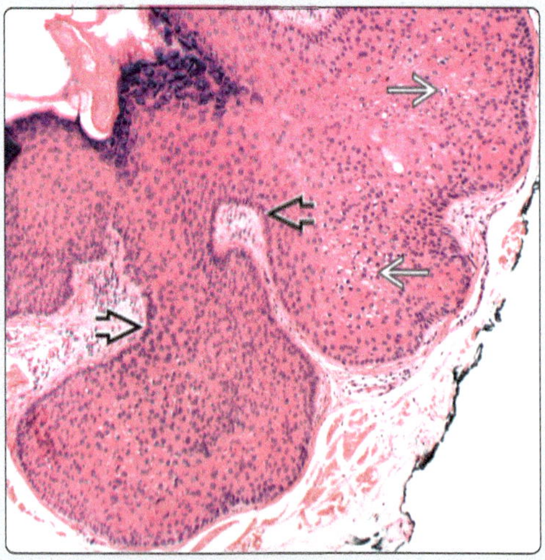

(Left) *Scanning magnification of a pilar sheath acanthoma shows a dilated follicular structure lined by a thickened squamous epithelium with endophytic, lobulated areas* ↷. **(Right)** *Higher magnification of the lobular areas shows acanthotic squamous epithelium with peripheral palisading* ⇨ *and scattered clear-staining cells* ⇨.

Pilar Sheath Acanthoma With Prominent Granular Layer

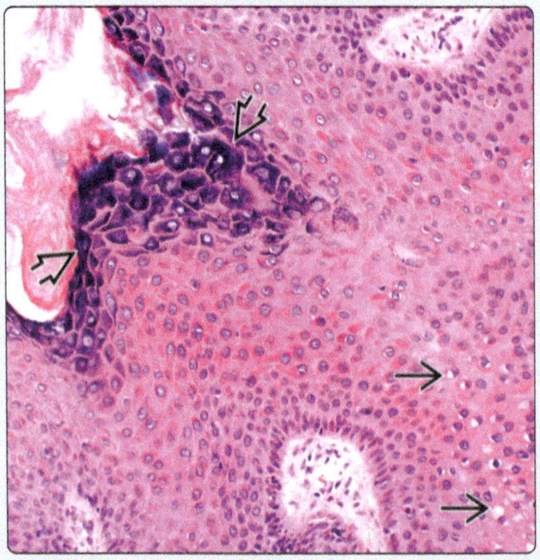

Pilar Sheath Acanthoma With Squamous Pearls

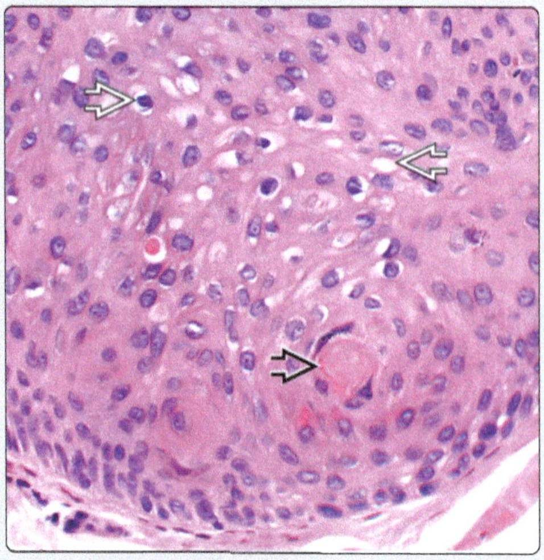

(Left) *High magnification of the epithelium shows a prominent granular layer* ⇨ *(consistent with infundibular keratinization). The cells are mildly enlarged and squamoid appearing, with scattered pale/clear cells* ⇨. **(Right)** *Foci of keratinization with squamous pearls* ⇨ *may be seen surrounded by bland squamoid to clear* ➡ *cells.*

TERMINOLOGY

Abbreviations

- Pilar sheath acanthoma (PSA)

Definitions

- Mature adnexal proliferation composed of thickened epithelium with enlarged pale-staining keratinocytes

ETIOLOGY/PATHOGENESIS

Unknown

- No known causes/associations

CLINICAL ISSUES

Epidemiology

- Incidence
  - Rare lesions
- Age
  - Usually occur in middle-aged to older adults
- Sex
  - Males and females equally affected

Site

- Most often occur on upper lip

Presentation

- Keratotic papular lesion with central pore-like area

Natural History

- Slow-growing, stable lesion
  - Often present for years

Treatment

- Options, risks, complications
  - Complete surgical excision is curative, but not necessary in most cases due to benign nature

Prognosis

- Excellent, benign behavior; no evidence of malignant transformation

MACROSCOPIC

General Features

- Superficial keratotic papule

Size

- Generally small, < 1 cm

MICROSCOPIC

Histologic Features

- Endophytic, lobular proliferation of enlarged, mature squamous cells with prominent acanthosis
  - Lobules typically surround central dilated follicular structure
  - Granular layer and foci of infundibular-type keratinization are present
  - Abortive follicles may be present
  - Peripheral palisading and thickened basement membrane may be seen (similar to tricholemmoma)
- Cells show abundant pale eosinophilic to clear-staining cytoplasm and small nuclei
- Lesion is usually superficial, well circumscribed, and noninfiltrative
- Mitotic figures absent to rare, limited to basilar layer

Predominant Cell/Compartment Type

- Adnexal cell showing outer root sheath differentiation

DIFFERENTIAL DIAGNOSIS

Dilated Pore of Winer

- Larger, more dilated follicular opening (comedone-like) than PSA
  - Filled with abundant keratin debris
- Does not show degree of acanthosis and clear cell features typical of PSA
- Small sebaceous glands and vellus hairs may attach to base (absent in PSA)

Trichofolliculoma

- Central dilated follicular structure with multiple small, immature radiating follicles
  - Central follicle opens to epidermal surface
- Fibrotic and cellular stroma (which is lacking in PSA)
- Sebaceous glands may be prominent in some cases (sebaceous trichofolliculoma or folliculosebaceous cystic hamartoma)

Inverted Follicular Keratosis

- Typically considered variant of irritated seborrheic keratosis
- Endophytic-appearing lesion composed of mature squamous keratinocytes
- Often shows numerous keratinizing pseudohorn cysts and squamous eddies
- Usually lacks pale to clear cells seen in PSA

Tumor of Follicular Infundibulum

- Proliferation of mature adnexal keratinocytes showing superficial plate-like formation with multiple epidermal attachments
- Cells show abundant pale- to clear-staining cytoplasm similar to PSA, but architectural features are different
- Peripheral palisading of tumor cells typically present

DIAGNOSTIC CHECKLIST

Pathologic Interpretation Pearls

- Endophytic proliferation of thickened epithelium with enlarged pale-staining keratinocytes

SELECTED REFERENCES

1. Bruscino N et al: Pilar sheath acanthoma simulating basal cell carcinoma. G Ital Dermatol Venereol. 149(1):155-6, 2014
2. Kushner JA et al: An unusual location of a pilar sheath acanthoma. Int J Trichology. 6(4):185-6, 2014
3. Choi YS et al: Pilar sheath acanthoma–report of a case with review of the literature. Yonsei Med J. 30(4):392-5, 1989
4. Lee JY et al: Pilar sheath acanthoma. Arch Dermatol. 123(5):569-70, 1987
5. Mehregan AH et al: Pilar sheath acanthoma. Arch Dermatol. 114(10):1495-7, 1978

KEY FACTS

TERMINOLOGY

- Inverted follicular keratosis (IFK)
- Benign tumor of follicular infundibulum, may be considered type of irritated seborrheic keratosis

ETIOLOGY/PATHOGENESIS

- Thought to arise from follicular infundibula, which explains downward proliferation of these lesions

CLINICAL ISSUES

- Common benign tumor found mostly in men
- 90% occur on head and neck
- Usually present as asymptomatic, solitary, dome-shaped or filiform, skin-colored papule
- Treatment not necessary, completely benign lesions

MICROSCOPIC

- Endophytic papillomatous proliferation of epithelium
  - Exophytic and exoendophytic growth pattern can be seen in some cases
- Numerous squamous eddies are typically present and are characteristic feature
- Overlying hyperkeratosis and parakeratosis usually present
- Mitotic figures present in basaloid cells
- No significant cytologic atypia or pleomorphism

TOP DIFFERENTIAL DIAGNOSES

- Irritated seborrheic keratosis (ISK)
  - ISK often has horizontal growth pattern, while IFK has endophytic growth pattern
- Well-differentiated squamous cell carcinoma
  - Cytologic atypia with pleomorphic cells present
  - Greater numbers of mitoses present, often atypical
- Tumor of follicular infundibulum
  - Shows more of a plate-like pattern parallel to epidermis

DIAGNOSTIC CHECKLIST

- Benign, endophytic epithelial proliferation with numerous squamous eddies is characteristic of IFK

Inverted Follicular Keratosis (IFK)

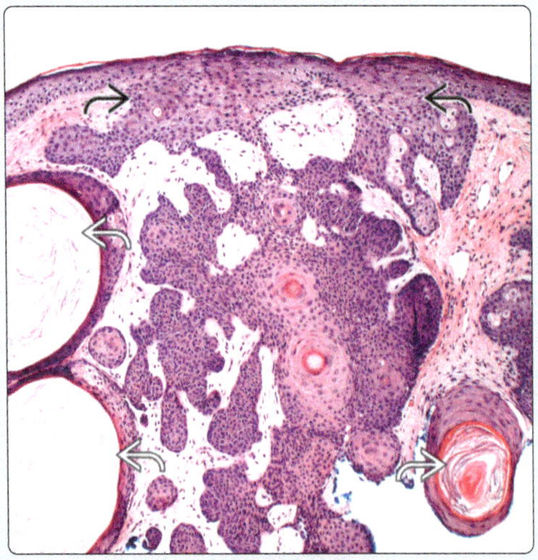

Higher Magnification of IFK

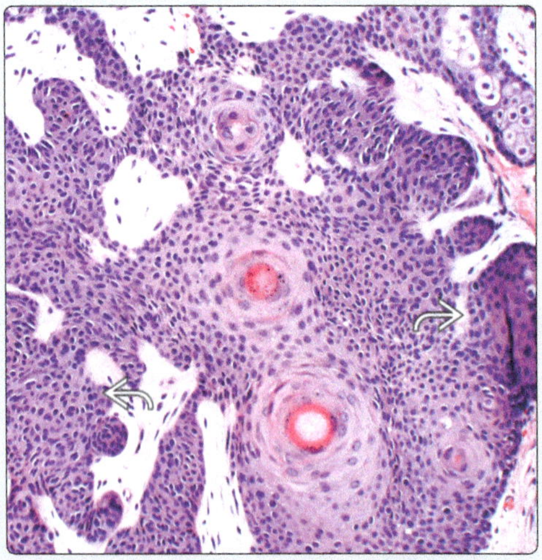

(Left) *Inverted follicular keratosis (IFK) is a well-circumscribed, endophytic epithelial proliferation. This tumor shows multiple connections to the epidermis, and multiple folliculocystic structures (similar to milia) are present.* **(Right)** *Higher magnification of the center of the lesion shows bland squamoid cells surrounding small follicular lumina and smaller peripheral, more basaloid-appearing cells.*

Traumatized IFK

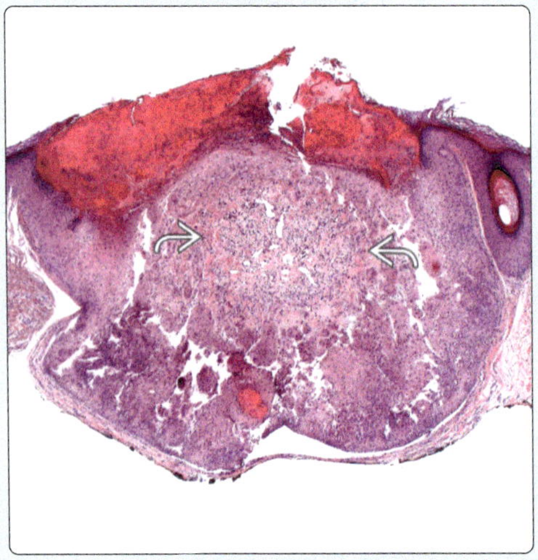

Traumatized IFK at Higher Magnification

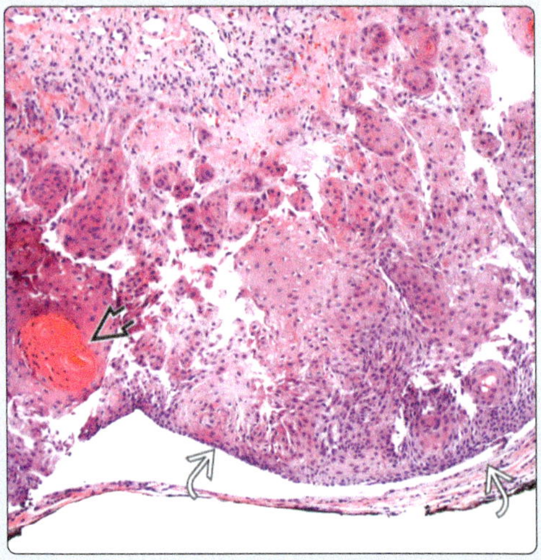

(Left) *Another example of IFK at low magnification shows a well-circumscribed, symmetric, endophytic epithelial proliferation. The overlying epidermis shows central erosion and dense serum crust overlying an area of healing granulation tissue, changes likely due to recent trauma.* **(Right)** *Higher magnification of the same case shows the well-circumscribed border of the lesion. Note the squamoid features and focal keratinization.*

TERMINOLOGY

Abbreviations

- Inverted follicular keratosis (IFK)

Synonyms

- Irritated seborrheic keratosis (SK) variant

Definitions

- Benign tumor of follicular infundibulum considered by many to be type of irritated/clonal SK

ETIOLOGY/PATHOGENESIS

Etiology

- Thought to arise from follicular infundibula, which explains downward proliferation of these lesions
- IFK is considered to be identical to SK derived from follicular infundibulum instead of surface epidermis
- Epithelium of follicular infundibulum has same histology and keratinization as surface epidermis

CLINICAL ISSUES

Epidemiology

- Incidence
  - Relatively common
- Age
  - Older adults
- Sex
  - More common in men

Site

- 90% occur on head and neck
  - Upper cutaneous lip and cheeks are most commonly affected

Presentation

- Usually present as asymptomatic, solitary, dome-shaped or filiform, skin-colored papule

Treatment

- Not necessary
- Usually biopsy for diagnosis removes entire lesion

Prognosis

- Excellent: Benign lesions

MICROSCOPIC

Histologic Features

- Usually endophytic papillomatous proliferation of epithelium
  - Exophytic and exoendophytic growth pattern can be seen
  - Composed predominately of squamous cells
  - Numerous squamous eddies are present and are characteristic feature
    - Squamous eddies are concentric layers of squamous cells with keratin at their centers
    - Presence of many squamous eddies is likely due to irritation of these lesions
  - Basaloid cells are often present at periphery of lesion
    - Mitotic figures often present in basaloid cells, but not atypical
- Overlying hyperkeratosis and parakeratosis
  - Prominent keratin-filled invagination
  - Cutaneous horn can be present

Cytologic Features

- Predominately squamous cells with basaloid cells at periphery of lesion
- No significant cytologic atypia or pleomorphism

DIFFERENTIAL DIAGNOSIS

Irritated Seborrheic Keratosis

- Many consider IFK to be the same as irritated seborrheic keratosis (ISK), except it is derived from follicular infundibulum
- Clinical
  - IFK often occurs on upper cutaneous lip or cheek
  - ISK shows variable location
- Histology
  - ISK often has horizontal growth pattern, while IFK has endophytic growth pattern
  - Bcl-2(+) dendritic cells present in increased numbers in suprabasilar areas of IFKs compared to ISKs

Well-Differentiated Squamous Cell Carcinoma (In Situ or Invasive)

- If squamous eddies are present, usually not as many as in IFKs
- Cytologic atypia with pleomorphic cells present
- Dyskeratotic cells and multiple mitotic figures usually present
- Bcl-2 positive dendritic cells present in increased numbers in suprabasilar areas of IFK compared to squamous cell carcinomas

Tumor of Follicular Infundibulum

- Typically shows plate-like pattern parallel to epidermis
- Benign proliferation of enlarged pale- to clear-staining squamous keratinocytes
- Peripheral palisading of basaloid cells present

DIAGNOSTIC CHECKLIST

Clinically Relevant Pathologic Features

- Age distribution

Pathologic Interpretation Pearls

- Benign, endophytic epithelial proliferation with numerous squamous eddies is characteristic of IFK

SELECTED REFERENCES

1. Mohamed M: Inverted follicular keratosis of the lip. Pan Afr Med J. 18:304, 2014
2. Armengot-Carbo M et al: Inverted follicular keratosis: dermoscopic and reflectance confocal microscopic features. Dermatology. 227(1):62-6, 2013
3. Noiles K et al: Are all seborrheic keratoses benign? Review of the typical lesion and its variants. J Cutan Med Surg. 12(5):203-10, 2008
4. Ko CJ et al: Bcl-2-positive epidermal dendritic cells in inverted follicular keratoses but not squamous cell carcinomas or seborrheic keratoses. J Cutan Pathol. 33(7):498-501, 2006
5. Mehregan AH: Inverted follicular keratosis is a distinct follicular tumor. Am J Dermatopathol. 5(5):467-70, 1983

Tricholemmoma

KEY FACTS

TERMINOLOGY

- Tricholemmoma (TL)
  - Benign clear cell adnexal proliferation with external root sheath differentiation
- Subtype: Desmoplastic tricholemmoma

ETIOLOGY/PATHOGENESIS

- Some cases are associated with Cowden syndrome (PTEN hamartoma syndrome)
  - Multiple tricholemmomas, hamartomas, and visceral tumors including breast and thyroid carcinomas
  - Mutations in *PTEN* gene on 10q23.31

CLINICAL ISSUES

- Relatively common tumors
- Usually occur in adults, although Cowden syndrome patients present at earlier age
- Most occur on face, especially nose and upper lip

MICROSCOPIC

- Lobular proliferation of mature squamoid cells with pale- to clear-staining cytoplasm
- Peripheral palisading of basaloid cells
- Cells are surrounded by thickened, glassy-appearing basement membrane
- Multiple broad connections to epidermis and follicles
- Desmoplastic tricholemmoma
  - Variant with prominent desmoplastic stroma
  - Typically in center of tumor, surrounded by conventional-appearing TL

TOP DIFFERENTIAL DIAGNOSES

- Tumor of follicular infundibulum
- Clear cell acanthoma
- Tricholemmal carcinoma
- Clear cell squamous cell carcinoma in situ (clear cell Bowen disease)
- Clear cell basal cell carcinoma

Clinical Photograph of Multiple Tricholemmomas

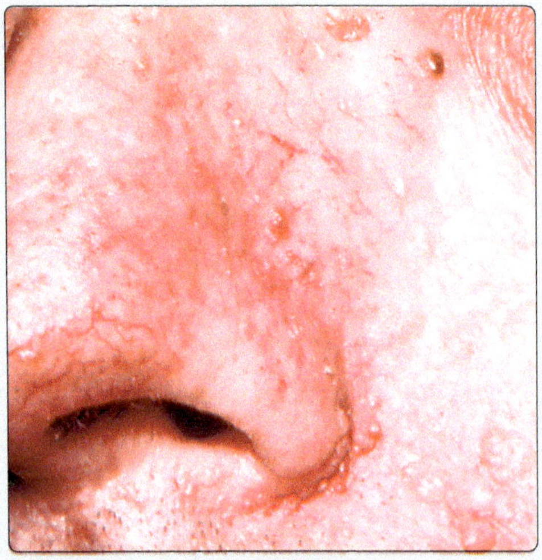

Superficial Tricholemmoma

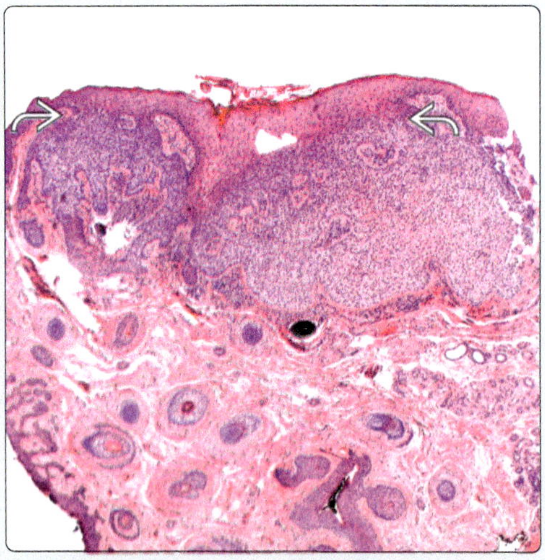

(Left) *Multiple tricholemmomas (TLs) are shown on and around the nose of a patient with Cowden syndrome. (Courtesy B. Hall, MD.)* **(Right)** *This is a small, superficial tricholemmoma on the eyelid showing multifocal epidermal attachments ➡. The tumor is composed of pale- to clear-staining epithelioid cells.*

Superficial Tricholemmoma

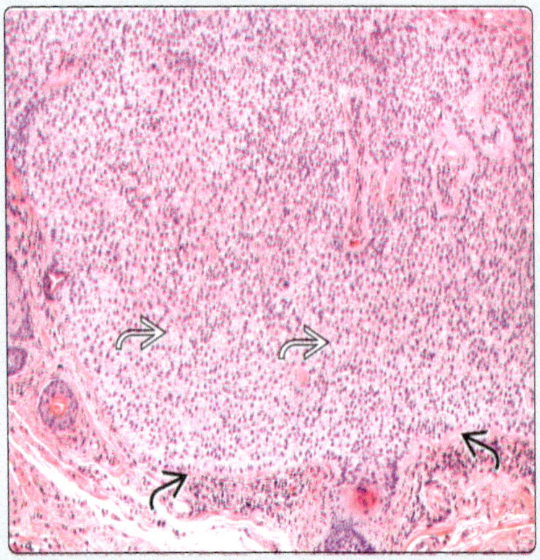

High Magnification of Tricholemmoma Basement Membrane

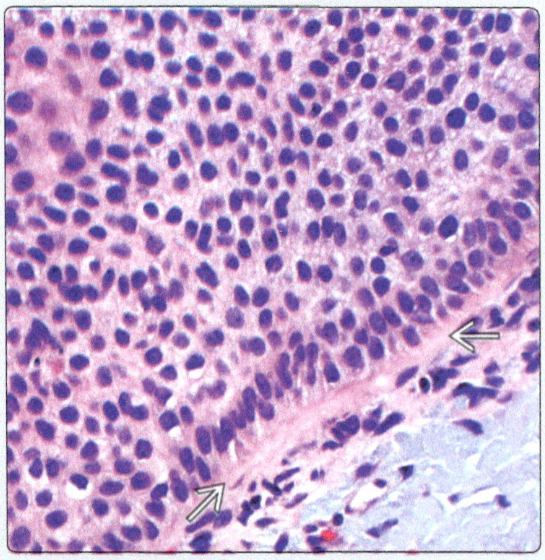

(Left) *Higher magnification of a superficial TL shows a lobular proliferation of small, pale- to clear-staining ➡ adnexal cells. Note the thickened basement membrane surrounding the tumor ➡.* **(Right)** *High magnification of the periphery of a TL shows bland-appearing small cells with pale to clear-staining cytoplasm and small nucleoli. The peripheral cells show palisading, and there is a thickened peripheral basement membrane ➡.*

TERMINOLOGY

Abbreviations

- Tricholemmoma (TL)
- Desmoplastic tricholemmoma (DTL)

Synonyms

- Trichilemmoma

Definitions

- Benign clear cell adnexal proliferation with external root sheath differentiation

ETIOLOGY/PATHOGENESIS

Unknown in Most Cases

- Some have considered TL to be related to HPV infection ("tricholemmal verrucae")
  - Not generally accepted, and most PCR studies for HPV have been negative

Genetic

- Some cases are associated with Cowden syndrome (PTEN hamartoma syndrome)
  - Characterized by multiple tricholemmomas, hamartomas, and visceral tumors including breast and thyroid carcinomas

CLINICAL ISSUES

Epidemiology

- Incidence
  - Relatively common tumors
- Age
  - Usually adults, although Cowden syndrome patients present at earlier age

Site

- Most occur on face, especially nose and upper lip

Presentation

- Small papular lesion
  - Usually flesh-colored

Treatment

- Surgical approaches
  - Usually not necessary, as these are benign tumors

Prognosis

- Excellent, no malignant potential

MICROSCOPIC

Histologic Features

- Lobular proliferation of mature squamoid cells with pale- to clear-staining cytoplasm
- Peripheral palisading of basaloid cells
  - Cells are surrounded by thickened, glassy-appearing basement membrane
- Squamous eddies and small foci of tricholemmal (pilar)-type keratinization often present
- Multiple broad connections to epidermis and follicles
  - Early lesions often surround follicle, consistent with follicular derivation

Subtype

- **Desmoplastic tricholemmoma**
  - Variant with prominent desmoplastic stroma
  - Typically in center of tumor
  - Can mimic invasive carcinoma

DIFFERENTIAL DIAGNOSIS

Clear Cell Acanthoma

- Psoriasiform epidermal acanthosis
- Epidermal cells show prominent clear cell changes, similar to TL, but
  - Clear cell acanthoma shows overlying hypogranulosis and parakeratosis
  - Lacks lobular configuration and thickened peripheral basement membrane

Tricholemmal Carcinoma

- Shows lobular proliferation of clear cells with peripheral palisading
- However, tricholemmal carcinoma also shows
  - Significant cytologic atypia, mitotic activity, infiltrative features, and may show necrosis
  - Desmoplastic areas at periphery, not in center of tumor (unlike DTL)

Tumor of Follicular Infundibulum

- Superficial, plate-like growth pattern parallel to epidermis
- Peripheral palisading and clear cells present, but
  - Tumor of follicular infundibulum (TFI) is more plate-like, less lobular than TL
  - TFI shows multiple anastomosing connections between tumor cells and with epidermis

Clear Cell Squamous Cell Carcinoma In Situ (Clear Cell Bowen Disease)

- Atypical intraepidermal proliferation of clear-staining keratinocytes
  - Prominent nuclear atypia with hyperchromasia and large nucleoli
  - Multiple mitotic figures, including atypical forms, typically present

Clear Cell Basal Cell Carcinoma

- Can occasionally show prominent clear cell features
- Peripheral palisading seen in both basal cell carcinoma (BCC) and TL, however
  - Prominent mitoses, apoptoses, and infiltrative feature characteristic of BCC
  - Tumor-stromal retraction artifact and mucinous stroma typical of BCC

SELECTED REFERENCES

1. Jha AK et al: Linear trichilemmoma following a blaschkoid pattern: a clinical dilemma. J Eur Acad Dermatol Venereol. 30(2):299-301, 2016
2. Tsai JH et al: Frequent activating HRAS mutations in trichilemmoma. Br J Dermatol. 171(5):1073-7, 2014
3. Cabral ES et al: Desmoplastic tricholemmoma of the eyelid misdiagnosed as sebaceous carcinoma: a potential diagnostic pitfall. J Cutan Pathol. 34 Suppl 1:22-5, 2007
4. Nelen MR et al: Novel PTEN mutations in patients with Cowden disease: absence of clear genotype-phenotype correlations. Eur J Hum Genet. 7(3):267-73, 1999
5. Headington JT: Tricholemmoma. To be or not to be? Am J Dermatopathol. 2(3):225-6, 1980

(Left) *Traumatized TL at low-power magnification shows epidermal erosion with dense serum crust and impetiginization overlying a symmetric, well-circumscribed, lobular neoplasm with epidermal attachments.* **(Right)** *This TL shows a well-circumscribed, lobular neoplasm with a thickened peripheral basement membrane ➢. At one side, the lesion shows focal desmoplastic features ➡.*

Traumatized Tricholemmoma

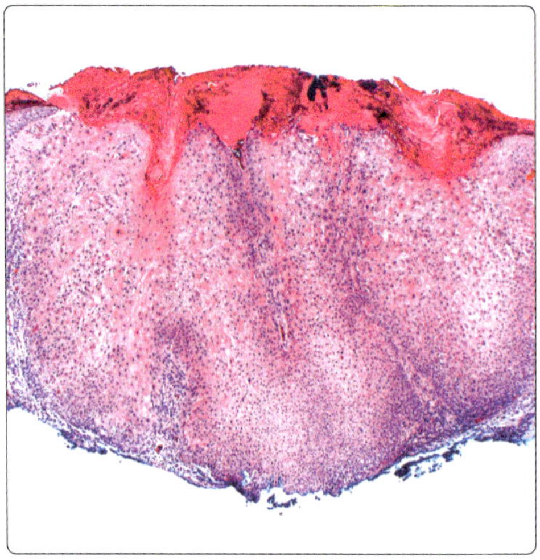

Tricholemmoma With Focal Desmoplastic Features

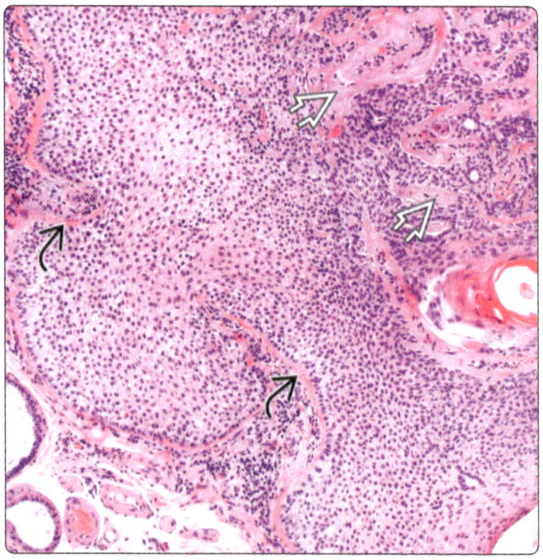

(Left) *This desmoplastic TL shows focal areas of infiltrative-appearing cells ➡ associated with a prominent hyalinized stroma in the center of a large, more conventional tumor.* **(Right)** *Higher magnification of desmoplastic TL shows areas of infiltrative-appearing cords and nests ➡ associated with a prominent hyalinized stroma.*

Desmoplastic Tricholemmoma

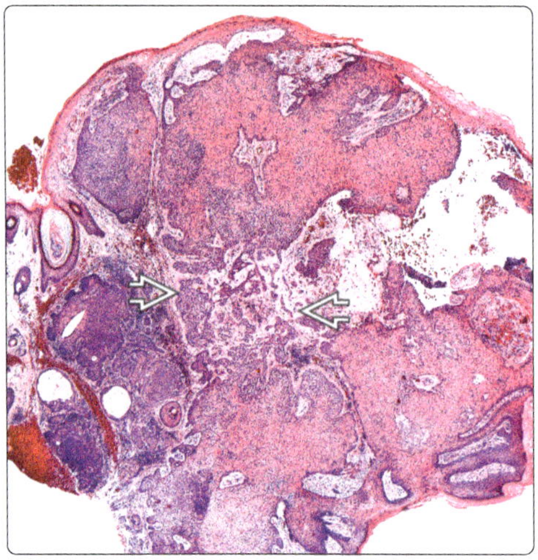

Desmoplastic Tricholemmoma

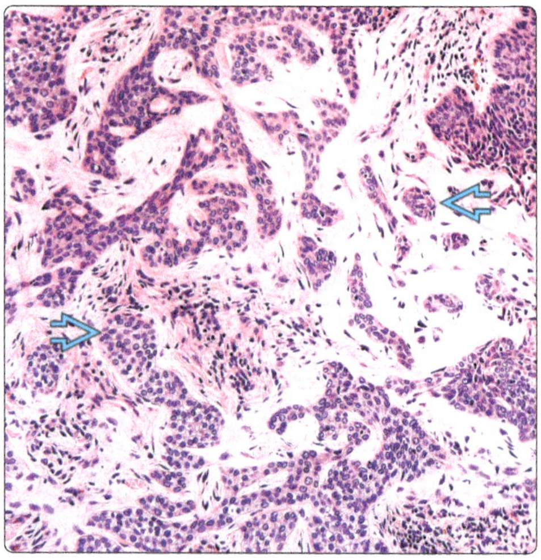

(Left) *High magnification of desmoplastic TL shows areas of infiltrative-appearing cords of eosinophilic-staining cells associated with a prominent hyalinized stroma ➡. This variant may be mistaken for an infiltrative carcinoma.* **(Right)** *Periodic acid-Schiff (PAS) stain without diastase digestion is usually strongly positive in TL due to cytoplasmic glycogenation.*

High Magnification of Desmoplastic Tricholemmoma

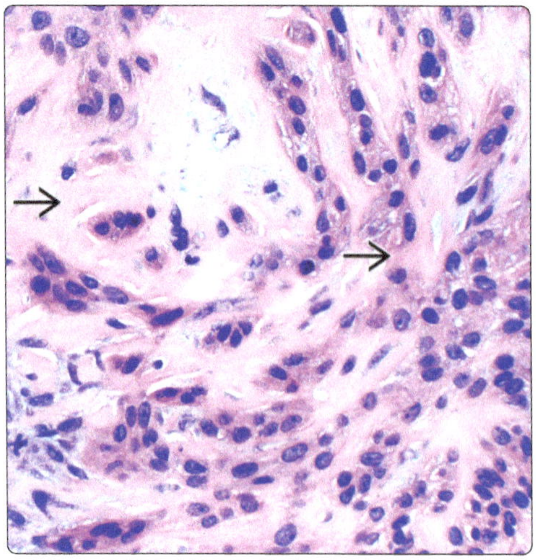

PAS Stain in Tricholemmoma

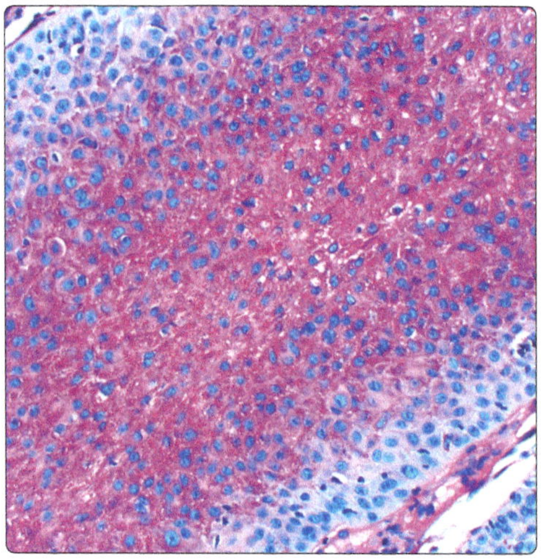

Differential Diagnosis: Clear Cell Acanthoma

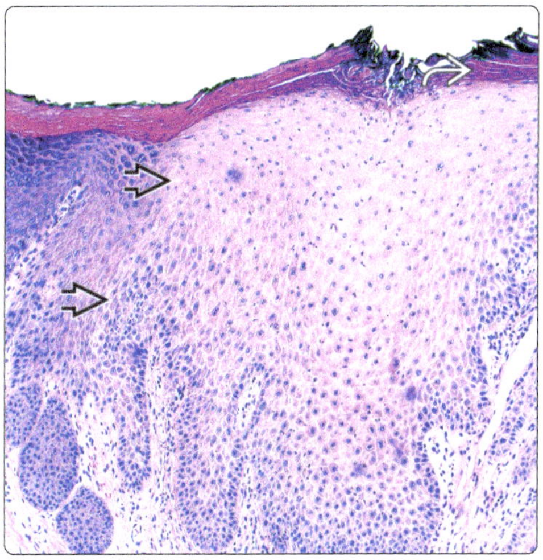

Differential Diagnosis: Tricholemmal Carcinoma

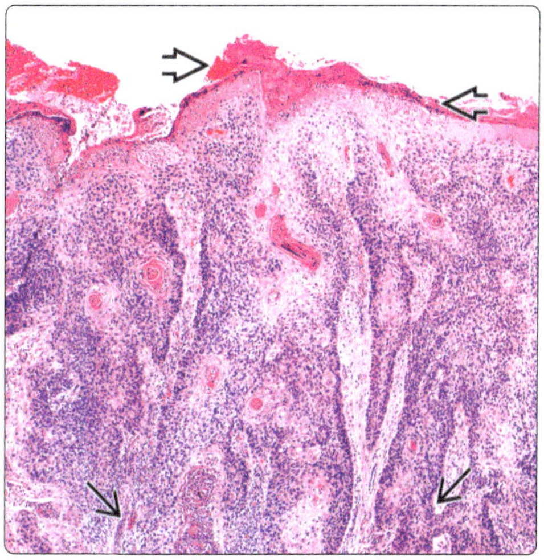

(Left) *Clear cell acanthoma shows psoriasiform acanthosis, parakeratosis, and a proliferation of bland-appearing pale eosinophilic to clear-staining keratinocytes. Note the sharp demarcation from the adjacent epidermis.* **(Right)** *Tricholemmal carcinoma is typically a larger tumor than TL and shows deep, irregular downgrowths of atypical basaloid to clear-staining cells. There is overlying epidermal erosion and serum crusting.*

Differential Diagnosis: Tricholemmal Carcinoma

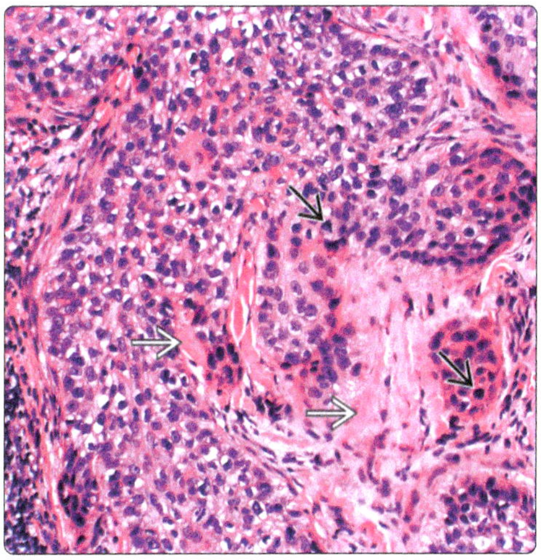

Differential Diagnosis: Tricholemmal Carcinoma

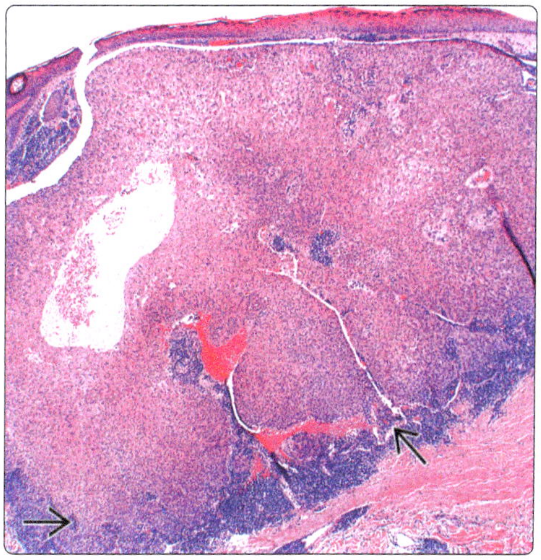

(Left) *High magnification of a tricholemmal carcinoma shows cytologic atypia, mitotic figures, and a hyalinized-appearing desmoplastic stroma.* **(Right)** *Another tricholemmal carcinoma shows a large, multilobulated, eosinophilic to clear cell neoplasm with irregular, jagged borders and relatively dense surrounding chronic inflammation.*

Differential Diagnosis: Tricholemmal Carcinoma

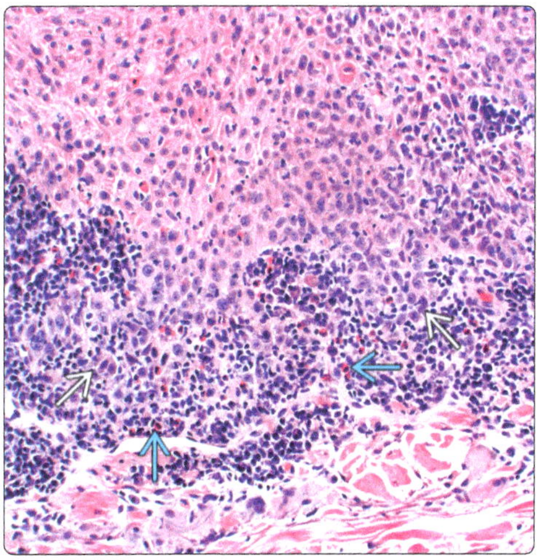

Differential Diagnosis: Clear Cell Squamous Cell Carcinoma

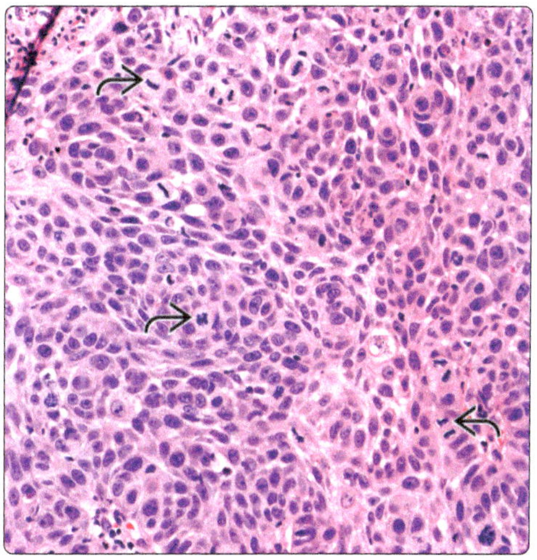

(Left) *Peripheral edge of tricholemmal carcinoma shows jagged borders, as opposed to the smooth, rounded borders and thickened basement membrane typical of TL. The lesion is associated with an inflammatory infiltrate including lymphocytes and numerous eosinophils.* **(Right)** *Invasive squamous cell carcinoma with clear cell features shows whorls of atypical pale- to clear-staining cells and numerous mitoses.*

KEY FACTS

TERMINOLOGY

- Tricholemmal carcinoma (TLC)
- Low-grade malignant tumor of clear-staining squamous cells with tricholemmal differentiation

CLINICAL ISSUES

- Rare, but may be underreported due to misclassification
- Occurs in sun-damaged skin of elderly people
- Most often presents in head and neck region
- Excellent prognosis, local recurrence potential but no confirmed metastatic cases

MICROSCOPIC

- Lobulated to nodular, predominantly dermal-based tumor
- Typically composed of proliferation of large clear cells with cytologic atypia
- Areas of tricholemmal (pilar)-type keratinization without intervening granular layer
- Peripheral palisading and thickened basement membrane often seen
- Mitotic figures usually abundant; necrosis may be seen

TOP DIFFERENTIAL DIAGNOSES

- Tricholemmoma
    - Usually smaller and more superficial than TLC
    - Lacks infiltrative features, cytologic atypia, and mitotic activity
- Clear cell squamous cell carcinoma (SCC)
    - Distinction from clear cell SCC may be subjective in some cases
    - However, conventional clear cell SCC does not show tricholemmal differentiation, peripheral palisading, or thickened basement membrane
- Clear cell basal cell carcinoma (BCC)
    - Most cases show areas of typical BCC composed of atypical basaloid cells in nodules, cords, or islands
- Sebaceous carcinoma

(Left) *Tricholemmal carcinoma (TLC) is a clear cell neoplasm that may show multiple attachments to the epidermis and overlying ulceration and crusting. Inset shows atypical cells with prominent nucleoli and multiple mitotic figures.* **(Right)** *Scanning magnification of a TLC shows a large, multilobulated eosinophilic to clear cell neoplasm with overlying erosions, irregular borders, and relatively dense surrounding chronic inflammation.*

Tricholemmal Carcinoma

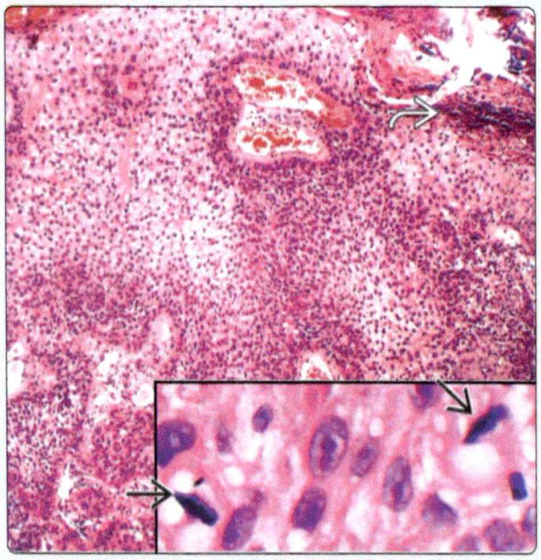

Low Magnification of TLC

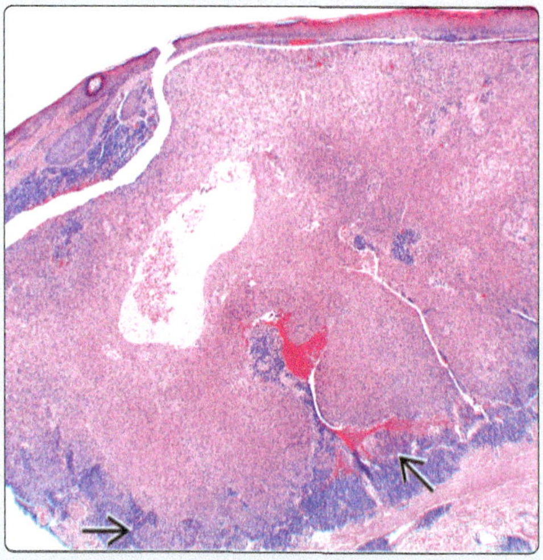

(Left) *Another example of TLC showing infiltrative lobules of atypical eosinophilic to clear-staining cells in the mid to deep dermis. Foci of tricholemmal keratinization are seen.* **(Right)** *High magnification of a TLC shows prominent atypia, mitotic figures, and a thickened basement membrane.*

Infiltrative Lobules in TLC

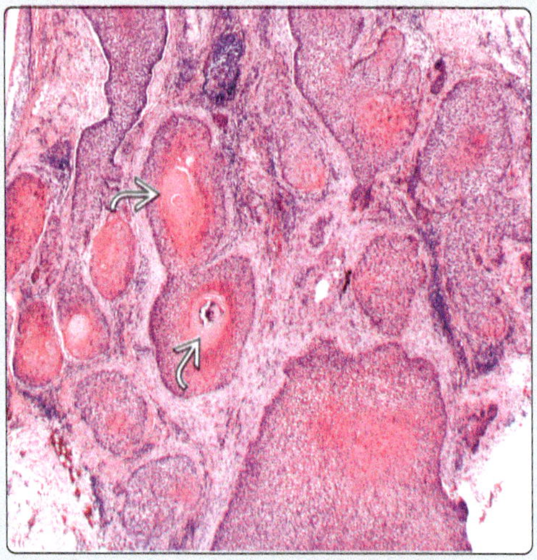

High Magnification of TLC With Multiple Mitoses

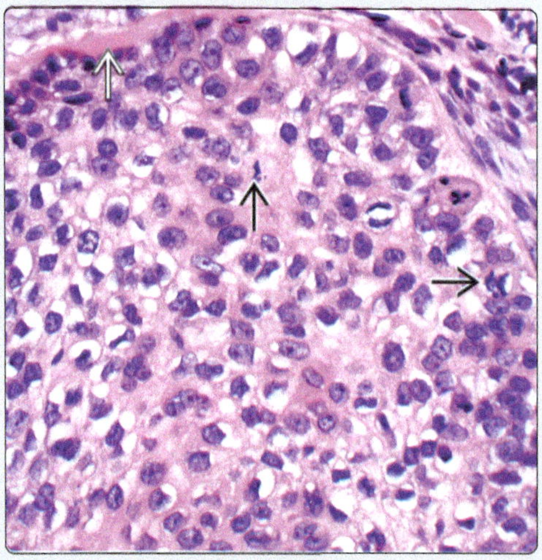

TERMINOLOGY

Abbreviations

- Tricholemmal carcinoma (TLC)

Synonyms

- Trichilemmal carcinoma
- Malignant tricholemmoma

Definitions

- Low-grade malignant tumor of clear-staining squamous cells with tricholemmal/outer root sheath differentiation
- Has been classified as low malignant potential variant of squamous cell carcinoma (SCC)

ETIOLOGY/PATHOGENESIS

Environmental Exposure

- Most cases likely due to ultraviolet light exposure
- Rare cases reportedly associated with radiation or immunosuppression

CLINICAL ISSUES

Epidemiology

- Incidence
  - Tumors rare, but may be underreported due to classification as clear cell SCC or other tumors
- Age
  - Occurs in elderly patients
- Sex
  - No definite gender predilection

Site

- Most often presents in head and neck region

Presentation

- Papule or nodule with overlying crusting &/or ulceration

Treatment

- Surgical approaches
  - Complete excision should be performed and is curative

Prognosis

- Excellent, local recurrence potential but no confirmed metastatic cases
  - Reported metastatic cases likely represent malignant proliferating tricholemmal/pilar tumors, not TLC

MACROSCOPIC

Size

- Generally small, < 2-3 cm

MICROSCOPIC

Histologic Features

- Lobulated to nodular tumor with dermal invasion
  - Composed of proliferation of large clear cells with cytologic atypia
    - Cells show nuclear hyperchromasia with prominent nucleoli and abundant clear-staining cytoplasm
    - Some cells may show prominent keratohyaline granules
  - Lobules may show connections to epidermis &/or hair follicles
  - Areas of tricholemmal (pilar)-type keratinization without intervening granular layer
  - Peripheral palisading and thickened basement membrane often seen
  - Mitotic figures usually abundant; necrosis may be present

Cytologic Features

- Large cells with nuclear hyperchromasia, prominent nucleoli, and abundant clear-staining cytoplasm

DIFFERENTIAL DIAGNOSIS

Tricholemmoma

- Usually smaller and more superficial than TLC
- Symmetric, well-circumscribed lobular proliferation
- Lacks significant cytologic atypia and mitotic activity

Clear Cell Squamous Cell Carcinoma

- TLC may be considered low-grade variant of clear cell SCC
- Therefore, distinction from clear cell SCC may be subjective in some cases
  - However, conventional clear cell SCC does not show tricholemmal differentiation, peripheral palisading, or thickened basement membrane
- Some cases of clear cell SCC are higher grade, and may behave aggressively, with metastatic disease
  - No well-documented cases of metastatic TLC reported

Clear Cell Basal Cell Carcinoma

- Most cases show areas of conventional basal cell carcinoma (BCC) with atypical basaloid cells in nodules, cords, or islands
- Presence of peripheral palisading seen in both TLC and BCC, but
  - Other features such as mucinous stroma and retraction artifact are lacking in TLC
  - Lobular architecture and thickened basement membrane are lacking in BCC

Sebaceous Carcinoma

- Composed of nodules &/or lobules of atypical clear cells, often with attachments to epidermis &/or hair follicles
- Cells typically show abundant multivacuolated cytoplasm with nuclear indentations, unlike uniformly clear-staining cytoplasm of TLC
- Lacks areas of tricholemmal keratinization and thickened basement membrane
- IHC shows positivity for EMA, androgen receptor, CAM5.2, and usually for CK7

SELECTED REFERENCES

1. Feng Z et al: Tricholemmal carcinoma of the head and neck region: a report of 15 cases. Oncol Lett. 7(2):423-426, 2014
2. Hamman MS et al: Management of trichilemmal carcinoma: an update and comprehensive review of the literature. Dermatol Surg. 40(7):711-7, 2014
3. Misago N: Controversial concepts: infundibular squamous cell carcinoma and tricholemmal carcinoma. Am J Dermatopathol. 35(4):523-4, 2013
4. Cassarino DS et al: Cutaneous squamous cell carcinoma: a comprehensive clinicopathologic classification. Part one. J Cutan Pathol. 33(3):191-206, 2006
5. Wong TY et al: Tricholemmal carcinoma. A clinicopathologic study of 13 cases. Am J Dermatopathol. 16(5):463-73, 1994

KEY FACTS

TERMINOLOGY

- Calcifying epithelioma of Malherbe

ETIOLOGY/PATHOGENESIS

- Derived from matrix of hair follicle

CLINICAL ISSUES

- Pilomatrixoma
  - Relatively common, rubbery to hard solitary tumor mostly seen in children and adolescents
  - Head and neck and upper limbs
- Pilomatrical carcinoma
  - Very rare, solitary tumor of elderly

MACROSCOPIC

- On gross sectioning, pilomatrixoma (PMX) often shows chalky material due to calcifications

MICROSCOPIC

- **Pilomatrixoma**
  - Well-circumscribed, dermal to subcutaneous tumor with mixture of basaloid and shadow cells
  - Lesion often surrounded by fibrous connective tissue capsule
  - Dystrophic calcification is frequently seen
  - Foreign-body giant cell reaction surrounding tumor is common
- **Pilomatrical carcinoma**
  - Ulcerated, asymmetrical, dermal to subcutaneous nodule
  - Poorly circumscribed, cellular, and infiltrative tumor
  - Numerous mitoses and tumor necrosis often present

TOP DIFFERENTIAL DIAGNOSES

- **Basal cell carcinoma**
  - Lacks shadow cells
  - Shows peripheral palisading and mucinous stroma
- **Merkel cell carcinoma**
- **Melanocytic matricoma**

Pilomatrixoma at Low Magnification

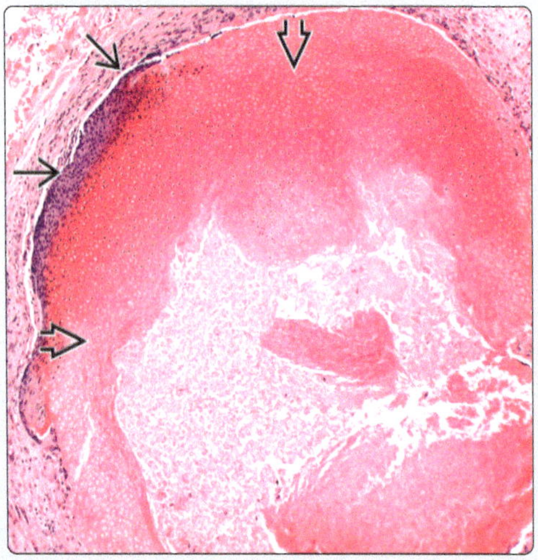

PMX: Basaloid and Ghost Cells

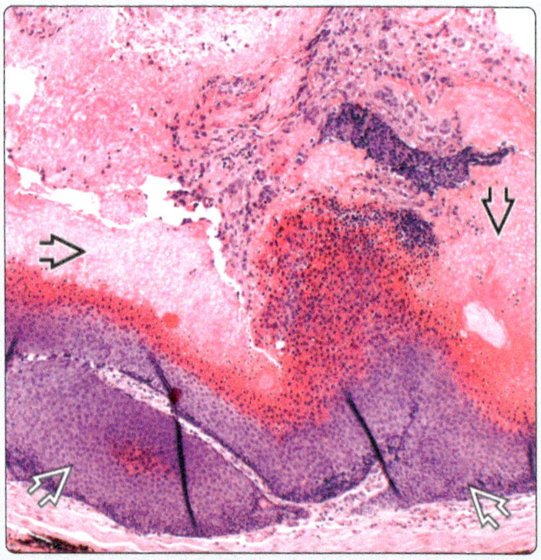

(Left) *Low magnification of a pilomatrixoma (PMX) shows a nodular-cystic dermal-based lesion with a thin, partial rim of peripheral basaloid cells → surrounding central collections of eosinophilic and shadow cells ⇩.* **(Right)** *Basaloid cells with variable thickness make up the periphery of the lesion ➡, and they merge gradually or abruptly with keratinizing eosinophilic cells called ghost or shadow cells ⇨.*

PMX at High Magnification

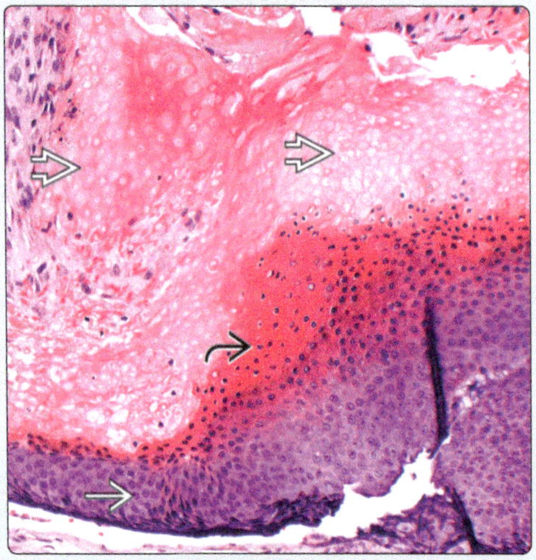

Foreign Body Giant Cell Reaction in PMX

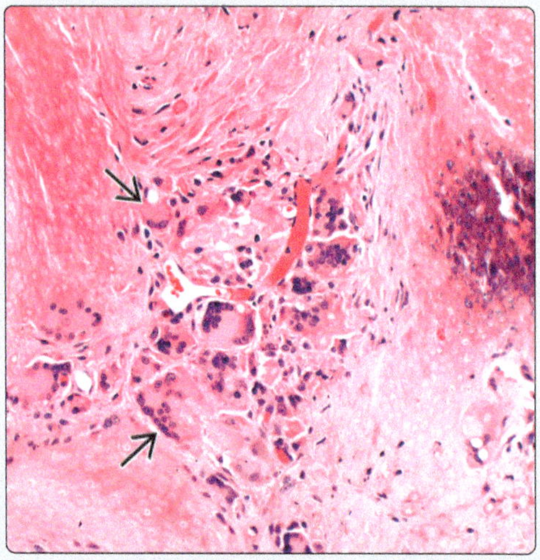

(Left) *Higher magnification shows the 2 cell types of PMX: Basaloid ➡ and shadow cells ➡. In this case, transitional cells ⇨ with pyknotic nuclei (prior to becoming shadow cells) are also seen.* **(Right)** *Foreign-body giant cell reaction → to keratin often surrounds ruptured areas in PMXs.*

TERMINOLOGY

Abbreviations

- Pilomatrixoma (PMX)

Synonyms

- PMX
  - Pilomatricoma
  - Calcifying epithelioma of Malherbe
  - Trichomatricoma
- Pilomatrical carcinoma
  - Matrical carcinoma
  - Malignant PMX
  - Pilomatrix carcinoma

Definitions

- PMX
  - Benign dermal &/or subcutaneous tumor
  - Derived from matrical portion of hair follicle, showing prominent ghost cells
- Pilomatrical carcinoma
  - Malignant counterpart of PMX

ETIOLOGY/PATHOGENESIS

Differentiation

- Derived from matrix of hair follicle

Genetics

- Mutations in the *CTNNB1* gene (encodes β-catenin) in both PMX and pilomatrical carcinomas
- Cysts of Gardner syndrome can show pilomatricoma-like changes

CLINICAL ISSUES

Epidemiology

- Incidence
  - PMX, relatively common
  - Pilomatrical carcinoma, very rare
- Age
  - PMX
    - Children and adolescents (1st and 2nd decade)
    - Rare in adults
  - Pilomatrical carcinoma
    - Elderly patients
- Sex
  - PMX
    - No gender predilection
  - Pilomatrical carcinoma
    - Male predominance (M:F = 5:1)

Site

- PMX and pilomatrical carcinoma
  - Head and neck and upper limbs

Presentation

- PMX
  - Solitary, rarely multiple
  - Rubbery or chalky hard
  - May be faceted, which lifts surface of skin
    - Tent sign is appearance of skin when lifted by underlying PMX
  - Rarely can perforate or rapidly enlarge
    - Rapid enlargement could be due to hemorrhage within tumor
- Pilomatrical carcinoma
  - Solitary
  - Usually occurs de novo
    - Rarely arises in preexisting PMX (usually large, longstanding tumor)
  - Recurrence after excision is common

Treatment

- Surgical approaches
  - PMX
    - Simple excision is curative
  - Pilomatrical carcinoma
    - Wide local excision
    - Radiation &/or chemotherapy for recurrence and nodal metastasis

Prognosis

- PMX
  - Excellent
  - Very rare malignant transformation to pilomatrical carcinoma
- Pilomatrical carcinoma
  - Local recurrence is common if not widely excised
  - Metastasis is rare
    - Rare cases have metastasized to lymph nodes, lung, and bone

MACROSCOPIC

General Features

- PMX
  - On gross sectioning, chalky material due to calcification often found

Size

- PMX: 0.5-3.0 cm
- Pilomatrical carcinoma: 0.6-10.0 cm (typically > 4 cm)

MICROSCOPIC

Histologic Features

- **PMX**
  - Well-circumscribed, dermal to subcutaneous nodule
  - 2 cell types: Basaloid cells and shadow cells
    - Basaloid cells with variable thickness make up periphery of lesion
      - Cells are small, homogeneous, and monotonous, and have scant cytoplasm and indistinct cellular borders
    - Basaloid cells merge gradually or abruptly with keratinizing eosinophilic cells, the so-called ghost or shadow cells
    - Ghost cells have abundant pink cytoplasm and open space at their center where nucleus was
    - Newer lesions usually have significant basaloid cells
    - Established lesions have predominately ghost cells

- Lesion often surrounded by fibrous connective tissue capsule
- Newer lesions may be cystic
- Dystrophic calcification is commonly seen
  - Calcium deposits are seen in about 75% of tumors (can be highlighted with von Kossa stain)
- Ossification is occasionally present
  - Seen in 15-20% of cases
  - Present in stroma near shadow cells
- Foreign-body giant cell reaction surrounding tumor is common
- Melanin might be present
  - Melanocytic matricoma is variant of PMX with prominent dendritic melanocytes

- **Pilomatrical carcinoma**
  - Often connected to epidermis
  - Ulcerated, asymmetrical, dermal to subcutaneous nodule
  - Poorly circumscribed, hypercellular, and infiltrative-apparent
  - Focal areas of true tumor necrosis
  - Basophilic cells with prominent nucleoli and numerous mitoses
  - Foci of shadow cells are helpful in diagnosis
  - Vascular/lymphatic invasion (rare)

Cytologic Features

- PMX
  - Basaloid cells
    - Deeply basophilic nuclei
    - Scant cytoplasm
    - Indistinct cell borders
    - Mitoses easily identified
  - Shadow cells
    - Central unstained areas where nuclei formerly resided
    - Abundant eosinophilic cytoplasm
    - Distinct cell borders
- Pilomatrical carcinoma
  - Basaloid cells
    - Pleomorphic with prominent nucleoli
    - Numerous and atypical mitoses
  - Shadow cells
    - Same features as in PMX

ANCILLARY TESTS

Immunohistochemistry

- β-catenin is strongly positive in vast majority of cases
- Cytoplasmic and nuclear staining for β-catenin, and nuclear staining for cyclin-D1 in basaloid cell population
- Keratins 5, 14, and 17 often positive in pilomatrical carcinomas, but negative in PMX

DIFFERENTIAL DIAGNOSIS

DDx of Pilomatrixoma

- **Basal cell carcinoma**
  - Lacks shadow cells
  - Often has mucinous stroma
  - Often shows connections with overlying epidermis
  - Less likely to have calcifications and ossifications, although they may be present in some cases
  - Does not commonly have granulomatous inflammation, typically seen in PMX due to reaction to keratin
- **Merkel cell carcinoma**
  - Lacks shadow cells
  - Tumor often shows foci of trabecular pattern that might be limited to periphery of lesion
  - Cells are often small, uniform, hyperchromatic-staining, and have vesicular nuclei with small nucleoli
  - CK20 stains tumoral cells in paranuclear dot-like pattern
- **Proliferating pilar/tricholemmal cyst**
  - On low power: Large symmetrical and well-circumscribed tumor, which may show cystic areas
  - Cells are squamoid with large eosinophilic cytoplasm, unlike basaloid small cells seen in PMX
  - Lacks shadow cells
- **Melanocytic matricoma**
  - Prominent pigment
  - Dendritic melanocytes present
  - Some consider this tumor to be variant of PMX with dendritic melanocytes and melanin pigment

DDx of Pilomatrical Carcinoma

- **Basal cell carcinoma with matrical differentiation**
  - Very rare and difficult to differentiate from pilomatrical carcinoma
  - Considered to be basal cell carcinoma derived from hair follicle epithelium
    - Shadow cells present
    - β-catenin can be positive in both tumors and is not helpful in differentiating them
- **Squamous cell carcinoma**
  - Cells show more abundant, eosinophilic cytoplasm with intercellular bridges
  - Keratinization more common, lacks shadow cells

DIAGNOSTIC CHECKLIST

Pathologic Interpretation Pearls

- PMXs are well-circumscribed dermal tumors with peripheral basaloid cells that merge into shadow cells and often show calcification
- Pilomatrical carcinomas are very rare and, in absence of shadow cells, can be difficult to diagnose

SELECTED REFERENCES

1. Zloto O et al: Periocular pilomatrixoma: a retrospective analysis of 16 cases. Ophthal Plast Reconstr Surg. 31(1):19-22, 2015
2. Battistella M et al: Skin tumors with matrical differentiation: lessons from hair keratins, beta-catenin and PHLDA-1 expression. J Cutan Pathol. 41(5):427-36, 2014
3. Herrmann JL et al: Pilomatrix carcinoma: 13 new cases and review of the literature with emphasis on predictors of metastasis. J Am Acad Dermatol. 71(1):38-43.e2, 2014
4. Del Sordo R et al: Basal cell carcinoma with matrical differentiation: expression of beta-catenin [corrected] and osteopontin. Am J Dermatopathol. 2007 Oct;29(5):470-4. Erratum in: Am J Dermatopathol. 30(3):317, 2008
5. Kim SH et al: Basal cell carcinoma with matrical differentiation. Yonsei Med J. 44(3):523-5, 2003
6. Haferkamp B et al: [Pilomatrix carcinoma in an unusual location. Case report and review of the literature.] Hautarzt. 50(5):355-9, 1999

Clinical Photograph of Pilomatrixoma

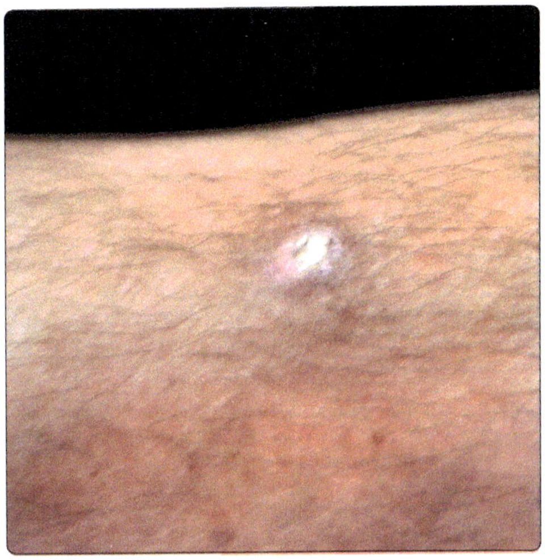

Pilomatrixoma: Basaloid and Ghost Cells

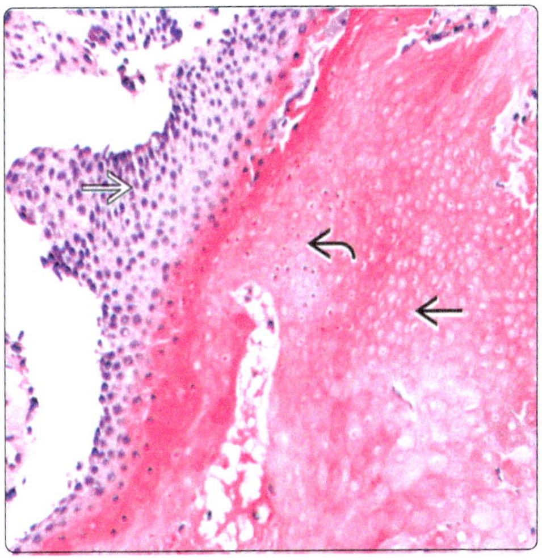

(Left) *This was a PMX which presented as a calcified nodule on the forearm of a young adult patient.* **(Right)** *The 2 cell types of a PMX are basaloid ➡ and shadow cells ➡. In this case, transitional cells ➡ with pyknotic nuclei prior to becoming shadow cells without nuclei are seen.*

Calcifications in Pilomatrixoma

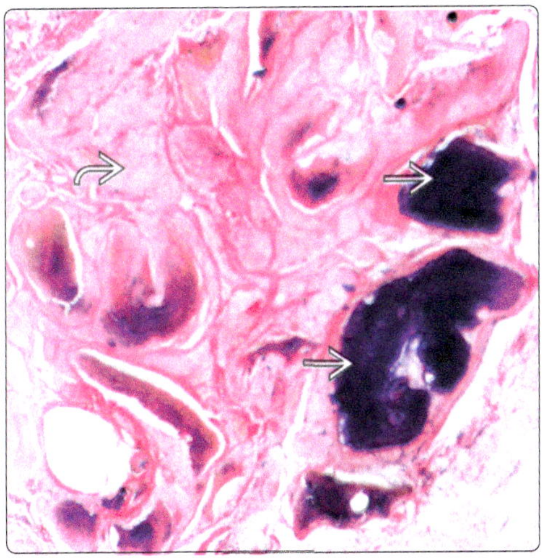

Pilomatrical Carcinoma

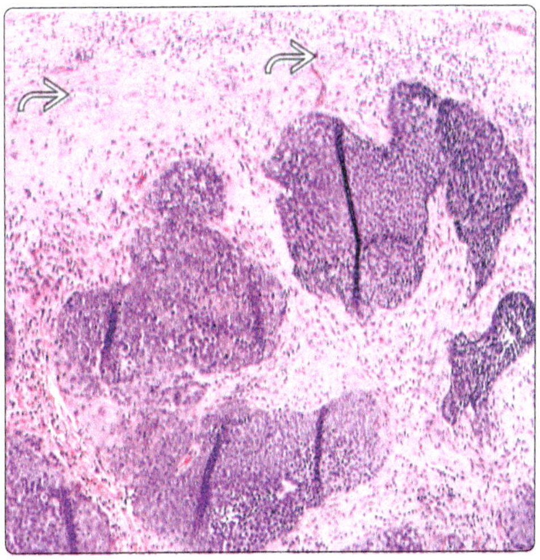

(Left) *In older, or so-called burned-out lesions, there are minimal to no basaloid cells, and the tumor is often composed only of shadow cells ➡ and large deposits of calcium ➡.* **(Right)** *Pilomatrical carcinomas typically show poor circumscription and an infiltrative pattern. The tumor is often composed predominately of basaloid cells, although larger, more squamoid-appearing cells can also be present ➡.*

Pilomatrical Carcinoma

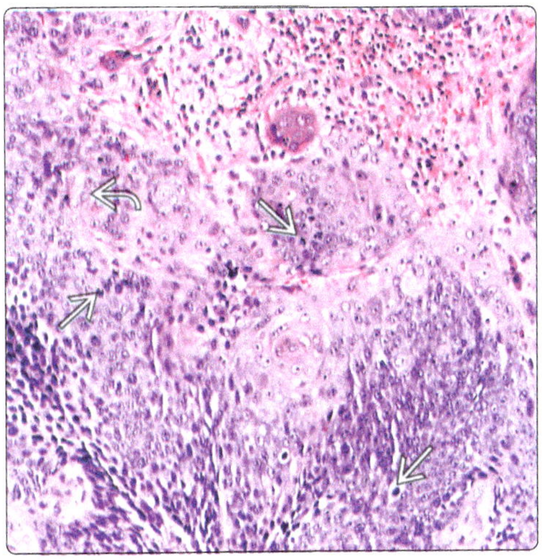

High Magnification of Pilomatrical Carcinoma

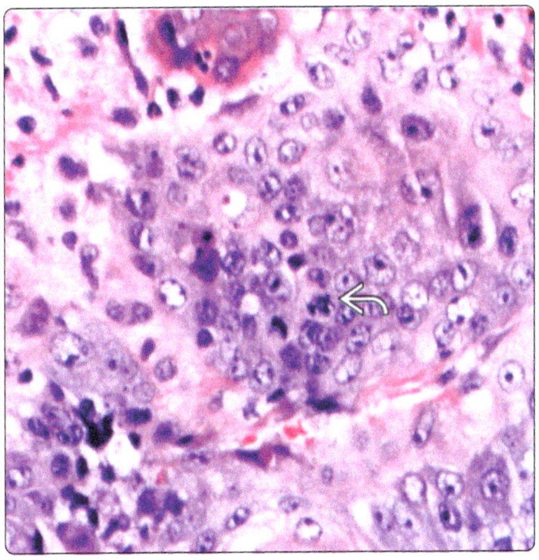

(Left) *The basaloid cells, as in PMX, show foci of monotonous cells with scant cytoplasm and indistinct cellular borders ➡. However, in pilomatrical carcinoma, the cells are markedly atypical and pleomorphic-appearing, and multiple mitotic figures are easily identified ➡.* **(Right)** *High magnification of pilomatrical carcinoma shows pleomorphic cells with prominent nucleoli and an atypical mitotic figure ➡. In the absence of shadow cells, it can be difficult to make this diagnosis.*

Fibrofolliculoma and Trichodiscoma

KEY FACTS

TERMINOLOGY

- Fibrofolliculoma (FF)
- Trichodiscoma (TD)
- Closely related hamartomas with follicular and mesenchymal differentiation
- TD likely represents late stage in evolution of fibrofolliculoma, showing stromal predominance

ETIOLOGY/PATHOGENESIS

- Multiple lesions are strongly correlated with Birt-Hogg-Dubé syndrome
  - High risk of renal cell carcinoma

CLINICAL ISSUES

- Typically present as multiple small papule(s) on face

MICROSCOPIC

- **FF** shows proliferation of thin, anastomosing epithelial cords
  - Numerous attachments to follicular structures and epidermis
  - Typically find central, dilated follicular structure
- **TD** is stromal-predominant lesion, may show only small/miniaturize follicle

TOP DIFFERENTIAL DIAGNOSES

- Tumor of follicular infundibulum
  - Superficial, plate-like proliferation of bland pale to clear squamoid cells
  - Anastomosing strands of epithelium present, but usually thicker than those in FF
- Inverted follicular keratosis
  - Endophytic epithelial proliferation with numerous squamous eddies
- Basal cell carcinoma, infundibulocystic type
  - Basal cell carcinoma shows areas of peripheral palisading and tumor-stromal retraction artifact

Clinical Photograph of Fibrofolliculoma

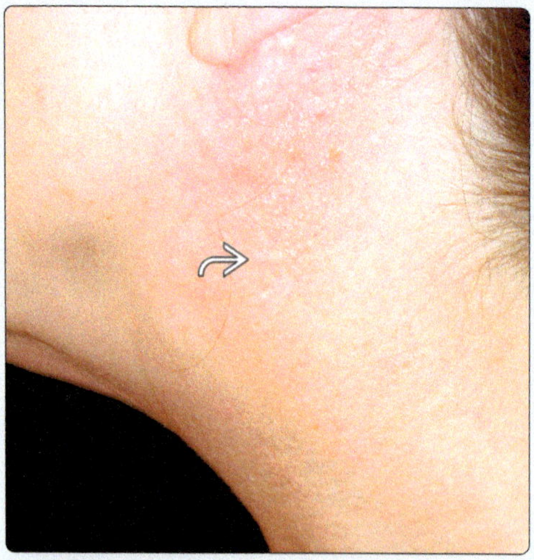

Fibrofolliculoma at Low Magnification

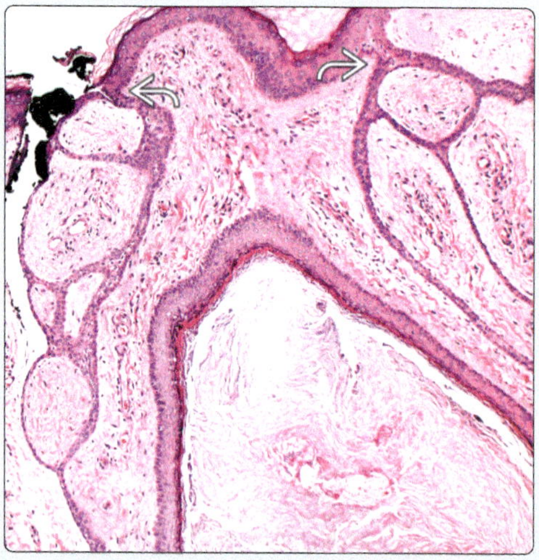

(Left) *Clinical photograph of a patient with Birt-Hogg-Dubé syndrome shows numerous small, flesh-colored papules on the lateral cheek and neck* ➔. *(Courtesy J. Wu, MD.)* **(Right)** *Fibrofolliculoma shows a central dilated (cystic) follicular structure with keratin debris. There are multiple thin, radiating epithelial strands attached to the overlying epidermis* ➔.

Fibrofolliculoma With Central Follicular Structure

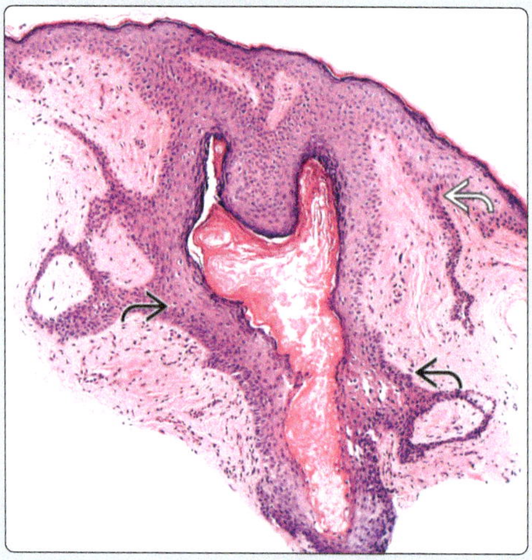

Trichodiscoma at Low Magnification

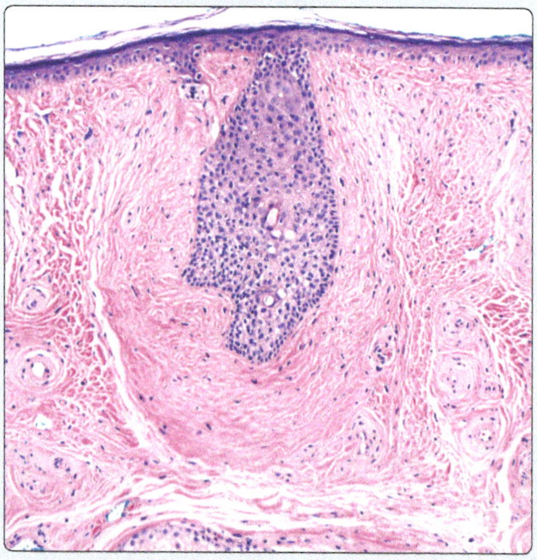

(Left) *Fibrofolliculoma shows a central follicular structure with a dilated lumen and thin, radiating epithelial strands attached to both the follicle* ➔ *and the epidermis* ➔. **(Right)** *Trichodiscoma is composed mostly of fibromyxoid stroma but will often demonstrate a residual miniaturized follicular structure if multiple deeper level sections are examined.*

TERMINOLOGY

Abbreviations

- Fibrofolliculoma (FF)
- Trichodiscoma (TD)

Synonyms

- Mantleoma (likely FF variant with sebaceous differentiation)

Definitions

- Closely related hamartomatous proliferations with follicular and mesenchymal differentiation
- Trichodiscoma likely represents late stage in evolution of FF showing stromal predominance

ETIOLOGY/PATHOGENESIS

Genetic Syndrome

- Multiple lesions are strongly correlated with Birt-Hogg-Dubé syndrome (BHD)
  - Due to mutations in folliculin (*FLCN*) gene
  - High risk of internal malignancies, especially renal cell carcinoma
  - Also predisposed to pulmonary cysts and pneumothoraces

CLINICAL ISSUES

Epidemiology

- Incidence
  - Very rare lesions
- Age
  - Usually present in young adults, especially in BHD syndrome
- Sex
  - More common in men

Site

- Facial area most common, but also may involve other head and neck sites, trunk, and arms

Presentation

- Small, asymptomatic papule(s) on face
  - Usually multiple (even hundreds), especially in BHD

Treatment

- Options, risks, complications
  - Excision is curative, but not necessary in most cases, given benign nature of these lesions
  - Work-up for underlying disease (including renal cell carcinoma) is indicated for patients suspected of having syndromic form

Prognosis

- Skin lesions are completely benign
- Patients with BHD syndrome have high incidence of internal organ involvement, which may be fatal

MICROSCOPIC

Histologic Features

- FF
  - Bland epithelial proliferation composed of thin, anastomosing cords
    - Numerous attachments to follicular structures and epidermis present
    - Cells are small, bland-appearing basaloid to squamoid cells
  - Typically central, dilated follicular structure is present
  - Fibromyxoid stroma, similar to TD, with decreased or lost elastic fibers
- TD
  - Stromal-predominant lesion
  - Consists of proliferation of small, bland-appearing fibroblastic cells within loose, fibromyxoid stroma
    - Elastic fibers markedly reduced or absent
  - Miniaturized peripheral follicular structure and epithelial strands usually can be identified
    - May need to examine multiple deeper level sections to identify

DIFFERENTIAL DIAGNOSIS

Tumor of Follicular Infundibulum

- Superficial, plate-like proliferation of bland pale to clear squamoid cells
- Anastomosing strands of epithelium present, but they are usually thicker than those in fibrofolliculoma
- Multiple follicles merge with undersurface of tumor
- Lacks fibromyxoid stroma of FF and TD

Inverted Follicular Keratosis

- Endophytic epithelial proliferation with numerous squamous eddies
  - Cells are larger and more squamoid-appearing than those in FF
- Typically shows multiple pseudohorn cysts, supporting theory that these are variants of irritated seborrheic keratoses
- Lacks fibromyxoid stroma of FF and TD

Basal Cell Carcinoma, Infundibulocystic Type

- Basal cell carcinoma shows areas of peripheral palisading and tumor-stromal retraction artifact
- Tumor cells are larger and more atypical, with hyperchromatic nuclei and multiple mitotic and apoptotic figures
- Mucinous stroma usually prominent (less fibromyxoid than that in FF and TD)

SELECTED REFERENCES

1. Bradley M et al: No association between Birt-Hogg-Dubé syndrome skin fibrofolliculomas and the first 10 described human polyomaviruses or human papillomaviruses. Virology. 468-470:244-7, 2014
2. Shvartsbeyn M et al: Perifollicular fibroma in Birt-Hogg-Dubé syndrome: an association revisited. J Cutan Pathol. 39(7):675-9, 2012
3. Menko FH et al: Birt-Hogg-Dubé syndrome: diagnosis and management. Lancet Oncol. 10(12):1199-206, 2009
4. Toro JR et al: BHD mutations, clinical and molecular genetic investigations of Birt-Hogg-Dubé syndrome: a new series of 50 families and a review of published reports. J Med Genet. 45(6):321-31, 2008
5. Schmidt LS: Birt-Hogg-Dubé syndrome, a genodermatosis that increases risk for renal carcinoma. Curr Mol Med. 4(8):877-85, 2004
6. Birt AR et al: Hereditary multiple fibrofolliculomas with trichodiscomas and acrochordons. Arch Dermatol. 113(12):1674-7, 1977

PART I

SECTION 4

Tumors and Tumor-Like Conditions With Sebaceous Differentiation

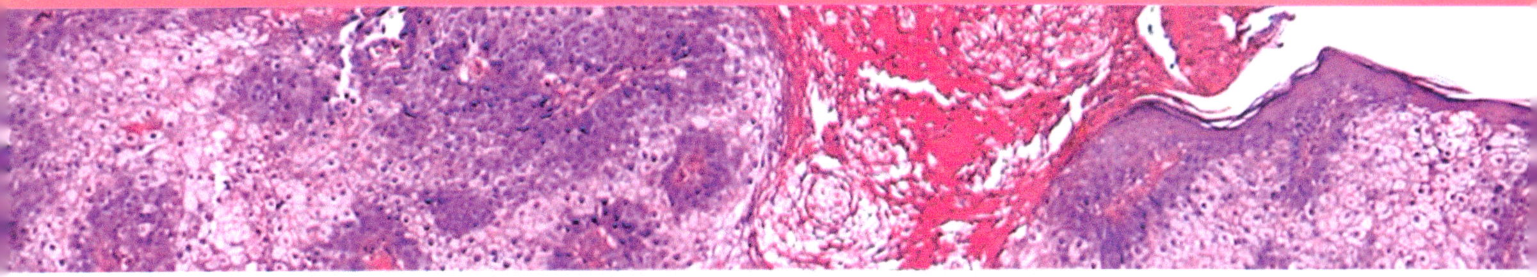

Sebaceous Hyperplasia

KEY FACTS

TERMINOLOGY

- Hyperplasia (overgrowth) of sebaceous glands

CLINICAL ISSUES

- Commonly on face
- Yellow to flesh-colored to slightly pink papule
- Often biopsied to rule out basal cell carcinoma

MICROSCOPIC

- Lobules of sebocytes arranged around infundibulum of central hair follicle
- 1 layer of basaloid cells compressed at periphery of sebocytes
- No cytologic atypia

TOP DIFFERENTIAL DIAGNOSES

- Sebaceous adenoma
  - Sebocytes in lobules, rimmed by more than 1 layer of basaloid cells
  - Often connecting directly to epidermal surface
- Ectopic sebaceous glands in other sites (e.g., nipple)
  - Often connect directly to epidermal surface
- Phymatous rosacea
  - Prominent sebaceous glands, edema, and fibrosis on different sites
  - Clinical history is key
- Sebaceous trichofolliculoma
  - Mature, central hair follicle, often producing hair shaft
  - Smaller, baby hair follicles and sebaceous glands radiating away from central follicle
- Folliculosebaceous cystic hamartoma
  - Central dilated infundibulum surrounded by hair follicles and sebaceous glands
- Sebaceous induction
  - Lobules of sebocytes connecting to epidermal surface
  - Most commonly seen above dermatofibroma

Sebaceous Hyperplasia

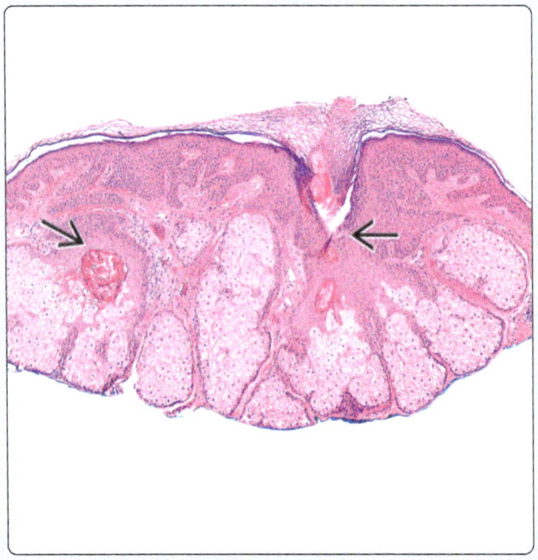

Sebaceous Hyperplasia Attached to Follicular Infundibulum

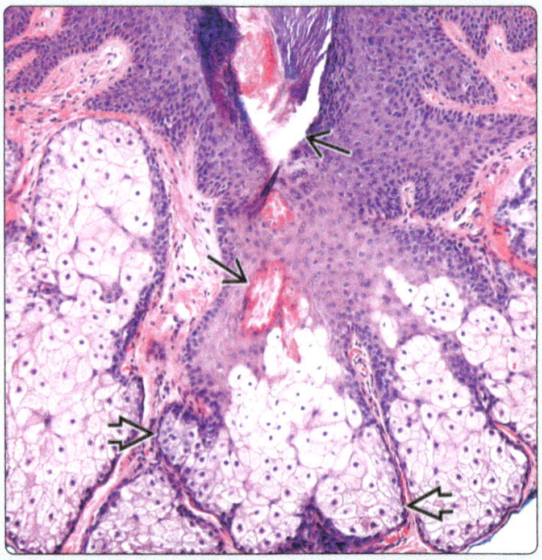

(Left) *Low-magnification view of sebaceous hyperplasia. There are normal-appearing lobules of sebocytes surrounding invaginations of epidermis that resemble the infundibula of hair follicles ➙.* **(Right)** *Lobules of sebocytes surround an invagination of epidermis ➙ that resembles the infundibulum of a hair follicle. The lobules of sebocytes are rimmed by a single compressed layer of small basaloid cells ➙.*

Sebaceous Hyperplasia at High Magnification

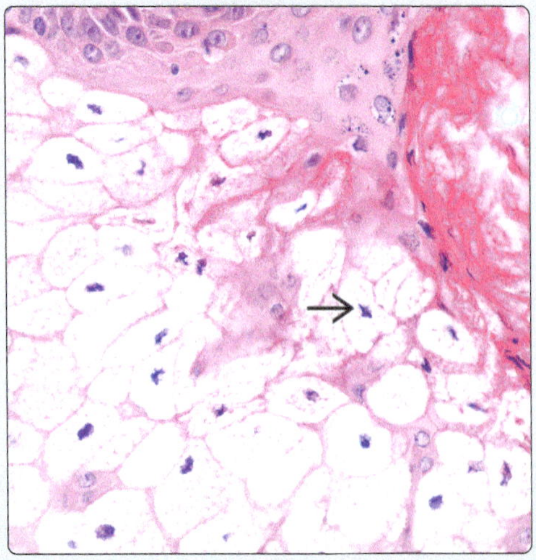

Sebaceous Hyperplasia at High Magnification

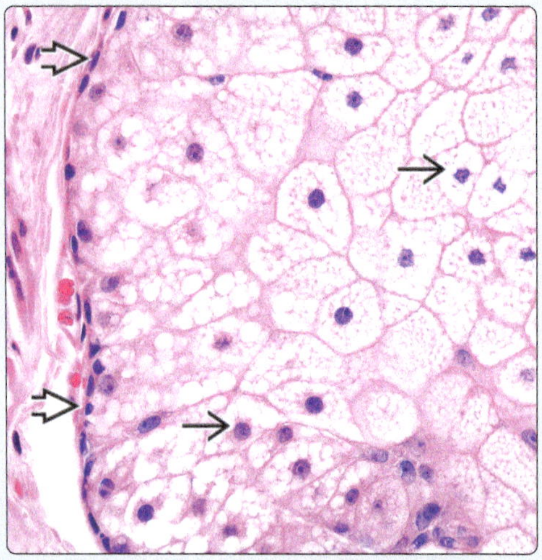

(Left) *High-power view of sebocytes shows bubbly cytoplasm and a central round or scalloped ➙ nucleus.* **(Right)** *High-magnification view of the edge of a lobule of sebocytes shows the central sebocytes ➙ with round to scalloped nuclei and bubbly cytoplasm, rimmed by a compressed layer of small, basaloid cells ➙.*

TERMINOLOGY

Definitions

- Hyperplasia (overgrowth) of sebaceous glands
- Plump lobules of sebaceous glands arranged around central follicular structures

CLINICAL ISSUES

Site

- Commonly on face
- Rarely on trunk or other sites

Presentation

- Yellow to flesh-colored to slightly pink papule
- Often there is central dell
- Telangiectasias may be present
- Often biopsied to rule out basal cell carcinoma

Laboratory Tests

- Generally not performed

Treatment

- Not necessary in most cases
- Biopsy (shave removal) may be curative
- Some studies suggest effective treatment with oral retinoids or lasers

Prognosis

- Benign lesions
- No malignant potential

MACROSCOPIC

Dermoscopic Findings

- Crown-like, thin, red vessels
- Vessels surround white to yellow globules

MICROSCOPIC

Histologic Features

- Lobules of sebocytes
  - Arranged around infundibula of central hair follicles
  - Rarely connect to epidermal surface
- Basaloid cells
  - 1 layer of basaloid cells compressed at periphery of sebocytes
  - Layers of basaloid cells not increased in number (as in adenomas)

Cytologic Features

- No cytologic atypia
- Sebocytes
  - Round to scalloped central nucleus
  - Abundant bubbly cytoplasm

DIFFERENTIAL DIAGNOSIS

Sebaceous Adenoma

- May have similar low-power architecture to sebaceous hyperplasia, but typically larger nodular aggregates
  - Sebocytes in lobules or around follicles
- Expanded layers of basaloid cells bordering sebocytes

Nevus Sebaceus

- Lobules of sebocytes directly connecting to hyperplastic epidermal surface
- Germinative (basaloid) cell layers not increased
- Abortive/vellus follicles may be present
- Apocrine glands may be present in deep dermis

Ectopic Sebaceous Glands in Other Sites

- Montgomery tubercles
  - Sebaceous glands on nipple
  - Lobules of sebocytes directly connecting to epithelial surface
- Fordyce spots
  - Sebaceous glands on mucosa
  - Lobules of sebocytes directly connecting to epithelial surface

Phymatous Rosacea

- Prominent sebaceous glands, edema, and fibrosis on different sites
  - Rhinophyma: Nose
  - Otophyma: Ear
  - Gnatophyma: Chin
  - Metophyma: Forehead
  - Blepharophyma: Eyelid
- Clinical history is key

Sebaceous Trichofolliculoma

- Central dilated follicular structure attached to epidermis
- Surrounding secondary hair follicles
- Sebaceous glands connecting to hair follicles

Folliculosebaceous Cystic Hamartoma

- Similar to sebaceous trichofolliculoma, but usually dermal based
- Central dilated infundibulum
  - Surrounding sebaceous glands and hair follicles
- Fibrocytic stroma

Sebaceous Induction

- Sebaceous glands connecting to epidermal surface
- May be seen above dermatofibromas

Juxtaclavicular Beaded Lines

- Hypertrophy of hair follicles and associated sebaceous glands on neck/upper trunk
- Clinical history is key

SELECTED REFERENCES

1. Simmons BJ et al: Light and laser therapies for the treatment of sebaceous gland hyperplasia a review of the literature. J Eur Acad Dermatol Venereol. ePub, 2015
2. Zeidi M et al: Sebaceous induction in dermatofibroma: a common feature of dermatofibromas on the shoulder. J Cutan Pathol. 42(6):400-5, 2015
3. Roma AA et al: Sebaceous hyperplasia of the vulva: a series of cases reporting no association with the Muir-Torre syndrome. Int J Gynecol Pathol. 33(4):437-42, 2014
4. Sato T et al: Linear sebaceous hyperplasia on the chest. Dermatol Pract Concept. 4(1):93-5, 2014
5. Gupta M et al: Otophyma: a rare and frequently misdiagnosed entity. Am J Otolaryngol. 31(3):199-201, 2010
6. Zalaudek I et al: How to diagnose nonpigmented skin tumors: a review of vascular structures seen with dermoscopy: part II. Nonmelanocytic skin tumors. J Am Acad Dermatol. 63(3):377-86; quiz 387-8, 2010
7. Eisen DB et al: Sebaceous lesions and their associated syndromes: part I. J Am Acad Dermatol. 61(4):549-60; quiz 561-2, 2009

Sebaceoma (Sebaceous Epithelioma)

KEY FACTS

TERMINOLOGY

- Sebaceous epithelioma is older term (discouraged)
- Benign proliferation of mature sebaceous cells with predominant basaloid cell population

ETIOLOGY/PATHOGENESIS

- Some cases are part of Muir-Torre syndrome (MTS)
  - Autosomal dominant disease due to mutations in mismatch repair genes *MLH1*, *MSH2*, *MSH6*
  - Multiple sebaceous tumors including sebaceous adenomas, less likely carcinomas and sebaceomas

CLINICAL ISSUES

- Rare tumors; typically occur in adults
- Most common on face
- Usually single but may be multiple, especially in MTS patients

MICROSCOPIC

- Nodular, dermal-based adnexal tumor
- Well circumscribed, noninfiltrative
- Composed mostly of basaloid cells
- Minor population of clear cells with multivacuolated cytoplasm, consistent with mature sebaceous cells
  - Show nuclear hyperchromasia with indentations
- Basaloid cells may show mild cytologic atypia and increased mitotic figures
- Sebaceous cells do not show significant atypia or mitotic activity

TOP DIFFERENTIAL DIAGNOSES

- Basal cell carcinoma with sebaceous differentiation
  - Basal cells show greater atypia and peripheral palisading
  - Mucinous stroma and retraction artifact often present (lacking in sebaceoma)
- Sebaceous adenoma
  - > 50% clear cells
- Sebaceous carcinoma
- Trichoblastoma with sebaceous differentiation

(Left) *Low magnification of a sebaceoma shows a dermal-based basaloid to clear cell neoplasm with peripheral basaloid cells surrounding clear cells, sebaceous secretions, and a focal cystic space.* **(Right)** *Higher magnification of sebaceoma shows a superficial, well-circumscribed lobule of predominantly basaloid cells with a smaller population of bland-appearing, mature sebaceous cells.*

Sebaceoma at Low Magnification

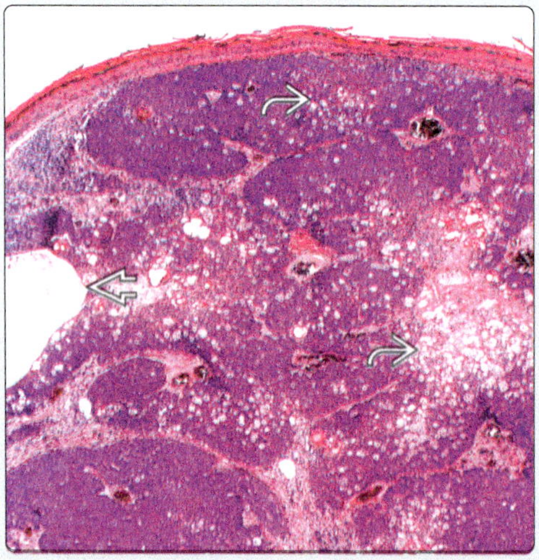

Sebaceoma at Higher Magnification

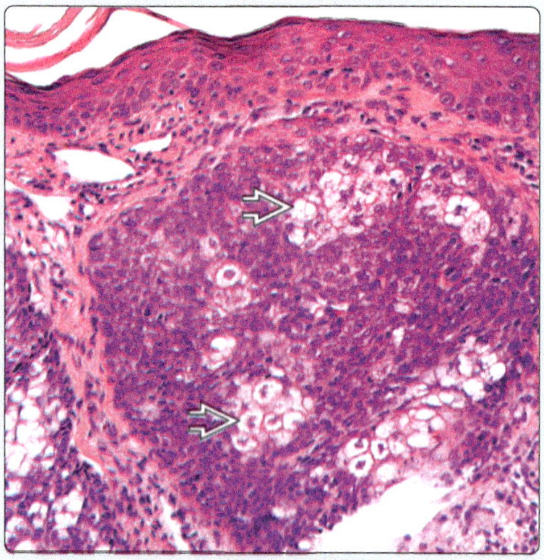

(Left) *High magnification of a sebaceoma shows a population of scattered, bland-appearing, multivacuolated clear cells demonstrating nuclear hyperchromasia and nuclear indentations, which are due to cytoplasmic lipids.* **(Right)** *This is an example of a sebaceoma with cystic areas, which shows a proliferation of predominantly basaloid and focal clear cells surrounding the cystic space.*

Sebaceoma at High Magnification

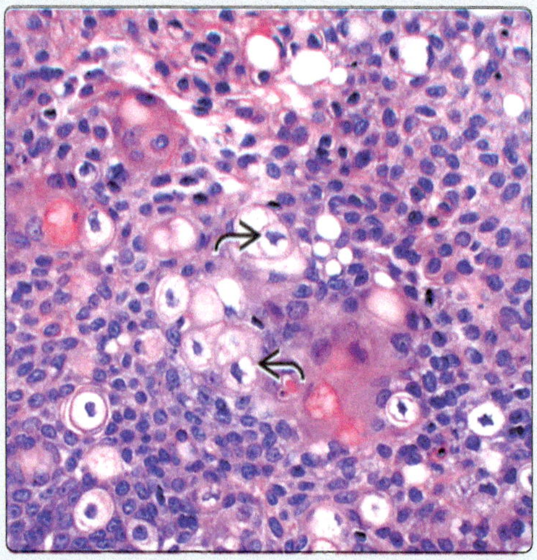

Cystic Sebaceoma

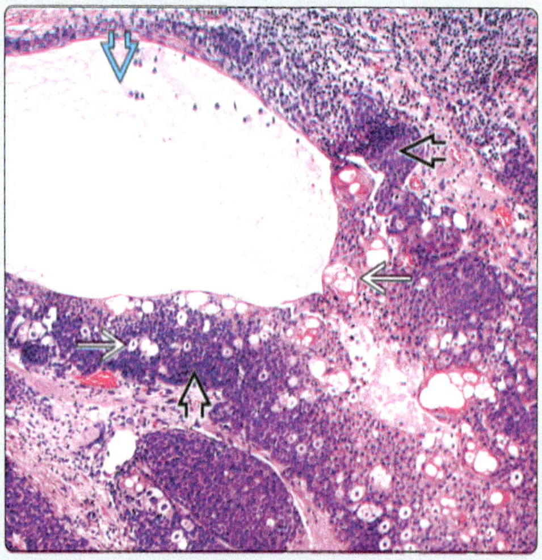

TERMINOLOGY

Synonyms

- Sebaceous epithelioma (older term, should be discouraged)

Definitions

- Benign proliferation of mature sebaceous cells associated with predominant basaloid cell population

ETIOLOGY/PATHOGENESIS

Unknown in Most Cases

- Some cases are part of Muir-Torre syndrome (MTS)
  - Autosomal dominant disease due to mutations in mismatch repair genes *MLH1*, *MSH2*, *MSH6*
  - Patients present with multiple sebaceous tumors, including sebaceous adenomas (most common), sebaceomas, and sebaceous carcinomas

CLINICAL ISSUES

Epidemiology

- Incidence
  - Rare tumors
- Age
  - Typically occur in adults

Site

- Often occur on face but may also present on trunk

Presentation

- Slow-growing papular to nodular lesion
  - Usually single, but may be multiple, especially in MTS

Treatment

- Surgical approaches
  - Complete conservative excision is curative

Prognosis

- Excellent; very low malignant potential

MICROSCOPIC

Histologic Features

- Nodular, dermal-based adnexal tumor
  - Usually located in mid to upper dermis
  - Well circumscribed, noninfiltrative appearing
  - May show association with hair follicle in some cases
  - Cysts and ductal-like structures often present
- Composed mostly of immature-appearing basaloid cells
  - Basaloid cells may show mild cytologic atypia and increased mitotic figures
  - Atypical mitoses should be absent
- Minority of tumor consists of clear cells with multivacuolated cytoplasm, consistent with mature sebaceous cells
  - Show nuclear hyperchromasia with indentations, typical of sebocytes
  - Sebaceous cells do not show significant atypia or mitotic activity
- **Rippled-pattern sebaceoma**: Rare variant showing palisading of basaloid nuclei

ANCILLARY TESTS

Immunohistochemistry

- EMA usually positive in clear cells; BER-EP4 negative (positive in basal cell carcinoma)
- Low p53, Ki-67 (higher in sebaceous carcinoma)

DIFFERENTIAL DIAGNOSIS

Basal Cell Carcinoma With Sebaceous Differentiation

- Basal cells show greater atypia and peripheral palisading
- Mucinous stroma and retraction artifact often present (lacking in sebaceoma)
- Some cases have previously been reported as sebaceous epithelioma, therefore, this term should not be used

Sebaceous Carcinoma

- Sebaceous cells show greater cytologic atypia and pleomorphism
- Mitotic figures usually numerous and often atypical
- Basaloid sebaceous carcinoma can be very difficult to separate from sebaceoma in some cases, especially in partial biopsies
  - If findings are not definitive in biopsy, complete excision should be recommended to allow for definitive diagnosis

Sebaceous Adenoma

- Mature sebaceous cells predominate over basaloid cells (> 50% clear cells)
- Basaloid cells confined to peripheral layers of sebaceous lobules
- Frequent attachment to hair follicles and epidermis

Trichoblastoma With Sebaceous Differentiation

- Typically larger, deeper dermal nodular lesions
- Sebaceous differentiation, when present, is very focal
- Areas of follicular differentiation, including papillary mesenchymal bodies and infundibulocystic structures with keratin debris

Superficial Epithelioma With Sebaceous Differentiation

- Very rare, solitary lesion that presents on face in older adults
- Superficial, plate-like proliferation with multiple attachments to epidermis (similar to tumor of follicular infundibulum)

SELECTED REFERENCES

1. Abreu Velez AM et al: Markers for sebaceoma show a spectrum of cell cycle regulators, tumor suppressor genes, and oncogenes. N Am J Med Sci. 7(6):275-80, 2015
2. Chuang HC et al: Desmoplastic sebaceoma arising from nevus sebaceus: a new variant. J Cutan Pathol. 41(6):509-12, 2014
3. Fan YS et al: Characteristic Ber-EP4 and EMA expression in sebaceoma is immunohistochemically distinct from basal cell carcinoma. Histopathology. 51(1):80-6, 2007
4. Cabral ES et al: Distinction of benign sebaceous proliferations from sebaceous carcinomas by immunohistochemistry. Am J Dermatopathol. 28(6):465-71, 2006
5. Troy JL et al: Sebaceoma. A distinctive benign neoplasm of adnexal epithelium differentiating toward sebaceous cells. Am J Dermatopathol. 6(1):7-13, 1984

(Left) *This sebaceoma showed prominent blood vessels and areas of hemorrhage ➡, findings which could suggest another adnexal tumor, such as spiradenoma at low magnification.* (Right) *Higher magnification of the same case shows a predominance of small basaloid cells, with a few scattered sebocytes ➡ present. Several small ductal structures are also seen ➡.*

Sebaceoma With Prominent Vascularity

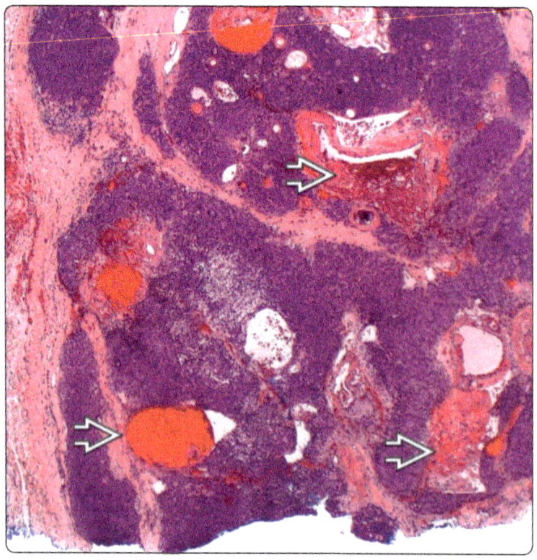

Sebaceoma With Prominent Vascularity at Higher Magnification

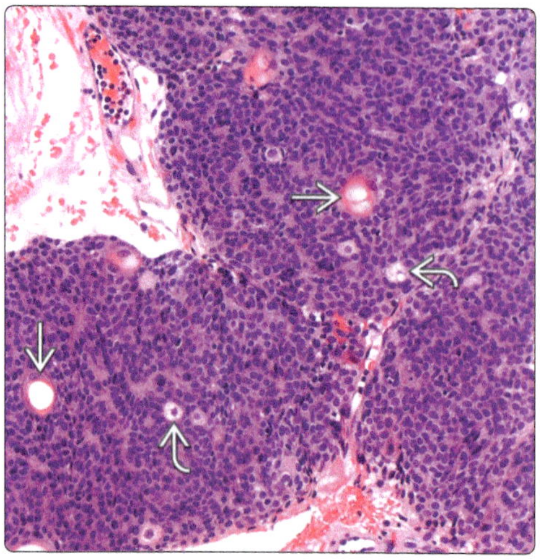

(Left) *High magnification of a sebaceoma shows a population of scattered, bland-appearing, multivacuolated clear cells ➡ demonstrating nuclear hyperchromasia and nuclear indentations. The basaloid cells show nuclear hyperchromasia and crowding, but no high-grade atypia.* (Right) *Podoplanin (D2-40) is often moderately to strongly positive in sebaceoma (especially in the basaloid cells ➡) but usually weak to absent in sebaceous carcinoma.*

Sebaceoma at High Magnification

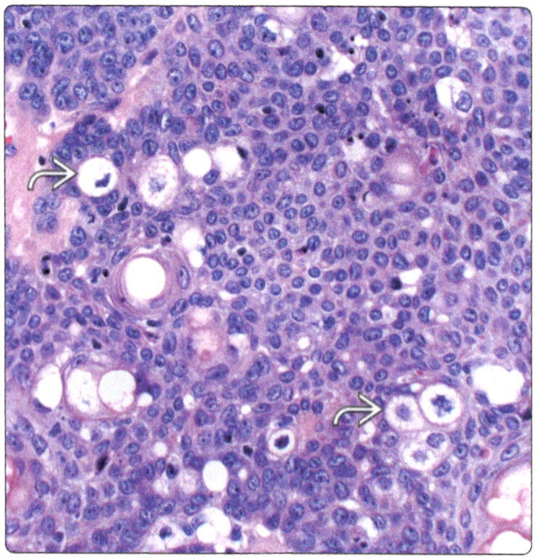

Podoplanin (D2-40) Immunohistochemistry in Sebaceoma

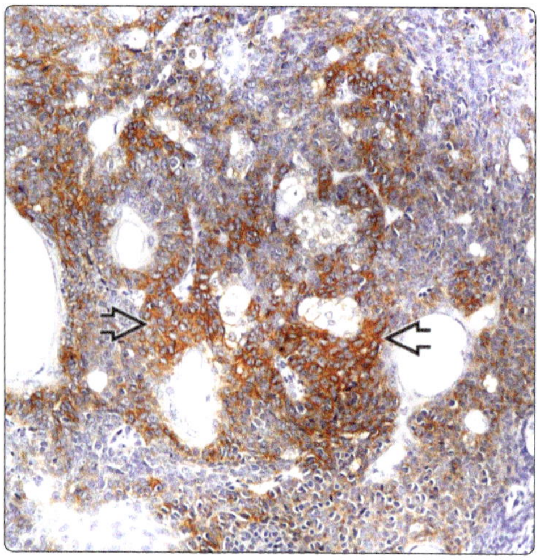

(Left) *Ki-67 highlights many of the peripheral basaloid cells ➡, but note its complete absence of staining in the large clear cells ➡ (which are also positive in sebaceous carcinoma). Both Ki-67 and p53 are typically low in sebaceomas but elevated in sebaceous carcinomas.* (Right) *Sebaceous adenoma is a benign sebaceous tumor characterized by a predominant population of enlarged bland, clear-staining multivacuolated sebocytes ➡, with only a minor component of peripheral, small basaloid cells ➡.*

Ki-67 Immunohistochemistry in Sebaceoma

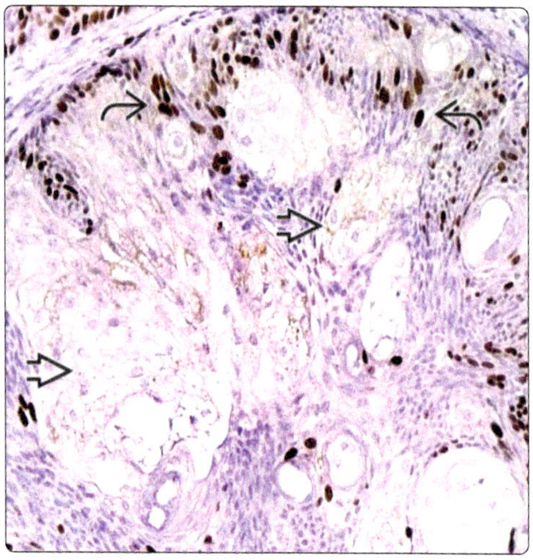

Differential Diagnosis: Sebaceous Adenoma

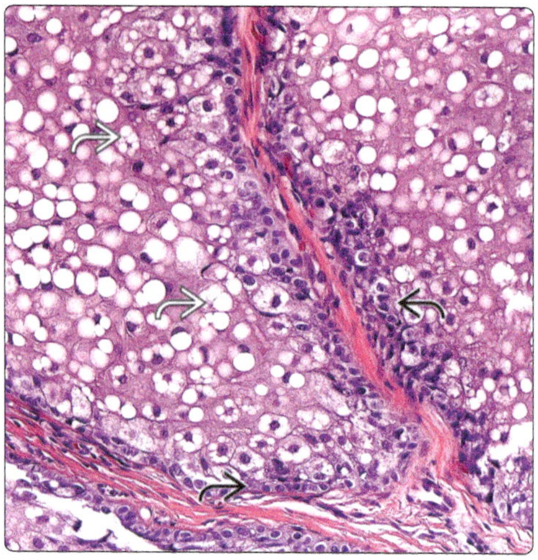

Differential Diagnosis: Basaloid Sebaceous Carcinoma

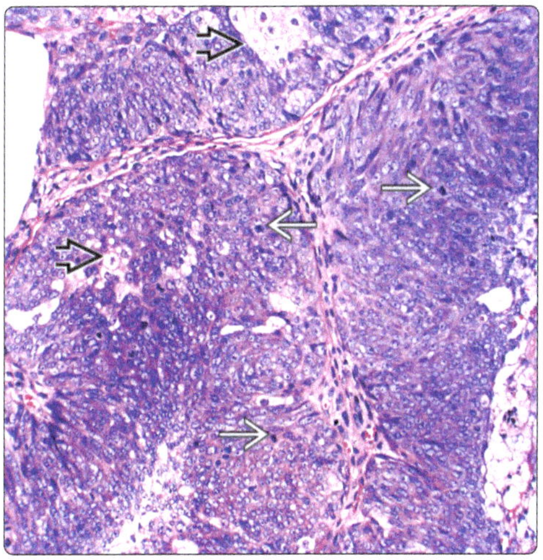

Differential Diagnosis: Basaloid Sebaceous Carcinoma

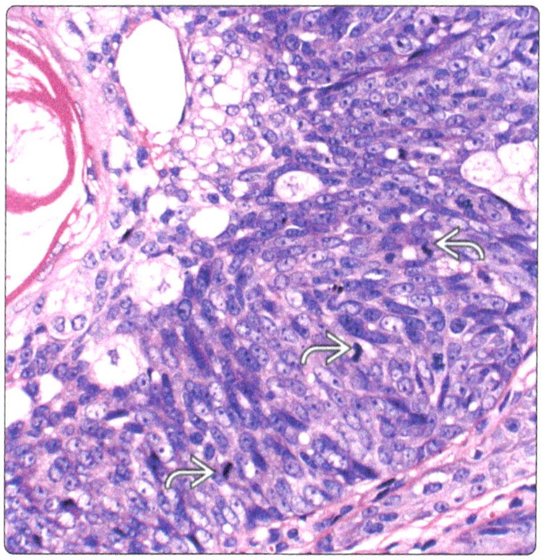

(Left) *Basaloid sebaceous carcinoma shows prominent nuclear crowding and hyperchromasia with increased mitotic figures in the basaloid population. Scattered, well-differentiated sebaceous cells are present.* **(Right)** *High magnification of a basaloid sebaceous carcinoma shows prominent nuclear atypia with hyperchromasia, irregular chromatin, enlarged nucleoli, and multiple mitotic figures.*

Differential Diagnosis: Sebaceous Carcinoma

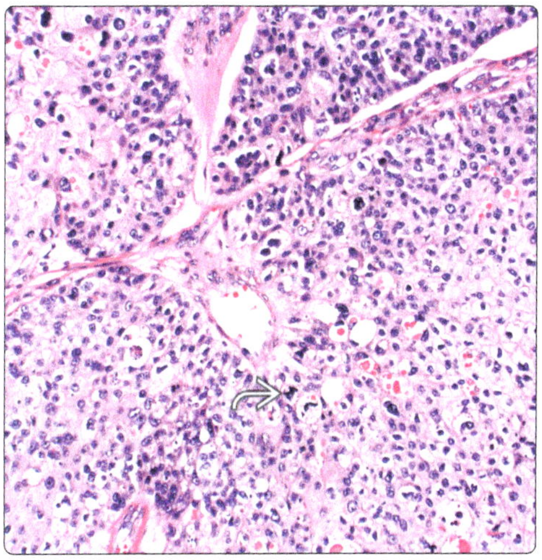

p53 Immunohistochemistry in Sebaceous Carcinoma

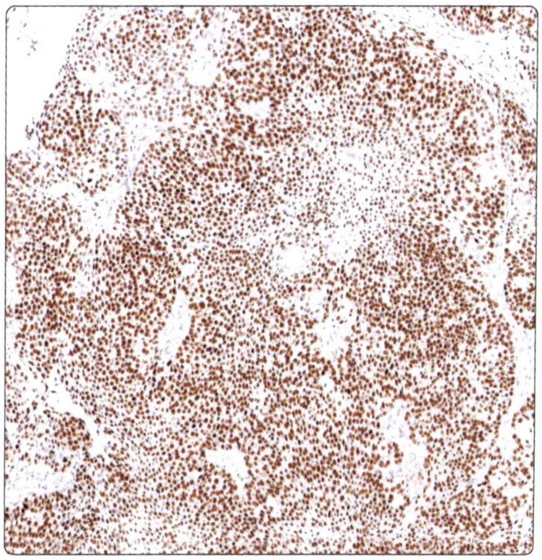

(Left) *High-grade sebaceous carcinoma shows larger basaloid to squamoid and clear cells with prominent nuclear atypia with hyperchromasia, enlarged nucleoli, and multiple mitotic figures.* **(Right)** *p53 shows very strong, diffuse, nuclear staining in a sebaceous carcinoma. Sebaceoma typically shows low p53 staining and a low nuclear proliferative rate by Ki-67 (< 20% of cells staining).*

Differential Diagnosis: Basal Cell Carcinoma

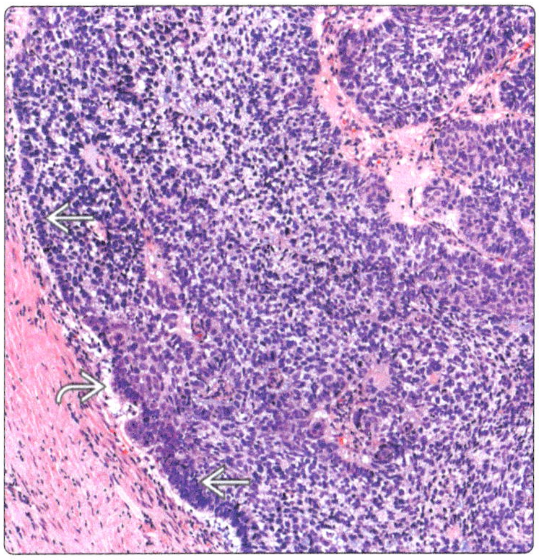

Differential Diagnosis: Basal Cell Carcinoma

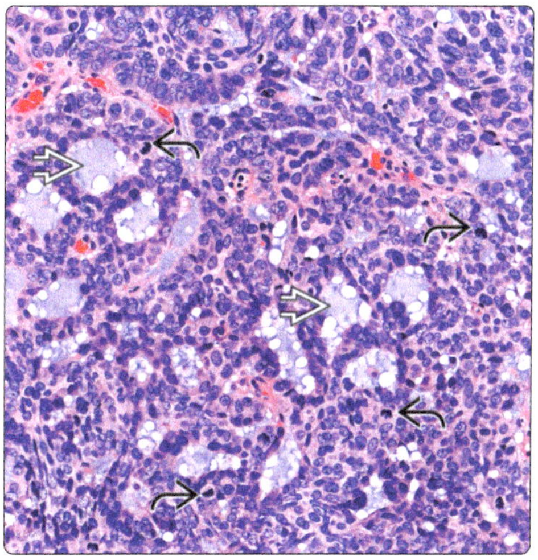

(Left) *Basal cell carcinoma (BCC) with clear cell features is shown. This is a nodular and adenoid-type BCC with areas of clear cell change. Note the peripheral palisading and tumor-stromal retraction artifact with mucinous material in the retraction space, findings lacking in sebaceoma.* **(Right)** *Higher magnification of BCC with adenoid features shows prominent pools of mucin within the tumor. Numerous mitotic figures are easily found.*

Sebaceous Adenoma

KEY FACTS

TERMINOLOGY

- > 50% of tumor is composed of mature sebocytes

CLINICAL ISSUES

- Often on head and neck, but any site possible
- Yellow, tan, to pink papule
- Even 1 sebaceous adenoma can be associated with Muir-Torre syndrome, which is association of sebaceous tumors or multiple keratoacanthomas with internal malignancy
- Immunohistochemistry (MSH2, MLH1, MLH6, PMS2) &/or microsatellite instability testing can be performed on tumor tissue

MICROSCOPIC

- Lobular downgrowth from epidermis
- Predominance (> 50%) of sebocytes
  - Located centrally within lobules
- Basaloid/germinative cells at periphery of lobules
- Cytologic atypia not prominent
- Presence of mitotic figure in germinative layer does not indicate malignant potential

ANCILLARY TESTS

- Sebocytes express EMA, podoplanin (D2-40), androgen receptor, and adipophilin

TOP DIFFERENTIAL DIAGNOSES

- Sebaceoma
  - Composed of > 50% germinative/basaloid cells
- Sebaceous hyperplasia
  - Superficial sebaceous lobules surrounding dilated follicle/pore
- Clear cell basal cell carcinoma
  - Lack of scalloped nuclei
  - Cytoplasm not truly bubbly

Scanning Magnification of a Sebaceous Adenoma

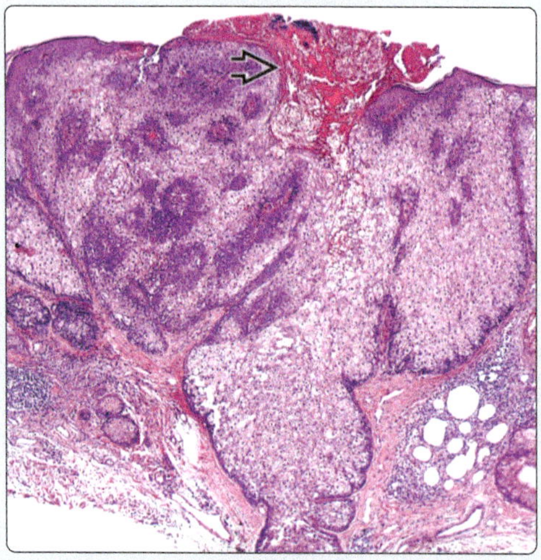

High Magnification of Sebaceous Adenoma

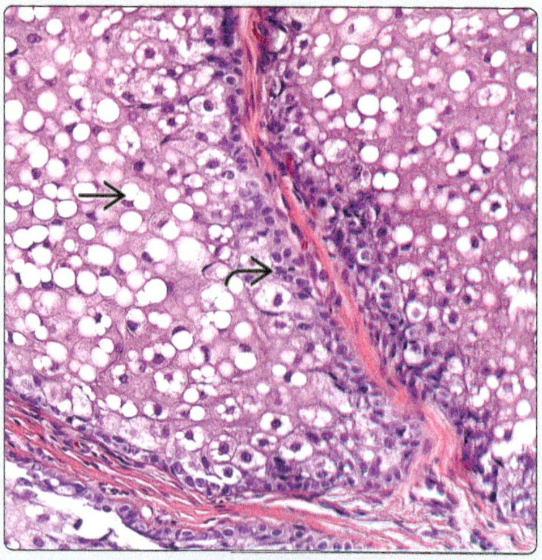

(Left) *In this low magnification of a large sebaceous adenoma, the tumor is a well-circumscribed, multilobular proliferation with multiple attachments to the epidermis and superficial holocrine necrosis.* **(Right)** *Sebocytes have a central, scalloped/crenulated nuclei with bubbly cytoplasm. Basaloid/germinative cells rim the sebocytes.*

Sebaceous Adenoma With Irregular Lobules

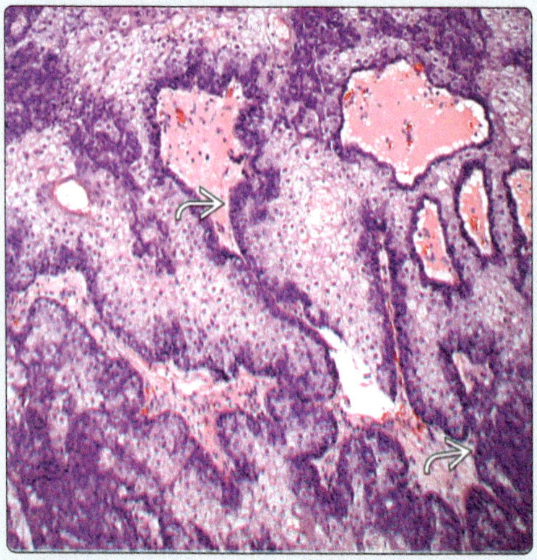

Traumatized Sebaceous Adenoma

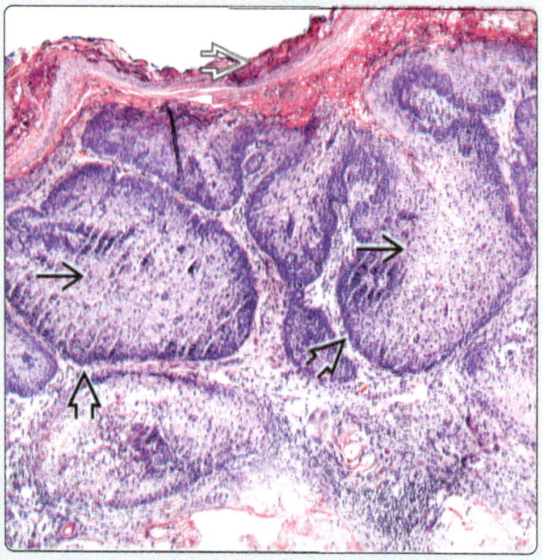

(Left) *This example of sebaceous adenoma shows a proliferation of small, irregularly-shaped sebaceous lobules composed of bland-appearing sebocytes surrounded by an expanded basaloid layer.* **(Right)** *This is an example of traumatized sebaceous adenoma, with overlying hemorrhage and serum crust. The lesion is composed of central sebocytes and peripheral basaloid cells. The basaloid cells form 1-3 layers at the periphery of lobules.*

TERMINOLOGY

Definitions

- Benign tumor
- > 50% of tumor is composed of mature sebocytes
- > 1 layer of basaloid/germinative cells at periphery of sebocyte-filled lobules

CLINICAL ISSUES

Site

- Often on head and neck, but any site possible

Presentation

- Yellow, tan, to pink papule

Treatment

- Reexcision not necessary

Prognosis

- Benign tumor
- No malignant potential

Associated Syndromes

- Even 1 sebaceous adenoma can be associated with Muir-Torre syndrome
  - Muir-Torre syndrome
    - Defined as association of sebaceous tumors (sebaceous adenoma, sebaceoma, sebaceous carcinoma) or multiple keratoacanthomas with internal malignancy
    - May be autosomal dominant; thus, syndrome has implications for screening of family members
    - Proportion of Muir-Torre cases are subset of Lynch (hereditary nonpolyposis colon cancer) syndrome
    - If desired, immunohistochemistry (MSH2, MLH1, possibly MLH6, PMS2) &/or microsatellite instability testing can be performed on tumor tissue

MICROSCOPIC

Histologic Features

- Lobular downgrowth from epidermis
- Predominance (> 50%) of mature sebocytes
- Basaloid/germinative cells at periphery of lobules form more than 1 layer
- Sebocytes arranged centrally, basaloid/germinative cells peripherally
- Cytologic atypia not prominent
- Presence of mitotic figure in germinative layer does not indicate malignant potential

Cytologic Features

- Sebocytes
  - Central, scalloped/crenulated nuclei
  - Bubbly, multivacuolated cytoplasm
- Basaloid/germinative cells
  - Round nuclei with small nucleoli
  - Minimal cytoplasm

ANCILLARY TESTS

Immunohistochemistry

- Sebocytes express EMA, podoplanin (D2-40), androgen receptor, and adipophilin
- Basaloid cells express cytokeratin 7

DIFFERENTIAL DIAGNOSIS

Sebaceoma

- Composed of > 50% germinative/basaloid cells
- < 50% sebocytes
- Sebocytes and germinative/basaloid cells often arranged haphazardly
- May or may not connect to epidermis

Sebaceous Hyperplasia

- Superficial sebaceous lobules surrounding dilated follicle/pore
- Lobules increased in number, but normal in size
- 1 layer of germinative/basaloid cells at periphery of sebocytes

Clear Cell Basal Cell Carcinoma

- Clear cells in variably sized islands
- Clear cells characterized by
  - Lack of scalloped nuclei
  - Cytoplasm not truly bubbly
- Some islands show peripheral palisading
- Typically express BER-EP4

Tricholemmoma

- Lobular downgrowth from epidermis
- Cells are pale/clear
- Clear cells lack scalloped nuclei and cytoplasm not truly bubbly
- Peripheral palisading with thickened basement membrane at periphery of lobules
- Surface may be papillated/verrucous

Nevus Sebaceus

- Lobular downgrowth of sebaceous glands from epidermis
- Absence of mature hair follicles
- Basaloid proliferations (i.e., trichoblastoma) may be present
- Apocrine glands may be present in deep dermis

Sebaceous Carcinoma

- Often larger, infiltrative tumors
- Basaloid/germinative cells generally predominate
- Often prominent cytologic atypia
- Numerous mitoses

SELECTED REFERENCES

1. Boennelycke M et al: Sebaceous neoplasms and the immunoprofile of mismatch-repair proteins as a screening target for syndromic cases. Pathol Res Pract. ePub, 2014
2. Roberts ME et al: A clinical scoring system to identify patients with sebaceous neoplasms at risk for the Muir-Torre variant of Lynch syndrome. Genet Med. 16(9):711-6, 2014
3. Ko CJ: Muir-Torre syndrome: facts and controversies. Clin Dermatol. 28(3):324-9, 2010
4. Shalin SC et al: Sebaceous neoplasia and the Muir-Torre syndrome: important connections with clinical implications. Histopathology. 56(1):133-47, 2010

KEY FACTS

TERMINOLOGY

- Aggressive adnexal carcinoma of sebaceous cells that often lacks clear cell features in poorly differentiated cases

ETIOLOGY/PATHOGENESIS

- Strong association with Muir-Torre syndrome if patients have multiple sebaceous tumors
    - Genes implicated include *MLH1*, *MSH2*, *MSH6*, *PMS2*

CLINICAL ISSUES

- Eyelids are most common site (~ 75% of cases)
- Mohs excision is effective in most cases
- Aggressive tumors with high incidence of metastasis (> 30%) and generally poor prognosis unless discovered early

MICROSCOPIC

- Dermal-based infiltrative, nodular to sheet-like tumor
- Often focal follicular &/or epidermal connections
- Well-differentiated tumors show clear cell changes
- Moderately and poorly differentiated tumors show few to rare clear cells
- Often show basaloid or squamoid features (leading to frequent misdiagnosis)
- Mitotic figures are usually abundant
- Areas of comedonecrosis are common

ANCILLARY TESTS

- EMA(+) in well-differentiated cases, but often lost in poorly differentiated tumors
- AR(+) in most cases, including poorly differentiated
- Other markers that may be positive include CAM5.2, BER-EP4, CK7 (~ 50% of cases), and CD10 (~ 50%)

TOP DIFFERENTIAL DIAGNOSES

- Clear cell squamous cell carcinoma
- Clear cell basal cell carcinoma
- Other primary cutaneous adnexal carcinomas
- Metastatic carcinoma to skin

Clinical Photograph

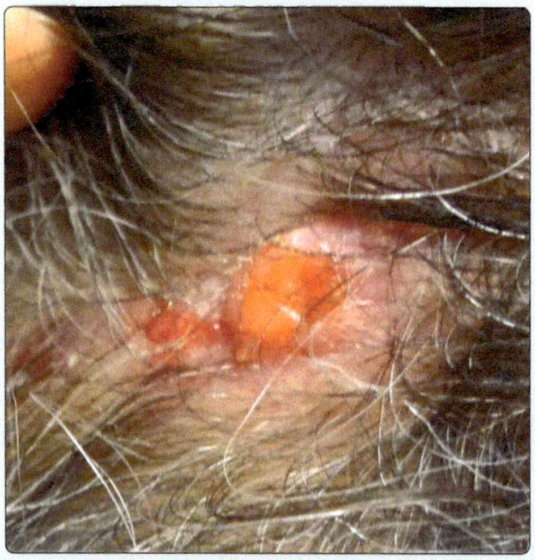

Scanning Magnification of Sebaceous Carcinoma

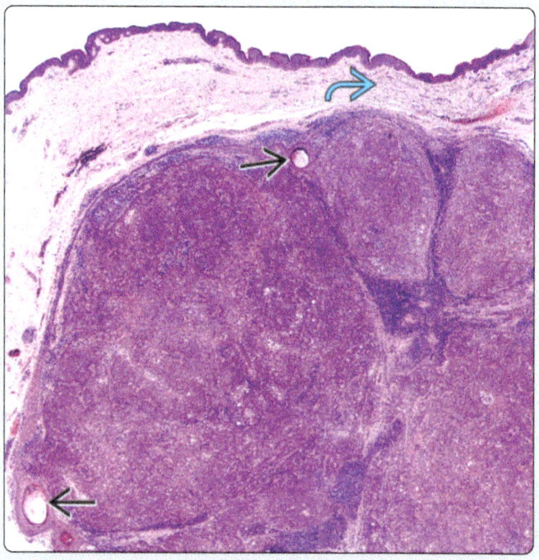

(Left) *This is a large, multinodular-appearing sebaceous carcinoma, which occurred on the scalp of an elderly patient.* **(Right)** *Scanning magnification of a sebaceous carcinoma shows a very large, nodular tumor in the dermis. Note the lack of epidermal attachments ➩; however, there are focal entrapped follicular structures ➙.*

Low Magnification of Sebaceous Carcinoma

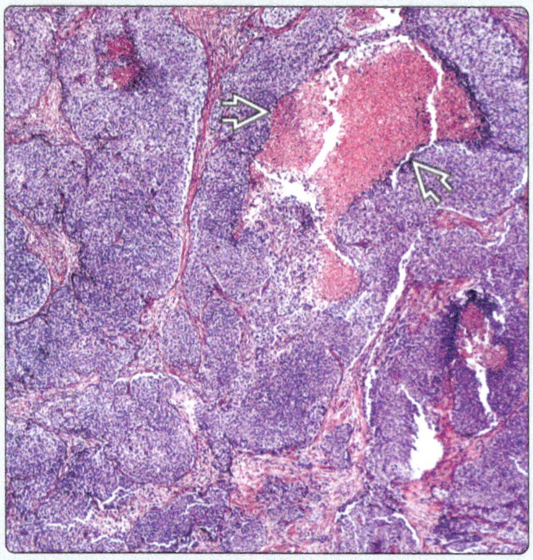

High Magnification of Sebaceous Carcinoma

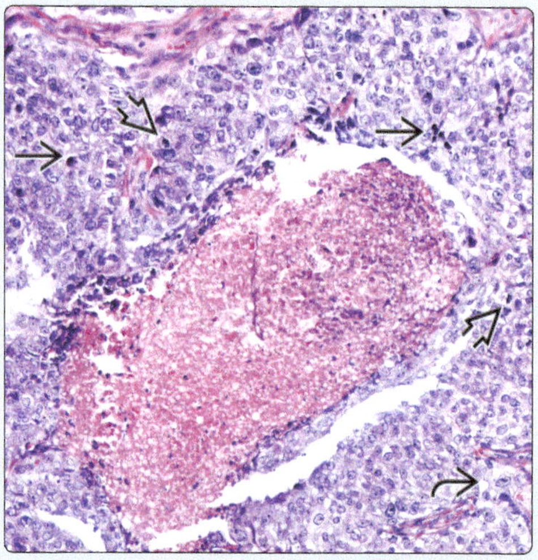

(Left) *Low-magnification view shows an atypical cellular, nodular, basaloid-appearing proliferation with large areas of comedonecrosis ➪.* **(Right)** *High magnification of an area of comedonecrosis is surrounded by atypical clear to basaloid cells with apoptotic bodies ➙ and mitoses ➪. Some of the cells show clear cytoplasmic vacuoles ➙.*

TERMINOLOGY

Definitions

- Malignant adnexal tumor of sebaceous cells
- Classically shows clear cell features, but often lacks them in poorly differentiated cases; may show basaloid or squamoid features, leading to high incidence of misdiagnosis

ETIOLOGY/PATHOGENESIS

Unknown in Most Cases

- Some cases likely due to solar (UV) damage, as most occur on sun-damaged skin of elderly

Genetic

- Strong association with Muir-Torre syndrome in patients who have multiple sebaceous tumors &/or multiple keratoacanthomas and internal organ malignancies
  - Genes implicated include *MLH1*, *MSH2*, *MSH6*, *PMS2*
    - Encode mismatch repair proteins
    - Mutations lead to microsatellite instability (MSI)
    - MSI assays and immunohistochemistry can be used to screen for Muir-Torre syndrome

CLINICAL ISSUES

Epidemiology

- Incidence
  - Uncommon tumors but 1 of the more common types of adnexal carcinoma
- Age
  - Most occur in elderly patients
- Sex
  - Females have slightly higher incidence

Site

- Eyelids are by far most common site (~ 75% of cases)
- Remainder of cases occur in other head and neck sites, followed by trunk, extremities

Presentation

- Nodular, firm, yellow-tan lesions
- Often ulcerated

Treatment

- Surgical approaches
  - Complete excision is necessary to ensure local removal
  - Mohs excision is reported to be effective in most cases
  - Sentinel lymph node biopsy may be useful for staging purposes

Prognosis

- Aggressive tumors with high incidence of metastasis (> 30% of cases) and generally poor prognosis unless discovered early

MACROSCOPIC

General Features

- Dermal-based firm, nodular lesion

Size

- Usually 1-4 cm

MICROSCOPIC

Histologic Features

- Dermal-based infiltrative, nodular to sheet-like tumor
- Often with focal follicular &/or epidermal connections
  - Pagetoid involvement of epidermis may be seen in up to 30% of cases
- Tumor consists of variably differentiated epithelioid cells
  - Clear cells often present but vary greatly in number
  - Well-differentiated tumors show prominent clear cell changes
    - Cells contain abundant cytoplasmic lipid, often producing multiple vacuoles and nuclear indentation
    - Nuclei are enlarged and vesicular or hyperchromatic-staining, with prominent nucleoli
  - Moderately and poorly differentiated tumors show few to rare clear cells
    - May be composed predominantly of basaloid or squamoid cells (leading to frequent misdiagnosis)
    - Show prominent cytologic atypia and pleomorphism
    - Mitotic figures, including atypical forms, are usually abundant
  - Areas of necrosis, with comedonecrosis pattern, are common
  - Lymphovascular invasion present in significant percentage of cases

Cytologic Features

- Enlarged, epithelioid cells with abundant cytoplasm and hyperchromatic or vesicular nuclei with enlarged nucleoli
  - Clear cells usually show cytoplasmic vacuoles and nuclear indentation
  - However, cells can also be basaloid (common) or squamoid (rare)

ANCILLARY TESTS

Histochemistry

- Sudan black B and oil red O (need frozen tissue)
  - Reactivity: Positive
  - Staining Pattern: Cytoplasmic staining
- Periodic acid-Schiff
  - Reactivity: Usually negative (indicating lack of glycogen)

Immunohistochemistry

- EMA is positive in most well-differentiated cases but is often negative in poorly differentiated tumors
  - EMA is negative in basal cell carcinoma (BCC) but often shows at least focal staining in squamous cell carcinoma (SCC)
  - EMA often highlights ductal structures in other adnexal carcinomas (i.e., porocarcinoma and hidradenocarcinoma) but not in sebaceous carcinoma
- AR is positive (nuclear staining) in most cases, including poorly differentiated carcinomas
  - SCC and most other primary cutaneous carcinomas are negative for AR
  - However, AR is often positive in BCC (> 60% of cases) and some metastatic carcinomas to skin
- HMWCKs (i.e., CK5/6 and CK903/34βE12) and p63 are typically strongly and diffusely positive

- Help to exclude metastatic tumors (most of which are negative for both of these markers) but do not distinguish from other primary cutaneous tumors
- D2-40 (podoplanin) is positive in subset of cases, especially in more basaloid sebaceous carcinomas
  - Can also highlight areas of lymphovascular invasion
- Other markers that may be positive include CAM5.2, BER-EP4, CK7 (~ 50% of cases), and CD10 (~ 50%)
- Negative for CEA-M, CK20, GCDFP-15, RCA/PRNA, TTF-1, S100
- Muir-Torre patients show loss of staining for *MLH1*, *MSH2*, &/or *MSH6*

Genetic Testing

- Muir-Torre syndrome in patients with multiple sebaceous tumors and internal organ carcinomas
  - Genes include *MLH1*, *MSH2*, *MSH6*, *PMS2*
  - Mutations lead to loss of mismatch repair capabilities
  - Can be identified directly through PCR for specific mutations or indirectly through MSI studies
    - MSI studies are less sensitive than PCR and immunohistochemistry

DIFFERENTIAL DIAGNOSIS

Squamous Cell Carcinoma

- SCC with clear cell features can be difficult to distinguish from sebaceous carcinoma in some cases
- Often associated with overlying actinic keratosis or SCC in situ (Bowen disease)
- Clear cells in SCC are due to either degenerative changes or glycogen accumulation
  - Lack cytoplasmic lipid and nuclear indentations
  - PAS (without diastase) is positive in cases with cytoplasmic glycogen (negative in sebaceous carcinoma)
- Areas of squamous eddies and keratinization typically present (only rarely seen in sebaceous carcinoma)
- Sebaceous carcinoma is usually diffusely positive for EMA (weak/focal in SCC) and AR (negative in SCC)

Basal Cell Carcinoma

- Most cases are not difficult to distinguish from sebaceous carcinoma
- However, some cases of sebaceous carcinoma are predominantly composed of basaloid cells
  - Usually, at least focal clear cells with sebaceous features are present
  - Lack peripheral palisading, mucinous stroma, and tumor-stromal retraction artifact of BCC
- Some cases of BCC are predominantly clear cell, **but**
  - Typically show at least focal areas of more conventional BCC with peripheral palisading and mucinous stroma
- Sebaceous carcinoma is usually diffusely positive for EMA (negative in BCC) and AR (often focally positive in BCC)

Other Primary Cutaneous Adnexal Carcinomas

- Porocarcinoma and hidradenocarcinoma with clear cell features may enter differential diagnosis in some cases
- Porocarcinoma shows multiple epidermal attachments, whereas hidradenocarcinoma is dermal-based tumor lacking epidermal connections
- Both tumors show at least focal ductal differentiation (rare in sebaceous carcinoma)
  - May be highlighted by EMA and CEA
- Sebaceous carcinoma is usually diffusely positive for EMA and AR

Metastatic Carcinomas to Skin

- Metastatic carcinomas with clear cell features should be considered in differential, especially if no epidermal or follicular connections are identified
- Metastatic clear cell renal cell carcinoma is most likely consideration
  - Prominent capillary-type vasculature typically present (lacking in sebaceous carcinoma)
  - Cells are typically relatively low-grade appearing
  - Show uniform cytoplasmic clearing rather than multivacuolization of sebaceous carcinoma
  - IHC: Positive for RCA/PRNA, pax-8, CD10 (positive in ~ 50% of sebaceous carcinomas); EMA is positive in both RCC and sebaceous carcinoma

DIAGNOSTIC CHECKLIST

Pathologic Interpretation Pearls

- Well-differentiated cells contain abundant cytoplasmic lipid, often producing multiple vacuoles and nuclear indentation
- Poorly differentiated cells often lack vacuoles and may appear basaloid or squamoid

SELECTED REFERENCES

1. Kyllo RL et al: Sebaceous carcinoma: review of the literature. Dermatol Surg. 41(1):1-15, 2015
2. Lee MJ et al: Increased gene copy number of HER2 and concordant protein overexpression found in a subset of eyelid sebaceous gland carcinoma indicate HER2 as a potential therapeutic target. J Cancer Res Clin Oncol. ePub, 2015
3. Misago N et al: Sebaceous carcinoma within ripple/carcinoid pattern sebaceoma. J Cutan Pathol. ePub, 2015
4. Tetzlaff MT et al: Distinct pathways in the pathogenesis of sebaceous carcinomas implicated by differentially expressed microRNAs. JAMA Ophthalmol. ePub, 2015
5. Boennelycke M et al: Sebaceous neoplasms and the immunoprofile of mismatch-repair proteins as a screening target for syndromic cases. Pathol Res Pract. ePub, 2014
6. Dasgupta T et al: A retrospective review of 1349 cases of sebaceous carcinoma. Cancer. 115(1):158-65, 2009
7. Buitrago W et al: Sebaceous carcinoma: the great masquerader: emgerging concepts in diagnosis and treatment. Dermatol Ther. 21(6):459-66, 2008
8. Yang HM et al: Immunohistochemical expression of D2-40 in benign and malignant sebaceous tumors and comparison to basal and squamous cell carcinomas. Am J Dermatopathol. 30(6):549-54, 2008
9. Cabral ES et al: Desmoplastic tricholemmoma of the eyelid misdiagnosed as sebaceous carcinoma: a potential diagnostic pitfall. J Cutan Pathol. 34 Suppl 1:22-5, 2007
10. Ho VH et al: Sentinel lymph node biopsy for sebaceous cell carcinoma and melanoma of the ocular adnexa. Arch Otolaryngol Head Neck Surg. 133(8):820-6, 2007
11. Cabral ES et al: Distinction of benign sebaceous proliferations from sebaceous carcinomas by immunohistochemistry. Am J Dermatopathol. 28(6):465-71, 2006
12. Curry ML et al: Muir-Torre syndrome: role of the dermatopathologist in diagnosis. Am J Dermatopathol. 26(3):217-21, 2004
13. Cohen PR et al: Association of sebaceous gland tumors and internal malignancy: the Muir-Torre syndrome. Am J Med. 90(5):606-13, 1991
14. Burgdorf WH et al: Muir-Torre syndrome. Histologic spectrum of sebaceous proliferations. Am J Dermatopathol. 8(3):202-8, 1986
15. Wolfe JT 3rd et al: Sebaceous carcinoma of the eyelid. Errors in clinical and pathologic diagnosis. Am J Surg Pathol. 8(8):597-606, 1984
16. Russell WG et al: Sebaceous carcinoma of meibomian gland origin. The diagnostic importance of pagetoid spread of neoplastic cells. Am J Clin Pathol. 73(4):504-11, 1980

Well-Differentiated Sebaceous Carcinoma

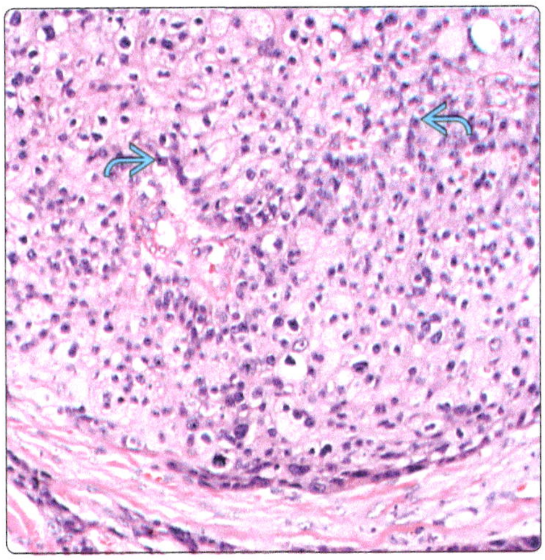

Well-Differentiated Sebaceous Carcinoma With Basaloid Features

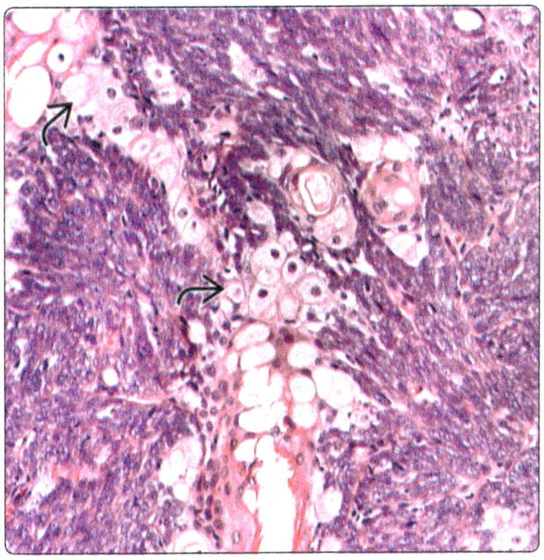

(Left) *This is an example of a well-differentiated sebaceous carcinoma composed of lobules of atypical pale to clear-staining cells. The cells show vesicular nuclei with enlarged nucleoli and abundant multivacuolated cytoplasm.* **(Right)** *This is a well-differentiated sebaceous carcinoma composed of oval to spindle-shaped basaloid cells surrounding collections of mature clear cells.*

High Magnification of Sebaceous Carcinoma

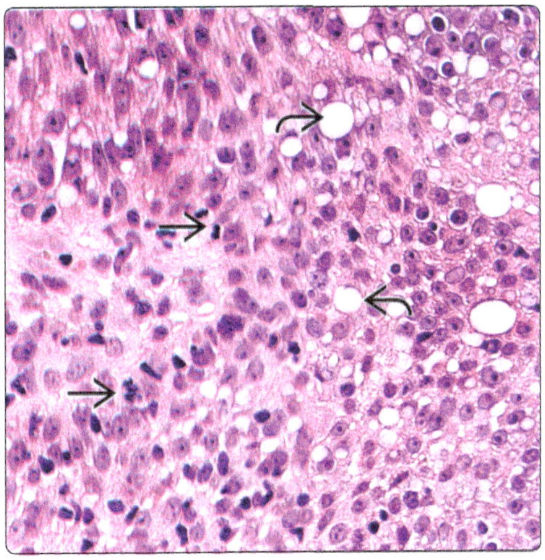

High Magnification of Sebaceous Carcinoma

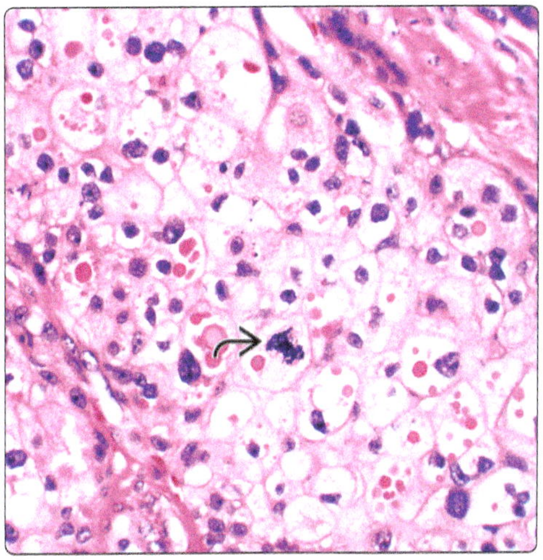

(Left) *High magnification of a moderately differentiated sebaceous carcinoma composed of atypical clear to basaloid cells with mitoses is shown. Many of the cells show multiple small to large clear cytoplasmic vacuoles.* **(Right)** *This is an example of a sebaceous carcinoma with abundant red blood cells, some of which appear to be within the cytoplasm of the atypical clear cells. However, the abundant vascularity of renal cell carcinoma is lacking. Note the central atypical mitotic figure.*

Poorly Differentiated Sebaceous Carcinoma

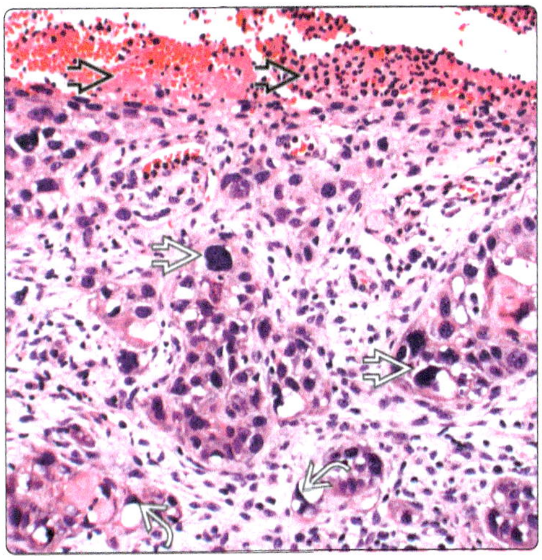

Sebaceous Carcinoma With Squamous Differentiation

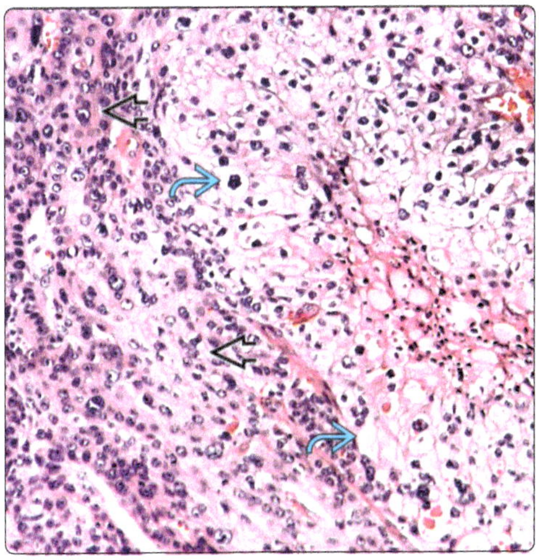

(Left) *Invasive poorly-differentiated sebaceous carcinoma shows markedly enlarged, atypical and pleomorphic-appearing cells. Note the overlying epidermal ulceration with serum crust and neutrophils. Some cells show nuclear indentations by cytoplasmic vacuoles.* **(Right)** *This sebaceous carcinoma shows areas of squamous differentiation adjacent to more typical areas with clear cell differentiation. This case was initially misdiagnosed as a clear cell squamous cell carcinoma.*

(Left) *Strong immunohistochemical staining for EMA, which is often positive in well- and moderately differentiated tumors and highlights the cytoplasmic membranes and intracytoplasmic vacuoles.* **(Right)** *AR immunohistochemistry is positive in most cases and shows moderate to strong diffuse nuclear staining in the majority of the tumor cells.*

EMA Immunohistochemistry in Sebaceous Carcinoma

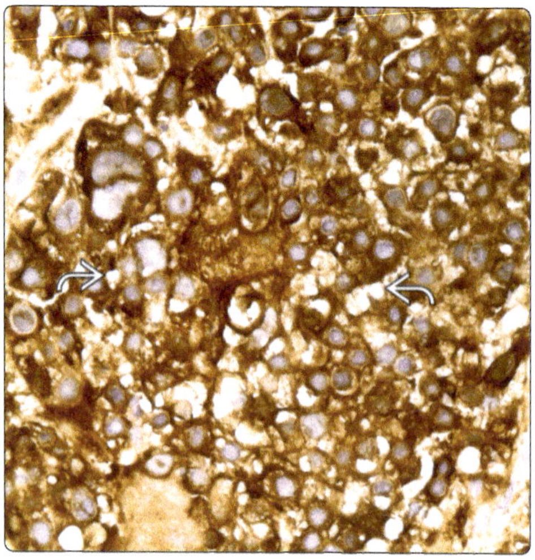

Androgen Receptor Staining in Sebaceous Carcinoma

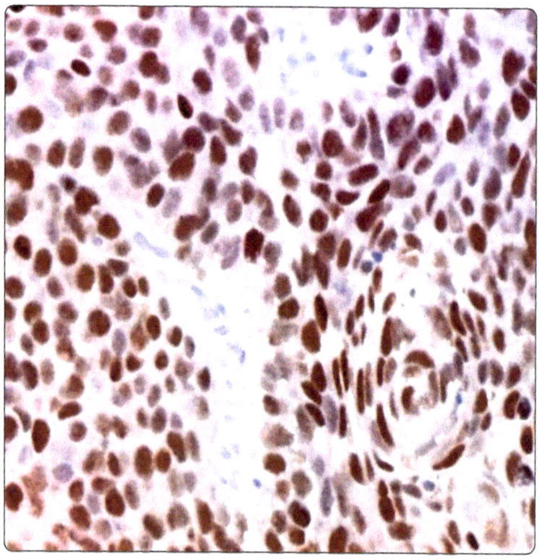

(Left) *CK7 may be positive but only in ~ 50% of cases. It often shows patchy, moderate to strong cytoplasmic staining, as in this case.* **(Right)** *D2-40 (podoplanin) is positive in some cases of sebaceous carcinoma, especially basaloid variants. This case shows strong cytoplasmic staining of many of the basaloid and spindled cells without significant staining of the well-differentiated clear cells.*

CK7 Staining in Sebaceous Carcinoma

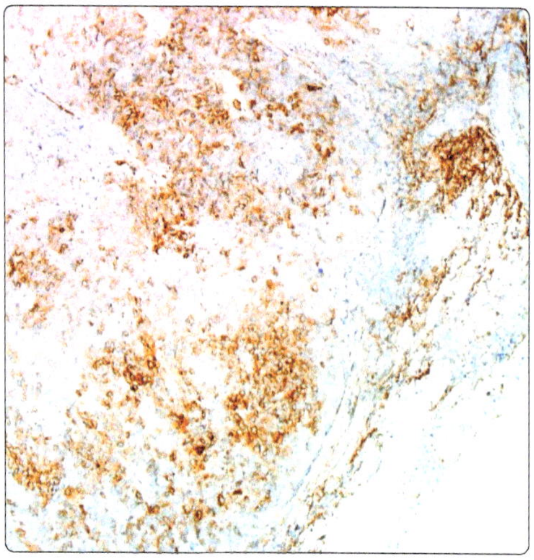

D2-40 Staining in Sebaceous Carcinoma

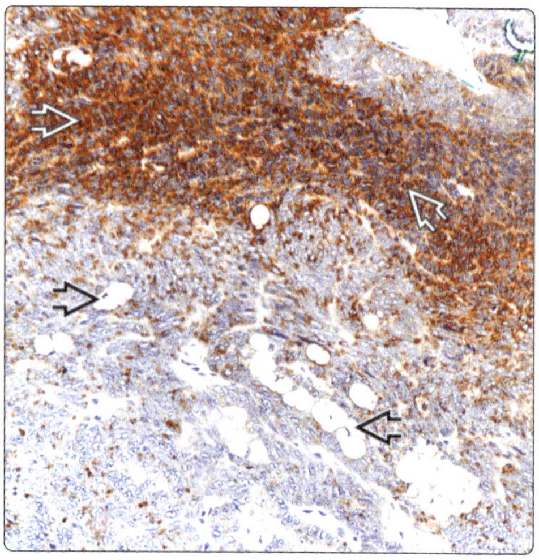

(Left) *Diffuse, strong nuclear staining for p53 is seen in this example of sebaceous carcinoma. p53 and Ki-67 are usually elevated in sebaceous carcinomas, and Bcl-2 is lost, compared with sebaceous adenomas and sebaceomas.* **(Right)** *Diffuse nuclear staining for Ki-67 is also seen in this sebaceous carcinoma, consistent with a high proliferative rate.*

Immunohistochemistry for p53 in Sebaceous Carcinoma

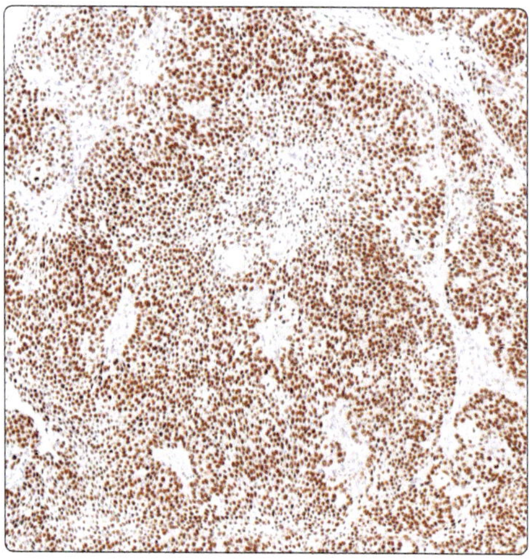

Immunohistochemistry for Ki-67 in Sebaceous Carcinoma

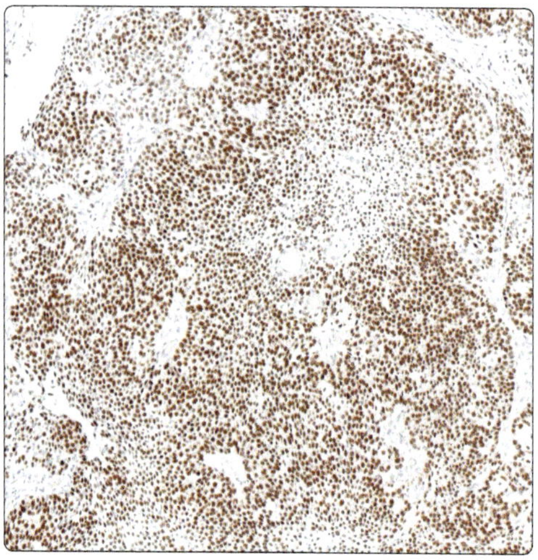

Differential Diagnosis: Atypical Sebaceoma

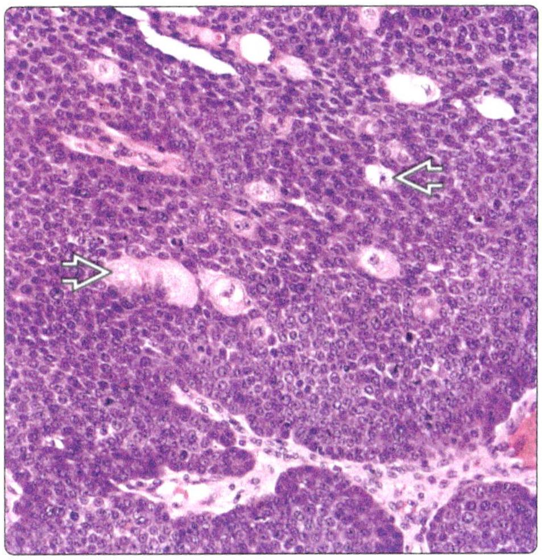

Differential Diagnosis: Atypical Sebaceoma at High Magnification

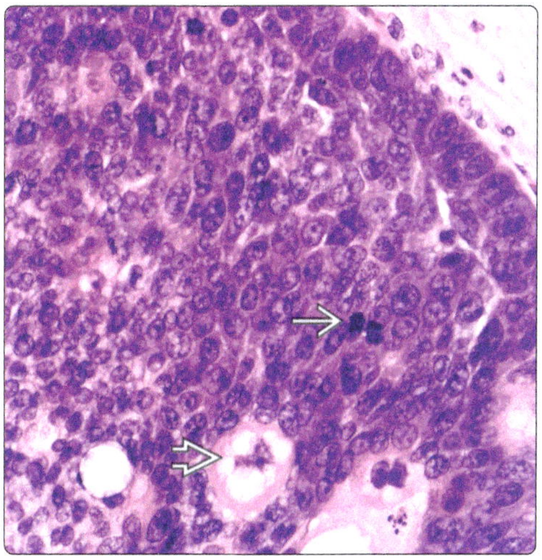

(Left) *This is an example of an atypical sebaceoma showing a basaloid population of enlarged, atypical cells with nuclear hyperchromasia surrounding several large clear cells* ➡ *with abundant, multivacuolated cytoplasm.* **(Right)** *High magnification of an atypical sebaceoma shows a basaloid population of enlarged, atypical cells with nuclear hyperchromasia and several large clear cells* ➡ *with abundant, multivacuolated cytoplasm. Mitotic figures are seen* ➡ *but can be quite numerous in some sebaceomas.*

Differential Diagnosis: Sebaceous Adenoma

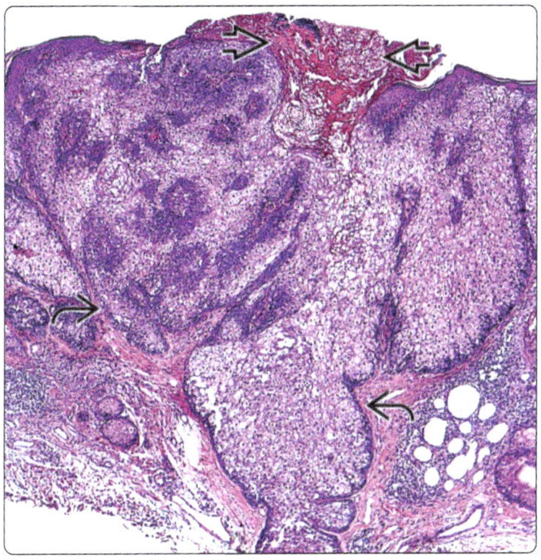

Differential Diagnosis: Sebaceous Adenoma at High Magnification

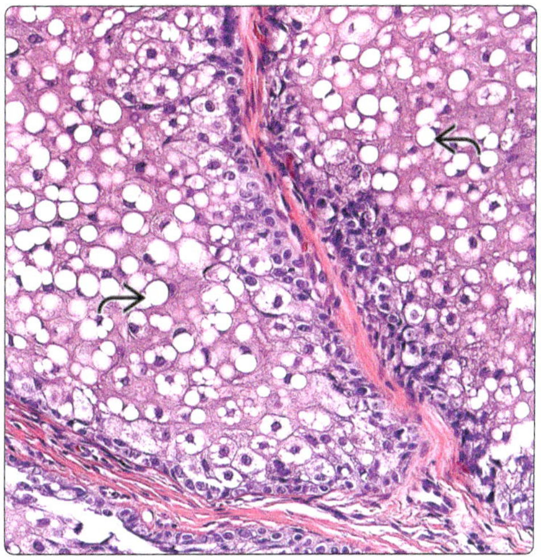

(Left) *Low magnification shows a large sebaceous adenoma. The tumor is a well-circumscribed fusing lobular proliferation with superficial holocrine necrosis* ➡ *(recapitulating normal sebaceous glands), composed of bland clear cells surrounded by a thin layer of basaloid cells* ➡*.* **(Right)** *High magnification of a sebaceous adenoma shows the bland cytologic appearance of the mature sebocytes and surrounding basaloid cells. Note the prominent intracytoplasmic lipid vacuoles* ➡*.*

Differential Diagnosis: Clear Cell Basal Cell Carcinoma

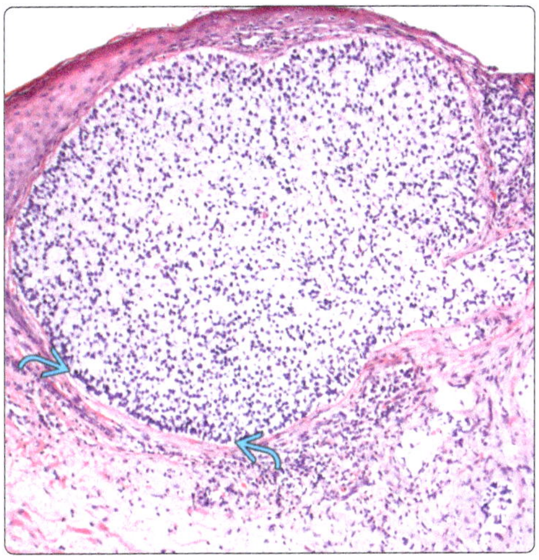

Differential Diagnosis: Clear Cell Basal Cell Carcinoma

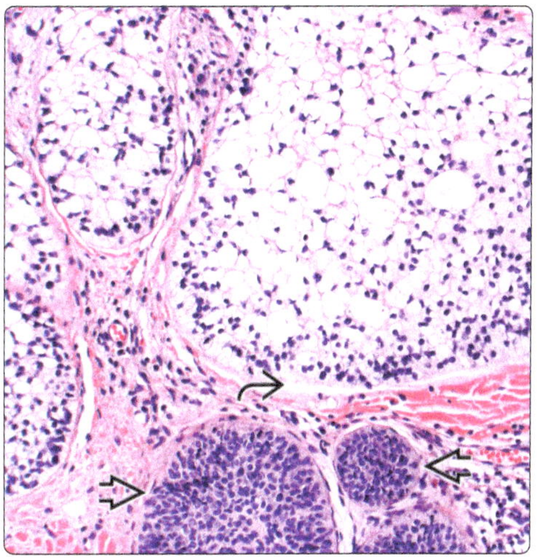

(Left) *Clear cell basal cell carcinoma (BCC) can mimic sebaceous carcinoma but usually shows uniform cytoplasmic clearing without the vacuoles and nuclear indentations seen in sebaceous carcinoma. Note the focal areas of peripheral palisading* ➡*.* **(Right)** *Clear cell BCC shows uniform cytoplasmic clearing without the vacuoles and nuclear indentations seen in sebaceous carcinoma. Note the focal retraction artifact* ➡ *and adjacent areas of conventional-type BCC* ➡*.*

PART I
SECTION 5

Neoplasms and Proliferations of Eccrine and Apocrine Sweat Glands

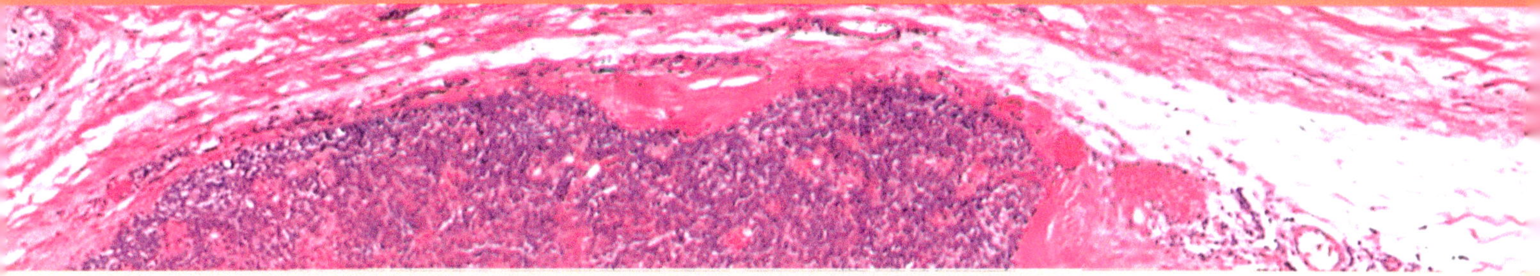

KEY FACTS

CLINICAL ISSUES

- Scalp
- Other locations include face, axilla, anogenital area, extremities, eyelids
  - Tumors in anogenital area may truly represent adenoma of anogenital mammary-like glands
  - Tumors in eyelid should be distinguished from endocrine mucin-producing sweat gland carcinoma
- F > M (2:1)
- Adult patients
- Nodule measuring < 2 cm
  - Sometimes pedunculated

MICROSCOPIC

- Circumscribed intradermal nodule
  - Subcutis may be involved
- Sometimes arises in association with nevus sebaceous and syringocystadenoma papilliferum
- Tubules of different size and shape
- Some cystically dilated
- Papillary projections devoid of fibrovascular cores
  - True papillae may be seen in cases associated with syringocystadenoma papilliferum
- Outer layer composed of myoepithelial cells
- Inner layer composed of apocrine cells
- Focal follicular or sebaceous differentiation may be rarely seen

ANCILLARY TESTS

- Luminal cells are positive for EMA and CEA
- Myoepithelial cells are positive for S100 and SMA

TOP DIFFERENTIAL DIAGNOSES

- Syringocystadenoma papilliferum
- Papillary eccrine adenoma
- Apocrine hamartoma
- Apocrine carcinoma
- Endocrine mucin-producing sweat gland carcinoma

Intradermal Tumor Without Epidermal Connection

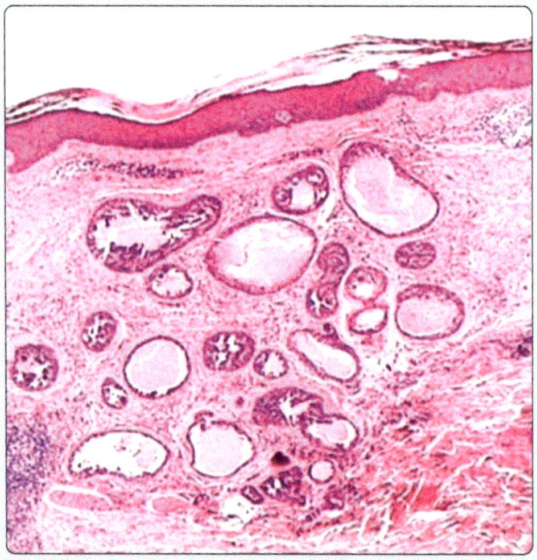

Cystically Dilated Tubules

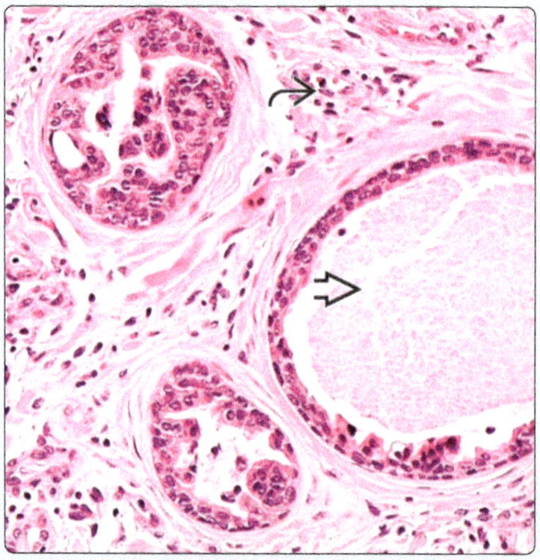

(Left) *Apocrine tubular adenoma is usually a well-circumscribed intradermal nodule composed of variably sized and shaped tubules. Some tubular structures are cystically dilated.* **(Right)** *The tubules may contain eosinophilic secretion and debris ⇨. The tubular structures are separated by a connective tissue stroma with few blood vessels ⇗ and scant chronic inflammation.*

Tubules Are Lined by Apocrine Cells

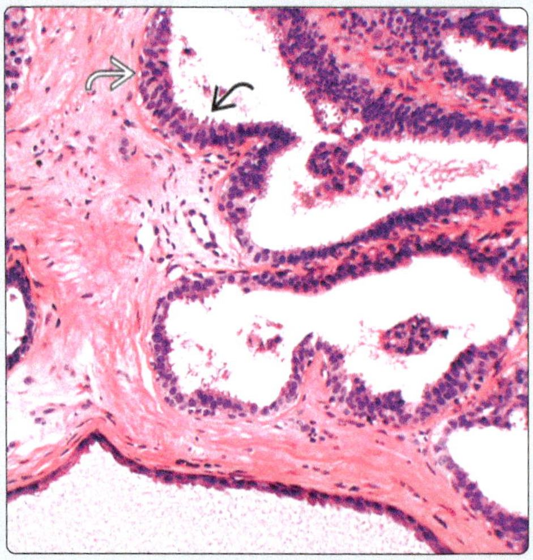

Apical Snouts in Tubular Apocrine Adenoma

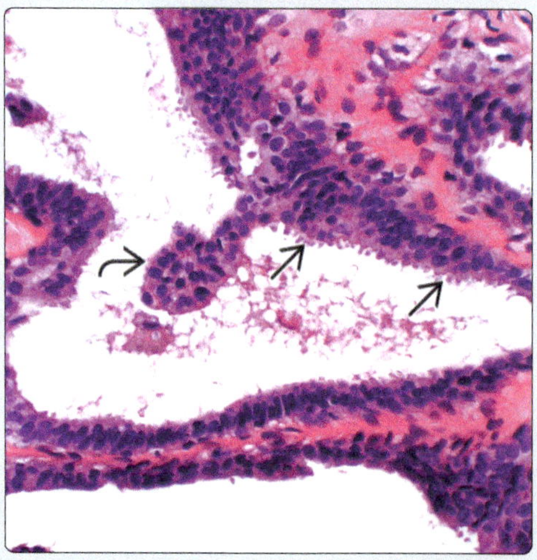

(Left) *The tubules are lined by at least 2 layers of cells. The outer layer is composed of small myoepithelial cells ⮕, and the luminal layer is composed of columnar apocrine cells ⇗ with apical snouts.* **(Right)** *Papillary projections ⇗ are common and usually devoid of fibrovascular cores. Note the decapitation secretions on the surface of the apocrine cells ⇨.*

TERMINOLOGY

Synonyms

- Tubular apocrine adenoma, apocrine adenoma, tubulopapillary hidradenoma, papillary tubular adenoma

Definitions

- Rare benign adnexal neoplasm with apocrine differentiation

CLINICAL ISSUES

Epidemiology

- Incidence
  - Rare tumor
- Age
  - Wide age distribution (range: 20-80 years)
- Sex
  - F > M (2:1)

Presentation

- Scalp nodule
  - Other locations include face, axilla, anogenital area, extremities, eyelids
- < 2 cm in diameter

Treatment

- Complete excision is curative

Prognosis

- Excellent

MACROSCOPIC

General Features

- Well-circumscribed intradermal nodule

Size

- < 2 cm in diameter
  - Larger lesions are exceptional

MICROSCOPIC

Histologic Features

- Intradermal nodule
  - Well circumscribed
  - Subcutaneous tissue may rarely be involved
  - Rarely tumor communicates with epidermis through ducts or infundibula of hair follicles
- Variable-sized tubules
  - Double or multilayered
  - Some cystically dilated
  - Some with papillary projections
    - Usually without fibrovascular cores
- Peripheral (outer) layer
  - Flattened to cuboidal myoepithelial cells
- Luminal (inner) layer
  - Lined by columnar cells with apocrine differentiation
  - Eosinophilic cytoplasm
  - Often showing decapitation secretion
  - Regular round to oval nuclei
  - Nuclear pleomorphism absent to minimal
  - Mitoses are very rare
- Eosinophilic proteinaceous material may be seen in lumen
- Connective tissue stroma
  - Scattered blood vessels and few inflammatory cells
- May arise in background of nevus sebaceous
  - Sometimes associated with syringocystadenoma papilliferum

Cytologic Features

- Apocrine cells with decapitation secretion (apical snouts and secretions)

ANCILLARY TESTS

Immunohistochemistry

- Luminal cells are positive for
  - EMA and CEA (surface expression)
  - HMFG-1 and GCDFP-15
- Myoepithelial cells are positive for
  - S100 and SMA

DIFFERENTIAL DIAGNOSIS

Syringocystadenoma Papilliferum

- Connects to epidermis
- Papillae with true fibrovascular cores
- Dense plasma cell-rich inflammatory infiltrate
- Some apocrine tubular adenomas arise in association with syringocystadenoma papilliferum

Papillary Eccrine Adenoma

- Lacks true apocrine differentiation
- Rare tumors may have mixed features of eccrine and apocrine tubular adenomas

Apocrine Hamartoma (Apocrine Nevus)

- Often affect axilla
- Excess of normal-appearing apocrine glands

Apocrine Carcinoma

- Infiltrative tumor
- Nuclear pleomorphism and numerous mitoses

Mucin-Producing Neuroendocrine Carcinoma

- Eyelid location
- Mucicarmine positive
- Positivity for at least 1 neuroendocrine marker

DIAGNOSTIC CHECKLIST

Pathologic Interpretation Pearls

- Apocrine tubular adenoma is well circumscribed
  - Infiltrative pattern should raise suspicion for apocrine carcinoma

SELECTED REFERENCES

1. Ito T et al: Tubular apocrine adenoma clinically and dermoscopically mimicking basal cell carcinoma. J Am Acad Dermatol. 71(2):e45-6, 2014
2. Mitsuishi T et al: Tubular apocrine adenoma of the nose. Eur J Dermatol. 21(1):132, 2011
3. Kazakov DV et al: Tubular adenoma and syringocystadenoma papilliferum: a reappraisal of their relationship. An interobserver study of a series, by a panel of dermatopathologists. Am J Dermatopathol. 29(3):256-63, 2007

Syringocystadenoma Papilliferum

KEY FACTS

TERMINOLOGY

- Syringocystadenoma papilliferum (SCP)

CLINICAL ISSUES

- ~ 1/2 present at birth or childhood
- Scalp most common location, followed by face
- Often associated with nevus sebaceus
- Benign tumors, but
  - Rare cases may transform to syringocystadenocarcinoma papilliferum
  - Rarely, basal cell carcinoma may develop within SCP

MICROSCOPIC

- Endophytic/exophytic adnexal tumors
  - Invaginations that communicate with epidermal surface
  - Invaginations have papillary architecture
- Papillary structures lined by glandular epithelium with double layer
  - Papillae communicate with duct-like structures in deeper aspects
  - Basal layer is flattened to cuboidal
  - Luminal layer usually columnar
- Characteristic stroma
  - Fibrovascular connective tissue within papillae
  - Numerous plasma cells admixed with some lymphocytes

TOP DIFFERENTIAL DIAGNOSES

- Hidradenoma papilliferum
  - Lacks connection with epidermis
  - Lacks plasma cells
- Tubular apocrine adenoma
  - Lacks epidermal attachment
- SCP/malignant syringocystadenoma
  - Architectural complexity
  - Cytologic atypia
  - Mitotic activity

Low-Power Image of Syringocystadenoma Papilliferum

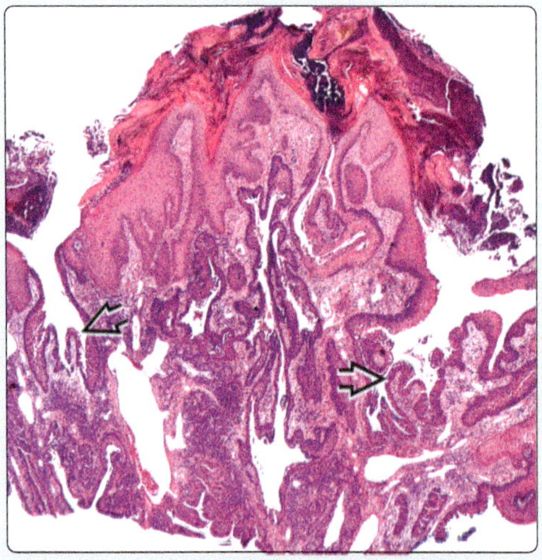

Syringocystadenoma Papilliferum With Transition From Squamous to Glandular Epithelium

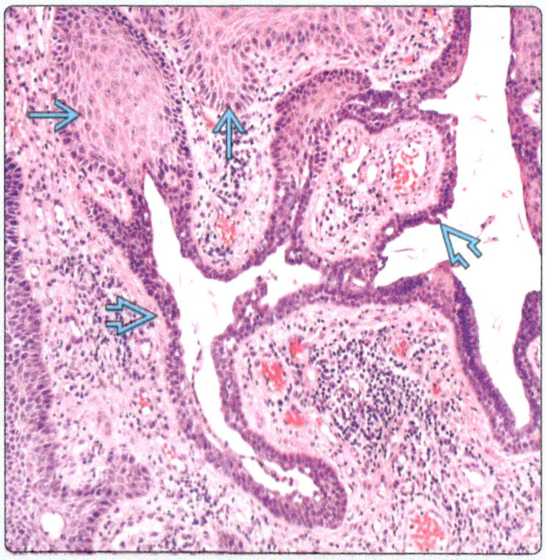

(Left) *Syringocystadenoma papilliferum has an endo/exophytic growth pattern with invaginations into the underlying dermis that have a papillary architecture.* **(Right)** *The superficial aspects of the imaginations are lined by squamous epithelium that transitions to glandular epithelium.*

Syringocystadenoma Papilliferum: High Magnification of Glandular Epithelium

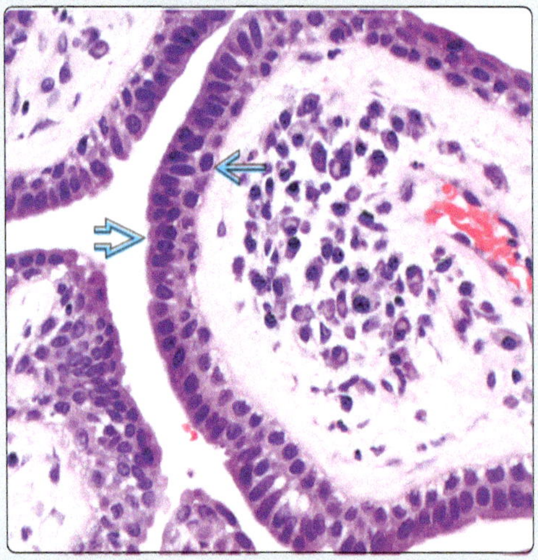

High Magnification of Apocrine Glandular Epithelium and Plasma Cells

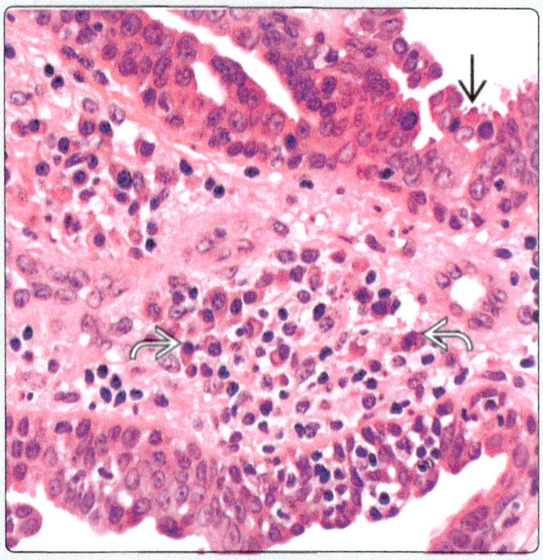

(Left) *The glandular component is composed of 2 cell layers with a basal myoepithelial layer and a columnar glandular layer.* **(Right)** *The glandular epithelium in this case shows evidence of apocrine differentiation, with focal apical snouts and secretions. The stroma contains numerous plasma cells.*

TERMINOLOGY

Abbreviations

- Syringocystadenoma papilliferum (SCP)

Definitions

- Benign adnexal tumor with endophytic and exophytic growth pattern

ETIOLOGY/PATHOGENESIS

Cytogenetics

- Subset of tumors show loss of heterozygosity for *PTCH1* (PTCH) &/or *CDKN2A* (P16), suggesting role for loss of these tumor suppressor genes in some cases

CLINICAL ISSUES

Epidemiology

- Age
  - ~ 1/2 present at birth or childhood

Presentation

- Scalp most common location, followed by face
- Solitary gray to dark brown papillomatous lesion
- Rarely multiple
- SCP seen in 5-19% of nevus sebaceus
  - 2nd most common tumor arising in nevus sebaceus after trichoblastoma
- Rarely associated with other neoplasms (e.g., tricholemmoma, apocrine hidrocystoma)

Treatment

- Surgical approaches
  - Simple excision is curative

Prognosis

- Benign
  - Rare cases may have associated basal cell carcinoma
  - Rarely transform to syringocystadenocarcinoma papilliferum

MICROSCOPIC

Histologic Features

- Endophytic/exophytic tumors
- Invaginations that communicate with epidermal surface
  - Superficial aspects lined by squamous epithelium transitioning to glandular epithelium
- Invaginations have papillary architecture
  - Papillary structures lined by glandular epithelium
    - Flattened to cuboidal myoepithelial basal layer
    - Luminal layer columnar; apocrine morphology common
    - Goblet cells occasionally present
    - May connect with duct-like structures in deeper aspects
- Characteristic stroma
  - Fibrovascular connective tissue within papillae
  - Numerous plasma cells admixed with some lymphocytes

ANCILLARY TESTS

Immunohistochemistry

- Glandular epithelium AE1/AE3, CAM5.2, EMA, and CEA (+)
  - Variably GCDFP-15(+), consistent with apocrine differentiation
- Myoepithelial layer positive for SMA, CK5/6, and p63

DIFFERENTIAL DIAGNOSIS

Hidradenoma Papilliferum

- Usually presents on vulva or perineum of women
- More delicate papillary architecture
- Usually does not communicate with surface epithelium
- Lacks plasma cell-rich stroma

Tubular Apocrine Adenoma

- Closely related tumors
- Tubular apocrine adenoma resembles SCP, however
  - Lacks epidermal attachments
  - Plasma cells not as common as in SCP

Syringocystadenocarcinoma Papilliferum/Malignant Syringocystadenoma

- Very rare tumors that present in adults
- May have history of rapid growth in longstanding lesion
- Recognizable precursor SCP usually present
- Malignant transformation: Multilayering of glandular epithelium, increased nuclear atypia and mitotic activity
  - May be in situ or invasive
  - In situ tumors have silhouette of SCP
  - Invasive tumors have invasive adenocarcinoma and sometimes squamous cell carcinoma

DIAGNOSTIC CHECKLIST

Pathologic Interpretation Pearls

- Usually presents on scalp of children
- Invaginations into underlying dermis
- Communicates with overlying epidermis
- Papillary architecture
- Papillae lined by glandular epithelium with double layer
- Numerous plasma cells in stroma

SELECTED REFERENCES

1. Shen AS et al: Activating mutations in the RAS/mitogen-activated protein kinase signaling pathway in sporadic trichoblastoma and syringocystadenoma papilliferum. Hum Pathol. 46(2):272-6, 2015
2. Satter E et al: Syringocystadenocarcinoma papilliferum with locoregional metastases. Dermatol Online J. 20(4):22335, 2014
3. Kazakov DV et al: Morphologic diversity of syringocystadenocarcinoma papilliferum based on a clinicopathologic study of 6 cases and review of the literature. Am J Dermatopathol. 32(4):340-7, 2010
4. Karg E et al: Congenital syringocystadenoma papilliferum. Pediatr Dermatol. 25(1):132-3, 2008
5. Laxmisha C et al: Linear syringocystadenoma papilliferum of the scalp. J Eur Acad Dermatol Venereol. 21(2):275-6, 2007
6. Rammeh-Rommani S et al: Syringocystadenoma papilliferum: report of 8 cases. Pathologica. 98(3):178-80, 2006
7. Böni R et al: Syringocystadenoma papilliferum: a study of potential tumor suppressor genes. Am J Dermatopathol. 23(2):87-9, 2001
8. Cribier B et al: Tumors arising in nevus sebaceus: a study of 596 cases. J Am Acad Dermatol. 42(2 Pt 1):263-8, 2000
9. Mammino JJ et al: Syringocystadenoma papilliferum. Int J Dermatol. 30(11):763-6, 1991

(Left) *Syringocystadenoma papilliferum often has a partially exophytic, as well as endophytic growth pattern. The overlying squamous epithelium shows acanthosis* ➡*, and the deeper aspects show glandular epithelium with papillae* ➡*.* **(Right)** *The tumor is characterized by invaginations with a papillary architecture that extend into the dermis.*

Syringocystadenoma Papilliferum With Exophytic and Endophytic Patterns

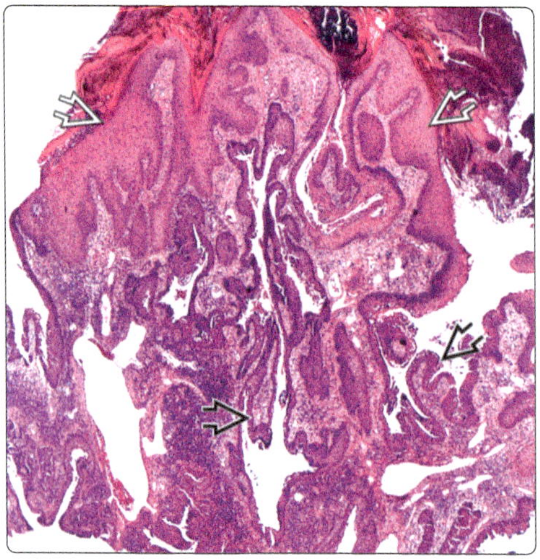

Endophytic Component With Papillary Architecture

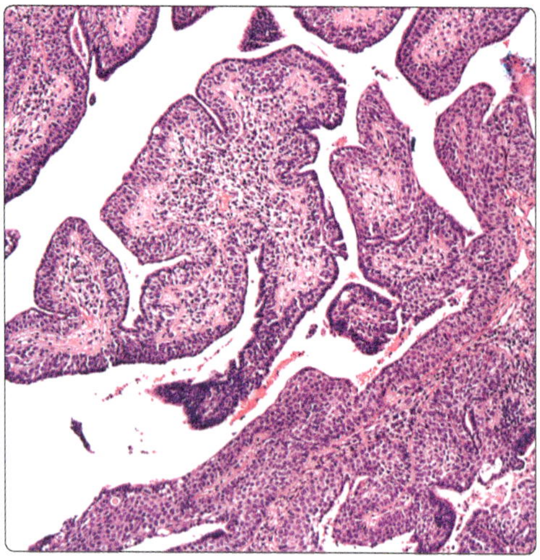

(Left) *The epithelium lining the papillae demonstrates a transition from squamous to glandular epithelium* ➡*. The stroma contains numerous plasma cells* ➡*.* **(Right)** *The stroma of syringocystadenoma papilliferum characteristically has numerous plasma cells* ➡*. The epithelium in this case has focal goblet cells* ➡*.*

Papillae of Syringocystadenoma Papilliferum

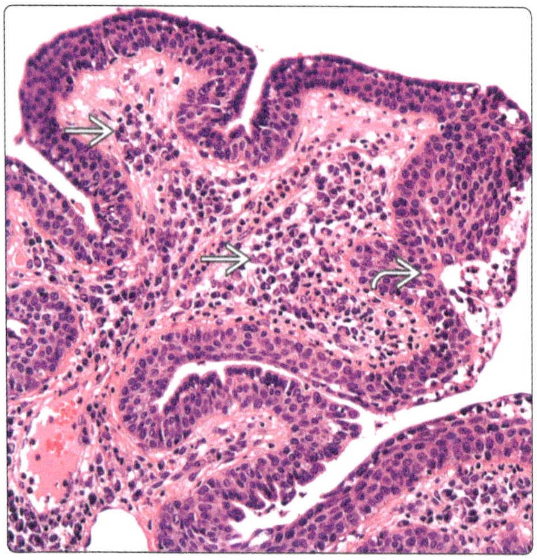

High-Power Image of Papillae and Stroma

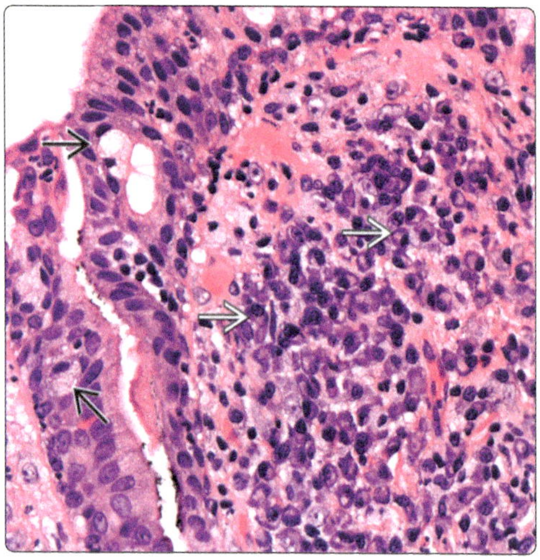

(Left) *This example of syringocystadenoma papilliferum has a predominantly endophytic growth pattern extending below the level of the adjacent epidermis. Note the overlying erosions with serum crust* ➡*, changes likely due to excoriation/trauma.* **(Right)** *The papillae are typically lined by squamous epithelium superficially* ➡ *that transitions to glandular epithelium more deeply* ➡*.*

Syringocystadenoma Papilliferum With Erosion and Serum Crust

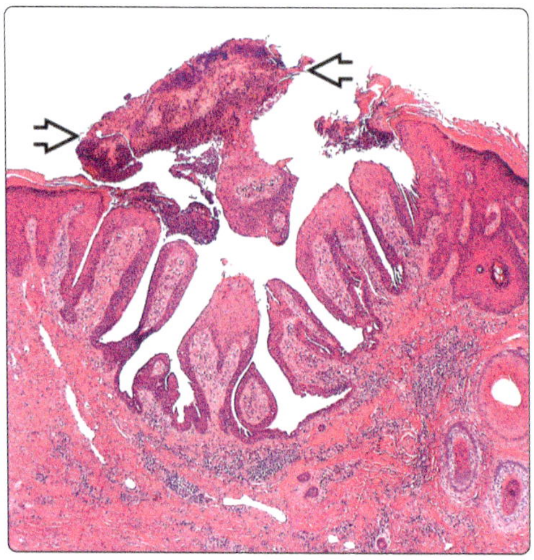

High Magnification of Syringocystadenoma Papilliferum Papillae

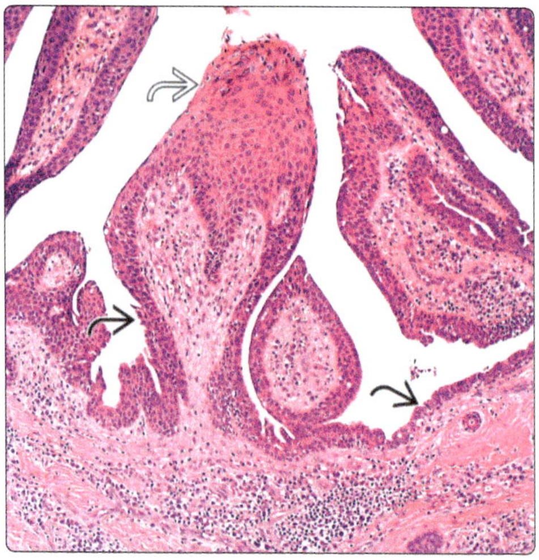

Malignant Syringocystadenocarcinoma Papilliferum

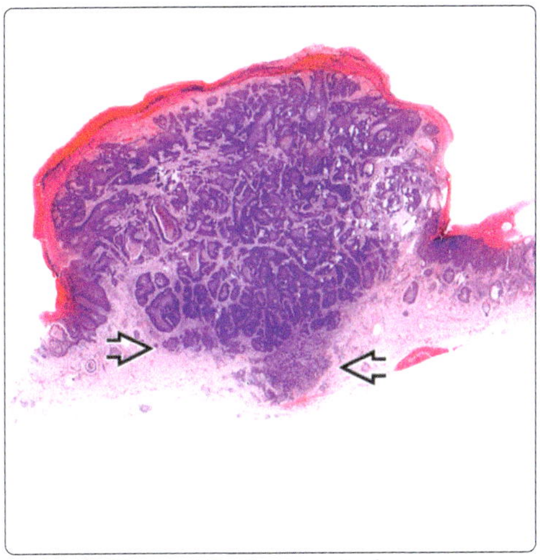

Benign Syringocystadenoma Papilliferum Area Associated With Malignant Syringocystadenoma Papilliferum

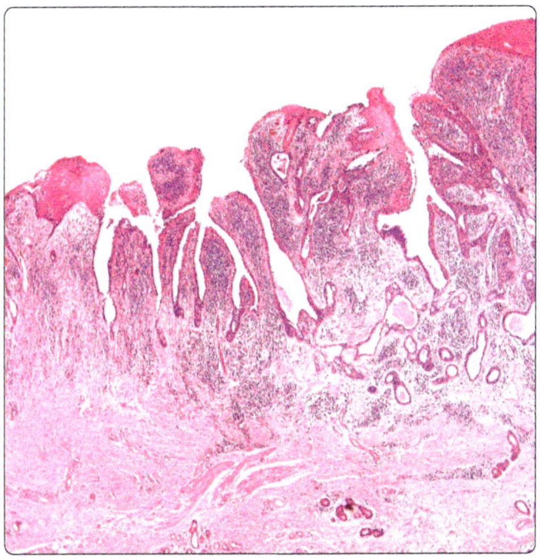

(Left) *Scanning image of a syringocystadenocarcinoma papilliferum shows a large, endophytic-appearing tumor with deep invasion into the dermis* ➡. **(Right)** *The periphery of the malignant syringocystadenoma papilliferum shows remnants of the precursor syringocystadenoma papilliferum.*

Malignant Syringocystadenoma Papilliferum With Squamoid and Glandular Components

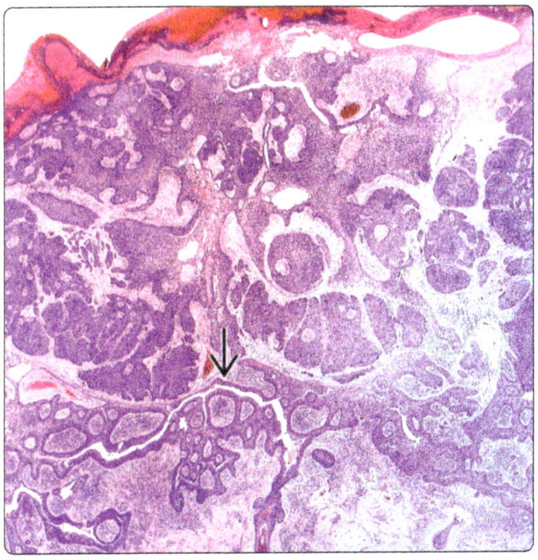

Intermediate Power Magnification of Squamous Cell Carcinoma Component

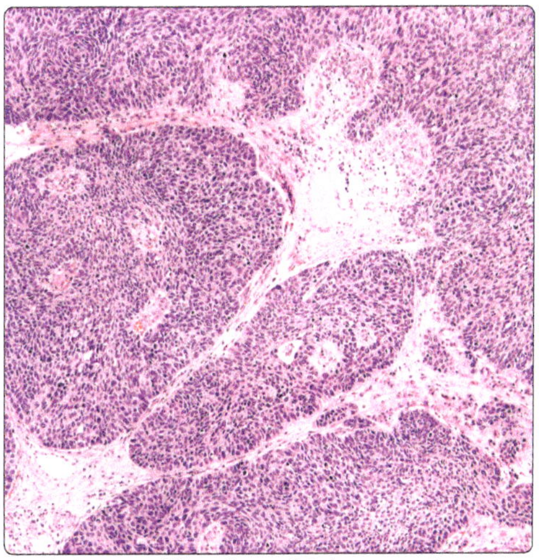

(Left) *This syringocystadenocarcinoma papilliferum demonstrates central areas of squamous cell carcinoma that transitions to an in situ adenocarcinoma component with a papillary architecture in the deeper aspects of the tumor* ➡. **(Right)** *In central areas of this malignant syringocystadenoma papilliferum, there are islands of tumor cells showing squamous differentiation.*

Adenocarcinoma Component in Malignant Syringocystadenoma Papilliferum

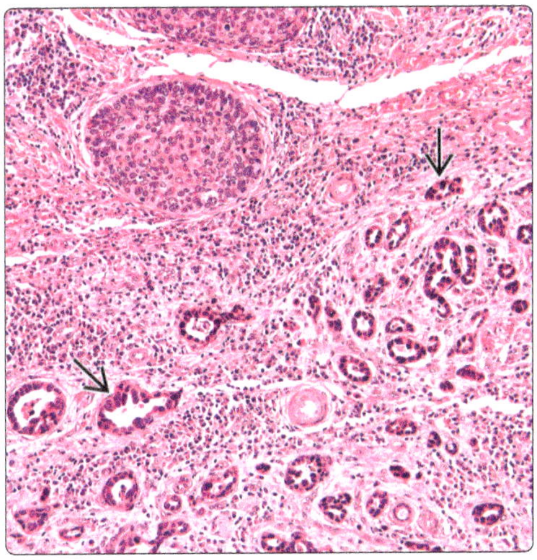

High Magnification of Adenocarcinoma Component in Malignant Syringocystadenoma Papilliferum

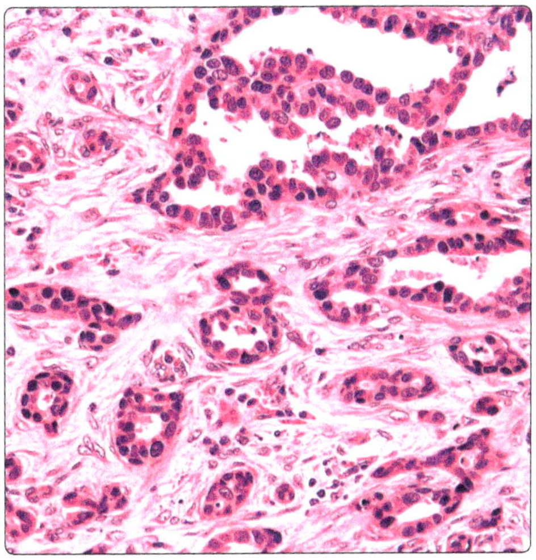

(Left) *The invasive adenocarcinoma component of syringocystadenocarcinoma papilliferum often loses the papillary architecture and shows infiltrative-appearing small ductal structure* ➡. **(Right)** *Invasive adenocarcinoma component of syringocystadenocarcinoma papilliferum is characterized by irregular glands lined by atypical cells with hyperchromatic nuclei. The invasive tumor has an irregular growth pattern and is surrounded by a desmoplastic stroma.*

Hidradenoma Papilliferum

KEY FACTS

TERMINOLOGY

- Papillary hidradenoma
- Well-circumscribed adenoma with apocrine differentiation

CLINICAL ISSUES

- Rare, benign tumor
- Vulvar or perianal area, almost always in women
- Extremely rare malignant transformation to hidradenocarcinoma papilliferum or aggressive adenosquamous carcinoma

MACROSCOPIC

- Solid or, rarely, cystic skin-colored papule
- Small, < 1 cm in most cases

MICROSCOPIC

- Well-circumscribed, dermal-based tumor
- No connections to epidermis in most cases
- Maze-like glandular spaces and papillary foldings
- Inner layer of columnar secretory cells
  - Apocrine differentiation is usually seen
  - Often with decapitation secretion
- Outer layer of cuboidal myoepithelial cells
- Variable degree of mitotic index

TOP DIFFERENTIAL DIAGNOSES

- Syringocystadenoma papilliferum (SCP)
  - Similar histologic features, indicating that these are likely closely related tumors
  - Epidermal connections much more common in SCP
- Tubular apocrine adenoma
  - Simpler lesions composed predominately of tubular structures
- Nipple adenoma (erosive adenomatosis of nipple, florid papillomatosis)
- Papillary eccrine adenoma
- Hidradenoma

Hidradenoma Papilliferum at Low Magnification

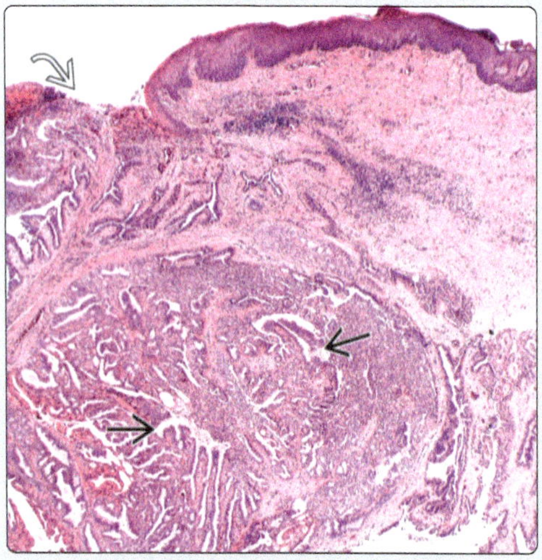

Hidradenoma Papilliferum With Branching Spaces

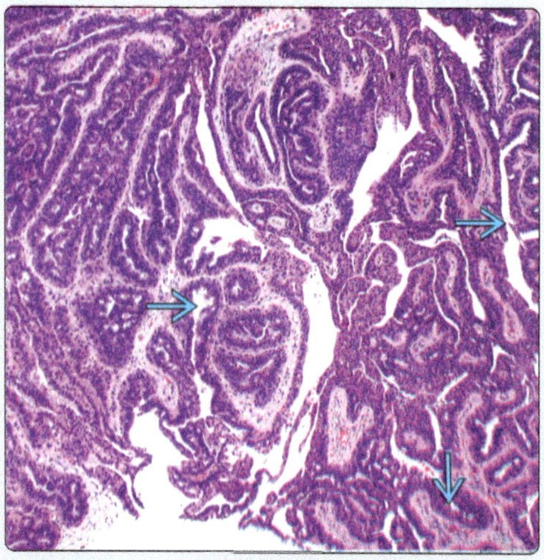

(Left) *Hidradenoma papilliferum (HP) is typically a well-circumscribed, dermal-based tumor. This case shows focal epidermal attachments with erosions, findings similar to those seen in syringocystadenoma papilliferum. Cystic and branching spaces can easily be identified on low power.* **(Right)** *This area of HP shows the cystic and branching ductal/glandular spaces, which can usually be easily identified on low power.*

Hidradenoma Papilliferum at Higher Magnification

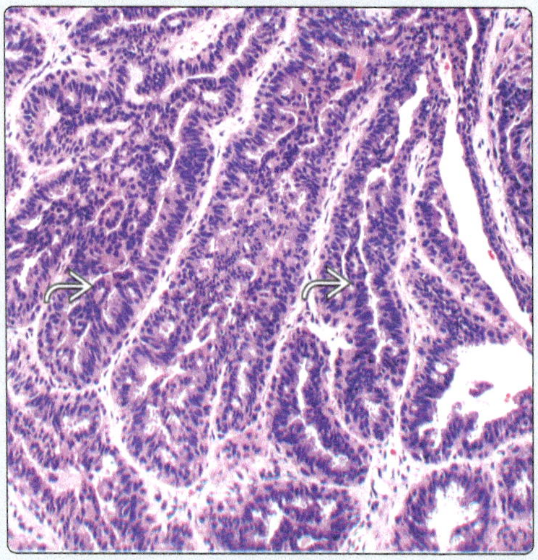

Hidradenoma Papilliferum at High Magnification

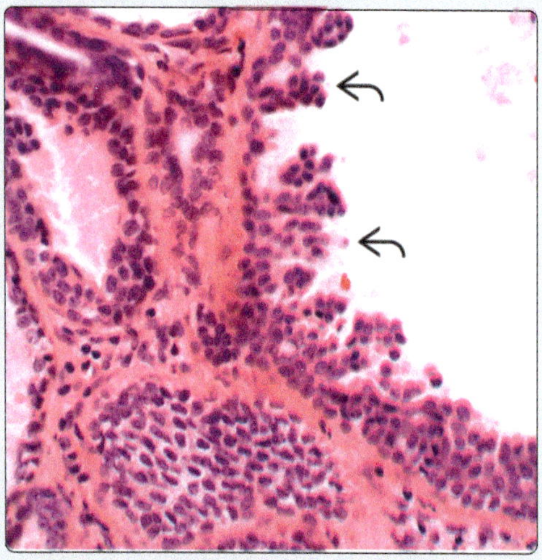

(Left) *Higher magnification of a HP shows the elongated, arborizing papillary structures lined by 2-3 cell layers of bland columnar luminal cells and underlying myoepithelial cells.* **(Right)** *H&E shows high magnification of a cystic area with evidence of apocrine differentiation. The surface-lining cells show apical snouts and secretions. Note the lack of cytologic atypia or pleomorphism.*

TERMINOLOGY

Abbreviations

- Hidradenoma papilliferum (HP)

Synonyms

- Papillary hidradenoma

Definitions

- Small, well-circumscribed, dermal-based adenoma with apocrine differentiation

CLINICAL ISSUES

Epidemiology

- Incidence
  - Rare
- Age
  - Adult
- Sex
  - Almost always women
- Ethnicity
  - No race predilection

Site

- Vulva or perianal region
  - Rarely other sites (and termed ectopic HP)

Treatment

- Conservative surgical excision

Prognosis

- Generally excellent
- Extremely rare malignant transformation to hidradenocarcinoma papilliferum or aggressive adenosquamous carcinoma

MACROSCOPIC

General Features

- Solid or, rarely, cystic skin-colored papule

Size

- Small, < 1 cm in most cases

MICROSCOPIC

Histologic Features

- Dermal-based, well-circumscribed tumor
  - Surrounded by fibrous capsule
- No connections to epidermis in most cases, but may be seen in some
  - If epidermal connections present, show associated erosions/ulceration (similar to syringocystadenoma papilliferum)
- Maze-like, arborizing glandular spaces
- Tubular and cystic structures
- Papillary folds
  - Often project into cystic spaces
- Inner layer of columnar apocrine secretory cells
  - Often with decapitation secretion
- Outer layer of cuboidal myoepithelial cells
- Cuboidal cells with eosinophilic cytoplasm and small nuclei present in 1/3 of cases
  - Resemble apocrine metaplasia seen in breast tissue
- Variable degree of mitotic index
  - High mitotic rate does not necessarily indicate malignancy (need to see cytologic atypia, pleomorphism, &/or infiltrative features)
- Minimal inflammation

Cytologic Features

- Benign apocrine secretory and myoepithelial cells

DIFFERENTIAL DIAGNOSIS

Syringocystadenoma Papilliferum

- Location is on head and neck
- Similar histologic features, indicating that these are likely closely related tumors; however
  - Epidermal connections are seen in syringocystadenoma papilliferum (SCP), but usually not in HP
  - Characteristic prominent plasma cell infiltrate present in SCP, rare in HP

Tubular Apocrine Adenoma

- Simpler lesions composed predominately of tubular structures
  - No maze-like glandular spaces
- No characteristic location

Nipple Adenoma (Erosive Adenomatosis of Nipple, Florid Papillomatosis)

- Location is on nipple
- Histology is similar to SCP and hidradenoma papilliferum

Papillary Eccrine Adenoma

- Rare tumors composed of small tubular structures with no decapitation secretion
  - Eccrine differentiation

Hidradenoma

- Nodular dermal-based tumor lacking epidermal connections
- More cellular; nodular to sheet-like collections of pale to clear-staining cells
  - Squamoid cells may also be present
- Lacks intricate, maze-like features of hidradenoma papilliferum

DIAGNOSTIC CHECKLIST

Pathologic Interpretation Pearls

- Small, dermal-based apocrine adenoma with maze-like appearance

SELECTED REFERENCES

1. McClain CM et al: Hidradenoma papilliferum associated with pregnancy: a case report. J Cutan Pathol. ePub, 2015
2. Kurashige Y et al: Hidradenoma papilliferum of the vulva in association with an anogenital mammary-like gland. J Dermatol. 41(5):411-3, 2014
3. Duhan N et al: Hidradenoma papilliferum of the vulva: case report and review of literature. Arch Gynecol Obstet. 284(4):1015-7, 2011
4. Vazmitel M et al: Hidradenoma papilliferum with a ductal carcinoma in situ component: case report and review of the literature. Am J Dermatopathol. 30(4):392-4, 2008
5. Vang R et al: Ectopic hidradenoma papilliferum: a case report and review of the literature. J Am Acad Dermatol. 41(1):115-8, 1999

Hidradenoma

KEY FACTS

CLINICAL ISSUES

- Solitary dermal nodule

MICROSCOPIC

- Architecture
  - Primarily solid
  - Primarily cystic
  - Solid and cystic
- Classically, does not connect to epidermis and is deep-seated
- Solid areas composed of varying proportion of
  - Clear cells
  - Poroid cells
  - Squamoid cells
  - Rarely mucinous cells
- Ducts with eosinophilic cuticles present in solid areas
- Cystic areas lined by cuboidal cells
  - Sometimes with evidence of decapitation secretion
- Stroma between solid islands &/or cystic areas is prominently hyalinized
- Well circumscribed
- Necrosis usually absent
- Prominent cytologic atypia not present
- Mitoses not numerous

TOP DIFFERENTIAL DIAGNOSES

- Metastatic renal cell carcinoma
- Other clear cell tumors
  - Basal cell carcinoma
  - Squamous cell carcinoma
- Other adnexal tumors
  - Lymphadenoma
  - Sebaceous adenoma
  - Cystadenoma
  - Sebaceoma
- Hidradenocarcinoma

Hidradenoma at Low Magnification

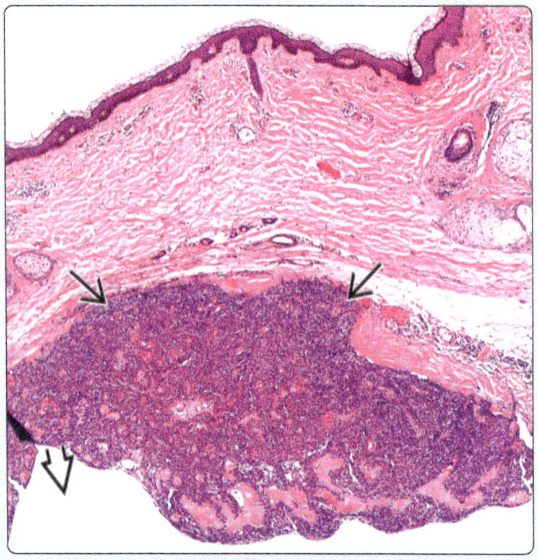

Hidradenoma: Characteristic Stroma, Cells, and Ducts

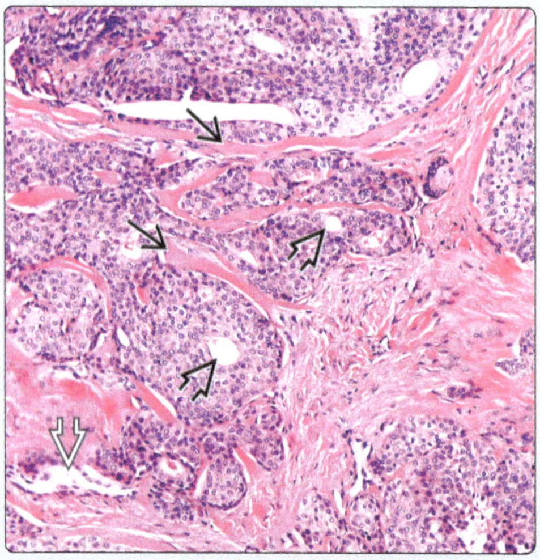

(Left) *Low-magnification view of a hidradenoma shows a dermal-based, nodular-appearing, solid to cystic tumor.* **(Right)** *Hidradenoma often has a prominent hyalinized stroma. Islands are composed of clear cells and poroid cells with some evidence of ductal and glandular differentiation.*

Hidradenoma: Poroid and Clear Cells

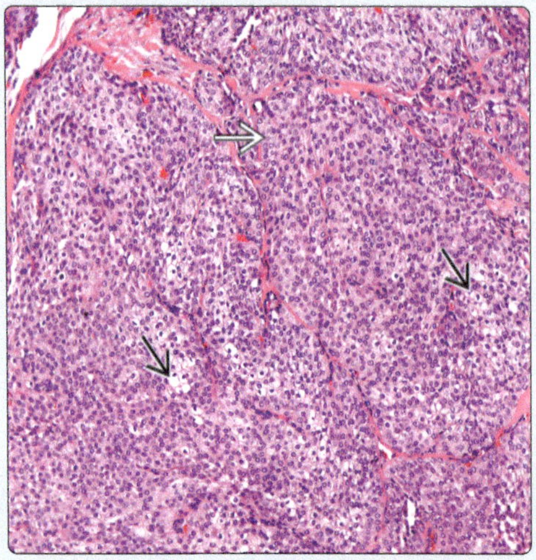

Hidradenoma: Poroid and Clear Cells

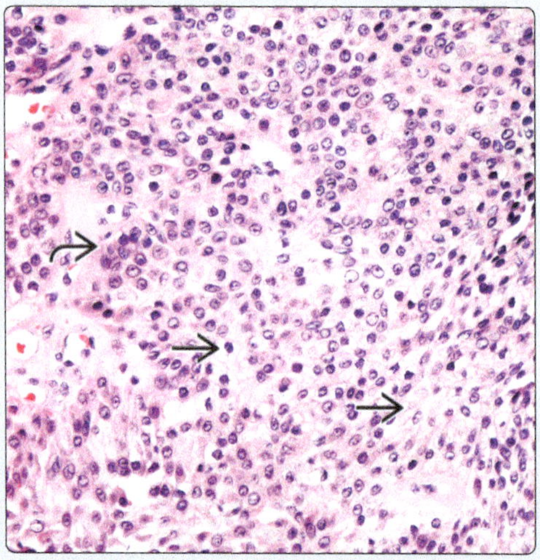

(Left) *This solid area of a hidradenoma is composed of small, bland-appearing clear cells and poroid cells. There is minimal cytologic atypia, an absence of necrosis, and mitoses are not prominent.* **(Right)** *Higher magnification of hidradenoma shows an admixture of clear cells and basaloid/poroid cells. The basaloid cells have minimal cytoplasm, which is eosinophilic to basophilic staining and round/oval nuclei. Mitoses and cytologic atypia are not present.*

TERMINOLOGY

Synonyms

- Clear cell hidradenoma, nodular hidradenoma, solid-cystic hidradenoma, cystic hidradenoma, eccrine acrospiroma, eccrine sweat gland adenoma, poroid hidradenoma, apocrine hidradenoma

Definitions

- Benign tumor showing apocrine or eccrine differentiation

CLINICAL ISSUES

Presentation

- Solitary dermal nodule

Treatment

- Excision is generally curative

Prognosis

- Benign with very low malignant potential; may rarely transform to hidradenocarcinoma

MICROSCOPIC

Histologic Features

- Well-circumscribed, dermal-based tumor (classically does not connect to epidermis and is deep-seated)
- May be primarily composed of solid areas, cystic areas, or both
- Solid areas composed of varying proportion of clear cells, poroid cells, squamoid cells, and, rarely, mucinous cells
- Ducts with eosinophilic cuticles present in solid areas
- Cystic areas lined by cuboidal cells, sometimes with evidence of decapitation secretion
- Stroma between solid islands &/or cystic areas is prominently hyalinized appearing
- Prominent cytologic atypia, numerous mitoses, necrosis not present
- Generally does not show infiltrative pattern

Cytologic Features

- Variable cell composition
  - Clear cells
    - Clear cytoplasm
    - Nuclei oval to round with small nucleoli
    - Contain glycogen and are PAS(+) (diastase sensitive)
  - Squamoid cells
    - Resemble keratinocytes with eosinophilic cytoplasm and well-demarcated, cytoplasmic borders
  - Poroid cells
    - Basaloid cells with little cytoplasm
    - Nuclei have blue outlines and single nucleoli or occasionally multiple small nucleoli

DIFFERENTIAL DIAGNOSIS

Metastatic Renal Cell Carcinoma

- Composed of clear cells arranged in variably sized islands
- Vascular pattern may be prominent
- Often extravasated erythrocytes numerous
- Generally does not show cystic areas
- More commonly CD10 and EMA (+); RCA(+)

Hidradenocarcinoma

- Cellular, atypical, nodular, dermal-based tumor
- Shows greater cytologic atypia and mitotic figures and often has infiltrative features

Clear Cell Basal Cell Carcinoma

- Composed of clear cells arranged in variably sized islands
- Some islands may have peripheral palisading
- Some foci of conventional basal cell carcinoma may be present
- Generally does not show cystic areas
- BER-EP4 and AR (+)

Clear Cell Squamous Cell Carcinoma

- Composed of clear cells arranged in variably sized islands
- Some foci of conventional squamous cell carcinoma may be present
- Absence of ductal differentiation
- Generally does not show cystic areas

Squamous Cell Carcinoma

- If hidradenoma has few clear cells and mostly squamoid cells, squamous cell carcinoma may enter differential
- Keratin pearls and epidermal connection often present
- Ductal/glandular differentiation and hyalinized stroma generally absent
- May be infiltrative

Lymphadenoma

- Jagged islands composed of clear cells with peripheral palisading
- Variably dense infiltrate of lymphocytes may obscure islands

Mixed Tumor of Skin

- May have islands of small basaloid cells that appear poroid
- Mixed tumors have different stroma: Chondroid to mucinous

Papillary Hidrocystoma (Cystadenoma)

- If hidradenoma is primarily cystic, cystadenoma enters differential
- Cystadenoma resembles traditional hidrocystoma, except there is increased cellularity and papillations

SELECTED REFERENCES

1. Luzar B et al: Perineural growth of benign cutaneous sweat gland tumors: a hitherto unrecognized phenomenon unassociated with malignancy. J Cutan Pathol. 42(11):878-83, 2015
2. Vasconcelos I et al: Hidradenoma of the breast: a source of diagnostic confusion. Breast J. 21(6):681-2, 2015
3. Nandeesh BN et al: A study of histopathologic spectrum of nodular hidradenoma. Am J Dermatopathol. 34(5):461-70, 2012
4. Battistella M et al: From hidroacanthoma simplex to poroid hidradenoma: clinicopathologic and immunohistochemic study of poroid neoplasms and reappraisal of their histogenesis. Am J Dermatopathol. 32(5):459-68, 2010
5. Yavel R et al: Hidradenomas and a hidradenocarcinoma of the scalp managed using Mohs micrographic surgery and a multidisciplinary approach: case reports and review of the literature. Dermatol Surg. 35(2):273-81, 2009
6. Biernat W et al: Phenotypic heterogeneity of nodular hidradenoma. Immunohistochemical analysis with emphasis on cytokeratin expression. Am J Dermatopathol. 18(6):592-6, 1996

(Left) *This hidradenoma shows both solid ⇒ and cystic areas ⇒. The lesion extends to the tissue margins, so circumscription cannot be assessed. However, necrosis is not evident, and there are no infiltrative features.* **(Right)** *This hidradenoma has an overall cystic architecture that is surrounded by fibrosis ⇒. The epithelial islands within the cystic space have tubular spaces ⇒ that are considered by some to be a marker of apocrine ductal differentiation.*

Hidradenoma: Solid and Cystic Features

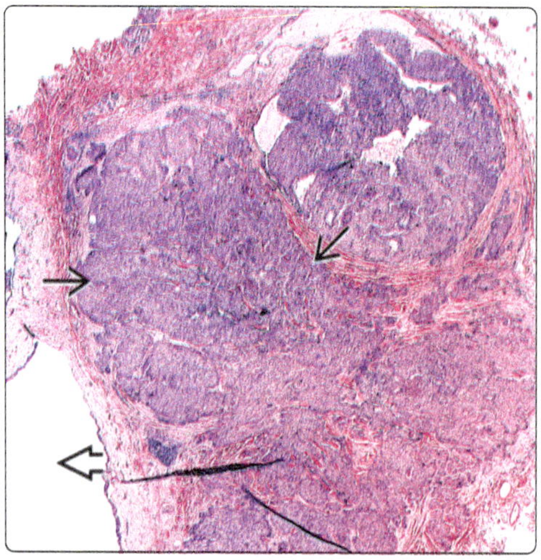

Hidradenoma With Cystic Architecture

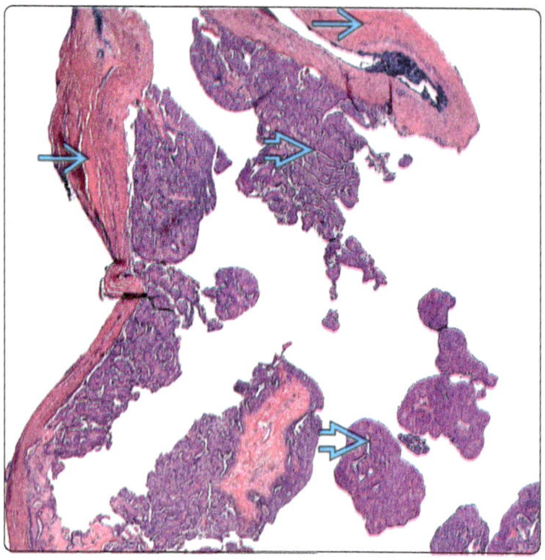

(Left) *Poroid cells ⇒, round and basaloid, are the classic cell type associated with hidradenoma.* **(Right)** *In addition to poroid cells, other cell types may be seen in hidradenoma in varying proportions. In this field, clear cells ⇒ and squamoid cells forming focal keratin pearls ⇒ are present.*

Hidradenoma: Solid Area Composed of Poroid Cells

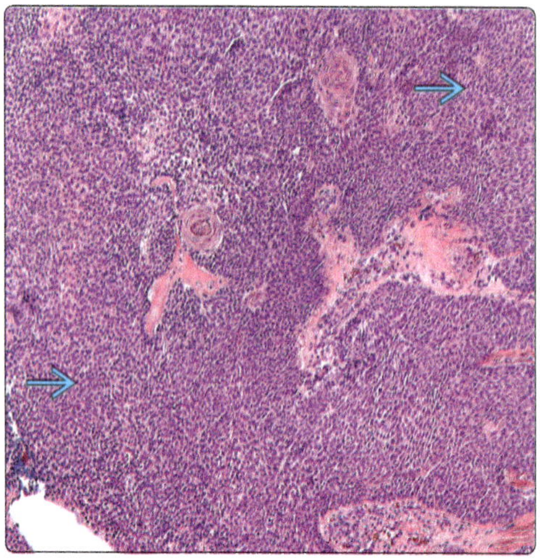

Hidradenoma: Clear and Squamoid Cells

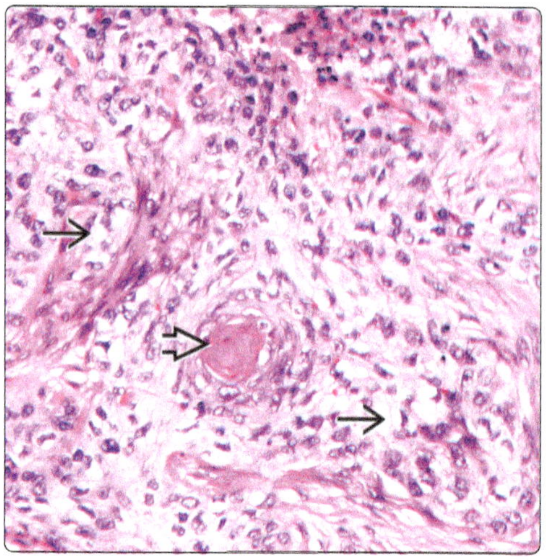

(Left) *This area of a hidradenoma shows an admixture of clear ⇒ and poroid cells ⇒. There is minimal cytologic atypia. Mitoses are not prominent, and necrosis is absent.* **(Right)** *High magnification of a more solid area of a mucinous hidradenoma shows scattered, goblet-like cells ⇒ with prominent cytoplasmic mucin.*

Hidradenoma With Clear Cells and Poroid Cells

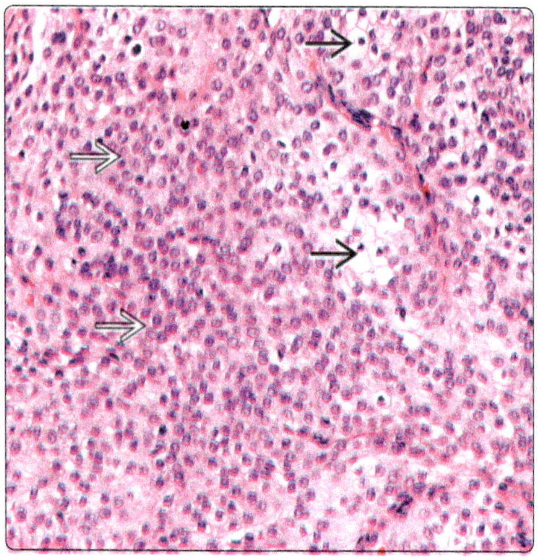

Hidradenoma With Mucinous Features

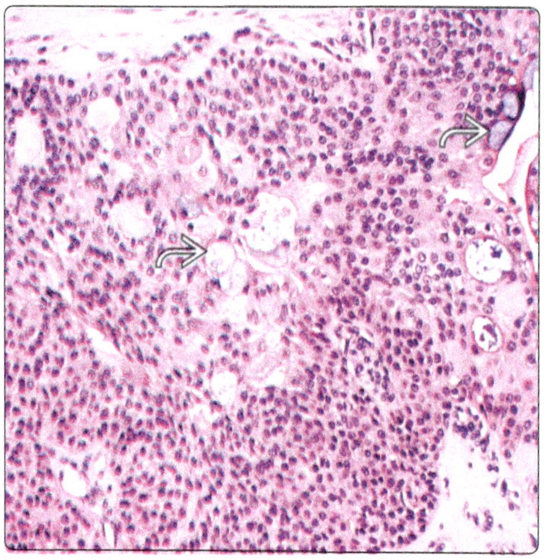

Acrospiroma

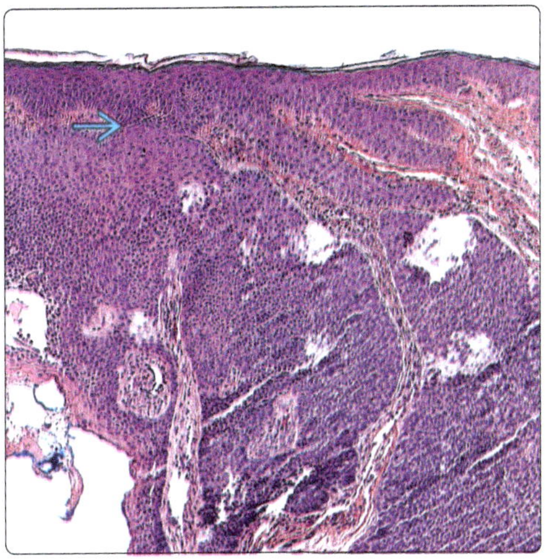

Differential Diagnosis: Mixed Tumor of Skin

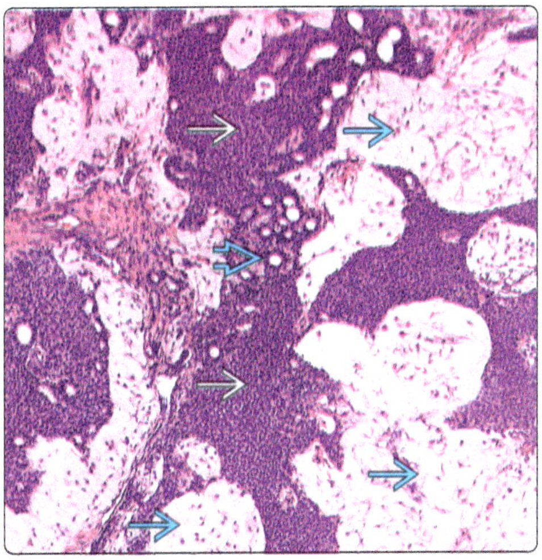

(Left) *Classically, hidradenoma is based in the dermis, but focal epidermal connections can be seen ➔, mimicking a poroma. Some experts advocate the term acrospiroma for tumors, such as this, that show overlapping features of poroma and hidradenoma.* **(Right)** *Mixed tumor of the skin has a characteristic mucinous ➔ to chondroid stroma. Epithelial islands have ductal differentiation ➔, and cytology can be poroid ➔, as in this example.*

Differential Diagnosis: Poroma

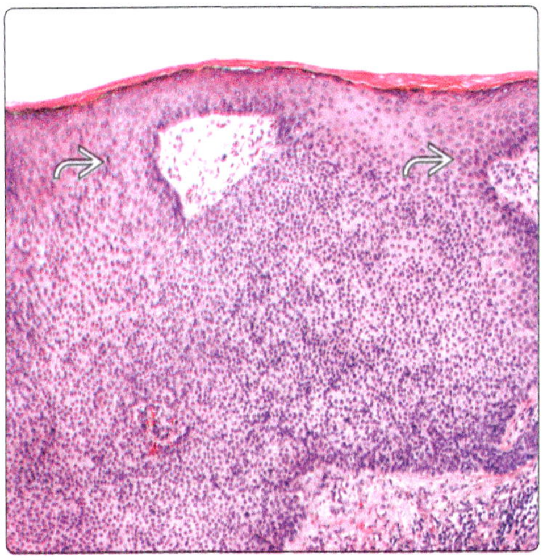

Poroma: Higher Magnification of Poroid Cells

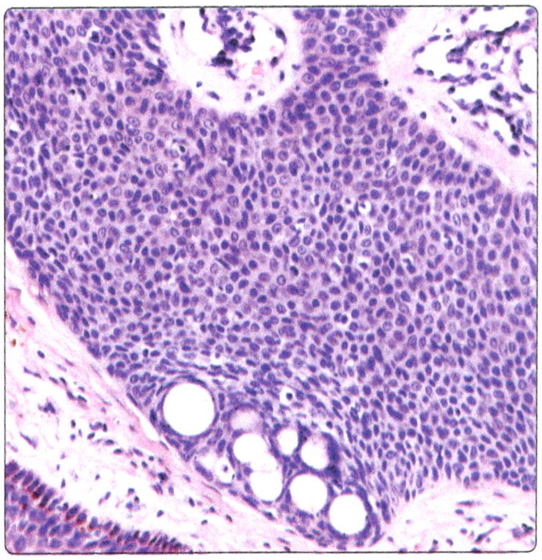

(Left) *Low magnification of a poroma shows basaloid to squamoid cells with thickened, anastomosing connections between the tumor cells and the overlying epidermis ➔. Although closely related tumors, hidradenomas are typically deeper seated, dermal-based tumors lacking epidermal connections.* **(Right)** *Poromas are composed of poroid cells with oval to round nuclei, small nucleoli, and indistinct cytoplasmic borders. Clear cell features are less common than in hidradenoma.*

Differential Diagnosis: Basal Cell Carcinoma Clear Cell Variant

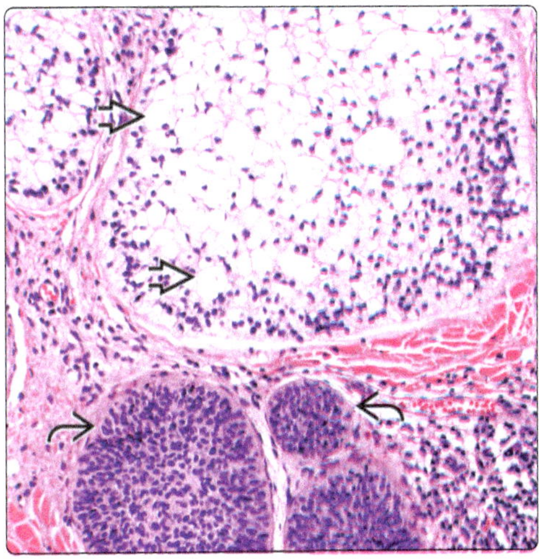

Differential Diagnosis: Metastatic Renal Cell Carcinoma

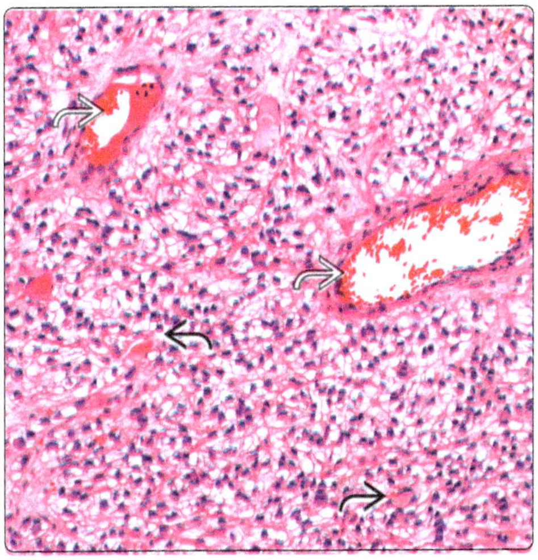

(Left) *Clear cell basal cell carcinoma (BCC) is composed of large cells with abundant clear cytoplasm ➔ and can mimic clear cell hidradenoma in some cases. However, areas of more conventional BCC ➔ are often present, as are seen in the lower corner of this field.* **(Right)** *Metastatic clear cell renal cell carcinoma (RCC) to the skin can present as a dermal nodule, mimicking clear cell hidradenoma. However, RCC shows numerous small ➔ to medium-sized blood vessels ➔, which are much sparser in hidradenoma.*

Hidradenocarcinoma

KEY FACTS

TERMINOLOGY

- Malignant acrospiroma, malignant hidradenoma
- Malignant adnexal tumor arising from, or showing areas similar to, hidradenoma

CLINICAL ISSUES

- Most frequently occurs on head and neck region
- Presents as nodule or mass lesion
- Excision is sometimes curative
- Mohs micrographic surgery may be best option to ensure clear margins
- Course can be aggressive
  - Local recurrences
  - Metastases

MICROSCOPIC

- Epithelial islands with interspersed glands/ducts
- Cells composing islands are variable
  - Clear
  - Poroid
  - Squamoid (less common)
  - Rarely mucinous
- Hyalinized stroma
  - Similar to hidradenoma
- Infiltrative growth pattern
  - Not well circumscribed, unlike hidradenoma
- Deep extension
- Perineural or vascular invasion may be present
- Ki-67 generally shows high proliferative index

TOP DIFFERENTIAL DIAGNOSES

- Hidradenoma
- Porocarcinoma
- Metastatic renal cell carcinoma
- Clear cell squamous cell carcinoma
- Clear cell basal cell carcinoma
- Sebaceous carcinoma

Hidradenocarcinoma: Low Magnification

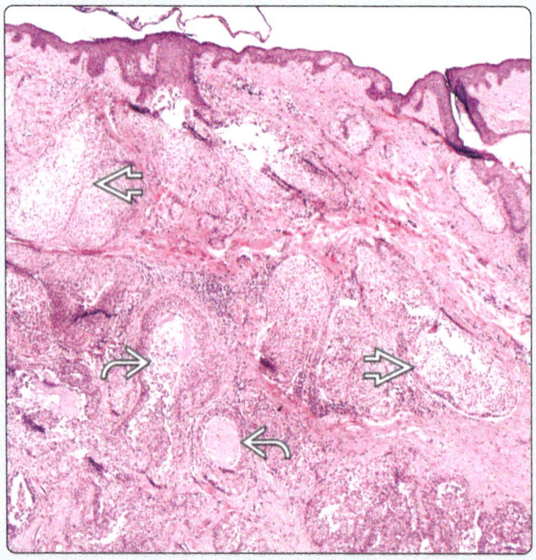

Hidradenocarcinoma: Areas of Necrosis

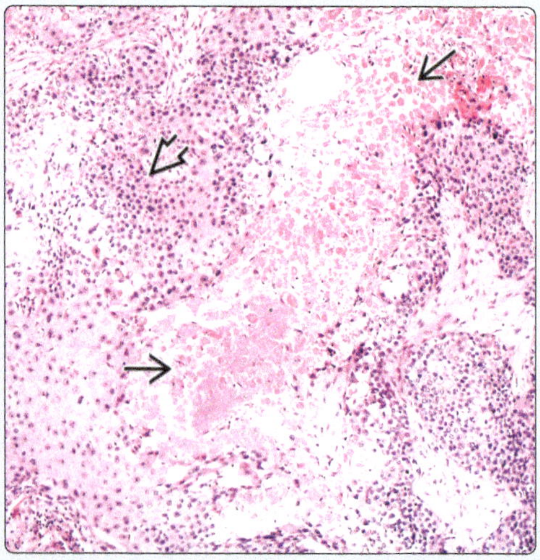

(Left) *Low magnification of a hidradenocarcinoma shows a dermal-based, atypical, multilobular neoplasm with clear cell features and cystic spaces containing mucinous material and cellular debris.* **(Right)** *Areas of squamous differentiation and prominent tumoral cell necrosis are present in this example of hidradenocarcinoma. Squamous differentiation is much less common than in porocarcinoma.*

Hidradenocarcinoma: Atypia and Mitoses

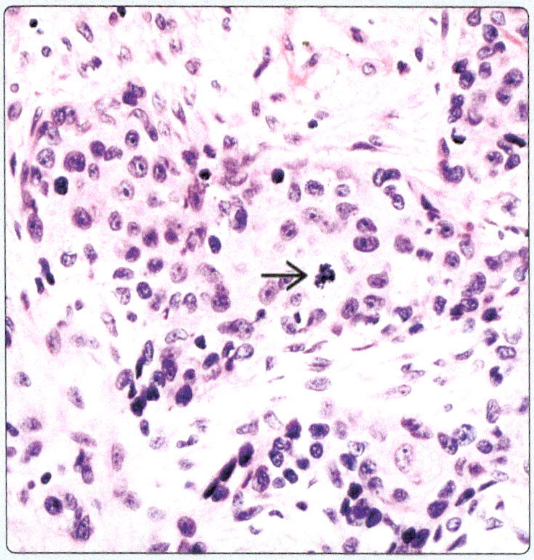

Hidradenocarcinoma: CEA Positivity

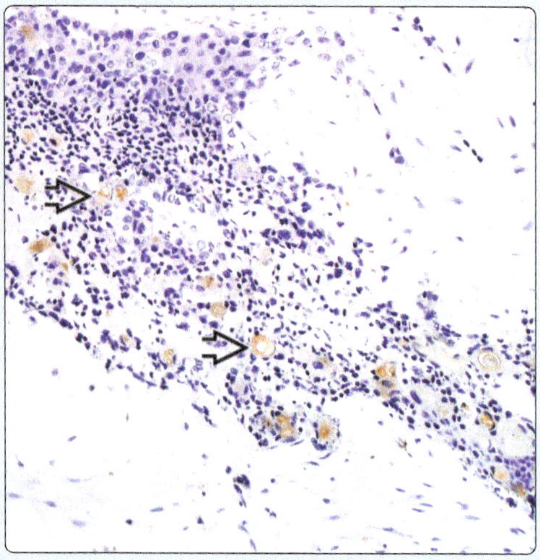

(Left) *Infiltrative islands of tumor cells in hidradenocarcinoma show cellular atypia, with enlarged nuclei and prominent nucleoli. There is also an atypical mitosis present.* **(Right)** *CEA highlights numerous small ductal lumina and their contents in this example of an infiltrative hidradenocarcinoma.*

TERMINOLOGY

Synonyms

- Malignant acrospiroma, malignant hidradenoma

Definitions

- Malignant adnexal tumor arising from, or showing areas similar to, hidradenoma

CLINICAL ISSUES

Site

- Most frequently in head and neck region

Presentation

- Nodule or mass

Treatment

- Surgical approaches
  - Wide, local excision of tumor
  - Mohs micrographic surgery may be best option to ensure clear margins
- Drugs
  - For metastatic hidradenocarcinoma, if surgery is not option
    - Various chemotherapeutic regimens reported
- Radiation
  - Variable response

Prognosis

- Excision may be curative
- Course can be aggressive
  - Local recurrences, metastatic disease (to lymph nodes, distant skin, internal organs)

MICROSCOPIC

Histologic Features

- Epithelial islands with interspersed glands/ducts
- Architecture may be predominantly solid islands; sometimes cystic areas present
  - Cells composing islands are variable
    - Clear, poroid, less commonly squamoid; rarely mucinous
- Hyalinized stroma
- Infiltrative growth pattern; not well-circumscribed
- Deep extension
- Necrosis may be evident
- Nuclear pleomorphism may be present
- Mitoses often seen
  - May see few to many
- Perineural or vascular invasion may be identified
- Area of tumor compatible with benign hidradenoma may be seen

Cytologic Features

- Often show high-grade cytologic atypia
- Some cases may be composed of relatively bland cells without prominent cytologic atypia
- Varying proportions of clear, poroid, and squamoid cells

ANCILLARY TESTS

Immunohistochemistry

- Positive with p63, CK5/6 (consistent with primary cutaneous tumor)
- CEA and EMA highlight glandular/ductal foci
- p53(+), and Ki-67 generally shows high proliferative index

DIFFERENTIAL DIAGNOSIS

Hidradenoma

- Nodular, well-circumscribed, dermal-based tumor
- Composed of varying proportion of clear cells, poroid cells, squamoid cells (less common than in porocarcinomas), and, rarely, mucinous cells
- Lacks high-grade atypia, necrosis, infiltrative features, and atypical mitoses

Porocarcinoma

- Invasive poroid neoplasm with anastomosing cords of tumor cells
- Typically shows multiple epidermal attachments (absent in hidradenocarcinoma)
- More frequent squamous differentiation and fewer clear cell features compared to hidradenocarcinoma

Metastatic Renal Cell Carcinoma

- Clear cells in variably sized islands; no true ductal differentiation present
- Prominence of small, capillary-type vessels and extravasated erythrocytes
- Hyalinized stroma absent
- Positive with EMA (cytoplasmic, not ductal), CAIX, RCA, and CD10

Clear Cell Squamous Cell Carcinoma

- Clear cells in variably sized nests and islands, poroid cells absent
- Dyskeratotic cells and areas of keratinization often present
- No true ductal differentiation present

Clear Cell Basal Cell Carcinoma

- Clear cells in variably sized islands, some with peripheral palisading
- Poroid cells absent, ductal differentiation absent to rare
- Positive with BER-EP4, Bcl-2

Sebaceous Carcinoma

- Invasive basaloid to squamoid tumor with interspersed clear cells with bubbly cytoplasm
- Ducts with pink cuticles may be present but are rare
- EMA (cytoplasmic staining), adipophilin, and AR staining are typically positive

SELECTED REFERENCES

1. Soni A et al: Current management approach to hidradenocarcinoma: a comprehensive review of the literature. Ecancermedicalscience. 9:517, 2015
2. Bhullar JS et al: Hidradenocarcinoma: a sinister diagnosis of a suspected benign condition. Am Surg. 80(12):1271-2, 2014
3. Wahl CE et al: Apocrine hidradenocarcinoma showing Paget's disease and mucinous metaplasia. J Cutan Pathol. 36(5):582-5, 2009
4. Hernández-Pérez E et al: Nodular hidradenoma and hidradenocarcinoma. A 10-year review. J Am Acad Dermatol. 12(1 Pt 1):15-20, 1985

Hidradenocarcinoma: Deep-Seated Tumor With Necrosis

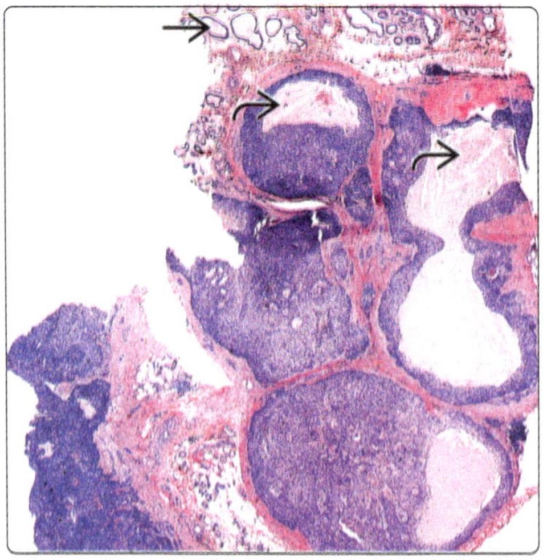

Hidradenocarcinoma: Perineural Invasion

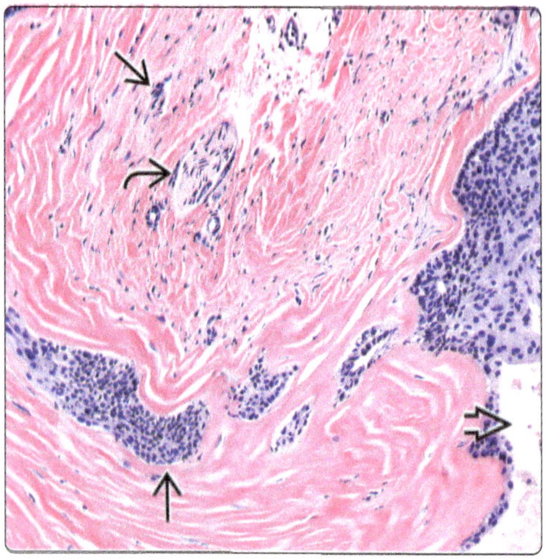

(Left) *Scanning magnification of a hidradenocarcinoma from the axilla shows normal apocrine glands → at the top of the photo. The tumor is deep-seated, has cystic areas containing necrotic cellular debris →, and is composed of basaloid and clear cells.* **(Right)** *Higher power view of a hidradenocarcinoma shows infiltrative islands → of cytologically atypical cells in a densely hyalinized stroma. There is focal perineural invasion →. Focal cystic spaces → are also seen at the edge of the field.*

Hidradenocarcinoma With Dense Nodular to Sheet-Like Areas

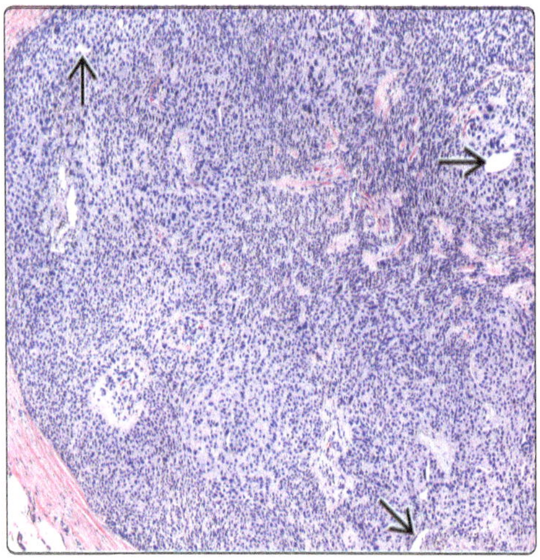

Hidradenocarcinoma: Infiltrative Cords

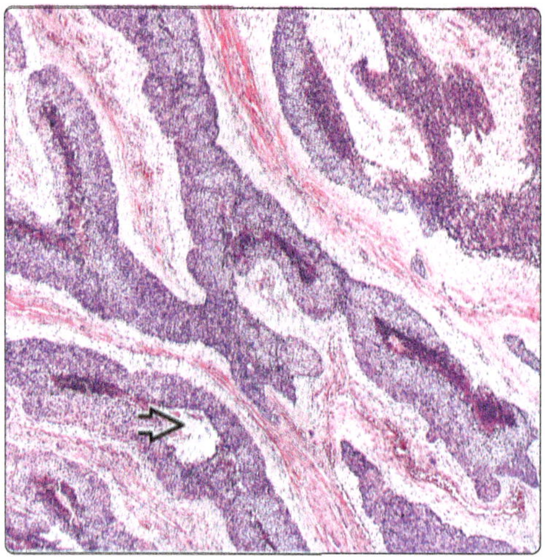

(Left) *Nodular hidradenocarcinoma at low magnification demonstrates a large tumor composed of sheets of cells showing prominent cytologic atypia, pleomorphism, and scattered ductal lumina →.* **(Right)** *Hidradenocarcinoma with an infiltrative, cord-like proliferation of basaloid to clear-staining cells also shows a focal cystic area containing mucinous material →.*

Hidradenocarcinoma: Mitoses, Necrosis, and Apoptosis

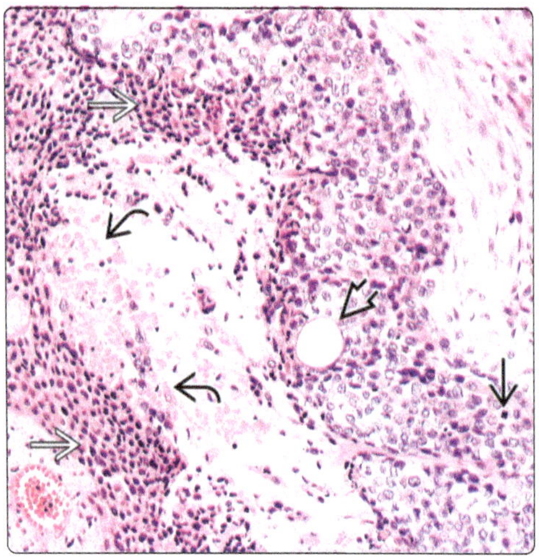

Mucinous Hidradenocarcinoma

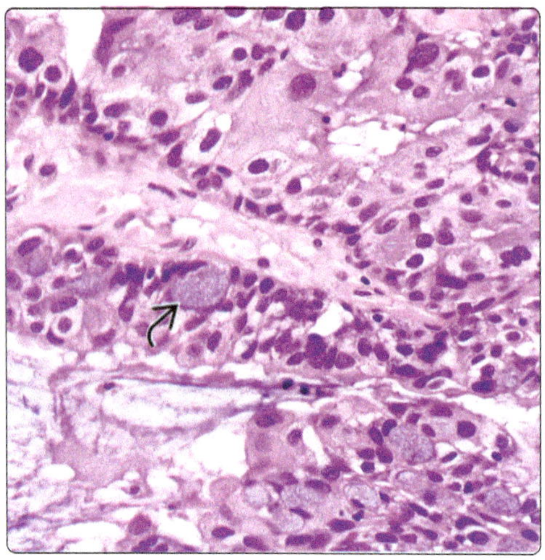

(Left) *High magnification of an area of hidradenocarcinoma with predominantly clear cell features and focal ductal differentiation → demonstrates mitotic figures →, clusters of apoptotic cells →, and necrotic cellular debris →.* **(Right)** *Mucinous features are rarely seen in hidradenocarcinoma. This case shows a proliferation of markedly enlarged and atypical-appearing, eosinophilic-staining cells with focal goblet cells showing cytoplasmic mucin →.*

Differential Diagnosis: Hidradenoma

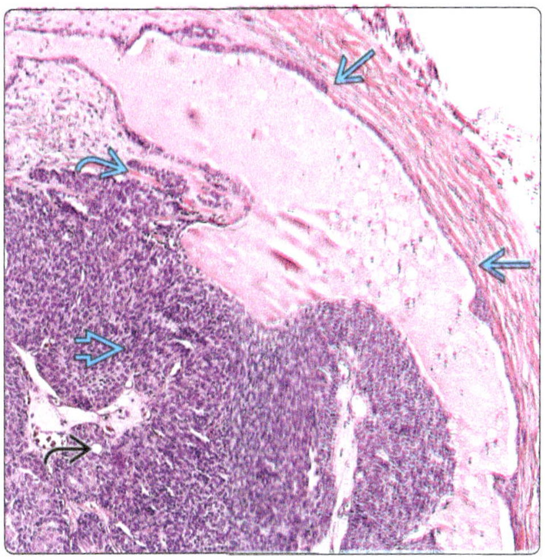

Differential Diagnosis: Hidradenoma With Typical Hyaline Stroma

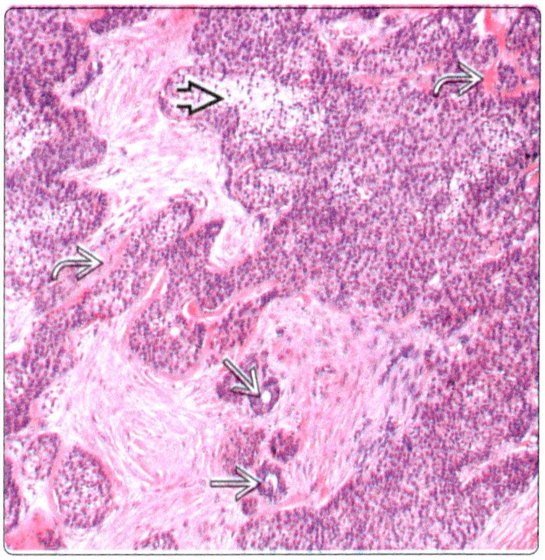

(Left) *In contrast to hidradenocarcinoma, hidradenomas are well circumscribed, typically composed of poroid to clear cells, and have hyaline stroma. Focal ductal differentiation is also seen.* **(Right)** *Low magnification of a hidradenoma shows hyalinized stroma, which can suggest an infiltrative tumor but is common in hidradenomas. The tumor cells are basaloid to focally clear staining. There is also focal ductal differentiation present.*

Hidradenoma With Mucinous Differentiation

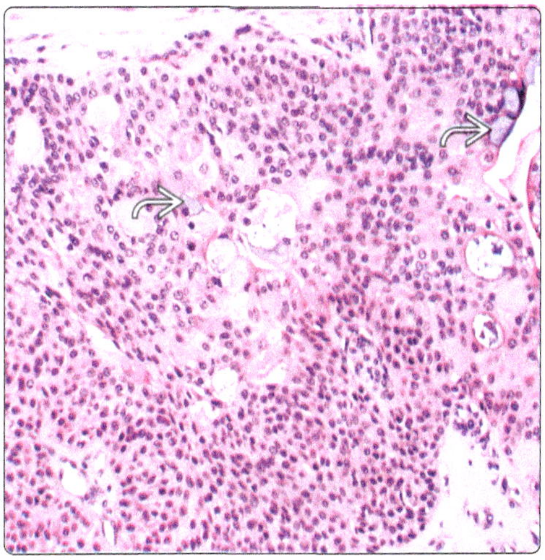

Hidradenocarcinoma With Mucinous Cells

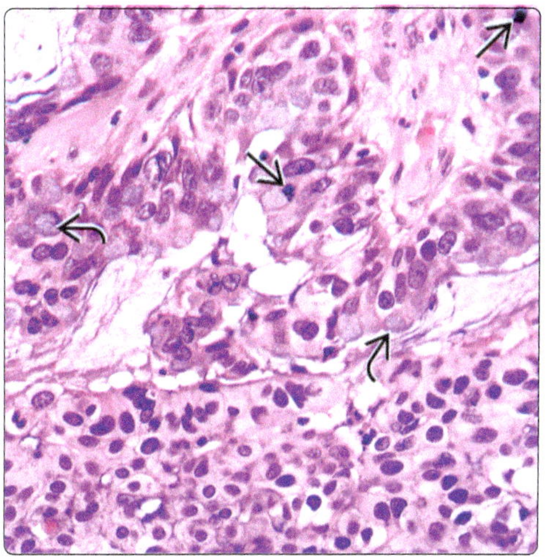

(Left) *Mucinous differentiation can be seen in a minority of cases of hidradenoma (and very rarely in hidradenocarcinoma). In this area, numerous goblet-like cells containing abundant cytoplasmic mucin are seen lining cystic spaces.* **(Right)** *Mucinous features are rarely seen in hidradenocarcinoma. This case shows a proliferation of markedly enlarged and atypical-appearing, eosinophilic-staining cells with focal cytoplasmic mucin. Several mitotic figures are present in this field.*

Hidradenocarcinoma With Pagetoid Spread

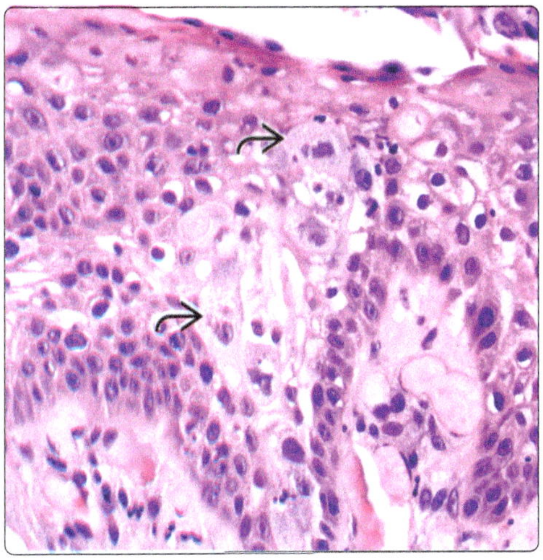

Differential Diagnosis: Porocarcinoma

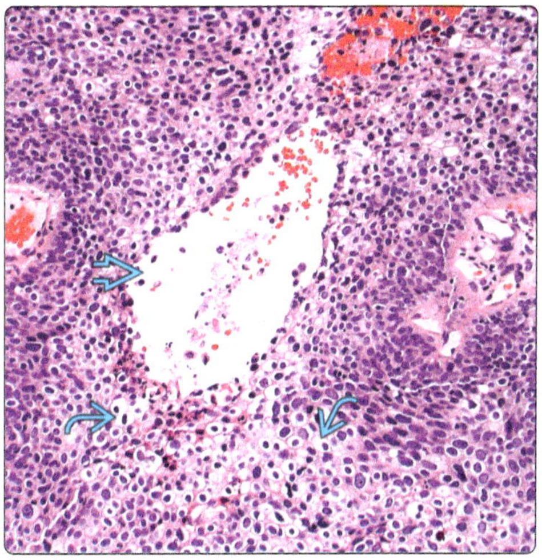

(Left) *Pagetoid spread in mucinous hidradenocarcinoma shows intraepidermal spread of atypical-appearing cells with abundant mucinous-appearing cytoplasm. This is a very rare finding that has been reported in only a few cases.* **(Right)** *Porocarcinoma and hidradenocarcinoma show overlapping features, including ductal/glandular spaces and atypical poroid and clear cells, which were prominent in this case. However, the tumor showed multiple overlying epidermal connections, findings typical of porocarcinoma.*

Poroma and Dermal Duct Tumor

KEY FACTS

TERMINOLOGY

- Eccrine poroma
- Apocrine poroma
- Hidroacanthoma simplex (intraepidermal poroma, syringoacanthoma)
- Benign adnexal proliferation with anastomosing cords of cells and ductal differentiation

CLINICAL ISSUES

- Relatively common tumors
- Usually occur in middle-aged adults
- Most common on the extremities, especially the palmar and plantar surfaces
- Solitary pink to reddish papular or nodular lesion
- Complete excision typically recommended to prevent recurrence and rare transformation to porocarcinoma
- Excellent prognosis in most cases; only rare transformation to porocarcinoma

MACROSCOPIC

- Generally < 1 cm but may be larger

MICROSCOPIC

- Symmetric, well-circumscribed tumor with multiple epidermal attachments (except in dermal duct tumor)
- Broad, anastomosing columns and thickened cords of tumor cells
- Ductal lumina typically well-formed, numerous
- Cells may be basaloid, squamoid, clear, or pigmented
- Mitotic figures may be present, and can be numerous in traumatized lesions

TOP DIFFERENTIAL DIAGNOSES

- Hidradenoma
- Irritated/clonal seborrheic keratosis
- Basal cell carcinoma
- Squamous cell carcinoma
- Porocarcinoma (malignant poroma)

Clinical Photograph of Poroma

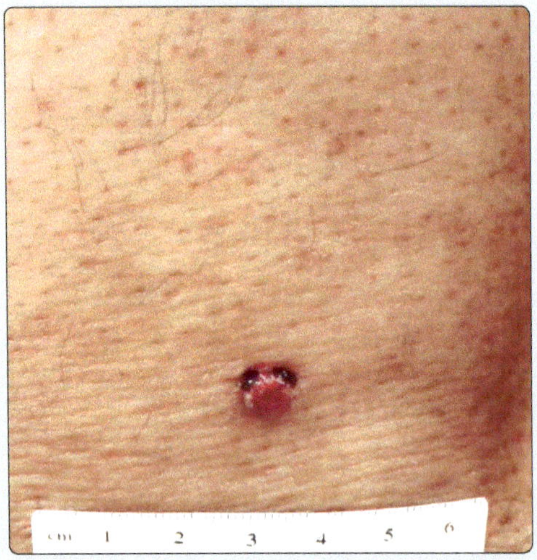

Poroma With Squamoid Features

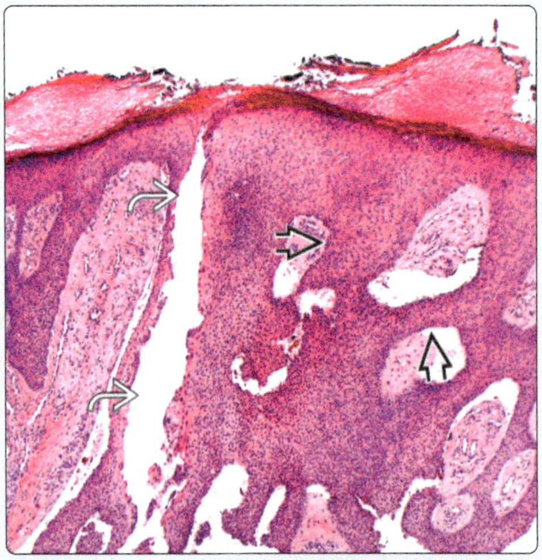

(Left) *Clinical photograph shows a traumatized poroma on the lower back of an adult male, which presented as an irritated polypoid lesion.* **(Right)** *Low magnification of a poroma with squamoid features shows a basaloid to squamoid-appearing neoplasm with multiple anastomosing connections between thickened cords of tumor cells and to epidermis. Note the ectatic ductal space on the left.*

Poroma With Clear Cell Features

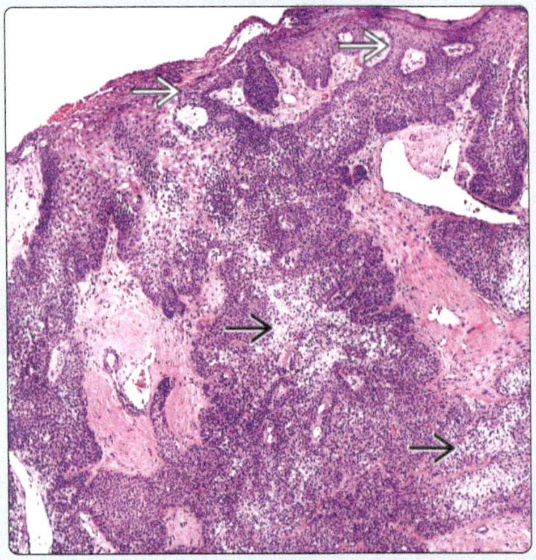

Higher Magnification of Clear Cell Poroma

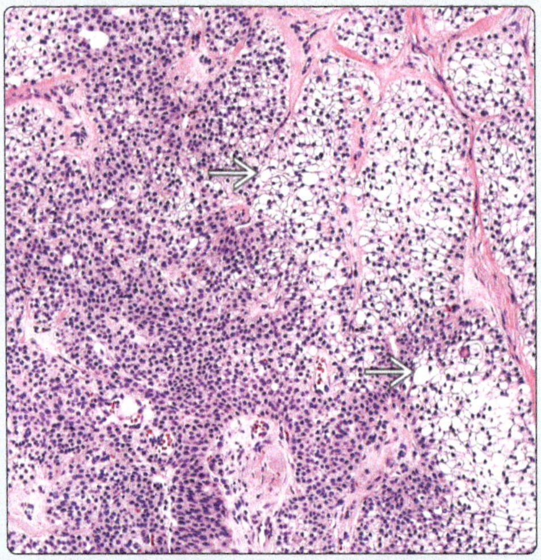

(Left) *Scanning magnification of a poroma with clear cell features shows a basaloid to clear cell neoplasm with multiple anastomosing connections between thickened cords of tumor cells and to epidermis.* **(Right)** *Higher magnification of a clear cell area of poroma shows a proliferation of small cells with abundant pale to clear-staining cytoplasm and small nuclei lacking atypia.*

TERMINOLOGY

Synonyms

- Apocrine poroma
- Eccrine poroma
- Hidroacanthoma simplex (intraepidermal poroma, syringoacanthoma)

Definitions

- Benign adnexal proliferation with anastomosing cords of tumor cells exhibiting ductal differentiation

ETIOLOGY/PATHOGENESIS

Unknown

- Formerly considered eccrine, but most cases likely of apocrine differentiation
  - May see sebaceous &/or follicular differentiation in apocrine cases

CLINICAL ISSUES

Epidemiology

- Incidence
  - Relatively common tumors
- Age
  - Usually occur in middle-aged adults
- Sex
  - Equal incidence in males and females

Site

- Most common on extremities, especially palmar and plantar surfaces

Presentation

- Solitary pink to reddish papular or nodular lesion

Natural History

- Stable lesions; do not usually regress

Treatment

- Surgical approaches
  - Complete conservative excision is curative

Prognosis

- Excellent; most cases do not show aggressive behavior

MACROSCOPIC

General Features

- Superficial, firm papule or nodule

Size

- Generally < 1 cm but may be larger

MICROSCOPIC

Histologic Features

- Symmetric, well-circumscribed tumor with multiple epidermal attachments
  - Intraepidermal component is typically sharply demarcated from adjacent normal epidermis
- Broad, anastomosing columns and thickened cords of tumor cells
- Ductal lumina small, but usually numerous
  - A few small cystic structures may also be present
- Composed of basaloid to squamoid-appearing cells
  - Most cells are small, cuboidal-shaped and have bland nuclei with uniform chromatin
  - Cells may also be clear or pigmented
- Mitotic figures may be present and can be numerous in traumatized lesions

Subtypes

- **Dermal duct tumor**
  - Similar-appearing tumor in dermis
  - Epidermal attachments often found if multiple deeper level sections examined
- **Hidroacanthoma simplex (intraepidermal poroma)**
  - Intraepidermal proliferation of nests of monotonous basaloid cells

DIFFERENTIAL DIAGNOSIS

Hidradenoma

- Closely related tumors (grouped together under "acrospiroma"), **but**
  - Typically deep dermal-based nodule lacking epidermal connections

Irritated/Clonal Seborrheic Keratosis

- Irritated seborrheic keratosis (SK) may occasionally mimic poroma (and hidroacanthoma simplex); **however**
  - SK shows follicular differentiation with keratinizing pseudohorn cysts, no ductal differentiation

Porocarcinoma (Malignant Poroma)

- Malignant poroid tumor; can be in situ or invasive
- Often arise in longstanding poroma
- Increased cytologic atypia, pleomorphism, and mitotic figures (including atypical forms)

Basal Cell Carcinoma

- Not difficult to separate from poroma except in some small, superficial biopsies
  - Areas of peripheral palisading, mucinous stroma, and tumor-stromal retraction artifact present

Squamous Cell Carcinoma

- Usually not difficult to separate from poroma except in small biopsies
  - Poromas show squamoid features in many cases
  - Greater cytologic atypia, dyskeratotic cells in squamous cell carcinoma (SCC)

SELECTED REFERENCES

1. Bloom BS et al: Collision tumor of eccrine poroma, seborrheic keratosis, and a viral wart. Dermatol Online J. 20(12), 2014
2. Sawaya JL et al: Poroma: a review of eccrine, apocrine, and malignant forms. Int J Dermatol. 53(9):1053-61, 2014
3. Mitsuishi T et al: Pigmented poroid neoplasm mimicking nodular melanoma. J Dermatol. 37(6):542-4, 2010
4. Galadari E et al: Malignant transformation of eccrine tumors. J Cutan Pathol. 14(1):15-22, 1987
5. Pylyser K et al: The histology of eccrine poromas: a study of 14 cases. Dermatologica. 167(5):243-9, 1983
6. Goldman P et al: Eccrine poroma; tumors exhibiting features of the epidermal sweat duct unit. AMA Arch Derm. 74(5):511-21, 1956

Poroma at Low Magnification

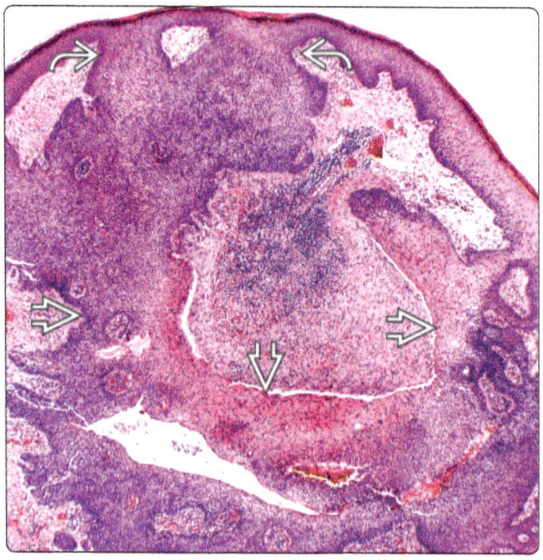

Poroma at High Magnification

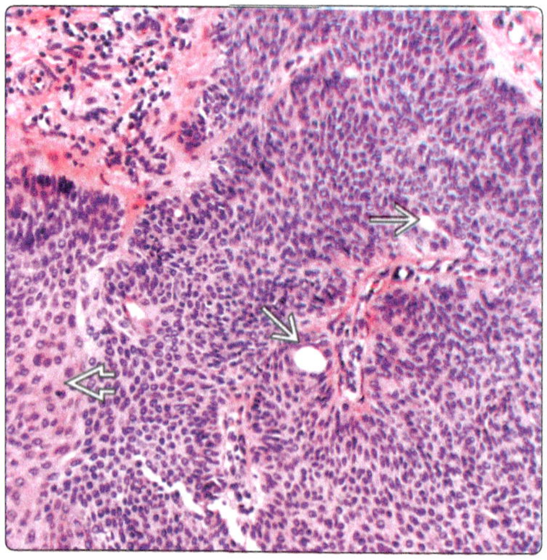

(Left) *Low magnification of a poroma shows a basaloid to squamoid tumor with multiple thickened, anastomosing connections between the tumor cords ➡ and to the overlying epidermis ➡.* **(Right)** *Higher magnification of a poroma shows a proliferation of small basaloid to focally squamoid ➡ cells forming thick, anastomosing cords. Note the scattered small ductal lumina ➡.*

Traumatized Poroma at Low Magnification

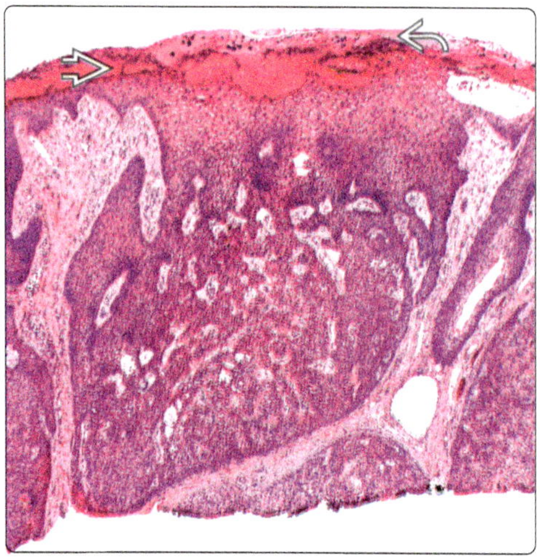

Traumatized Poroma at High Magnification

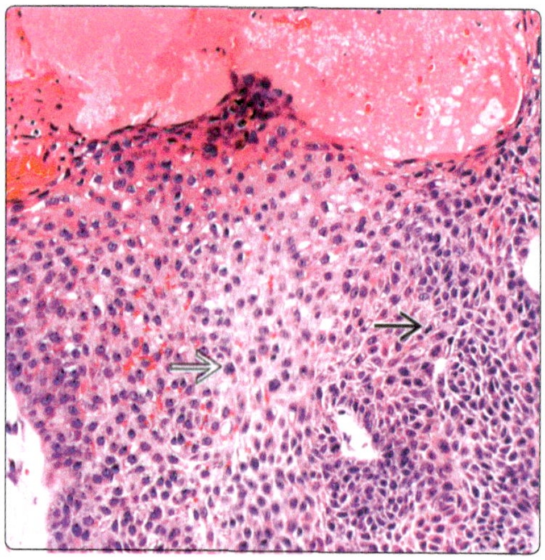

(Left) *Traumatized poroma shows overlying erosion, dense serum crusting ➡, and impetiginization ➡. Reactive atypia may be seen in cases with recent irritation/trauma.* **(Right)** *Higher magnification of a traumatized poroma shows mild nuclear enlargement and hyperchromasia ➡, as well as a few (nonatypical) mitotic figures ➡, consistent with reactive changes due to irritation/trauma.*

Pigmented Poroma

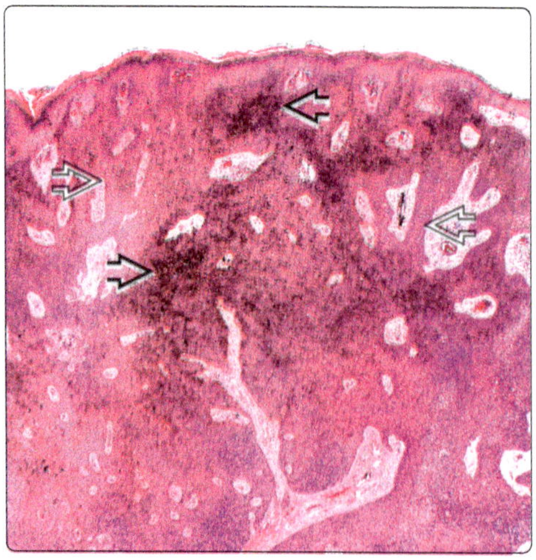

Pigmented Poroma at Higher Magnification

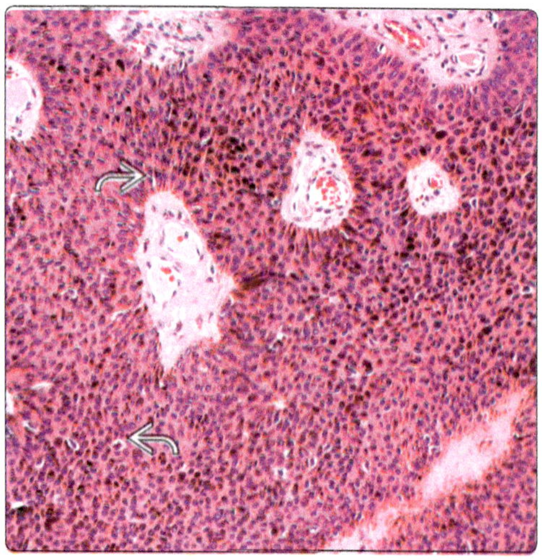

(Left) *Pigmented poroma is not an uncommon variant. Although many of the cells are darkly pigmented ➡, it otherwise shows features typical of poroma, being composed of basaloid to squamoid cells forming multiple thickened, anastomosing connections between the tumor cords ➡.* **(Right)** *High magnification of a pigmented poroma shows a bland-appearing population of small basaloid to squamoid cells with prominent cytoplasmic pigmentation. Colonizing melanocytes ➡ are present.*

CK5/6 Immunohistochemistry in Poroma

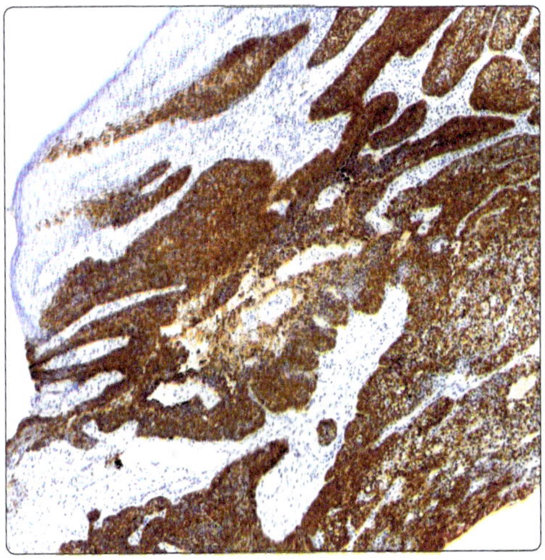

Ki-67 Immunohistochemistry in Poroma

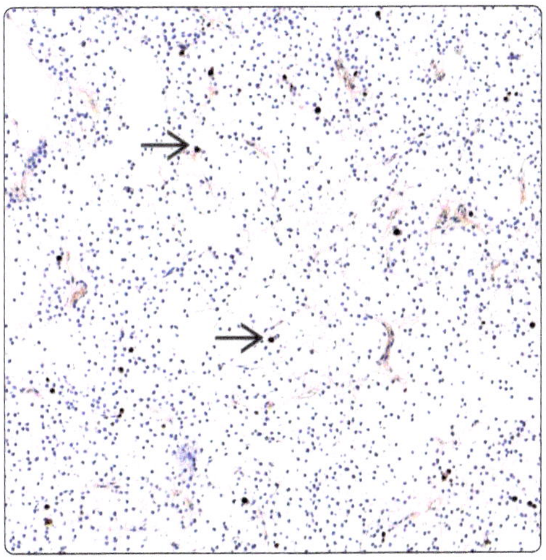

(Left) *High molecular weight cytokeratins including CK5/6 and CK903/34βE12 are typically strongly and diffusely positive in poroma and porocarcinoma, similar to most adnexal tumors.* **(Right)** *Ki-67 highlights scattered nuclei* → *in a poroma, consistent with a low nuclear proliferative rate (< 5% in most cases).*

Differential Diagnosis: Nodular Hidradenoma

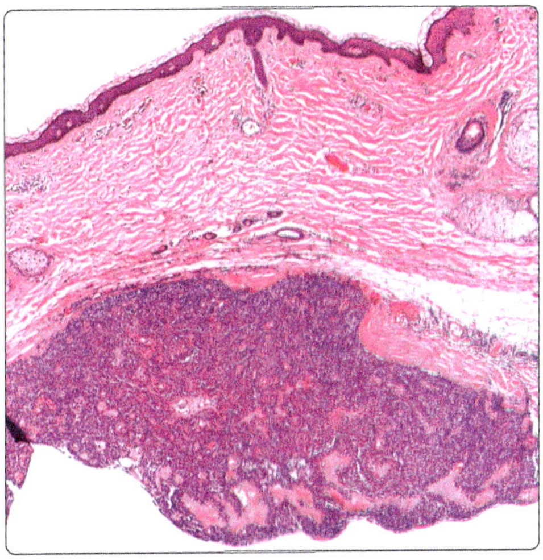

Differential Diagnosis: Nodular Hidradenoma

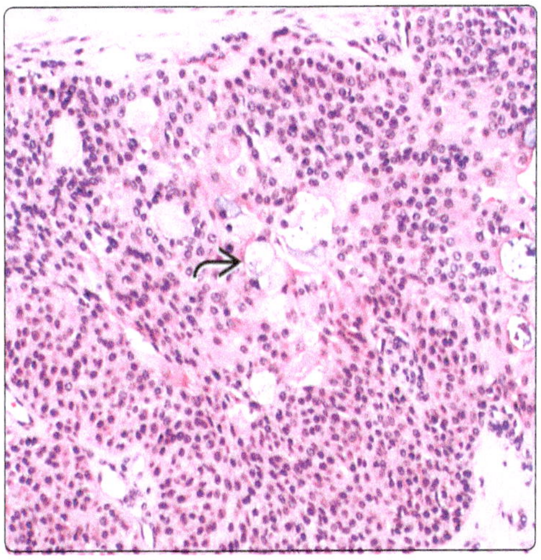

(Left) *Nodular-cystic hidradenoma is a closely related tumor (and may be grouped together under the term acrospiroma), but it is typically situated deeper in the dermis, often shows clear cell features, and lacks connections to the epidermis.* **(Right)** *High magnification of a hidradenoma shows pale eosinophilic to clear-staining cells and focal mucinous metaplasia with goblet cells* →*. This is not an uncommon finding in hidradenomas but is extremely rare in poromas.*

Differential Diagnosis: Sarcomatoid Porocarcinoma

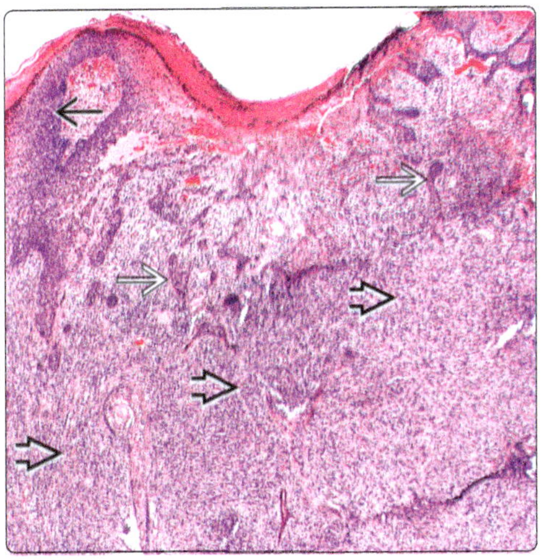

Differential Diagnosis: Sarcomatoid Porocarcinoma

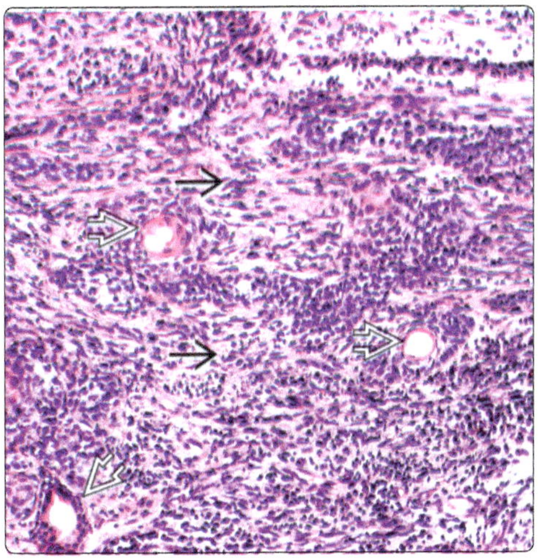

(Left) *Scanning magnification of sarcomatoid porocarcinoma shows an in situ component* → *with areas of ulceration that is overlying an invasive tumor composed of epithelial islands* → *surrounded by poorly differentiated spindle cells* →*.* **(Right)** *Invasive porocarcinoma with sarcomatoid features shows scattered, well-differentiated ductal structures* → *that are surrounded by infiltrative atypical spindle cells* →*.*

KEY FACTS

TERMINOLOGY

- Malignant poroma

ETIOLOGY/PATHOGENESIS

- May arise from malignant transformation of longstanding poroma

CLINICAL ISSUES

- Rare tumors
- Usually occur in elderly patients
- Acral surfaces most common
- Significant rate of metastasis (up to 50% of cases)
- Complete surgical excision is recommended to ensure complete removal
    - Mohs surgery reported to be effective

MICROSCOPIC

- Epidermal-based atypical adnexal tumor with anastomosing cords of tumor cells
- Most cases are invasive, but some may be completely intraepidermal (porocarcinoma in situ)
- Cells are usually basaloid, but may show clear cell, squamoid, or spindle cell features
- Mitotic figures are usually numerous and may be atypical
- Rare sarcomatoid variants have been reported, with invasive spindle cell component

ANCILLARY TESTS

- Ductal/glandular lumina usually positive for EMA and CEA-m
- Tumor cells are usually diffusely positive for pancytokeratins, high molecular weight cytokeratins (i.e., CK5/CK6), and p63

TOP DIFFERENTIAL DIAGNOSES

- Poroma
- Hidradenoma and hidradenocarcinoma
- Squamous cell carcinoma
- Basal cell carcinoma

(Left) *This is an example of an invasive, well-differentiated porocarcinoma. Note the focal epidermal attachments ➡ and clear cell features ➡. Focal squamoid differentiation is also seen ➡.* **(Right)** *Higher magnification of well-differentiated porocarcinoma shows collections of pale eosinophilic to clear-staining cells showing cytologic atypia and multiple mitotic figures ➡.*

Well-Differentiated Porocarcinoma

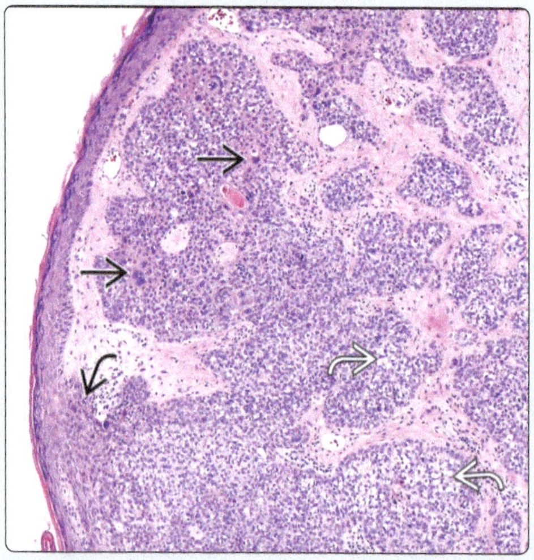

Well-Differentiated Porocarcinoma at Higher Magnification

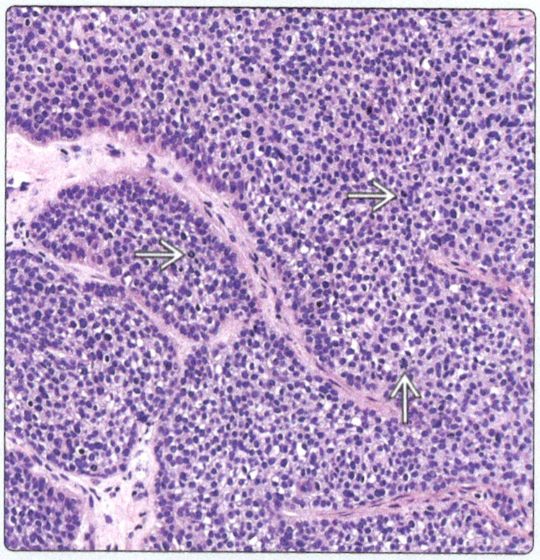

(Left) *Scanning magnification of porocarcinoma shows an situ component ➡ overlying an invasive tumor composed of epithelial islands ➡ surrounded by poorly differentiated spindle cells ➡.* **(Right)** *Invasive porocarcinoma with sarcomatoid features. Note the scattered well-differentiated ductal structures ➡, which are surrounded by infiltrative atypical spindle cells ➡.*

Invasive Sarcomatoid Porocarcinoma

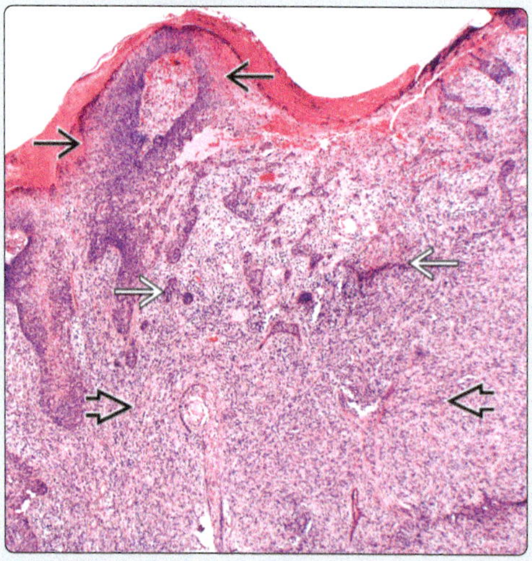

Invasive Sarcomatoid Porocarcinoma at Higher Magnification

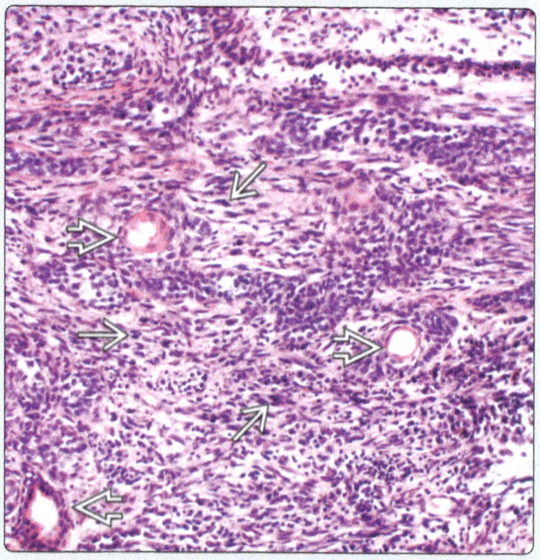

TERMINOLOGY

Synonyms

- Malignant poroma

Definitions

- Malignant adnexal tumor with ductal differentiation

ETIOLOGY/PATHOGENESIS

Unknown

- May arise from malignant transformation of longstanding poroma
- Rare cases have been reported in nevus sebaceus

CLINICAL ISSUES

Epidemiology

- Incidence
  - Rare tumors; ~ 200 cases reported
- Age
  - Usually occur in elderly patients

Site

- Predilection for extremities
  - Acral surfaces most common

Presentation

- Plaque or polypoid tumor

Treatment

- Surgical approaches
  - Complete surgical excision is recommended to ensure complete removal
    - Mohs surgery reported to be effective

Prognosis

- Significant rate of metastasis (up to 40-50% reported, usually to lymph nodes)

MACROSCOPIC

Size

- Typically large tumors, several cm

MICROSCOPIC

Histologic Features

- Epidermal-based atypical adnexal tumor with anastomosing cords of tumor cells
  - Most cases are invasive, but some show only intraepidermal growth (porocarcinoma in situ)
- Ductal structures are typically found and are often numerous in well-differentiated cases
- Cells are usually basaloid but may show clear cell or squamoid features
- Rare sarcomatoid variants have been reported, with invasive spindle cell component
- Mitotic figures usually numerous and may be atypical

Cytologic Features

- Cells show cytologic atypia, with enlarged, hyperchromatic-staining nuclei and prominent nucleoli

ANCILLARY TESTS

Immunohistochemistry

- Immunohistochemistry usually not necessary but can be useful to confirm diagnosis
  - Ductal/glandular lumina usually positive for EMA and CEA-m
    - Squamous cell carcinoma and basal cell carcinoma lack luminal staining
  - Tumor cells are usually diffusely positive for pancytokeratins, high molecular weight cytokeratins (i.e., CK5/CK6), and p63
    - Metastatic tumors to skin are typically negative for CK5/CK6 and p63

DIFFERENTIAL DIAGNOSIS

Poroma

- May be difficult to distinguish from porocarcinoma on superficial shave biopsy
  - Particularly if tumor is traumatized &/or inflamed and shows reactive changes
- Epidermal-based neoplasm with multiple anastomosing cords of tumor cells
- Lacks dermal invasion, significant cytologic atypia, and necrosis
- Mitoses often present but not numerous or atypical

Hidradenoma and Hidradenocarcinoma

- Dermal-based tumors without prominent anastomosing connections (unlike poroma and porocarcinoma)
- Usually nodular, well-circumscribed tumors, although hidradenocarcinomas are usually infiltrative
- Clear cell change more common and squamoid features less common than in poroid neoplasms

Squamous Cell Carcinoma

- Invasive epithelial tumor composed of large squamoid cells with abundant eosinophilic cytoplasm
- Squamoid variant of porocarcinoma may be difficult to distinguish from squamous cell carcinoma (SCC), **but**
  - SCC lacks ductal structures (can be highlighted with EMA and CEA)
  - Porocarcinoma shows more anastomosing tumor cords

Basal Cell Carcinoma

- Most cases easily distinguishable
- Basal cell carcinoma shows peripheral palisading, mucinous stroma, and tumor-stroma retraction artifact
- Porocarcinoma shows more anastomosing cords and at least focal ductal structures

SELECTED REFERENCES

1. Le MD et al: Biphasic sarcomatoid porocarcinoma. Am J Dermatopathol. ePub, 2015
2. Riera-Leal L et al: Eccrine porocarcinoma: epidemiologic and histopathologic characteristics. Int J Dermatol. 54(5):580-6, 2015
3. Song SS et al: Mohs micrographic surgery for eccrine porocarcinoma: an update and review of the literature. Dermatol Surg. 41(3):301-6, 2015
4. Mahomed F et al: The squamous variant of eccrine porocarcinoma: a clinicopathological study of 21 cases. J Clin Pathol. 61(3):361-5, 2008
5. Gschnait F et al: Eccrine porocarcinoma. J Cutan Pathol. 7(6):349-53, 1980

Cylindroma

KEY FACTS

TERMINOLOGY

- Turban tumor (clinical term for multiple tumors on head)
- Benign, dermal-based adnexal tumor with distinctive jigsaw puzzle pattern

ETIOLOGY/PATHOGENESIS

- Familial cases associated with Brooke-Spiegler syndrome
- Mutation of *CYLD* found in both sporadic and familial cases

CLINICAL ISSUES

- Marked female predominance (F:M = 9:1)
- 90% present on head and neck

MICROSCOPIC

- Dermal-based tumor, circumscribed but not encapsulated
- Composed of multiple nodules/lobules of basaloid cells
- Tumor lobules have complex pattern, appearing to fit together in jigsaw puzzle pattern
- Tumor lobules surrounded by dense eosinophilic basement membrane material
- Lobules have 2 cell types: Small basaloid cells and larger pale cells
- Focal ductal lumen formation
- Globules of hyaline basement membrane material often present in interior of tumor nodules

TOP DIFFERENTIAL DIAGNOSES

- Spiradenoma
  - Can have areas indistinguishable from cylindroma
  - Usually encapsulated
  - Tumor stroma has prominent vasculature
- Malignant cylindroma/cylindrocarcinoma
- Basal cell carcinoma
  - Peripheral palisading with tumor-stroma retraction
- Trichoblastoma
  - Tumor lobule surrounded by fibroblastic stroma; not thick basement membrane

(Left) *Cylindroma is typically a dermal-based, well-circumscribed but unencapsulated tumor without connections to the overlying dermis.* **(Right)** *This low-power image of cylindroma demonstrates the jigsaw puzzle arrangement of the tumor lobules filling the dermis.*

Classic Cylindroma

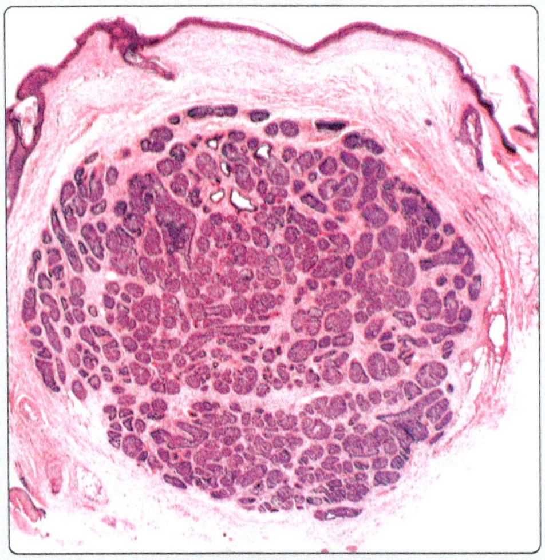

Superficial Portion of Cylindroma

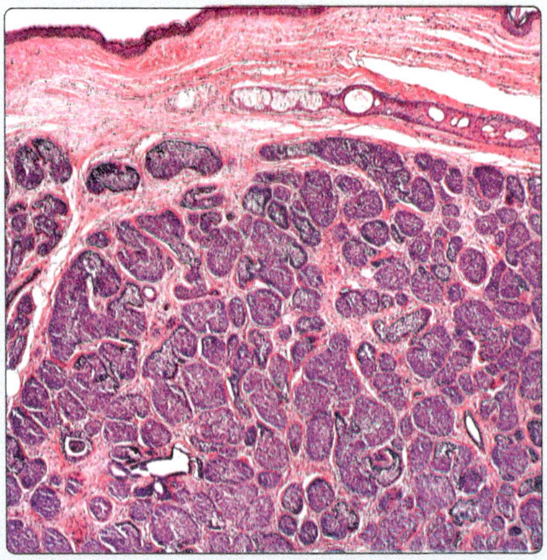

(Left) *The tumor lobules are surrounded by a dense, eosinophilic basement membrane ⇨ and show intratumoral hyalinized globules ➡.* **(Right)** *This higher power image demonstrates how the tumor lobules fit together in an irregular jigsaw puzzle pattern. Note the prominent basement membranes surrounding the tumor lobules that are characteristic of cylindroma.*

Cylindroma With Hyalinized Membranes

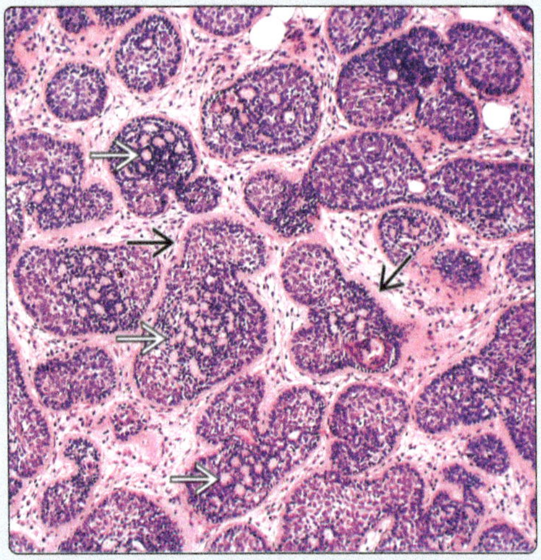

Cylindroma at High Magnification

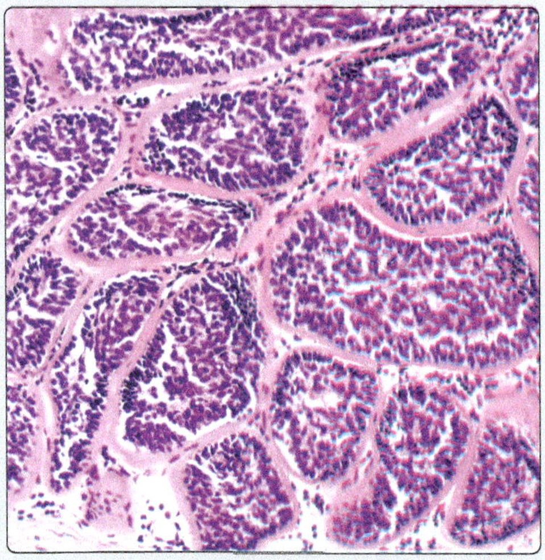

TERMINOLOGY

Synonyms

- Dermal cylindroma
- Turban tumor (clinical term for multiple tumors on head)

Definitions

- Benign, dermal-based adnexal tumor with distinctive jigsaw puzzle pattern
- May show apocrine differentiation in most cases (formerly considered eccrine)

ETIOLOGY/PATHOGENESIS

Loss of Heterozygosity of Tumor Suppressor Gene *CYLD*

- Mutation of *CYLD* found in both sporadic and familial cases

Sporadic or Familial

- Familial cases associated with Brooke-Spiegler syndrome
  - a.k.a., familial cylindromatosis or turban tumor syndrome
  - Autosomal dominant
  - Predilection for women
  - Eccrine spiradenomas and trichoepitheliomas often present

CLINICAL ISSUES

Epidemiology

- Incidence
  - Common adnexal tumor of sweat glands
- Age
  - Usually early adulthood
- Sex
  - Marked female predominance (F:M = 9:1)

Site

- 90% present on head and neck; 60% on scalp

Presentation

- Dermal mass

Treatment

- Surgical approaches
  - Complete excision is curative

Prognosis

- Benign; may recur if incompletely excised
- Rare transformation to malignant cylindroma (cylindrocarcinoma), usually in large, longstanding tumors

MICROSCOPIC

Histologic Features

- Usually located in upper dermis
- No attachments to epidermis
- Circumscribed but not encapsulated
- Multiple nodules/lobules of basaloid cells surrounded by dense eosinophilic basement membrane
- Tumor lobules have complex pattern, where tumor lobules appear to fit together in irregular jigsaw puzzle-like pattern
- Tumor lobules have 2 cell types
  - Outer, small basaloid cells with small hyperchromatic nuclei
  - Inner cells have larger oval vesicular nuclei
  - Tumor cells positive for CK6, CK7, CK19, and EMA
  - Basaloid myoepithelial cells positive for SMA, calponin, and S100
- Focal ductal lumen formation
  - Lumina positive for CEA and EMA
- Globules of PAS(+), diastase resistant, hyaline basement membrane material often present in tumor lobules
- Mitotic figures rare

DIFFERENTIAL DIAGNOSIS

Spiradenoma

- Encapsulated tumor composed of nodules of small basophilic tumor cells
- Significant histologic overlap with cylindroma
  - 2 cell types essentially same as cylindroma
  - Tumor nodules can have thickened basement membrane
  - Tumor nodules can have globules of hyaline material
  - Can have areas indistinguishable from cylindroma
  - Essentially same immunophenotype as cylindroma
- Ductal lumen formation more frequent
- Tumor stroma has prominent vasculature and often hemorrhage

Malignant Cylindroma/Cylindrocarcinoma

- Rare tumor
- Infiltrative growth with loss of jigsaw pattern
- Loss of thickened basement membrane and biphasic cell population of cylindroma
- Overt cytologic atypia and frequent mitotic figures

Basal Cell Carcinoma

- Attachments to epidermis often present
- Peripheral palisading with mucin and tumor-stroma retraction
- Lacks jigsaw pattern and duct formation
- Lacks thickened basement membrane
- Mitotic and apoptotic figures often abundant

Trichoblastoma

- Dermal-based lobules of basaloid epithelium, circumscribed but not encapsulated
- Peripheral palisading surrounded by fibroblastic stroma
- No thickened hyalinized basement membranes
- Papillary mesenchymal bodies

SELECTED REFERENCES

1. Dubois A et al: CYLD genetic testing for Brooke-Spiegler syndrome, familial cylindromatosis and multiple familial trichoepitheliomas. PLoS Curr. 7, 2015
2. Kazakov DV et al: Morphologic diversity of malignant neoplasms arising in preexisting spiradenoma, cylindroma, and spiradenocylindroma based on the study of 24 cases, sporadic or occurring in the setting of Brooke-Spiegler syndrome. Am J Surg Pathol. 33(5):705-19, 2009
3. Scheinfeld N et al: Identification of a recurrent mutation in the CYLD gene in Brooke-Spiegler syndrome. Clin Exp Dermatol. 28(5):539-41, 2003
4. van der Putte SC: The pathogenesis of familial multiple cylindromas, trichoepitheliomas, milia, and spiradenomas. Am J Dermatopathol. 17(3):271-80, 1995
5. Crain RC et al: Dermal cylindroma (dermal eccrine cylindroma). Am J Clin Pathol. 35:504-15, 1961

Cylindroma With Subcutaneous Involvement

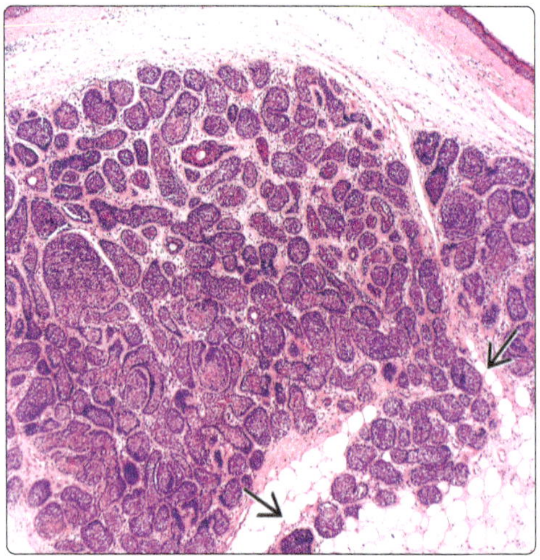

Cylindroma Showing Ductal Areas

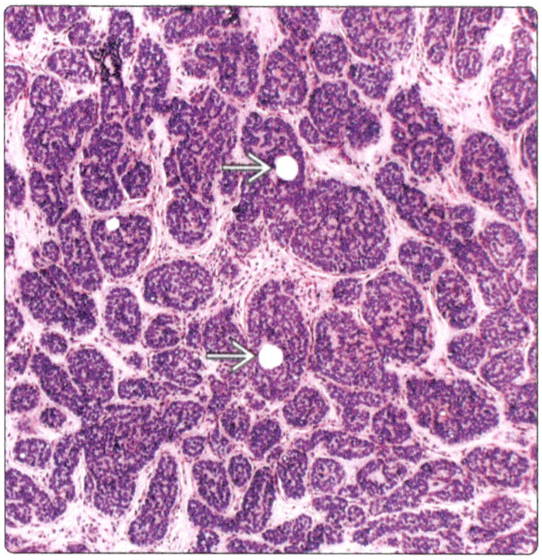

(Left) *Some otherwise typical-appearing cylindromas extend into the subcutaneous fat* →. **(Right)** *Duct lumen* → *formation is present. The presence of true lumina can aid in the distinction of cylindroma from basal cell carcinoma. Lumen formation is often a focal finding.*

Cylindroma: Cytologic Features

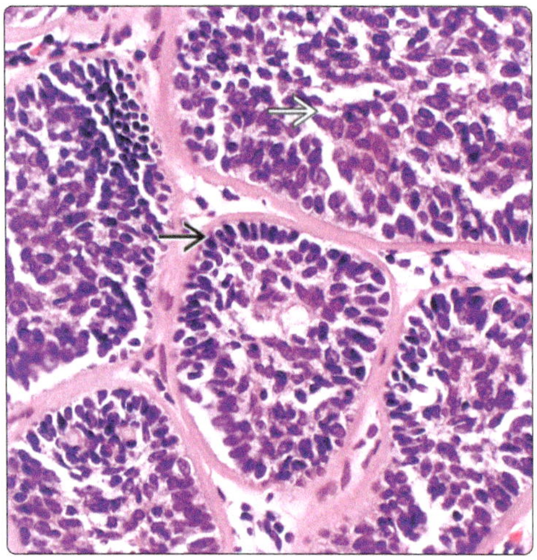

PAS-D Stain in Cylindroma

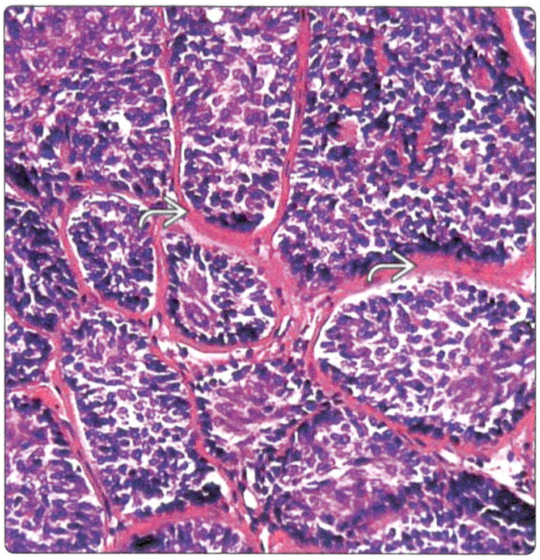

(Left) *The smaller basaloid cells are usually at the periphery* → *and may demonstrate peripheral palisading. The larger cells* → *have more cytoplasm and a larger, pale-staining nucleus. They are typically in the central portion of the tumor lobule.* **(Right)** *PAS stain with diastase digestion shows strong, pink staining of the hyalinized membranes* → *surrounding the tumor nests and lobules.*

Cylindroma With Nodular Area

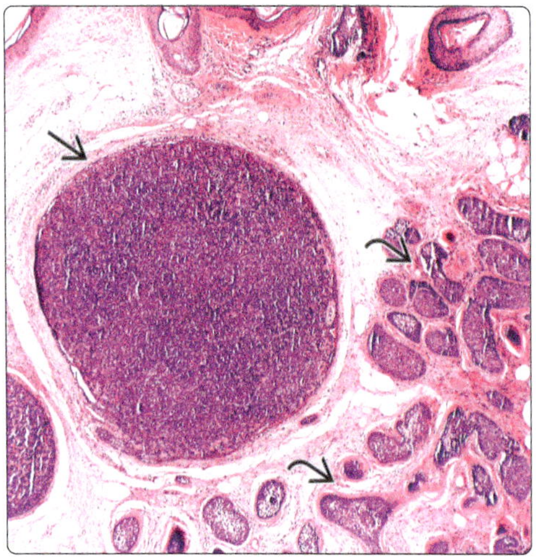

Cylindroma With Focal Retraction Artifact

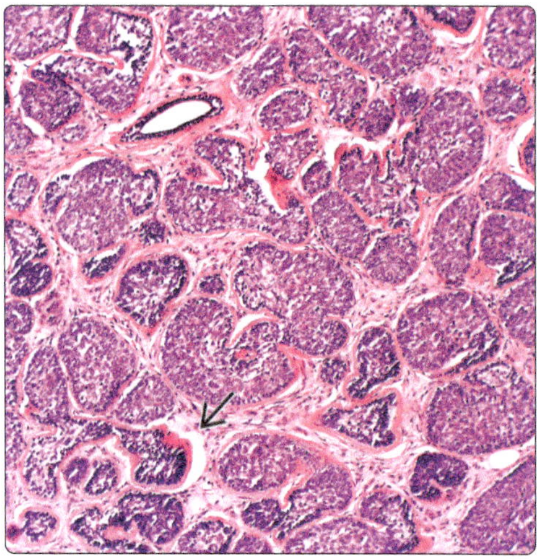

(Left) *Occasional cylindromas will have discrete nodules* → *without the classic jigsaw-like growth pattern. The right portion of the image demonstrates the more typical growth pattern* →. **(Right)** *Some cylindromas will have retraction artifact* → *separating the tumor from the surrounding stroma. However, note that the thick basement membrane is still attached to the tumor lobule; this helps distinguish the tumor from basal cell carcinoma.*

Differential Diagnosis: Spiradenoma

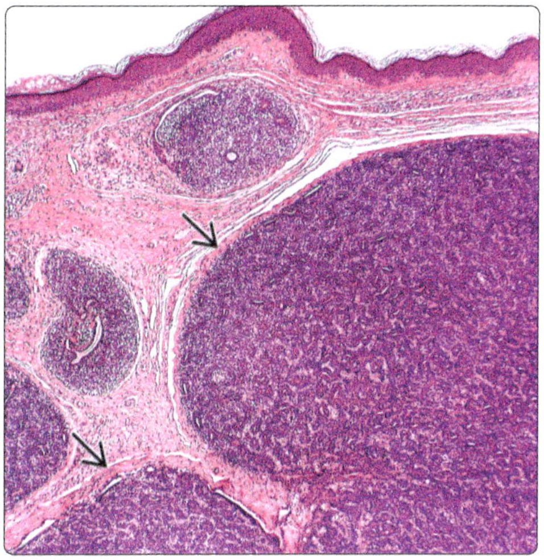

Differential Diagnosis: Spiradenoma

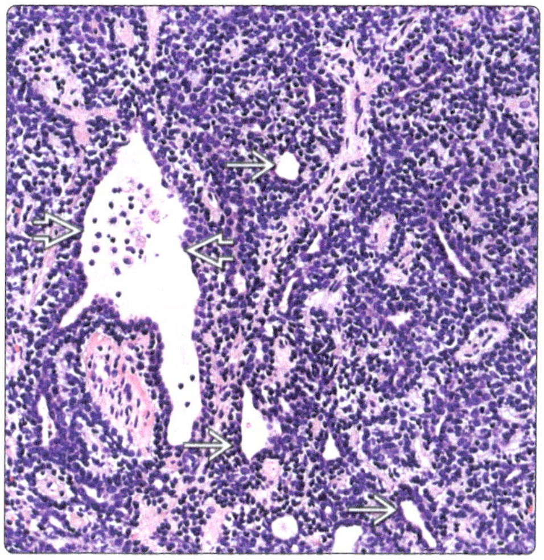

(Left) *Spiradenoma has overlapping features with cylindroma but is characterized by multiple cellular basophilic lobules in the dermis, often with a surrounding fibrous capsule, which is lacking in cylindroma.* **(Right)** *Higher magnification of spiradenoma shows a proliferation of small blue cells and lymphocytes surrounding a dilated glandular lumen and multiple small ductal lumina, which are more numerous than in cylindromas.*

Differential Diagnosis: Basal Cell Carcinoma

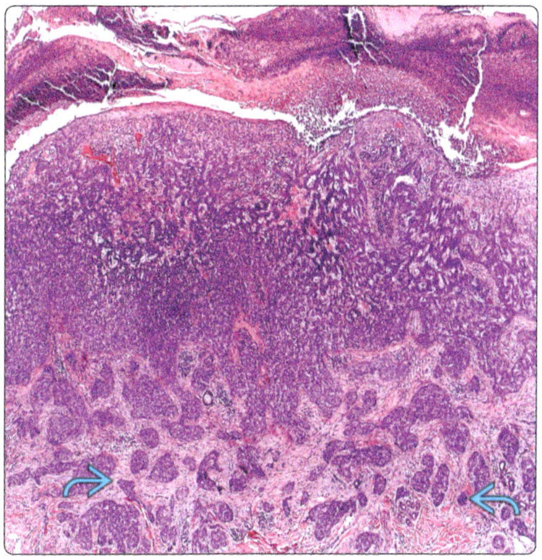

Differential Diagnosis: Nodular-Type Basal Cell Carcinoma

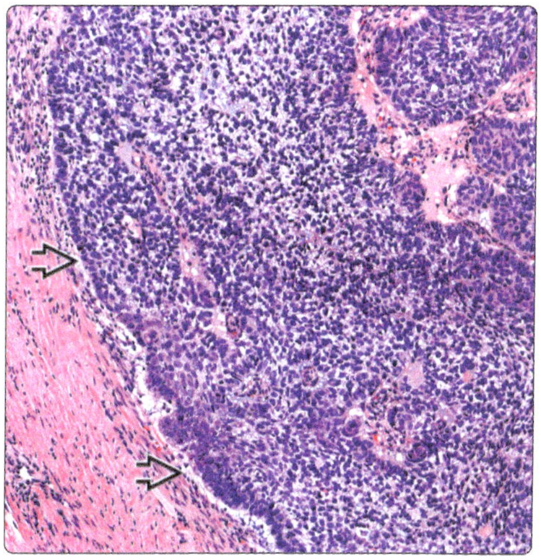

(Left) *This is a large, nodular and micronodular type basal cell carcinoma (BCC). Note the overlying erosions with dense serum crust, and the deeply invasive micronodules.* **(Right)** *Histologic section of a nodular-type basal cell carcinoma shows a proliferation of atypical basaloid cells with peripheral palisading and prominent retraction artifact, findings that are lacking in cylindromas.*

Differential Diagnosis: Cylindrocarcinoma

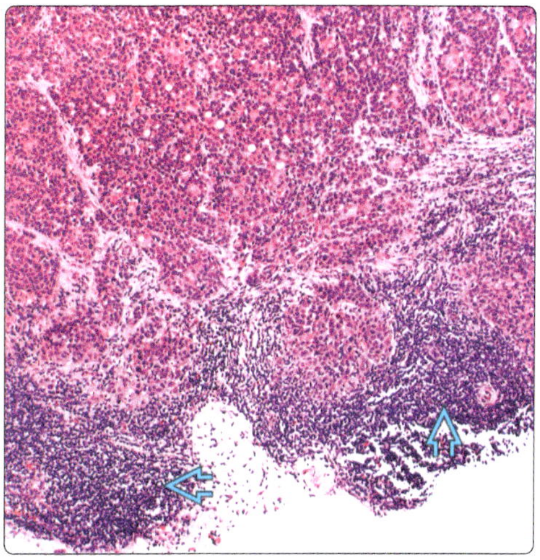

Differential Diagnosis: Cylindrocarcinoma

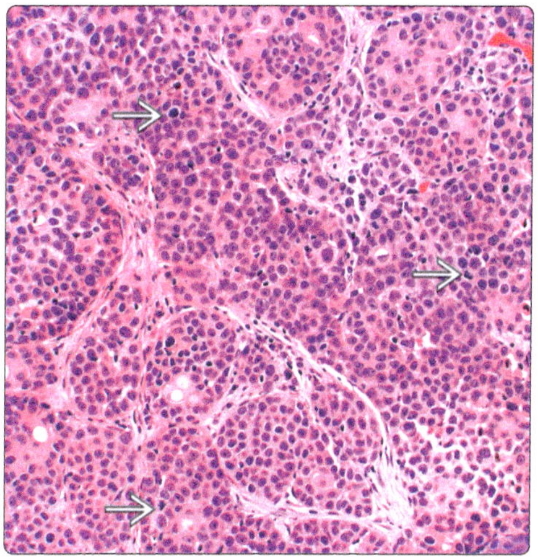

(Left) *Cylindrocarcinoma is a rare malignant tumor which can arise in a large, longstanding cylindroma, and is characterized by infiltrative islands of atypical adnexal cells. Note the relatively dense surrounding lymphoid infiltrate.* **(Right)** *Higher magnification of cylindrocarcinoma shows enlarged, atypical epithelioid cells with hyperchromatic nuclei and more abundant eosinophilic-staining cytoplasm than that seen in cylindroma. Multiple mitotic figures are present.*

Spiradenoma

KEY FACTS

TERMINOLOGY

- Eccrine spiradenoma
- Benign adnexal tumor composed of nodules of basaloid cells with ductal differentiation

ETIOLOGY/PATHOGENESIS

- Familial cases associated with autosomal dominant Brooke-Spiegler syndrome

CLINICAL ISSUES

- Most common in young adults but can present at any age
- Upper 1/2 of body most commonly involved
- Dermal mass/nodule, < 2 cm in size
- Often tender or painful lesion

MICROSCOPIC

- Basophilic tumor lobules/nodules in dermis
- Tumor may be partially encapsulated
- Biphasic with 2 cell types
  - Small cells with scant cytoplasm and small hyperchromatic nuclei; typically at periphery of tumor lobules
  - Larger cells with eosinophilic cytoplasm and oval, vesicular nuclei; typically in centers of tumor lobules
- Focal to diffuse duct lumen formation
- Tumor lobules associated with vascularized stroma, hemorrhage may be present

TOP DIFFERENTIAL DIAGNOSES

- Cylindroma
  - Significant overlap with spiradenoma and may have combined tumors
  - Cylindroma has jigsaw puzzle pattern
- Spiradenocarcinoma (malignant spiradenoma)
  - Associated with precursor spiradenoma
- Basal cell carcinoma
  - Peripheral palisading with tumor-stroma retraction
- Merkel cell carcinoma

(Left) *Low magnification of a spiradenoma shows a dermal-based tumor characterized by irregularly-shaped nodules and smaller lobules → in the dermis.* **(Right)** *Spiradenoma is characterized by circumscribed, cellular basophilic nodules or lobules in the dermis. The tumor lobules often have a surrounding fibrous capsule →.*

Spiradenoma at Low Magnification

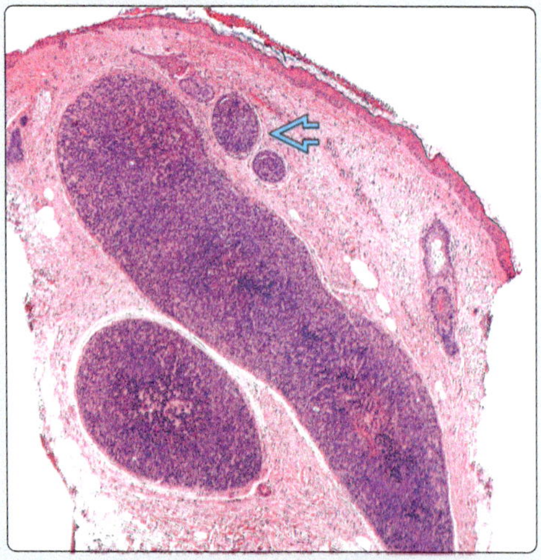

Spiradenoma With Large Dermal Nodules

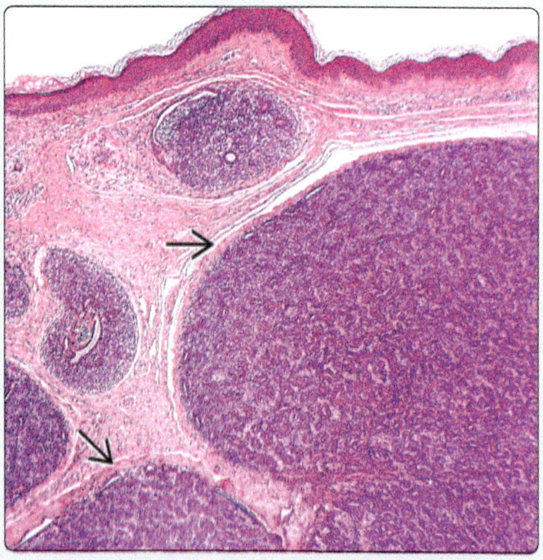

(Left) *The stroma in this case is edematous and highlights the associated capillary vasculature →.* **(Right)** *The tumor is composed of a biphasic population of smaller basaloid cells and larger pale cells. Duct lumen formation → is present and may be focal or relatively prominent, as in this case.*

Spiradenoma With Edematous Stroma

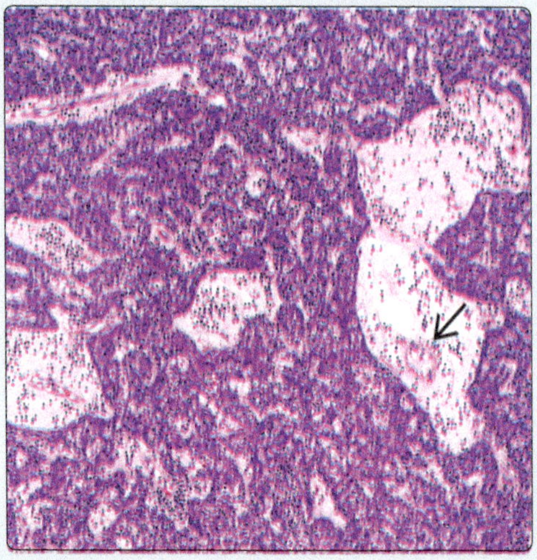

Spiradenoma at High Magnification

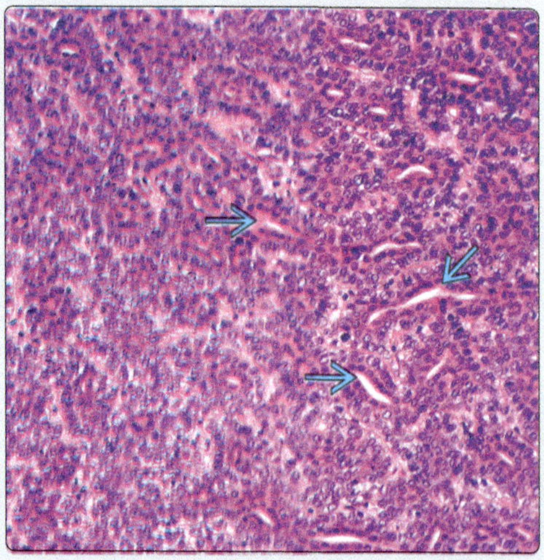

TERMINOLOGY

Synonyms

- Eccrine spiradenoma

Definitions

- Benign adnexal tumor composed of nodules of basaloid cells with ductal differentiation
- May have apocrine or eccrine differentiation

ETIOLOGY/PATHOGENESIS

Genetic Syndrome

- Familial cases associated with autosomal dominant Brooke-Spiegler syndrome
  - a.k.a. familial cylindromatosis or turban tumor syndrome
  - Multiple cylindromas, but can also have spiradenomas and trichoepitheliomas

CLINICAL ISSUES

Epidemiology

- Age
  - Most common in young adults but can present at any age

Site

- Upper 1/2 of body most commonly involved; > 75% present on ventral surface

Presentation

- Dermal mass/nodular lesion
  - Often tender or painful, may have bluish color
  - Usually solitary but may be multiple
    - Multiple lesions may be part of Brooke-Spiegler syndrome

Treatment

- Surgical approaches
  - Complete surgical excision is curative

Prognosis

- Benign, but local recurrence may occur; very rare malignant transformation

MACROSCOPIC

General Features

- Dermal-based, bluish nodule

Size

- Typically small, < 1-2 cm

MICROSCOPIC

Histologic Features

- Basophilic tumor nodules in dermis
- Tumor lobules may be partially encapsulated
- Biphasic appearance with 2 cell types
  - Peripheral small cells with scant cytoplasm and small hyperchromatic nuclei
  - Central larger cells with eosinophilic cytoplasm and oval, vesicular nuclei ± distinct nucleolus
- Focal duct lumen formation
  - Highlighted by stains for EMA and CEA
- Tumor lobules sometimes surrounded by thickened basement membrane, similar to cylindroma
- Tumor lobules associated with vascularized stroma, hemorrhage sometimes present
- Mitotic activity absent to rare

ANCILLARY TESTS

Immunohistochemistry

- Tumor cells positive for cytokeratins 7, 8, and 18 (CAM5.2), CK5/6, and p63; EMA and CEA highlight ducts
- Some immunoreactivity for SMA, calponin, and S100, consistent with myoepithelial differentiation

DIFFERENTIAL DIAGNOSIS

Cylindroma

- Significant overlap; may have combined tumors or areas that are indistinguishable
  - Combined tumors more common in Brooke-Spiegler patients
- Cylindromas have distinct jigsaw puzzle pattern
- Lobules surrounded by dense hyalinized membranes

Spiradenocarcinoma (Malignant Spiradenoma)

- Associated with precursor spiradenoma
- Infiltrative, not circumscribed
- Prominent atypia and numerous mitotic figures
- Variable tumor necrosis

Basal Cell Carcinoma

- Attachments to epidermis often present
- Peripheral palisading with tumor-stroma retraction
- Lacks ductal differentiation
- Mitotic and apoptotic figures often present

Merkel Cell Carcinoma

- Lacks biphasic pattern of 2 cell types
- More cytologic atypia and high mitotic rate
- Positive for CK20 and neuroendocrine markers

DIAGNOSTIC CHECKLIST

Pathologic Interpretation Pearls

- Basophilic tumor nodules in dermis
- Biphasic: Peripheral small and central larger cells
- Vascular stroma

SELECTED REFERENCES

1. Sellheyer K: Spiradenoma and cylindroma originate from the hair follicle bulge and not from the eccrine sweat gland: an immunohistochemical study with CD200 and other stem cell markers. J Cutan Pathol. ePub, 2014
2. Mahalingam M et al: Expression of stem-cell markers (cytokeratin 15 and nestin) in primary adnexal neoplasms-clues to etiopathogenesis. Am J Dermatopathol. 32(8):774-9, 2010
3. Plaza JA et al: Value of p63 and podoplanin (D2-40) immunoreactivity in the distinction between primary cutaneous tumors and adenocarcinomas metastatic to the skin: a clinicopathologic and immunohistochemical study of 79 cases. J Cutan Pathol. 37(4):403-10, 2010
4. Bumgardner AC et al: Trichoepitheliomas and eccrine spiradenomas with spiradenoma/cylindroma overlap. Int J Dermatol. 44(5):415-7, 2005
5. Wright S et al: Multiple familial eccrine spiradenoma with cylindroma. Acta Derm Venereol. 70(1):79-82, 1990
6. Mambo NC: Eccrine spiradenoma: clinical and pathologic study of 49 tumors. J Cutan Pathol. 10(5):312-20, 1983

(Left) *Spiradenoma is characterized by circumscribed basophilic tumor nodules or lobules in the dermis. The tumor lobules often have a fibrous capsule.* **(Right)** *The tumor is composed of 2 cell types: Small cells with scant cytoplasm and hyperchromatic nuclei, and larger cells with oval vesicular nuclei →. Scattered lymphocytes are also present throughout the tumor ↪.*

Spiradenoma at Low Magnification

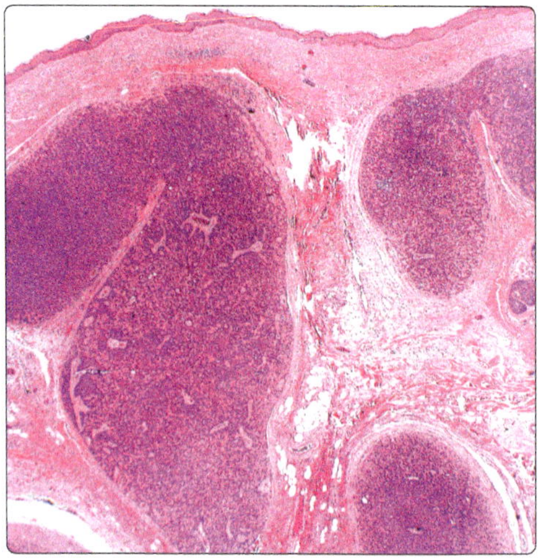

High Magnification With Lymphocytes

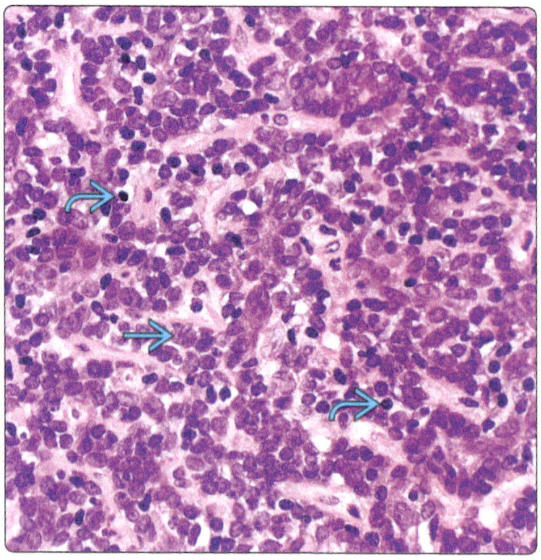

(Left) *High magnification of a spiradenoma with a very prominent hyalinized stroma. Note the focal duct formation surrounded by cells with vesicular nuclei ↪.* **(Right)** *This case has overlapping features of spiradenoma and cylindroma. The tumor lobules on the left → have a jigsaw-like pattern reminiscent of cylindroma, while the right side demonstrates circumscribed nodules ⇨ more typical of spiradenoma.*

Spiradenoma Hyalinized Stroma

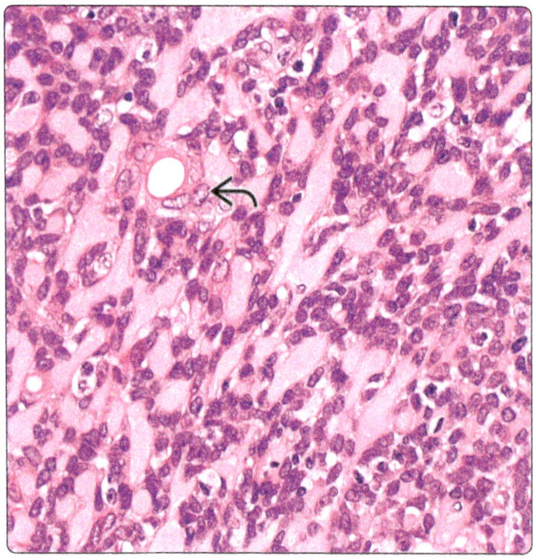

Combined Spiradenoma and Cylindroma

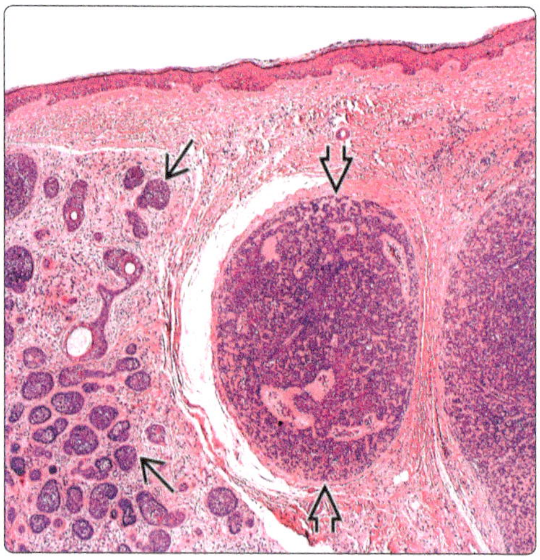

(Left) *Higher magnification shows cylindroma ⇨ and spiradenoma ⇨ side by side. The jigsaw-like basaloid nodules with eosinophilic mantle ↪ on the left distinguishes cylindromatous component from the spiradenomatous element on the right.* **(Right)** *Cylindromas are closely related tumors, but typically demonstrate the characteristic jigsaw puzzle-like arrangement of the tumor lobules (which are usually smaller than those in spiradenoma) filling the dermis.*

Combined Spiradenoma and Cylindroma

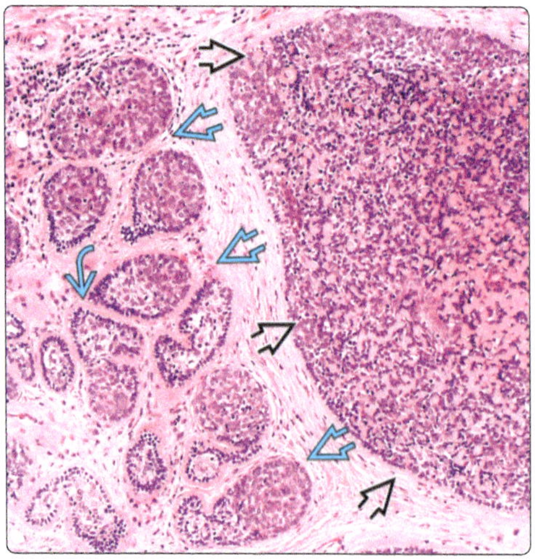

Differential Diagnosis: Cylindroma

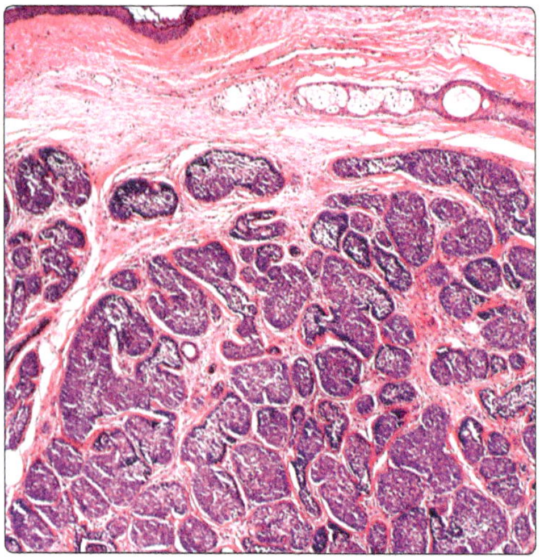

Differential Diagnosis: Cylindroma

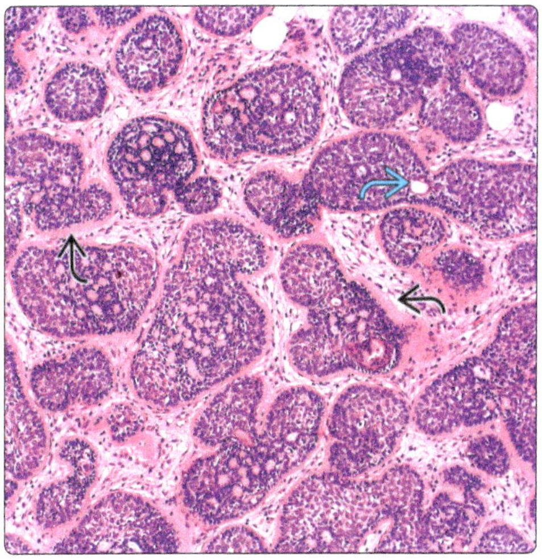

Differential Diagnosis: Cylindroma

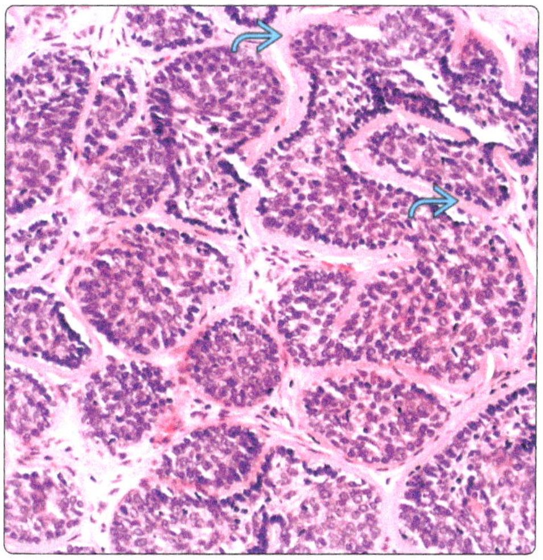

(Left) *Cylindroma shows a proliferation composed of irregular lobules of basaloid cells with focal ductal lumina, and surrounded by dense hyalinized membranous material.* **(Right)** *Higher magnification of cylindroma shows a proliferation composed of irregular lobules composed of small, bland-appearing basaloid cells, which are surrounded by dense hyalinized membranous material.*

Differential Diagnosis: Spiradenocarcinoma

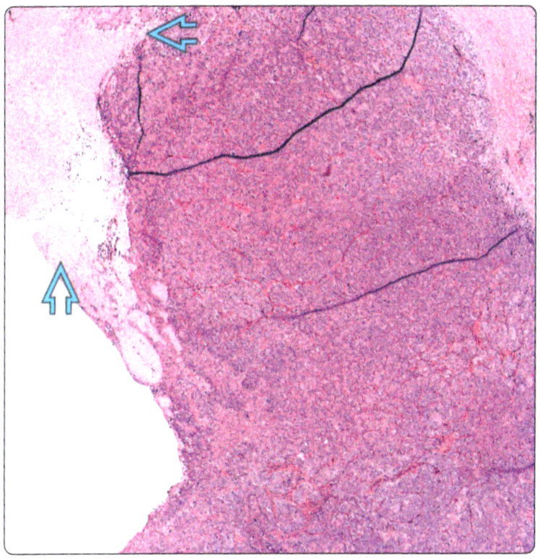

Differential Diagnosis: Spiradenocarcinoma

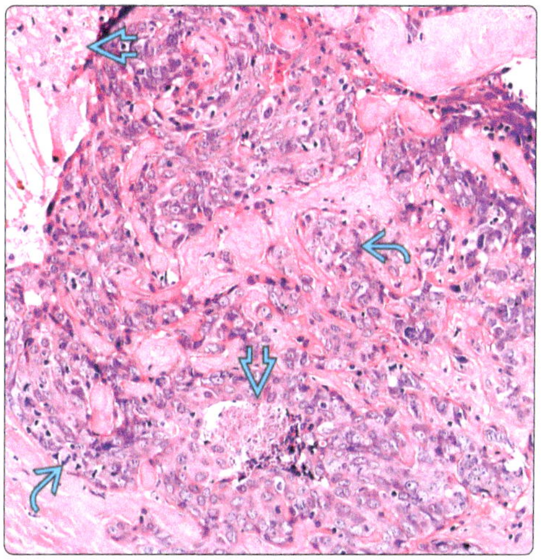

(Left) *Spiradenocarcinoma is a very rare adnexal carcinoma that may arise in large, longstanding spiradenomas. This is a very cellular tumor composed of nodular to sheet-like collections of basaloid cells with a large area of tumor necrosis.* **(Right)** *Spiradenocarcinoma at high-power magnification shows infiltrative nests and cords of markedly enlarged and atypical-appearing cells. Note the presence of mitoses and tumor necrosis.*

Differential Diagnosis: BCC

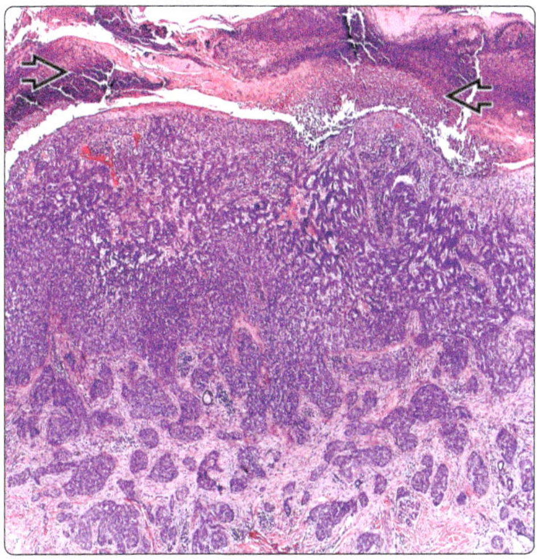

Differential Diagnosis: BCC

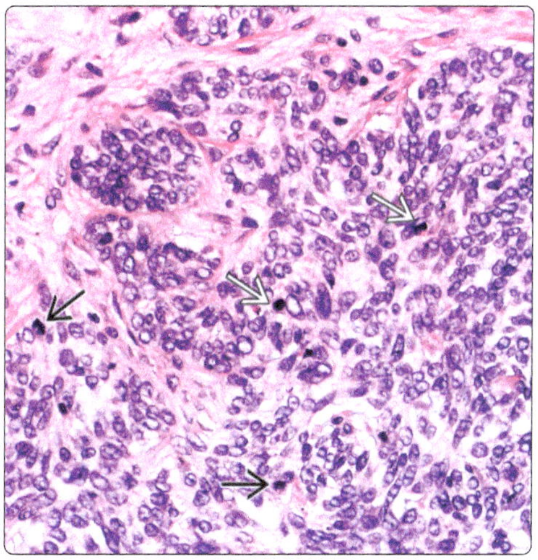

(Left) *Histologic section of a nodular and micronodular-type basal cell carcinoma (BCC) shows a proliferation of atypical basaloid cells with epidermal attachments and overlying ulceration and dense serum crusting, findings which are lacking in spiradenomas and spiradenocarcinomas.* **(Right)** *High magnification of BCC shows a proliferation of atypical basaloid cells with high nuclear:cytoplasmic ratios and numerous apoptotic and mitotic figures.*

Adenoid Cystic Carcinoma

KEY FACTS

TERMINOLOGY

- Adenoid cystic carcinoma (ACC)
- Rare adnexal tumor showing prominent cribriform pattern and perineural invasion

ETIOLOGY/PATHOGENESIS

- May be related to chronic solar damage in some cases

CLINICAL ISSUES

- Typically occur in adults
- Slow-growing, skin-colored nodule
- Prognosis: Up to 70% of cases reported to recur (due to perineural invasion)
  - Only a few cases have metastasized, usually to lymph nodes and lungs

MACROSCOPIC

- Usually a few centimeters, can be up to 8 cm

MICROSCOPIC

- Composed of infiltrative lobules, islands, and cords of basaloid cells
  - Numerous cystic and ductular spaces with prominent cribriform pattern
- Cells are typically small, relatively monomorphic appearing, and cuboidal shaped

ANCILLARY TESTS

- Epithelial cells stain positive with EMA, CEA-m, and cytokeratins (low and high molecular weight keratins)
- S100, p63, GFAP, SMA, MSA, and calponin often stain peripheral cells, consistent with myoepithelial differentiation

TOP DIFFERENTIAL DIAGNOSES

- Basal cell carcinoma (BCC)
- Metastatic adenoid cystic carcinoma
- Other primary cutaneous adnexal tumors

(Left) *Adenoid cystic carcinoma (ACC) at low magnification shows a dermal-based basaloid neoplasm with numerous cribriform spaces ➡ containing basophilic mucin and showing a prominent Swiss cheese-like pattern.* **(Right)** *Higher magnification of ACC shows relatively bland basaloid cells surrounding the ductal lumina containing prominent collections of blue mucinous material.*

Adenoid Cystic Carcinoma

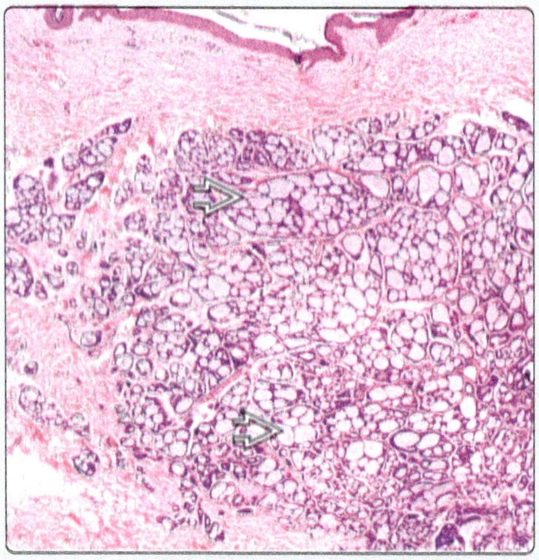

Adenoid Cystic Carcinoma With Prominent Mucin

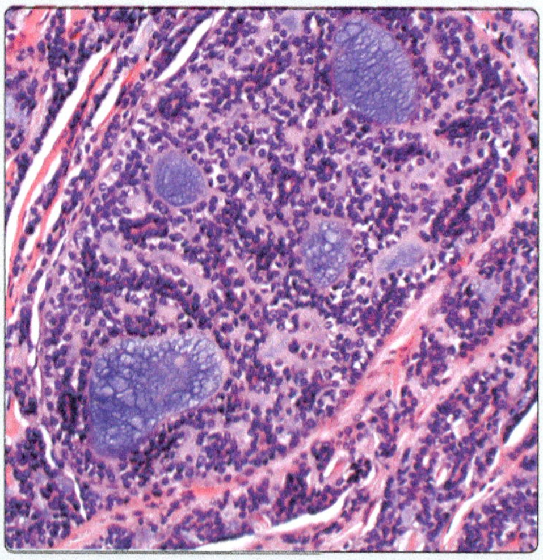

(Left) *ACC frequently shows perineural invasion, which accounts for its high local recurrence rate. Here, a large central nerve ➡ is surrounded by multiple tumor cords and ducts.* **(Right)** *ACC typically demonstrates expression of myoepithelial markers including SMA (shown here), MSA, calponin, cytokeratins, S100, and GFAP.*

Adenoid Cystic Carcinoma With Perineural Invasion

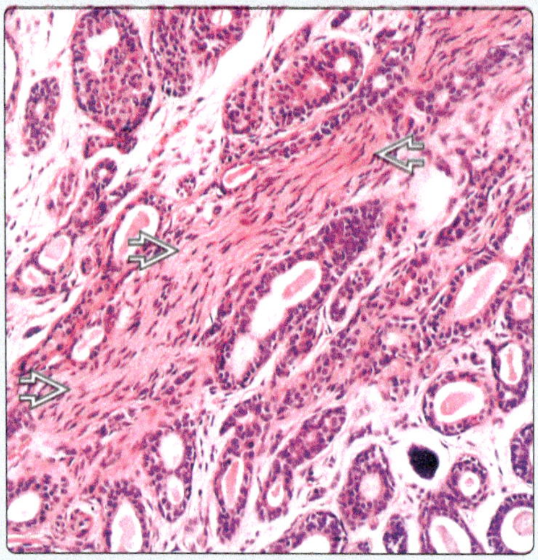

SMA Immunohistochemistry in ACC

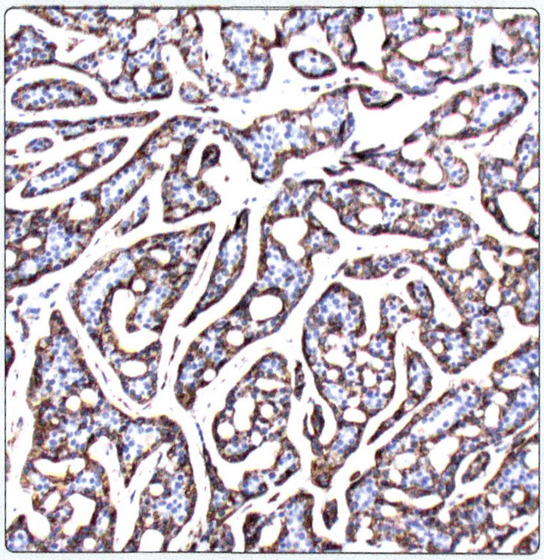

TERMINOLOGY

Abbreviations

- Adenoid cystic carcinoma (ACC)

Synonyms

- Primary cutaneous adenoid cystic carcinoma

Definitions

- Rare adnexal tumor showing prominent cribriform pattern and perineural invasion

ETIOLOGY/PATHOGENESIS

Unknown

- May be related to chronic sun damage in some cases

CLINICAL ISSUES

Epidemiology

- Incidence
  - Rare tumors
- Age
  - Typically occur in adults

Presentation

- Dermal mass
  - Slow-growing, skin-colored nodule

Treatment

- Surgical approaches
  - Complete and wider excision is necessary to prevent recurrence given high incidence of perineural invasion
  - Mohs surgery may be effective to minimize recurrence

Prognosis

- Up to 70% of cases have been reported to recur (due to perineural invasion)
- Only a few cases have metastasized, usually to lymph nodes and lungs

MACROSCOPIC

Size

- Usually a few centimeters, can be up to 8 cm

MICROSCOPIC

Histologic Features

- Poorly circumscribed dermal-based tumor
- Composed of lobules, islands, and cords of basaloid cells with numerous cystic and ductular spaces
  - Typically shows prominent cribriform pattern, similar to that seen in adenoid cystic carcinoma of salivary glands and breast
  - Spaces are filled with mucinous material that stains with mucicarmine, Alcian blue, and colloidal iron
  - Cells are typically small, relatively monomorphic appearing, and cuboidal shaped
  - Mitotic figures are usually not prominent
- Perineural invasion is very common
  - Multiple sections should be examined if it is not initially identified

Cytologic Features

- Nuclei are typically hyperchromatic-staining with small nucleoli

ANCILLARY TESTS

Immunohistochemistry

- ACC stains positive with EMA, CEA-m, and cytokeratins, including low and high molecular weight keratins
- S100, p63, GFAP, and muscle markers including SMA, MSA, and calponin often stain peripheral cells, consistent with myoepithelial differentiation

DIFFERENTIAL DIAGNOSIS

Basal Cell Carcinoma

- Can show adenoid cystic carcinoma-like features (adenoid-type basal cell carcinoma)
- Should have areas of peripheral palisading, tumor-stromal retraction, and mucinous stroma

Metastatic Adenoid Cystic Carcinoma

- Shows essentially identical histologic features
- Very rarely metastatic, but must be excluded based on clinical history and imaging studies

Other Primary Cutaneous Adnexal Tumors

- Cylindroma
  - Composed of irregularly shaped nests and islands of basaloid cells surrounded by dense basement membranes
  - Does not show prominent degree of cystic/ductal spaces seen in ACC
- Spiradenoma
  - Large nodules composed of biphasic population of small, hyperchromatic-staining basaloid cells and larger clear cells
  - Often associated with dilated vascular spaces and numerous lymphocytes scattered throughout tumor
- Both tumors lack perineural invasion

SELECTED REFERENCES

1. Dores GM et al: Primary cutaneous adenoid cystic carcinoma in the United States: incidence, survival, and associated cancers, 1976 to 2005. J Am Acad Dermatol. 63(1):71-8, 2010
2. Singh A et al: Primary cutaneous adenoid cystic carcinoma with distant metastasis: a case report and brief literature review. Indian J Dermatol Venereol Leprol. 76(2):176-9, 2010
3. Xu YG et al: Cutaneous adenoid cystic carcinoma with perineural invasion treated by mohs micrographic surgery-a case report with literature review. J Oncol. 2010:469049, 2010
4. Doganay L et al: Primary cutaneous adenoid cystic carcinoma with lung and lymph node metastases. J Eur Acad Dermatol Venereol. 18(3):383-5, 2004
5. Matsumura T et al: Adenoid cystic carcinoma of the skin--an immunohistochemical and ultrastructural study. J Dermatol. 20(3):164-70, 1993
6. Bergman R et al: A comparative immunohistochemical study of adenoid cystic carcinoma of the skin and salivary glands. Am J Dermatopathol. 13(2):162-8, 1991
7. Wick MR et al: Primary adenoid cystic carcinoma of the skin. a clinical, histological, and immunocytochemical comparison with adenoid cystic carcinoma of salivary glands and adenoid basal cell carcinoma. Am J Dermatopathol. 8(1):2-13, 1986
8. Cooper PH et al: Primary cutaneous adenoid cystic carcinoma. Arch Dermatol. 120(6):774-7, 1984

Primary Cutaneous Mucinous Carcinoma

KEY FACTS

TERMINOLOGY

- Primary cutaneous mucinous carcinoma (PCMC)
- a.k.a. mucinous carcinoma, mucinous eccrine carcinoma, endocrine mucin producing carcinoma
- Malignant tumor with characteristic histology of epithelial islands "floating" in pools of mucin

CLINICAL ISSUES

- Very rare tumor, commonly on eyelids
- Slow-growing, asymptomatic, solitary, reddish papule, ulcer, or cyst
- Up to 36% local recurrence and up to 15% metastasis to regional lymph nodes or distant metastasis

MICROSCOPIC

- Well-circumscribed, dermal-based tumor with occasional extension to subcutaneous or deeper tissue
- Strands of fibrous tissue divide tumor into different compartments
- Within compartments, epithelial cells in nests and cords appear to float in large pools of mucin

ANCILLARY TESTS

- CK5/6 and p63 at least focally positive and favor cutaneous primary
- CK7 is typically positive; CK20 is negative
- ER, PR, and GCDFP-15 are often positive but not useful in excluding metastatic breast carcinoma

TOP DIFFERENTIAL DIAGNOSES

- Metastatic mucinous carcinoma
  - Mucinous breast carcinoma
  - Mucinous colonic carcinoma
- Other primary cutaneous tumors with mucin
  - Basal cell carcinoma
  - Adenoid cystic carcinoma

Low Magnification of Primary Cutaneous Mucinous Carcinoma

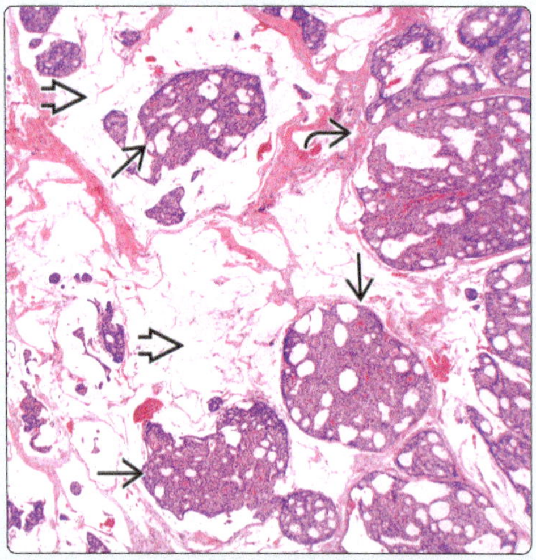

Intermediate Magnification of Primary Cutaneous Mucinous Carcinoma

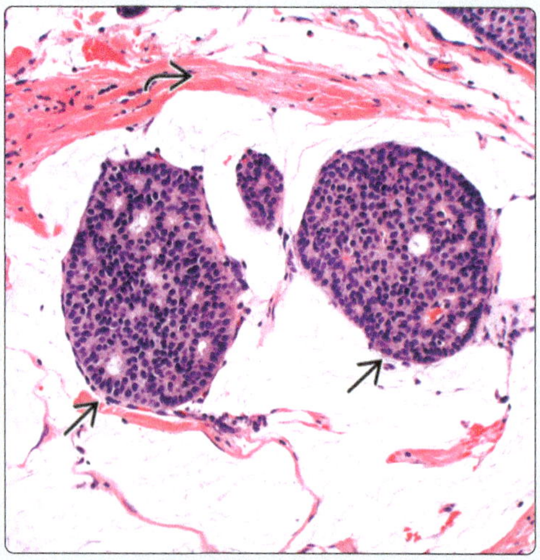

(Left) *Low-power view of primary cutaneous mucinous carcinoma (PCMC) shows islands of epithelial cells → floating in pools of mucin ⇨. Fibrous septa ↪ are present between some of the epithelial islands.* **(Right)** *Medium-power view of PCMC shows islands of epithelial cells → in pools of mucin. Fibrous septa ↪, which characteristically divide the tumor into compartments, are present.*

High Magnification of Primary Cutaneous Mucinous Carcinoma

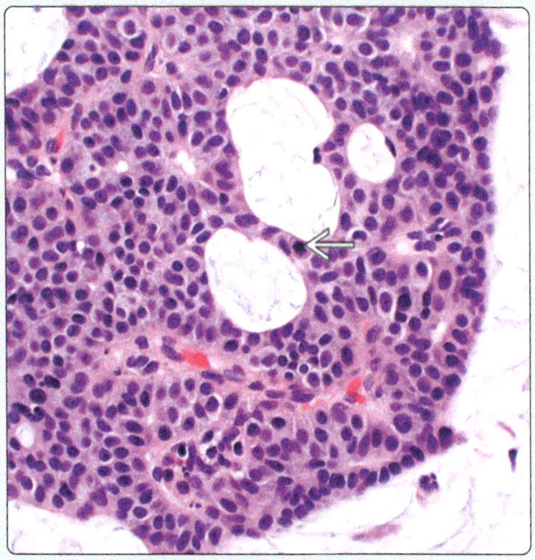

ER Immunohistochemistry in Primary Cutaneous Mucinous Carcinoma

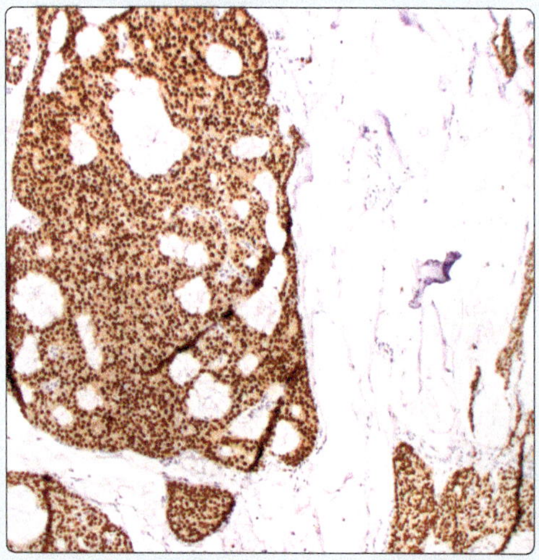

(Left) *Higher magnification shows uniform cells with hyperchromatic nuclei and eosinophilic cytoplasm. An occasional mitotic figure is identified ➡, but necrosis and marked cytologic atypia are not present.* **(Right)** *ER shows strong and diffuse nuclear staining in almost 100% of the tumor cells. This is a useful finding in excluding a metastatic mucinous colonic carcinoma, but it is not useful in excluding a metastatic breast carcinoma.*

TERMINOLOGY

Abbreviations

- Primary cutaneous mucinous carcinoma (PCMC)

Synonyms

- Mucinous carcinoma, mucinous eccrine carcinoma, endocrine mucin producing carcinoma

Definitions

- Malignant cutaneous tumor with classic histology of epithelial islands "floating" in pools of mucin

CLINICAL ISSUES

Epidemiology

- Sex
  - Men affected more often than women

Presentation

- Very rare tumor
- Occurs in adults and elderly
- Commonly on face, especially on eyelids
- Slow-growing, asymptomatic, solitary reddish papule, nodule, or cyst

Treatment

- Surgical approaches
  - Wide local excision, ± dissection of regional lymph nodes
  - Mohs micrographic surgery
  - Chemotherapy and radiation have not been helpful in recurrent tumors

Prognosis

- Up to 36% local recurrence and up to 15% metastasis to regional lymph nodes or distant metastasis

MACROSCOPIC

Size

- 0.5-7 cm; rare larger lesions

MICROSCOPIC

Histologic Features

- Highly distinct low-power histologic appearance
  - Composed of epithelial cells in nests and cords present in large pools of mucin
- Well-circumscribed, dermal-based tumor with occasional extension into subcutaneous tissues
- Occasional overlying ulceration
- Strands of fibrous tissue divide tumor into different compartments
- Epithelial component
  - Usually denser at tumor periphery
  - Nests and cords of epithelial cells with ductal and tubular spaces
  - Glandular or tubular spaces have mucin
  - Cribriform pattern can be seen
- Mucinous component
  - Strongly positive with PAS, mucicarmine, and colloidal iron

ANCILLARY TESTS

Immunohistochemistry

- CK7 positive, CK20 negative
- ER, PR, and GCDFP-15 are often positive but are not useful in excluding metastatic breast carcinoma
- CK5/6 and p63 are typically positive
  - p63 can only show very focal staining in some cases
  - May indicate presence of myoepithelial differentiation
- Chromogranin and synaptophysin usually positive

DIFFERENTIAL DIAGNOSIS

Metastatic Mucinous Carcinoma

- **Metastasis from breast and colon are most likely**
- Exclusion of metastatic visceral carcinoma by histology alone is essentially impossible
- Definitive diagnosis of PCMC should be made only after thorough work-up for visceral carcinoma is found to be negative
- Histologic features that can help distinguish PCMC from metastatic mucinous carcinoma (MMC)
  - Tumor cells in MMC infiltrate surrounding collagen bundles
  - Epithelial tumor cells in MMC show higher degree of atypia
  - Presence of myoepithelial cells can help in identifying PCMC
- Immunohistochemical stains may be of some help in distinguishing PCMC from MMC
  - CK5/6 and p63 staining favor primary over metastatic MCC
  - CK20 and CDX-2 staining are consistent with metastasis from colon/gastrointestinal tract
  - Breast carcinoma is much more difficult to separate from PCMC
    - CK7, GCDFP-15, and ER/PR staining is seen in both PCMC and metastatic mucinous breast carcinoma

Other Primary Cutaneous Tumors With Prominent Mucin

- Basal cell carcinoma
  - Shows focal stromal mucin but not nearly as prominent as that in PCMC
  - Tumor-stromal retraction artifact, peripheral palisading, and numerous mitoses and apoptoses typically present
- Adenoid cystic carcinoma
  - Prominent cribriform appearance
  - Mucin present in ductal lumina but not prominent in stroma (as in PCMC)

SELECTED REFERENCES

1. Fernandez-Flores A et al: Endocrine mucin-producing sweat gland carcinoma: a study of three cases and CK8, CK18 and CD5/6 immunoexpression. J Cutan Pathol. 42(8):578-86, 2015
2. Levy G et al: Immunohistochemical techniques to compare primary vs. metastatic mucinous carcinoma of the skin. J Cutan Pathol. 37(4):411-5, 2010
3. Qureshi HS et al: Primary cutaneous mucinous carcinoma: presence of myoepithelial cells as a clue to the cutaneous origin. Am J Dermatopathol. 26(5):353-8, 2004
4. Ohnishi T et al: Immunohistochemical analysis of cytokeratin and human milk fat globulin expression in mucinous carcinoma of the skin. J Cutan Pathol. 29(1):38-43, 2002

Primary Cutaneous Mucinous Carcinoma at Low Magnification

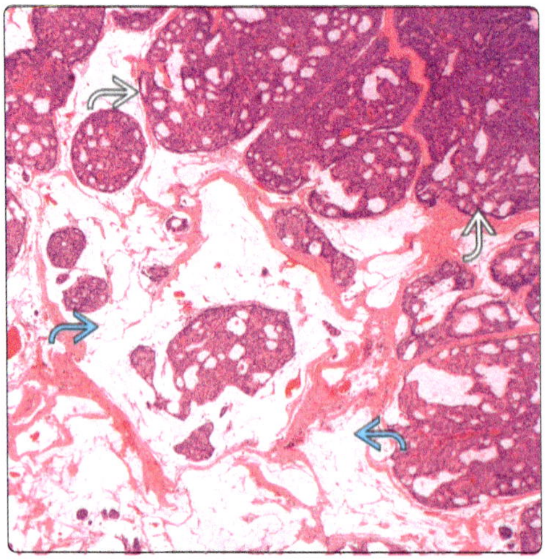

Primary Cutaneous Mucinous Carcinoma With More Cellular Areas

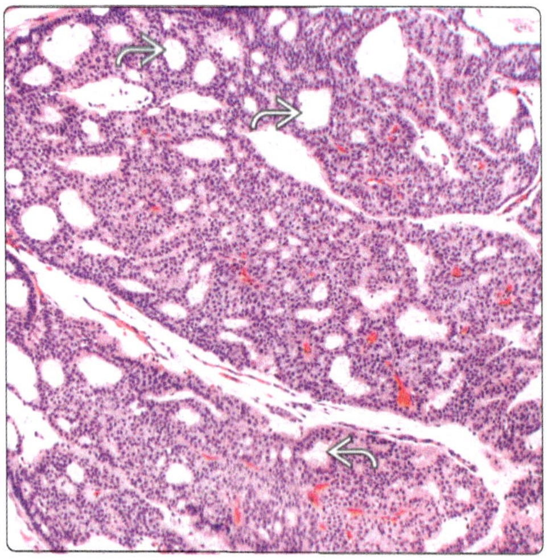

(Left) *PCMC shows a nodular, cellular proliferation of cells in the upper right and more prominent myxoid areas on the lower left.* **(Right)** *More cellular areas are typically present at the periphery of the tumor and are composed of nodular collections of basophilic tumor cells surrounding multiple ductal lumina.*

Primary Cutaneous Mucinous Carcinoma With Cribriform Areas

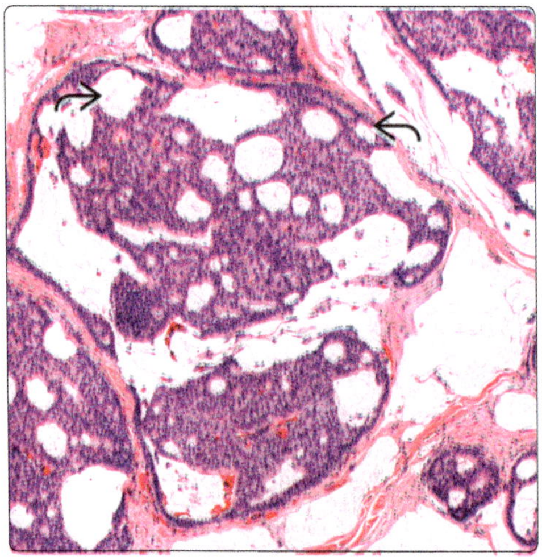

High Magnification of Primary Cutaneous Mucinous Carcinoma

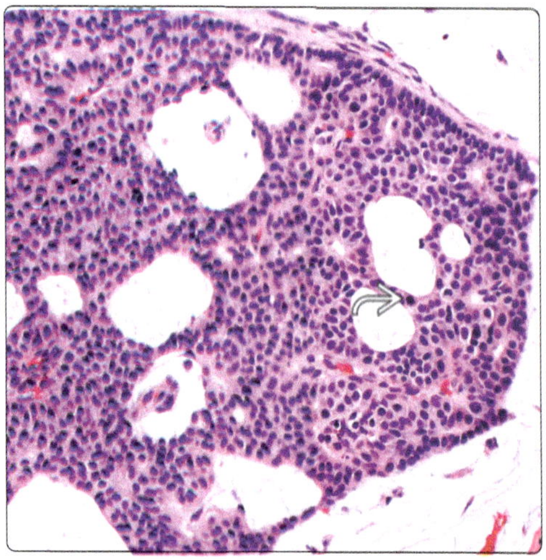

(Left) *Intermediate magnification of PCMC shows cribriforming ductal structures containing mucin.* **(Right)** *Higher magnification shows the relatively bland, monomorphous appearance of the tumor cells. Rare mitotic figures can sometimes be seen.*

Differential Diagnosis: Metastatic Colonic Carcinoma

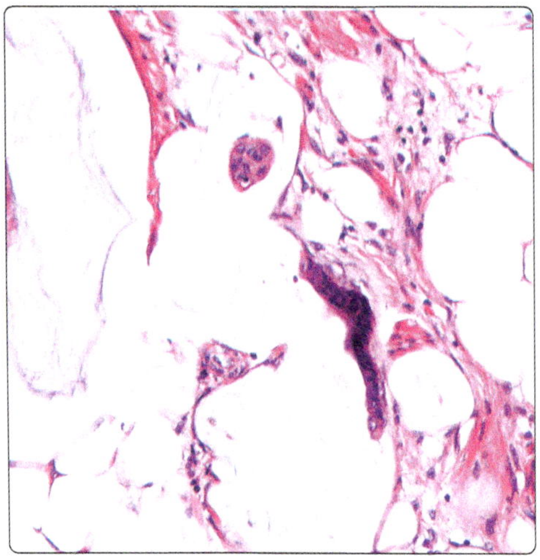

High Magnification of Metastatic Colonic Mucinous Carcinoma

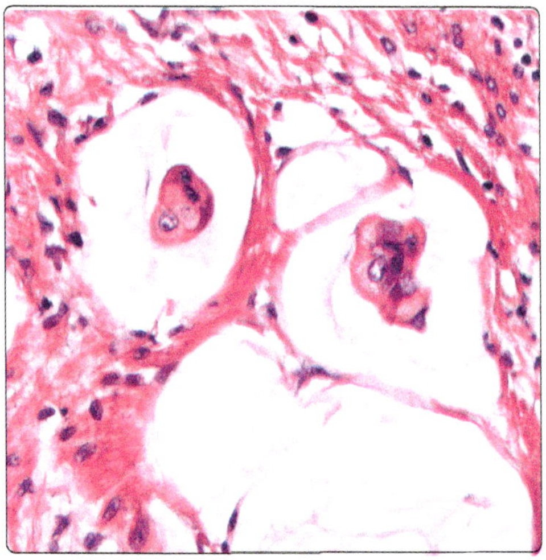

(Left) *Metastatic mucinous carcinoma of the colon or appendix can appear histologically identical to PCMC and can only be excluded by immunohistochemistry for markers such as CK20 and CDX-2.* **(Right)** *High magnification shows small clusters of atypical epithelial cells floating in pools of mucin. This case shows greater cytologic atypia than is typically seen.*

CK5/6 Immunohistochemistry in Primary Cutaneous Mucinous Carcinoma

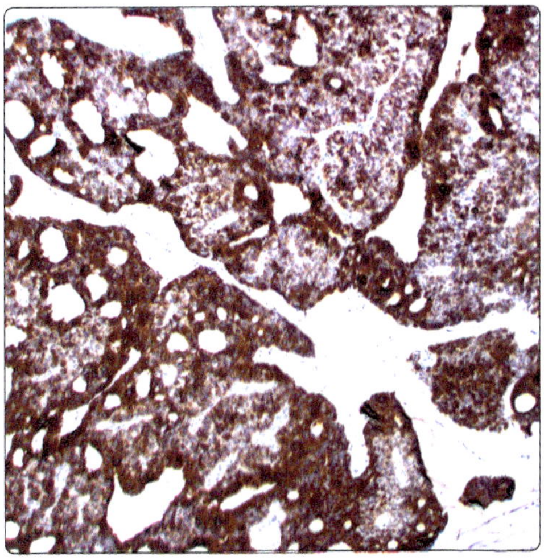

p63 Immunohistochemistry in Primary Cutaneous Mucinous Carcinoma

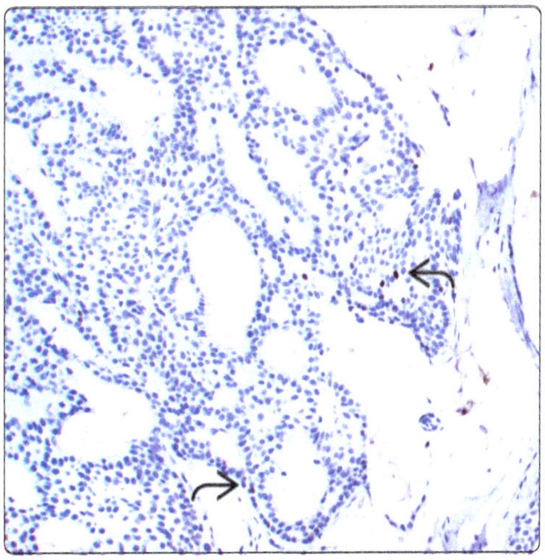

(Left) *CK5/6 shows strong staining of many of the cells, especially around the periphery of the tumor, possibly indicating myoepithelial cells. This finding can help distinguish PCMC from metastatic mucinous carcinoma, which is typically negative for this marker.* **(Right)** *p63 shows only very focal nuclear staining in a few cells in some cases of PCMC.*

GCDFP-15 Immunohistochemistry in Primary Cutaneous Mucinous Carcinoma

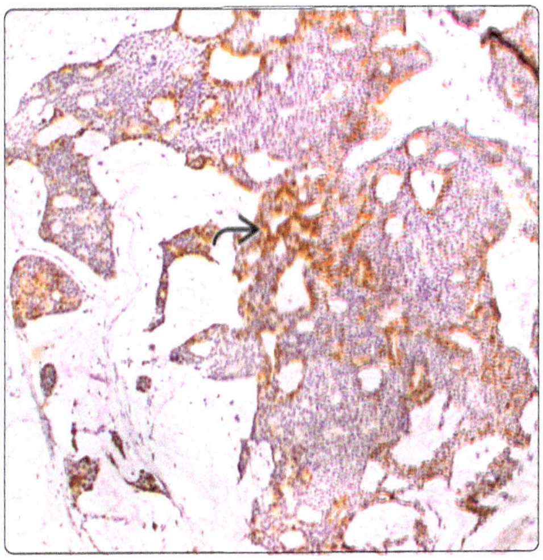

PAS-D Staining in Primary Cutaneous Mucinous Carcinoma

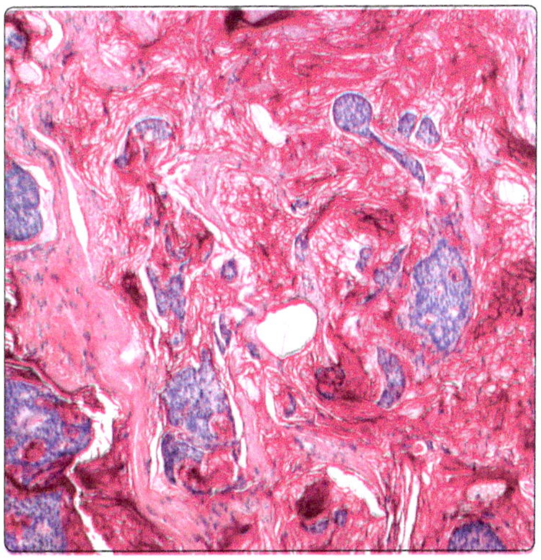

(Left) *GCDFP-15 shows patchy, peripheral-positive staining in a subset of the tumor cells, a finding that is also typical of PCMC but not helpful in excluding a metastatic mucinous breast carcinoma.* **(Right)** *PAS staining with diastase shows strong and diffuse purplish/reddish staining of the pools of mucin in PCMC.*

Metastatic Mucinous Carcinoma

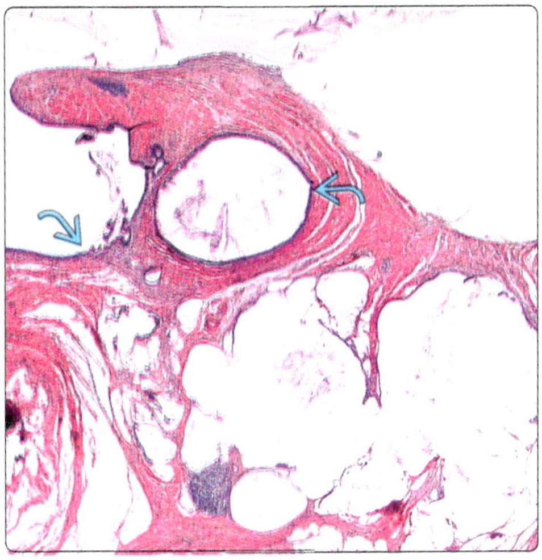

CDX-2 in Metastatic Mucinous Carcinoma

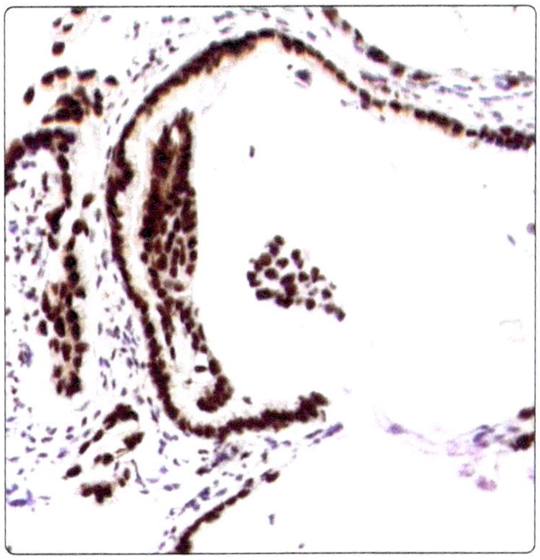

(Left) *This is an example of a metastatic mucinous pancreatic carcinoma to the skin. The tumor shows pools of mucin surrounded by a thin lining of tumor cells, rather than the cells floating in pools of mucin, which is typically seen in PCMC.* **(Right)** *CDX-2 in a metastatic mucinous pancreatic carcinoma to the skin shows strong and diffuse nuclear staining. This marker is not expressed in PCMC and is strong evidence for a metastatic tumor of gastrointestinal origin.*

Apocrine Carcinoma (Apocrine Adenocarcinoma)

KEY FACTS

CLINICAL ISSUES

- Axilla and anogenital region are most common sites, but other sites are described
- No history of breast carcinoma
- Indolent or aggressive course

MICROSCOPIC

- Dermal/subcutaneous tumor
- Tubular, papillary, cord-like, solid, or complex interconnecting glandular patterns
- May have cribriform pattern to islands
- Cells often hyperchromatic/pleomorphic
- Glandular areas lined by cells showing decapitation secretion
- Infiltrative growth pattern

TOP DIFFERENTIAL DIAGNOSES

- Metastatic breast carcinoma
  - History of breast carcinoma
  - May be indistinguishable histologically and immunohistochemically from apocrine carcinoma
- Primary cutaneous adenoid cystic carcinoma
  - Cribriform pattern within islands that are relatively uniform in size/shape and not interconnected
  - Deeply infiltrative, almost always with perineural invasion
- Tubular apocrine adenoma
  - Well circumscribed, noninfiltrative
  - Tubular islands with evidence of decapitation secretion
  - Islands not crowded together
  - Minimal cytologic atypia
  - Often myoepithelial cell layer present
- Hidradenocarcinoma
  - Larger solid and cystic nodules, infiltrative
  - Admixture of cell types: Clear, squamoid, poroid, mucinous
  - Hyalinized stroma

Apocrine Carcinoma at Scanning Magnification

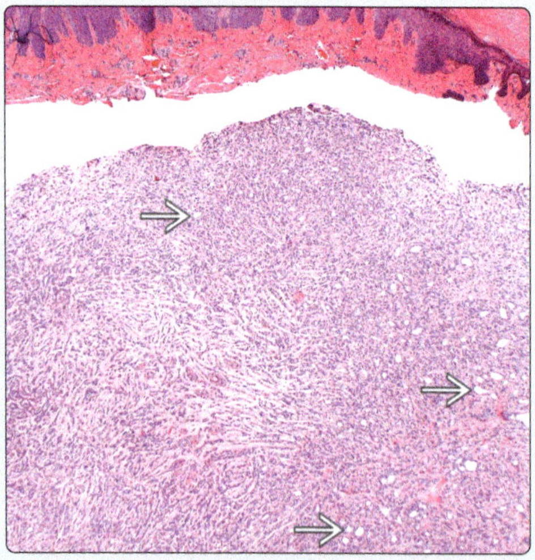

Apocrine Carcinoma With Prominent Snouts and Secretions

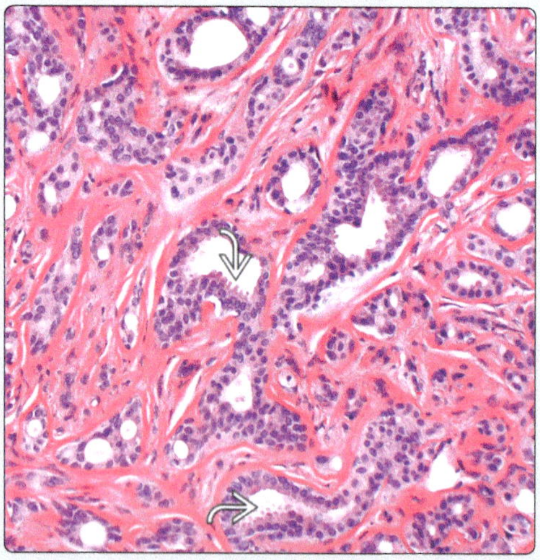

(Left) *Low magnification shows a densely cellular dermal proliferation of packed glands and ductal structures, with many lumina* → *easily identified.* **(Right)** *Higher magnification of the ductal/glandular structures shows enlarged, cuboidal to columnar-shaped cells with prominent apical snouts and secretions* →*, typical of apocrine differentiation.*

Apocrine Carcinoma With Perineural Invasion

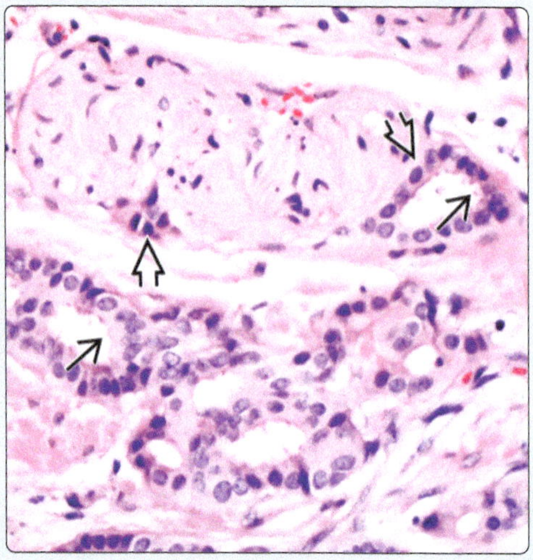

Immunohistochemistry for GCDFP-15

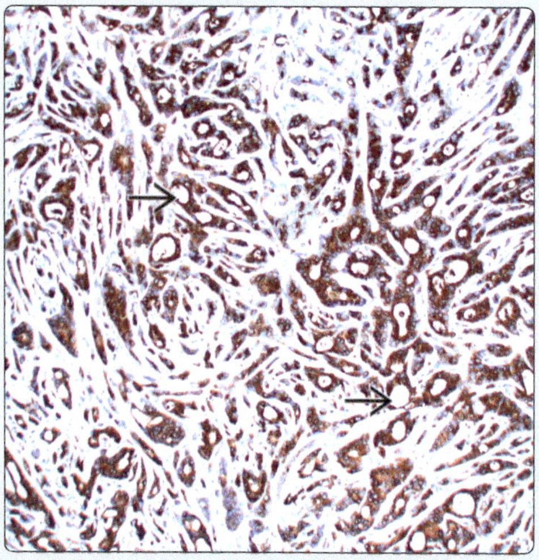

(Left) *High-magnification view of apocrine carcinoma with perineural invasion* → *shows glands lined by cuboidal cells surrounding a nerve. Focal snouts and secretions of cytoplasm* → *are present within the lumina.* **(Right)** *Apocrine carcinoma stains diffusely with GCDFP-15. The islands are crowded together, and lumina* → *can be seen in many of the islands.*

TERMINOLOGY

Synonyms

- Cribriform apocrine carcinoma

Definitions

- Malignant tumor with apocrine differentiation

CLINICAL ISSUES

Site

- Axilla and anogenital regions are most common sites, but other sites described

Presentation

- Dermal nodule, often asymptomatic
- May present within nevus sebaceus
- No history of breast carcinoma

Treatment

- Wide local excision; role of chemotherapy or radiotherapy unclear

Prognosis

- Variable: Indolent or aggressive course (local recurrences common, metastasis to lymph nodes or other internal organs in 25% or more of reported cases)

MICROSCOPIC

Histologic Features

- Dermal tumor composed of islands, cords, and ductal/glandular structures
- May extend into subcutaneous tissue
- Surface may be ulcerated
- Pagetoid spread may be present
- Variable architecture of islands: Tubular, papillary, solid, complex
- Islands generally interconnecting
- May have cribriform pattern in areas
- Glandular areas lined by cells showing decapitation secretion
- Cells often atypical and pleomorphic appearing, mitoses often present with variable necrosis
- Infiltrative growth pattern; vascular invasion may be present

Cytologic Features

- Eosinophilic, granular cytoplasm
- Hyperchromatic nuclei

ANCILLARY TESTS

Immunohistochemistry

- Generally positive with GCDFP-15; often positive with estrogen receptor and androgen receptor
- Negative or only patchy staining with mammaglobin

DIFFERENTIAL DIAGNOSIS

Metastatic Breast Carcinoma

- History of primary breast carcinoma
- May be indistinguishable histologically and immunohistochemically from apocrine carcinoma
  - ER, PR, and GCDFP-15 are all typically positive in both tumors
  - However, strong diffuse staining of majority of cells with mammaglobin supports breast carcinoma

Primary Cutaneous Adenoid Cystic Carcinoma

- Cribriform pattern within islands that are relatively uniform in size/shape and not interconnected
- Deeply infiltrative, almost always with perineural invasion

Tubular Apocrine Adenoma

- Well circumscribed, noninfiltrative
- Tubular islands with evidence of decapitation secretion
- Islands not crowded together
- Cytologic atypia not prominent
- Often myoepithelial cell layer present around islands

Hidradenocarcinoma

- Larger solid and cystic nodules, infiltrative
- Admixture of cell types: Clear, squamoid, poroid, mucinous
- Hyalinized stroma

Microcystic Adnexal Carcinoma

- Horn cysts often present superficially
- Middermal islands may be solid or tubular
- Deeply infiltrative tubular cords with perineural invasion
- Cytologic atypia often not prominent

Papillary Eccrine Adenoma

- Well circumscribed, not infiltrative
- Islands with papillations
- Islands not crowded together
- Cytologic atypia not prominent
- Often myoepithelial cell layer present around islands

DIAGNOSTIC CHECKLIST

Clinically Relevant Pathologic Features

- No history of breast carcinoma

Pathologic Interpretation Pearls

- Dermal/subcutaneous tumor with variable architecture
  - Tubular, papillary, cord-like, solid, cribriform, or complex interconnecting glandular patterns
- Cells often hyperchromatic and pleomorphic appearing
- Infiltrative growth pattern

SELECTED REFERENCES

1. Seong MK et al: Primary apocrine sweat gland carcinomas of the axilla: a report of two cases and a review of the literature. World J Surg Oncol. 13:59, 2015
2. Guo J et al: Cutaneous apocrine carcinoma in groin with bilateral lymph node metastasis: a case report and review of the literature. Int J Clin Exp Pathol. 7(11):8266-70, 2014
3. Llamas-Velasco M et al: Apocrine intraductal carcinoma in situ in nevus sebaceus: two case reports. J Cutan Pathol. 41(12):944-9, 2014
4. Fernandez-Flores A: Podoplanin immunostaining in cutaneous apocrine carcinoma and in cutaneous metastasis from the breast. Appl Immunohistochem Mol Morphol. 18(6):573-4, 2010
5. Maury G et al: [Unusual axillary apocrine carcinoma of the skin: histological diagnostic difficulties.] Ann Dermatol Venereol. 137(8-9):555-9, 2010
6. Rütten A et al: Primary cutaneous cribriform apocrine carcinoma: a clinicopathologic and immunohistochemical study of 26 cases of an under-recognized cutaneous adnexal neoplasm. J Am Acad Dermatol. 61(4):644-51, 2009
7. Robson A et al: Primary cutaneous apocrine carcinoma: a clinico-pathologic analysis of 24 cases. Am J Surg Pathol. 32(5):682-90, 2008

Digital Papillary Adenocarcinoma

KEY FACTS

TERMINOLOGY

- Digital papillary adenocarcinoma (DPA)
- Formerly known as aggressive DPA and aggressive digital papillary adenoma (misnomer, as all are considered malignant)
- Malignant sweat gland tumor that typically presents on digits of young adult patients

CLINICAL ISSUES

- Young to middle-aged adult men
- Papular or nodular lesion on digit
- Often slowly growing and painless (leading to delayed diagnosis)
- Complete and wide excision or amputation
  - Associated with low recurrence and metastatic rates

MICROSCOPIC

- Multinodular solid or cystic tumor based in dermis
- Solid areas composed of dense collections of cells with focal ductal lumina
- Cystic/glandular areas with papillary projections often seen (although may be focal or absent in some cases)
- Mitotic figures often seen; can be numerous
- Focal necrosis may be present

TOP DIFFERENTIAL DIAGNOSES

- Eccrine carcinoma
  - Head and neck location
  - More infiltrative, small cords and nests of basophilic cells
- Apocrine carcinoma
  - Axillary and groin locations
  - Infiltrative lobules, nests, and cords of eosinophilic-staining cells
- Apocrine adenoma
- Spiradenoma
- Cylindroma

Digital Papillary Adenocarcinoma

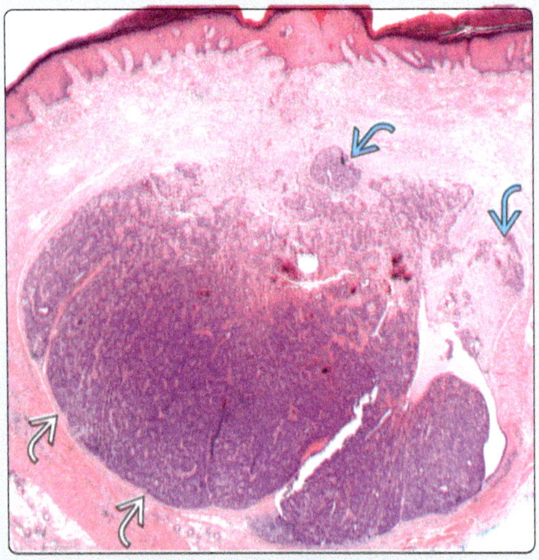

Intermediate Magnification of Nodular Area

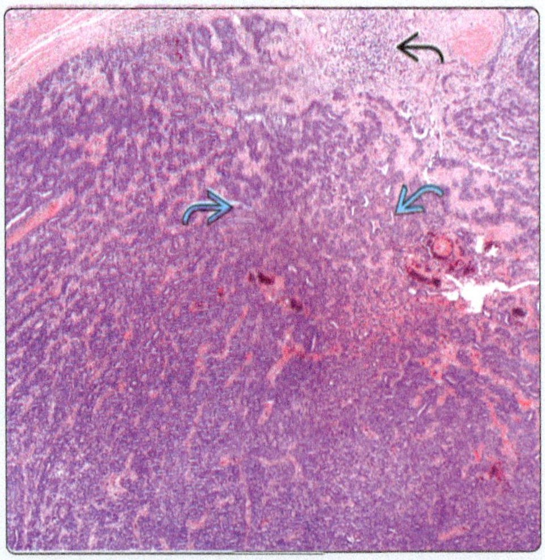

***(Left)** Digital papillary adenocarcinoma shows a nodular, basaloid tumor in the mid to deep dermis. Although the tumor is relatively well-circumscribed in most areas, there are other areas that appear more infiltrative. **(Right)** This nodular area is composed of crowded basaloid cells forming irregular cords and focal ductal lumina. There is surrounding stromal sclerosis and inflammation.*

High Magnification of Cellular Area

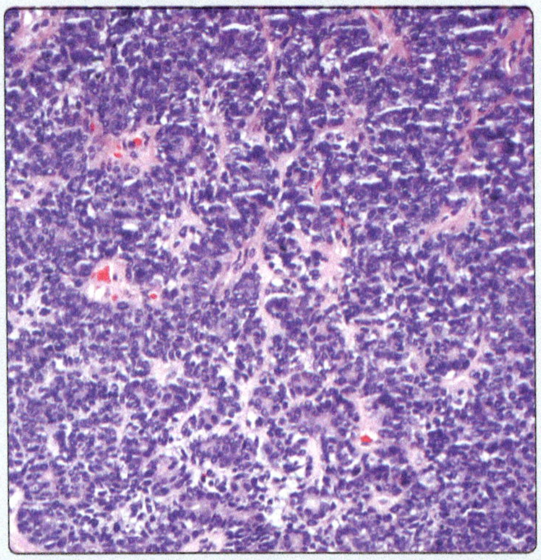

High Magnification of Glandular Area

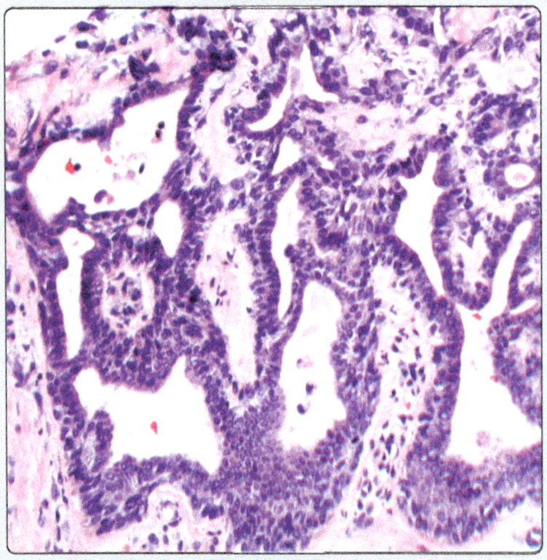

***(Left)** This more cellular area is composed of irregular, anastomosing cords of crowded basaloid cells showing nuclear hyperchromasia. **(Right)** This focus is composed of irregular, anastomosing glandular structures lined by cuboidal epithelial cells. Although the cells are small and relatively bland appearing, they show nuclear crowding and hyperchromasia.*

TERMINOLOGY

Abbreviations

- Digital papillary adenocarcinoma (DPA)

Synonyms

- Aggressive DPA
- Aggressive digital papillary adenoma (misnomer, as all are considered malignant)

Definitions

- Malignant sweat gland tumor that typically presents on digits of young adult patients

CLINICAL ISSUES

Epidemiology

- Incidence
  - Rare tumors
- Age
  - Young to middle-aged adults (mean age: 43 years)
    - Some cases also reported in children
- Sex
  - Most cases occur in men

Presentation

- Papular or nodular lesion on digit
  - Typically present on distal finger (most commonly) or toe but some cases on proximal digit/webspace
  - Often slowly growing and painless (leading to delayed diagnosis)

Treatment

- Complete and wide excision or amputation
- Sentinel lymph node biopsy has been advocated, given significant incidence of metastasis
  - However, most metastases involve lungs

Prognosis

- Wide excision or amputation associated with low recurrence and metastatic rates
  - However, some cases present with metastatic disease
  - Metastatic disease can also develop years after initial diagnosis, so long-term follow-up required

MACROSCOPIC

General Features

- Dermal nodular or nodular-cystic lesion

MICROSCOPIC

Histologic Features

- Multinodular solid or cystic tumor based in dermis
  - Subcutaneous invasion often seen
- Solid areas composed of dense collections of cells with focal ductal lumina
- Cystic/glandular areas with papillary projections often seen (although may be focal or absent in some cases)
- Composed of small cuboidal-shaped cells with nuclear hyperchromasia and eosinophilic-staining cytoplasm
- Mitotic figures often seen, can be numerous
- Necrosis may be present, usually focal
- Stroma varies from thin fibrous septa to dense hyalinized collagen

ANCILLARY TESTS

Immunohistochemistry

- Positive for cytokeratins, including pankeratin and high-molecular-weight keratins
- CEA and EMA highlight ductal/glandular lumens
- SMA, calponin, and p63 may highlight myoepithelial layer

DIFFERENTIAL DIAGNOSIS

Eccrine Carcinoma

- Most commonly occurs on scalp and head and neck, not digits
- Infiltrative small cords and nests of basaloid cells with nuclear hyperchromasia (not large nodulocystic collections of DPA)

Apocrine Carcinoma

- Typically occurs in axillary and groin region, not digits
- Composed mostly of smaller infiltrative lobules, nests and cords of eosinophilic-staining tumor cells

Apocrine Adenoma

- Small, well-circumscribed, noninfiltrative tumor
- Lacks significant atypia and mitotic activity

Spiradenoma

- Large basophilic tumor nodules associated with thickened basement membranes
- Biphasic tumor cell population of small, dark cells and larger, pale-staining cells

Cylindroma

- Irregular, jigsaw puzzle-like pattern of nests and lobules
- Associated with prominent thickened basement membranes and droplets of hyalinized material within lobules

SELECTED REFERENCES

1. Bell D et al: Next-generation sequencing reveals rare genomic alterations in aggressive digital papillary adenocarcinoma. Ann Diagn Pathol. 19(6):381-4, 2015
2. Kempton SJ et al: Aggressive digital papillary adenocarcinoma: case report of a positive sentinel lymph node and discussion of utility of sentinel lymph node biopsy. Ann Plast Surg. 75(1):34-6, 2015
3. Chen S et al: Papillary adenocarcinoma in situ of the skin: report of four cases. Dermatol Pract Concept. 4(2):23-8, 2014
4. Scolyer RA et al: Digital papillary adenocarcinoma: a tumour that should be considered in the differential diagnosis of neoplasms involving the digits. Pathology. 45(1):55-61, 2013
5. Suchak R et al: Cutaneous digital papillary adenocarcinoma: a clinicopathologic study of 31 cases of a rare neoplasm with new observations. Am J Surg Pathol. 36(12):1883-91, 2012
6. Chi CC et al: Aggressive digital papillary adenocarcinoma: a silent malignancy masquerading as acquired digital fibrokeratoma. Am J Clin Dermatol. 8(4):243-5, 2007
7. Duke WH et al: Aggressive digital papillary adenocarcinoma (aggressive digital papillary adenoma and adenocarcinoma revisited). Am J Surg Pathol. 24(6):775-84, 2000
8. Malafa MP et al: Sentinel node biopsy for staging of aggressive digital papillary adenocarcinoma. Dermatol Surg. 26(6):580-3, 2000
9. Kao GF et al: Aggressive digital papillary adenoma and adenocarcinoma. A clinicopathological study of 57 patients, with histochemical, immunopathological, and ultrastructural observations. J Cutan Pathol. 14(3):129-46, 1987

(Left) *Histologic examination shows a nodular, cellular, deep dermal neoplasm with scattered spaces, consistent with ductal/glandular differentiation.* **(Right)** *This area of the tumor shows a focus of comedonecrosis, which may be seen in a minority of cases. Note the scattered ductal lumina also present in this field.*

Digital Papillary Adenocarcinoma at Scanning Magnification

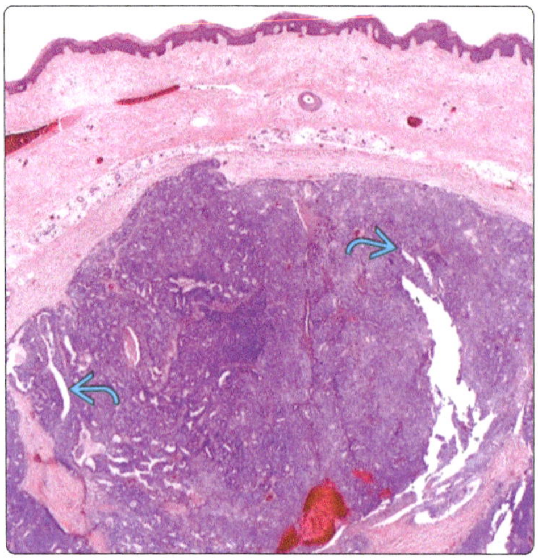

Digital Papillary Adenocarcinoma With Focal Comedonecrosis

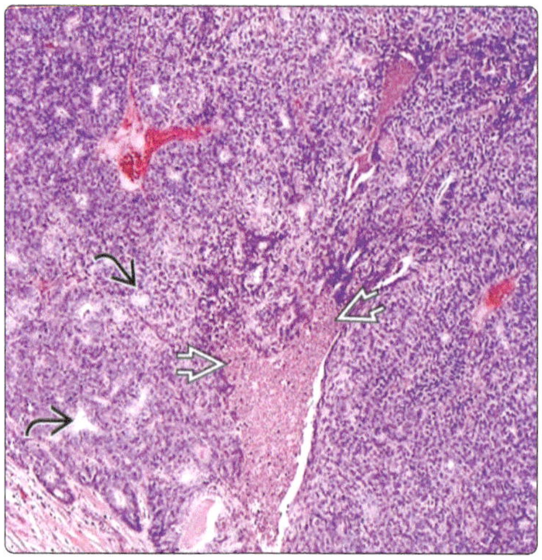

(Left) *Although the mitotic rate is variable, it can be quite high in some cases, as shown here. Multiple mitoses are easily identified in this field.* **(Right)** *High-molecular-weight cytokeratins, such as CK5/6, are typically strongly positive in digital papillary adenocarcinoma, consistent with a primary cutaneous tumor.*

High Magnification of Cellular Area With Mitoses

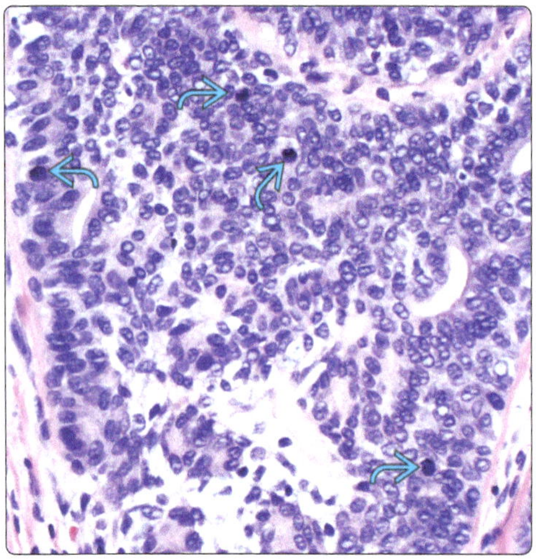

CK5/6 Is Strongly Positive in Digital Papillary Adenocarcinoma

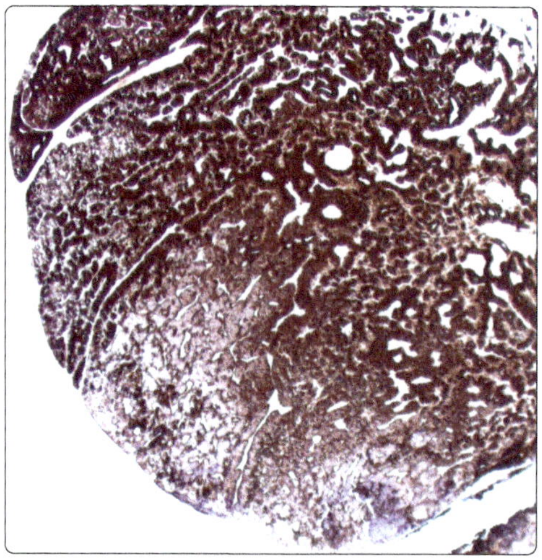

(Left) *EMA strongly highlights numerous ductal/glandular lumina in digital papillary adenocarcinoma.* **(Right)** *GCDFP-15 strongly highlights the ductal lumina, a finding consistent with apocrine differentiation.*

EMA/MUC1 Stain in Digital Carcinoma

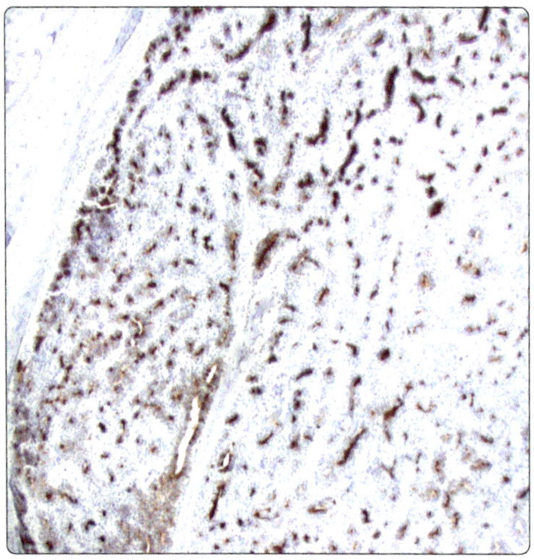

GCDFP-15 Highlights Ductal Lumina

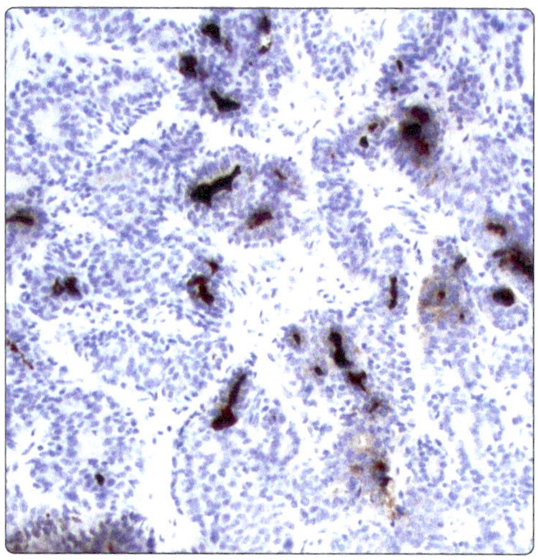

Nodular Digital Papillary Adenocarcinoma at Low Magnification

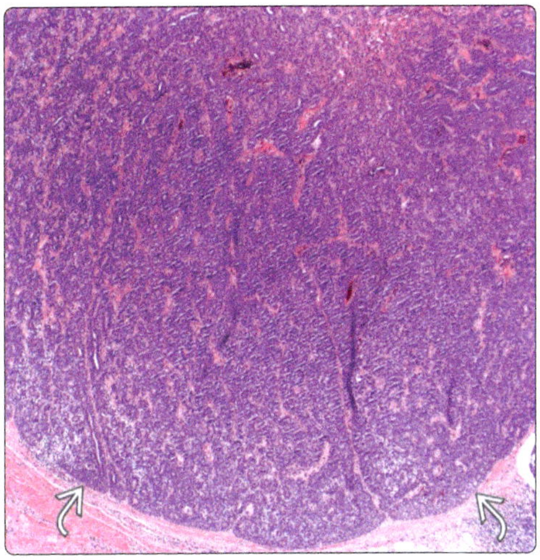

Digital Papillary Adenocarcinoma With Cystic Features

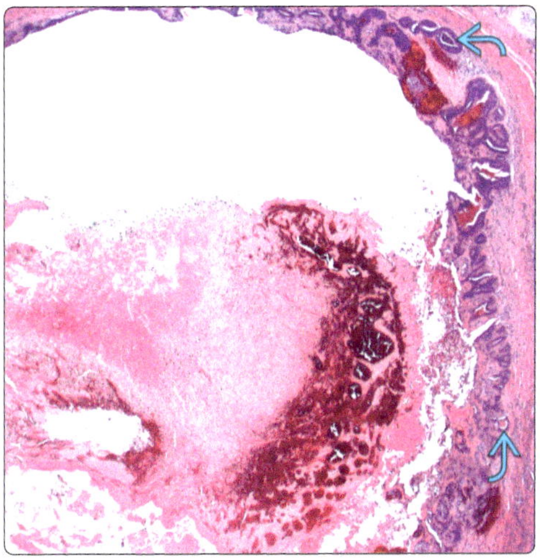

(Left) *This image shows a nodular basaloid tumor in the mid to deep dermis. Although the tumor is relatively well circumscribed in most areas, there is prominent cellularity and nuclear hyperchromasia.* **(Right)** *Although most tumors are nodular, cystic spaces can also be seen. This tumor showed areas with large cystic spaces lined by atypical basaloid cells forming ductal and papillary structures.*

Differential Diagnosis: Spiradenoma

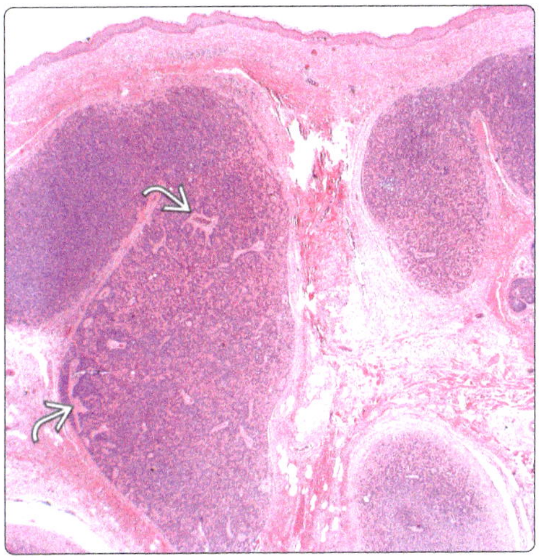

Differential Diagnosis: Spiradenocarcinoma

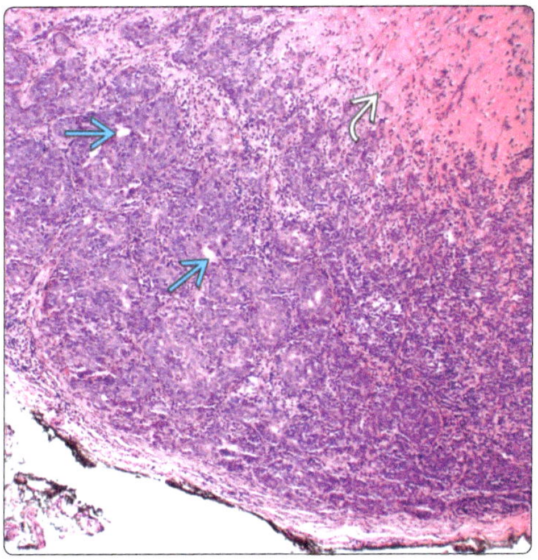

(Left) *Spiradenoma is another nodular, dermal-basaloid tumor, which can enter the differential diagnosis at low magnification. However, it shows a more hyalinized stroma, which can be seen around the blood vessels even at this magnification.* **(Right)** *Spiradenocarcinoma is also a nodular, atypical basaloid dermal neoplasm but typically shows areas of hyalinized stroma and multiple small ductal lumina lacking papillary areas.*

Differential Diagnosis: Cylindroma

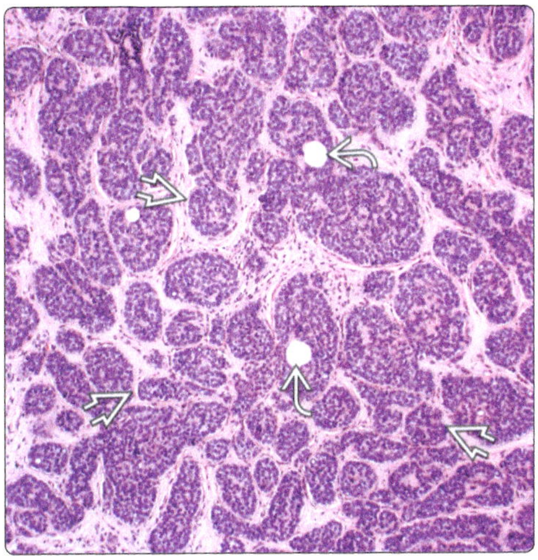

Differential Diagnosis: Cylindrocarcinoma

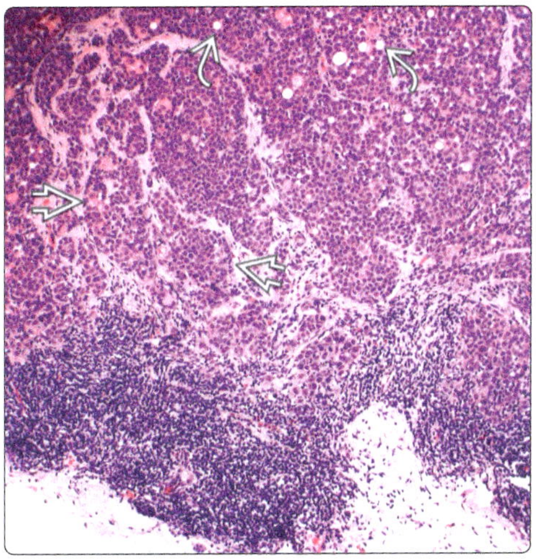

(Left) *Another dermal-based nodular adnexal tumor that could enter the differential diagnosis is cylindroma. However, note the numerous small nests in a jigsaw puzzle-like pattern, surrounded by a hyalinized stroma, as well as multiple small ductal lumina.* **(Right)** *Cylindrocarcinoma is another rare adnexal carcinoma that can be considered in the differential but also lacks papillary features. Note the irregular, jigsaw puzzle-like pattern in areas, as well as multiple small ductal lumina.*

KEY FACTS

TERMINOLOGY

- Synonyms
  - Eccrine angiomatous hamartoma
    - Sweating angiomatous hamartoma
    - Functioning sudoriparous angiomatous hamartoma
  - Porokeratotic eccrine ostial and dermal duct nevus
    - Porokeratotic eccrine duct and hair follicle nevus

CLINICAL ISSUES

- Congenital or develop in childhood; may present in adulthood

MICROSCOPIC

- Eccrine angiomatous hamartoma
  - Eccrine glands normal (occasionally enlarged) or increased in number
  - Endothelial cell-lined, thin-walled vascular spaces intimately admixed with eccrine glands
- Coccygeal polypoid eccrine nevus
  - Polypoid shape; increased number of eccrine glands
- Porokeratotic eccrine ostial and dermal duct nevus
  - Cornoid lamellae (tiers of parakeratosis over diminished granular layer) above acrosyringeal ducts &/or hair follicles
- Eccrine nevus
  - Increased number or size of eccrine glands
  - No increase in vessels; not polypoid

TOP DIFFERENTIAL DIAGNOSES

- Eccrine angiomatous hamartoma
  - Eccrine nevus
- Eccrine nevus
  - Normal eccrine glands
- Coccygeal polypoid eccrine nevus
  - Skin tag/acrochordon or soft fibroma
- Porokeratotic eccrine ostial and dermal duct nevus
  - Porokeratosis
  - Inflammatory linear verrucous epidermal nevus

Clinical Photograph of Porokeratotic Eccrine Ostial and Dermal Duct Nevus

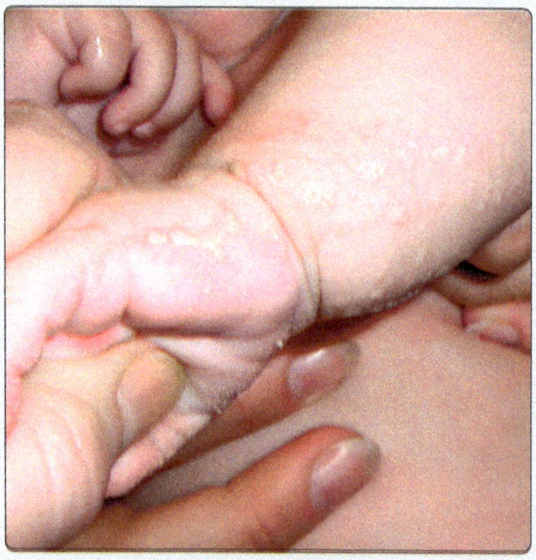

Porokeratotic Eccrine Ostial and Dermal Duct Nevus

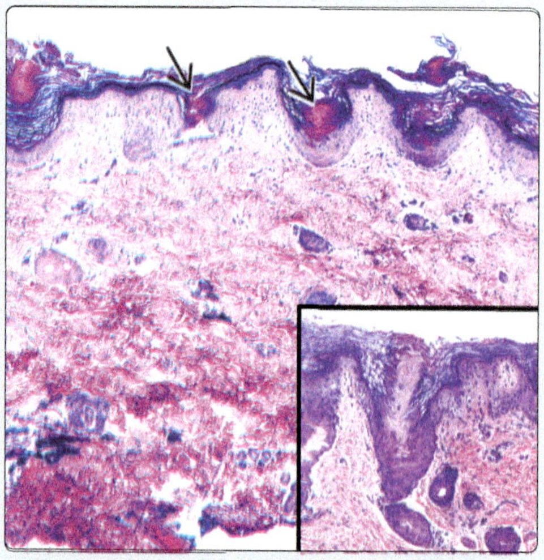

(Left) *This is a porokeratotic eccrine ostial and dermal duct nevus with light pink, hyperkeratotic streaks following Blaschko lines. There are focal spines. (Courtesy J. McNiff, MD, and R. Antaya, MD.)* **(Right)** *Biopsy of porokeratotic eccrine ostial and dermal duct nevus shows tiers of parakeratosis (cornoid lamellae) ➔ overlying acrosyringeal ostia. The inset shows another example with a cornoid lamella. (Courtesy J. McNiff, MD.)*

Eccrine Angiomatous Hamartoma

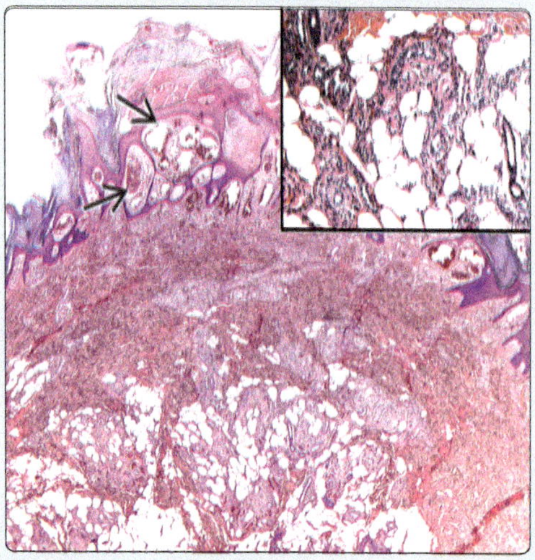

Coccygeal Polypoid Eccrine Nevus

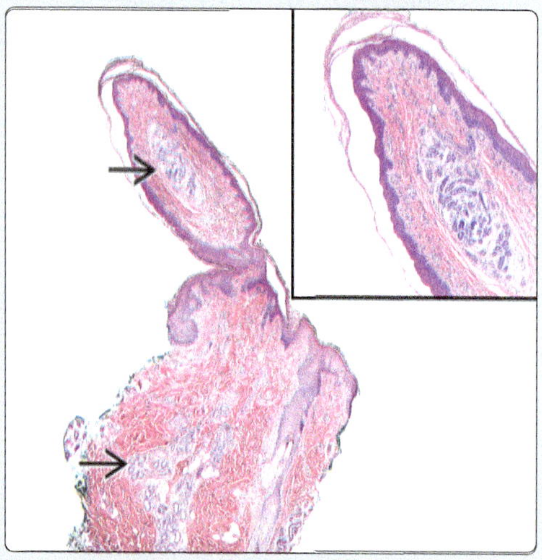

(Left) *In eccrine angiomatous hamartoma, the epidermis is often normal; this example has an overlying verrucous hemangioma ➔. In the lower dermis, eccrine glands are intimately admixed with fat and vessels (as seen in the inset). (Courtesy of A. Galan, MD.)* **(Right)** *Coccygeal polypoid eccrine nevus is polypoid; increased numbers of eccrine glands ➔ are in the dermis (highlighted in the inset).*

TERMINOLOGY

Synonyms

- Eccrine angiomatous hamartoma
  - Sweating angiomatous hamartoma
  - Sudoriparous angioma
  - Functioning sudoriparous angiomatous hamartoma
- Porokeratotic eccrine ostial and dermal duct nevus
  - Porokeratotic eccrine duct and hair follicle nevus
  - Porokeratotic adnexal ostial nevus

Definitions

- Often congenital lesions with prominent component of eccrine glands

CLINICAL ISSUES

Presentation

- **Eccrine angiomatous hamartoma**
  - Congenital or develops in childhood; may present in adulthood
  - Occasionally familial
  - Symptoms/signs
    - May be asymptomatic; may be hyperhidrotic or painful
    - Tends to grow slowly over time
    - Hypertrichosis may be evident
  - Macule or plaque (0.3-11.0 cm), generally solitary
    - Occasionally papular or nodular, rarely surface is verrucous or hyperkeratotic
    - Variable color: Red, blue, yellow, purple, or brown
    - Overlying telangiectasias may be present
  - Commonly on palms/soles or extremities, but other sites described
- **Eccrine nevus**
  - Rarely congenital; usually develops in childhood or adulthood
  - Solitary or multiple (may follow Blaschko lines)
  - Nondescript macule/patch; may display hyperhidrosis
- **Coccygeal polypoid eccrine nevus**
  - Often congenital; skin tag-like papule over coccygeal area
  - Generally asymptomatic
- **Porokeratotic eccrine ostial and dermal duct nevus**
  - Often congenital
  - May be solitary and localized to palms/soles and adjacent limb
  - May be generalized, following Blaschko lines
    - Rarely associated with systemic abnormalities (e.g., deafness)
  - Tend to be asymptomatic
  - Rarely spontaneously involute
  - Rarely may develop malignancy

Treatment

- Conservative excision not necessary, but may be performed if symptomatic (e.g., hyperhidrotic)

MICROSCOPIC

Histologic Features

- **Eccrine angiomatous hamartoma**
  - Epidermis
    - May be normal
    - Or may display hyperkeratosis, acanthosis, &/or papillomatosis
  - Dermal eccrine glands appear normal (occasionally enlarged), or may be increased in numbers
  - Adipose tissue, hair follicles, &/or mucin may be increased
  - Endothelial cell-lined, thin-walled vascular spaces intimately admixed with eccrine glands
  - Papillary and upper reticular dermis may show increased vessels, sometimes resembling an angioma (i.e., verrucous hemangioma or angiokeratoma-like)
  - Immunohistochemistry
    - Eccrine glands stain as normal (positive with CK7, CEA-M, EMA)
    - Vascular structures stain with CD31 and other vascular markers
- **Eccrine nevus**
  - Increased number &/or size of eccrine glands
  - Mucin may be increased (if so, termed mucinous eccrine nevus)
  - No increase in vessels; not polypoid
- **Coccygeal polypoid eccrine nevus**
  - Polypoid shape
  - Dermis contains increased number of eccrine glands
  - No increase in vessels or nerves
- **Porokeratotic eccrine ostial and dermal duct nevus**
  - Cornoid lamellae (tiers of parakeratosis over diminished granular layer) overlying acrosyringeal ducts &/or hair follicles

DIFFERENTIAL DIAGNOSIS

Eccrine Angiomatous Hamartoma

- Eccrine nevus
  - Shows enlargement of eccrine glands, lacks increase in vessels

Eccrine Nevus

- Normal eccrine glands
  - In eccrine nevus, eccrine glands are often enlarged

Coccygeal Polypoid Eccrine Nevus

- Skin tag/acrochordon or soft fibroma
  - Polypoid shape
  - No increase in eccrine glands in dermis

Porokeratotic Eccrine Ostial and Dermal Duct Nevus

- Porokeratosis
  - Cornoid lamellae are not centered over acrosyringeal ducts
- Inflammatory linear verrucous epidermal nevus
  - Hyperkeratosis alternating with orthokeratosis, acanthotic epidermis
  - True cornoid lamellae absent

SELECTED REFERENCES

1. Sanusi T et al: Eccrine angiomatous hamartoma: a clinicopathological study of 26 cases. Dermatology. 231(1):63-9, 2015
2. Masferrer E et al: Porokeratotic eccrine ostial and dermal duct naevus: report of 10 cases. J Eur Acad Dermatol Venereol. 24(7):847-51, 2010

Papillary Eccrine Adenoma

KEY FACTS

TERMINOLOGY

- Papillary eccrine adenoma (PEA)
- Rare benign adnexal tumor with eccrine differentiation
- Most authorities separate PEAs from tubular apocrine adenomas

CLINICAL ISSUES

- Rare tumors
- Presentation: Slowly growing firm or hard nodules
- Site: Distal extremity
- More common in women
- Prognosis: Excellent

MICROSCOPIC

- Circumscribed, symmetrical dermal tumor with rare connections to epidermis
- Ducts lined by ≥ 2 layers of cuboidal cells
- Dilated glandular structures of various sizes
- Microcysts may be present
- Inner layer often forms 1 or multiple papillae of variable complexity
- Some lumina contain eosinophilic amorphous material
- Foci of loosely arranged spindled cells and hyalinized collagen present in stroma

ANCILLARY TESTS

- Epithelial cells often show S100, CEA, and EMA reactivity

TOP DIFFERENTIAL DIAGNOSES

- Tubular apocrine adenoma
  - Evidence of apocrine glandular differentiation
- Aggressive digital papillary adenocarcinoma
  - Larger nodular tumor with ductal structures
  - More cellular and shows infiltrative features
- Metastatic adenocarcinoma
  - Cytologic atypia and mitoses usually prominent

Papillary Eccrine Adenoma

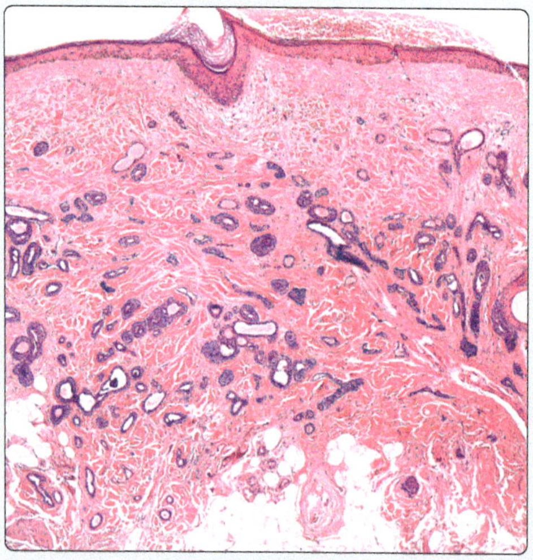

Papillary Eccrine Adenoma at Higher Magnification

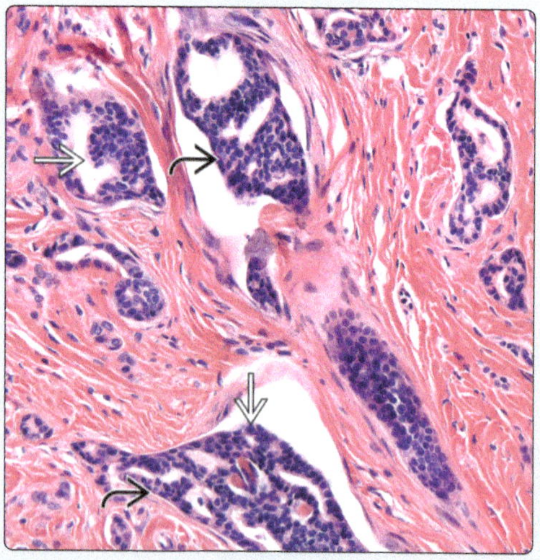

(Left) *Low-power examination shows a dermal adnexal tumor with variably sized ductal and glandular spaces associated with a fibrous stroma.* **(Right)** *On high magnification, the glands show low-cuboidal eccrine cells ➡ and areas with cribriforming and papillary projection of variable complexity ➡. (Courtesy J. McNiff, MD.)*

Papillary Eccrine Adenoma at High Magnification

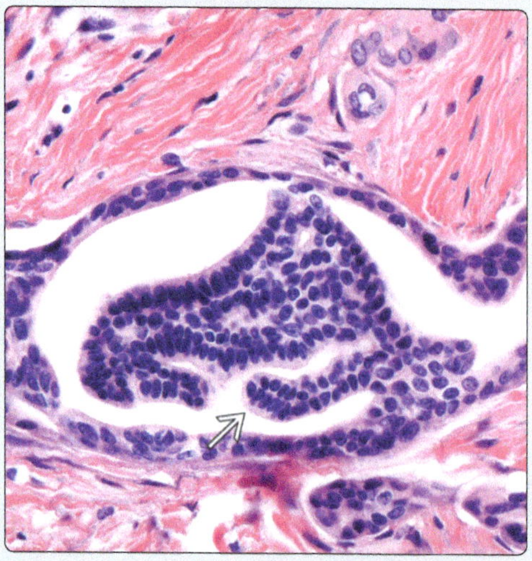

Immunohistochemistry for p63

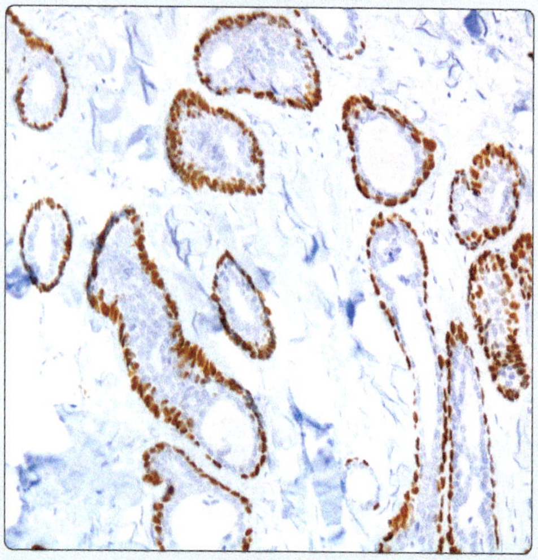

(Left) *High magnification shows uniform, small cuboidal cells lining the glands and forming papillary projections ➡. (Courtesy J. McNiff, MD.)* **(Right)** *p63 immunohistochemistry shows strong staining of the peripheral myoepithelial cell layer, consistent with a benign tumor. (Courtesy J. McNiff, MD.)*

TERMINOLOGY

Abbreviations

- Papillary eccrine adenoma (PEA)

Synonyms

- Tubulopapillary hidradenoma with eccrine differentiation

Definitions

- Rare benign adnexal tumor with evidence of eccrine derivation/differentiation
  - In the past, many cases with apocrine features were included in this category
  - However, most authorities now separate PEAs from tubular apocrine adenomas

CLINICAL ISSUES

Epidemiology

- Incidence
  - Rare
- Sex
  - Women
- Ethnicity
  - More common in Africans/African Americans

Site

- Distal extremity
  - Other sites include trunk and head and neck

Presentation

- Firm or hard nodule
- Asymptomatic
  - Occasionally tender
- Slowly growing

Treatment

- Surgical approaches
  - Treatment is not usually necessary
  - If treatment is desired, simple excision is optimal treatment
  - Mohs micrographic surgery
    - May be done in cases where possibility of aggressive digital papillary adenocarcinoma cannot be ruled out due to superficial nature of biopsy

Prognosis

- Excellent
- Can recur if partially removed

MICROSCOPIC

Histologic Features

- Circumscribed, symmetric-appearing dermal tumor
- Rare connections to epidermis
- Dilated ductal and glandular structures of various sizes
- Microcysts from dilated ducts may be present
- Inner layer often forms 1 or multiple papillae of variable complexity
- Ducts are lined by ≥ 2 layers of cuboidal cells
- Some lumina contain eosinophilic amorphous material
- Rare keratin-filled cysts
- Lesion embedded in dense fibrous stroma
- Stroma often forms bands around ducts
- Foci of loosely arranged spindled cells and hyalinized collagen present in stroma
- Rare histologic features
  - Focal squamous differentiation
  - Clear cell change
  - Epidermal connections of ducts
  - Follicular and sebaceous differentiation
  - Proliferation of nerves within stroma
  - Human papillomavirus-like epidermal changes
- Term "tubulopapillary hidradenoma" is used for lesions with both eccrine and apocrine differentiation

Cytologic Features

- Cuboidal to columnar cells

ANCILLARY TESTS

Immunohistochemistry

- Epithelial cells often show S100, CEA, and EMA reactivity

DIFFERENTIAL DIAGNOSIS

Tubular Apocrine Adenoma

- Similar histology as PEA, but with evidence of apocrine glandular differentiation
- Shows decapitation secretion
- Some consider PEA and tubular apocrine adenoma to be synonymous, but most separate these entities

Aggressive Digital Papillary Adenocarcinoma

- Predominately in young adult males
- Larger nodular tumor with ductal structures
- More cellular and shows infiltrative features
- Cytologic atypia and increased mitoses usually present
- High recurrence rate

Metastatic Adenocarcinoma

- Usually large, nodular, and infiltrative tumor
- Cytologic atypia and mitoses usually prominent

DIAGNOSTIC CHECKLIST

Pathologic Interpretation Pearls

- Dermal-based adnexal tumor with variably dilated eccrine ducts
- Projection of papillae into lumen of ducts

SELECTED REFERENCES

1. Asgari M et al: Papillary eccrine adenoma should not be mistaken for aggressive digital papillary adenocarcinoma. Clin Exp Dermatol. 39(2):223-4, 2014
2. Blasini W et al: Papillary eccrine adenoma in association with cutaneous horn. Am J Clin Dermatol. 8(3):179-82, 2007
3. Mizuoka H et al: Papillary eccrine adenoma: immunohistochemical study and literature review. J Cutan Pathol. 25(1):59-64, 1998
4. Hattori N et al: Papillary tubular adenoma with marked tubular vacuolization. J Dermatol. 24(12):777-80, 1997
5. Ishiko A et al: Is tubular apocrine adenoma a distinct clinical entity? Am J Dermatopathol. 15(5):482-7, 1993
6. Falck VG et al: Papillary eccrine adenoma. A tubulopapillary hidradenoma with eccrine differentiation. Am J Dermatopathol. 8(1):64-72, 1986

KEY FACTS

TERMINOLOGY

- Benign ductal proliferation in superficial dermis

ETIOLOGY/PATHOGENESIS

- Eruptive syringomas may be due to autoimmune destruction of acrosyringium

CLINICAL ISSUES

- Predilection for eyelids
- Often multiple, small, skin-colored to translucent papules
- More common in females, Asians, and Down syndrome patients
- Variants include giant, solitary, plaque, linear, disseminated, and eruptive
- Clear cell variant associated with diabetes mellitus
- Benign tumors with excellent prognosis
  - Treatment is not necessary in most cases
  - Syringoid eccrine carcinomas are likely de novo tumors, and not derived from syringomas

MICROSCOPIC

- Small ducts, nests, and cords of pale eosinophilic to clear cells in superficial dermis
- Ducts lined by 1 or 2 layers of cuboidal cells
- Tadpole-like pattern often seen, with comma-like tails
- Fibrotic stroma

TOP DIFFERENTIAL DIAGNOSES

- Desmoplastic trichoepithelioma
  - Presents as single lesion rather than multiple, as is often seen with syringomas
  - Lacks true ductal differentiation
- Microcystic adnexal carcinoma
  - Larger, more infiltrative tumor that extends into deep dermis or subcutaneous tissue
- Morpheaform basal cell carcinoma
  - Often presents in sun-damaged skin of elderly as single lesion that is indurated
  - Cytologic atypia and mitoses present

Clinical Photograph of Multiple Syringomas

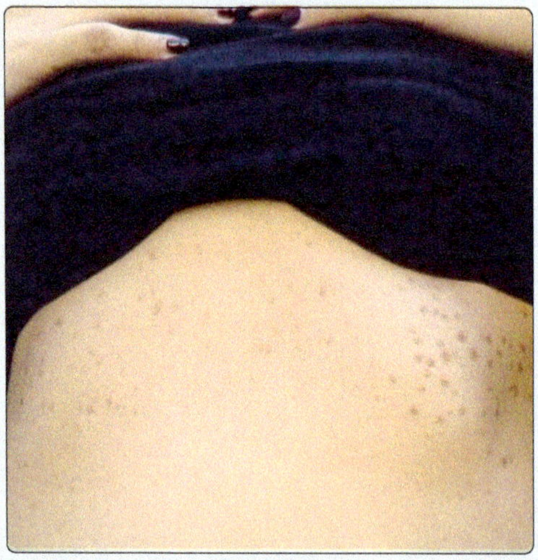

Low Magnification of Syringoma

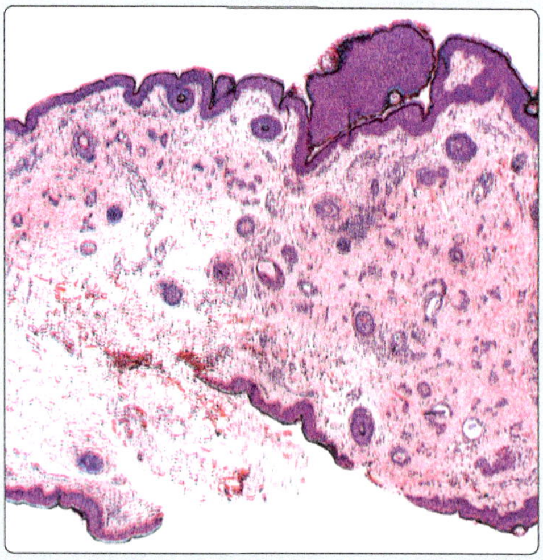

(Left) *This is a young adult female patient who presented with numerous reddish/brown-appearing syringomas on her chest and abdomen.* **(Right)** *Low magnification of a typical syringoma shows basaloid nests and strands of small epithelial cells admixed with small ducts.*

Higher Magnification of Syringoma

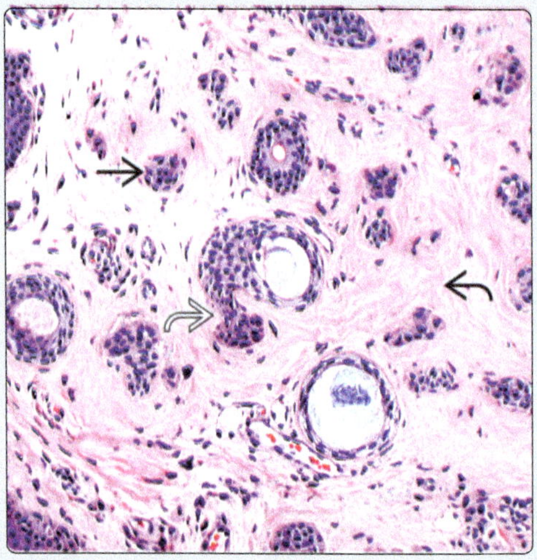

Clustered Ducts in Syringoma

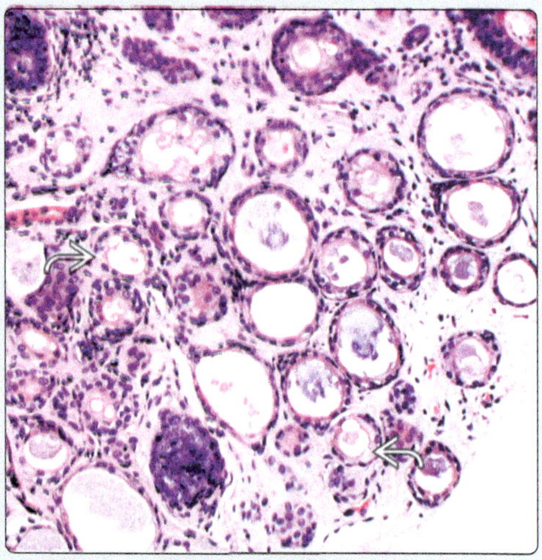

(Left) *Higher magnification shows small ducts, one with a tadpole-like shape ➡, solid nests ➡, and strands of epithelial cells in a fibrotic stroma ➡.* **(Right)** *This section shows a higher power view of a cellular area of an otherwise classic syringoma. Note the pale to clear-staining cells ➡ lining well-differentiated ductal structures.*

TERMINOLOGY

Definitions

- Benign eccrine ductal proliferation in superficial dermis

ETIOLOGY/PATHOGENESIS

Etiology

- Eruptive syringomas may be due to autoimmune destruction of acrosyringium

CLINICAL ISSUES

Epidemiology

- Incidence
  - Relatively common tumors
- Age
  - Puberty to old age
- Sex
  - More common in females
- Ethnicity
  - More common in Asians

Site

- Commonly head and neck
  - Predilection for eyelids
  - Rare sites include: Vulva, penis, buttocks, hands, and feet

Presentation

- Often multiple, small, skin-colored to translucent papules
- Asymptomatic
  - Rarely pruritic, which is worse with perspiration
- Rare clinical variants
  - Giant, solitary, plaque, linear, disseminated, and eruptive
  - Clear cell variant associated with diabetes mellitus
- More common in Down syndrome patients
- Can rarely be seen in Brooke-Spiegler syndrome

Treatment

- Treatment is not necessary
- If cosmetically bothersome: Cryotherapy, chemical peels, electrosurgical destruction, excision, and laser ablation are some options

Prognosis

- Benign; excellent prognosis
  - Malignant transformation is extremely rare, if it even exists
  - Syringoid eccrine carcinomas are likely de novo tumors, and not derived from syringomas

MICROSCOPIC

Histologic Features

- Small ducts, nests, cords, and cysts lined by pale eosinophilic to clear-staining cells in superficial dermis
- Ducts and cysts lined by 1 or 2 layers of small, bland-appearing cuboidal cells
- Some ducts have tadpole-like appearance with comma-like tails
- Dilated ducts may have eosinophilic contents
- Horn cysts can rarely be present
- Fibrotic stroma
- Clear cell variant
  - Epithelial cells lining ducts with clear cytoplasm
  - Clear cell change might only be focal finding
- Immunohistochemistry: Cells stain positive with CEA, EMA, and cytokeratins 1, 5, 10, 11, 19
- Rare variants
  - Syringoma admixed with benign melanocytes
  - Presence of dense plasmacytic inflammation within stroma

Cytologic Features

- Bland-appearing small cuboidal cells

DIFFERENTIAL DIAGNOSIS

Desmoplastic Trichoepithelioma

- Presents as single lesion rather than multiple, as is often seen with syringomas
- Often shows multiple basaloid islands, as well as superficial keratinizing horn cysts
- May show focal papillary mesenchymal bodies
- Lacks true ductal differentiation
- Does not express CEA and EMA, unlike syringomas

Microcystic Adnexal Carcinoma

- Often presents as single lesion
- Larger, more infiltrative tumor that extends into deep dermis or subcutaneous tissue
- Perineural invasion is common
- Superficial portion of tumor shows follicular differentiation, with keratinizing infundibulocystic structures
- May be difficult to differentiate microcystic adnexal carcinoma from syringoma in a small, superficial biopsy

Morpheaform Basal Cell Carcinoma

- Often presents in sun-damaged skin of the elderly as single lesion that is indurated
  - Syringomas are often multiple and have skin-colored appearance
- Retraction of tumor cells from stroma is often seen
- Cytologic atypia and mitoses present
- Ductal differentiation only very rarely present in basal cell carcinoma

Metastatic Adenocarcinoma

- Much less likely consideration in differential diagnosis
- Scalp and trunk are most common sites
- Larger and more infiltrative tumors
- Cytologic atypia and mitosis are usually prominent

SELECTED REFERENCES

1. Wallace JS et al: An important mimicker: plaque-type syringoma mistakenly diagnosed as microcystic adnexal carcinoma. Dermatol Surg. 40(7):810-2, 2014
2. Akoglu G et al: Vulvar nonclear cell syringoma associated with pruritus and diabetes mellitus. Case Rep Dermatol Med. 2013:418794, 2013
3. Uede K et al: Brooke-Spiegler syndrome associated with cylindroma, trichoepithelioma, spiradenoma, and syringoma. J Dermatol. 31(1):32-8, 2004
4. Cassarino DS et al: Puzzling penile papules. Int J Dermatol. 42(12):954-6, 2003
5. Patrizi A et al: Syringoma: a review of twenty-nine cases. Acta Derm Venereol. 78(6):460-2, 1998
6. Furue M et al: Clear-cell syringoma. Association with diabetes mellitus. Am J Dermatopathol. 6(2):131-8, 1984

Syringofibroadenoma

KEY FACTS

TERMINOLOGY

- Syringofibroadenoma (SFA)
- Also known as eccrine syringofibroadenoma (of Mascaro), acrosyringeal adenomatosis
- Rare benign proliferation of eccrine ductal origin

CLINICAL ISSUES

- Commonly on extremities
- More common in women
- Usually solitary, hyperkeratotic plaque
- Sometimes multiple, diffuse, or zosteriform
  - Multiple lesions can be associated with rare genetic syndromes
- Excellent prognosis in vast majority of cases
- Treatment: Usually not necessary, but some suggest simple excision or destruction due to rare possible risk of malignant transformation

MICROSCOPIC

- Vertically oriented, slender, interconnected basaloid epithelial cords extending from epidermis
- Lumina formation can be present
- Embedded in fibrovascular stroma

TOP DIFFERENTIAL DIAGNOSES

- Basal cell carcinoma (fibroepithelioma of Pinkus variant)
  - Thin anastomosing cords of basaloid cells with palisading
  - Mucinous stroma and tumor-stroma retraction artifact usually seen
- Poroma
  - Thicker anastomosing cords of small, cuboidal-shaped epithelioid cells
- Hidroacanthoma simplex (poroma variant)
  - Intraepidermal proliferation that lacks anastomosing architecture of SFA
- Acrosyringeal nevus
  - Likely represents variant of SFA

Syringofibroadenoma

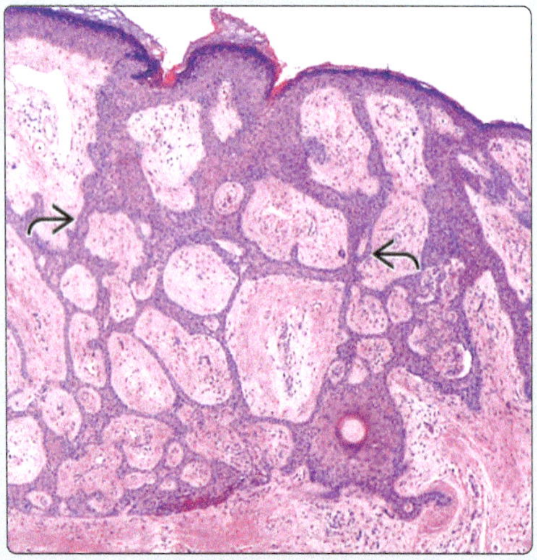

Syringofibroadenoma With Ductal Lumina

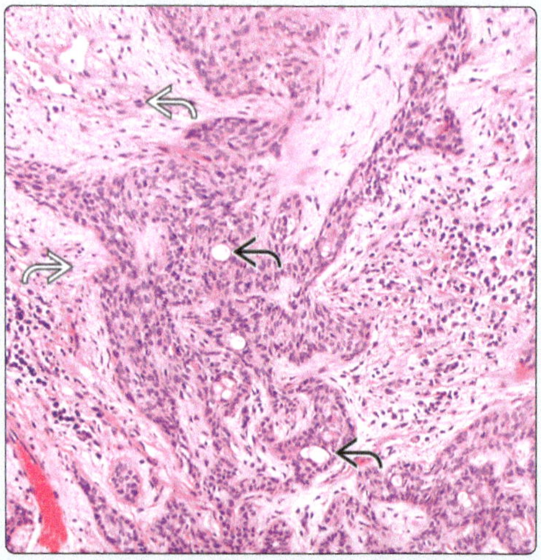

(Left) *Seen arising from multiple points along the epidermis are thin, anastomosing cords ➜ of uniform epithelial cells embedded in a fibrovascular stroma, findings typical of syringofibroadenoma (SFA).* **(Right)** *Epithelial strands of acrosyringeal cells show focal ductal formation ➜. The lesion is associated with a fibrovascular stroma ➜, a characteristic finding of SFA.*

Differential Diagnosis: Fibroepithelioma of Pinkus (BCC Variant)

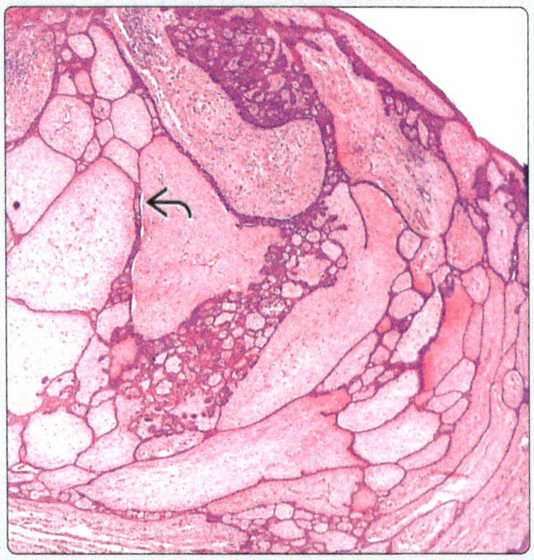

Differential Diagnosis: Poroma

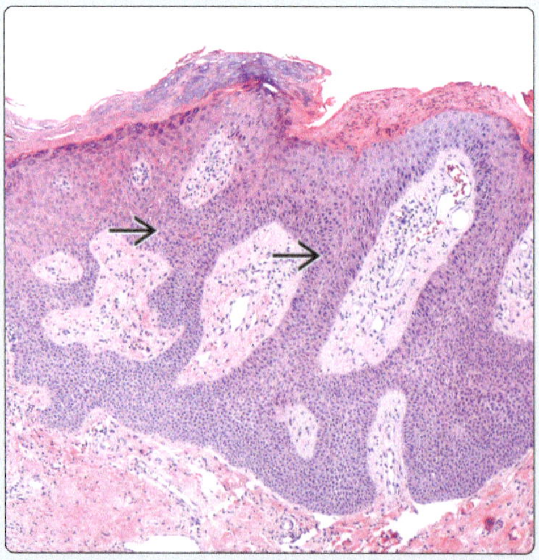

(Left) *Fibroepithelioma of Pinkus type of basal cell carcinoma (BCC) shows thin anastomosing strands of epithelial cells arranged in a net-like pattern in a myxoid stroma. Focal tumor-stromal clefting ➜ is seen.* **(Right)** *Poroma shows thicker anastomosing cords of epithelial cells extending from the epidermis ➜; the cells are generally smaller and more monotonous-appearing than in SFA.*

TERMINOLOGY

Abbreviations

- Syringofibroadenoma (SFA)

Synonyms

- Eccrine SFA (of Mascaro), acrosyringeal adenomatosis

Definitions

- Rare benign proliferation of eccrine ductal origin

CLINICAL ISSUES

Epidemiology

- Age
  - Commonly in elderly
- Sex
  - More common in women

Site

- Commonly on extremities
- Rare locations include face, trunk, and nails

Presentation

- Clinical presentation
  - Usually solitary, hyperkeratotic plaque
  - Sometimes multiple, diffuse, or zosteriform
    - Terms acrosyringeal adenomatosis, eccrine syringofibroadenomatosis, and acrosyringeal nevus are used to identify this clinical variation
  - Multiple SFA associated with hidrotic ectodermal dysplasia (Clouston syndrome)
  - Multiple SFA associated with Schöpf-Schulz-Passarge syndrome
    - Rare ectodermal dysplasia
  - Multiple SFA associated with familial ophthalmologic abnormalities
  - Reactive eccrine syringofibroadenomatosis
    - Rarely develop as reactive process in association with unrelated inflammatory conditions or tumors
    - Usually on acral sites
    - Lichen planus, bullous pemphigoid, burn scars, diabetic foot ulcer, leprosy, and squamous cell carcinoma are some associated conditions

Treatment

- Treatment is usually not necessary
- Some suggest simple excision or destruction due to rare possible risk of malignant transformation

Prognosis

- Excellent
- Rare reports of malignant transformation

MICROSCOPIC

Histologic Features

- Vertically oriented, slender, interconnected basaloid epithelial cords extending from epidermis into dermis
- Epithelial cords contain ducts and cystic structures
  - Ducts are lined with cuboidal cells resembling eccrine ducts
- Basaloid cells are smaller than adjacent keratinocytes
- Lesion is embedded in fibrovascular stroma
- Mild superficial lymphocytic infiltrate can be seen
  - Lacks prominent plasma cell infiltrate reported in acrosyringeal nevus
- Clear cell SFA is rare variant

Cytologic Features

- Small cuboidal cells lacking atypia

ANCILLARY TESTS

Immunohistochemistry

- Luminal cells are highlighted by EMA, CEA
- Cytokeratin stains have been inconsistent and are not helpful

DIFFERENTIAL DIAGNOSIS

Basal Cell Carcinoma: Fibroepithelioma of Pinkus Variant

- Thin anastomosing cords of basaloid cells
- Peripheral palisading, typical of basal cell carcinoma
- Tumor-stromal clefting artifact
- Loose myxoid stroma

Poroma

- Thicker anastomosing epithelioid cords
- More uniform, smaller epithelial cells
- Loose stroma

Hidroacanthoma Simplex (Poroma Variant)

- Intraepidermal proliferation that lacks anastomosing architecture of SFA
- Proliferation of basaloid and clear cells with ducts

Acrosyringeal Nevus

- Some consider this entity to be variant of SFA
- Strong PAS positivity of acrosyringeal keratinocytes
- Prominent plasma cell infiltrate

Syringofibroadenocarcinoma

- Only rare reported cases
- Foci of malignant transformation in association with SFA
- Development of reactive SFA within carcinoma instead of malignant transformation is possibility

DIAGNOSTIC CHECKLIST

Pathologic Interpretation Pearls

- Thin, anastomosing, benign epithelial proliferation in fibrovascular stroma

SELECTED REFERENCES

1. Andrade AC et al: Clouston syndrome associated with eccrine syringofibroadenoma. An Bras Dermatol. 89(3):504-6, 2014
2. Shalin SC et al: Clear cell acanthoma with changes of eccrine syringofibroadenoma: reactive change or clue to etiology? J Cutan Pathol. 40(12):1021-6, 2013
3. Bjarke T et al: Carcinoma and eccrine syringofibroadenoma: a report of five cases. J Cutan Pathol. 30(6):382-92, 2003
4. Komine M et al: Eccrine syringofibroadenoma (Mascaro): an immunohistochemical study. Am J Dermatopathol. 22(2):171-5, 2000

KEY FACTS

TERMINOLOGY

- Syringoid carcinoma, syringoid eccrine carcinoma, eccrine syringomatous carcinoma, eccrine epithelioma
- Malignant adnexal tumor with eccrine differentiation somewhat resembling syringoma

CLINICAL ISSUES

- Very rare tumors
- Typically present as plaque on scalp
- Locally aggressive
- Only rare lymph node metastasis

MICROSCOPIC

- Dermal-based tumor; attachments to epidermis are very rare
- Composed of basaloid epithelium with uniform hyperchromatic nuclei
- Forms epithelial strands with lumen formation
- May have hand mirror shape similar to syringoma
- Infiltrative growth pattern
- Perineural invasion common
- No keratocyst formation

ANCILLARY TESTS

- Lumina highlighted by EMA &/or CEA

TOP DIFFERENTIAL DIAGNOSES

- Microcystic adnexal carcinoma
  - Presence of keratocysts allows for distinction (absent in eccrine carcinoma)
- Adenoid cystic carcinoma
  - Cribriform architecture allows distinction (generally absent in eccrine carcinoma)
- Infiltrative basal cell carcinoma
  - Lacks true lumen formation
    - Typically negative for EMA and CEA
  - Often has epidermal attachments
  - May have other basal cell carcinoma subtypes

Eccrine Carcinoma With Deep Invasion

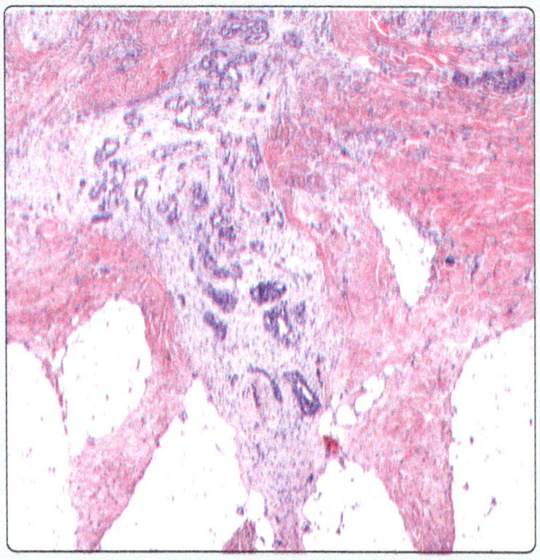

Eccrine Carcinoma With Subcutaneous Invasion

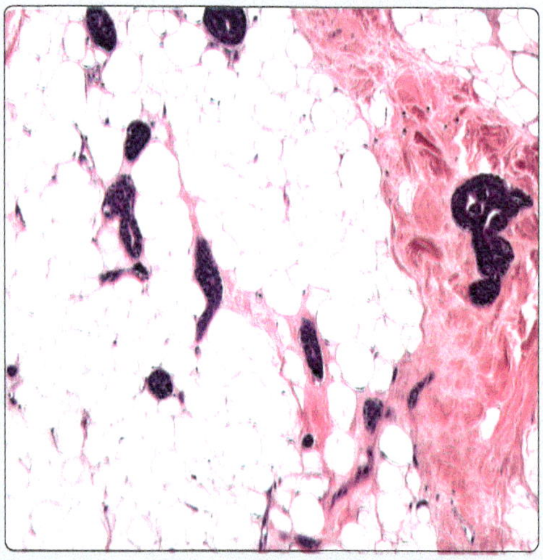

(Left) *Eccrine carcinoma is a dermal-based tumor composed of infiltrating ducts/glands associated with a sclerotic stroma. The tumor is often deeply infiltrative, with invasion into the deep dermis and subcutaneous adipose tissue in most cases.* **(Right)** *Eccrine carcinoma is very infiltrative and often extends into the underlying subcutaneous fat, as in this case.*

Eccrine Carcinoma at Higher Magnification

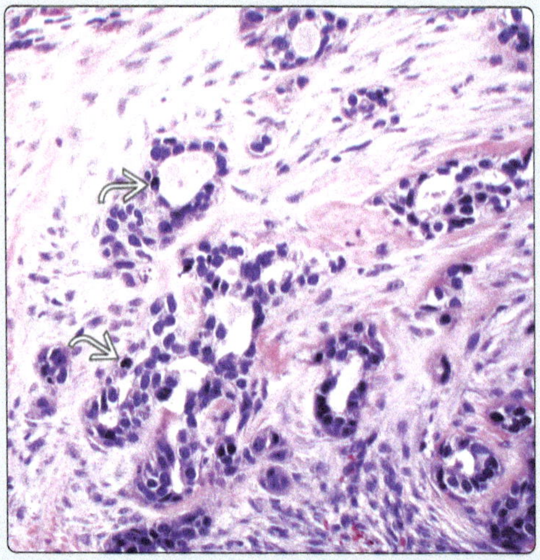

Eccrine Carcinoma With Perineural Invasion

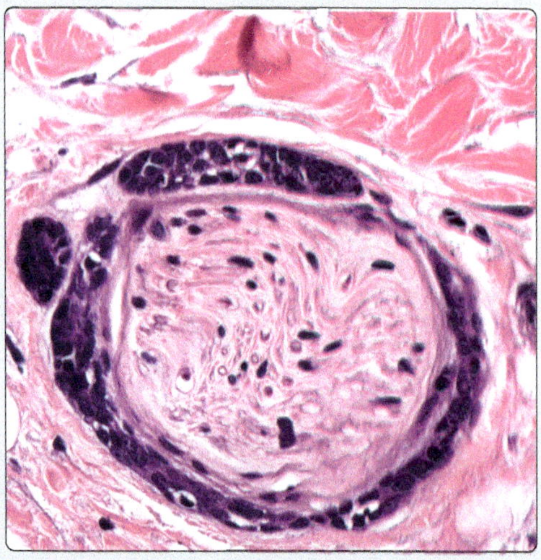

(Left) *Higher magnification of the infiltrative ducts shows significant atypia, with nuclear hyperchromasia, crowding, and a few mitotic figures* ➩. **(Right)** *Perineural invasion is a common and expected finding in many eccrine carcinomas.*

TERMINOLOGY

Synonyms

- Syringoid carcinoma, syringoid eccrine carcinoma, eccrine syringomatous carcinoma, eccrine epithelioma

Definitions

- Malignant adnexal tumor with eccrine differentiation somewhat resembling syringoma
  - No evidence of association with or development from syringomas
- Some authorities group these tumors with microcystic adnexal carcinoma (MAC)

CLINICAL ISSUES

Epidemiology

- Incidence
  - Very rare tumors
- Age
  - Usually present in middle-aged patients
- Sex
  - More common in women (3:1)

Site

- Most common on scalp
- May also present on face, neck, trunk, or extremities

Presentation

- Typically present as plaque or nodule
  - May present as painful lesion ± alopecia
  - May be present for many years before diagnosis

Treatment

- Surgical approaches
  - Wide excision

Prognosis

- Locally aggressive
  - Multiple episodes of local recurrence common
- Rare lymph node metastasis

MICROSCOPIC

Histologic Features

- Based in dermis; attachment to epidermis is very rare
- Infiltrative growth pattern
  - May involve subcutis and underlying skeletal muscle
  - Perineural invasion common
- Tumor composed of basaloid epithelium
  - Tumor cells have relatively uniform hyperchromatic nuclei
    - Nuclear atypia usually relatively mild
  - Mitotic rate low
  - Occasionally have clear cytoplasm due to glycogen
    - Glycogen can be highlighted with PAS stain (without diastase)
- Tumor forms epithelial strands with lumen formation
  - May have hand mirror shape similar to syringoma
  - May also have cyst formation
- No keratocyst formation
- No squamous differentiation

ANCILLARY TESTS

Immunohistochemistry

- Immunohistochemistry may be useful to confirm diagnosis
  - Lumina highlighted by EMA &/or CEA
  - Tumor cells positive for p63, high and low molecular weight cytokeratins
    - Can help to exclude metastatic carcinoma to skin
  - May show focal immunoreactivity for S100

DIFFERENTIAL DIAGNOSIS

Microcystic Adnexal Carcinoma

- MAC has similar growth pattern and may be closely related to eccrine carcinoma
- Presence of keratocysts allows distinction (absent in eccrine carcinoma)

Squamoid Eccrine Ductal Carcinoma

- Very rare tumors with basaloid ductal elements and areas of squamous differentiation
- May actually represent unusual squamoid variant of MAC

Adenoid Cystic Carcinoma

- Cribriform architecture classically seen (typically absent in eccrine carcinoma)
- Ductal lumina filled with mucinous and basement membrane-like material

Infiltrative Basal Cell Carcinoma

- Lacks true lumen formation
- Often shows mucinous stroma and tumor-stromal retraction artifact
- Often admixed with other basal cell carcinoma patterns
  - i.e., nodular, micronodular, or superficial multicentric
- Connections to overlying epidermis often present

DIAGNOSTIC CHECKLIST

Pathologic Interpretation Pearls

- Infiltrative growth pattern of basaloid ductal structures key to diagnosis

SELECTED REFERENCES

1. Frouin E et al: Anatomoclinical study of 30 cases of sclerosing sweat duct carcinomas (microcystic adnexal carcinoma, syringomatous carcinoma and squamoid eccrine ductal carcinoma). J Eur Acad Dermatol Venereol. 29(10):1978-94, 2015
2. Lorente-Luna M et al: Eccrine carcinoma: the role of Mohs micrographic surgery and a review of the literature. Actas Dermosifiliogr. ePub, 2015
3. Ballardini P et al: Metastatic syringoid eccrine carcinoma of the nipple. Int Med Case Rep J. 5:45-8, 2012
4. Sidiropoulos M et al: Syringoid eccrine carcinoma: a clinicopathological and immunohistochemical study of four cases. J Clin Pathol. 64(9):788-92, 2011
5. Kavand S et al: "Squamoid eccrine ductal carcinoma": an unusual low-grade case with follicular differentiation. Are these tumors squamoid variants of microcystic adnexal carcinoma? Am J Dermatopathol. 31(8):849-52, 2009
6. Chhibber V et al: Ductal eccrine carcinoma with squamous differentiation: apropos a case. J Cutan Pathol. 34(6):503-7, 2007
7. Wildemore JK et al: Mohs surgery for malignant eccrine neoplasms. Dermatol Surg. 30(12 Pt 2):1574-9, 2004
8. Ramos D et al: Clear cell syringoid carcinoma: an ultrastructural and immunohistochemical study. Am J Dermatopathol. 22(1):60-4, 2000
9. Dave VK: Eccrine sweat gland carcinoma with metastases. Br J Dermatol. 86(1):95-7, 1972

Squamoid Eccrine Ductal Carcinoma

KEY FACTS

TERMINOLOGY

- Squamoid eccrine ductal carcinoma (SEDC)
- Rare carcinoma with evidence of both ductal and squamous differentiation

ETIOLOGY/PATHOGENESIS

- May be associated with solar damage or immunosuppression

CLINICAL ISSUES

- Aggressive local recurrences, but no metastases reported to date
- Wide local excision is recommended to ensure complete removal

MICROSCOPIC

- Deeply infiltrative-appearing lobules, nests, and cords of cells
- Mixed population of smaller basaloid adnexal cells and larger squamoid cells
  - Adnexal cells show small hyperchromatic nuclei and scant amounts of cytoplasm
  - Squamoid cells show larger nuclei, prominent nucleoli, and abundant eosinophilic-staining cytoplasm
- Both cell types can surround ductal lumina
- Evidence of follicular differentiation can be seen
  - Suggests that these may represent squamoid variants of microcystic adnexal carcinoma

ANCILLARY TESTS

- Diffusely positive for cytokeratins and p63
- Focally positive for EMA and CEA (ductal structures)

TOP DIFFERENTIAL DIAGNOSES

- Squamous cell carcinoma
- Microcystic adnexal carcinoma
- Eccrine (syringoid/syringomatous) carcinoma
- Porocarcinoma

Squamoid Eccrine Ductal Carcinoma

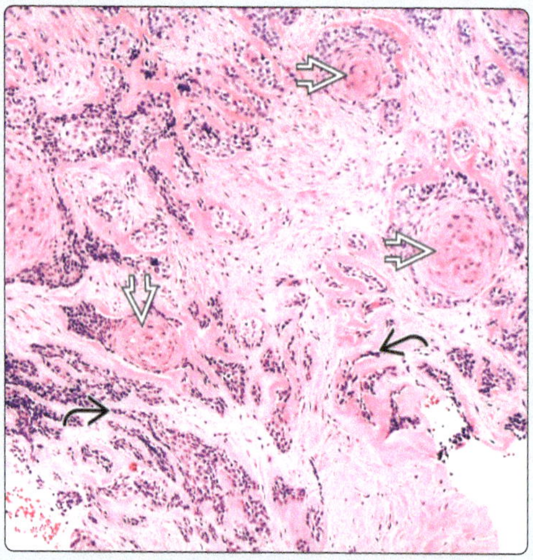

High Magnification of Squamoid Eccrine Ductal Carcinoma With Pale to Clear Squamoid Cells

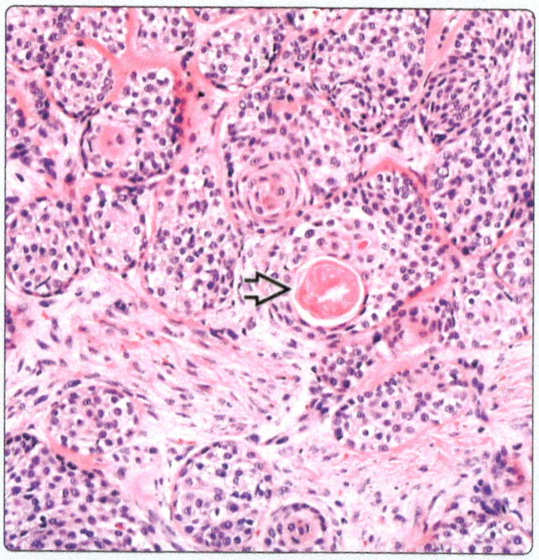

(Left) *Squamoid eccrine ductal carcinoma (SEDC) shows a proliferation of both enlarged, squamoid cells forming islands ➡, and smaller, more cord-like collections of basaloid cells ➡.* **(Right)** *SEDC shows a nested proliferation of enlarged pale to clear squamoid cells surrounding a well-formed ductal lumina ➡.*

High Magnification of Squamoid Eccrine Ductal Carcinoma

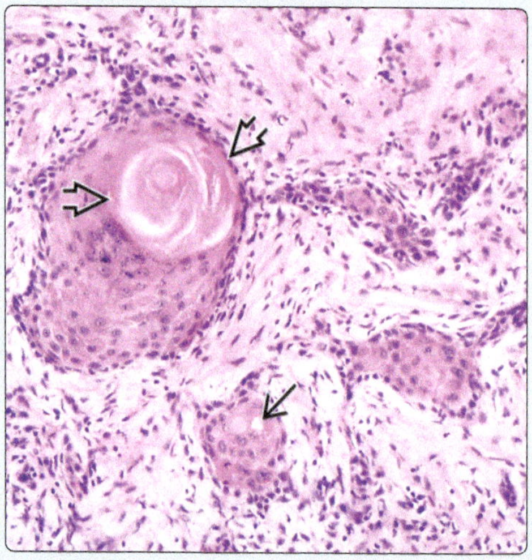

CEA-M Immunohistochemistry

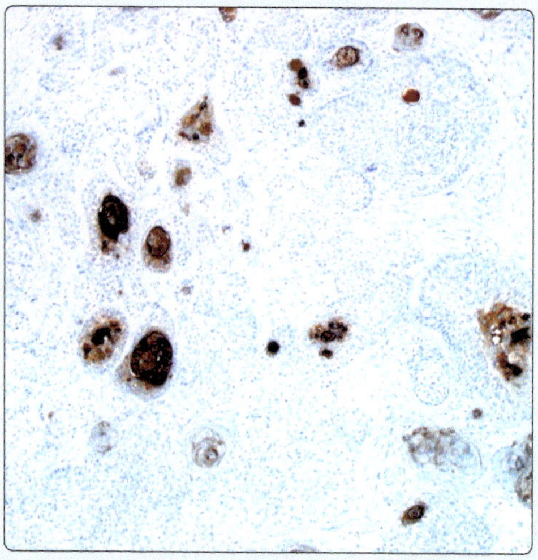

(Left) *High magnification of a predominantly squamoid area shows collections of large cells with abundant eosinophilic cytoplasm surrounding keratinizing cystic spaces ➡ and small ductal lumina ➡.* **(Right)** *Immunohistochemistry for CEA-M shows strong and diffuse luminal staining in the ductal structures.*

TERMINOLOGY

Abbreviations

- Squamoid eccrine ductal carcinoma (SEDC)

Synonyms

- Ductal eccrine carcinoma with squamous differentiation

Definitions

- Rare adnexal carcinoma with both ductal and squamous differentiation

ETIOLOGY/PATHOGENESIS

Unknown

- May be associated with solar damage or immunosuppression

CLINICAL ISSUES

Epidemiology

- Incidence
  - Very rare tumors; only 12 cases reported to date
- Age
  - Usually adult patients

Site

- Head and neck region or extremities

Presentation

- Nodular lesion

Treatment

- Surgical approaches
  - Wide local excision is recommended to ensure complete removal
  - Mohs micrographic surgery has also been reported to be effective in few cases

Prognosis

- Aggressive local recurrences, but no metastases reported to date

MICROSCOPIC

Histologic Features

- Dermal-based invasive tumor
  - Composed of infiltrative-appearing lobules, nests, and cords of cells
  - Mixed population of smaller basaloid adnexal cells and larger squamoid cells
    - Adnexal cells show small hyperchromatic nuclei and scant amounts of cytoplasm
    - Squamoid cells show larger nuclei with prominent nucleoli and abundant eosinophilic-staining cytoplasm
    - Both cell types can surround ductal lumina
  - Evidence of follicular differentiation can be seen
    - Scattered infundibulocystic keratinizing structures can be present
    - Other evidence of follicular differentiation can include external root sheath (tricholemmal) differentiation
    - Suggests possibility that these may represent squamoid variants of microcystic adnexal carcinoma
    - Many authorities now consider that microcystic adnexal carcinoma shows follicular and apocrine, rather than eccrine, differentiation

ANCILLARY TESTS

Immunohistochemistry

- Diffusely positive for cytokeratins (CK7, CK17, CK5/6) and p63
- Focally positive for EMA and CEA (highlight ductal structures)

DIFFERENTIAL DIAGNOSIS

Squamous Cell Carcinoma

- Invasive tumor composed of large, atypical epithelioid cells with dense eosinophilic-staining cytoplasm
  - Degree of differentiation varies (well to moderately to poorly differentiated)
- SEDC lacks high-grade atypia and overlying AK or squamous cell carcinoma (SCC) in situ (present in majority of SCC cases)
- SCC lacks ductal differentiation

Microcystic Adnexal Carcinoma

- Typically presents on face of young adult patients
- More prominent superficial folliculocystic differentiation typically present
- SEDC may represent squamoid variant of microcystic adnexal carcinoma; therefore, distinction may be academic

Eccrine (Syringoid/Syringomatous) Carcinoma

- Often regarded as higher grade variant of MAC lacking superficial folliculocystic differentiation
- Monotonous proliferation of ductal structures deeply invading dermis and subcutis
- Lined by basaloid cells, not squamoid cells of SEDC

Porocarcinoma

- More common tumors, often occur in acral sites
- May show prominent squamous differentiation, however
  - Superficial portion of tumor often shows attachments to overlying epidermis and intraepidermal (pagetoid) involvement

SELECTED REFERENCES

1. Cardoso JC et al: Malignant sweat gland tumours: an update. Histopathology. 67(5):589-606, 2015
2. Chan H et al: Squamoid eccrine ductal carcinoma of the scalp. Australas J Dermatol. ePub, 2015
3. Frouin E et al: Anatomoclinical study of 30 cases of sclerosing sweat duct carcinomas (microcystic adnexal carcinoma, syringomatous carcinoma and squamoid eccrine ductal carcinoma). J Eur Acad Dermatol Venereol. 29(10):1978-94, 2015
4. Sidiropoulos M et al: Syringoid eccrine carcinoma: a clinicopathological and immunohistochemical study of four cases. J Clin Pathol. 64(9):788-92, 2011
5. Terushkin E et al: Squamoid eccrine ductal carcinoma: a case report and review of the literature. Am J Dermatopathol. 32(3):287-92, 2010
6. Kavand S et al: "Squamoid eccrine ductal carcinoma": an unusual low-grade case with follicular differentiation. Are these tumors squamoid variants of microcystic adnexal carcinoma? Am J Dermatopathol. 31(8):849-52, 2009
7. Kim YJ et al: Mohs micrographic surgery for squamoid eccrine ductal carcinoma. Dermatol Surg. 31(11 Pt 1):1462-4, 2005
8. Herrero J et al: Squamoid eccrine ductal carcinoma. Histopathology. 32(5):478-80, 1998
9. Wong TY et al: Squamoid eccrine ductal carcinoma. Histopathology. 30(3):288-93, 1997

Microcystic Adnexal Carcinoma

KEY FACTS

TERMINOLOGY

- Microcystic adnexal carcinoma
- Synonyms: Sclerosing sweat duct carcinoma, syringoid carcinoma
- Low-grade malignant adnexal tumor with follicular and ductal differentiation

ETIOLOGY/PATHOGENESIS

- Some cases may be related to solar damage (UV radiation) or radiation therapy

CLINICAL ISSUES

- Most common on face
- Indurated, plaque-like lesion
- High incidence of local recurrence but only very rare metastases
- Usually occur in middle-aged to older adults
- Treatment: Mohs excision is effective and likely optimal approach in most cases

MICROSCOPIC

- Bland-appearing, dermal-based adnexal tumor
- Deeply invasive and not well circumscribed
- Perineural invasion often present in deeper areas
- Superficially, typically consists of folliculocystic elements
- Deeply, consists of infiltrative cords and ductal structures lined by bland-appearing cells
- Lymph nodes only very rarely involved

ANCILLARY TESTS

- Luminal cells often positive for EMA and CEA [negative in trichoepithelioma and basal cell carcinoma (BCC)]
- Low proliferative rate by Ki-67, low levels of p53 and Bcl-2 (high in BCC)

TOP DIFFERENTIAL DIAGNOSES

- Desmoplastic trichoepithelioma
- Syringoma
- Desmoplastic basal cell carcinoma

MAC on Cheek

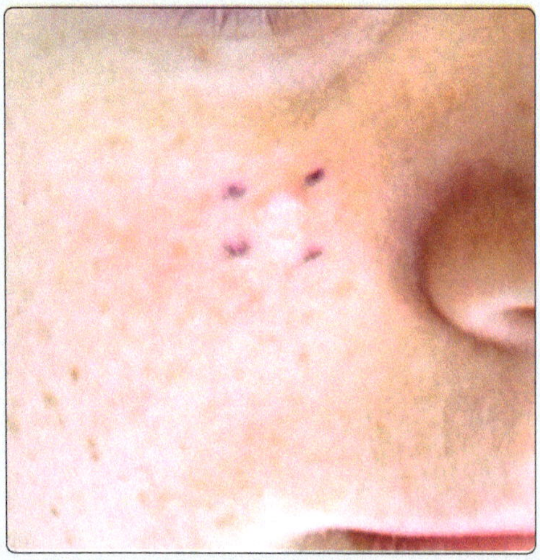

MAC at Low Magnification

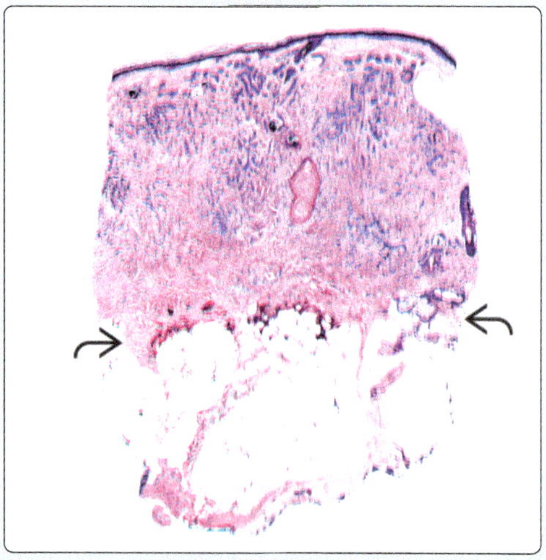

(Left) *Clinical photograph of microcystic adnexal carcinoma (MAC) on the cheek of a middle-aged woman shows a flesh-colored papular to plaque-like lesion.* **(Right)** *Scanning magnification of a microcystic adnexal carcinoma shows a diffusely infiltrative neoplasm in the dermis and extending into the dermal-subcutaneous interface ➙.*

MAC at Higher Magnification

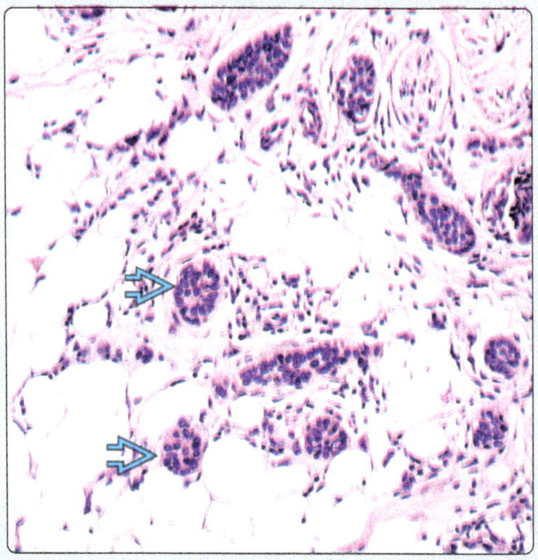

Perineural Invasion in MAC

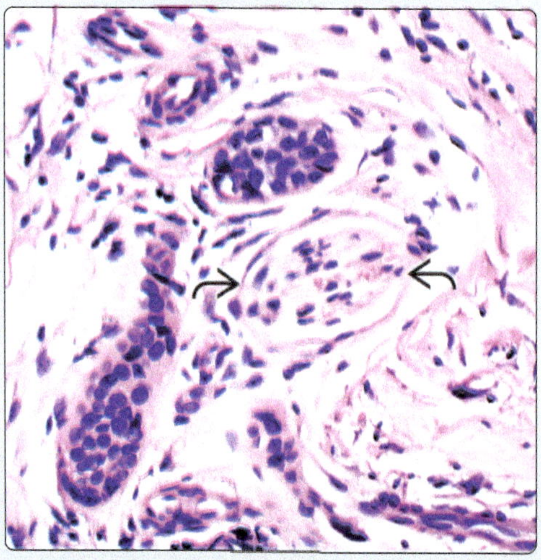

(Left) *Higher magnification of the deep area of MAC shows infiltrative tumor nests ➩ and cords invading into the subcutaneous adipose tissue.* **(Right)** *High magnification of a deep area of MAC shows tumor cell aggregates closely approaching a nerve ➙.*

TERMINOLOGY

Abbreviations

- Microcystic adnexal carcinoma (MAC)

Synonyms

- Sclerosing sweat duct carcinoma

Definitions

- Low-grade malignant adnexal tumor with follicular and ductal differentiation

ETIOLOGY/PATHOGENESIS

Environmental Exposure

- Some cases may be related to solar damage (UV radiation) or radiation therapy
  - Higher incidence reported on left side of face, which receives greater solar exposure during driving

CLINICAL ISSUES

Epidemiology

- Age
  - Usually occur in middle-aged to older adults

Site

- Most common on face
  - Upper lip is most common site
- Can also occur on scalp, trunk, extremities, axillae, and groin

Presentation

- Indurated, plaque-like, or nodular lesion

Treatment

- Surgical approaches
  - Complete excision with clear margins
  - Mohs excision is effective and likely optimal approach in most cases

Prognosis

- High incidence of local recurrence (up to 50%), but only very rare metastases
  - Metastases have been reported to local lymph nodes, but may represent local, deep invasion, rather than true metastasis

MACROSCOPIC

Size

- Typically measure ≥ 1 cm in diameter

MICROSCOPIC

Histologic Features

- Bland-appearing, dermal-based adnexal tumor
- Deeply invasive and not well circumscribed
- Perineural invasion often present in deeper areas
- Superficially, typically consists of follicular elements
  - Well-differentiated infundibulocystic structures
  - Smaller basaloid nests and islands, similar to trichoepithelioma
- Deeply, consists of infiltrative cords and ductal structures
  - Cells are small, cuboidal-shaped, and bland-appearing
  - Associated with desmoplastic stroma
  - Invade into subcutaneous adipose tissue, even fascia and skeletal muscle

ANCILLARY TESTS

Immunohistochemistry

- Positive for pan cytokeratin, high molecular weight keratins, and often CK7
- Luminal cells often positive for EMA and CEA [negative in trichoepithelioma and basal cell carcinoma (BCC)]
- Low proliferative rate by Ki-67 (high in BCC)
- Low levels of p53 and Bcl-2 (high in BCC)

DIFFERENTIAL DIAGNOSIS

Desmoplastic Trichoepithelioma

- Histologically appears almost identical to superficial portion of MAC
- Typically shows more basaloid-appearing nests and islands
- Lacks deep subcutaneous and perineural invasion
  - Therefore, it is virtually impossible to completely exclude MAC on superficial shave biopsy

Syringoma

- Usually superficial, noninfiltrative ductal proliferation
  - Ductal structures often show tadpole-like projections
- Lacks evidence of follicular differentiation (typical of MAC)
- No deep or perineural invasion

Desmoplastic Basal Cell Carcinoma

- Infiltrative small nests and cords of atypical basaloid cells
- BCC usually shows multiple apoptotic and mitotic figures, which are absent in MAC
- Focal mucinous stroma and tumor-stromal retraction artifact may be present

DIAGNOSTIC CHECKLIST

Pathologic Interpretation Pearls

- Superficial folliculocystic structures and deeper infiltrative cords and ductal elements
- Perineural invasion often present in deeper areas
- Need deep biopsy or excision to distinguish from desmoplastic trichoepithelioma

SELECTED REFERENCES

1. Evangelista MT et al: Comparative analysis of cytokeratin 15, TDAG51, cytokeratin 20 and androgen receptor in sclerosing adnexal neoplasms and variants of basal cell carcinoma. J Cutan Pathol. 42(11):824-31, 2015
2. Frouin E et al: Anatomoclinical study of 30 cases of sclerosing sweat duct carcinomas (microcystic adnexal carcinoma, syringomatous carcinoma and squamoid eccrine ductal carcinoma). J Eur Acad Dermatol Venereol. 29(10):1978-94, 2015
3. McKinley LH et al: Microcystic adnexal carcinoma: review of a potential diagnostic pitfall and management. Cutis. 93(3):162-5, 2014
4. Kavand S et al: "Squamoid eccrine ductal carcinoma": an unusual low-grade case with follicular differentiation. Are these tumors squamoid variants of microcystic adnexal carcinoma? Am J Dermatopathol. 31(8):849-52, 2009
5. Gabillot-Carré M et al: Microcystic adnexal carcinoma: report of seven cases including one with lung metastasis. Dermatology. 212(3):221-8, 2006
6. Smith KJ et al: Microcystic adnexal carcinoma: an immunohistochemical study including markers of proliferation and apoptosis. Am J Surg Pathol. 25(4):464-71, 2001
7. Goldstein DJ et al: Microcystic adnexal carcinoma: a distinct clinicopathologic entity. Cancer. 50(3):566-72, 1982

MAC at Low Magnification

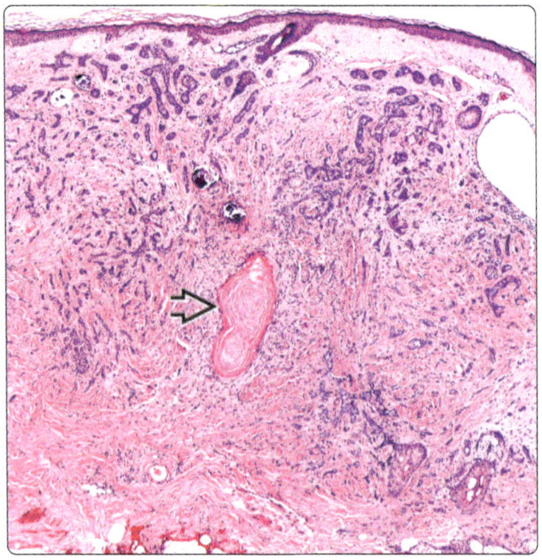

MAC at Intermediate Magnification

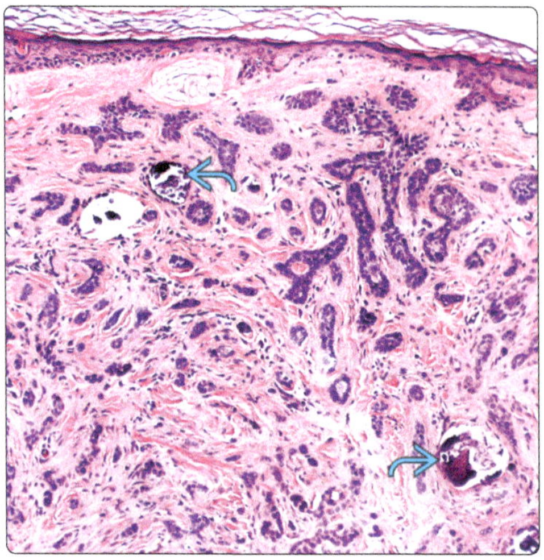

(Left) *Low magnification of MAC shows a dermal-based infiltrative basaloid neoplasm with focal calcifications and a large keratinizing cystic structure ➡.* **(Right)** *Superficial portion of MAC at intermediate power shows a proliferation of basaloid cords and nests in a sclerotic stroma. Prominent calcifications are present ➡.*

MAC at High Magnification

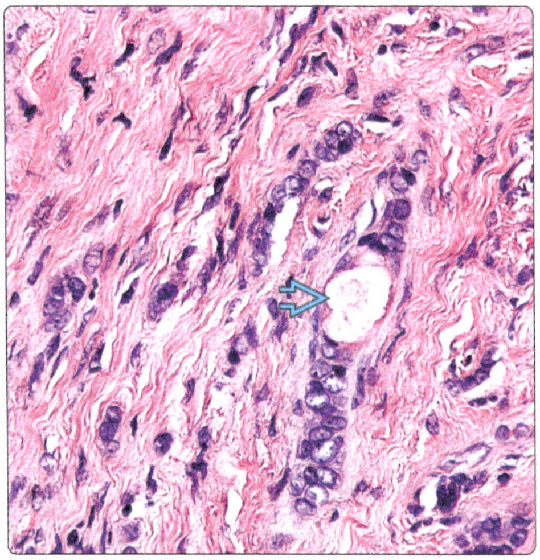

Perineural Invasion in MAC

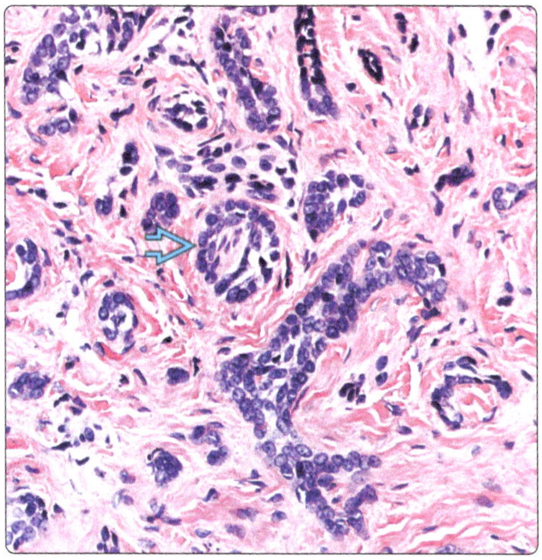

(Left) *High magnification of MAC shows the relatively bland appearance of the tumor cells, which show round to oval nuclei with uniform chromatin and inconspicuous to small nucleoli. Note the focal well-formed ductal lumen ➡.* **(Right)** *High magnification of MAC shows the relatively bland-appearing cells forming small cords in a desmoplastic stroma. Note the focal perineural invasion ➡.*

CEA-M Immunohistochemical Staining in MAC

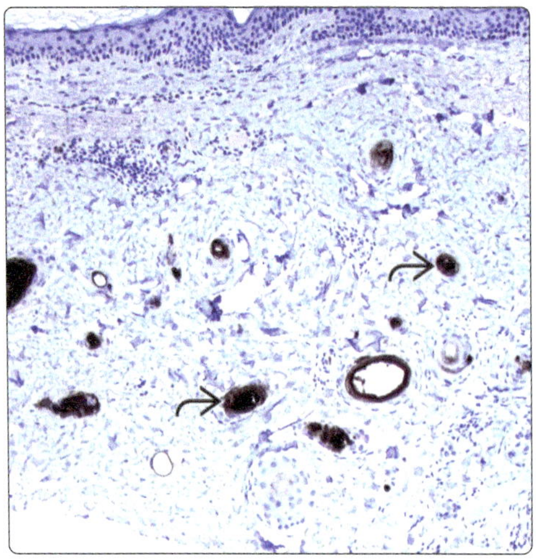

Ki-67 Immunohistochemical Staining in MAC

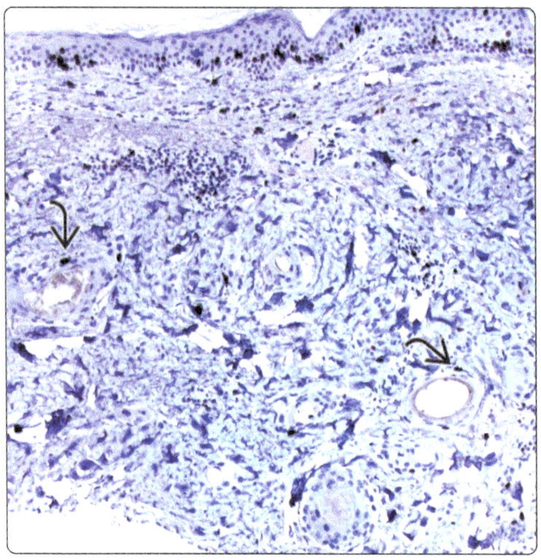

(Left) *CEA-M immunohistochemistry shows strong staining of the ductal luminal cells and secretions ➡ in this MAC, consistent with true ductal/glandular differentiation [which is not seen in desmoplastic trichoepithelioma (DTE), basal cell carcinoma (BCC), and squamous cell carcinoma(SCC)].* **(Right)** *This Ki-67 immunohistochemical stain highlights a very low proliferative rate, with only a few scattered tumor cell nuclei ➡ staining, consistent with the low growth rate of this tumor.*

Differential Diagnosis: DTE

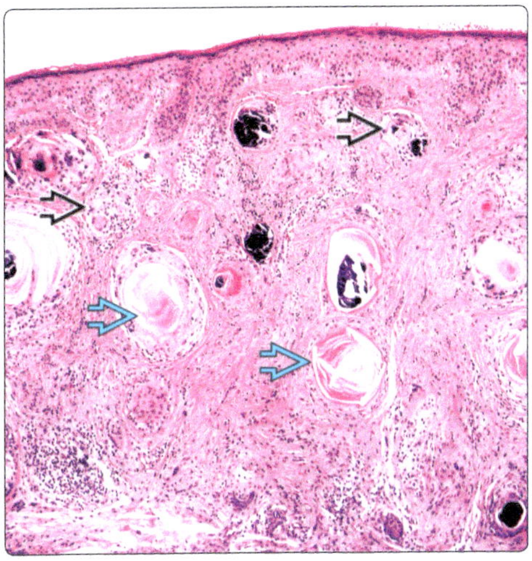

Differential Diagnosis: DTE at Higher Magnification

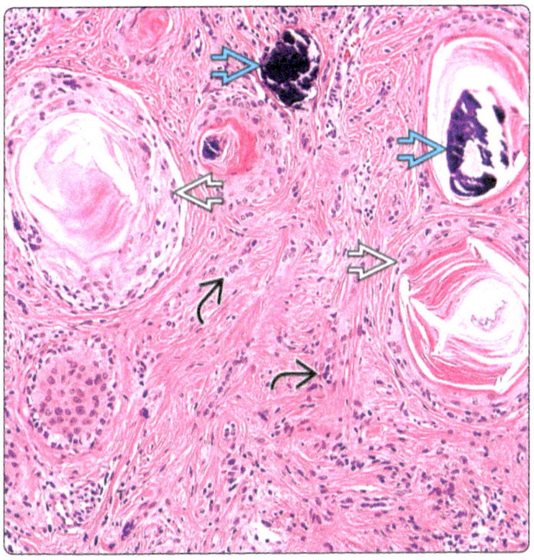

(Left) *Low magnification of a DTE shows multiple keratinizing cystic spaces and calcifications with areas of granulomatous inflammation.* **(Right)** *Higher magnification of a DTE shows multiple keratinizing cystic spaces and calcifications. There are also small, infiltrating epithelial cords associated with a surrounding desmoplastic stroma.*

Differential Diagnosis: DTE at High Magnification

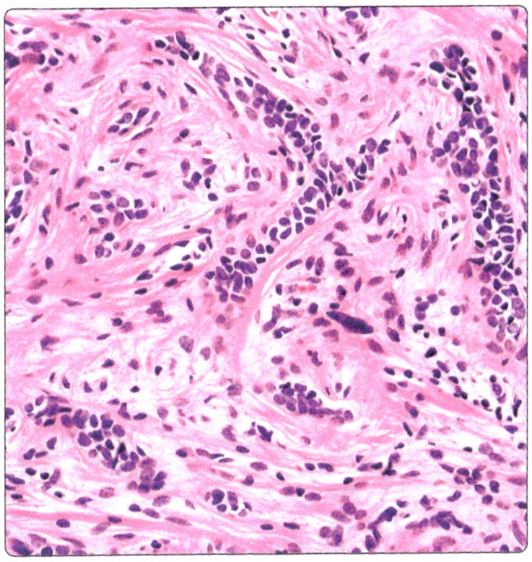

Differential Diagnosis: BCC

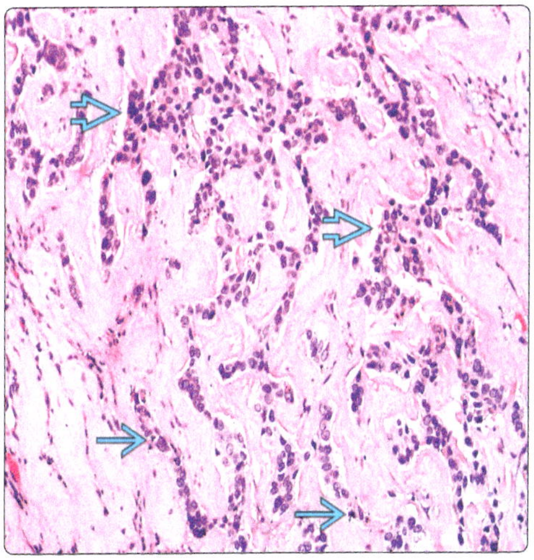

(Left) *High magnification of a DTE shows the small, bland, ductal structures in the deeper aspect of the tumor. The ductal structures in MAC are similar-appearing, but DTE does not deeply invade the subcutis or show perineural invasion.* **(Right)** *Desmoplastic BCC shows infiltrative cords of atypical cells with scattered apoptotic bodies, which are usually absent in MAC. Note the focal mucinous stroma and tumor-stromal retraction artifact.*

Differential Diagnosis: SCC

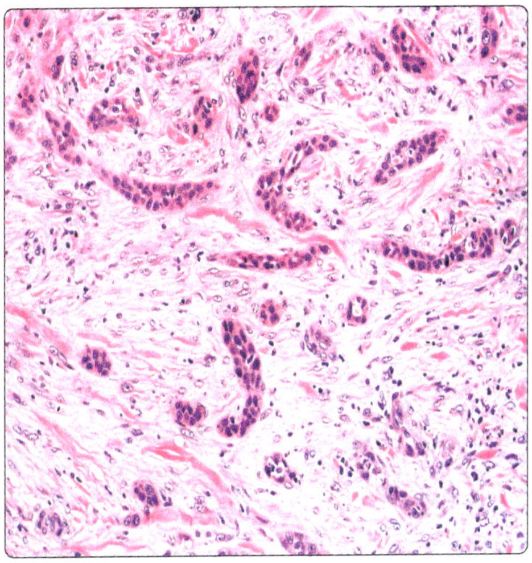

Differential Diagnosis: ACC

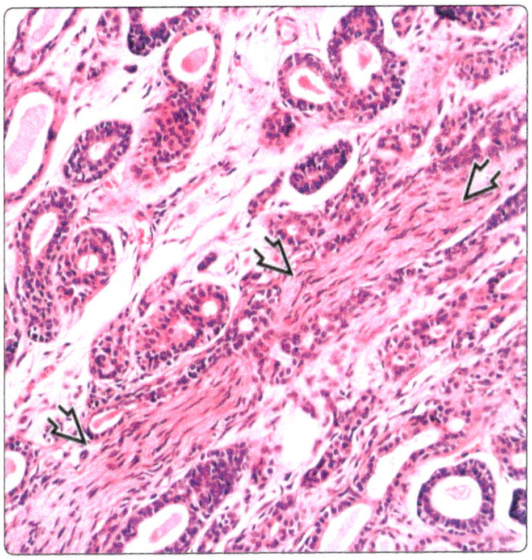

(Left) *Infiltrative SCC with cord-like structures associated with a desmoplastic stroma can mimic desmoplastic/morpheaform BCC or, less likely, MAC.* **(Right)** *Adenoid cystic carcinoma (ACC) frequently shows perineural invasion, similar to MAC; however, ACC lacks follicular differentiation and shows a prominent cribriforming pattern. Here, a large nerve is surrounded by multiple tumor cords and ducts.*

KEY FACTS

TERMINOLOGY

- Well-circumscribed benign epithelial tumor in chondromyxoid matrix
- Cutaneous mixed tumor

CLINICAL ISSUES

- Head and neck
- Skin-colored, asymptomatic, dermal to subcutaneous tumors
- Rare
- Middle-aged to elderly
- Very rare malignant transformation

MICROSCOPIC

- Very rare malignant transformation
- Epithelial cells embedded in myxoid, chondroid, or fibrous stroma
- Tumor shows eccrine and apocrine differentiation
- Ductal structures of variable size and shape present
- Ducts lined by 2 layers of cuboidal cells and peripheral layer of myoepithelial cells
- Chondrocyte-like cells commonly seen
- Inner cuboidal cells express CK, EMA, and CEA
- Outer myoepithelial cells express vimentin, S100, and NSE
- Chondrocyte-like cells in lacunae secrete hyaline cartilage and are S100 positive
- Mucin is Alcian blue, mucicarmine, and aldehyde-fuchsin-positive and hyaluronidase resistant

TOP DIFFERENTIAL DIAGNOSES

- Malignant chondroid syringoma
- Chondroid lipoma
- Extraskeletal chondroma (cutaneous cartilaginous tumor)
- Pleomorphic adenoma (mixed tumor of salivary gland)
- Myoepithelioma

Chondroid Syringoma/Cutaneous Mixed Tumor Low Magnification

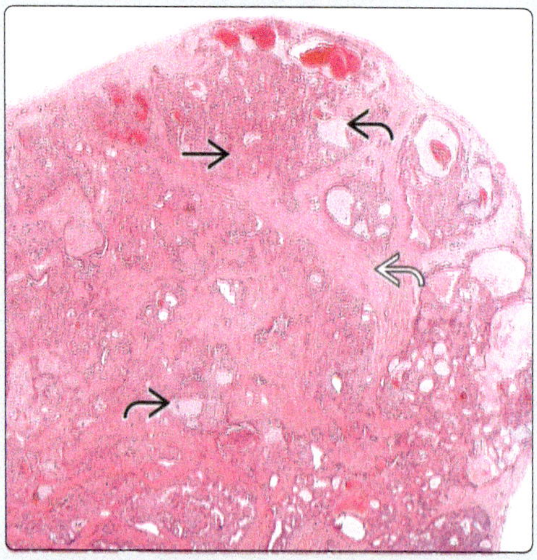

Cutaneous Mixed Tumor With Ductal Lumina and Myxoid Stroma

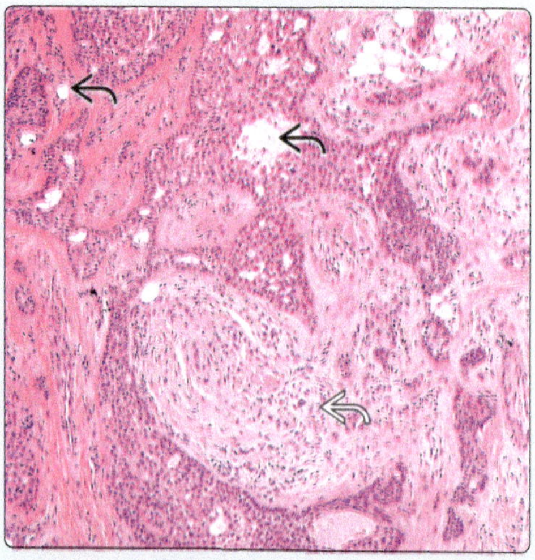

(Left) *Low magnification shows a well-circumscribed tumor composed of epithelial islands ➙ with easily identifiable glandular/ductal structures ➙ embedded in a myxoid and hyaline ➙ stroma.* **(Right)** *Small ducts ➙ lined by cuboidal cells are a common finding. The classic abundant myxoid and cartilaginous stroma is also seen ➙.*

Cutaneous Mixed Tumor at High Magnification

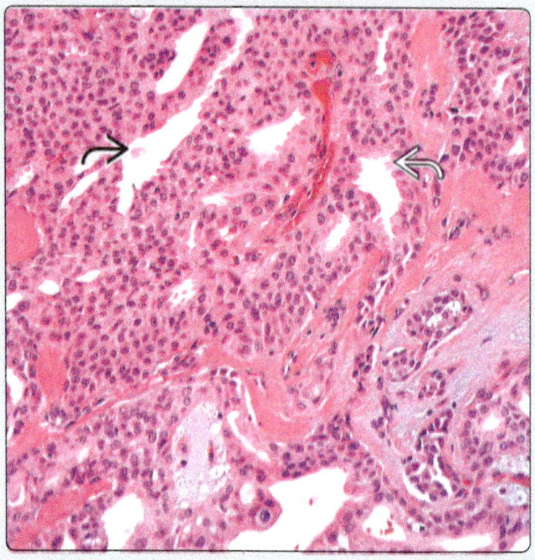

Cutaneous Mixed Tumor Composed of Basaloid Cells

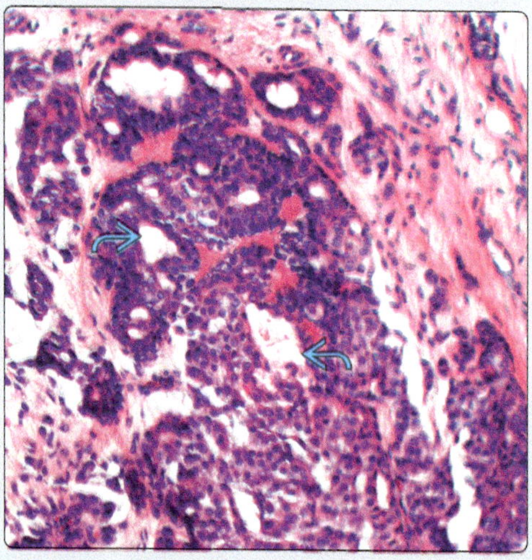

(Left) *Ductal structures ➙ with some foci of decapitation secretion ➙ are present in the epithelial component.* **(Right)** *This chondroid syringoma is composed mostly of small, cuboidal-shaped basaloid cells surrounding multiple ductal lumina ➙.*

TERMINOLOGY

Abbreviations

- Cutaneous mixed tumor (CMT)

Synonyms

- Apocrine mixed tumor
- Eccrine mixed tumor
- Mixed tumor of folliculosebaceous-apocrine complex

Definitions

- Well-circumscribed benign epithelial tumor with chondromyxoid matrix

CLINICAL ISSUES

Epidemiology

- Incidence
  - Rare
- Age
  - Middle-aged to elderly
- Sex
  - Male predominance
- Ethnicity
  - No ethnic predilection

Site

- Head and neck sites are most common
- Extremities and trunk

Presentation

- Skin-colored, asymptomatic, dermal to subcutaneous tumors

Natural History

- Slow growth

Treatment

- Surgical excision

Prognosis

- Excellent
  - Very rare malignant transformation

MACROSCOPIC

Size

- 0.5-3.0 cm

Sections to Be Submitted

- Representative sections of grossly different-appearing areas should be submitted

MICROSCOPIC

Histologic Features

- Well-circumscribed dermal to subcutaneous tumor
- Composed of proliferation of epithelial cells embedded in myxoid, chondroid, or fibrous stroma
- Apocrine ducts within tumor can be seen
  - Many authors consider CMT to be predominately tumor of apocrine origin
- Differentiation toward different parts of folliculosebaceous-apocrine complex reported
  - Focal areas of matrical or sebaceous differentiation may rarely be seen
- Eccrine differentiation may be present in some cases
- Large amounts of adipose tissue are seen in what are called lipomatous mixed tumors
- Calcification and ossification are rare focal findings
- Due to shrinkage of stroma, fibroblasts and epithelial cells within stroma are surrounded by halos and appear similar to cells of cartilage
- Epithelial component
  - Epithelial cells can be arranged singly, in small and large clusters, or in solid cords
  - Ductal structures are of variable size and shape
  - CMTs have been divided into 2 types according to ductal structures by some
    - Tumors with tubular, branching lumina
    - Tumors with small, tubular lumina
  - Cystic dilation and branching of ducts is common
  - PAS(+), amorphous, eosinophilic material (collagenous spherulosis) can be seen in tubular lumina
  - Larger ducts lined by 2 layers of cuboidal cells and peripheral layer of myoepithelial cells
  - Some CMT composed predominantly of small ducts and small epithelial clusters
  - Small ducts lined by single layer of cuboidal cells
  - Extension of epithelial cells of smaller ducts into stroma may give comma-like shape, similar to syringomas
  - Keratinous cysts are occasionally present
  - Epithelial cells in some CMTs show plasmacytoid appearance
    - These cells have abundant hyalin in cytoplasm, which displaces nuclei to periphery
    - Tumors with predominately hyaline cells are termed hyaline-rich CMT
  - Epithelial component occasionally shows metaplastic changes
    - Squamous metaplasia is most common
    - Mucinous, oxyphilic, columnar, and hobnail metaplasia can be seen
    - Cytoplasmic vacuolization and clear cell changes may be present
  - Rare cases of intravascular involvement of tumor have been reported
    - This finding is currently considered to be benign feature
    - Metastases were not observed on follow-up of these patients
- Stroma is abundant and may vary from myxoid to chondroid, hyalinized, fibroid, or mixture of these
  - Stellate, fibroblast-like cells are present in stroma of early lesions
  - Older lesions show signet ring-like fat cells and cells that appear to be chondrocytes
  - Chondrocyte-like cells in lacunae secrete hyaline cartilage
- Rare histologic variants include tumors with clear cell changes, pseudorosette structures, prominent cribriform areas, osseous metaplasia, tyrosine crystals, and physaliphorous-like cells
- Atypical mixed tumor

- This designation rarely given to tumors with borderline features between benign mixed tumor and malignant mixed tumor
- Predominately of hyalin-rich cell type
- Pushing border and epithelial cells with cytologic atypia seen
- No lymph node or distant metastases on follow-up
- Electron microscopy
  - Ductal and secretory lumina present
  - Myoepithelial cells present

Cytologic Features

- Benign-appearing epithelial cells with hyperchromatic nuclei and scant cytoplasm
- Rare cases show abundant, hyaline-rich cytoplasm
- Abundant fibroblasts are seen in myxoid stroma of younger lesions
- In older lesions, chondrocyte-like cells with lacunae that produce cartilaginous matrix are present

ANCILLARY TESTS

Immunohistochemistry

- Inner cuboidal cells express CK, EMA, and CEA
- Myoepithelial cells express smooth muscle markers (e.g., actin, calponin), CKs, EMA, S100, NSE, and vimentin
- Chondrocyte-like cells are S100 positive
- Stromal mucin is Alcian blue, mucicarmine, and aldehyde-fuchsin positive and hyaluronidase resistant
  - It is mostly sulfated acid mucopolysaccharides or chondroitin sulfate
- Chondromyxoid matrix is positive for collagen IV, laminin, fibronectin, and tenascin
- Type II collagen, found in cartilage, may be positive in stromal or epithelial component

DIFFERENTIAL DIAGNOSIS

Malignant Mixed Tumor (Malignant Chondroid Syringoma)

- More common on extremities than head and neck
- More frequent in women
- Asymmetrical appearance at low magnification
- Infiltrative borders
- Atypia of epithelial component showing mitoses and nuclear pleomorphism
- Nuclear atypia is not prominent feature in some tumors
- Tumor necrosis
- About 45% metastasize to regional lymph nodes, and 45% distant metastases are reported
- This tumor is not typically considered to arise from its benign CMT counterpart
  - Only in few cases have there been benign CMT adjacent to malignant chondroid syringoma

Myoepithelioma

- Rare primary cutaneous tumors considered closely related to chondroid syringomas
- Composed of pure myoepithelial population
  - Lack epithelial elements with ductal differentiation of chondroid syringoma

Chondroid Lipoma

- Predominately occurs in females
- Frequently occurs on extremities
- Deep subcutaneous to intramuscular location
- Presents as larger tumor than CMT
- No epithelial cells or glands present
- Lacks epithelial markers
- Mature lipocytes and multivacuolated lipoblast-like cells in chondromyxoid stroma

Extraskeletal Chondroma (Cutaneous Cartilaginous Tumor)

- Predominately occurs on hands and feet
- Largely composed of hypocellular mature hyaline cartilage
- Cystic degeneration is common
- Calcification is often present
- No epithelial or glandular component
- Lacks epithelial markers

Pleomorphic Adenoma (Mixed Tumor of Salivary Gland)

- Tumor arises in salivary glands and not skin
- Most common tumor of parotid gland
- Although benign, tumor can recur after resection and can invade adjacent tissue
- Histology is essentially same as CMT
- Chromosomal translocations between chromosomes 3 and 8 often found
- Radiographic studies in addition to tissue sampling may be useful
  - US, MR, and CT scans are helpful in areas difficult to biopsy
  - Fine-needle aspiration used as diagnostic tool

DIAGNOSTIC CHECKLIST

Pathologic Interpretation Pearls

- Epithelial strands, cords with glandular spaces in myxoid/cartilaginous stroma
- Small, medium-sized, or large ductal structures
- Hyalinized stroma

SELECTED REFERENCES

1. Bedir R et al: Chondroid syringomas: an immunohistopatological analysis. G Ital Dermatol Venereol. ePub, 2015
2. Naujokas A et al: SOX-10 expression in cutaneous myoepitheliomas and mixed tumors. J Cutan Pathol. 41(4):353-63, 2014
3. Kazakov DV et al: Cutaneous apocrine mixed tumor with intravascular tumor deposits: a diagnostic pitfall. Am J Dermatopathol. 33(8):775-9, 2011
4. Constantinescu MB et al: Chondroid syringoma with tyrosine crystals: case report and review of the literature. Am J Dermatopathol. 32(2):171-4, 2010
5. Kazakov DV et al: Apocrine mixed tumor of the skin ("mixed tumor of the folliculosebaceous-apocrine complex"). Spectrum of differentiations and metaplastic changes in the epithelial, myoepithelial, and stromal components based on a histopathologic study of 244 cases. J Am Acad Dermatol. 57(3):467-83, 2007
6. Ohata C et al: Lipomatous apocrine mixed tumor of the skin. Am J Dermatopathol. 25(2):138-41, 2003
7. Nakayama H et al: Hyaline cell-rich chondroid syringoma: epithelial nature of the hyaline cells. Jpn J Clin Oncol. 26(4):237-42, 1996
8. Mills SE: Mixed tumor of the skin: a model of divergent differentiation. J Cutan Pathol. 11(5):382-6, 1984

Cutaneous Mixed Tumor With Atypia at Low Magnification

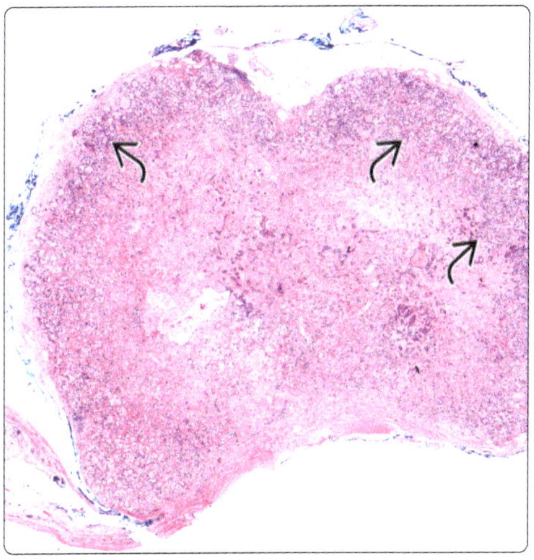

Cutaneous Mixed Tumor With Atypia at High Magnification

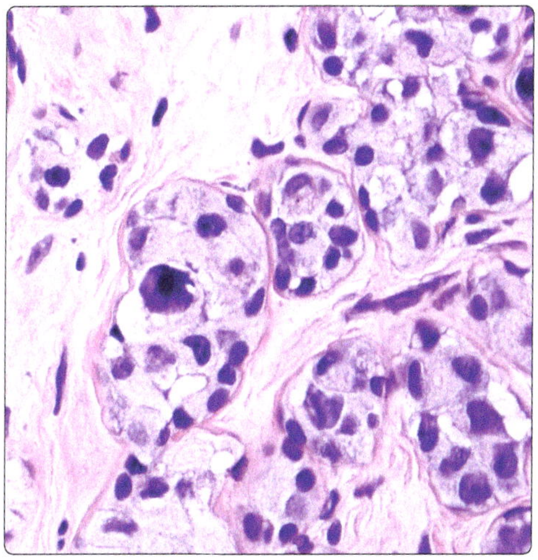

(Left) *This lesion was relatively symmetric and well-circumscribed-appearing at low magnification, but there are more cellular areas at the periphery ↗ of the tumor, which showed atypia on higher magnification.* **(Right)** *High magnification shows foci of markedly atypical and pleomorphic-appearing cells within some of the ductal structures. These cells were surrounded by a myoepithelial layer, findings suspicious for a rare carcinoma in situ arising in a cutaneous mixed tumor (CMT).*

Cutaneous Mixed Tumor With Tyrosine Crystals

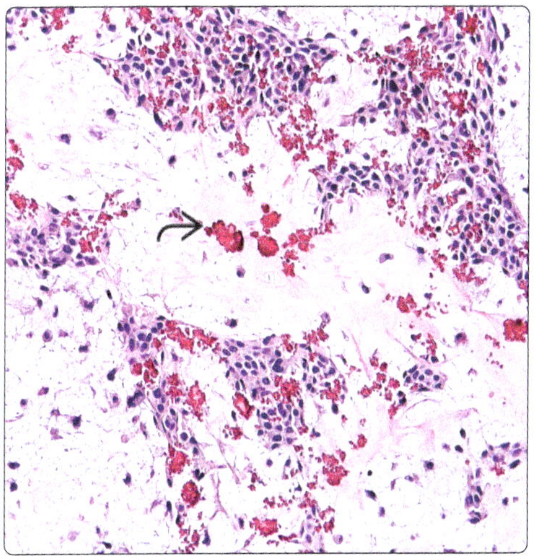

Cutaneous Mixed Tumor With Tyrosine Crystals

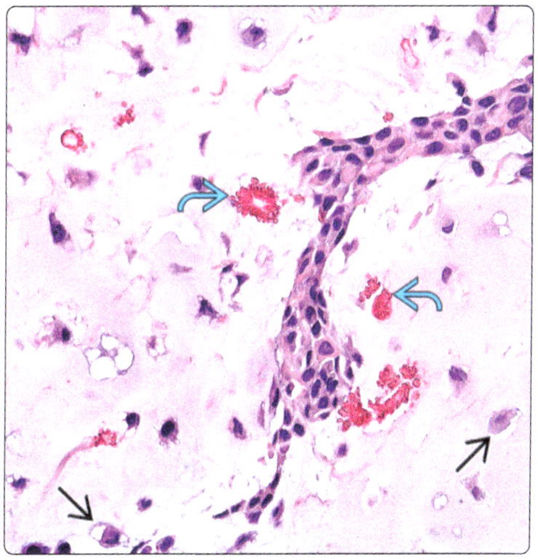

(Left) *This CMT shows islands of basaloid epithelial cells in a myxoid and cartilaginous stroma with scattered tyrosine crystals ↗, a rare finding that may also be seen in salivary gland mixed tumors.* **(Right)** *Chondrocyte-like cells → with perinuclear halos are seen within a cartilaginous stroma adjacent to a thin epithelial structure and tyrosine crystals ↗.*

S100 Immunohistochemistry in Cutaneous Mixed Tumor

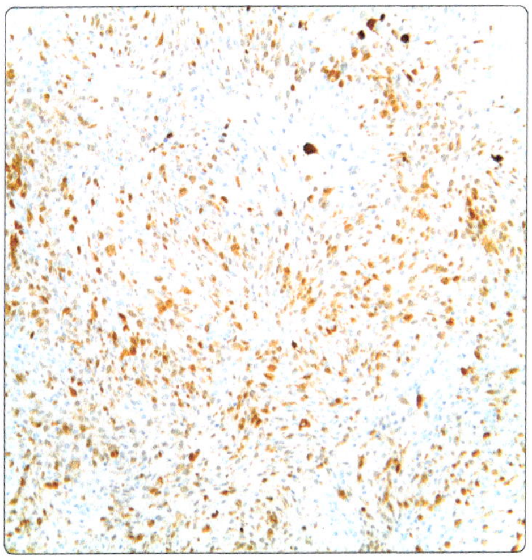

EMA Immunohistochemistry in Cutaneous Mixed Tumor

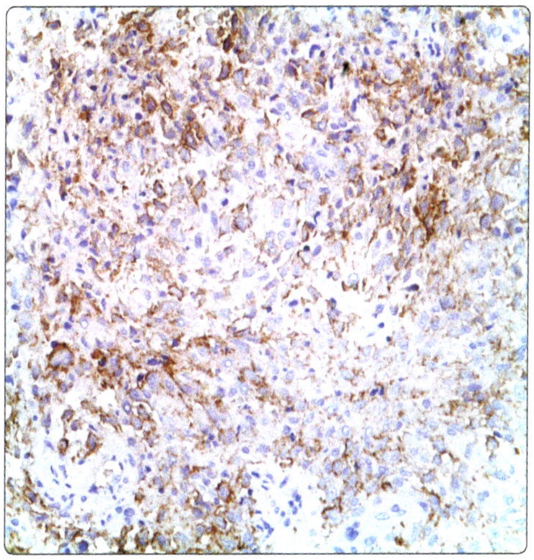

(Left) *The myoepithelial component of CMT is strongly positive for S100.* **(Right)** *CMT shows relatively weak to moderate positive staining with EMA.*

Malignant Mixed Tumor

KEY FACTS

TERMINOLOGY

- Malignant mixed tumor (MMT)
- Malignant chondroid syringoma

CLINICAL ISSUES

- Slow-growing tumor on extremities and trunk
- Local recurrence, regional and distant metastasis occur
- Most often occur on extremities and trunk
- Rarely, occurs from malignant transformation of mixed tumor of skin
- Wide excision with clear margins is primary treatment

MICROSCOPIC

- Histologic appearances vary greatly
- Composed of epithelial and chondroid/myxoid stromal components
- Epithelial component tends to predominate at periphery of lesion
- Epithelial component shows carcinomatous features and benign-appearing islands
  - Glandular differentiation is often present; not as common as in benign mixed tumor of skin
  - Irregular nests, cords, and sheets of cuboidal or polygonal cells
  - Foci of highly atypical cells with hyperchromatic nuclei and numerous mitotic figures
- Some cases may show frankly malignant stromal cells (i.e., true carcinosarcoma)
- Infiltration of surrounding tissue, vascular invasion, and necrosis are helpful diagnostic features
- Rarely, features of associated benign mixed tumor can be seen

TOP DIFFERENTIAL DIAGNOSES

- Cutaneous mixed tumor
- Biphasic synovial sarcoma

(Left) *Malignant mixed tumor (MMT) ➡ arising in a longstanding benign mixed tumor (well-circumscribed nodule on the left ➡) shows a large, asymmetrical, lobular, and infiltrative tumor invading from the dermis into the subcutaneous tissue.* **(Right)** *Marked infiltrative features with deep dermal and perineural ➡ invasion is observed.*

MMT at Low Magnification

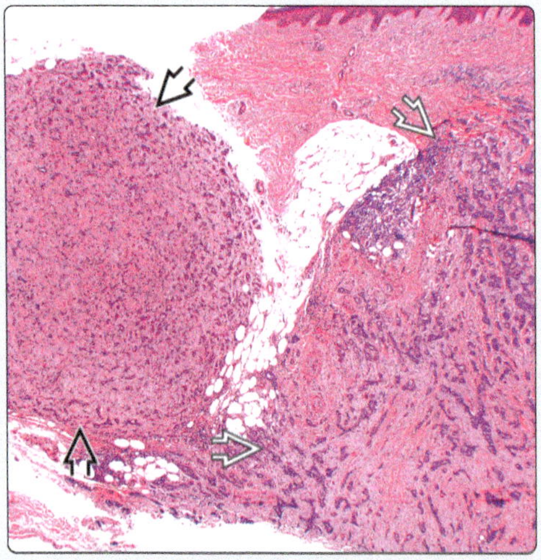

MMT With Perineural Invasion

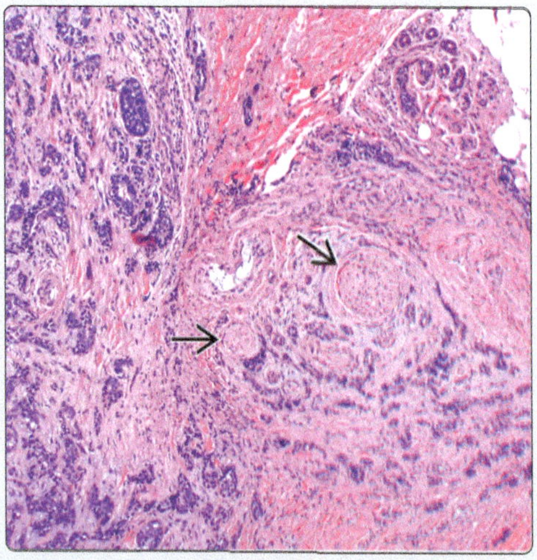

(Left) *High magnification of an epithelial area shows infiltrative cords of cells, which demonstrate marked cytologic atypia with enlarged, hyperchromatic-staining nuclei surrounding small ductal lumina ➡.* **(Right)** *The epithelial component of the tumor is strongly highlighted by a HMWCK (CK5-CK6) stain.*

MMT at High Magnification

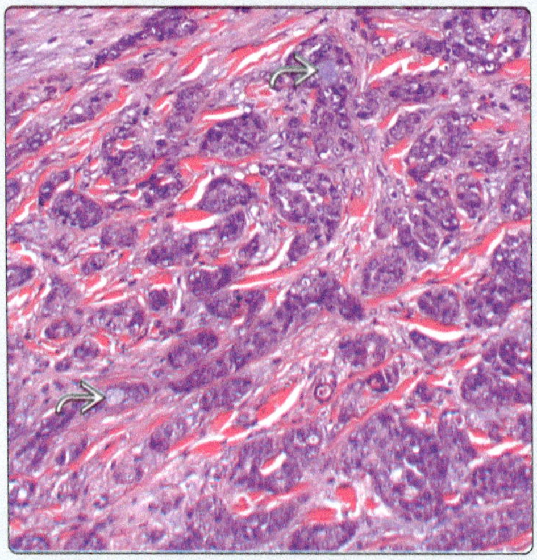

HMWCK (CK5-CK6) Immunohistochemistry in MMT

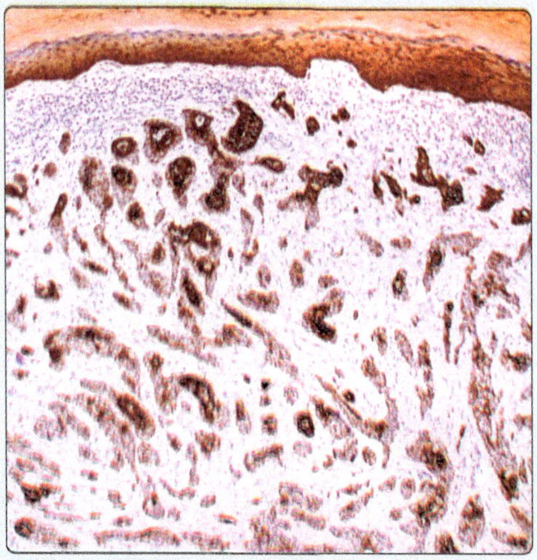

TERMINOLOGY

Abbreviations

- Malignant mixed tumor (MMT)

Synonyms

- Malignant chondroid syringoma
- Malignant apocrine mixed tumor

Definitions

- Rare variant of malignant tumor derived from adnexal ductal/gland and myoepithelial cells

CLINICAL ISSUES

Presentation

- Most often on extremities and trunk
- More common in women
  - F:M ratio ~ 2:1
- Average age at time of diagnosis is 5th decade
- Slow-growing, skin-colored tumor
- Slow protracted growth phase followed by rapid growth
- Rarely, malignant transformation from mixed tumor of skin
  - Most tumors begin with anaplastic changes

Treatment

- Surgical approaches
  - Wide excision with broad margin is primary treatment
- Adjuvant therapy
  - Effectiveness of chemotherapy is not established
- Radiation
  - Effectiveness of radiotherapy is not established; however, it might be helpful since tumors have propensity to form satellite lesions

Prognosis

- Biologic behavior of MMT varies: Local recurrence, metastasis (regional lymph node to distant viscera)
- Bone and lung are most common sites for distant metastases
- Up to 39% of cases were found to have metastatic lesions, and 22% died of disease
- Tumor loses chondroid stroma and often metastasizes as adenocarcinoma

MICROSCOPIC

Histologic Features

- Histologic appearances vary greatly
- It is often large, lobulated tumor in dermis &/or subcutaneous tissue
- Composed of both epithelial and mesenchymal component
  - Epithelial component tends to be predominately at periphery of lesion
    - Irregular nests, cords, and sheets of cuboidal or polygonal cells
    - Glandular differentiation is often present; not as common as in benign mixed tumor of skin
    - Foci of highly atypical cells with hyperchromatic nuclei and numerous mitotic figures are often present
    - Areas with moderate nuclear atypia or lacking morphologic criteria of malignancy are also common
    - Infiltration of surrounding tissue, vascular invasion, and necrosis are helpful diagnostic features
- Stroma is myxoid, chondroid, or hyalinized and is most abundant at center of lesion
  - Spindled mesenchymal cells are observed in stroma
  - Some cases may show frankly malignant stromal cells (i.e., true carcinosarcoma)
- Satellite tumor nodules might be present
- Rarely, features of associated benign mixed tumor can be seen
- MMT can easily be misdiagnosed due to its rare occurrence

Cytologic Features

- Epithelial cells with glandular differentiation and carcinomatous features

ANCILLARY TESTS

Immunohistochemistry

- Epithelial cells express cytokeratins (CK-PAN, HMWCKs such as CK5-CK6) and p63
- Chondroid and myoepithelial areas are often S100, actin, calponin, and vimentin positive

DIFFERENTIAL DIAGNOSIS

Benign Cutaneous Mixed Tumor

- Often small, symmetric, nodular dermal-based tumor
- Lacks features of malignancy
  - i.e., infiltration of surrounding tissue, cytologic atypia of epithelial cells, tumor necrosis, and perineural or vascular invasion
- Glandular areas are more abundant in benign lesions

Biphasic Synovial Sarcoma

- Commonly found in deep, intramuscular soft tissue
- Biphasic histology including epithelial and spindle cells
- S100 is rarely positive

DIAGNOSTIC CHECKLIST

Pathologic Interpretation Pearls

- Malignant epithelial tumor with glandular differentiation embedded in chondroid/myxoid stroma

SELECTED REFERENCES

1. Jo VY: Myoepithelial tumors: an update. Surg Pathol Clin. 8(3):445-66, 2015
2. Tural D et al: Facial localization of malignant chondroid syringoma: a rare case report. Case Rep Oncol Med. 2013:907980, 2013
3. Takahashi H et al: Malignant chondroid syringoma with bone invasion: a case report and review of the literature. Am J Dermatopathol. 26(5):403-6, 2004
4. Barnett MD et al: Recurrent malignant chondroid syringoma of the foot: a case report and review of the literature. Am J Clin Oncol. 23(3):227-32, 2000
5. Bates AW et al: Atypical mixed tumor of the skin: histologic, immunohistochemical, and ultrastructural features in three cases and a review of the criteria for malignancy. Am J Dermatopathol. 20(1):35-40, 1998
6. Trown K et al: Malignant mixed tumor of the skin (malignant chondroid syringoma). Pathology. 26(3):237-43, 1994
7. Steinmetz JC et al: Malignant chondroid syringoma with widespread metastasis. J Am Acad Dermatol. 22(5 Pt 1):845-7, 1990

PART I
SECTION 6
Metastatic Tumors

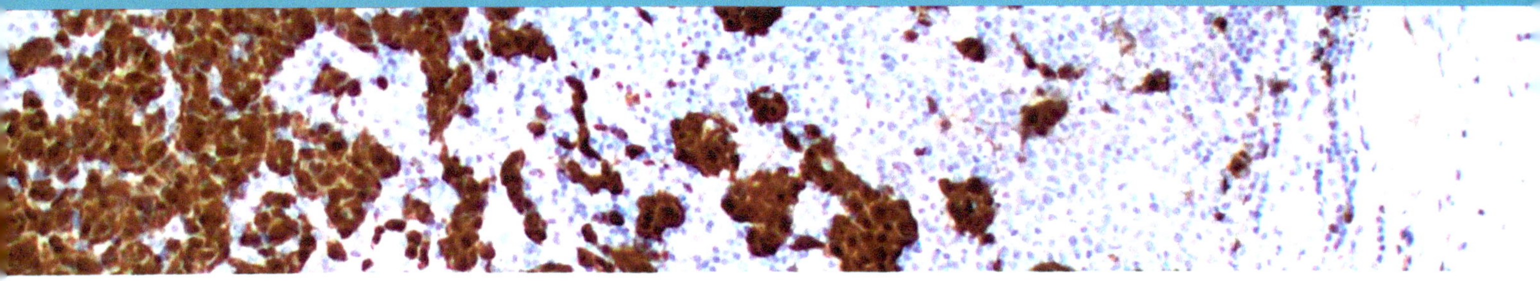

Metastatic Skin Tumors

KEY FACTS

CLINICAL ISSUES

- Melanoma
  - Skin metastases: Nodule, often pigmented, may be ulcerated, multiple or solitary
  - Nodal metastases: Usually in regional lymph nodes
  - Blue nevus-like melanoma: Blue macule/papule, often near original site of primary melanoma
  - Survival often < 3 years, but varies
- Squamous cell carcinoma and basal cell carcinoma
  - Nonspecific nodule(s), often pink to red
- Merkel cell carcinoma
  - Nodal &/or distant metastasis common
- Dermatofibrosarcoma protuberans
  - Essentially only the fibrosarcomatous variant

MICROSCOPIC

- Metastatic melanoma
  - Cutaneous metastases generally lack epidermal component (rare epidermotropism)
  - Nodal metastases
    - Micrometastasis often detected with use of stains, i.e., S100, SOX10, Melan-A, HMB-45, MiTF
- Blue nevus-like metastatic melanoma
  - Virtually identical to blue nevus; history may be key clue to diagnosis
  - May see some mitoses, atypical epithelioid melanocytes, and peripheral inflammation

TOP DIFFERENTIAL DIAGNOSES

- All metastatic skin tumors
  - Primary skin tumor (rather than metastasis from tumor elsewhere in skin)
- Nodal metastasis of melanoma
  - Nodal nevus [typically small, subcapsular; p16(+), weak/negative HMB-45, low proliferation rate with Ki-67]
- Merkel cell carcinoma
  - Other metastatic small cell neuroendocrine tumors [should be CK20(-)]

Clinical Photograph of Metastatic Melanoma

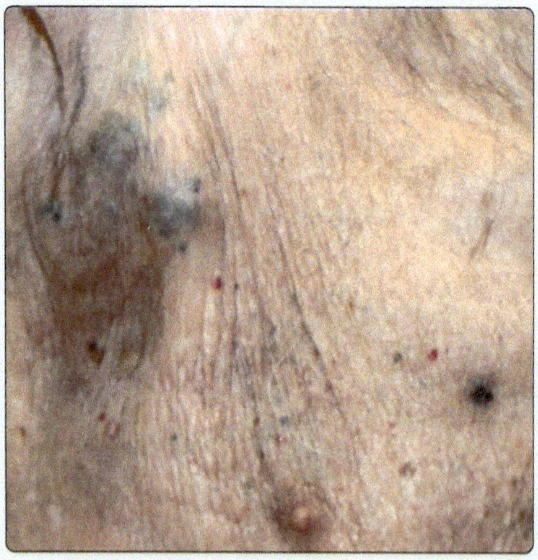

Metastatic Melanoma to Dermis

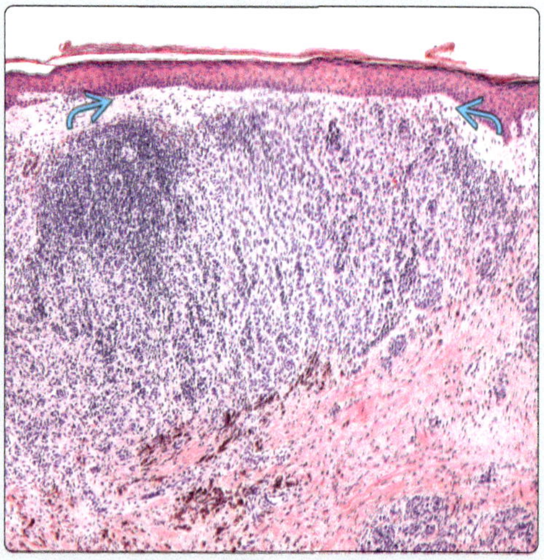

(Left) *Melanoma metastases are often blue-black in color. Typically, they are located in somewhat close proximity to the original primary. (Courtesy Yale Dermatology Residents' Slide Collection.)* **(Right)** *This metastatic melanoma shows dermal invasion, with lack of epidermal involvement (note the presence of a thin grenz zone →). The tumor is composed of infiltrative nests and cords of atypical cells with melanin pigment in the dermis.*

Metastatic Merkel Cell Carcinoma

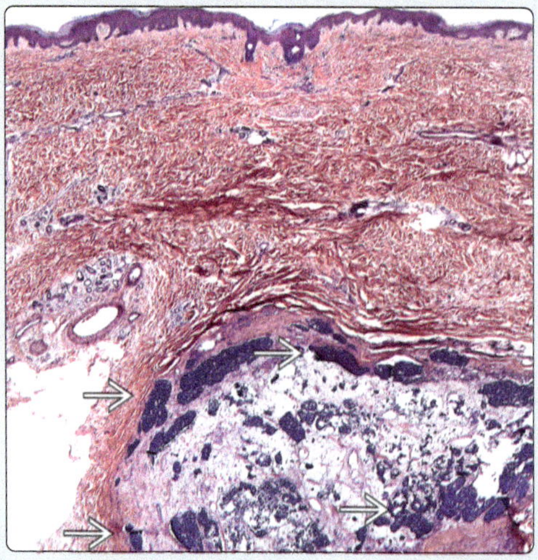

Metastatic Sebaceous Carcinoma

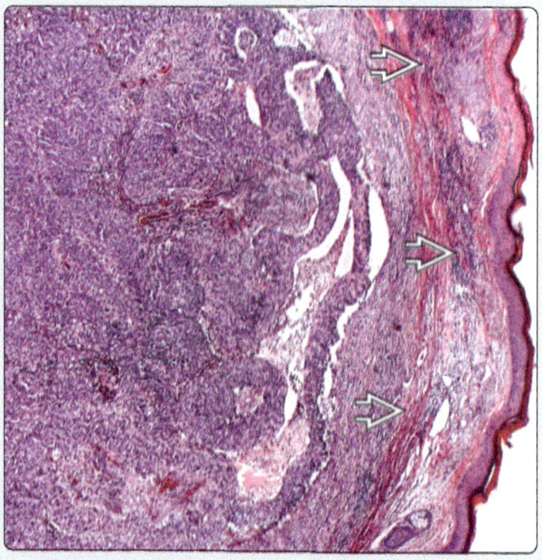

(Left) *Other primary skin tumors can also metastasize to the skin. This is an example of metastatic Merkel cell carcinoma. There are islands → composed of small, dark blue cells in the deep dermis.* **(Right)** *This is an example of a metastatic poorly differentiated sebaceous carcinoma to the skin of the cheek. Note the broad grenz zone separating the tumor from the epidermis →.*

TERMINOLOGY

Definitions

- Metastatic tumor originating from skin

CLINICAL ISSUES

Presentation

- Melanoma
  - Cutaneous metastases
    - Nodule or papule, often pigmented, may be ulcerated, multiple or solitary
    - Rarely presenting sign of disease; occasionally primary tumor site cannot be determined
  - Nodal metastases
    - Most commonly in regional, draining lymph nodes
  - Distant metastases
    - Any site, including bone, gastrointestinal tract, lung, brain
  - Blue nevus-like melanoma
    - Blue macule/papule, often near original site of primary melanoma
- Merkel cell carcinoma
  - Spreads to lymph nodes in up to 50-75% of cases
  - Distant metastasis (e.g., liver, lungs, bone, brain) in up to 30-50% of cases
- Squamous cell carcinoma (SCC)
  - Nonspecific nodules, often pink to red, rarely zosteriform pattern
- Basal cell carcinoma (BCC)
  - Very rarely metastasizes to other sites (lymph nodes, bone, parotid, lungs, other internal organs)
  - Usually only in very large, deeply invasive, recurrent tumors
- Dermatofibrosarcoma protuberans (DFSP)
  - Essentially only fibrosarcomatous cases; often history of multiple local recurrences
  - Rarely metastasizes
    - Lung most common site; also lymph nodes, bone, soft tissue
- Many other cutaneous malignancies may metastasize
  - Adnexal carcinomas
    - Sebaceous carcinoma: Relatively high incidence of metastasis
    - Apocrine and eccrine carcinomas
    - Aggressive digital papillary adenocarcinoma (typically to lungs)
    - Microcystic adnexal carcinoma (extremely rare, with history of multiple recurrences)

Prognosis

- Melanoma: Survival often < 3 years, but varies
- Merkel cell carcinoma: Survival at 5 years: 59% for regional metastasis, 25% for distant metastasis

MICROSCOPIC

Histologic Features

- Melanoma
  - Nodal metastases
    - Micrometastases may be detected with use of stains: S100, SOX10, MART-1/Melan-A, HMB-45
  - Cutaneous metastases
    - Generally lack epidermal component (only very rare epidermotropism)
    - Often similar histologic features to primary tumor
  - Distant metastases
    - Often similar histology to primary tumor
  - Blue nevus-like metastatic melanoma
    - Virtually identical to blue nevus; history may be major clue to diagnosis
    - Histopathologic clues include mitoses, atypical epithelioid melanocytes, and peripheral inflammation
- Merkel cell carcinoma
  - Anastomosing bands/sheets of cells, often in lower dermis/subcutaneous
  - Cells with indistinct cytoplasmic borders, little cytoplasm, salt and pepper chromatin; numerous mitoses
  - CK20, chromogranin, synaptophysin (+); TTF-1(-)
- SCC
  - May be poorly differentiated; in such cases, staining with HMWCK &/or p63 is helpful
  - More aggressive variants, such as desmoplastic SCC and adenosquamous carcinoma, are more likely to metastasize
- BCC
  - Typical histologic features of BCC with peripheral palisading, retraction artifact, mucinous stroma often seen
- DFSP
  - Often has fibrosarcomatous component

DIFFERENTIAL DIAGNOSIS

Metastatic Cutaneous Tumors to Skin

- Primary tumor needs to be considered; primary tumors often have epidermal connections &/or in situ component (melanoma and SCC), or are located more superficially in dermis (BCC and Merkel cell carcinoma)
- Clinical history and examination findings may be key for diagnosis

Nodal Metastasis of Melanoma

- Nodal nevus
  - Generally small and subcapsular, but rarely parenchymal
  - Often p16(+), weak/negative HMB-45, low proliferation rate with Ki-67

Metastatic Merkel Cell Carcinoma

- Metastatic small cell carcinoma of lung [CK20(-); CK7 and TTF-1 (+)] and other neuroendocrine tumors

SELECTED REFERENCES

1. Bae JM et al: Metastatic melanomas of unknown primary show better prognosis than those of known primary: a systematic review and meta-analysis of observational studies. J Am Acad Dermatol. 72(1):59-70, 2015
2. Kotteas EA et al: Neuroendocrine Merkel cell nodal carcinoma of unknown primary site: management and outcomes of a rare entity. Crit Rev Oncol Hematol. 94(1):116-21, 2015
3. Brougham ND et al: The incidence and risk factors of metastasis for cutaneous squamous cell carcinoma–implications on the T-classification system. J Surg Oncol. 110(7):876-82, 2014
4. McCusker M et al: Metastatic basal cell carcinoma: prognosis dependent on anatomic site and spread of disease. Eur J Cancer. 50(4):774-83, 2014
5. Hussein MR: Skin metastasis: a pathologist's perspective. J Cutan Pathol. 37(9):e1-20, 2010

Metastatic Melanoma to Skin

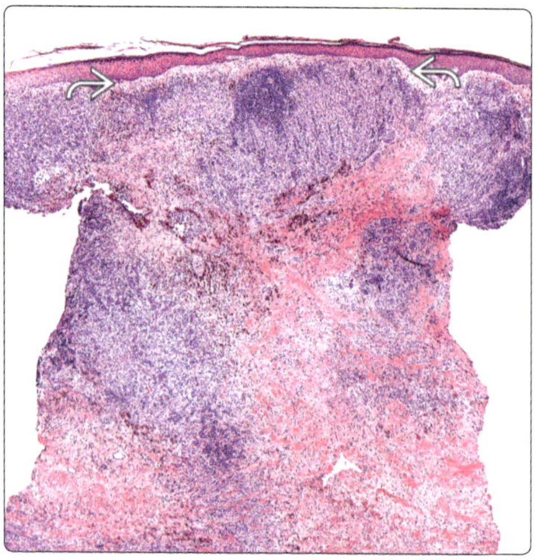

Metastatic Melanoma: High Magnification

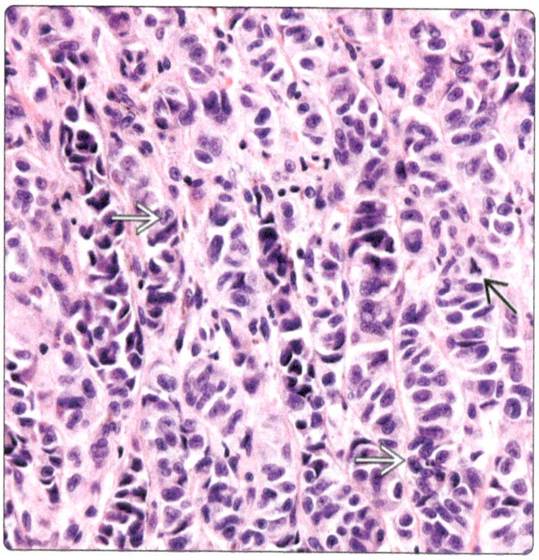

(Left) *This metastatic melanoma shows extensive involvement of the dermis. There is a slight grenz zone present and no evidence of epidermotropism identified.* **(Right)** *Higher magnification view of metastatic melanoma shows nests of atypical, hyperchromatic-staining cells with marked pleomorphism. There are enlarged nucleoli and mitoses are evident.*

Metastatic Merkel Cell Carcinoma With Lymphatic Invasion

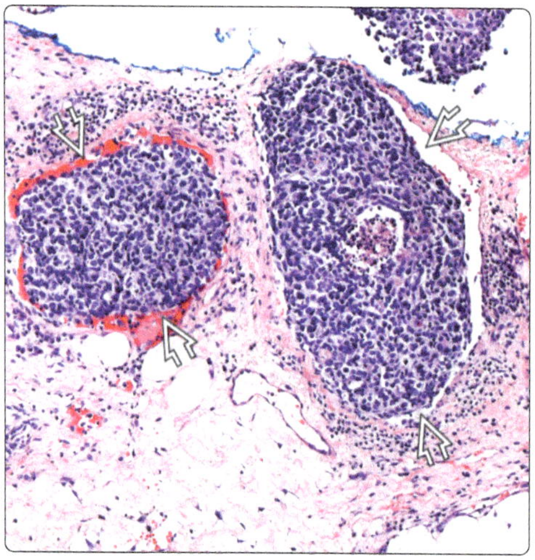

Metastatic Merkel Cell Carcinoma at High Magnification

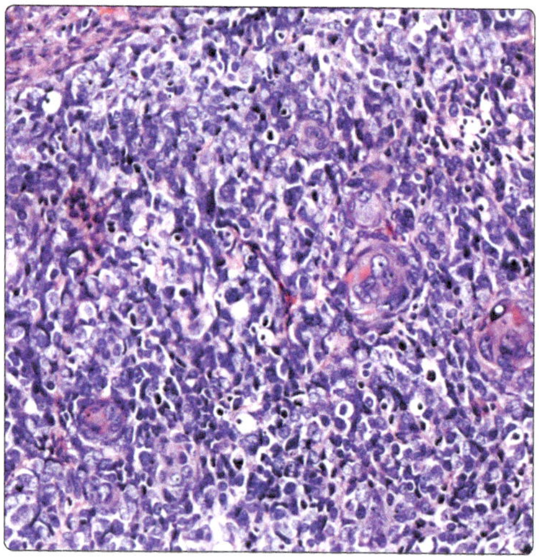

(Left) *This is an example of a metastatic Merkel cell carcinoma to the subcutaneous soft tissue showing prominent lymphovascular invasion.* **(Right)** *This is a higher magnification view of metastatic Merkel cell carcinoma showing cohesive clusters of cells with large nuclei and scant amounts of cytoplasm. The cells have salt and pepper chromatin, typical of neuroendocrine tumors.*

Metastatic Merkel Cell Carcinoma: CK20 Staining

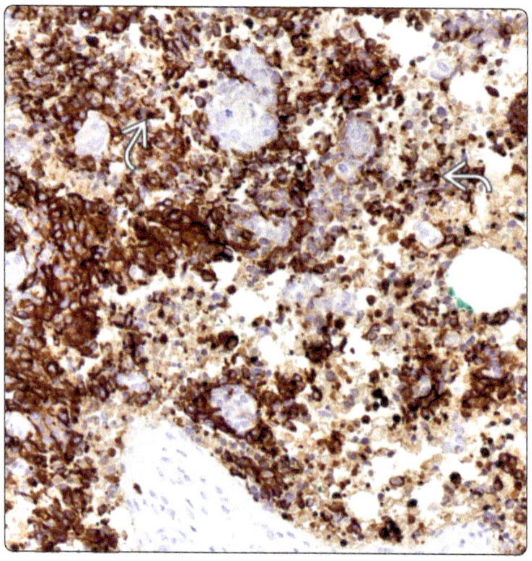

Metastatic Merkel Cell Carcinoma: Synaptophysin Staining

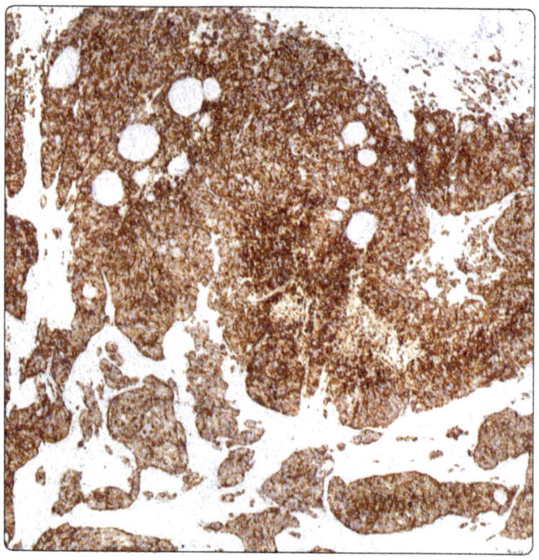

(Left) *Metastatic Merkel cell carcinoma shows strong and diffuse positivity with CK20, with many of the cells showing a perinuclear dot-like pattern.* **(Right)** *Metastatic Merkel cell carcinoma shows strong and diffuse positive staining for the neuroendocrine marker synaptophysin.*

Metastatic Melanoma to Skin

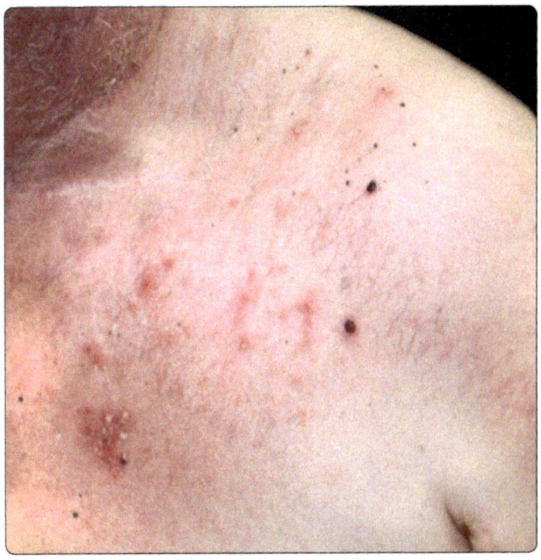

Metastatic Melanoma Involving Lymph Node

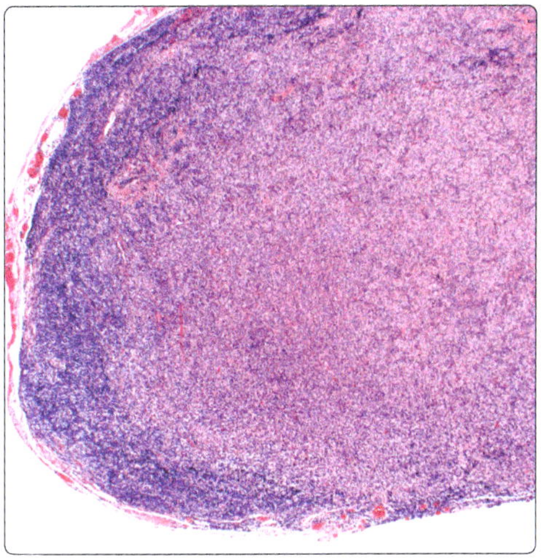

(Left) *This patient with a history of melanoma on the chest had an unusual presentation of metastatic melanoma, with numerous 1- to 3-mm black-red papules on the upper chest and shoulder region.* **(Right)** *This example of metastatic melanoma shows diffuse replacement of a lymph node by the tumor cells.*

Metastatic Melanoma to Lymph Node

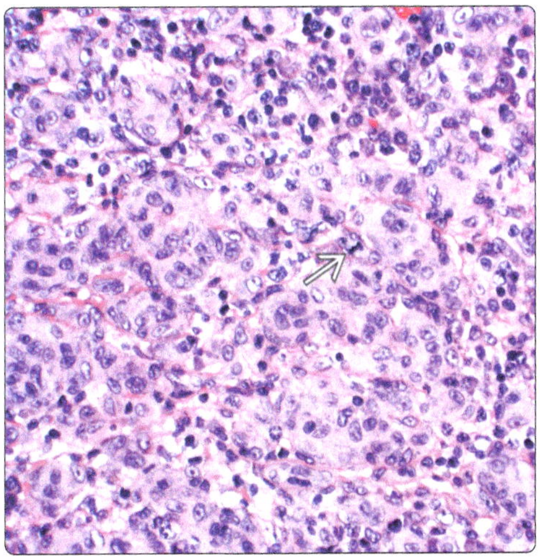

Metastatic Melanoma to Lymph Node: S100 Staining

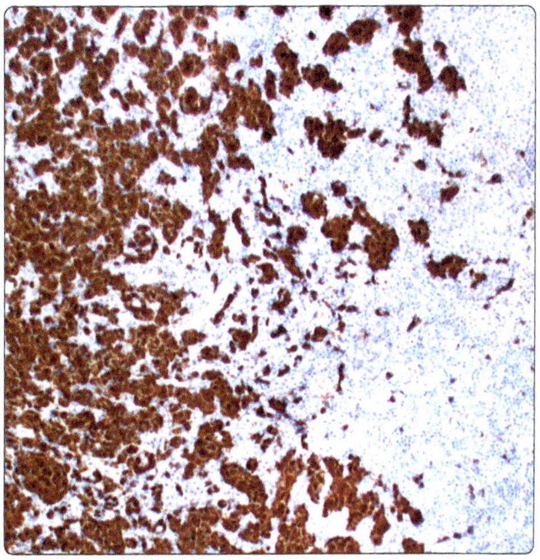

(Left) *This is a higher magnification view of metastatic melanoma replacing a lymph node. The cells are somewhat nested and show hyperchromatic-staining nuclei with pleomorphism and large, purple nucleoli. Mitotic figures are present* ➡*.* **(Right)** *This is an S100 immunohistochemical stain of metastatic melanoma diffusely infiltrating a lymph node.*

Metastatic Melanoma to Lymph Node: HMB-45 Staining

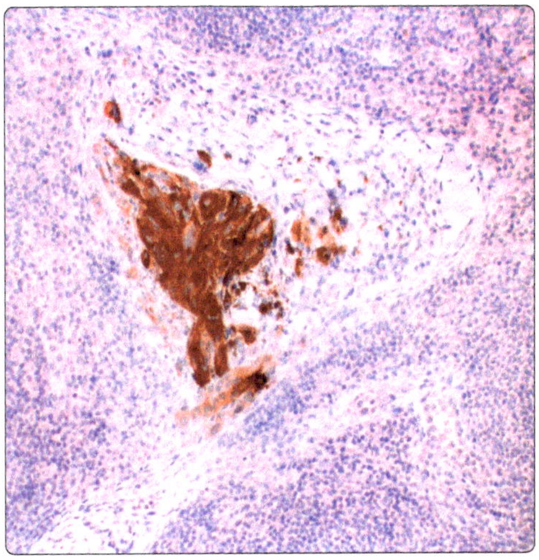

Metastatic Melanoma to Lymph Node: Melan-A Staining

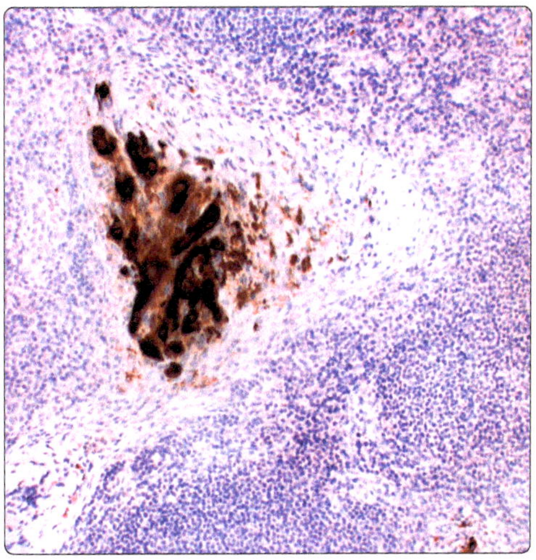

(Left) *This is an example of a micrometastasis of melanoma in a lymph node. Immunohistochemical stains including HMB-45 are helpful in identifying these tumor cells; HMB-45 is less sensitive but more specific than S100, making use of a panel of immunostains the optimal approach.* **(Right)** *This micrometastasis is also strongly Melan-A positive; this marker is slightly less sensitive than S100 but more specific.*

KEY FACTS

CLINICAL ISSUES

- Cutaneous metastases often located near primary tumor site
- Incidence rate of ~ 2-10% in patients with internal malignancy
- Breast cancer metastasizes to skin most frequently
- In most cases, skin metastases present after primary tumor has been diagnosed
- Very poor prognosis

MICROSCOPIC

- Many metastases represent adenocarcinoma
  - Irregular collections of cells, often with lumina

ANCILLARY TESTS

- Organ-specific markers include PSA, TTF-1, CDX-2, and RCC
- Cytokeratin 7 (CK7) and cytokeratin 20 (CK20)
  - Traditionally, these stains helpful in narrowing down origin of metastatic carcinoma
- Cytokeratin 5/cytokeratin 6, p63, podoplanin/D2-40
  - Positivity with these stains supports primary cutaneous origin over metastasis

TOP DIFFERENTIAL DIAGNOSES

- Metastatic adenocarcinoma
  - Primary adnexal tumors of skin
    - Generally positive with p63, cytokeratin 5/cytokeratin 6, podoplanin
- Metastatic renal cell carcinoma
  - Clear cell hidradenoma
  - Hidradenocarcinoma
- Metastatic small cell carcinoma of lung
  - Main differential is with primary cutaneous Merkel cell carcinoma

Metastatic Lung Adenocarcinoma

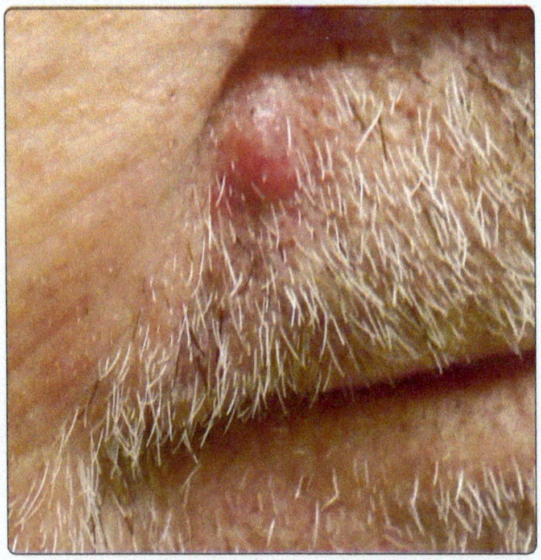

Metastatic Lung Adenocarcinoma

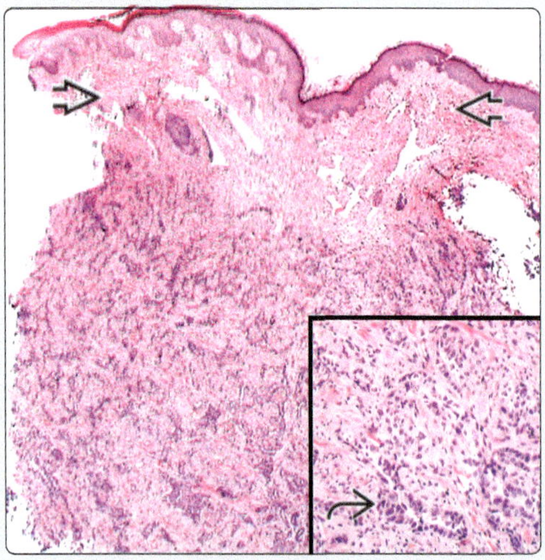

(Left) *This is a patient with a history of lung adenocarcinoma who presented with a nodular lesion in the nasolabial area.* **(Right)** *Diffusely infiltrating the dermis are irregular, jagged islands of epithelial cells. Note the absence of epidermal or superficial dermal involvement. Higher magnification shows glandular lumina lined by markedly enlarged and atypical-appearing epithelial cells with columnar features.*

Metastatic Small Intestinal Carcinoma

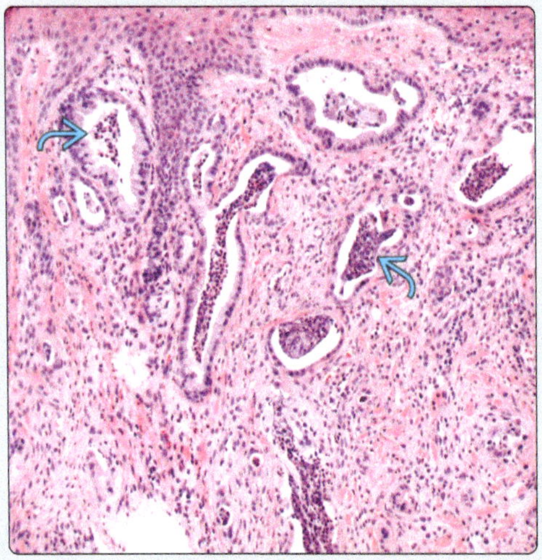

Metastatic Colonic Carcinoma to Scalp

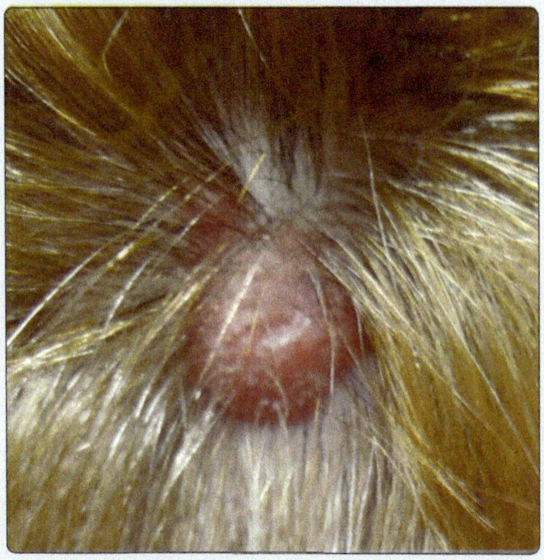

(Left) *This is an example of a rare metastatic small intestinal (duodenal primary) carcinoma to the skin. Similar to colon carcinoma, there are large glandular spaces associated with collections of intraluminal neutrophils.* **(Right)** *This is a nodular lesion on the scalp of an elderly patient who had a history of colon carcinoma.*

ETIOLOGY/PATHOGENESIS

Mode of Metastasis

- Hematogenous spread
- Lymphatic spread
- Direct extension from primary tumor
- Accidental implantation during surgical procedure
  - Described with oral cavity, laryngeal, lung, mesothelioma, renal cell, colorectal cancers, and others

CLINICAL ISSUES

Epidemiology

- Sex
  - Male: Primary tumor most often lung, colon
  - Female: Primary tumor most often breast, colon

Site

- Cutaneous metastases often located near primary tumor site
  - Breast and lung carcinoma: Chest wall
  - Genitourinary carcinoma: Abdominal wall, rarely genitalia
  - Oral cavity: Head and neck
- Scalp
  - Tumors with predilection to metastasize to scalp: Thyroid, breast, kidney, lung
- Umbilicus: Sister Mary Joseph nodule
  - Associated with adenocarcinoma of stomach, pancreas, ovary, and others

Presentation

- General points
  - Incidence rate of ~ 2-10% in patients with internal malignancy
  - Rare among skin tumors (~ 2% of all skin tumors)
  - Patients generally of age 60 yr or above, but exceptions occur
    - In neonates, neuroblastoma or other small round blue cell tumors may metastasize to skin
  - Skin metastases usually present within 2-3 yr of diagnosis of primary
  - Breast cancer metastasizes to skin most frequently
  - Other internal cancers with not infrequent skin metastases include lung, colorectal, ovarian, head and neck, renal cell carcinoma (RCC), and gastrointestinal cancer
- Signs/symptoms
  - Appearance
    - Generally red-pink, 1-3 cm firm nodule
    - Deeper purple or vascular appearance has been described for RCC metastasis
    - Multiple or solitary, clustered or randomly distributed
    - May be movable or fixed, sometimes ulcerated
  - Asymptomatic or painful
- Special clinical variants
  - Inflammatory (erysipeloid) carcinoma
    - Lymphatic spread of carcinoma
    - Warm, red, tender plaque; resembles erysipelas
    - Most commonly associated with breast carcinoma, but also may be due to other carcinomas (i.e., colon, prostate) and melanoma
  - Carcinoma telangiectodes
    - Secondary to breast carcinoma
    - Plaque of coalescing telangiectasias and erythematous papules
  - Carcinoma en cuirasse
    - Secondary to breast carcinoma
    - Skin hardened and leathery
  - Superior vena cava syndrome
    - Can be secondary to lung carcinoma
    - Obstruction of superior vena cava leads to edema, cyanosis, plethora of head/neck; subcutaneous vessels may be prominent
  - Sister Mary Joseph nodule
    - Classically described as red nodule on umbilicus, most commonly due to gastric carcinoma
  - Alopecia neoplastica
    - Localized patches of alopecia on scalp secondary to metastatic disease in dermis

Laboratory Tests

- Ovarian cancer
  - High CA-125 suggestive of advanced disease; CA 19-9 may be elevated
- Colon cancer
  - CEA may be used to monitor disease
- Gastric cancer
  - CA 19-9 may be elevated
- Prostate cancer
  - PSA often elevated

Natural History

- Skin metastases are rarely presenting clue to internal malignancy
- In most cases, skin metastases present after primary tumor has been diagnosed

Treatment

- In advanced disease, excision of metastases may be palliative
- Other treatment options dependent on type of tumor and extent of disease (e.g., chemotherapy or radiation)
  - Chemotherapy
    - Traditional drugs (e.g., anthracyclines, taxanes)
    - Trend is to test tissue for molecular targets, and if positive, use targeted treatment (e.g., trastuzumab in Her2/neu(+) breast cancer, tamoxifen in estrogen receptor positive cancers)

Prognosis

- Poor overall survival
  - 1 study cites range of 1-34 months

MICROSCOPIC

Histologic Features

- Many metastases represent adenocarcinoma: Irregular collections of cells in dermis, often forming lumina
  - Breast
    - Glandular differentiation may be virtually absent in high-grade cases

- Cytologically atypical cells may be seen infiltrating in single file (Indian file) pattern between collagen bundles (lobular carcinoma)
- Inflammatory carcinoma: Cytologically atypical cells in clusters within lymphatic vessels
- Cells are often positive with GCDFP-15, CEA, CK7, mammaglobin, ER/PR
  - Colon
    - Dirty necrosis (neutrophils and degenerating cells in glandular lumina) may be evident
    - Glandular differentiation often obvious with columnar cells lining lumina
  - Gastric
    - Signet ring cells may be present
  - Ovarian
    - Psammoma bodies and papillations may be present
- Mucinous carcinoma
  - Primary mucinous carcinoma of skin can mimic metastatic mucinous carcinoma (typically of breast, colon)
  - Immunohistochemical stains may not be helpful (especially versus breast, i.e., ER, PR, GCDFP-15 often positive)
- Metastatic RCC
  - Clear cells, often bland, in nests and forming ducts
  - Stroma with rich vascularity and numerous extravasated erythrocytes
- Metastatic squamous cell carcinoma (SCC)
  - Lacks epidermal connections
  - Often secondary to primary of lung or head and neck
  - TTF-1 positivity rarely seen in metastases from lung
- Neuroblastoma and other small round blue cell tumors
  - Small, hyperchromatic cells, rosettes may be present
  - Positive with neuron-specific enolase &/or CD99 (Ewing/PNET)

ANCILLARY TESTS

Immunohistochemistry

- Markers suggestive of particular primary
  - Thyroid transcription factor-1 (TTF-1)
    - Positive in lung adenocarcinoma, small cell carcinoma, and rarely SCC
    - Positive in thyroid cancers
    - Negative in primary cutaneous Merkel cell carcinoma
  - Prostate specific antigen (PSA): Positive in metastatic prostate cancer
  - CDX-2: Positive in colonic carcinoma and mucinous carcinomas of pancreas, intestine, ovary
  - Thyroglobulin: Positive in papillary and follicular thyroid carcinoma
  - Calcitonin: Positive in medullary thyroid carcinoma
  - RCC-antigen (PCRNA): Positive in RCC
- Cytokeratin 7 (CK7) and cytokeratin 20 (CK20)
  - Traditionally, these stains helpful in narrowing down origin of metastatic adenocarcinoma
  - CK7 positive, CK20 negative
    - Breast carcinoma, lung carcinoma, ovarian adenocarcinoma
  - CK7 negative, CK20 positive
    - Colon carcinoma (although ~ 15% of primary colon cancer negative for CK20; also ~ 15% positive for CK7)
  - CK7 positive, CK20 positive
    - Pancreatic carcinoma
    - Transitional RCC and bladder carcinoma
    - Some gastric carcinomas
- Cytokeratin 5/cytokeratin 6 and p63
  - Diffuse positivity with these 2 stains supports primary adnexal cutaneous origin over metastatic adenocarcinoma
  - Important exception: Primary mucinous carcinoma of skin stains poorly with these markers
- Podoplanin (D2-40)
  - Generally positive in primary cutaneous adnexal tumors
  - Negative in metastatic adenocarcinomas
- CD10
  - Staining with CD10 is supportive of RCC
  - Also positive in some sebaceous carcinomas, and, rarely, clear cell hidradenomas
- Other stains
  - Useful stains reported in literature include calretinin, TAG72, WT1, BER-EP4, MUCs

DIFFERENTIAL DIAGNOSIS

Metastatic Adenocarcinoma

- Primary adnexal tumors of skin
  - May show well-differentiated areas with characteristic features
  - Generally diffusely positive with p63 and CK5/CK6, Podoplanin/D2-40

Lobular Breast Carcinoma

- Infiltrating cords of cells create busy dermis pattern
  - Differential can include granuloma annulare, dermatofibroma, leukemia cutis

Metastatic RCC

- Main differential is with clear cell hidradenoma and hidradenocarcinoma
  - Generally negative with CD10 and RCC-antigen
  - Vessels and extravasated erythrocytes not prominent
  - Hyalinized stroma
  - Other clues: Ducts lined by eosinophilic cuticles, squamoid differentiation, poroid differentiation

Metastatic Small (Oat) Cell Carcinoma of Lung

- Main differential is with primary cutaneous Merkel cell carcinoma
- Small cell carcinoma is TTF-1(+), CK7(+), CK20(-)

SELECTED REFERENCES

1. Nashan D et al: Cutaneous metastases from internal malignancies. Dermatol Ther. 23(6):567-80, 2010
2. Plaza JA et al: Value of p63 and podoplanin (D2-40) immunoreactivity in the distinction between primary cutaneous tumors and adenocarcinomas metastatic to the skin: a clinicopathologic and immunohistochemical study of 79 cases. J Cutan Pathol. 37(4):403-10, 2010

Metastatic Colon Carcinoma

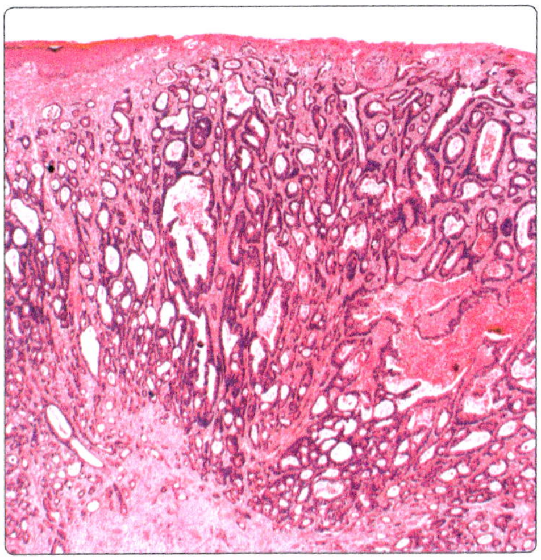

Metastatic Renal Cell Carcinoma

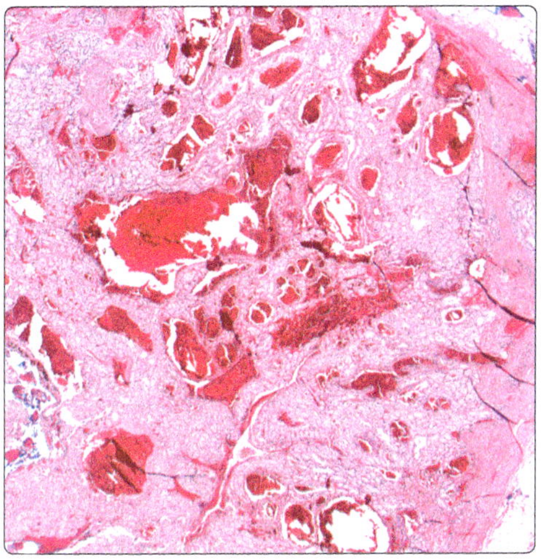

(Left) *Histologic examination of the lesion at low magnification shows metastatic colon carcinoma with overlying ulceration. The tumor is composed of variably sized ductal and glandular structures with irregular lumina lined by columnar cells.* **(Right)** *This low-power image shows diffuse dermal replacement by collections of clear cells with pools of extravasated erythrocytes, consistent with metastatic RCC. These tumors are typically positive with CD10, EMA, CAIX, and RCC-antigen.*

Metastatic Renal Cell Carcinoma at High Magnification

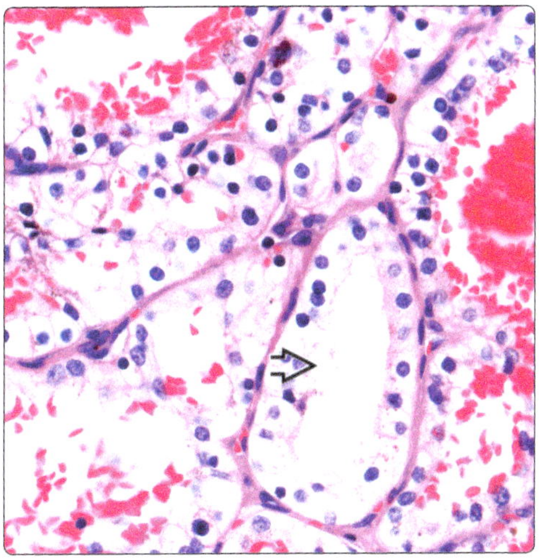

Metastatic Small Cell Carcinoma of Lung

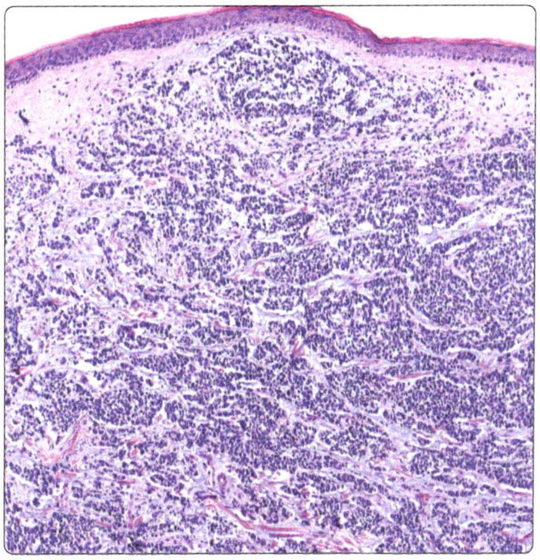

(Left) *Higher magnification of metastatic renal cell carcinoma shows collections of clear cells forming lumina. Extravasated erythrocytes are prominent.* **(Right)** *Metastatic small cell carcinoma of lung to the skin is shown. The dermis is diffusely infiltrated by small cells, which show prominent nuclear hyperchromasia and a high N:C ratio, similar to Merkel cell carcinoma.*

TTF-1 Staining in Metastatic Small Cell Carcinoma of Lung

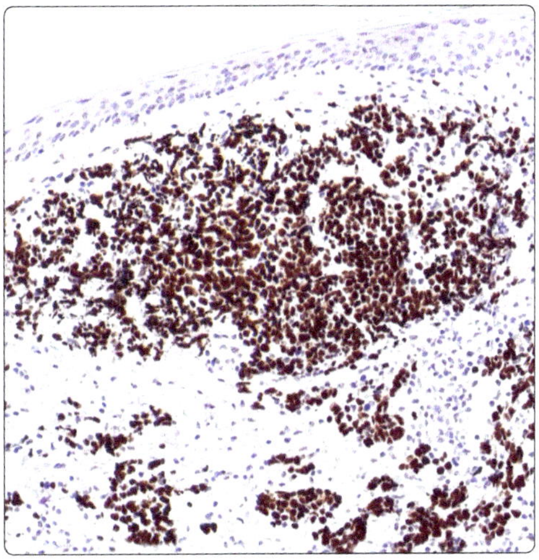

Carcinoma Erysipelatoides

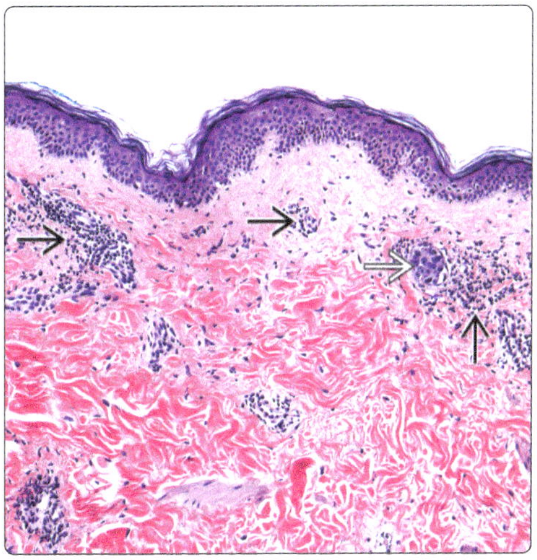

(Left) *Metastatic small cell carcinoma of the lung stains with TTF-1, distinguishing it from Merkel cell carcinoma, which is uniformly TTF-1 negative. In general, metastatic carcinomas from the lung show nuclear positivity with TTF-1, and are also usually CK7(+)/CK20(-) (unlike Merkel cell carcinoma).* **(Right)** *This example of carcinoma erysipelatoides (metastatic breast carcinoma) shows a perivascular lymphocytic inflammatory infiltrate. Within one of the lymphatic vessels, there is a cluster of atypical cells.*

Carcinoma Erysipelatoides at High Magnification

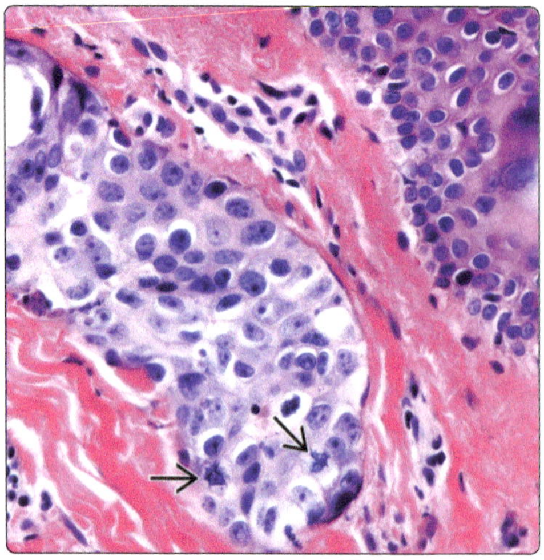

Metastatic Breast Ductal Carcinoma

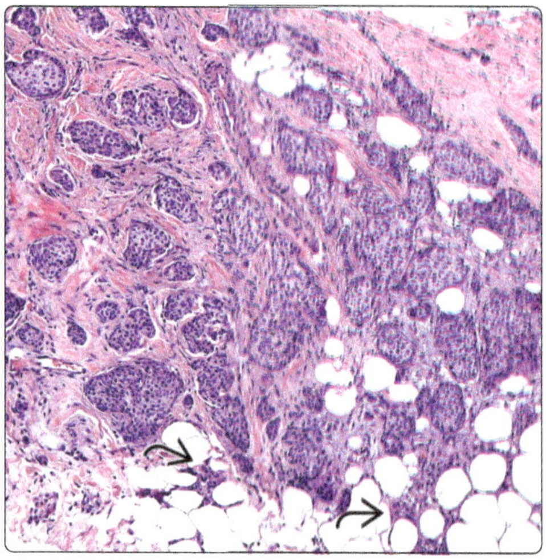

(Left) *High-magnification view of carcinoma erysipelatoides is shown. In this section, clustered atypical cells with multiple mitotic figures more prominently fill a superficial lymphatic vessel. Part of the epidermis is visible in the right upper corner.* **(Right)** *This is a metastatic breast carcinoma with ductal features, composed of large, infiltrative nests of cells in the deep dermis and invading into the superficial adipose tissue.*

Metastatic Breast Ductal Carcinoma

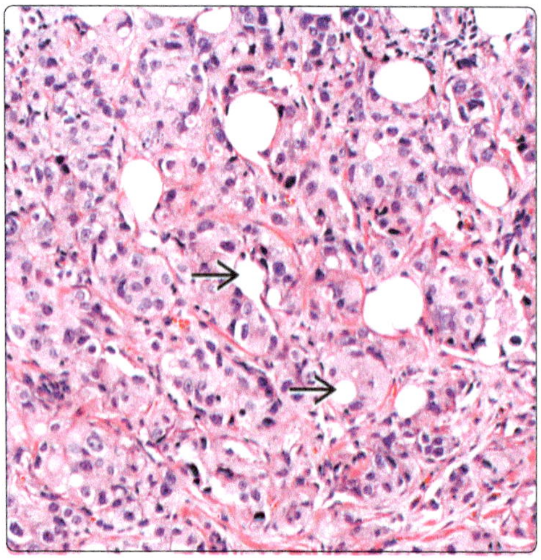

Metastatic Lobular Breast Carcinoma

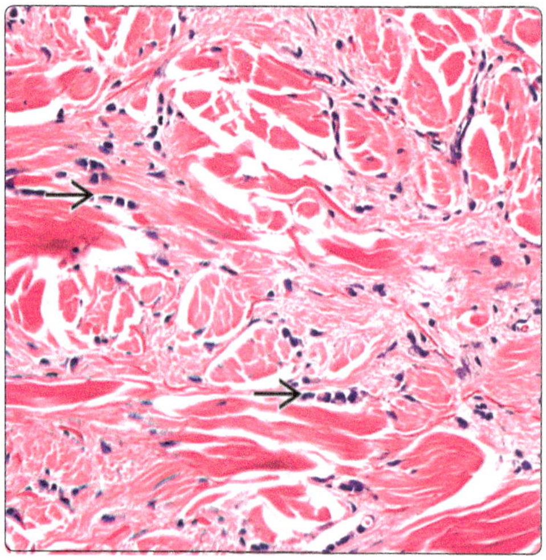

(Left) *High magnification of a metastatic high-grade ductal breast carcinoma, with circular islands of cells forming central lumina. The cells comprising the islands are markedly atypical, with nuclear hyperchromasia and prominent nucleoli.* **(Right)** *Cases of lobular breast carcinoma often show diffuse infiltration of the dermis with atypical, hyperchromatic, single cells; the cells show a linear filing pattern through the collagen.*

GCDFP Staining in Metastatic Ductal Carcinoma of Breast

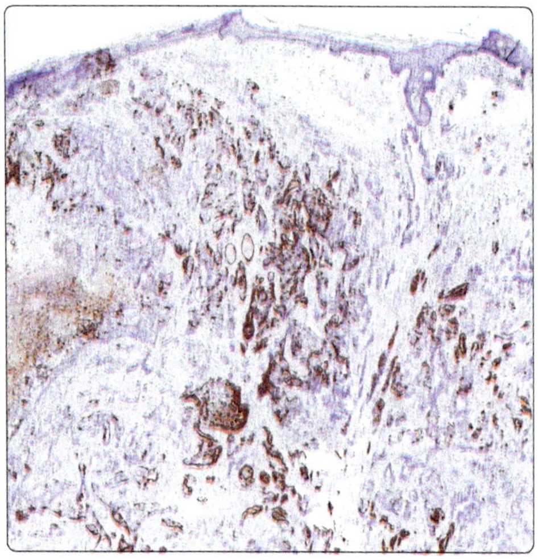

Metastatic Small Intestinal Carcinoma

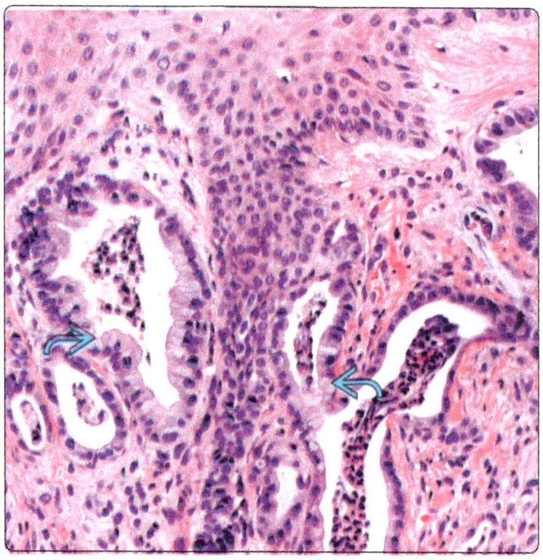

(Left) *Metastatic ductal carcinoma of the breast at low magnification shows moderate positive staining with GCDFP-15. This case was also CK7 positive and positive for estrogen and progesterone receptors.* **(Right)** *High magnification shows atypical glands closely abutting the epidermis. The cells are cuboidal to columnar-shaped, and many show prominent cytoplasmic mucin droplets.*

Metastatic Small Intestinal Carcinoma: CK-PAN

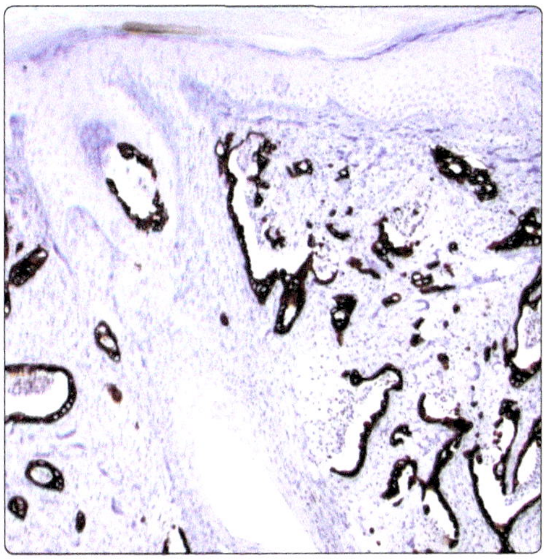

Metastatic Gastric Carcinoma

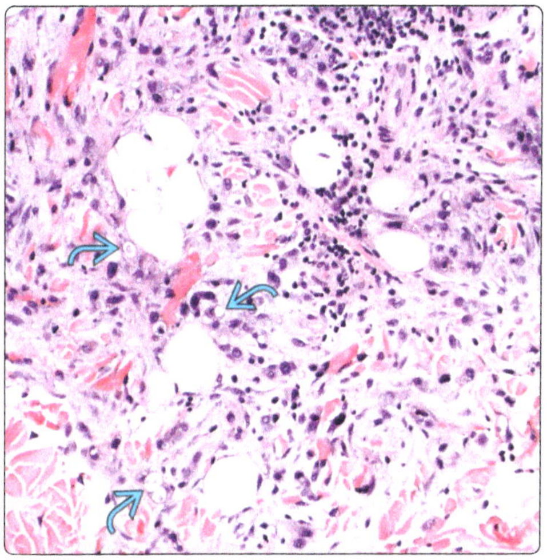

(Left) *Pancytokeratin and CK7 were strongly positive in this case. CK7 is often positive in upper gastrointestinal tract tumors such as gastric and duodenal carcinoma. Colonic carcinomas, in contrast, are typically CK7(-)/CK20(+).* **(Right)** *This is metastatic gastric carcinoma, which first presented as a skin metastasis in an older adult patient. The dermis is diffusely infiltrated by atypical oval to epithelioid-shaped cells associated with mucin. Cells with intracytoplasmic vacuoles are seen.*

CK7 in Metastatic Gastric Carcinoma

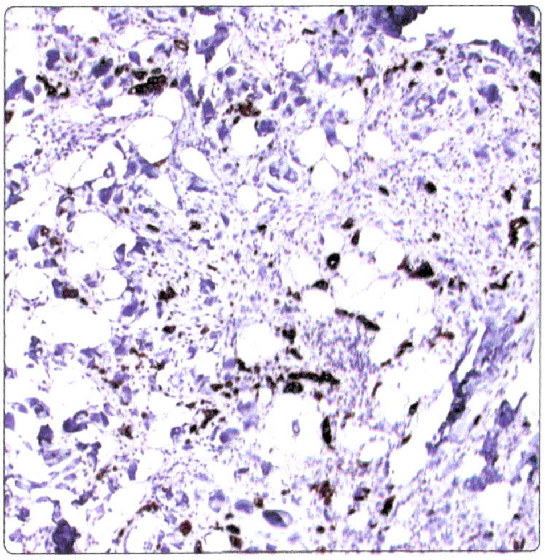

Metastatic Pancreaticobiliary Carcinoma

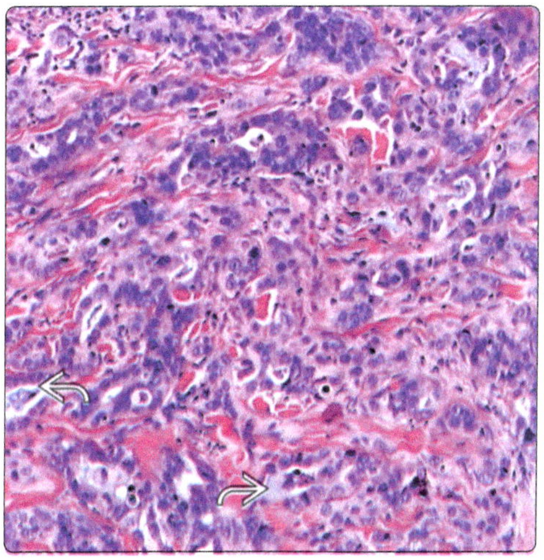

(Left) *CK7 shows strong and diffuse cytoplasmic staining in this metastatic gastric carcinoma. EMA and CDX2 were also positive.* **(Right)** *This is an example of metastatic high-grade pancreaticobiliary carcinoma. There are clusters and tubules of atypical cells forming glandular clusters with small lumina containing mucinous secretions. The stroma is sclerotic.*

Metastatic Glioblastoma Multiforme

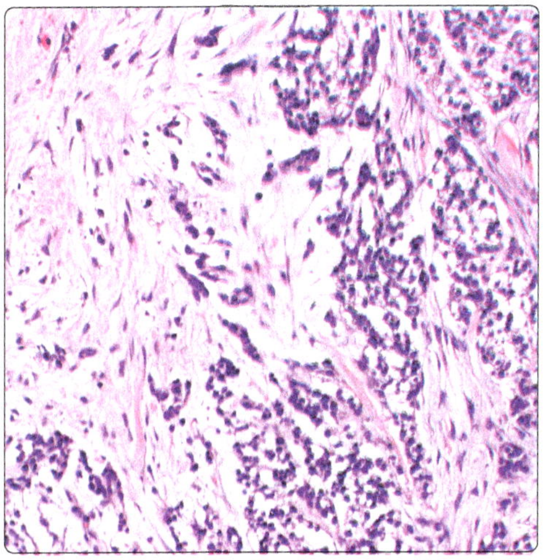

Sister Mary Joseph Nodule

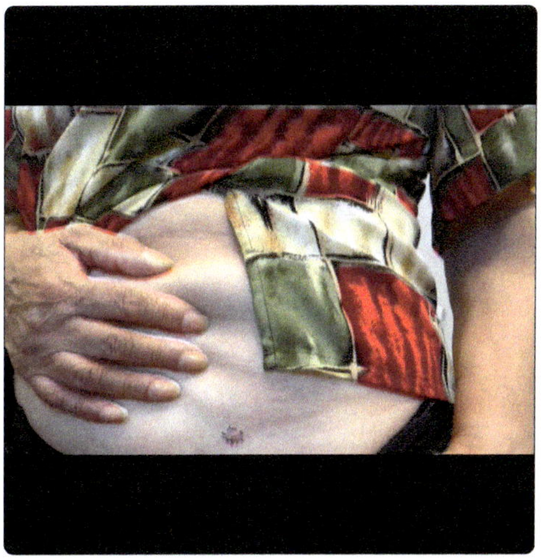

(Left) *This is an example of a rare metastatic glioblastoma multiforme to the skin of the scalp. Hyperchromatic oval to spindle-shaped cells show indistinct cytoplasmic borders with a fibrillary background. The cells typically stain with GFAP.* **(Right)** *Metastases to the skin can present as an umbilical nodule.*

PART I

SECTION 7

Fibrous and "Fibrohistiocytic" Tissue Tumors

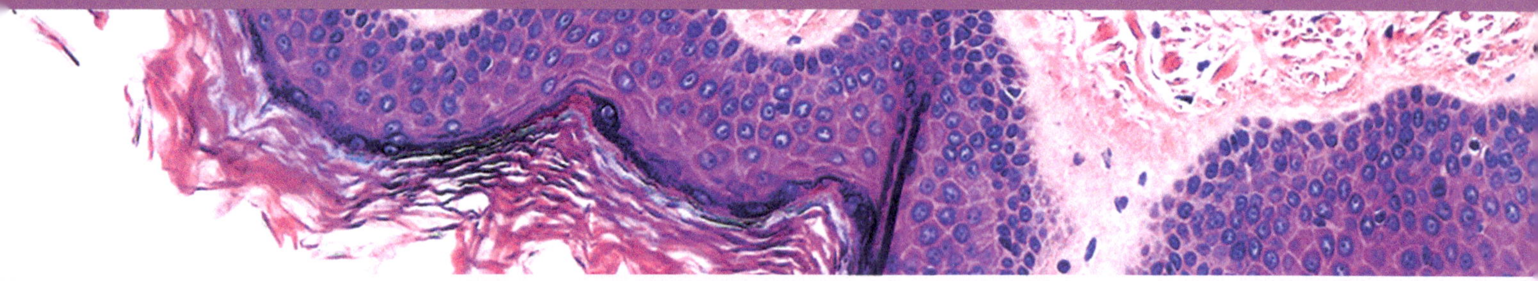

Benign Fibrous and "Fibrohistiocytic" Tissue Tumors

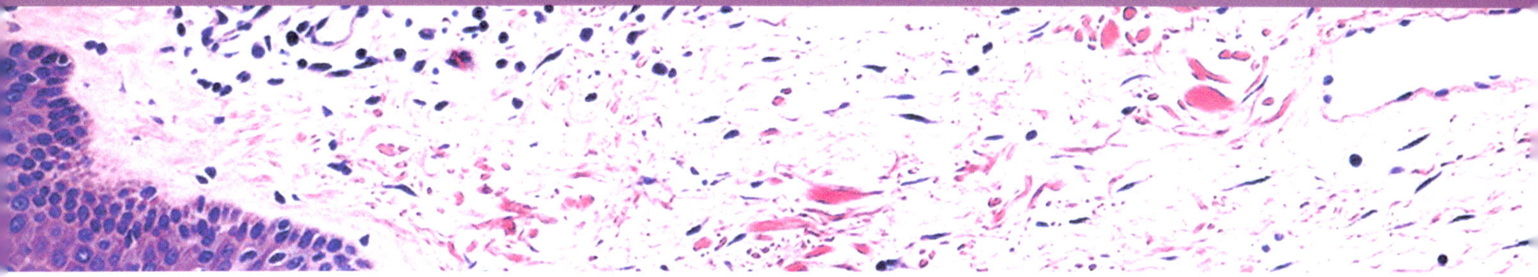

Atypical and Malignant Fibrous and "Fibrohistiocytic" Tissue Tumors

Fibroepithelial Polyps (Acrochordons)

KEY FACTS

TERMINOLOGY

- Skin tag, soft fibroma

CLINICAL ISSUES

- Very common lesions
- Usually affect adults
  - > 50 years old
- Single or multiple
- Neck, axilla, groin
- Association with
  - Diabetes
  - Obesity
  - Hypertension

MICROSCOPIC

- Thin to acanthotic squamous epithelium
  - May show papillomatosis and horn cysts
    - Such lesions most likely represent polypoid seborrheic keratosis
- Fibrovascular core is composed of loose to dense connective tissue
  - Variable amount of blood vessels
  - Devoid of adnexal structures
  - Mature adipocytes may be present (fibrolipoma)
- Many different benign and malignant tumors may arise in acrochordon-like lesion
  - This is especially true in locations such as eyelids, axilla, groin, neck
  - 30% of skin tag growths contain melanocytic nevi
  - Lymphomatoid papulosis, lymphomas, and melanomas have been described in acrochordon-like lesions

TOP DIFFERENTIAL DIAGNOSES

- Seborrheic keratosis
- Nevus lipomatosus superficialis
- Pleomorphic fibroma

Slightly Acanthotic Epidermis Lining Acrochordon

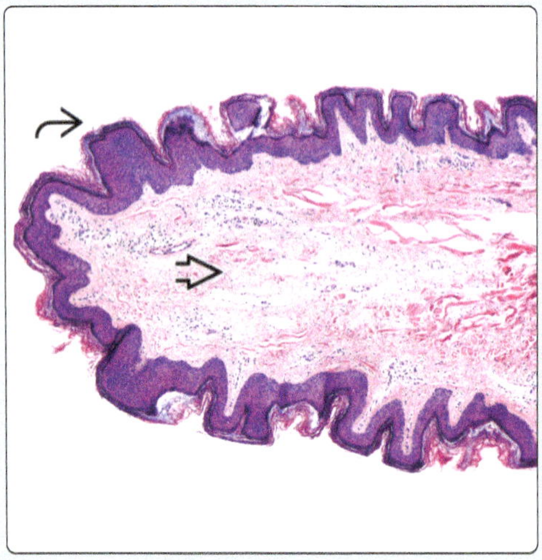

Loose Connective Tissue in Fibroepithelial Polyp

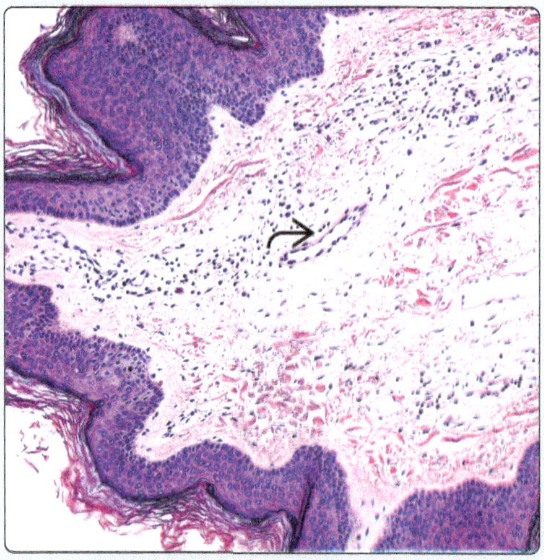

(Left) *Acrochordon characterized by a core of loose connective tissue devoid of adnexal structures ➡ is covered by squamous epithelium ➡.* **(Right)** *The fibrovascular core in this fibroepithelial polyp is composed of loose connective tissue with scattered vessels ➡ and a few inflammatory cells.*

Mature Fat in Fibrolipoma

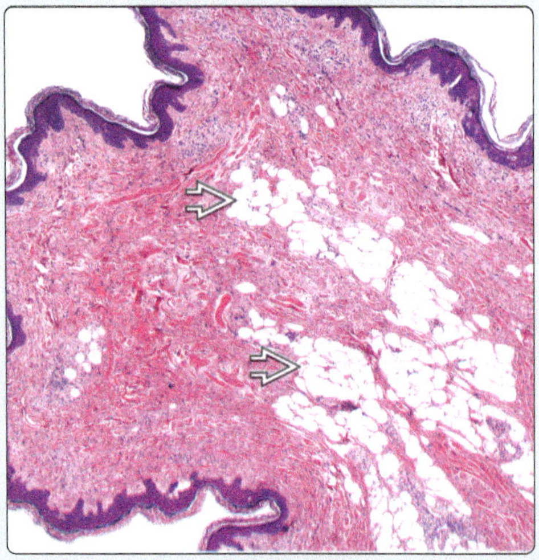

Seborrheic Keratosis With Features of Skin Tag

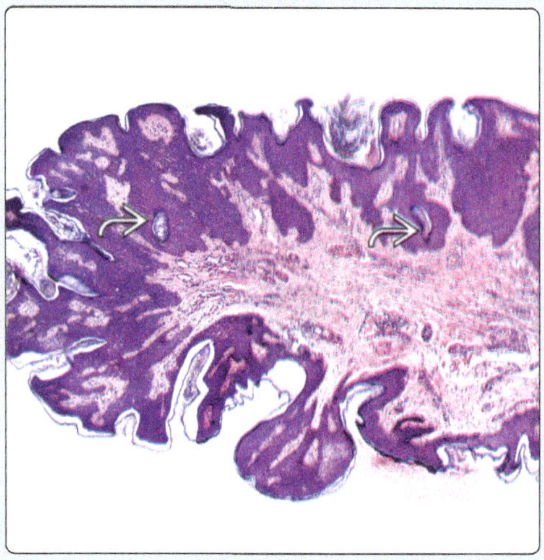

(Left) *Fibrolipoma (nevus lipomatosus superficialis) with polypoid features is shown. Some would consider this a skin tag containing mature adipose tissue ➡ in its fibrovascular core. Such lesions are considered acrochordons containing adipose tissue by some authors.* **(Right)** *Skin tag-like growth with acanthotic and papillomatous epithelium shows a few horn pseudocysts ➡. Such lesions most likely represent seborrheic keratoses that, in special locations (e.g., axillae), have polypoid features.*

TERMINOLOGY

Synonyms

- Skin tag, soft fibroma, fibrolipoma (with adipose tissue)

ETIOLOGY/PATHOGENESIS

May Be Associated With

- Obesity
- Diabetes
- Acromegaly
- Colonic polyps (controversial)

CLINICAL ISSUES

Epidemiology

- Incidence
  - Very common
- Age
  - Adults
    - > 50 years old
- Sex
  - Predilection for females
    - Obese patients

Site

- Neck, axilla, eyelid
- Inguinal and perianal lesions are frequent
- Lymphedematous fibroepithelial polyps of glans penis and prepuce have been described

Presentation

- Furrowed papules
  - 1-2 mm
  - Usually multiple
  - Especially on neck and axilla
- Filiform lesions
  - < 5 mm
  - Solitary or multiple
  - Variable location
- Pedunculated (bag-like) polyps
  - > 1 cm
  - Solitary
  - Lower trunk, buttocks
  - Some of these lesions represent fibrolipomas

Treatment

- Surgical approaches
  - Shave excision is curative

Prognosis

- Excellent

MACROSCOPIC

General Features

- Papular, filiform, or pedunculated

Size

- Ranges from few millimeters to few centimeters
  - Most measure < 1 cm

MICROSCOPIC

Histologic Features

- Squamous epithelium
  - Thin to acanthotic
  - Papillomatosis and horn pseudocysts may be present
    - Most such lesions likely represent seborrheic keratoses with polypoid/pedunculated features
- Connective tissue stalk
  - Loose to dense connective tissue with variable amount of blood vessels
  - Mature adipocytes may be present
    - Such lesions represent fibrolipomas (similar to nevus lipomatosus superficialis)
- In special locations (e.g., eyelids, axillae, and neck) different lesions (e.g., nevi, neurofibromas, and seborrheic keratoses) may be polypoid and clinically present as skin tags
- Many different benign and malignant tumors have been described arising in acrochordon
  - Basal cell carcinoma, melanoma, atypical lipomatous tumors, etc.

DIFFERENTIAL DIAGNOSIS

Seborrheic Keratosis

- May show polypoid appearance, especially in sites such as axilla and groin
- Usually show more epidermal acanthosis and pseudohorn cysts

Nevus Lipomatosus Superficialis

- Fibroadipose tissue present in superficial dermis but flatter lesion than fibrolipoma
- Usually present in hips &/or buttocks region

Pleomorphic Fibroma

- Acrochordon-like lesions containing atypical stromal cells
- May represent variant of fibroepithelial polyp with ancient changes

Polypoid Melanocytic Nevus

- Acrochordon-like growths containing nevus cells
- Usually intradermal nevi

DIAGNOSTIC CHECKLIST

Pathologic Interpretation Pearls

- Skin polyp with thin squamous epithelium and fibrovascular core without adnexal structures

SELECTED REFERENCES

1. Akpinar F et al: Association between acrochordons and the components of metabolic syndrome. Eur J Dermatol. 22(1):106-10, 2012
2. Kollitz KM et al: An acrochordon-like melanoma metastasis. Arch Dermatol. 148(1):136-7, 2012
3. McClain CM et al: Mycosis fungoides involving an acrochordon: a case report. J Cutan Pathol. 39(12):1131-4, 2012
4. Aksoy B et al: Basal cell carcinoma in a skin tag. Eur J Dermatol. 18(5):605-6, 2008
5. Fetsch JF et al: Lymphedematous fibroepithelial polyps of the glans penis and prepuce: a clinicopathologic study of 7 cases demonstrating a strong association with chronic condom catheter use. Hum Pathol. 35(2):190-5, 2004
6. Banik R et al: Skin tags: localization and frequencies according to sex and age. Dermatologica. 174(4):180-3, 1987

Keloid and Cellular Scar

KEY FACTS

TERMINOLOGY

- Scar with keloidal collagen
- Scar with prominent thickened and eosinophilic bundles of collagen

CLINICAL ISSUES

- Earlobe is most common site
- Scar that grows beyond original wound
- More common in patients of African lineage; least common in Caucasians
- Persistence and recurrence are common, but no risk of malignancy
- Treatment: Complete excision, accompanied by steroid injections or radiotherapy to decrease risk of recurrence

MICROSCOPIC

- Dense proliferation of thickened, hyalinized collagen bundles in dermis
- Decreased vessels compared to conventional and hypertrophic scars
  - Superficial telangiectatic vessels often present
  - May be associated with mild chronic inflammation
- Increased fibroblasts, lymphocytes, and mast cells usually present

TOP DIFFERENTIAL DIAGNOSES

- Hypertrophic scar
  - Lacks characteristic hyalinized collagen bundles of keloid
- Nodular fasciitis
  - May rarely show focal keloidal collagen but should have background of typical loose stroma
- Desmoplastic melanoma
  - Rarely may enter differential diagnosis if no history of trauma or previous biopsy/surgery
- Dermatofibroma
- Keloidal atypical fibroxanthoma

Clinical Photograph of Multiple Keloids

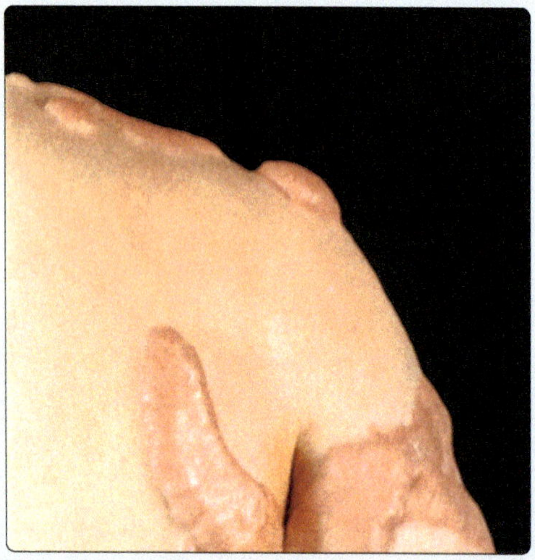

Scanning Magnification of Keloid

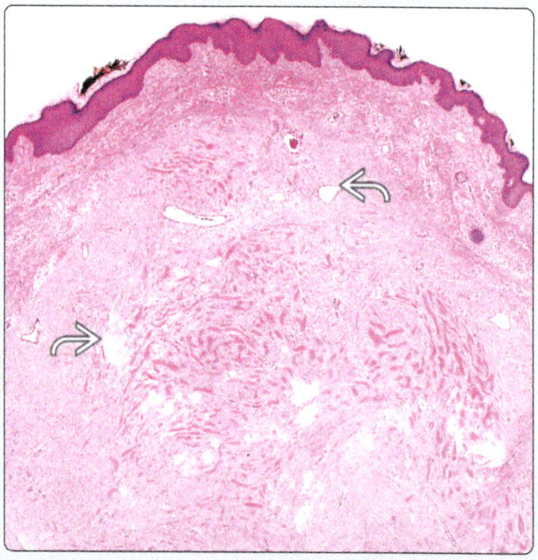

(Left) *Clinical photograph shows multiple keloids on the shoulder and upper arm of this patient.* **(Right)** *Scanning magnification of a keloid shows a polypoid skin lesion with dense dermal collagen. Note the mild epidermal hyperplasia and telangiectatic vessels ➦.*

High Magnification of Keloidal Collagen

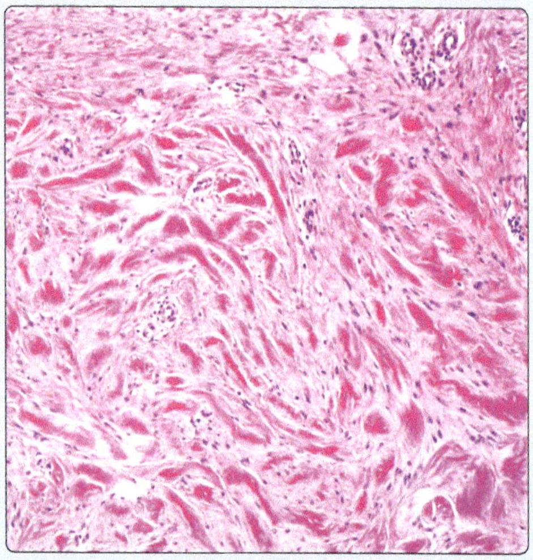

Keloid With Telangiectasia

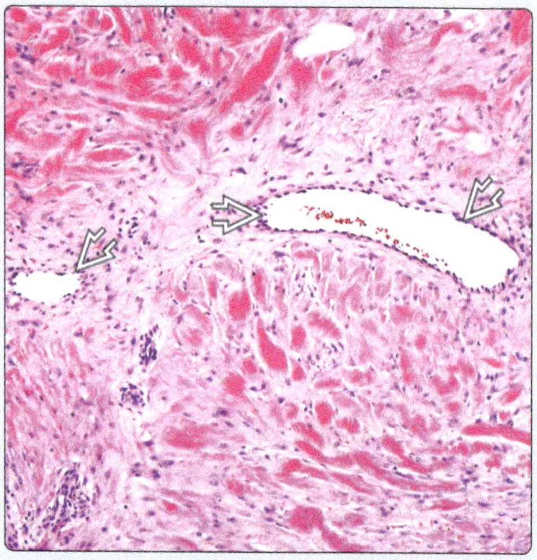

(Left) *High-power examination of a keloid shows a proliferation of thickened, hyalinized eosinophilic collagen bundles with increased numbers of stromal fibroblasts. Collagen bundles are randomly oriented and unevenly distributed.* **(Right)** *Superficial portion of keloid shows telangiectatic vessels ➡ surrounded by thickened collagen bundles.*

TERMINOLOGY

Synonyms

- Scar with keloidal collagen

Definitions

- Scar with prominent thickened and eosinophilic bundles of collagen extending beyond original wound

ETIOLOGY/PATHOGENESIS

Unknown, Possibly Genetic

- Fibroblasts from keloids show decreased apoptosis
- Many cytokines implicated in stimulating fibroblasts, including TGF-β, heat shock proteins, and IL-15

CLINICAL ISSUES

Epidemiology

- Age
  - Most common in patients < 30 yr
- Ethnicity
  - More common in patients of African lineage; least common in Caucasians

Site

- Earlobe is most common site
  - Typically follows ear piercing or other trauma

Presentation

- Nodule/mass lesion is most common
- Scar that grows beyond confines of original wound
- Often erythematous, pruritic lesions with predilection for earlobe

Treatment

- Options, risks, complications
  - Potentially disfiguring with high risk of recurrence
- Surgical approaches
  - Complete excision, accompanied by concurrent steroid injections or radiotherapy to decrease risk of recurrence
- Drugs
  - Direct injection of steroids is often first-line treatment

Prognosis

- Persistence and recurrence are common, but no risk of malignancy

MACROSCOPIC

General Features

- Large, nodular, dermal-based lesion with firm, white cut surface

MICROSCOPIC

Histologic Features

- Dense proliferation of thickened, hyalinized collagen bundles in dermis
- May be background of conventional or hypertrophic scar with smaller collagen bundles and perpendicular vessels
- Decreased vessels compared to conventional and hypertrophic scars
  - Superficial telangiectatic vessels often present
  - Associated with mild chronic inflammation
- Overlying epidermis shows atrophy in most cases, may show hyperplasia in some cases
- Increased fibroblasts, lymphocytes, and mast cells usually present

Predominant Pattern/Injury Type

- Fibrosis, thickened collagen bundles

Predominant Cell/Compartment Type

- Fibroblast

DIFFERENTIAL DIAGNOSIS

Hypertrophic Scar

- Lacks characteristic hyalinized collagen bundles of keloid
- Has more small, perpendicularly oriented vessels; lacks telangiectasia
- Overlapping cases may be seen and may be diagnosed as hypertrophic scar with focal keloidal collagen

Dermatofibroma

- Rare cases can show keloidal collagen
- Usually only focal finding in otherwise typical dermatofibroma

Nodular Fasciitis

- May rarely show focal keloidal collagen
- Background shows classic features of nodular fasciitis with loose, tissue culture appearance
- Zonation with cellular, myxoid, and more fibrous areas

Desmoplastic Melanoma

- Unlikely, but rarely may enter differential diagnosis if no history of trauma or previous biopsy/surgery
- Reexcision specimens of desmoplastic melanoma may show keloidal collagen
- S100 immunohistochemical stain should be positive

Keloidal Atypical Fibroxanthoma

- Rare cases of atypical fibroxanthoma may show keloidal collagen
- Pleomorphic cells trapped within hyalinized keloidal collagen bands

DIAGNOSTIC CHECKLIST

Pathologic Interpretation Pearls

- Nodular, elevated lesion compared to adjacent skin
- Thickened, hyalinized eosinophilic collagen bundles

SELECTED REFERENCES

1. Heurung A et al: Multiple pruritic and reticulated keloid-like plaques since childhood. Pediatr Dermatol. 32(4):549-50, 2015
2. Park TH et al: Do histopathologic parameters affect the rate of recurrence in auricular keloid patients? J Craniofac Surg. 26(7):e571-3, 2015
3. Kim J et al: Keloidal atypical fibroxanthoma: a case series. J Cutan Pathol. 36(5):535-9, 2009
4. Wolfram D et al: Hypertrophic scars and keloids--a review of their pathophysiology, risk factors, and therapeutic management. Dermatol Surg. 35(2):171-81, 2009
5. Köse O et al: Keloids and hypertrophic scars: are they two different sides of the same coin? Dermatol Surg. 34(3):336-46, 2008
6. Thompson LD et al: Nodular fasciitis of the external ear region: a clinicopathologic study of 50 cases. Ann Diagn Pathol. 5(4):191-8, 2001
7. Kuo TT et al: Keloidal dermatofibroma: report of 10 cases of a new variant. Am J Surg Pathol. 22(5):564-8, 1998

Desmoplastic Fibroblastoma

KEY FACTS

TERMINOLOGY

- Rare benign fibrous soft tissue neoplasm occurring mainly in men and consisting of paucicellular arrays of stellate and spindle-shaped fibroblasts
- Synonym: Collagenous fibroma

CLINICAL ISSUES

- Usually in older adults (5th to 6th decades) as slow-growing, painless mass
- Male preponderance
- Most occur in subcutaneous tissue, but up to 25% involve skeletal muscle
- Most common in proximal extremity

MICROSCOPIC

- Generally well circumscribed, although may infiltrate adjacent soft tissues
- Characteristically hypocellular
- Patternless distribution of bland spindled and stellate-shaped cells
- Hypovascular fibrous or fibromyxoid stroma
- Mitotic figures rare; no necrosis

ANCILLARY TESTS

- Variably SMA(+)
- Negative for CD34
- Cytogenetics: Reciprocal translocation t(2;11)(q31;q12) reported in a few cases

TOP DIFFERENTIAL DIAGNOSES

- Fibromatosis
- Neurofibroma
- Nodular fasciitis
- Elastofibroma
- Fibroma of tendon sheath
- Calcifying fibrous pseudotumor

Desmoplastic Fibroblastoma

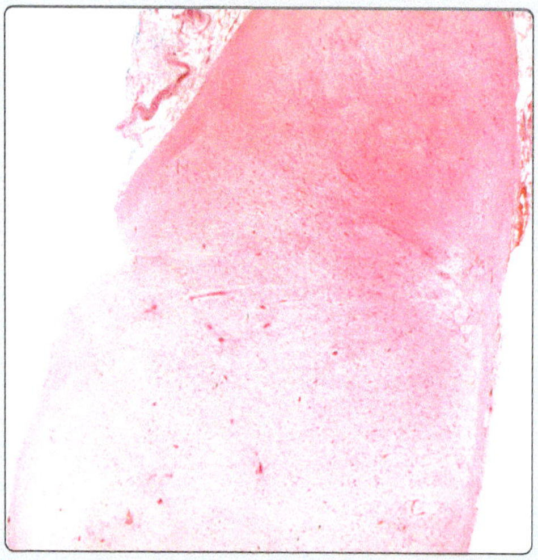

Desmoplastic Fibroblastoma With Deep Extension

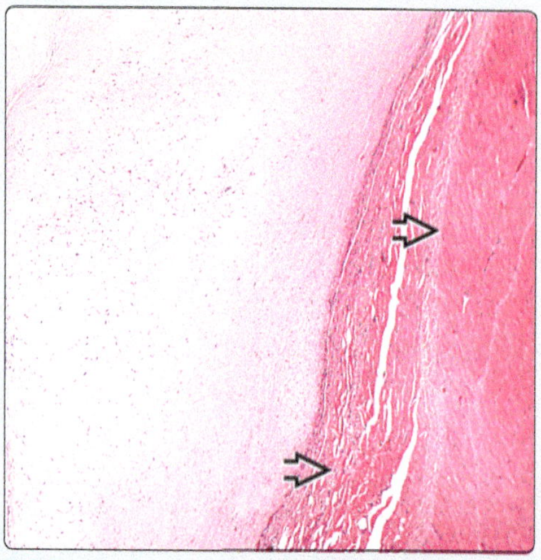

***(Left)** Low-magnification examination of a desmoplastic fibroblastoma is shown. The lesion is a well-circumscribed ovoid or fusiform mass. The characteristic hypocellularity is apparent at low power. **(Right)** Although most desmoplastic fibroblastomas are subcutaneous, some involve skeletal muscle ➾, to which this lesion closely abuts.*

Fibroblastoma With Spindled and Stellate Fibroblasts

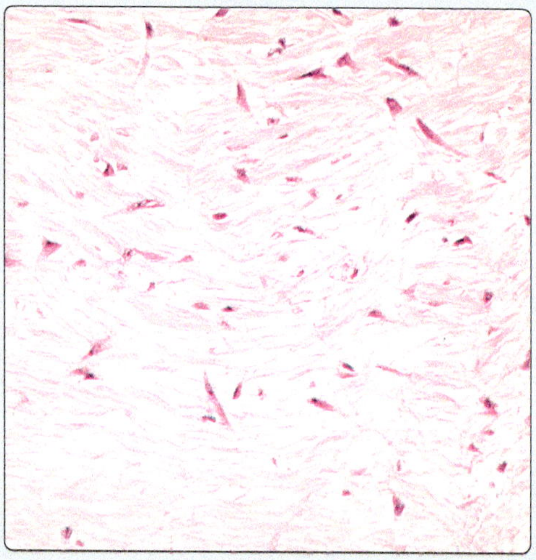

Fibroblastoma Myxoid Stroma

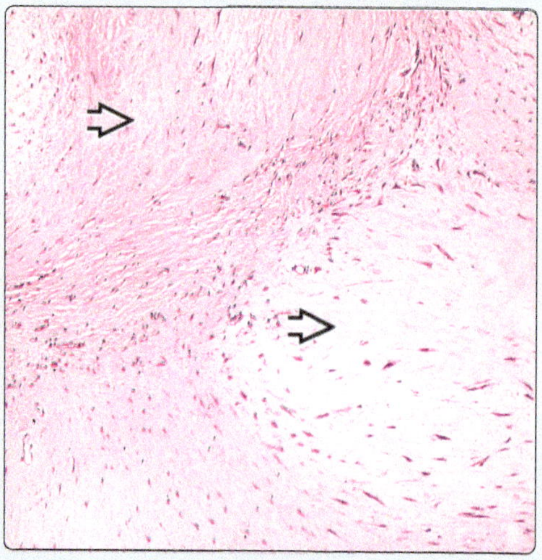

***(Left)** High magnification shows stroma that is densely collagenous and contains spindle and stellate fibroblasts in patternless distributions. The vessels are inconspicuous. **(Right)** This image of desmoplastic fibroblastoma shows the sparsely cellular nature of the lesion. The stroma can be myxoid ➾ in some cases. Although cells may be plump, no true atypia is seen, and mitotic figures are rare or absent.*

TERMINOLOGY

Synonyms

- Collagenous fibroma

Definitions

- Rare benign fibrous soft tissue neoplasm occurring mainly in men and consisting of paucicellular arrays of stellate and spindle fibroblasts

CLINICAL ISSUES

Epidemiology

- Age
  - All ages, but particularly older adults (5th-6th decades)
- Sex
  - M > F

Site

- Most occur in subcutaneous tissue
  - Up to 25% involve skeletal muscle
- Most common in upper extremity (shoulder, upper arm, forearm), followed by lower extremity
- Rare in head and neck

Presentation

- Slow growing
- Painless mass

Treatment

- Simple complete excision

Prognosis

- Benign
- Does not recur or metastasize

MACROSCOPIC

General Features

- Firm, well-circumscribed, lobulated mass
- White or gray cut surface
- No necrosis or hemorrhage

Size

- Often small (< 4 cm)
  - Range: 1.5-20.0 cm

MICROSCOPIC

Histologic Features

- Generally well circumscribed, although may focally infiltrate adjacent soft tissues
- Sparsely cellular
- Patternless proliferation of bland spindle or stellate cells
- Hypovascular fibrous or fibromyxoid stroma
- Mitotic figures very rare
- No necrosis

ANCILLARY TESTS

Immunohistochemistry

- Variable SMA(+)
- Negative for CD34, desmin, S100

Cytogenetics

- Reciprocal translocation t(2;11)(q31;q12) reported in 2 cases
  - Same translocation has also been reported in 1 case of fibroma of tendon sheath

DIFFERENTIAL DIAGNOSIS

Fibromatosis

- More infiltrative and cellular
- Cells in loose fascicles
- Prominent vascular pattern

Neurofibroma

- Cell nuclei are usually angulated or wavy-appearing
- Strongly S100(+)

Nodular Fasciitis (Late Stage)

- Foci of increased cellularity
- Chronic inflammation, extravasated red cells
- *USP6* rearrangements

Elastofibroma

- Typically located in subscapular region
- Fragmented elastic fibers

Fibroma of Tendon Sheath

- Peritendinous locations, particularly of hands

Calcifying Fibrous Pseudotumor

- Children and young adults
- Psammomatous calcifications
- Lymphoplasmacytic infiltrate

Low-Grade Fibromyxoid Sarcoma (Evans Tumor)

- More common in deep soft tissues
- Often larger and more cellular; may show hyalinizing rosette formation
- MUC4(+)
- Characteristic translocations t(7;16) and t(11;16)

SELECTED REFERENCES

1. Nagaraja V et al: Desmoplastic fibroblastoma presenting as a parotid tumour: a case report and review of the literature. Head Neck Pathol. 7(3):285-90, 2013
2. Macchia G et al: FOSL1 as a candidate target gene for 11q12 rearrangements in desmoplastic fibroblastoma. Lab Invest. 92(5):735-43, 2012
3. Nishio J et al: Translocation t(2;11) is characteristic of collagenous fibroma (desmoplastic fibroblastoma). Cancer Genet. 204(10):569-71, 2011
4. Watanabe H et al: Desmoplastic fibroblastoma (collagenous fibroma). J Dermatol. 35(2):93-7, 2008
5. Bernal K et al: Translocation (2;11)(q31;q12) is recurrent in collagenous fibroma (desmoplastic fibroblastoma). Cancer Genet Cytogenet. 149(2):161-3, 2004
6. Miettinen M et al: Collagenous fibroma (desmoplastic fibroblastoma): a clinicopathologic analysis of 63 cases of a distinctive soft tissue lesion with stellate-shaped fibroblasts. Hum Pathol. 29(7):676-82, 1998
7. Nielsen GP et al: Collagenous fibroma (desmoplastic fibroblastoma): a report of seven cases. Mod Pathol. 9(7):781-5, 1996
8. Evans HL: Desmoplastic fibroblastoma. A report of seven cases. Am J Surg Pathol. 19(9):1077-81, 1995

Pleomorphic Fibroma

KEY FACTS

TERMINOLOGY

- Pleomorphic fibroma
- Benign dermal-based neoplasm composed of pleomorphic-appearing myofibroblasts

ETIOLOGY/PATHOGENESIS

- May be related to ischemia, trauma, or degenerative changes

CLINICAL ISSUES

- Slow-growing skin nodule
- Typically occur on trunk, extremities, or head and neck region
- Usually dome-shaped or polypoid-appearing
- Benign, but may show local recurrence if incompletely excised

MICROSCOPIC

- Well-circumscribed, dome-shaped, or polypoid hypocellular proliferation of dermal spindle cells
- Cells are predominantly spindle-shaped, also with stellate and multinucleated cells
- Show enlarged, hyperchromatic-staining nuclei with small nucleoli, scant amounts of eosinophilic cytoplasm
- Mitotic figures rare or absent
- Stroma typically composed of hyalinized-appearing collagen fibers
- Myxoid areas may be present

ANCILLARY TESTS

- Typically positive for actin, CD34, and vimentin; variable positivity for FXIIIA reported

TOP DIFFERENTIAL DIAGNOSES

- Sclerotic fibroma
- Dermatofibroma
- Fibrous papule (angiofibroma)
- Atypical fibroxanthoma

Pleomorphic Fibroma at Scanning Magnification

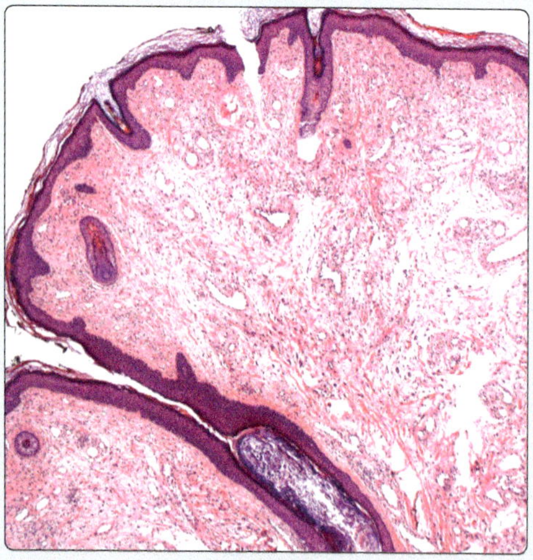

Pleomorphic Fibroma With Spindled and Multinucleated Cells

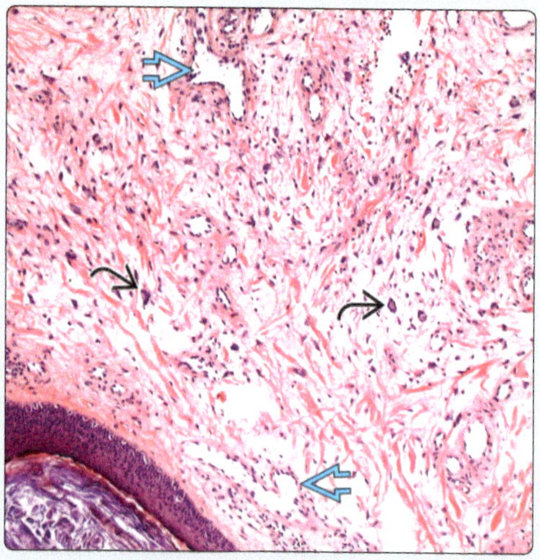

(Left) *Scanning magnification shows a polypoid (skin tag-like) lesion with a fibromyxoid and vascular stroma. Pleomorphic fibroma is usually solitary and occurs on the trunk, head and neck region, or extremities.* **(Right)** *Intermediate-power examination shows areas of collagenous and vascularized stroma containing the pleomorphic, hyperchromatic-staining spindled and multinucleated cells.*

Pleomorphic Fibroma Higher Magnification

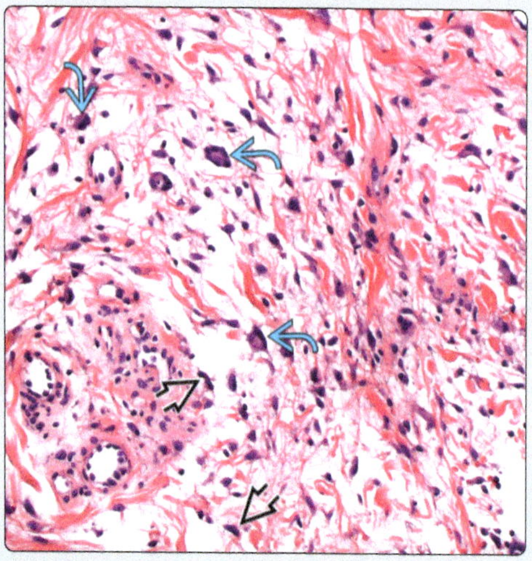

Pleomorphic Fibroma: CD34 Immunohistochemistry

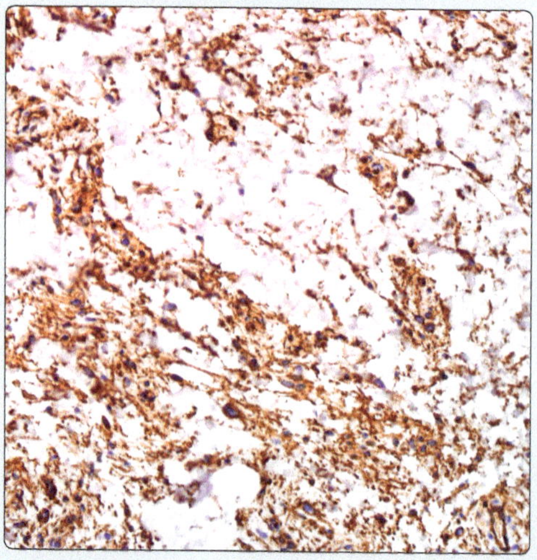

(Left) *High-power examination shows a population of enlarged, hyperchromatic-staining oval, spindled, stellate, and multinucleated cells set in a fibromyxoid stroma. No mitoses are seen.* **(Right)** *CD34 immunohistochemistry shows strong and diffuse staining of the spindled and multinucleated cells.*

TERMINOLOGY

Abbreviations

- Pleomorphic fibroma (PF)

Definitions

- Benign dermal-based neoplasm composed of pleomorphic-appearing myofibroblasts

ETIOLOGY/PATHOGENESIS

Unknown

- Some cases may be related to ischemia, trauma, or degenerative changes

CLINICAL ISSUES

Presentation

- Slow-growing skin nodule
  - Usually dome-shaped or polypoid-appearing
  - Flesh-colored and nonulcerated
- Typically occur on trunk, extremities, or head and neck region

Treatment

- Surgical approaches
  - Complete conservative excision curative

Prognosis

- Benign tumors with excellent prognosis
- May show local recurrence if incompletely excised

MACROSCOPIC

Size

- 0.4-1.6 cm

MICROSCOPIC

Histologic Features

- Well-circumscribed, dome-shaped, or polypoid hypocellular proliferation of dermal spindle cells
- Lesional cells are predominantly spindle-shaped, also with stellate and multinucleated cells
- Cells show enlarged, hyperchromatic-staining nuclei with small nucleoli, scant amounts of eosinophilic cytoplasm
- Mitotic figures rare or absent
  - No atypical mitoses should be seen
- Stroma typically composed of hyalinized-appearing collagen fibers
  - Some cases show overlapping features with sclerotic fibroma
    - These cases show storiforming of hyalinized collagen bundles with collagen clefts
- Myxoid areas may be present
  - Can be prominent/diffuse in some cases (myxoid pleomorphic fibroma)

Cytologic Features

- Enlarged spindled to stellate-shaped cells with irregular, hyperchromatic-staining nuclei

Predominant Cell/Compartment Type

- Fibroblast/myofibroblast

ANCILLARY TESTS

Immunohistochemistry

- Typically positive for actin-sm, CD34, and vimentin
- FXIIIA variably positive

DIFFERENTIAL DIAGNOSIS

Sclerotic Fibroma

- Shows characteristic storiform pattern of thickened, hyalinized-appearing collagen bundles with clefts between them
- Some cases show overlapping features with PF, with population of enlarged, pleomorphic-appearing spindled cells
  - Therefore, some believe that PF is variant of sclerotic fibroma, but this is not well accepted

Dermatofibroma

- Usually does not show degree of pleomorphism seen in PF, although rare cases may (atypical dermatofibroma/"dermatofibroma with monster cells")
- More typical dermatofibroma areas should be present at periphery of tumor
  - Collagen trapping, histiocytoid cells, and overlying epidermal hyperplasia usually present
- CD34 typically negative, unlike PF

Fibrous Papule (Angiofibroma)

- Small, dome-shaped papule that shows dermal fibrosis and blood vessels with telangiectasia
- Scattered, enlarged, mildly pleomorphic-appearing fibroblasts may be present
- CD34(-), FXIIIA usually positive

Atypical Fibroxanthoma

- Highly cellular and atypical-appearing dermal-based tumor associated with solar elastosis
- Mitotic figures easily found in most cases, including atypical forms
- CD34(-); nonspecific markers, including CD68, CD10, and CD99, are usually positive

DIAGNOSTIC CHECKLIST

Pathologic Interpretation Pearls

- Hypocellular dermal proliferation of spindled, stellate, and multinucleated cells
- Cells appear pleomorphic and hyperchromatic but lack mitotic activity

SELECTED REFERENCES

1. Nakamura Y et al: A case of pleomorphic fibroma of the skin presenting as intradermal nodule. Am J Dermatopathol. 37(2):175-6, 2015
2. Brenn T: Pleomorphic dermal neoplasms: a review. Adv Anat Pathol. 21(2):108-30, 2014
3. Al-Zaid T et al: Pleomorphic fibroma and dermal atypical lipomatous tumor: are they related? J Cutan Pathol. 40(4):379-84, 2013
4. Mahmood MN et al: Solitary sclerotic fibroma of skin: a possible link with pleomorphic fibroma with immunophenotypic expression for O13 (CD99) and CD34. J Cutan Pathol. 30(10):631-6, 2003
5. Pitt MA et al: Myxoid cutaneous pleomorphic fibroma. Histopathology. 25(3):300, 1994
6. Kamino H et al: Pleomorphic fibroma of the skin: a benign neoplasm with cytologic atypia. A clinicopathologic study of eight cases. Am J Surg Pathol. 13(2):107-13, 1989

Sclerotic Fibroma

KEY FACTS

TERMINOLOGY
- Storiform collagenoma
- Benign, dermal-based fibroblastic proliferation

ETIOLOGY/PATHOGENESIS
- May be related to trauma
- Some cases may represent regressed dermatofibromas
- Multiple lesions are associated with Cowden syndrome

CLINICAL ISSUES
- Excellent prognosis; may locally recur, but no metastatic potential

MICROSCOPIC
- Circumscribed, unencapsulated dermal nodule
- Composed of thickened, hyalinized-appearing collagen bundles in storiform/whorled pattern
- Prominent clefts often seen between collagen bundles
- Occasional cases may show large, bizarre-appearing cells (pleomorphic sclerotic fibroma)
- Pacinian collagenoma is rare variant with onion skinning

ANCILLARY TESTS
- IHC generally not necessary, but cells should stain for FXIIIA, CD34 (focally), and vimentin

TOP DIFFERENTIAL DIAGNOSES
- Dermatofibroma
  - Typically does not show prominent storiforming of collagen, although it may be focally present in rare cases
- Pleomorphic fibroma
  - Pleomorphic cells are more prominent, and storiforming pattern of collagen should be absent
- Collagenous fibroma
  - Densely collagenous or fibromyxoid stroma; lacks prominent storiforming of collagen
- Acral fibrokeratoma (subungual and periungual fibroma)

Sclerotic Fibroma at Scanning Magnification

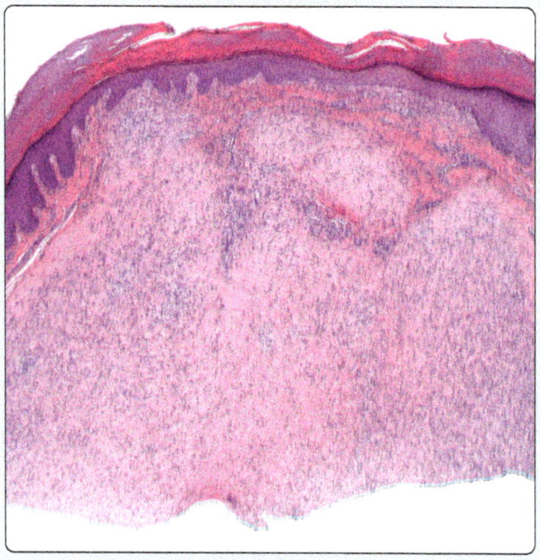

Sclerotic Fibroma With Storiforming Collagen

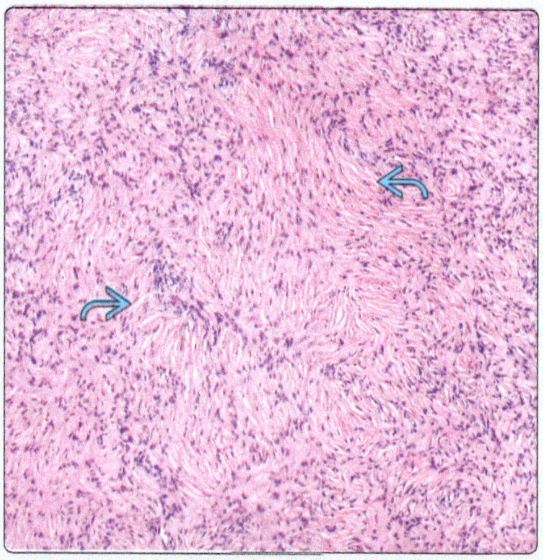

(Left) *Scanning magnification view shows a dermal-based nodular fibroblastic proliferation with storiforming of collagen.* **(Right)** *Higher magnification of the lesion shows prominent areas of storiforming collagen bundles separated by small clefts ➚, imparting a typical plywood-like pattern.*

Inflamed and Traumatized Sclerotic Fibroma

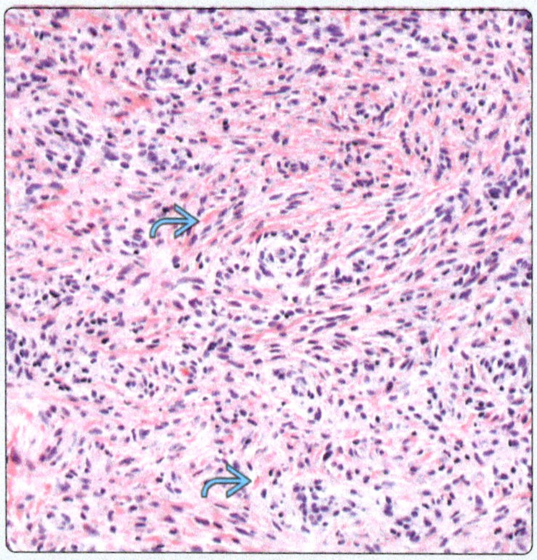

FXIIIA Immunohistochemistry in Sclerotic Fibroma

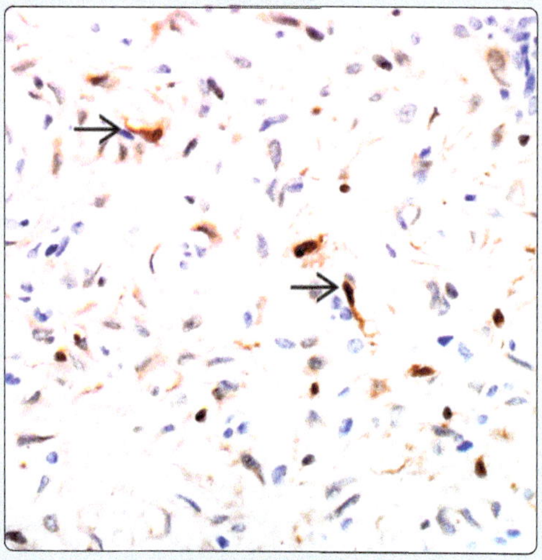

(Left) *This lesion showed overlying evidence of trauma and mixed, predominantly lymphocytic inflammation in the dermis. However, there are sclerotic collagen bundles ➚ with clefts and a vaguely storiforming appearance.* **(Right)** *FXIIIA immunohistochemistry shows staining of scattered spindle cells ➙.*

TERMINOLOGY

Synonyms

- Storiform collagenoma
- Pleomorphic sclerotic fibroma

Definitions

- Benign, dermal-based fibroblastic proliferation with storiforming bundles of collagen

ETIOLOGY/PATHOGENESIS

Unknown

- May be related to trauma
- Some cases may represent regressed dermatofibromas

Genetic Syndrome

- Multiple lesions are associated with Cowden syndrome, consistent with genetic influence

CLINICAL ISSUES

Epidemiology

- Age
  - May occur at any age, including in infants and elderly
- Sex
  - Roughly equal incidence in male and female patients

Site

- Presents most commonly on face, extremities, and trunk

Presentation

- Slow-growing, flesh-colored papule or nodule

Treatment

- Surgical approaches
  - Complete conservative excision is curative

Prognosis

- Excellent; may locally recur, but no metastatic potential

MACROSCOPIC

General Features

- Dermal nodule with firm, yellow-tan surface

Size

- Typically 0.5-3.0 cm

MICROSCOPIC

Histologic Features

- Circumscribed, unencapsulated dermal nodule
- Composed of thickened, hyalinized-appearing collagen bundles in storiform/whorled pattern
  - Prominent clefts often seen between collagen bundles
- Cells are typically small, bland, spindled to stellate-shaped fibroblasts
- Occasional cases may show large, bizarre-appearing cells (pleomorphic sclerotic fibroma or giant cell collagenoma), similar to pleomorphic fibroma
  - These cells do not show infiltrative features or increased mitotic activity
- Pacinian collagenoma is rare variant with onion skinning, mimicking pacinian corpuscle

Predominant Cell/Compartment Type

- Fibroblast

ANCILLARY TESTS

Immunohistochemistry

- Generally not necessary, but cells will typically stain for FXIIIA, CD34 (focally), and vimentin
- Ki-67 staining may highlight a few scattered nuclei, but overall staining is low

DIFFERENTIAL DIAGNOSIS

Dermatofibroma

- Typically does not show prominent storiforming of collagen, although it may be focally present in rare cases
- Areas of conventional dermatofibroma with collagen trapping and histiocytic cells should be present
  - Some cases may show overlapping features, leading some investigators to believe that sclerotic fibromas are involuting dermatofibromas

Pleomorphic Fibroma

- Clinically resembles skin tag
- Pleomorphic cells are more prominent, and storiforming pattern of collagen should be absent

Collagenous Fibroma

- Usually subcutaneous tumor with only rare dermal involvement
- Densely collagenous or fibromyxoid stroma; lacks prominent storiforming of collagen

Acral Fibrokeratoma (Subungual and Periungual Fibroma)

- Usually shows overlying hyperkeratosis and acanthosis
- Proliferation of thick collagen bundles, often vertically oriented

DIAGNOSTIC CHECKLIST

Pathologic Interpretation Pearls

- Dermal nodule of thickened, hyalinized-appearing collagen bundles in storiform/whorled pattern

SELECTED REFERENCES

1. Stocchero GF: Storiform collagenoma: case report. Einstein (Sao Paulo). 13(1):103-5, 2015
2. Pernet C et al: Solitary sclerotic fibroma of the skin: a possible clue for Cowden syndrome. Eur J Dermatol. 22(2):278-9, 2012
3. Nakashima K et al: Solitary sclerotic fibroma of the skin: morphological characterization of the 'plywood-like pattern'. J Cutan Pathol. 35 Suppl 1:74-9, 2008
4. González-Vela MC et al: Sclerotic fibroma-like dermatofibroma: an uncommon distinctive variant of dermatofibroma. Histol Histopathol. 20(3):801-6, 2005
5. Chen TM et al: Pleomorphic sclerotic fibroma: a case report and literature review. Am J Dermatopathol. 24(1):54-8, 2002
6. Hanft VN et al: Expression of CD34 in sclerotic ("plywood") fibromas. Am J Dermatopathol. 22(1):17-21, 2000
7. Martín-López R et al: Pleomorphic sclerotic fibroma. Dermatology. 198(1):69-72, 1999
8. Requena L et al: Multiple sclerotic fibromas of the skin. A cutaneous marker of Cowden's disease. J Cutan Pathol. 19(4):346-51, 1992
9. Rapini RP et al: Sclerotic fibromas of the skin. J Am Acad Dermatol. 20(2 Pt 1):266-71, 1989

Fibromatosis

KEY FACTS

TERMINOLOGY

- Deep fibromatosis: Desmoid tumor
- Palmar fibromatosis (Dupuytren contracture), plantar fibromatosis (Ledderhose disease), penile fibromatosis (Peyronie disease)
- Myofibroblastic proliferations with infiltrative growth pattern that show local recurrences but not metastasis

CLINICAL ISSUES

- Palmar fibromatosis
- Deep fibromatosis
- Recurrences common for both superficial and deep fibromatoses, but deaths only from deep fibromatoses
- Increased incidence in familial adenomatous polyposis

MICROSCOPIC

- Sweeping fascicles of myofibroblasts
- Smooth nuclear membranes and small nucleoli in most cells
- Occasional cells with stellate cytoplasmic contours
- Small but conspicuous vessels
- Gaping, thin-walled vessels with perivascular sclerosis often feature of mesenteric fibromatosis

ANCILLARY TESTS

- β-catenin (+) (nuclear), especially in deep lesions, SMA(+); desmin (-), keratins (-), CD117(+/-)

TOP DIFFERENTIAL DIAGNOSES

- Scar
- Tenosynovial giant cell tumor (giant cell tumor of tendon sheath, pigmented villonodular tenosynovitis)
- Leiomyoma and leiomyosarcoma
- Clear cell sarcoma
- Epithelioid sarcoma
- Low-grade fibromyxoid sarcoma

Fibromatosis, Clinical Image

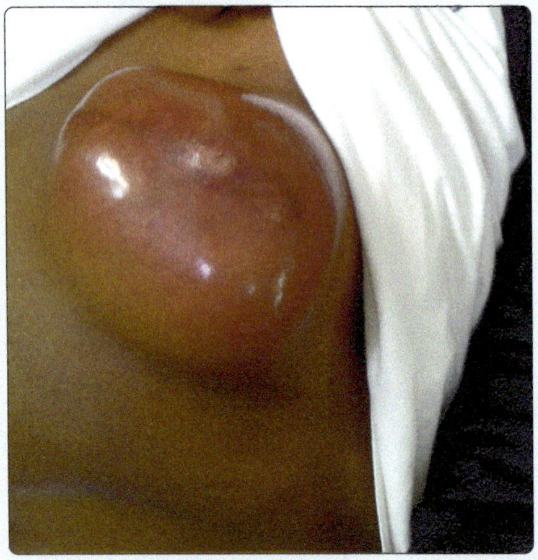

Fibromatosis, Low Magnification

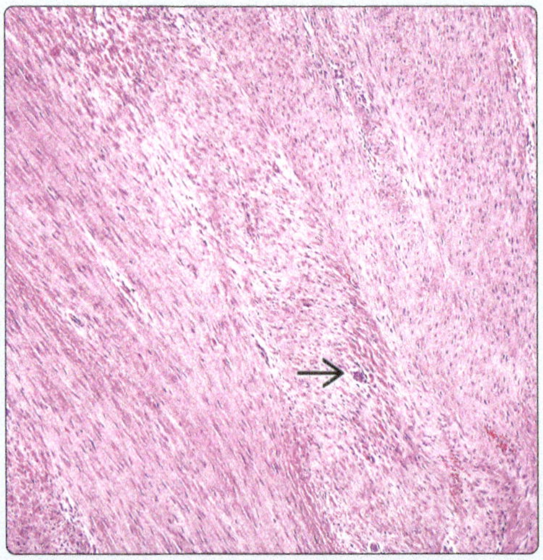

(Left) *This fibromatosis is unusually superficial and arose in the chest wall of a young adult. These tumors are typically deep (deep fascia or within muscle).* **(Right)** *This image of a deep-type fibromatosis shows sweeping fascicles of spindle cells separated by regularly spaced collagen. Even at this magnification, small vessels are readily apparent* ⇨.

Fibromatosis, Gross Specimen

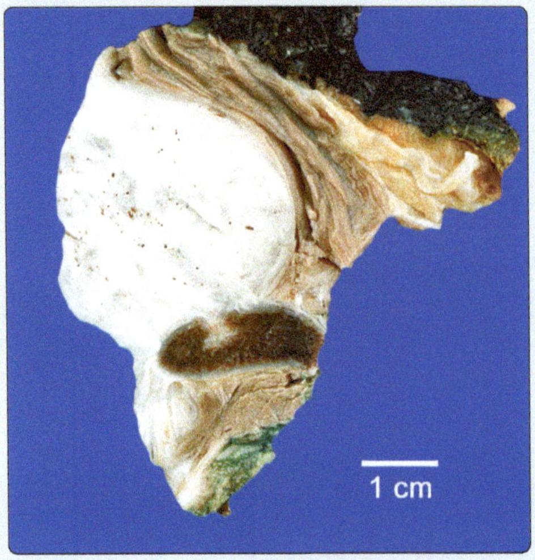

Fibromatosis, Neck

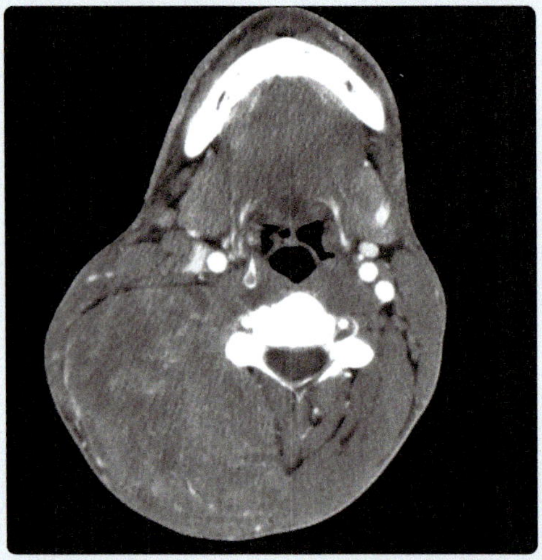

(Left) *This gross photograph shows a large, deep fibromatosis of the shoulder that has eroded into the scapula. Superficial portions of such lesions can be encountered on skin biopsies.* **(Right)** *This radiologic image shows a large fibromatosis of the head and neck in an elderly alcoholic man. Although more arise in the shoulder girdles (or in the abdominal wall in young women), the head and neck is a common location for fibromatoses.*

TERMINOLOGY

Synonyms

- Deep fibromatosis: Aggressive fibromatosis, desmoid tumor
- Superficial fibromatoses: Palmar fibromatosis (Dupuytren contracture, Dupuytren disease), plantar fibromatosis (Ledderhose disease), penile fibromatosis (Peyronie disease), knuckle pads

Definitions

- **Palmar fibromatosis**: Nodular myofibroblastic proliferation of volar surface of hand that is prone to local persistence but does not metastasize
- **Plantar fibromatosis**: Nodular myofibroblastic proliferation of plantar surface of foot that is prone to local persistence but does not metastasize
- **Peyronie disease**: Penile fibrous lesion causing various deformities; initially pain with erection, erectile dysfunction
- **Knuckle pads**: Well-circumscribed thickening of skin over metacarpophalangeal and, more commonly, proximal interphalangeal joints
- **Deep fibromatosis**: Myofibroblastic proliferation of deep soft tissues with infiltrative growth pattern; prone to local recurrences but does not metastasize

CLINICAL ISSUES

Epidemiology

- Incidence
  - Palmar fibromatosis
    - 4-6% of Caucasian adults > 50 years of age; reports of up to 75% of Celtic male patients
    - Uncommon in nonwhites; marked male predominance
  - Plantar fibromatosis
    - 1-2 per 100,000 persons per year (Northern Europe)
    - Most patients 30-50 years of age; slight male predominance
  - Penile fibromatosis
    - ~ 3.5% of white men > 50 years of age
  - Deep fibromatosis
    - 2.40-4.43 new cases per 100,000 persons per year (Scandinavian data)
  - Knuckle pads (rare)

Presentation

- Superficial fibromatoses present as nodular lesions on palms, soles, knuckles, or penis
  - Variable tenderness
- Deep fibromatoses present as firm large masses, typically with intramuscular component
  - Relationship to age and gender
    - In children and older adults, no gender predominance: Lesions of shoulders, chest wall, back, thigh, head, and neck
    - In women in childbearing years: Abdominal wall
      - May also arise in shoulder girdles, chest wall, back, thigh, head, and neck
  - Usually clinically concerning for sarcomas based on large size, deep location
- Familial adenomatous polyposis-associated lesions
  - Risk of fibromatoses is 2.56/1,000 person/year; comparative risk is 852x that of general population
  - Patients have numerous colon adenomas and must undergo colectomy to forestall development of colorectal carcinoma
- Occasionally associated with scar ("cicatricial fibromatosis")

Treatment

- Superficial fibromatoses treated by excision
- Nonsurgical treatments for penile lesions: Verapamil, colchicine, Potaba, L-carnitine, and liposomal superoxide dismutase
- Deep fibromatoses treated by wide excision; for unresectable lesions, radiation, chemotherapy, hormone therapy
  - Clear surgical margins are key to successful outcome
  - Multiple recurrences are common
  - Usually they are diagnosed on needle biopsy to plan treatment and exclude sarcomas preoperatively

Prognosis

- Recurrences common for both superficial and deep fibromatoses
- Occasional deaths from deep fibromatoses

MICROSCOPIC

Histologic Features

- Sweeping fascicles of myofibroblasts with nuclei regularly spaced
  - Smooth nuclear membranes
  - Delicate nucleoli in most cells
  - Cells with stellate cytoplasm in keeping with myofibroblastic differentiation (as opposed to bipolar cytoplasm such as in smooth muscle tumors)
- Uniformly distributed collagen, some cases with keloid-like collagen
  - Some cases have myxoid zones but retain uniform distribution of nuclei
  - Lack of uniform distribution of nuclei raises possibility of low-grade fibromyxoid sarcoma
- Prominent vascular pattern
  - Small but conspicuous vessels
  - Smooth muscle in vessel walls if more eosinophilic than cytoplasm of lesional cells
- Minimal background inflammation
  - Occasional lymphoid cells
- Scattered giant cells (especially plantar fibromatoses)
  - When deep fibromatoses infiltrate skeletal muscle, damaged skeletal myocytes appear similar to giant cells

ANCILLARY TESTS

Immunohistochemistry

- β-catenin (+) (nuclear, especially in deep lesions), SMA(+), desmin (-), keratins (-) (usually), CD117(+/-) (pitfall in mesenteric lesions)
  - Occasional keratin and calretinin expression can be diagnostic pitfall
- Many lesions express hormone receptors (estrogen or progesterone receptor)

Genetic Testing

- Deep fibromatoses may harbor *APC* or *CTNNB1* (gene that encodes for β-catenin) mutations
    - In general, *APC* mutations are detected in familial lesions and *CTNNB1* mutations in sporadic lesions

DIFFERENTIAL DIAGNOSIS

Scar

- Disorganized myofibroblastic proliferation without nodular configuration; β-catenin negative

Tenosynovial Giant Cell Tumor (Giant Cell Tumor of Tendon Sheath, Pigmented Villonodular Tenosynovitis)

- Usually involves fingers and toes of middle-aged women (localized type)
- Rounded cells, giant cells, foamy macrophages, hemosiderin, CD68(+), clusterin (+)
- Diffuse type (pigmented villonodular tenosynovitis) classically affects knee area synovium of young women
    - Locally aggressive, rare malignant transformation or malignant-type behavior
- Benign behavior

Leiomyoma and Leiomyosarcoma

- Perpendicularly oriented fascicles of spindle cells with brightly eosinophilic cytoplasm, blunt-ended nuclei, paranuclear vacuoles, none to few mitoses (leiomyoma), bland cytologic features (leiomyoma) or scattered mitoses (leiomyosarcoma), and atypical nuclei (leiomyosarcoma)
- Actin, desmin, calponin, H-caldesmon (+); S100, CD34, β-catenin (-)
- Outcome for leiomyosarcomas depends on size, depth, grade

Clear Cell Sarcoma

- Most involve hands and feet of young adults
- Packeted arrangement of spindle cells, scattered giant cells
    - S100, HMB-45, Melan-A (+); *EWSR1-ATF1* gene fusion
- Nuclei are uniform (generally case for sarcomas associated with characteristic translocations and gene fusions)
    - Large nucleoli are characteristic
    - Pale/clear to eosinophilic-staining cytoplasm
- Some cases have melanin
- Giant cells can be pitfall (can be mistaken for tenosynovial giant cell tumor)
- Behave as high-grade sarcomas
- Should not be regarded as "melanoma of soft parts" since these behave as per sarcomas rather than as per melanomas

Epithelioid Sarcoma

- Most involve distal upper extremity
- Epithelioid cells arranged around necrotic zones, reminiscent of granulomatous inflammation
    - Cytokeratins, EMA, CD34 (+); loss of nuclear INI1
- Low-grade behavior in most cases: Recurrences common
    - With better awareness in pathology community, prognosis is better than in past
    - Exception: Proximal type is high grade
        - Tend to arise in trunk and limb girdles
        - Highly cellular and aggressive neoplasms

Low-Grade Fibromyxoid Sarcoma

- Deep lesions without gender predilection
- Disorganized and swirled arrangement of fibroblastic cells with hyperchromatic nuclei, variable myxoid background, cellularity similar to that of fibromatosis
- Express MUC4 on immunolabeling, but S100, desmin, CD34, β-catenin (-); occasionally actin, claudin-1, epithelial membrane antigen (+); pitfall with perineurioma, *FUS-CREB3L2* fusion
- Good outcome overall with early recognition and treatment
- Sclerosing epithelioid fibrosarcoma can be regarded as high-grade counterpart and behaves aggressively

SELECTED REFERENCES

1. Arbajian E et al: Recurrent EWSR1-CREB3L1 gene fusions in sclerosing epithelioid fibrosarcoma. Am J Surg Pathol. 38(6):801-8, 2014
2. Cates JM et al: Surgical resection margins in desmoid-type fibromatosis: a critical reassessment. Am J Surg Pathol. 38(12):1707-14, 2014
3. Fisher C et al: Aggressive fibromatosis. Pathology. 46(2):135-40, 2014
4. Colombo C et al: CTNNB1 45F mutation is a molecular prognosticator of increased postoperative primary desmoid tumor recurrence: an independent, multicenter validation study. Cancer. 119(20):3696-702, 2013
5. Barak S et al: Immunoreactivity for calretinin and keratins in desmoid fibromatosis and other myofibroblastic tumors: a diagnostic pitfall. Am J Surg Pathol. 36(9):1404-9, 2012
6. Guzzetta AA et al: Epithelioid sarcoma: one institution's experience with a rare sarcoma. J Surg Res. 177(1):116-22, 2012
7. Doyle LA et al: MUC4 is a highly sensitive and specific marker for low-grade fibromyxoid sarcoma. Am J Surg Pathol. 35(5):733-41, 2011
8. Bhattacharya B et al: Nuclear beta-catenin expression distinguishes deep fibromatosis from other benign and malignant fibroblastic and myofibroblastic lesions. Am J Surg Pathol. 29(5):653-9, 2005
9. Evans HL: Multinucleated giant cells in plantar fibromatosis. Am J Surg Pathol. 26(2):244-8, 2002
10. Montgomery E et al: Superficial fibromatoses are genetically distinct from deep fibromatoses. Mod Pathol. 14(7):695-701, 2001
11. Reitamo JJ et al: The desmoid tumor. I. Incidence, sex-, age- and anatomical distribution in the Finnish population. Am J Clin Pathol. 77(6):665-73, 1982

Familial Adenomatous Polyposis, Colectomy Specimen

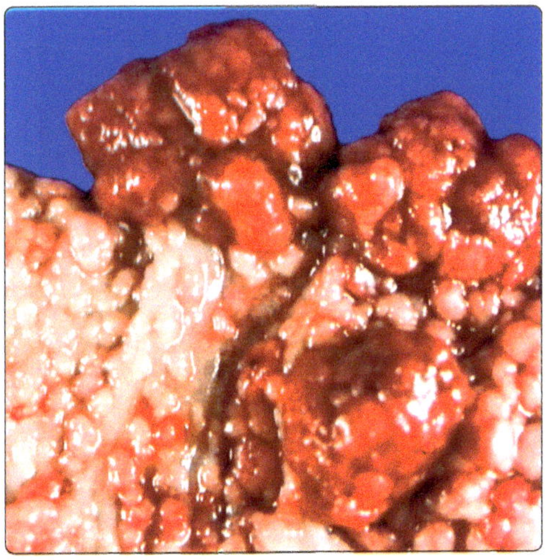

Palmar Fibromatosis (Dupuytren Contracture)

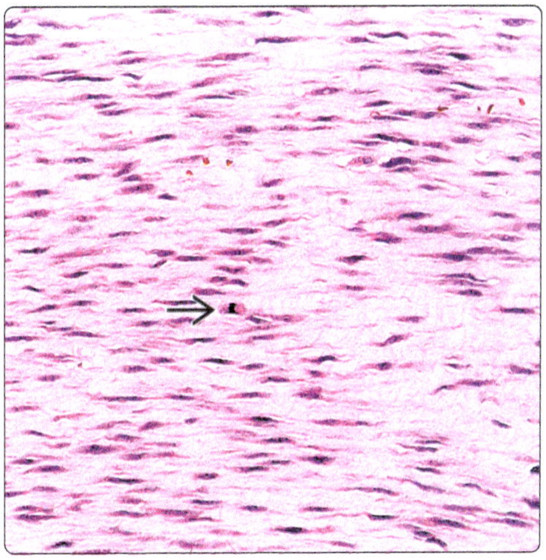

(Left) *Gross photograph shows a colectomy sample from a patient with familial adenomatous polyposis (FAP). FAP patients often have fibromatoses (mesenteric) in addition to their colon polyps.* **(Right)** *High magnification shows a mitosis in palmar fibromatosis ⮕. Mitotic activity can be encountered in both palmar and plantar fibromatoses and should not lead to concern for malignancy.*

Plantar Fibromatosis

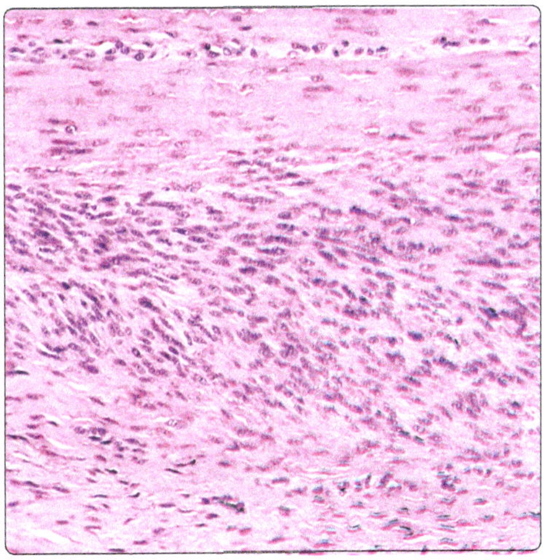

Plantar Fibromatosis, Giant Cell

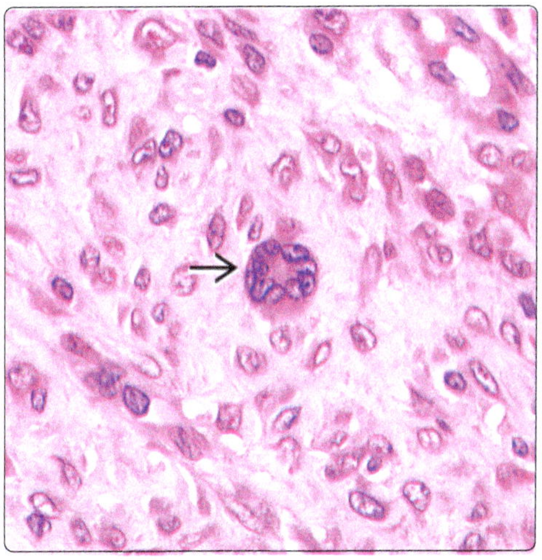

(Left) *Plantar fibromatosis, such as this, can be fairly large and have pockets of enhanced cellularity, leading to misidentification as a sarcoma. Superficial fibromatoses can show β-catenin immunolabeling but lack β-catenin and APC gene mutations.* **(Right)** *High magnification shows a giant cell in plantar fibromatosis ⮕. Such cells can also occur in palmar lesions and can cause confusion with a tenosynovial giant cell tumor and clear cell sarcoma.*

Peyronie Disease

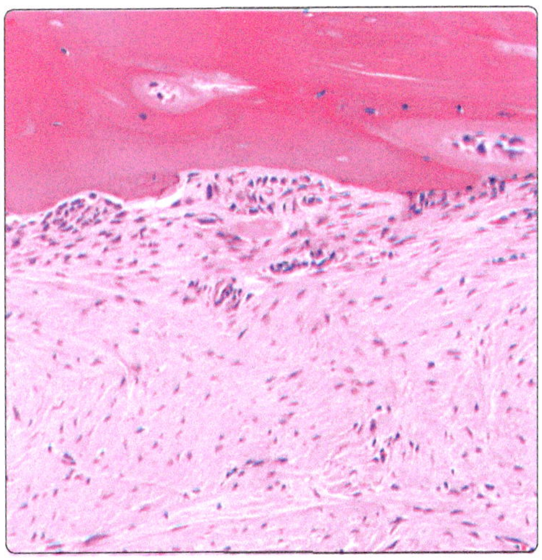

Deep Fibromatosis With Small Vessel

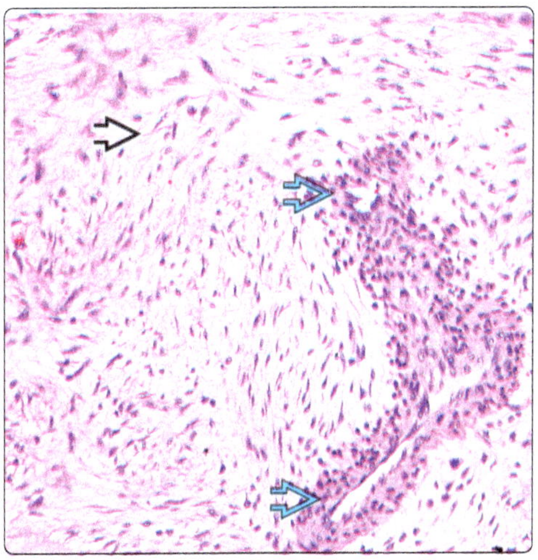

(Left) *This is an example of Peyronie disease (penile fibromatosis) that has ossified. Peyronie disease consists of a fibrous proliferation of the tunica albuginea, resulting in a palpable scar and penile curvature, hinging, narrowing, shortening, and painful erections.* **(Right)** *This image shows a deep fibromatosis with a small vessel. The vascular smooth muscle ⮕ appears more eosinophilic than the myofibroblastic lesional cells, some of which have stellate cytoplasmic contours ⮕.*

(Left) *High magnification of a deep fibromatosis demonstrates cells that contain nuclei with single delicate nucleoli ⇒ and bipolar or stellate cytoplasm. Collagen is evenly distributed in most examples but is occasionally keloid-like.* **(Right)** *β-catenin shows nuclear staining in a fibromatosis, a reflection of either APC or CTNNB1 mutations in most fibromatoses.*

Fibromatosis, High Magnification

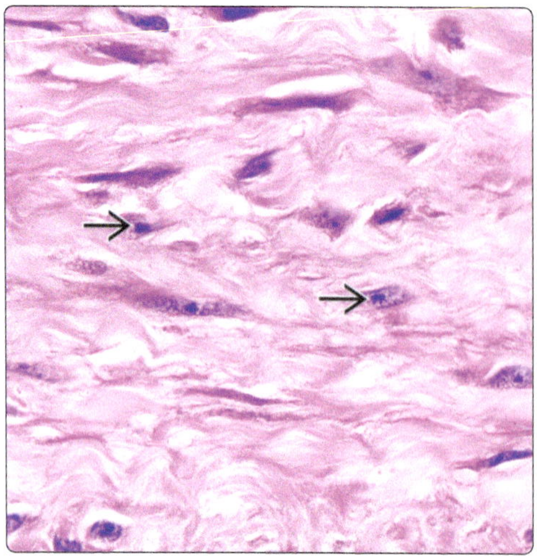

Fibromatosis, β-catenin Immunolabeling

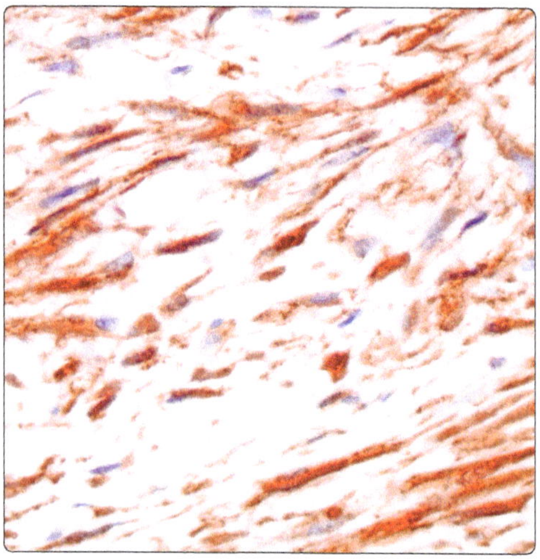

(Left) *CD117 shows strong labeling in a deep fibromatosis. This particular example displays more prominent staining than most fibromatoses, and this finding can result in misdiagnosis as a (metastatic) gastrointestinal stromal tumor. Fibromatoses lack KIT mutations and have minimal response to imatinib.* **(Right)** *This example of a low-grade fibromatosis appears gelatinous, although some tumors of this type appear more sclerotic.*

Fibromatosis, CD117 Expression

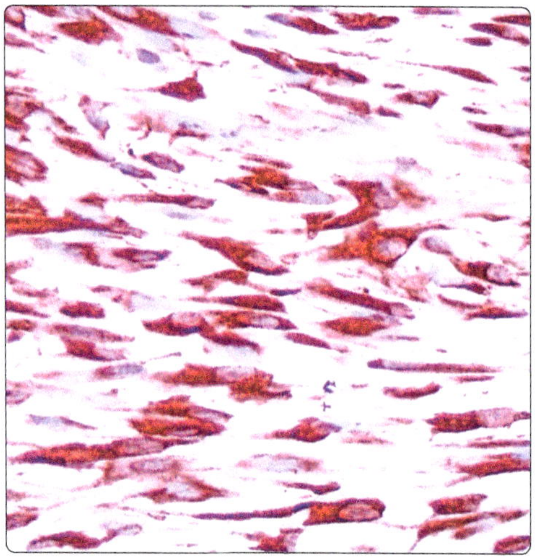

Differential Diagnosis: Low-Grade Fibromyxoid Sarcoma, Gross Image

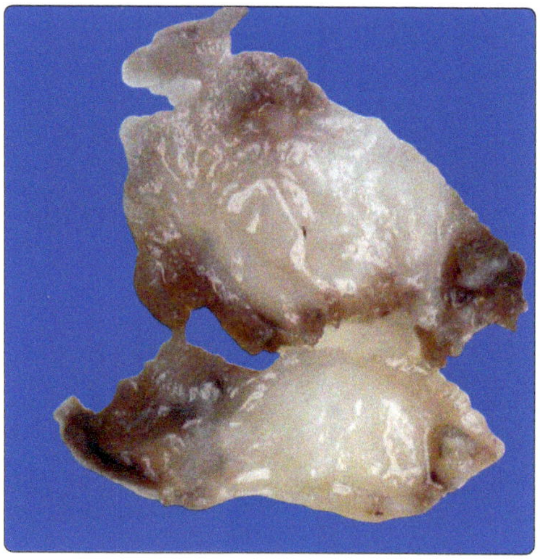

(Left) *Although low-grade fibromyxoid sarcoma can appear similar to a fibromatosis at low magnification, it differs by featuring a less uniformly fascicular low-power appearance. Note the myxoid zones ⇨.* **(Right)** *On high magnification, low-grade fibromyxoid sarcoma consists of cells that are far more hyperchromatic than those of a fibromatosis. These lesions lack nuclear β-catenin and have a characteristic translocation, t(7;16) (q32-34;p11), with a FUS/CREB3L2 fusion gene.*

Differential Diagnosis: Low-Grade Fibromyxoid Sarcoma

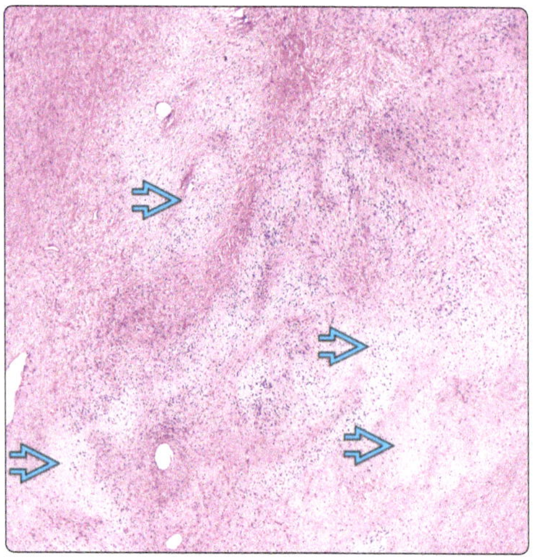

Low-Grade Fibromyxoid Sarcoma

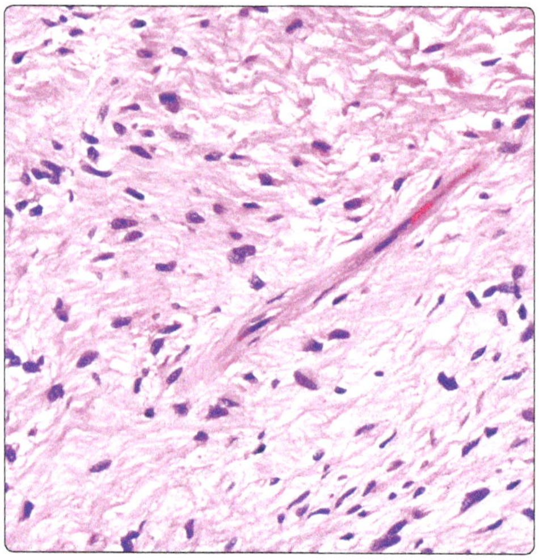

Low-Grade Fibromyxoid Sarcoma, Needle Biopsy

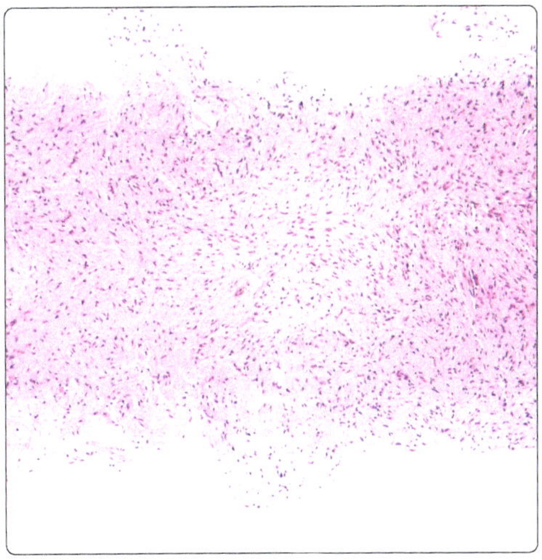

Low-Grade Fibromyxoid Sarcoma

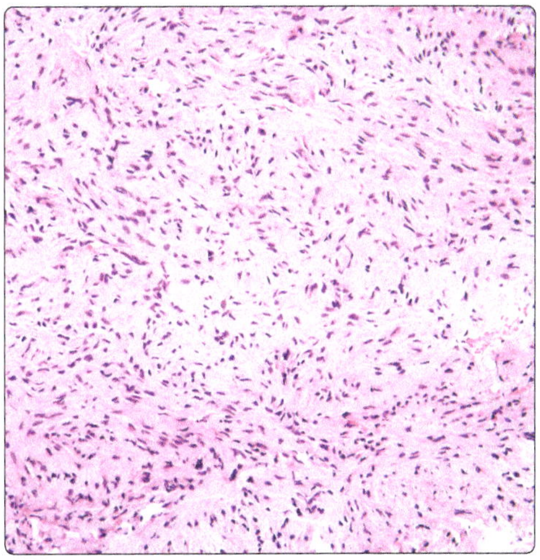

(Left) *This lesion has uniform cellularity, akin to a fibromatosis, but has a whorled appearance at low magnification, rather than the sweeping fascicles typical of fibromatosis.* **(Right)** *The nuclei in this low-grade fibromyxoid sarcoma are small but feature hyperchromatic nuclei, in contrast to the pale nuclei that characterize fibromatosis.*

Low-Grade Fibromyxoid Sarcoma, MUC4 Stain

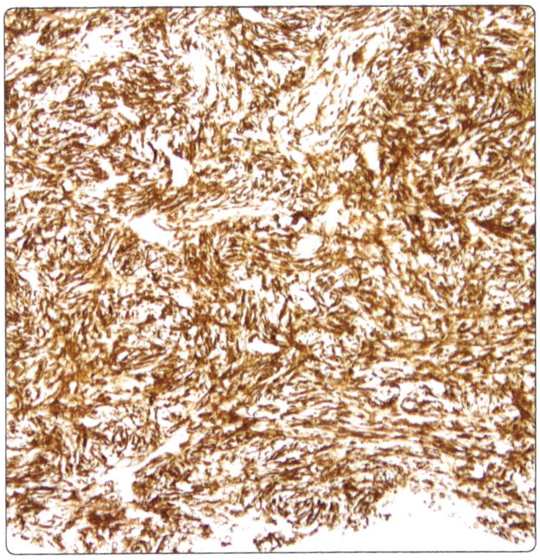

Differential Diagnosis: Leiomyosarcoma

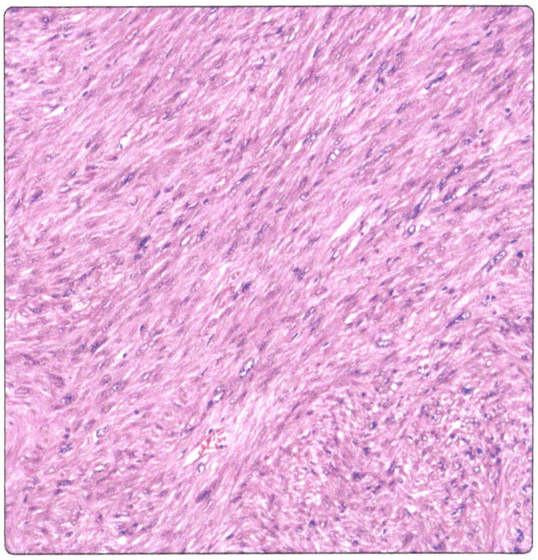

(Left) *MUC4 immunolabeling can be very useful in confirming the impression of low-grade fibromyxoid sarcoma. There is strong cytoplasmic labeling.* **(Right)** *This image shows a spindle cell tumor, consistent with leiomyosarcoma. The lesional nuclei are larger and more hyperchromatic than those of fibromatoses, and the cytoplasm is strikingly eosinophilic.*

Leiomyosarcoma

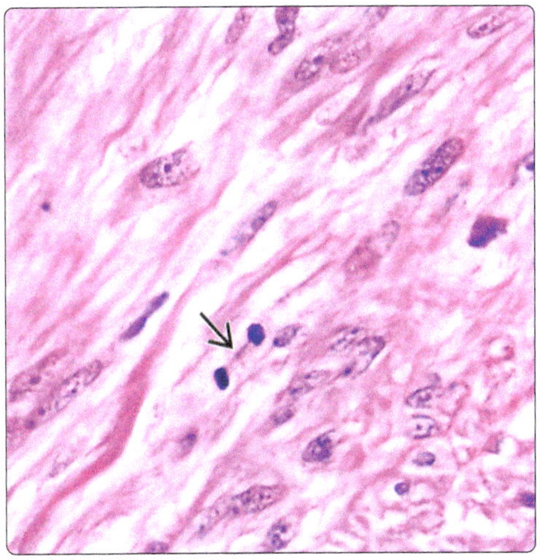

Leiomyosarcoma

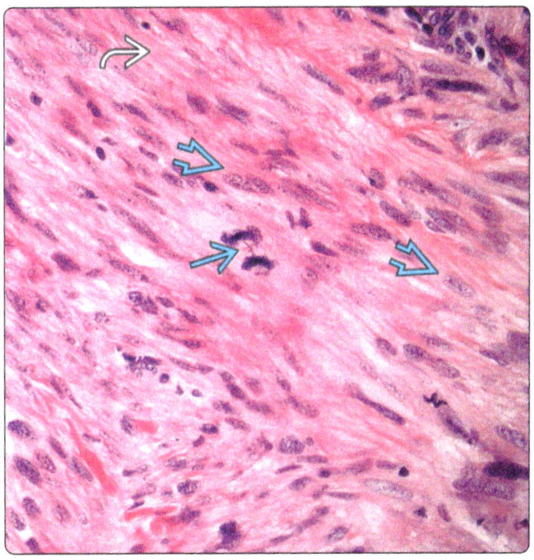

(Left) *High magnification of a leiomyosarcoma demonstrates that the nuclear chromatin is coarser than that in fibromatoses. There is an anaphase bridge ➙, a feature of chromosomally unstable tumors (in contrast to the lack of anaphase bridges in tumors with characteristic mutations or translocations).* **(Right)** *This leiomyosarcoma features an anaphase bridge ➙ as well as blunt-ended nuclei ➙ and fibrillary cytoplasm ➙.*

Juvenile Hyaline Fibromatosis

KEY FACTS

TERMINOLOGY

- Juvenile hyaline fibromatosis
- Related disorder: Infantile systemic hyalinosis

CLINICAL ISSUES

- Autosomal recessive transmission
- Infantile presentation of lesions of scalp, face, neck, retroauricular areas
  - Gingival hypertrophy
- Cutaneous papules and plaques

MICROSCOPIC

- Uniform round to spindle cells
  - Some in clear spaces
- No significant cellular pleomorphism
- No mitoses or necrosis
- Homogeneous, hyalinized, pale, eosinophilic intercellular matrix
  - PAS(+); diastase resistant
- Blood vessels sparse

TOP DIFFERENTIAL DIAGNOSES

- Fibrodysplasia (myositis) ossificans progressiva
  - Rare, autosomal dominant disease
  - Lesions appear similar to those of myositis ossificans
- Infantile myofibromatosis
  - Multiple lesions presenting in infancy
  - Can involve bones, soft tissues, and viscera
- Desmoid-type fibromatosis
  - Large masses of deep soft tissues, usually solitary
- Calcifying aponeurotic fibroma
  - Distal extremities of infants and children
  - Solitary lesions
- Nuchal fibrocartilaginous tumor
  - Solitary lesion of adults

Juvenile Hyaline Fibromatosis, Low Magnification

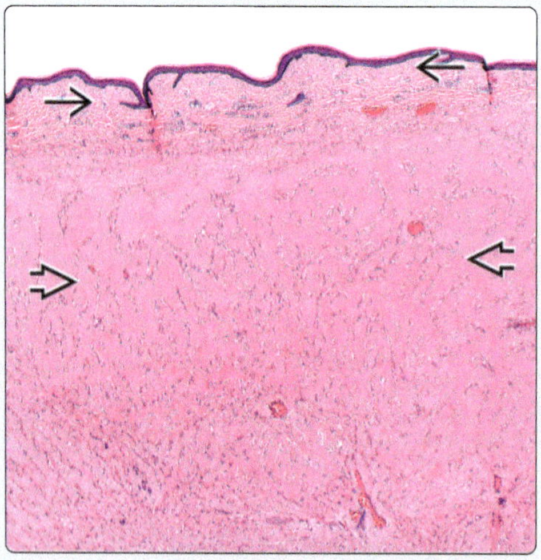

Juvenile Hyaline Fibromatosis, High Magnification

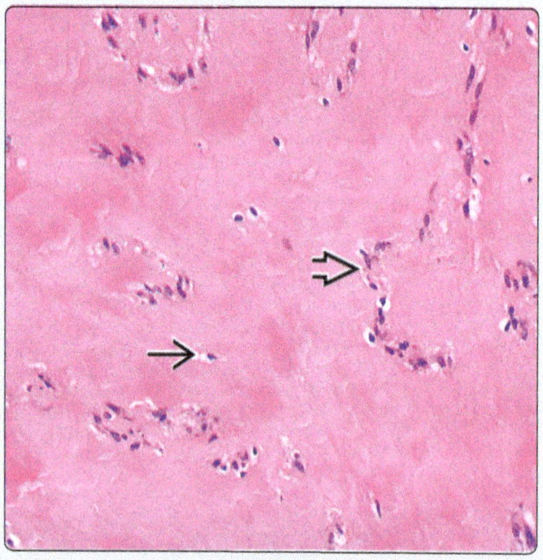

(Left) *Low magnification shows juvenile hyaline fibromatosis of the face in the deep dermis ⇨. There is a tumor-free (grenz) zone ➡ between the epidermis and the lesional tissue.* **(Right)** *Higher magnification shows scattered lesional cells in homogeneous-appearing dense eosinophilic stroma. The cells are small and uniform, arranged in short, curved cords ⇨. Some nuclei appear in spaces ➡.*

Juvenile Hyaline Fibromatosis, Cellular Phase

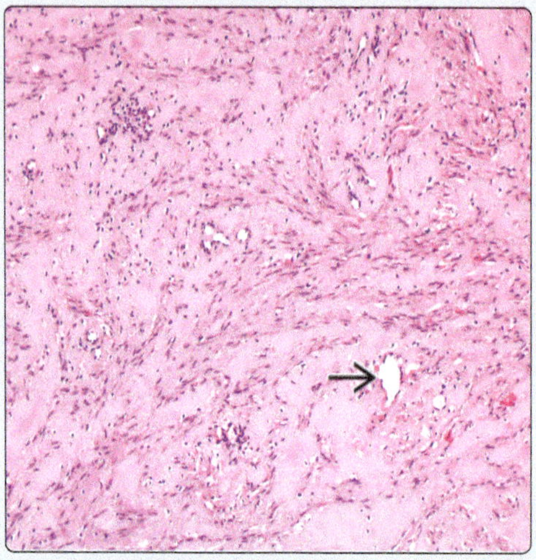

Juvenile Hyaline Fibromatosis, Cytologic Features

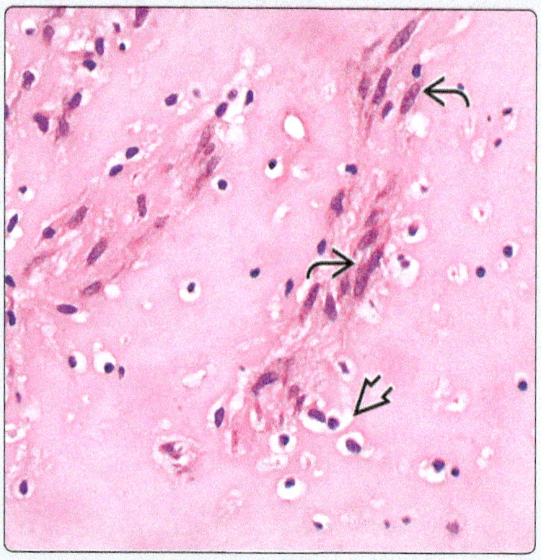

(Left) *A cellular example of juvenile hyaline fibromatosis with branching cords of spindle cells is shown. Note the occasional thin-walled dilated blood vessel ➡.* **(Right)** *High magnification shows numerous cells with clear cytoplasm ⇨ resembling chondrocytes and small clusters of spindle cells ↪. Note the absence of pleomorphism and mitotic activity.*

TERMINOLOGY

Abbreviations

- Juvenile hyaline fibromatosis (JHF)

Synonyms

- Related disorder: Infantile systemic hyalinosis (ISH)
  - Suggested synonym: Hyaline fibromatosis syndrome

Definitions

- Rare autosomal recessive disorder (often found in consanguineous populations) characterized by multiple skin papules and early onset

ETIOLOGY/PATHOGENESIS

Genetic Disorder

- Mutations in *ANTXR2* in both juvenile hyaline fibromatosis and infantile systemic hyalinosis
  - Same gene also termed *CMP2* (encoding capillary morphogenesis gene 2 protein)
- Autosomal recessive transmission (encountered in populations with consanguinity)

CLINICAL ISSUES

Presentation

- Juvenile hyaline fibromatosis
  - Infantile presentation of lesions of scalp, face, neck, retroauricular areas, and perineal region and gingival hypertrophy
  - Joint contractures and motion limitation
  - Osteolytic lesions, mainly in phalanges and distal portions of long bones; cortical defects in subset of patients
- Infantile systemic hyalinosis
  - More severe end of clinical spectrum of mutations in *ANTXR2*
    - Hyaline changes are seen in multiple viscera as well as in skin
    - More prominent than those described in JHF
    - Affected individuals usually die in 1st years of life as result of complications of visceral involvement
  - Infiltration of intestines leads to malabsorption

MACROSCOPIC

Skin and Gingival Lesions

- Plaques and papules of skin
- Larger lesions form soft tissue masses
- Gingival hyperplasia

Systemic Lesions

- Infiltration of small bowel and colon, forming masses

MICROSCOPIC

Histologic Features

- Histologic findings in both JHF and ISH are indistinguishable
  - Round to spindle cell proliferation composed of bland fibroblasts often lying in clear spaces and simulating chondrocyte lacunae
  - No significant cellular pleomorphism or mitoses
  - Homogeneous, hyalinized, dense eosinophilic intercellular matrix
  - PAS positive; diastase-resistant stromal material
  - Displaces normal components of dermis and lamina propria of gingival and intestinal mucosa
  - Early lesions can lack classic hyalinized stroma

DIFFERENTIAL DIAGNOSIS

Fibrodysplasia (Myositis) Ossificans Progressiva

- Rare, autosomal dominant disease
  - Characterized by soft tissue ossification at multiple sites and skeletal abnormalities of digits and cervical spine
  - Short great toes
- No gender predominance
- Trauma (accidental or surgical) results in painful soft tissue lesions
  - Progressive ossification of lesions over 2-3 months
- Lesions appear similar to those of myositis ossificans
  - Mitotically active myofibroblasts
  - Variable ossification depending on age of lesions

Infantile Myofibromatosis

- Multiple lesions presenting in infancy
  - Can involve bones, soft tissues, and viscera
    - Pulmonary involvement is poor prognostic feature
- Biphasic lobulated lesions
  - Central myoid nodules composed of short oval to spindle-shaped cells
  - Peripheral hemangiopericytoma-like zones

Desmoid-Type Fibromatosis

- Large tumors of deep soft tissues, usually solitary
- Cellular fascicular lesions
- Associated with familial adenomatous polyposis
- Nuclear immunoreactivity for β-catenin (in deep cases)

Calcifying Aponeurotic Fibroma

- Distal extremities of infants and children
- Solitary lesions
- Stippled calcifications and fibrous areas

Nuchal Fibrocartilaginous Tumor

- Solitary lesion of adults
- Associated with prior neck injury
- Posterior aspect of base of neck
  - Junction of nuchal ligament and deep cervical fascia
- Fibrocartilaginous tissue forming mass

SELECTED REFERENCES

1. Jaouad IC et al: Hyaline fibromatosis syndrome with mutation c.1074delT of the CMG2 gene: a case report. J Med Case Rep. 8:291, 2014
2. Nofal A et al: Juvenile hyaline fibromatosis and infantile systemic hyalinosis: a unifying term and a proposed grading system. J Am Acad Dermatol. 61(4):695-700, 2009
3. Tanaka K et al: Abnormal collagen deposition in fibromas from patient with juvenile hyaline fibromatosis. J Dermatol Sci. 55(3):197-200, 2009
4. Antaya RJ et al: Juvenile hyaline fibromatosis and infantile systemic hyalinosis overlap associated with a novel mutation in capillary morphogenesis protein-2 gene. Am J Dermatopathol. 29(1):99-103, 2007
5. Hanks S et al: Mutations in the gene encoding capillary morphogenesis protein 2 cause juvenile hyaline fibromatosis and infantile systemic hyalinosis. Am J Hum Genet. 73(4):791-800, 2003
6. Rahman N et al: The gene for juvenile hyaline fibromatosis maps to chromosome 4q21. Am J Hum Genet. 71(4):975-80, 2002

Angiofibroma and Related Lesions

KEY FACTS

CLINICAL ISSUES

- Fibrous papule (FP)
  - Solitary, dome-shaped, flesh-colored papules on nose or central face
- Adenoma sebaceum: Angiofibromas associated with tuberous sclerosis
  - Grouped papules or nodules with butterfly distribution on central face
- May clinically mimic basal cell carcinoma

MICROSCOPIC

- Involves superficial dermis
- Scattered bland, spindled to stellate, and multinucleated fibroblasts
- Rare cases with epithelioid or clear cells
- Dense collagenous stroma
- Absence of solar elastosis
- Ectatic thin-walled blood vessels
- **Clear cell FP**
  - Tumor cells have abundant clear vacuolated cytoplasm
- **Epithelioid FP**
  - Sheets and small groups of epithelioid tumor cells
- **Granular cell FP**
  - Tumor cells have abundant granular cytoplasm

TOP DIFFERENTIAL DIAGNOSES

- Dermatofibroma
  - More cellular with collagen trapping
- Scar
  - Horizontal arrangement of fibroblasts
- Xanthogranuloma
  - Foamy histiocytes with admixed inflammatory cells
- Epithelioid cell histiocytoma
  - Rare on face
  - Epidermal collarette
- Intradermal nevus
  - Nested pattern; melanocytic markers positive

(Left) *Fibrous papule (FP) is characterized by a dome-shaped lesion with ectatic thin-walled blood vessels ➡ and a dense collagenous stroma.* **(Right)** *This higher power image of an FP demonstrates the relatively hypocellular proliferation of bland spindled to stellate fibroblasts, small ectatic vessels, and dense collagenous stroma.*

Fibrous Papule at Low Magnification

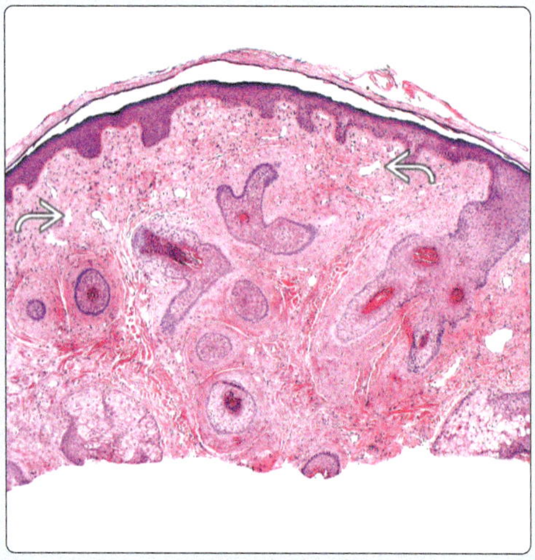

Higher Magnification of Fibrous Papule

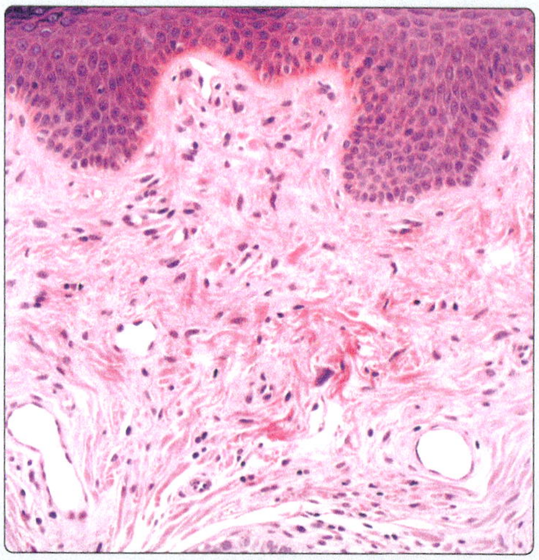

(Left) *This example of clear cell FP is composed of epithelioid cells with abundant clear-staining cytoplasm ➡. The lesion also has an associated mildly collagenous stroma and a few small, dilated vessels ➡.* **(Right)** *Epithelioid FP is more cellular and shows a proliferation of round cells with eosinophilic cytoplasm ➡.*

Clear Cell Variant of Fibrous Papule

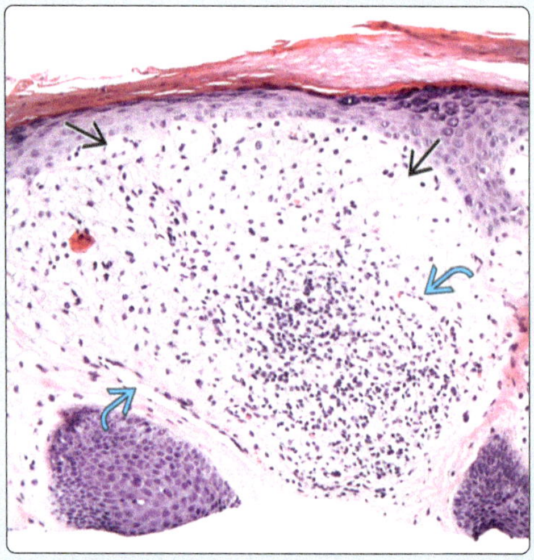

Epithelioid Variant of Fibrous Papule

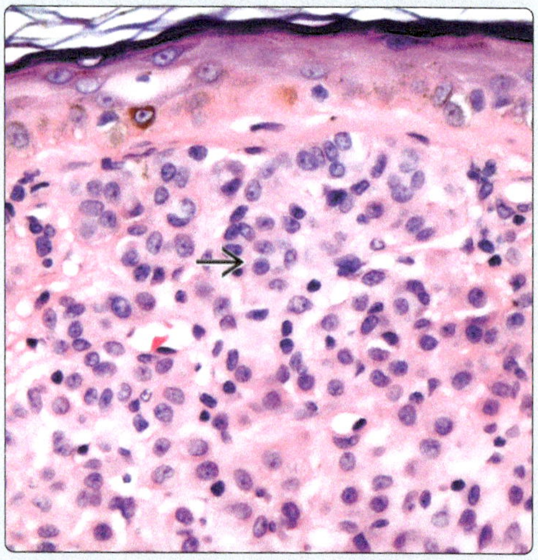

TERMINOLOGY

Synonyms

- Fibrous papule (FP), adenoma sebaceum, acral angiofibroma, pearly penile papule

Definitions

- Angiofibroma encompasses group of benign mesenchymal tumors characterized by spindled to stellate fibroblasts, dense collagenous stroma, and ectatic blood vessels
  - May be related to proliferation of papillary dermal elements

CLINICAL ISSUES

Presentation

- FP
  - Middle-aged patients
  - Solitary, dome-shaped, flesh-colored papules on nose or central face
    - May clinically mimic basal cell carcinoma
- **Adenoma sebaceum**
  - Angiofibromas associated with tuberous sclerosis
    - Tuberous sclerosis: Autosomal dominant inheritance, but most cases sporadic
    - Mutations in *TSC1* or *TSC2*
  - Term is misnomer, as there is no proliferation of sebaceous glands
  - Grouped papules or nodules with butterfly distribution on central face
- **Pearly penile papules**
  - Grouped or linear white papules on coronal margin &/or sulcus of penis

Treatment

- No treatment necessary
- Excision or laser therapy can be used in some cases

Prognosis

- Benign, no malignant potential

MICROSCOPIC

Histologic Features

- Involves superficial dermis
- Scattered bland, spindled to stellate-shaped, and multinucleated fibroblasts
- Dense collagen
  - Elastic tissue absent in collagenous stroma
- Ectatic thin-walled blood vessels
  - May have concentric perivascular fibrosis
- Scant perivascular lymphocytic infiltrate may be present
- Variants
  - **Clear cell FP**
    - Tumor cells have abundant clear vacuolated cytoplasm
    - Otherwise resembles conventional FP
  - **Epithelioid FP**
    - Sheets and small groups of epithelioid tumor cells
    - Increased small blood vessels
    - Collagenous stroma
  - **Granular cell FP**
    - Tumor cells have granular eosinophilic cytoplasm

ANCILLARY TESTS

Immunohistochemistry

- Not needed for diagnosis
- Positive for vimentin; variably positive for CD34, factor XIIIA, CD68, NKI/C3
  - Negative for cytokeratins, S100, HMB-45, melan-A/MART-1

DIFFERENTIAL DIAGNOSIS

Dermatofibroma

- Uncommon on face
- Storiform proliferation of spindled cells with overlying epidermal hyperplasia
- More cellular
  - Polymorphous population of spindled cells, histiocytes, multinucleated cells
- Peripheral collagen trapping

Scar

- More organized with horizontally oriented fibroblasts and vertically oriented blood vessels
- Effacement of rete peg architecture often present

Xanthogranuloma

- Composed of foamy histiocytes, Touton giant cells, and infiltrate that usually includes eosinophils

Epithelioid Cell Histiocytoma

- Rare on face; often with epidermal collarette

Intradermal Nevus

- Cohesive nests of melanocytes
- Positive for S100 and melanocytic markers

Cellular Neurothekeoma

- More cellular, nested proliferation of epithelioid to spindled cells with fibrous septa

DIAGNOSTIC CHECKLIST

Pathologic Interpretation Pearls

- Dense collagenous stroma with absence of solar elastosis clue to diagnosis

SELECTED REFERENCES

1. Mandato VD et al: Cellular angiofibroma in women: a review of the literature. Diagn Pathol. 10:114, 2015
2. Schaberg KB et al: A fibrous papule with abundant CD34-immunoreactive ganglion-like multinucleated giant cells: a case report and review of the literature. Dermatol Online J. 21(7), 2015
3. Borkowska J et al: Tuberous sclerosis complex: tumors and tumorigenesis. Int J Dermatol. 50(1):13-20, 2011
4. Chiang YY et al: Clear cell fibrous papule: report of a case mimicking a balloon cell nevus. J Cutan Pathol. 36(3):381-4, 2009
5. Jacyk WK et al: Fibrous papule of the face with granular cells. Dermatology. 216(1):56-9, 2008
6. Kucher C et al: Epithelioid fibrous papule - a new variant. J Cutan Pathol. 34(7):571-5, 2007
7. Bansal C et al: Histologic variants of fibrous papule. J Cutan Pathol. 32(6):424-8, 2005
8. Lee AN et al: Clear cell fibrous papule with NKI/C3 expression: clinical and histologic features in six cases. Am J Dermatopathol. 27(4):296-300, 2005

Acral Fibrokeratoma

KEY FACTS

TERMINOLOGY

- Acquired digital fibrokeratoma
- Acquired periungual fibrokeratoma
- Benign, dome-shaped, relatively hypocellular mesenchymal tumor that usually presents on digits

ETIOLOGY/PATHOGENESIS

- Subset of cases associated with tuberous sclerosis

CLINICAL ISSUES

- Relatively rare lesions
- Usually present in adults
- Most cases are solitary
- Multiple lesions associated with tuberous sclerosis

MICROSCOPIC

- Dome-shaped to elongated silhouette
- Epidermis is hyperkeratotic and acanthotic
- Relatively hypocellular proliferation of fibroblasts
- Vertically oriented thick collagen bundles

TOP DIFFERENTIAL DIAGNOSES

- Cellular digital fibroma
  - More cellular than acral fibrokeratoma
  - Fascicles of spindled cells
  - Lacks vertically oriented collagen bundles
  - CD34(+)
- Superficial acral fibromyxoma
  - More cellular lesion
  - Loose storiform to fascicular growth pattern
  - Lacks vertically oriented collagen bundles
- Supernumerary digit
  - Clinically resembles acral fibrokeratoma
  - Disorganized nerve bundles in dermis
- Dermatofibroma
  - Also more cellular than acral fibrokeratoma
  - Storiform pattern
  - Peripheral collagen trapping

Acral Fibrokeratoma at Low Magnification

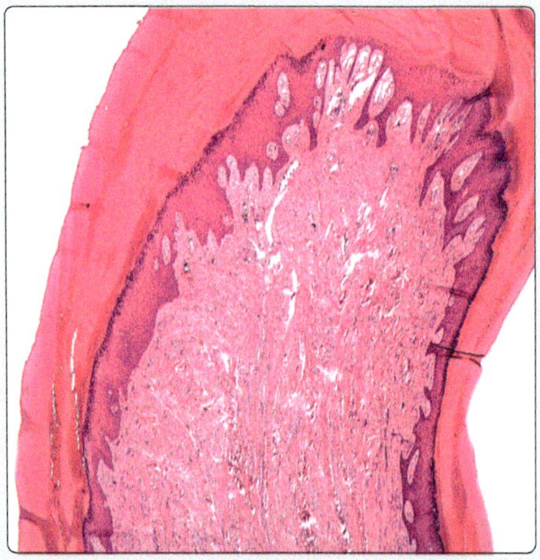

Superficial Portion of Acral Fibrokeratoma

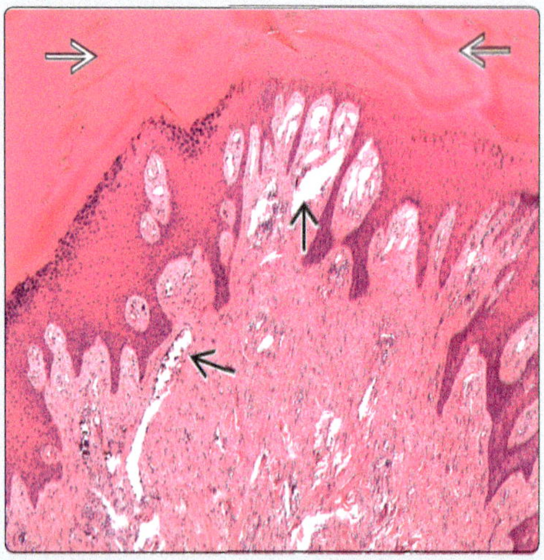

(Left) *Acral fibrokeratoma is a protuberant, pedunculated lesion covered by a hyperkeratotic, variably acanthotic epidermis.* **(Right)** *The epidermis overlying acral fibrokeratoma demonstrates thick, compact hyperkeratosis ⇨. In the superficial dermis, there may be dilated blood vessels ⇨. Note the absence of adnexal structures.*

Dermal Spindle Cells in Acral Fibrokeratoma

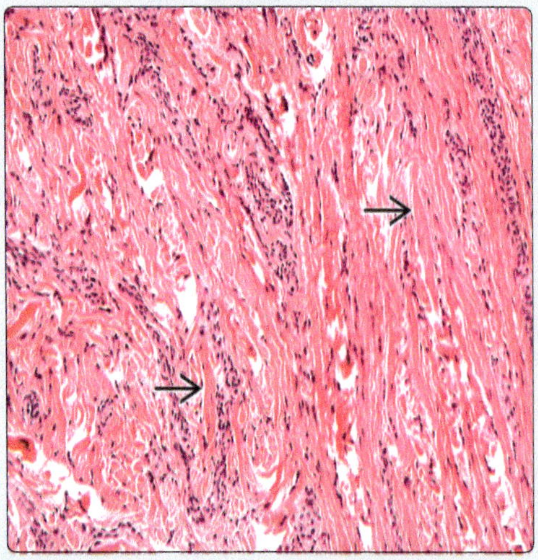

Acral Fibrokeratoma at High Magnification

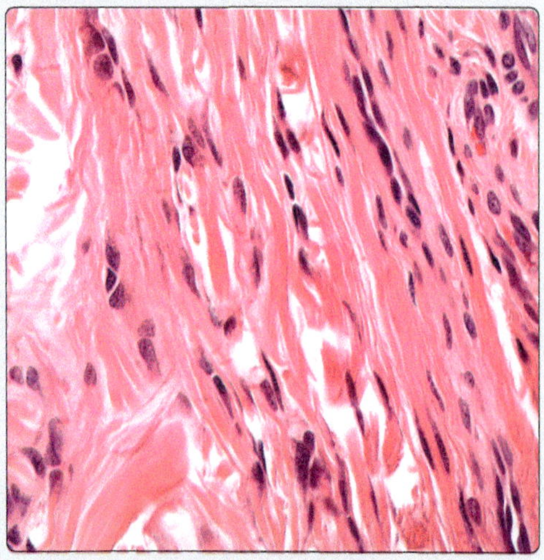

(Left) *Acral fibrokeratoma is characterized by a relatively hypocellular fibroblastic proliferation and thickened, vertically oriented collagen bundles ⇨ in the dermis.* **(Right)** *High-power examination demonstrates the bland fibroblasts and vertically oriented, thickened collagen bundles.*

TERMINOLOGY

Synonyms

- Acquired digital fibrokeratoma
- Acquired periungual fibrokeratoma
- Garlic clove fibroma
- Subungual fibroma of tuberous sclerosis

Definitions

- Benign, dome-shaped, relatively hypocellular mesenchymal tumor that usually presents on digits

ETIOLOGY/PATHOGENESIS

Genetic Syndrome

- Subset of cases associated with tuberous sclerosis
- Mutation of *TSC1* or *TSC2*

CLINICAL ISSUES

Epidemiology

- Incidence
  - Relatively rare lesions
- Age
  - Present in adults most commonly
- Sex
  - Men more commonly affected

Site

- Fingers or toes

Presentation

- Usually solitary
- Dome-shaped to elongated hyperkeratotic papule on digit
- Multiple lesions associated with tuberous sclerosis
  - Often in clusters
  - Ungual location
  - Develop in adolescence

Treatment

- Surgical approaches
  - Simple excision for solitary lesions

Prognosis

- Benign

MICROSCOPIC

Histologic Features

- Dome-shaped to elongated silhouette at lower magnification
- Epidermis is hyperkeratotic and acanthotic
- Relatively hypocellular dermal proliferation of fibroblasts
- Vertically oriented, thickened collagen bundles
- May have dilated capillaries superficially
- Absence of adnexal structures in affected dermis

ANCILLARY TESTS

Immunohistochemistry

- Typically FXIIIA(+)
- Usually CD34(-)

DIFFERENTIAL DIAGNOSIS

Cellular Digital Fibroma

- Polypoid lesion affecting digits
- More cellular with fascicles of bland spindled cells
- Lacks vertically oriented collagen bundles
- Immunohistochemistry shows CD34 positivity

Superficial Acral Fibromyxoma

- Toes are affected > fingers
- Loose storiform to fascicular growth pattern
- Myxoid to collagenous matrix
- Lacks vertically oriented collagen bundles
- CD34(+); often EMA(+)

Accessory Digit

- Also known as supernumerary digit
- Polypoid lesion usually at ulnar base of 5th finger
- Clinical overlap with digital fibrokeratoma
- Disorganized nerves and Meissner corpuscles
  - Resembles traumatic neuroma

Infantile Digital Fibromatosis (Inclusion Body Fibromatosis)

- Presents in first 2 yr of life
- Fascicles of fibroblasts
- Eosinophilic perinuclear inclusions classically present
  - Stains positively with PTAH, trichrome
  - Immunohistochemistry positive for actin, desmin

Dermatofibroma/Fibrous Histiocytoma

- Rarely presents on digits
- Storiform arrangement of fibroblastic and histiocytoid cells
- Peripheral collagen trapping
- Lacks vertically oriented collagen bundles

DIAGNOSTIC CHECKLIST

Pathologic Interpretation Pearls

- Acral location
- Hypocellular fibroblastic proliferation
- Vertically oriented collagen bundles
- Lacks storiform growth pattern

SELECTED REFERENCES

1. Göktay F et al: Multibranched acquired periungual fibrokeratomas with confounding histopathologic findings resembling papillomavirus infection: a report of two cases. J Cutan Pathol. 42(9):652-6, 2015
2. Boffeli TJ et al: Acral fibrokeratoma of the foot treated with excision and trap door flap closure: a case report. J Foot Ankle Surg. 53(4):449-52, 2014
3. Guitart J et al: Cellular digital fibromas: what about superficial acral fibromyxoma? J Cutan Pathol. 33(11):762-3; author reply 764, 2006
4. McNiff JM et al: Cellular digital fibromas: distinctive CD34-positive lesions that may mimic dermatofibrosarcoma protuberans. J Cutan Pathol. 32(6):413-8, 2005
5. Kakurai M et al: Giant acquired digital fibrokeratoma. J Am Acad Dermatol. 48(5 Suppl):S67-8, 2003
6. Fetsch JF et al: Superficial acral fibromyxoma: a clinicopathologic and immunohistochemical analysis of 37 cases of a distinctive soft tissue tumor with a predilection for the fingers and toes. Hum Pathol. 32(7):704-14, 2001
7. Cahn RL: Acquired periungual fibrokeratoma. A rare benign tumor previously described as the garlic-clove fibroma. Arch Dermatol. 113(11):1564-8, 1977
8. Hare PJ et al: Acquired (digital) fibrokeratoma. Br J Dermatol. 81(9):667-70, 1969

KEY FACTS

TERMINOLOGY

- Dermatofibroma (DF)
- Benign, limited proliferation of histiocytic & fibroblastic cells in dermis

ETIOLOGY/PATHOGENESIS

- Evidence supports both neoplastic & reactive pathogenesis
- Tumor may be preceded by local trauma, including insect bite, in some cases

CLINICAL ISSUES

- Affects all ages; most common in young/middle-aged adults
- Excellent prognosis in vast majority of cases
- Metastasis & death in rare cases of cellular & atypical DF

MICROSCOPIC

- Dermal-based proliferation of typically bland, spindled to histiocytoid-appearing cells
- Collagen trapping at periphery
- Overlying epithelial basilar induction with hyperpigmentation
- Early lesions typically show more histiocytes & lymphocytes
- Established lesions show greater cellularity & spindled cells

ANCILLARY TESTS

- FXIIIA(+), CD163(+), CD68(+), CD34(-)

TOP DIFFERENTIAL DIAGNOSES

- Dermatofibrosarcoma protuberans
  - Deep subcutaneous extension & fat entrapment
  - CD34(+), CD163(-), & FXIIIA(-)
- Atypical fibroxanthoma
  - Highly atypical spindled & epithelioid cells
- Basal cell carcinoma, superficial-multicentric type
- Angiosarcoma & Kaposi sarcoma

Clinical Photograph of Lesion on Lower Leg

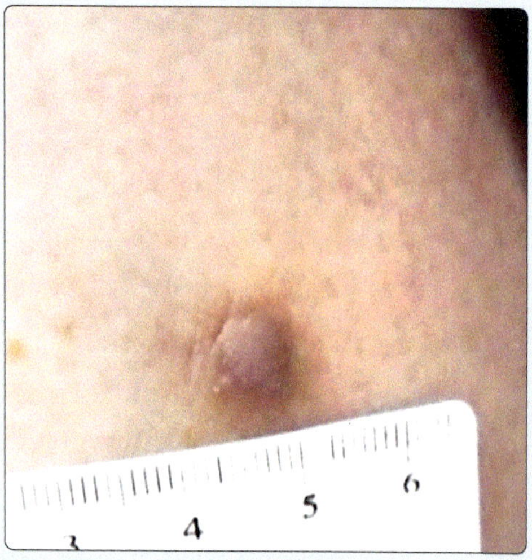

Dermatofibroma at Low Magnification

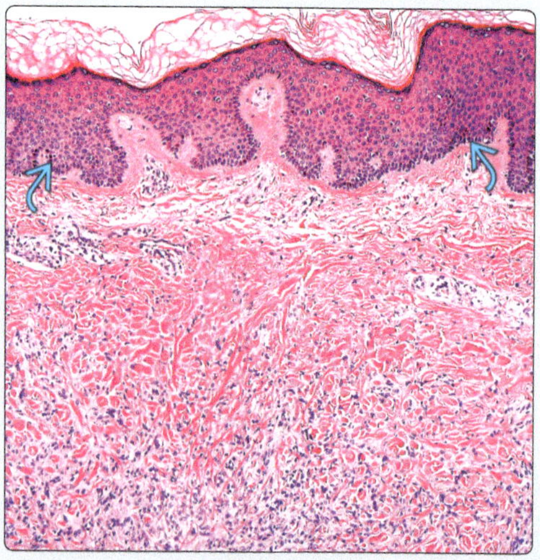

(Left) *This is a dermatofibroma (DF) on the lower leg of an adult patient, which is a common presentation of this lesion. Note the light reddish/brown appearance of the lesion.* **(Right)** *Classic DF shows a dermal-based proliferation of bland spindled to histiocytic-appearing cells associated with a grenz zone and overlying epidermal hyperplasia and basilar pigmentation* ↪*.*

High Magnification With Collagen Entrapment

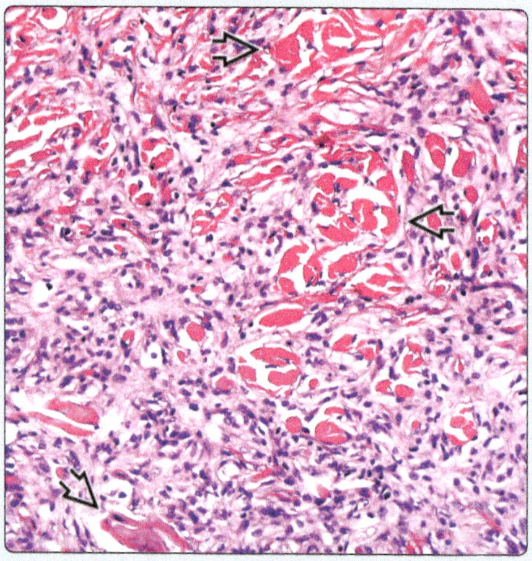

Lipidized Dermatofibroma at High Magnification

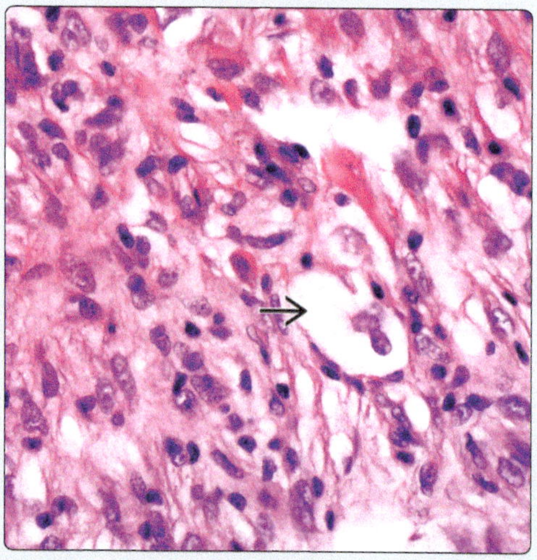

(Left) *Higher power examination of a classic DF shows a proliferation of bland spindled to histiocytoid cells entrapping numerous hyalinized balls of collagen* ⇨*.* **(Right)** *Lipidized DF shows proliferation of bland histiocytoid cells and scattered multivacuolated cells with nuclear indentation simulating lipoblasts* →*.*

TERMINOLOGY

Abbreviations

- Dermatofibroma (DF)
- Fibrous histiocytoma (FH)

Synonyms

- Cutaneous FH
- Sclerosing hemangioma
- Histiocytoma
- Epithelioid cell histiocytoma (ECH)

Definitions

- Common, benign, localized proliferation of mesenchymal cells in dermis
- Lineage not well defined, although commonly referred to as fibrohistiocytic

ETIOLOGY/PATHOGENESIS

Unknown

- Evidence supports both reactive & neoplastic pathogenesis
  - Histiocytic population may be clonal; fibroblast/myofibroblastic population may be polyclonal (reactive)
- Tumor may be preceded by local trauma, including insect bite, in some cases
  - However, no inciting event identified in majority of cases

CLINICAL ISSUES

Epidemiology

- Incidence
  - Common tumors in most populations
- Age
  - All ages; most common in 4th & 5th decades
- Sex
  - Affects males & females equally

Site

- Typically occurs on distal extremities, but may present at any cutaneous site

Presentation

- Firm, isolated, flesh-colored subcutaneous papule or nodule
  - New DFs are typically pink (vascular); older DFs are brown (overlying epidermal hyperplasia with basilar pigmentation)
- Multiple DFs may occur in immunosuppressed populations
- Dimpling sign when in vivo DF is pinched by fingers

Treatment

- Complete excision is curative
  - Often not necessary for most types of DF

Prognosis

- Excellent in vast majority of cases
  - Local recurrence potential significant (up to 30%) with cellular variant
  - Metastasis & death from rare cellular & atypical tumors reported
    - Usually large & deep lesions

MACROSCOPIC

General Features

- Firm, circumscribed, but nonencapsulated dermal-based tumor
- White to yellow cut surface
- Can have cystic changes & hemorrhage

MICROSCOPIC

Histologic Features

- Dermal-based proliferation of typically bland, spindled to histiocytoid-appearing cells
  - Either spindled (fibroblastic) or histiocytoid cells may predominate
  - Early lesions typically show more histiocytes & lymphocytes
  - Established lesions show greater cellularity & spindled cells
  - Older lesions show more fibrosis
  - Spindled cells show elongated eosinophilic cytoplasmic processes
  - Histiocytic-type cells are larger, epithelioid-shaped, & have abundant pale vacuolated cytoplasm
  - Cytologic atypia & pleomorphism are usually minimal but can be focally present
- Tumors are grossly circumscribed but microscopically have irregular, often jagged borders
- Collagen trapping at periphery
  - Spheres of intensely eosinophilic collagen (so-called collagen balls) separated by bands of pale fibrohistiocytic cells
- Grenz zone
  - Tumor often spares band of superficial papillary dermis
- Folliculosebaceous induction & basilar epidermal hyperplasia overlying DF
  - Can mimic basal cell carcinoma (BCC) if basilar induction is marked
- Adjacent adnexal hyperplasia
- Overlying epidermal hyperplasia with basilar hyperpigmentation is common, occasional melanocytic hyperplasia
  - So-called dirty feet or dirty-sock sign

Histologic Subtypes

- **Aneurysmal (hemosiderotic/sclerosing hemangioma variant)**
  - Pseudovascular spaces, hemosiderin, reactive spindled & epithelioid cells
    - May mimic vascular tumor, including Kaposi sarcoma & angiosarcoma
  - Aneurysmal DF can show some cytologic atypia but lacks high-grade atypia & shows only few mitoses
- **Cellular**
  - Uncommon, often large, deeply penetrating tumors
    - May show overlap with atypical DF
    - Occasional mitoses & multinucleated cells are seen
    - Up to 12% of cases may show focal central necrosis
  - Most likely subtype to recur (up to 30% in some studies)
    - Complete conservative excision often suggested to prevent recurrence

- **ECH**
  - Nodular to sheet-like, well-circumscribed proliferation in papillary dermis
    - Often has associated epidermal collarette
  - Clinical & histologic mimic of intradermal Spitz nevus, but negative for melanocytic markers
- **Atypical/pseudosarcomatous/DF with monster cells**
  - Shows population of atypical cells with nuclear hyperchromasia & prominent nucleoli, often with abundant cytoplasm
    - Mitotic figures are sparse; usually not atypical in appearance
  - Some cases have been reported to metastasize
    - Complete excision should be recommended
- **Lipidized**
  - Often large tumors; typically present in ankle region
  - Numerous large foamy cells are present, with few hemosiderin-containing cells
  - Stromal hyalinization is typically present, which may be wiry or keloidal in appearance
- Many other rare variants described, including granular cell, clear cell, histiocytic/xanthomatous, osteoclastic, myxoid, keloidal/scar-like, palisading, deep penetrating (may mimic dermatofibrosarcoma protuberans), & lichenoid

ANCILLARY TESTS

Immunohistochemistry

- FXIIIA(+), CD10(+), CD163(+), HMGA1/HMGA2(+)
  - CD68 also often positive but may be weak; typically highlights histiocytic-appearing cells
  - Actin-sm often positive; may indicate myofibroblastic differentiation
- CD34 typically negative but may show focal staining, especially at periphery of lesion
- Nestin (-), S100(-), MART-1/Melan-A (-), HMB-45(-), MSA(-), desmin (-)

DIFFERENTIAL DIAGNOSIS

Dermatofibrosarcoma Protuberans

- Shows monotonous proliferation of spindled cells
- Typically extends deeply along septa of subcutaneous fat with honeycombing fat entrapment
  - Typically CD34(+), nestin (+), CD10(-), CD163(-), HMGA1/HMGA2(-), FXIIIA(+/-)

Basal Cell Carcinoma, Superficial-Multicentric Type

- In superficial biopsies, BCC may be difficult to distinguish from benign follicular induction overlying DF
  - CK20 highlights Merkel cells in basal layer overlying DF; these cells are typically absent in BCC

Angiosarcoma

- Aneurysmal variant of DF can have atypical cells, pseudovascular spaces, & mitoses
  - Aneurysmal DF is negative for vascular markers, including CD31 & CD34

Kaposi Sarcoma

- Nodular/tumor stage Kaposi sarcoma shows cellular spindle cell proliferation
- Slit-like vascular spaces & extravasated red blood cells are often present
  - Immunohistochemistry shows CD31 & HHV8 positivity

Atypical Fibroxanthoma

- Dermal nodule composed of highly atypical spindled & pleomorphic epithelioid cells
- Typically occurs in heavily sun-damaged skin (especially head & neck area) of elderly patients
  - Both atypical fibroxanthoma & DF are typically positive for nonspecific markers, including CD68, CD10, & vimentin
  - FXIIIA may show greater positivity in DF

DIAGNOSTIC CHECKLIST

Clinically Relevant Pathologic Features

- Cellularity & atypia
- Tumor size (more aggressive cases typically large & deep)

Pathologic Interpretation Pearls

- Collagen balls classically seen
- Basilar epidermal induction with hyperpigmentation
- Occasional adnexal & melanocytic hyperplasia

SELECTED REFERENCES

1. Şenel E et al: Clinical, histopathological, dermatoscopic and digital microscopic features of dermatofibroma: a retrospective analysis of 200 lesions. J Eur Acad Dermatol Venereol. 29(10):1958-66, 2015
2. Charli-Joseph Y et al: DNA copy number changes in tumors within the spectrum of cellular, atypical, and metastasizing fibrous histiocytoma. J Am Acad Dermatol. 71(2):256-63, 2014
3. Doyle LA et al: Metastasizing "benign" cutaneous fibrous histiocytoma: a clinicopathologic analysis of 16 cases. Am J Surg Pathol. 37(4):484-95, 2013
4. Fernandez-Flores A et al: Mitosis in dermatofibroma: a worrisome histopathologic sign that does not necessarily equal recurrence. J Cutan Pathol. 35(9):839-42, 2008
5. Gleason BC et al: Deep "benign" fibrous histiocytoma: clinicopathologic analysis of 69 cases of a rare tumor indicating occasional metastatic potential. Am J Surg Pathol. 32(3):354-62, 2008
6. Kim HJ et al: Stromelysin-3 expression in the differential diagnosis of dermatofibroma and dermatofibrosarcoma protuberans: comparison with factor XIIIa and CD34. Br J Dermatol. 157(2):319-24, 2007
7. Sachdev R et al: Expression of CD163 in dermatofibroma, cellular fibrous histiocytoma, and dermatofibrosarcoma protuberans: comparison with CD68, CD34, and Factor XIIIa. J Cutan Pathol. 33(5):353-60, 2006
8. Mahmoodi M et al: Anti-cytokeratin 20 staining of Merkel cells helps differentiate basaloid proliferations overlying dermatofibromas from basal cell carcinoma. J Cutan Pathol. 32(7):491-5, 2005
9. Hui P et al: Clonal analysis of cutaneous fibrous histiocytoma (dermatofibroma). J Cutan Pathol. 29(7):385-9, 2002
10. Kaddu S et al: Atypical fibrous histiocytoma of the skin: clinicopathologic analysis of 59 cases with evidence of infrequent metastasis. Am J Surg Pathol. 26(1):35-46, 2002
11. Massone C et al: Multiple eruptive dermatofibromas in patients with systemic lupus erythematosus treated with prednisone. Int J Dermatol. 41(5):279-81, 2002
12. Chen TC et al: Dermatofibroma is a clonal proliferative disease. J Cutan Pathol. 27(1):36-9, 2000
13. Ammirati CT et al: Multiple eruptive dermatofibromas in three men with HIV infection. Dermatology. 195(4):344-8, 1997
14. Li DF et al: Dermatofibroma: superficial fibrous proliferation with reactive histiocytes. A multiple immunostaining analysis. Cancer. 74(1):66-73, 1994
15. Altman DA et al: Differential expression of factor XIIIa and CD34 in cutaneous mesenchymal tumors. J Cutan Pathol. 20(2):154-8, 1993
16. Santa Cruz DJ et al: Aneurysmal ("angiomatoid") fibrous histiocytoma of the skin. Cancer. 47(8):2053-61, 1981

Basaloid Hyperplasia Overlying Dermatofibroma

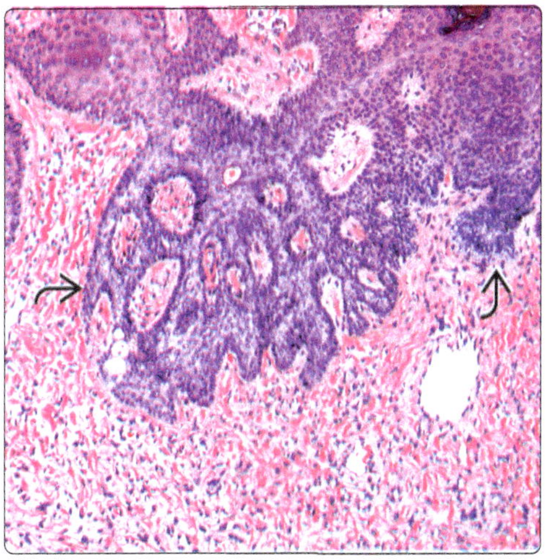

Cellular Dermatofibroma/Fibrous Histiocytoma

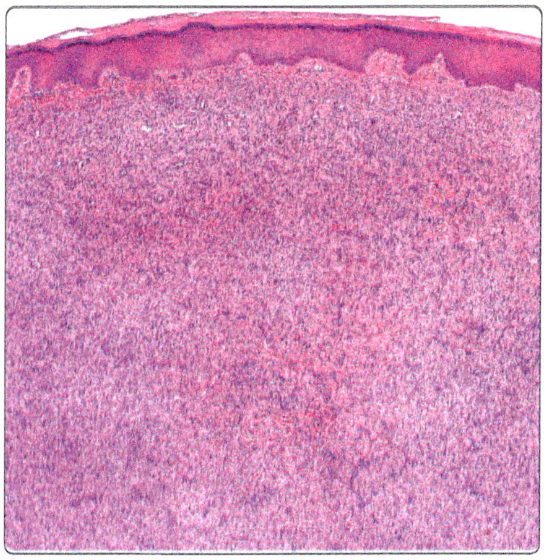

(Left) *The overlying epidermis often shows acanthosis and basilar hyperplasia, which, in some cases, can be exuberant enough to mimic a basal cell carcinoma (BCC). Such cases can be misdiagnosed as BCC on a small, superficial shave biopsy.* **(Right)** *Low-power view of a cellular DF shows a dense proliferation of spindled and histiocytic-appearing cells with nuclear hyperchromasia.*

Cellular and Histiocytic Variant of Dermatofibroma

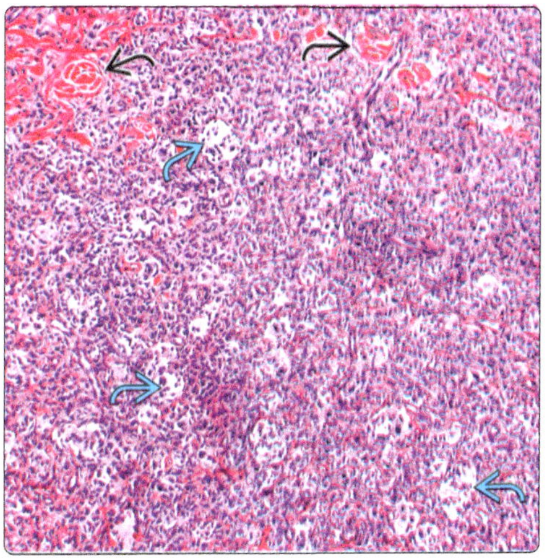

Cellular Dermatofibroma With Atypia

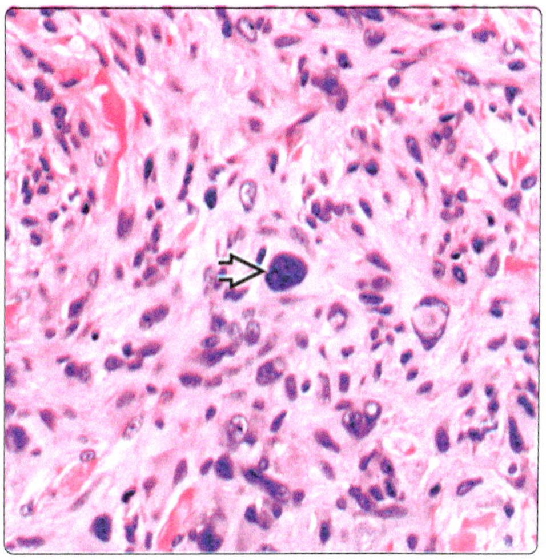

(Left) *This example of cellular DF shows multiple collections of large, pale- to clear-staining histiocytic cells. Note the prominent hyalinized balls of collagen at the periphery of the tumor.* **(Right)** *Higher power view of a cellular DF with focal atypia (or so-called DF with monster cells) shows scattered, bizarre-appearing cells with enlarged, irregular, hyperchromatic-staining nuclei.*

Aneurysmal Fibrous Histiocytoma

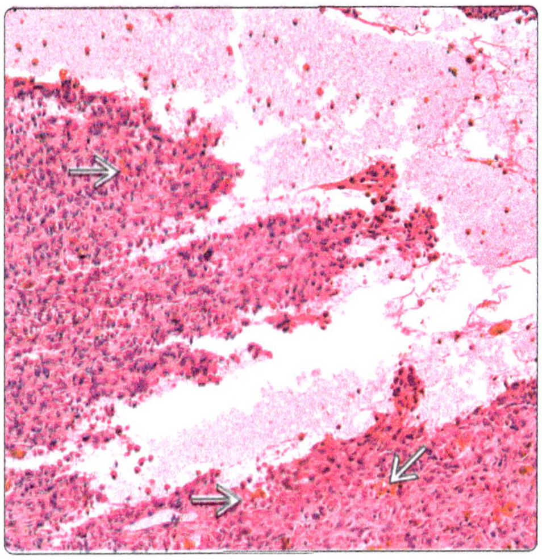

Aneurysmal Fibrous Histiocytoma at High Magnification

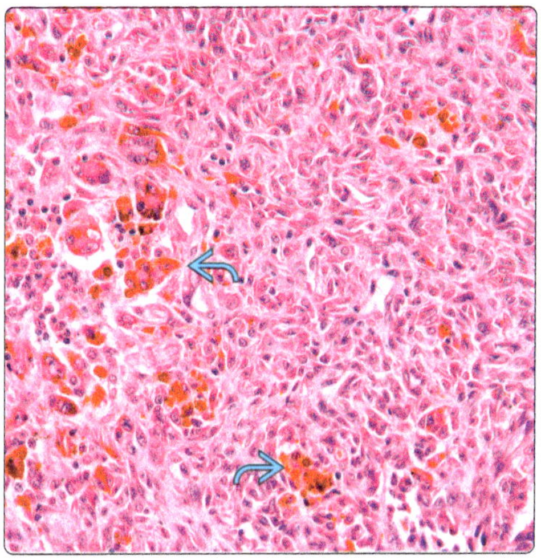

(Left) *An example of an aneurysmal fibrous histiocytoma (FH) shows large, irregular, blood-filled spaces and prominent hemosiderin deposition.* **(Right)** *Higher magnification of an aneurysmal FH shows numerous hemosiderin-laden macrophages.*

(Left) *Histiocytic-predominant DF shows a proliferation of large, epithelioid-appearing cells with abundant pale/vacuolated cytoplasm and scattered small, entrapped collagen bundles* ⇨. **(Right)** *High-power examination of histiocytic DF shows a proliferation of large cells with abundant pale to vacuolated cytoplasm* ↝ *and bland-appearing nuclei.*

Histiocytic-Predominant Dermatofibroma

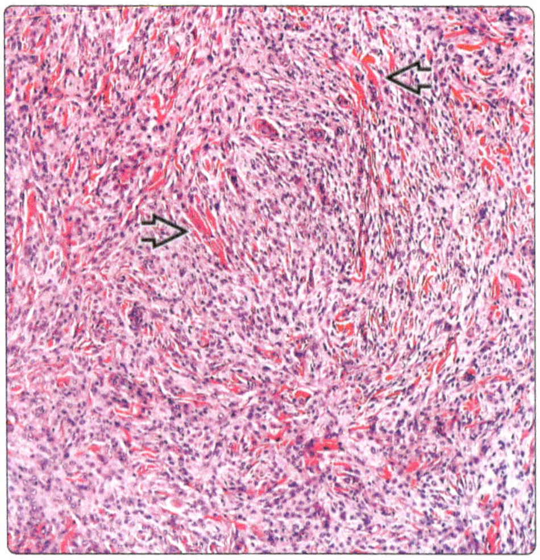

Histiocytic Dermatofibroma at High Magnification

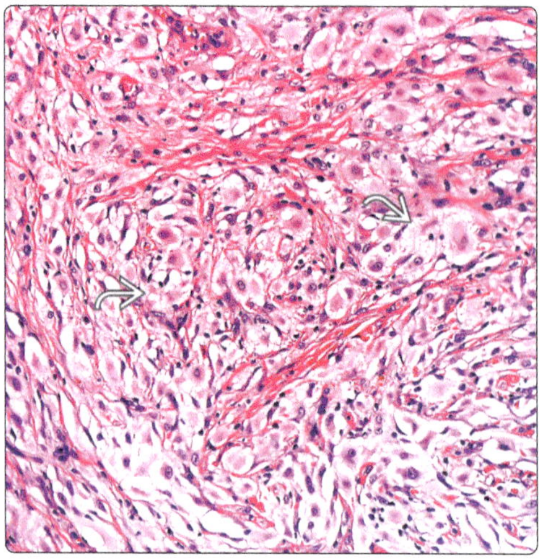

(Left) *Scanning magnification of a scar-like DF with prominent thickened, keloidal collagen bundles* ⇨ *is shown.* **(Right)** *Higher power view of scar-like DF shows dense and glassy-appearing bundles of keloidal collagen* ⇨.

Scar-Like Dermatofibroma

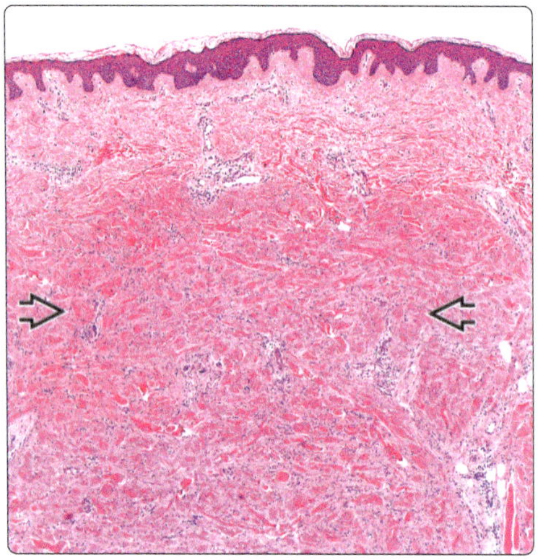

Scar-Like Dermatofibroma at Higher Magnification

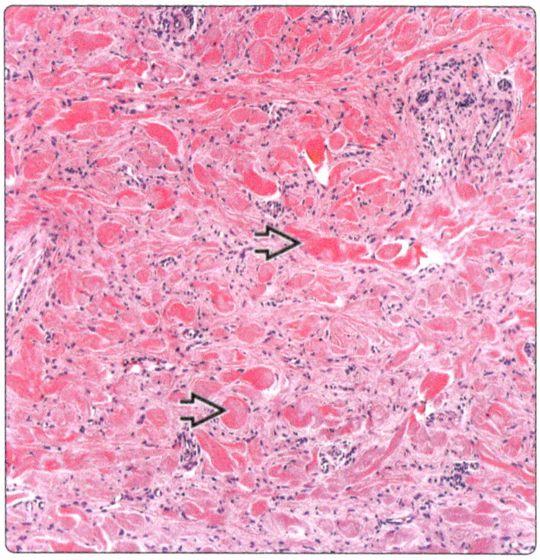

(Left) *Low magnification of a dermatofibrosarcoma protuberans (DFSP) shows deep dermal and subcutaneous involvement by a very cellular spindle cell tumor with prominent honeycombing fat entrapment* ⇨. **(Right)** *DFSP typically shows strong and diffuse CD34 staining, unlike DF, which is usually negative, or shows only focal/patchy staining at the periphery of the tumor.*

Differential Diagnosis: Dermatofibrosarcoma Protuberans

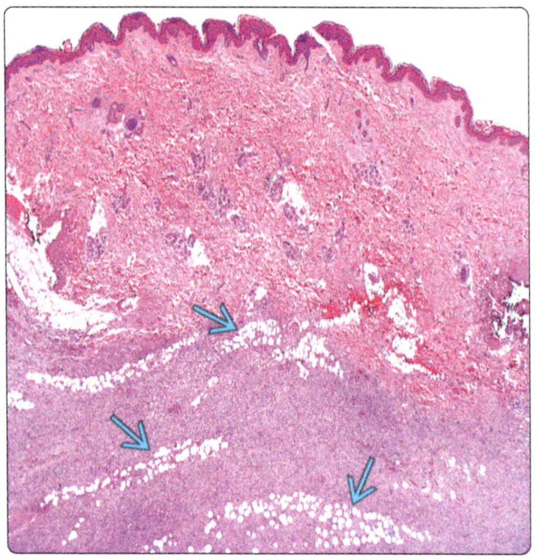

CD34 Immunohistochemistry in Dermatofibrosarcoma Protuberans

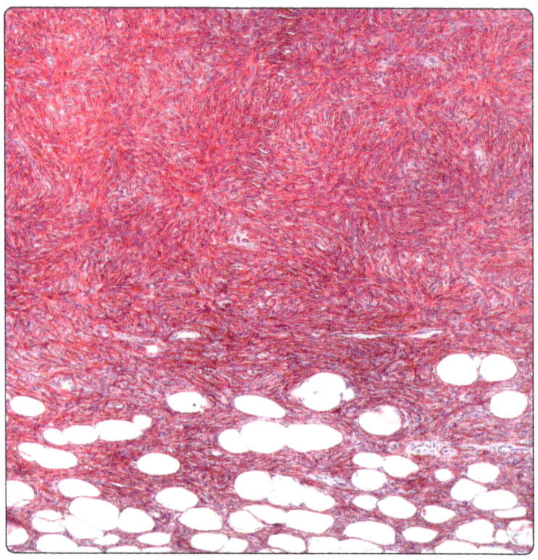

Fibrosarcoma Arising in Dermatofibroma

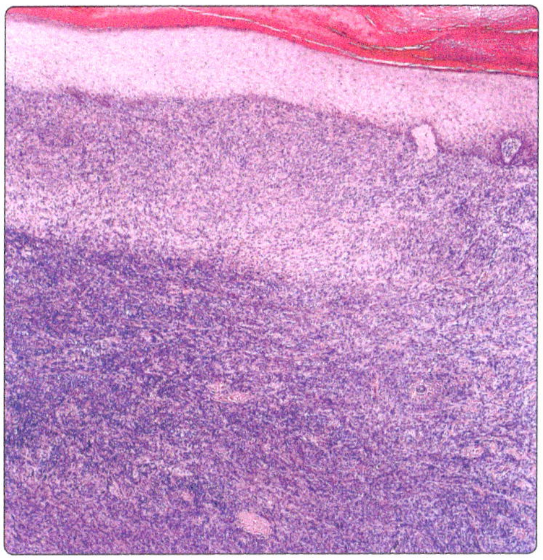

Fibrosarcoma Arising in Dermatofibroma

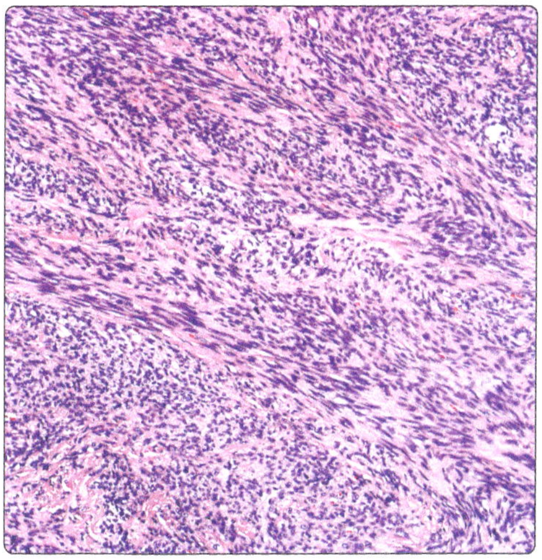

(Left) *Low-power view of a large and highly cellular spindle cell tumor with atypia is shown. The tumor fills the dermis and presses directly against the epidermis (loss of the normal grenz zone).* **(Right)** *Higher power view shows quite marked atypia and a focal fascicular growth pattern, consistent with a low-grade sarcoma (i.e., fibrosarcoma) arising in a cellular FH.*

FXIIIA Immunohistochemistry in Dermatofibroma

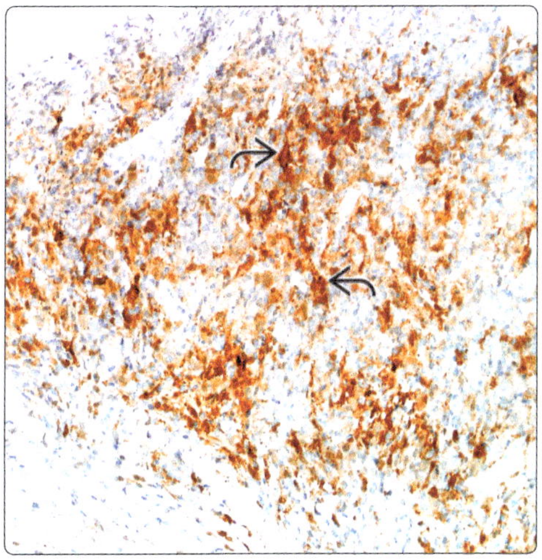

FXIIIA Immunohistochemistry in Dermatofibroma

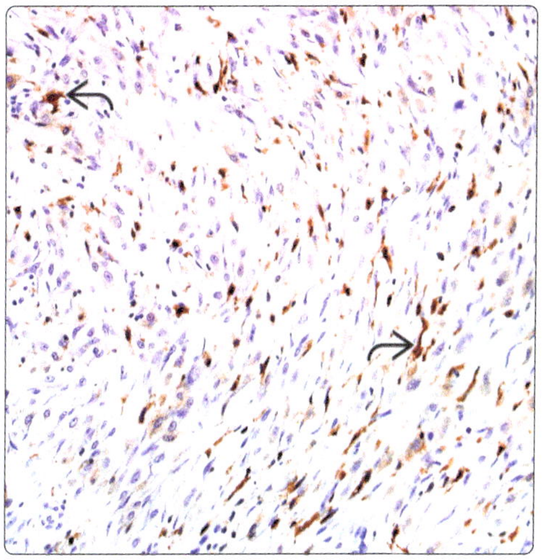

(Left) *Strongly positive FXIIIA staining of many of the spindled and dendritic-appearing tumor cells ↷ is seen in some cases of DF.* **(Right)** *Weakly positive FXIIIA stain in another case shows weak staining of the spindled cells and stronger staining of scattered dermal dendritic cells ↷.*

CD163 Immunohistochemistry in Dermatofibroma

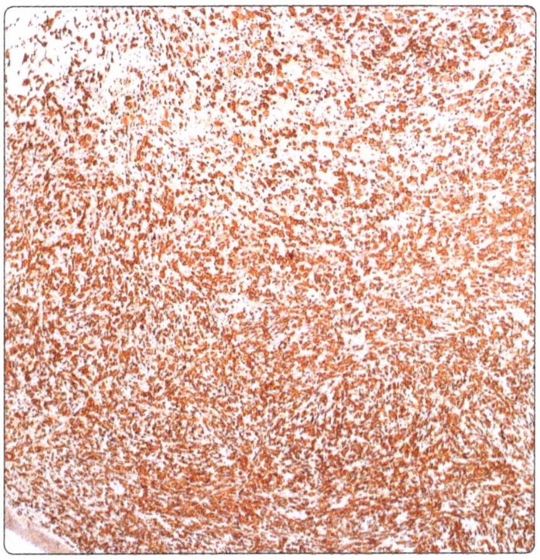

CD34 Immunohistochemistry in Dermatofibroma

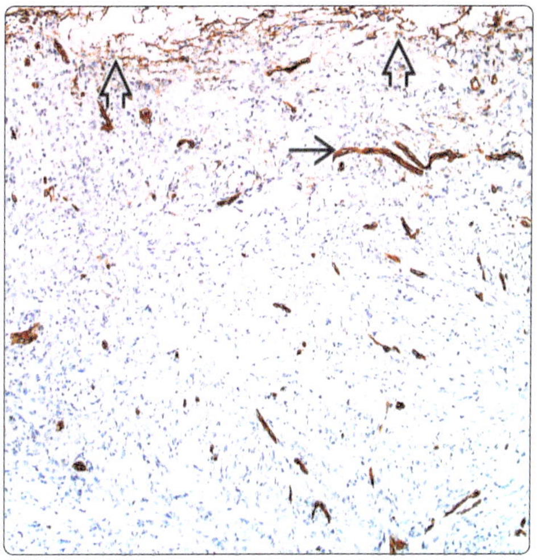

(Left) *CD163 immunohistochemistry shows strong and diffuse staining in a cellular and histiocytic-type DF. CD163 is a more sensitive marker and usually shows stronger staining than FXIIIA.* **(Right)** *CD34 strongly highlights vessels ⇨ and shows weak background staining of some of the peripheral stroma ⇧ but is negative within the tumoral cells.*

Epithelioid Cell Histiocytoma

KEY FACTS

TERMINOLOGY

- Epithelioid cell histiocytoma
- Epithelioid histiocytoma variant of dermatofibroma
- Dermal-based benign fibrohistiocytic tumor, which can mimic melanocytic, vascular, epithelial, or other histiocytic lesions

CLINICAL ISSUES

- Rare tumors
- Usually occur in young adults (mean age ~ 40 yr)
- Most cases occur on extremities
- Typically present as erythematous dermal nodule
- Excellent prognosis; no malignant potential reported

MICROSCOPIC

- Dermal-based nodular fibrohistiocytic proliferation
- Shows symmetry and relatively sharp circumscription
- Most cases are surrounded by epidermal collarette
- Composed of monomorphic proliferation of enlarged, epithelioid to polygonal-appearing cells
- Show round to oval nuclei, uniform vesicular chromatin, small nucleoli, and abundant eosinophilic-staining cytoplasm

ANCILLARY TESTS

- Cells are typically positive for fibrohistiocytic markers including CD68, FXIIIA
- CD31 can also be positive (consistent with histiocytic differentiation)

TOP DIFFERENTIAL DIAGNOSES

- Dermatofibroma
  - More polymorphic population, often including giant cells, foamy, and hemosiderin-laden macrophages
- Spitz nevus
  - Often composed of proliferation of mixed spindled and epithelioid cells
- Epithelioid angiomatous nodule

(Left) *Low magnification of an epithelioid histiocytoma (ECH) shows a nodular, dermal-based tumor surrounded by an epidermal collarette ➢. Note the prominent superficial blood vessels with telangiectasia ➡.* **(Right)** *Higher magnification of ECH shows a population of moderately enlarged, oval to epithelioid-appearing cells with eosinophilic-staining cytoplasm. Multiple telangiectatic intratumoral vessels are also seen ➡.*

ECH

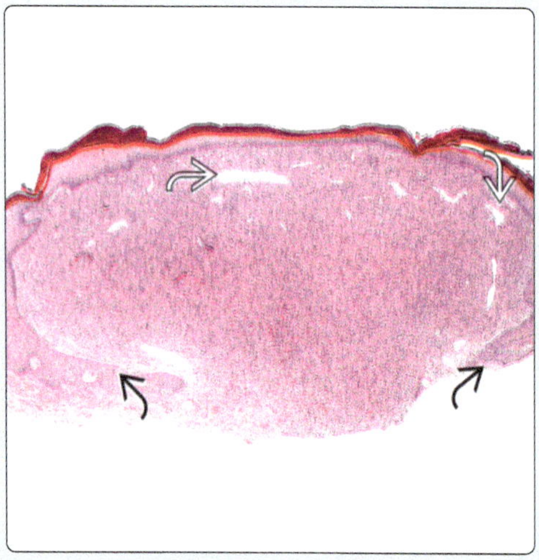

ECH at Higher Magnification

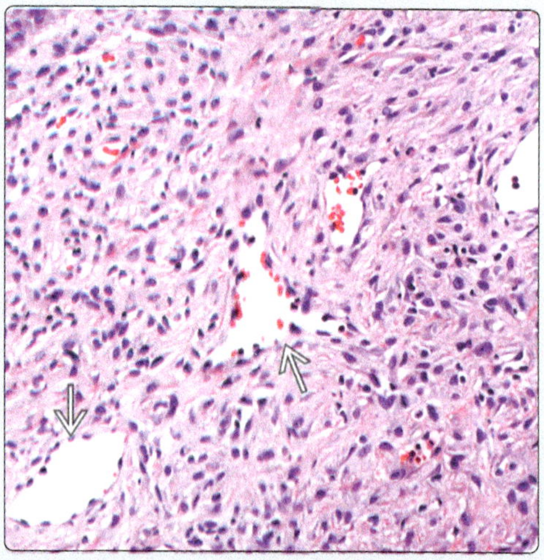

(Left) *High magnification of ECH shows the epithelioid-appearing cells with eosinophilic staining to focally vacuolated ➢ cytoplasm. Many of the cells show small nucleoli ➡. (Courtesy E. J. Glusac, MD.)* **(Right)** *Immunohistochemistry for CD10 shows strong and diffuse staining in this ECH, similar to other types of dermatofibroma/fibrous histiocytoma.*

ECH at High Magnification

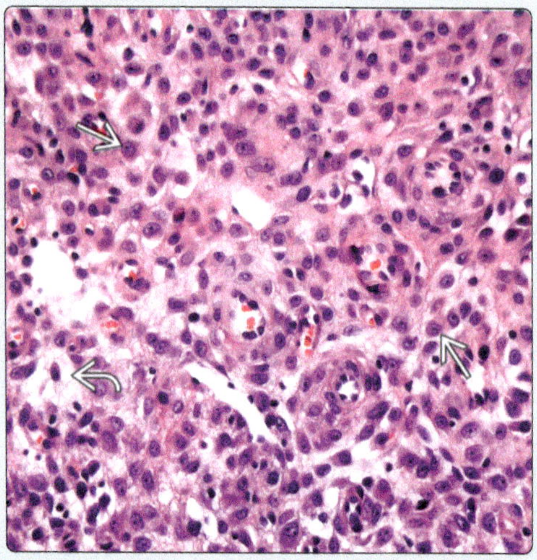

CD10 Immunohistochemistry in ECH

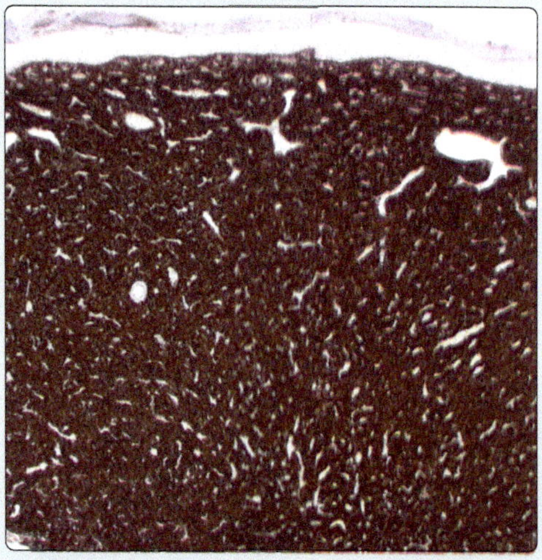

TERMINOLOGY

Abbreviations

- Epithelioid cell histiocytoma (ECH)

Synonyms

- Epithelioid histiocytoma variant of dermatofibroma

Definitions

- Dermal-based benign fibrohistiocytic tumor, which can mimic melanocytic, vascular, epithelial, or other histiocytic lesions

ETIOLOGY/PATHOGENESIS

Unknown

- May arise from activated dermal dendrocytes

CLINICAL ISSUES

Epidemiology

- Incidence
  - Rare tumors
- Age
  - Usually occur in young adults (mean age ~ 40 yr)
- Sex
  - Slightly more common in male patients

Site

- Most cases occur on extremities
  - Lower extremity > upper
- May also present on trunk, head, and neck region

Presentation

- Dermal nodule
- Erythematous

Treatment

- Surgical approaches
  - Conservative excision is curative

Prognosis

- Excellent; no malignant potential reported

MACROSCOPIC

Size

- 0.5-2.0 cm in greatest diameter

MICROSCOPIC

Histologic Features

- Dermal-based nodular proliferation
  - Shows symmetry and relatively sharp circumscription
  - Often surrounded by epidermal collarette
  - Typically centered in papillary dermis
  - Cellular versions based in reticular dermis
- Composed of monomorphic proliferation of enlarged, epithelioid to polygonal-appearing cells
  - Show round to oval nuclei, uniform vesicular chromatin, small nucleoli, and abundant eosinophilic-staining cytoplasm
  - Lack of (or rare) giant cells, foamy or hemosiderin-laden macrophages
- Dermal fibrosis and prominent vascularity usually present
- Mild background inflammatory infiltrate

ANCILLARY TESTS

Immunohistochemistry

- Cells are typically positive for fibrohistiocytic markers including CD10, CD68, and FXIIIA
- CD31 can be positive (reflecting histiocytic, rather than endothelial, differentiation)
- Recent studies have reported ALK positivity (corresponding to *ALK* gene rearrangement)

DIFFERENTIAL DIAGNOSIS

Dermatofibroma

- Conventional dermatofibroma shows more diffuse, poorly demarcated fibrohistiocytic proliferation
- Prominent collagen trapping and overlying epidermal hyperplasia typically seen
- More polymorphic population, often including giant cells, foamy and hemosiderin-laden macrophages

Spitz Nevus

- Often composed of proliferation of mixed spindled and epithelioid cells, but purely epithelioid variants can mimic ECH
- Typically junctional and intradermal proliferation (ECH is purely dermal) in most cases
- Melanocytic markers including S100, HMB-45, and MART-1/Melan-A strongly positive

Epithelioid Angiomatous Nodule

- Rare dermal-based nodular vascular proliferation
- May represent variant of epithelioid hemangioma (angiolymphoid hyperplasia with eosinophilia)
- Composed of enlarged epithelioid endothelial cells and scattered small blood vessels
  - Cells show frequent intracytoplasmic vacuoles
- Positive for vascular markers including CD31 and CD34

SELECTED REFERENCES

1. Jedrych J et al: Epithelioid cell histiocytoma of the skin with clonal ALK gene rearrangement resulting in VCL-ALK and SQSTM1-ALK gene fusions. Br J Dermatol. 172(5):1427-9, 2015
2. Rabkin MS et al: Granular cell variant of epithelioid cell histiocytoma. Am J Dermatopathol. 34(7):766-9, 2012
3. Wilk M et al: Dermatofibroma with intracytoplasmic eosinophilic globules--another case with features overlapping between epithelioid cell histiocytoma and dermal nodular fasciitis. J Cutan Pathol. 38(2):254-5, 2011
4. Cangelosi JJ et al: Unusual presentation of multiple epithelioid cell histiocytomas. Am J Dermatopathol. 30(4):373-6, 2008
5. Lee J: Epithelioid cell histiocytoma with granular cells (another nonneural granular cell neoplasm). Am J Dermatopathol. 29(5):475-6, 2007
6. Busam KJ et al: Immunohistochemical distinction of epithelioid histiocytic proliferations from epithelioid melanocytic nevi. Am J Dermatopathol. 22(3):237-41, 2000
7. Glusac EJ et al: Epithelioid cell histiocytoma: a simulant of vascular and melanocytic neoplasms. Am J Dermatopathol. 21(1):1-7, 1999
8. Singh Gomez C et al: Epithelioid benign fibrous histiocytoma of skin: clinico-pathological analysis of 20 cases of a poorly known variant. Histopathology. 24(2):123-9, 1994
9. Jones EW et al: Epithelioid cell histiocytoma: a new entity. Br J Dermatol. 120(2):185-95, 1989

Dermatomyofibroma

KEY FACTS

TERMINOLOGY

- Myofibroblastic tumor with features overlapping with dermatofibroma
- Also known as plaque-like dermal fibromatosis

ETIOLOGY/PATHOGENESIS

- May be related to trauma in some cases

CLINICAL ISSUES

- Rare tumor
- Usually occurs in young adults
- Slow-growing plaque or nodule
- Most cases present in shoulder and axillary regions

MACROSCOPIC

- Usually 1-2 cm in size but occasionally much larger

MICROSCOPIC

- Dermal-based spindle cell proliferation
- Overlying epidermal hyperplasia, similar to dermatofibroma, is often seen
- Usually located in reticular dermis but may show involvement of superficial subcutis
- Tumor is composed of broad fascicles of elongated monomorphous spindle cells oriented parallel to surface
- Nuclei bland and tapered
- Elastic fibers are typically increased in numbers and fragmented; may be highlighted with elastic stains

TOP DIFFERENTIAL DIAGNOSES

- Dermatofibroma
  - Lacks parallel orientation of tumor cells to epidermis
- Hypertrophic scar
  - Dense proliferation of thickened collagen with vertically oriented vessels
- Leiomyoma
  - Fascicles of spindle cells not typically oriented parallel to epidermis, actins are positive

Dermatomyofibroma

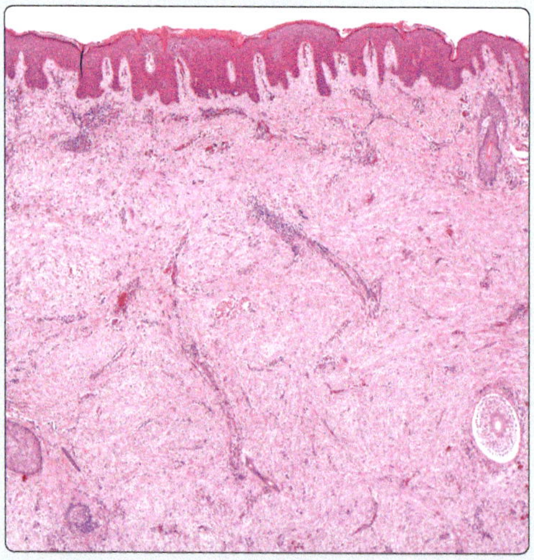

Dermatomyofibroma With Fascicles of Spindle Cells

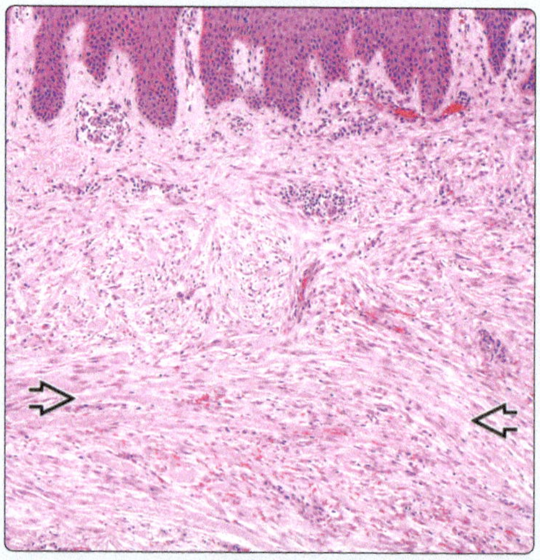

(Left) *Scanning magnification of a dermatomyofibroma shows a dermal-based, plaque-like spindle proliferation with overlying epidermal hyperplasia, similar to a dermatofibroma.* **(Right)** *Higher magnification shows a proliferation of bland spindle cells arranged in fascicles, largely running parallel to the epidermis and associated with focal collagen trapping ⇨.*

Dermatomyofibroma at Higher Magnification

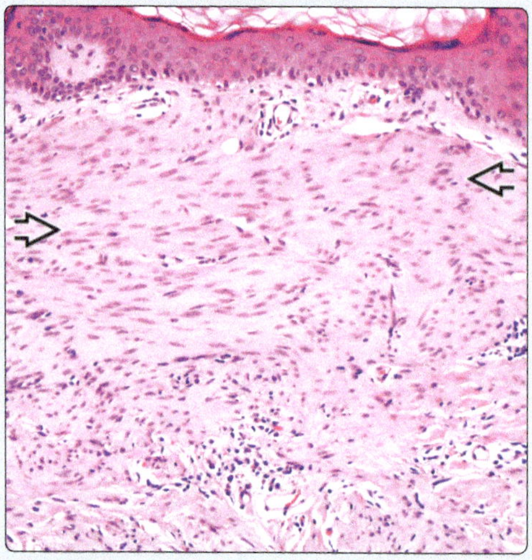

Dermatomyofibroma at High Magnification

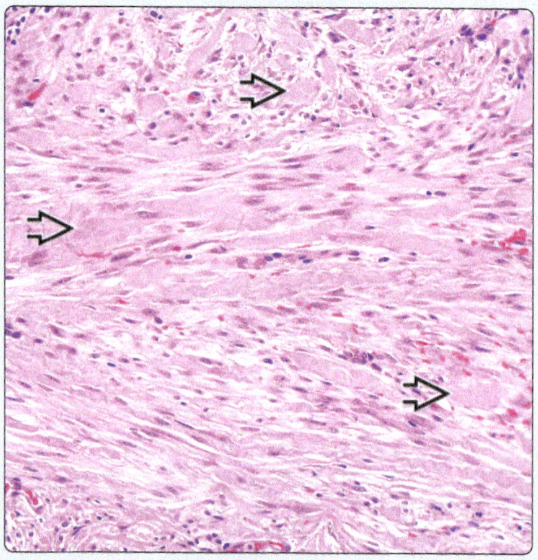

(Left) *Higher magnification shows the superficial portion of the lesion with parallel arrays of spindle cells ⇨ closely approaching the epidermis.* **(Right)** *High-power examination shows bland cytologic features of the elongated myofibroblastic cells. There is also associated collagen trapping ⇨.*

TERMINOLOGY

Synonyms

- Plaque-like dermal fibromatosis

Definitions

- Myofibroblastic tumor with many features similar to dermatofibroma

ETIOLOGY/PATHOGENESIS

Unknown

- May be related to trauma in some cases

CLINICAL ISSUES

Epidemiology

- Incidence
  - Rare tumor
- Age
  - Usually occurs in young adults
- Sex
  - Typically female patients (M:F = 1:8)

Site

- Most cases present in shoulder and axillary regions
  - Also may occur on trunk, head, and neck

Presentation

- Slow-growing indurated plaque or nodule
  - Often red-brown in color
- Rarely, may present as multiple lesions

Treatment

- Surgical approaches
  - Complete surgical excision is curative

Prognosis

- Excellent
  - No malignant potential, but may continue to enlarge if not completely removed

MACROSCOPIC

General Features

- Small, dermal-based nodule

Size

- Usually 1-2 cm in size, but occasionally much larger

MICROSCOPIC

Histologic Features

- Dermal-based, plaque-like spindle cell proliferation oriented parallel to epidermis
  - Usually located in reticular dermis, but may show involvement of superficial subcutis
  - Adnexal structures are usually preserved
  - Overlying epidermal hyperplasia, similar to dermatofibroma, is often seen
- Tumor is composed of broad fascicles of elongated monomorphous spindle cells
  - Nuclei bland and tapered
  - Uniform chromatin
  - Small nucleoli
  - Cytoplasm eosinophilic, poorly delineated
- Mitotic figures are rare and not atypical
- Elastic fibers are typically increased in numbers and fragmented
  - Can highlight with elastic stains

Predominant Cell/Compartment Type

- Fibroblast, myofibroblast

ANCILLARY TESTS

Immunohistochemistry

- Tumor cells variably positive for smooth muscle actin (SMA)
- Cells are negative for muscle-specific actin (MSA), desmin, S100, CD34, and FXIIIA

DIFFERENTIAL DIAGNOSIS

Dermatofibroma

- Lacks parallel orientation of tumor cells to epidermis
- Shows more prominent collagen trapping and overlying epidermal hyperplasia

Hypertrophic Scar

- Dense proliferation of thickened collagen with vertically oriented vessels
- Adnexal structures are lost, as opposed to preserved in dermatomyofibroma

Leiomyoma

- Fascicles of spindle cells not typically oriented parallel to epidermis
- Shows strong smooth muscle differentiation with SMA, MSA, and desmin staining

Dermatofibrosarcoma Protuberans

- Plaque-like variant can show histologic features similar to dermatomyofibroma
- In dermatofibrosarcoma protuberans, CD34 is typically strongly positive and SMA is negative

DIAGNOSTIC CHECKLIST

Pathologic Interpretation Pearls

- Dermal-based, plaque-like proliferation composed of broad fascicles of elongated monomorphous spindle cells oriented parallel to surface

SELECTED REFERENCES

1. Romaní J et al: Dermatomyofibroma on the nape of the neck: a report of 2 pediatric cases. Actas Dermosifiliogr. 105(3):315-7, 2014
2. Sim JH et al: Development of dermatomyofibroma in a male infant. Ann Dermatol. 23 Suppl 1:S72-4, 2011
3. Gomez-Moyano E et al: Two cases of dermatomyofibroma (plaque-like dermal fibromatosis). Int J Dermatol. 49(8):914-7, 2010
4. Mentzel T et al: Dermatomyofibroma: clinicopathologic and immunohistochemical analysis of 56 cases and reappraisal of a rare and distinct cutaneous neoplasm. Am J Dermatopathol. 31(1):44-9, 2009
5. Viglizzo G et al: A unique case of multiple dermatomyofibromas. Clin Exp Dermatol. 33(5):622-4, 2008
6. Mentzel T et al: Dermatomyofibroma: additional observations on a distinctive cutaneous myofibroblastic tumour with emphasis on differential diagnosis. Br J Dermatol. 129(1):69-73, 1993
7. Kamino H et al: Dermatomyofibroma. A benign cutaneous, plaque-like proliferation of fibroblasts and myofibroblasts in young adults. J Cutan Pathol. 19(2):85-93, 1992

KEY FACTS

TERMINOLOGY

- Benign superficial fibrous lesion occurring during first 2 years of life

ETIOLOGY/PATHOGENESIS

- No conclusive familial or syndromic associations
- Rare cases reported in tuberous sclerosis patients, patients with Williams syndrome, patients with Proteus syndrome, and synchronously with desmoid fibromatosis

CLINICAL ISSUES

- Congenital in up to 25% of cases
- M > F
- Occurs in deep dermis or subcutis
  - Typically in upper torso but at variety of sites
  - ~ 20% in groin area
- Complete excision is curative
  - Can recur if incompletely excised

MICROSCOPIC

- 3 components in organoid growth pattern
  - Intersecting bands of mature fibrous tissue, comprising spindle-shaped myofibroblasts and fibroblasts
  - Nests of immature round, ovoid, or spindle cells within loose stroma
  - Interspersed mature fat
- About half of cases show pseudoangiomatous zones

ANCILLARY TESTS

- **Immunolabeling not needed for diagnosis**

TOP DIFFERENTIAL DIAGNOSES

- Fibromatosis
  - Large deep masses that often infiltrate skeletal muscle
- Infantile fibromatosis/lipofibromatosis
- Myofibroma
- Inclusion body fibromatosis (infantile digital fibromatosis)
- Embryonal rhabdomyosarcoma

Fibrous Hamartoma of Infancy: Gross Specimen

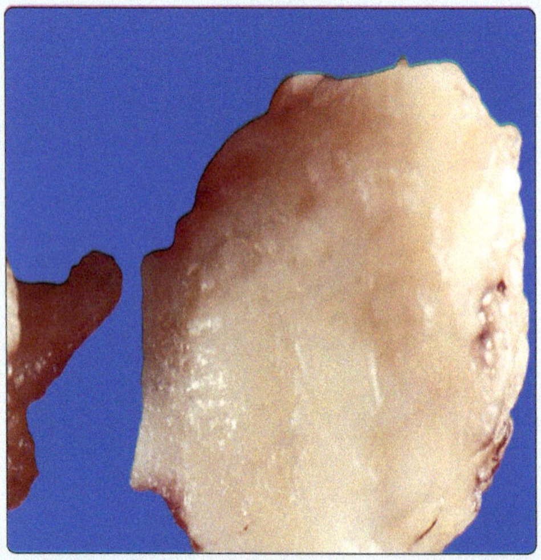

Fibrous Hamartoma of Infancy at Low Magnification

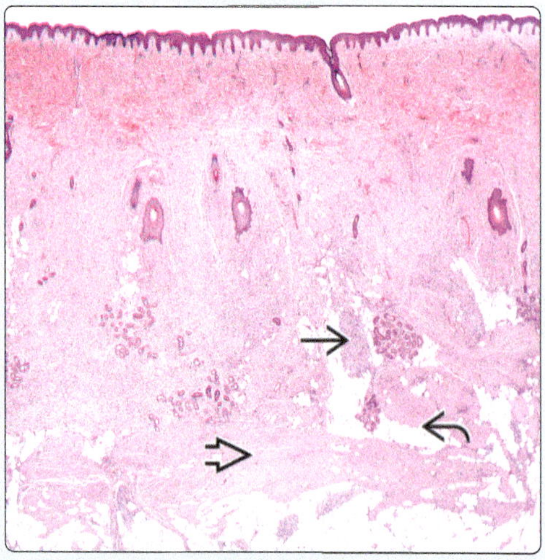

(Left) *This is a gross specimen from a fibrous hamartoma of infancy (FHI). It is a small lesion (2-3 cm) with a firm, tan cut surface.* **(Right)** *This FHI expands the deep dermis and superficial submucosa consisting of eosinophilic fibrous zones ➡, more basophilic areas ➡, and fat ➡.*

Fibrous Hamartoma of Infancy With Fat, Fibrous Tissue, and Spindle Cells

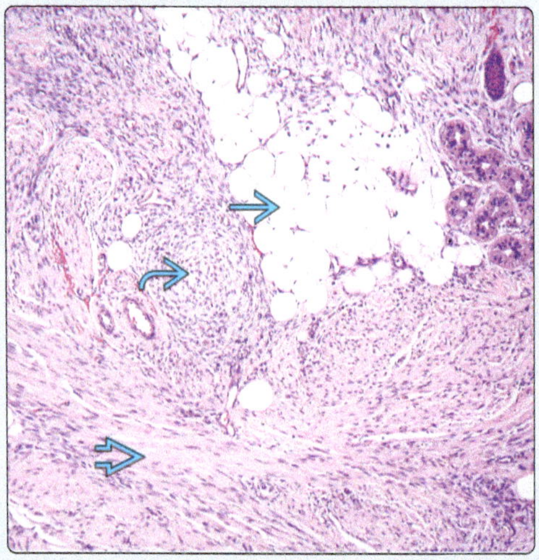

Fibrous Hamartoma of Infancy at Higher Magnification

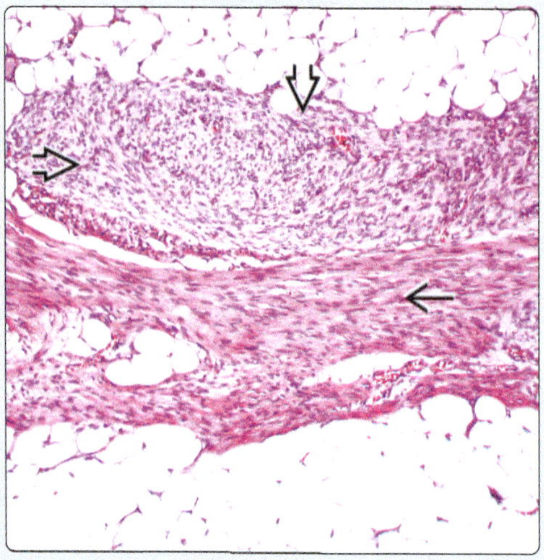

(Left) *This example shows all the components of FHI, namely fat ➡, fibrous tissue resembling a fibromatosis ➡, and more primitive-appearing cells ➡. These tumors are benign.* **(Right)** *This field demonstrates nodules of immature round to ovoid cells ➡, both present within mature fat and abutting the fibrous trabeculae ➡.*

TERMINOLOGY

Abbreviations

- Fibrous hamartoma of infancy (FHI)

Definitions

- Benign superficial fibrous lesion occurring in first 2 years of life
  - Some examples detected in older children, but almost 90% arise in first 2 years of life

ETIOLOGY/PATHOGENESIS

Developmental Anomaly

- No conclusive familial or syndromic associations
  - Rare cases reported in patients with
    - Tuberous sclerosis
    - Williams syndrome
    - Proteus syndrome
    - Desmoid fibromatosis as synchronous tumor

CLINICAL ISSUES

Epidemiology

- Age
  - Infants and children up to 2 years
    - Up to 25% present at birth
  - Rarely arise in older children (reported up to 19 years old)
- Sex
  - M > F

Site

- Deep dermis or subcutis
- Most occur in upper body, especially axillary fold
  - Other sites include upper arm, shoulder, forearm, groin, thigh, chest wall, back, neck, and scalp
  - ~ 20% arise in groin area and can be concerning for embryonal rhabdomyosarcoma
- Usually solitary
  - Rarely multiple synchronous nodules

Presentation

- Rapidly enlarging mass
- Painless and often freely mobile

Natural History

- Rapid growth, which slows but does not regress

Treatment

- Complete local excision curative
  - Only occasional recurrences

Prognosis

- Excellent but can recur if incompletely excised
  - ~ 15% reported to recur owing to incomplete excision

IMAGING

General Features

- Usually nonspecific, but occasionally admixed adipose tissue can appear distinctive and suggest diagnosis

MACROSCOPIC

General Features

- Poorly defined, variegated surface
- Admixture of firm white fibrous tissue and fat
  - Some examples grossly appear purely fibrous
- Sometimes overlying skin changes (e.g., altered pigmentation)

Size

- Most up to 5 cm, but larger lesions reported
- Mean size: 3-4 cm

MICROSCOPIC

Histologic Features

- 3 distinct components in varying amounts
- Organoid growth pattern
  - Intersecting bands and trabeculae of mature fibrous tissue, comprising spindle-shaped myofibroblasts and fibroblasts
  - Nests and whorls of immature round, ovoid, or spindle cells in loose stroma
  - Interspersed mature fat
  - Lymphocytes and patent capillaries often within mesenchyme
  - ~ 1/2 of cases show pseudoangiomatous pattern in sclerotic zones
    - Appears similar to pseudoangiomatous hyperplasia in breast lesions

ANCILLARY TESTS

Immunohistochemistry

- Vimentin in both fibrous and primitive areas
- Actin and rarely CD34 or desmin in fibrous areas
- S100 in adipose tissue component
- All components negative for HMB-45
- Angiomatous pattern zones are CD34 positive
  - Negative for CD31 and D2-40
- Ki-67 labeling present in nuclei of primitive zones and pseudoangiomatous zones in various amounts
- BCL2 staining in immature zones and pseudoangiomatous zones
- **Immunolabeling not needed for diagnosis**

Genetic Testing

- Alterations reported
  - Reciprocal t(2;3)(q31;q21)
  - Complex t(6;12;8)(q25;q24.3;q13)
  - Rearrangements involving chromosomes 1, 2, 4, 17
  - Raises possibility of FHI being neoplastic rather than hamartomatous

Electron Microscopy

- Fibroblasts and myofibroblasts in fascicular areas
- Primitive mesenchymal cells in immature areas
- Irregular collagen fibers among mature fat

DIFFERENTIAL DIAGNOSIS

Fibromatosis

- Large, deep-seated masses that often infiltrate skeletal muscle
  - Classic location is shoulder girdle
  - Abdominal wall classic location in young women (these tumors express estrogen receptor)
- Equal gender incidence in childhood
  - Female predominance in young adults
  - Equal gender incidence in elderly persons
- No primitive oval cell component
  - Uniform proliferation with monotonous cellularity
- β-catenin positive in nuclei
  - Usually corresponds to mutations but to *APC* gene mutations in patients with familial adenomatous polyposis
- Many examples express actin (myofibroblastic differentiation)
- Usually CD34 and desmin negative
- Benign but prone to local recurrences

Infantile Fibromatosis/Lipofibromatosis

- Deep-seated lesions
- Predilection for distal extremities
- Can occur in older children (up to early 2nd decade) but often in babies or congenital
- No primitive oval cell component
  - Adipose tissue and fibroblastic proliferation
  - In areas where fibroblastic and fat zones merge; can simulate lipoblasts
- Prone to local recurrences owing to infiltrative growth pattern

Myofibroma

- Localized form can be found at all ages
  - Solitary lesion
- Systemic form in infants
  - Multiple lesions
  - Poor prognosis in patients with multiple pulmonary lesions
- Nodular proliferations of myofibroblastic cells (actin positive, desmin negative)
- Hemangiopericytoma-like areas
  - Biphasic pattern with hypocellular nodular myoid areas and cellular hemangiopericytoma-like areas

Inclusion Body Fibromatosis (Infantile Digital Fibromatosis)

- Arises in digits of infants (usually detected in 1st year of life)
- Prone to local recurrence but benign
- ~ 1/3 congenital
- Fibroblastic lesion of fingers and toes
- Spindle cells and cytoplasmic inclusions that correspond to actin filaments

Lipoblastoma

- Trunk and extremities most common sites
- 90% found in first 3 years of life
- Rare examples in older children
- Slight male predominance
- Lobulated architecture
- Immature adipocytes (lipoblasts) in areas with rich vascularity
  - These areas mature to mature fat if the lesion is left in place
- Alterations of *PLAG1* gene on chromosome 8
  - Various fusions (such as *COL3A1*, *RAB2A)*
- Diffuse form (lipoblastomatosis) more aggressive
- Benign but can be confused with myxoid liposarcoma
- Lacks the fusions of *FUS* (TUS) and *DDIT3* (CHOP) that characterize myxoid liposarcoma

Embryonal Rhabdomyosarcoma

- Occurs in older children but can arise in genital region of infants (botryoid type)
  - Botryoid form has cambium layer of malignant cells proliferating just beneath epithelium
- Cytologic atypia and mitoses present
- Desmin (+), myogenin, MYOD1(+)
  - Myogenin labeling can be focal
- Not translocation sarcoma (in contrast to alveolar rhabdomyosarcoma)

Infantile Fibrosarcoma

- Clinically tends to mimic hemangiomas
- Most patients have good outcome following excision
- Cells in sheets and intersecting fascicles
  - Highly cellular lesion
  - Some examples have herringbone pattern
- Lack of organoid pattern
- *ETV6/NTRK3* fusion

SELECTED REFERENCES

1. Yu G et al: Fibrous hamartoma of infancy: a clinical pathological analysis of seventeen cases. Int J Clin Exp Pathol. 8(3):3374-7, 2015
2. Lee S et al: Ultrasonographic features of fibrous hamartoma of infancy. Skeletal Radiol. 43(5):649-53, 2014
3. Saab ST et al: Fibrous hamartoma of infancy: a clinicopathologic analysis of 60 cases. Am J Surg Pathol. 38(3):394-401, 2014
4. Stensby JD et al: Benign fibrous hamartoma of infancy: a case of MR imaging paralleling histologic findings. Skeletal Radiol. 43(11):1639-43, 2014
5. Trivedi D et al: Fibrous tumor of the superior oblique tendon in Proteus syndrome. J AAPOS. 17(4):420-2, 2013
6. Tassano E et al: Cytogenetic characterization of a fibrous hamartoma of infancy with complex translocations. Cancer Genet Cytogenet. 201(1):66-9, 2010
7. Rougemont AL et al: A complex translocation (6;12;8)(q25;q24.3;q13) in a fibrous hamartoma of infancy. Cancer Genet Cytogenet. 171(2):115-8, 2006
8. Lakshminarayanan R et al: Fibrous hamartoma of infancy: a case report with associated cytogenetic findings. Arch Pathol Lab Med. 129(4):520-2, 2005
9. Popek EJ et al: Fibrous hamartoma of infancy in the genital region: findings in 15 cases. J Urol. 152(3):990-3, 1994
10. Sotelo-Avila C et al: Subdermal fibrous hamartoma of infancy: pathology of 40 cases and differential diagnosis. Pediatr Pathol. 14(1):39-52, 1994
11. Efem SE et al: Clinicopathological features of untreated fibrous hamartoma of infancy. J Clin Pathol. 46(6):522-4, 1993
12. Michal M et al: Fibrous hamartoma of infancy. A study of eight cases with immunohistochemical and electron microscopical findings. Pathol Res Pract. 188(8):1049-53, 1992
13. Groisman G et al: Fibrous hamartoma of infancy: an immunohistochemical and ultrastructural study. Hum Pathol. 22(9):914-8, 1991

Fibrous Hamartoma of Infancy at Low Magnification

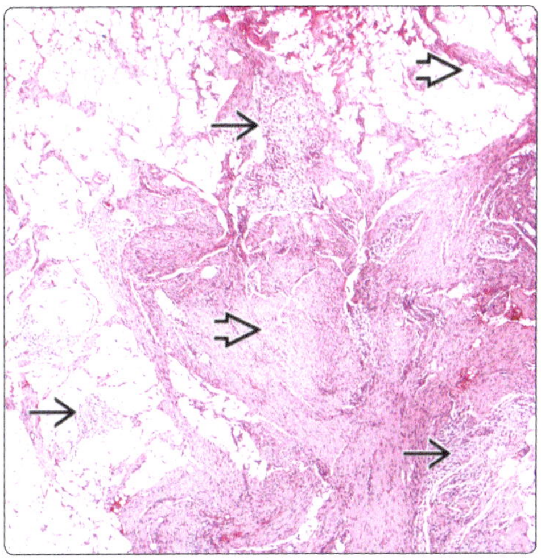

Fibrous Hamartoma of Infancy

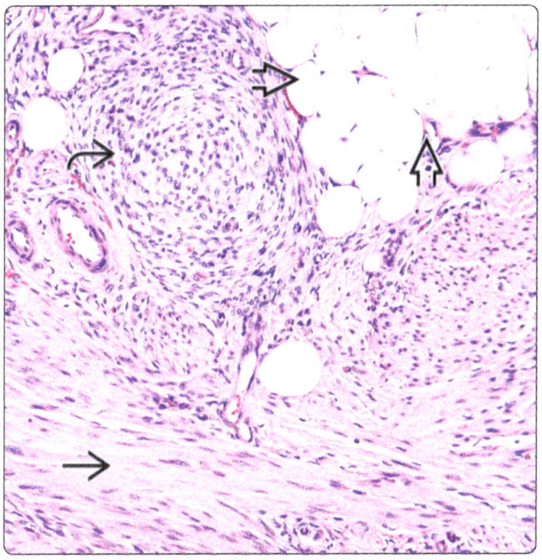

(Left) *Low magnification of FHI is shown. The lesion is poorly defined, with nodules of rounded to ovoid cells ⇨ and fibrous bands of spindle cells → admixed with mature fat.* **(Right)** *This field shows the 3 key components of FHI. The so-called primitive cells are on the upper left ↷, intimately admixed with the fibrous → and fat ⇨ elements.*

Fibrous Hamartoma of Infancy: Oval Cells

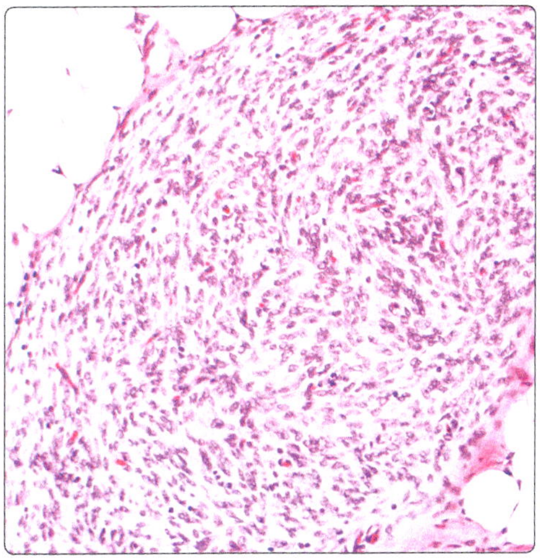

Fibrous Hamartoma of Infancy With Myxoid Stroma

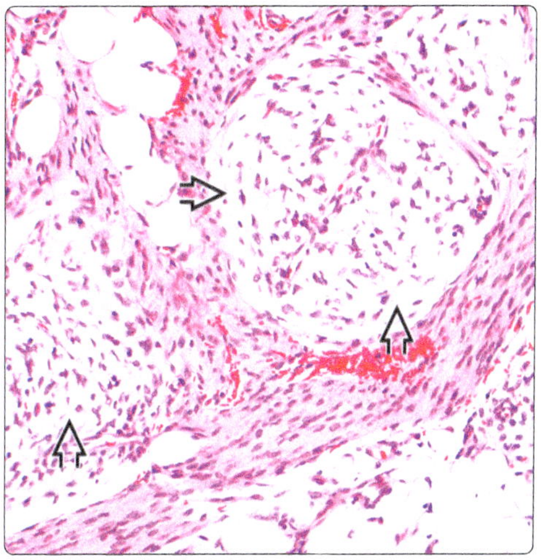

(Left) *This zone shows sheets of immature cells with bland, ovoid vesicular nuclei. Mitotic figures are absent.* **(Right)** *High magnification shows the 3 components of FHI. There is prominent myxoid stroma within the nodules ⇨. No cellular atypia is seen in any of the elements.*

Fibrous Hamartoma of Infancy: Vessels

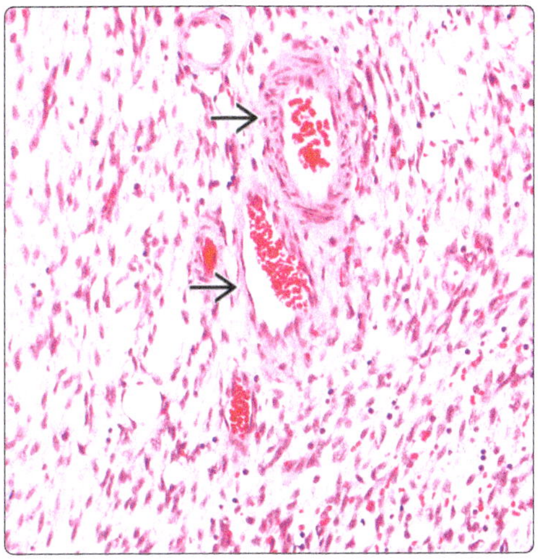

Fibrous Hamartoma of Infancy: Pseudoangiomatous Pattern

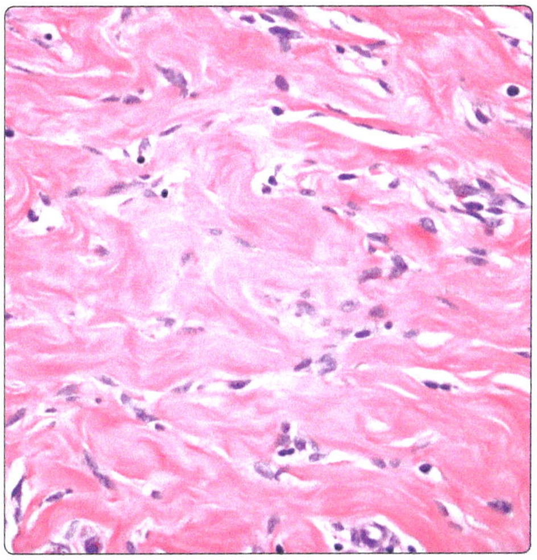

(Left) *High magnification of an FHI shows that the myxoid zones are often oriented around small veins →.* **(Right)** *Many examples of FHI show a pseudoangiomatous pattern. This component is CD34 reactive but does not express other vascular markers (D2-40, CD31).*

Differential Diagnosis: Myofibroma

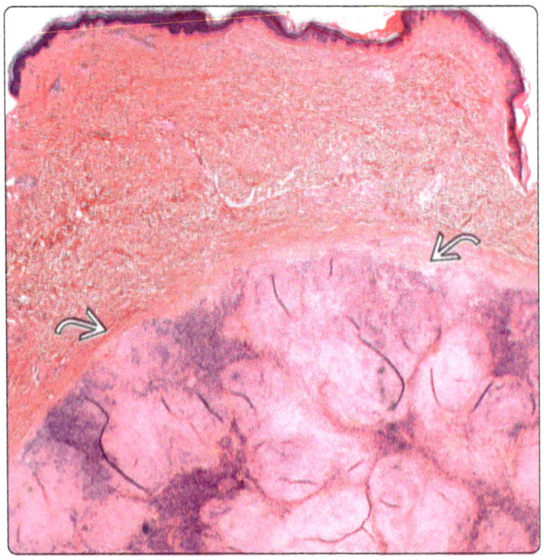

Differential Diagnosis: Myofibroma at Higher Magnification

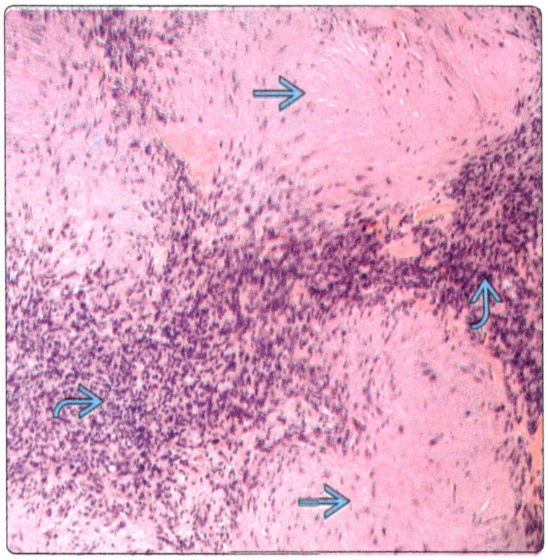

(Left) *Myofibroma is a benign myofibroblastic tumor that may arise in the deep dermis or subcutaneous tissue. It is composed of well-circumscribed nodules → of spindle cells with a myxohyalinized to chondroid-appearing stroma.* **(Right)** *Higher magnification shows the hypocellular lobules of myoid cells → surrounded by more cellular spindle cell areas → (hemangiopericytomatous zones).*

Differential Diagnosis: Myofibroma at Higher Magnification

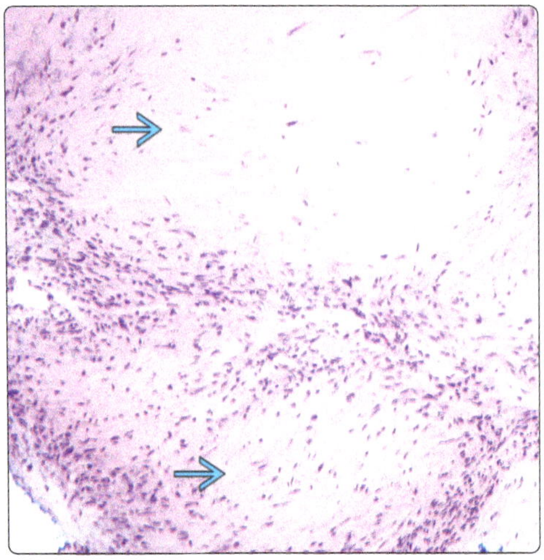

Differential Diagnosis: Infantile Digital Fibromatosis/Inclusion Body Fibromatosis

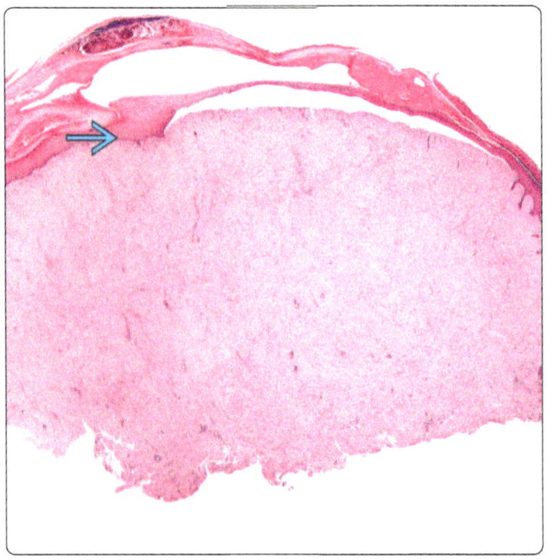

(Left) *High magnification of the lobules of myoid cells → is shown. In contrast to FHI, these lesions are biphasic (myoid lobules and hemangiopericytomatous zones) rather than triphasic (fat, fibrous zones, and primitive cells).* **(Right)** *These lesions arise on the digits of babies and proliferate up to the overlying skin →. At low power, they resemble deep fibromatosis.*

Differential Diagnosis: Infantile Digital Fibromatosis at Higher Magnification

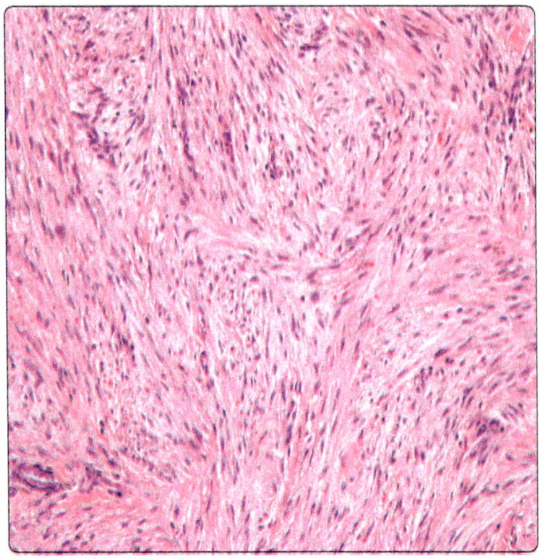

Differential Diagnosis: Infantile Digital Fibromatosis at High Magnification

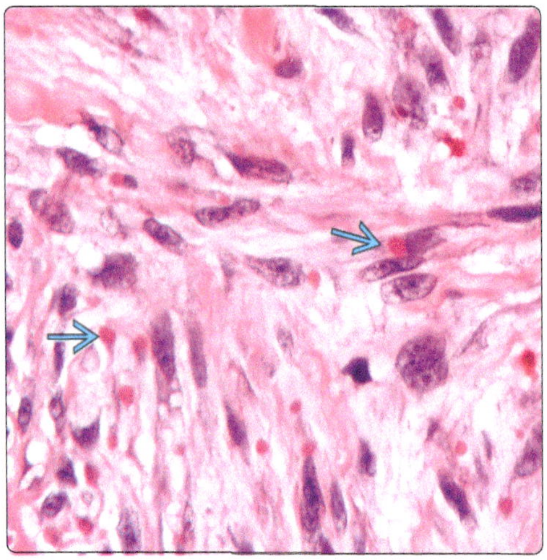

(Left) *The tumor has a pale eosinophilic appearance at intermediate magnification. The characteristic inclusion bodies are not discernible at this magnification. Note the vague storiform pattern.* **(Right)** *Note the brightly eosinophilic inclusion bodies →. Ultrastructurally, they correspond to actin filaments, which can be demonstrated by immunolabeling as well.*

Differential Diagnosis: Deep Fibromatosis (Desmoid Tumor)

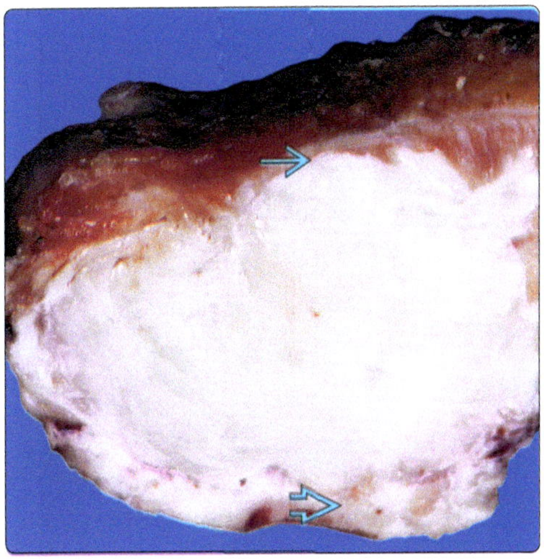

Differential Diagnosis: Deep Fibromatosis (Desmoid Tumor)

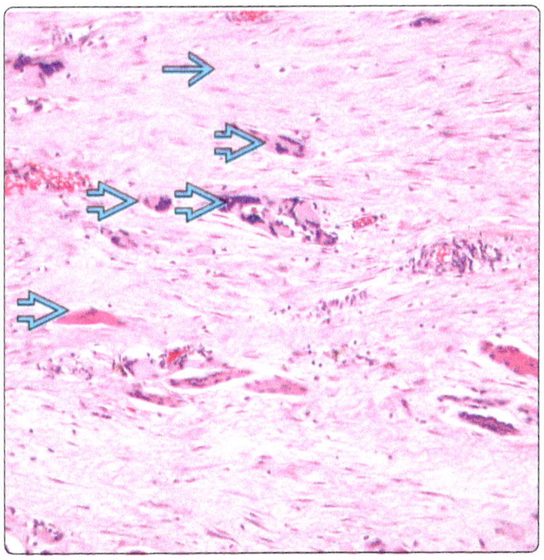

(Left) *This is a large, deep mass that was clinically recurrent. It has a firm cut surface and shows an infiltrative pattern ➡ at the bottom of the field. However, in some areas, the lesion is deceptively well marginated ➡.* **(Right)** *The lesion is pale ➡ and consists of myofibroblastic cells. There is entrapped damaged skeletal muscle ➡ in the field, which appears brightly eosinophilic.*

Differential Diagnosis: Deep Fibromatosis at High Magnification

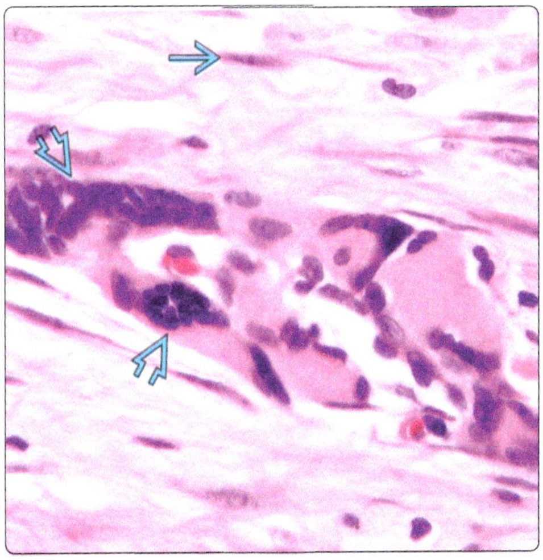

Differential Diagnosis: Fibromatosis With β-Catenin Expression

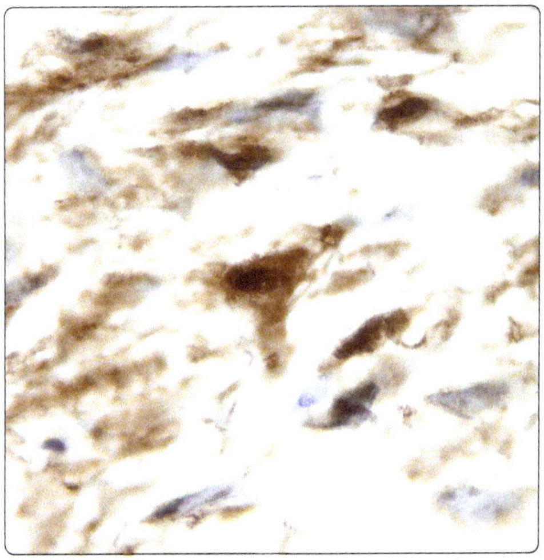

(Left) *High magnification shows the delicate nuclear membrane and small, round nucleoli in fibromatosis ➡. Note the damaged skeletal myocytes with multinucleating ➡. Their nuclei coalesce to create an alarming appearance, but they are devoid of mitotic activity.* **(Right)** *Note the nuclear labeling that characterizes fibromatosis. Cytoplasmic or membranous labeling alone does not confirm the interpretation of desmoid fibromatosis.*

Differential Diagnosis: Embryonal Rhabdomyosarcoma, Mucosal Biopsy

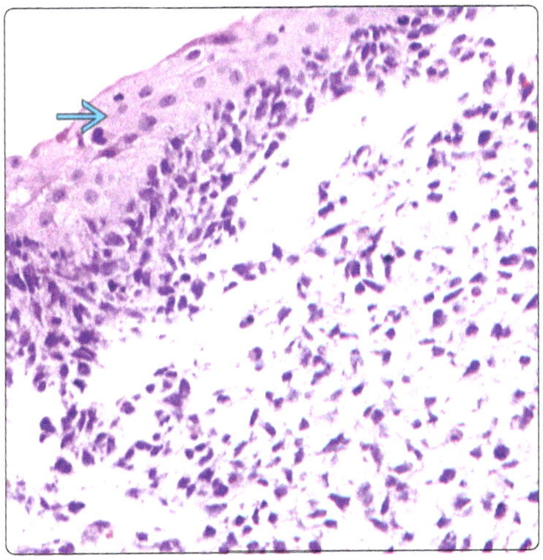

Differential Diagnosis: Myogenin Immunolabeling in Embryonal Rhabdomyosarcoma

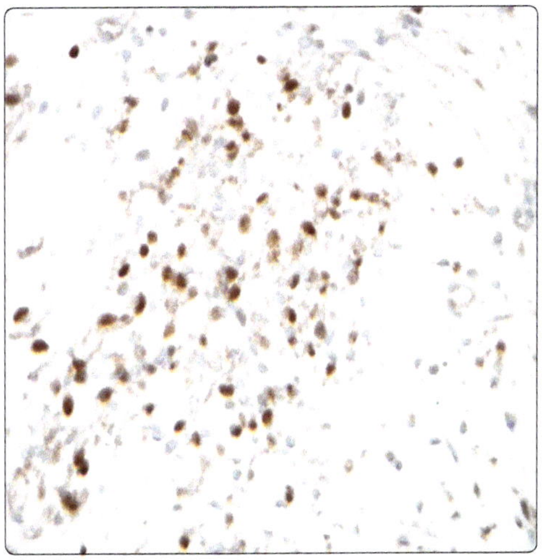

(Left) *This is a bladder lesion (the overlying epithelium shows squamous features ➡). The malignant cells are larger and more hyperchromatic than those in the primitive component of FHI.* **(Right)** *Not every nucleus labels, which is typical in embryonal rhabdomyosarcoma. In contrast, alveolar rhabdomyosarcomas usually display diffuse nuclear labeling with myogenin antibodies.*

KEY FACTS

TERMINOLOGY

- Benign proliferation of fibroblasts and myofibroblasts containing scattered eosinophilic inclusion bodies that occur on digits of young children

CLINICAL ISSUES

- Rare fibroblastic/myofibroblastic neoplasm
- Occurs usually in 1st year of life
- Dorsal aspects of hands or feet
- Presents with digital enlargement
- Dome-shaped swelling overlying phalanges or interphalangeal joints
- Extradigital soft tissues (i.e., arm, breast) are extremely rarely affected
- May recur locally, but excellent prognosis
- May show spontaneous regression
- Local excision with preservation of function

MACROSCOPIC

- Ill-defined neoplasms

MICROSCOPIC

- Infiltrating fascicles
- Uniform spindle-shaped tumor cells
- No significant cytologic atypia
- Pale eosinophilic, fibrillary cytoplasm
- Intracytoplasmic eosinophilic spherical inclusions
- Inclusions are trichrome positive

ANCILLARY TESTS

- Spindled cells show features of myofibroblasts
- Expression of actins, desmin, calponin, and CD99
  - No nuclear β-catenin labeling but cytoplasmic labeling common
- Inclusions show granular &/or filamentous features by EM
- Cytoplasmic filaments extend onto inclusions

Infantile Digital Fibromatosis/Inclusion Body Fibromatosis

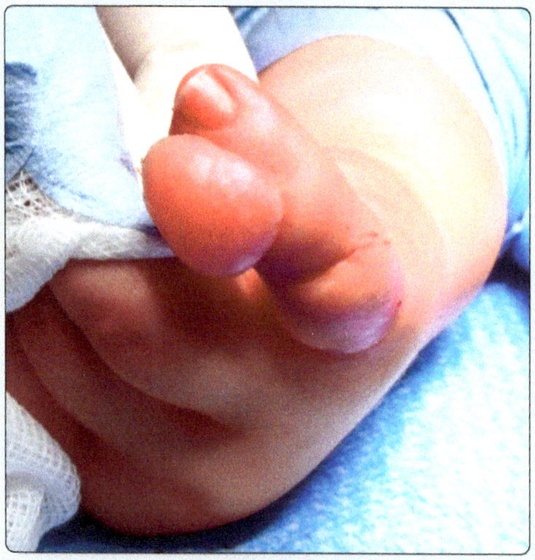

Infantile Digital Fibromatosis, Low Magnification

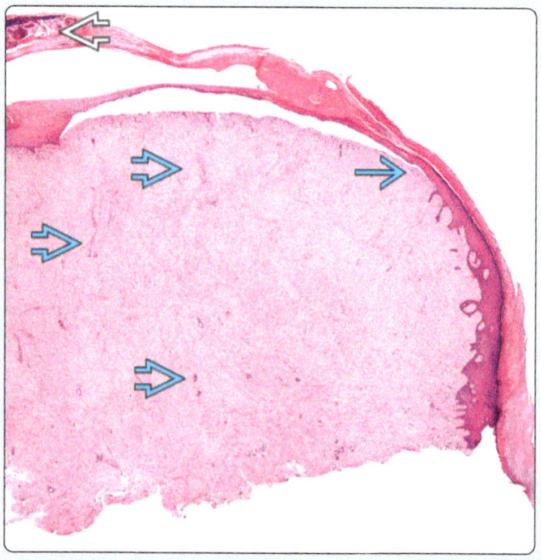

(Left) *Clinical examination of infantile digital fibromatosis shows an exophytic, dome-shaped superficial neoplasm, which presents in infants and small children.* **(Right)** *At low magnification, the lesion is plastered against the overlying skin ⇨. Because it is pale, tiny capillaries ⇨ are readily apparent even at low magnification. This example has a surface erosion with exudate ➡.*

Infantile Digital Fibromatosis, Storiform Architecture

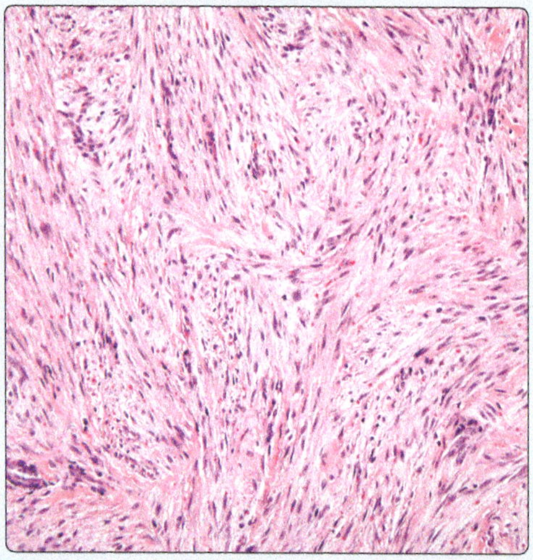

Infantile Digital Fibromatosis, Cytologic Features

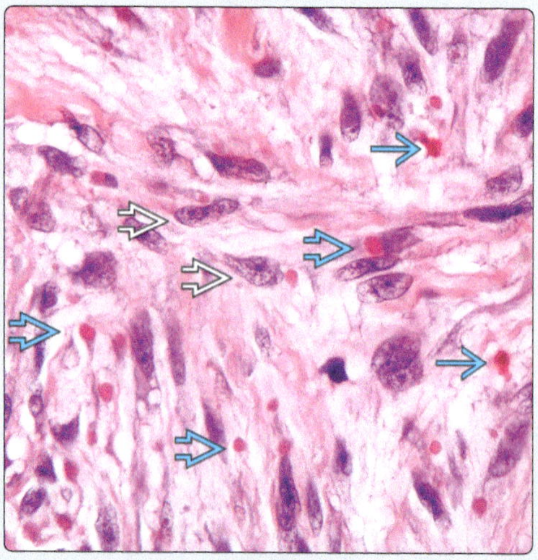

(Left) *Note the storiform pattern of this tumor at intermediate magnification. The process is myofibroblastic, so it is not as brightly eosinophilic as a smooth muscle tumor.* **(Right)** *Note the eosinophilic inclusion bodies ⇨, which consist of actin filaments. They are not as eosinophilic as erythrocytes →. This image also shows the delicate nuclear chromatin in the myofibroblastic cells ➡ of the lesion. Most of the nuclei display delicate nucleoli.*

TERMINOLOGY

Synonyms

- Infantile digital fibromatosis
  - Infantile digital fibroma
- Inclusion body fibromatosis (term used by World Health Organization)

Definitions

- Benign proliferation of fibroblasts and myofibroblasts, containing scattered eosinophilic spherical inclusions, that arises on digits (both fingers and toes) of young children

CLINICAL ISSUES

Epidemiology

- Incidence
  - Rare fibroblastic/myofibroblastic neoplasm
- Age
  - Most cases occur in 1st year of life, occasional cases in older children
  - Very rare in adult patients
- Sex
  - M = F

Site

- Dorsal aspects of hands or feet most common
- Rarely synchronous or asynchronous involvement of > 1 digit
- Thumb or great toe is only very rarely affected
- Extradigital soft tissues (i.e., arm, breast) are only extremely rarely affected

Presentation

- Digital enlargement
- Dome-shaped swelling overlying phalanges or interphalangeal joints
- Nontender nodules
- Rarely erosion of bone

Natural History

- May recur locally
- May regress spontaneously
- No progression
- No metastases

Treatment

- Surgical approaches
  - Local excision with preservation of function

Prognosis

- Excellent overall prognosis
- May recur locally
- May show spontaneous regression
- Main prognostic indicator is adequacy of primary excision

MACROSCOPIC

General Features

- Ill-defined neoplasm
- Dermal-based neoplasm with gray-white, indurated cut surface covered by intact skin
- No areas of hemorrhage
- No areas of necrosis

Size

- Nodules of variable size
  - Usually measure < 2 cm

MICROSCOPIC

Histologic Features

- Dermal tumor composed of infiltrating fascicles and sheets of spindle cells
- Uniform-appearing spindle-shaped fibroblasts and myofibroblasts
- No significant cytologic atypia
- Elongated spindled nuclei
- Pale eosinophilic, fibrillary cytoplasm
- Intracytoplasmic eosinophilic spherical inclusions
  - Often show perinuclear localization
  - Lack of refringence helps in distinction from erythrocytes
  - Stain red with Masson trichrome
  - PAS(-)
- Rare mitoses
- Variable amounts of extracellular collagen

Predominant Pattern/Injury Type

- Fascicular
- Infiltrative

Predominant Cell/Compartment Type

- Myofibroblast

ANCILLARY TESTS

Immunohistochemistry

- Tumor cells are typically actin positive, desmin negative
  - Some cases may show focal desmin staining

Electron Microscopy

- Spindled cells show features of myofibroblasts
- Tumor cells contain rough endoplasmic reticulum and cytoplasmic aggregates of filaments
- Scattered dense bodies
- Inclusions show granular &/or filamentous features
- Cytoplasmic filaments extend onto inclusions

DIFFERENTIAL DIAGNOSIS

Dermatofibroma

- Often presents on extremities, but not usually on digits
- Acanthotic, hyperpigmented epidermis
- Stellate appearance with irregular borders
- Storiform growth pattern
- Tumor cells surround hyalinized collagen bundles
- Admixture of plump spindled and histiocytoid tumor cells
- May show multinucleated giant cells
- May contain hemosiderin deposits
- Lack of cytoplasmic inclusions

Pilar Leiomyoma

- Adult patients, typically not on digits
- Lobules and bundles of spindled cells
- Bright eosinophilic, fibrillary cytoplasm with perinuclear vacuoles

Immunohistochemistry

Antibody	Reactivity	Staining Pattern	Comment
Actin-sm	Positive	Cytoplasmic inclusion	Parallel positivity beneath cell membrane; eosinophilic globules are variably positive
Desmin	Negative	Cytoplasmic	Most cases negative, but can be focally positive
Calponin	Positive	Cytoplasmic	
CD99	Positive	Cytoplasmic	
Caldesmon	Negative		
S100	Negative		
β-catenin	Negative	Cytoplasmic	Can display nonspecific cytoplasmic labeling, but no nuclear staining
CD34	Negative		

- Spindle-shaped, blunt-ended nuclei
- Lack of cytoplasmic inclusions
- Actin and desmin positive

Neurofibroma

- Usually adult patients
- Elongated spindled tumor cells
- Spindled to wavy or wrinkled-appearing nuclei
- Lack of cytoplasmic inclusions
- S100 strongly positive
- Muscle markers negative

Extraneural Spindle Cell Perineurioma

- Usually adult patients
- Elongated spindled tumor cells
- May show perivascular accentuation
- Lack of cytoplasmic inclusions
- EMA(+)
- Muscle markers negative

Dermatomyofibroma

- Does not occur in 1st years of life
- Does not occur on fingers and toes
- Plaque-like dermal neoplasms
- Bundles of spindle cells oriented parallel to epidermis
- Tumor cells grow around preexisting adnexal structures
- Lack of cytoplasmic inclusions
- Increased number of fragmented elastic fibers

Superficial Acral Fibromyxoma

- Usually in adults
- Typically involves fingers and toes
- Varying myxoid and collagenous stroma
- Lack of cytoplasmic inclusions
- No/focal expression of actins
- Frequent expression of EMA

Desmoid Fibromatosis

- Involves proximal extremities, trunk
- Occurs usually in deep soft tissues
- Locally aggressive
- High rate of local recurrences
- Nuclear expression of β-catenin
- Numerous vessels
- Perivascular edema

Superficial Solitary Fibrous Tumor

- Typically adults
- Usually well-circumscribed, nodular neoplasms
- Varying cellularity
- Numerous hemangiopericytoma-like blood vessels
- No/focal expression of actins
- Usually homogeneous CD34 and Bcl-2 expression

Myofibroma

- Can affect children and adults
- Multinodular growth
- Biphasic growth
    - Small undifferentiated mesenchymal cells associated with hemangiopericytoma-like vessels
    - Mature, spindled, eosinophilic myofibroblasts
- Myxohyaline stroma
- Lack of cytoplasmic inclusions

DIAGNOSTIC CHECKLIST

Clinically Relevant Pathologic Features

- Organ distribution
- Age distribution

Pathologic Interpretation Pearls

- Ill-defined dermal neoplasms
- Proliferation of fibroblastic/myofibroblastic tumor cells
- Bland cytology of neoplastic cells
- Tumor cells contain characteristic cytoplasmic inclusions
- Expression of actins

SELECTED REFERENCES

1. Henderson H et al: Anti-calponin 1 antibodies highlight intracytoplasmic inclusions of infantile digital fibromatosis. Histopathology. 64(5):752-5, 2014
2. Quick T et al: Case report of an ulcerated infantile digital fibromatosis in an older child. The lump to spot in the child's hand (a spot not to lump in with the others). J Hand Surg Eur Vol. 39(8):888-9, 2014
3. Laskin WB et al: Infantile digital fibroma/fibromatosis: a clinicopathologic and immunohistochemical study of 69 tumors from 57 patients with long-term follow-up. Am J Surg Pathol. 33(1):1-13, 2009
4. Niamba P et al: Further documentation of spontaneous regression of infantile digital fibromatosis. Pediatr Dermatol. 24(3):280-4, 2007
5. Choi KC et al: Infantile digital fibromatosis. Immunohistochemical and immunoelectron microscopic studies. J Cutan Pathol. 17(4):225-32, 1990
6. Bhawan J et al: A myofibroblastic tumor. Infantile digital fibroma (recurrent digital fibrous tumor of childhood). Am J Pathol. 94(1):19-36, 1979

Infantile Digital Fibromatosis

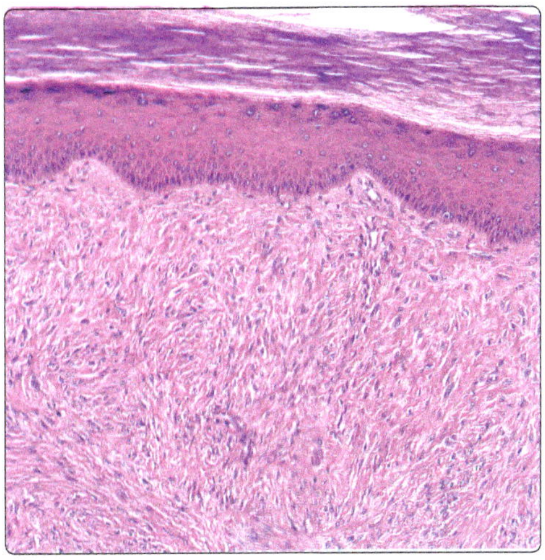

Infantile Digital Fibromatosis, Higher Magnification

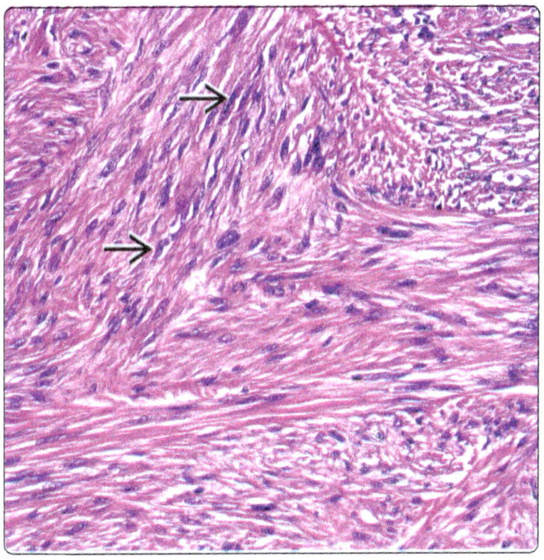

(Left) *Histology of digital fibromatosis shows a moderately cellular spindle cell neoplasm of the superficial dermis. There is no grenz zone between the lesion and the overlying squamous epithelium.* **(Right)** *The neoplasm shows ill-defined fascicles composed of cytologically bland-appearing, spindled fibroblasts and myofibroblasts with pale eosinophilic cytoplasm and elongated, spindle-shaped nuclei →.*

Infantile Digital Fibromatosis, Low Magnification

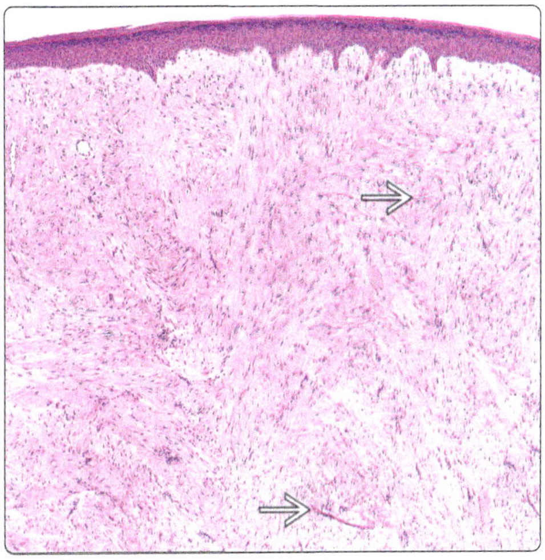

Infantile Digital Fibromatosis, Inclusion Bodies

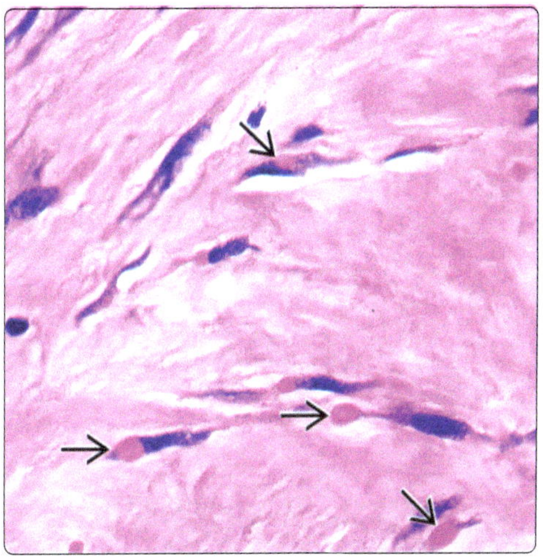

(Left) *A relatively hypocellular spindle cell neoplasm is seen in this case. The neoplastic cells are set in a collagenous stroma. Since the proliferating cells are pale, the delicate stromal capillaries are readily identified →.* **(Right)** *High magnification shows numerous cytoplasmic inclusions → in this case. The background in this field is heavily collagenized. The inclusions, believed in the past to reflect viral material, are now known to contain actin filaments.*

Infantile Digital Fibromatosis, Actin Stain

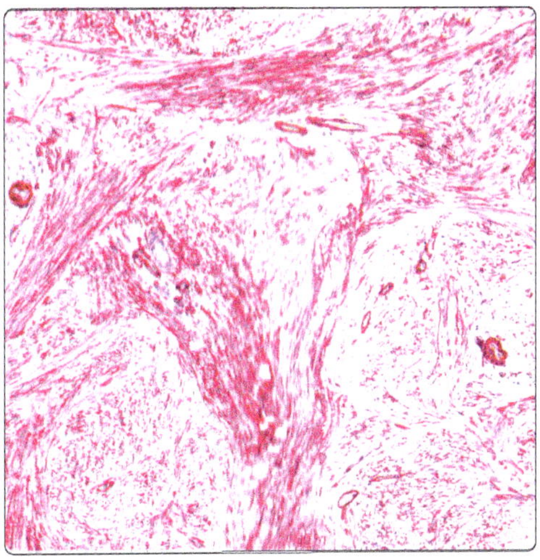

Infantile Digital Fibromatosis, Desmin Stain (Focal)

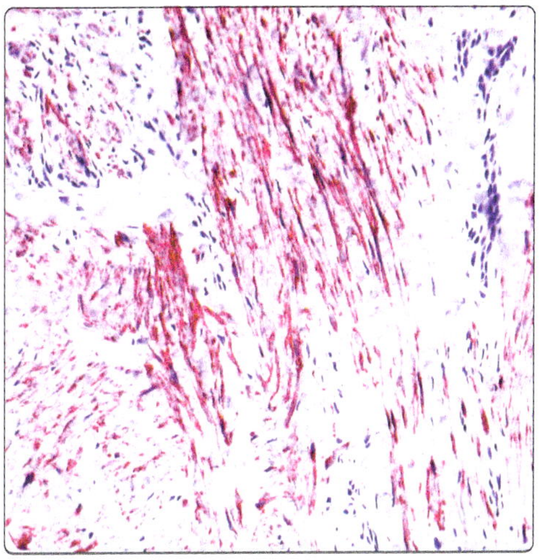

(Left) *Neoplastic cells in digital fibromatosis stain positively for actin-sm in most cases. This feature indicates myofibroblastic differentiation rather than true smooth muscle differentiation. Desmin stains are usually, but not invariably, negative. In general, it is not necessary to perform immunostaining on these lesions, as their routine histologic features (with inclusion bodies) are diagnostic.* **(Right)** *In some cases, focal expression of desmin may be present.*

Angiomyofibroblastoma

KEY FACTS

TERMINOLOGY

- Benign genital stromal tumor composed of fibroblasts oriented around a prominent capillary vasculature

CLINICAL ISSUES

- Occurs in women between 35-60 years (median: 46 years)
- Vulva and vagina most common sites
- Slow-growing, painless mass
- Treatment: Simple local excision
- Benign

MACROSCOPIC

- Superficial, well-circumscribed, solid mass

MICROSCOPIC

- Nonencapsulated
- Alternating zones of cellularity
- Prominent vascular component
- Plump epithelioid, ovoid, or plasmacytoid tumor cells with eosinophilic cytoplasm
  - Cells characteristically cluster around thin-walled capillaries
- In postmenopausal patients, cells are more spindled, and overall cellularity is low
- Mature adipose tissue component in minority of cases
- Some cases show morphologic overlap with cellular angiofibroma

ANCILLARY TESTS

- Desmin (+), ER(+), PR(+)
- Usually CD34(-) and SMA(-)

TOP DIFFERENTIAL DIAGNOSES

- Deep (aggressive) angiomyxoma
- Cellular angiofibroma
- Fibroepithelial stromal polyp

AMFB at Low Magnification

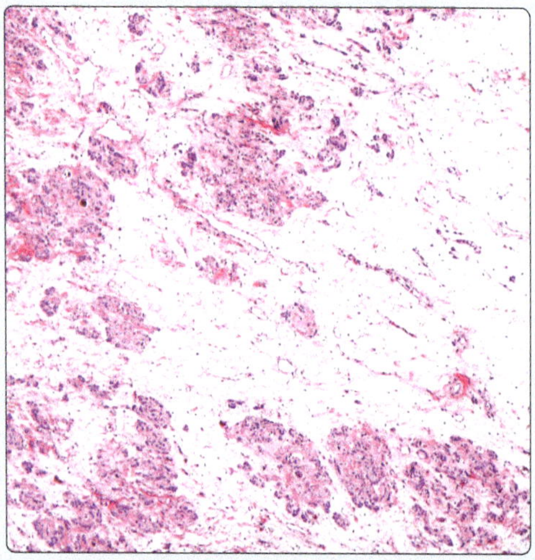

AMFB With Fibrous Areas

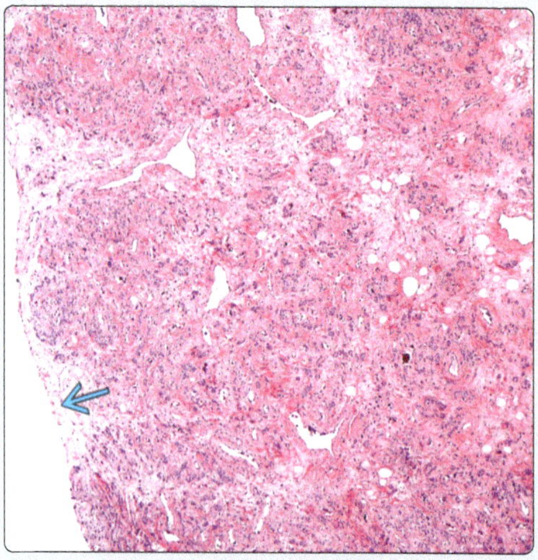

(Left) *Angiomyofibroblastoma (AMFB) is a distinctive, benign neoplasm of the lower female genital tract. At low magnification, the classic morphologic pattern is that of irregular zones of cellularity within a myxoid or fibrous stroma.* **(Right)** *Some areas of AMFB are less myxoid and more fibrous, as seen here. Note the sharp circumscription →, a feature seen in most examples.*

AMFB With Alternating Zones of Cellularity

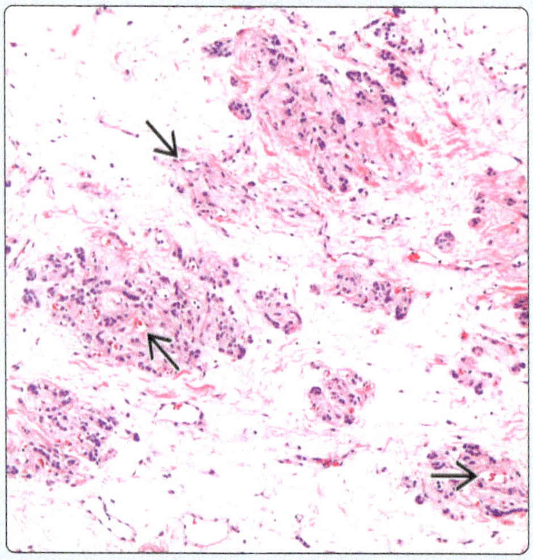

Perivascular Organization in AMFB

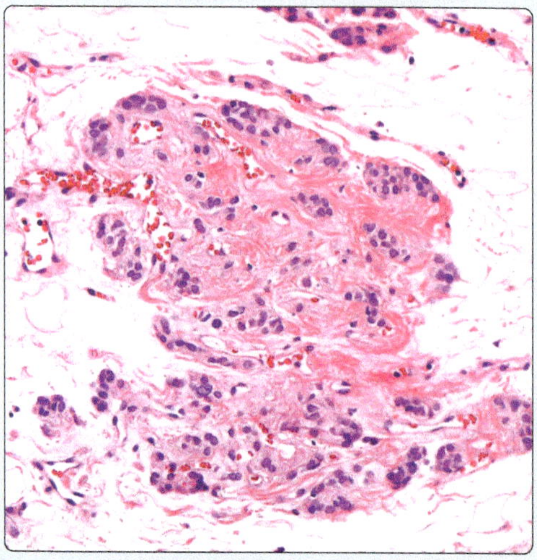

(Left) *The neoplastic cells of AMFB are characteristically clustered around small, thin-walled capillary channels →, which can often be recognized by the presence of intraluminal erythrocytes. The intervening myxoid stroma is hypocellular.* **(Right)** *In classic cases of AMFB, the tumor cells are epithelioid, ovoid, or plasmacytoid-appearing, and form small nests or clusters around capillary channels. This perivascular orientation is characteristic of this tumor.*

TERMINOLOGY

Abbreviations

- Angiomyofibroblastoma (AMFB)

Definitions

- Benign genital stromal tumor composed of fibroblasts oriented around a prominent capillary vasculature

CLINICAL ISSUES

Epidemiology

- Age
  - Generally 35-60 years (median: 46 years)
- Sex
  - Affects women almost exclusively

Site

- Vulva (most common) and vagina
- Rarely perineum or inguinal region

Presentation

- Slow-growing, painless mass
  - Often mistaken clinically for Bartholin cyst

Treatment

- Simple local excision

Prognosis

- Benign
- Very rare recurrences reported

MACROSCOPIC

General Features

- Well-circumscribed solid mass
- Tan-white coloration
- Rubbery or mucoid cut surface

Size

- Usually < 5 cm

MICROSCOPIC

Histologic Features

- Nonencapsulated
- Alternating zones of cellularity
  - Hypocellular zones often myxoid or edematous
- Prominent vascular component
  - Numerous thin-walled capillaries
- Plump epithelioid, ovoid, or plasmacytoid tumor cells with eosinophilic cytoplasm
  - Singly or in cords or small nests
  - Cells characteristically cluster around thin-walled capillaries
  - Cells may show multinucleation
- Mast cells common
- In postmenopausal patients
  - Often less cellular
  - Cells are more spindled than epithelioid
  - Increased stromal collagen
- Mature adipose tissue component in minority of cases
- Some cases of AMFB show morphologic overlap with cellular angiofibroma
- Very rare reports describing malignant transformation

ANCILLARY TESTS

Immunohistochemistry

- Desmin (+)
- Often ER(+) and PR(+)
- Usually CD34(-) and SMA(-)
- Negative for keratin and S100

DIFFERENTIAL DIAGNOSIS

Deep (Aggressive) Angiomyxoma

- Often large and deeply located
- Infiltrative margins
- Uniform cellularity (lacks perivascular orientation of AMFB)
- Contains medium to large-sized vessels
  - Overall less vascular than AMFB
- Lacks epithelioid cells
- Aberrations involving 12q13-15 (*HMGA2*)

Cellular Angiofibroma

- Some cases may show considerable overlap with AMFB
  - May appropriately classify as "benign genital stromal tumor"
- More uniformly cellular
  - May show formation of short fascicles
- Contains medium-sized vessels, often with hyalinization
  - Overall less vascular than AMFB
- Lacks epithelioid cells with perivascular orientation
- Often CD34(+)
- Most cases desmin (-)
- Loss of *RB1* (13q14)

Fibroepithelial Stromal Polyp

- Young to middle-aged women
- Typically very superficial and polypoid
  - Overlying squamous epithelium
  - No grenz zone
- Stellate and multinucleate cells are characteristic
  - Often located beneath epithelial surface at epithelial-stromal interface
- Some cases are associated with pregnancy
  - May contain bizarre nuclear atypia and mitoses (pseudosarcomatous stromal polyp)
- Desmin (+), ER(+), PR(+)

SELECTED REFERENCES

1. Luis PP et al: Lipomatous variant of angiomyofibroblastoma involving the vulva: report of 3 cases of an extremely rare neoplasm with discussion of the differential diagnosis. Int J Gynecol Pathol. 34(2):204-7, 2015
2. Schoolmeester JK et al: Genital soft tissue tumors. J Cutan Pathol. 42(7):441-51, 2015
3. Magro G et al: Vulvovaginal angiomyofibroblastomas: morphologic, immunohistochemical, and fluorescence in situ hybridization analysis for deletion of 13q14 region. Hum Pathol. 45(8):1647-55, 2014
4. Kairi-Vassilatou E et al: Angiomyofibroblastoma of the vulva: a clinicopathological and immunohistochemical analysis of a rare benign mesenchymal tumor. Eur J Gynaecol Oncol. 32(3):353-5, 2011
5. Nucci MR et al: Vulvovaginal soft tissue tumours: update and review. Histopathology. 36(2):97-108, 2000
6. Laskin WB et al: Angiomyofibroblastoma of the female genital tract: analysis of 17 cases including a lipomatous variant. Hum Pathol. 28(9):1046-55, 1997

(Left) *In addition to small clusters and nests, the tumor cells in AMFB may show a linear, corded growth pattern ⇨. This pattern may mimic the growth of lobular carcinoma of the breast or a Sertoli cell tumor.* **(Right)** *A component of mature adipose tissue is seen in a minority (~ 10%) of cases of AMFB. These tumors have been referred to as lipomatous AMFB when the fat is prominent.*

Cording Growth in AMFB

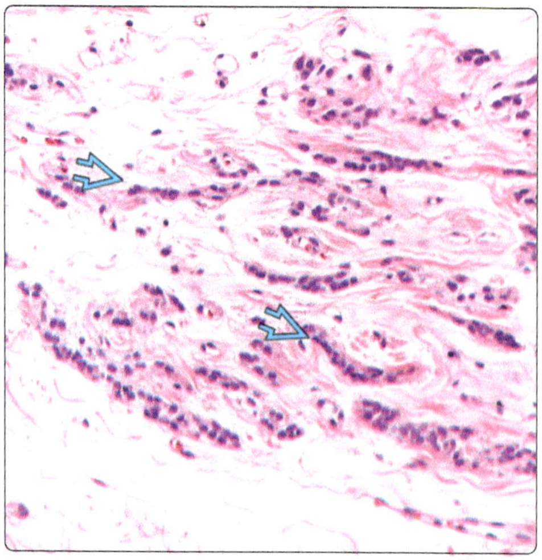

Mature Adipose Tissue in AMFB

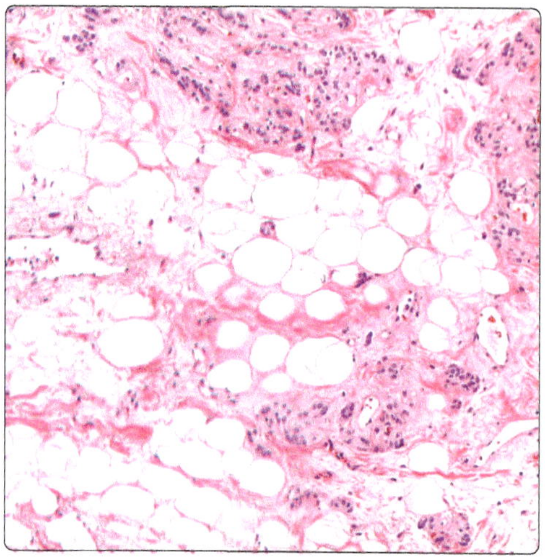

(Left) *A mild, chronic, inflammatory infiltrate ⇨ may be seen in AMFB and tends to be accentuated around the vessels. Mast cells are also a common finding.* **(Right)** *The tumor cell nuclei of AMFB are cytologically bland and may show small, inconspicuous nucleoli. Multinucleated forms → are not uncommon. Mitoses are rare.*

Chronic Inflammatory Infiltrate in AMFB

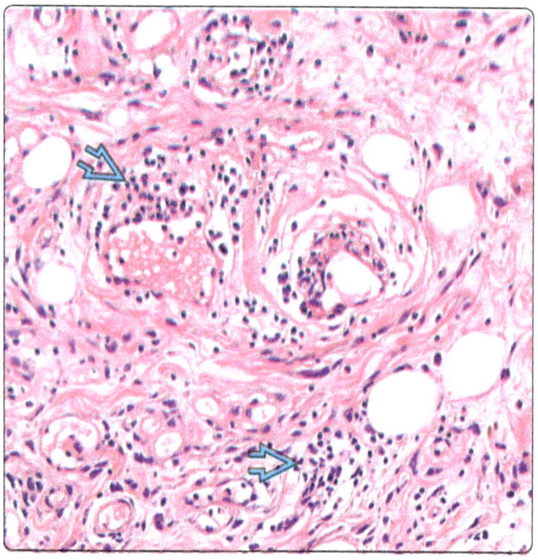

Epithelioid Cytomorphology in AMFB

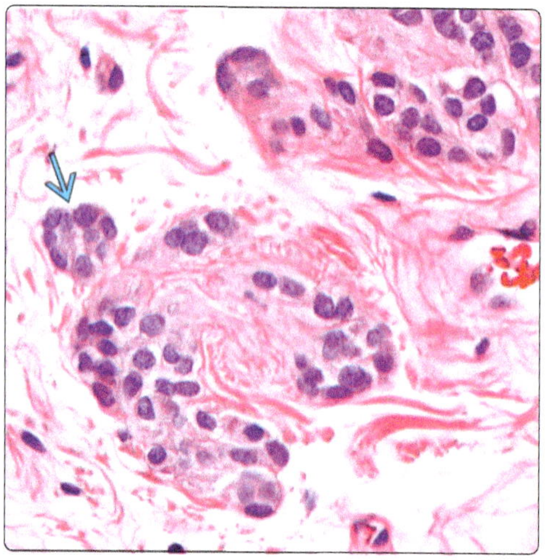

(Left) *In rare cases of AMFB, larger dilated vessels forming an ectatic staghorn pattern may be apparent. This finding is generally nonspecific, but it may raise the consideration of a solitary fibrous tumor.* **(Right)** *Although the vast majority of vessels in AMFB are thin-walled capillaries, larger thicker-walled vessels are occasionally seen.*

Vasculature in AMFB

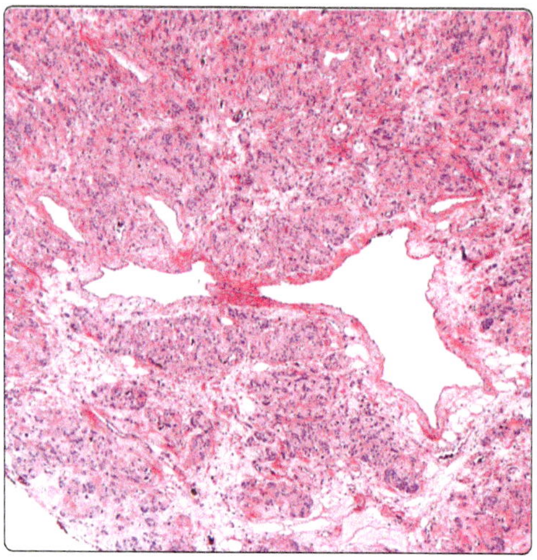

Vasculature in AMFB

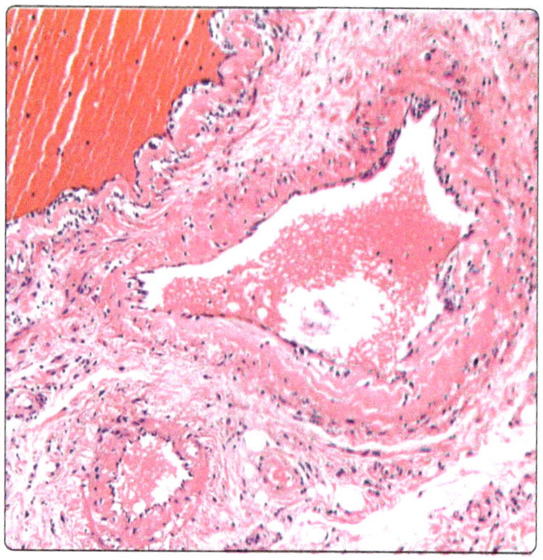

Postmenopausal Changes in AMFB

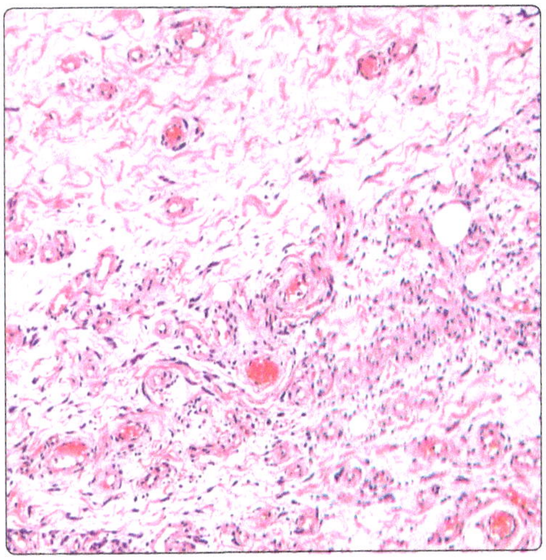

Postmenopausal Changes in AMFB

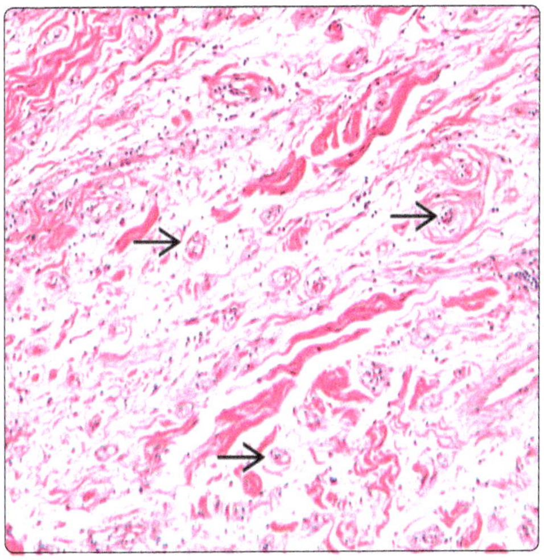

(Left) *In postmenopausal patients, AMFB often shows a drop in cellularity, as well as a tendency for the tumor cells to be more spindled and less epithelioid-shaped. Note, however, that the perivascular orientation is still maintained.* **(Right)** *Some examples of postmenopausal AMFB are markedly hypocellular and may show prominent collagen or hyalinization. Note the numerous thin-walled capillary channels* ➙.

Postmenopausal Changes in AMFB

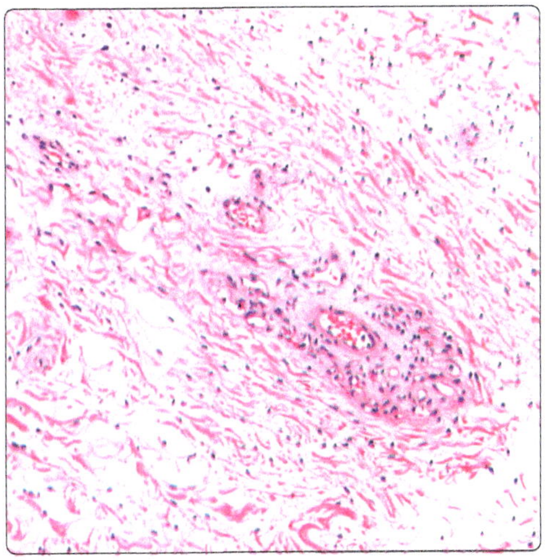

Desmin Expression in AMFB

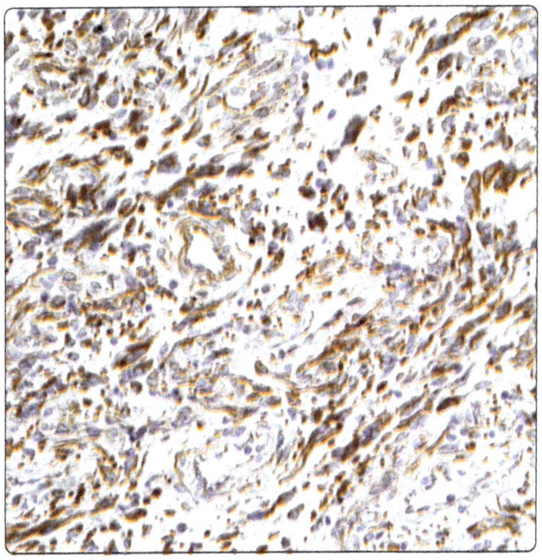

(Left) *This image of AMFB in a postmenopausal patient demonstrates a marked drop in overall cellularity but also shows how the tumor cells (more spindled rather than epithelioid) congregate around the capillary channels.* **(Right)** *The tumor cells of AMFB usually show diffuse expression of desmin. Estrogen receptor and progesterone receptor stains are often positive as well. CD34 is usually negative.*

Differential Diagnosis: Cellular Angiofibroma

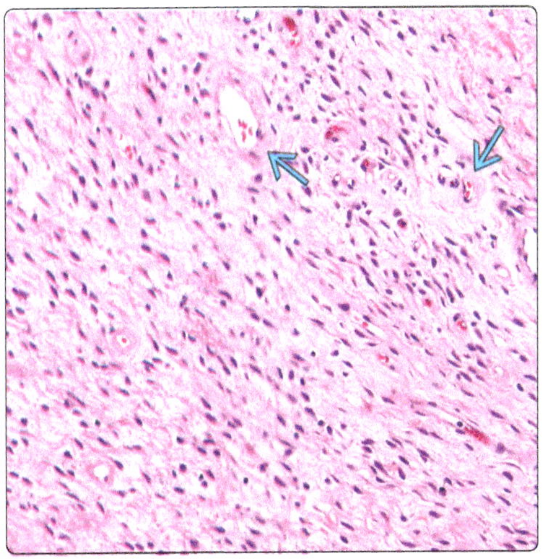

Differential Diagnosis: Deep (Aggressive) Angiomyxoma

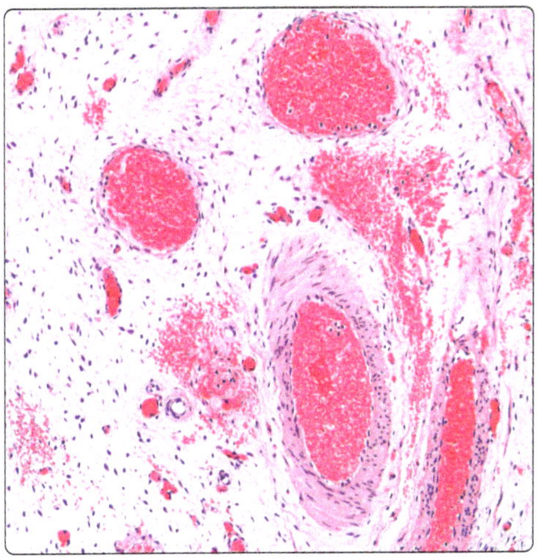

(Left) *In contrast to AMFB, cellular angiofibroma is more uniformly cellular. The vessels are often of a larger caliber and usually show at least focal hyalinization* ➙. *CD34 is also typically expressed.* **(Right)** *Deep angiomyxoma differs from AMFB in that it is often larger, more deeply located, and demonstrates a prominent component of medium to large-sized, thick-walled vessels. The uniform hypocellularity and myxoedematous stroma are also characteristic.*

Multinucleate Cell Angiohistiocytoma

KEY FACTS

TERMINOLOGY

- Proliferation of vessels and multinucleated stromal cells

ETIOLOGY/PATHOGENESIS

- May be nonneoplastic reactive process

CLINICAL ISSUES

- Usually occurs in female patients > 40 yr old
- Most cases have been reported on legs or hands
- Typically present as multiple grouped papules
- May rarely be generalized
- Excellent prognosis, no malignant potential described

MICROSCOPIC

- Increased numbers of superficial small to telangiectatic vessels
- Proliferation of enlarged, angulated multinucleated cells
- Nuclear hyperchromasia and mild atypia present
- No infiltrative features identified
- Do not show slit-like spaces suggestive of Kaposi sarcoma
- Lack of, or only rare, mitotic figures

ANCILLARY TESTS

- Multinucleated cells are typically positive for FXIIIA and vimentin
- Stromal cells are positive for FXIIIA, vimentin, and lysozyme

TOP DIFFERENTIAL DIAGNOSES

- Giant cell angioblastoma
  - Concentric arrays of spindle cells around small vessels
- Pleomorphic fibroma
  - Atypical-appearing multinucleated pleomorphic fibroblasts present
- Kaposi sarcoma
  - Proliferation of atypical spindle cells and slit-like blood vessels

Multinucleate Cell Angiohistiocytoma

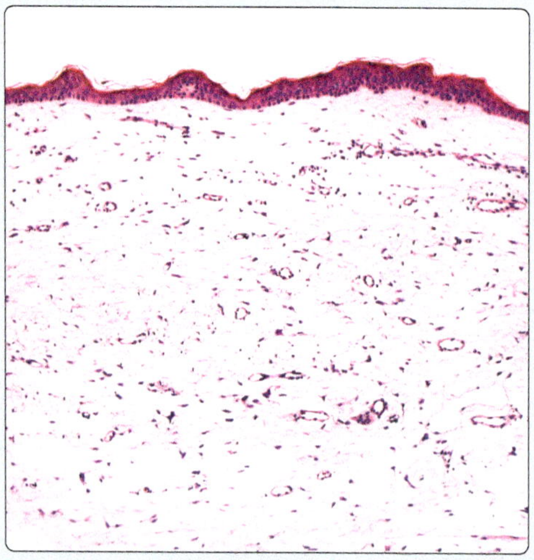

Multinucleate Cell Angiohistiocytoma at Higher Magnification

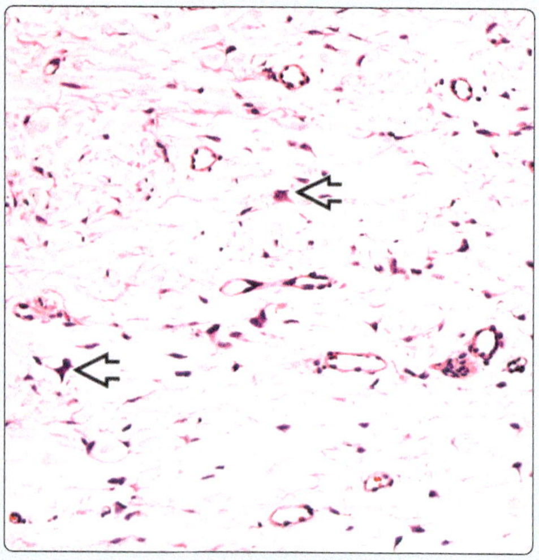

(Left) *Low-power examination of multinucleate cell angiohistiocytoma shows a dermal-based proliferation of small vessels with focal telangiectasia and increased numbers of stromal cells.* **(Right)** *Higher power view shows a proliferation of numerous small blood vessels and scattered enlarged, angulated mononuclear and multinucleated ⇨ stromal cells.*

Multinucleate Cell Angiohistiocytoma: High Magnification of Multinucleated Cells

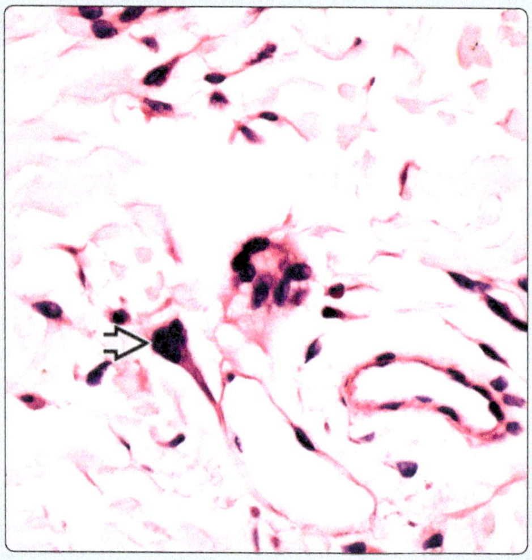

FXIIIA Immunohistochemistry

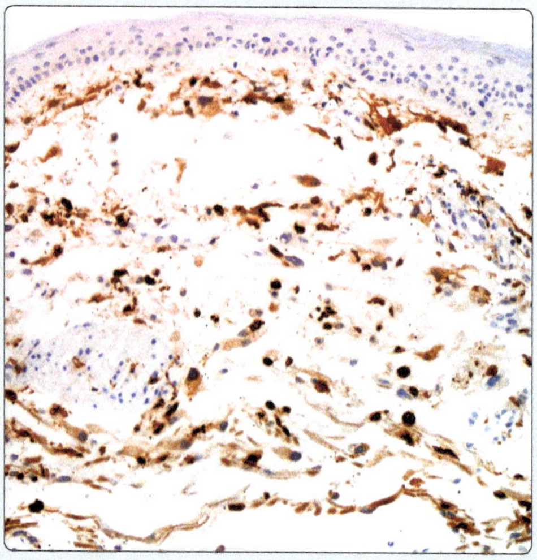

(Left) *High-power examination of the multinucleated cells shows clumping or a wreath-like arrangement of the hyperchromatic nuclei ⇨.* **(Right)** *FXIIIA immunohistochemistry shows strong cytoplasmic staining of most of the lesional cells.*

TERMINOLOGY

Abbreviations

- Multinucleate cell angiohistiocytoma (MCAH)

Definitions

- Proliferation of vessels and multinucleated stromal cells

ETIOLOGY/PATHOGENESIS

Unknown

- May actually represent nonneoplastic reactive process
- Some authors consider MCAH variant of dermatofibroma

CLINICAL ISSUES

Epidemiology

- Age
  - Usually presents in patients > 40 yr old
- Sex
  - Typically occurs in female patients

Site

- Most cases have been reported on legs (calves and thighs) or hands
  - Others sites rarely described, including oral mucosa

Presentation

- Multiple grouped round to oval papules
  - Usually described as red to violet lesions
  - May rarely be generalized
  - Rarely, may coalesce into 1 large annular lesion
- May be asymptomatic or pruritic

Prognosis

- Excellent, no malignant potential described
- Treatment not necessary; some lesions may regress spontaneously

MACROSCOPIC

General Features

- Well-circumscribed, nonencapsulated dermal-based lesion

MICROSCOPIC

Histologic Features

- Increased numbers of superficial small to telangiectatic vessels in reticular dermis
  - Endothelial cells show hyperchromatic nuclei
  - Do not show slit-like spaces suggestive of Kaposi sarcoma
- Proliferation of enlarged, angulated multinucleated cells
  - Cells contain 3-10 nuclei, which may be arranged in ring or aggregated together
  - Nuclear hyperchromasia and mild atypia present
    - However, no frank atypia or pleomorphism
  - Lack of, or only rare, mitotic figures
- No infiltrative features should be identified
- Surrounding stroma may show mild inflammatory infiltrate
  - Consists of lymphocytes, plasma cells, mast cells, and neutrophils

Predominant Pattern/Injury Type

- Vascular and fibrohistiocytic

ANCILLARY TESTS

Immunohistochemistry

- Multinucleated cells are typically positive for FXIIIA and vimentin
  - CD68 staining is variably positive
- Stromal cells are positive for FXIIIA, vimentin, and lysozyme
- Vessels are positive for CD31, CD34, and FVIIIRAg; HHV8 is negative

DIFFERENTIAL DIAGNOSIS

Giant Cell Angioblastoma

- Exceptionally rare tumor, present at birth or shortly thereafter
- Concentric arrays of spindle cells around small vessels

Pleomorphic Fibroma

- Polypoid lesion, likely related to fibroepithelial polyp
- Large, atypical-appearing multinucleated pleomorphic fibroblasts present
- Proliferation of small vessels not prominent, as in MCAH

Kaposi Sarcoma

- Proliferation of atypical spindle cells and slit-like blood vessels
- Chronic infiltrate with plasma cells usually present
- Multinucleate cells not identified
- Immunoreactive for HHV8 (nuclear staining)

DIAGNOSTIC CHECKLIST

Pathologic Interpretation Pearls

- Proliferation of enlarged, angulated multinucleated cells associated with numerous small vessels
  - Cells show 3-10 nuclei, which may be arranged in ring or clumped together

SELECTED REFERENCES

1. Frew JW: Multinucleate cell angiohistiocytoma: clinicopathological correlation of 142 cases with insights into etiology and pathogenesis. Am J Dermatopathol. 37(3):222-8, 2015
2. Wilk M et al: Generalized eruptive histiocytosis with features of multinucleate cell angiohistiocytoma. Am J Dermatopathol. ePub, 2015
3. Doshi-Chougule BN et al: Multinucleate cell angiohistiocytoma with hypertrophic nerves. J Cutan Pathol. 40(12):1048-53, 2013
4. Rawal YB et al: Multinucleate cell angiohistiocytoma: an uncommon mucosal tumour. Clin Exp Dermatol. 34(3):333-6, 2009
5. Puig L et al: Multinucleate cell angiohistiocytoma: a fibrohistiocytic proliferation with increased mast cell numbers and vascular hyperplasia. J Cutan Pathol. 29(4):232-7, 2002
6. Chang SN et al: Generalized multinucleate cell angiohistiocytoma. J Am Acad Dermatol. 35(2 Pt 2):320-2, 1996
7. Shapiro PE et al: Multinucleate cell angiohistiocytoma: a distinct entity diagnosable by clinical and histologic features. J Am Acad Dermatol. 30(3):417-22, 1994
8. Jones WE et al: Multinucleate cell angiohistiocytoma: an acquired vascular anomaly to be distinguished from Kaposi's sarcoma. Br J Dermatol. 122(5):651-63, 1990
9. Smolle J et al: Multinucleate cell angiohistiocytoma: a clinicopathological, immunohistochemical and ultrastructural study. Br J Dermatol. 121(1):113-21, 1989

Giant Cell Tumor of Tendon Sheath

KEY FACTS

TERMINOLOGY

- Synonyms: Localized-type tenosynovial giant cell, nodular tenosynovitis, localized pigmented villonodular synovitis (PVNS)
- Benign soft tissue tumor of synovial origin
- Arises from tendon sheath, intraarticular site, or bursa

ETIOLOGY/PATHOGENESIS

- Neoplastic growth
- Balanced translocation involving 1p13 (*CSF1* gene)
  - CSF1 overexpression by neoplastic stromal cells
  - Autocrine activation of neoplastic cells via CSF1R
  - Recruitment and activation of intratumoral macrophages via CSF1R

CLINICAL ISSUES

- 2nd most common tumor of hand
- Any age; peak: 3rd-4th decade
- Digits (85%)
- Around large joints (10%)
- Benign but recurs locally (15-20%)
- Intraarticular tumors called localized PVNS

MACROSCOPIC

- Average size: 1.1 cm (range: 0.5-6.0 cm)

MICROSCOPIC

- Well-demarcated nodular lesion
- Multinodular with fibrous septa
- Polymorphous population of epithelioid cells, macrophages, and osteoclast-like giant cells
- Stromal fibrosis
- Average mitotic rate: 5 per 10 figures/high-power field)

TOP DIFFERENTIAL DIAGNOSES

- Diffuse-type tenosynovial giant cell tumor (PVNS)
- Giant cell tumor of soft tissue
- Fibroma of tendon sheath
- Dermatofibroma

Clinical Presentation of GCTTS

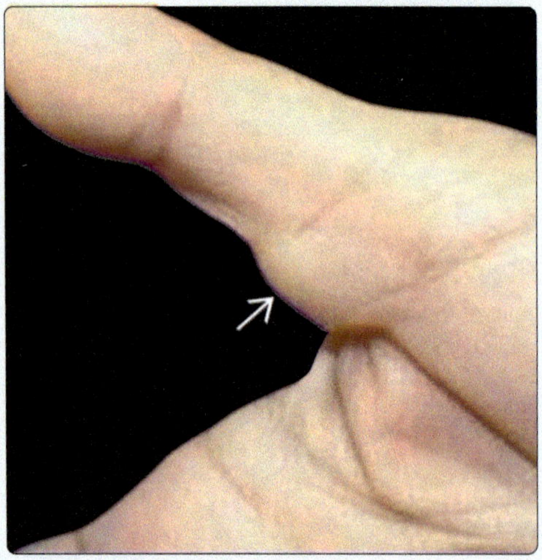

Gross Appearance of GCTTS

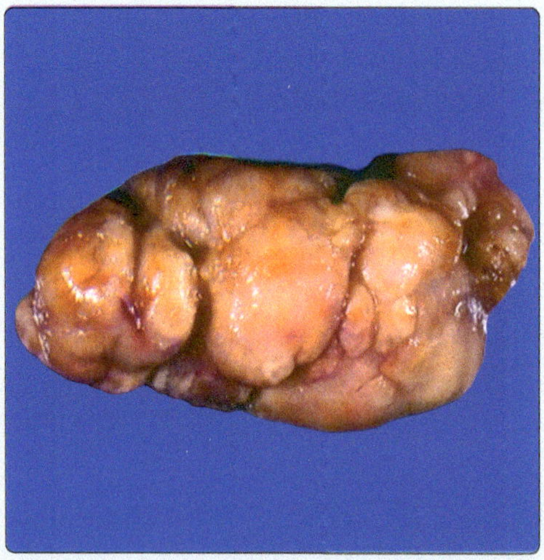

(Left) *Giant cell tumor of tendon sheath giant cell tumor of tendon sheath (GCTTS) typically presents as a painless, slow-growing mass that arises from a tendon sheath, most often on the volar aspect of a finger, such as this thumb mass ➡.* **(Right)** *Grossly, GCTTS is well demarcated, yellow to red-brown, and typically has a lobular configuration with surface clefting as depicted. Average size is 1.1 cm, ranging from 0.5-6.0 cm.*

Superficial Dermal GCTTS

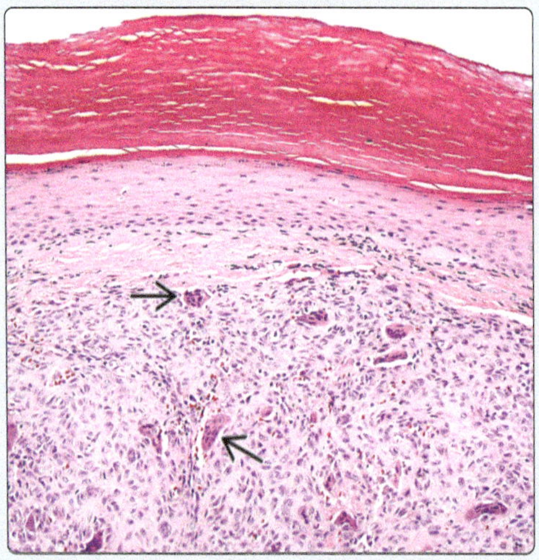

GCTTS at High Magnification

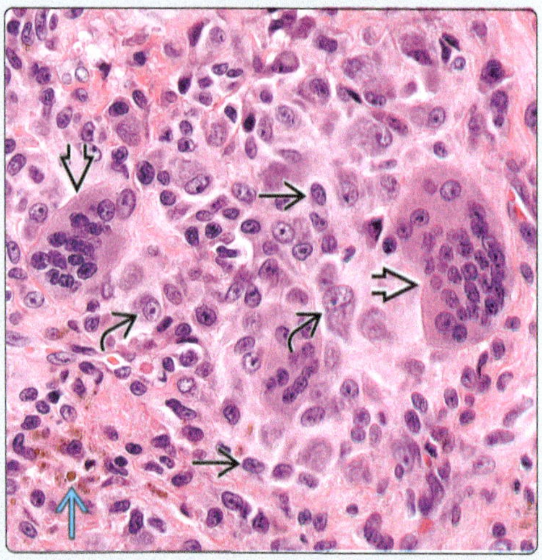

(Left) *In this example of GCTTS, the tumor involves the superficial dermis, mimicking a dermatofibroma. Unlike GCTTS, however, dermatofibroma does not contain prominent osteoclast-like giant cells ➡.* **(Right)** *High magnification shows a polymorphous cell population including large epithelioid cells with abundant eosinophilic cytoplasm and eccentric vesicular nuclei ➡, mononuclear stromal cells with smaller round or reniform nuclei ➡, and osteoclast-like giant cells ➡. Note the hemosiderin deposits ➡.*

TERMINOLOGY

Abbreviations

- Giant cell tumor of tendon sheath (GCTTS)

Synonyms

- Localized-type tenosynovial giant cell tumor
- Nodular tenosynovitis
- Localized pigmented villonodular synovitis (PVNS)
  - Intraarticular forms

Definitions

- Benign soft tissue neoplasm of synovial origin
  - Polymorphous cell population
    - Large epithelioid cells
    - Macrophages
    - Osteoclast-like giant cells
  - Well circumscribed, noninvasive

ETIOLOGY/PATHOGENESIS

Histogenesis

- Neoplastic growth
  - Balanced translocation involving 1p13 (*CSF1* gene) in many tumors
    - *COL6A3-CSF1* fusion transcripts often present
    - CSF1 overexpression by neoplastic stromal cells
    - Autocrine activation of neoplastic cells via CSF1R
    - Recruitment and activation of intratumoral macrophages and osteoclasts via CSF1R
- Synoviocytic differentiation
  - Positive for clusterin

CLINICAL ISSUES

Epidemiology

- Incidence
  - 2nd most common tumor of hand
    - Ganglion cyst most common
- Age
  - Wide age spectrum
    - Peak: 3rd-4th decade
- Sex
  - M < F (1:2)

Site

- Digits (85%)
  - Especially fingers (75%)
  - Tendon sheath
    - Usually volar
    - Often adjacent to interphalangeal joint
- Around large joints (10%)
  - Ankle
  - Knee
  - Wrist
  - Elbow
- Unusual sites
  - Scapular region
  - Brachial plexus
  - Cervicothoracic junction
- Within bursae
- Intraarticular GCTTS
  - Also called localized PVNS
  - Knee most common site
  - Complete excision usually curative

Presentation

- Painless mass
- Slow growing
- Uncommon findings
  - Triggering
  - Carpal and ulnar tunnel syndromes
  - Multifocal cases

Treatment

- Complete local excision

Prognosis

- Benign but recurs locally (15-20%)
- Risk factors for recurrence
  - Degenerative joint disease
  - Distal phalanx
  - Interphalangeal joint of thumb
  - Osseous erosion

IMAGING

Radiographic Findings

- Soft tissue mass
- Cortical bony erosion (10%)
  - Rarely invades bone to mimic primary bone tumor

MR Findings

- Lobulated mass with low T1 and T2 signal

MACROSCOPIC

General Features

- Well circumscribed
- Partially encapsulated
- Lobular configuration
  - Surface clefting
  - Sometimes grooved along tendon interface
- Variegated cut surface: Tan, red-brown, yellow

Size

- Average: 1.1 cm (range: 0.5-6.0 cm)
  - Large joint tumors often larger than digital tumors (average: 2 cm)

MICROSCOPIC

Histologic Features

- Well demarcated
- Multinodular with fibrous septa
- Stromal fibrosis
  - Can be extensive
  - Can mimic osteoid
- Hemosiderin deposits
- Dyscohesive areas render pseudoglandular appearance
- Cleft-like spaces lined by synoviocytes
- Distal tumors can invade dermis

Cytologic Features

- Polymorphous cell population
  - Large epithelioid cells
    - Abundant, eccentric, eosinophilic cytoplasm
      - Often contain hemosiderin pigment
    - Vesicular, round nuclei with prominent nucleoli
  - Histiocytes with pale cytoplasm and round or reniform nuclei
  - Osteoclast-like multinucleated giant cells
    - Can be sparse in some tumors
  - Xanthoma cells
  - Hemosiderin-laden macrophages
- Mitotic rate 1-20 per 10 high-power fields (average: 5 per 10 high-power fields)

ANCILLARY TESTS

Immunohistochemistry

- Epithelioid cells are clusterin (+)
- Histiocytes are CD68(+)
- Osteoclast-like giant cells are CD68(+), CD45(+), TRAP(+)
- Scattered desmin (+) cells in 50% of cases

DIFFERENTIAL DIAGNOSIS

Diffuse-Type Tenosynovial Giant Cell Tumor (PVNS)

- Microscopically similar to GCTTS
- Diffuse intraarticular tumors form villonodular masses
- Large joints; knee most common site
- Diffuse extraarticular tumors invade adjacent tissues
- Often have fewer giant cells and less lobular architecture

Giant Cell Tumor of Soft Tissue

- More uniform, less polymorphous mononuclear stromal cell population
- Osteoclast-like giant cell component prominent
- Less stromal fibrosis
- Often encased by shell of bone

Fibroma of Tendon Sheath

- Lacks hemosiderin and multinucleated giant cells
- Peripheral thin-walled vessels &/or clefts
- Usually occurs in fingers
- GCTTS may show diffuse fibrosis mimicking fibroma of tendon sheath

Dermatofibroma

- Rare in digits
- Can show multinucleated histiocytic cells but lacks osteoclast-like giant cells
- GCTTS can sometimes invade skin

Plexiform Fibrohistiocytic Tumor

- Often has osteoclast-like giant cells
- Plexiform architecture but can be nodular
- Involves dermis and subcutis
- Rare in acral extremities
- Usually children and young adults

Giant Cell Tumor of Bone

- Identical histology to giant cell tumor of soft tissue
- Primary osseous tumor but can invade soft tissue

SELECTED REFERENCES

1. Qin JR et al: Diffuse-type giant cell tumor of the tendon sheath in the temporal region incidentally diagnosed due to a temporal tumor: a report of two cases and review of the literature. Oncol Lett. 10(2):1179-1183, 2015
2. Vargaonkar G et al: Giant cell tumor of the tendon sheath around the foot and ankle. A report of three cases and a literature review. J Am Podiatr Med Assoc. 105(3):249-54, 2015
3. Beytemür O et al: Localized giant cell tenosynovial tumor seen in the knee joint. Case Rep Orthop. 2014:840243, 2014
4. Ding Y et al: Tenosynovial giant cell tumors lacking giant cells: report of diagnostic pitfalls. Ann Clin Lab Sci. 44(2):222-7, 2014
5. Panagopoulos I et al: Novel CSF1-S100A10 fusion gene and CSF1 transcript identified by RNA sequencing in tenosynovial giant cell tumors. Int J Oncol. 44(5):1425-32, 2014
6. Ye JM et al: Tenosynovial giant cell tumour of brachial plexus. J Clin Neurosci. 21(6):1070-2, 2014
7. Yoshimoto T et al: Hepatoid tenosynovial giant cell tumor - a rare morphologic variant case report. Pathol Res Pract. 210(10):694-7, 2014
8. Atik E et al: Tenosynovial giant cell tumor in an unusual localization. Acta Orthop Traumatol Turc. 47(2):139-41, 2013
9. Di Grazia S et al: Giant cell tumor of tendon sheath: study of 64 cases and review of literature. G Chir. 34(5-6):149-52, 2013
10. Fukuda A et al: Tenosynovial giant cell tumor arising on the scapular region. Case Rep Dermatol. 5(3):267-71, 2013
11. Lanzinger WD et al: Giant cell tumor of the tendon sheath. J Hand Surg Am. 38(1):154-7; quiz 157, 2013
12. van der Heijden L et al: A multidisciplinary approach to giant cell tumors of tendon sheath and synovium--a critical appraisal of literature and treatment proposal. J Surg Oncol. 107(4):433-45, 2013
13. Ho CY et al: Giant cell tumor of tendon sheath: cytomorphologic and radiologic findings in 41 patients. Diagn Cytopathol. 40 Suppl 2:E94-8, 2012
14. Lucas DR: Tenosynovial giant cell tumor: case report and review. Arch Pathol Lab Med. 136(8):901-6, 2012
15. Okutan O et al: Tenosynovial giant cell tumor in the cervico-thoracic junction. Turk Neurosurg. 22(6):769-71, 2012
16. Kim HS et al: Localized tenosynovial giant cell tumor in both knee joints. Skeletal Radiol. 39(9):923-6, 2010
17. Boland JM et al: Clusterin is expressed in normal synoviocytes and in tenosynovial giant cell tumors of localized and diffuse types: diagnostic and histogenetic implications. Am J Surg Pathol. 33(8):1225-9, 2009
18. Darwish FM et al: Giant cell tumour of tendon sheath: experience with 52 cases. Singapore Med J. 49(11):879-82, 2008
19. Murphey MD et al: Pigmented villonodular synovitis: radiologic-pathologic correlation. Radiographics. 28(5):1493-518, 2008
20. Möller E et al: Molecular identification of COL6A3-CSF1 fusion transcripts in tenosynovial giant cell tumors. Genes Chromosomes Cancer. 47(1):21-5, 2008
21. Cupp JS et al: Translocation and expression of CSF1 in pigmented villonodular synovitis, tenosynovial giant cell tumor, rheumatoid arthritis and other reactive synovitides. Am J Surg Pathol. 31(6):970-6, 2007
22. Dines JS et al: Long-term follow-up of surgically treated localized pigmented villonodular synovitis of the knee. Arthroscopy. 23(9):930-7, 2007
23. Jafarian F et al: Plexiform fibrohistiocytic tumor in three children. Pediatr Dermatol. 23(1):7-12, 2006
24. West RB et al: A landscape effect in tenosynovial giant-cell tumor from activation of CSF1 expression by a translocation in a minority of tumor cells. Proc Natl Acad Sci U S A. 103(3):690-5, 2006
25. Nilsson M et al: Molecular cytogenetic mapping of recurrent chromosomal breakpoints in tenosynovial giant cell tumors. Virchows Arch. 441(5):475-80, 2002
26. Reilly KE et al: Recurrent giant cell tumors of the tendon sheath. J Hand Surg Am. 24(6):1298-302, 1999
27. Enzinger FM et al: Plexiform fibrohistiocytic tumor presenting in children and young adults. An analysis of 65 cases. Am J Surg Pathol. 12(11):818-26, 1988
28. Ushijima M et al: Giant cell tumor of the tendon sheath (nodular tenosynovitis). A study of 207 cases to compare the large joint group with the common digit group. Cancer. 57(4):875-84, 1986
29. Chung EB et al: Fibroma of tendon sheath. Cancer. 44(5):1945-54, 1979

Gross Cut Surface of GCTTS

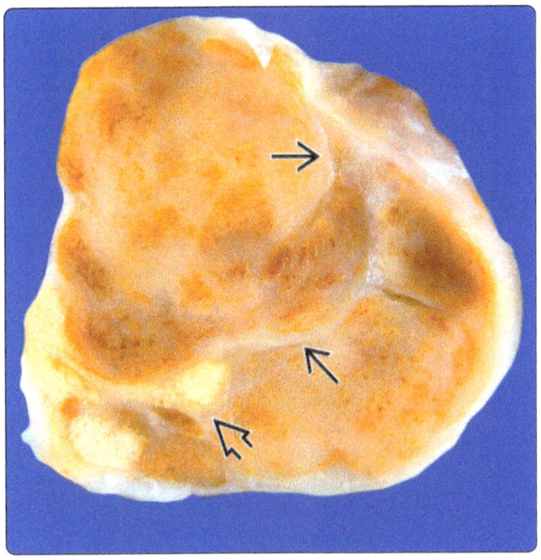

Radiographic Appearance of GCTTS

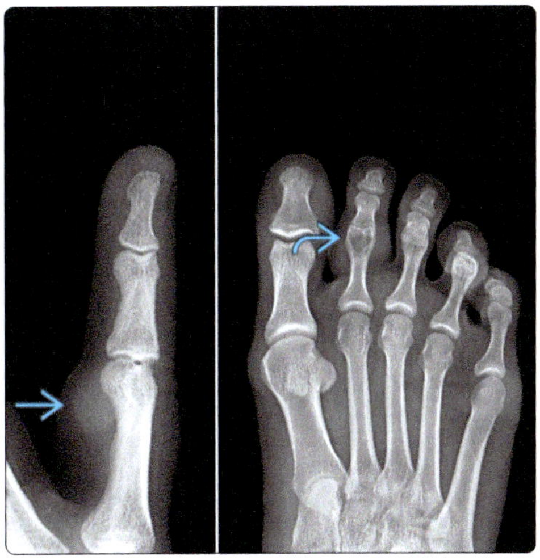

(Left) *GCTTS is well circumscribed, encapsulated, and multinodular. Fibrous septa divide it into nodules. The cut surface is variegated with gold, tan, red-brown, and yellow areas. Bright yellow areas represent xanthoma cells.* **(Right)** *Radiographically, it appears as a soft tissue density most often on the volar side of a finger. Approximately 10% erode the bony cortex as shown. Rare tumors invade medullary bone, mimicking a primary bone tumor, such as this 2nd toe tumor.*

Mixed Cell Population of GCTTS

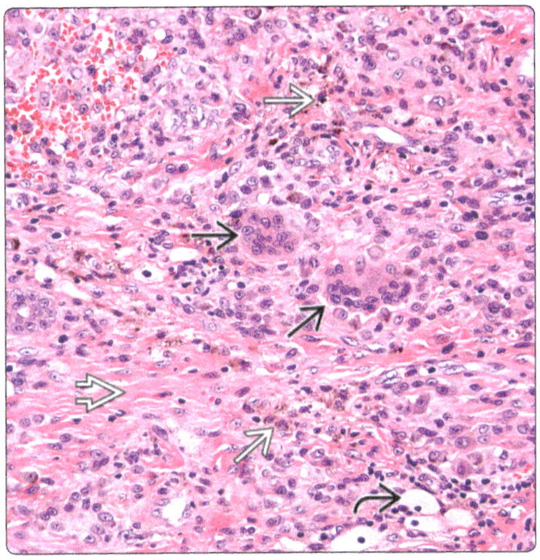

High Magnification of GCTTS

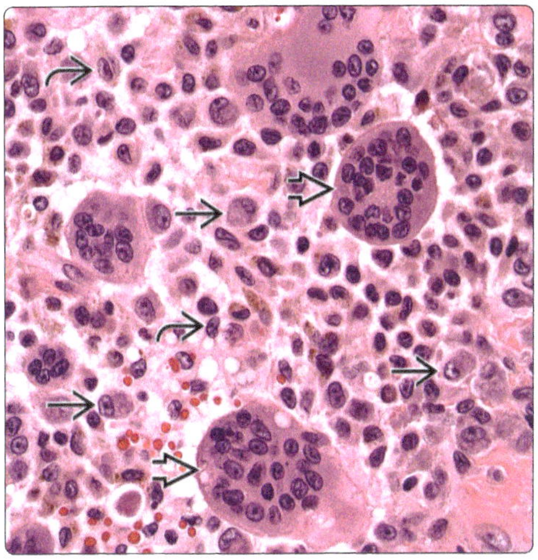

(Left) *GCTTS has a mixture of mononuclear stromal cells, multinucleated giant cells, and macrophages, including xanthoma cells. Stromal fibrosis and hemosiderin deposits are very common.* **(Right)** *This high-power view depicts large epithelioid cells with eccentric cytoplasm (believed to be the neoplastic element), macrophages with smaller round to reniform nuclei, and osteoclast-like giant cells.*

Xanthoma Cells in GCTTS

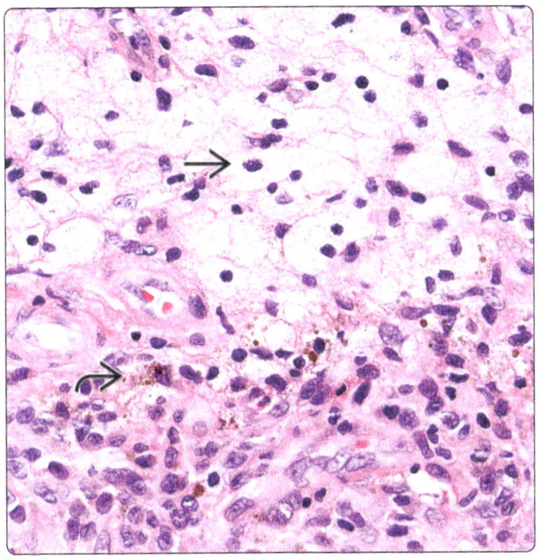

Prominent Hemosiderin Deposition

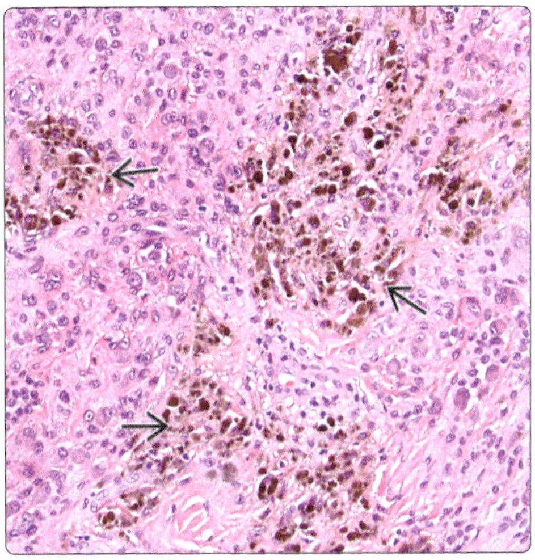

(Left) *Sheets and clusters of xanthoma cells are very common in GCTTS. Xanthoma cells (foamy macrophages) have copious, finely vacuolated cytoplasm and small central nuclei as depicted. Hemosiderin-laden macrophages are also common.* **(Right)** *Some tumors have very extensive hemosiderin deposition, as depicted in this case.*

(Left) *Occasionally, fibrosis can be very extensive, affecting large areas of a tumor. This low-power micrograph shows diffuse stromal fibrosis that entraps mononuclear cells and multinucleated giant cells* ➔. **(Right)** *Stromal fibrosis is usually present in GCTTS but highly variable in its extent. In some tumors, fibrosis consists of lace-like hyalinized collagen that resembles osteoid* ➔.

Stromal Fibrosis GCTTS

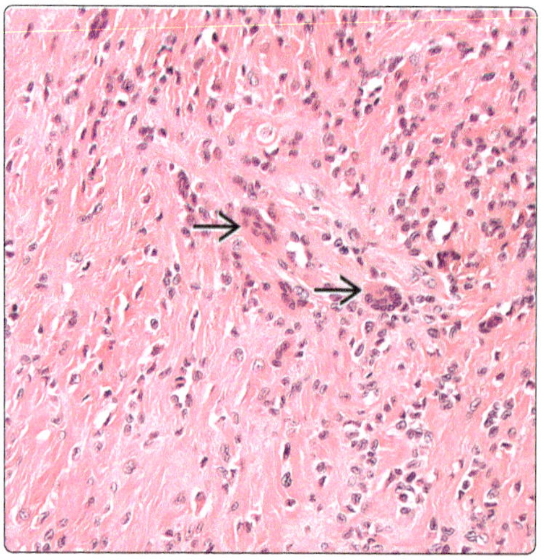

Osteoid-Like Fibrosis in GCTTS

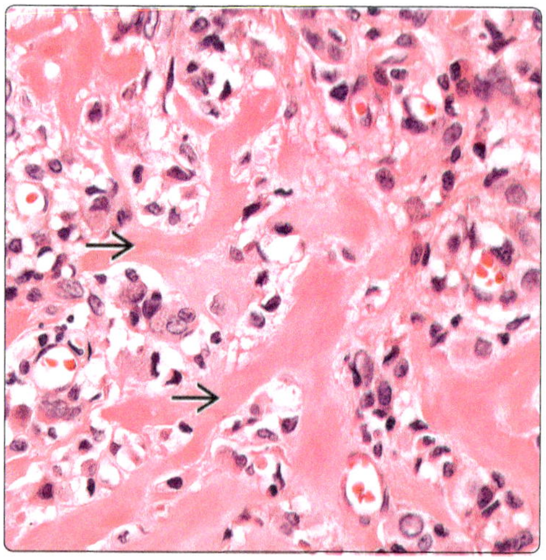

(Left) *Areas of cellular dyscohesion are not uncommon in GCTTS. In some tumors, it can be so pronounced as to form cystic spaces* ➔*, creating a pseudoglandular pattern.* **(Right)** *Occasionally, GCTTS can have very few giant cells, as in this example, which consists of a uniform population of mononuclear stromal cells with round nuclei.*

Pseudoglandular Pattern

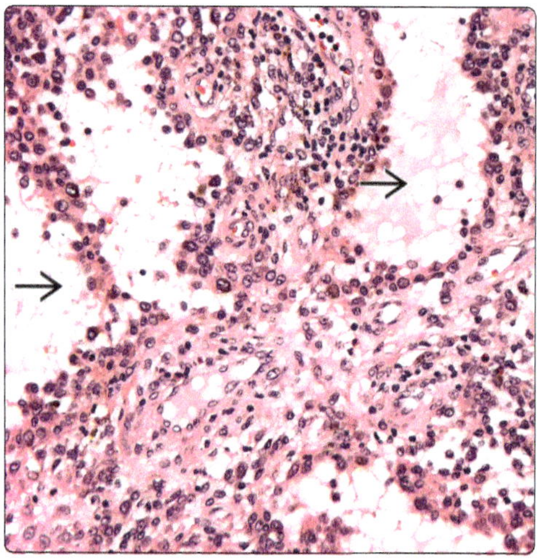

GCTTS Without Giant Cells

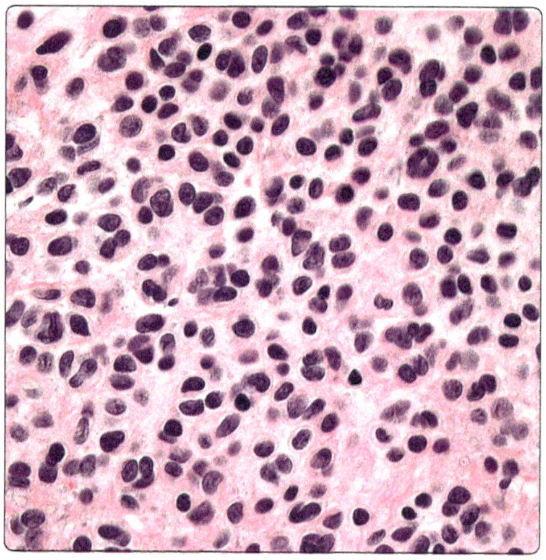

(Left) *Some GCTTSs contain sheets of the large epithelioid cells with abundant eosinophilic-staining cytoplasm and eccentric vesicular nuclei. Note the intracytoplasmic hemosiderin deposits* ➔. **(Right)** *The large epithelioid cells are positive for clusterin* ➔*, indicating synoviocytic differentiation. By contrast, infiltrating macrophages and giant cells* ↪ *are negative.*

Epithelioid Cells in GCTTS

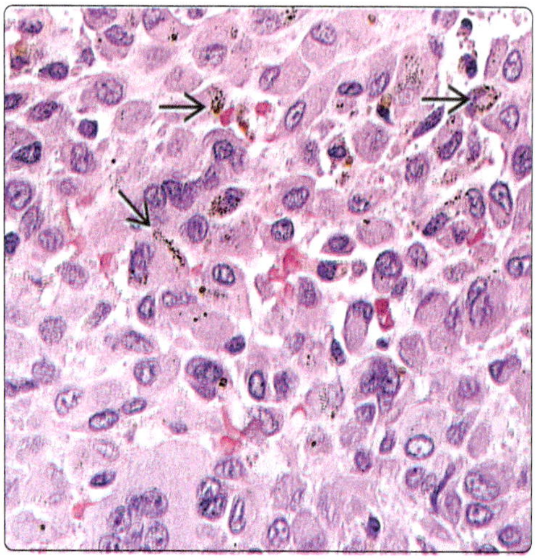

Clusterin Immunostain

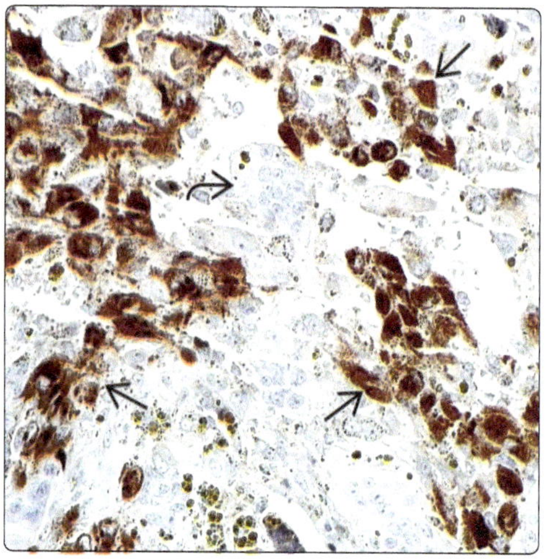

Lobular Architecture of GCTTS

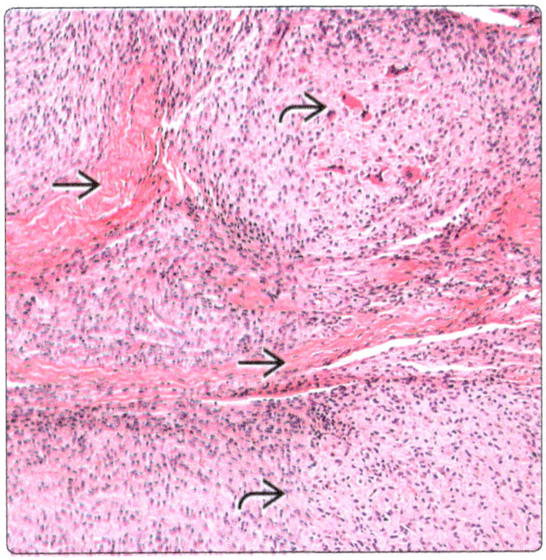

Brisk Mitotic Activity in GCTTS

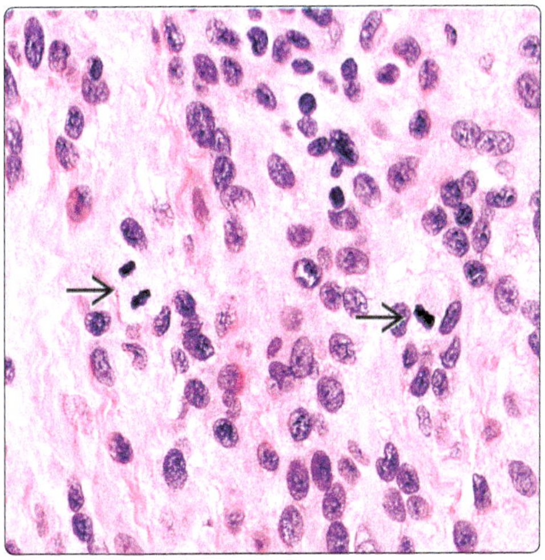

(Left) *GCTTS has a lobular/multinodular architecture as illustrated by this low-power micrograph. Note the long, thick fibrous septa ➔ that divide the tumor into nodules ➚.* **(Right)** *Mitotic activity ranges from 1 to 20 mitoses ➔ per 10 high-power fields (average 5 per 10 high-power fields). Brisk mitotic activity, therefore, is not uncommon in these lesions and by itself does not suggest malignancy.*

Giant Cells in GCTTS

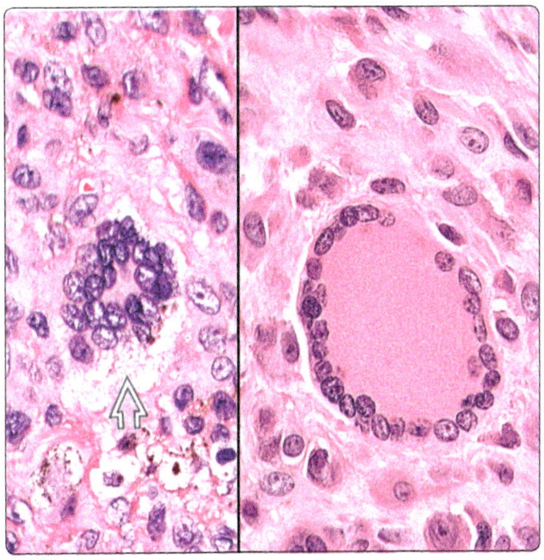

Superficial Cutaneous Involvement

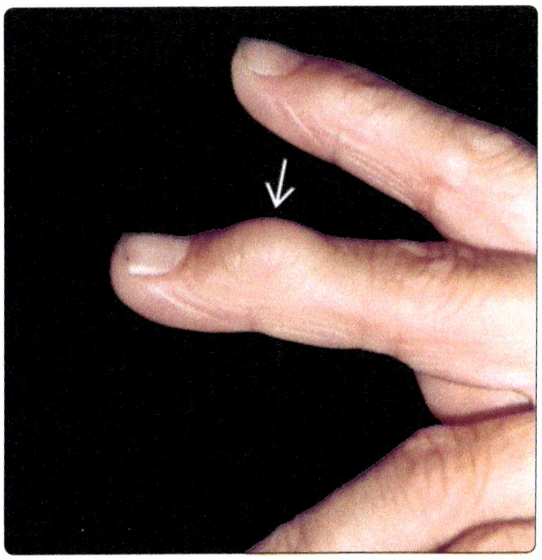

(Left) *Although osteoclast-like multinucleated giant cells are most common, occasionally GCTTS can have Touton-like (left, with a rim of foamy cytoplasm ➔ surrounding the ring of nuclei) or Langhans-type (right, with a partial ring of peripheral nuclei) giant cells.* **(Right)** *In a distal acral location, GCTTS can adhere to and invade the overlying skin, as depicted ➔ by this tumor of the middle finger.*

Intraarticular Growth on MR

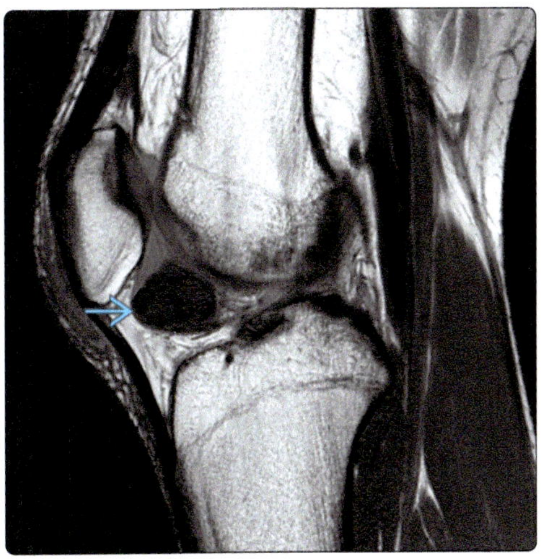

Gross Specimen With Intraarticular Growth

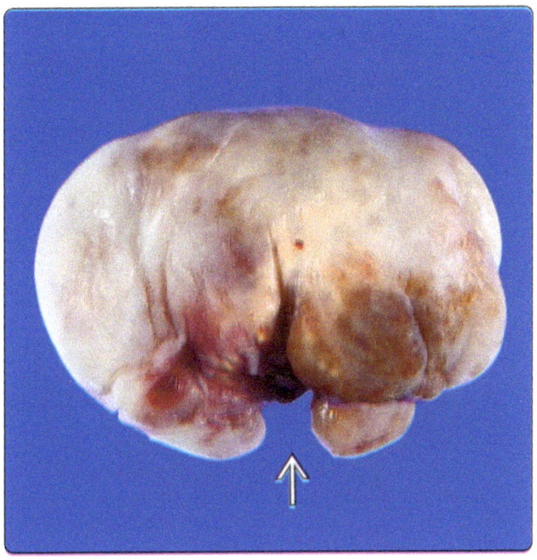

(Left) *Localized intraarticular GCTTS (or localized pigmented villonodular synovitis) forms a well-demarcated tumor within the joint space. Knee is the most common site, as depicted in this MR ➔.* **(Right)** *Grossly, intraarticular tumors are well circumscribed and form pedunculated or sessile polypoid masses attached to the synovial surface by a stalk ➔ (inverted here). Unlike diffuse tumors (PVNS), localized tumors rarely recur following complete excision and have an excellent prognosis.*

Myofibroma and Myofibromatosis

KEY FACTS

TERMINOLOGY

- Benign neoplasms composed of lobules of myoid cells separated by vascularized zones (biphasic pattern)
  - Solitary form (myofibroma)
  - Multicentric form (myofibromatosis)
- Synonyms: Infantile myofibromatosis, congenital generalized fibromatosis
  - Continuum with lesions termed myopericytoma and infantile hemangiopericytoma

CLINICAL ISSUES

- Most common from birth to 2 years
- Most solitary examples in subcutaneous tissues of head and neck
- Simple excision for solitary lesions
- Outcome for multicentric form is function of involved sites
  - Extensive lung involvement poor prognostic factor

MICROSCOPIC

- Biphasic pattern classic
- Myoid nodules separated by cellular pockets with hemangiopericytoma-like vascular pattern
- Variable amounts of each component may be present
- Most cases have minimal atypia and mitotic activity
- Spindle cell areas
  - Often prominent beneath ulcerated mucosal surfaces

ANCILLARY TESTS

- Usually label with α-actin and calponin, but negative to focal desmin, caldesmon
- Negative for S100 and cytokeratins
- Mutations detected in *PDGFRB, NOTCH3, NDRG4* in myofibromatosis

TOP DIFFERENTIAL DIAGNOSES

- Smooth muscle tumors
- Fibromatosis

(Left) *This punch biopsy shows a deep-seated dermal tumor. Note the prominent lobulations and a biphasic pattern, consisting of myoid nodules ➙ and intervening hemangiopericytomatous ⇨ zones.* **(Right)** *This example of cutaneous myofibroma has prominent hemangiopericytomatous zones ⇨.*

Myofibroma at Scanning Magnification

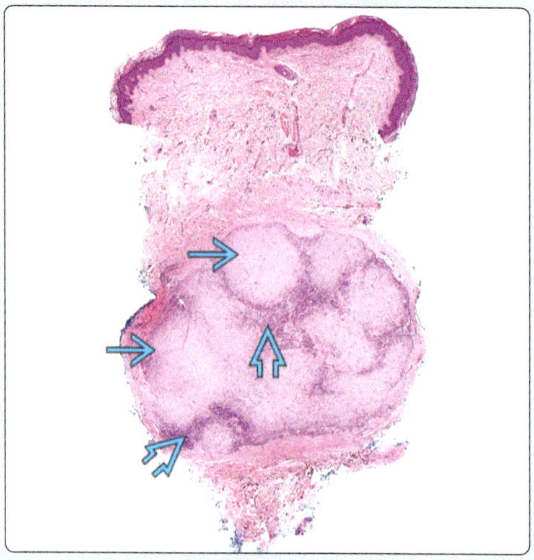

Myofibroma With Hemangiopericytomatous Areas

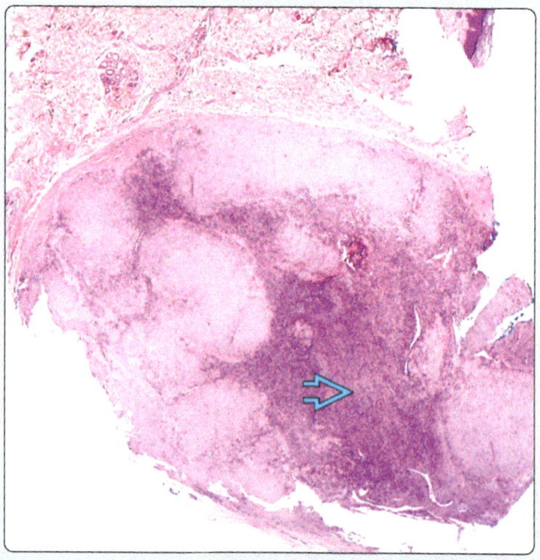

(Left) *Higher magnification shows the myoid lobules separated by more cellular areas. The myoid cells show cytoplasmic eosinophilia →.* **(Right)** *Higher magnification shows the hemangiopericytoma-like component of a myofibroma.*

Myofibroma, Higher Magnification of Myoid Lobules

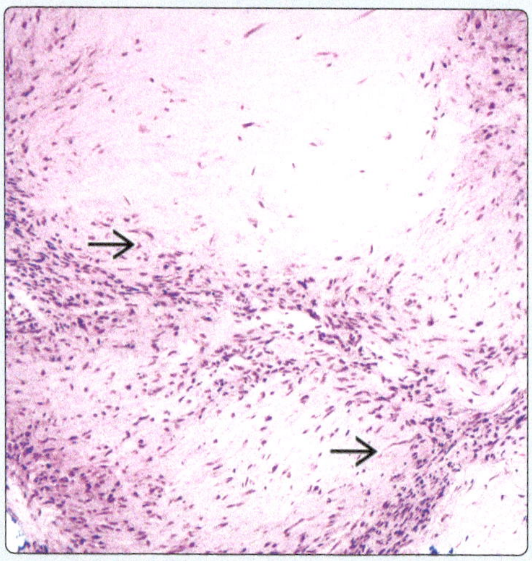

Myofibroma, Hemangiopericytomatous Zone

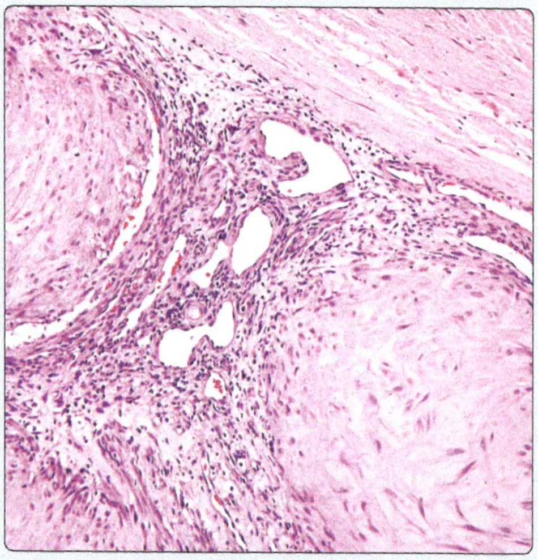

TERMINOLOGY

Synonyms

- Infantile myofibromatosis, congenital generalized fibromatosis
  - Continuum with lesions termed myopericytoma and infantile hemangiopericytoma

Definitions

- Benign neoplasms composed of lobules of myoid cells separated by vascularized zones (biphasic pattern)
  - Solitary form (myofibroma)
  - Multicentric form (myofibromatosis)

CLINICAL ISSUES

Epidemiology

- Incidence
  - Solitary form rare but more common than multicentric form
  - Multicentric form extremely rare
  - Rare familial cases
- Age
  - Wide age range (neonates to elderly)
  - Most common from birth to 2 years
- Sex
  - Male predominance

Site

- Most solitary examples in subcutaneous tissues of head and neck
  - Trunk, extremities
  - Occasional skeletal example, especially skull
- Multicentric form usually involves soft tissue and bone
  - Usually long bones
  - Visceral sites
    - Gastrointestinal tract
    - Liver, kidney, pancreas

Presentation

- Asymptomatic skin nodules with purplish color (solitary form)
- Visceral lesions with site-specific presentations
- Bone lesions seen as multiple elongated radiolucencies in metaphysis

Treatment

- Simple excision for solitary lesions
- Selective excisions for multicentric form

Prognosis

- Excellent for solitary form
- Outcome for multicentric form is function of involved sites
  - Extensive lung involvement poor prognostic factor

MICROSCOPIC

Histologic Features

- Most lesions well marginated
  - Can be locally infiltrative with intravascular and osseous extension and foci of necrosis
- Biphasic pattern
  - Myoid nodules separated by cellular pockets with hemangiopericytoma-like vascular pattern
  - Variable amounts of each component
  - Most cases have minimal atypia and mitotic activity
- Spindle cell areas
  - Prominent beneath ulcerated mucosal surfaces
- Myoid nodules
  - Pink cytoplasm and round to tapered nuclei
  - Myxoid change or hyalinization
- Hemangiopericytoma-like areas
  - Cellular but with minimal mitotic activity
  - Round cells similar to glomus cells

ANCILLARY TESTS

Immunohistochemistry

- Usually label with α-actin and calponin but not desmin or caldesmon
- Negative for S100 and cytokeratins

Genetic Testing

- Mutations detected in *PDGFRB, NOTCH3, NDRG4* in myofibromatosis

DIFFERENTIAL DIAGNOSIS

Smooth Muscle Tumors

- Not lobulated
- Perpendicularly oriented fascicles of spindle-shaped cells with cigar-shaped nuclei
- Express actins, desmin, caldesmon

Fibromatosis

- Highly infiltrative growth pattern; sweeping fascicles of myofibroblasts
- Express actins, usually not desmin; nuclear β-catenin labeling
- *CTNNB1* (gene that encodes for β-catenin) and *APC* mutations

Hemangiopericytoma

- No myoid areas
- Infantile form on continuum with myofibroma

Myoepithelioma

- Epithelioid neoplasm with immunolabeling for epithelial markers, myoid markers, and S100 akin to myoepithelial cells

Myofibroblastoma

- Not biphasic, with immunolabeling for both CD34 and desmin

SELECTED REFERENCES

1. Linhares ND et al: Exome sequencing identifies a novel homozygous variant in NDRG4 in a family with infantile myofibromatosis. Eur J Med Genet. 57(11-12):643-8, 2014
2. Cheung YH et al: A recurrent PDGFRB mutation causes familial infantile myofibromatosis. Am J Hum Genet. 92(6):996-1000, 2013
3. Lee JW: Mutations in PDGFRB and NOTCH3 are the first genetic causes identified for autosomal dominant infantile myofibromatosis. Clin Genet. 84(4):340-1, 2013
4. Smith KJ et al: Cutaneous myofibroma. Mod Pathol. 2(6):603-9, 1989
5. Chung EB et al: Infantile myofibromatosis. Cancer. 48(8):1807-18, 1981

Myofibroma, Vascular and Myoid Zones

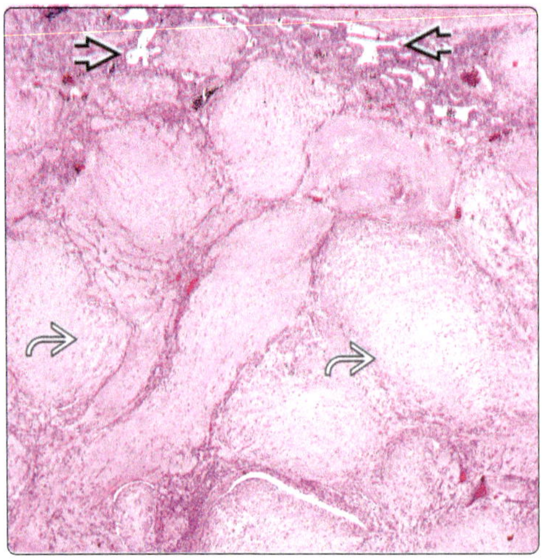

Myofibroma, Higher Magnification of Periphery of Myoid Lobule

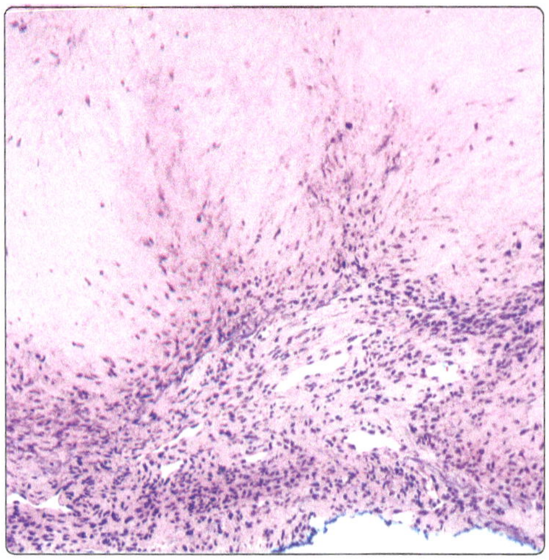

(Left) *This cutaneous myofibroma shows a prominent lobular configuration. Note the biphasic appearance: The upper portion of the field shows a prominent hemangiopericytomatous vascular pattern ⇨, whereas the lower portion shows the myoid lobules ↷.* **(Right)** *Many vessels are typically present at the periphery of a myoid lobule in a myofibroma. The stroma has a chondromyxoid appearance.*

Myofibroma at Scanning Magnification

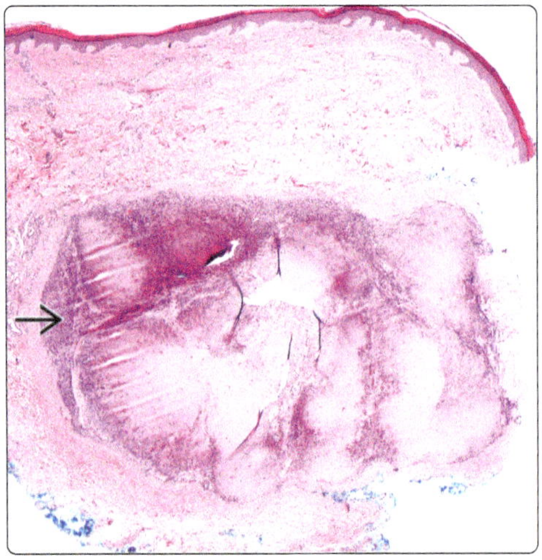

Myofibroma, High Magnification of Myoid Cells

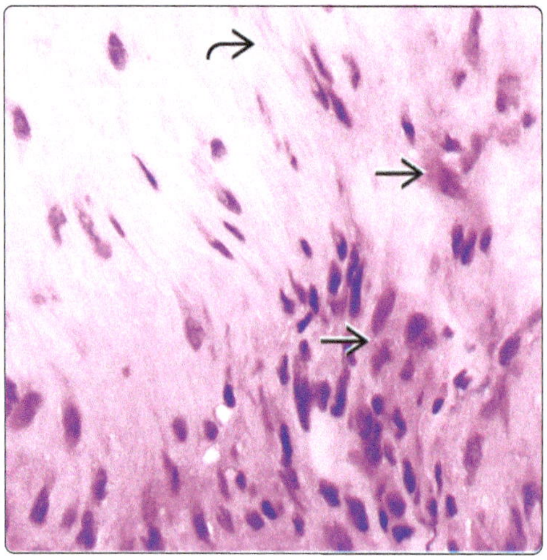

(Left) *Scanning magnification shows a cutaneous myofibroma in the dermis. Note the multilobulated appearance. In this example, the darker hemangiopericytoma-like component is at the periphery → of the tumor.* **(Right)** *High magnification shows the myoid cells in a myofibroma. Many of the cells have prominent cytoplasmic eosinophilia →, and there are delicate amphophilic cytoplasmic processes ↷.*

Myofibroma, Bone Invasion

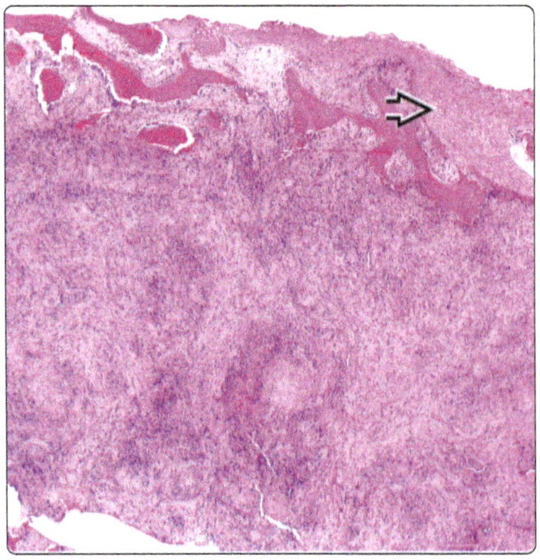

Myofibroma, Spindled Area

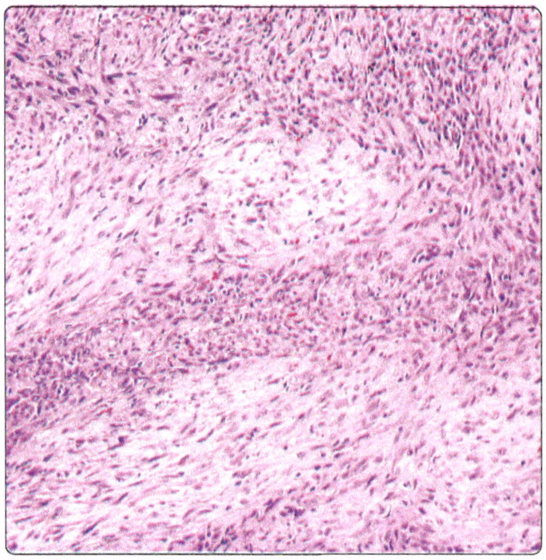

(Left) *This is an example of a skeletal myofibroma. There is a vaguely lobulated appearance, and the tumor is infiltrative at the periphery. There is also focal necrosis ⇨.* **(Right)** *High magnification shows a myofibroma of the parotid region of a child. The spindle cells are arranged in nodules.*

Myofibroma, Intravascular Extension

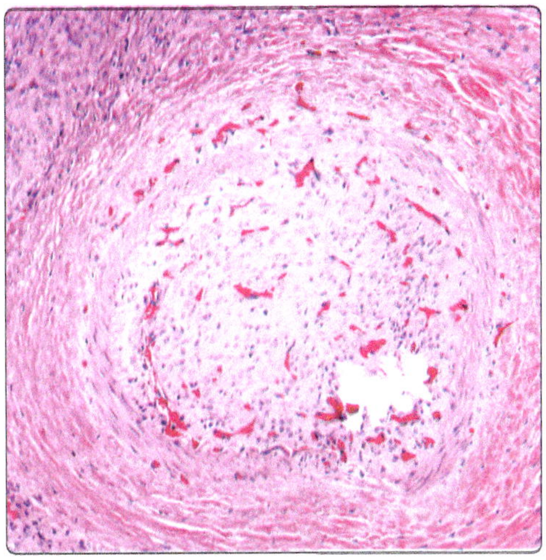

Myofibroma, Actin Expression

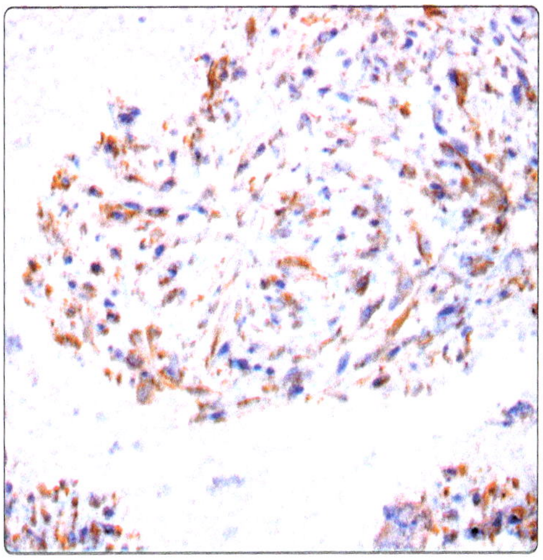

(Left) *Histologic examination shows vascular space invasion in a myofibroma. This feature can lead to an erroneous interpretation of malignancy.* **(Right)** *Actin-HHF-35 shows cytoplasmic labeling in a myofibroma.*

Cutaneous Myofibroma/Myopericytoma

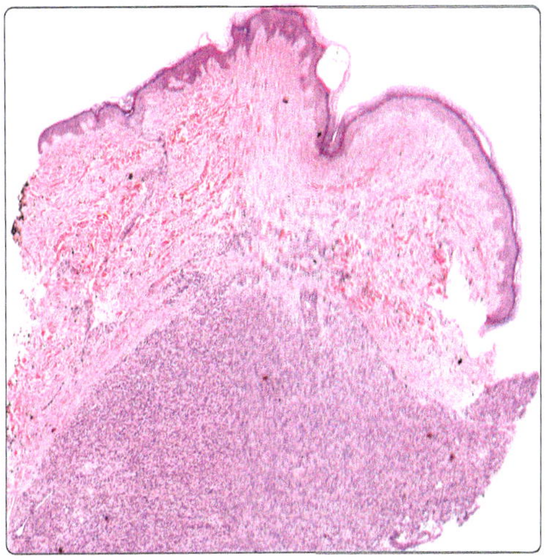

Myofibroma/Myopericytoma

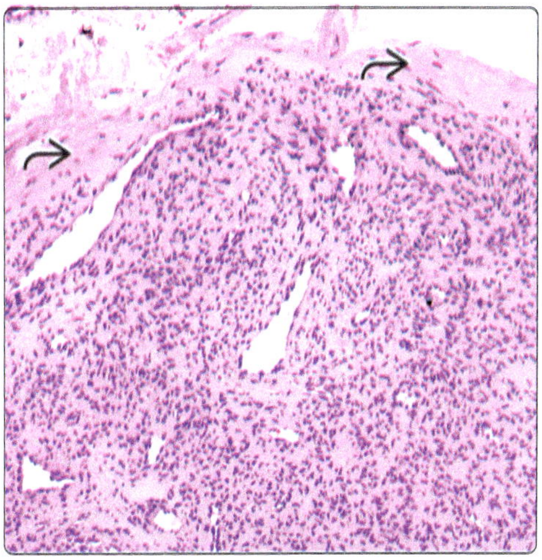

(Left) *Low magnification shows a dermal-based lesion that has a predominance of hemangiopericytoma-like areas. This lesion should be regarded as myopericytoma, a tumor that is on a continuum with myofibroma.* **(Right)** *Higher magnification of a cutaneous myofibroma/myopericytoma is shown. Subtle myoid features can be appreciated, particularly at the edge of the nodule ↪.*

Glomangiopericytoma

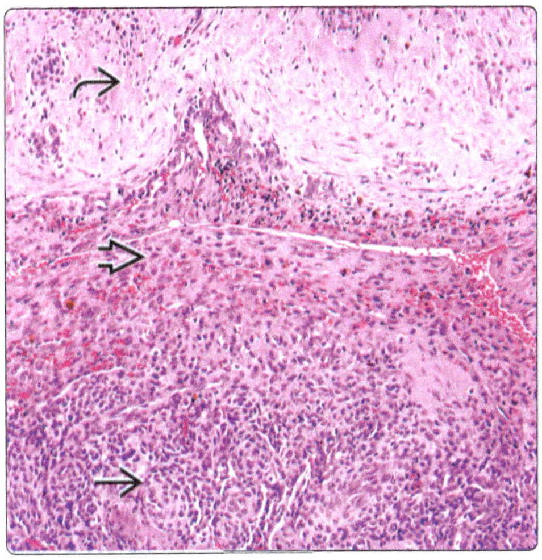

Myopericytoma

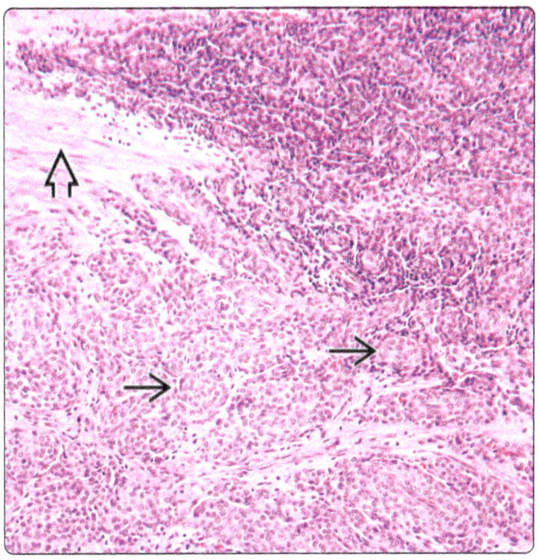

(Left) *A lesion with myoid ↪, whorled hemangiopericytomatous →, and glomus cell ⇨ areas is shown. Such a lesion would be classified as a glomangiopericytoma.* **(Right)** *Another field from a myopericytoma shows cellular areas that may appear alarming but have negligible mitotic activity. Note the myoid area ⇨ and whorled areas →.*

Differential Diagnosis: Myoepithelioma

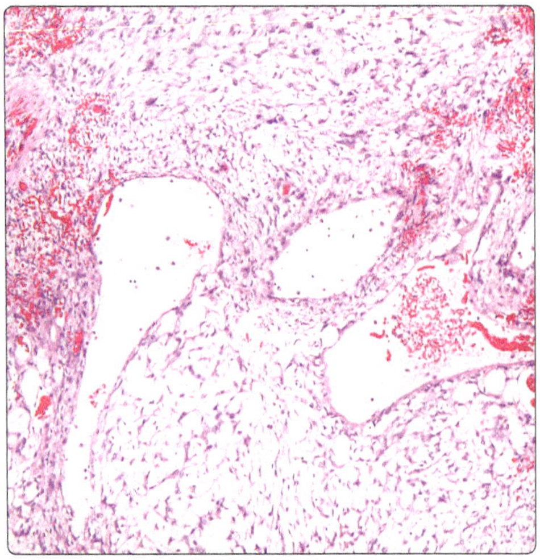

Differential Diagnosis: Myoepithelioma, High Magnification

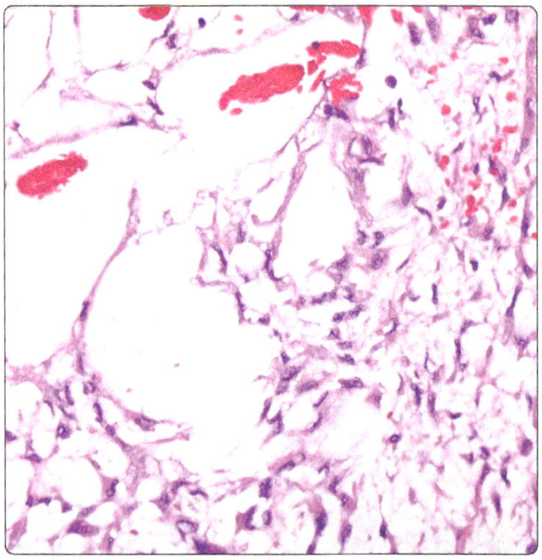

(Left) These tumors tend to be lobulated but not biphasic like myofibromas. This example has cystic spaces. These tumors are thought to be related to cutaneous mixed tumors. (Right) Note the eosinophilic myoid cytoplasm in this image. There are no overtly malignant features, and such tumors generally behave indolently.

Differential Diagnosis: Myoepithelioma, Cellular Variant

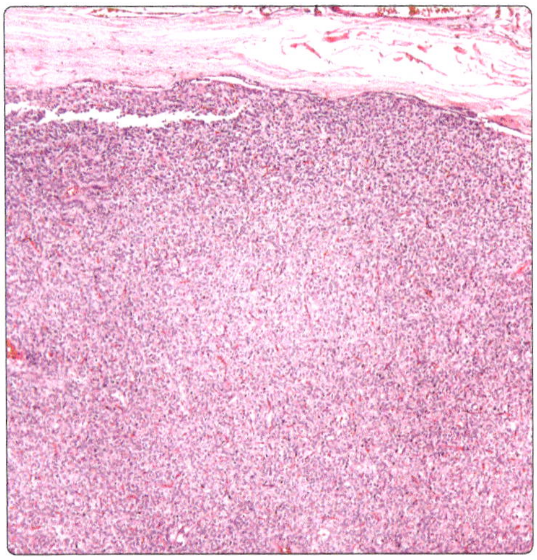

Differential Diagnosis: Myoepithelioma, S100 Staining

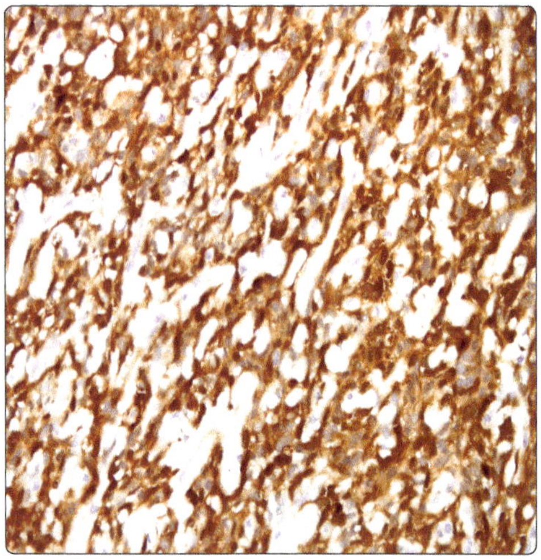

(Left) This tumor is solid (rather than biphasic like a myofibroma) and consists of cells with monotonous uniform nuclei. (Right) Note the strong nuclear and cytoplasmic labeling with S100, akin to that seen in myoepithelial cells.

Differential Diagnosis: Myoepithelioma, Keratin Immunostaining

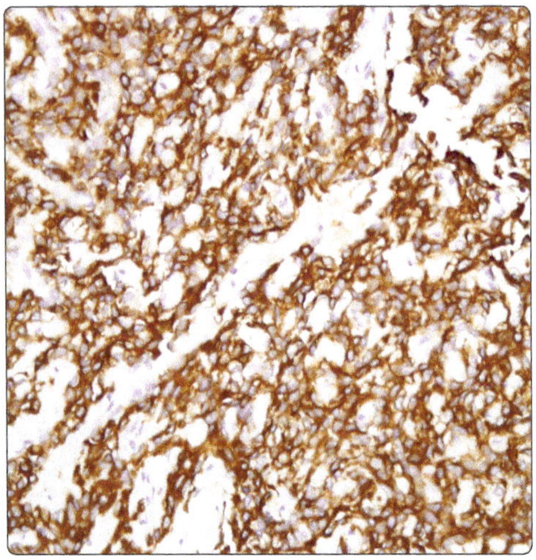

Differential Diagnosis: Myoepithelioma, Smooth Muscle Actin Immunolabeling

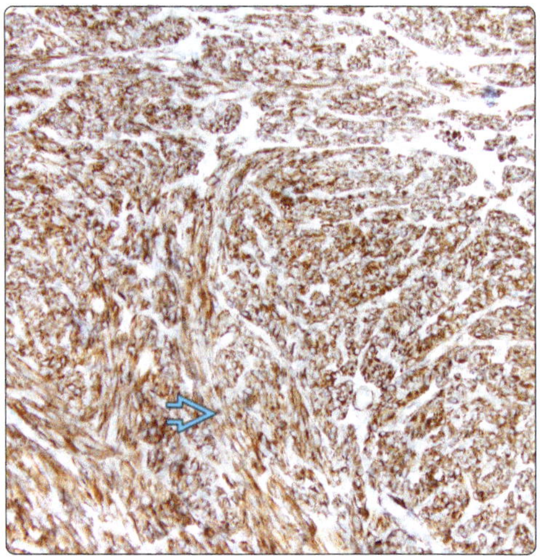

(Left) This example shows strong keratin expression. Note the uniform nuclei on the hematoxylin counterstain. (Right) The staining appears fibrillary ⇨ in parts of the tumor. Most myoepitheliomas express keratin and S100, but actin expression is less common.

Differential Diagnosis: Myofibroblastoma, Extramammary Type

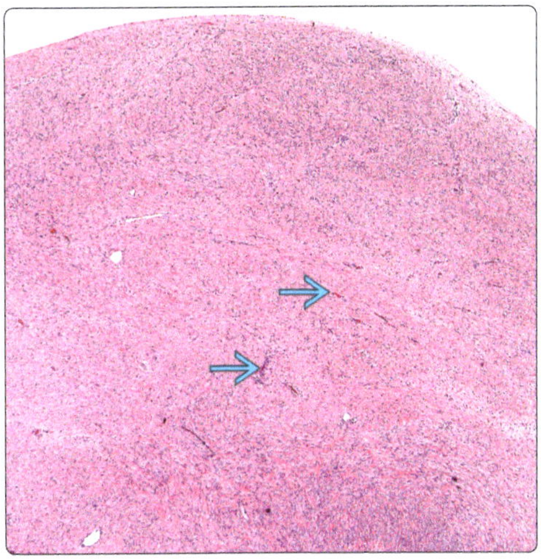

Differential Diagnosis: Myofibroblastoma, Cytologic Features

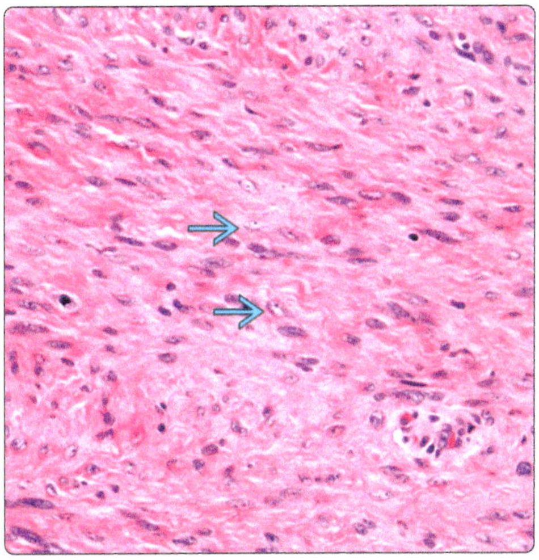

(Left) *This tumor is monophasic, composed of bland spindle cells. The tumor is pale on H&E stains, so delicate capillaries → appear conspicuous at low magnification.* **(Right)** *Note the bland nuclei with delicate nuclear membranes and inconspicuous nucleoli →.*

Differential Diagnosis: Myofibroblastoma, Extramammary, CD34 Staining

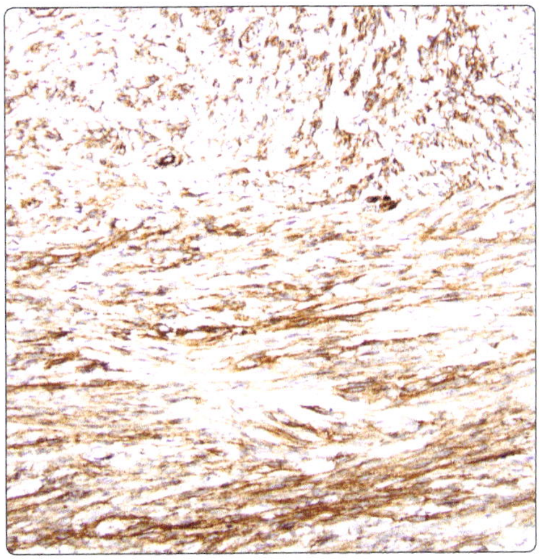

Differential Diagnosis: Myofibroblastoma, Extramammary, Desmin Staining

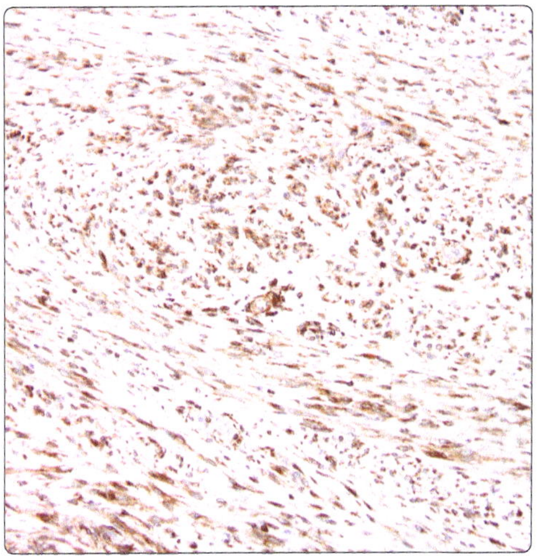

(Left) *These tumors express desmin and CD34, both of which are usually negative in myofibromas.* **(Right)** *The staining is weaker than that usually encountered in leiomyomas. Desmin is not usually reactive in myofibromas.*

Palisaded Myofibroblastoma of Lymph Node

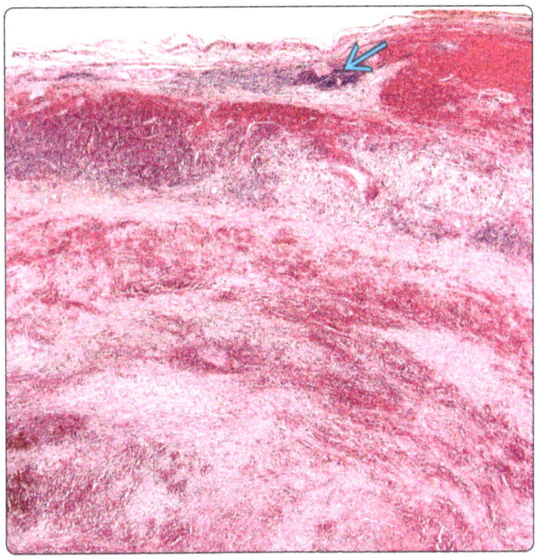

Palisaded Myofibroblastoma of Lymph Node

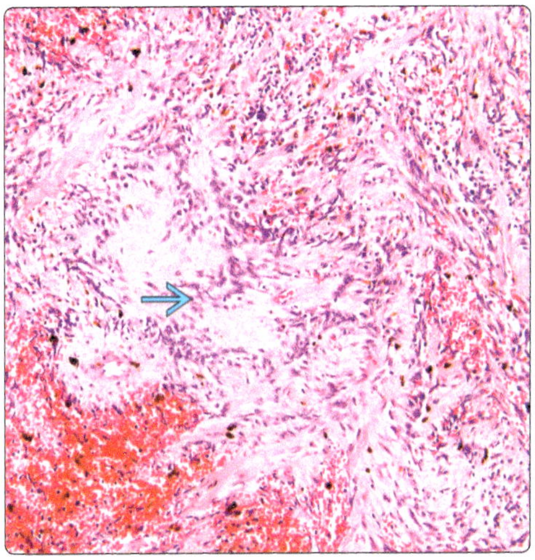

(Left) *Note the peripheral cuff of lymph node tissue →. Such tumors tend to be hemorrhagic and may mimic Kaposi sarcoma. The same tumors have also been described as "intranodal hemorrhagic spindle-cell tumor with amianthoid fibers."* **(Right)** *Note the hemorrhagic appearance and palisaded nuclei →. These lesions display cytoplasmic actin expression (but usually not desmin) and also show nuclear β-catenin labeling. They are nonreactive with S100 and HHV8 antibodies.*

Cutaneous Myxoma and Angiomyxoma

KEY FACTS

TERMINOLOGY

- Superficial angiomyxoma
- Benign mesenchymal proliferation of spindled to stellate fibroblasts in abundant myxoid stroma

ETIOLOGY/PATHOGENESIS

- May be associated with Carney complex
  - a.k.a. NAME (nevi, atrial myxomas, myxoid neurofibromas, and ephelides) and LAMB (lentigines, atrial myxomas, and blue nevi) syndromes
  - If patient has multiple cutaneous myxomas, should consider Carney complex

CLINICAL ISSUES

- Uncommon lesions, which typically present in adults
- Papule, nodule, or polypoid lesion
- Benign but local recurrence common (up to ~ 20%)
- Excision is curative

MICROSCOPIC

- Relatively hypocellular proliferation of bland, spindled to stellate fibroblasts
- Abundant myxoid stroma
- Many thin-walled blood vessels present
- Perivascular neutrophils common
- May have associated epithelial proliferation, usually resulting from entrapped adnexal structures

TOP DIFFERENTIAL DIAGNOSES

- Focal dermal mucinosis
  - Lacks associated vasculature
- Myxoid dermatofibrosarcoma protuberans
  - More uniformly cellular
- Myxoid neurofibroma
  - May show abundant myxoid stroma, but areas of collagenous stroma also present
- Myxoid neurothekeoma (dermal nerve sheath myxoma)
- Superficial acral fibromyxoma

Cutaneous Myxoma

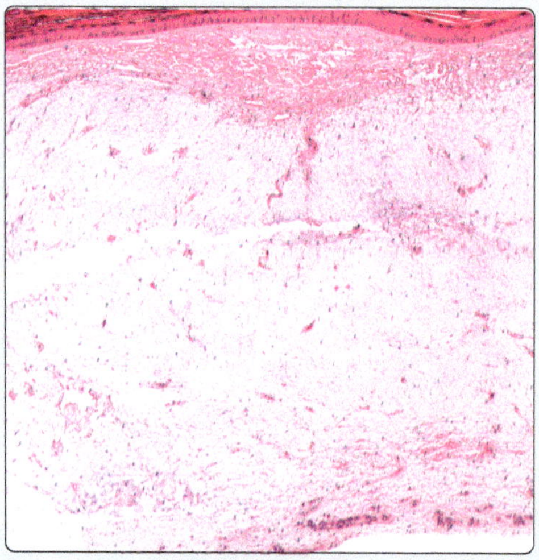

Cutaneous Myxoma With Prominent Myxoid Stroma and Vessels

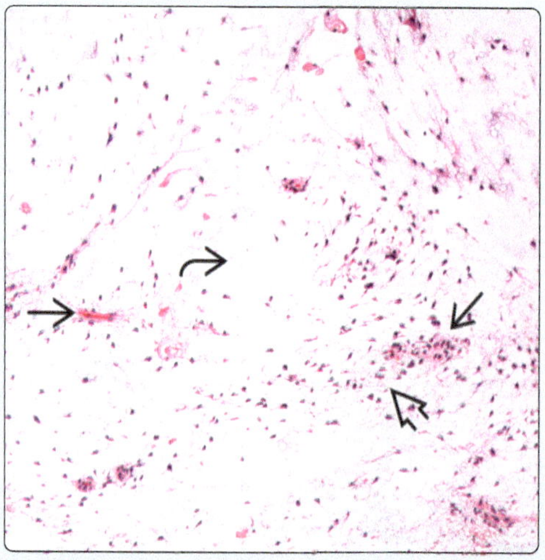

(Left) *Cutaneous myxomas are dermal-based tumors characterized by a hypocellular proliferation of bland, spindled cells and abundant myxoid stroma.* **(Right)** *Intermediate magnification shows that the spindled cells are associated with a capillary vasculature → . Often, there are subtly more cellular ↷ and less cellular ⇨ areas.*

Cutaneous Myxoma With Basaloid Proliferation

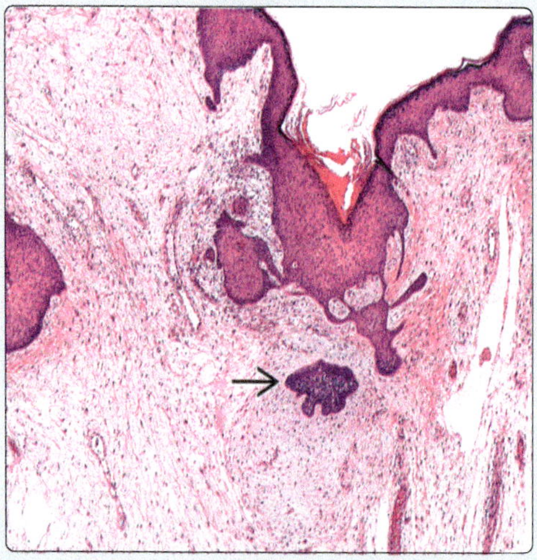

High Magnification of Myxoma With Stromal Neutrophils

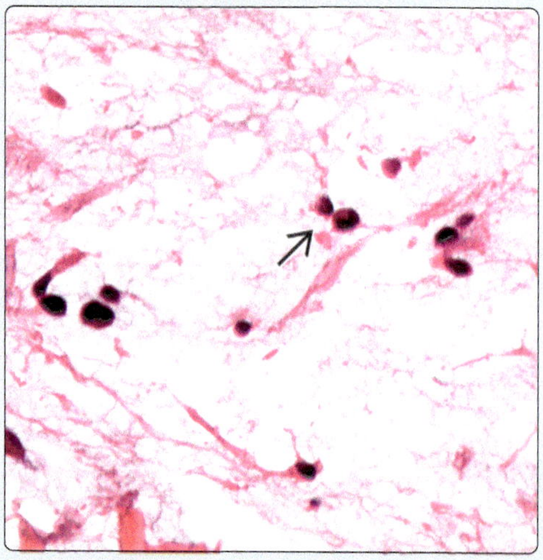

(Left) *Angiomyxomas may induce a superficial proliferation of basaloid epithelium →, similar to dermatofibroma.* **(Right)** *Stromal neutrophils → are often present within cutaneous myxomas.*

TERMINOLOGY

Synonyms

- Superficial angiomyxoma

Definitions

- Benign, mesenchymal proliferation of spindled to stellate fibroblasts in abundant myxoid stroma

ETIOLOGY/PATHOGENESIS

Some Cases Associated With Carney Complex

- Carney complex
  - a.k.a. NAME (nevi, atrial myxomas, myxoid neurofibromas, and ephelides) and LAMB (lentigines, atrial myxomas, and blue nevi) syndromes
  - Multiple cutaneous myxomas
  - Endocrine overactivity
  - Psammomatous melanotic schwannoma

CLINICAL ISSUES

Epidemiology

- Incidence
  - Relatively uncommon lesions
- Age
  - Present in adults in most cases

Presentation

- Papule, nodule, or polypoid lesion

Treatment

- Surgical approaches: Simple excision is curative

Prognosis

- Benign
  - Local recurrence common (up to ~ 20%)
  - No risk of metastasis

MICROSCOPIC

Histologic Features

- Dermal-based tumor that may extend into subcutis
- Poorly circumscribed, multinodular growth pattern
- Relatively hypocellular proliferation of bland spindled to stellate-shaped fibroblasts
  - Cellularity is not uniform
    - Subtle variations in cellularity with relatively more and less cellular areas
- Abundant myxoid stroma
- Many thin-walled blood vessels
- Stromal neutrophils in ~ 50% of cases
- May have associated epithelial proliferation
  - May demonstrate basaloid proliferation in overlying epidermis (similar to dermatofibroma)
  - Rarely associated with benign adnexal tumors
  - Usually result of proliferation of entrapped adnexal tumors

DIFFERENTIAL DIAGNOSIS

Focal Cutaneous Mucinosis

- Dermal mucin between collagen bundles of reticular dermis
- Lacks multinodular growth pattern
- No prominent tumor-associated vasculature
- Lacks secondary epithelial proliferation

Myxoid Dermatofibrosarcoma Protuberans

- Randomly arranged spindled to stellate cells in myxoid stroma
- More uniform cellularity
- Areas of conventional myxoid dermatofibrosarcoma protuberans present in > 60% of cases
- Areas with fat infiltration always at least focally present
- Stromal neutrophils less common than in angiomyxoma
- Usually strongly CD34(+) by immunohistochemistry

Myxoid Neurofibroma

- Sometimes have abundant myxoid stroma, but areas of collagenous stroma also invariably present
- Tumor cells have wavy/comma-shaped nuclei
- Positive for S100

Myxoid Neurothekeoma (Nerve Sheath Myxoma)

- Distinctly nested growth of spindled cells in myxoid stroma
- Nests separated by fibrous septa
- Positive for S100

Perineurioma

- Swirling growth pattern
- Spindled cells with delicate, elongated cytoplasmic processes
- Positive for EMA

Superficial Acral Fibromyxoma

- Stroma fibrous and myxoid, rather than purely myxoid
- Spindled cells may have vaguely storiform pattern
- Almost exclusively occurs on acral surfaces

DIAGNOSTIC CHECKLIST

Pathologic Interpretation Pearls

- Hypocellular tumor with abundant myxoid stroma
  - Subtle variations in cellularity present
- Tumor-associated vasculature
- Associated stromal neutrophils can be clue

SELECTED REFERENCES

1. Correa R et al: Carney complex: an update. Eur J Endocrinol. 173(4):M85-97, 2015
2. Rodríguez Bandera AI et al: Cutaneous embolism of an atrial myxoma. Australas J Dermatol. 56(3):218-20, 2015
3. Satter EK: Solitary superficial angiomyxoma: an infrequent but distinct soft tissue tumor. J Cutan Pathol. 36 Suppl 1:56-9, 2009
4. Pérez Tato B et al: Superficial angiomyxoma with trichofolliculoma. Ann Diagn Pathol. 12(5):375-7, 2008
5. Mehregan DR et al: Epidermal basaloid proliferation in cutaneous myxomas. J Cutan Pathol. 30(8):499-503, 2003
6. Calonje E et al: Superficial angiomyxoma: clinicopathologic analysis of a series of distinctive but poorly recognized cutaneous tumors with tendency for recurrence. Am J Surg Pathol. 23(8):910-7, 1999

Superficial Acral Fibromyxoma

KEY FACTS

TERMINOLOGY

- Synonyms: Digital fibromyxoma, cellular digital fibroma
- Benign fibroblastic neoplasm that occurs in hands and feet, particularly nail bed region

CLINICAL ISSUES

- Most common > 40 yr
- Male predilection
- Vast majority arise in fingers and toes
  - Particularly in or near nail bed
- Solitary, slowly growing, and often long-standing lesion
- Treatment: Complete excision
- Excellent prognosis
- Low rate of recurrence, usually related to incomplete excision

MACROSCOPIC

- Usually < 5 cm (median: 1.5 cm)

MICROSCOPIC

- Moderately cellular proliferation of spindled to stellate fibroblastic cells in randomly arranged loose fascicles or storiform arrays
- Nuclear atypia minimal to absent
- Rare mitoses; no necrosis
- Variable myxoid, myxocollagenous, or collagenous stroma
- Mast cells common

ANCILLARY TESTS

- CD34(+)
- Negative for S100, desmin, keratin, claudin-1

TOP DIFFERENTIAL DIAGNOSES

- Dermatofibroma (fibrous histiocytoma)
- Perineurioma
- Acquired digital fibrokeratoma
- Dermatofibrosarcoma protuberans
- Myxoid neurofibroma

(Left) *Superficial acral fibromyxoma (SAF), also referred to as digital fibromyxoma, is a benign fibroblastic tumor that shows a marked predilection for the fingers and toes, particularly the nail bed region. Histologically, it is characterized by bland spindled and stellate cells arranged in random loose fascicles and storiform arrays within a variable myxoid to fibrous stroma.* **(Right)** *Some areas of SAF feature prominent stromal collagen, as depicted.*

SAF

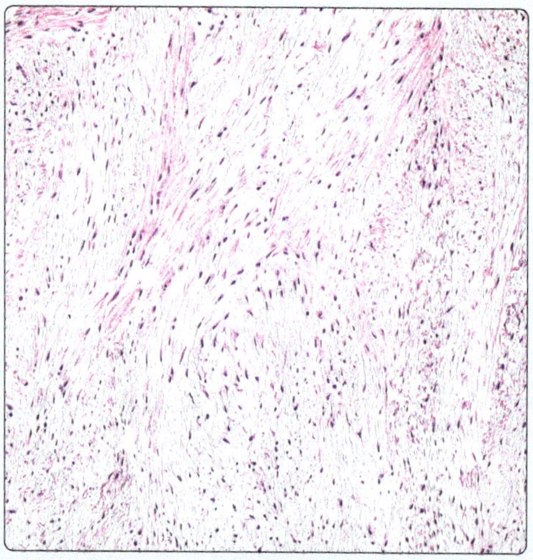

Prominent Collagen in SAF

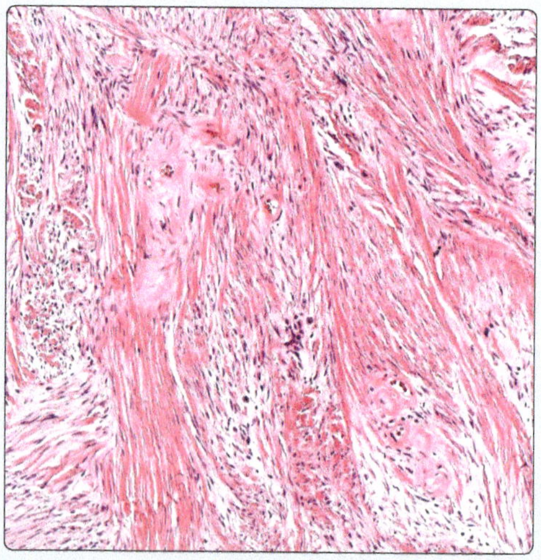

(Left) *SAF may also demonstrate a loose arrangement of cells in a more vascularized stroma, somewhat resembling perineurioma. Despite its usual dermal origin, in some cases, SAF shows superficial extension into subcutaneous fat* ➙*.* **(Right)** *CD34 expression is seen in most cases of SAF, but the extent of this positivity varies. Focal EMA and SMA may also be seen in rare cases. S100, claudin-1, desmin, and keratins are negative.*

Loose Storiform Growth in SAF

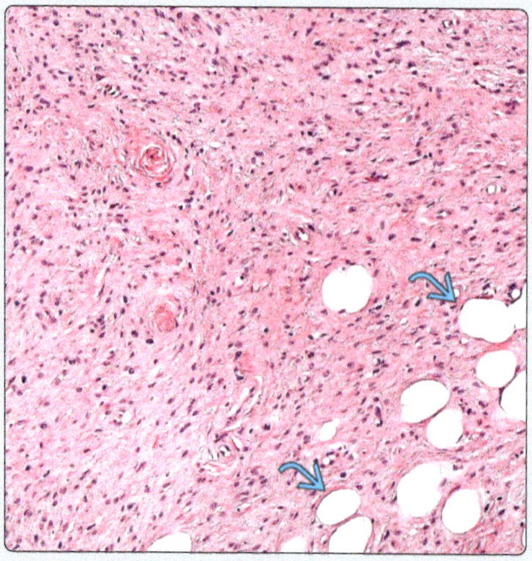

CD34 Expression in SAF

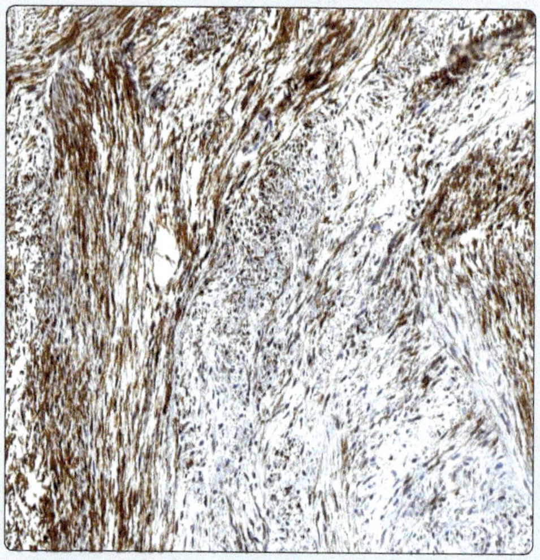

TERMINOLOGY

Abbreviations

- Superficial acral fibromyxoma (SAF)

Synonyms

- Acral fibromyxoma
- Digital fibromyxoma

Definitions

- Benign fibroblastic neoplasm that occurs in hands and feet, particularly nail bed region

CLINICAL ISSUES

Epidemiology

- Incidence
  - Rare
- Age
  - Wide age range
    - Most common > 40 yr
- Sex
  - Male predilection

Site

- Almost exclusively on hands and feet
  - Vast majority in fingers and toes
    - Particularly subungual or periungual region (nail bed)

Presentation

- Solitary, slowly growing, and often longstanding lesion
  - Associated with pain in up to 40-50% of cases
- Superficial, dermal based

Treatment

- Complete excision

Prognosis

- Excellent prognosis
- Recurrences have been reported in up to 22%
  - Usually related to incomplete excision
- No reported case of metastasis or progression

MACROSCOPIC

General Features

- May appear dome-shaped, polypoid, or verrucoid
- Overlying epidermis intact or ulcerated
- Rare tumors can erode underlying bone

Size

- Usually < 5 cm (median: 1.5 cm)

MICROSCOPIC

Histologic Features

- Dermal-based nodular, lobular, or irregular/infiltrative growth
  - Superficial involvement of subcutis and fat in some tumors
- Moderately cellular proliferation of spindled to stellate fibroblastic cells in randomly arranged loose fascicles or storiform arrays
  - Nuclear atypia generally minimal to absent
    - Rare cases with scattered pleomorphic nuclei
  - Occasional multinucleated cells
  - Few cases may show increased cellularity
- Variable myxoid, myxocollagenous, or collagenous stroma
- Small blood vessels common
- Mast cells common
- Rare mitoses; no necrosis

ANCILLARY TESTS

Immunohistochemistry

- CD34(+)
- Occasional focal reactivity for EMA, SMA
- Negative for S100, desmin, cytokeratins, claudin-1

DIFFERENTIAL DIAGNOSIS

Dermatofibroma (Fibrous Histiocytoma)

- Peripheral collagen trapping
- Chronic inflammation, foamy histiocytes common
- Generally negative for CD34 and EMA

Perineurioma

- Can show morphologic overlap with SAF
- Whorled (perivascular) growth pattern often prominent
- Claudin-1 (+)
- Also EMA(+) and variable CD34(+)

Acquired Digital Fibrokeratoma

- Characteristic clinical appearance
- Hyperkeratotic dome-shaped lesion

Dermatofibrosarcoma Protuberans

- Prominent infiltration of subcutaneous fat
- Characteristic prominent storiform growth pattern
- Strong and diffuse CD34(+)
- t(17;22) with *COL1A1-PDGFB* fusion

Myxoid Neurofibroma

- Elongated wrinkled or buckled nuclei
- Loose fascicular or storiform growth uncommon
- S100(+)

Superficial Angiomyxoma

- Lobular growth
- Blood vessels with slightly fibrosed walls
- Prominent myxoid stroma with perivascular neutrophils

SELECTED REFERENCES

1. Sawaya JL et al: Superficial acral fibromyxoma. Int J Dermatol. 54(5):499-508, 2015
2. Schwager ZA et al: Superficial acral fibromyxoma and other slow-growing tumors in acral areas. Cutis. 95(2):E15-9, 2015
3. Hollmann TJ et al: Digital fibromyxoma (superficial acral fibromyxoma): a detailed characterization of 124 cases. Am J Surg Pathol. 36(6):789-98, 2012
4. Al-Daraji WI et al: Superficial acral fibromyxoma: a clinicopathological analysis of 32 tumors including 4 in the heel. J Cutan Pathol. 35(11):1020-6, 2008
5. Prescott RJ et al: Superficial acral fibromyxoma: a clinicopathological study of new 41 cases from the U.K.: should myxoma (NOS) and fibroma (NOS) continue as part of 21st-century reporting? Br J Dermatol. 159(6):1315-21, 2008
6. Fetsch JF et al: Superficial acral fibromyxoma: a clinicopathologic and immunohistochemical analysis of 37 cases of a distinctive soft tissue tumor with a predilection for the fingers and toes. Hum Pathol. 32(7):704-14, 2001

KEY FACTS

TERMINOLOGY

- Rare, dermal-based clear cell tumor of unknown derivation

ETIOLOGY/PATHOGENESIS

- Very rare tumors of unknown etiology

CLINICAL ISSUES

- Extremely rare
- Reported in adults > age 35
- Presents as cutaneous nodule
- Most cases have been reported on lower extremities
- Prognosis uncertain, given their rarity, but appear to be benign or low-grade tumors

MICROSCOPIC

- Nodular dermal-based proliferation of large clear cells with epidermal involvement
- Cytologically, cells are usually bland-appearing, with vesicular nuclei and abundant clear cytoplasm
- Tumors may focally infiltrate subcutaneous adipose tissue
- Lateral borders are typically poorly circumscribed, but deep border is smooth and rounded

ANCILLARY TESTS

- Reportedly positive for NKI-C3/CD63 in all cases
- Negative for CD34, FXIIIA, melanocytic (S100, Melan-A, HMB-45), smooth muscle, and epithelial (cytokeratins) markers

TOP DIFFERENTIAL DIAGNOSES

- Perivascular epithelioid cell tumor
- Clear cell fibrous papule
- Clear cell sarcoma
- Clear cell squamous cell carcinoma and tricholemmal carcinoma
- Paraganglioma-like dermal melanocytic tumor

DDCCMT

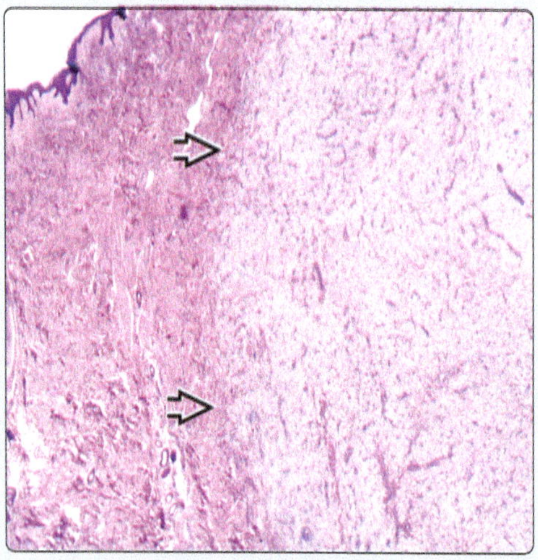

DDCCMT at Higher Magnification

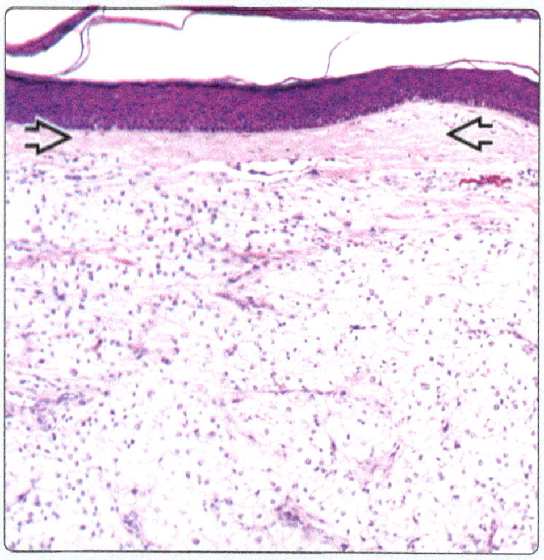

(Left) *Low-power examination shows a dermal-based clear cell tumor with a nonencapsulated lateral border ⇒. (Courtesy A. Lazar, MD, PhD.)* **(Right)** *Higher magnification examination shows a dermal-based clear cell tumor with a thin grenz zone ⇒ separating it from the overlying epidermis. (Courtesy A. Lazar, MD, PhD.)*

DDCCMT at High Magnification

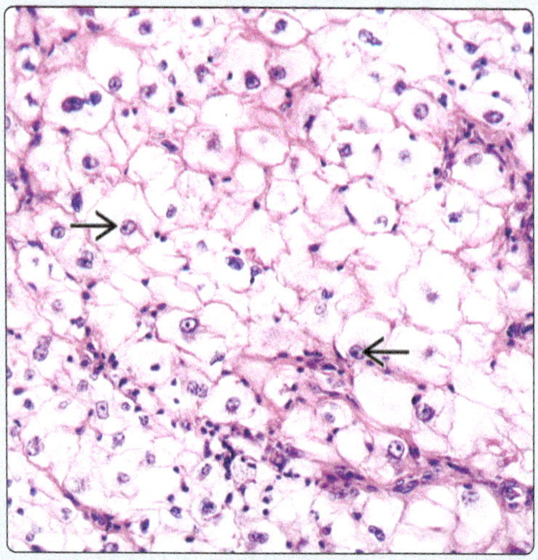

DDCCMT: Cytologic Features

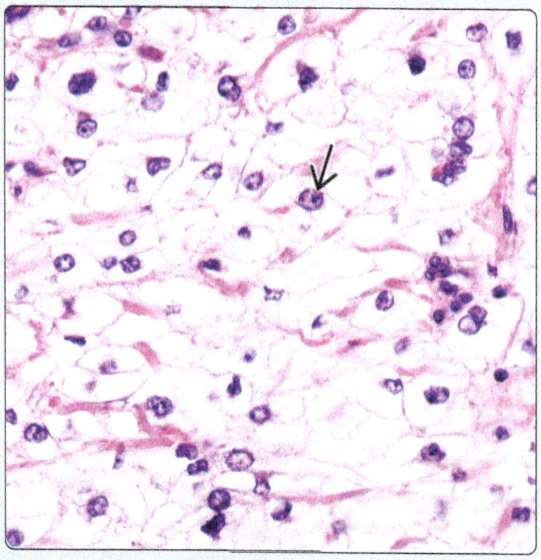

(Left) *High magnification shows the relatively bland cytologic features of the large clear cells with vesicular nuclei, focally enlarged nucleoli ⇒, and abundant clear cytoplasm. (Courtesy A. Lazar, MD, PhD.)* **(Right)** *Higher magnification shows relatively bland cytologic features of large clear cells, which show enlarged nuclei with vesicular chromatin and focally prominent nucleoli ⇒. Cytoplasm is predominantly clear to focally granular-appearing. (Courtesy A. Lazar, MD, PhD.)*

TERMINOLOGY

Abbreviations

- Distinctive dermal clear cell mesenchymal tumor (DDCCMT)

Synonyms

- Distinctive dermal clear cell mesenchymal neoplasm

Definitions

- Rare, dermal-based clear cell tumor of unclear derivation

ETIOLOGY/PATHOGENESIS

Unknown

- Very rare tumors of unknown etiology

CLINICAL ISSUES

Epidemiology

- Incidence
  - Extremely rare
- Age
  - Reported in adults over age 35

Site

- Most cases have occurred on lower extremities

Presentation

- Cutaneous nodule

Treatment

- Surgical approaches
  - Complete conservative excision should be encouraged

Prognosis

- Uncertain, given their rarity, but appear to be benign or low-grade tumors

MACROSCOPIC

General Features

- Nonencapsulated, poorly circumscribed reticular dermal-based nodule

Size

- 0.5-3.0 cm in greatest dimension

MICROSCOPIC

Histologic Features

- Dermal-based tumor composed of nodules of large clear cells
  - Tumors may focally infiltrate subcutaneous adipose tissue
  - Lateral borders are typically poorly circumscribed, but deep border is smooth and rounded
  - No evidence of nesting or junctional involvement
- Cytologically, cells are usually bland-appearing with vesicular nuclei and abundant clear cytoplasm
  - Some cases may show cytologic atypia and pleomorphism with increased numbers of mitoses
  - No cytoplasmic pigmentation

ANCILLARY TESTS

Immunohistochemistry

- Reportedly positive for NKI-C3/CD63 in all cases
- Variable positivity for CD68 and vimentin
- Negative for CD34, FXIIIA, and melanocytic (S100, HMB-45, MART-1/Melan-A), smooth muscle (actin-sm, desmin), and epithelial (cytokeratins) markers

DIFFERENTIAL DIAGNOSIS

Perivascular Epithelioid Cell Tumor (PEComa)

- Rare soft tissue tumor, which may occasionally present in skin
- Tumor cells typically show clear, palely eosinophilic, or granular cytoplasm
- Associated with many small vessels
- Immunoreactivity for melanocytic markers, especially HMB-45, as well as actin-sm

Clear Cell Fibrous Papule

- More superficial, often in papillary dermis with dome-shaped appearance
- Cells may show staining for CD68 and FXIIIA

Clear Cell Sarcoma

- Packets of atypical spindled clear cells surrounded by fibrous stroma
- S100 and other melanocytic markers, such as HMB-45, MART-1/Melan-A, &/or tyrosinase typically positive
- Usually deep soft tissue tumor, may rarely involve dermis

Clear Cell Squamous Cell Carcinoma and Tricholemmal Carcinoma

- Should show more cytologic atypia and abundant mitoses than DDCCMT
- Focal epidermal attachments and areas of keratinization and dyskeratotic cells often present
- Positive for cytokeratins, especially high molecular weight (CK5/CK6, CK903, etc.), and p63

Paraganglioma-Like Dermal Melanocytic Tumor

- Packets of cells with clear to eosinophilic-staining cytoplasm
- Melanocytic markers, including S100, HMB-45, and MART-1/Melan-A, are positive

DIAGNOSTIC CHECKLIST

Pathologic Interpretation Pearls

- Dermal-based proliferation composed of nodules of large clear cells with relatively bland cytologic features

SELECTED REFERENCES

1. Cheng N et al: Clear cell proliferations of the skin. Adv Anat Pathol. 22(3):181-93, 2015
2. Gavino AC et al: Atypical distinctive dermal clear cell mesenchymal neoplasm arising in the scalp. J Cutan Pathol. 35(4):423-7, 2008
3. Liegl B et al: Primary cutaneous PEComa: distinctive clear cell lesions of skin. Am J Surg Pathol. 32(4):608-14, 2008
4. Lee AN et al: Clear cell fibrous papule with NKI/C3 expression: clinical and histologic features in six cases. Am J Dermatopathol. 27(4):296-300, 2005
5. Lazar AJ et al: Distinctive dermal clear cell mesenchymal neoplasm: clinicopathologic analysis of five cases. Am J Dermatopathol. 26(4):273-9, 2004

KEY FACTS

TERMINOLOGY

- Nodular fasciitis (NF): Rapidly growing myofibroblastic proliferation that is often cellular and mitotically active but behaves in benign fashion
- Intravascular fasciitis: Rare variant of NF arising in association with small- and medium-sized vessels
- Cranial fasciitis: Variant of NF involving soft tissues of scalp and underlying skull in infants
- Proliferative fasciitis/myositis: Subcutaneous (fasciitis) or intramuscular (myositis) proliferation of ganglion-like cells in background of myofibroblasts similar to those seen in NF
- Ischemic fasciitis: Proliferation composed of zones of fat and fibrinoid necrosis with ingrowth of capillaries, fibroblasts, and myofibroblasts
- Myositis/panniculitis ossificans: Pseudosarcomatous, bone-producing lesion triggered by trauma

CLINICAL ISSUES

- Excellent prognosis: All these lesions are benign and typically do not recur even after incomplete excision
- Recurrence should prompt rereview of prior sample to ensure initial diagnosis was correct

MICROSCOPIC

- Myofibroblastic differentiation results in expression of "smooth muscle" immunohistochemical markers

TOP DIFFERENTIAL DIAGNOSES

- Fibrous histiocytoma (dermatofibroma)
- Neurofibroma
- Fibromatosis
- Malignant fibrous histiocytoma (undifferentiated pleomorphic sarcoma)
- Leiomyosarcoma
- Kaposi sarcoma

(Left) *This gross specimen example shows bone formation* ➔. **(Right)** *The appearance of many examples of nodular fasciitis is similar to that of granulation tissue, although there is not a consistent history of trauma reported in most cases.*

Myositis Ossificans, Gross Image

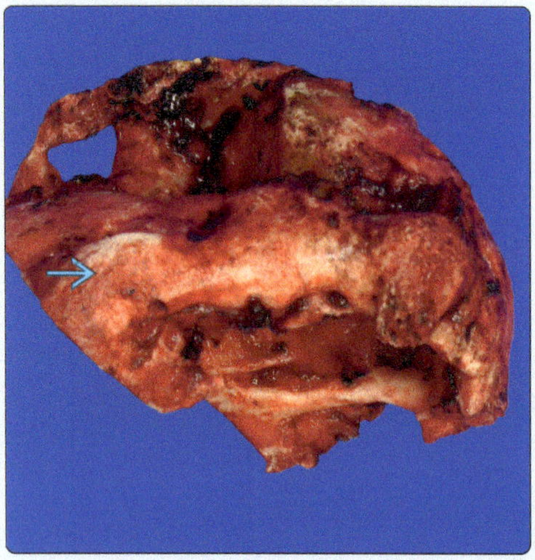

Nodular Fasciitis, Granulation Tissue-Like Pattern

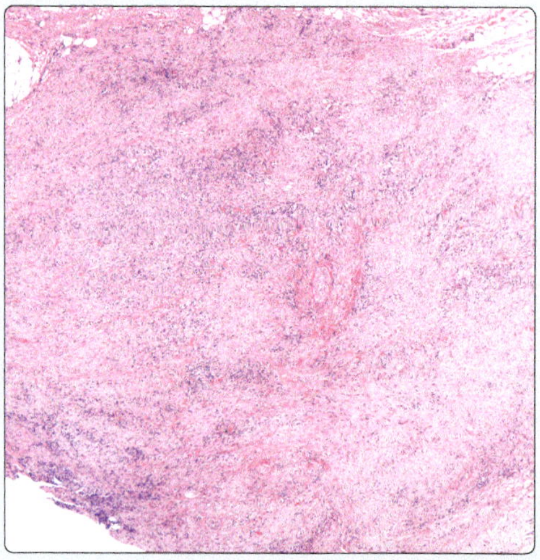

(Left) *This classic image of nodular fasciitis shows a myofibroblastic lesion with a storiform pattern, cystic spaces, scattered lymphocytes* ➔, *and extravasated erythrocytes.* **(Right)** *Proliferative fasciitis features the same background spindled myofibroblastic cells as nodular fasciitis* ➔, *with the addition of ganglion cell-like fibroblasts* ➔. *The latter are not true ganglion cells.*

Nodular Fasciitis, Storiform Pattern

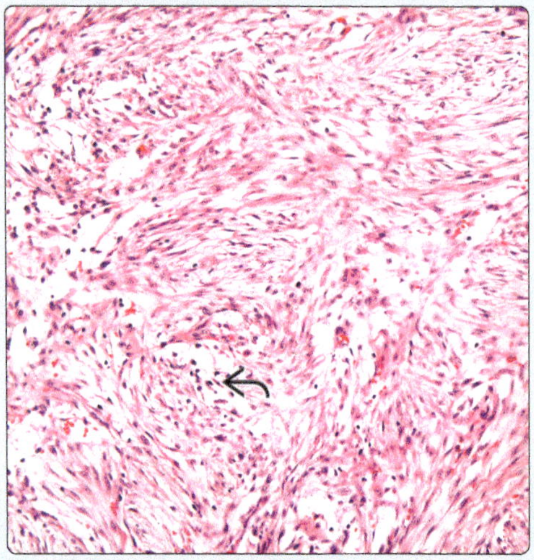

Proliferative Fasciitis, Ganglion-Like Cells

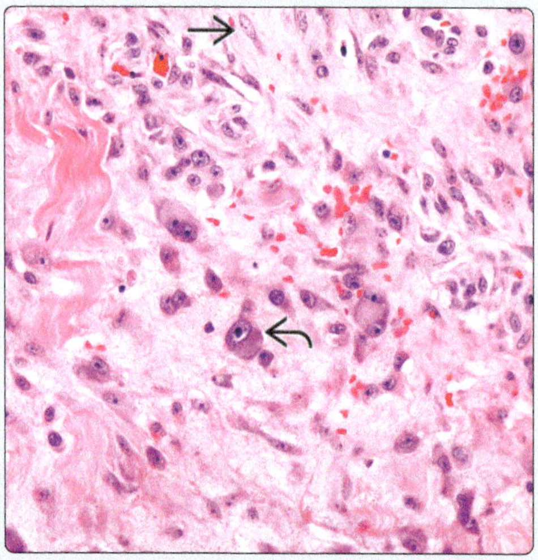

TERMINOLOGY

Abbreviations

- Nodular fasciitis (NF)

Synonyms

- Pseudosarcomatous fasciitis (NF)
- Subcutaneous pseudosarcomatous fibromatosis (NF)
- Atypical decubital fibroplasia (ischemic fasciitis)

Definitions

- **NF**: Rapidly growing, myofibroblastic, mass-forming proliferation that is often cellular and mitotically active but behaves in benign fashion
- **Intravascular fasciitis**: Rare variant of NF arising in association with small- and medium-sized vessels
- **Cranial fasciitis**: Variant of NF involving soft tissues of scalp and underlying skull in infants
- **Proliferative fasciitis/myositis**: Tumefactive subcutaneous (fasciitis) or intramuscular (myositis) proliferation featuring ganglion-like fibroblasts in background of myofibroblasts similar to those seen in NF
- **Ischemic fasciitis**: Pseudosarcomatous proliferation composed of zones of fat and fibrinoid necrosis with zonal ingrowth of capillaries, fibroblasts, and myofibroblasts
  - Initially described as tumefactive pressure sore arising over bony prominences in debilitated patients, but some examples do not fit this profile
- **Myositis/panniculitis ossificans**: Pseudosarcomatous, bone-producing lesion triggered by trauma

CLINICAL ISSUES

Epidemiology

- Incidence
  - All are uncommon; NF is most common among them
- Age
  - NF: Most patients are in their 3rd and 4th decades
  - Intravascular fasciitis: Most patients are in their 3rd and 4th decades
  - Cranial fasciitis: Infants in peripartum period
  - Proliferative fasciitis: Middle-aged and older adults; rare in children
  - Ischemic fasciitis: Elderly patients typical
- Sex
  - No predilection

Site

- NF: Classic site is forearm
- Intravascular fasciitis: Classic sites are distal extremities (especially fingers) and head and neck
- Cranial fasciitis: Head
- Proliferative fasciitis: Classic site is forearm
- Ischemic fasciitis: Classic sites are overlying sacral promontory or greater trochanter
- Myositis/panniculitis ossificans: Usually in proximal lower extremities

Presentation

- All of these pseudosarcomatous processes present as mass lesions, usually painless
  - Most lesions: 1-3 cm
  - Ischemic fasciitis lesions can be large

Treatment

- Simple excision is curative

Prognosis

- Excellent; all of these lesions are benign and typically do not recur
- Recurrence should prompt review of prior sample to ensure that initial diagnosis was correct

IMAGING

General Features

- Imaging generally shows well-marginated subcutaneous process
  - Exception: Proliferative fasciitis tracks along connective tissue septa

MACROSCOPIC

General Features

- Well-marginated but unencapsulated lesions
- White to gelatinous cross section
- Ischemic fasciitis can feature areas of hemorrhage

Size

- Most 2-3 cm (exception is ischemic fasciitis, which can attain large size)

MICROSCOPIC

Histologic Features

- **NF**
  - Loose storiform pattern with tissue culture appearance, variable myxoid stroma, cystic spaces, strands of keloid-like collagen
  - Osteoclast-like giant cells common (see in most lesions if sought; can be enhanced by CD68 staining)
  - Scattered lymphocytes but negligible plasma cells
  - Extravasated erythrocytes unassociated with hemosiderin deposition
  - 3 reported forms: Myxoid, cellular, fibrous
    - Loose correlation with duration of lesions
    - Myxoid lesions often have been resected within 10 days of coming to clinical attention
    - Cellular and fibrous forms more longstanding; some lesions show mixed patterns
  - Myofibroblastic differentiation results in expression of "smooth muscle" immunohistochemical markers
    - Lesions can thus be mistaken for leiomyosarcoma when mitotically active
- **Intravascular fasciitis**
  - Similar features to NF, except has intravascular component
    - Often associated extravascular component encountered
  - Abundant osteoclast-like giant cells
  - Prominent mitotic activity can result in incorrect diagnosis of intravascular leiomyosarcoma
- **Cranial fasciitis**
  - Lesion of infancy sometimes attributed to birth trauma
  - Similar morphology to that of NF but more myxoid

- Some reported lesions are probably instead fibromatoses
- **Proliferative fasciitis**
  - Predominantly plump stellate to spindled fibroblasts and myofibroblasts
  - Extravasated erythrocytes
  - Background myofibroblasts
  - Large ganglion-like fibroblasts
    - Macronucleoli, abundant amphophilic cytoplasm
    - Not true ganglion cells; no Nissl substance
  - Pediatric examples
    - Ganglion-like cells predominate
    - Exuberant mitotic activity
    - Mistaken for rhabdomyosarcomas in the past
    - Lack skeletal muscle markers (MYOD1, myogenin)
- **Ischemic fasciitis**
  - Ill-defined, focally myxoid masses
  - Lobular configuration
  - Most centered in deep subcutis
  - Few extend into skeletal muscle or tendon/aponeurosis; overlying skin typically intact
  - Zones of fibrinoid necrosis and myxoid stroma
  - Necrotic zones rimmed by ingrowing ectatic, thin-walled vessels
  - Atypical enlarged degenerating fibroblasts with abundant basophilic cytoplasm, large hyperchromatic nuclei, prominent nucleoli
  - Occasional mitoses, including atypical forms

DIFFERENTIAL DIAGNOSIS

Fibrous Histiocytoma (Dermatofibroma)

- Mostly in differential diagnosis of NF
- Storiform pattern in cellular examples
- Collagen trapping usually prominent
- Abundant background changes (foamy histiocytes, hemosiderin, plasma cells)
- Overlying epidermal hyperplasia
- Factor XIII and CD10 (+); variable actin expression
- Tend to recur locally when incompletely excised

Neurofibroma

- Wavy/angulated nuclei
- Shredded appearing collagen, nuclei "plastered" against collagen fibrils
- Myxoid change, mast cells
- S100(+), variable CD34(+)
- Benign behavior

Fibromatosis

- Large, deep, infiltrative lesions
- Shoulder girdle, abdomen (in women in childbearing years), head and neck
- Sweeping fascicles of myofibroblasts
- Uniform collagen deposition
- Prominent vascular pattern
- Express actin (myofibroblastic), show nuclear β-catenin labeling
- Prone to local recurrences

Kaposi Sarcoma

- Immunocompromised patients and elderly patients
- In setting of AIDS/HIV, often in skin and mucosal surfaces of upper 1/2 of body
- In elderly, in distal lower extremity
- All examples associated with HHV-8
- Hyperchromatic-staining spindle cells
- Extravasated erythrocytes, hemosiderin, plasma cells, hyaline globules
- Immunoreactivity: Positive for CD34, CD31, HHV8
- Most behave indolently; some regress

Malignant Fibrous Histiocytoma (Undifferentiated Pleomorphic Sarcoma)

- Deep lesions in 6th and 7th decades
- Storiform pattern
- Marked atypia, pleomorphism, atypical mitoses

Embryonal Rhabdomyosarcoma

- Mostly in differential diagnosis of proliferative fasciitis in children
- Genital region/head and neck of young children
- Enhanced cellularity beneath mucous membranes (cambium layer)
- Atypical nuclei often without prominent nucleoli
- Expresses skeletal muscle markers on immunolabeling

Well-Differentiated Liposarcoma (Atypical Lipomatous Tumor)

- Mostly in differential diagnosis for ischemic fasciitis
- Large, deep lesions of proximal extremities and retroperitoneum
- Mature-appearing adipose tissue lesion with relatively homogeneous low-power appearance
- Lobules of fat separated by fibrous bands containing enlarged hyperchromatic nuclei
- Occasional lipoblasts (not required for diagnosis)

Leiomyosarcoma

- Wide range of clinical presentations
- Perpendicularly oriented fascicles
- Brightly eosinophilic-staining cytoplasm
- Hyperchromatic nuclei with blunt ends
- Paranuclear vacuoles
- Immunolabeling: Actin, desmin, calponin, and caldesmon all reactive
- Outcome relates to stage and site

Pleomorphic Rhabdomyosarcoma

- In differential diagnosis of proliferative fasciitis in adults
- Highly aggressive tumors of deep proximal extremities of older adults
- Markedly pleomorphic cells
- Skeletal muscle immunophenotype

SELECTED REFERENCES

1. Oliveira AM et al: USP6-induced neoplasms: the biologic spectrum of aneurysmal bone cyst and nodular fasciitis. Hum Pathol. 45(1):1-11, 2014

Nodular Fasciitis: More Cellular Example

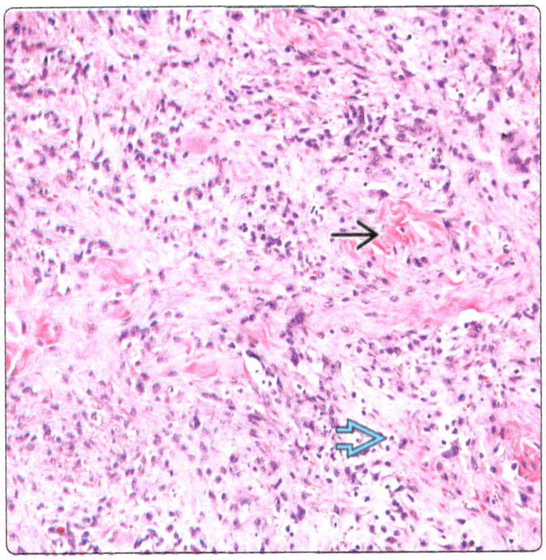

Nodular Fasciitis, Cytologic Features

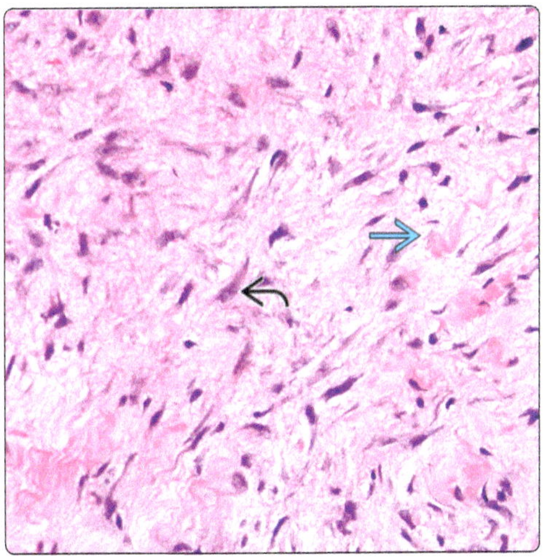

(Left) *This example is relatively cellular and expressed strong actin but not desmin, a profile typical of nodular fasciitis. This example also shows keloid-like collagen* → *and scattered lymphocytes* ⇨*, but no hemosiderin or plasma cells.* **(Right)** *The myofibroblastic cells have a stellate appearance. They are interspersed between fragments of keloid-like collagen* ⇨*. Each nucleus features a delicate nucleolus* ↶*, a feature shared with fibromatosis. This forearm lesion was from a 20-year-old man.*

Nodular Fasciitis, Keloid-Like Collagen

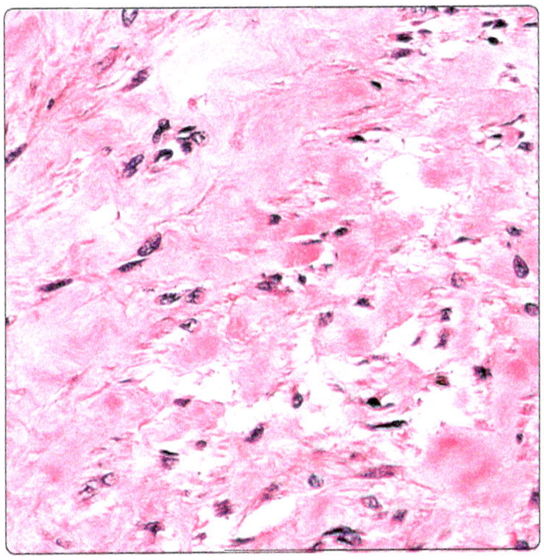

Nodular Fasciitis, Osteoclast-Like Giant Cell

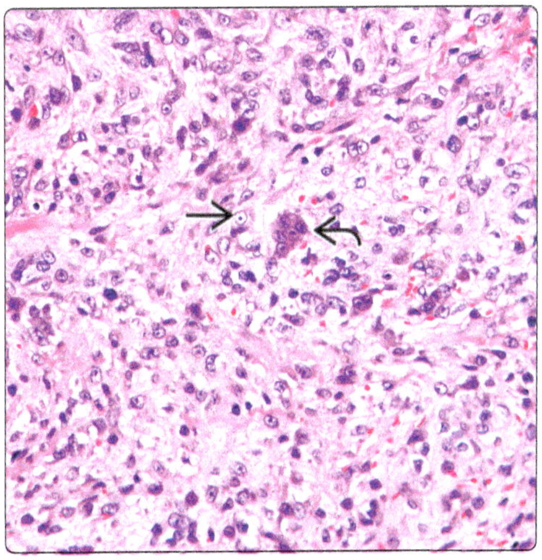

(Left) *This field shows an example with striking keloid-like collagen. Some observers believe this suggests that the lesion has been present for months.* **(Right)** *An osteoclast-like giant cell is present in the center of the field* ↶*. Otherwise, the tumor is composed of uniform spindle cells with delicate chromatin. Most of the cells contain small nucleoli* →*.*

Nodular Fasciitis, Osteoclast-Like Giant Cells

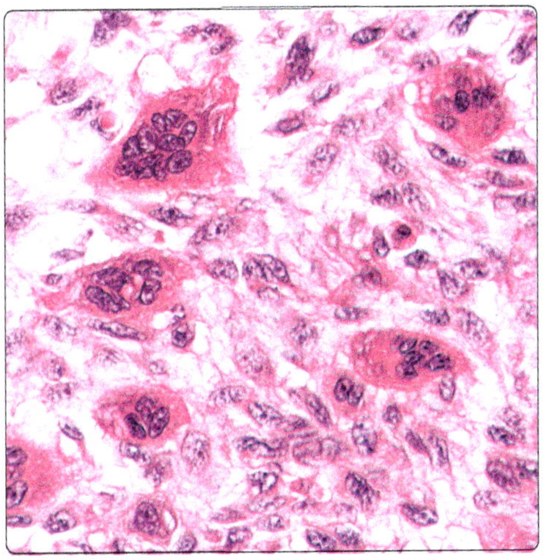

Nodular Fasciitis, SMA Immunostain

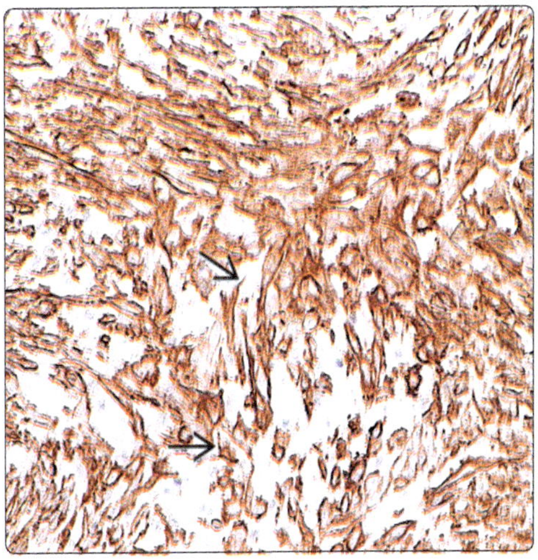

(Left) *Some examples contain numerous osteoclast-like giant cells. This appearance is reminiscent of that of giant cell tumor of tendon sheath. However, in contrast to giant cell tumor of tendon sheath, hemosiderin deposition is not a feature of nodular fasciitis.* **(Right)** *SMA is strongly reactive, as nodular fasciitis is a myofibroblastic lesion. This can lead to misinterpretation as a leiomyosarcoma. The stain highlights the stellate appearance of the cytoplasm* → *of the cells, which differs from the bipolar cytoplasm of smooth muscle tumors.*

(Left) *This field shows the typical constellation of features of nodular fasciitis: An osteoclast-like giant cell* ↷*, keloid-like collagen, numerous myofibroblasts with pale chromatin, and extravasated erythrocytes* →*.* **(Right)** *At low magnification, proliferative fasciitis is striking for tracking along fibrous connective tissue septa in the subcutaneous tissue. The center of the lesion shows some thickened, keloid-like collagen* ⇨*.*

Nodular Fasciitis, Cytologic Features

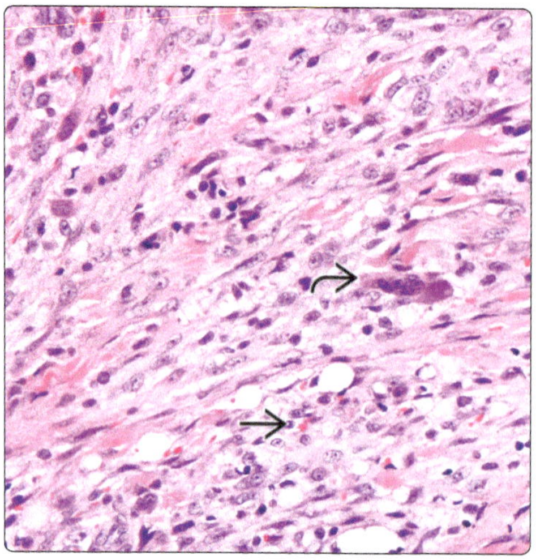

Proliferative Fasciitis, Architectural Features

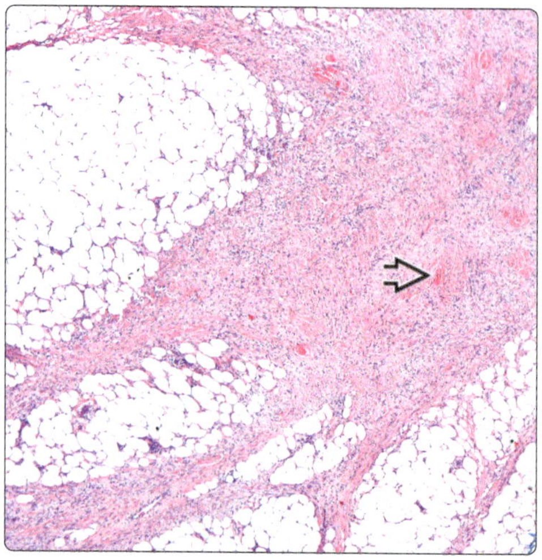

(Left) *At this magnification of proliferative fasciitis, a background of cells similar to those of nodular fasciitis is present, but larger ganglion-like fibroblasts* → *can also be seen. Note the paucicellular appearance at the center of the lesion* ⇨*.* **(Right)** *This image shows several large ganglion-like cells of proliferative fasciitis* → *in a background of smaller cells that are more like those seen in nodular fasciitis. There are also extravasated erythrocytes* ⇨*.*

Proliferative Fasciitis, Zonation

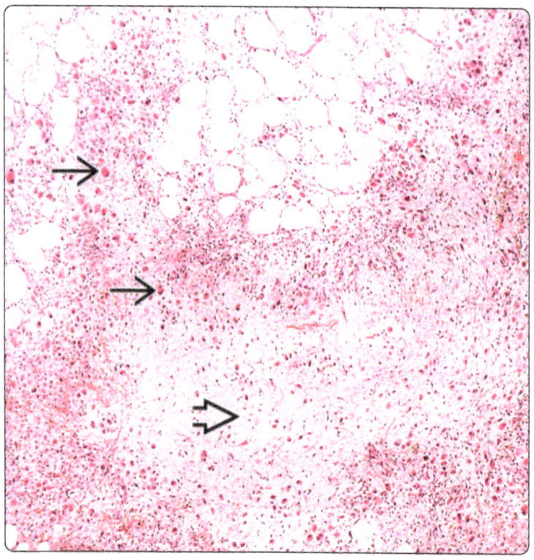

Proliferative Fasciitis, Ganglion-Like Cells

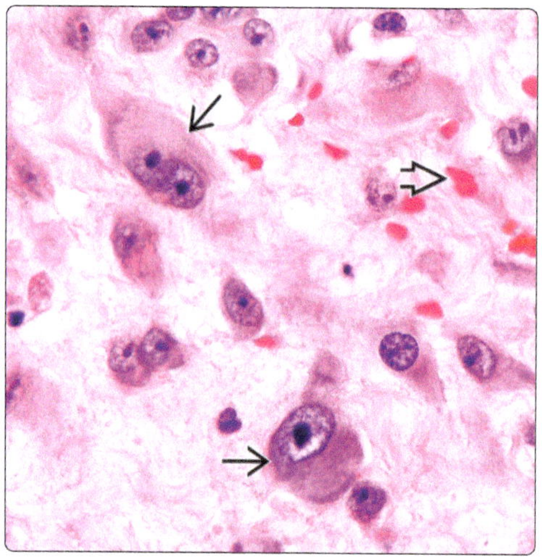

(Left) *Proliferative myositis is akin to proliferative fasciitis but is centered in skeletal muscle* ↶*. Ganglion-like cells* ⇨ *are apparent at this magnification. Like nodular fasciitis, proliferative fasciitis/myositis displays a backdrop of lymphocytes* →*.* **(Right)** *Ganglion-like cells* ⇨ *are the key element of proliferative myositis, but the background cells* → *are identical to those of nodular fasciitis. Scattered lymphocytes* ↶ *are present.*

Proliferative Myositis, Infiltration Between Muscle Cells

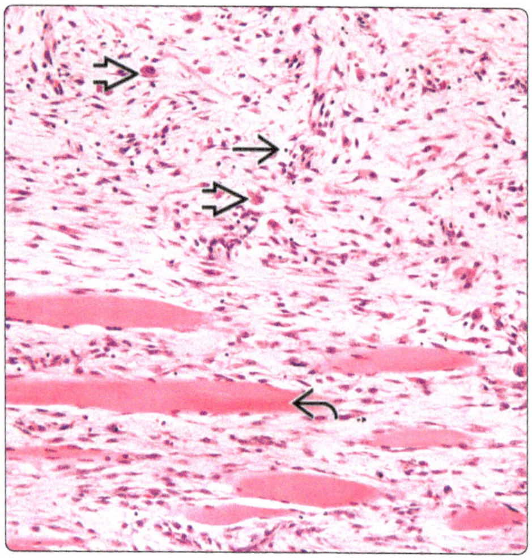

Proliferative Myositis at Higher Magnification

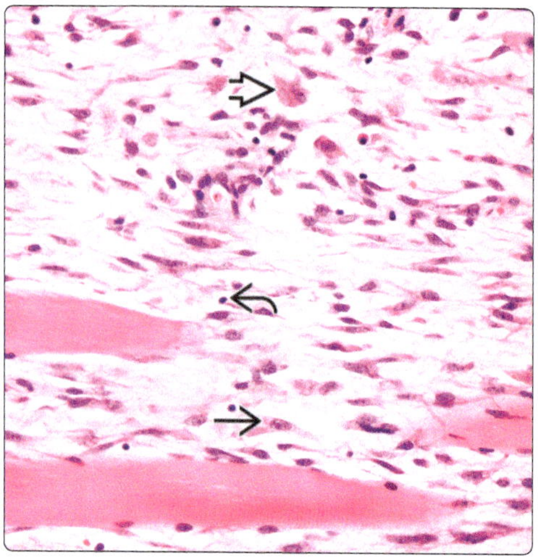

Intravascular Fasciitis, Intraoperative Image

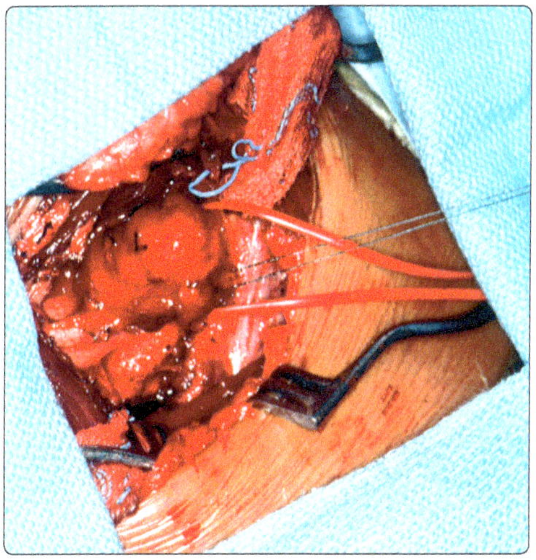

Intravascular Fasciitis in Capillary

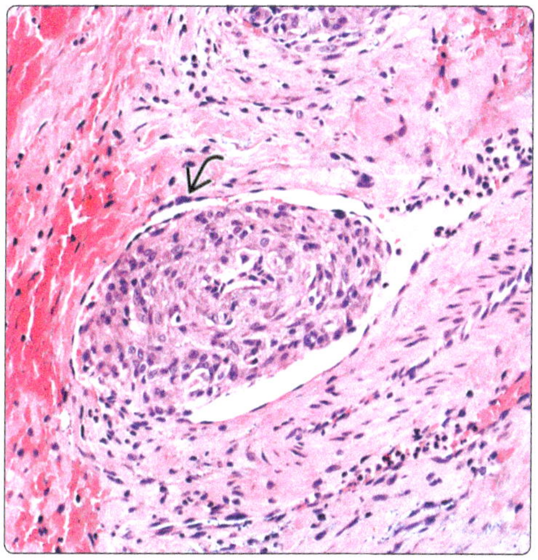

(Left) *This intraoperative image is of an example of intravascular fasciitis obstructing the brachial artery. The patient gave a history of falling asleep slumped over a wooden chair. Intraoperatively, the surgeon interpreted this 3-cm mass as a sarcoma.* **(Right)** *Note that the nuclei of intravascular fasciitis are paler than those of the endothelial cells → in the involved capillary. This feature is a clue that the process is pseudosarcomatous rather than sarcomatous.*

Intravascular Fasciitis, Osteoclast-Like Giant Cell

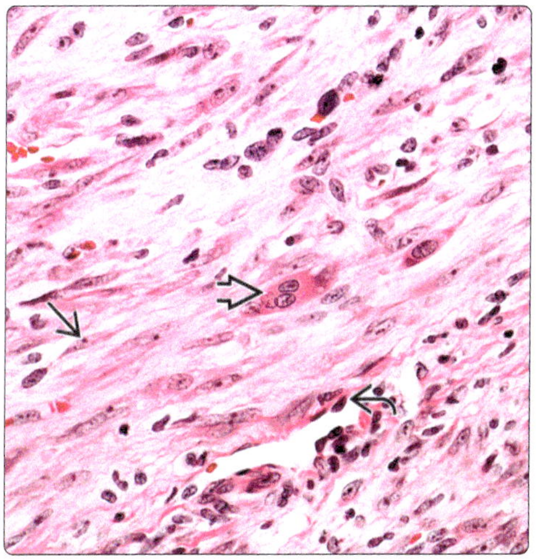

Intravascular Fasciitis, Movat Stain

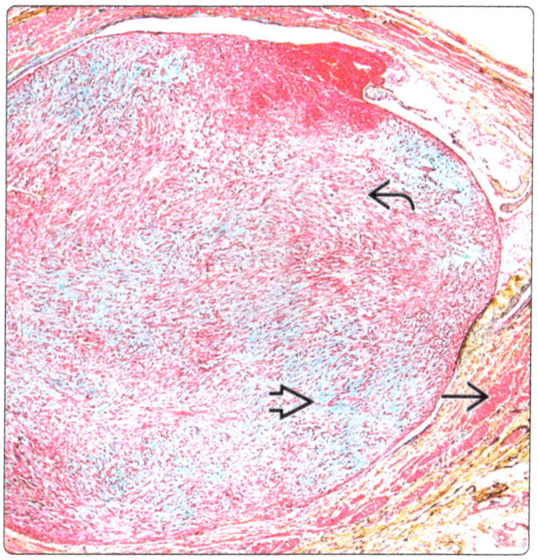

(Left) *Osteoclast-like giant cells → are often a prominent feature of intravascular fasciitis. The background cells are paler than the endothelial cells →. As in nodular fasciitis, the individual cells have uniform, small nucleoli →.* **(Right)** *Movat stain in intravascular fasciitis shows a reddish color → that is less striking than the vessel containing the process →, accompanied by fibroblastic zones that appear bluish →. These qualities indicate that the lesion is myofibroblastic.*

Intravascular Fasciitis, Cytologic Features

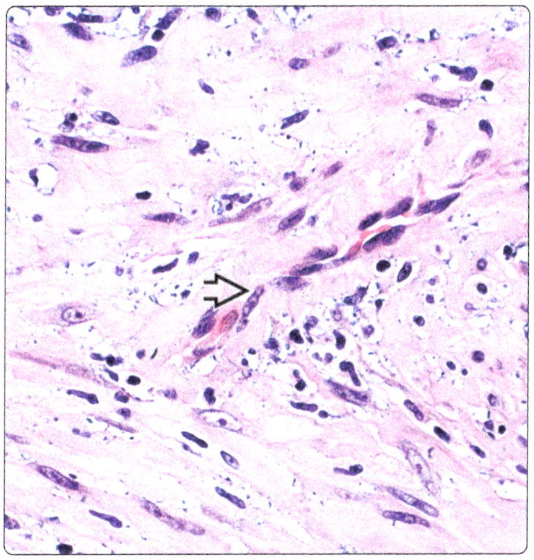

Ischemic Fasciitis

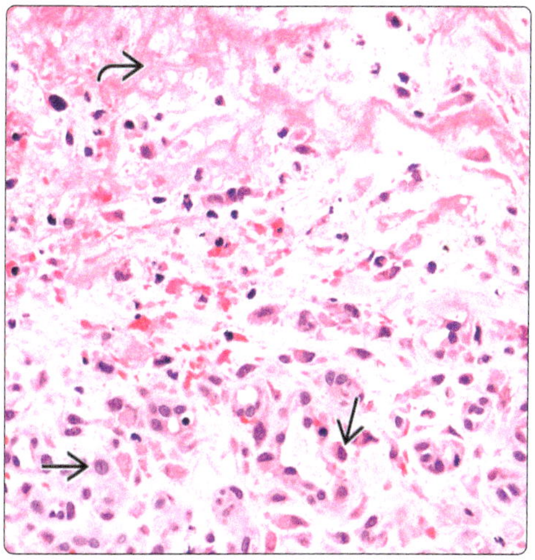

(Left) *This image demonstrates the comparison between endothelial cells and lesional cells of intravascular fasciitis. The benign endothelial cells → are darker-staining.* **(Right)** *This example of ischemic fasciitis shows fibrinoid necrosis →. Enlarged fibroblasts are found in the viable portion →.*

Ischemic Fasciitis, Gross Image

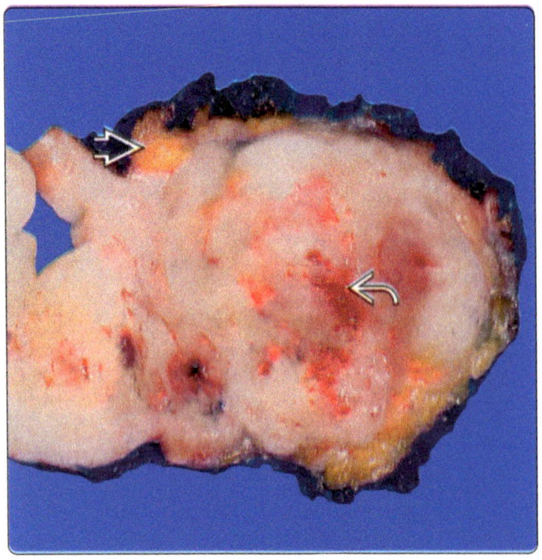

Ischemic Fasciitis, Architectural Features

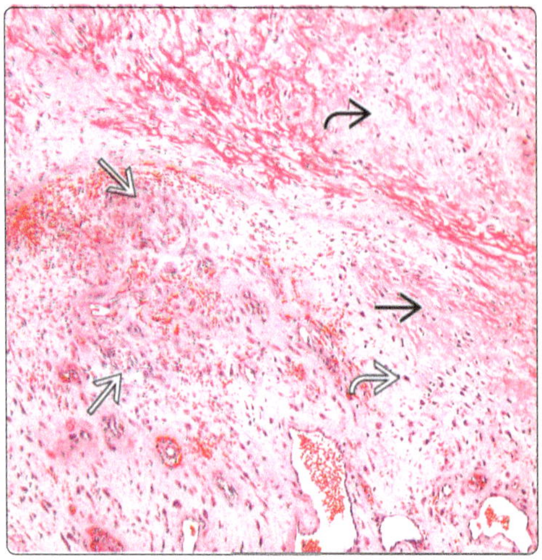

(Left) *Ischemic fasciitis (atypical decubital fibroplasia) generally involves subcutaneous fat and has a hemorrhagic center.* **(Right)** *In this example of ischemic fasciitis (atypical decubital fibroplasia), the top of the field and the right side show zones of fibrinoid necrosis. A more cellular area containing ingrowing fibroblasts and vessels is at the left of the field. Even at this low magnification, there appear to be enlarged nuclei.*

Ischemic Fasciitis: High Magnification

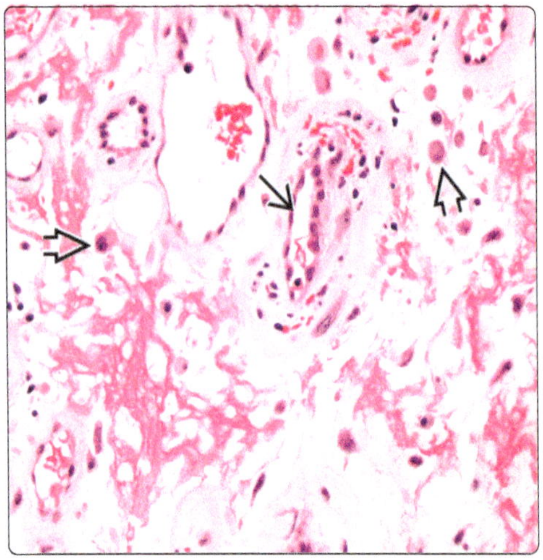

Ischemic Fasciitis, Cytologic Features

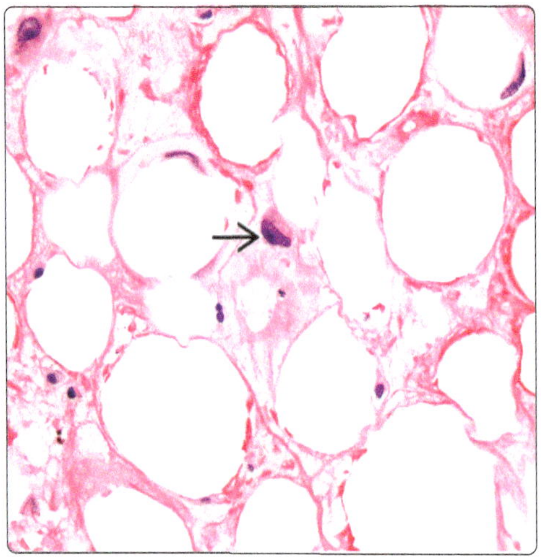

(Left) *This image from a case of ischemic fasciitis is from the interface between an area of fibrinoid necrosis and a viable area. There are prominent capillaries and a few enlarged fibroblasts, with appearances similar to those encountered in proliferative fasciitis.* **(Right)** *Note the enlarged fibroblast in this example of ischemic fasciitis (atypical decubital fibroplasia). The cell has a conspicuous nucleolus and is seen in a background of fat with fibrinoid necrosis.*

Panniculitis Ossificans, Low Magnification

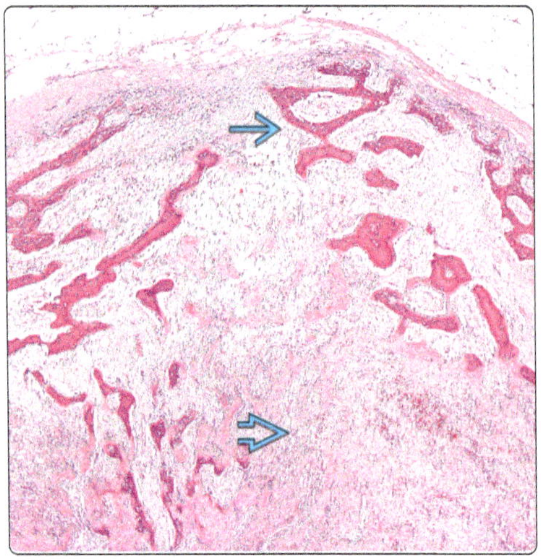

Panniculitis Ossificans, Early Bone Formation

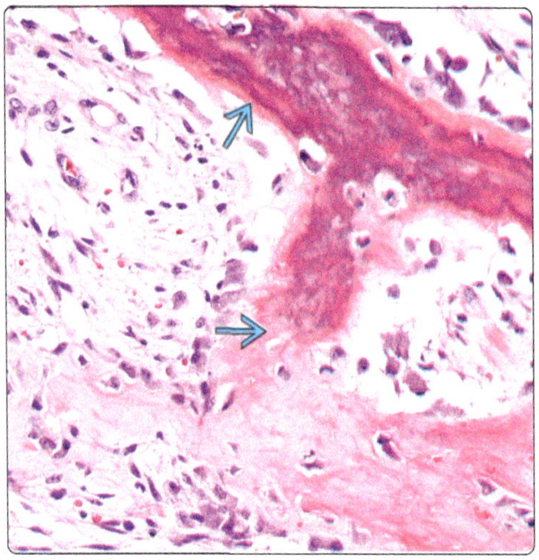

(Left) *The bone in the lesion is at the periphery, whereas the central portion is more cellular, with a similar appearance to those of nodular fasciitis.* **(Right)** *This image shows the interface between the early bone formation and the cellular zone.*

Differential Diagnosis: Fibrous Histiocytoma/ Dermatofibroma

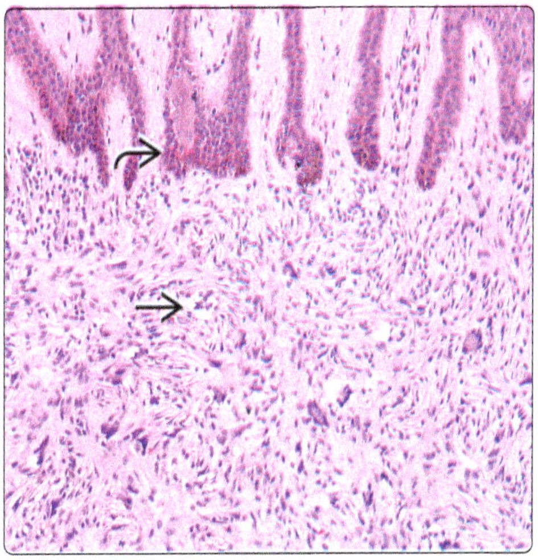

Differential Diagnosis: Neurofibroma

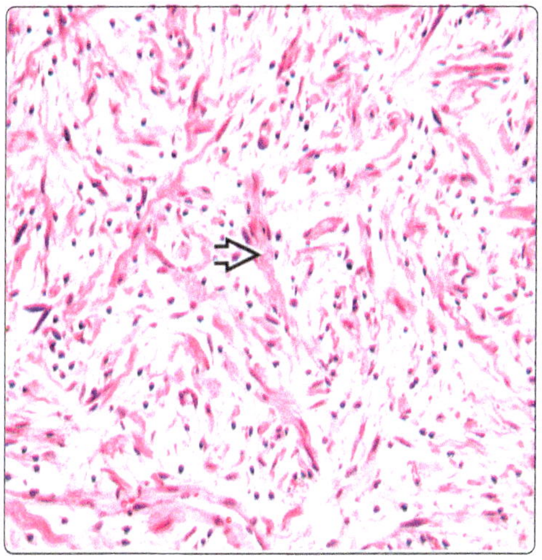

(Left) *Fibrous histiocytoma/dermatofibroma shows overlying epidermal hyperplasia with basilar hyperpigmentation ↪, and the lesion contains foamy histiocytes →, in contrast to the osteoclast-like giant cells in nodular fasciitis.* **(Right)** *Neurofibromas feature prominent wiry collagen, and the lesional cell nuclei often appear tightly plastered against the collagen ⇨. This pattern of collagen is very different from the keloid-like collagen in nodular fasciitis.*

Differential Diagnosis: Fibromatosis, Fascicular Pattern

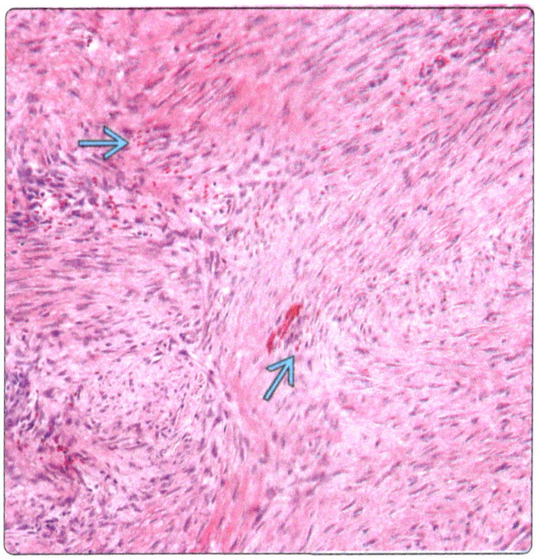

Differential Diagnosis: Hyalinizing Spindle Cell Tumor With Giant Rosettes

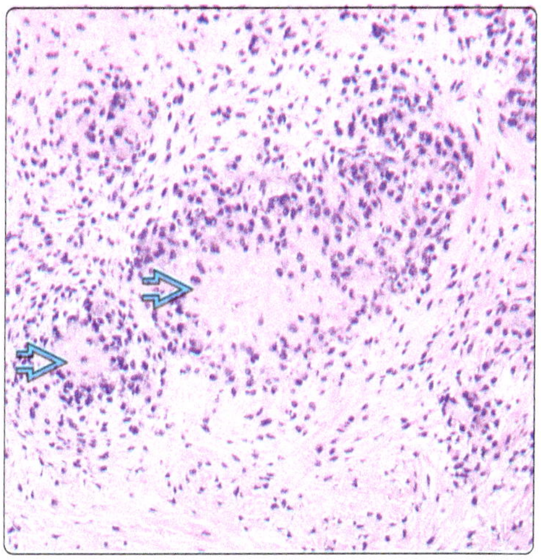

(Left) *Fibromatoses are characterized by evenly spaced nuclei separated by collagen. Extravasated erythrocytes → can be encountered, as in nodular fasciitis, but they are not a prominent feature; there are typically few inflammatory cells.* **(Right)** *This tumor is a variant of low-grade fibromyxoid sarcoma and shares the molecular alterations. Note the rosettes ⇨. The background lesion is indistinguishable from low-grade fibromyxoid sarcoma.*

Differential Diagnosis: Low-Grade Fibromyxoid Sarcoma

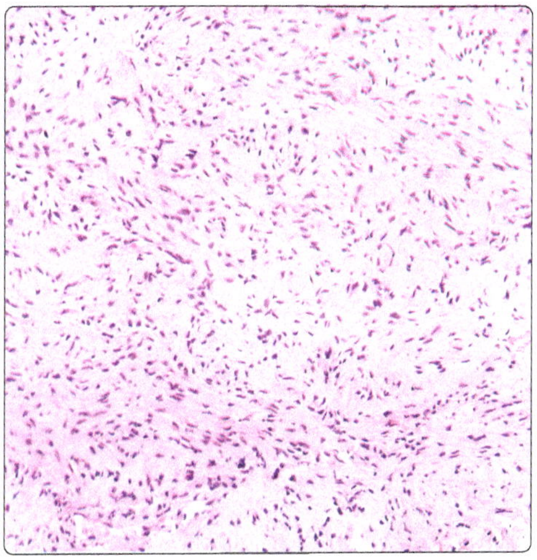

Differential Diagnosis: Low-Grade Fibromyxoid Sarcoma, Cytologic Features

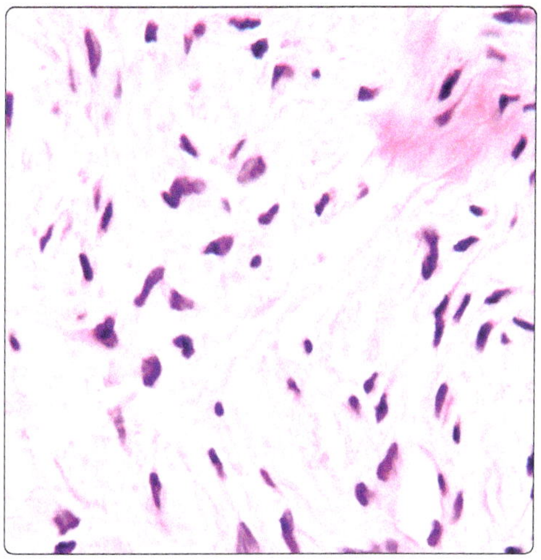

(Left) *The nuclei are arranged more haphazardly than those of fibromatosis.* **(Right)** *The nuclei are small but hyperchromatic. Note the lack of identifiable nucleoli.*

Angiomatoid Fibrous Histiocytoma

KEY FACTS

TERMINOLOGY

- Distinctive, rarely metastasizing mesenchymal neoplasm composed of nodules and sheets of spindled and histiocytoid cells
  - Often demonstrates pseudoangiomatous spaces and peripheral lymphoplasmic cuff

CLINICAL ISSUES

- Predominantly children and young adults
- Most often arises in superficial extremities
- Constitutional symptoms in subset (e.g., fever, malaise, anemia)
- Treatment: Wide local excision with follow-up
- Up to 15% recur locally
- Rare cases metastasize (< 5%)

MICROSCOPIC

- Fibrous pseudocapsule with lymphoplasmacytic cuff (80% of cases)
- Sheets, nodules, and aggregates of ovoid to spindled cells
- Most cells are cytologically bland with vesicular nuclei; mitoses infrequent
  - Scattered cells with nuclear hyperchromasia and pleomorphism are common
- Variably sized, blood-filled pseudovascular spaces in majority of cases

ANCILLARY TESTS

- Desmin (+) in 50-60% of cases
- Variable, nonspecific expression of EMA, CD68, CD99, SMA
- Molecular: t(2:22) with *EWSR1-CREB1* fusion most common

TOP DIFFERENTIAL DIAGNOSES

- Aneurysmal fibrous histiocytoma
- Undifferentiated pleomorphic sarcoma
- Nodal metastasis
- Follicular dendritic cell sarcoma
- Granulomatous lesions

AFH

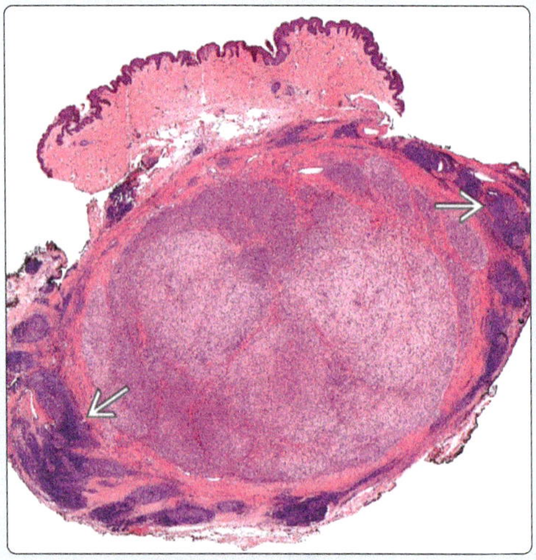

AFH With Nodular/Lobular Growth

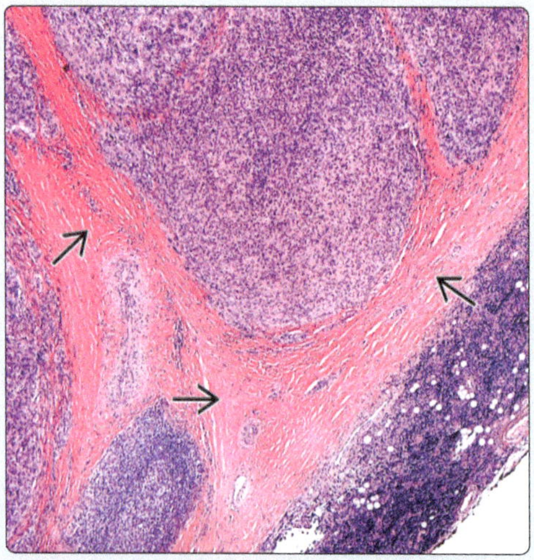

(Left) *Angiomatoid fibrous histiocytoma (AFH) usually occurs in the subcutaneous tissue or deep dermis of the extremities. Most examples demonstrate a fibrous pseudocapsule associated with a patchy chronic inflammatory infiltrate ➡. The overall pattern may mimic a lymph node metastasis.* **(Right)** *Many cases of AFH show a multinodular or lobular growth pattern. The fibrous septa are extensions of the characteristic fibrous pseudocapsule ➡ surrounding the tumor.*

AFH With Lymphoplasmacytic Cuff

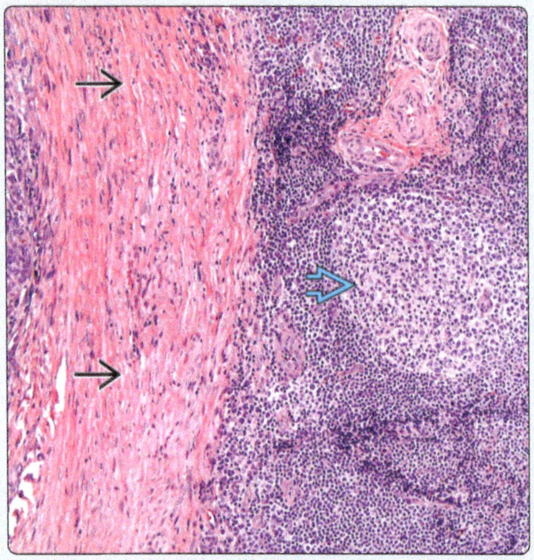

High Magnification of Lymphoplasmacytic Cuff

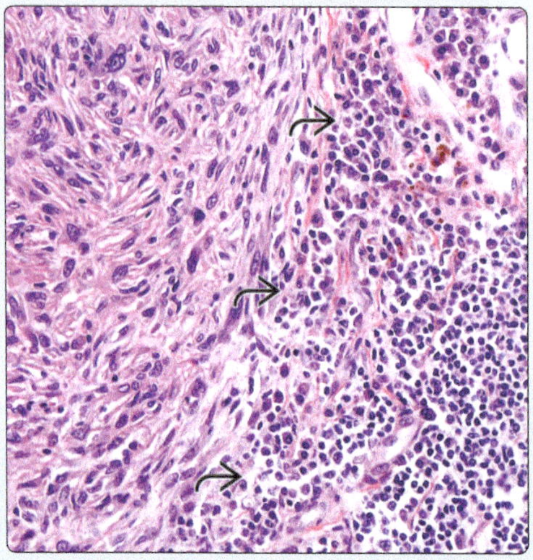

(Left) *The majority of cases of AFH have a lymphoplasmacytic cuff of varying extent and thickness in and around the pseudocapsule ➡. Reactive germinal centers ➡ may also be seen, further simulating the appearance of a lymph node containing metastatic tumor.* **(Right)** *The chronic inflammatory infiltrate ➡ that makes up the characteristic peripheral cuff of AFH is composed of a mixture of nonclonal B and T lymphocytes and polytypic plasma cells.*

TERMINOLOGY

Abbreviations

- Angiomatoid fibrous histiocytoma (AFH)

Synonyms

- Angiomatoid "malignant" fibrous histiocytoma
  - Term "malignant" removed due to relatively indolent clinical behavior

Definitions

- Distinctive, rarely metastasizing mesenchymal neoplasm composed of nodules and sheets of spindled and histiocytoid cells
  - Often demonstrates pseudoangiomatous spaces and peripheral lymphoplasmic cuff

ETIOLOGY/PATHOGENESIS

Lineage Uncertain

- Postulated nodal fibroblastic reticulum cell differentiation
- Myoid, myofibroblastic, endothelial, or histiocytic differentiation not proven

CLINICAL ISSUES

Epidemiology

- Incidence
  - Rare
- Age
  - Predominantly children and young adults
  - Rare in adults > 40 years
    - More likely to arise in extrasomatic locations
- Sex
  - Slight female predilection

Site

- Most common in superficial extremities (deep dermis and subcutis)
  - Rarely arise in deep soft tissue
- Also trunk and head/neck, including scalp
- Rare extrasomatic cases reported in lung, bone, mediastinum, retroperitoneum, brain, ovary, and vulva

Presentation

- Slowly growing, painless mass
  - Rapid growth uncommon and likely attributable to intratumoral hemorrhage
- Constitutional symptoms in subset (e.g., fever, malaise, anemia)
  - May be more common in extrasomatic tumors
  - Possibly related to tumoral cytokine production

Treatment

- Wide surgical excision
- Radiotherapy and chemotherapy may be indicated for rare metastatic or unresectable tumors
- Indefinite long-term clinical follow-up recommended

Prognosis

- Majority of lesions are clinically indolent
- Regional recurrence rate up to 15%
  - Higher rate reported in extrasomatic tumors (up to 33%)
  - May be related to site (difficulty of excision) and tumors showing infiltrative margins
- Rare metastasis (< 5% of reported cases)
  - Most frequently to regional lymph nodes
  - Very rare reports of death due to late distant metastases
- At present, no firm morphologic or clinical indicators of behavior

MACROSCOPIC

General Features

- Well-circumscribed tumor
- Lobulated or multinodular
- Blood-filled cystic cavities may be apparent grossly

Size

- Usually small (2-4 cm)

MICROSCOPIC

Histologic Features

- Uni- or multinodular growth
- Fibrous pseudocapsule
  - Contains patchy, dense peripheral lymphoplasmacytic cuff in up to 80%
- Sheets, nodules, and aggregates of ovoid to spindled cells
  - Variety of patterns: Loose swirling, storiform, short fascicles
- Majority of cells are cytologically bland with vesicular nuclei
  - Scattered cells with conspicuous nuclear pleomorphism or atypia are common and likely degenerative
  - Minority of cases show diffuse nuclear pleomorphism
- Fibrosclerotic to myxoid stroma
- Mitotic figures usually infrequent
  - Rare cases may show conspicuous mitotic activity or isolated atypical mitoses
- Variably sized, blood-filled pseudoangiomatous spaces in majority of cases
  - Lined by tumor cells, not endothelial cells
  - Scattered osteoclast-like giant cells common near these areas
- Stromal chronic inflammatory infiltrate may be present
  - May contain variable number of eosinophils
- Less common and exceptional features
  - Myxoid/reticular, clear cell, epithelioid, small cell, and focal palisading patterns
  - Rhabdoid morphology, pulmonary edema-like foci, hyalinized vessels, hemangioendothelioma-like foci

ANCILLARY TESTS

Immunohistochemistry

- Desmin (+) in 50-60% of cases
  - Varies from focal to diffuse cytoplasmic
  - Dendritic process-like staining in many cases
  - Scattered desmin (+) cells may be present within peripheral lymphoid proliferation
- Variable and nonspecific expression of EMA, CD68, CD99, SMA, calponin
- Negative for myogenin, MYOD1, CD31, and S100
  - Isolated reports of focal CD34, CD21, and keratin expression

Molecular Genetics

- 3 characteristic chromosomal translocations identified
  - t(2:22)(q33:q12); *EWSR1-CREB1*
    - Most common overall (90% of cases)
  - t(12:22)(q13:q12); *EWSR1-ATF1*
    - More common in extrasomatic cases of AFH
  - t(12:16)(q13:p11); *FUS-ATF1*
    - Infrequent
- *EWSR1-ATF1* and *EWSR1-CREB1* also identified in clear cell sarcoma of soft tissue and malignant gastrointestinal neuroectodermal tumor

DIFFERENTIAL DIAGNOSIS

Aneurysmal Fibrous Histiocytoma

- Morphologic variant of benign fibrous histiocytoma (dermatofibroma)
- Dermal localization, often with overlying epidermal changes
- No pseudocapsule or lymphoplasmacytic cuff
- Peripheral collagen trapping often present
- Mixed cell population, including chronic inflammatory cells, siderophages, and giant cells
- Negative for desmin

Undifferentiated Pleomorphic Sarcoma (Malignant Fibrous Histiocytoma)

- Older age group
- Mostly large, deeply located masses
- Often profound nuclear atypia
- Atypical mitoses and tumor necrosis are common

Nodal Metastasis

- Metastatic melanoma in particular can mimic AFH
- Arises in regions populated by lymph nodes
- True nodal architecture present
  - Subcapsular and medullary sinuses
- History of malignancy may or may not be present

Follicular Dendritic Cell Sarcoma

- Most arise in lymph nodes
- Infiltrating lymphocytes are common
- CD21(+), CD23(+), CD35(+), EMA(+)
- Negative for desmin

Granulomatous Lesions

- Lack solid growth pattern of AFH
  - Granulomas are usually dispersed and discrete or irregular and confluent
- Large granulomas often show central necrosis and lack cystic hemorrhage
- May contain foreign body-type giant cells
- Predisposing factors may be noted clinically (exposure to infectious agents, etc.)
- CD68(+), CD168(+)
- Negative for desmin

Rhabdomyosarcoma

- May be confused with AFH due to age and desmin (+)
- Morphologic appearance depends upon specific subtype
- Myogenin (+), MYOD1(+)

Kaposi Sarcoma (Nodular)

- May involve lymph nodes
- Predisposing factors often present (AIDS history)
- Moderately cellular neoplasm of spindled endothelial cells
- CD34(+), CD31(+), D2-40(+), HHV8(+)
- Negative for desmin

Spindle Cell Hemangioma

- Distal extremities, particularly acral
- No pseudocapsule or lymphoplasmacytic cuff
- Resembles cavernous hemangioma with cellular septa composed of spindle cells
- CD31(+), CD34(+), SMA(+)
- Negative for desmin

Intranodal Palisaded Myofibroblastoma

- Occurs in lymph nodes, predominantly in inguinal region in male patients
- Fascicles of spindle cells with nuclear palisading and amianthoid fibers characteristic
- SMA(+); desmin (-)

Nodular Fasciitis

- Lacks thick fibrous pseudocapsule and lymphoplasmacytic cuff
- Spindle and stellate myofibroblasts with tissue culture appearance
- SMA(+); desmin (-) (rarely focal)
- *MYH9-USP6* fusion

SELECTED REFERENCES

1. Justin Wong SB et al: Angiomatoid fibrous histiocytoma with prominent myxoid stroma: a case report and review of the literature. Am J Dermatopathol. 37(8):623-31, 2015
2. Shi H et al: Clinicopathological features of angiomatoid fibrous histiocytoma: a series of 21 cases with variant morphology. Int J Clin Exp Pathol. 8(1):772-8, 2015
3. Thway K et al: Angiomatoid fibrous histiocytoma: the current status of pathology and genetics. Arch Pathol Lab Med. 139(5):674-82, 2015
4. Thway K et al: Angiomatoid fibrous histiocytoma: comparison of fluorescence in situ hybridization and reverse transcription polymerase chain reaction as adjunct diagnostic modalities. Ann Diagn Pathol. 19(3):137-42, 2015
5. Bohman SL et al: Angiomatoid fibrous histiocytoma: an expansion of the clinical and histological spectrum. Pathology. 46(3):199-204, 2014
6. Kao YC et al: Angiomatoid fibrous histiocytoma: clinicopathological and molecular characterisation with emphasis on variant histomorphology. J Clin Pathol. 67(3):210-5, 2014
7. Schaefer IM et al: Myxoid variant of so-called angiomatoid "malignant fibrous histiocytoma": clinicopathologic characterization in a series of 21 cases. Am J Surg Pathol. 38(6):816-23, 2014
8. Chen G et al: Angiomatoid fibrous histiocytoma: unusual sites and unusual morphology. Mod Pathol. 24(12):1560-70, 2011
9. Matsumura T et al: Angiomatoid fibrous histiocytoma including cases with pleomorphic features analysed by fluorescence in situ hybridisation. J Clin Pathol. 63(2):124-8, 2010
10. Thway K: Angiomatoid fibrous histiocytoma: a review with recent genetic findings. Arch Pathol Lab Med. 132(2):273-7, 2008
11. Fanburg-Smith JC et al: Angiomatoid "malignant" fibrous histiocytoma: a clinicopathologic study of 158 cases and further exploration of the myoid phenotype. Hum Pathol. 30(11):1336-43, 1999
12. Costa MJ et al: Angiomatoid malignant fibrous histiocytoma. A follow-up study of 108 cases with evaluation of possible histologic predictors of outcome. Am J Surg Pathol. 14(12):1126-32, 1990

AFH With Bland Nuclear Features

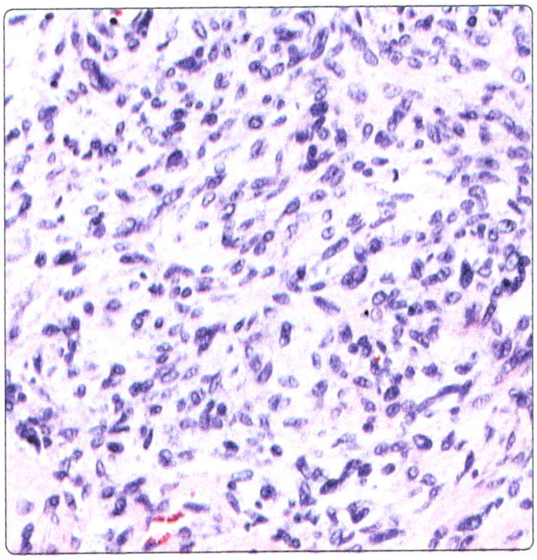

AFH With Rare Mitosis

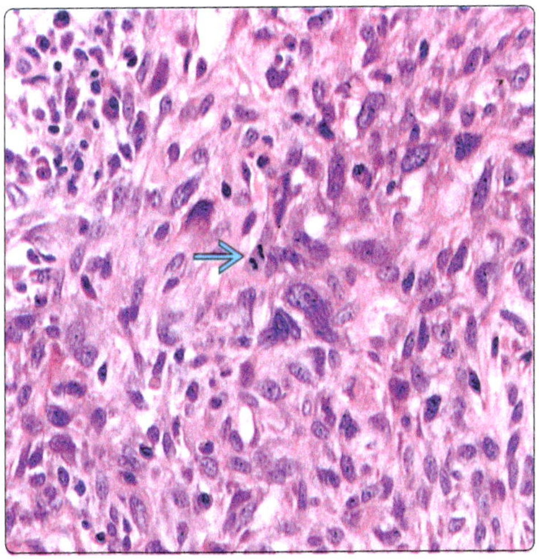

(Left) *In a typical case of AFH, the tumor cells are spindled to ovoid with generally bland nuclei containing pale or vesicular chromatin with small nucleoli and showing minimal to mild pleomorphism. They often appear histiocytoid. The overall cellularity varies widely from case to case.* **(Right)** *The mitotic rate in AFH is generally low, and mitotic figures → are often small and difficult to find. In rare cases, they are more numerous, but this does not appear to affect prognosis. In exceptional cases, atypical mitotic figures may be identified.*

AFH With Focal Nuclear Atypia

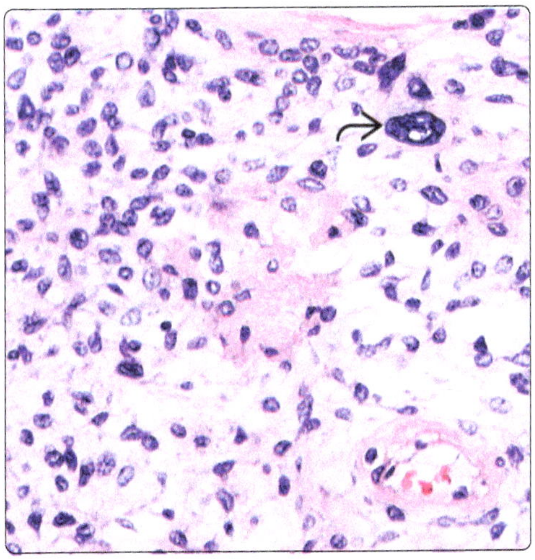

AFH With Marked Nuclear Atypia

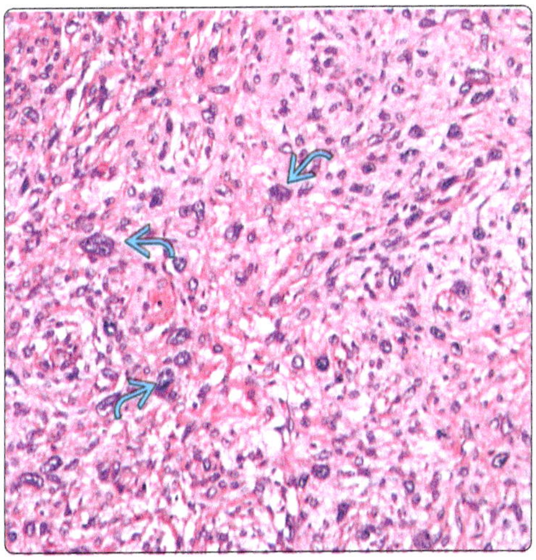

(Left) *It is common for AFH to contain scattered tumor cells ↗ with nuclear enlargement, hyperchromasia, and pleomorphism. Intranuclear pseudoinclusions may be identified. These changes are likely degenerative in nature.* **(Right)** *In some cases, pleomorphic tumor cells ↗ are more prominent in number and distribution. Coupled together with an increase in cellularity, these cases may be misdiagnosed as an undifferentiated pleomorphic sarcoma. Notably, however, mitotic activity is disproportionately low.*

High Magnification Showing Nuclear Grooves

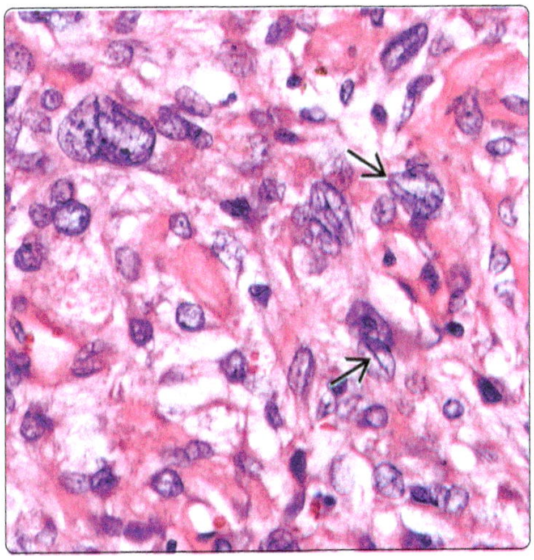

Pseudovascular Spaces in AFH

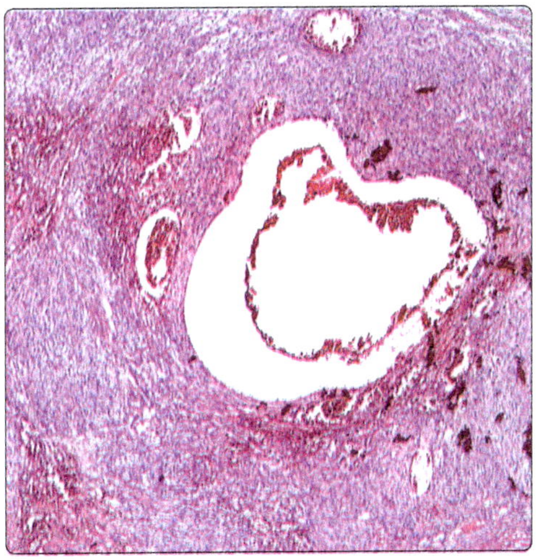

(Left) *Nuclear irregularity with the presence of grooves → or folds is not an uncommon finding in AFH and may even be quite prominent in rare cases.* **(Right)** *Most cases of AFH show at least focal hemorrhage and often the formation of dilated blood-filled spaces, similar to what is seen in the unrelated aneurysmal fibrous histiocytoma. These spaces may predominate in rare cases, clinically and pathologically simulating a hematoma. Thorough histologic examination is required in these cases.*

(Left) *The dilated vascular spaces seen in AFH are not true vessels or cysts, as they lack endothelial and epithelial linings, respectively, but rather are lined by tumor cells. Osteoclast-like giant cells ➡ are commonly identified near these spaces and, very rarely, may be numerous.* **(Right)** *Osteoclast-like giant cells ➡ are generally infrequent in AFH and may be sparsely scattered throughout the tumor; however, when present, they are most typically identified adjacent to or near hemorrhagic foci and pseudovascular spaces.*

Pseudovascular Space Lining in AFH

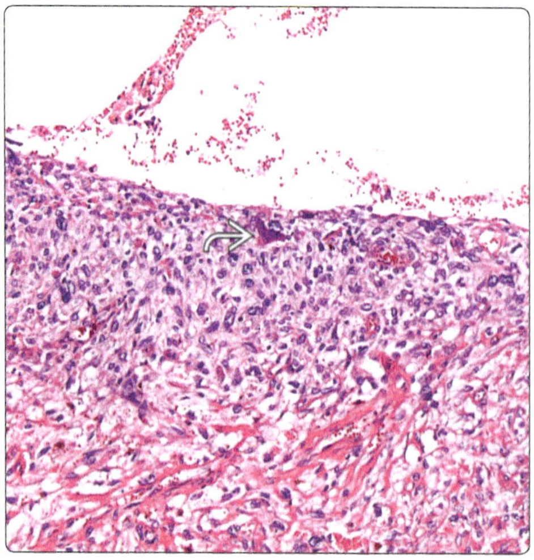

Osteoclast-Like Giant Cells

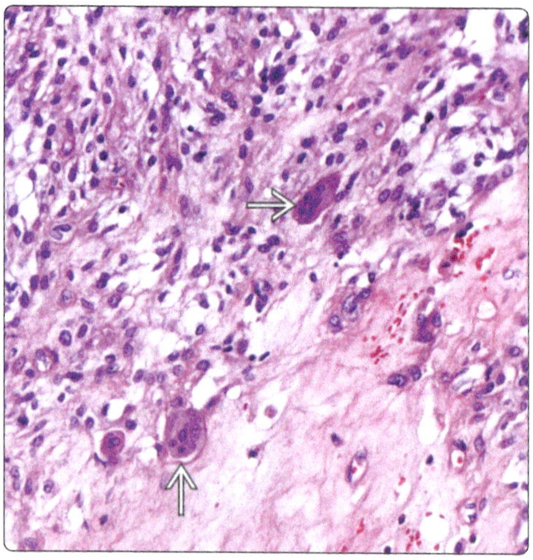

(Left) *Hemosiderin pigment ➡ is a common finding in AFH and varies in distribution from case to case. It is most commonly seen around regions of hemorrhage and pseudovascular space formation and may be seen in the stroma or within the cytoplasm of the tumor cells.* **(Right)** *The overall growth pattern of AFH varies widely from one tumor to the next, as does the cellularity. Tumor cells may form sheets, short fascicles, loose storiform arrays, or a variety of other unusual patterns.*

Hemosiderin Deposition in AFH

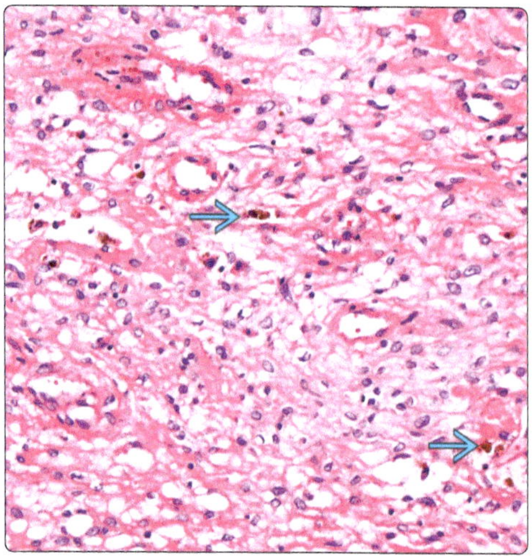

AFH With Variable Architecture

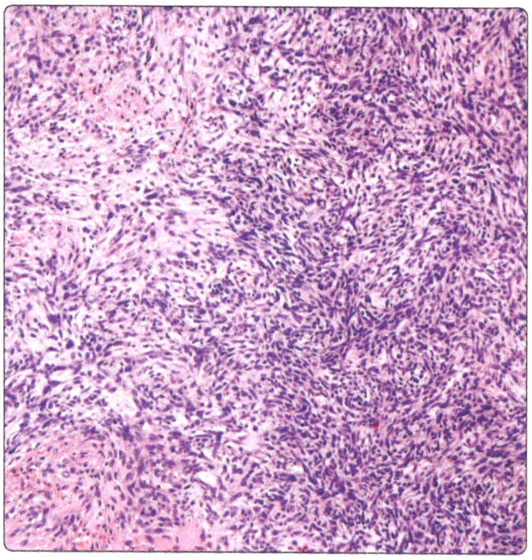

(Left) *The growth pattern in this AFH shows a mixture of short irregular fascicles and a vague, loose storiform architecture. It also contained regions of prominent myxoid stromal change (not shown).* **(Right)** *Myxoid stromal change is uncommon in AFH and, when present, varies from focal to diffuse in extent. Even when these changes are diffuse, other typical pathologic features of AFH, such as the characteristic pseudocapsule and inflammatory cuff, can usually be identified to aid in a correct diagnosis.*

AFH With Loose Storiform Growth

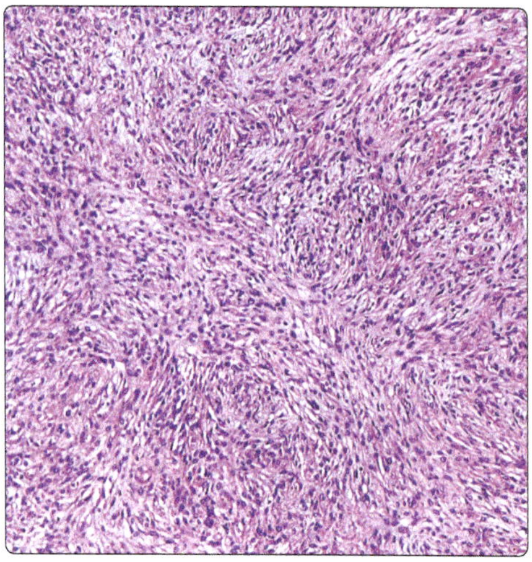

AFH With Myxoid Stromal Change

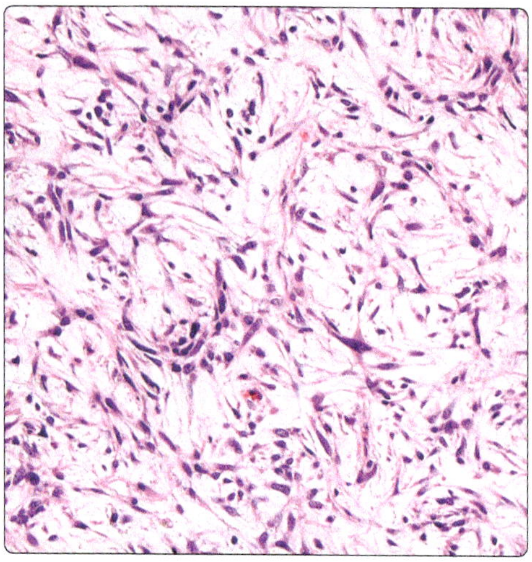

AFH With Myxoid/Reticulated Pattern

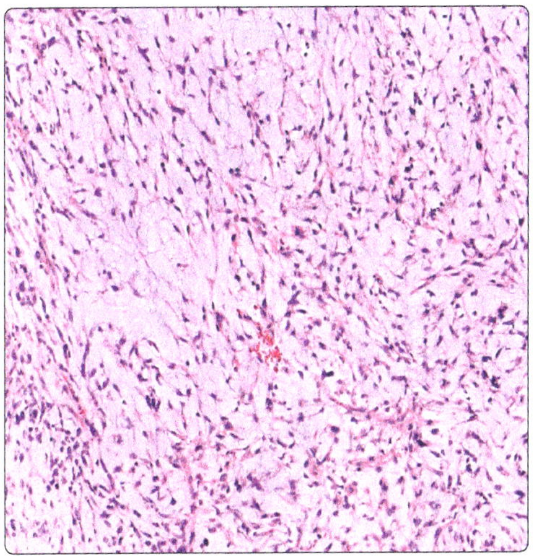

AFH With Pulmonary Edema-Like Pattern

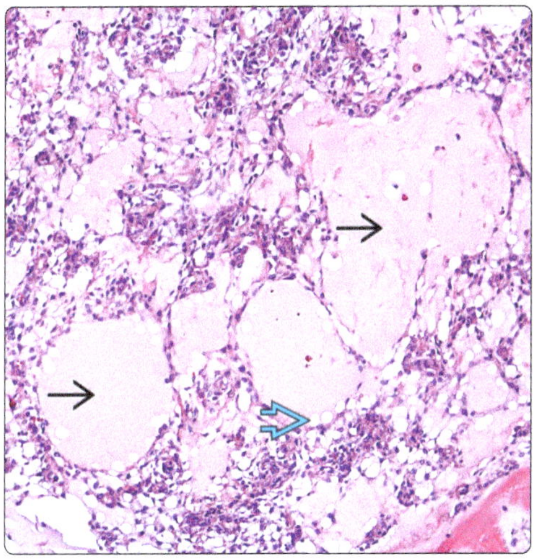

(Left) *In some cases of myxoid AFH, the cells are small, spindled to stellate, and form an interconnecting, reticulated growth pattern. This morphology may cause confusion with other myxoid neoplasms, particularly extraskeletal myxoid chondrosarcoma.* **(Right)** *Variably dilated, cyst-like foci ➡ containing homogeneous eosinophilic material may be seen in AFH (similar to myxoid liposarcoma). This appearance is reminiscent of edema filling pulmonary alveoli. Scattered vacuolar forms are also seen at the periphery ⇨.*

Prominent Vasculature in AFH

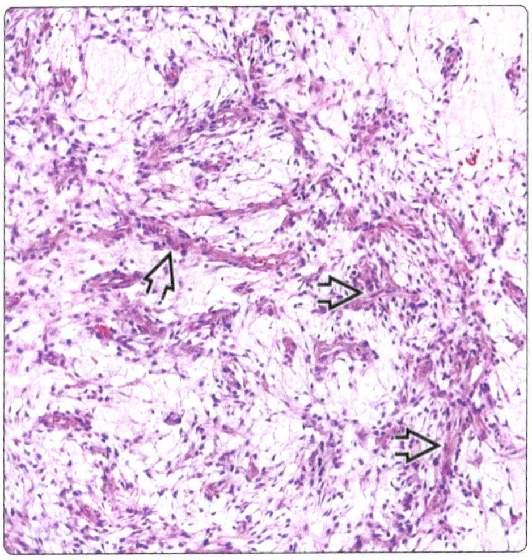

Stromal Hyalinization in AFH

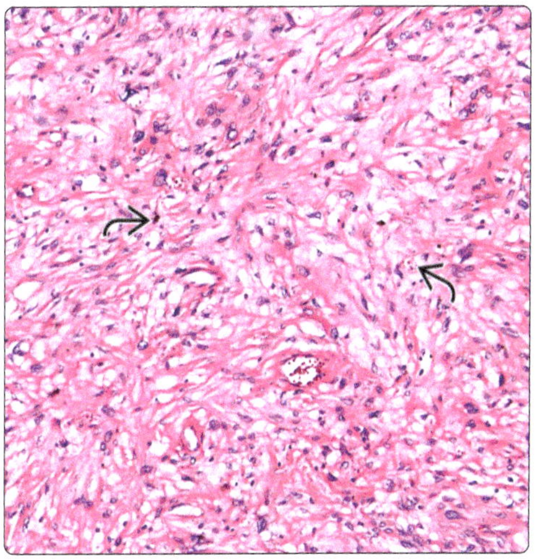

(Left) *A rare finding in some cases of myxoid AFH are thin-walled branching vessels ⇨ with a "curvilinear" appearance, similar to that seen in low-grade fibromyxoid sarcoma and myxofibrosarcoma. Other, more typical areas of AFH may be present and should be sought out.* **(Right)** *AFH may show regions of stromal hyalinization or hypocellularity, which can vary from focal to extensive. Chronic inflammatory cells are often identified within the stroma, as is hemosiderin ↷.*

Stromal Sclerosis in AFH

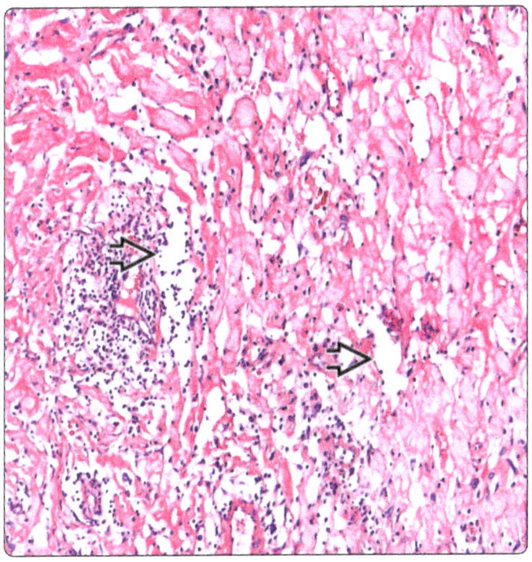

Hemangioendothelioma-Like Foci

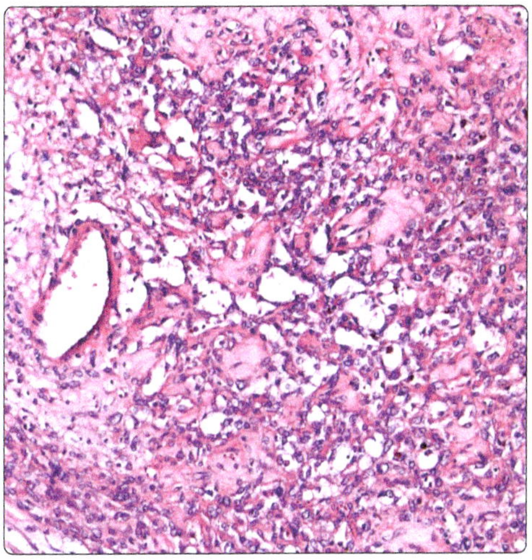

(Left) *In extreme cases, extensive stromal sclerosis may lead to diagnostic difficulties. In particular, tissue separation artifact ⇨ may lead to an appearance suggestive of a vascular neoplasm or even a nonneoplastic sclerosing process.* **(Right)** *This unusual case of AFH showed foci containing irregular stromal clefts between tumor cells, imparting a hemangioendothelioma-like appearance. Erythrocytes may even be seen within some of these clefts, further mimicking a vascular lesion.*

(Left) *Occasional cases of AFH demonstrate areas of tight whorling or storiform growth ➨, mimicking soft tissue perineurioma. Immunohistochemical expression of EMA in AFH may further confound the issue.* **(Right)** *A mixed chronic inflammatory infiltrate is usually present to some degree in AFH; however, it varies from subtle to prominent. Most of the constituent inflammatory cells are lymphocytes ➙ and plasma cells, but eosinophils may also be present.*

Whorled Perineurioma-Like Growth in AFH

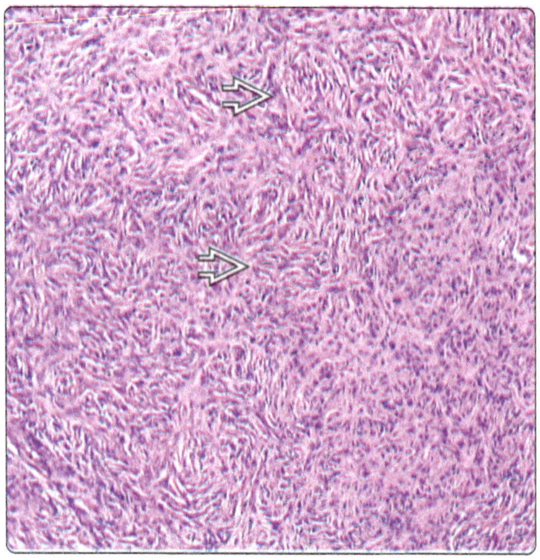

Stromal Inflammation in AFH

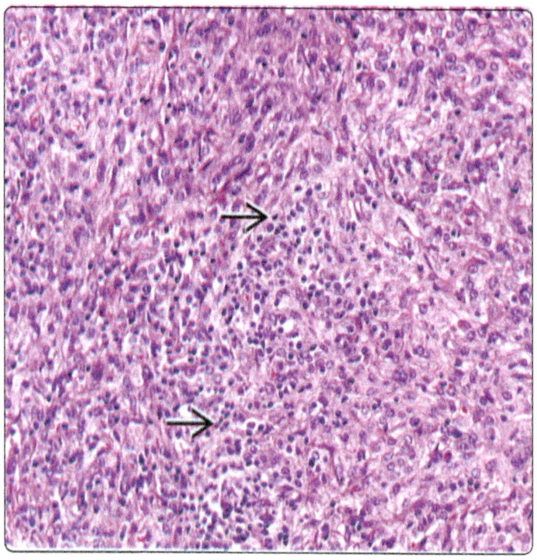

(Left) *Eosinophils ➨ are not a common finding in AFH and are usually sparsely distributed, but in very rare cases they can be surprisingly abundant.* **(Right)** *Small cell morphology may also be seen and is characterized by tumor cells with minimal cytoplasm and increased nuclear density. When nuclear monomorphism is prominent, this morphology may resemble Ewing sarcoma, a major pitfall, given that both tumors may express CD99 and show EWSR1 gene fusions.*

Stromal Eosinophils

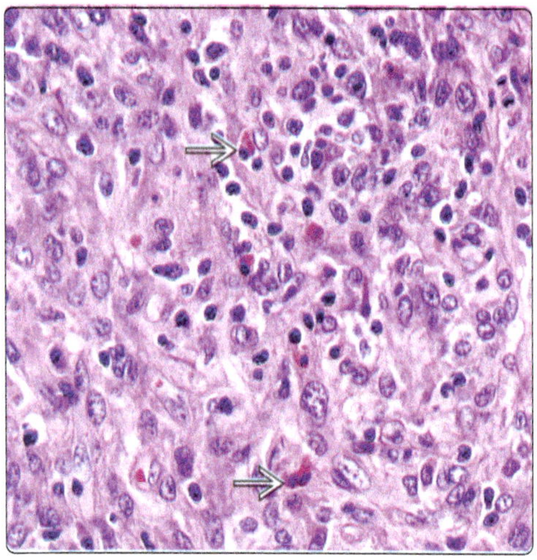

Small Cell Morphology

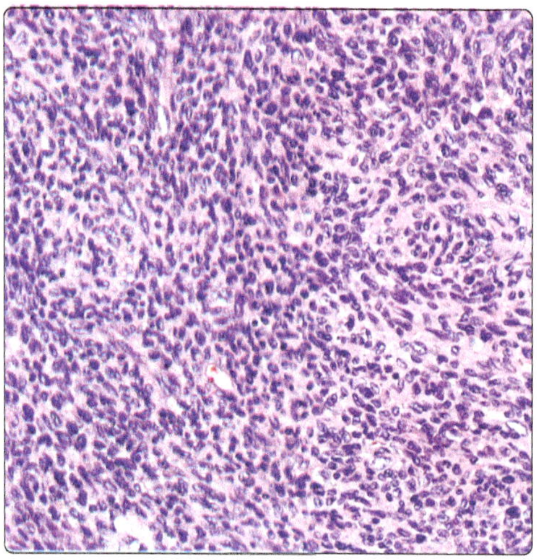

(Left) *A conspicuous short fascicular growth pattern may rarely be seen in AFH and, in combination with small cell morphology and nuclear monomorphism, may resemble other more aggressive tumors, such as synovial sarcoma.* **(Right)** *Focal vascular hyalinization ➙ may be seen in some cases of AFH and can simulate the Antoni B zones of schwannoma. In some reported cases, this finding has been associated with focal nuclear palisading, further mimicking schwannoma.*

Fascicular Growth Pattern

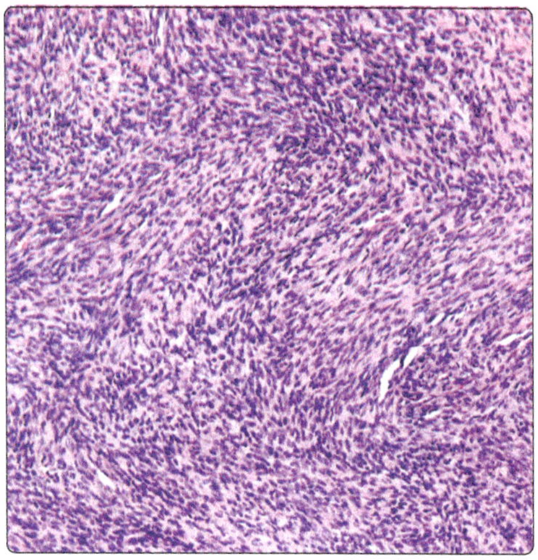

Rare Vascular Hyalinization

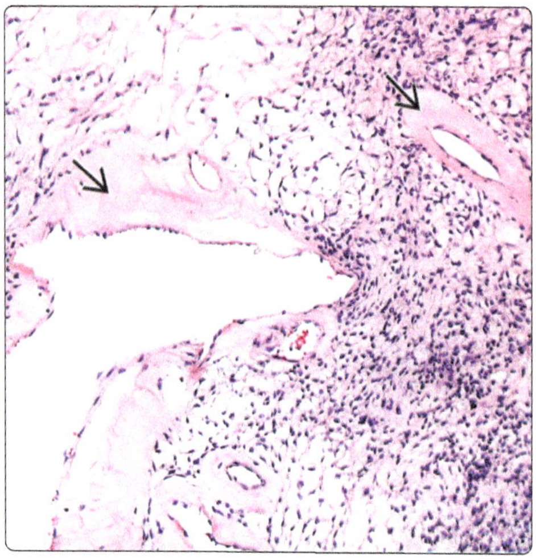

Carcinoma-Like Morphology in AFH

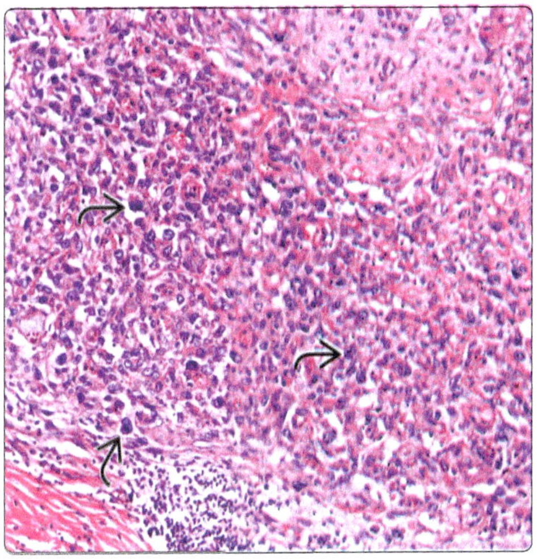

Rhabdoid-Like Morphology

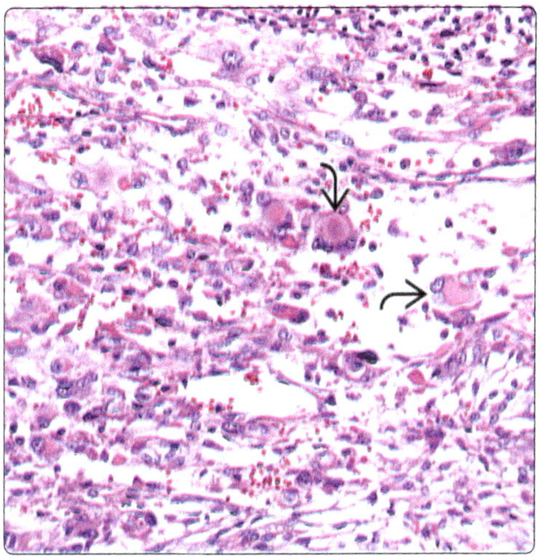

(Left) *This image shows AFH with sheet-like areas of larger eosinophilic tumor cells with atypia and pleomorphism →, somewhat mimicking a poorly differentiated carcinoma. A background of stromal sclerosis or fibromyxoid change can also complicate the issue.* **(Right)** *Epithelioid tumor cells → with dense glassy, eosinophilic cytoplasm and eccentric nuclei, resembling rhabdomyoblasts, are a rare finding in AFH. Given the usual age of the patient, care should be taken to avoid a misdiagnosis of rhabdomyosarcoma.*

Hyaline Eosinophilic Globules

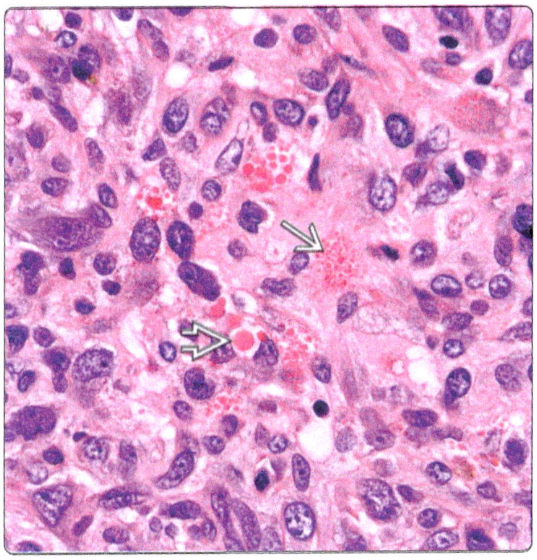

Predominantly Cystic AFH

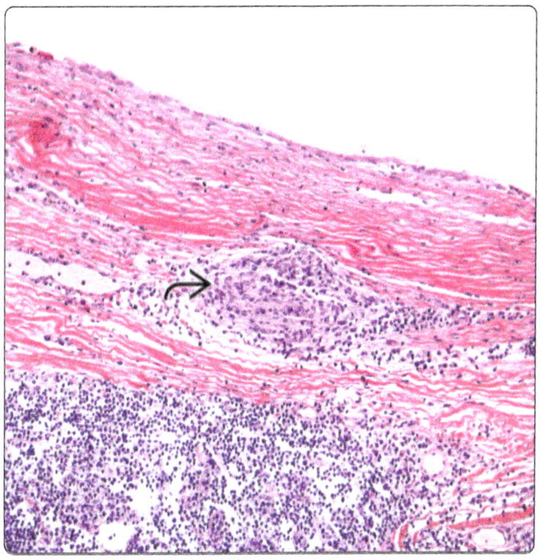

(Left) *Intracytoplasmic eosinophilic globules are a rare finding in AFH and vary from tiny clusters → to larger, pale globules →. The latter form resembles the hyaline globules seen in Kaposi sarcoma.* **(Right)** *Some cases of AFH are extensively cystic and may appear to be a large blood cyst with a collagenous pseudocapsule, thus closely mimicking a hematoma. However, close inspection of the fibrous capsule and inflammatory infiltrate often reveals small nodules → of diagnostic tumor cells.*

Small Tumor Nodules in AFH

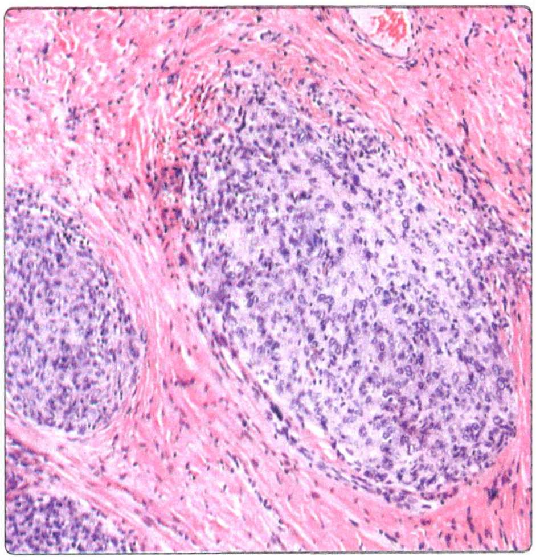

Desmin Expression in AFH

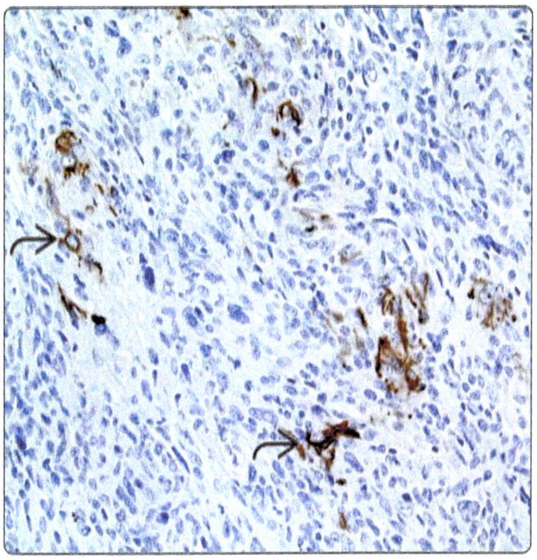

(Left) *Small nodules or nests of tumor cells may appear isolated in zones of sclerosis or within the fibrous pseudocapsule. On a limited biopsy, these foci may closely resemble granulomas.* **(Right)** *Approximately half of cases of AFH show expression of desmin within the tumor cells, which varies from focal to extensive, and often shows areas of stellate, dendritic process-like staining →. Isolated desmin (+) cells may be identified in the peripheral lymphoplasmacytic infiltrate as well.*

Plexiform Fibrohistiocytic Tumor

KEY FACTS

TERMINOLOGY

- Rarely metastasizing dermal-subcutaneous mesenchymal neoplasm composed of variable mixture of fibroblasts and histiocyte-like cells

CLINICAL ISSUES

- Children and young adults
- Most common in upper extremity
  - Most arise at dermal-subcutaneous interface
- Also lower extremity, trunk, head, and neck
- Painless, slow-growing mass or plaque
- Treatment: Wide surgical excision with negative margins
- Local recurrence in up to 40%
- Low metastatic potential (6%)

MACROSCOPIC

- Multinodular, poorly delineated, tan-white
- Usually < 3 cm (range: 0.3-8.5 cm)

MICROSCOPIC

- Poorly circumscribed with infiltrative growth pattern
- Morphologically subdivided into 3 types (fibroblastic, histiocytic, mixed)
- Fascicles of spindled fibroblastic cells
- Nodules or aggregates of epithelioid histiocytoid cells
  - Osteoclast-like giant cells common
- Multinodular and plexiform growth
- Low mitotic rate; usually no cellular pleomorphism

ANCILLARY TESTS

- (Myo)fibroblasts SMA(+); histiocytes CD68(+) and CD163(+)
- Negative for S100, CD34, desmin, keratin, MITF

TOP DIFFERENTIAL DIAGNOSES

- Cellular neurothekeoma
- Giant cell tumor of soft tissue
- Fibromatosis
- Low-grade myofibroblastic sarcoma

Plexiform Fibrohistiocytic Tumor

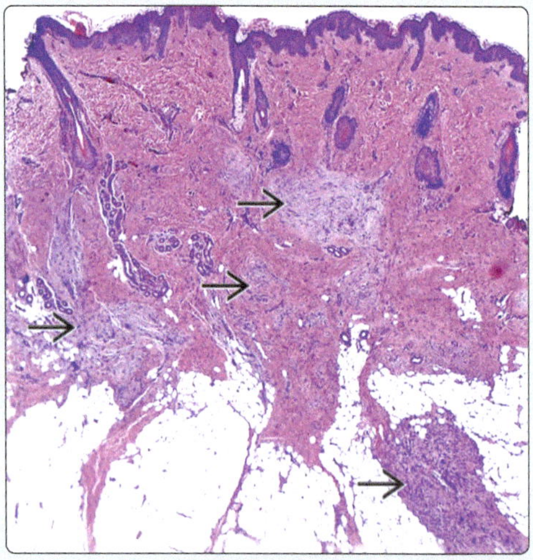

Infiltrative Growth in Plexiform Fibrohistiocytic Tumor

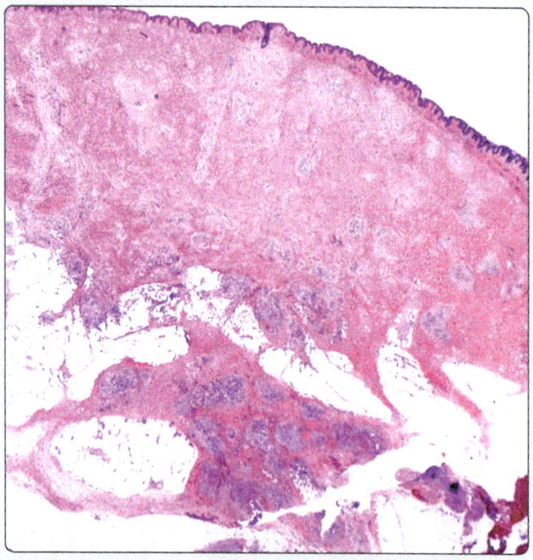

(Left) *Plexiform fibrohistiocytic tumor (PFHT) is an unusual, infiltrative mesenchymal neoplasm ➡ that typically arises near the dermal-subcutaneous junction, as depicted. Tumors are characterized by fascicles or sheets of spindled fibroblasts &/or nests of histiocytoid cells in a nodular and plexiform growth pattern.* **(Right)** *Most cases of PFHT are infiltrative and characteristically show extensions or projections of tumor into the subcutaneous adipose tissue.*

Mixed-Type Plexiform Fibrohistiocytic Tumor

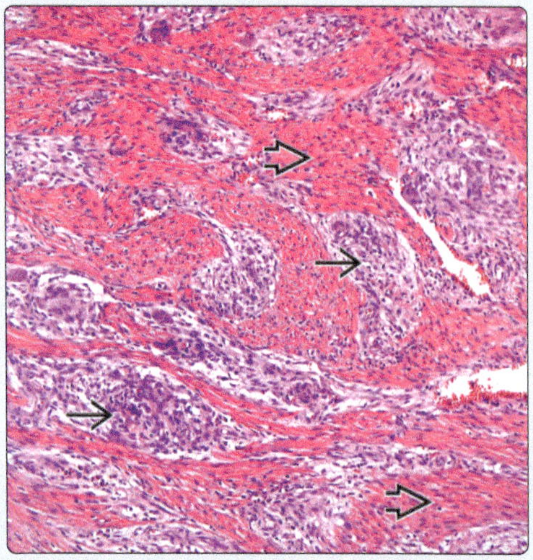

Histiocytoid Nests in Plexiform Fibrohistiocytic Tumor

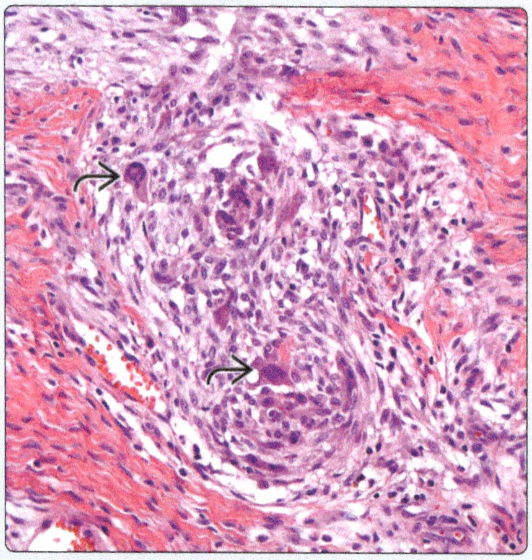

(Left) *The mixed subtype of PFHT shows a complex mixture of nests ➡ of histiocytoid cells with short fascicles of bland spindled cells ⇨.* **(Right)** *The characteristic nests and aggregates of PFHT, when present, contain plump to epithelioid mononuclear histiocytoid cells. Multinucleated giant cells ↪ may or may not be present.*

TERMINOLOGY

Abbreviations

- Plexiform fibrohistiocytic tumor (PFHT)

Definitions

- Rarely metastasizing dermal-subcutaneous mesenchymal neoplasm composed of variable mixture of fibroblasts and histiocyte-like cells

CLINICAL ISSUES

Epidemiology

- Incidence
  - Rare
- Age
  - Most common in children and young adults
    - Overall wide range: 1-77 years

Site

- Upper extremity (particularly forearm and hand)
- Also lower extremity, trunk, head and neck
- Most arise at dermal-subcutaneous interface
  - May also be purely dermal or subcutaneous
    - Subcutaneous tumors may involve skeletal muscle

Presentation

- Painless, slow-growing mass or plaque

Treatment

- Wide surgical excision or reexcision with negative margins
- Examination of regional lymph nodes may be warranted
- Indefinite clinical follow-up recommended

Prognosis

- Local recurrence in up to 40%
- Low metastatic potential (6%)
  - Regional lymph nodes
  - Systemic metastases very rare (lung)

MACROSCOPIC

General Features

- Multinodular, poorly delineated, tan-white

Size

- Usually < 3 cm (range: 0.3-8.5 cm)

MICROSCOPIC

Histologic Features

- Most are located near dermal-subcutaneous interface
- Poorly circumscribed with infiltrative growth pattern
  - Adnexa often spared
- Morphologically subdivided into 3 types
  - Fibroblastic
    - Predominantly spindled fibroblastic cells
    - Plexiform to infiltrative fascicular growth
      - Ray-like extensions into subcutis
    - Chronic inflammatory infiltrate common
  - Histiocytic
    - Epithelioid histiocytoid cells
    - Cannonball-like, multinodular growth
      - Nodules may show hemorrhage
    - Osteoclast-like giant cells common
  - Mixed type
    - Histiocytoid nodules separated by fascicles
- Cellular and nuclear pleomorphism are usually absent
- Stromal can show dense hyalinization or myxoid change
  - Rare metaplastic bone formation
- Usually low mitotic rate (very rare atypical mitoses)
- Necrosis absent
- Rare focal lymphovascular invasion

ANCILLARY TESTS

Immunohistochemistry

- (Myo)fibroblastic cells are SMA(+), at least focally
- Histiocytes are CD68(+) and CD163(+)
- Negative for S100, CD34, desmin, keratin
- Negative for MITF (may be focally positive)

DIFFERENTIAL DIAGNOSIS

Cellular Neurothekeoma

- Can show significant morphologic overlap with PFHT
  - Entities may be closely related
- 1/3 of cases arise in head/neck
- MITF(+), usually diffuse

Giant Cell Tumor of Soft Tissue

- Prominent nodularity with abundant osteoclast-like giant cells
- Lacks infiltrative spindle cell component
- Peripheral shell of woven bone in 50%

Fibromatosis

- Lacks nodules of histiocytoid and osteoclast-like giant cells
- Characteristic elongated stromal vasculature
- Nuclear β-catenin (+)

Low-Grade Myofibroblastic Sarcoma

- Most common in head/neck and extremities
- Usually arise in deep subcutaneous tissue or skeletal muscle
- Highly infiltrative, often with checkerboard pattern
- At least focal nuclear enlargement, hyperchromasia

SELECTED REFERENCES

1. Fox MD et al: Expression of MiTF may be helpful in differentiating cellular neurothekeoma from plexiform fibrohistiocytic tumor (histiocytoid predominant) in a partial biopsy specimen. Am J Dermatopathol. 34(2):157-60, 2012
2. Luzar B et al: Cutaneous fibrohistiocytic tumours - an update. Histopathology. 56(1):148-65, 2010
3. Jaffer S et al: Neurothekeoma and plexiform fibrohistiocytic tumor: mere histologic resemblance or histogenetic relationship? Am J Surg Pathol. 33(6):905-13, 2009
4. Moosavi C et al: An update on plexiform fibrohistiocytic tumor and addition of 66 new cases from the Armed Forces Institute of Pathology, in honor of Franz M. Enzinger, MD. Ann Diagn Pathol. 11(5):313-9, 2007
5. Remstein ED et al: Plexiform fibrohistiocytic tumor: clinicopathologic analysis of 22 cases. Am J Surg Pathol. 23(6):662-70, 1999
6. Fisher C: Atypical plexiform fibrohistiocytic tumour. Histopathology. 30(3):271-3, 1997
7. Enzinger FM et al: Plexiform fibrohistiocytic tumor presenting in children and young adults. An analysis of 65 cases. Am J Surg Pathol. 12(11):818-26, 1988

(Left) *Osteoclast-like multinucleated giant cells ↪ are often seen within the histiocytoid nodules in PFHT; however, they are absent in a subset of cases. Note also the cells at the periphery of the nests may be spindled → and appear to encircle the plumper epithelioid cells ⇒.* **(Right)** *The histiocytoid nodules of PFHT may lack multinucleated giant cells, as depicted here. In the histiocytic subtype, this absence of giant cells may lead to an overall impression of cellular neurothekeoma, an entity that may be related to PFHT.*

Multinucleated Giant Cells in Plexiform Fibrohistiocytic Tumor

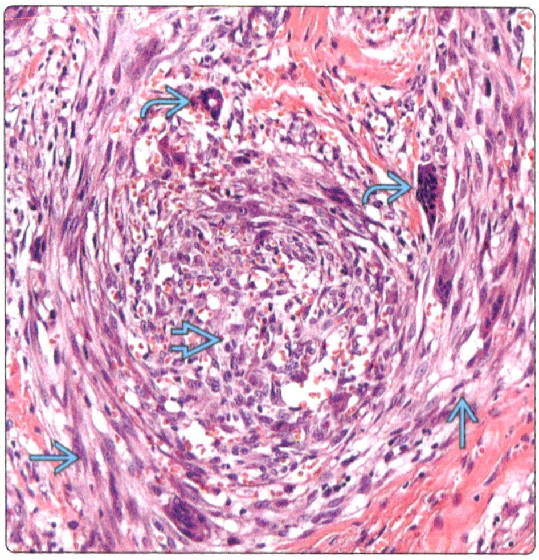

Histiocytoid Nodules in Plexiform Fibrohistiocytic Tumor

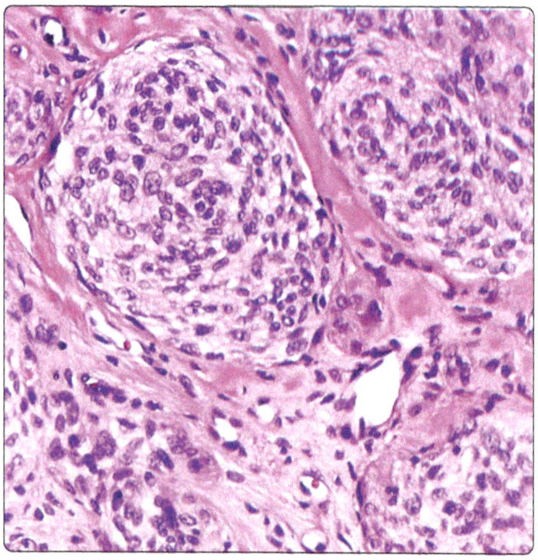

(Left) *Hemorrhage may be seen within PFHT and is often localized to histiocytoid nodules and nests, particularly if osteoclast-like multinucleated giant cells are present. This appearance can lead to consideration of a soft tissue giant cell tumor.* **(Right)** *The fibroblastic component of PFHT is characterized by fascicles and sheets → of spindled cells within a variably collagenous stroma. Histiocytoid nodules ⇒ ± giant cells are also seen in mixed subtypes.*

Intranodular Hemorrhage in Plexiform Fibrohistiocytic Tumor

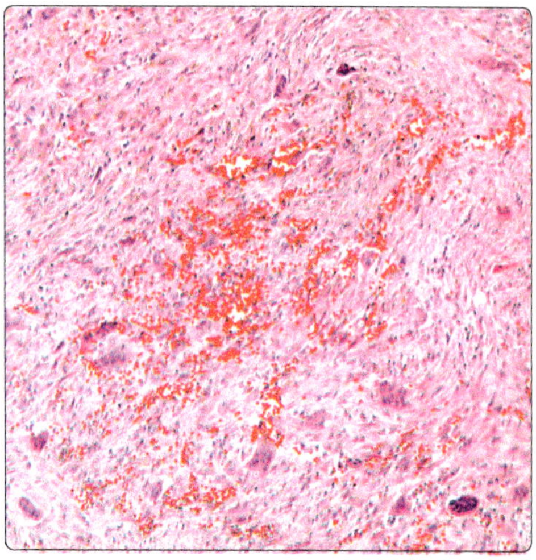

Fibroblastic Component in Plexiform Fibrohistiocytic Tumor

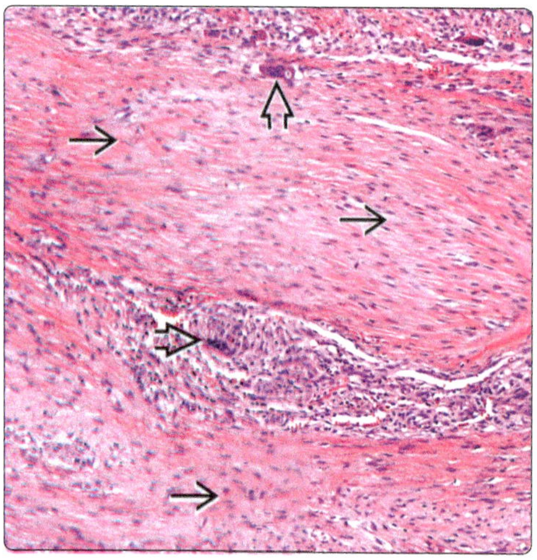

(Left) *The spindled fibroblastic cells of PFHT are generally cytologically banal and are associated with a variable amount of stromal collagen. In some cases, the stroma can be densely hyalinized or even focally myxoid.* **(Right)** *This case of PFHT shows areas of fibroblastic morphology with densely hyalinized stroma.*

Fibroblastic Component in Plexiform Fibrohistiocytic Tumor

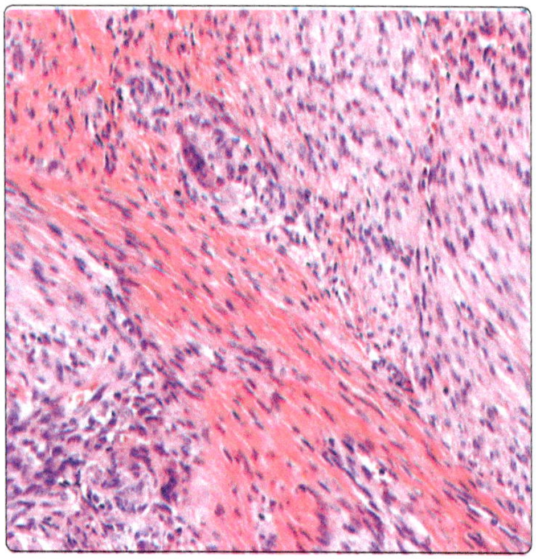

Fibroblastic Component in Plexiform Fibrohistiocytic Tumor

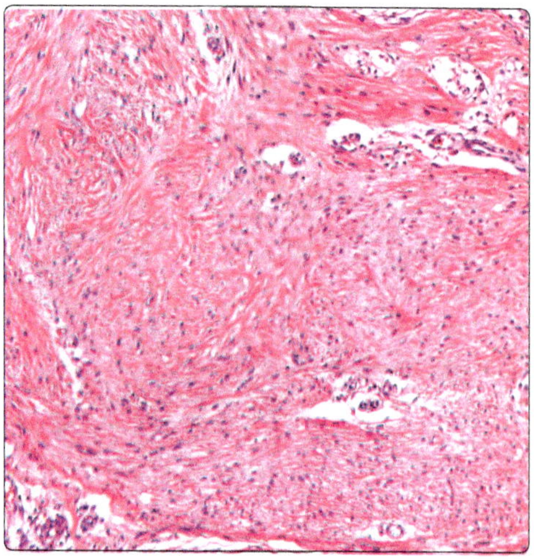

Cytologic Features of Plexiform Fibrohistiocytic Tumor

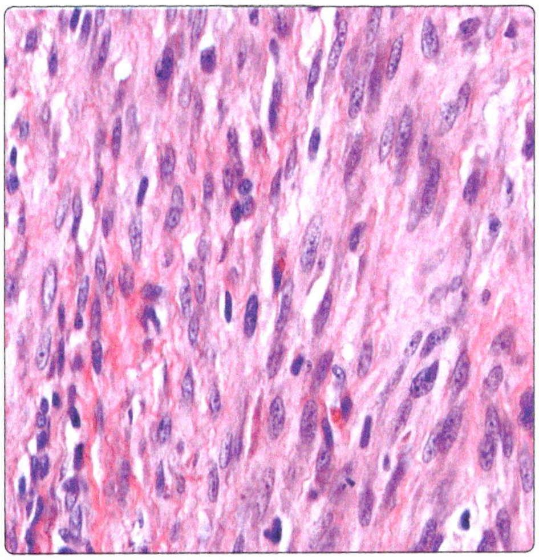

Fibroblastic-Type Plexiform Fibrohistiocytic Tumor

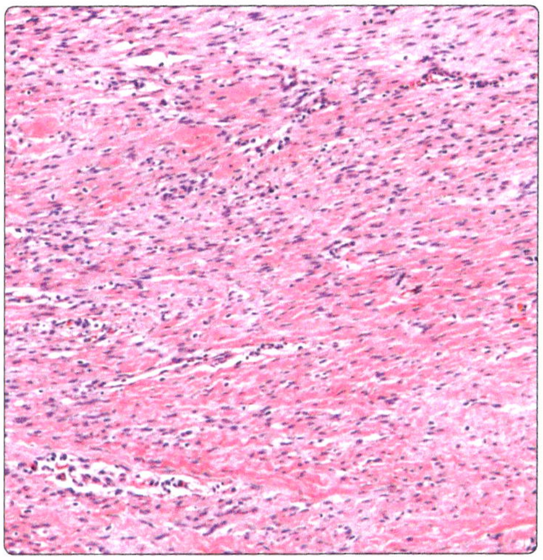

(Left) *The lesional cells of PFHT usually lack significant cytologic atypia, and mitotic activity is often low. Rare tumors, however, can show nuclear pleomorphism &/or rare atypical mitoses.* **(Right)** *The fibroblastic subtype of PFHT is composed predominantly or entirely of short fascicles and sheets of bland spindle cells, with few to no histiocytic nests. Together with the infiltrative growth pattern, this subtype morphologically resembles fibromatosis.*

Histiocytic-Type Plexiform Fibrohistiocytic Tumor

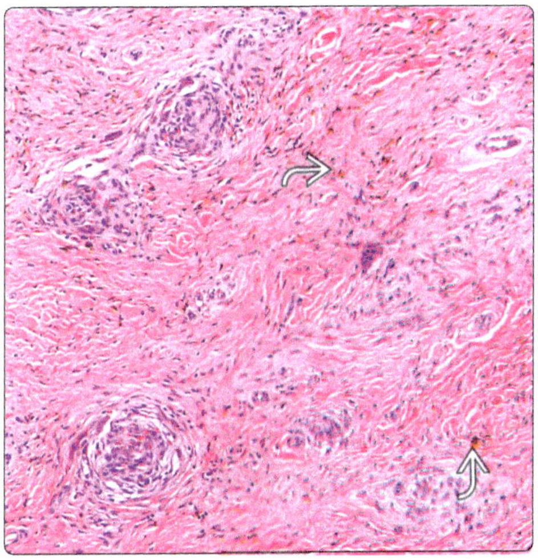

Infiltrative Growth Pattern in Plexiform Fibrohistiocytic Tumor

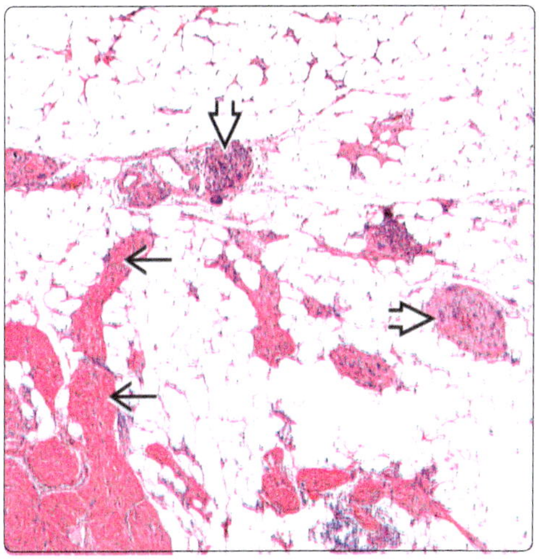

(Left) *The histiocytic subtype of PFHT is composed of infiltrating clusters and nests of plump histiocytoid cells ± giant cells. The surrounding connective tissue may appear reactive and contain inflammatory cells &/or hemosiderin pigment.* **(Right)** *Infiltrative growth is characteristic of PFHT, and the fibroblastic component, if present, often projects out into surrounding tissues as finger-like or ray-like extensions. Isolated nodules of histiocytoid cells and giant cells may also be seen within fat.*

Increased Cellularity in Plexiform Fibrohistiocytic Tumor

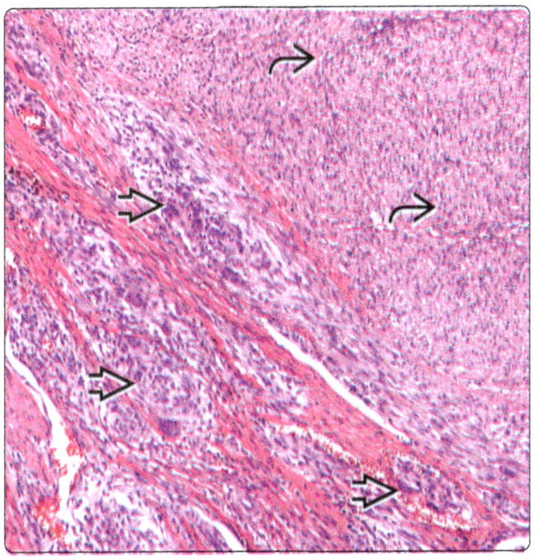

Increased Cellularity in Plexiform Fibrohistiocytic Tumor

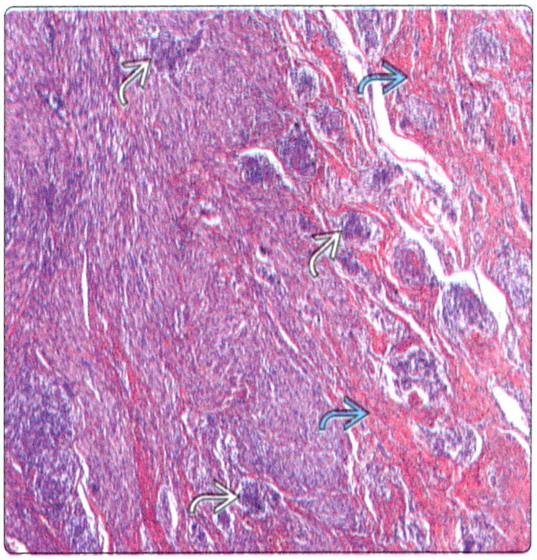

(Left) *Rare cases of PFHT show an increase in cellularity in the spindled fibroblastic component that may be easily mistaken for frank sarcoma. Note the compressed histiocytic nodules, some of which contain osteoclast-like giant cells and hemorrhage.* **(Right)** *Image of a cellular example of PFHT shows a mixture of fibroblastic elements and histiocytoid nodules.*

Dermatofibrosarcoma Protuberans

KEY FACTS

TERMINOLOGY

- Dermatofibrosarcoma protuberans (DFSP)
- Low-grade malignant spindle cell tumor of skin characteristically showing prominent storiforming

CLINICAL ISSUES

- Typically occurs in young adults
- Excellent prognosis in most cases
- Relatively low recurrence rate
- Very low metastatic rates (in cases with fibrosarcomatous transformation)

MICROSCOPIC

- Dermal and subcutaneous involvement
- Cells arrayed in storiform or cartwheel patterns
- Proliferation of monomorphic spindle-shaped cells
- Lesional cells lack significant pleomorphism
- Mitoses usually infrequent (< 4/10 HPF)
  - Atypical mitoses usually absent
- **Bednar tumor**
  - Pigmented DFSP with scattered benign melanocytes
- **Giant cell fibroblastoma**
  - Proliferation of bland spindled cells and giant cells with nuclear hyperchromasia lining pseudovascular spaces

ANCILLARY TESTS

- CD34 is most reliable marker, typically strongly and diffusely positive
  - May be weak and focal in some cases
- FXIIIA is typically negative
  - Focal staining, usually at periphery or in scattered dendritic cells

TOP DIFFERENTIAL DIAGNOSES

- Cellular dermatofibroma/fibrous histiocytoma
- Indeterminate fibrohistiocytic lesion
- Fibrosarcoma (including transformation in DFSP)
- Leiomyosarcoma

(Left) *Dermatofibrosarcoma protuberans (DFSP) is often characterized clinically by an exophytic, multinodular growth with areas of interposed flattening or atrophy.* **(Right)** *Low magnification of a DFSP shows deep dermal and subcutaneous ➡ involvement by a cellular spindle cell tumor with fat entrapment. Epidermis is separated from tumor by thin grenz zone ➡. (Courtesy T. Mentzel, MD.)*

Clinical Photograph of DFSP

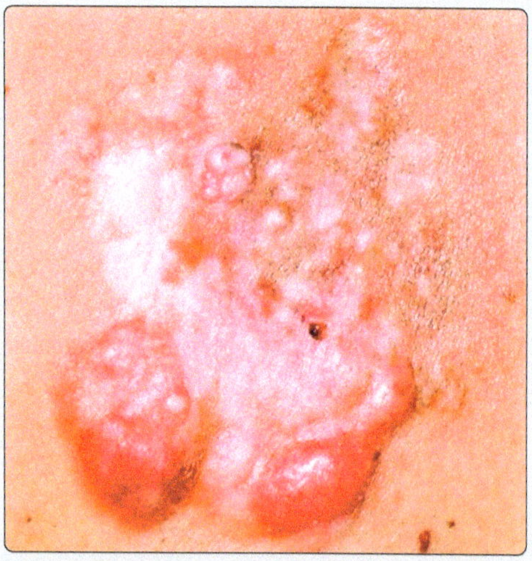

Low Magnification of DFSP

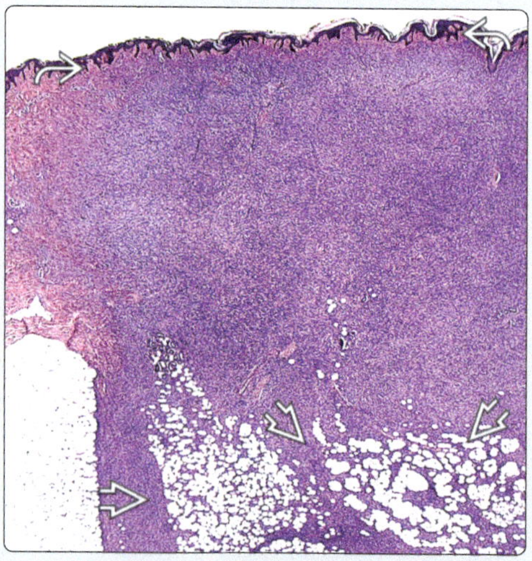

(Left) *Cellular and more atypical area of DFSP shows a proliferation of densely packed atypical spindle cells with storiforming. A few adipocytes ➡ are surrounded (entrapped) by the neoplastic population.* **(Right)** *Fibrosarcomatous transformation in a DFSP is diagnosed when there is increased cellularity, cytologic atypia, and multiple mitotic figures ➡. The tumor is also arranged in a much more fascicular or herringbone architecture than a typical DFSP.*

Higher Magnification of DFSP

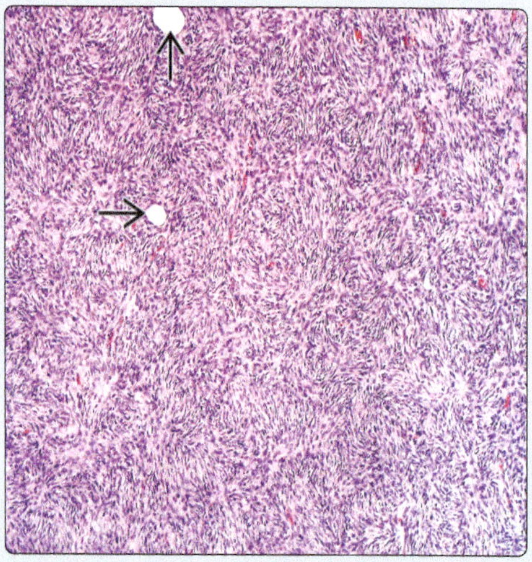

Fibrosarcomatous Transformation in DFSP

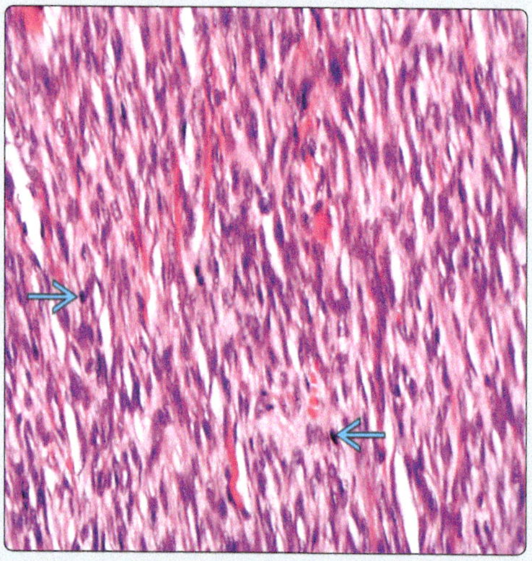

TERMINOLOGY

Abbreviations

- Dermatofibrosarcoma protuberans (DFSP)

Synonyms

- Bednar tumor (pigmented DFSP)

Definitions

- Low-grade malignant spindle cell tumor of skin characteristically showing prominent storiforming

ETIOLOGY/PATHOGENESIS

Unknown in Most Cases

- Rare cases reportedly associated with previous trauma, burns, or arsenic exposure

Genetics

- Rearrangements of collagen 1A1 *(COL1A1)*/platelet-derived growth factor B (*PDGFB*)
- Characteristic t(17;22) detected in most cases
  - Can be detected by FISH or PCR studies for fusion protein

CLINICAL ISSUES

Epidemiology

- Incidence
  - Uncommon tumors
- Age
  - Typically occurs in young adults
- Sex
  - Male predominance

Site

- Most often present on trunk or extremities
- Rarely occur on head and neck

Presentation

- Dermal and subcutaneous nodular/multinodular or plaque-like mass

Natural History

- Slowly progressive, locally aggressive tumor

Treatment

- Optimal treatment is complete surgical excision
- Imatinib has been used for locally extensive and metastatic disease

Prognosis

- Excellent in most cases
- Local recurrences in up to 30% of cases
- Very low metastatic potential (and essentially only in cases with fibrosarcomatous transformation)

MACROSCOPIC

General Features

- Polypoid, multinodular, or bosselated-appearing tumor
  - Rare cases may be atrophic-appearing
- Cut surface usually gray-white
- May show hemorrhage and cystic changes

MICROSCOPIC

Histologic Features

- Spindle cell tumor with deep dermal and subcutaneous involvement
- Proliferation of monomorphic spindle-shaped cells
- Arrayed in storiform or cartwheel patterns
- Lesional cells typically lack significant atypia and pleomorphism
  - Elongated spindle-shaped nuclei
  - Mild nuclear hyperchromasia, small to inconspicuous nucleoli
  - Moderate amounts of eosinophilic cytoplasm
- Mitoses are usually infrequent (< 4/10 HPF) and not atypical
  - Increased mitoses and atypical forms are seen with fibrosarcomatous change
- Necrosis is usually absent
- Adnexal structures entrapped but not obliterated
- Subcutaneous areas typically show honeycombing fat entrapment
- Myxoid stromal change may be prominent in some cases

Cytologic Features

- Elongated spindle-shaped cells with hyperchromatic-staining nuclei, small or absent nucleoli, and eosinophilic-staining cytoplasm

Variants

- **Bednar tumor**
  - Pigmented DFSP due to intratumoral population of benign melanocytes
  - No prognostic significance
- **Giant cell fibroblastoma**
  - Clinical: Occurs in children and young adults
  - Histologic features are distinctive
    - Proliferation of spindled cells and giant cells with nuclear hyperchromasia
    - Pseudovascular spaces lined by giant cells
  - Mutations involving *COL1A1/PDGFRB* (*PDGFR*) (same as in DFSP)

ANCILLARY TESTS

Immunohistochemistry

- Useful to confirm diagnosis, although often not necessary
  - CD34 is most reliable marker
    - Typically, strongly and diffusely positive
    - May be weak and focal in some cases
  - FXIIIA is usually negative [positive in dermatofibroma (DF)]
    - May show focal staining, usually at periphery or in scattered dendritic cells
  - CD68, CD10, lysozyme, and chymotrypsin are typically negative
    - These markers are relatively nonspecific (but positive in DF and atypical fibroxanthoma)

Genetic Testing

- t(17;22): Rearrangement of collagen 1A1 (*COL1A1*)/platelet-derived growth factor B (*PDGFB*)

Immunohistochemistry

Antibody	Reactivity	Staining Pattern	Comment
CD34	Positive	Cell membrane & cytoplasm	Usually strongly and diffusely positive
FXIIIA	Negative		May see focal staining of scattered single cells
CD68	Negative		May see focal staining of entrapped histiocytes
CD163	Negative		Strongly positive in dermatofibroma
S100	Negative		Rarely positive in pigmented cells (Bednar tumor)

DIFFERENTIAL DIAGNOSIS

Cellular Dermatofibroma/Fibrous Histiocytoma

- More pleomorphic cell types
  - Both small spindle-shaped fibroblastic cells and larger histiocytoid-appearing cells
- No prominent storiforming
- May show superficial, jagged involvement of fat
  - No deep, honeycombing fat entrapment as in DFSP
- FXIIIA(+), CD68(+), CD163(+), and CD10(+); CD34(-)
  - CD34 may be focally positive, usually at periphery

Fibrosarcoma (Including Transformation in DFSP)

- Areas of increased cellularity, atypia, and mitoses (> 5/10 HPF)
- Spindle cells typically arrayed in prominent fascicles with herringbone appearance
  - Intersecting fascicles at 45° angles
- Usually see loss of CD34 expression in fibrosarcomatous areas

Indeterminate Fibrohistiocytic Lesion

- Cellular fibrohistiocytic tumor with features intermediate between DF and DFSP
- Often shows at least focal involvement of subcutis with fat entrapment
- CD34 and FXIIIA both usually positive
  - CD34 may only be weak/focal
- Lack *COL1A/PDGFB* translocation

Fibromatosis

- Proliferation of elongated spindle cells associated with dense collagenous stroma
- Small blood vessels associated with extravasated red blood cells
- Often deeply infiltrates soft tissues, but lacks honeycombing fat entrapment of DFSP
- β-catenin (+) and actin (SMA)(+); CD34(-)

Solitary Fibrous Tumor

- CD34(+) spindle cell proliferation, but lacks storiforming of DFSP
- More common in soft tissues; only rarely occurs in skin
- Composed of patternless proliferation of spindle cells associated with thickened, ropy collagen bundles and "staghorn" vessels

Leiomyosarcoma

- Long fascicles of enlarged, atypical, eosinophilic-staining spindle cells
- Usually shows more cytologic atypia, pleomorphism, and multiple mitoses
- Lacks storiforming pattern of DFSP
- Actin and desmin positive; CD34 typically negative

Atypical Fibroxanthoma

- Occurs in sun-damaged skin of elderly (typically head and neck region)
- Dermal-based proliferation of markedly atypical and pleomorphic-appearing tumor cells
- Usually shows mixture of spindle-shaped and epithelioid cells with tumor giant cells
  - However, some cases can be mostly composed of spindle cells
    - But cells show higher grade atypia and lack storiforming pattern of DFSP

Spindle Cell/Desmoplastic Melanoma

- Typically shows greater atypia, pleomorphism, and nuclear hyperchromasia
- Lacks areas of storiforming
- Overlying melanoma in situ present in majority of cases (> 70%)
- S100(+); other melanocytic markers often negative

DIAGNOSTIC CHECKLIST

Clinically Relevant Pathologic Features

- Fibrosarcomatous transformation
- Margins: Tumors with positive margins much more likely to recur

SELECTED REFERENCES

1. Kreicher KL et al: Incidence and survival of primary dermatofibrosarcoma protuberans in the United States. Dermatol Surg. 42 Suppl 1:S24-31, 2016
2. Nakamura I et al: A novel chromosomal translocation associated with COL1A2- PDGFB gene fusion in dermatofibrosarcoma protuberans: PDGF expression as a new diagnostic tool. JAMA Dermatol. 151(12):1330-1337, 2015
3. Saiag P et al: Diagnosis and treatment of dermatofibrosarcoma protuberans. European consensus-based interdisciplinary guideline. Eur J Cancer. 51(17):2604-8, 2015
4. Llombart B et al: Dermatofibrosarcoma protuberans: clinical, pathological, and genetic (COL1A1-PDGFB) study with therapeutic implications. Histopathology. 54(7):860-72, 2009
5. Paradisi A et al: Dermatofibrosarcoma protuberans: wide local excision vs. Mohs micrographic surgery. Cancer Treat Rev. 34(8):728-36, 2008
6. Maire G et al: A clinical, histologic, and molecular study of 9 cases of congenital dermatofibrosarcoma protuberans. Arch Dermatol. 143(2):203-10, 2007
7. Mentzel T et al: Myxoid dermatofibrosarcoma protuberans: clinicopathologic, immunohistochemical, and molecular analysis of eight cases. Am J Dermatopathol. 29(5):443-8, 2007
8. Abrams TA et al: Targeted therapy for dermatofibrosarcoma protuberans. Curr Oncol Rep. 8(4):291-6, 2006

Recurrent DFSP

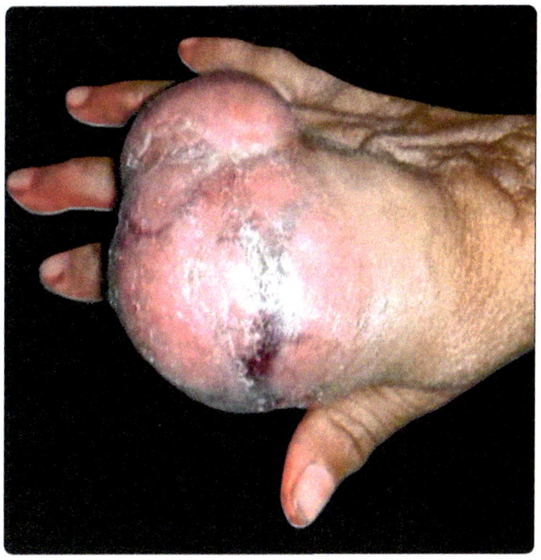

Scanning Magnification of DFSP

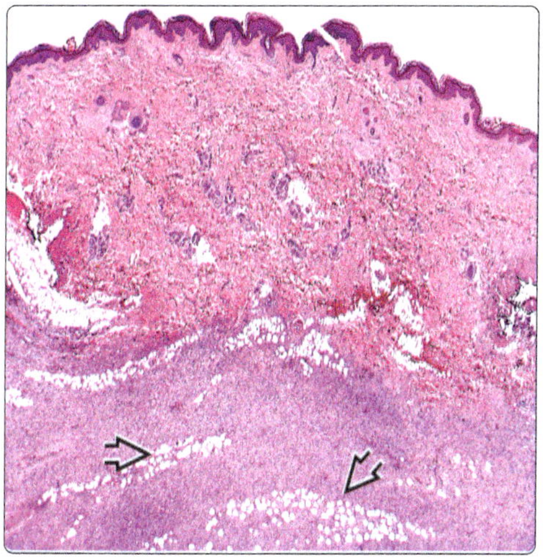

(Left) *Clinical photograph shows a case of a recurrent DFSP with diffuse, nodular involvement of the distal hand. (Courtesy T. Mentzel, MD.)* **(Right)** *Scanning magnification view of a DFSP shows deep dermal and subcutaneous involvement by a cellular spindle cell tumor with fat entrapment ⮚. The epidermis and superficial dermis are unremarkable.*

Prominent Honeycombing Fat Entrapment

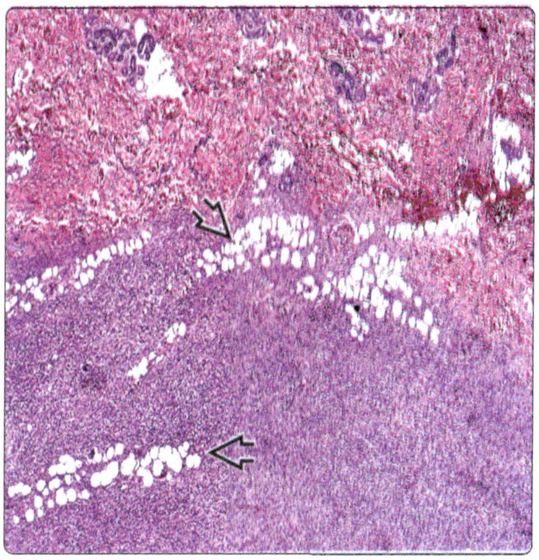

Prominent Fat Entrapment

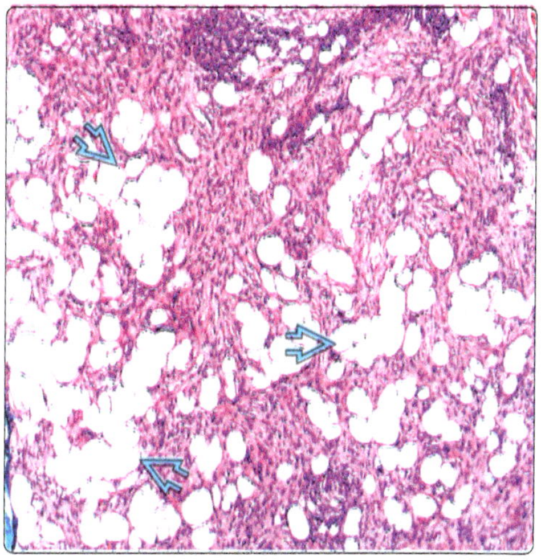

(Left) *Deep dermal and subcutaneous involvement by a DFSP shows prominent honeycombing ⮚ fat entrapment. The neoplasm is cellular, giving a blue appearance to the proliferation on low power. The borders of the tumor are irregular.* **(Right)** *The deep subcutaneous tissues of this DFSP highlight the significant fat entrapment ⮚. The neoplastic cells are cytologically bland, and mitotic figures are not easily identified.*

Entrapped Adnexal Glands

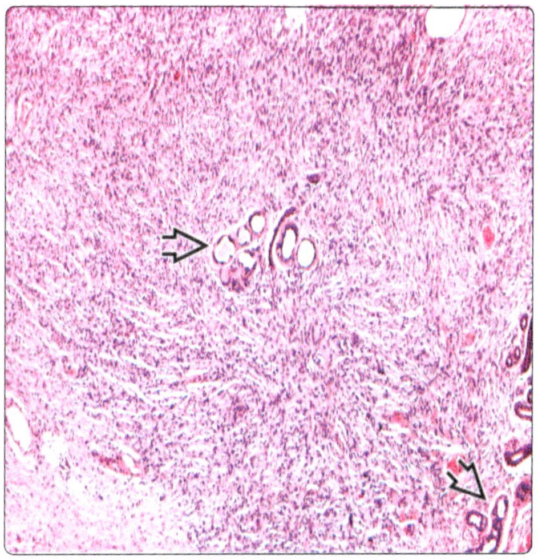

Pigmented DFSP (Bednar Tumor)

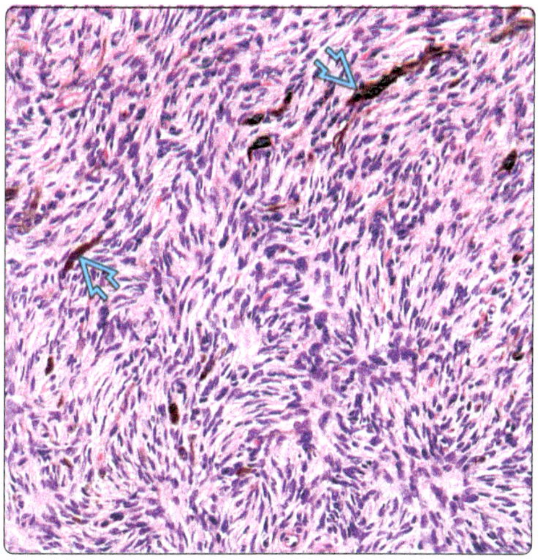

(Left) *On low power, there are a number of adnexal glands that are entrapped ⮚ by the cellular, vaguely storiform neoplastic proliferation. However, there is no destruction of these adnexal structures by the tumor.* **(Right)** *In addition to the spindled tumor cells, scattered elongated pigmented (melanin-containing) cells are seen ⮚ in Bednar tumors. The finding is of no prognostic significance, and similar cells can be found in fibrosarcomatous DFSP and in giant cell fibroblastoma.*

Superficial (Atrophic) Plaque-Like DFSP

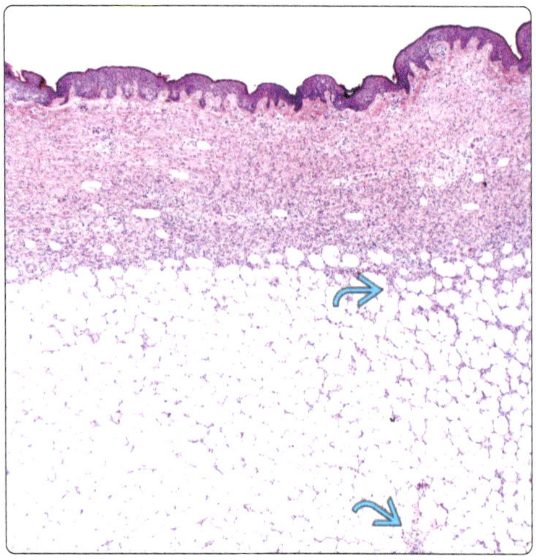

Superficial (Atrophic) Plaque-Like DFSP

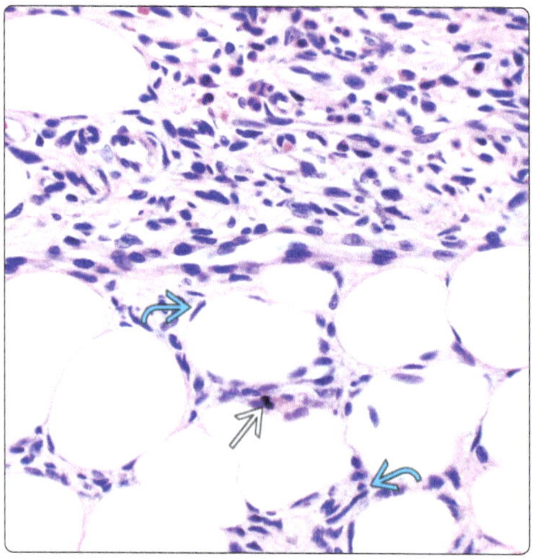

(Left) *This is an example of a rare superficial (atrophic) plaque-like DFSP. Although the dermis is atrophic-appearing, it is diffusely infiltrated by a spindle neoplasm, which also extends deeply into the fat ➜.* **(Right)** *High magnification of the fat involvement in plaque-like DFSP is shown. The adipocytes are infiltrated and focally entrapped by the spindle cells ➜. Note the rare mitotic figure present ➜.*

DFSP With Myxoid Stroma

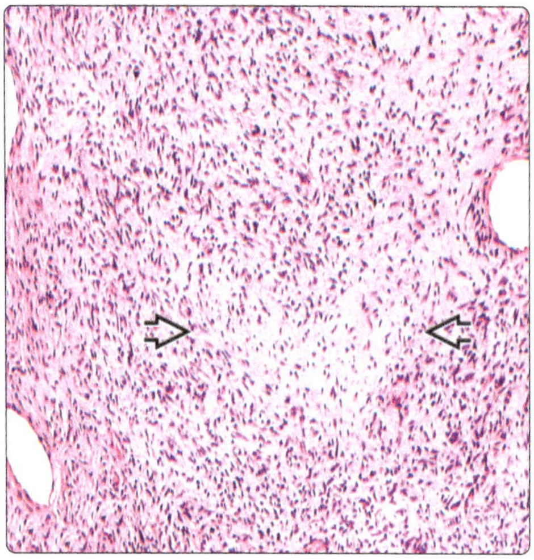

High Magnification of DFSP With Myxoid Stroma

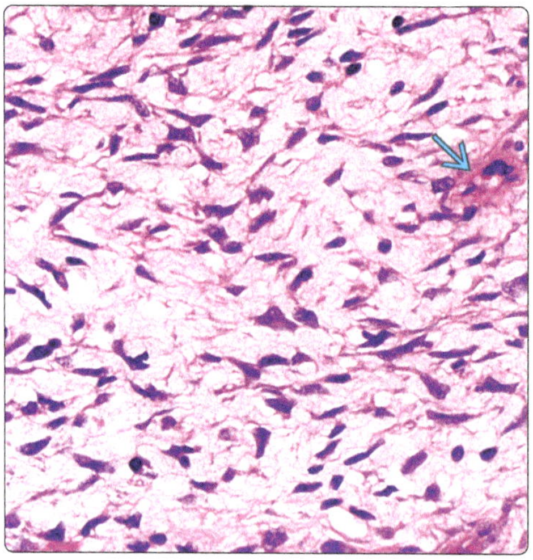

(Left) *Areas of myxoid stromal change may be seen in a minority of cases of DFSP. The myxoid changes give a lighter stromal appearance ➜ to a tumor that is otherwise usually quite densely cellular.* **(Right)** *High magnification of a myxoid DFSP shows stellate and spindle cells in a myxoid stroma. There is a residual storiform pattern, although the cells are widely separated by the stromal material. A blood vessel is seen with a mildly thickened wall ➜. (Courtesy T. Mentzel, MD.)*

DFSP Variant: Giant Cell Fibroblastoma

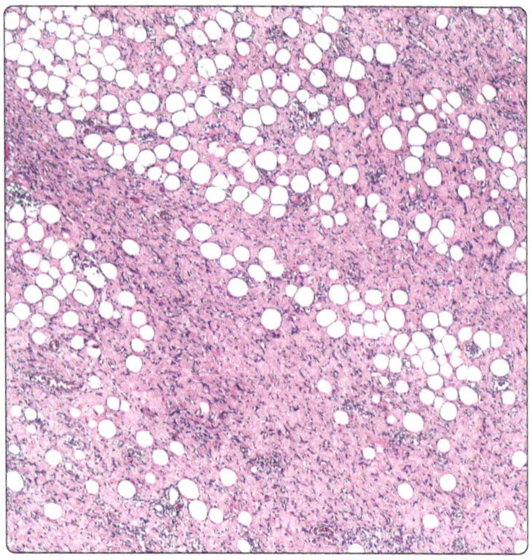

DFSP Variant: Giant Cell Fibroblastoma

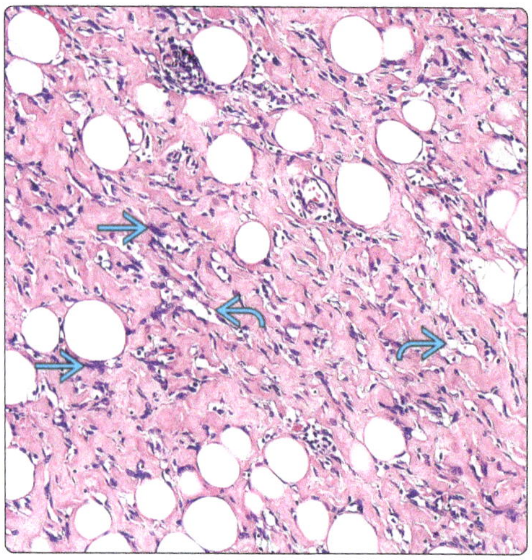

(Left) *Diffuse infiltration of subcutaneous tissue is seen in many examples of giant cell fibroblastoma (GCFB), such as this case, which shows honeycombing fat entrapment, similar to DFSP.* **(Right)** *Higher magnification of GCFB shows diffuse infiltration of subcutaneous tissue by spindle-shaped to multinucleated cells ➜ with nuclear hyperchromasia. Note the pseudovascular spaces ➜, which are typical of this tumor. (Courtesy T. Mentzel, MD.)*

CD34 Immunohistochemistry in DFSP

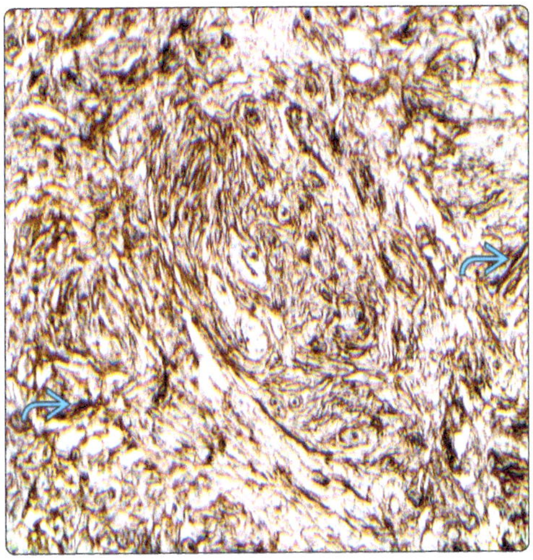

FXIIIA Immunohistochemistry in DFSP

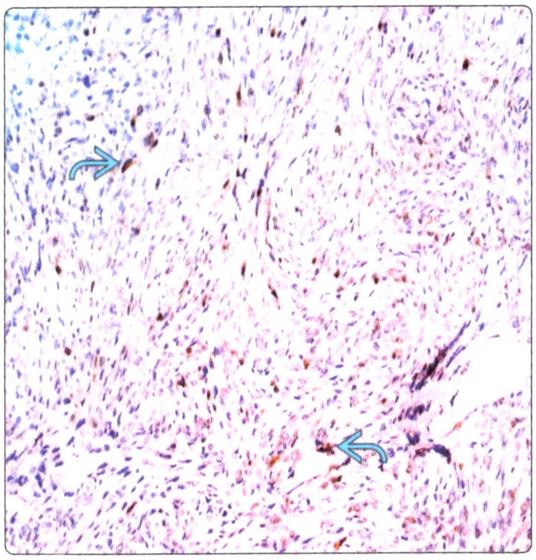

(Left) *Strong immunohistochemical staining for CD34 is shown in nearly all of the tumor spindle cells in a typical DFSP. Vessels will also be highlighted with the stain ➜, a good internal control.* **(Right)** *Immunohistochemistry for FXIIIA typically shows only scattered positive entrapped fibroblasts or dendritic cells ➜, but the majority of the spindle cells are negative.*

CD34 Staining in Giant Cell Fibroblastoma

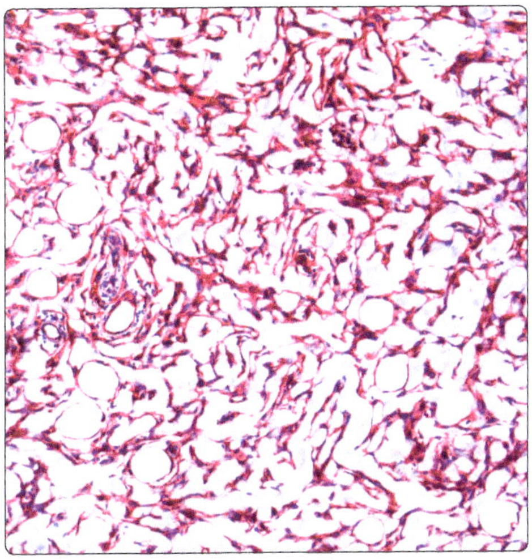

Loss of CD34 Staining in Fibrosarcomatous DFSP

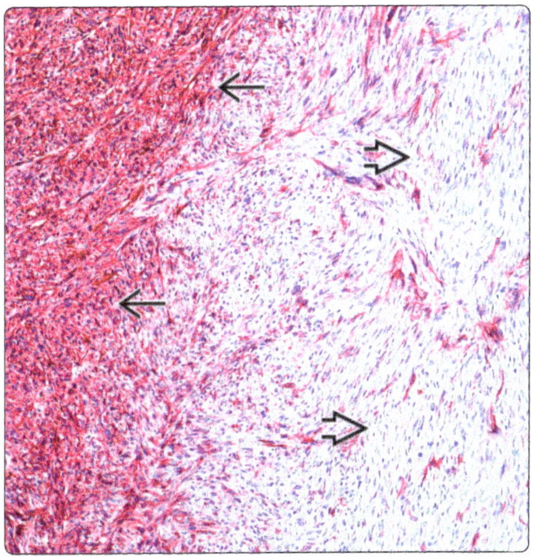

(Left) *GCFB shows strong and diffuse CD34 staining in the spindle cells and multinucleated giant cells. (Courtesy T. Mentzel, MD.)* **(Right)** *Loss of CD34 expression ➜ is seen in areas of fibrosarcomatous DFSP, compared with the residual adjacent dermatofibrosarcoma ➜. However, some cases retain diffuse CD34 immunoreactivity. (Courtesy T. Mentzel, MD.)*

Differential Diagnosis: Cellular and Histiocytic Dermatofibroma

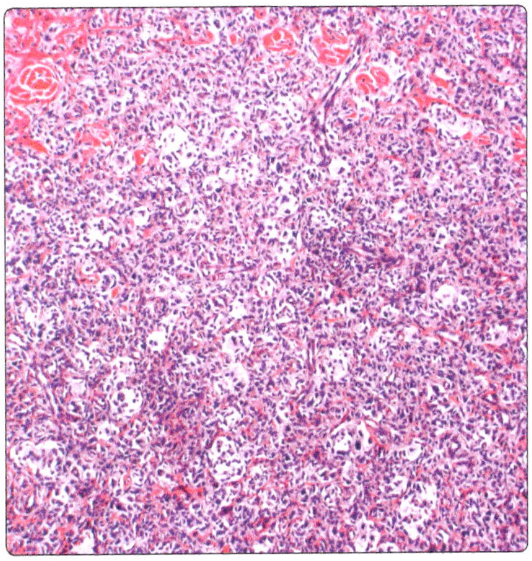

CD163 Staining in Cellular and Histiocytic Dermatofibroma

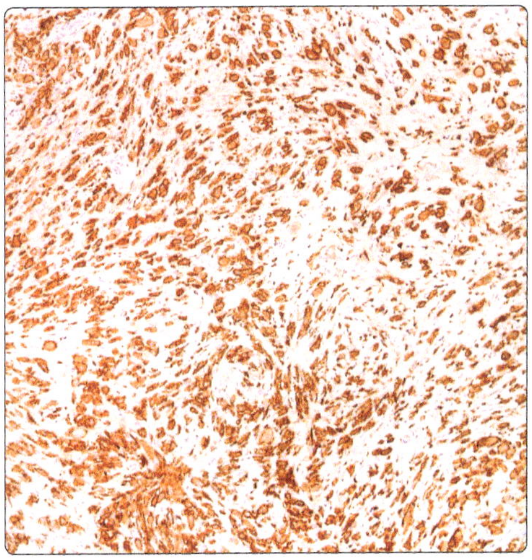

(Left) *Cellular and histiocytic dermatofibroma (DF) shows diffuse dermal involvement by a predominantly spindle cell tumor with scattered larger, clear-staining cells, consistent with histiocytic differentiation.* **(Right)** *CD163 shows strong and diffuse staining of the histiocytic and spindled cells in a cellular and histiocytic variant of DF. This marker is typically negative in DFSP.*

Atypical Fibroxanthoma

KEY FACTS

TERMINOLOGY

- Superficial malignant fibrous histiocytoma/pleomorphic sarcoma
- Dermal-based, low-grade mesenchymal neoplasm showing no specific lineage of differentiation

CLINICAL ISSUES

- Mass lesion, may be ulcerated or bleeding
- Often rapidly growing tumor in head and neck region of elderly adult
- Rate of local recurrence is low (< 10% reported)

MICROSCOPIC

- Highly atypical and pleomorphic dermal-based proliferation of spindled to epithelioid-appearing cells
- Scattered large, bizarre-appearing multinucleated cells often seen
- Variants include spindle cell, clear cell, granular, chondroid, and osteoid
- Numerous mitoses, including highly atypical forms, easily found

ANCILLARY TESTS

- Immunohistochemistry is key in confirming diagnosis
  - Essential to exclude other, more specific diagnoses
- Negative for melanocytic markers, cytokeratins (especially HMWCKs), p63, muscle (except for SMA), and vascular markers
- Positive for nonspecific markers including CD10, CD68, CD99, and vimentin

TOP DIFFERENTIAL DIAGNOSES

- Sarcomatoid carcinoma (typically squamous cell carcinoma)
- Spindle cell melanoma
- Leiomyosarcoma
- Rarely, other sarcomas

Clinical Image of AFX on Ear

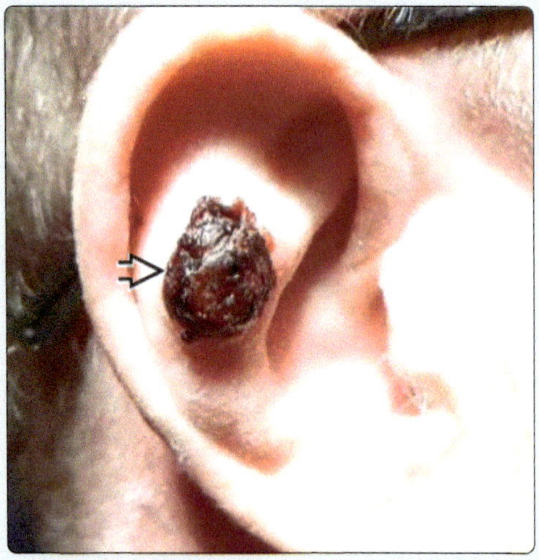

Clear Cell AFX at Low Magnification

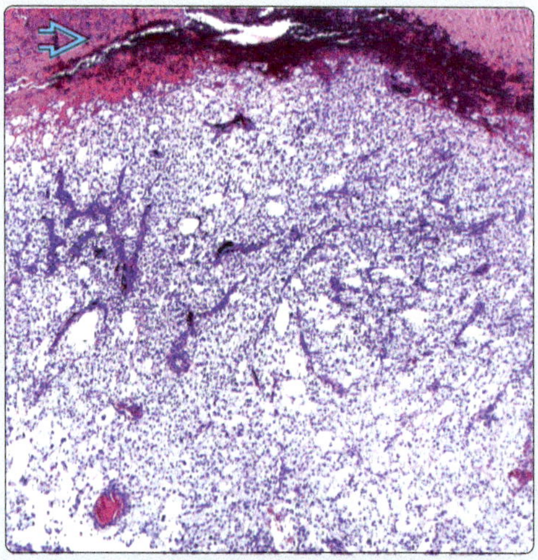

(Left) *Clinical photograph shows a large, nodular tumor on the ear of an elderly patient. The surface is diffusely ulcerated and covered with serum crust ⇒.* **(Right)** *Clear cell atypical fibroxanthoma (AFX) is a rare variant of AFX, which can be confused with other clear cell tumors. This example shows diffuse overlying ulceration with dense serum crust ⇒.*

Higher Magnification of Clear Cell AFX

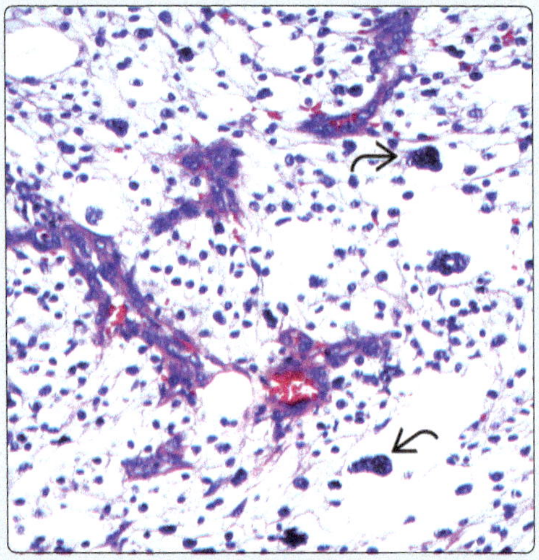

CD10 Immunohistochemical Stain in AFX

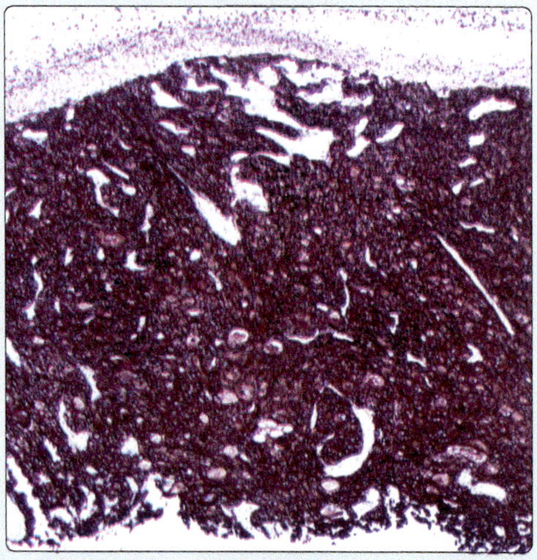

(Left) *Higher power examination shows a proliferation of markedly enlarged and atypical-appearing histiocytic cells with abundant pale to vacuolated cytoplasm. Note the large, pleomorphic multinucleated cells ↗ present.* **(Right)** *CD10 shows very strong and diffuse staining in this clear cell AFX.*

TERMINOLOGY

Abbreviations

- Atypical fibroxanthoma (AFX)

Synonyms

- Superficial pleomorphic sarcoma

Definitions

- Dermal-based, low-grade mesenchymal neoplasm showing no specific lineage of differentiation
  - Should be negative for markers of melanocytic (i.e., S100, SOX10) and epithelial (i.e., cytokeratins and p63) differentiation

ETIOLOGY/PATHOGENESIS

Environmental Exposure

- Likely related to UV exposure, as most cases occur in elderly patients in sun-damaged skin
- Some cases reported following radiation therapy
- May also be increased in immunosuppressed patients (i.e., renal transplant patients)

CLINICAL ISSUES

Epidemiology

- Age
  - Typically occurs in elderly patients
  - Rare cases in children with xeroderma pigmentosum or Li-Fraumeni syndrome
- Sex
  - May have slight male predominance

Site

- Head and neck in general is most commonly affected area
  - Scalp is most common location
- Uncommonly, occurs on trunk or extremities

Presentation

- Skin nodule, asymptomatic in most cases
  - Often rapidly growing lesion
  - Dermal-based lesion
  - Often shows overlying ulceration or hemorrhage/crusting
- Regional lymph node metastases may be found in small number of cases

Natural History

- Progressive lesion; does not regress without treatment

Treatment

- Surgical approaches
  - Complete and wide surgical excision
    - Mohs surgery is also effective
  - Unresectable or metastatic cases may be treated with chemoradiation

Prognosis

- Very good in most cases
- Rate of local recurrence is low (< 10% reported)
- Vast majority of cases do not metastasize
  - Cases with subcutaneous involvement can metastasize

MACROSCOPIC

General Features

- Large, nodular, unencapsulated, dermal-based tumor

Size

- < 2 cm in greatest dimension in most cases

MICROSCOPIC

Histologic Features

- Nodular, dermal-based proliferation of atypical, pleomorphic-appearing spindled and epithelioid-shaped cells
  - Cells are markedly enlarged and often bizarre-appearing
  - Show atypical, hyperchromatic-staining nuclei
    - Irregular nuclear borders and prominent nucleoli
  - Cytoplasm of tumor cells is abundant, eosinophilic, and sometimes pale to clear/vacuolated-appearing
  - Variants include spindle cell, clear cell, granular cell, chondroid, and osteoid
- Scattered large, bizarre-appearing multinucleated giant cells typically present
- Numerous mitoses, including highly atypical forms, easily found
- No evidence of associated/overlying carcinoma or melanoma in situ
  - Often separated from epidermis by thin grenz zone
- No evidence of epithelial (squamous, ductal, or glandular) or melanocytic differentiation should be identifiable

Cytologic Features

- Frankly atypical and pleomorphic-appearing spindle-shaped to epithelioid cells
- Multinucleated tumor giant cells with prominent nuclear atypia

ANCILLARY TESTS

Immunohistochemistry

- Immunohistochemistry is key in confirming diagnosis
  - Essential to exclude other, more specific diagnoses
- Negative for melanocytic markers, cytokeratins (especially HMWCKs), p63, p40, muscle (except for SMA, which is typically focal/weak) and vascular markers
- Positive for nonspecific markers, including CD10, CD68 (may be focal/weak), CD99, and vimentin

DIFFERENTIAL DIAGNOSIS

Sarcomatoid Carcinoma

- Typically squamous cell carcinoma, but poorly differentiated adnexal carcinomas and metastatic poorly differentiated carcinomas should also be considered
- Positive: High molecular weight cytokeratins (CK5/6, CK903/34βE12), p63 and p40
  - May or may not show staining for pancytokeratin, AE1/AE3, EMA, and CAM5.2 (low molecular weight CKs)

Pleomorphic, Spindle Cell, and Desmoplastic Melanoma

- Overlying junctional component/melanoma in situ is present in majority of cases (> 70%)

Immunohistochemistry Table

Antibody	Reactivity	Staining Pattern	Comment
CD10	Positive	Cell membrane & cytoplasm	Usually strongly and diffusely positive (nonspecific)
CD68	Positive	Cell membrane & cytoplasm	Usually positive, may be weak/focal (nonspecific)
CK-PAN	Negative		Positive control staining of epidermis and adnexal structures
CK-HMW-NOS	Negative		Positive control staining of epidermis and adnexal structures
p63	Negative	Nuclear	Rare cases reportedly positive; must be CK negative
S100	Negative		Entrapped dendritic cells positive
Melan-A	Negative		Junctional melanocytes serve as positive control
HMB-45	Negative		Junctional melanocytes serve as positive control
Desmin	Negative		Muscular vessels are positive
CD34	Negative		Highlights stromal vessels
CD31	Negative		Highlights stromal vessels
Actin-sm	Equivocal	Cytoplasmic	May be weakly positive in some cases, likely indicating myofibroblastic differentiation
MITF	Equivocal	Nuclear	Rare cases may be weakly/focally positive

- S100 and SOX10 positive; MART-1/Melan-A, HMB-45, tyrosinase, and MITF may be negative
    - Scattered S100(+) dendritic cells are present in AFX, may be numerous in some cases, and should not be misinterpreted as melanoma

Leiomyosarcoma

- Proliferation of atypical spindle cells with elongated, blunt-ended, or cigar-shaped nuclei
- Cells show abundant eosinophilic-staining cytoplasm and perinuclear vacuoles
- Positive: MSA, SMA, desmin (most cases, although up to 30% can be negative)
    - Focal/weak cytoplasmic/membranous SMA may be seen in some AFXs, likely indicating myofibroblastic differentiation

Other Sarcomas

- Much less likely considerations, but differential may include both primary and metastatic sarcomas
- **Angiosarcoma**
    - Irregular, anastomosing vascular spaces; CD31(+), CD34(+)
- **Malignant peripheral nerve sheath tumor**
    - Usually deep-seated lesions, but can rarely involve dermis
    - S100(+) in 50-70% of cases, usually focal to weak, may show CD56(+), nestin (+)
- **Fibrosarcoma (FS)**
    - Usually arises in dermatofibrosarcoma protuberans (DFSP) in dermis or superficial subcutis
    - Prominent herringbone pattern in FS areas, storiforming in DFSP areas
    - DFSP shows strong CD34(+) (may be negative in fibrosarcoma areas)

DIAGNOSTIC CHECKLIST

Clinically Relevant Pathologic Features

- Depth of involvement (subcutaneous invasion implies more aggressive behavior, and such cases are typically diagnosed as malignant fibrous histiocytoma/pleomorphic sarcoma)

Pathologic Interpretation Pearls

- Poorly differentiated malignancy, often shows bizarre tumor cells and nonspecific immunohistochemistry findings

SELECTED REFERENCES

1. Tardío JC et al: Pleomorphic dermal sarcoma: a more aggressive neoplasm than previously estimated. J Cutan Pathol. 43(2):101-12, 2016
2. Koch M et al: Atypical fibroxanthoma - histological diagnosis, immunohistochemical markers and concepts of therapy. Anticancer Res. 35(11):5717-35, 2015
3. Wang WL et al: Metastatic atypical fibroxanthoma: a series of 11 cases including with minimal and no subcutaneous involvement. Am J Dermatopathol. 37(6):455-61, 2015
4. Bedir R et al: Clear cell atypical fibroxantoma: a rare variant of atypical fibroxanthoma and review of the literature. J Clin Diagn Res. 8(6):FD09-11, 2014
5. Němejcová K et al: Granular cell variant of atypical fibroxanthoma. A case report. Cesk Patol. 50(1):34-37, 2014
6. Tallon B et al: MITF positivity in atypical fibroxanthoma: a diagnostic pitfall. Am J Dermatopathol. 36(11):888-91, 2014
7. Kanner WA et al: CD10, p63 and CD99 expression in the differential diagnosis of atypical fibroxanthoma, spindle cell squamous cell carcinoma and desmoplastic melanoma. J Cutan Pathol. 37(7):744-50, 2010
8. New D et al: Atypical fibroxanthoma with regional lymph node metastasis: report of a case and review of the literature. Arch Dermatol. 146(12):1399-404, 2010
9. Gleason BC et al: Utility of p63 in the differential diagnosis of atypical fibroxanthoma and spindle cell squamous cell carcinoma. J Cutan Pathol. 36(5):543-7, 2009
10. Hultgren TL et al: Immunohistochemical staining of CD10 in atypical fibroxanthomas. J Cutan Pathol. 34(5):415-9, 2007
11. Ríos-Martín JJ et al: Granular cell atypical fibroxanthoma: report of two cases. Am J Dermatopathol. 29(1):84-7, 2007
12. Seavolt M et al: Atypical fibroxanthoma: review of the literature and summary of 13 patients treated with mohs micrographic surgery. Dermatol Surg. 32(3):435-41; discussion 439-41, 2006
13. Fretzin DF et al: Atypical fibroxanthoma of the skin. A clinicopathologic study of 140 cases. Cancer. 31(6):1541-52, 1973

AFX With Ulceration, Hemorrhage, and Hemosiderin

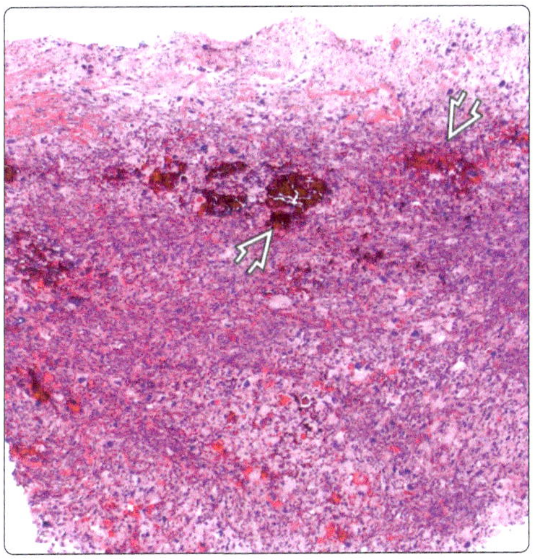

Higher Magnification of AFX With Hemorrhage and Hemosiderin

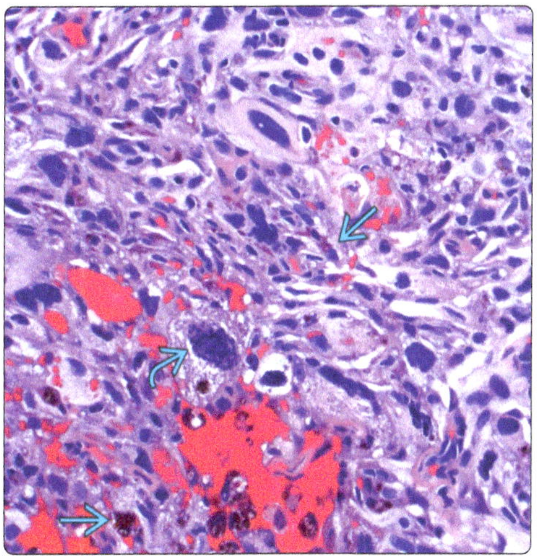

(Left) *This case of AFX shows diffuse loss of the epidermis overlying an atypical dermal tumor associated with prominent areas of sclerotic collagen, hemorrhage, and hemosiderin deposition, findings mimicking an aneurysmal dermatofibroma.* **(Right)** *Higher magnification of the same case shows markedly enlarged, pleomorphic, and atypical-appearing cells, with an atypical mitosis. Note the hemorrhage and hemosiderin deposits.*

Low Magnification of AFX

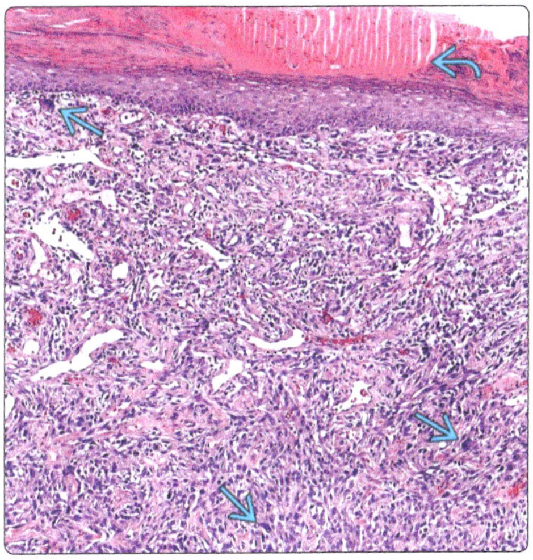

Spindle Cell Variant of AFX

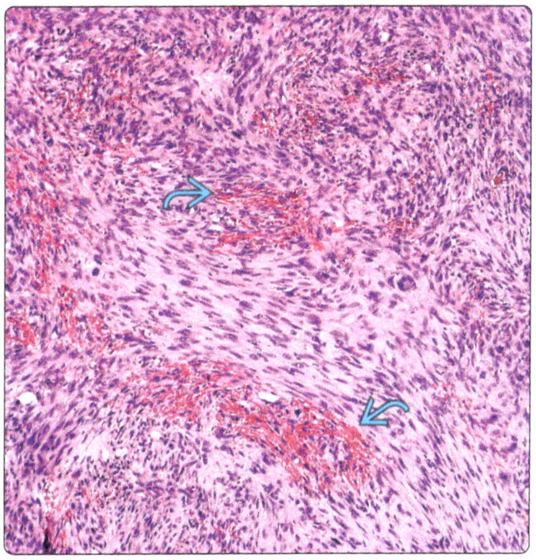

(Left) *Low magnification of AFX shows a cellular and sheet-like, dermal-based proliferation of atypical spindle-shaped and pleomorphic cells associated with telangiectatic vessels. The epidermis shows dense overlying serum crusting.* **(Right)** *This spindle cell variant of AFX shows a proliferation of atypical, hyperchromatic-staining spindle cells forming dense, short fascicles. There are prominent areas of hemorrhage, which could raise suspicion for an angiosarcoma in this case.*

High Magnification of Spindle Cell AFX

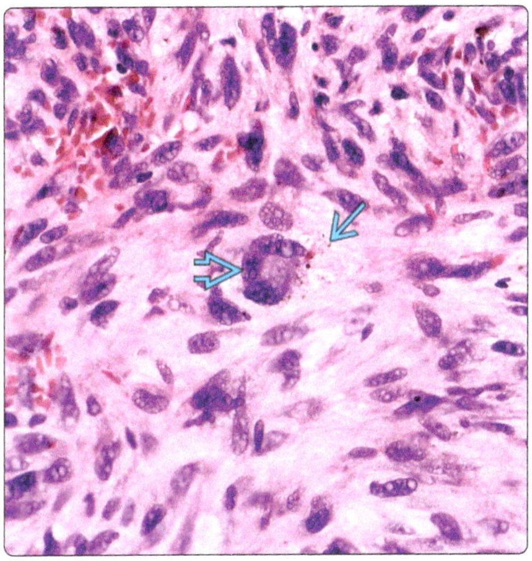

High Magnification With Atypical Mitoses

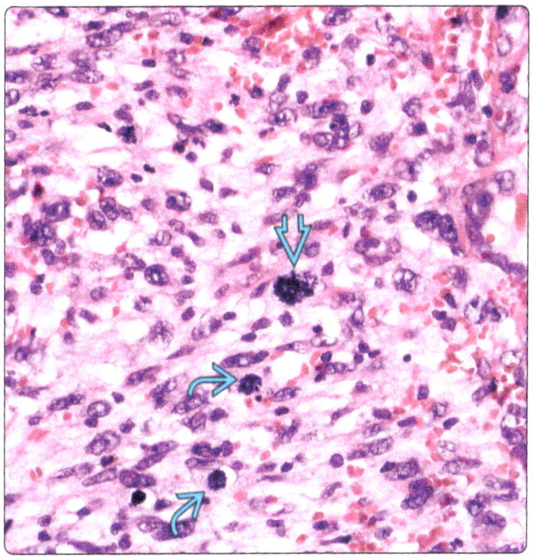

(Left) *High magnification of the same case shows a proliferation of highly atypical and pleomorphic-appearing spindled and multinucleated tumor cells focally containing hemosiderin.* **(Right)** *High magnification of another example of AFX shows highly atypical cells with numerous mitoses, including frankly atypical forms.*

Chondroid Variant of AFX

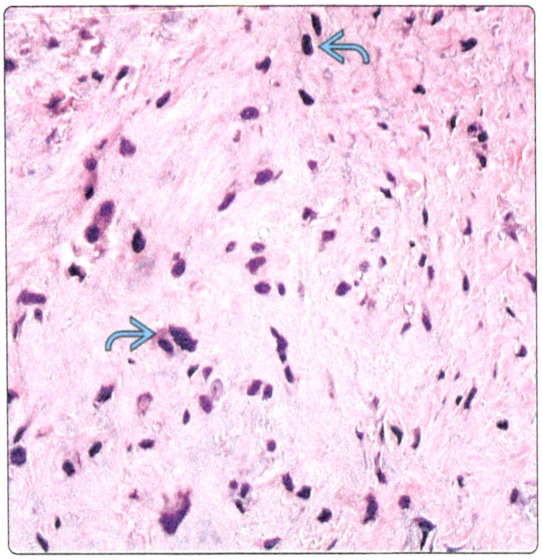

Granular Cell Variant of AFX

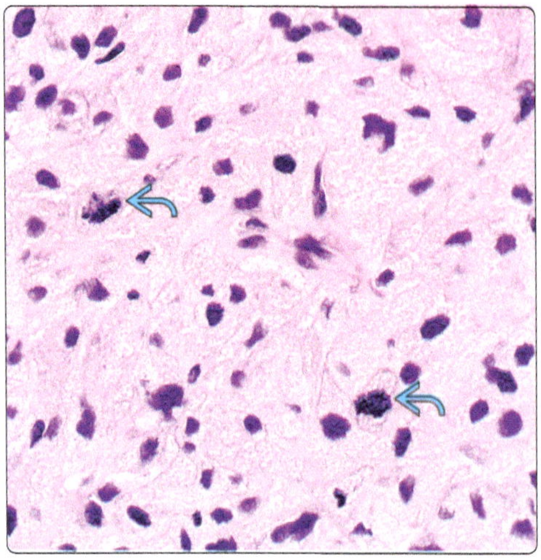

(Left) *An example of the rare chondroid variant of AFX shows an unusual hypocellular tumor with atypical, hyperchromatic-staining cells ↶ scattered in a chondromyxoid-appearing stroma.* **(Right)** *High magnification of an example of the granular cell variant of AFX shows large, bizarre-appearing histiocytoid cells containing abundant granular cytoplasm, similar to a malignant granular cell tumor. Mitoses ↶ are easily found.*

High Molecular Weight Cytokeratin Staining in AFX

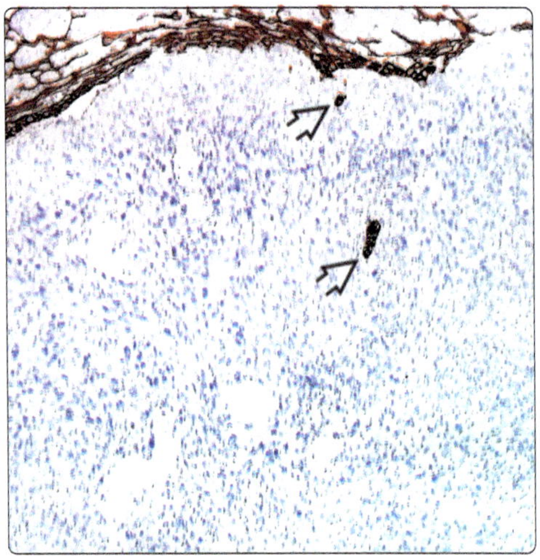

S100 Immunohistochemical Stain in AFX

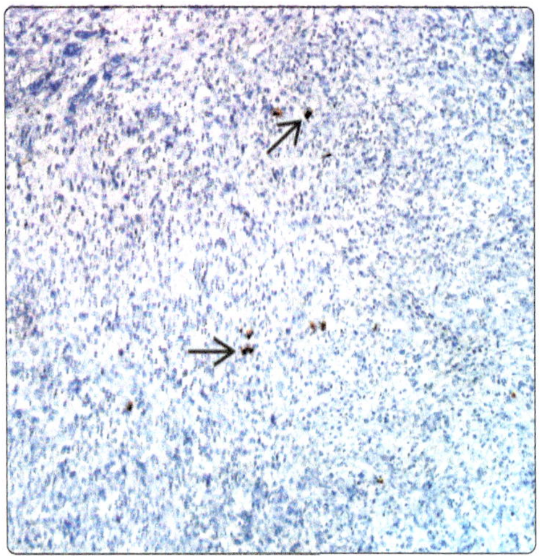

(Left) *High molecular weight cytokeratin immunohistochemical stain shows positivity within the epidermis and adnexal ducts ⇨ but is negative within the tumor cells.* **(Right)** *S100 immunohistochemistry shows no staining of the tumor cells but highlights a few scattered small intradermal dendritic cells →.*

Smooth Muscle Actin Stain in AFX

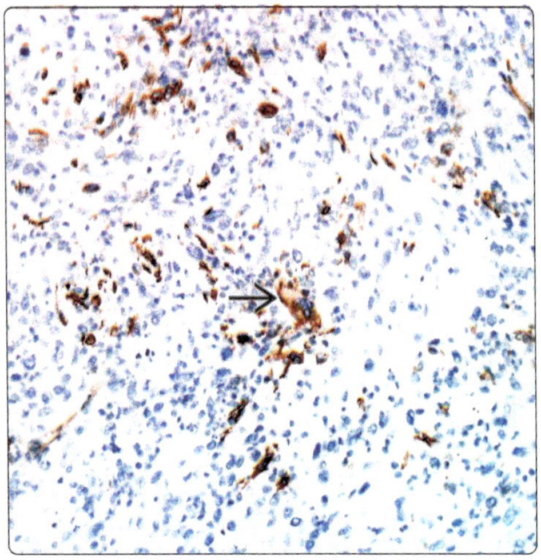

CD34 Immunohistochemical Stain in AFX

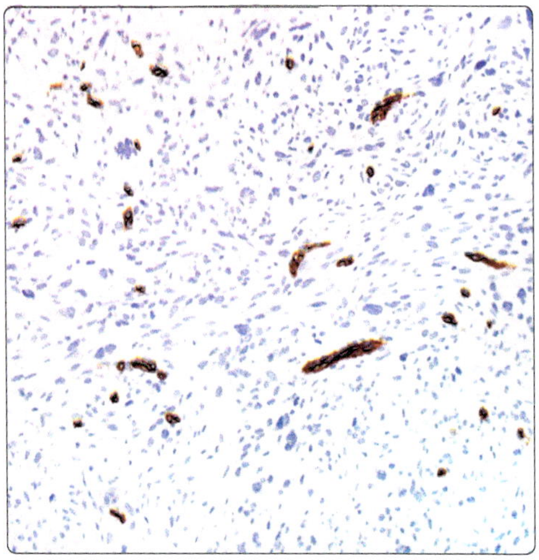

(Left) *Smooth muscle actin stain shows scattered weakly positive cytoplasmic staining →, likely indicating myofibroblastic differentiation.* **(Right)** *CD34 immunohistochemical stain shows strong positive staining of small blood vessels but is negative within the tumor cells (CD31 shows an identical pattern).*

Differential Diagnosis: Melanoma

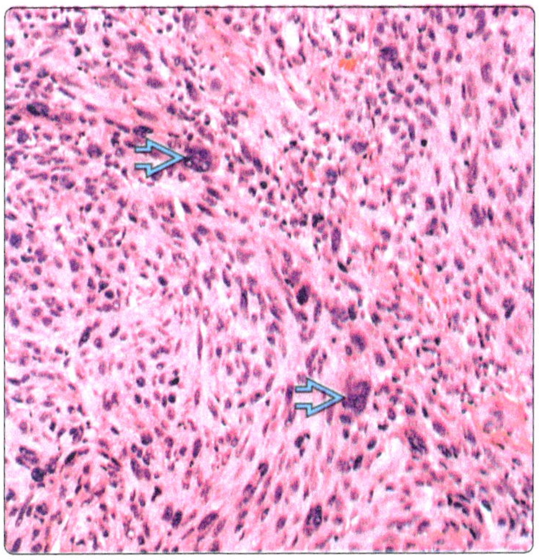

Differential Diagnosis: Melanoma S100 Immunohistochemical Stain

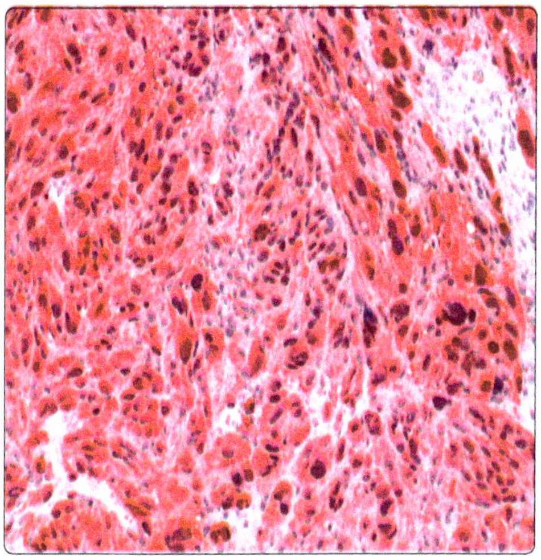

(Left) *Melanoma should always be considered in the differential diagnosis with AFX, especially spindle cell/desmoplastic and metastatic melanomas, which can lack epidermal attachments and show striking atypia and pleomorphism, including multinucleated tumor giant cells. This case lacks pigmentation.* **(Right)** *S100 immunohistochemistry shows diffuse, strong nuclear and cytoplasmic staining in a pleomorphic melanoma. This finding would exclude the possibility of AFX.*

Differential Diagnosis: Poorly Differentiated SCC

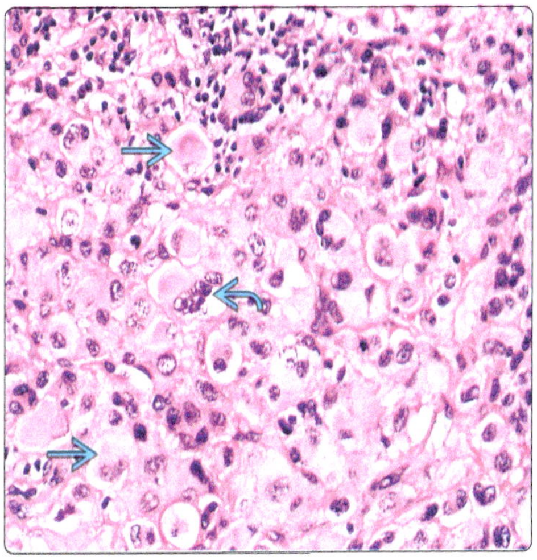

Differential Diagnosis: SCC p63 Stain

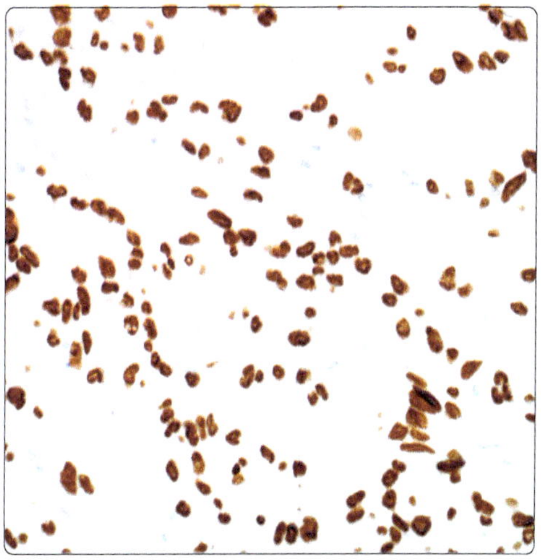

(Left) *This is a poorly differentiated squamous cell carcinoma (SCC) composed of atypical epithelioid cells with abundant pale to eosinophilic-staining cytoplasm. Scattered pleomorphic multinucleated tumor cells can be seen in some cases of SCC.* **(Right)** *This is a high-magnification view of a p63 stain in a poorly differentiated SCC. HMWCK and p63 are the most sensitive markers for poorly differentiated and spindle cell SCC and are typically negative in AFX.*

Differential Diagnosis: Leiomyosarcoma

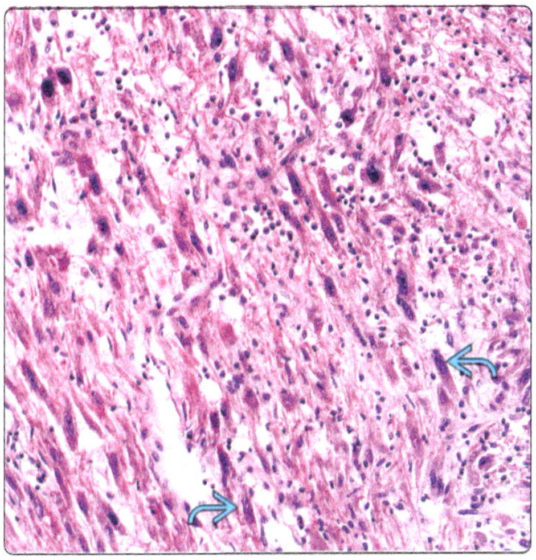

Differential Diagnosis: Leiomyosarcoma Desmin Stain

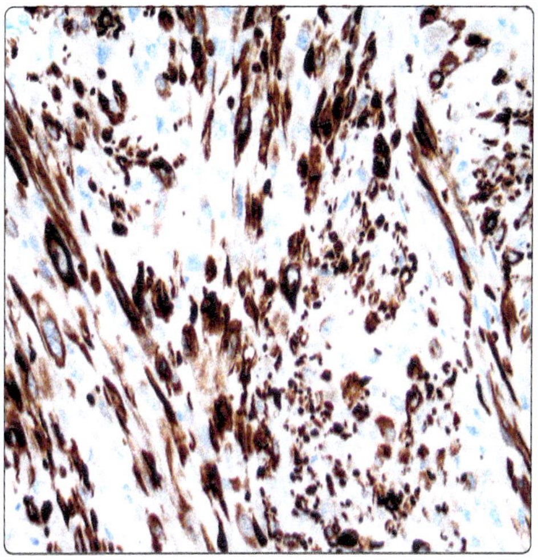

(Left) *Leiomyosarcoma is composed of highly atypical spindle-shaped cells with oval to elongated, cigar-shaped nuclei and abundant eosinophilic-staining cytoplasm.* **(Right)** *Desmin immunostain shows strong cytoplasmic labeling in this leiomyosarcoma. Most cases are positive for both SMA and desmin, although up to 30% of cases can be desmin negative.*

Pleomorphic Dermal Sarcoma

KEY FACTS

TERMINOLOGY

- Pleomorphic sarcoma exhibiting morphologic similarity to atypical fibroxanthoma but also aggressive growth characteristics
  - Deep subcutaneous/fascial/muscular extension, necrosis, &/or lymphovascular invasion
  - Shows no identifiable line of differentiation (i.e., diagnosis of exclusion)
- Synonyms: Superficial malignant fibrous histiocytoma, undifferentiated pleomorphic sarcoma of skin

CLINICAL ISSUES

- Older and elderly adults (most > 50 yr)
- Male predilection
- Usually affects head region, particularly scalp
- Treatment: Complete surgical resection with negative margins
- Local recurrences in up to 30% of cases
- Metastases in 10-20% of cases

MACROSCOPIC

- Median: 2.5 cm

MICROSCOPIC

- Poorly marginated, usually with deep tissue extension
- Prominent cytologic and nuclear atypia and mitotic activity
- Frequent coagulative necrosis
- Lymphovascular invasion in some cases

ANCILLARY TESTS

- Negative for keratins, S100, desmin, CD34, most others
- Immunohistochemical best utilized to exclude other diagnoses

TOP DIFFERENTIAL DIAGNOSES

- Atypical fibroxanthoma
- Carcinoma, melanoma
- Angiosarcoma
- Other superficial pleomorphic sarcomas

PDS

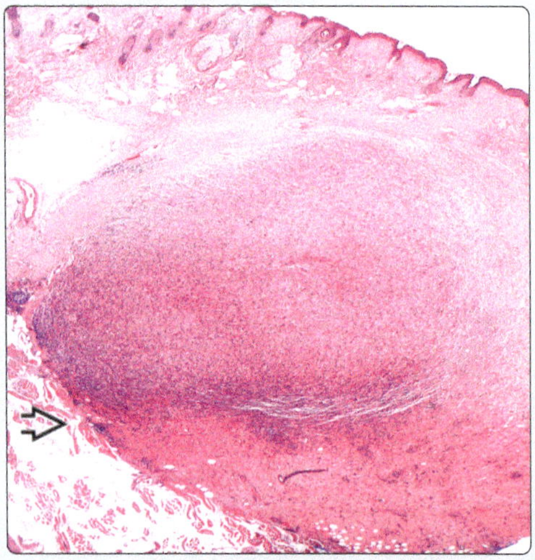

PDS With Resemblance to Atypical Fibroxanthoma

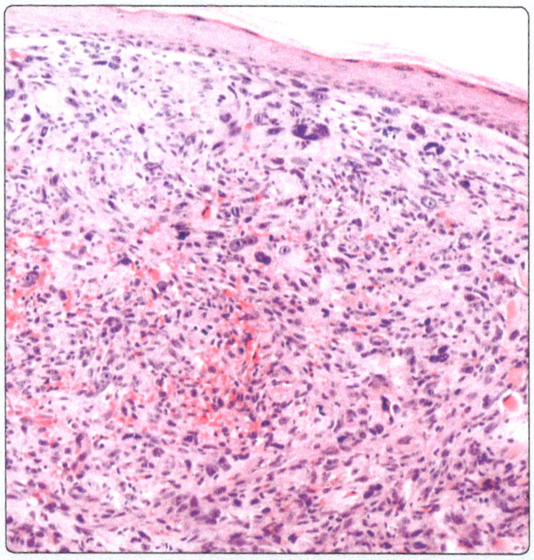

(Left) *Pleomorphic dermal sarcoma (PDS) originates superficially in the dermis, as depicted, but usually shows deeper extension with involvement of the subcutis, fascia, &/or underlying muscle.* **(Right)** *PDS shows histomorphologic features similar to atypical fibroxanthoma (AFX), and these 2 entities can be indistinguishable on a superficial/partial biopsy. The presence of deep tissue extension, necrosis, or lymphovascular invasion would be most consistent with the former.*

PDS With Marked Nuclear Atypia

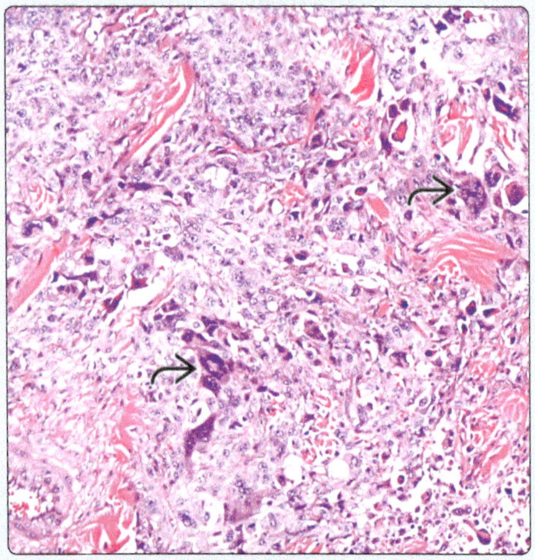

PDS With Coagulative Necrosis

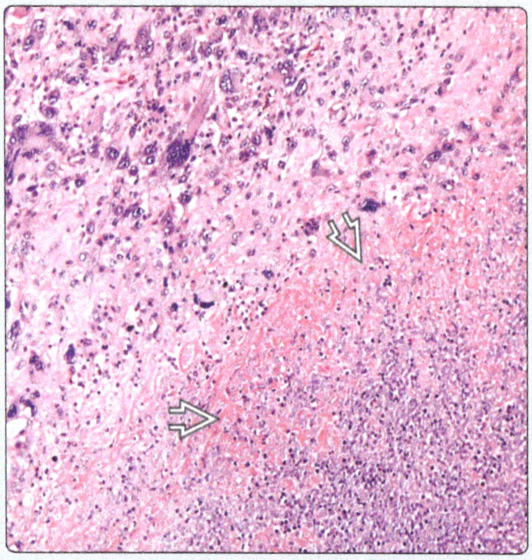

(Left) *Nuclear and cytologic atypia is often prominent and diffuse in PDS, as depicted, similar to its counterpart in deep soft tissues (undifferentiated pleomorphic sarcoma). Multinucleated tumor giant cells are common, as are atypical mitotic figures.* **(Right)** *Coagulative tumor necrosis is common in PDS but varies in amount and distribution. The presence of necrosis in a pleomorphic dermal neoplasm favors PDS over AFX, assuming that carcinoma, melanoma, and other tumors are first excluded.*

TERMINOLOGY

Abbreviations

- Pleomorphic dermal sarcoma (PDS)

Synonyms

- Superficial malignant fibrous histiocytoma
- Undifferentiated pleomorphic sarcoma of skin

Definitions

- Pleomorphic sarcoma exhibiting morphologic similarity to atypical fibroxanthoma (AFX), but also demonstrating aggressive growth characteristics
  - Deep subcutaneous/fascial/muscular extension, necrosis, &/or lymphovascular invasion
  - Shows no identifiable line of differentiation (i.e., diagnosis of exclusion)

ETIOLOGY/PATHOGENESIS

Environmental Exposure

- History of long-term sun exposure usually exists

CLINICAL ISSUES

Epidemiology

- Incidence
  - Rare
- Age
  - Older and elderly adults (most > 50 yr)
- Sex
  - Male predilection

Site

- Usually head region, particularly scalp

Presentation

- Rapid growth common

Treatment

- Complete surgical resection with clear margins
- Chemotherapy may be utilized for metastatic disease

Prognosis

- Local recurrences in up to 30% of cases
  - Likely related to incomplete excision
- Metastases in up to 10-20% of cases
  - Cutaneous sites, lymph nodes, lung reported
- Overall better prognosis than deeply situated, conventional undifferentiated pleomorphic sarcoma

MACROSCOPIC

General Features

- Nodular or plaque-like growth

Size

- Median: 2.5 cm

MICROSCOPIC

Histologic Features

- Surrounding/overlying skin frequently shows solar elastosis
- Poorly marginated
  - Extension beyond dermis is important feature
    - May invade only into deep subcutaneous fat, or may also involve underlying fascia/muscle
- Surface ulceration common
- Shows similar morphologic features and spectrum as AFX
  - Storiform, fascicular, or patternless arrangement of highly atypical spindled &/or polygonal cells
    - Marked nuclear pleomorphism in most cases
      - Bizarre nuclei &/or multinucleation (tumor giant cells) common
      - Abundant mitoses, often with abnormal forms
- Coagulative necrosis is common
- Collagenous stroma that may be focally myxoid or hyalinized
- Lymphovascular invasion &/or perineural involvement not uncommon
- Rare findings: Osteoclast-like giant cells, pseudoangiomatous features
- No discernible microscopic evidence of any specific form of differentiation (e.g., lipoblasts, bone formation, epithelial structures)

ANCILLARY TESTS

Immunohistochemistry

- Negative for keratins, S100, SOX10, desmin, CD34, myogenin, p63, myogenin, ERG, CD31
- Focal expression of some markers (particularly SMA, CD34, EMA) may occur and is likely nonspecific
- Main purpose of immunohistochemistry is to exclude other diagnoses

DIFFERENTIAL DIAGNOSIS

Atypical Fibroxanthoma

- Usually small (< 1 cm) , well marginated, and symmetrical
- Can be cytomorphologically indistinguishable from PDS
- Lacks necrosis, deep tissue invasion, lymphovascular invasion

Carcinoma, Melanoma, Lymphoma

- Can be excluded through immunohistochemistry and often clinical history

Angiosarcoma

- Poorly differentiated tumors may lack vasoformation
- Strong expression of vascular markers (CD31, CD34, ERG)

Other Superficial Pleomorphic Sarcomas

- Includes myxofibrosarcoma, leiomyosarcoma, pleomorphic liposarcoma, rhabdomyosarcoma, and others
- Thorough sampling and careful scrutiny is necessary to identify characteristic histologic findings that support these other diagnoses
- Immunohistochemistry is often invaluable

SELECTED REFERENCES

1. Tardío JC et al: Pleomorphic dermal sarcoma: a more aggressive neoplasm than previously estimated. J Cutan Pathol. 43(2):101-12, 2016
2. Miller K et al: Pleomorphic dermal sarcoma: adverse histologic features predict aggressive behavior and allow distinction from atypical fibroxanthoma. Am J Surg Pathol. 36(9):1317-26, 2012

Adult-Type Fibrosarcoma

KEY FACTS

TERMINOLOGY

- Sarcoma composed of spindle cells resembling fibroblasts
  - Most tumors classified as fibrosarcoma in older literature now reclassified as other entities
  - Must lack features of well-defined fibrosarcoma subtypes and other entities
    - Diagnosis of exclusion
  - Lacks significant nuclear pleomorphism
    - Tumors with marked pleomorphism classified as undifferentiated pleomorphic sarcoma

CLINICAL ISSUES

- Very rare if strictly defined [except for cases arising in dermatofibrosarcoma protuberans)
- Most arise in deep soft tissues of extremities in adults
- Treatment: Wide surgical resection
- Limited prognostic data using modern strict diagnostic criteria
- 50% overall mortality

MICROSCOPIC

- Uniform hyperchromatic spindle cells in herringbone fascicles
- Lacks characteristic features of other defined entities

ANCILLARY TESTS

- Negative for keratin, EMA, S100, desmin, most others
- Lacks molecular signatures of other defined sarcomas

TOP DIFFERENTIAL DIAGNOSES

- Fibrosarcomatous dermatofibrosarcoma protuberans
- Undifferentiated pleomorphic sarcoma
- Synovial sarcoma
- Malignant peripheral nerve sheath tumor
- Desmoid fibromatosis
- Cellular dermatofibroma
- Low-grade myofibroblastic sarcoma
- Leiomyosarcoma

Adult-Type FS

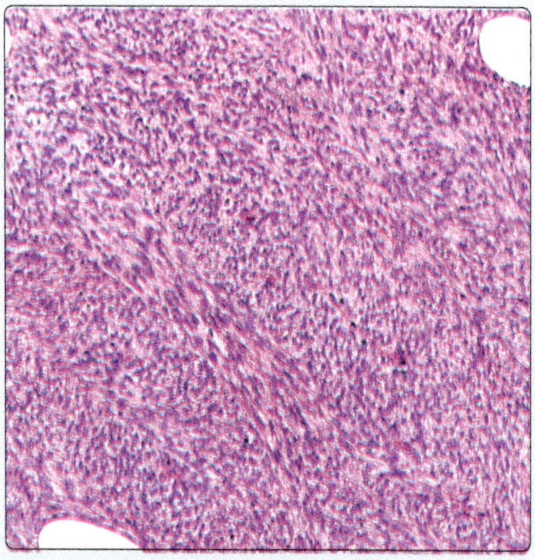

Fascicular Herringbone Pattern in FS

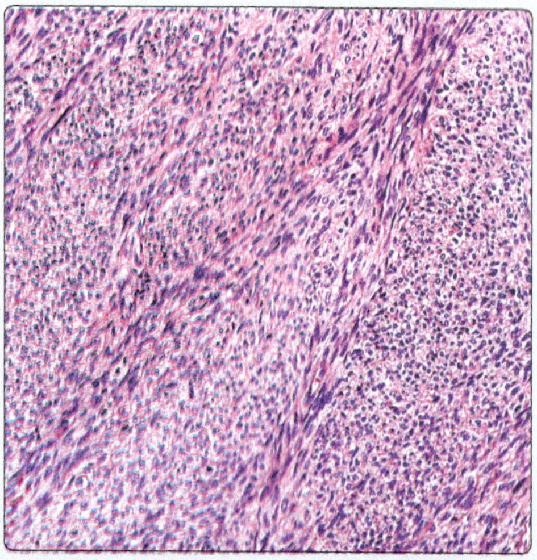

(Left) *The rare adult-type fibrosarcoma (FS) should be diagnosed only after all morphologically similar entities have been rigorously excluded. Strictly defined cases demonstrate prominent fascicular growth by spindled tumor cells lacking significant nuclear pleomorphism. (Courtesy K. Fritchie, MD.)* **(Right)** *Relatively uniform spindle cells are arranged in prominent fascicles that intersect at acute angles giving rise to the characteristic herringbone pattern. (Courtesy K. Fritchie, MD.)*

FS Arising in Dermatofibrosarcoma Protuberans

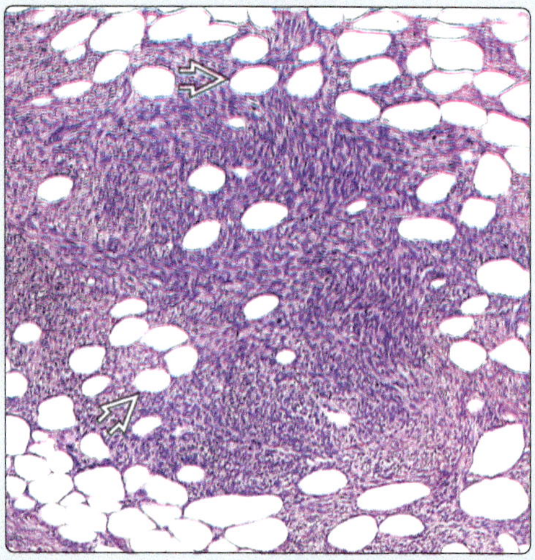

Higher Magnification of FS Arising in Dermatofibrosarcoma Protuberans

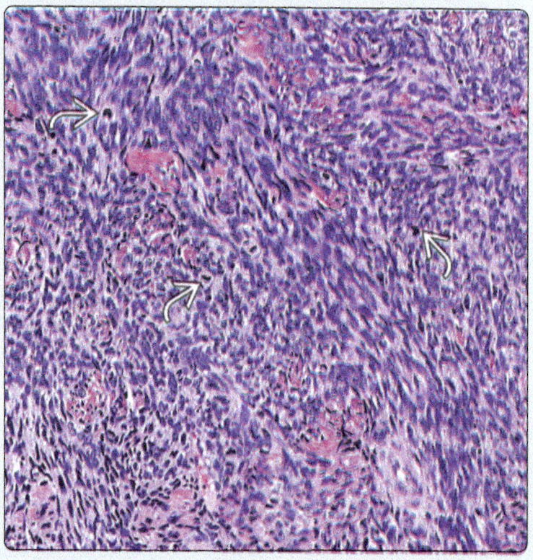

(Left) *This is an example of FS arising in a dermatofibrosarcoma protuberans (DFSP), the most common scenario in which FS is seen in the skin/subcutaneous tissue. Note the background of honeycombing fat entrapment, typical of DFSP ➡.* **(Right)** *Higher magnification of a cellular area of FS arising in DFSP shows significant nuclear atypia, pleomorphism, and multiple mitotic figures ➡.*

TERMINOLOGY

Definitions

- Sarcoma composed of spindle cells resembling fibroblasts
  - Vast majority of tumors classified as fibrosarcoma in older literature now reclassified as other entities
  - Currently, very rare entity, except for cases arising in dermatofibrosarcoma protuberans (DFSP)
  - Diagnosis should only be made with extreme caution
- Lacks features of well-defined fibrosarcoma subtypes
- Pleomorphic high-grade fibroblastic sarcomas are currently classified as undifferentiated pleomorphic sarcoma (PS)

CLINICAL ISSUES

Epidemiology

- Incidence
  - Very rare (if strictly defined)
    - Most cases arise in DFSP in skin/superficial subcutis
- Age
  - Median: 50 years

Presentation

- Usually deep mass of lower extremity but may occur anywhere
  - Subset arise in subcutis

Treatment

- Wide surgical resection

Prognosis

- Only 2 modern studies using strict diagnostic criteria
  - Most older series represent wide variety of sarcoma types (by current criteria); thus, unreliable data
- Overall, 50% mortality from locally aggressive growth &/or distant metastasis
  - Low-grade tumors appear to have better prognosis

MACROSCOPIC

General Features

- Smaller lesions are often circumscribed, but larger lesions may be infiltrative

Size

- Median size: 6.5 cm (range: 2-17 cm)

MICROSCOPIC

Histologic Features

- Elongated hyperchromatic fusiform/spindle cells with little cytoplasm
  - Relatively uniform: Only mild-moderate pleomorphism allowed
    - If severe pleomorphism, better classified as PS
  - Variable mitotic rate but present in most cases
- Fascicles arranged in characteristic herringbone pattern
- Parallel collagen fibers between cells (variable)
- Hypocellular or myxoid areas may mimic fibromatosis
  - Usually focal; other areas show typical fibrosarcoma
- Lacks features of other defined fibrosarcoma subtypes
  - Low-grade fibromyxoid sarcoma, sclerosing epithelioid fibrosarcoma
  - Myxofibrosarcoma, infantile fibrosarcoma

ANCILLARY TESTS

Immunohistochemistry

- May express focal smooth actin-HHF-35
- Most other markers negative: Keratins, EMA, S100, desmin, CD34, etc.

Genetic Testing

- No known characteristic molecular abnormality
- Lacks molecular findings of other well-defined sarcomas

DIFFERENTIAL DIAGNOSIS

Fibrosarcomatous Transformation in Dermatofibrosarcoma Protuberans

- Identical histologic features to adult-type fibrosarcoma
- Often shows areas of classic low-grade DFSP
- Variable CD34(+) but can be absent
- Characteristic t(17;22)

Cellular Dermatofibroma

- Majority in dermis/subcutis
- Fibrosarcoma-like foci (cellular fascicles, mitoses) but also has typical dermatofibroma areas

Undifferentiated Pleomorphic Sarcoma

- Sheets of markedly pleomorphic cells
- Severe nuclear atypia

Malignant Peripheral Nerve Sheath Tumor

- Often has evidence of neural origin
  - Arises in nerve, in neurofibroma, or within setting of neurofibromatosis type 1
- Perivascular cuffing by plumper tumor cells
- Focal/patchy S100(+) in 1/2 of cases; may be absent

Low-Grade Myofibroblastic Sarcoma

- Often show highly infiltrative growth
- Cells tend to have more cytoplasm than in adult-type fibrosarcoma
- Multifocal SMA(+), focal desmin (+)

Leiomyosarcoma

- Nuclear pleomorphism common
- Usually diffuse SMA(+); variable desmin (+)

Synovial Sarcoma

- Cells more monotonous and ovoid, fascicles less organized
- May contain epithelial structures (biphasic type)
- Focal cytokeratin (+) &/or EMA(+) in majority
- Strong, diffuse nuclear TLE1(+)
- Characteristic t(X;18)

SELECTED REFERENCES

1. Bahrami A et al: Adult-type fibrosarcoma: a reevaluation of 163 putative cases diagnosed at a single institution over a 48-year period. Am J Surg Pathol. 34(10):1504-13, 2010
2. Hansen T et al: Low-grade fibrosarcoma–report on 39 not otherwise specified cases and comparison with defined low-grade fibrosarcoma types. Histopathology. 49(2):152-60, 2006

Myxofibrosarcoma

KEY FACTS

TERMINOLOGY

- Myxofibrosarcoma (MFS)
- MFS represents spectrum of malignant fibroblastic neoplasms with variably myxoid stroma and characteristic elongated curvilinear vessels

CLINICAL ISSUES

- 1 of most common sarcomas in elderly patients
- Majority arises in limbs, including limb girdles
  - Lower > upper extremities
- 2/3 of cases arise in dermal/subcutaneous tissues
- Local, often repeated, recurrences in up to 50-60% of cases (unrelated to histologic grade)
- Intermediate- and high-grade malignant neoplasms may develop metastases in 30-35% of cases

MACROSCOPIC

- Superficially located neoplasms consist of multiple variably gelatinous or firmer nodules
- Deep-seated neoplasms often present as single mass with myxoid cut surfaces

MICROSCOPIC

- Broad spectrum of cellularity, cytologic atypia, and proliferative activity reflected by 3 grades of malignancy
- Multinodular growth, spindled and stellate atypical fibroblastic cells
- Myxoid stroma with elongated, curvilinear, thin-walled vessels
- Often pseudolipoblasts are present

TOP DIFFERENTIAL DIAGNOSES

- Myxoid dermatofibrosarcoma protuberans
- Myxoid liposarcoma
- Low-grade fibromyxoid sarcoma (Evans tumor)
- Myxoinflammatory fibroblastic sarcoma
- Myxoid malignant peripheral nerve sheath tumor

(Left) *A case of low-grade myxofibrosarcoma is shown with myxoid, gelatinous cut surfaces. (Courtesy T. Mentzel, MD.)* **(Right)** *Scanning magnification view shows a superficial, low-grade myxofibrosarcoma involving the subcutis and deep dermis. Numerous elongated, thin vessels ⇨ are easily identified in a prominent myxoid stroma.*

Gross Photograph of Myxofibrosarcoma

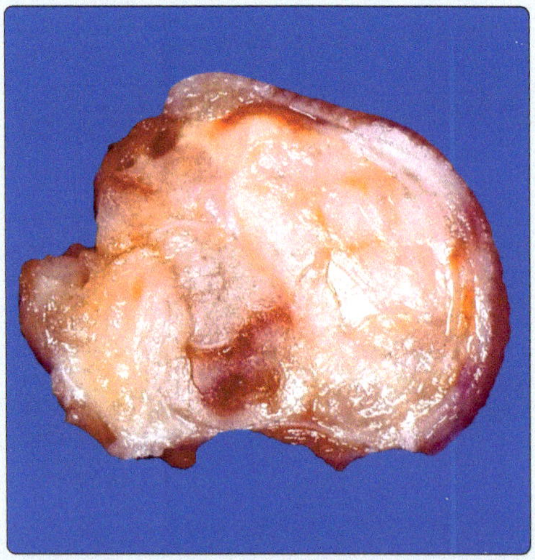

Superficial Myxofibrosarcoma

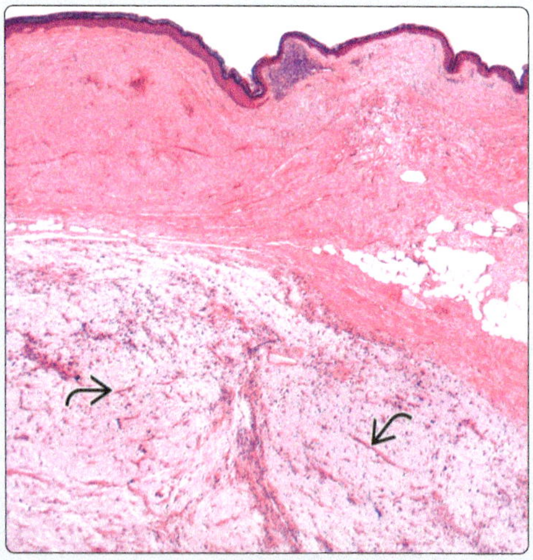

(Left) *Myxofibrosarcoma is characterized by a variable cellularity and is composed of atypical fibroblastic cells that are set in a prominent myxoid stroma with numerous elongated curvilinear vessels* ⇨. **(Right)** *This more cellular neoplasm is composed of atypical, epithelioid-shaped tumor cells with abundant eosinophilic cytoplasm and round, vesicular nuclei. This case represents a rare epithelioid cell variant of myxofibrosarcoma.*

Myxofibrosarcoma With Cellular and Myxoid Areas

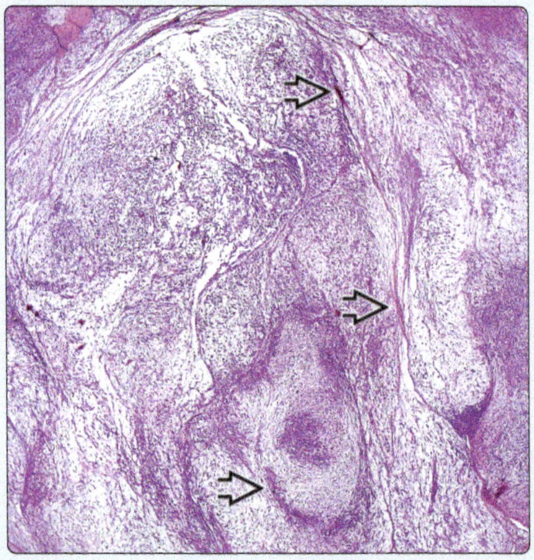

High-Grade Myxofibrosarcoma

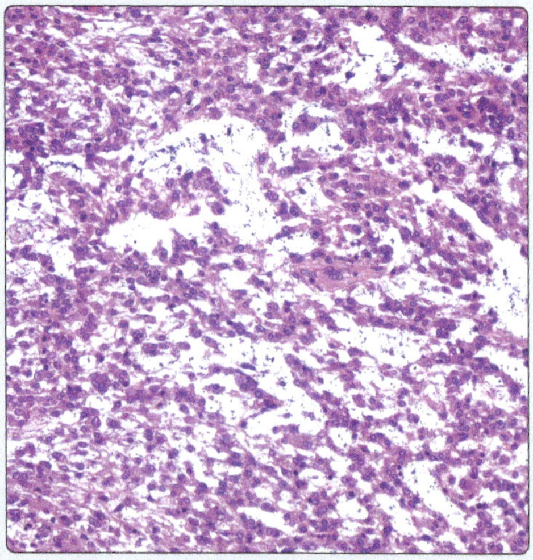

TERMINOLOGY

Abbreviations

- Myxofibrosarcoma (MFS)

Synonyms

- Myxoid malignant fibrous histiocytoma

Definitions

- MFS represents spectrum of malignant fibroblastic neoplasms with variably myxoid stroma and characteristic elongated curvilinear vessels

CLINICAL ISSUES

Epidemiology

- Incidence
  - 1 of most common sarcomas in elderly patients
- Age
  - Affects mainly patients in 6th-8th decades
- Sex
  - Slight male predominance

Site

- Majority arise in limbs and limb girdles
  - Lower > upper extremities
- Rarely on trunk, head and neck region
- 2/3 of cases arise in dermal/subcutaneous tissues

Presentation

- Painless mass
- Slow growing

Treatment

- Surgical approaches
  - Complete and wide excision

Prognosis

- Local, often repeated, recurrences in up to 50-60% of cases (unrelated to histologic grade)
- Low-grade MFS usually does not metastasize
- Intermediate- and high-grade MFS may develop metastases in 30-35% of cases
- Overall 5-year survival is 60-70%

MACROSCOPIC

General Features

- Superficially located neoplasms consist of multiple variably gelatinous or firmer nodules
- Deep-seated neoplasms often present as single mass with myxoid cut surfaces

MICROSCOPIC

Histologic Features

- Broad spectrum of cellularity, cytologic atypia, and proliferative activity
- Multinodular growth with prominent myxoid stroma
- Elongated, curvilinear, thin-walled blood vessels
- Foci of inflammatory cells may be present
- Low-grade MFS
  - Hypocellular neoplasms
  - Scattered spindle-shaped tumor cells
  - Ill-defined eosinophilic cytoplasm
  - Enlarged hyperchromatic nuclei
- Intermediate-grade MFS
  - More cellular and pleomorphic than low-grade MFS
  - No solid areas or necrosis
- High-grade MFS
  - Large areas of solid sheets and cellular fascicles
  - Spindled and pleomorphic tumor cells
  - Bizarre, multinucleated tumor giant cells
  - Numerous, often atypical mitoses
  - Areas of tumor necrosis may be present

DIFFERENTIAL DIAGNOSIS

Myxoid Dermatofibrosarcoma Protuberans

- Often diffuse infiltration of dermis and subcutis with honeycombing fat entrapment
- No prominent cytologic atypia
- Homogeneous expression of CD34

Myxoid Liposarcoma

- Frequently in deep soft tissues of lower extremity
- Small, undifferentiated round tumor cells and vacuolated lipoblasts
- Usually lack prominent cytologic atypia
- Delicate, plexiform vascular pattern

Low-Grade Fibromyxoid Sarcoma (Evans Tumor)

- Mainly in deep soft tissues
- Bland spindled tumor cells in alternating myxoid and fibrous stroma

Myxoinflammatory Fibroblastic Sarcoma

- Frequently arises in subcutaneous tissues of hands, wrists, feet, and ankles
- Spindled, polygonal, and bizarre ganglion-like tumor cells with huge, inclusion-like nucleoli
- Prominent mixed inflammatory infiltrate

Myxoid Malignant Peripheral Nerve Sheath Tumor

- Fascicular arrangement of spindle-shaped tumor cells
- Often perivascular whorling of tumor cells
- In ~ 1/2 of cases, focal expression of S100

DIAGNOSTIC CHECKLIST

Pathologic Interpretation Pearls

- Spectrum of variably cellular atypical fibroblastic neoplasms
- Myxoid stromal changes with characteristic elongated curvilinear blood vessels

SELECTED REFERENCES

1. Cates JM et al: Cell cycle and apoptosis regulatory proteins, proliferative markers, cell signaling molecules, CD209, and decorin immunoreactivity in low-grade myxofibrosarcoma and myxoma. Virchows Arch. 467(2):211-6, 2015
2. Nascimento AF et al: Epithelioid variant of myxofibrosarcoma: expanding the clinicomorphologic spectrum of myxofibrosarcoma in a series of 17 cases. Am J Surg Pathol. 31(1):99-105, 2007
3. Mansoor A et al: Myxofibrosarcoma presenting in the skin: clinicopathological features and differential diagnosis with cutaneous myxoid neoplasms. Am J Dermatopathol. 25(4):281-6, 2003
4. Mentzel T et al: Myxofibrosarcoma. Clinicopathologic analysis of 75 cases with emphasis on the low-grade variant. Am J Surg Pathol. 20(4):391-405, 1996

Gross Specimen of Myxofibrosarcoma

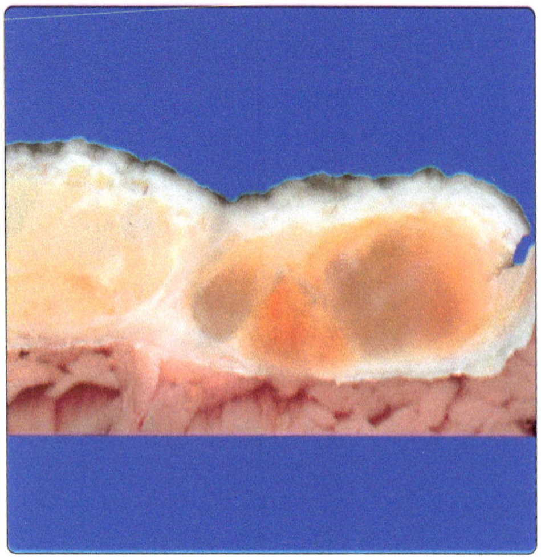

Low-Grade Myxofibrosarcoma With Thin-Walled Vessels

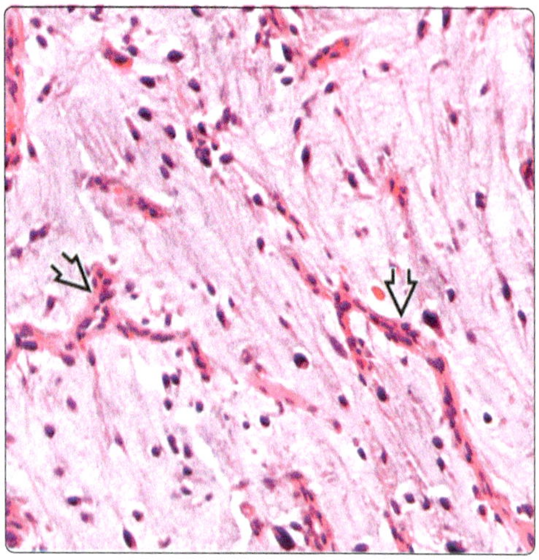

(Left) *Grossly, myxofibrosarcoma often shows a multinodular growth pattern with gelatinous-appearing cut surfaces. (Courtesy T. Mentzel, MD.)* **(Right)** *Higher magnification of a low-grade myxofibrosarcoma shows prominent, elongated, thin-walled blood vessels ⇨ with scattered atypical, spindle-shaped cells in a background of prominent mucinous stroma.*

Low-Grade Myxofibrosarcoma

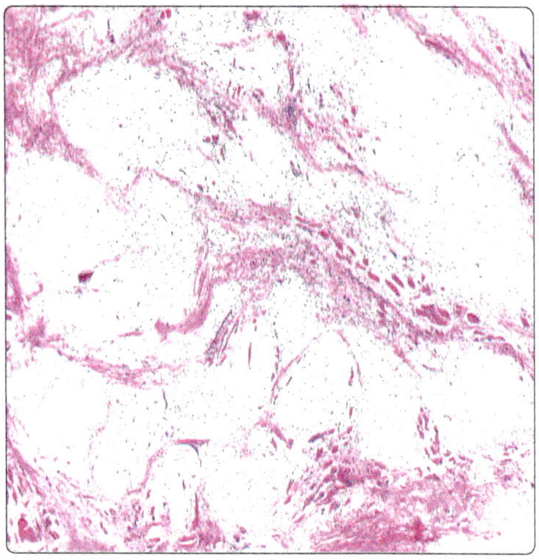

Low-Grade Myxofibrosarcoma

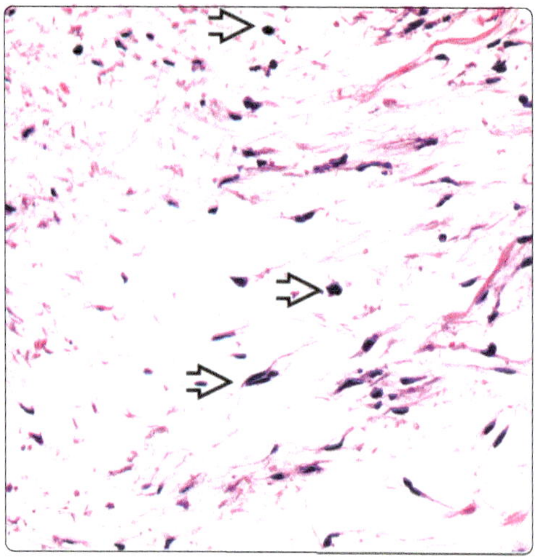

(Left) *Low-power view of a low-grade myxofibrosarcoma shows a deep-seated intramuscular tumor. Note the characteristic multinodular growth and the presence of thin fibrous septa. (Courtesy T. Mentzel, MD.)* **(Right)** *Despite low cellularity, cases of low-grade myxofibrosarcoma are composed of atypical fibroblastic tumor cells showing enlarged and hyperchromatic-staining nuclei ⇨. (Courtesy T. Mentzel, MD.)*

Intermediate-Grade Myxofibrosarcoma

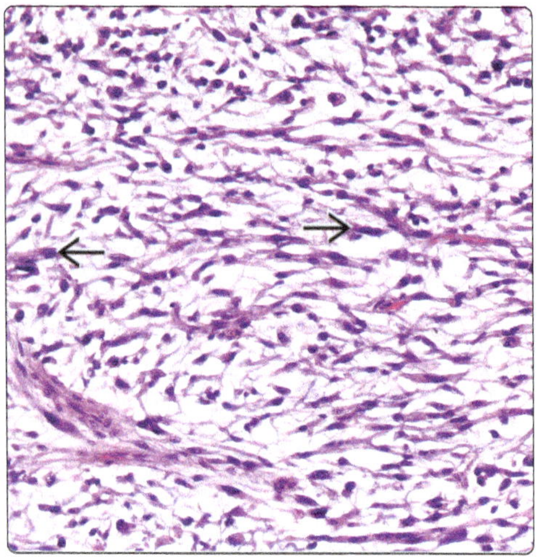

Intermediate-Grade Myxofibrosarcoma

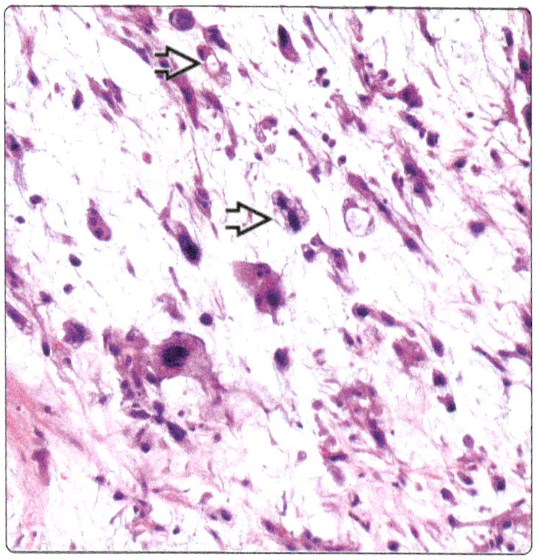

(Left) *Cases of intermediate-grade myxofibrosarcoma show increased cellularity with numerous atypical, spindle-shaped fibroblastic tumor cells that demonstrate nuclear hyperchromasia ⇨. (Courtesy T. Mentzel, MD.)* **(Right)** *High-power view of an intermediate-grade myxofibrosarcoma shows atypical tumor cells with enlarged hyperchromatic-staining nuclei. Note the scattered multivacuolated pseudolipoblasts ⇨. (Courtesy T. Mentzel, MD.)*

High-Grade Myxofibrosarcoma With Necrosis

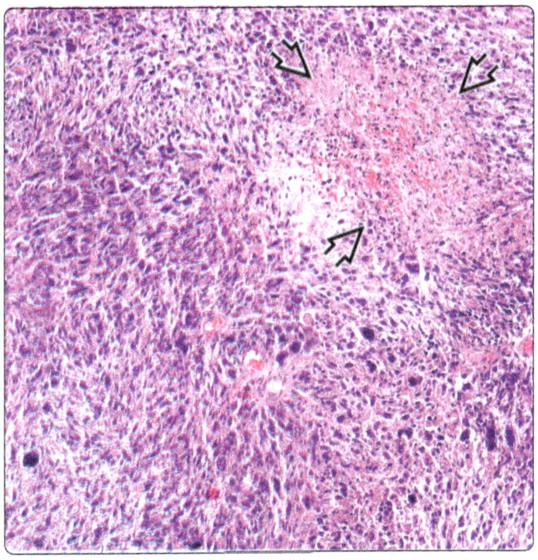

High-Grade Myxofibrosarcoma With Myoid Features

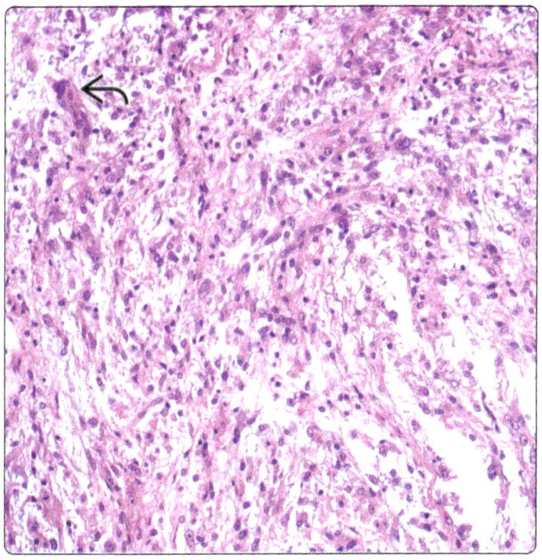

(Left) *Cases of high-grade myxofibrosarcoma show features of a high-grade pleomorphic sarcoma with increased proliferative activity and areas of tumor necrosis* →*. (Courtesy T. Mentzel, MD.)* **(Right)** *Multinucleated tumor giant cells containing abundant eosinophilic cytoplasm, mimicking a myogenic neoplasm, are seen in this example of a high-grade malignant myxofibrosarcoma* →*. (Courtesy T. Mentzel, MD.)*

High-Grade Myxofibrosarcoma: Cytology

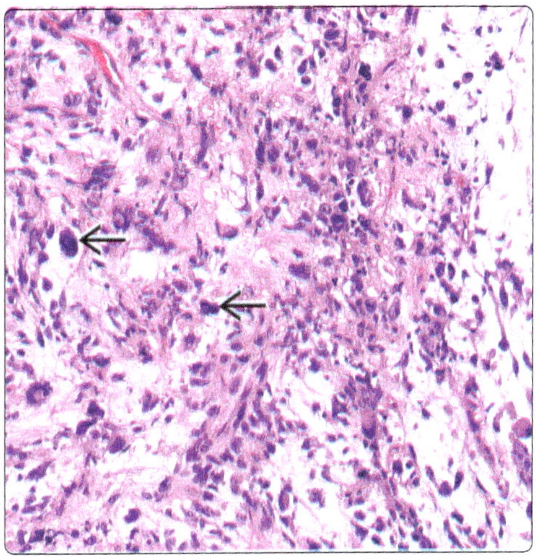

High-Grade Myxofibrosarcoma: Cytology

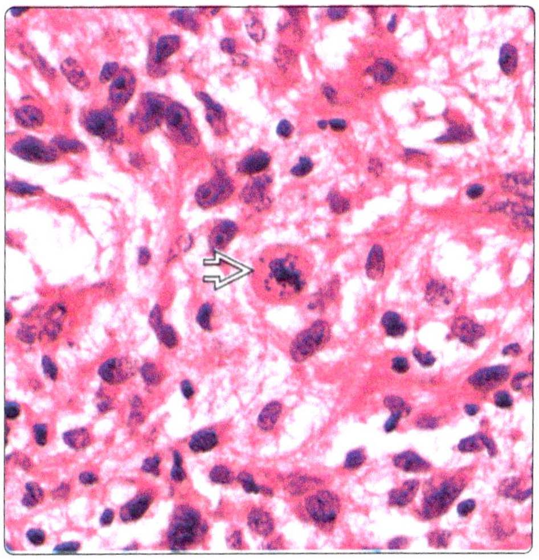

(Left) *High magnification of a high-grade malignant myxofibrosarcoma shows prominent cytologic atypia with enlarged, hyperchromatic-staining nuclei* →*. (Courtesy T. Mentzel, MD.)* **(Right)** *Higher magnification of another example of high-grade myxofibrosarcoma shows prominent cytologic atypia, nuclear hyperchromasia, irregular nuclear contours, and mitotic activity* →*.*

Alcian Blue Stain in Myxofibrosarcoma

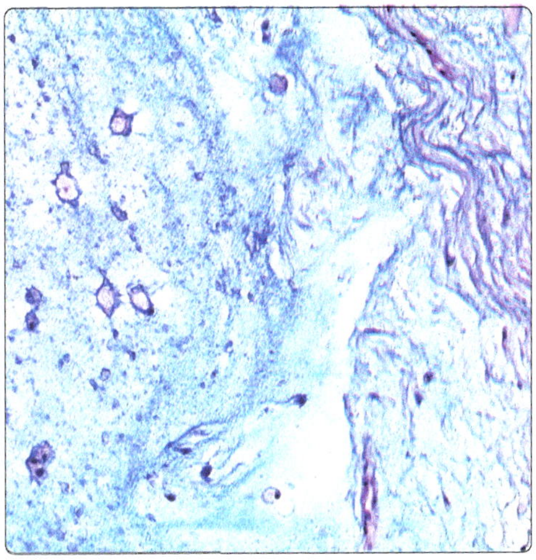

Immunohistochemical Stain for CD34

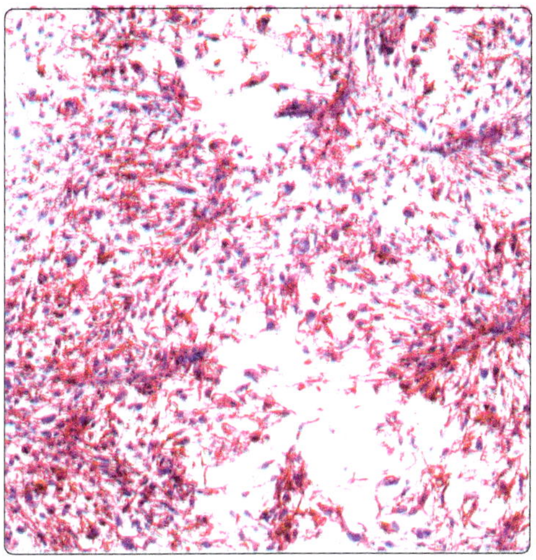

(Left) *Alcian blue staining reveals the presence of abundant mucin in the stroma and also in the cytoplasm of the neoplastic cells in this case of low-grade myxofibrosarcoma. (Courtesy T. Mentzel, MD.)* **(Right)** *The immunohistochemical expression of CD34, in some cases, confirms the fibroblastic line of differentiation in these neoplasms. (Courtesy T. Mentzel, MD.)*

Superficial Low-Grade Fibromyxoid Sarcoma

KEY FACTS

TERMINOLOGY

- Subset of low-grade fibromyxoid sarcoma (LGFMS) arising in dermis &/or subcutaneous tissue
  - Histologically and genetically identical to conventional deep LGFMS

CLINICAL ISSUES

- Appear to represent 10-20% of reported cases of LGFMS
- Often adults (typically 3rd-4th decade), but wide range
  - Up to 1/3 arise in children and adolescents
- Most common in extremities (especially lower limb), buttock, and trunk
- Treatment: Complete surgical excision
- Better outcome reported than in deep forms of LGFMS
- Local recurrence uncommon; no metastases reported

MACROSCOPIC

- Well-defined mass, most often in subcutis
- Median 4.2 cm (occasionally > 10 cm)

MICROSCOPIC

- Identical cytomorphologic features and spectrum as conventional LGFMS
- Variant morphology includes component of distinct collagen rosette-like structures

ANCILLARY TESTS

- Diffuse MUC4(+) characteristic
- Negative for keratins, S100, SMA, desmin
- Molecular: *FUS* rearrangements with *CREB3L2* or *CREB3L1*

TOP DIFFERENTIAL DIAGNOSES

- Nodular fasciitis
- Fibromatosis
- Perineurioma
- Neurofibroma
- Cellular myxoma
- Dermatofibrosarcoma protuberans
- Myxofibrosarcoma

(Left) *Low-grade fibromyxoid sarcoma (LGFMS) is classically characterized by admixed fibrocollagenous* ➔ *and looser, myxoid* ↷ *zones. Most cases arise in deep locations, but a minority occur superficially in the subcutis or less likely dermis.* **(Right)** *The collagenous zones of LGFMS tend to show relatively low cellularity, as depicted. On a limited biopsy, care must be taken to avoid misinterpretation as a benign process. Cytologically, the cells usually show mild to no atypia.*

LGFMS

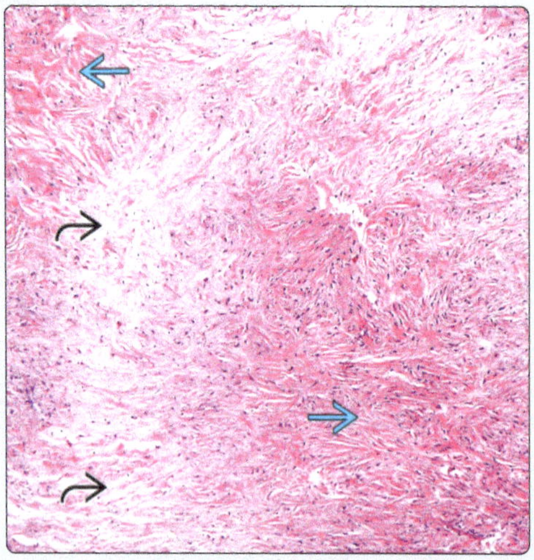

Collagenous Zones in LGFMS

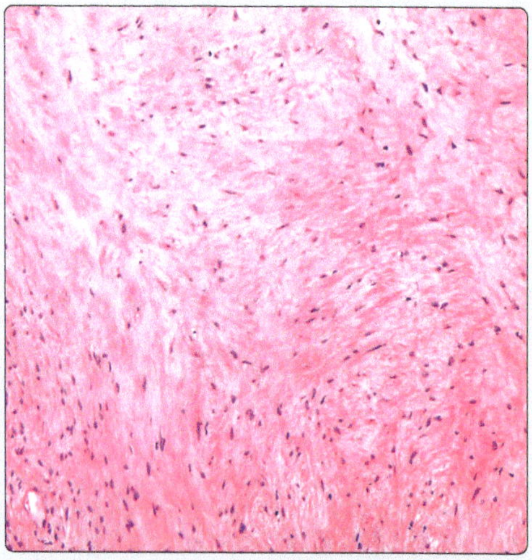

(Left) *The myxoid zones of LGFMS are often more cellular than the fibrocollagenous zones and tend to feature a more prominent stromal vasculature, as depicted here.* **(Right)** *A distinctive morphologic variant of LGFMS contains a variable number of rosette-like structures with hyalinized collagenous cores* ↷*. These tumors were originally described as hyalinizing spindle cell tumor with giant rosettes.*

Myxoid Zones in LGFMS

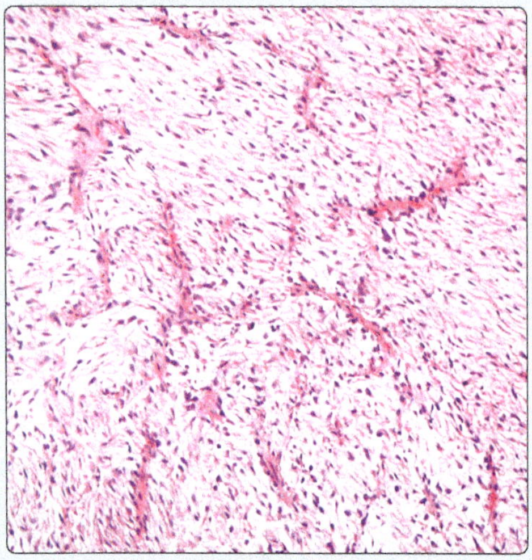

Hyalinizing Rosette-Like Structures

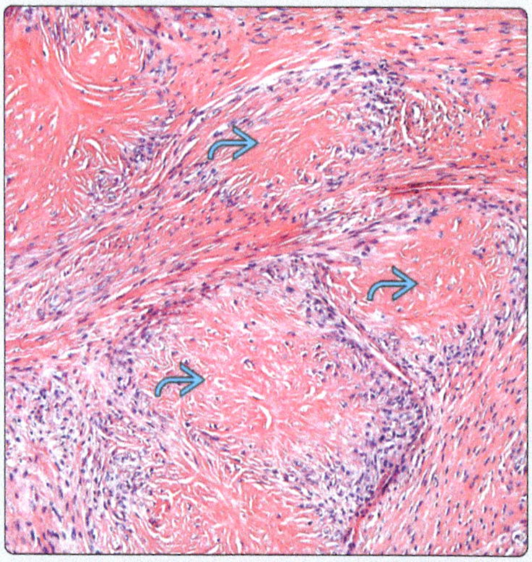

TERMINOLOGY

Abbreviations

- Low-grade fibromyxoid sarcoma (LGFMS)

Synonyms

- Evan tumor
- Hyalinizing spindle cell tumor with giant rosettes

Definitions

- Subset of low-grade fibromyxoid sarcoma arising in dermis &/or subcutaneous tissue
  - Histologically and genetically identical to conventional deep LGFMS

CLINICAL ISSUES

Epidemiology

- Incidence
  - Appear to represent 10-20% of reported cases of LGFMS
  - Probably underreported in literature
- Age
  - Often adults (typically 3rd-4th decade) but wide range
    - Up to 1/3 arise in children and adolescents

Site

- Most common in extremities (especially lower limb), buttock, and trunk

Presentation

- Usually slow-growing, painless mass

Treatment

- Complete surgical excision
- Long-term clinical follow-up is recommended

Prognosis

- Better outcome reported than in deep forms of LGFMS
- Local recurrence uncommon
- No metastases yet reported

MACROSCOPIC

General Features

- Well-defined mass, most often in subcutis
- White fibrous to myxoid cut surface

Size

- Median 4.2 cm (occasionally > 10 cm)

MICROSCOPIC

Histologic Features

- Usually well circumscribed, ± fibrous pseudocapsule
- Identical cytomorphologic features and spectrum as conventional LGFMS
  - Low to moderately cellular arrays of bland fibroblasts in whorled or loosely fascicular arrangements
    - Minimal to mild nuclear atypia characteristic
    - Mitoses rare
  - Collagenous or myxoid matrix, often in distinct zones
    - Vascularity often prominent in myxoid zones
  - Ischemic necrosis may be present (not coagulative)
- Variant morphology includes component of distinct collagen rosette-like structures

ANCILLARY TESTS

Immunohistochemistry

- Diffuse MUC4(+) characteristic
- Rare focal or weak expression of CD34, EMA, or claudin-1
- Negative for keratins, S100, SMA, desmin

Molecular Genetics

- Characteristic molecular signatures in both superficial and deeper tumors
  - Rearrangements of *FUS* gene (chr. 16) with either *CREB3L2* (chr. 7) or *CREB3L1* (chr. 11)

DIFFERENTIAL DIAGNOSIS

Nodular Fasciitis

- Clinical presentation: Small but rapidly growing lesion
- Spindle and stellate fibroblasts with tissue culture-like appearance
- Extravasated erythrocytes, giant cells common
- SMA(+)

Fibromatosis

- Sweeping fascicles of myofibroblastic cells
- Superficial forms arise in hands and feet; deep forms usually arise in muscle or mesentery
- Lacks distinctive zonal arrangement of collagenous and myxoid stroma in LGFMS

Perineurioma

- Elongated spindle cells with bipolar processes
- Perivascular whorls and storiform arrays common
- EMA(+), claudin-1(+), variable CD34(+)
- MUC4(-)

Neurofibroma

- Cells with elongated, wavy-appearing nuclei
- S100(+)

Cellular Myxoma

- Diffuse myxoid stroma containing very bland cells
- Lack of pronounced fibrous zones
- MUC4(-)

Myxofibrosarcoma

- Most common in elderly patients
- Atypical hyperchromatic nuclei and mitoses common
- More prominent myxoid stroma

Dermatofibrosarcoma Protuberans

- Infiltrative growth pattern
- Tight storiform growth pattern in conventional areas
- Myxoid zones often show prominent vascularity
- Diffuse, strong CD34(+)

SELECTED REFERENCES

1. Sedrak MP et al: Low-grade fibromyxoid sarcoma with nuclear pleomorphism arising in the subcutis of a child. J Cutan Pathol. 41(2):134-8, 2014
2. Billings SD et al: Superficial low-grade fibromyxoid sarcoma (Evans tumor): a clinicopathologic analysis of 19 cases with a unique observation in the pediatric population. Am J Surg Pathol. 29(2):204-10, 2005

Myxoinflammatory Fibroblastic Sarcoma

KEY FACTS

TERMINOLOGY

- Acral myxoinflammatory fibroblastic sarcoma, inflammatory myxohyaline tumor

CLINICAL ISSUES

- Slow-growing infiltrative mass usually affecting distal extremities (hands and feet) of adults
- Recurrences are common, but metastases are rare

MICROSCOPIC

- Poorly marginated tumor with fibrosis, hyalinization, myxoid stroma, and inflammatory components
  - Inflammatory component shows variable mixtures of lymphoplasmacytic cells, eosinophils, neutrophils, and histiocytes
- Areas with prominent myxoid change
- Scattered enlarged atypical tumor cells, some with macronucleoli
  - Cells with macronucleoli resemble Reed-Sternberg cells
- Fibroblasts often vacuolated (pseudolipoblasts)
- Low mitotic rate
- Lesional cells are fibroblasts ultrastructurally

ANCILLARY TESTS

- Variable expression of CD34, CD68, EGFR, CD163, CD117, EMA
- Negative CD15, CD30, CD45 in cells with macronucleoli
- Rearrangements of *TGFBR3* &/or *MGEA5* reported, but their presence in these tumors is subject of debate

TOP DIFFERENTIAL DIAGNOSES

- Extranodal Hodgkin disease
- Pigmented villonodular tenosynovitis
- Hemosiderotic fibrohistiocytic lipomatous lesion
- Viral infection
- Myxofibrosarcoma

Myxoinflammatory Fibroblastic Sarcoma: Gross Specimen

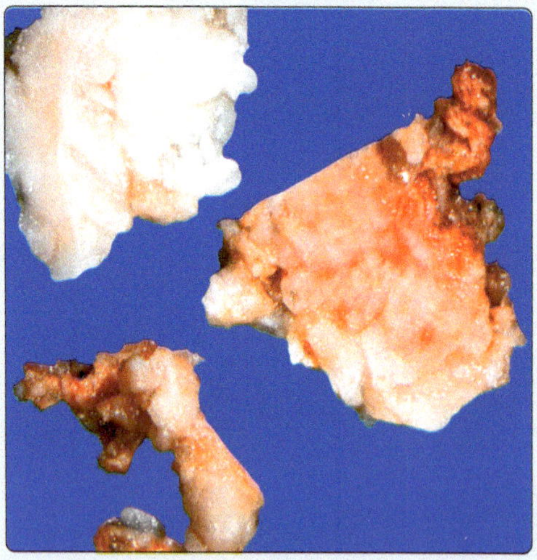

Myxoinflammatory Fibroblastic Sarcoma, Low Magnification

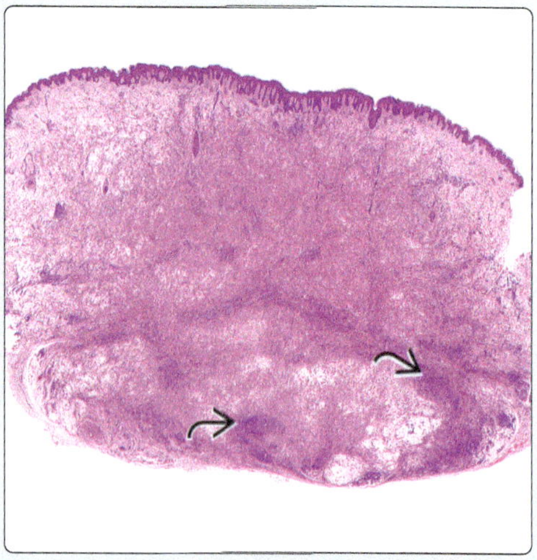

(Left) *This is a gross example of a myxoinflammatory fibroblastic sarcoma (MIFS). This lesion was highly infiltrative but was clinically mistaken for pigmented villonodular tenosynovitis.* **(Right)** *This MIFS is superficial and shows a myxoinflammatory expansion of the subcutaneous fat. Such neoplasms can also be associated with tendons and have an infiltrative appearance. A prominent lymphoid infiltrate ➔ is present throughout the neoplasm.*

Myxoinflammatory Fibroblastic Sarcoma, Low Magnification

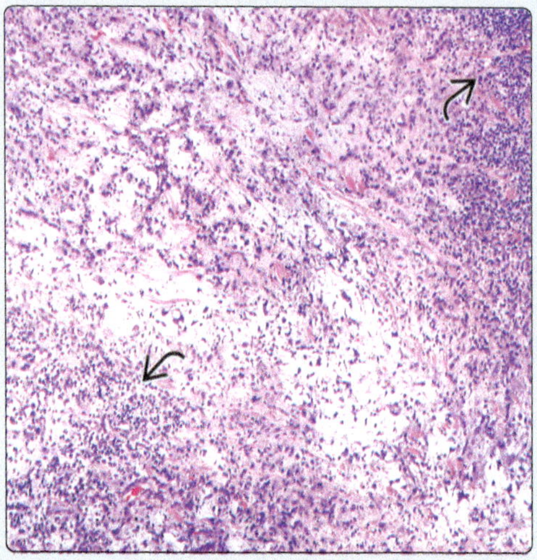

Myxoinflammatory Fibroblastic Sarcoma: Atypical Mitotic Figure

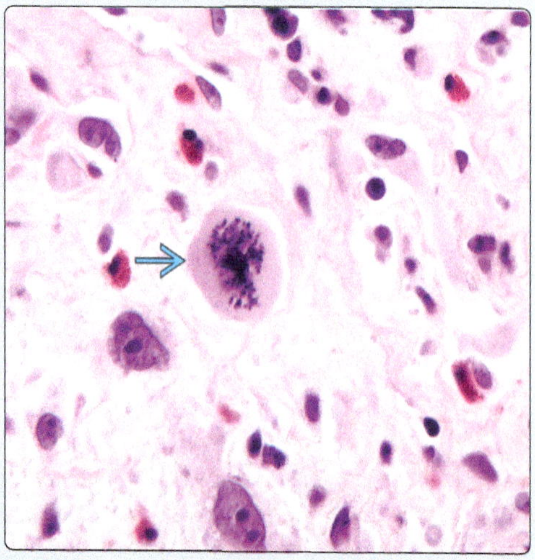

(Left) *At scanning magnification, MIFS displays a generous inflammatory background and scattered myxoid zones. Lymphoid cells are prominent at the edges of the field ➔.* **(Right)** *Finding atypical mitoses ➔ in these tumors is unusual for a translocation sarcoma, but rearrangements TGFBR3 &/or MGEA5 have been reported in some cases.*

TERMINOLOGY

Synonyms

- Acral myxoinflammatory fibroblastic sarcoma (MIFS)
- Inflammatory myxohyaline tumor of distal extremities (with virocyte or Reed-Sternberg-like cells)

Definitions

- Low-grade fibroblastic sarcoma characterized by typical acral presentation and inflammatory background, often rich in eosinophils

CLINICAL ISSUES

Presentation

- Slow-growing infiltrative mass usually affecting distal extremities (hands and feet) of adults
  - Subset of lesions presents in axial rather than acral sites
- Lesions are often present for years before patients seek medical attention
- Often clinically mistaken for pigmented villonodular tenosynovitis

Prognosis

- Recurrences are common, especially in examples with prominent atypical nuclei, but metastases are rare
  - Metastases in only ~ 1% of cases

MACROSCOPIC

General Features

- Highly infiltrative
- Can involve both superficial and deep soft tissues

Size

- 1-10 cm
- Most lesions measure 3-4 cm

MICROSCOPIC

Histologic Features

- Poorly marginated tumor with fibrosis, hyalinization, myxoid stroma, and inflammatory components
  - Various lesions have different proportions of each component
- Variable background of lymphoplasmacytic cells, eosinophils, neutrophils, and histiocytes
- Lesional cells are fibroblasts ultrastructurally
- Scattered enlarged atypical fibroblasts, some with macronucleoli
  - Cells with macronucleoli resemble Reed-Sternberg cells
- Areas with prominent myxoid change
  - Fibroblasts often vacuolated ("pseudolipoblasts")
  - These areas resemble myxofibrosarcoma (malignant fibrous histiocytoma)
- Low mitotic rate
  - Low proliferative index by Ki-67
  - Atypical mitoses may be encountered

ANCILLARY TESTS

Immunohistochemistry

- Variable expression of CD34, CD68, EGFR, CD163, CD117, EMA
- Negative CD15, CD30, CD45 in cells with macronucleoli
- No demonstration of various viral agents
  - Cases have been tested for Epstein Barr virus and for cytomegalovirus (CMV) and herpes simplex virus (HSV)

Genetic Testing

- Rearrangements of *TGFBR3* &/or *MGEA5* have been reported
  - Same rearrangements have been reported in hemosiderotic fibrolipomatous tumor (HFLT), pleomorphic hyalinizing angiectatic tumor
  - Same rearrangements have been reported in rare tumors allegedly showing features of both HFLT and MIFS termed hybrid HFLT-MIFS
  - Initially myxoinflammatory fibroblastic sarcoma was associated with t(1;10)
  - Subject of controversy in literature
- Probably MIFS in fact lacks rearrangements of *TGFBR3* &/or *MGEA5* when strict morphologic criteria are used
- Additional studies will be needed to clarify genetics of these tumors

DIFFERENTIAL DIAGNOSIS

Extranodal Hodgkin Disease

- Patients usually have history of nodal disease
- Usually no myxoid areas
- Background mostly lymphoid cells; neutrophils not common
- Reed-Sternberg cells label with CD15 and CD30 and are lymphoid rather than fibroblastic
- Managed as per lymphomas

Pigmented Villonodular Tenosynovitis

- Also termed tenosynovial giant cell tumor, diffuse type
- Often presents in knee joint area of young women
- Proliferated around joint space
- Proliferation of uniform rounded cells
- Hemosiderin, histiocytes, lymphoplasmacytic cells
  - Usually contain giant cells
- Eosinophils and neutrophils not feature
- Not myxoid
- No atypical large nuclei
  - No macronucleoli

Hemosiderotic Fibrohistiocytic Lipomatous Lesion/Hemosiderotic Fibrolipomatous Tumor

- Classically involves feet
- May form spectrum with both myxoinflammatory fibroblastic sarcoma and with pleomorphic hyalinizing angiectatic tumor
  - No metastases have been recorded for either hemosiderotic fibrohistiocytic lipomatous lesion or pleomorphic hyalinizing angiectatic tumor
- Tracks along connective tissue septa
- Spindle cells, abundant hemosiderin, histiocytes
- No cells with macronucleoli

- No eosinophils
- Strongly CD34(+)
- Can recur locally
  - Difficult to remove totally based on infiltrative growth pattern

Viral Infection

- Usually involves internal organs and lymph nodes
- Viral cytopathic effect consists of nuclear [CMV and HSV or cytoplasmic (CMV) inclusions]
- CMV effect best seen in stromal cells
- HSV effect often seen in epithelial cells
- Agents can be demonstrated by immunohistochemistry or molecular testing
- Usually eosinophils are not feature of inflammation
  - Some cases feature prominent monohistiocytic cells

Myxofibrosarcoma

- Usually in proximal extremities of older persons
- Typically superficial and lobulated rather than infiltrative; inflammatory cells minor component
- Richly vascular
  - Curvilinear vessels are reminiscent of those in myxoid liposarcoma
- Abundance of myxoid stroma
- No hyalinized zones
- Shows morphologic overlap with myxoinflammatory fibroblastic sarcoma by featuring large atypical cells embedded in myxoid matrix

Epithelioid Sarcoma

- Distal extremities of adults
- Neoplastic cells surround zones of necrosis
  - Appearance mimics granulomatous process
- Minimal inflammation
- Pankeratin, EMA(+), CK5/6(-), CD34(+/-); loss of nuclear INI1
- Aggressive: Metastases to regional nodes as well as systemic metastases and death
  - Outcome is improved by prompt aggressive surgical intervention
  - Amputation often required for management

Clear Cell Sarcoma (Melanoma of Soft Parts)

- Distal extremities of adults
- Often centered in tendons or aponeuroses
- Packeted groups of uniform cells with macronucleoli
- S100(+), HMB-45(+), Melan-A(+), MITF1(+)
- Characteristic translocation and gene fusion between *EWSR1* (EWS) and *ATF1* genes
- Behaves as high-grade sarcoma

SELECTED REFERENCES

1. Michal M et al: Pleomorphic hyalinizing angiectatic tumor revisited: all tumors manifest typical morphologic features of myxoinflammatory fibroblastic sarcoma, further suggesting 2 morphologic variants of a single entity. Ann Diagn Pathol. 20:40-3, 2016
2. Michal M et al: High-grade myxoinflammatory fibroblastic sarcoma: a report of 23 cases. Ann Diagn Pathol. 19(3):157-63, 2015
3. Carter JM et al: TGFBR3 and MGEA5 rearrangements in pleomorphic hyalinizing angiectatic tumors and the spectrum of related neoplasms. Am J Surg Pathol. 38(9):1182-992, 2014
4. Laskin WB et al: Myxoinflammatory fibroblastic sarcoma: a clinicopathologic analysis of 104 cases, with emphasis on predictors of outcome. Am J Surg Pathol. 38(1):1-12, 2014
5. Marušić Z et al: Hybrid myxoinflammatory fibroblastic sarcoma/hemosiderotic fibrolipomatous tumor of the ankle following repeated trauma. Pathol Int. 64(4):195-7, 2014
6. Solomon DA et al: Hemosiderotic fibrolipomatous tumor, not an entirely benign entity. Am J Surg Pathol. 37(10):1627-30, 2013
7. Weiss VL et al: Myxoinflammatory fibroblastic sarcoma in children and adolescents: clinicopathologic aspects of a rare neoplasm. Pediatr Dev Pathol. 16(6):425-31, 2013
8. Subhawong TK et al: Pleomorphic hyalinizing angiectatic tumor: imaging findings. Skeletal Radiol. 41(12):1621-6, 2012
9. Wei S et al: Complex analysis of a recurrent pleomorphic hyalinizing angiectatic tumor of soft parts. Hum Pathol. 43(1):121-6, 2012
10. Antonescu CR et al: Consistent t(1;10) with rearrangements of TGFBR3 and MGEA5 in both myxoinflammatory fibroblastic sarcoma and hemosiderotic fibrolipomatous tumor. Genes Chromosomes Cancer. 50(10):757-64, 2011
11. Elco CP et al: Hybrid myxoinflammatory fibroblastic sarcoma/hemosiderotic fibrolipomatous tumor: report of a case providing further evidence for a pathogenetic link. Am J Surg Pathol. 34(11):1723-7, 2010
12. Moretti VM et al: Early pleomorphic hyalinizing angiectatic tumor: precursor or distinct lesion? Orthopedics. 33(7):516, 2010
13. Hallor KH et al: Two genetic pathways, t(1;10) and amplification of 3p11-12, in myxoinflammatory fibroblastic sarcoma, haemosiderotic fibrolipomatous tumour, and morphologically similar lesions. J Pathol. 217(5):716-27, 2009
14. Kovarik CL et al: Acral myxoinflammatory fibroblastic sarcoma: case series and immunohistochemical analysis. J Cutan Pathol. 35(2):192-6, 2008
15. Wettach GR et al: Cytogenetic analysis of a hemosiderotic fibrolipomatous tumor. Cancer Genet Cytogenet. 182(2):140-3, 2008
16. Ida CM et al: Myxoinflammatory fibroblastic sarcoma showing t(2;6)(q31;p21.3) as a sole cytogenetic abnormality. Cancer Genet Cytogenet. 177(2):139-42, 2007
17. Luzar B et al: Hemosiderotic fibrohistiocytic lipomatous lesion: early pleomorphic hyalinizing angiectatic tumor? Pathol Int. 56(5):283-6, 2006
18. Kazakov DV et al: Hemosiderotic fibrohistiocytic lipomatous lesion: clinical correlation with venous stasis. Virchows Arch. 447(1):103-6, 2005
19. Folpe AL et al: Pleomorphic hyalinizing angiectatic tumor: analysis of 41 cases supporting evolution from a distinctive precursor lesion. Am J Surg Pathol. 28(11):1417-25, 2004
20. Jurcić V et al: Myxoinflammatory fibroblastic sarcoma: a tumor not restricted to acral sites. Ann Diagn Pathol. 6(5):272-80, 2002
21. Lambert I et al: Acral myxoinflammatory fibroblastic sarcoma with unique clonal chromosomal changes. Virchows Arch. 438(5):509-12, 2001
22. Marshall-Taylor C et al: Hemosiderotic fibrohistiocytic lipomatous lesion: ten cases of a previously undescribed fatty lesion of the foot/ankle. Mod Pathol. 13(11):1192-9, 2000
23. Meis-Kindblom JM et al: Acral myxoinflammatory fibroblastic sarcoma: a low-grade tumor of the hands and feet. Am J Surg Pathol. 22(8):911-24, 1998
24. Montgomery EA et al: Inflammatory myxohyaline tumor of distal extremities with virocyte or Reed-Sternberg-like cells: a distinctive lesion with features simulating inflammatory conditions, Hodgkin's disease, and various sarcomas. Mod Pathol. 11(4):384-91, 1998

Myxoinflammatory Fibroblastic Sarcoma, Lobulations

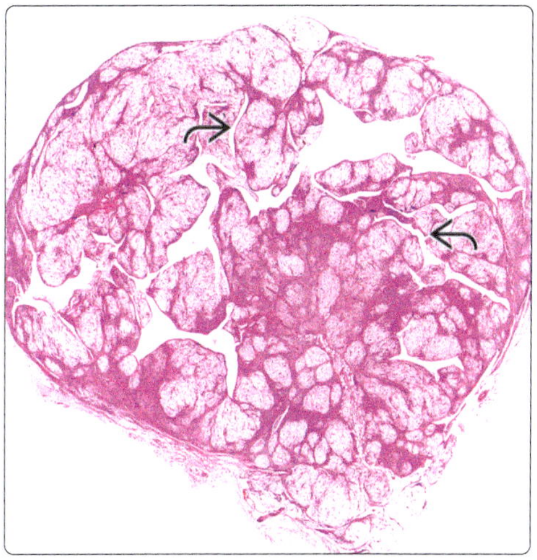

Myxoinflammatory Fibroblastic Sarcoma, Myxoid Zones

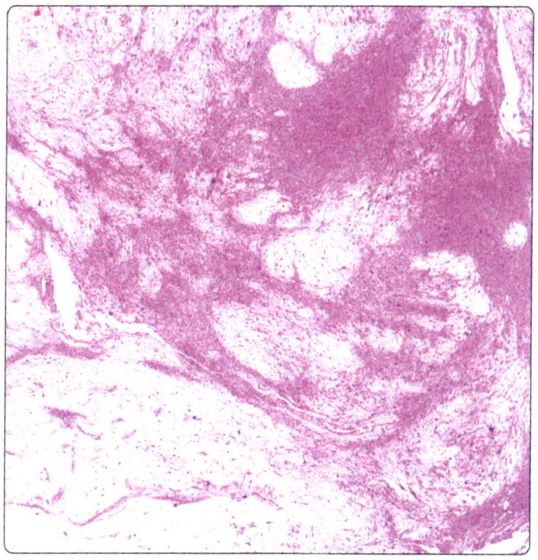

(Left) *This image shows a MIFS at low magnification. This lesion is characterized by myxoid areas alternating with fibrous areas, and it also has prominent cleft-like spaces →.* **(Right)** *This MIFS has pockets of myxoid matrix interspersed with more solid fibroinflammatory zones.*

Myxoinflammatory Fibroblastic Sarcoma, Inflammatory and Myxoid Areas

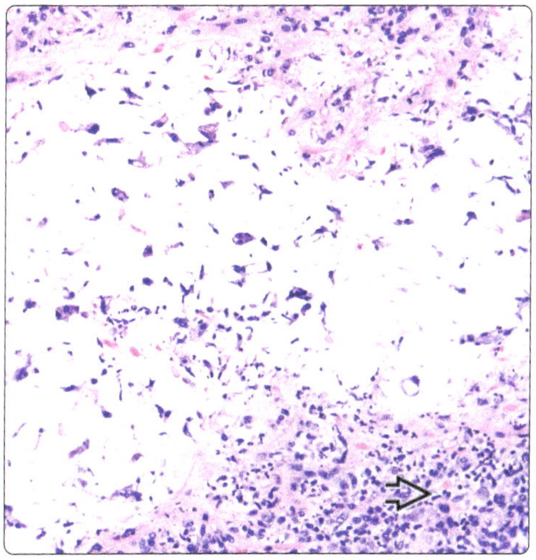

MIFS, Reed-Sternberg-Like Cell

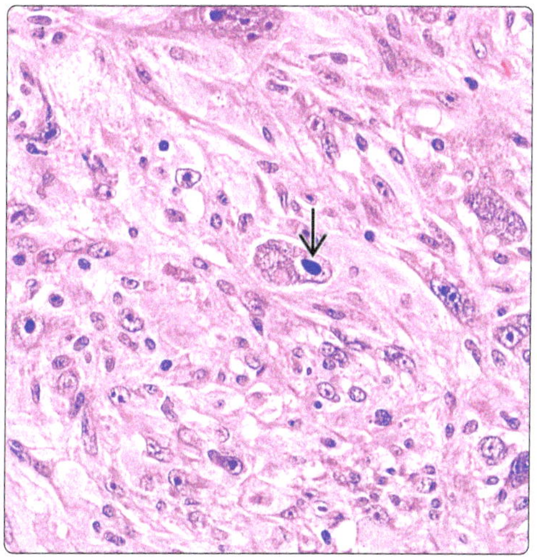

(Left) *Higher power of MIFS shows the junction of a myxoid area with an inflammatory area. The cells suspended in the myxoid matrix are enlarged and hyperchromatic. Note the lymphocytes in the lower right portion of the image →.* **(Right)** *High magnification shows markedly atypical enlarged epithelioid cells. In this field, the cells also display a granular cytoplasmic appearance. The cell in the center has a striking macronucleolus →.*

Myxoinflammatory Fibroblastic Sarcoma, Myxofibrosarcoma-Like Zone

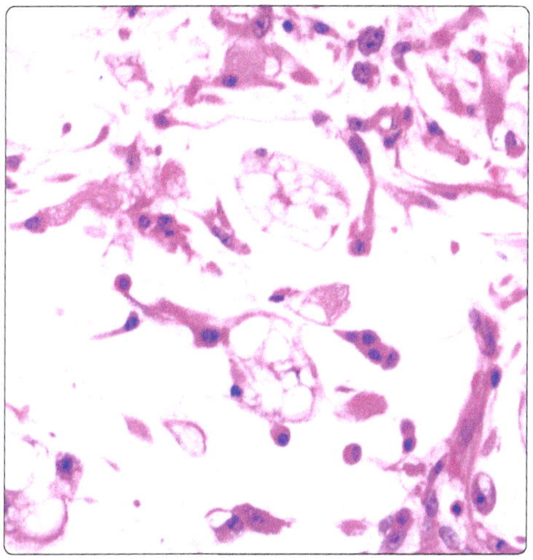

Myxoinflammatory Fibroblastic Sarcoma: Cytologic Features

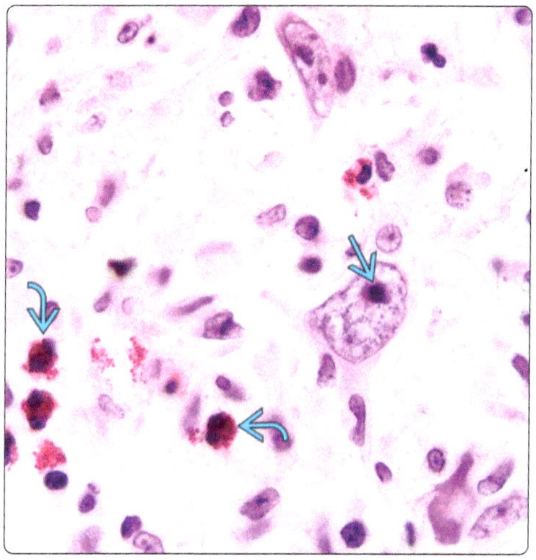

(Left) *This MIFS shows abundant myxoid matrix. In this field, the neoplasm appears similar to myxofibrosarcoma (myxoid malignant fibrous histiocytoma) but lacks the rich vascular pattern of myxofibrosarcoma and has inflammatory cells.* **(Right)** *Cells such as this, with macronucleoli →, are frequently encountered in MIFS. Since they are accompanied by inflammation, including eosinophils →, the findings can suggest Hodgkin disease.*

Myxoinflammatory Fibroblastic Sarcoma, Hyalinized Zone

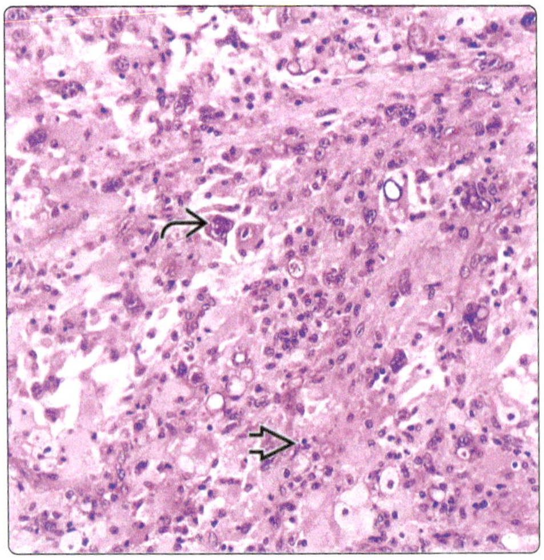

Myxoinflammatory Fibroblastic Sarcoma, Macronucleoli

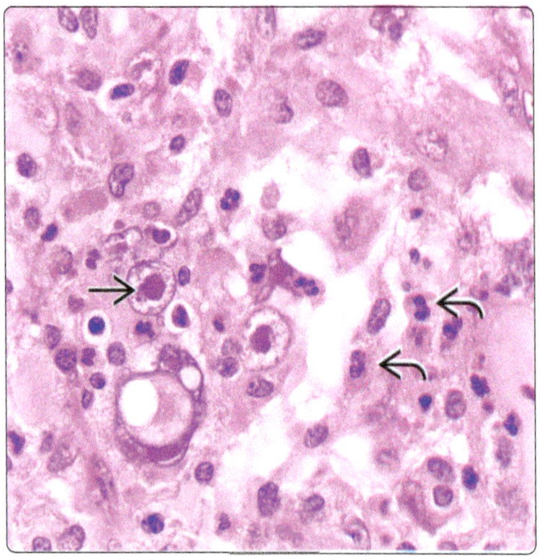

(Left) *This is a hyalinized portion of a MIFS. Based on areas such as this, these neoplasms were initially described as inflammatory myxohyaline tumors. Note the cells with macronucleoli* ⇨ *and the scattered lymphoid cells in the background* ⇨. **(Right)** *The fibroblasts in MIFS often have macronucleoli* ⇨. *Paired with the frequent eosinophils in many examples* ⇨, *the presence of the prominent nucleoli in many cells can lead to a misinterpretation of Hodgkin disease.*

Myxoinflammatory Fibroblastic Sarcoma, Myxoid Matrix

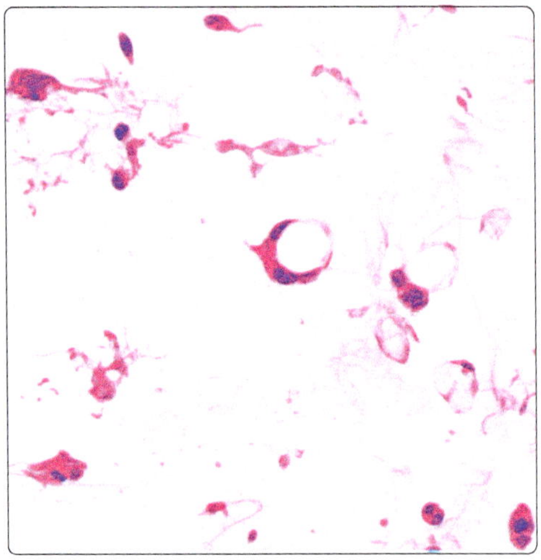

Myxoinflammatory Fibroblastic Sarcoma With Pseudolipoblasts

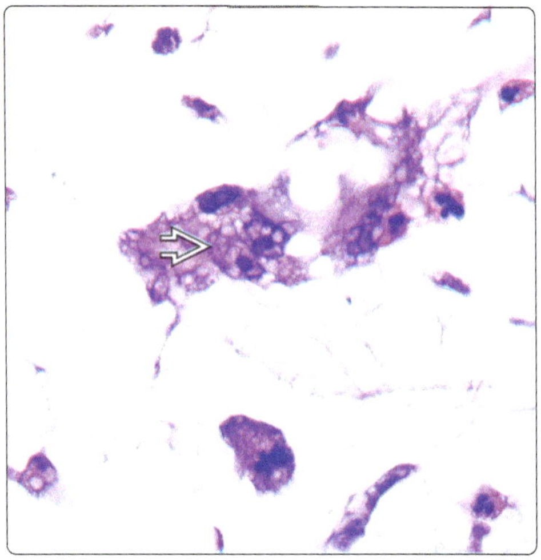

(Left) *This MIFS is characterized by cells with hyperchromatic nuclei and mucinous cytoplasmic vacuoles embedded in a myxoid mucopolysaccharide matrix.* **(Right)** *High magnification shows a myxoid focus in a MIFS. The cell in the center* ➡ *with a pair of nuclei with macronucleoli and abundant multivacuolated cytoplasm is reminiscent of a lipoblast.*

Myxoinflammatory Fibroblastic Sarcoma, Hyalinized Zone

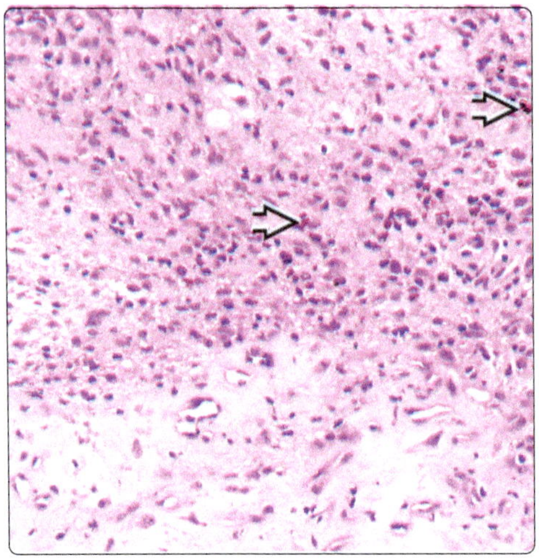

Myxoinflammatory Fibroblastic Sarcoma, CD34 Expression

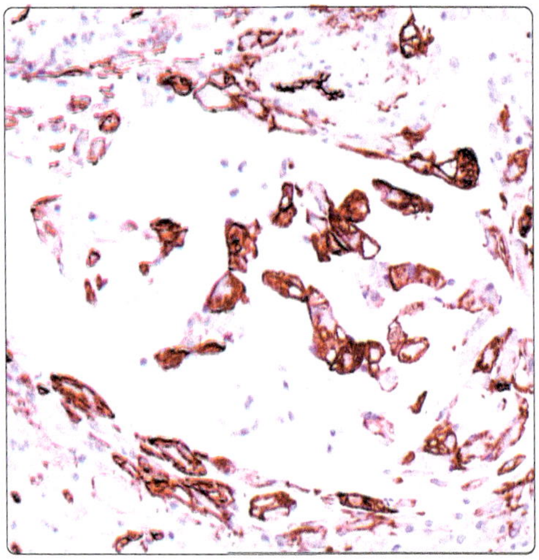

(Left) *This particular example of MIFS has fairly abundant hemosiderin deposition* ⇨. *The lower portion of the field has a hyalinized appearance.* **(Right)** *CD34 expression is commonly found in MIFS. Focal keratin expression in MIFS can suggest epithelioid sarcoma as well, but there is retention of INI1.*

Differential Diagnosis: Myxofibrosarcoma, Low Magnification

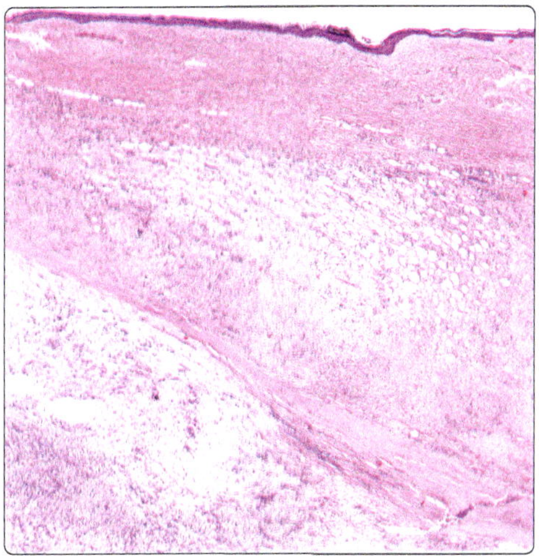

Differential Diagnosis: Myxofibrosarcoma, High Magnification

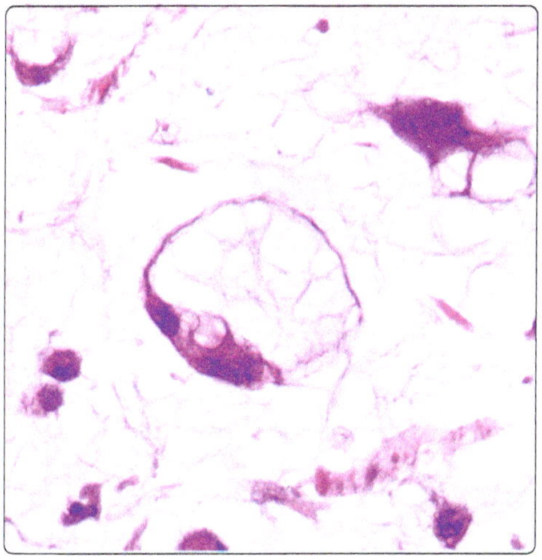

(Left) *This superficial lesion arose in the thigh. It appears similar to MIFS but differs by being richly vascular and by lacking prominent inflammation.* **(Right)** *This atypical fibroblast from a myxofibrosarcoma appears similar to the cells in MIFS and contains abundant mucopolysaccharides, which are also present in the stroma surrounding the cell.*

Differential Diagnosis: Pigmented Villonodular Tenosynovitis

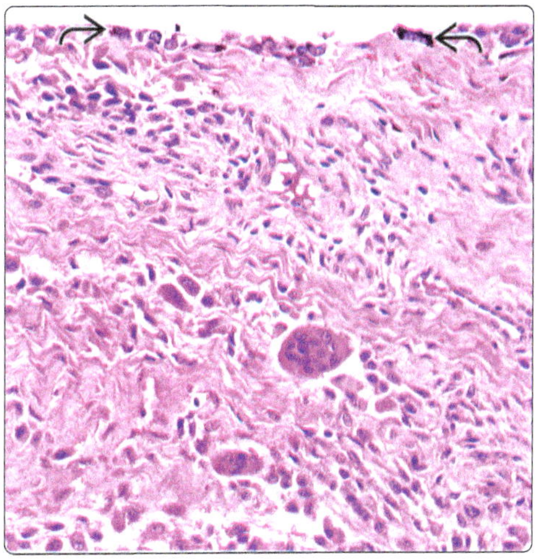

Differential Diagnosis: Pigmented Villonodular Tenosynovitis

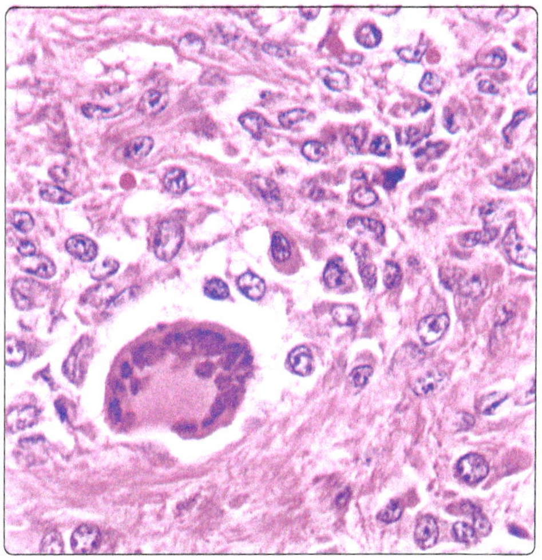

(Left) *Pigmented villonodular tenosynovitis appears similar to MIFS clinically but differs histologically, consisting of giant cells and uniform mononucleate cells. Note the layer of pigmented synovium on the surface* ➔. **(Right)** *At high magnification, pigmented villonodular tenosynovitis features multinucleated giant cells, uniform cells with single nuclei, and hemosiderin. These lesions often affect the knee joint.*

Hemosiderotic Fibrohistiocytic Lipomatous Lesion

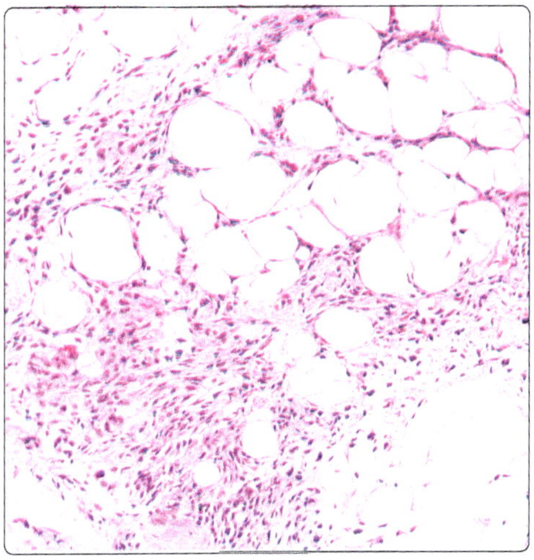

Hemosiderotic Fibrohistiocytic Lipomatous Lesion/Hemosiderotic Fibrolipomatous Tumor: Iron Stain

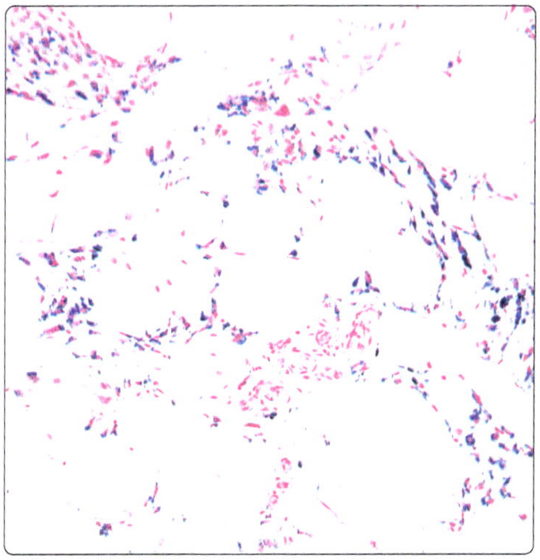

(Left) *Hemosiderotic fibrohistiocytic lipomatous lesion (hemosiderotic fibrolipomatous tumor), shown here, may form a spectrum with both MIFS and with pleomorphic hyalinizing angiectatic tumor. It typically arises on the foot and consists of CD34(+) reactive spindle cells, fat, and abundant hemosiderin, which is often inconspicuous on routine H&E stains but readily apparent on iron staining.* **(Right)** *Hemosiderotic fibrohistiocytic lipomatous lesion often shows abundant iron on iron stains.*

Epithelioid Sarcoma

KEY FACTS

TERMINOLOGY

- Distinctive malignant mesenchymal neoplasm that often shows epithelioid cytomorphology and demonstrates evidence of epithelial differentiation
  - Classic epithelioid sarcoma (ES) most commonly affects adolescents and young adults and arises in distal extremities
  - Proximal-type ES tends to affect older age groups (median: 40 years), arises in proximal locations, and is often more clinically aggressive

CLINICAL ISSUES

- Classic ES may appear clinically as nonhealing ulcer
- Clinically aggressive sarcoma
  - High rate of recurrence and metastases
    - Metastases to lymph nodes, lung, and skin

MICROSCOPIC

- Classic ES
  - Nodules with central necrosis (granuloma-like)
  - Epithelioid and spindled cells with eosinophilic cytoplasm and uniform, irregular, mildly atypical nuclei
  - Rare predominantly spindled tumors (fibroma-like ES)
- Proximal-type ES
  - Large, cellular nodules of large polygonal cells with prominent macronucleoli
  - Rhabdoid morphology common

ANCILLARY TESTS

- Keratin (+); CD34(+) in 50%
- Complete loss of nuclear INI1 protein expression
- Molecular: High frequency of *SMARCB1* (INI1) deletion (22q11)

TOP DIFFERENTIAL DIAGNOSES

- Granulomatous processes, carcinoma or melanoma, extrarenal rhabdoid tumor, epithelioid angiosarcoma

Epithelioid Sarcoma

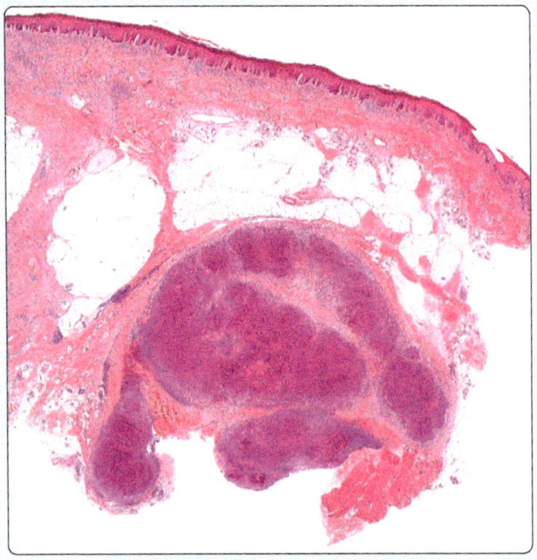

Pseudogranulomatous Morphology

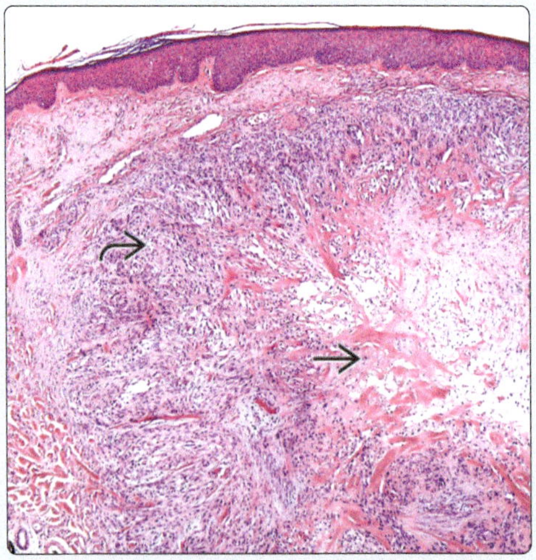

(Left) *Epithelioid sarcoma (ES) is a distinctive malignant mesenchymal neoplasm of uncertain differentiation that classically arises in the subcutaneous tissues on the distal extremities of adolescents and young adults.* **(Right)** *The nodules of ES ↪ often demonstrate centralized necrosis →, imparting an appearance reminiscent of a necrotizing granulomatous process, such as an infection or necrobiotic granulomatous dermatitis.*

Classic Epithelioid Sarcoma

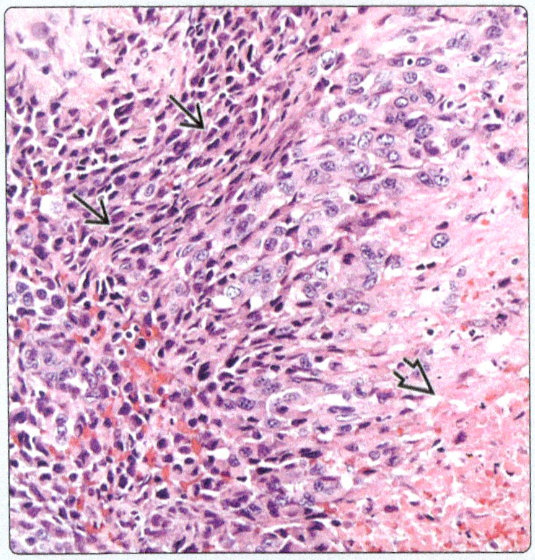

Immunohistochemistry for EMA

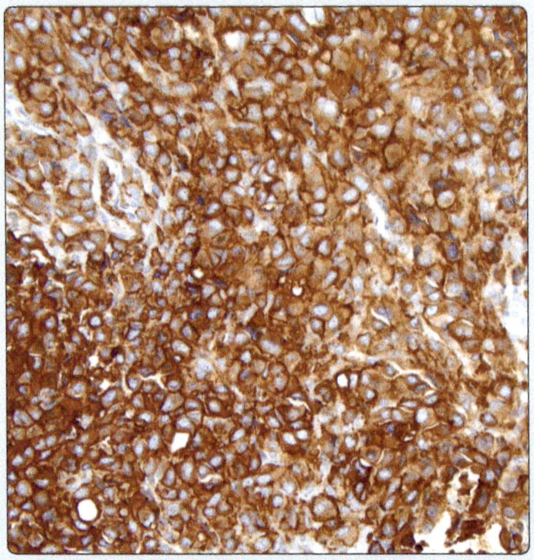

(Left) *The classic type of ES is composed of small- to medium-sized epithelioid cells with eosinophilic cytoplasm. Admixed small spindled cells → can also be identified and often appear more conspicuous at the periphery of a nodule. Note the central tumor necrosis ⇨.* **(Right)** *ES is notable among mesenchymal tumors for its expression of epithelial markers, including most keratins and EMA. CD34 is coexpressed in 50% of cases. Complete loss of nuclear INI1 is also characteristic of ES cells.*

TERMINOLOGY

Abbreviations

- Epithelioid sarcoma (ES)

Definitions

- Distinctive malignant mesenchymal neoplasm that often shows epithelioid cytomorphology and demonstrates evidence of epithelial differentiation
  - Classic ES most commonly affects adolescents and young adults and arises in distal extremities
  - Proximal-type ES tends to affect older age groups, arises in proximal locations, and is often more clinically aggressive

CLINICAL ISSUES

Epidemiology

- Incidence
  - Rare
    - Accounts for ~ 1% of all soft tissue sarcomas
    - Classic ES is more common than proximal-type ES
- Age
  - Classic ES
    - Adolescents and young adults (median: 26 years)
  - Proximal-type ES
    - Affects middle-aged to older adults (median: 40 years)
- Sex
  - More frequent in male patients (both types)

Site

- Classic ES
  - Most common in distal extremities, especially hand, wrist, forearm, lower leg
  - Also head and neck, genital sites
- Proximal-type ES
  - Proximal limb girdles
  - Perineum, pelvis, mediastinum
  - Trunk

Presentation

- Classic ES
  - Slow-growing, often painless
  - Often small, indurated dermal or subcutaneous nodule(s)
    - Can appear to track up limb
  - May appear as nonhealing ulcer
    - Can closely mimic infection clinically
    - Raised "sealing wax" margins
- Proximal-type ES
  - Subcutaneous or deep soft tissue mass
  - Can appear and grow more rapidly than classical ES

Treatment

- Wide surgical excision and reexcision
  - Amputation in some cases
- Chemotherapy can be palliative but currently of limited therapeutic benefit
  - Preclinical models suggest possible therapeutic benefit of EGFR-TK, mTOR, and c-MET inhibitors

Prognosis

- Clinically aggressive sarcoma
  - > 70% recur
    - Successive recurrences often extend more proximally in limbs
  - ~ 50% metastasize
    - Lymph nodes and lungs
    - Also skin and other soft tissue sites
  - 5-year survival (70%), 10-year survival (40%)
- Proximal-type ES has worse prognosis
  - Up to 75% metastasize
  - 5-year survival (35-65%)
- Adverse prognostic factors
  - Proximal location
  - Male patients
  - Size > 5 cm
  - Localization to deep soft tissue sites

MACROSCOPIC

General Features

- Uni- or multinodular firm lesion
- Tan/white/gray cut surface
- Hemorrhage and necrosis common in proximal-type ES

Size

- Classic ES: Usually < 5 cm
- Proximal-type ES: Wide range (1-20 cm)

MICROSCOPIC

Histologic Features

- Classic ES
  - Dermal/subcutaneous nodule(s), ± central necrosis
    - Can simulate granulomatous process at low magnification
    - Peripheral infiltration of connective tissue is common
    - Deeply extending lesions often involve and track along tendons/aponeuroses
  - Small- to medium-sized epithelioid cells with eosinophilic cytoplasm
    - Irregular but uniform, mildly atypical nuclei with small nucleoli
    - Admixed cells with spindled morphology common (particularly at periphery)
      - May rarely predominate (termed fibroma-like variant of ES)
      - Can show storiform growth
  - Variable mitotic activity, often low
  - Mixed chronic inflammatory infiltrate common
  - Other findings
    - Densely hyalinized collagenous stroma
    - Rare myxoid change
    - Osteoclast-like giant cells, calcification, metaplastic bone formation
    - Pseudogland formation
    - Pseudovascular morphology
- Proximal-type ES
  - More infiltrative with less defined peripheral borders
  - Multiple large nodules

- Sheets of large polygonal cells with abundant eosinophilic cytoplasm
  - Rhabdoid morphology common
- Vesicular nuclei with prominent macronucleoli
- Mitoses common
- Necrosis and hemorrhage common

ANCILLARY TESTS

Immunohistochemistry

- Positive for high- and low-molecular weight keratins, EMA, vimentin
  - However, negative for CK5/6
- Positive for CD34 in 50%
- Positive for ERG in 40% of cases; positive for GLUT1 in 50% of cases
- Complete loss of nuclear INI1 protein expression
- Negative for CD31, S100, p63, desmin, FLI-1, PROX1

Molecular Genetics

- High frequency of *SMARCB1* (INI1) deletion (22q11)
  - Both classic and proximal-type ES

DIFFERENTIAL DIAGNOSIS

Granulomatous Processes

- Particularly granuloma annulare
- Lacks infiltrative or invasion growth
- Lacks coagulative tumor cell necrosis
- Negative for keratin and EMA
- Retained nuclear INI1 expression

Squamous Cell Carcinoma

- Overlying in situ component may be identifiable
- Prior clinical history may be present
- Usually more pleomorphic than ES
- Positive for CK5/6 and p63
- Negative for CD34
- Retained nuclear INI1 expression

Extrarenal Rhabdoid Tumor

- Can show significant morphologic overlap with proximal-type ES
- Most common in infants and young children
- Positive for keratin but less prominent than in ES
- Consistent loss of nuclear INI1 expression
- Mutation of *SMARCB1* gene

Melanoma

- Junctional component or prior clinical history may be present
- Usually larger, more pleomorphic cells than classic ES
- Positive for S100, SOX10; variably positive for HMB-45 or MART-1
- Retained nuclear INI1 expression

Epithelioid Angiosarcoma

- Can show significant morphologic overlap with proximal-type ES
- Foci of vasoformation often present at least focally
- Positive for CD31, CD34, FLI-1
- May be positive for keratin, though usually not diffuse
- Retained nuclear INI1 expression

Pseudomyogenic (Epithelioid Sarcoma-Like) Hemangioendothelioma

- Commonly involves multiple tissue planes
- Predominantly spindled morphology
- Neutrophilic infiltrate characteristic
- Positive for keratin, CD31
- Negative for CD34
- Retained nuclear INI1 expression

Malignant Myoepithelioma (Myoepithelial Carcinoma)

- Can show morphologic overlap with proximal-type ES
- Myxoid stroma common
- Positive for keratin, EMA, S100
- Loss of nuclear INI1 expression in subset of cases

Cellular Fibrous Histiocytoma (Dermatofibroma)

- Can show morphologic overlap with predominantly spindled forms of ES
- Negative for keratin
- Retained nuclear INI1 expression

SELECTED REFERENCES

1. Asano N et al: Prognostic value of relevant clinicopathologic variables in epithelioid sarcoma: a multi-institutional retrospective study of 44 patients. Ann Surg Oncol. 22(8):2624-32, 2015
2. Coates SJ et al: Epidermotropic metastatic epithelioid sarcoma: a potential diagnostic pitfall. J Cutan Pathol. 41(8):672-6, 2014
3. Folpe AL: Selected topics in the pathology of epithelioid soft tissue tumors. Mod Pathol. 27 Suppl 1:S64-79, 2014
4. Imura Y et al: Combined targeting of mTOR and c-MET signaling pathways for effective management of epithelioid sarcoma. Mol Cancer. 13:185, 2014
5. Stockman DL et al: ERG and FLI1 protein expression in epithelioid sarcoma. Mod Pathol. 27(4):496-501, 2014
6. Miettinen M et al: ERG expression in epithelioid sarcoma: a diagnostic pitfall. Am J Surg Pathol. 37(10):1580-5, 2013
7. Sullivan LM et al: Epithelioid sarcoma is associated with a high percentage of SMARCB1 deletions. Mod Pathol. 26(3):385-92, 2013
8. Jones RL et al: Role of palliative chemotherapy in advanced epithelioid sarcoma. Am J Clin Oncol. 35(4):351-7, 2012
9. Xie X et al: Combining EGFR and mTOR blockade for the treatment of epithelioid sarcoma. Clin Cancer Res. 17(18):5901-12, 2011
10. Flucke U et al: Myxoid epithelioid sarcoma: a diagnostic challenge. A report on six cases. Histopathology. 57(5):753-9, 2010
11. Chbani L et al: Epithelioid sarcoma: a clinicopathologic and immunohistochemical analysis of 106 cases from the French sarcoma group. Am J Clin Pathol. 131(2):222-7, 2009
12. Hornick JL et al: Loss of INI1 expression is characteristic of both conventional and proximal-type epithelioid sarcoma. Am J Surg Pathol. 33(4):542-50, 2009
13. Jawad MU et al: Prognostic factors for survival in patients with epithelioid sarcoma: 441 cases from the SEER database. Clin Orthop Relat Res. 467(11):2939-48, 2009
14. Orrock JM et al: INI1 and GLUT-1 expression in epithelioid sarcoma and its cutaneous neoplastic and nonneoplastic mimics. Am J Dermatopathol. 31(2):152-6, 2009
15. Fisher C: Epithelioid sarcoma of Enzinger. Adv Anat Pathol. 13(3):114-21, 2006
16. Miettinen M et al: Epithelioid sarcoma: an immunohistochemical analysis of 112 classical and variant cases and a discussion of the differential diagnosis. Hum Pathol. 30(8):934-42, 1999
17. Guillou L et al: "Proximal-type" epithelioid sarcoma, a distinctive aggressive neoplasm showing rhabdoid features. Clinicopathologic, immunohistochemical, and ultrastructural study of a series. Am J Surg Pathol. 21(2):130-46, 1997

Cytologic Features of Epithelioid Sarcoma

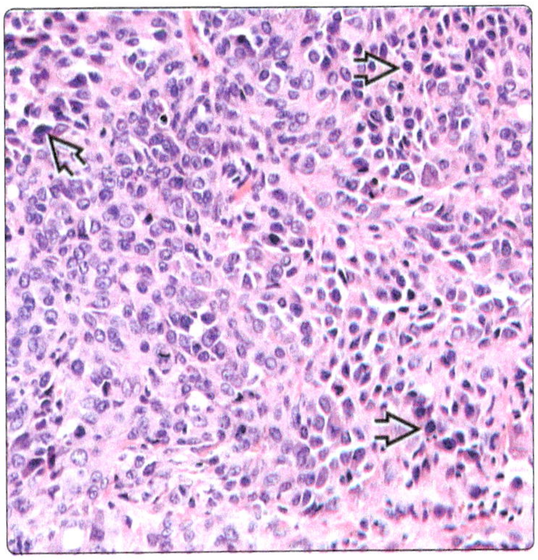

Typical Cytology of Epithelioid Sarcoma

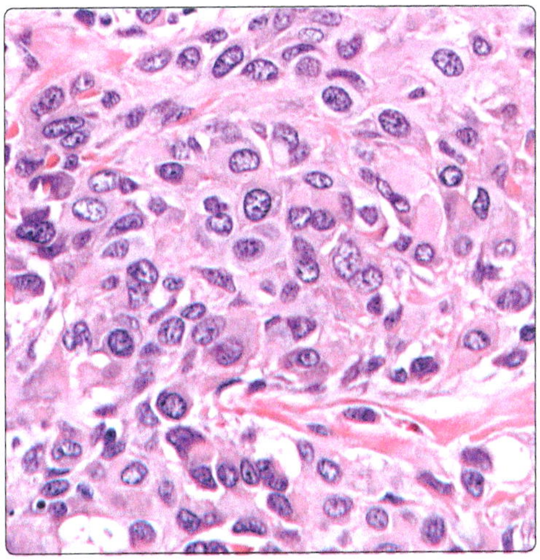

(Left) *The lesional cells of ES show eosinophilic cytoplasm and contain mildly atypical but relatively uniform nuclei. Significant nuclear pleomorphism is very uncommon in this tumor. Note that some cells are compressed and appear to have darker cytoplasm and more hyperchromatic nuclei.* **(Right)** *Most cases show large, epithelioid-shaped cells with round to oval nuclei and abundant amounts of eosinophilic-staining cytoplasm. Mitotic activity varies but is often low in classic forms.*

Spindled Morphology in Epithelioid Sarcoma

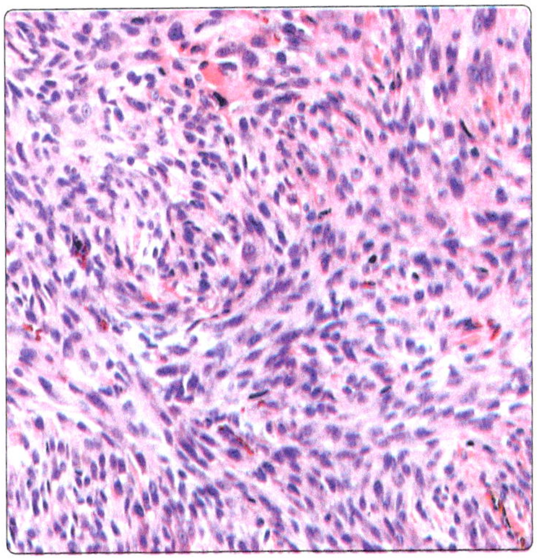

Infiltrative Growth Pattern in Epithelioid Sarcoma

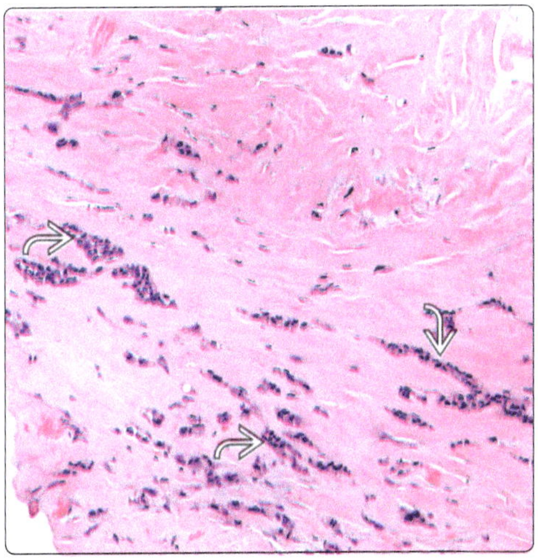

(Left) *Admixed tumor cells with a spindled rather than epithelioid morphology are common in ES. Occasionally, this morphology is more prominent, and a vague storiform or fascicular growth pattern may be seen.* **(Right)** *Most cases of ES show infiltrative growth at the periphery of the main tumor mass. Small nests and cords of cells within fibrotic connective tissue, as depicted here, can mimic infiltrating carcinoma.*

Stromal Hyalinization/Sclerosis in Epithelioid Sarcoma

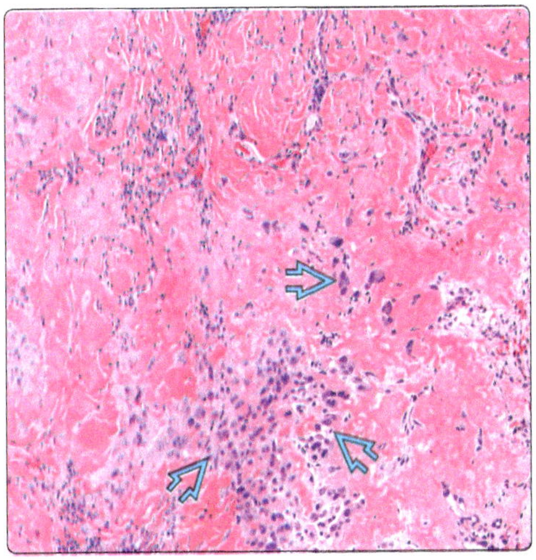

Osteoid-Like Collagen in Epithelioid Sarcoma

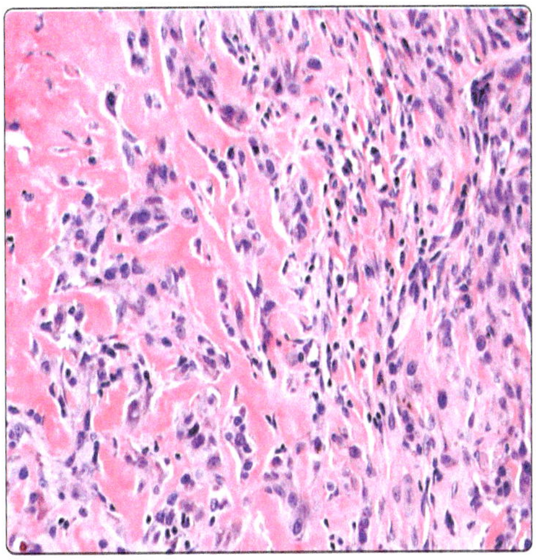

(Left) *Some cases of ES show prominent stromal hyalinization or sclerosis, as seen here. Entrapped tumor cells may appear singly or as irregular clusters, aggregates, or cords.* **(Right)** *Hyalinized stromal collagen may appear as irregular, thickened bundles, imparting an appearance reminiscent of osteoid deposition in osteosarcoma.*

(Left) *A chronic inflammatory infiltrate may be seen in ES and can rarely be so prominent as to obscure the underlying neoplasm. Lymphocytes are predominantly seen in this image.* **(Right)** *In contrast to the classic type, the proximal-type variant of ES usually shows a larger, more solid and cellular, nodular growth pattern. Clinically, this form of ES generally affects an older age group and arises in proximal locations.*

Chronic Inflammatory Infiltrate in Epithelioid Sarcoma

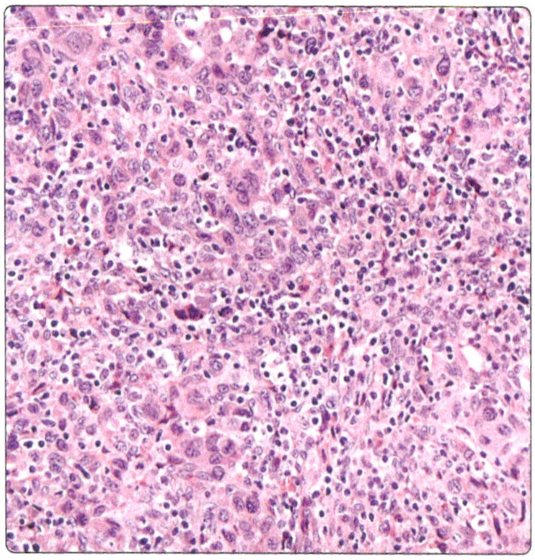

Proximal-Type Epithelioid Sarcoma

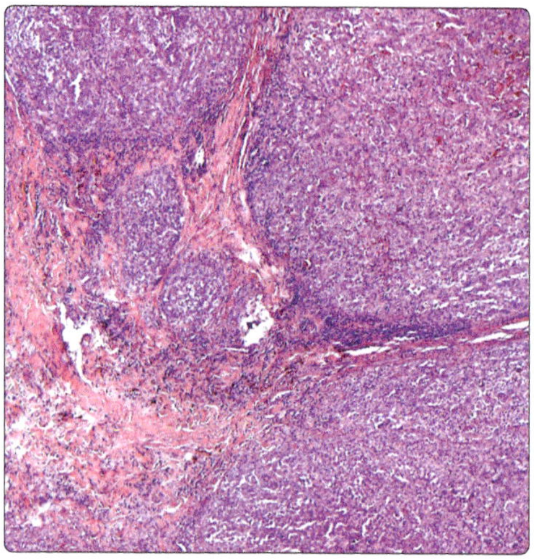

(Left) *The cells of proximal-type ES are larger and plumper than those of classic ES and show more abundant eosinophilic cytoplasm. Vesicular nuclei with prominent macronucleoli are characteristic of this variant and aid in its histologic recognition.* **(Right)** *Rhabdoid cytomorphology is not uncommon in proximal-type ES and can lead to significant morphologic overlap with malignant extrarenal rhabdoid tumor; however, the clinical scenarios for these 2 entities are often very different.*

Macronucleoli in Proximal-Type Epithelioid Sarcoma

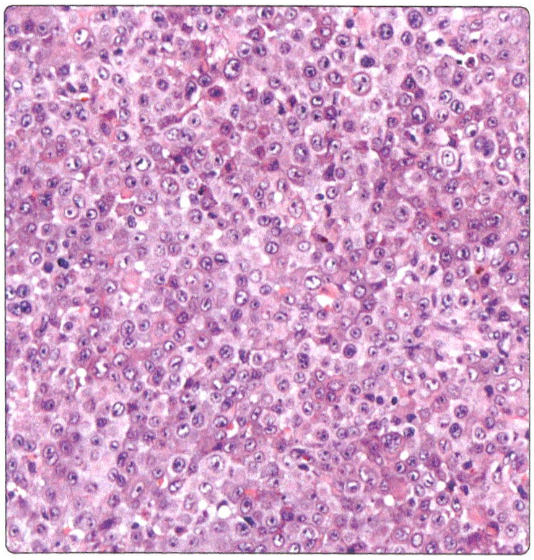

Rhabdoid Cytomorphology in Proximal-Type Epithelioid Sarcoma

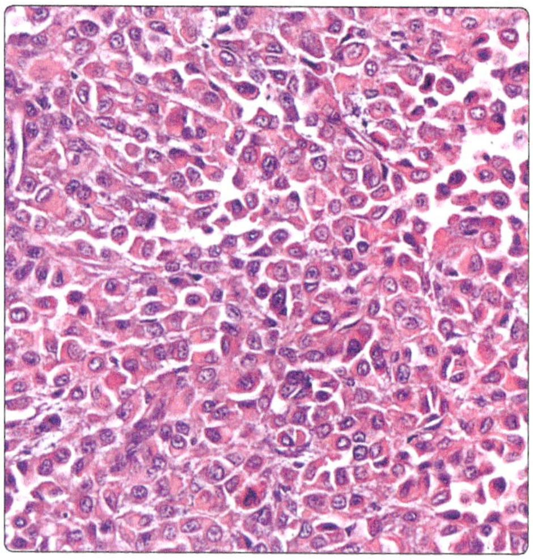

(Left) *Heterotopic bone formation ➡ is a rare finding in ES and may be focal or prominent. It is often woven in composition but can also be lamellar.* **(Right)** *Rare cases of ES may contain a population of reactive multinucleated osteoclast-like giant cells ➡ scattered within otherwise typical lesional cells (proximal-type ES in this image). This is usually a focal finding.*

Heterotopic Bone Formation

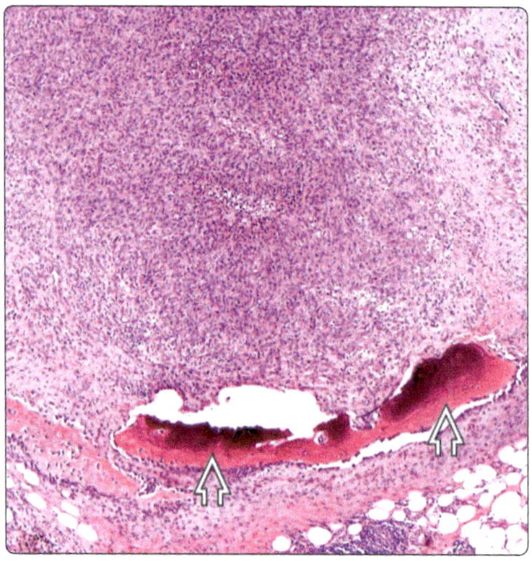

Osteoclast-Like Giant Cells

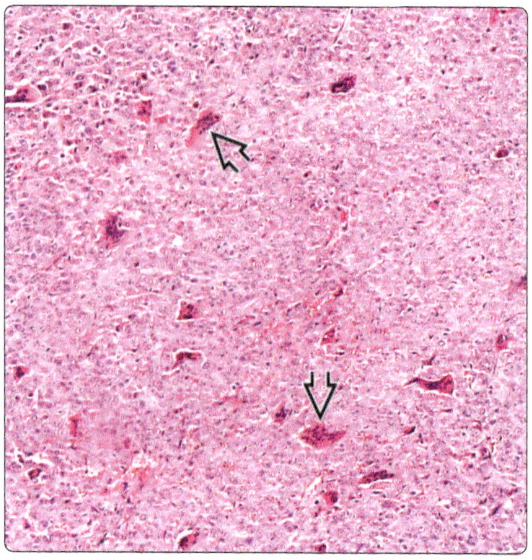

Pseudoglandular Foci in Epithelioid Sarcoma

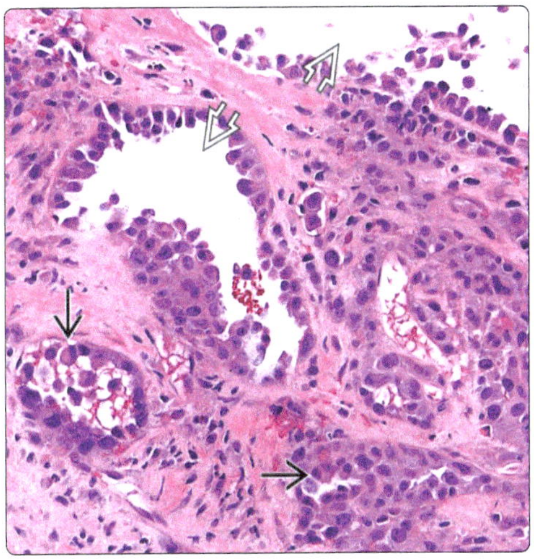

Pseudovascular Morphology in Epithelioid Sarcoma

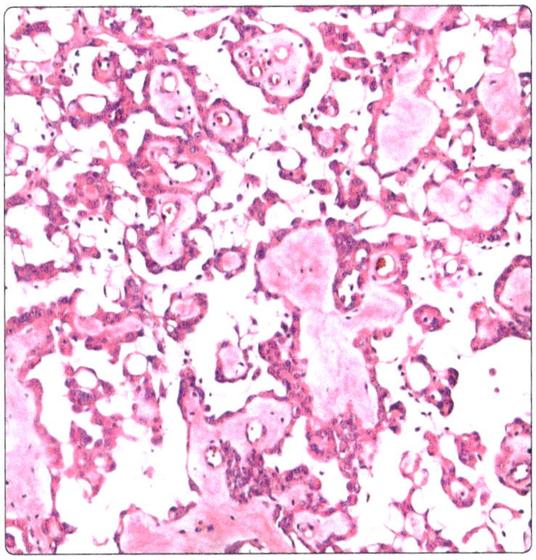

(Left) *Central loss of cellular cohesion in ES can lead to a pseudoglandular appearance. Note the larger lesional cells with prominent nucleoli and scattered rhabdoid forms, identifying this tumor as a proximal-type ES.* **(Right)** *A loosely dyscohesive, pseudovascular pattern is a rare finding in ES but can resemble angiosarcoma. The absence of CD31 &/or FLI1 expression in ES is helpful in the distinction.*

Proximal Myxoid Stroma in Epithelioid Sarcoma

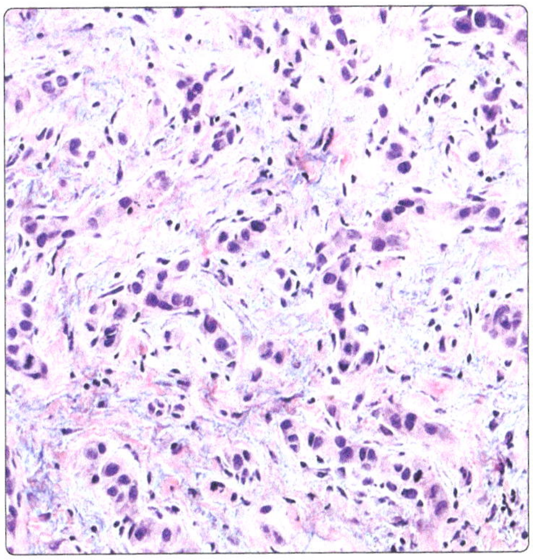

Rare Fibroma-Like Variant of Epithelioid Sarcoma

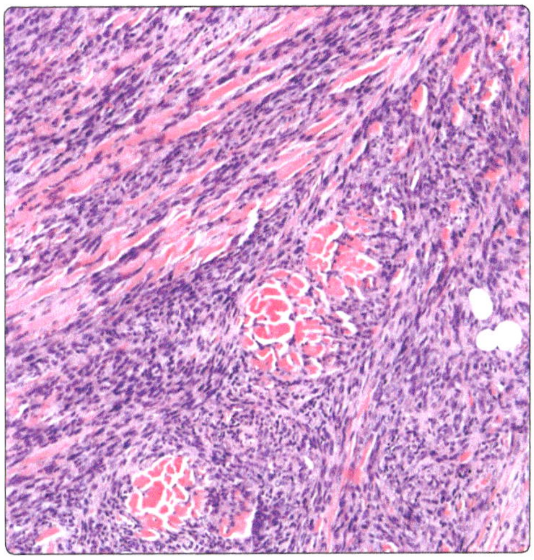

(Left) *Myxoid stromal change is a very rare finding in ES and is usually focal if present. Exceptional cases show diffuse myxoid change.* **(Right)** *Although spindled tumor cells are common in classic ES, rare tumors show a predominant or exclusive spindled morphology. This variant has been described as fibroma-like ES and may lead to consideration of cellular fibrous histiocytoma.*

Lymph Node Metastasis

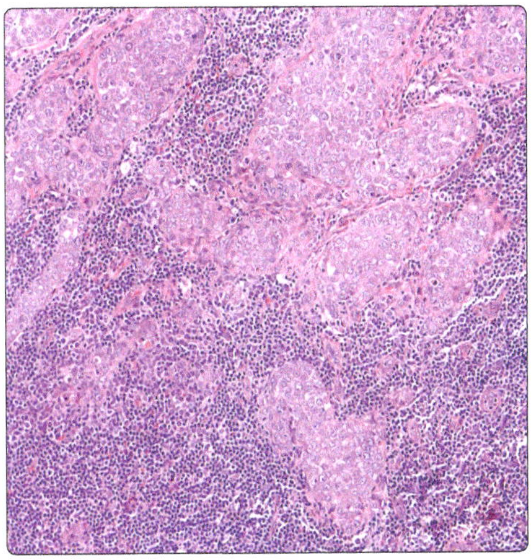

Cutaneous Metastasis

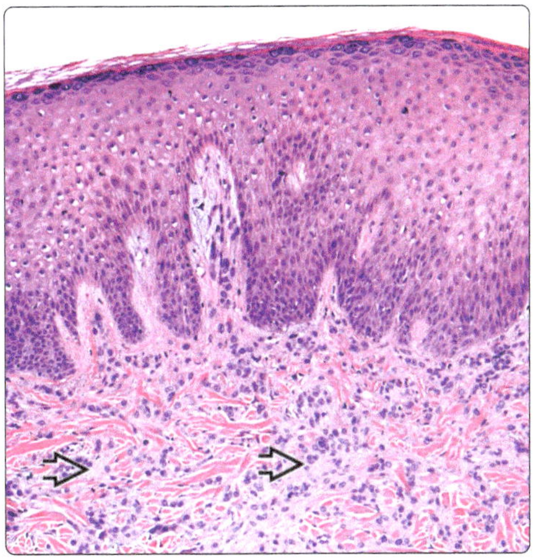

(Left) *ES is 1 of the few mesenchymal neoplasms that is well known to metastasize to lymph nodes. Spread to the lungs is also common. Overall, metastasis occurs in up to 50% of cases.* **(Right)** *Cutaneous and soft tissue metastases are not uncommon in ES and may present as small nodules or bumps that do not immediately raise clinical suspicion for malignancy. In some cases, the relatively bland cytologic features may lead to tumor cells getting overlooked.*

PART I
SECTION 8

Vascular and Perivascular Tumors and Pseudotumors

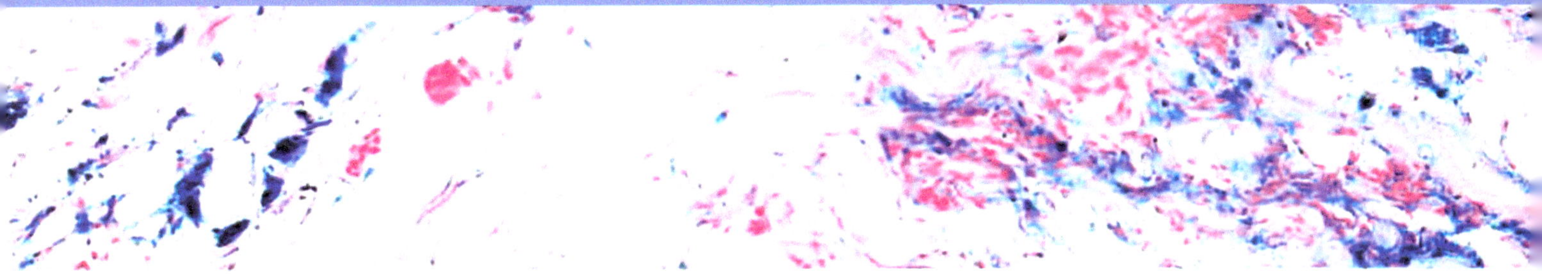

KEY FACTS

TERMINOLOGY

- Congenital vascular malformations
- Nevus flammeus: Group of congenital vascular malformations

CLINICAL ISSUES

- Port-wine stain: Usually involves head and neck
- Sturge-Weber syndrome: Port-wine stain involving ophthalmic branch of trigeminal nerve
- Klippel-Trenaunay-Weber syndrome
  - Port-wine stain usually involving extremity
  - Underlying venous and lymphatic malformations
  - Limb overgrowth with hypertrophy of soft tissue and bone
- Blue rubber bleb nevus syndrome
  - Multiple blue-colored, rubbery hemangiomas of skin
  - Usually resemble cavernous hemangiomas
  - Gastrointestinal tract frequently involved
- Maffucci syndrome
  - Multiple hemangiomas of dermis and subcutis and enchondromas
    - Cavernous, capillary, and spindle cell hemangiomas common
    - Enchondromas most commonly affecting metacarpals and phalanges
  - Associated with mutations in isocitrate dehydrogenase
    - Usually isocitrate dehydrogenase-1
  - Chondrosarcomas develop in 15-30%
  - Increased risk of pancreatic, ovarian, and central nervous system malignancies

MICROSCOPIC

- Dilated, blood-filled capillaries
  - Confined to papillary dermis in salmon patch
  - Involve deeper dermis in port-wine stain
- May have cavernous vessels

Port-Wine Stain

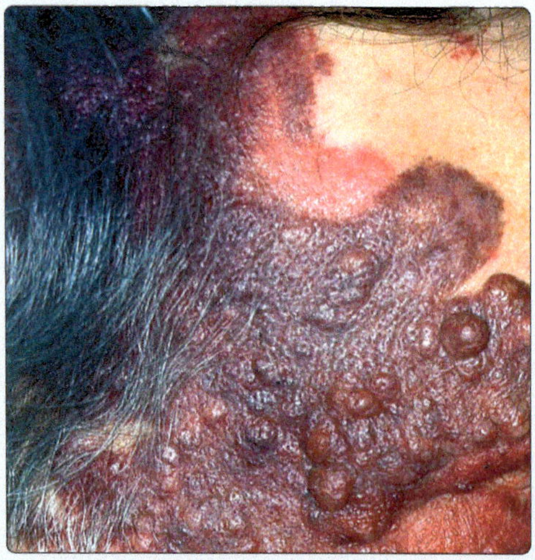

Klippel-Trenaunay Syndrome

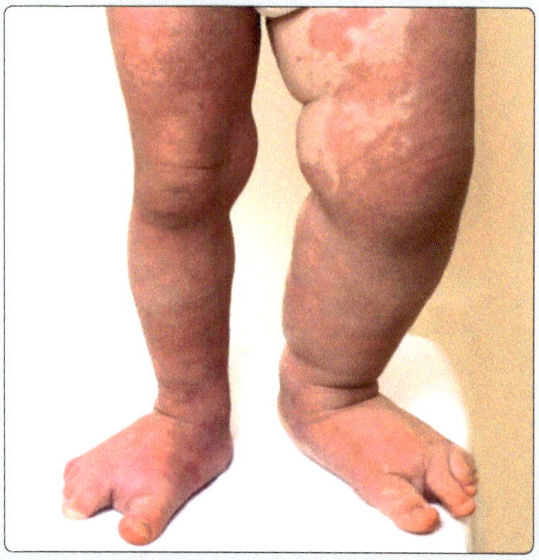

(Left) *Port-wine stain is a vascular hamartoma that usually presents on the head and neck. As the patient ages, it often becomes thicker and more nodular. (Courtesy A. Vidimos, MD.)* **(Right)** *Klippel-Trenaunay syndrome is an extensive port-wine stain affecting an extremity associated with limb overgrowth. (Courtesy A. Vidimos, MD.)*

Vascular Hamartoma

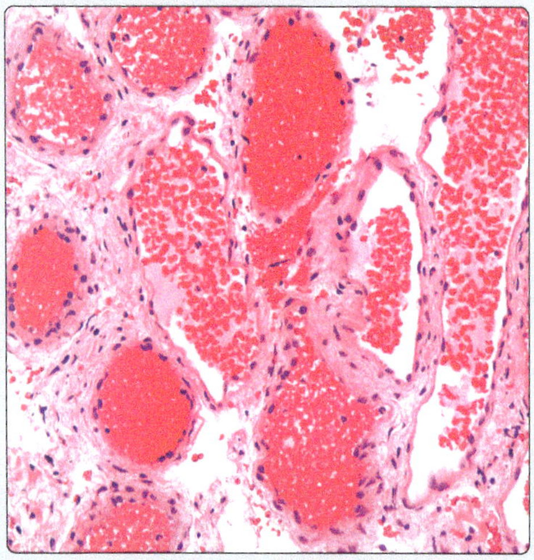

Leptomeningeal Involvement in Sturge-Weber Syndrome

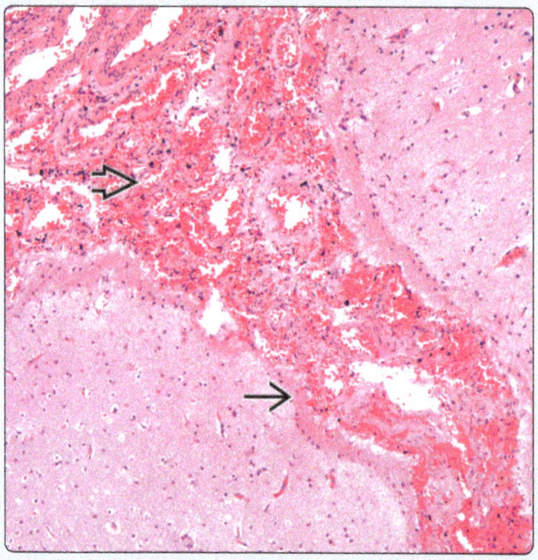

(Left) *Vascular hamartomas are usually characterized by closely packed, dilated, thin-walled blood vessels.* **(Right)** *In Sturge-Weber syndrome, an associated vascular hamartoma ➾ involving the ipsilateral meninges → may be present.*

TERMINOLOGY

Synonyms

- Congenital vascular malformations
- Sturge-Weber syndrome: Encephalotrigeminal angiomatosis
- Klippel-Trenaunay-Weber syndrome: Angioosteohypertrophy, hemangiectatic hypertrophy

Definitions

- Nevus flammeus: Group of congenital vascular malformations

ETIOLOGY/PATHOGENESIS

Developmental Anomaly

- Vascular malformations present at birth
  - Klippel-Trenaunay-Weber syndrome may be associated with t(8;14)(q22.3;q13)

CLINICAL ISSUES

Presentation

- Present at birth usually in head and neck area but may involve extremities or trunk
- Port-wine stain
  - Present in 0.3% of all births
  - Usually in head and neck, but any location may be affected
  - May be segmental
  - Usually starts as flat, pink lesions
  - Typically not apparent histologically until patients are ~ 10 years old
  - Grows with patient and becomes darker and thicker with time
- Salmon patch
  - Present in ~ 40% of population at birth
  - Presents as pink macule on head and neck
  - Majority fade within 1st year of life
- Sturge-Weber syndrome
  - Port-wine stain involving ophthalmic branch of trigeminal nerve and 1 of following
    - Ipsilateral vascular abnormality of leptomeninges
    - Ipsilateral vascular abnormality of choroid
- Klippel-Trenaunay-Weber syndrome
  - Men and women equally affected
  - Port-wine stain usually involving extremity
  - Underlying venous and lymphatic malformations
  - Limb overgrowth with hypertrophy of soft tissue and bone
  - Varicose veins
  - May be associated with high-output cardiac failure
- Cobb syndrome
  - Present at birth but may not be recognized initially
  - Port-wine stain in dermatomal distribution
  - Associated with underlying spinal arteriovenous hemangioma or venous hemangioma
  - May have with neurologic symptoms (e.g., weakness) from underlying spinal vascular tumor
- Blue rubber bleb nevus syndrome
  - Presents at birth or early childhood
  - Multiple blue-colored, rubbery hemangiomas of skin
  - Usually resemble cavernous hemangiomas
  - Gastrointestinal tract frequently involved
  - Sometimes painful
  - Lesions do not regress
  - May develop iron deficiency anemia from gastrointestinal hemorrhage
- Maffucci syndrome
  - Presents in childhood
  - Associated with mutations in isocitrate dehydrogenase
  - Cavernous, capillary, and spindle cell hemangiomas
  - Multiple enchondromas, most commonly affecting metacarpals and phalanges
  - May have associated skeletal deformities
  - Chondrosarcomas develop in 15-30%
  - Increased risk of pancreatic, ovarian, and central nervous system malignancies

Treatment

- Surgical approaches
  - Variable surgical approaches that depend on individual case
  - Laser treatment

Prognosis

- Benign but some associated with increased risk of secondary malignancy or high-output cardiac failure

MICROSCOPIC

Histologic Features

- All show similar features
  - Dilated, blood-filled capillaries
    - Confined to papillary dermis in salmon patch
    - Involve deeper dermis in port-wine stain
  - May have cavernous vessels
    - In Maffucci syndrome and blue rubber bleb nevus
    - Often present in deep dermis and involving subcutis
  - May resemble arteriovenous malformation
  - Cobb syndrome lesion resembles verrucous hemangioma
  - Immunohistochemistry: CD31(+), CD34(+), WT1(-) (except arteriovenous malformation)

DIFFERENTIAL DIAGNOSIS

Acquired Hemangiomas, Arteriovenous Hemangioma, Verrucous Hemangioma

- Histology may be indistinguishable; key difference is clinical presentation

SELECTED REFERENCES

1. Piram M et al: Sturge-Weber syndrome in patients with facial port-wine stain. Pediatr Dermatol. 29(1):32- 2011
2. Redondo P et al: Diagnosis and management of extensive vascular malformations of the lower limb Part I. Clinical diagnosis. J Am Acad Dermatol. 65(5):893-906, 2011
3. Dilmé-Carreras E et al: Cobb syndrome: case report and review of the literature. Dermatology. 221(2):110-2, 2010
4. Wong CH et al: Blue rubber bleb nevus syndrome: a clinical spectrum with correlation between cutaneous and gastrointestinal manifestations. J Gastroenterol Hepatol. 18(8):1000-2, 2003

Arteriovenous Hemangioma (Malformation)

KEY FACTS

TERMINOLOGY

- Cirsoid aneurysm
- Acral arteriovenous tumor
- Benign, vascular tumor composed of thick- and thin-walled blood vessels

CLINICAL ISSUES

- Occur in adults; equally common in males and females
- Usually involves face, especially lip
- Presents as solitary, dark red papule or nodule
- Stable vascular proliferations that do not regress

MACROSCOPIC

- Small (< 1 cm in most cases)

MICROSCOPIC

- Circumscribed tumor in dermis
- Vessels closely aggregated together
- Ectatic, thin- and thick-walled blood vessels
- Thicker blood vessels have muscular walls resembling arteries
- Vessels lined by single layer of flattened endothelial cells
- Bland endothelial cells lacking nuclear atypia or pleomorphism

TOP DIFFERENTIAL DIAGNOSES

- Deep arteriovenous malformation
- Capillary hemangioma
  - Lacks thick-walled vessels
- Cavernous hemangioma
  - Ectatic, thin-walled vessels
- Venous hemangioma
- Venous lake
  - Single, dilated, thin-walled vessel
- Angioleiomyoma
  - Syncytial proliferation of vascular smooth muscle

Low-Power Image of Arteriovenous Hemangioma

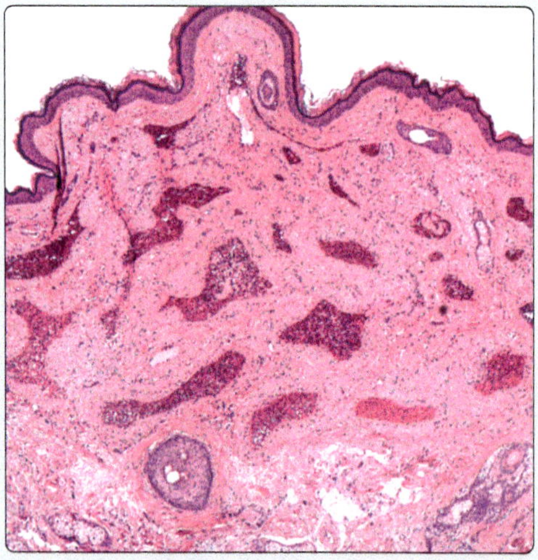

Arteriovenous Hemangioma in Superficial Dermis

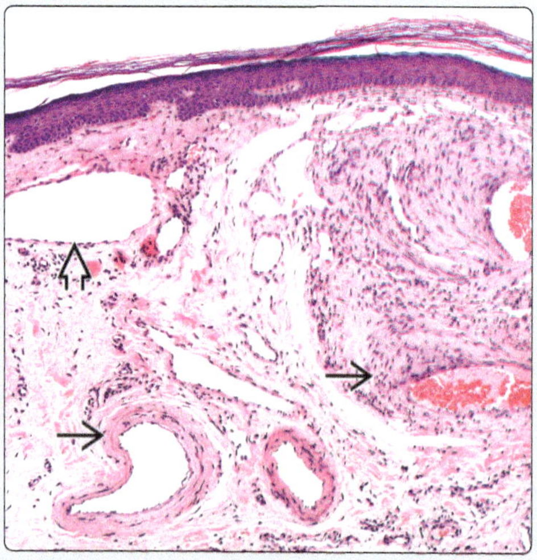

(Left) *Low magnification of a superficial arteriovenous hemangioma shows a tumor that is mostly composed of thick-walled vessels.* **(Right)** *Arteriovenous hemangioma is composed of a circumscribed proliferation of thick-walled muscular vessels that resemble arteries and thin-walled ectatic veins.*

Higher Magnification Demonstrating Thin- and Thick-Walled Vessels

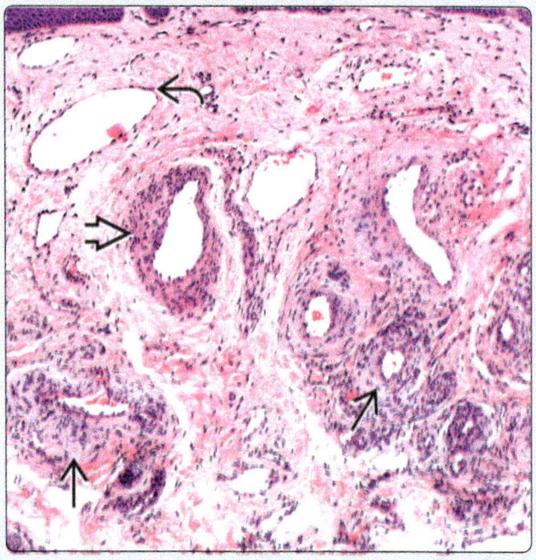

Arteriovenous Hemangioma With Focal Thrombi

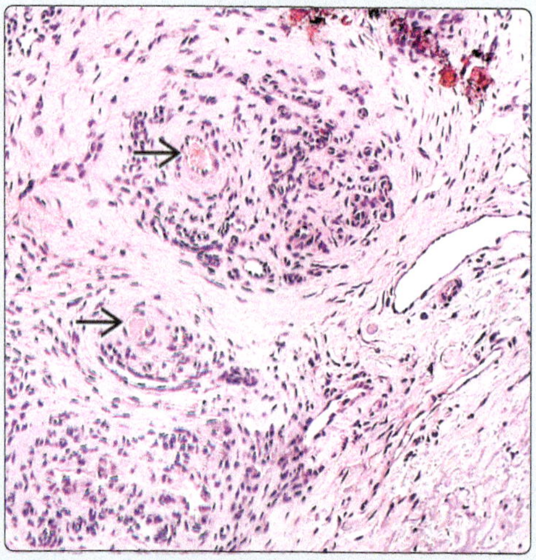

(Left) *Arteriovenous hemangioma is classically composed of a combination of thick- and thin-walled vessels. The thick-walled vessels often have degenerative changes resulting in myxoid stroma surrounding the vessel.* **(Right)** *Fibrin thrombi are sometimes present in the lumina of some of the thick-walled vessels, as shown here.*

TERMINOLOGY

Synonyms

- Cirsoid aneurysm
- Cirsoid hemangioma
- Acral arteriovenous tumor

Definitions

- Benign vascular tumor composed of thick- and thin-walled blood vessels

CLINICAL ISSUES

Epidemiology

- Incidence
  - Uncommon lesions
- Age
  - Present in adults
    - Usually in 5th-6th decades
- Sex
  - Women and men affected equally

Site

- Usually involves face
  - Especially lip
  - Rarely oral cavity
- Extremities: Acral arteriovenous tumors

Presentation

- Solitary, dark red papule or nodule

Natural History

- Stable vascular proliferations that do not regress

Treatment

- Surgical approaches
  - Simple excision

Prognosis

- Benign

MACROSCOPIC

Size

- Small (< 1 cm in most cases)

MICROSCOPIC

Histologic Features

- Circumscribed vascular tumor in dermis
  - Vessels closely aggregated together
- Ectatic thin- and thick-walled blood vessels
  - Most thick-walled vessels lack true internal elastic lamina on elastic stains, indicating they are more likely veins
- Vessels lined by single layer of flattened endothelial cells
- May have thrombi
- Dystrophic calcification occasionally present in vascular walls

Cytologic Features

- No nuclear atypia or pleomorphism

DIFFERENTIAL DIAGNOSIS

Deep Arteriovenous Malformation

- Usually presents on extremities in children
- Similar histologic appearance
- Involves deeper soft tissue than arteriovenous hemangioma

Capillary Hemangioma

- Clustered proliferation of capillary-like blood vessels
- Large feeder vessel supplies each lobule
- Lacks thick-walled vessels
- Mitotic figures may be present, especially in juvenile and pyogenic granuloma forms

Venous Hemangioma

- Proliferation composed of enlarged, thick-walled vascular spaces
- Dilated lumen with thrombi or phleboliths
- Cystically dilated vessels may mimic cavernous hemangioma

Cavernous Hemangioma

- Ectatic, thin-walled vessels
- May represent dilated veins with attenuated smooth muscle layers

Venous Lake

- Solitary, thin-walled, ectatic vessel

Angioleiomyoma

- Well-circumscribed, nodular tumor composed of vascular smooth muscle punctuated by focal vascular lumina
- Syncytial proliferation of smooth muscle
- Lacks distinctly separate vessels

Acquired Digital Arteriovenous Malformation

- Presents on fingertips
- Composed of superficial thick- and thin-walled vessels but less aggregated than arteriovenous hemangioma

Angiosarcoma

- Architecturally complex vessels with anastomosing network of neoplastic vessels
- Cytologic atypia and mitotic activity present

SELECTED REFERENCES

1. Clemens RK et al: Vascular malformations revisited. Vasa. 44(1):5-22, 2015
2. Larralde M et al: Capillary malformation-arteriovenous malformation: a clinical review of 45 patients. Int J Dermatol. 53(4):458-61, 2014
3. Yoon NY et al: An acral arteriovenous tumor arising within a facial port-wine stain. Int J Dermatol. 53(3):e226-8, 2014
4. Bekhor PS et al: Acquired digital arteriovenous malformation: ultrasound imaging and response to long-pulsed neodymium:yttrium-aluminum-garnet treatment. J Am Acad Dermatol. 56(5 Suppl):S122-4, 2007
5. Park CO et al: Treatment of unusual vascular lesions: usefulness of sclerotherapy in lymphangioma circumscriptum and acquired digital arteriovenous malformation. Dermatol Surg. 31(11 Pt 1):1451-3, 2005
6. Kadono T et al: Acquired digital arteriovenous malformation: a report of six cases. Br J Dermatol. 142(2):362-5, 2000
7. Poyton HG et al: Cirsoid aneurysm secondary to an arteriovenous fistula of the facial artery and vein. Oral Surg Oral Med Oral Pathol. 37(3):474-9, 1974
8. Biberstein HH et al: A cirsoid aneurysm in the skin; a case report. Dermatologica. 113(3):129-41, 1956
9. Burston H: Recurrent swelling of the tongue due to cirsoid aneurysm (angioma). AMA Arch Otolaryngol. 62(1):90-2, 1955

KEY FACTS

TERMINOLOGY

- Benign vascular tumors composed of blood vessels lined by plump to flattened endothelial cells with no atypia

ETIOLOGY/PATHOGENESIS

- May be congenital (infantile/juvenile hemangiomas)

CLINICAL ISSUES

- Capillary hemangioma is most common subtype of hemangioma
- Juvenile hemangiomas occur in infancy
- Capillary and cavernous hemangiomas in adults occur more commonly in women
- Pyogenic granuloma occurs on skin and mucosal surfaces and is often ulcerated
- Cavernous hemangiomas present as birthmarks
- Venous hemangiomas are rare and present in adulthood
- Juvenile capillary hemangiomas regress spontaneously with time

MICROSCOPIC

- Nodules of small, capillary-sized vessels in lobular pattern in capillary hemangioma
- Large, cystically dilated vessels filled with blood in cavernous hemangioma
- Large, thick-walled veins in venous hemangioma
- Lining endothelium in all lesions does not typically show atypia
- Thrombosis (± Masson tumor/change), hemorrhage, and calcifications may be present
    - Especially in venous and cavernous hemangiomas

TOP DIFFERENTIAL DIAGNOSES

- Arteriovenous malformation
- Kaposi sarcoma
- Reactive granulation tissue

Red Papule

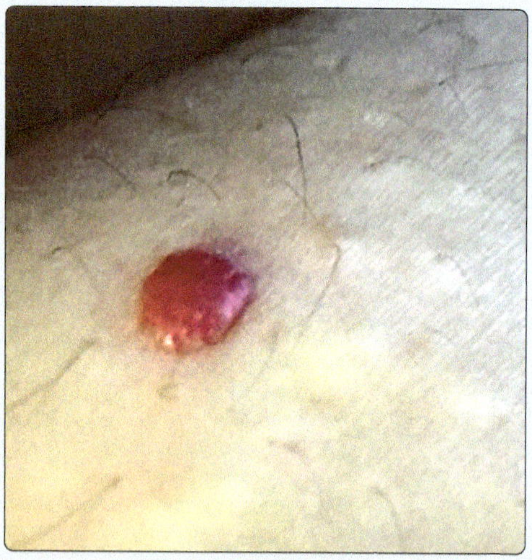

Collarette Formation in Lobular Capillary Hemangioma

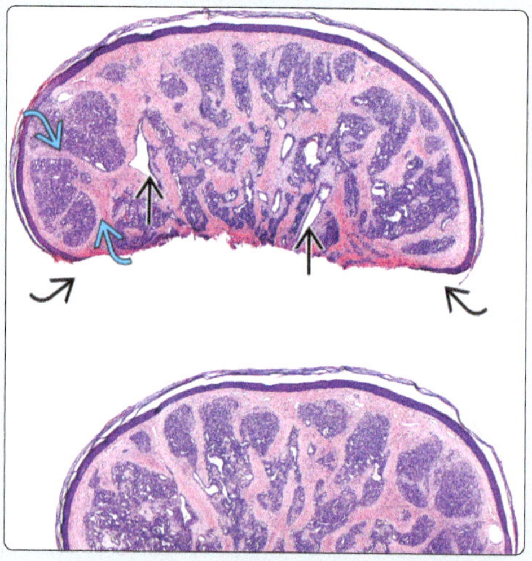

(Left) *Lobular capillary hemangioma is an exophytic bright red papule and may be ulcerated in some lesions.* **(Right)** *On low-power, an exophytic configuration with collarette formation is noted ↗. Note the lobular configuration of blood vessels separated by fibrous septa ↗. Several telangiectatic spaces → are also seen.*

Central Dilated Vessels Lobular Capillary Hemangioma

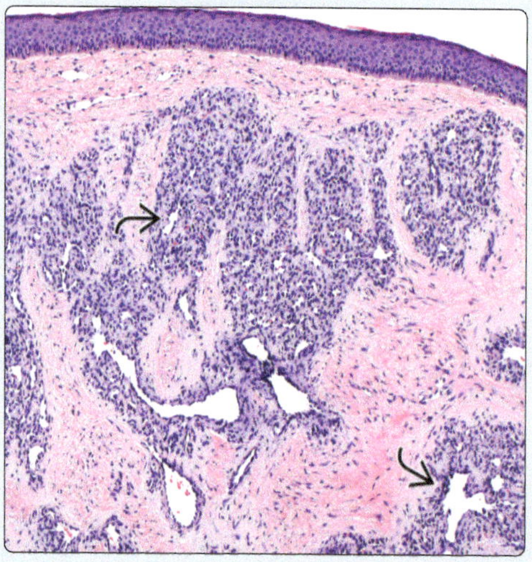

Low Mitotic Activity

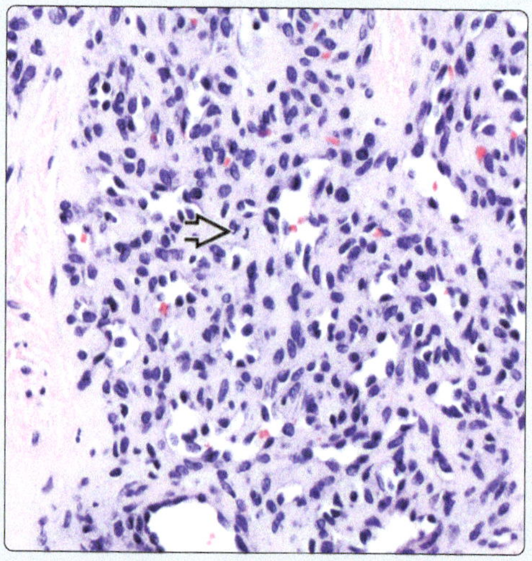

(Left) *The lobules, lacking evident capillary-sized lumina, emanate from central larger and dilated vessels ↗.* **(Right)** *Rare mitotic figures ⇒ in lobular capillary hemangioma should not raise concern for malignancy.*

TERMINOLOGY

Abbreviations

- Lobular capillary hemangioma (LCH)
- Venous hemangioma (VH)
- Cavernous hemangioma (CH)

Synonyms

- LCH also known as pyogenic granuloma

Definitions

- Benign, lobular proliferation of blood vessels of varying cross-sectional diameter lined by plump to flattened endothelial cells without cytological atypia
- Because of capillary histopathology, there are a number of variants classified under capillary hemangioma
  - Can range from acquired elastotic hemangioma to spindle cell hemangioma

ETIOLOGY/PATHOGENESIS

Developmental Anomaly

- Venous hemangiomas may represent vascular malformations
  - Malformation is more appropriate terminology

CLINICAL ISSUES

Epidemiology

- Age
  - LCH or VH: Any age
  - CH: Infants and children; mirrors infantile hemangioma
- Sex
  - Capillary and cavernous hemangiomas in adults occur more commonly in women

Site

- LCH: Head and neck, oral mucous membrane, and limbs
  - Even in gastrointestinal tract and other organs
- VH: Oral mucosa, trunk, and upper extremity
- CH: Head and neck
  - Sinusoidal hemangioma, uncommon variant, can present as subcutaneous nodules on trunk (breast) or limbs of middle-aged women

Presentation

- LCH: Red or bluish nodule, prone to ulceration or bleeding
  - Polypoid friable lesions that bleed easily and are often ulcerated
  - Can be multiple, either disseminated or localized
- VH: Blue, soft nodule to plaque
  - Compressible and fills with dependency
  - Can have segmental distribution
- CH: Red or blue plaque
  - Rarely clinically associated with
    - Consumption coagulopathy (Kasabach-Merritt syndrome)
    - Multiple enchondromas (Maffucci syndrome)
    - Hemangiomas in alimentary tract (blue rubber bleb nevus syndrome)

Natural History

- LCH may or may not undergo complete spontaneous regression
  - Can recur even after shave biopsy
- CH may rapidly involute

Treatment

- Surgical approaches
  - Simple excision for VH or CH are curative
  - LCH treated by shave biopsy

Prognosis

- Excellent for all 3

IMAGING

General Features

- In suspected VH cases, best imaged using T2 MR, especially if extensive

MACROSCOPIC

General Features

- Elevated, nodular, red-purple lesions
- Usually involve skin or subcutaneous tissue
- Discoloration may not be obvious in deep-seated lesions
- Recurrences may be sessile

MICROSCOPIC

Histologic Features

- **Lobular capillary hemangioma**
  - Typically exophytic with collarette formation overlying lobular, dermal tumor
    - Composed of numerous small capillaries, radiating from larger, more central vessels
    - Flat to plump endothelial cells with little or no cytological atypia
  - Surface epithelium may be atrophic or ulcerated
  - Mitotic figures may be present
  - Can be markedly inflamed
  - Rarely, LCH can exist in intravascular location
    - Similar to conventional form minus inflammation
- **Venous hemangioma**
  - Large-caliber, convoluted, and interconnected anomalous venous channels, dissecting surrounding connective tissue
  - Dilated lumen with organized thrombi or phleboliths
  - Masson's papillary endothelial hyperplasia may be observed
  - These abnormally dilated blood vessels have continuous flat endothelium and thin basement membrane
    - Walls have discontinuous media due to foci with relative lack or absence of smooth muscle cells
  - Can closely resemble CH
    - Needs clinicopathologic correlation to resolve this differential diagnosis
- **Cavernous hemangioma**
  - Nonlobular, poorly demarcated proliferation of numerous dilated vessels
  - Large, cystically dilated vessels filled with blood
  - Lined by flat endothelium without cytological atypia

- Organizing thrombi and Masson tumor-like change may be present
- Recanalizing thrombi may create sinusoidal pattern (sinusoidal hemangioma)
- CH, especially its adult variant (sinusoidal hemangioma), can resemble angiosarcoma (AS)
  - AS is more superficial and shows dissection of papillary of reticular collagen
    - AS has infiltrative growth pattern with endothelial atypia, multilayering, and mitoses
  - Sinusoidal hemangioma is typically located in subcutaneous compartment

ANCILLARY TESTS

Immunohistochemistry

- For VH- or CH-like lesions, may consider lymphatic and blood vascular endothelial markers to identify lymphatic &/or vascular components
  - D2-40 (podoplanin) highlights lymphatic spaces
  - CD31 highlights mostly blood vessels but some lymphatic spaces (and some histiocytes)
  - CD34 highlights blood vessels and dermal dendrocytes
- If lesion with VH- or CH-like histopathology shows that lesional vascular spaces are positive for podoplanin, CD31, and CD34, consider venous-lymphatic malformation

Genetic Testing

- Somatic activating *RAS* mutation found in LCH

DIFFERENTIAL DIAGNOSIS

Arteriovenous Malformation

- May mimic venous hemangioma
- Unlike arteriovenous malformations, elastic stain shows absence of internal elastic lamina in venous hemangioma

Kaposi Sarcoma

- Angiomatous form of Kaposi sarcoma may be mistaken for LCH
  - LCH is well circumscribed and shows lobular arrangement
- Spindle cell proliferation with slit-like spaces
- Nuclear immunoreactivity for HHV8

Reactive Granulation Tissue

- Lacks lobular architecture of capillaries seen in LCH
- Vascular proliferation is haphazard

Angiosarcoma

- May resemble sinusoidal hemangioma, especially in breast
- Angiosarcoma shows dissecting pattern with intraparenchymal location

DIAGNOSTIC CHECKLIST

Pathologic Interpretation Pearls

- Lobular architecture of blood vessels is typical of LCH
- Cavernous or venous hemangiomas may show Masson tumor-like changes
  - Look for intravascular thrombi
  - Look for papillary endothelial hyperplasia

SELECTED REFERENCES

1. Lim YH et al: Somatic activating RAS mutations cause vascular tumors including pyogenic granuloma. J Invest Dermatol. 135(6):1698-700, 2015
2. Barrick B et al: Agminated pyogenic granuloma-like growth arising in a congenital hemangioma. JAMA Dermatol. 150(7):781-3, 2014
3. Prates FV et al: Multiple erythematous, shiny papules in a child. Int J Dermatol. 53(12):1423-4, 2014
4. Sammut SJ et al: Pyogenic granuloma as a cutaneous adverse effect of vemurafenib. N Engl J Med. 371(13):1265-7, 2014
5. Martorell-Calatayud A et al: Definition of the features of acquired elastotic hemangioma reporting the clinical and histopathological characteristics of 14 patients. J Cutan Pathol. 37(4):460-4, 2010
6. Dadras SS et al: Angiogenesis and lymphangiogenesis of skin cancers. Hematol Oncol Clin North Am. 18(5):1059-70, viii, 2004
7. Hong YK et al: Lymphatic reprogramming of blood vascular endothelium by Kaposi sarcoma-associated herpesvirus. Nat Genet. 36(7):683-5, 2004
8. Wong CH et al: Blue rubber bleb nevus syndrome: a clinical spectrum with correlation between cutaneous and gastrointestinal manifestations. J Gastroenterol Hepatol. 18(8):1000-2, 2003
9. Maguiness S et al: Kasabach-merritt syndrome. J Cutan Med Surg. 6(4):335-9, 2002
10. Requena L et al: Acquired elastotic hemangioma: A clinicopathologic variant of hemangioma. J Am Acad Dermatol. 47(3):371-6, 2002
11. Jackson R: The natural history of strawberry naevi. J Cutan Med Surg. 2(3):187-9, 1998
12. Coffin CM et al: Vascular tumors in children and adolescents: a clinicopathologic study of 228 tumors in 222 patients. Pathol Annu. 28 Pt 1:97-120, 1993
13. Calonje E et al: Sinusoidal hemangioma. A distinctive benign vascular neoplasm within the group of cavernous hemangiomas. Am J Surg Pathol. 15(12):1130-5, 1991
14. Rutgers JL et al: The expression of endothelial cell surface antigens by AIDS-associated Kaposi's sarcoma. Evidence for a vascular endothelial cell origin. Am J Pathol. 122(3):493-9, 1986
15. Mills SE et al: Lobular capillary hemangioma: the underlying lesion of pyogenic granuloma. A study of 73 cases from the oral and nasal mucous membranes. Am J Surg Pathol. 4(5):470-9, 1980
16. Girard C et al: Arteriovenous hemangioma (arteriovenous shunt). A clinicopathological and histochemical study. J Cutan Pathol. 1(2):73-87, 1974
17. MARTIN LW et al: Hemangiomas in infants and children. Am J Surg. 101:571-80, 1961
18. MACCOLLUM DW et al: Hemangiomas in infancy and childhood; a report based on 6479 cases. Surg Clin North Am. 1647-63, 1956

Cherry Angioma

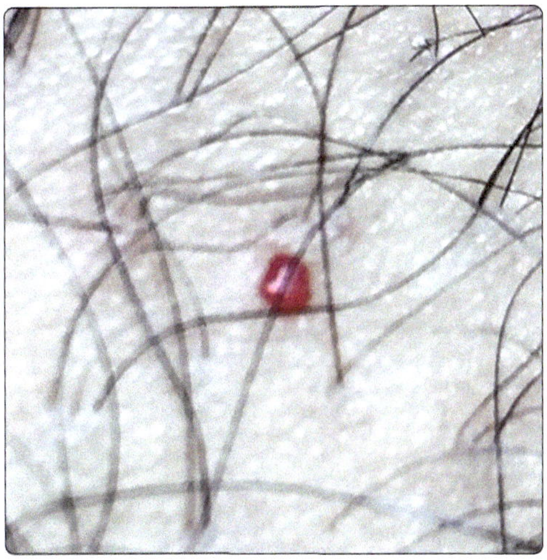

Cherry Angioma, Scanning Magnification

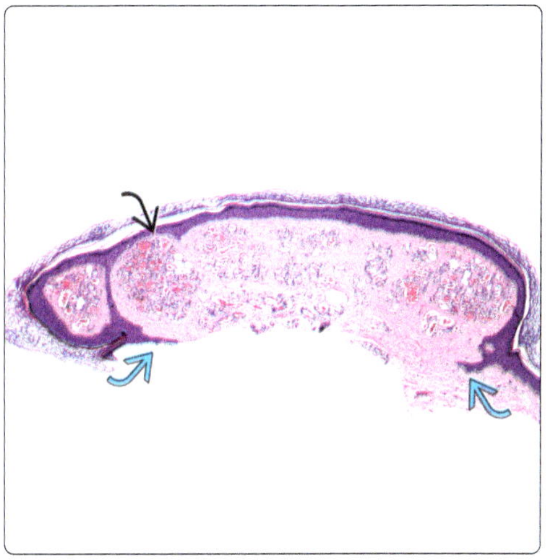

(Left) *A pin-point, 2- to 3-mm, bright red macule or papule is characteristic of cherry angioma.* **(Right)** *Under low-power magnification, lobular configuration* ⇗ *and collarette formation* ⇗ *can resemble a lobular capillary hemangioma (which this may be considered a variant of).*

Capillary-Sized Lobules in Cherry Angioma

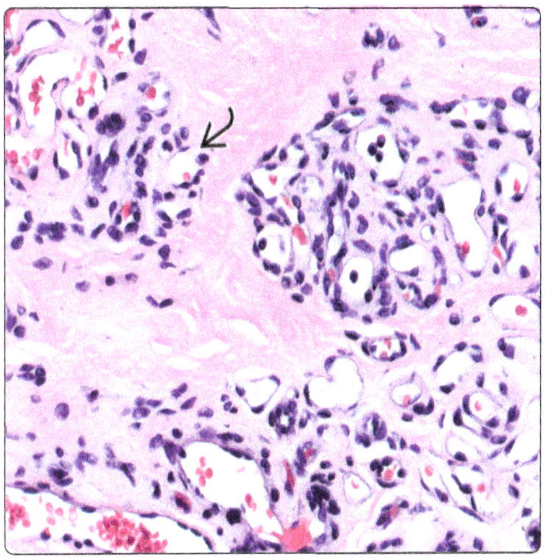

Acquired Elastotic Hemangioma

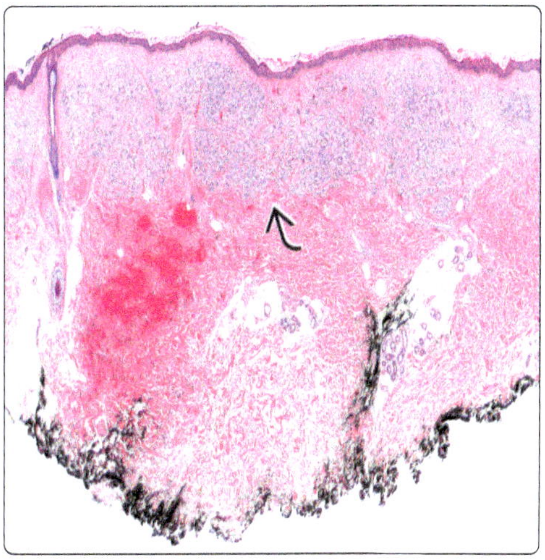

(Left) *Higher magnification shows that widely patent, capillary-sized blood vessels* ⇗ *are evident.* **(Right)** *Low power view shows that acquired elastotic hemangioma is a plaque-like tumor, set in the superficial dermis* ⇗*.*

Acquired Elastotic Hemangioma

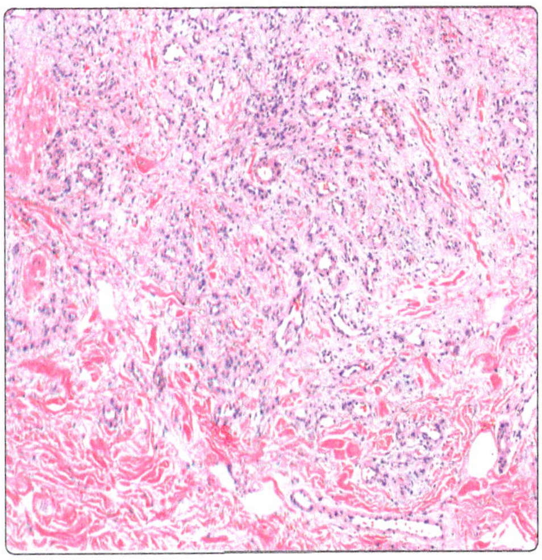

Acquired Elastotic Hemangioma

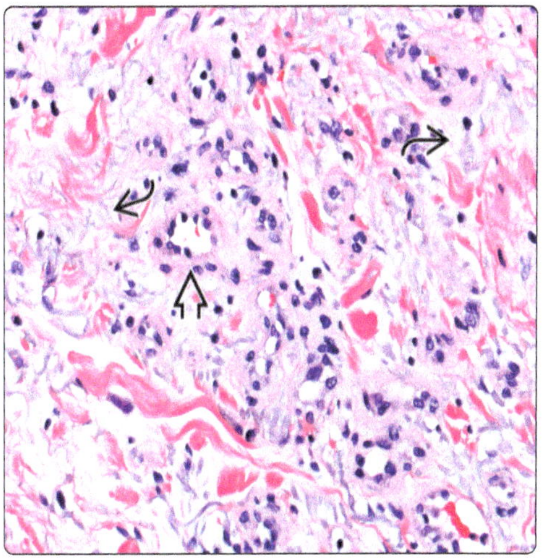

(Left) *Low magnification shows the capillary-sized blood vessels separated by solar elastosis.* **(Right)** *Thick, blue elastotic fibers are evident* ⇗ *among lesional vessels* ⇒ *at higher magnification.*

(Left) *Superficial venous hemangioma can be somewhat papular with a deep dermal component. The tumor is composed of cystically dilated blood-filled vessels.* **(Right)** *The deep dermal component is well circumscribed and noninvasive, coming to close proximity of underlying skeletal muscle.*

Venous Hemangioma

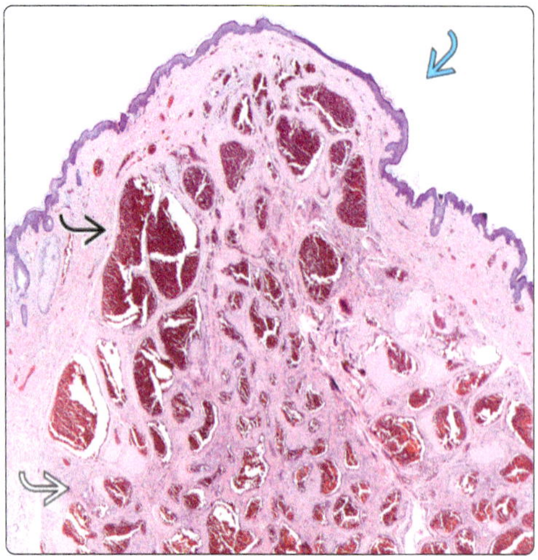

Well-Defined Edge in Venous Hemangioma

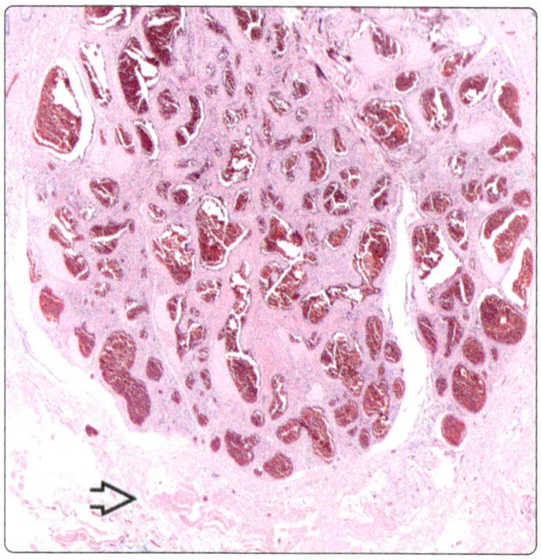

(Left) *High-power examination reveals large-caliber venous structures lined by flat endothelium and filled with blood.* **(Right)** *In a deeper aspect, there is a nodular collection of thick-walled blood vessels. The lack of an internal elastic lamina in these proliferating vessels is helpful in distinguishing a venous hemangioma from arteriovenous (hemangioma) malformation.*

Venous Hemangioma

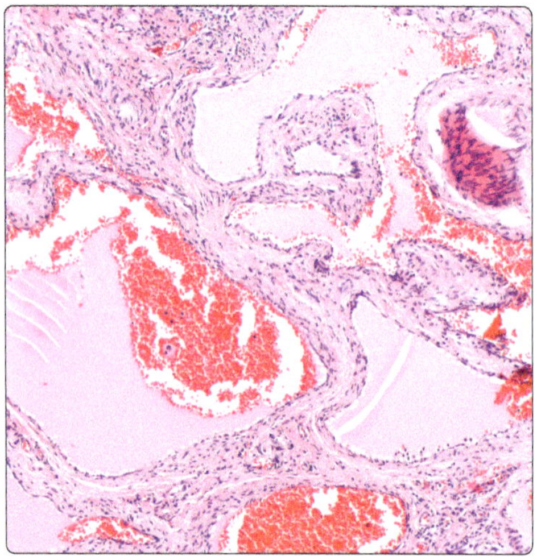

Venous Hemangioma

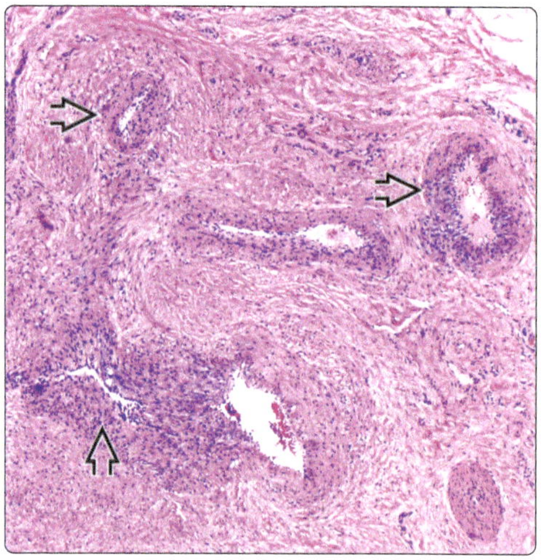

(Left) *The smooth muscle layer surrounding the veins in venous hemangioma may be variable in thickness and not well formed. Cystically dilated veins in venous hemangiomas may mimic a cavernous hemangioma.* **(Right)** *The cut surface of cavernous hemangioma is typically spongy in appearance with cystic spaces of variable size filled with blood. Large, thick-walled blood vessels are seen.*

Venous Hemangioma

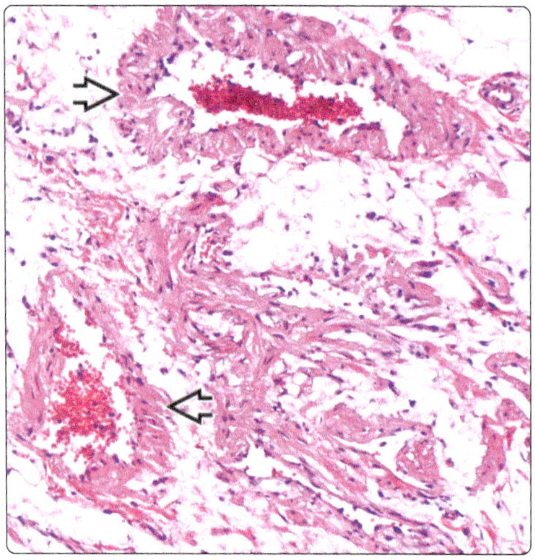

Cavernous Hemangioma Spongy Appearance

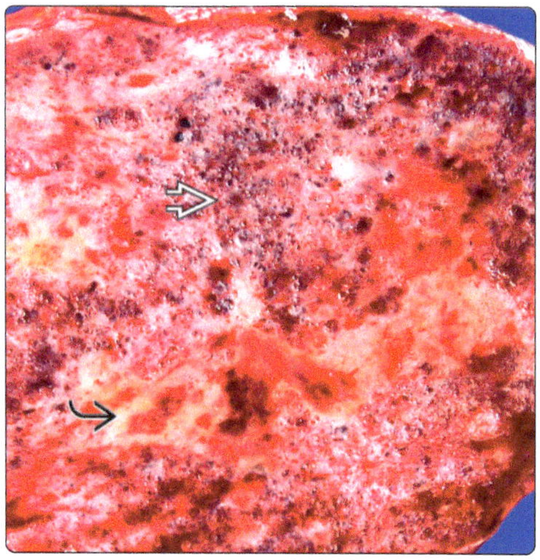

Cavernous Hemangioma

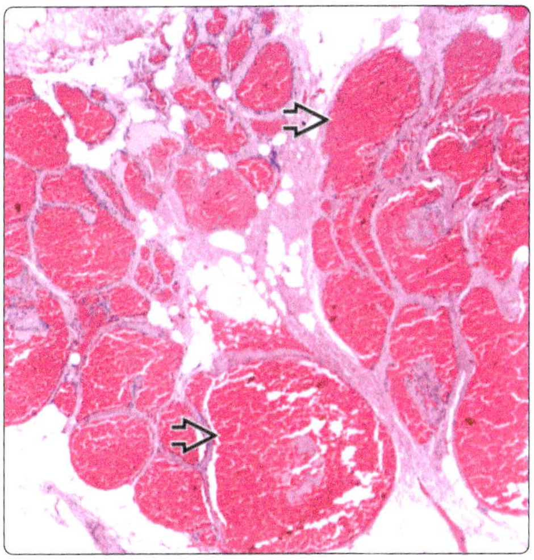

Cavernous Hemangioma

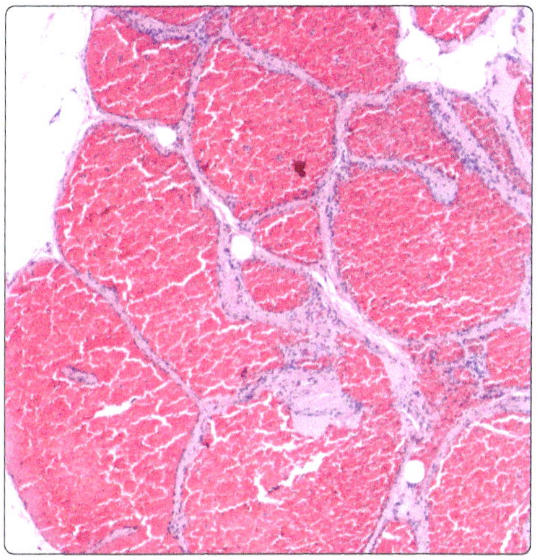

(Left) *Cavernous hemangioma is well-circumscribed, composed of lobules of cystically dilated vascular spaces filled with blood.* **(Right)** *The endothelial cells lining the cystically dilated blood vessels are flat and attenuated in appearance and show no nuclear cytological atypia.*

Cavernous Hemangioma

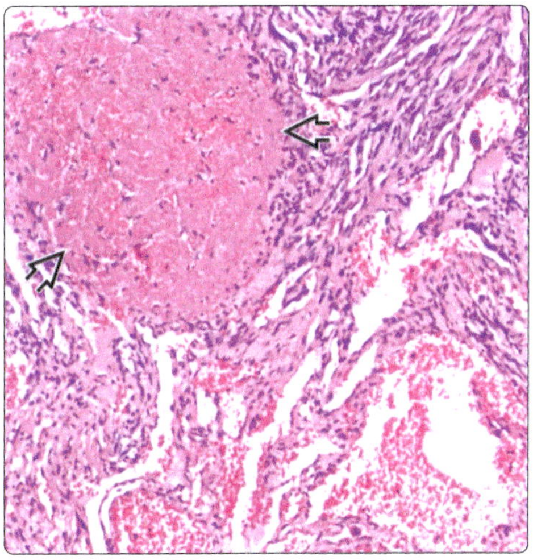

Thrombi Formed in Cavernous Hemangioma

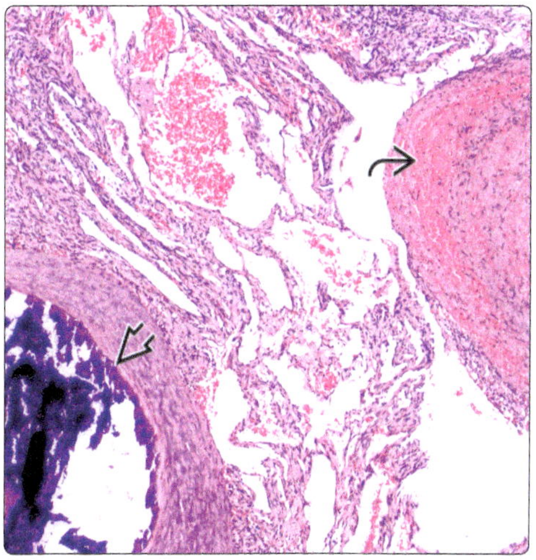

(Left) *Large collections of blood within these cavernous spaces increases predisposition to thrombus formation, which may undergo reorganization to Masson tumor (intravascular papillary endothelial hyperplasia)-like changes.* **(Right)** *Large intralesional thrombi may also undergo calcification and be apparent on imaging studies as phleboliths. A noncalcified thrombus is also present in this example of cavernous hemangioma.*

Sinusoidal Hemangioma

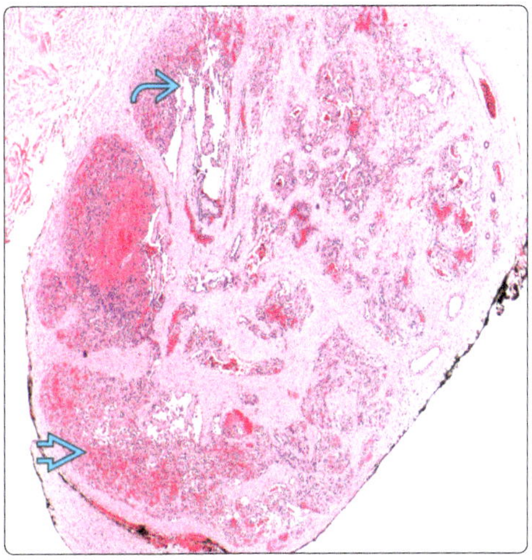

Sinusoidal Hemangioma

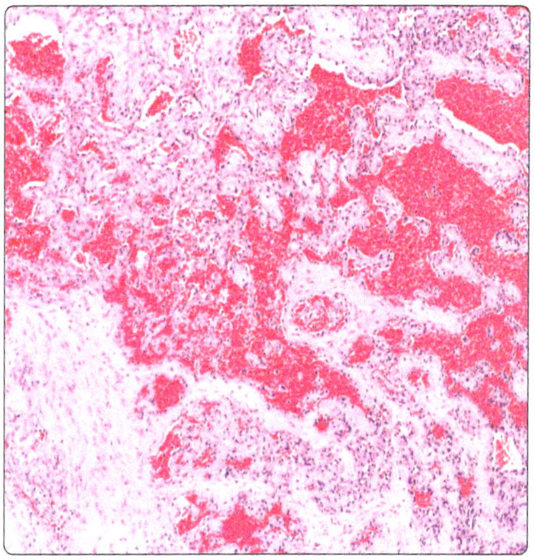

(Left) *The lesion is composed of gaping, markedly dilated, intercommunicating, back-to-back, congested vascular channels with very thin walls, giving rise to a typical sieve-like appearance.* **(Right)** *The intercommunicating, back-to-back, congested vascular channels with very thin walls are evident.*

Infantile (Juvenile) Hemangioma

KEY FACTS

TERMINOLOGY

- Juvenile hemangioma
- Vascular neoplasm of infancy with characteristic onset, rapid growth, and spontaneous involution
- Does not include congenital hemangiomas, as they are clinically, histologically, and immunohistochemically distinct from infantile hemangiomas
- Rapidly involuting congenital hemangioma
- Noninvoluting congenital hemangioma

CLINICAL ISSUES

- Most common tumor of infancy
- Appears within 1st few weeks of life
- Rapidly enlarges over several months
- Hemangiomas typically achieve 80% of their final size by end of early proliferative phase, which occurs at mean age of 3.2 months
- Regresses over several years

MICROSCOPIC

- Multiple lobules composed of tightly packed small- to medium-sized capillaries
- Lobules are separated by normal stroma
- Plump endothelial cells that line small vascular spaces in early lesions
- Progressive interstitial fibrosis in older lesions

ANCILLARY TESTS

- GLUT1 is most useful marker for diagnosis, expressed during all phases of infantile hemangioma
- LYVE-1 is highly expressed during proliferative phase but is decreased during involution

TOP DIFFERENTIAL DIAGNOSES

- Pyogenic granuloma
- Arteriovenous malformation
- Tufted angioma
- Kaposiform hemangioendothelioma

Clinical Photograph

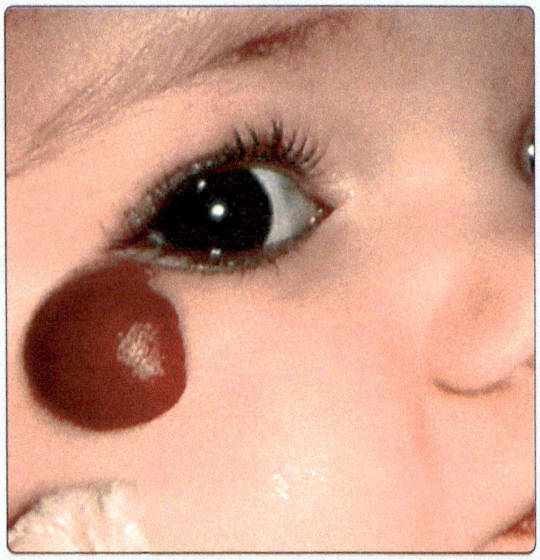

Infantile Hemangioma: Lobular Growth

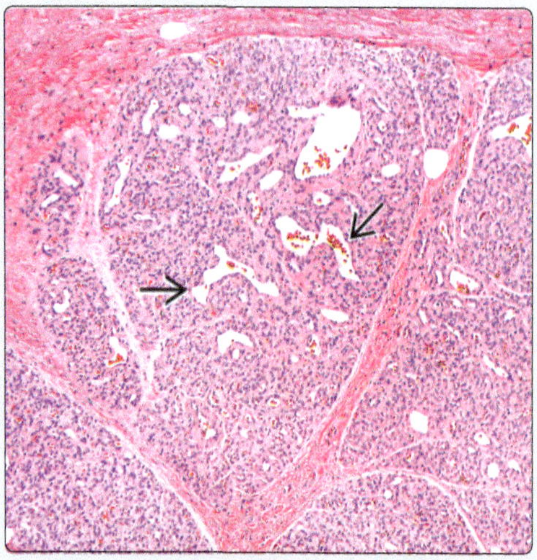

(Left) *Photograph shows a medium-sized infantile hemangioma on the face of a female infant. Most of these lesions are located in the head and neck region. (Courtesy J. Hall, MD.)* **(Right)** *Low-power examination reveals multiple lobules composed of tightly packed capillaries, separated by fibrous septa. Note the scattered, centrally located feeding and draining vessels* ➔.

Facial Infantile Hemangioma

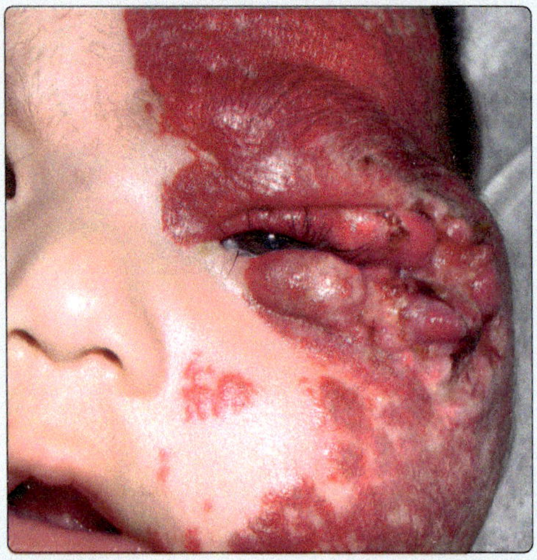

Infantile Hemangioma: Ulcerated

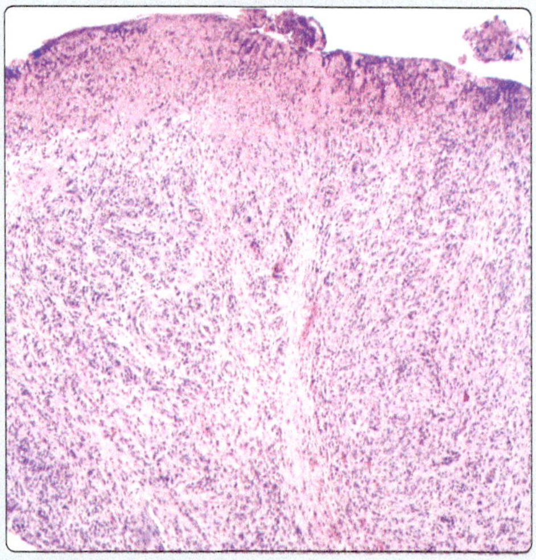

(Left) *Facial infantile hemangioma is seen in a patient with PHACES (posterior fossa malformations, hemangiomas, arterial and cardiac anomalies, eye abnormalities, and sternal cleft raphe). (Courtesy S. Yashar, MD.)* **(Right)** *The skin overlying infantile hemangioma may ulcerate, resembling an inflamed granulation tissue or pyogenic granulomas. The sharp separation between the 2 nodules of proliferating capillaries is a useful diagnostic clue.*

TERMINOLOGY

Synonyms

- Hemangioma of infancy
- Juvenile hemangioma
- Cellular hemangioma of infancy
- Strawberry nevus/hemangioma

Definitions

- Benign proliferations of endothelial tissue; represent most common tumors arising in neonatal period
- Vascular neoplasm of infancy with characteristic onset, rapid growth, and spontaneous involution
- Does not include congenital hemangiomas, as they are clinically, histologically, and immunohistochemically distinct from infantile hemangiomas
  - Both below are negative for GLUT1 and Lewis-Y antigen
    - Rapidly involuting congenital hemangioma
    - Noninvoluting congenital hemangioma

CLINICAL ISSUES

Epidemiology

- Incidence
  - Most common tumor of infancy
  - Affects ~ 4% of children
- Sex
  - F > M
- Ethnicity
  - Caucasians more frequently affected

Site

- Skin and subcutis
  - Head and neck (60%)
  - Extremities, trunk, and genitals
- Viscera

Presentation

- Appears within 1st few weeks after birth
  - Blanched telangiectatic area

Natural History

- Rapidly enlarges over several months
  - Maximum size usually achieved by 6-12 months
- Hemangiomas typically achieve 80% of their final size by end of early proliferative phase
  - Occurs at mean age of 3.2 months
- Regresses over several years
  - 75-90% involute by age 7 years

Treatment

- Options, risks, complications
  - Propranolol
  - Corticosteroids
  - Pulsed dye laser
  - Surgical excision
  - Watchful waiting
    - Small innocuous lesions
  - Interferon-α
    - Restricted to life-threatening lesions
  - Topical imiquimod

Prognosis

- Excellent; all eventually spontaneously regress

MACROSCOPIC

General Features

- Crimson-colored multinodular mass
- Can start out as flat red or purple patch, frequently less than 5 cm in diameter
- Then gradually enlarges and develops raised surface

MICROSCOPIC

Histologic Features

- Multiple lobules composed of tightly packed small- to medium-sized capillaries
- Early lesions
  - Plump endothelial cells that line small vascular spaces
  - Inconspicuous vascular lumina
  - Distinct lobules separated by normal stroma
  - Moderate mitotic activity and scattered mast cells
- Mature lesions
  - Small vessels lined by flattened endothelial cells
  - Zonal maturation begins at periphery
- Regressing lesions
  - Progressive and diffuse interstitial fibrosis
  - Increased apoptotic bodies and mast cells
- End-stage lesions
  - Scattered residual vessels
  - Fibrofatty background

Predominant Cell/Compartment Type

- By immunohistochemistry and electron microscopy, tumor lobule is composed of
  - Endothelial cells
  - Pericytic cells
  - Fibroblasts
  - Mast cells

ANCILLARY TESTS

Immunohistochemistry

- Shares unique immunoprofile with placental vasculature by expressing (absent in cutaneous vasculature)
  - GLUT1 (expressed during all 3 phases of infantile hemangioma)
    - GLUT1 is also positive in hepatic infantile hemangioma but negative in hepatic vascular malformations
    - Helpful in classifying hepatic vascular lesions in pediatric patients
  - FcgammaRII
  - Lewis-Y antigen
  - Merosin
- Endothelial cells express LYVE-1 during proliferative phase
- Lesional vessels and tumor are negative for PROX1
  - Look for PROX1(+) lymphatic endothelial nuclei as internal positive control
  - PROX1 negativity is in contrast to kaposiform hemangioendothelioma/tufted angioma
    - Helps resolve differential diagnosis of infantile hemangioma and kaposiform hemangioendothelioma/tufted angioma

Immunohistochemical Profile

Antibody	Reactivity	Staining Pattern	Comment
VEGF	Positive	Cytoplasmic	Intense staining in early lesions
CD31	Positive	Cell membrane	Lost after fully involuted
CD34	Positive	Cell membrane	Lost after fully involuted
Actin-sm	Positive	Cytoplasmic	Stains pericytes
FVIIIRAg	Positive	Cell membrane & cytoplasm	Lost after fully involuted
GLUT1	Positive	Cell membrane	Not expressed in other vascular neoplasms, expressed during all phases
LYVE-1	Positive	Cell membrane	Expresses during proliferative phase and not involution
PROX1	Negative	Nuclear & cytoplasmic	Distinguishes IH from KHE/TA

IH = infantile hemangioma; KHE = kaposiform hemangioendothelioma; TA = tufted angioma.

DIFFERENTIAL DIAGNOSIS

Pyogenic Granuloma

- Another type of lobular capillary hemangioma
- Polypoid red mass surrounded by epidermal collarette
- Nodules of small capillaries subserved by feeder vessel

Arteriovenous Malformation

- Dilated, often thick-walled vessels within papillary and reticular dermis
  - May resemble infantile hemangioma during involution

Tufted Angioma

- Small capillaries in prominent clustered or cannonball pattern
- Peripheral, dilated, and crescent-shaped vessels
  - Shares many histological and immunohistochemical features with kaposiform hemangioendothelioma
- Endothelial nuclei are positive for PROX1

Granulation Tissue

- Fibroblastic stromal cells and collagenous matrix with small capillaries and inflammatory cells
- Haphazard proliferation of blood vessels and even some lymphatics

Kaposiform Hemangioendothelioma

- Infiltrating sheets of slender spindled endothelial cells
- Peripheral, dilated, and crescent-shaped vessels
- Endothelial nuclei are positive for PROX1

DIAGNOSTIC CHECKLIST

Clinically Relevant Pathologic Features

- Presence of ulceration does not denote malignancy
- Normal-appearing mitoses are expected during proliferative phase
  - Mitoses should not raise suspicion for malignancy
- Finding of perineural invasion (rare) does not equal malignancy

Pathologic Interpretation Pearls

- When in proliferative phase, presence of expansile lobules is helpful
- Presence of feeding and draining blood vessels

SELECTED REFERENCES

1. Léauté-Labrèze C et al: A randomized, controlled trial of oral propranolol in infantile hemangioma. N Engl J Med. 372(8):735-46, 2015
2. Lee PW et al: Characteristics of noninvoluting congenital hemangioma: a retrospective review. J Am Acad Dermatol. 70(5):899-903, 2014
3. Liang MG et al: Infantile and congenital hemangiomas. Semin Pediatr Surg. 23(4):162-7, 2014
4. Munden A et al: Prospective study of infantile haemangiomas: incidence, clinical characteristics and association with placental anomalies. Br J Dermatol. 170(4):907-13, 2014
5. Prey S et al: Mast cells as possible targets of propranolol therapy: an immunohistological study of beta-adrenergic receptors in infantile haemangiomas. Histopathology. 65(3):436-9, 2014
6. Le Huu AR et al: Expression of prox1, lymphatic endothelial nuclear transcription factor, in Kaposiform hemangioendothelioma and tufted angioma. Am J Surg Pathol. 34(11):1563-73, 2010
7. Suh KY et al: Infantile hemangiomas with minimal or arrested growth: a retrospective case series. Arch Dermatol. 146(9):971-6, 2010
8. Toledo-Alberola F et al: Abortive hemangiomas. Description of clinical and pathological findings with special emphasis on dermoscopy. Eur J Dermatol. 20(4):497-500, 2010
9. Corella F et al: Abortive or minimal-growth hemangiomas: Immunohistochemical evidence that they represent true infantile hemangiomas. J Am Acad Dermatol. 58(4):685-90, 2008
10. North PE et al: Vascular tumors of infancy and childhood: beyond capillary hemangioma. Cardiovasc Pathol. 15(6):303-17, 2006
11. Dadras SS et al: Infantile hemangiomas are arrested in an early developmental vascular differentiation state. Mod Pathol. 17(9):1068-79, 2004
12. Mo JQ et al: GLUT1 endothelial reactivity distinguishes hepatic infantile hemangioma from congenital hepatic vascular malformation with associated capillary proliferation. Hum Pathol. 35(2):200-9, 2004
13. North PE et al: A unique microvascular phenotype shared by juvenile hemangiomas and human placenta. Arch Dermatol. 137(5):559-70, 2001
14. North PE et al: GLUT1: a newly discovered immunohistochemical marker for juvenile hemangiomas. Hum Pathol. 31(1):11-22, 2000
15. Calonje E et al: Pseudomalignant perineurial invasion in cellular ('infantile') capillary haemangiomas. Histopathology. 26(2):159-64, 1995
16. Gonzalez-Crussi F et al: Cellular hemangiomas ("hemangioendotheliomas") in infants. Light microscopic, immunohistochemical, and ultrastructural observations. Am J Surg Pathol. 15(8):769-78, 1991
17. MACCOLLUM DW et al: Hemangiomas in infancy and childhood; a report based on 6479 cases. Surg Clin North Am. 1647-63, 1956

Submucosal Infantile Hemangioma: Proliferative Phase

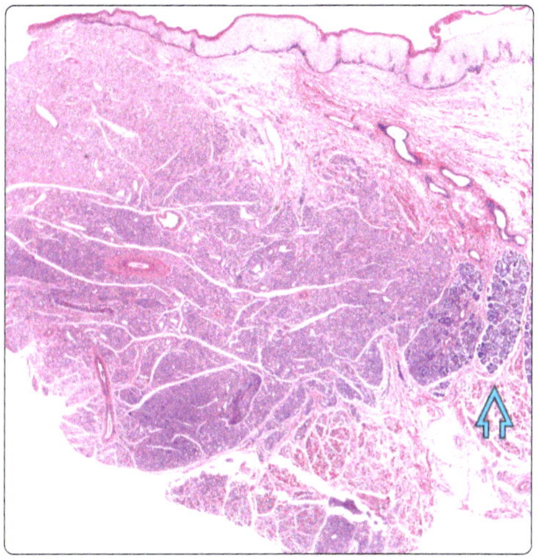

Submucosal Infantile Hemangioma: Proliferative Phase

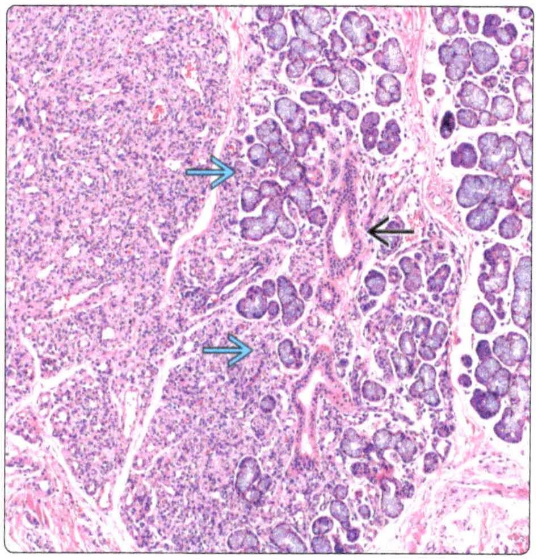

(Left) *Submucosal infantile hemangioma shows expansive, lobular proliferation of tightly packed capillary-size vessels. Mucous salivary glands are seen to the lower right.* **(Right)** *Focally, the lesional vessels infiltrate the in between salivary glands. The mucinous acini and salivary ducts remain intact.*

Submucosal Infantile Hemangioma: Proliferative Phase

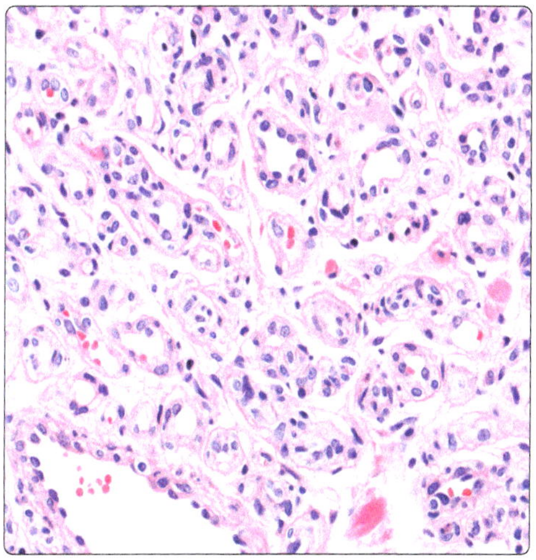

Infantile Hemangioma: Proliferative Phase, Spanning Dermis

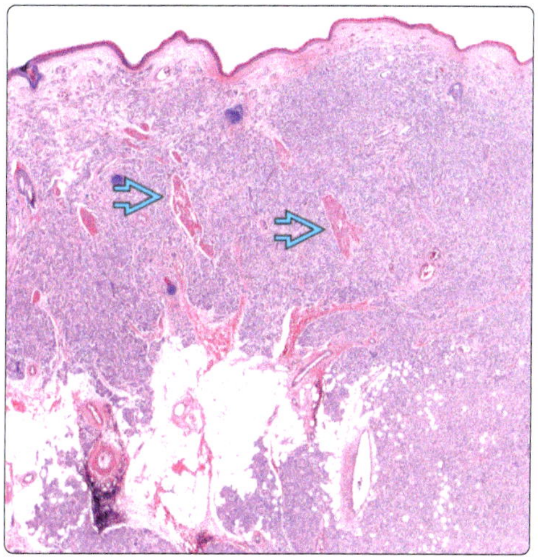

(Left) *Higher power examination shows capillary-sized blood vessels within a lobule lined by plump endothelial cells in this infantile hemangioma in proliferative phase.* **(Right)** *Another example of infantile hemangioma in the proliferative phase spans the facial dermal skin. The lesional vessels extend from the superficial dermis to the subcutis, sparing pilar muscles.*

Infantile Hemangioma: Proliferative Phase

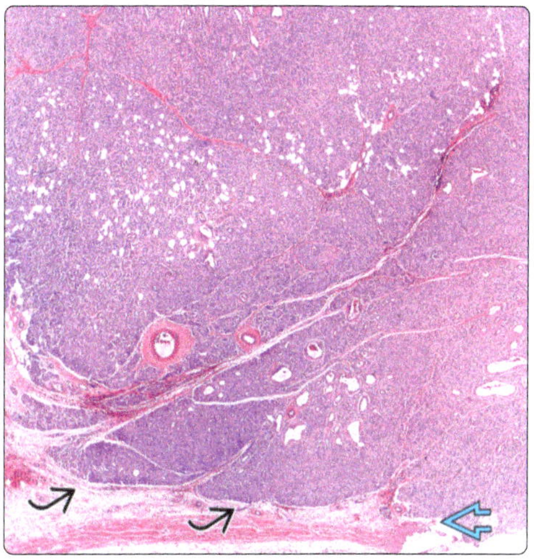

Infantile Hemangioma: Proliferative Phase at Intermediate Magnification

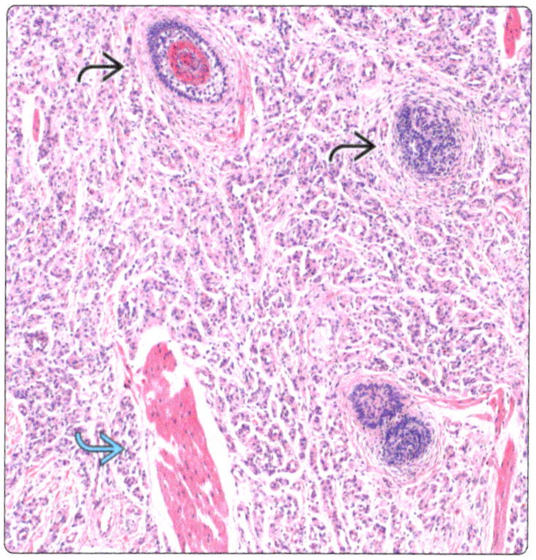

(Left) *Low magnification shows the same lesion with deep extension of the tumor abutting the skeletal muscle layer. Note the well-circumscribed tumor edge.* **(Right)** *The adnexa and pilar muscle bundles are preserved in this intermediate-power image.*

(Left) *Well-defined lobules delineated by fibrous septa are characteristic for infantile hemangioma. Note the feeding and draining vessels within the lobules.* **(Right)** *The lesional vessels wrap around a nerve bundle in infantile hemangioma, proliferative phase.*

Infantile Hemangioma: Proliferative Phase at Higher Magnification

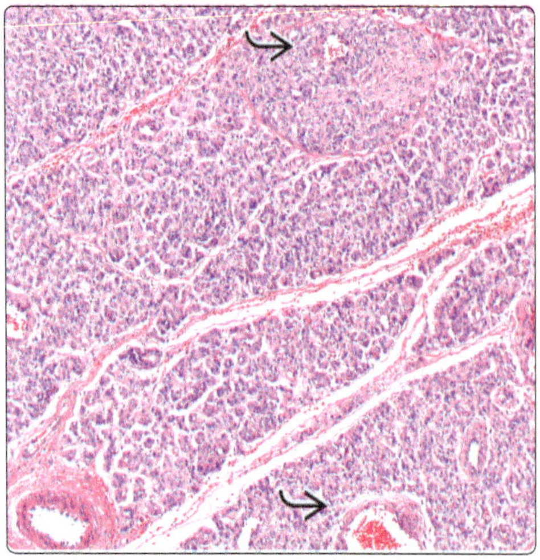

Pseudomalignant Perineural Invasion in Infantile Hemangioma

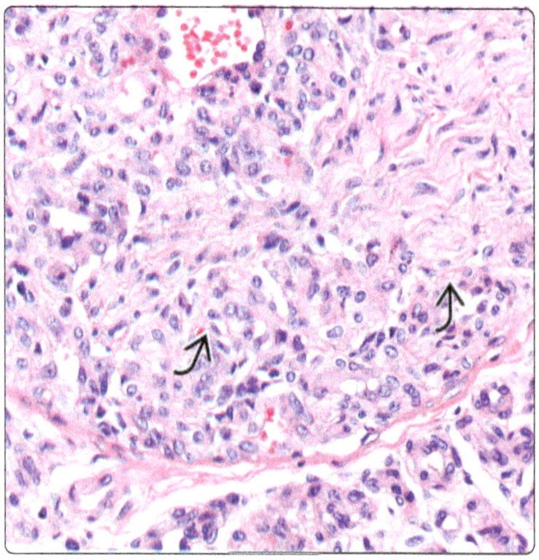

(Left) *Immunofluorescence using anti-LYVE-1 antibody shows marked expression (red) in the lobules of an infantile hemangioma in the proliferating phase.* **(Right)** *During involution, the lobules of plump capillaries are replaced by fibrofatty residuum. Feeding and draining vessels remain. These are too large and superficial to be the nascent arteries/veins at this site.*

LYVE-1 Expression in Infantile Hemangioma: Proliferative Phase

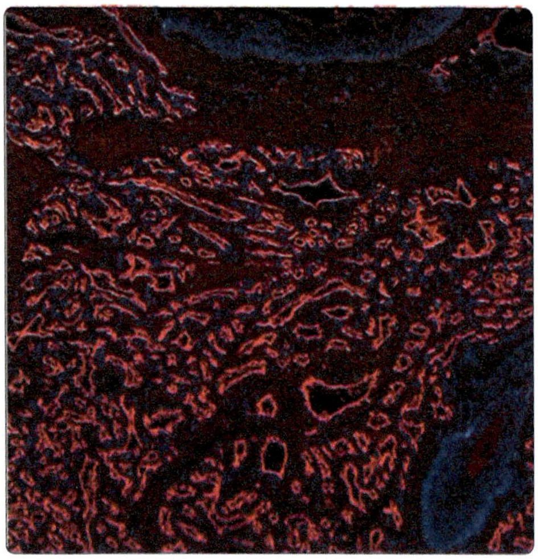

Involuting Infantile Hemangioma

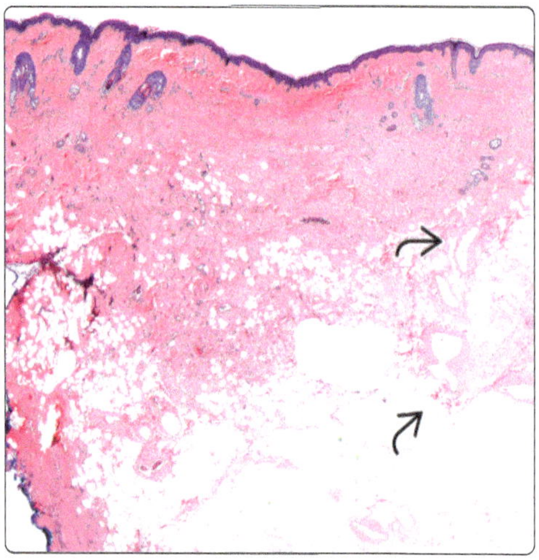

(Left) *A closer examination shows the residual capillary-sized lesional vessels in between adipose tissue and skeletal muscle.* **(Right)** *Larger caliber feeding and draining vessels are evident among the fibroadipose tissue residuum.*

Involuting Infantile Hemangioma

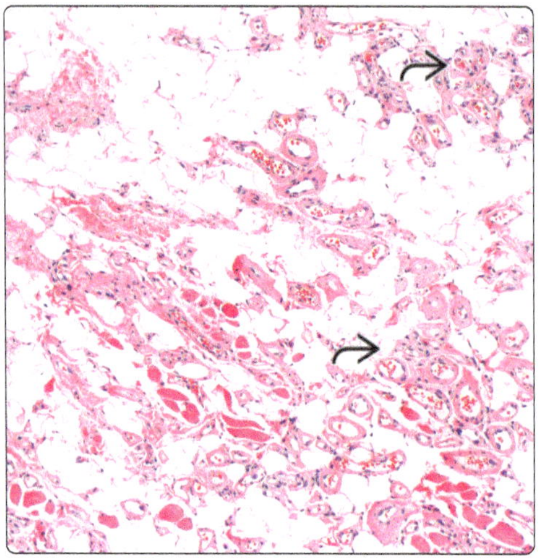

Involuting Infantile Hemangioma

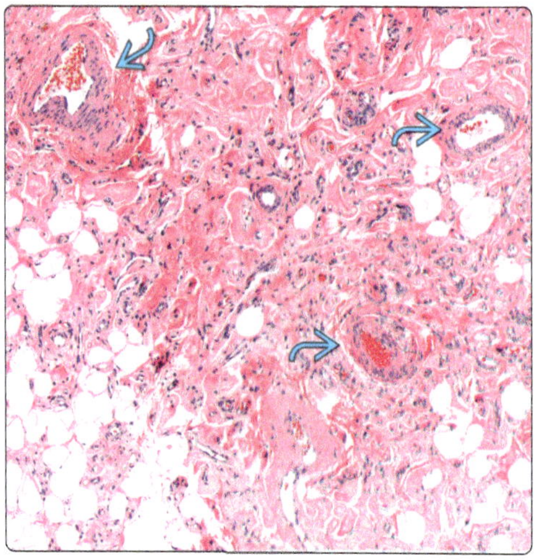

Involuting Infantile Hemangioma: Mast Cells

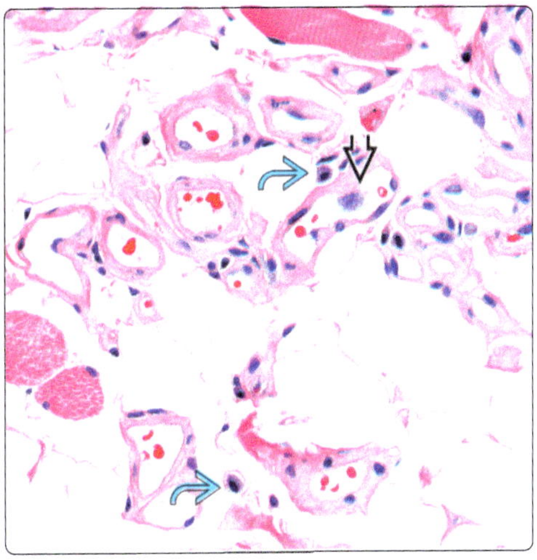

GLUT1 in Involuting Infantile Hemangioma

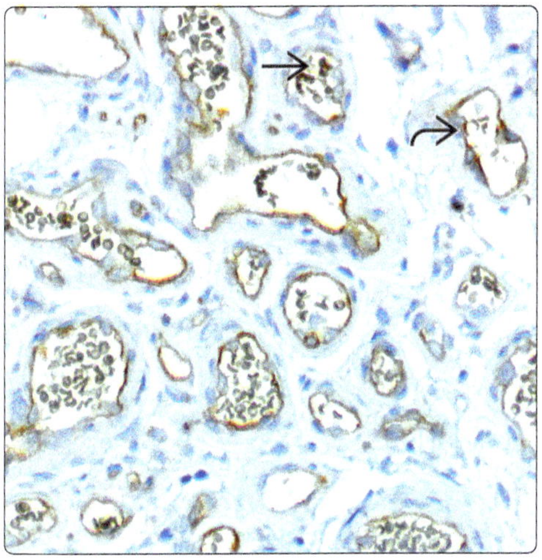

(Left) *Lone capillary-sized vessels remain showing some cytological atypia of endothelial nuclei related to senescence* ➙. *Mast cells* ➙ *are seen during the involution.* **(Right)** *Immunostaining confirms the presence of GLUT1(+) endothelial cells lining the residual lesional vessels* ➙ *in this involuting infantile hemangioma. Note that LYVE-1 expression (not shown) is decreased during involution. Note that the glucose transporter is normally expressed on the erythrocyte membrane* ➙. *This is not overstaining.*

Infantile Hemangioma: Proliferative Phase at Low Magnification

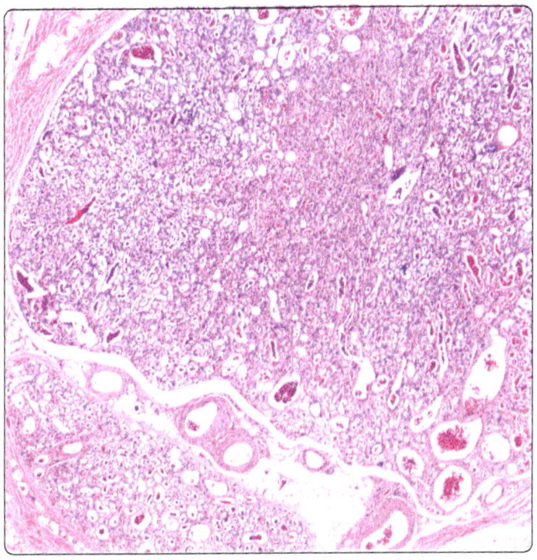

Infantile Hemangioma: Proliferative Phase at Higher Magnification

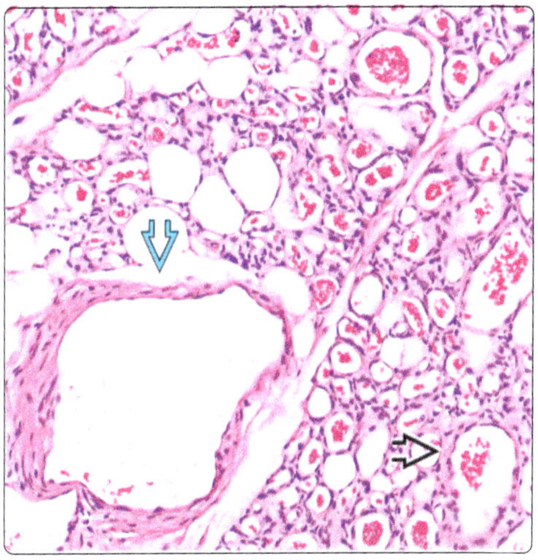

(Left) *Another example of infantile hemangioma in proliferative phase shows the well-circumscribed lobules composed of capillary-sized vessels with variable lumina.* **(Right)** *Each lobule is supplied by a large feeder vessel* ➙ *and drained by draining vessels* ➙. *The capillary lumina may be inconspicuous in early lesions but become more apparent as the lesion matures.*

Infantile Hemangioma: Proliferative Phase at High Magnification

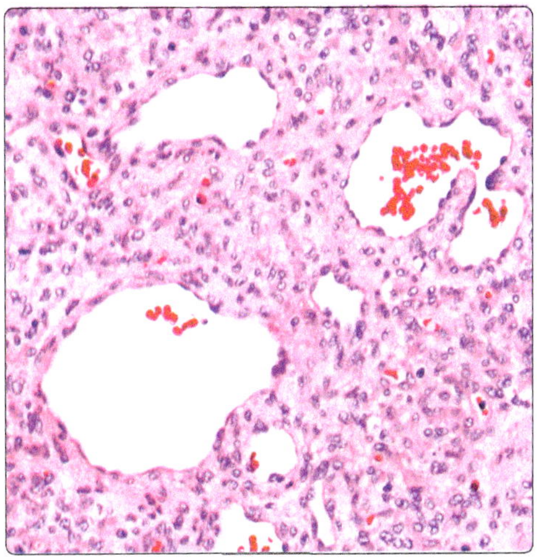

Cellular Area in Infantile Hemangioma: Proliferative Phase

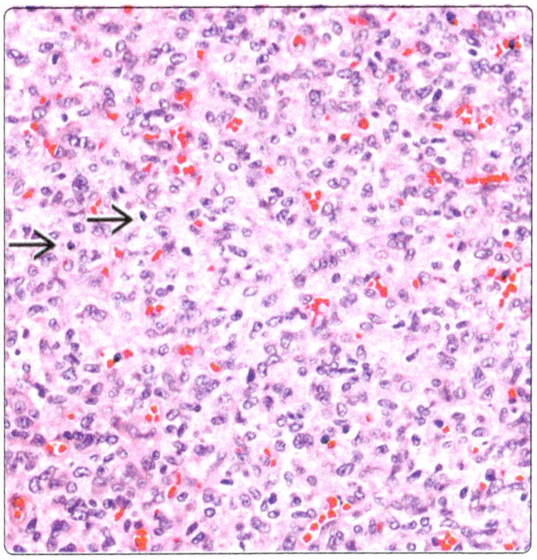

(Left) *The central feeding vessels with dilated lumina lined by flattened endothelial cells are shown.* **(Right)** *Early lesions, as illustrated, are composed of plump endothelial cells with inconspicuous vascular lumina. Numerous mitoses may also be present* ➙.

KEY FACTS

TERMINOLOGY
- Sinusoidal hemangioma
- Cavernous hemangioma (variant)
- Acquired vascular lesion in adults; features similar to venous malformation

CLINICAL ISSUES
- Rare lesions
- Typically occur in adults, more common in females
- Present as painless bluish or red nodule
  - Subcutaneous or dermal mass
- Excellent prognosis, no malignant potential
- Complete excision is curative but not necessary given benign nature of lesions

MICROSCOPIC
- Well-circumscribed vascular proliferation
- Vessels are thin-walled and closely packed, with little intervening stroma
- Lining cells are small endothelial cells with nuclear hyperchromasia
- Pseudopapillary pattern may be seen (due to tangential sectioning)
- Mitotic figures typically not seen
- Thrombosis may occur and be associated with intravascular papillary endothelial hyperplasia (Masson tumor/change)
- Calcifications rarely seen

TOP DIFFERENTIAL DIAGNOSES
- Arteriovenous hemangioma (malformation)
  - Usually occurs on lips, perioral skin, or nose of older adult males
- Venous malformation (cavernous hemangioma)
  - Occurs in children, usually present at birth
- Cherry angioma
  - Much more common, small superficial lesions occurring in adults
- Glomeruloid hemangioma

Sinusoidal Hemangioma in Superficial Dermis

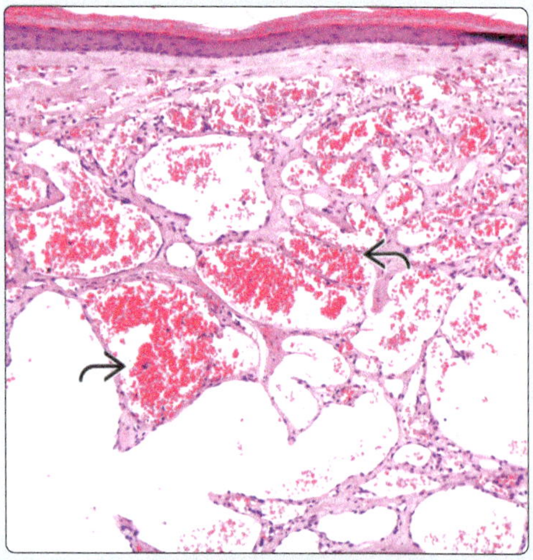

Sinusoidal Hemangioma With Dilated Vascular Spaces

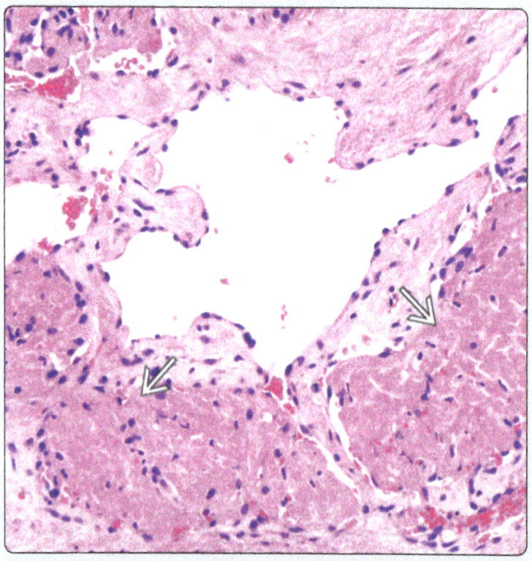

(Left) *Low-magnification histologic examination shows the superficial portion of a cutaneous sinusoidal hemangioma (SH) involving the papillary and reticular dermis with large, dilated vascular spaces, some of which are filled with red blood cells* ➩. **(Right)** *Higher magnification shows sinusoidal vascular spaces with large areas of thrombosis* ➡, *a finding often seen in SH.*

Sinusoidal Hemangioma With Thrombosis

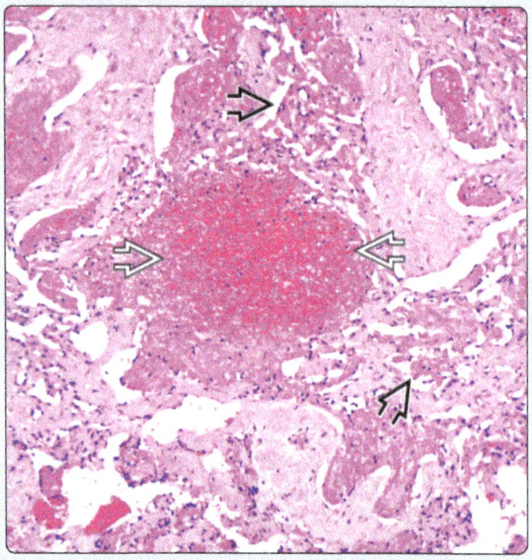

Sinusoidal Hemangioma: Cytologic Features

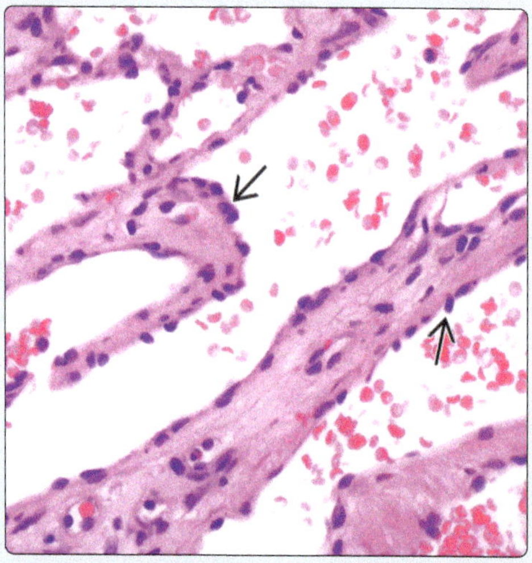

(Left) *Another example of an SH shows hemorrhage and thrombosis* ➡ *with adjacent areas of papillary endothelial hyperplasia (Masson change)* ➩. **(Right)** *High-magnification examination demonstrates the cytologic features of the endothelial cells, which show small, uniform-appearing round to oval nuclei with hyperchromasia* ➩.

TERMINOLOGY

Abbreviations

- Sinusoidal hemangioma

Synonyms

- Cavernous hemangioma (variant)

Definitions

- Acquired vascular lesion in adults; features similar to cavernous hemangioma/venous malformation

ETIOLOGY/PATHOGENESIS

Unknown

- May represent reactive vascular proliferation rather than true neoplastic process

CLINICAL ISSUES

Epidemiology

- Incidence
    - Rare
- Age
    - Typically occurs in adults
- Sex
    - More common in females

Site

- Often occurs on extremities, trunk, or breast

Presentation

- Subcutaneous or dermal mass
    - Solitary, painless, bluish (deep) or red (superficial) nodule
        - Freely movable

Treatment

- Surgical approaches
    - Complete excision is curative, but not necessary given benign nature of lesions

Prognosis

- Excellent, no malignant potential

MACROSCOPIC

Size

- Typically < 2.0 cm

MICROSCOPIC

Histologic Features

- Proliferation of numerous thin-walled anastomosing vessels
    - Well-circumscribed proliferation of vessels in sinusoidal pattern
    - Vessels are thin-walled and closely packed, with little intervening stroma
        - Occasional cases may show smooth muscle in vessel walls
        - Pseudopapillary pattern may be seen (due to tangential sectioning)
        - Thrombosis may occur and be associated with intravascular papillary endothelial hyperplasia (Masson tumor)
    - Lining cells are small endothelial cells with nuclear hyperchromasia
    - Mitotic figures typically not seen
    - Calcifications may rarely be present

Cytologic Features

- Nuclei are hyperchromatic but show regular borders and uniform chromatin

DIFFERENTIAL DIAGNOSIS

Arteriovenous Hemangioma (Malformation)

- Typically occurs on lips, perioral skin, or nose of older adult males
- Proliferation of large, thick-walled blood vessels with smooth muscle in their walls, which mostly represent veins
- Feeder vessel (ascending muscular artery) may be present in some cases

Venous Malformation (Cavernous Hemangioma)

- Occurs in children, usually present at birth
- Often larger and more poorly circumscribed than sinusoidal hemangioma
- Does not show as closely packed vessels or ramified pattern

Cherry Angioma

- Very common, small papular lesions occurring in adults
- Superficial papillary dermal lesions, as opposed to sinusoidal hemangioma (which is typically deep dermal or subcutaneous)

Glomeruloid Hemangioma

- Associated with Castleman syndrome and polyneuropathy, organomegaly, endocrinopathy, monoclonal paraproteinemia, and skin lesions (POEMS) syndrome
- Typically present as multiple, eruptive lesions on trunk and limbs
- Dilated vascular spaces filled by grape-like clusters of capillaries, reminiscent of renal glomeruli

DIAGNOSTIC CHECKLIST

Pathologic Interpretation Pearls

- Closely packed lobular proliferation of vessels in deep dermis or subcutis

SELECTED REFERENCES

1. Park K et al: Sinusoidal haemangioma: are ultrasonographic features helpful? Clin Exp Dermatol. 40(6):691-4, 2015
2. Song BH et al: A case of sinusoidal hemangioma with lipoma. Ann Dermatol. 23(Suppl 2):S250-3, 2011
3. Ban M et al: Giant sinusoidal hemangioma revealing diffuse ancient change: hyalinization and organized thrombi. Int J Dermatol. 49(5):589-90, 2010
4. Nakamura M et al: Calcifying sinusoidal haemangioma on the back. Br J Dermatol. 141(2):377-8, 1999
5. Calonje E et al: New entities in cutaneous soft tissue tumours. Pathologica. 85(1095):1-15, 1993
6. Calonje E et al: Sinusoidal hemangioma. A distinctive benign vascular neoplasm within the group of cavernous hemangiomas. Am J Surg Pathol. 15(12):1130-5, 1991

Tufted Angioma

KEY FACTS

TERMINOLOGY

- Acquired tufted angioma
- Angioblastoma (of Nakagawa)
- Multiple cannonball-like cellular collections of small vessels in dermis

ETIOLOGY/PATHOGENESIS

- Most cases sporadic; rare familial case described

CLINICAL ISSUES

- Rare tumors
- Occur in children and young adults
- Slowly growing erythematous macules and plaques
- May be associated with Kasabach-Merritt syndrome

MACROSCOPIC

- Reddish-brown nonencapsulated dermal lesion
- Typically small papules but may be large plaque

MICROSCOPIC

- Scattered lobular collections of small capillary-type vessels throughout dermis; may involve subcutis
- Have typical **cannonball appearance** at low-power examination
- Cleft-like lumina often present around capillary tufts; may impart glomeruloid appearance
- Cells are oval to spindle-shaped
- Mitoses may be present, but cells lack significant cytologic atypia
- Hemosiderin deposition may be seen

TOP DIFFERENTIAL DIAGNOSES

- Glomeruloid hemangioma
- Infantile (juvenile) hemangioma
- Lobular capillary hemangioma
- Targetoid hemosiderotic hemangioma (hobnail hemangioma)
- Kaposi sarcoma

Acquired Tufted Angioma at Scanning Magnification

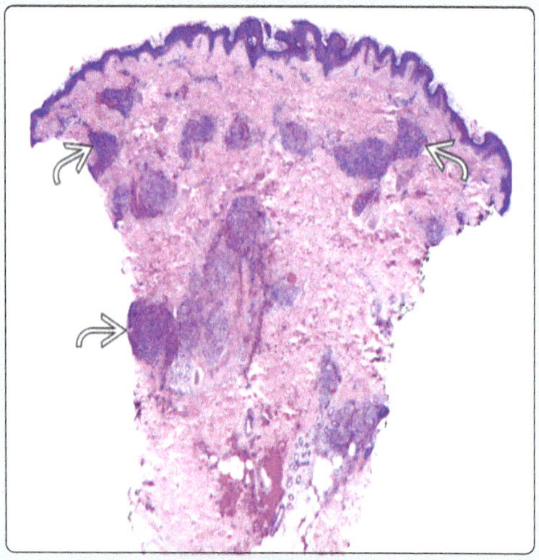

Acquired Tufted Angioma: Lobular Cluster of Vessels

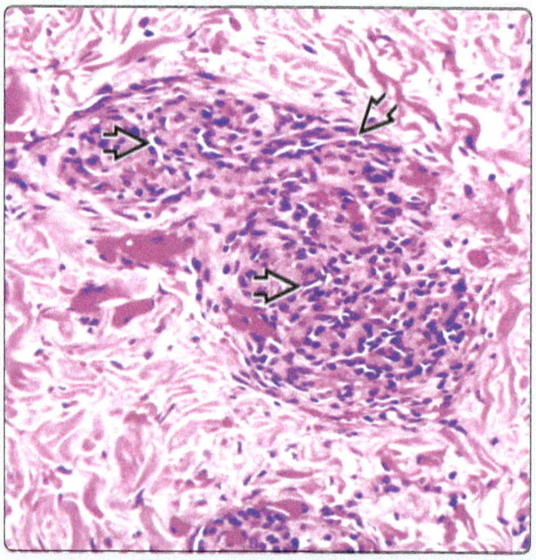

(Left) *Scanning magnification of acquired tufted angioma (ATA) shows scattered lobular collections of vessels ➡ in the superficial and deep dermis. The lobules bulge into dilated vessels, with a few peripheral semilunar spaces identified.* **(Right)** *Higher magnification of ATA shows a lobular cluster of blood vessels lined by small, oval to spindle-shaped cells. Lumina are collapsed and slit-like ➡.*

Acquired Tufted Angioma at High Magnification

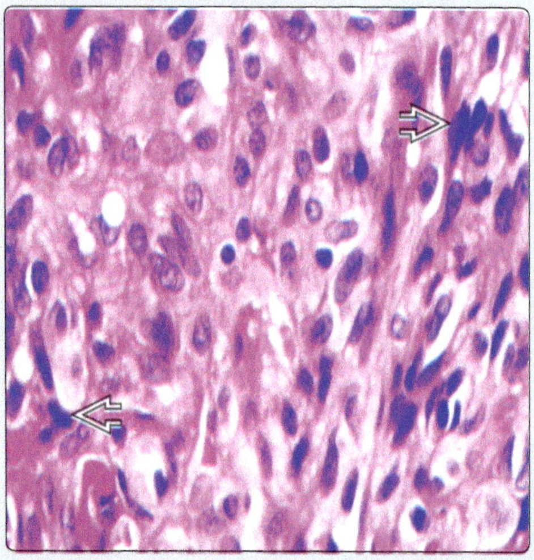

Acquired Tufted Angioma at Low Magnification

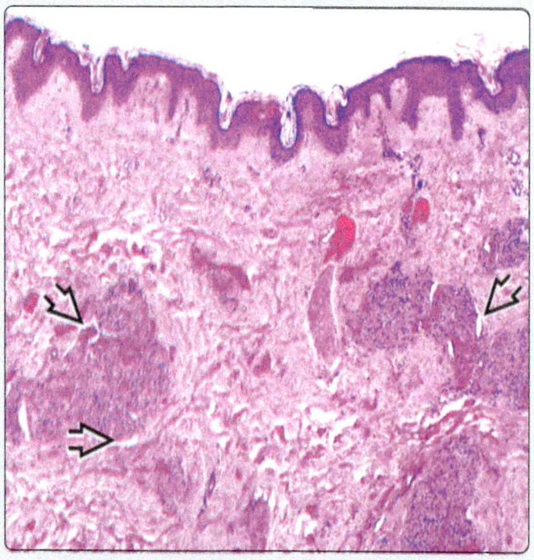

(Left) *High-power view shows bland cytologic features of the tufted angioma endothelial cells. Some of the cells show mild nuclear hyperchromasia ➡, but no significant cytologic atypia is identified.* **(Right)** *Scanning magnification of another ATA shows scattered dermal lobular collections of vessels. The lobules bulge into dilated vessels, with a few peripheral semilunar spaces identified ➡.*

TERMINOLOGY

Synonyms

- Acquired tufted angioma (ATA)
- Tufted hemangioma
- Angioblastoma (of Nakagawa)
- Progressive capillary hemangioma

Definitions

- Multiple cannonball-like, scattered cellular collections of small vessels in dermis

ETIOLOGY/PATHOGENESIS

Unknown

- Most cases sporadic; rare familial case described
- Some cases associated with pregnancy or liver transplantation

CLINICAL ISSUES

Epidemiology

- Incidence
  - Rare tumors
- Age
  - Children and young adults

Site

- Neck, shoulders, and upper trunk most common

Presentation

- Slow growing
  - Erythematous macules and plaques

Prognosis

- Excellent; completely benign behavior
- May be associated with Kasabach-Merritt syndrome (consumptive coagulopathy)

MACROSCOPIC

General Features

- Reddish-brown nonencapsulated dermal lesion

Size

- Typically small papules, but may be large plaque

MICROSCOPIC

Histologic Features

- Multiple scattered lobular collections of small capillary-type vessels throughout dermis
  - Have typical **cannonball appearance** at low-power examination
  - Collections are larger in mid- and lower dermis
  - Cleft-like lumina often present around capillary tufts; may impart glomerular-like appearance
  - Capillaries may be so closely packed that lumina can be inconspicuous
  - Cells are oval to spindle-shaped
  - May show nuclear hyperchromasia but lack significant cytologic atypia
  - A few mitoses may be present
- Hemosiderin deposition may be seen
- Inflammation typically not present
- Subcutaneous tissue typically not involved

DIFFERENTIAL DIAGNOSIS

Glomeruloid Hemangioma

- Usually associated with Castleman disease or polyorganomegaly, endocrinopathy, M-protein, skin changes (POEMS syndrome)
- Smaller capillary-like collections inside vascular spaces with clefts around them
- Cytoplasmic globules, which are PAS(+) (immunoglobulin aggregates)

Infantile (Juvenile) Hemangioma

- Cellular dermal nodules composed of lobular collections of oval endothelial cells
- Vascular lumina often small and slit-like, become larger later-stage lesions

Lobular Capillary Hemangioma

- Shows exophytic appearance and epidermal collarette, often ulcerated and acutely inflamed (i.e., pyogenic granuloma)
- Proliferation of small capillary-type blood vessels typically arranged in a few larger nodular collections rather than multiple smaller dispersed collections seen in ATA

Targetoid Hemosiderotic Hemangioma (Hobnail Hemangioma)

- Superficial dilated vessels and smaller, narrow, deeper vessels lined by plump (hobnailed) cells
- Extravasated red blood cells and prominent stromal hemosiderin deposition

Kaposi Sarcoma

- Proliferation of interlacing bundles of spindle cells forming slit-like vascular spaces
- Cytoplasmic hyalinized globules, plasma cells, and hemosiderin deposits typically present
- HHV8(+) by immunohistochemistry

DIAGNOSTIC CHECKLIST

Pathologic Interpretation Pearls

- Scattered cannonball-like lobular collections of small capillary-type vessels throughout dermis

SELECTED REFERENCES

1. Pesapane F et al: A case of acquired tufted angioma in adulthood. An Bras Dermatol. 90(3 Suppl 1):16-8, 2015
2. Omori M et al: Acquired tufted angioma in pregnancy showing expression of estrogen and progesterone receptors. Eur J Dermatol. 23(6):898-9, 2013
3. Arai E et al: Usefulness of D2-40 immunohistochemistry for differentiation between kaposiform hemangioendothelioma and tufted angioma. J Cutan Pathol. 33(7):492-7, 2006
4. Ishikawa K et al: The spontaneous regression of tufted angioma. A case of regression after two recurrences and a review of 27 cases reported in the literature. Dermatology. 210(4):346-8, 2005
5. Wong SN et al: Tufted angioma: a report of five cases. Pediatr Dermatol. 19(5):388-93, 2002
6. Igarashi M et al: The relationship between angioblastoma (Nakagawa) and tufted angioma: report of four cases with angioblastoma and a literature-based comparison of the two conditions. J Dermatol. 27(8):537-42, 2000
7. Padilla RS et al: Acquired "tufted" angioma (progressive capillary hemangioma). A distinctive clinicopathologic entity related to lobular capillary hemangioma. Am J Dermatopathol. 9(4):292-300, 1987

Glomeruloid Hemangioma

KEY FACTS

TERMINOLOGY

- Glomeruloid angioma
- Glomeruloid hemangioma
- Benign proliferation of small vessels mimicking renal glomeruli

ETIOLOGY/PATHOGENESIS

- Association with polyneuropathy, organomegaly, endocrinopathy, M-protein, skin changes (POEMS) or multicentric Castleman syndrome in most cases

CLINICAL ISSUES

- Rare tumors
- More common in Asians (especially Japanese)
- Multiple red to purple eruptive papules (POEMS syndrome)
- Excellent prognosis, no malignant potential

MICROSCOPIC

- Vessels show distinctive grape-like clusters, mimicking renal glomeruli
- Endothelial cells are mildly enlarged and many show cytoplasmic eosinophilic globules
- Cytoplasmic globules (immunoglobulins) are PAS(+)
- Endothelial cells may show nuclear hyperchromasia but no significant cytologic atypia
- Few mitoses, lack of necrosis or infiltrative features

TOP DIFFERENTIAL DIAGNOSES

- Acquired tufted hemangioma (angioblastoma)
- Lobular capillary hemangioma (pyogenic granuloma)
- Targetoid hemosiderotic hemangioma (hobnail hemangioma)
- Kaposi sarcoma

DIAGNOSTIC CHECKLIST

- Dermal proliferation of vessels showing distinctive glomeruloid groups mimicking renal glomeruli

Glomeruloid Hemangioma at Scanning Magnification

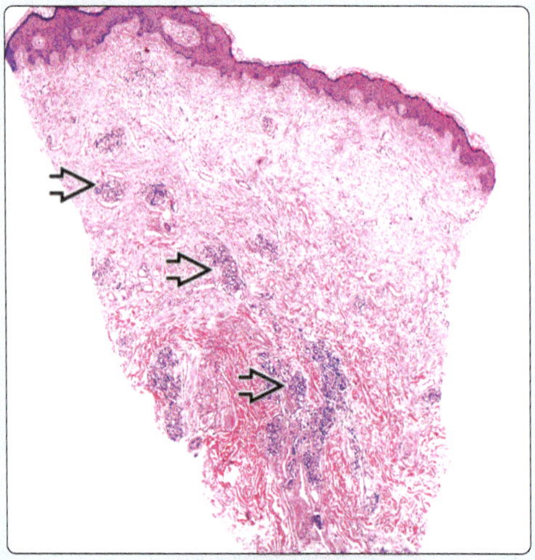

Glomeruloid Hemangioma at Higher Magnification

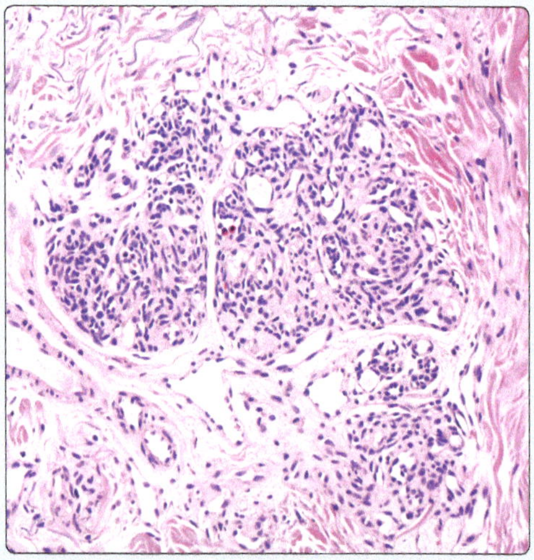

(Left) *Scanning magnification view of a glomeruloid hemangioma shows small clusters of vessels in the mid to deep dermis* ⇨. **(Right)** *Higher magnification shows the grape-like pattern of clustered small vessels, mimicking renal glomeruli.*

Glomeruloid Hemangioma With Grape-Like Vascular Clusters

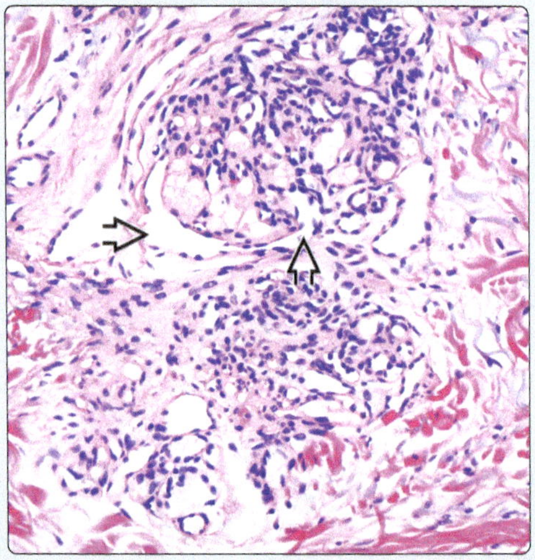

Glomeruloid Hemangioma at High Magnification

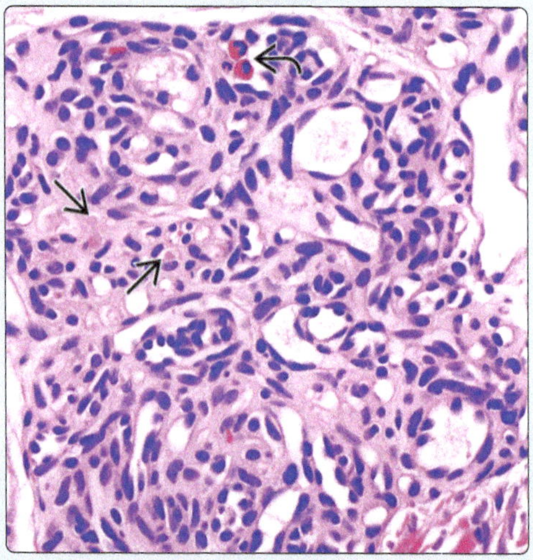

(Left) *High-power view of a glomeruloid hemangioma shows small, grape-like clusters of vessels projecting into vascular lumina (with peripheral crescentic spaces* ⇨ *present).* **(Right)** *High magnification of the vessels in a glomeruloid hemangioma shows endothelial cells with oval to spindle-shaped nuclei. Cytoplasmic eosinophilic globules are present focally* → *. A few intraluminal eosinophils are also present* ↩ *.*

TERMINOLOGY

Abbreviations

- Glomeruloid hemangioma

Synonyms

- Glomeruloid angioma

Definitions

- Benign proliferation of small vessels mimicking renal glomeruli

ETIOLOGY/PATHOGENESIS

Paraneoplastic Syndrome

- Association with polyneuropathy, organomegaly, endocrinopathy, M-protein, skin changes (POEMS) syndrome or multicentric Castleman disease in most cases

Unknown

- Rare cases not associated with POEMS syndrome

CLINICAL ISSUES

Epidemiology

- Incidence
  - Rare tumors
- Sex
  - More common in females
- Ethnicity
  - More common in Asians (Japanese)

Site

- Trunk and extremities

Presentation

- Multiple red to purple eruptive papules (POEMS syndrome)
  - Most patients also have diffuse skin hyperpigmentation
- Single lesions reported in patients without POEMS

Treatment

- Surgical approaches
  - Excision is curative, but not necessary in most cases
- Adjuvant therapy
  - Treatment of underlying plasma cell disorder may lead to regression of lesions

Prognosis

- Excellent, no malignant potential

MACROSCOPIC

General Features

- Dermal-based, well-circumscribed unencapsulated lesions

Size

- Small, typically only few millimeters

MICROSCOPIC

Histologic Features

- Dermal-based proliferation of dilated spaces containing small capillary-type vessels
- Vessels show distinctive grape-like clusters projecting into lumina, mimicking renal glomeruli
- Endothelial cells are mildly enlarged, and many show cytoplasmic eosinophilic globules
  - Cytoplasmic globules (secondary lysosomes containing immunoglobulins) are PAS(+)
- Endothelial cells may show nuclear hyperchromasia but do not show significant cytologic atypia
- Few mitoses, no necrosis or infiltrative features

DIFFERENTIAL DIAGNOSIS

Acquired Tufted Hemangioma (Angioblastoma)

- Slowly spreading macules and plaques in young children and adults
- Multiple dermal and subcutaneous vascular lobules composed of spindled and polygonal-shaped cells
- Some cases may show overlapping features with glomeruloid hemangioma

Lobular Capillary Hemangioma (Pyogenic Granuloma)

- Often shows polypoid configuration with epidermal collarette
- Lobular proliferation typically associated with ulceration, edema, and acute inflammation

Targetoid Hemosiderotic Hemangioma (Hobnail Hemangioma)

- Superficial dilated vessels and smaller, narrow, deeper vessels lined by plump (hobnailed) cells
- Extravasated red blood cells and prominent stromal hemosiderin deposition

Kaposi Sarcoma

- Clinical history distinctive [HIV(+) with multiple lesions or lower extremity lesion in elderly Mediterranean male]
- Cords or fascicles of spindled cells with slit-like lumina associated with hemosiderin deposition and plasma cells
- HHV8(+) (not reported in glomeruloid hemangioma)

DIAGNOSTIC CHECKLIST

Pathologic Interpretation Pearls

- Dermal proliferation of vessels showing distinctive glomeruloid groups or clusters mimicking renal glomeruli

SELECTED REFERENCES

1. Dispenzieri A: POEMS syndrome: Update on diagnosis, risk-stratification, and management. Am J Hematol. 90(10):951-62, 2015
2. Gupta J et al: Glomeruloid hemangioma in normal individuals. Indian J Dermatol. 58(2):160, 2013
3. Jacobson-Dunlop E et al: Glomeruloid hemangiomas in the absence of POEMS syndrome. J Cutan Pathol. 39(4):402-3, 2012
4. Forman SB et al: Glomeruloid hemangiomas without POEMS syndrome: series of three cases. J Cutan Pathol. 34(12):956-7, 2007
5. Perdaens C et al: POEMS syndrome characterized by glomeruloid angioma, osteosclerosis and multicentric Castleman disease. J Eur Acad Dermatol Venereol. 20(4):480-1, 2006
6. Rongioletti F et al: Glomeruloid hemangioma. A cutaneous marker of POEMS syndrome. Am J Dermatopathol. 16(2):175-8, 1994
7. Chan JK et al: Glomeruloid hemangioma. A distinctive cutaneous lesion of multicentric Castleman's disease associated with POEMS syndrome. Am J Surg Pathol. 14(11):1036-46, 1990

Angiolymphoid Hyperplasia With Eosinophilia

KEY FACTS

TERMINOLOGY

- Angiolymphoid hyperplasia with eosinophilia or epithelioid hemangioma
- Benign vascular tumor with well-formed, immature blood vessels, most of which are lined by plump, epithelioid (histiocytoid) endothelial cells with prominent inflammatory component, rich in eosinophils

CLINICAL ISSUES

- Wide range; mean: 3rd to 5th decades
- F > M
- Head (scalp, ears) most commonly affected
- Nodule or mass in subcutaneous tissues (**not** lymph nodes), present for up to 12 months
- Pink to red-brown (hyperpigmented), dome-shaped papules or nodules
- Excision, but recurrences, regrowth, or persistence after surgery requires follow-up

MICROSCOPIC

- Multiple lobules of inflammatory elements with increased vascularity on low power
- Proliferation of small, immature capillary-type to medium vessels usually without lumina
- Endothelial cells are enlarged with epithelioid or histiocytic appearance
  - Endothelial cells may have cytoplasmic vacuolization
  - May have solid appearance
- Many eosinophils, lymphocytes, and mast cells, although eosinophil number can vary greatly

TOP DIFFERENTIAL DIAGNOSES

- Papillary endothelial hyperplasia
- Kimura disease
- Angiosarcoma
- Metastatic papillary thyroid carcinoma

Subepithelial Vascular Proliferation

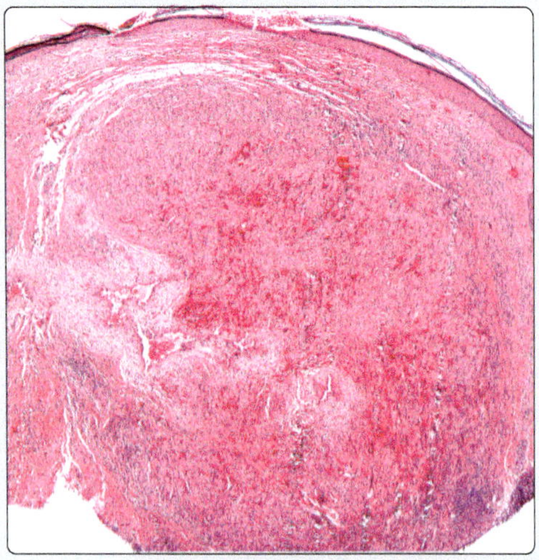

Vascular Proliferation With Eosinophils

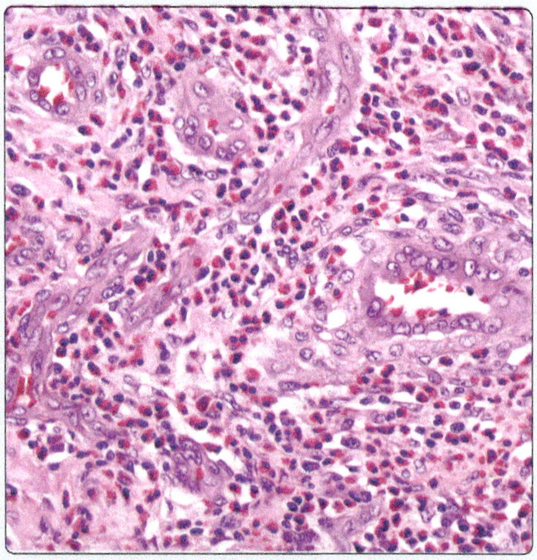

(Left) *Hematoxylin and eosin shows an intact surface epithelium with a richly vascularized stroma containing lymphoid elements. Eosinophils are present, imparting a bright red appearance at this low magnification.* **(Right)** *There are sheets of eosinophils in the background stroma. The vascular spaces are lined by endothelial cells that are enlarged and prominent. There is no atypia and no anastomosing.*

High Endothelial Cells

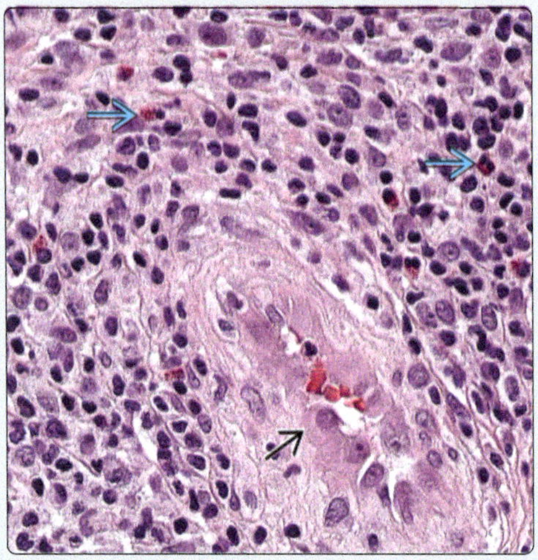

Endothelial Hyperplasia

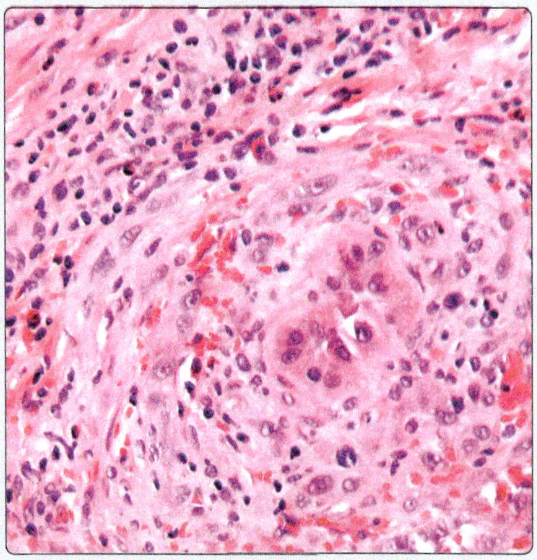

(Left) *The endothelial cells* → *are enlarged and partly occlude the lumen. Eosinophils* → *are noted in the background. Sometimes the eosinophils are inconspicuous.* **(Right)** *Hematoxylin and eosin shows endothelial hyperplasia with a thickened vessel wall and increased inflammatory cells, including eosinophils, in the surrounding tissue. Note the extravasated erythrocytes.*

TERMINOLOGY

Abbreviations

- Angiolymphoid hyperplasia with eosinophilia

Synonyms

- Epithelioid hemangioma

Definitions

- Benign vascular tumor with well-formed, immature blood vessels, most of which are lined by plump, epithelioid (histiocytoid) endothelial cells with prominent inflammatory component, especially eosinophils

ETIOLOGY/PATHOGENESIS

Reactive

- History of trauma; larger vessels show damage with prominent inflammatory component

Neoplastic

- May represent benign neoplasm, with evidence of clonal T-cell population in some cases

CLINICAL ISSUES

Epidemiology

- Age
  - Wide range; mean: 3rd to 5th decades
- Sex
  - F > M
- Ethnicity
  - **Not** increased in Asian patients (i.e., **not** Kimura disease)

Site

- Head (scalp, ears) most commonly affected
  - Digits next most common

Presentation

- Nodule or mass in subcutaneous tissues (**not** lymph nodes), present for up to 12 months
- Pain &/or pruritus; easily excoriate or bleed
- Pink to red-brown (hyperpigmented), dome-shaped papules or nodules
- Nodules may be multiple, ultimately coalescing
- Rarely may spontaneously regress/involute

Laboratory Tests

- Peripheral blood eosinophilia in some patients
- **No** elevated IgE levels

Treatment

- Excision, but recurrences, regrowth, or persistence after surgery requires follow-up

Prognosis

- Excellent, although with frequent recurrence

MACROSCOPIC

General Features

- May resemble lymph node due to circumscription and peripheral inflammation

Size

- Mean: 0.5-2 cm; rarely > 5 cm

MICROSCOPIC

Histologic Features

- Multiple lobules of inflammatory elements with increased vascularity on low power
- Surface usually intact but can be excoriated
- Proliferation of small, immature capillary-type to medium vessels usually without lumina
- May be attached to or associated with larger vessels
- May have solid appearance
- Endothelial cells are enlarged with epithelioid or histiocytic appearance
- Endothelial cells may have cytoplasmic vacuolization
- Endothelial nuclei are enlarged
- Many eosinophils, lymphocytes, and mast cells, although eosinophil number can vary greatly
- Lymphoid follicles sparse and poorly formed

ANCILLARY TESTS

Immunohistochemistry

- Endothelial cells **positive** for CD31, CD34, FLI-1, FVIIIRAg
- Actin (+) vascular muscle walls
- IgE(+) mast cells, but no IgE on follicular dendritic cells
  - Mast cells have IgE receptors but are distinct from follicular dendritic cells

DIFFERENTIAL DIAGNOSIS

Papillary Endothelial Hyperplasia

- Reactive process limited to intravascular space(s)
- Papillary projections of enlarged endothelial cells

Kimura Disease

- Asian men with large, disfiguring preauricular lymph node masses; peripheral eosinophilia
- Reactive lymphoid follicles with follicular lysis, eosinophilic abscesses, polykaryocytes, and IgE deposition

Angiosarcoma

- Highly atypical, mitotically active, freely anastomosing endothelial proliferation
- Usually shows necrosis and hemorrhage

Metastatic Papillary Thyroid Carcinoma

- Epithelioid cells with intranuclear cytoplasmic inclusions in lymphoid stroma
- **Positive**: TTF-1, thyroglobulin, pax-8

SELECTED REFERENCES

1. San Nicoló M et al: Angiolymphoid hyperplasia with eosinophilia of the external ear: case report and review of the literature. Eur Arch Otorhinolaryngol. 270(10):2775-7, 2013
2. Rahman A et al: Auricular angiolymphoid hyperplasia with eosinophilia. J Coll Physicians Surg Pak. 21(10):623-5, 2011
3. Sun ZJ et al: Epithelioid hemangioma in the oral mucosa: a clinicopathological study of seven cases and review of the literature. Oral Oncol. 42(5):441-7, 2006
4. Kempf W et al: Angiolymphoid hyperplasia with eosinophilia: evidence for a T-cell lymphoproliferative origin. Hum Pathol. 33(10):1023-9, 2002
5. Sharp JF et al: Angiolymphoid hyperplasia with eosinophilia. J Laryngol Otol. 104(12):977-9, 1990

Hobnail (Targetoid Hemosiderotic) Hemangioma

KEY FACTS

TERMINOLOGY

- Hobnail hemangioma
- Targetoid hemosiderotic hemangioma
- Benign vascular proliferation, typically wedge-shaped, showing intravascular papillae and hobnailed endothelial cells

ETIOLOGY/PATHOGENESIS

- Postulated to represent traumatized lymphangioma or hemangioma

CLINICAL ISSUES

- Uncommon tumors
- Occur mostly in young to middle-aged adults
- Typically present on lower extremities; also may occur on upper extremities, rarely in oral cavity
- Often pigmented due to hemosiderin deposition
- May show halo (targetoid appearance) in minority of cases
- Complete excision is curative but not necessary

MICROSCOPIC

- Vascular proliferation with wedge-shaped appearance in dermis
- Superficial vessels are dilated and thin walled
- Deeper vessels are progressively smaller, may show collapsed lumens
- Vessels are lined by small, bland-appearing endothelial cells with hobnail appearance
- Hemorrhage and hemosiderin deposition are typically prominent

TOP DIFFERENTIAL DIAGNOSES

- Progressive lymphangioma
- Kaposi sarcoma
- Microvenular hemangioma
- Retiform hemangioendothelioma

(Left) *Low-magnification view of a hobnail hemangioma (HH) demonstrates superficial dilated vascular spaces → in the papillary dermis with deeper small blood vessels and stromal hemosiderin deposits →.* **(Right)** *Higher power examination of the superficial portion of an HH shows superficial dilated vessels lined by small endothelial cells with nuclear hyperchromasia protruding into the lumina →.*

Hobnail Hemangioma

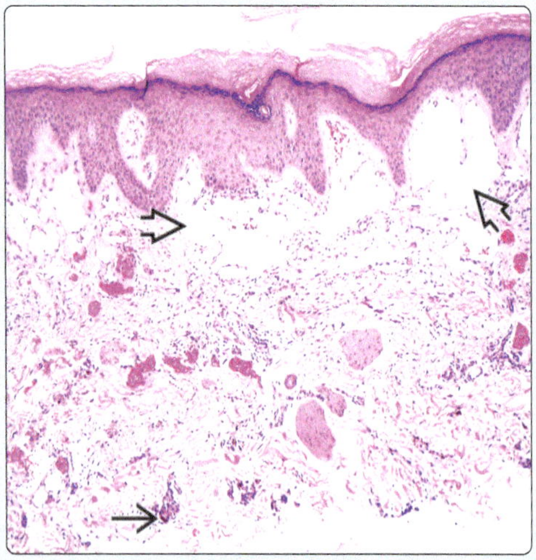

Higher Magnification of Superficial HH

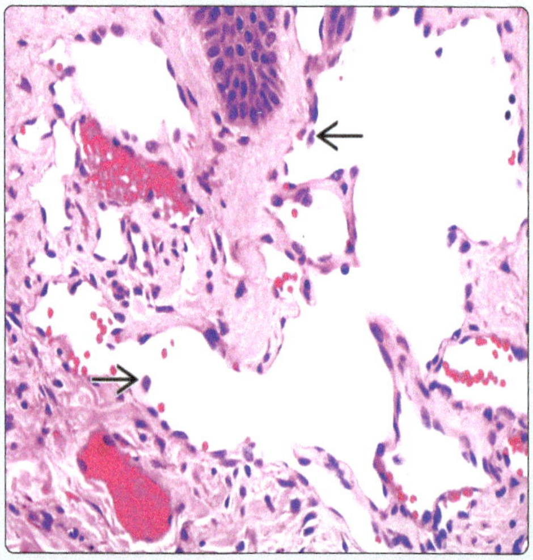

(Left) *Histologic examination of the deeper aspect of the lesion shows small, thin-walled blood vessels → and prominent hemosiderin deposition in the stroma →.* **(Right)** *This is an example of a more cellular HH composed of many closely apposed vessels in the superficial dermis, many of which show very small, compressed lumens →. Hobnailed endothelial cells can be appreciated in some of the vessels →.*

Deeper Vessels and Hemosiderin Deposits in HH

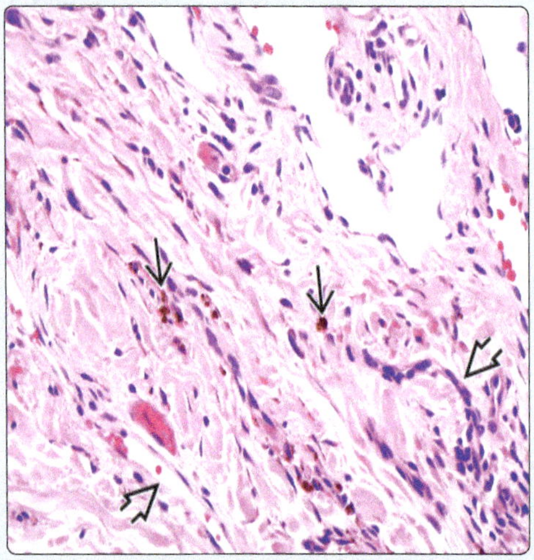

More Cellular Example of HH

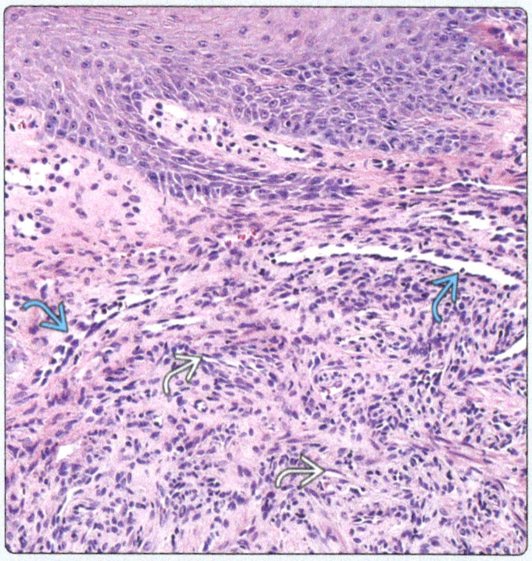

Hobnail (Targetoid Hemosiderotic) Hemangioma

TERMINOLOGY

Abbreviations

- Hobnail hemangioma (HH)

Synonyms

- Targetoid hemosiderotic hemangioma (clinical term)

Definitions

- Benign vascular proliferation, typically wedge-shaped, showing intravascular papillae and hobnailed endothelial cells

ETIOLOGY/PATHOGENESIS

Unknown

- Trauma has been implicated in some cases
  - Postulated to represent traumatized lymphangioma or hemangioma

CLINICAL ISSUES

Epidemiology

- Incidence
  - Uncommon tumors
- Age
  - Young to middle-aged adults
- Sex
  - More common in males

Site

- Typically present on lower extremities; also may occur on upper extremities, rarely in oral cavity

Presentation

- Skin papule or nodule
  - Often pigmented due to hemosiderin deposition
  - May show halo (targetoid appearance) in minority of cases

Treatment

- Surgical approaches
  - Complete excision is curative but not necessary, given benign nature

Prognosis

- Excellent, with no tendency for local recurrence

MACROSCOPIC

General Features

- Dermal-based reddish brown lesion with hemorrhage

Size

- Small, usually < 2 cm

MICROSCOPIC

Histologic Features

- Vascular proliferation with wedge-shaped appearance
- Superficial vessels are dilated and thin walled
  - Some vessels may resemble lymphatics
  - Focal papillary projections with fibrous cores may be present
  - Vessels are lined by small, bland-appearing endothelial cells with hobnail appearance
    - Nuclei project into lumina
  - Mitoses should not be present
- Deeper vessels are progressively smaller and show narrow/collapsed lumina
- Hemorrhage and hemosiderin deposition are typically prominent
- Inflammation is usually minimal

Cytologic Features

- Bland, plump endothelial cells with uniform-appearing nuclei

DIFFERENTIAL DIAGNOSIS

Progressive Lymphangioma

- Thin-walled, dilated superficial vascular spaces with narrower deeper vessels
- Lacks hobnail endothelial cell morphology and hemosiderin deposition of HH

Kaposi Sarcoma

- Shows proliferation of slit-like spaces lined by atypical spindle cells
- Typically lacks superficial dilated vascular spaces and hobnail cells of HH
- HHV8(+) by immunohistochemistry

Microvenular Hemangioma

- Proliferation of small, round to slit-like, thin-walled vessels involving reticular dermis
- Lacks superficial dilated vascular spaces, hobnail cells, and hemosiderin deposition of HH

Retiform Hemangioendothelioma

- Dermal and subcutaneous tumor characterized by proliferation of arborizing vessels lined by hobnailed endothelial cells
- Typically prominent lymphoid infiltrate, which is lacking in HH
- HH is typically more superficial, and deeper vessels are smaller and compact

DIAGNOSTIC CHECKLIST

Pathologic Interpretation Pearls

- Wedge-shaped vascular proliferation
- Dilated superficial vessels, deeper small/collapsed vessels
- Intravascular papillae and hobnailed endothelial cells
- Prominent hemosiderin deposition

SELECTED REFERENCES

1. AbuHilal M et al: Hobnail hemangioma (superficial hemosiderotic lymphovascular malformation) in children: a series of 6 pediatric cases and review of the literature. J Cutan Med Surg. ePub, 2015
2. Joyce JC et al: Superficial hemosiderotic lymphovascular malformation (hobnail hemangioma): a report of six cases. Pediatr Dermatol. 31(3):281-5, 2014
3. Kim DS et al: Multiple hobnail hemangiomas. Int J Dermatol. 53(4):e240-2, 2014
4. Fernandez-Flores A et al: Clinical changes in "true" hobnail hemangioma during menstruation. Bratisl Lek Listy. 109(3):141-3, 2008
5. Guillou L et al: Hobnail hemangioma: a pseudomalignant vascular lesion with a reappraisal of targetoid hemosiderotic hemangioma. Am J Surg Pathol. 23(1):97-105, 1999

Spindle Cell Hemangioma

KEY FACTS

TERMINOLOGY

- Formerly called spindle cell hemangioendothelioma

ETIOLOGY/PATHOGENESIS

- Some cases associated with Maffucci syndrome, Klippel-Trenaunay syndrome, varicosities, and congenital lymphedema

CLINICAL ISSUES

- Subcutaneous mass
- Usually acral location
- Sometimes multifocal
- Local recurrence in 50-60% of cases
- No metastatic potential
- Associated with Maffucci syndrome in some cases
- Young adults
- Distal extremities

MICROSCOPIC

- Dilated vessels often with focal thrombi
- Solid spindled cell areas
- Vacuolated endothelial cells, so-called blister cells
- Often partially intravascular

ANCILLARY TESTS

- Positive for CD31, CD34, ERG
- Negative for HHV8
- Mutations in isocitrate dehydrogenase present in > 70% of cases

TOP DIFFERENTIAL DIAGNOSES

- Kaposi sarcoma
- Kaposiform hemangioendothelioma
- Epithelioid hemangioendothelioma
- Organizing thrombus/intravascular papillary endothelial hyperplasia (Masson tumor)

Spindle Cell Hemangioma

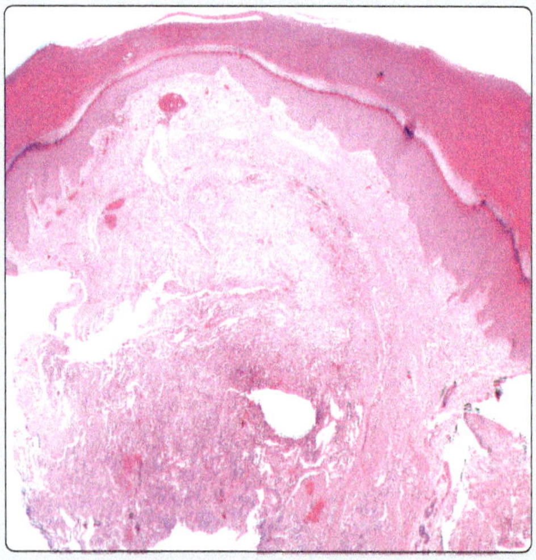

Spindle Cell Hemangioma Arising Within Vessel

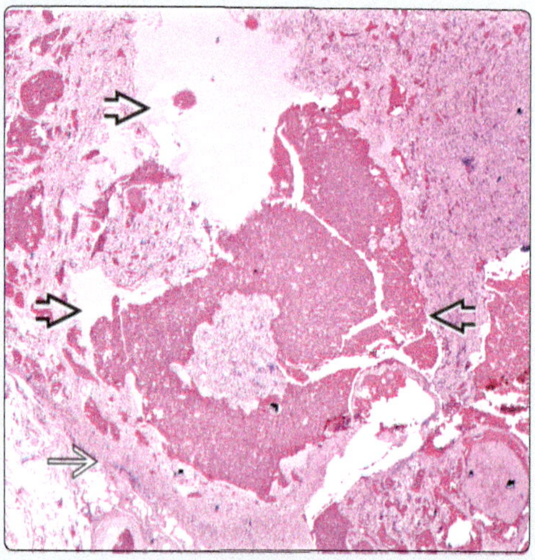

(Left) *Low magnification shows a noncircumscribed lesion in the dermis and subcutis composed of an admixture of thin-walled dilated blood vessels and sheets of spindle cells.* **(Right)** *Low magnification of a spindle cell hemangioma shows a well-circumscribed intravascular tumor with ectatic vascular spaces ⇨ and a cellular spindle cell proliferation. There is a remnant of a preexisting vessel at the periphery ➡.*

Spindle Cells in Spindle Cell Hemangioma

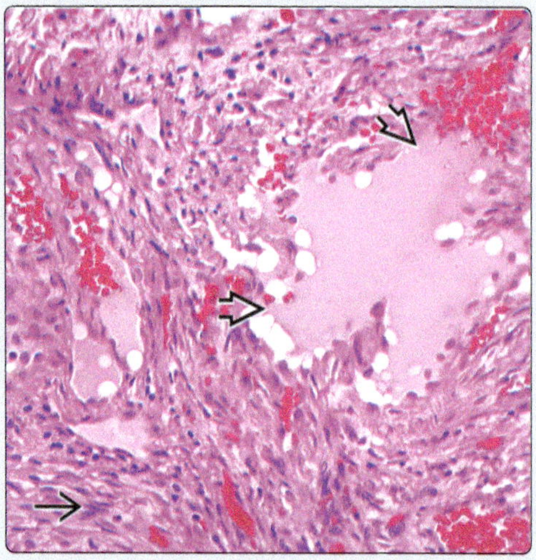

High-Power Image of Spindle Cell Hemangioma

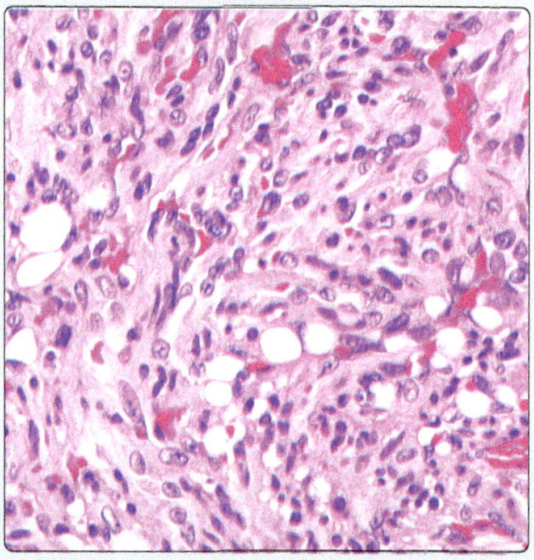

(Left) *High magnification of spindle cell hemangioma shows straight/curved fascicles of uniform spindle cells ➡ with irregularly shaped vascular spaces ⇨ and small areas of hemorrhage.* **(Right)** *High magnification shows the spindled tumor cells and the characteristic vacuolated endothelial cells (so-called blister cells).*

TERMINOLOGY

Synonyms

- Formerly known as spindle cell hemangioendothelioma

Definitions

- Benign vascular tumor characterized by cavernous vascular spaces and spindled cell areas

ETIOLOGY/PATHOGENESIS

Unknown

- Some cases associated with Maffucci syndrome, Klippel-Trenaunay syndrome, varicosities, and congenital lymphedema

CLINICAL ISSUES

Epidemiology

- Age
  - Young adults

Site

- Distal extremities
  - Acral location most common

Presentation

- Subcutaneous mass
  - Sometimes multifocal

Treatment

- Surgical approaches
  - Excision

Prognosis

- Local recurrence in 50-60%
- No metastatic potential

MICROSCOPIC

Histologic Features

- Dilated vessels often with focal thrombi
  - Cavernous thin-walled vascular spaces
- Solid spindled cell areas
  - May resemble Kaposi sarcoma
- Vacuolated endothelial cells, so-called blister cells
- ~ 50% are intravascular tumors

Cytologic Features

- Oval to spindle-shaped hyperchromatic-staining nuclei

Predominant Pattern/Injury Type

- Circumscribed dermal/subcutaneous nodular spindle cell tumor

Predominant Cell/Compartment Type

- Endothelial cell

ANCILLARY TESTS

Immunohistochemistry

- Positive for CD31, CD34, ERG
- Negative for HHV8

Genetic Testing

- Mutations in isocitrate dehydrogenase (IDH) present in > 70% of cases
- IDH1 > IDH2
- Same mutation seen in in patients with Maffucci syndrome

DIFFERENTIAL DIAGNOSIS

Kaposi Sarcoma

- Patch stage
  - Irregular vessels and atypical spindle cells dissecting through collagen
- Plaque/tumor stage
  - More cellular areas with fascicles of spindled cells and slit-like vascular lumina
- Immunoreactive for HHV8 latent nuclear antigen

Kaposiform Hemangioendothelioma

- Almost exclusively in children
- Dilated vessels
- Solid spindled cell areas
- Glomeruloid nests of rounded endothelial cells
- Associated with Kasabach-Merritt phenomenon

Epithelioid Hemangioendothelioma

- Nodules and cords of epithelioid endothelial cells
- Vacuolated endothelial cells
- Myxohyaline-hyaline stroma
- Lacks cavernous vascular spaces

Organizing Thrombus/Intravascular Papillary Endothelial Hyperplasia (Masson Tumor)

- Less prominent spindle cell proliferation
- Lacks so-called blister cells
- Papillary architecture of endothelial cells overlying fibrin cores

DIAGNOSTIC CHECKLIST

Pathologic Interpretation Pearls

- Combination of ectatic vessels, spindled cells, and vacuolated endothelial cells (blister cells) are key features
- At least partially intravascular in ~ 1/2 of cases

SELECTED REFERENCES

1. Kurek KC et al: R132C IDH1 mutations are found in spindle cell hemangiomas and not in other vascular tumors or malformations. Am J Pathol. 182(5):1494-500, 2013
2. Pansuriya TC et al: Somatic mosaic IDH1 and IDH2 mutations are associated with enchondroma and spindle cell hemangioma in Ollier disease and Maffucci syndrome. Nat Genet. 43(12):1256-61, 2011
3. Lyons LL et al: Kaposiform hemangioendothelioma: a study of 33 cases emphasizing its pathologic, immunophenotypic, and biologic uniqueness from juvenile hemangioma. Am J Surg Pathol. 28(5):559-68, 2004
4. Perkins P et al: Spindle cell hemangioendothelioma. An analysis of 78 cases with reassessment of its pathogenesis and biologic behavior. Am J Surg Pathol. 20(10):1196-204, 1996
5. Fletcher CD et al: Spindle cell haemangioendothelioma: a clinicopathological and immunohistochemical study indicative of a non-neoplastic lesion. Histopathology. 18(4):291-301, 1991
6. Weiss SW et al: Spindle cell hemangioendothelioma. A low-grade angiosarcoma resembling a cavernous hemangioma and Kaposi's sarcoma. Am J Surg Pathol. 10(8):521-30, 1986

Microvenular Hemangioma

KEY FACTS

TERMINOLOGY

- Microvenular hemangioma (MVH)
- Microcapillary angioma
- Slowly growing, benign vascular proliferation composed of small, thin vessels

CLINICAL ISSUES

- Young to middle-aged adults
- Typically occur on upper extremities, especially forearms
- Slow-growing papule or nodule

MICROSCOPIC

- Poorly circumscribed dermal proliferation of small blood vessels that diffusely involve reticular dermis
- Branching vessels typically present
- Most vessels show narrow or collapsed lumina
- Endothelial cells may be slightly enlarged but lack significant cytologic atypia
- Tufted groups of vessels may be seen in deep dermis
- Background of dermal sclerosis
- Usually lacks inflammation and hemosiderin

TOP DIFFERENTIAL DIAGNOSES

- Kaposi sarcoma
    - Often shows thin-walled vessels, but also has irregular, slit-like vascular spaces lined by atypical spindle cells
- Targetoid hemosiderotic hemangioma (hobnail hemangioma)
    - While deeper, small vessels are similar to those in MVH, superficial vessels are larger and more dilated
- Stasis changes and stasis dermatitis
    - Superficial proliferation of small, thick-walled blood vessels
- Early scar

DIAGNOSTIC CHECKLIST

- Benign vascular proliferation composed of small, collapsed vessels

(Left) *Histologic section shows increased numbers of small blood vessels in the superficial dermis with irregular branching ⇨ and narrow lumina.* **(Right)** *Another example of microvenular hemangioma (MVH) shows a proliferation of small blood vessels with thin walls and small to collapsed lumina ⇨ associated with a dense, sclerotic stroma.*

Microvenular Hemangioma

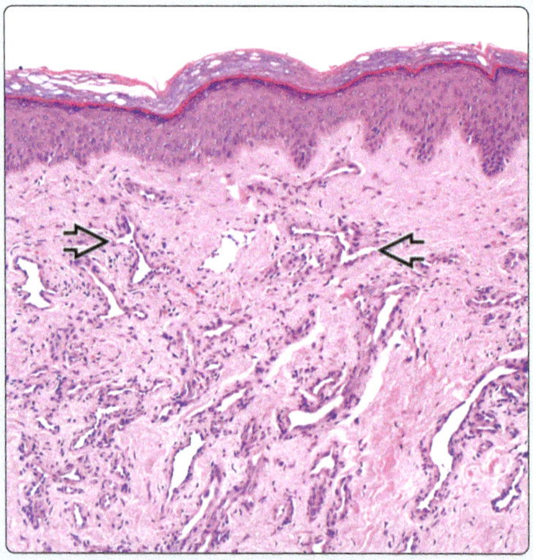

MVH With Small, Branching Vessels

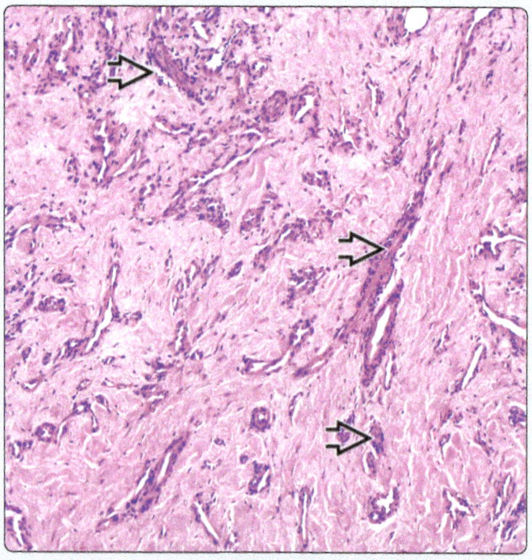

(Left) *High-power examination shows bland cytologic features of the endothelial cells, with small, hyperchromatic-staining nuclei ⇨. No necrosis or mitoses are present.* **(Right)** *Higher magnification of MVH shows small, thin branching vessels associated with sclerotic collagen bundles ⇨.*

MVH at High Magnification

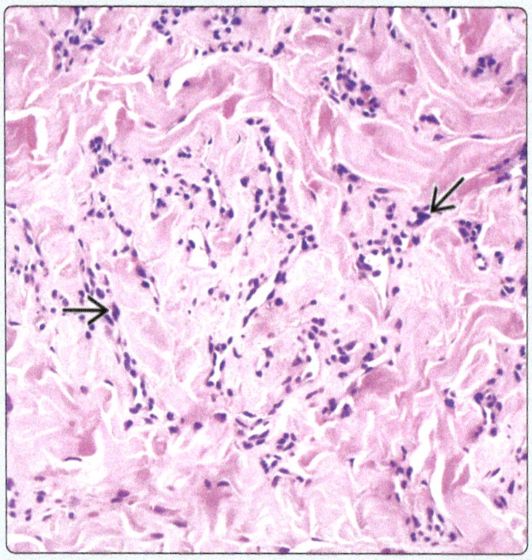

Microvenular Hemangioma With Small Vessels and Sclerotic Stroma

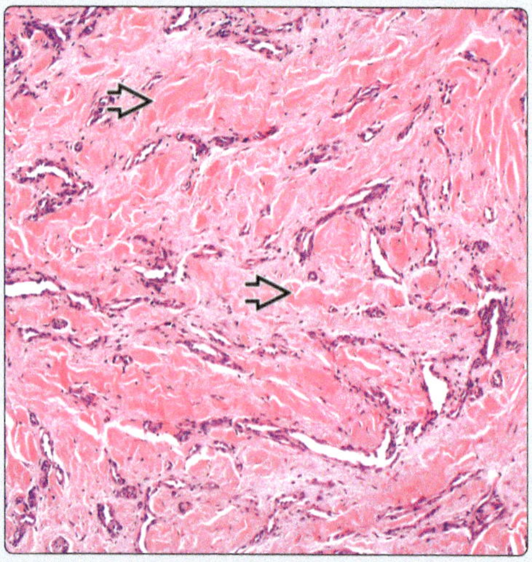

TERMINOLOGY

Abbreviations

- Microvenular hemangioma (MVH)

Synonyms

- Microcapillary angioma

Definitions

- Slowly growing, benign vascular proliferation composed of small, collapsed vessels

ETIOLOGY/PATHOGENESIS

Unknown

- In most cases

Hormonal Influence

- Some cases reportedly related to pregnancy or contraceptives

CLINICAL ISSUES

Epidemiology

- Age
  - Young to middle-aged adults
- Sex
  - Occurs in both males and females about equally

Site

- Typically occurs on trunk or upper extremities, especially forearms

Presentation

- Slow-growing papule or nodule

Natural History

- Often present for only few weeks to months at presentation

Treatment

- Surgical approaches
  - Simple excision is curative but not necessary, as these are benign lesions

Prognosis

- Excellent

MACROSCOPIC

Size

- Small, typically < 1 cm

MICROSCOPIC

Histologic Features

- Poorly circumscribed dermal proliferation of small blood vessels that diffusely involve reticular dermis
  - Branching vessels typically present
  - Most vessels show narrow or collapsed lumina
    - Few erythrocytes may be present within lumina
  - Endothelial cells may be slightly enlarged but lack significant cytologic atypia
  - Some cases may show large epithelioid cells resembling those seen in epithelioid (histiocytoid) hemangiomas
- Tufted groups of vessels may be seen in deep dermis
- Background of dermal sclerosis
- Inflammation and hemosiderin deposition typically lacking

Cytologic Features

- Endothelial cells may be enlarged, but show bland nuclei without significant atypia or pleomorphism

DIFFERENTIAL DIAGNOSIS

Kaposi Sarcoma

- May show thin-walled vessels but typically also has irregular, slit-like vascular spaces lined by atypical spindle cells
- Plasma cells and hyaline globules are lacking in MVH
- HHV8(+) by immunohistochemistry

Targetoid Hemosiderotic Hemangioma (Hobnail Hemangioma)

- While deeper small vessels are similar to those in MVH, superficial vessels are larger and more dilated
- Hobnailed endothelial cells project into vascular lumina
- Hemosiderin deposition is typically very prominent

Stasis Changes and Stasis Dermatitis

- Superficial proliferation of small, thick-walled blood vessels
- Show prominent hemosiderin deposition throughout dermis (lacking in MVH)
- Often show more inflammation and overlying spongiosis (stasis dermatitis)
- Clinical presentation distinctive: Lower extremities of elderly adults

Early Scar

- Angiogenesis in early scars may mimic MVH
  - But vessels more vertically oriented
- Typically greater fibrosis, inflammation, extravasated red blood cells, and hemosiderin deposition in scars

DIAGNOSTIC CHECKLIST

Pathologic Interpretation Pearls

- Benign vascular proliferation composed of small, collapsed vessels
- Branching vessels typically present
- Endothelial cells may be enlarged but lack cytologic atypia
- Background of dermal sclerosis

SELECTED REFERENCES

1. Ai DF et al: Multiple microvenular hemangioma: A case report. Oncol Lett. 7(1):275-277, 2014
2. Napekoski KM et al: Microvenular hemangioma: a clinicopathologic review of 13 cases. J Cutan Pathol. 41(11):816-22, 2014
3. Trindade F et al: Microvenular hemangioma-an immunohistochemical study of 9 cases. Am J Dermatopathol. 34(8):810-2, 2012
4. Fernandez-Flores A: Lack of expression of podoplanin by microvenular hemangioma. Pathol Res Pract. 204(11):817-21, 2008
5. Chang SE et al: Microvenular hemangioma in a boy with acute myelogenous leukemia. Pediatr Dermatol. 20(3):266-7, 2003
6. Kim YC et al: Microvenular hemangioma. Dermatology. 206(2):161-4, 2003
7. Rikihisa W et al: Microvenular haemangioma in a patient with Wiskott-Aldrich syndrome. Br J Dermatol. 141(4):752-4, 1999
8. Hunt SJ et al: Microvenular hemangioma. J Cutan Pathol. 18(4):235-40, 1991

Verrucous Hemangioma

KEY FACTS

TERMINOLOGY

- Vascular tumor with superficial verrucous appearance

ETIOLOGY/PATHOGENESIS

- Most likely congenital lymphovascular malformation

CLINICAL ISSUES

- Presents in children
- Dark blue nodule
- Surface has warty appearance
- Most common on extremities
- Cobb syndrome
  - Verrucous hemangioma on midline of back
  - Associated with underlying spinal cord vascular malformation

MICROSCOPIC

- Epidermis is acanthotic and papillomatous
- Cavernous vascular spaces superficially
  - May appear to extend into epidermis due to very superficial location in dermal papillae, similar to angiokeratoma
- Dilated capillaries
- Vascular proliferation involves superficial and deep dermis
  - Vascular spaces lined by bland, flattened endothelial cells

ANCILLARY TESTS

- Positive for GLUT-1, CD31, and CD34
- Negative for WT1, podoplanin (D2-40), and PROX-1

TOP DIFFERENTIAL DIAGNOSES

- Angiokeratoma
  - Vascular proliferation is restricted to superficial dermis
- Lymphangioma
- Hamartomatous vascular lesions
- Pyogenic granuloma (lobular capillary hemangioma)

Verrucous Hemangioma Displaying Papillomatous Epidermal Surface

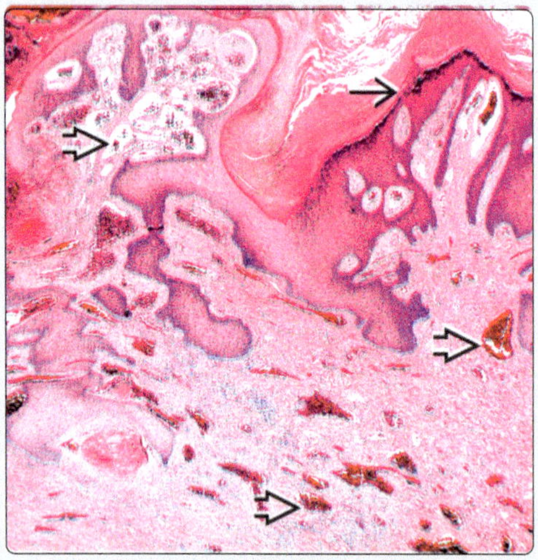

Ectatic Vessels Herniating Into Overlying Epidermis

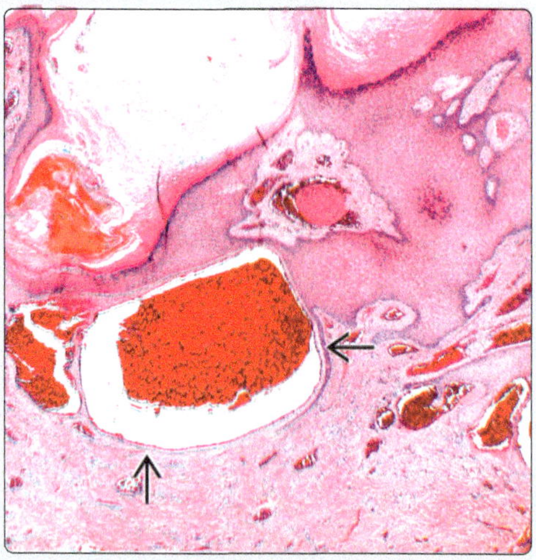

(Left) *In this low-power image, verrucous hemangioma has an acanthotic papillomatous epidermis* → *and ectatic dermal blood vessels* ⇨ *involving both the superficial and deep dermis.* **(Right)** *In addition to the verrucous-like epidermal changes, this case demonstrates cavernous vascular spaces* → *in close apposition to the epidermis, resembling an angiokeratoma.*

Verrucous Hemangioma With Thrombosis

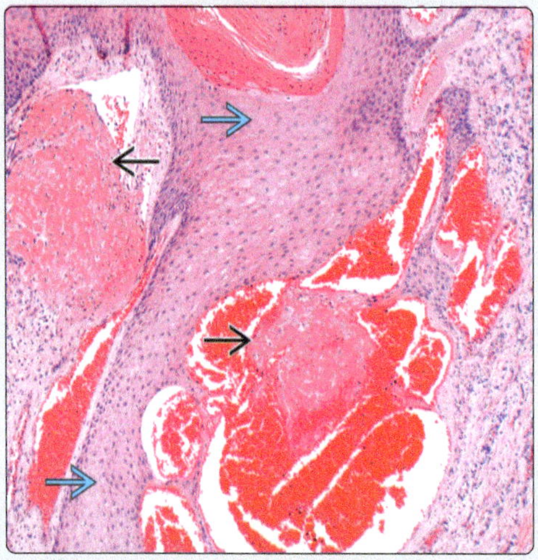

Deep Aspect of Verrucous Hemangioma

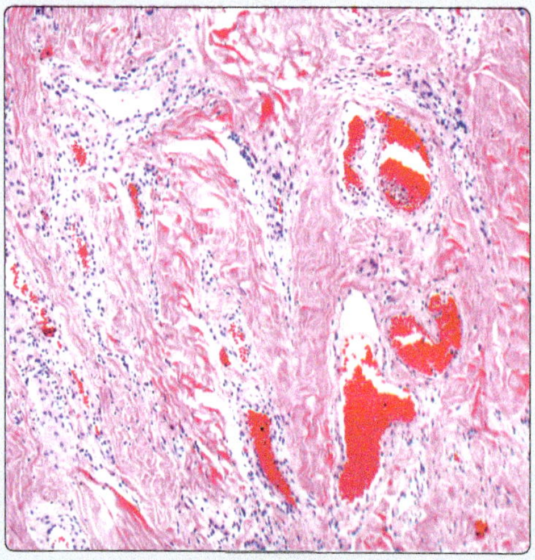

(Left) *The superficial cavernous vascular spaces may undergo thrombosis* →*. Note the intimately associated verrucous epidermal hyperplasia* →*.* **(Right)** *In addition to involvement of the superficial dermis, verrucous hemangioma has a vascular proliferation of small to dilated vessels extending into the deep dermis or even the subcutaneous adipose tissue (not shown in this field).*

TERMINOLOGY

Definitions

- Vascular tumor with superficial verrucous appearance

ETIOLOGY/PATHOGENESIS

Developmental Anomaly

- Most likely congenital lymphovascular malformation

CLINICAL ISSUES

Epidemiology

- Incidence
  - Very rare lesion
- Age
  - Present in children
    - At birth or early childhood
    - Only very rare cases present in adults
- Sex
  - No gender predilection

Presentation

- Dark blue papule or nodule
  - Usually solitary
  - May develop satellite lesions over time
  - Rare linear form
- Surface has warty appearance
  - Becomes more verrucous-appearing over time
- Most common on extremities
  - Lower extremities > upper extremities
- Cobb syndrome
  - Verrucous hemangioma on midline of back
  - Associated with spinal cord vascular malformation

Treatment

- Surgical approaches
  - Simple excision
    - Radiologic examination should be performed on midline back lesions to help exclude Cobb syndrome
  - Laser removal

Prognosis

- Benign
  - Local recurrence common
    - Related to involvement of deep dermis

MICROSCOPIC

Histologic Features

- Epidermis is acanthotic and papillomatous
  - Early lesions may be less verrucous in appearance
- Composed of dilated capillaries
- Cavernous vascular spaces are present superficially
  - May appear to extend into epidermis due to very superficial location in dermal papillae, similar to angiokeratoma
- Vascular proliferation involves superficial and deep dermis
  - Vascular spaces lined by bland, flattened endothelial cells
  - Deeper spaces include mixture of small, capillary-type and larger, cavernous, thin-walled vessels

ANCILLARY TESTS

Immunohistochemistry

- Positive for CD31, CD34
- Positive for GLUT-1
  - Immunoreactivity is evident in deeply located blood vessels in subcutaneous adipose tissue
- Negative for WT1, podoplanin (D2-40), and PROX-1

DIFFERENTIAL DIAGNOSIS

Angiokeratoma

- Superficial resemblance is striking
- Key difference is distribution of vascular proliferation
  - In angiokeratoma, restricted to superficial dermis
  - In verrucous hemangioma, extends into deep dermis

Lymphangioma

- May be superficial and deep
- Lacks verrucous epidermal changes of verrucous hemangioma
- Lymphatic valves present

Hamartomatous Vascular Lesions

- Usually lack verrucous epidermal changes
- Different clinical presentations, often associated with syndromes and present in head and neck region

Pyogenic Granuloma (Lobular Capillary Hemangioma)

- Polypoid lesion but lacks verrucous epidermal changes
- Often ulcerated and inflamed with numerous lymphocytes and neutrophils present
- Lobular proliferation of closely packed capillaries with less ectatic vessels
- Epidermal collarette not seen in verrucous hemangioma

DIAGNOSTIC CHECKLIST

Pathologic Interpretation Pearls

- Verrucous epidermal appearance
- Capillaries and cavernous vascular spaces
- Involvement of superficial and deep dermis

SELECTED REFERENCES

1. Clairwood MQ et al: Verrucous hemangioma: a report of two cases and review of the literature. J Cutan Pathol. 38(9):740-6, 2011
2. Al Dhaybi R et al: Differentiation of vascular tumors from vascular malformations by expression of Wilms tumor 1 gene: evaluation of 126 cases. J Am Acad Dermatol. 63(6):1052-7, 2010
3. Lara-Corrales I et al: Verrucous hemangioma: a challenging vascular lesion. J Cutan Med Surg. 14(3):144-6, 2010
4. Brown A et al: Verrucous lymphovascular malformation versus verrucous hemangioma: controversial nomenclature. Cutis. 81(5):390-6, 2008
5. Tennant LB et al: Verrucous hemangioma revisited. Pediatr Dermatol. 23(3):208-15, 2006
6. Hayashi H et al: Linear verrucous haemangioma on the abdomen. Acta Derm Venereol. 84(1):79-80, 2004
7. Clinton TS et al: Cobb syndrome associated with a verrucous (angiokeratomalike) vascular malformation. Cutis. 71(4):283-7, 2003
8. Rossi A et al: Verrucous hemangioma and angiokeratoma circumscriptum: clinical and histologic differential characteristics. J Dermatol Surg Oncol. 15(1):88-91, 1989
9. Imperial R et al: Verrucous hemangioma. A clinicopathologic study of 21 cases. Arch Dermatol. 96(3):247-53, 1967

Angiokeratoma

KEY FACTS

TERMINOLOGY

- Ectatic superficial dermal blood vessels associated with reactive epidermal hyperplasia

CLINICAL ISSUES

- Solitary and multiple angiokeratomas
  - Usually on extremities
- Angiokeratoma of Fordyce
  - Elderly men
  - Multiple lesions, often on scrotum
- Angiokeratoma of Mibelli
  - Childhood
  - Warty lesions over bony prominences of acral locations
- Angiokeratoma corporis diffusum
  - Associated with Anderson-Fabry disease
- Angiokeratoma circumscriptum
  - Presents in children
  - Least common subtype

MICROSCOPIC

- Marked ectasia of papillary dermal blood vessels
- Vessels herniate into epidermis, resulting in appearance of intraepidermal vessels
- Hemorrhage in stratum corneum common
- May have evidence of thrombosis and intravascular papillary endothelial hyperplasia
- Reactive epidermal changes: Acanthosis, hyperkeratosis, and elongation of rete ridges around ectatic vessels

TOP DIFFERENTIAL DIAGNOSES

- Verrucous hemangioma
  - Verrucous epidermal hyperplasia
  - Superficial and deep vascular proliferation
- Pyogenic granuloma (lobular capillary hemangioma)
  - Polypoid lesion with epidermal collarette
  - Granulation tissue-like dermal vascular proliferation

Clinical Image of Angiokeratomas

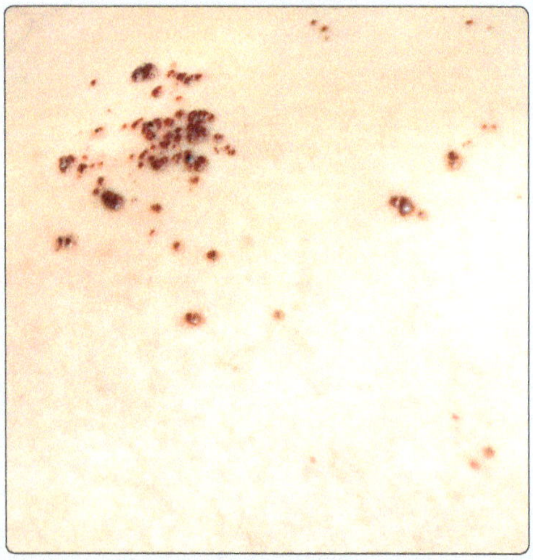

Angiokeratoma at Low Magnification

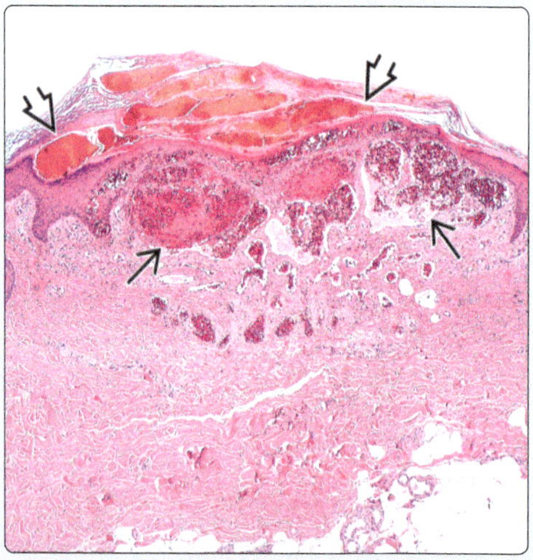

(Left) *Clinical image demonstrates numerous grouped angiokeratomas in a patient with Anderson-Fabry disease.* **(Right)** *Angiokeratomas are characterized by ectatic vessels → in the superficial dermis that appear to herniate into the epidermis. There is often overlying hemorrhage ⇨, epidermal acanthosis, and frequently compact hyperkeratosis.*

Angiokeratoma With Epidermal Acanthosis and Hyperkeratosis

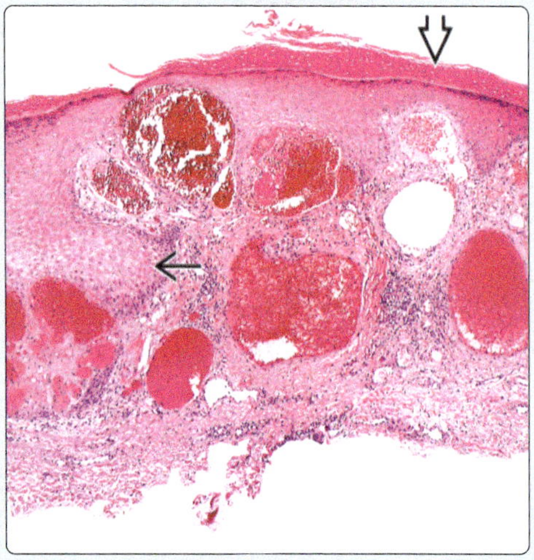

Angiokeratoma at High Magnification

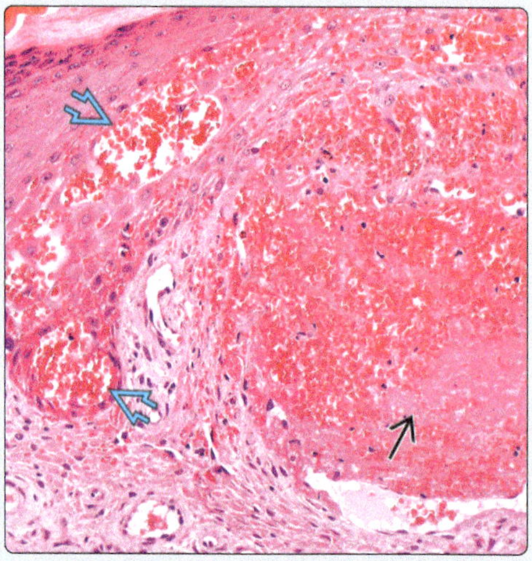

(Left) *The epidermis overlying angiokeratomas typically demonstrates acanthosis → and compact hyperkeratosis ⇨. Numerous, dilated, superficial dermal blood vessels are also seen in this field.* **(Right)** *The vessels of angiokeratoma herniate up into the epidermis ⇨. The vessels frequently undergo thrombosis, and in this case demonstrates an early thrombus characterized by fibrin → admixed with erythrocytes.*

TERMINOLOGY

Definitions

- Ectatic superficial dermal blood vessels associated with reactive epidermal hyperplasia

CLINICAL ISSUES

Presentation

- 5 clinical variants
  - **Solitary and multiple angiokeratoma**
    - Usually solitary
    - Multiple lesions may have zosteriform presentation
    - Wide age range
    - Usually on extremities
  - **Angiokeratoma of Fordyce**
    - Elderly men
    - Solitary or multiple papules on scrotum
  - **Angiokeratoma of Mibelli**
    - Presents in childhood and adolescence
    - Warty lesions over bony prominences of acral locations
  - **Angiokeratoma corporis diffusum**
    - Associated with Anderson-Fabry disease: X-linked recessive disorder of α-galactosidase A
    - Multiple, often clustered papules
    - Bathing suit distribution
    - M > F
    - May also be associated with deficiency of α-L-fucosidase, β-galactosidase, β-mannosidase, α-N-acetylgalactosaminidase, or neuraminidase
  - **Angiokeratoma circumscriptum**
    - Least common variant
    - Usually presents in children
    - Plaque composed of grouped papules &/or nodules
    - Trunk or extremities

Treatment

- Surgical approaches
  - Simple excision of solitary lesions
  - Excision may not be practical for multiple lesions
  - Laser treatment also may be used
- Drugs
  - Enzyme replacement therapy for patients with Anderson-Fabry disease or other heritable enzyme deficiencies
- May follow clinically

Prognosis

- Benign, no risk for transformation to malignancy

MACROSCOPIC

General Features

- Red to blue superficial dermal papules or plaques

MICROSCOPIC

Histologic Features

- Marked ectasia of papillary dermal blood vessels
  - Blood vessels lined by flattened, bland-appearing endothelial cells
  - May have evidence of thrombosis and intravascular papillary endothelial hyperplasia (Masson tumor/change)
  - Blood vessels herniate into overlying epidermis
    - Can result in appearance that vessels are within epidermis
- Reactive epidermal changes
  - Irregular acanthosis
  - Variable hyperkeratosis
  - Elongation of rete pegs that encircle dermal blood vessels
  - May have epidermal collarette
- Angiokeratomas associated with Anderson-Fabry disease
  - May have lipid vacuoles in endothelial cells, pericytes, and fibroblasts
  - PAS(+), Sudan black (+) granules may be seen in endothelial cells on frozen sections
  - Electron microscopy may show characteristic lamellar cytoplasmic granules

DIFFERENTIAL DIAGNOSIS

Verrucous Hemangioma

- Presents at birth or in childhood
- Verrucous epidermal hyperplasia
- Superficial and deep vascular proliferation, which is not limited to papillary dermis, as in angiokeratoma

Pyogenic Granuloma (Lobular Capillary Hemangioma)

- Polypoid lesion with epidermal collarette
- Granulation tissue-like dermal vascular proliferation
- Lacks epidermal acanthosis and hyperkeratosis
- Vascular proliferation more florid than angiokeratoma

DIAGNOSTIC CHECKLIST

Clinically Relevant Pathologic Features

- Ectatic vessels limited to superficial dermis
- Acanthotic epidermis, vessels may appear to extend into epidermis, often with surrounding collarette

SELECTED REFERENCES

1. Baumgartner J et al: Extensive angiokeratoma circumscriptum - successful treatment with 595-nm variable-pulse pulsed dye laser and 755-nm long-pulse pulsed alexandrite laser. J Cosmet Laser Ther. 1-14, 2016
2. Ghosh SK et al: Multiple giant angiokeratoma of Fordyce on the shaft of the penis masquerading as keratoacanthoma. An Bras Dermatol. 90(3 Suppl 1):150-2, 2015
3. McFaddin C et al: Linear acral pseudolymphomatous angiokeratoma of children with associated nail dystrophy. Dermatol Online J. 21(7), 2015
4. Saeb-Lima M et al: Thrombotic phenomena in angiokeratoma can evolve into spontaneous involution of the lesions: a report of two cases. J Cutan Pathol. ePub, 2015
5. O'Mahony C et al: Angiokeratomas - When is a few too many? Int J STD AIDS. 25(5):378-9, 2014
6. Albano LM et al: Angiokeratoma: a cutaneous marker of Fabry's disease. Clin Exp Dermatol. 35(5):505-8, 2010
7. Goldman L et al: Thrombotic angiokeratoma circumscriptum simulating melanoma. Arch Dermatol. 117(3):138-9, 1981
8. Kint JA: Fabry's disease: alpha-galactosidase deficiency. Science. 167(922):1268-9, 1970
9. Haye KR et al: Angiokeratoma of Mibelli. Acta Derm Venereol. 41:56-60, 1961

Venous Lake

KEY FACTS

TERMINOLOGY

- Capillary aneurysm
- Type of telangiectasia characterized by ectatic superficial blood vessel in superficial dermis

CLINICAL ISSUES

- Usually presents in elderly patients
- More common in Caucasians
  - Related to chronic actinic damage
- Head and neck
- Especially common on lip
- Can clinically mimic melanoma
- Often multiple
- Laser treatment

MICROSCOPIC

- Ectatic vessel in upper dermis
- Usually single dilated vessel
  - Lined by single layer of bland endothelial cells
- Vessel may collapse after biopsy and not appear ectatic
- Vessel may be thrombosed
- Background of solar elastosis

TOP DIFFERENTIAL DIAGNOSES

- Hemangioma
  - Multiple not single vessels
- Pyogenic granuloma
  - Lobular proliferation of capillaries (type of lobular capillary hemangioma)
  - Often overlying epidermal ulceration and serum crust with acute inflammation
- Angiokeratoma
  - Vessels herniate into overlying epidermis
- Lymphangioma
  - Ectatic lymphatic channels
  - Have lymphatic valves
- Angiosarcoma
- Kaposi sarcoma

Clinical Image of Venous Lake

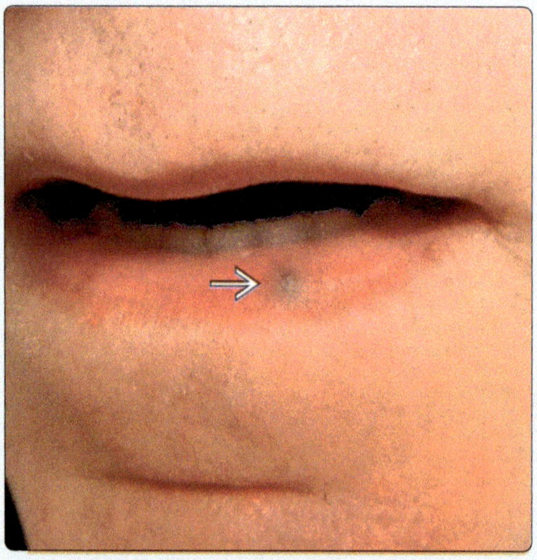

Low Magnification of Venous Lake

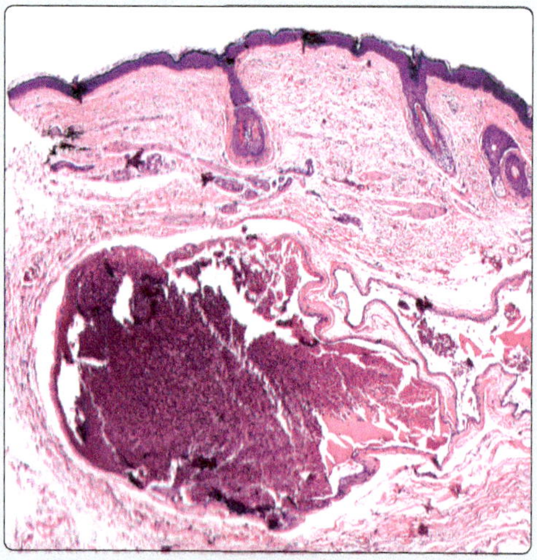

(Left) *Venous lake presents as a dark blue papule ➡ on the sun-damaged skin of elderly patients. It is especially common on the lip.* **(Right)** *Venous lake is characterized by a single large, ectatic vessel in actinically damaged skin.*

High Magnification of Venous Lake

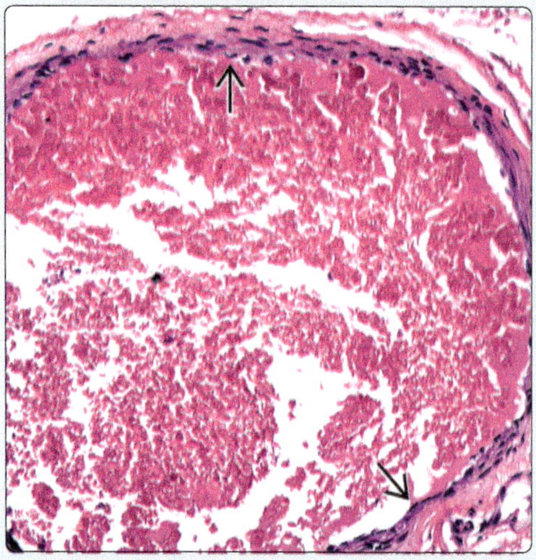

Venous Lake With Thrombus

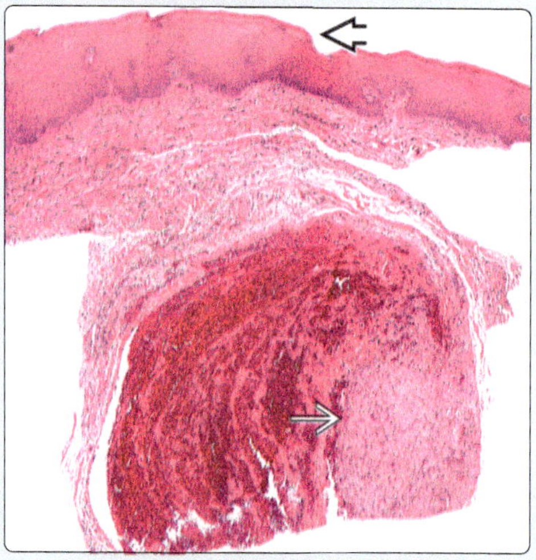

(Left) *The vessel of a venous lake is lined by flattened endothelial cells ⇨ that lack atypia.* **(Right)** *This is an example of a venous lake presenting on the lip (note the squamous mucosa ⇨ overlying the lesion), one of the most common locations. The vessel has a partial thrombus ➡ filling its lumen, consistent with Masson change.*

TERMINOLOGY

Synonyms

- Capillary aneurysm

Definitions

- Type of telangiectasia characterized by ectatic superficial blood vessel in superficial dermis

ETIOLOGY/PATHOGENESIS

Chronic Sun Damage

- Results in inadequate stromal support for affected vessel, resulting in marked ectasia

CLINICAL ISSUES

Epidemiology

- Incidence
  - Relatively common lesions
- Age
  - Usually in elderly patients
- Ethnicity
  - More common in Caucasians

Presentation

- Usually presents in sun-damaged skin of elderly patients
- Dark blue papules
- Often multiple
- Head and neck
  - Especially common on lip
- Can mimic melanoma clinically

Treatment

- Surgical approaches
  - Simple excision is curative
- Laser treatment
- Can be managed expectantly

Prognosis

- Benign

MICROSCOPIC

Histologic Features

- Ectatic vessel in upper dermis
  - Usually single, large, dilated vessel with relatively thin, muscular wall
  - Vessel may collapse after biopsy and not appear ectatic
  - Vessel is lined by flattened endothelial cells
  - May be thrombosed and show papillary endothelial hyperplasia (Masson change/tumor)
- Solar elastosis typically present

Cytologic Features

- Bland endothelial cells with uniform, round to oval nuclei, inconspicuous nucleoli

DIFFERENTIAL DIAGNOSIS

Hemangioma

- Capillary hemangiomas are composed of multiple small, capillary-type vessels
- Cavernous hemangiomas are composed of multiple large, thin-walled, dilated vessels
- Venous hemangiomas are similar to cavernous hemangiomas but are composed of large, thick-walled, dilated vessels

Pyogenic Granuloma

- 1 type of lobular capillary hemangioma
- Epidermal collarette and ulceration with acute inflammation often present (absent in venous lake)
- Lobular proliferation of capillaries resembling granulation tissue, rather than single dilated vessel

Angiokeratoma

- Superficial, dilated, thin-walled vessels
- Appear to extend into epidermis on low-power examination
- Show overlying epidermal acanthosis and hyperkeratosis

Arteriovenous Hemangioma

- May mimic venous hemangioma with large, thick-walled vessels
- Elastic stain shows presence of elastic lumina in some of vessels

Lymphangioma

- Ectatic lymphatic channels
  - Often larger spaces superficially, progressing to narrower channels deeper in dermis (absent in venous lake)
  - Lymphatic vessels of superficial dermis have valves, unlike venous lake

Kaposi Sarcoma

- Proliferation of small, irregular vascular spaces lined by spindle-shaped endothelial cells (absent in venous lake)
- Stroma often shows hemosiderin deposition and plasma cells
- Positive for HHV8 by immunohistochemistry

Angiosarcoma

- Usually composed of multiple large, irregularly shaped, anastomosing vessels, unlike venous lake, which is single dilated vessel
- Lined by enlarged, atypical epithelioid or spindle-shaped cells
- Pleomorphism and mitoses often prominent (lacking in venous lake)

DIAGNOSTIC CHECKLIST

Pathologic Interpretation Pearls

- Single dilated blood vessel in upper dermis of sun-damaged skin

SELECTED REFERENCES

1. Becher GL et al: Treatment of superficial vascular lesions with the KTP 532-nm laser: experience with 647 patients. Lasers Med Sci. 29(1):267-71, 2014
2. Astner S et al: Preliminary evaluation of benign vascular lesions using in vivo reflectance confocal microscopy. Dermatol Surg. 36(7):1099-110, 2010
3. Requena L et al: Cutaneous vascular anomalies. Part I. Hamartomas, malformations, and dilation of preexisting vessels. J Am Acad Dermatol. 37(4):523-49; quiz 549-52, 1997

Papillary Endothelial Hyperplasia (Masson Tumor)

KEY FACTS

TERMINOLOGY

- Benign, reactive, intravascular papillary endothelial proliferation
- Masson tumor
- Vegetant intravascular hemangioendothelioma
- Intravascular angiomatosis
- Intravascular papillary endothelial hyperplasia
- Papillary endothelial hyperplasia (PEH)

CLINICAL ISSUES

- Wide site distribution; located in deep dermis or subcutaneous tissue
- Common sites include: Head and neck, fingers, trunk

MACROSCOPIC

- Small, cystic lesions with red-purple discoloration

MICROSCOPIC

- Circumscribed lesion with pseudocapsule
- Fibrin thrombus
- Papillary structures lined by endothelial cells
- Intravascular location
- Significant nuclear pleomorphism is absent

TOP DIFFERENTIAL DIAGNOSES

- Angiosarcoma
  - PEH lacks nuclear atypia, tumor cell necrosis, and mitotic activity present in angiosarcoma
- Hemangioma
- PEH-like changes may occur in hemangiomas complicated by thrombosis
- Arteriovenous malformation (AVM)
  - PEH-like changes may occur in background of AVM
- Hematoma
- Venous lymphatic malformation (VLM)
  - In VLM, there are lobules of abnormally dilated vessels, some with lymphatic morphology

Well-Circumscribed Vascular Proliferation

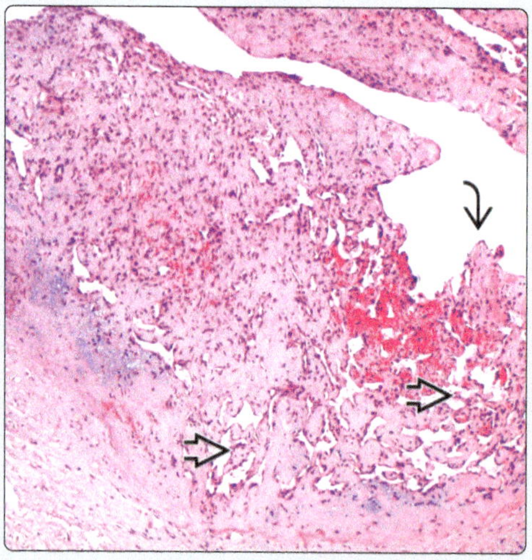

Fibrin Thrombi Seen in PEH

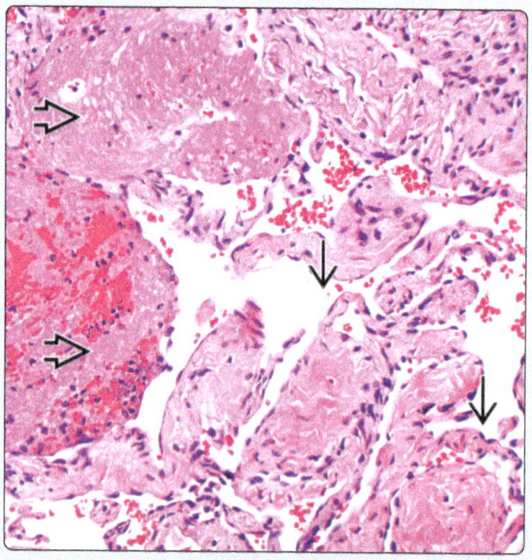

(Left) *Papillary endothelial hyperplasia (PEH) is a well-circumscribed reactive lesion in which papillary fronds ⇨ lined by a single layer of endothelial cells proliferate within a vascular lumen ↷.* **(Right)** *Fibrin thrombi ⇨ are apparent in early stages, and with time are replaced by papillary fronds with a fibrous core lined by a single layer of banal-appearing endothelial cells → characteristic of PEH.*

PEH With Single Layer of Flat Endothelium

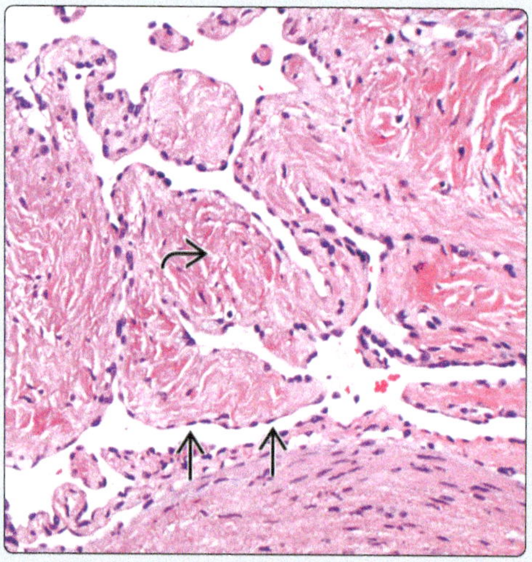

Some Cases of PEH Can Resemble Angiosarcoma

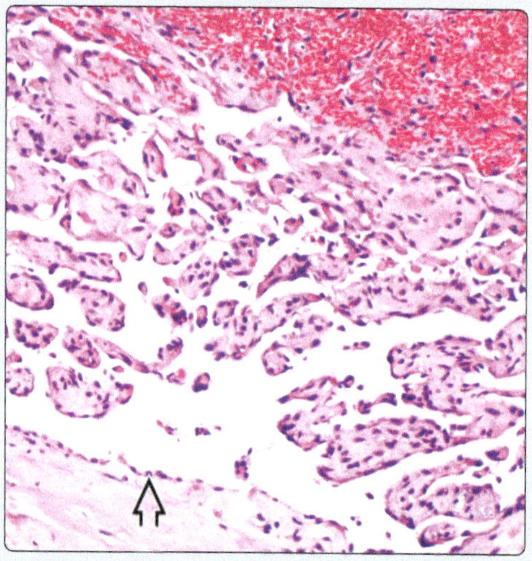

(Left) *The lined endothelium → is a single layer of evenly spaced, banal-appearing flat cells wrapping around the fibrotic core ↷.* **(Right)** *PEH can be mistaken for the dissecting vascular spaces seen in low-grade angiosarcoma. Note the bland endothelial lining ⇨ of the blood vessel lumen and intravascular location.*

TERMINOLOGY

Abbreviations

- Papillary endothelial hyperplasia (PEH)

Synonyms

- Masson tumor
- Vegetant intravascular hemangioendothelioma
- Intravascular angiomatosis
- Intravascular papillary endothelial hyperplasia

Definitions

- Benign, reactive, and papillary endothelial proliferation within vessel

ETIOLOGY/PATHOGENESIS

Reactive Vascular Proliferation

- Manifestation of organizing intravascular thrombus
- PEH-like changes may be present in preexisting hemangiomas or vascular malformations

CLINICAL ISSUES

Site

- Wide distribution
- Common sites include: Head and neck, fingers, trunk

Presentation

- Painless mass
- Located in deep dermis &/or subcutaneous tissue

Treatment

- Excision is not necessary but is curative

Prognosis

- Excellent
- Cases with underlying hemangioma or vascular malformation may recur

MACROSCOPIC

General Features

- Cystic mass with red-purple discoloration
- Often surrounded by pseudocapsule

Size

- Mostly small (< 2 cm)

MICROSCOPIC

Histologic Features

- Circumscribed lesion with pseudocapsule
  - Residual smooth muscle or elastic lamina of preexisting vessel may be apparent
- Fibrin thrombus
- Papillary structures lined by endothelial cells
  - Endothelial cells in single layer
  - Papillae form anastomosing network
- Papillary cores may consist of fibrin or fibrous connective tissue
- Intravascular location
- Vessel rupture may lead to extension of papillary endothelial proliferation into adjacent soft tissue
- Rare examples of extravascular variant in soft tissue have been reported
  - Represent reactive endothelial proliferation in organizing hematoma

Cytologic Features

- Nuclei lining papillae may appear plump or hobnailed in appearance
  - However, significant nuclear pleomorphism is absent

ANCILLARY TESTS

Electron Microscopy

- Differentiated endothelial cells line papillae
  - Luminal micropinocytotic vesicles
  - Tight junctions and basal lamina
  - Weibel-Palade bodies
- Undifferentiated &/or pericytic cells present within papillary cores

DIFFERENTIAL DIAGNOSIS

Angiosarcoma

- PEH is intraluminal process, unlike angiosarcoma, which is infiltrative
- Even PEH cases with soft tissue extension have bulk of lesion confined to vascular lumen
- PEH lacks nuclear atypia, tumor cell necrosis, and mitotic activity present in angiosarcoma

Hemangioma

- PEH-like changes may occur in hemangiomas complicated by thrombosis

Arteriovenous Malformation

- PEH-like changes may occur in background of arteriovenous malformation
- Important to recognize since these may recur

Hematoma

- Soft tissue hematomas may have foci of PEH
- May be mistaken for angiosarcoma

Venous Lymphatic Malformation

- May show foci of papillary hyperplasia, mimicking PEH
- In venous lymphatic malformation, there are lobules of abnormally dilated vessels, some with lymphatic morphology
  - In PEH, there is typically well-circumscribed lesion, preexisting vessel showing papillary hyperplasia

DIAGNOSTIC CHECKLIST

Clinically Relevant Pathologic Features

- Tissue distribution
  - Intravascular process

Pathologic Interpretation Pearls

- Intravascular papillary proliferation lined by endothelial cells without significant nuclear atypia

SELECTED REFERENCES

1. Pegado PF et al: Intravascular papillary endothelial hyperplasia (Masson tumor) mimicking a sarcoma and developing from an arteriovenous hemodialysis fistula. Skeletal Radiol. 44(6):859-62, 2015

(Left) *Low magnification shows a deceptively dissecting pattern; however, the depth of invasion tumor is well defined* →. **(Right)** *The second 1/2 of the same lesion shows that the deceptively dissecting process ends with a sharp border* →.

Well-Defined Border

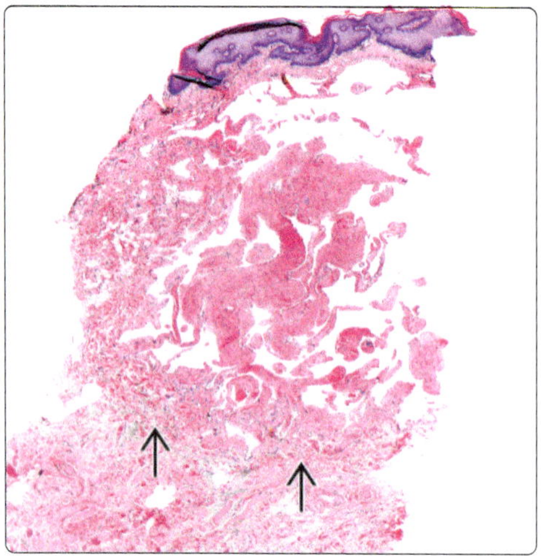

May Appear to Be Dissecting but Well Defined

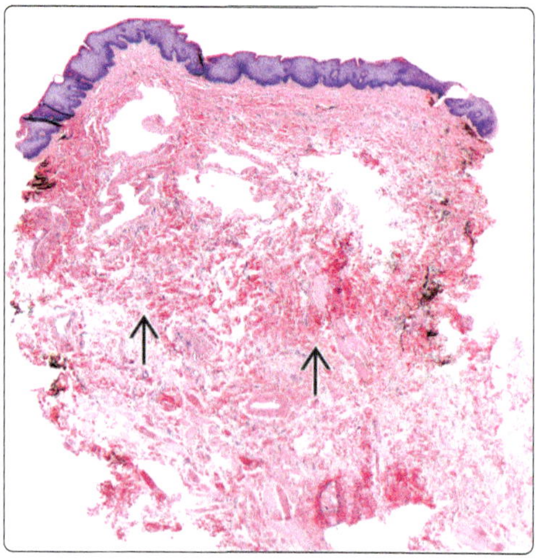

(Left) *A single layer of endothelial cells* → *line the papillary fronds in PEH. The endothelial cells may be plump and swollen but do not show significant nuclear atypia. The nuclei are hyperchromatic and the chromatin appear smudged.* **(Right)** *Foci of papillary endothelial proliferations can be seen in angiosarcomas, as shown in this example. Note the ill-defined pattern of collagen dissection* ↪ *and marked nuclear cytological atypia* →. *Collagen dissection extends beyond the central, papillary focus.*

High-Power Examination of PEH

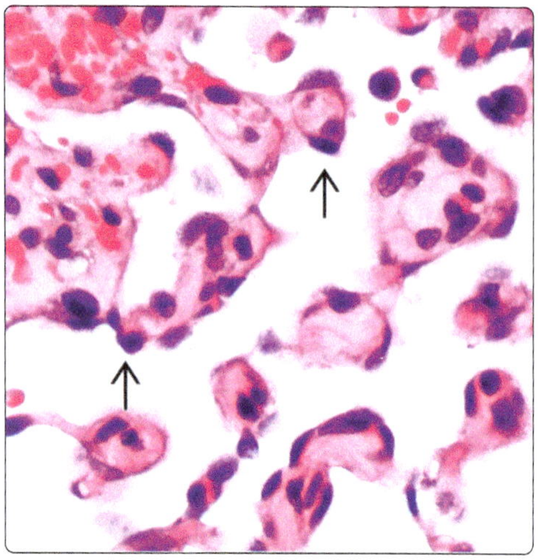

Angiosarcoma for Comparison

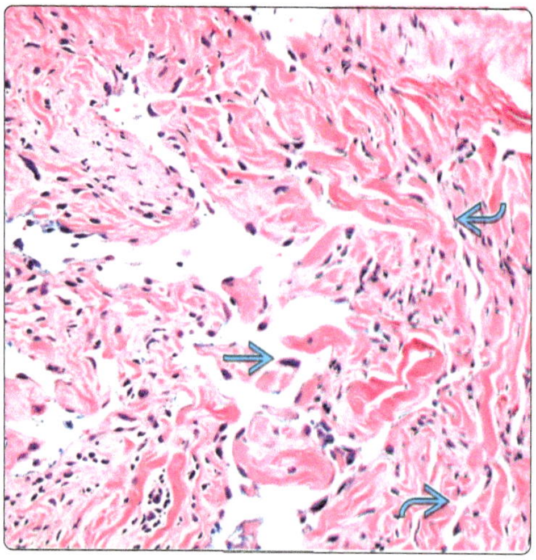

(Left) *Desmin immunostain highlights remnants of smooth muscle* → *in the blood vessel wall and confirms the intravascular location of PEH. The papillae are negative for desmin as expected* ↪. **(Right)** *Immunostaining for CD31 diffusely outlines the endothelium-lined papilla.*

Desmin Highlights Blood Vessels

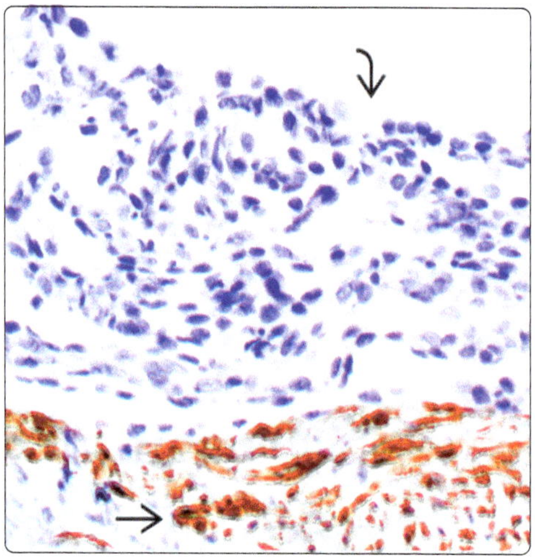

CD31 Immunostains Endothelium

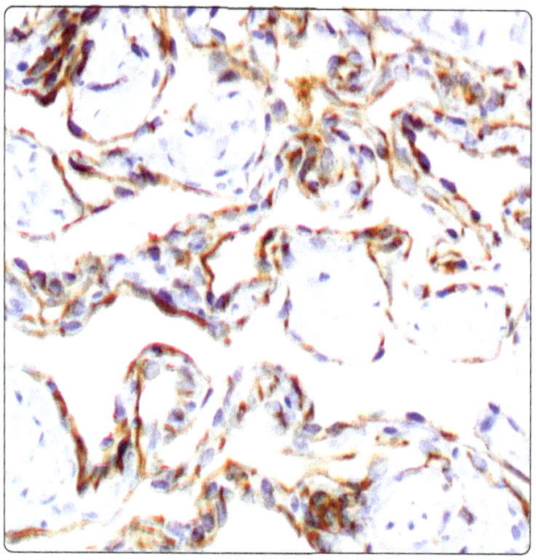

High-Power Examination

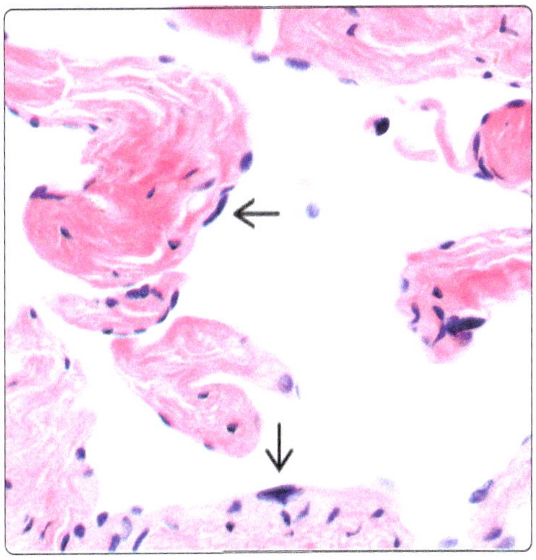

Well-Preserved Adnexae

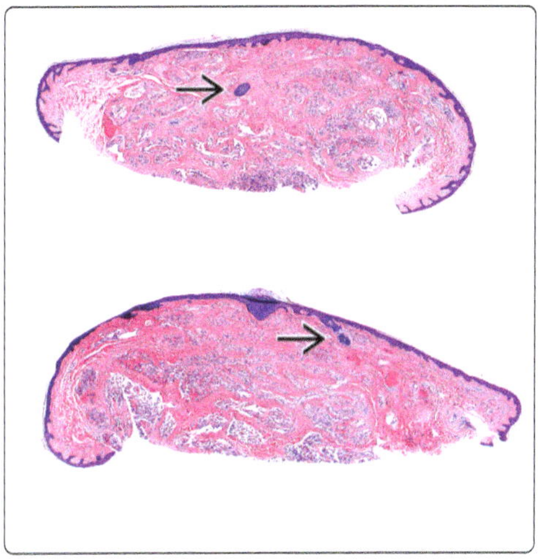

(Left) *The lining endothelial cells appear to have smudged chromatin* → *and are devoid of cytological atypia. No multilayering of these cells is noted.* **(Right)** *Under low magnification, the dermis is expanded by a well-circumscribed vascular proliferation. The adnexa* → *are pushed to the side but are well preserved. These features are distinct from an ill-defined, destructive vascular proliferation like angiosarcoma.*

Defined Border

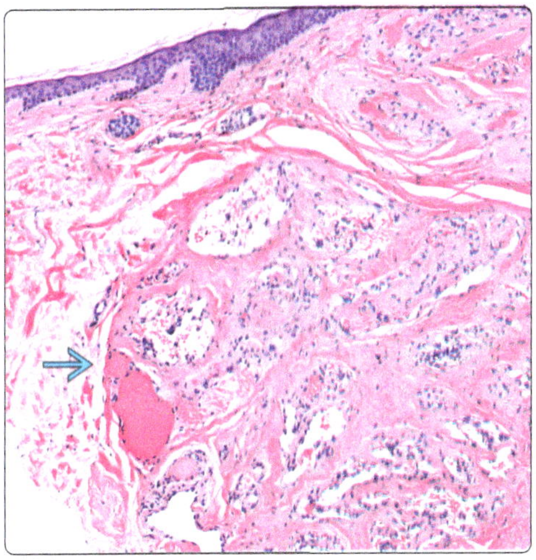

High Power Shows Intraluminal Fibrin

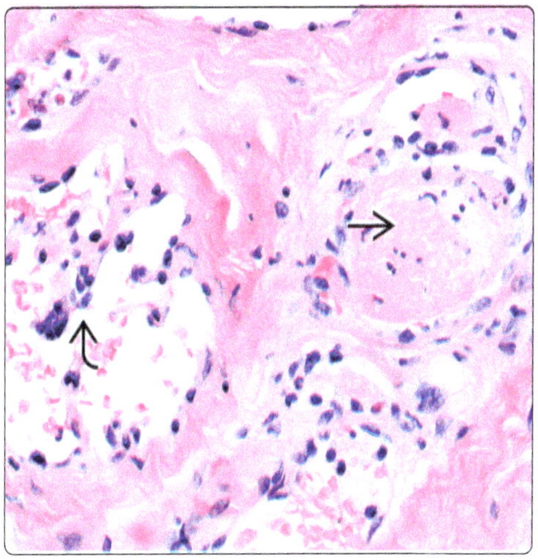

(Left) *PEH is well circumscribed as demonstrated by the sharp edge* →*, in contrast to the adjacent, unremarkable dermis.* **(Right)** *Fibrin-plugged vascular space* → *is seen adjacent to an area of intravascular papillary proliferation* ↗*.*

Thin Papillae and Fibrotic Cores

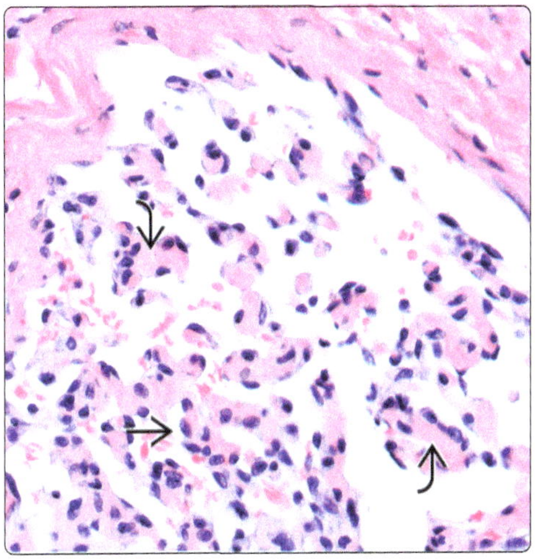

Mimics Kaposi Sarcoma

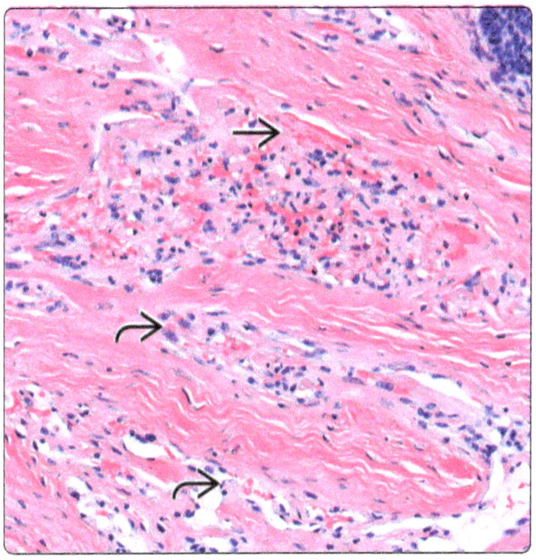

(Left) *Higher magnification of a papillary area reveals more delicate, thin papillae with a small foci of fibrotic cores* ↗*. The lining endothelium is evenly spaced with banal cytology* →*.* **(Right)** *Another focus of the same lesion shows that the slit-like, poorly formed vascular spaces* ↗ *can mimic Kaposi sarcoma (KS), especially with extravasated erythrocytes* →*. In such challenging cases, immunostaining for HHV8 is recommended to exclude KS.*

Glomus Tumors

KEY FACTS

TERMINOLOGY

- Perivascular mesenchymal neoplasm composed of cells closely resembling modified smooth muscle cells of normal glomus body
  - Considered to fall on morphologic spectrum with myopericytoma, myofibroma, and angioleiomyoma

CLINICAL ISSUES

- Most common in young adults (20-40 years)
- Female predilection in subungual tumors
- Most common in distal extremities (particularly nail bed)
- Typically small, red-blue nodule, often solitary and painful
- Most arise in skin or subcutis
- Treatment: Complete surgical excision
- Excellent prognosis in conventional glomus tumor (GT)
- Malignant GT is clinically aggressive

MACROSCOPIC

- Most are < 1 cm in size

MICROSCOPIC

- Typically solid nests of round cells closely associated with variably sized blood vessels
  - Characteristic centralized, rounded, uniform nuclei
- Hyalinized to myxoid stroma
- No mitotic activity or necrosis
- Variants: Glomangioma, glomangiomyoma, glomangiomatosis, symplastic GT
- Malignant forms exist but are very rare

ANCILLARY TESTS

- SMA(+), caldesmon (+)
- Negative for desmin, S100, keratin, synaptophysin

TOP DIFFERENTIAL DIAGNOSES

- Myopericytoma
- Benign adnexal tumors
- Dermal melanocytic nevus
- Paraganglioma

(Left) *This is an example of a subungual glomangioma on the thumb (the nail has been avulsed prior to biopsy).* **(Right)** *Glomus tumor (GT) is a rare benign tumor that may arise almost anywhere, but shows a predilection for the distal extremities, particularly under the nail bed (subungual). It is histologically characterized by sheets and nests of uniform, round to epithelioid cells arranged around a conspicuous vasculature.*

Clinical Photograph of Subungual Glomangioma

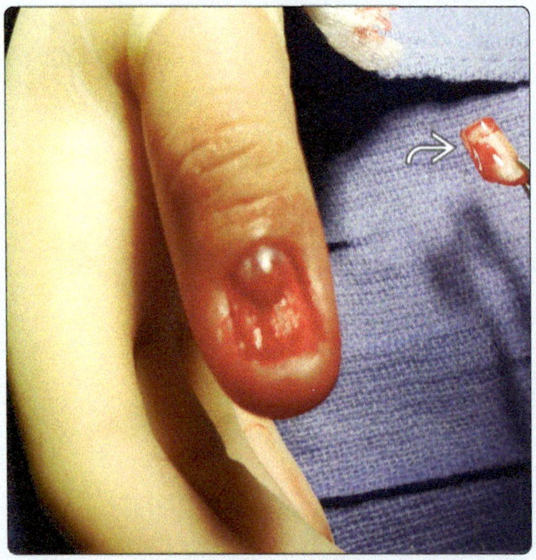

Glomus Tumor at Low Magnification

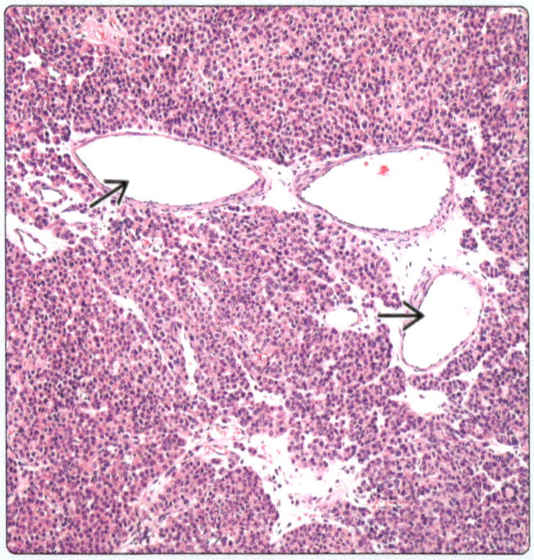

(Left) *The distinctive nuclei in GT are strikingly monomorphic and feature a sharply defined, round nuclear contour. They are often described as being "punched out." Cytoplasmic borders vary in prominence, and may be easy or difficult to visualize, depending upon the individual tumor. Mitotic figures are absent.* **(Right)** *Strong, diffuse cytoplasmic expression of SMA is characteristic of GT. Caldesmon is also typically positive. Desmin is negative.*

Monotonous Nuclei in Glomus Tumor

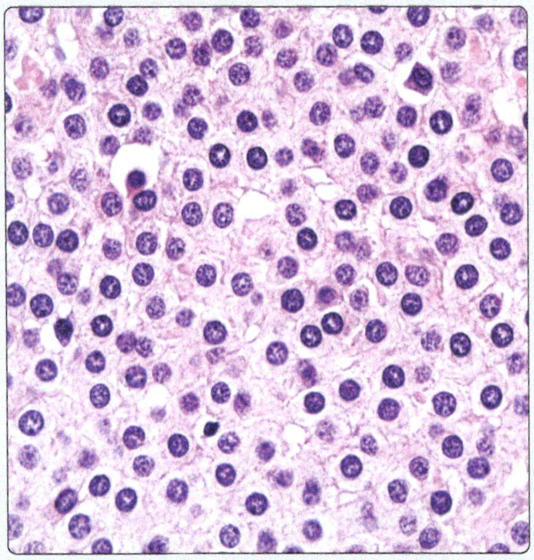

SMA Expression in Glomus Tumor

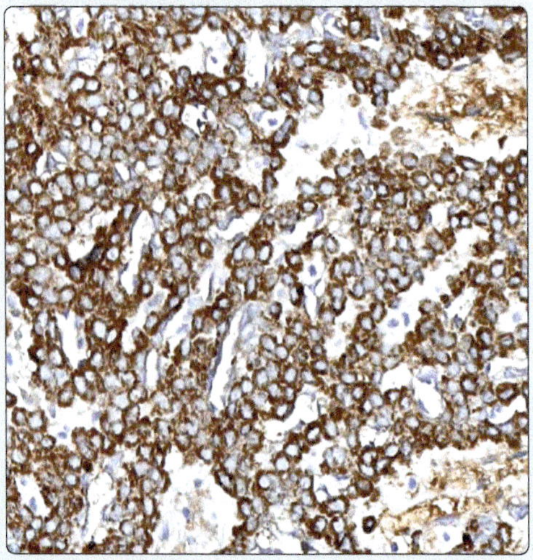

TERMINOLOGY

Abbreviations

- Glomus tumor (GT)

Definitions

- Perivascular mesenchymal neoplasm composed of cells closely resembling modified smooth muscle cells of normal glomus body
  - Considered to fall on morphologic spectrum with myopericytoma, myofibroma, and angioleiomyoma
- Several morphologic variants exist, including glomangioma (glomuvenous malformation), glomangiomyoma, glomangiomatosis, and symplastic GT

ETIOLOGY/PATHOGENESIS

Small Subsets Are Inherited

- Often feature multiple lesions
- Multiple familial GT
  - Inactivation of *GLMN* gene
- Neurofibromatosis type 1 (NF1)
  - Biallelic inactivation of *NF1* gene

CLINICAL ISSUES

Epidemiology

- Incidence
  - Rare
    - Malignant GT extremely rare
- Age
  - Most common in young adults (20-40 years)
    - Overall wide age range
    - Glomangioma variant more common in childhood
- Sex
  - Female predilection in subungual tumors

Site

- Overall wide distribution
- Most common in distal extremities
  - Particularly subungual location
- Rarely in other anatomic locations, including visceral organs (particularly GI tract), bone, mediastinum

Presentation

- Typically small, red-blue nodule, often solitary
  - Multiple in up to 10% of cases
    - Multifocality also seen within setting of NF1
- Most arise in skin or subcutis
  - Rarely in deep soft tissues
- Usually painful
  - Long history of pain
  - Pain with exposure to cold &/or tactile stimulation

Treatment

- Complete surgical excision
- Clinical follow-up for malignant GT and GT of uncertain malignant potential

Prognosis

- Excellent prognosis in conventional GT
  - < 10% recur locally
  - Includes symplastic forms, glomangiomatosis, and other variants
- Malignant GT is clinically aggressive
  - Metastases and death of patients in up to 40% of cases
- Large, visceral GT have potential for aggressive behavior regardless of histology

MACROSCOPIC

General Features

- Red-blue nodular lesions

Size

- Most are < 1 cm
  - Deeper lesions may be larger

MICROSCOPIC

Histologic Features

- Well circumscribed ± fibrous pseudocapsule
  - Small nests of glomus cells associated with small vessels may be identified around periphery of main tumor
- Typically solid nests of cells within highly vascularized stroma
  - Vessels range from small to large and ectatic (staghorn appearance)
  - Tumor cells arranged around vessels, often as cuffs
  - Diffuse nodular, sheet-like appearance in highly cellular tumors
- Characteristic small, round, uniform tumor cells with pale eosinophilic to amphophilic cytoplasm
  - Each cell contains single centralized small, round, uniform nucleus
    - Sometimes described as "punched out"
    - Absence of nuclear atypia and significant mitotic activity
  - Occasionally cases feature oncocytic or epithelioid cytomorphology
  - Each cell surrounded by basal lamina
- Hyalinized to myxoid stroma
- No necrosis
- Rare intravascular growth

Morphologic Variants

- Glomangioma (glomuvenous malformation)
  - 20% of cases
  - Less well circumscribed
  - Large, gaping veins surrounded by clusters of glomus cells
    - Resembles vascular spaces of cavernous hemangioma
    - Secondary thrombosis may occur
- Symplastic GT
  - Prominent degenerative atypia in form of marked nuclear hyperchromasia and pleomorphism
    - Lacks mitotic activity and necrosis
    - Lacks other atypical features (e.g., large size, deep location)
  - Otherwise typical features of GT
- Glomangiomyoma
  - Typical GT or glomangioma with additional component of spindled cells resembling smooth muscle
  - Rare

- Glomangiomatosis
  - Diffuse, infiltrative growth pattern resembling angiomatosis
  - Nests of glomus cells around vessels
  - Very rare

Malignant Glomus Tumor (Glomangiosarcoma)

- Preexisting conventional GT may or may not be present
- Criteria for malignancy
  - Tumors showing marked nuclear atypia **and** any degree of mitotic activity, **or**
  - Tumor showing atypical mitotic figures
- 2 main morphologies
  - Spindled cells in bundles or fascicles
  - Sheets of small round cells with high grade nuclei
  - Mitoses frequent

Glomus Tumor of Uncertain Malignant Potential

- Reserved for tumors that do not fulfill above criteria for malignancy but that show at least 1 atypical feature other than nuclear pleomorphism
- Also includes deeply situated tumors that are > 2 cm

ANCILLARY TESTS

Immunohistochemistry

- SMA(+), caldesmon (+)
- Variable CD34(+)
- Abundant pericellular type IV collagen (+)
- Negative for desmin, S100, keratin, synaptophysin

Molecular Genetics

- NOTCH gene rearrangements (*NOTCH1*, *NOTCH2*, or *NOTCH3*) reported in recent series of benign and malignant GTs
  - 1 case of *NOTCH3-MIR143* fusion reported
- *BRAF* (V600E) and *KRAS* (G12A) mutations reported in some cases of sporadic GT

DIFFERENTIAL DIAGNOSIS

Myopericytoma

- Exists on morphologic spectrum with GT
- Pure forms lack uniform round cell component of GT
- Characteristic perivascular concentric growth of ovoid to spindled tumor cells

Benign Adnexal Tumors

- e.g., nodular hidradenoma, spiradenoma
- Epithelial, ductal/glandular, or sebaceous differentiation should be identifiable
- Keratins (+)
- Negative for SMA

Paraganglioma

- Deceptively termed glomus tympanicum in ear and glomus jugulare in neck
- Prominent nested Zellballen growth pattern common
- Synaptophysin (+), chromogranin (+)
- S100(+) in sustentacular cells
- Negative for SMA

Dermal Melanocytic Nevus

- Nests of melanocytic cells, ± pigmentation
- Intranuclear pseudoinclusions common
- Cells lack close association with blood vessels
- Expression of melanocytic markers (e.g., S100, melan-A)
- Negative for SMA, caldesmon

Angioleiomyoma

- Predominantly composed of bundles of mature, eosinophilic smooth muscle cells
- Lacks prominent uniform round cell component of GT
- SMA(+), desmin (+)
- Often painful

Carcinoid Tumor

- Visceral organs
- Can show close architectural overlap with GT
- Speckled or salt and pepper chromatin pattern
- Negative for SMA
- Keratin (+), synaptophysin (+), chromogranin (+)

SELECTED REFERENCES

1. Mravic M et al: Clinical and histopathological diagnosis of glomus tumor: an institutional experience of 138 cases. Int J Surg Pathol. ePub, 2015
2. Kumar MG et al: Glomus tumors in individuals with neurofibromatosis type 1. J Am Acad Dermatol. 71(1):44-8, 2014
3. Mosquera JM et al: Novel MIR143-NOTCH fusions in benign and malignant glomus tumors. Genes Chromosomes Cancer. 52(11):1075-87, 2013
4. Chakrapani A et al: BRAF and KRAS mutations in sporadic glomus tumors. Am J Dermatopathol. 34(5):533-5, 2012
5. Sheehan JP et al: Gamma Knife surgery for the management of glomus tumors: a multicenter study. J Neurosurg. 117(2):246-54, 2012
6. Lamba G et al: Malignant glomus tumor of kidney: the first reported case and review of literature. Hum Pathol. 42(8):1200-3, 2011
7. Brems H et al: Glomus tumors in neurofibromatosis type 1: genetic, functional, and clinical evidence of a novel association. Cancer Res. 2009 Sep 15;69(18):7393-401. Epub 2009 Sep 8. Erratum in: Cancer Res. 69(20):8216, 2009
8. Semaan MT et al: Current assessment and management of glomus tumors. Curr Opin Otolaryngol Head Neck Surg. 16(5):420-6, 2008
9. Brouillard P et al: Four common glomulin mutations cause two thirds of glomuvenous malformations ("familial glomangiomas"): evidence for a founder effect. J Med Genet. 42(2):e13, 2005
10. De Chiara A et al: Malignant glomus tumour: a case report and review of the literature. Sarcoma. 7(2):87-91, 2003
11. Brouillard P et al: Mutations in a novel factor, glomulin, are responsible for glomuvenous malformations ("glomangiomas"). Am J Hum Genet. 70(4):866-74, 2002
12. Mentzel T et al: CD34-positive glomus tumor: clinicopathologic and immunohistochemical analysis of six cases with myxoid stromal changes. J Cutan Pathol. 29(7):421-5, 2002
13. Calvert JT et al: Additional glomangioma families link to chromosome 1p: no evidence for genetic heterogeneity. Hum Hered. 51(3):180-2, 2001
14. Folpe AL et al: Atypical and malignant glomus tumors: analysis of 52 cases, with a proposal for the reclassification of glomus tumors. Am J Surg Pathol. 25(1):1-12, 2001
15. Takata H et al: Treatment of subungual glomus tumour. Hand Surg. 6(1):25-7, 2001
16. Boon LM et al: A gene for inherited cutaneous venous anomalies ("glomangiomas") localizes to chromosome 1p21-22. Am J Hum Genet. 65(1):125-33, 1999
17. Hiruta N et al: Malignant glomus tumor: a case report and review of the literature. Am J Surg Pathol. 21(9):1096-103, 1997
18. Van Geertruyden J et al: Glomus tumours of the hand. A retrospective study of 51 cases. J Hand Surg [Br]. 21(2):257-60, 1996
19. Pulitzer DR et al: Epithelioid glomus tumor. Hum Pathol. 26(9):1022-7, 1995
20. Haque S et al: Multiple glomus tumors of the stomach with intravascular spread. Am J Surg Pathol. 16(3):291-9, 1992
21. Gould EW et al: Locally infiltrative glomus tumors and glomangiosarcomas. A clinical, ultrastructural, and immunohistochemical study. Cancer. 65(2):310-8, 1990

Variable Stromal Hyalinization in Glomus Tumor

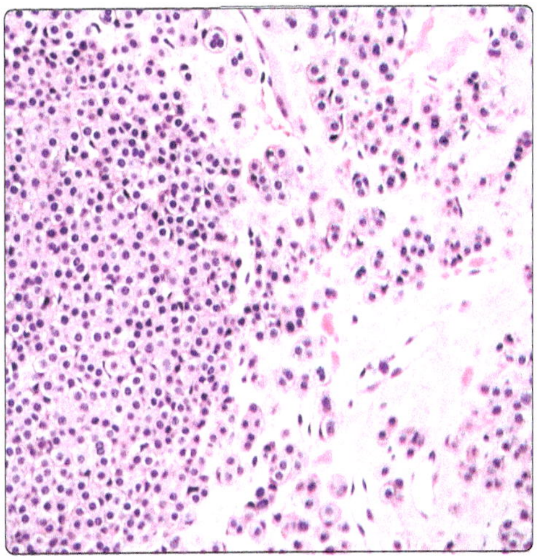

Peritumoral Glomus Proliferations

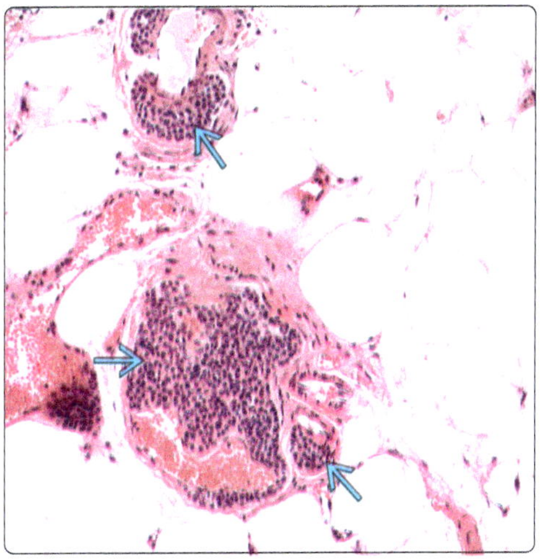

(Left) *The stroma in GT varies from hyalinized to myxoid. Some zones of prominent hyalinization or sclerosis can feature tumor cells arranged singly or in a small aggregate or cords (right).* **(Right)** *In some cases of GT, small vessels at the periphery of the tumor may contain a subtle or conspicuous glomus cell proliferation →. This finding can be diagnostically helpful in distinguishing a solid GT from an adnexal tumor.*

Sheet-Like Growth in Glomus Tumor

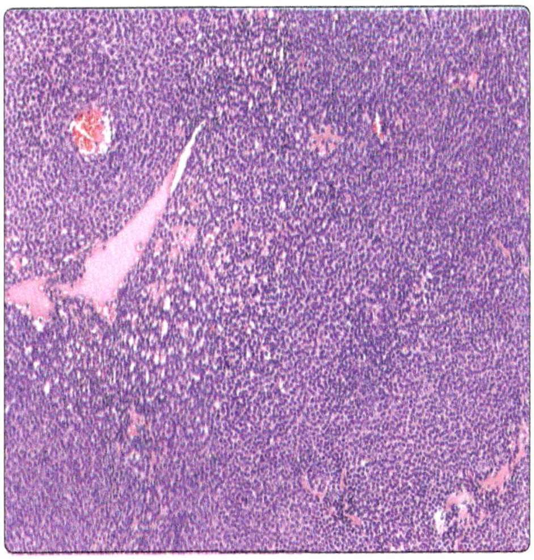

Glomus Tumor Vasculature

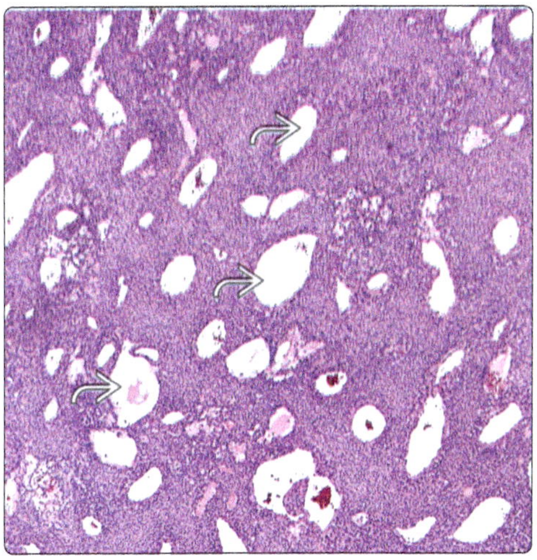

(Left) *Some GTs may feature a strikingly solid growth pattern with a less prominent vasculature, as depicted. These tumors can closely mimic a cutaneous adnexal neoplasm.* **(Right)** *The stromal vasculature ➡ can be very prominent in some cases of GT and may also adopt irregular or staghorn shapes. This morphology can lead to consideration of a cellular solitary fibrous tumor (previously termed hemangiopericytoma).*

Pericellular Type IV Collagen in Glomus Tumor

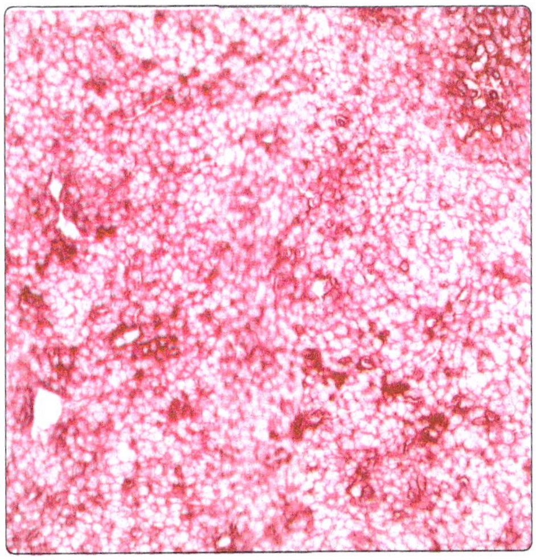

Oncocytic Change in Glomus Tumor

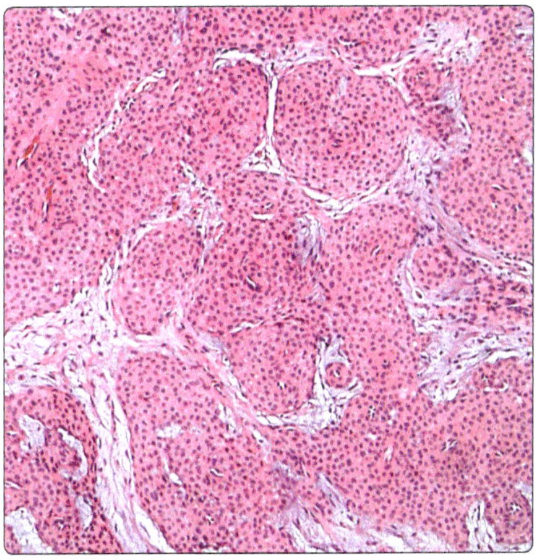

(Left) *Although not widely utilized in general practice, a collagen IV (or laminin) immunostain can nicely highlight the pericellular basement membrane material characteristic of GT.* **(Right)** *Oncocytic change is an occasional finding in GT and is characterized by tumor cells with abundant granular cytoplasm, as depicted here. This particular tumor also features a myxoid stroma.*

(Left) *Glomangioma is a variant of GT that features larger, dilated vascular spaces lined by characteristic tumor cells. Compared to conventional GT, glomangioma is often less well circumscribed and is more common in children and familial cases.* **(Right)** *The large dilated spaces of glomangioma are always lined by arrays of neoplastic glomus cells; however, this lining can vary widely in thickness from field to field.*

Glomangioma

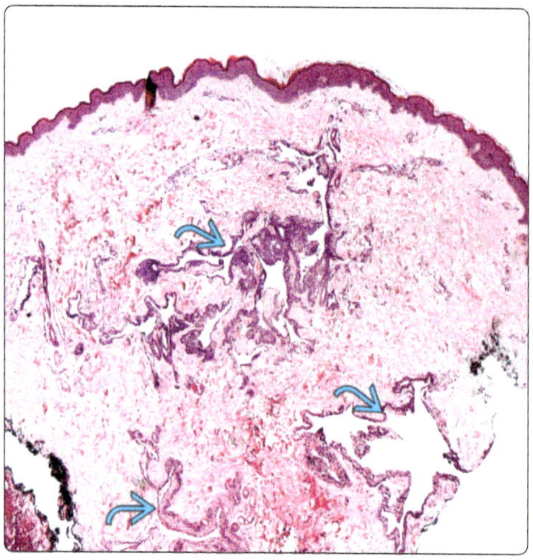

Prominent Dilated Vessels in Glomangioma

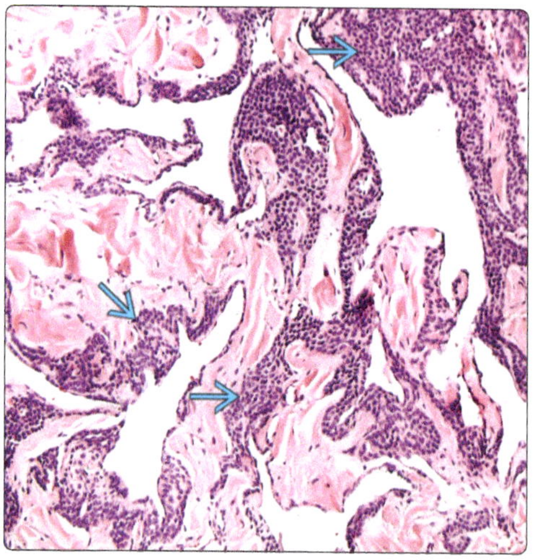

(Left) *As shown in this image, vascular spaces in glomangioma may be markedly expanded and closely resemble those of cavernous hemangioma. However, the glomus cell lining is distinctive. Also note that large thrombi or phleboliths may be present in some cases.* **(Right)** *Rare cases of GT (or any of its other variants) may contain scattered pleomorphic nuclei, suggesting malignancy. Mitoses and other atypical features are absent, however. These changes are likely degenerative in nature.*

Cavernous Vascular Pattern in Glomangioma

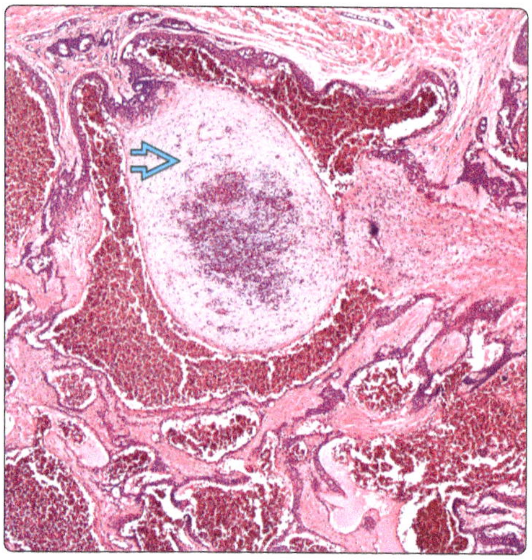

Symplastic Glomangioma

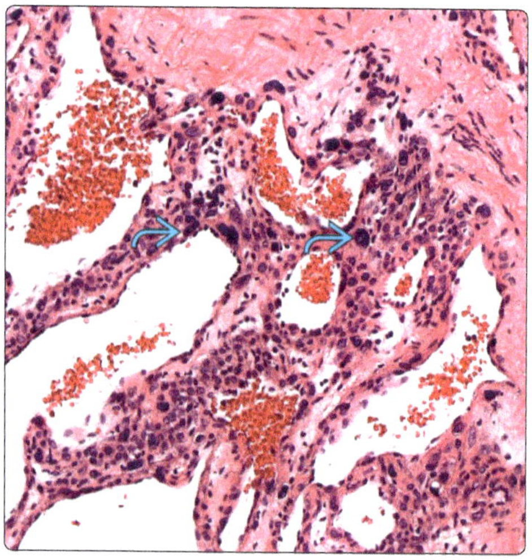

(Left) *Glomangiomyoma is a variant of GT that features a smooth muscle component in addition to areas of otherwise conventional-appearing GT or glomangioma. Note the small areas of rounded glomus cells.* **(Right)** *Glomangiomatosis is a rare, benign, diffuse variant of GT that resembles the pattern seen in angiomatosis; however, small vessels in glomangiomatosis feature glomus cell proliferations.*

Glomangiomyoma

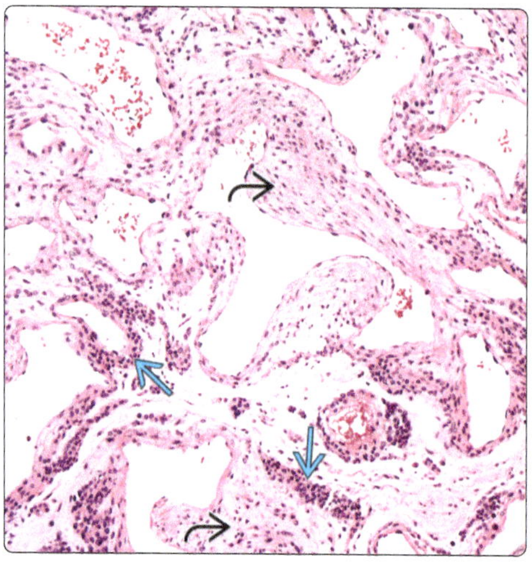

Glomangiomatosis

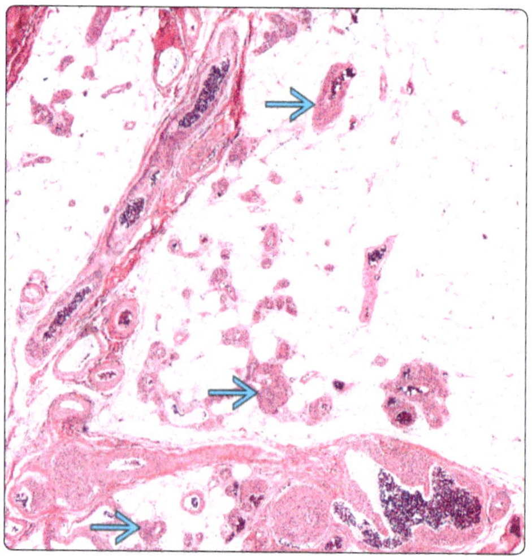

Interface Between Benign and Malignant Glomus Tumor

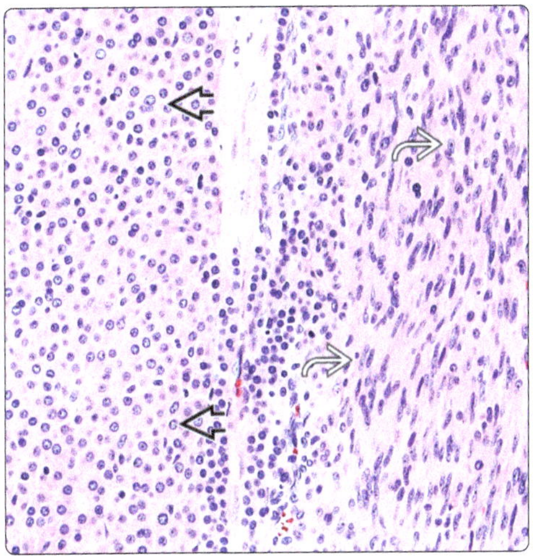

Malignant Spindle Cell Morphology

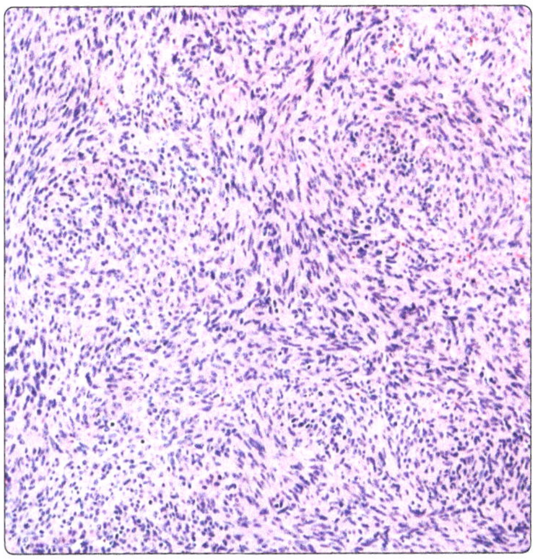

(Left) *Malignant GT is very rare. A preexisting component of conventional benign-appearing GT may or may not be present. In the latter situation, immunohistochemistry is often needed to support the diagnosis.* **(Right)** *The spindled morphology of malignant GT often resembles other spindle cell sarcomas, such as leiomyosarcoma. Short fascicles and whorls are common. Mitoses are usually numerous.*

Malignant Round Cell Morphology

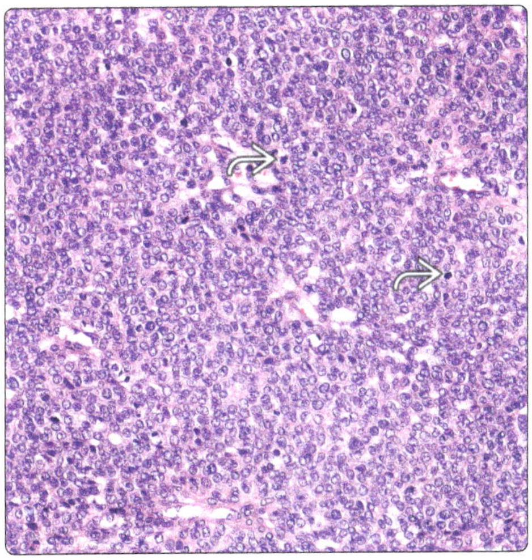

Nuclear Atypia and Mitoses in Malignant Glomus Tumor

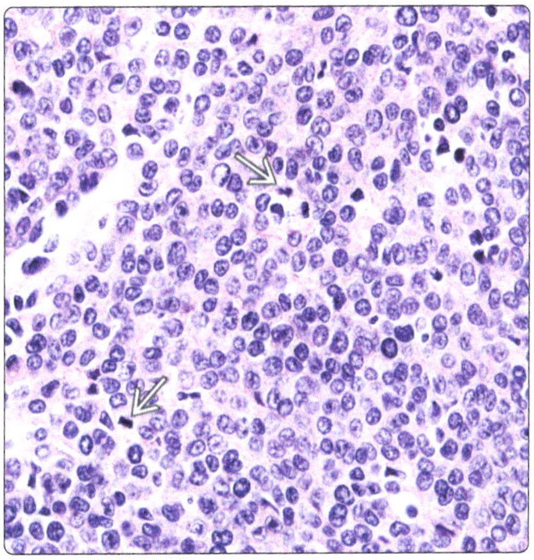

(Left) *The round cell morphology of malignant GT mimics somewhat conventional GT in architecture; however, the nuclei often show a high degree of atypia and mitoses are easily identified.* **(Right)** *Malignant GT with a round cell pattern shows increased nuclear atypia, including prominent nucleoli in some cases. Note the mitoses.*

Nuclear Pleomorphism in Malignant Glomus Tumor

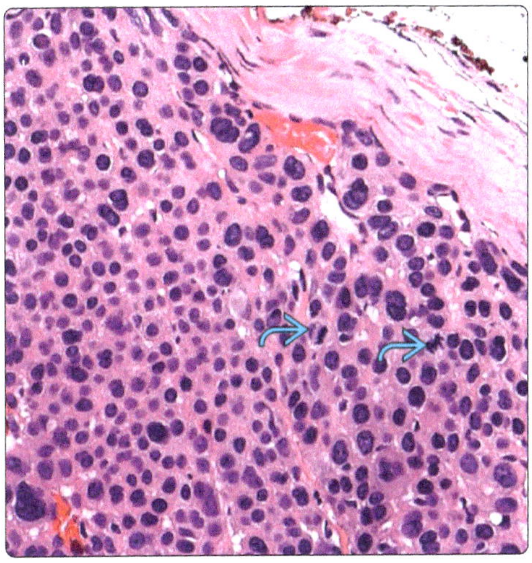

Vascular Invasion in Malignant Glomus Tumor

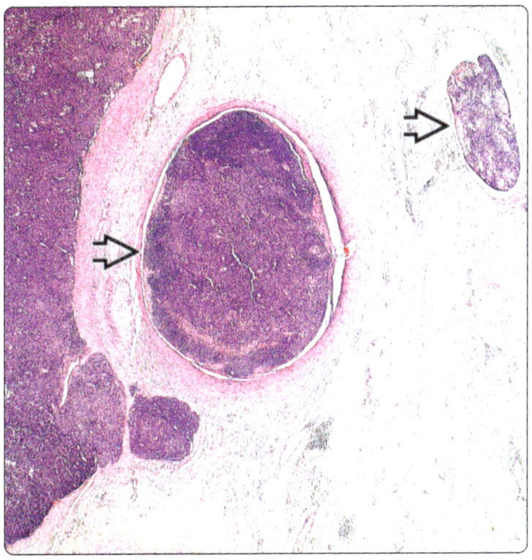

(Left) *Some cases of malignant GT feature marked nuclear pleomorphism &/or hyperchromasia. Distinction from symplastic GT is possible through identification of other atypical features, including multiple mitoses.* **(Right)** *Malignant GT can show a more prominent multinodular growth pattern compared to conventional GT. Vascular invasion may also be seen.*

Lymphangioma and Superficial Lymphangioma

KEY FACTS

TERMINOLOGY

- Lymphangioma circumscriptum (LC) (superficial lymphangioma)
- Lymphangiomatosis (systemic angiomatosis)
- Cystic lymphangioma (cystic hygroma)
- Deep lymphangioma (cavernous lymphangioma)

ETIOLOGY/PATHOGENESIS

- Most cases considered developmental malformations/hamartomas, **not** true neoplasms
- Associated with trisomies and other genetic syndromes, including Turner (cystic hygroma), Noonan, and Maffucci

CLINICAL ISSUES

- More common in children (6% of benign childhood tumors); present at birth or within first 2 years of life
- Typically presents as large, slow-growing, painless mass (deep lymphangioma) or as multiple small, grouped, superficial vesicular lesions (LC)
- Excellent prognosis in most cases, although may be fatal if involving mediastinum or internal organs
- Recurrence rate high if removal incomplete

MICROSCOPIC

- Variably sized anastomosing vascular spaces lined by small, bland endothelial cells
- Often contain abundant proteinaceous debris, scattered lymphocytes, and erythrocytes
- Walls show stromal fibrosis (older lesions) and may contain smooth muscle
- Endothelial cells are small with uniform, bland-appearing, oval to flattened, hyperchromatic nuclei

TOP DIFFERENTIAL DIAGNOSES

- Hemangiomas
- Progressive lymphangioma
- Secondary lymphangiectasia
- Atypical vascular proliferation

(Left) *Clinical photograph shows a large, deep lymphangioma (cystic hygroma) on the lateral neck of a child.* **(Right)** *This example of a superficial lymphangioma shows widely dilated spaces in the superficial dermis. The lumina show several papillary projections ⇨ with slightly fibrinous cores lined by small, hyperchromatic-staining endothelial cells.*

Large, Deep Lymphangioma

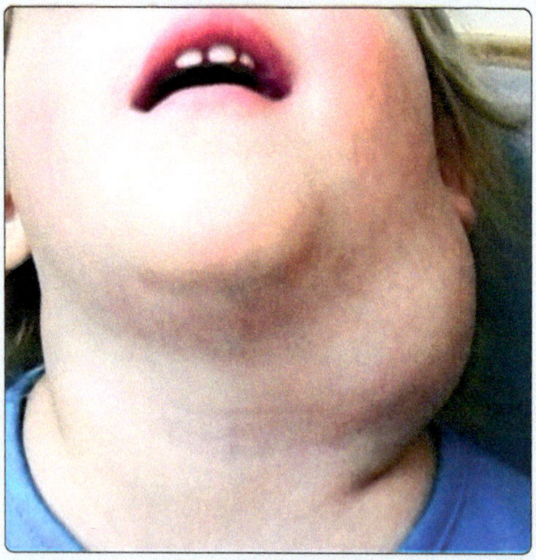

Superficial Lymphangioma

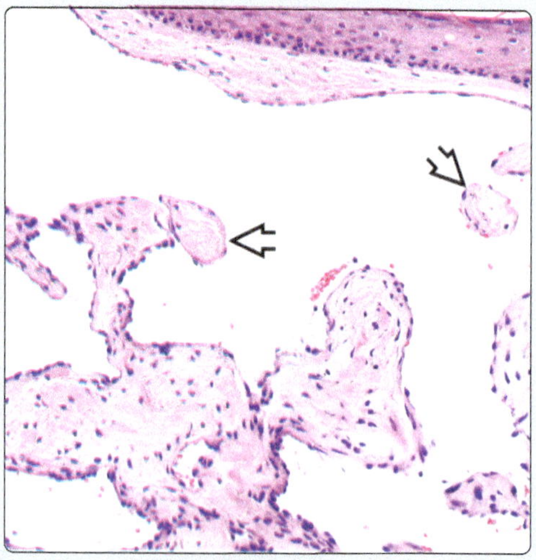

(Left) *Deep lymphangioma shows large vascular channels filled with proteinaceous material, a few lymphocytes, and scattered erythrocytes ⇨.* **(Right)** *This example of a deep lymphangioma shows multiple dilated endothelial-lined channels with small collections of lymphocytes → within the lumina, along with fluid and erythrocytes.*

Deep Lymphangioma

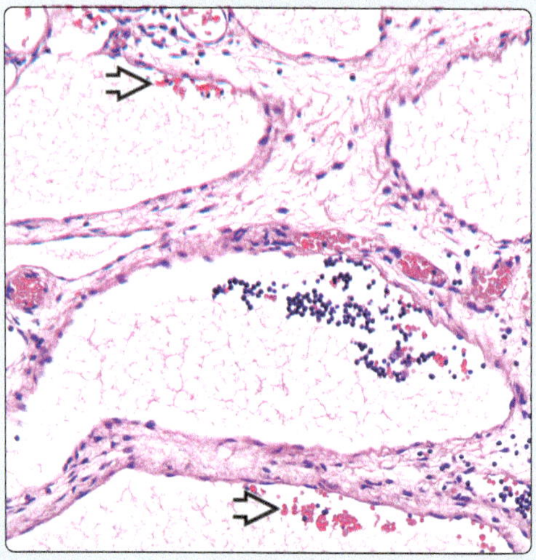

Deep Lymphangioma

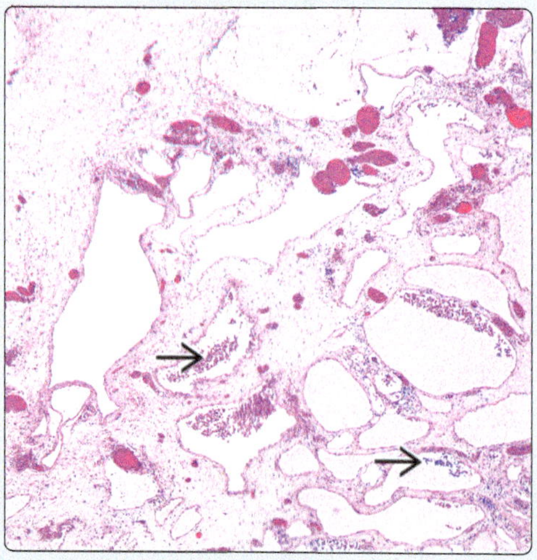

TERMINOLOGY

Synonyms

- Lymphangioma circumscriptum (LC) (superficial cutaneous lymphangioma)
- Lymphangiomatosis (LS) (generalized lymphangioma, systemic angiomatosis)
- Cystic lymphangioma (cystic hygroma)
- Deep lymphangioma (cavernous lymphangioma)
- Lymphatic malformation

Definitions

- Proliferation of lymphatic vessels
  - Superficial (lymphangioma circumscription)
  - Deep (cavernous lymphangioma)
  - Diffusely involve most organ systems (LS)

ETIOLOGY/PATHOGENESIS

Developmental Anomaly

- Most cases are considered developmental or congenital malformations/hamartomas, **not** true neoplasms
  - Maldevelopment during embryonic lymphangiogenesis most likely etiology
    - Leads to sequestered lymphatics that fail to communicate with normal lymphovascular system
  - May be due to maternal infections or substance abuse
  - LS considered congenital in most cases

Genetics

- Associated with genetic syndromes, including Turner syndrome (cystic hygroma), Noonan syndrome, Maffucci syndrome, trisomies 13, 18, 21
- Mutations in *VEGFR-C*, *VEGFR3*, *PROX1*, *FOXC2*, and *SOX18* genes implicated

Acquired

- Rare acquired cases occur in adults
  - Likely associated with infection or trauma

CLINICAL ISSUES

Epidemiology

- Incidence
  - More common in children: Estimated 6% of benign childhood tumors
- Age
  - Often present at birth or within first 2 years of life (~ 90% of cases)
  - LS usually presents within first 2 decades of life
- Sex
  - Intraabdominal lymphangiomas have slight male predominance
  - LS has no gender predilection

Site

- Head and neck most common site for cystic lymphangiomas
  - Usually posterior triangle but can occur in anterior triangle
  - Also occur in axillae, abdomen, and internal organs
- Cavernous type more frequent in oral cavity, upper trunk, limbs, and abdominal sites
  - Intraabdominal lymphangiomas occur in mesentery, omentum, and retroperitoneum
- LC: Axillary folds, neck, and trunk are most common sites
- LS: Can affect any organ system but often involves bones, soft tissues, and skin

Presentation

- Cystic mass lesion; may be superficial or deep
  - Typically presents as large, slow-growing, painless mass (deep lymphangioma) or as multiple small, grouped, superficial vesicular lesions (LC)
  - LS presents with numerous cystic lesions, both superficial and deep
- Soft and fluctuant swellings on palpation
- Intraabdominal cases may present with abdominal distension, mass on palpation
  - May also develop abdominal obstruction, volvulus, and infarction
- Generalized LS: Depends on affected site
  - Bone: Pathologic fractures
  - Lungs: Dyspnea, wheezing due to chylothorax, chylous ascites
  - Spleen: Splenomegaly, left upper quadrant pain

Treatment

- Surgical approaches
  - May be indicated in large, deep lesions, especially if symptomatic
  - LS not amenable to surgical excision
- Drugs
  - Intralesional injection of sclerosing agents, including bleomycin and OK-432 (Picibanil)

Prognosis

- Excellent in most cases, although LS may be fatal if involving mediastinum or internal organs, especially lungs
- Recurrence rate high with incomplete removal
- No malignant transformation reported

IMAGING

Ultrasonographic Findings

- Unilocular or multilocular anechoic mass
- Can be used in utero to detect cystic lymphangioma (associated with hydrops fetalis, Turner syndrome, and high death rate)

CT Findings

- Nonenhancing cystic lesions with homogeneous attenuation
- Visceral and osseous lesions often show contrast enhancement
- May displace surrounding organs

MACROSCOPIC

General Features

- Multiple cystic spaces with clear to whitish fluid

MICROSCOPIC

Histologic Features

- Variably sized anastomosing vascular spaces lined by small, bland endothelial cells
- Dilated lumina
  - Often contain abundant proteinaceous debris, scattered lymphocytes, and erythrocytes
- Walls show stromal fibrosis (older lesions) and occasional myxoid change
  - Often contain lymphoid infiltrates
    - May show occasional reactive germinal centers
  - Mast cells are common
  - Hemosiderin deposition in stroma may be seen
- Large vessels may contain smooth muscle in their walls
- Cavernous hemangiomas have infiltrative margins and often extend into surrounding tissues

Cytologic Features

- Endothelial cells are small with uniform, bland-appearing, oval to flattened, hyperchromatic nuclei

Predominant Pattern/Injury Type

- Cystic, macroscopic

Predominant Cell/Compartment Type

- Lymphatics

ANCILLARY TESTS

Immunohistochemistry

- Endothelial lining cells show variable positivity with vascular markers CD31, CD34, and FVIIIRAg
- Newer lymphatic markers, including podoplanin (D2-40), VEGFR-3, and LYVE-1, typically positive

DIFFERENTIAL DIAGNOSIS

Hemangiomas

- Most cases show smaller vascular spaces with more red blood cells, less proteinaceous material, and fewer lymphocytes
- Often well-circumscribed, noninfiltrative borders

Progressive Lymphangioma

- Form of cutaneous lymphangioma with distinct clinical findings
  - Typically presents on lower extremities of adults as slow-growing patches or plaques
- Histologic findings very similar to other forms of lymphangioma
  - Superficially dilated spaces that become progressively smaller with deep extension

Secondary Lymphangiectasia

- May be due to local factors, such as obstruction (e.g., due to tumor), scarring, or previous radiation therapy
- Identical histologic findings; can only be distinguished by clinical history or other findings (if present)

Atypical Vascular Proliferation

- Radiation-induced lesion; most frequent in breast
- Clinically, presents as multiple small vesicles in radiation field
- Irregularly dilated vascular spaces lined by atypical endothelial cells

Lymphangioma-Like Kaposi Sarcoma

- Usually shows at least focal areas of more typical Kaposi sarcoma
  - Infiltrative slit-like spaces lined by hyperchromatic spindle-shaped cells
  - Stromal hemosiderin deposition and inflammatory infiltrate containing plasma cells
- HHV8 positivity is diagnostic

Angiosarcoma/Lymphangiosarcoma

- Atypical vascular proliferation showing irregular, anastomosing vascular spaces
- Poorly circumscribed, infiltrative neoplasm
- Endothelial cells typically show epithelioid or spindle cell features, prominent nuclear enlargement, and atypia with enlarged nucleoli
  - Endothelial multilayering often present
  - Mitotic figures easily identified

DIAGNOSTIC CHECKLIST

Clinically Relevant Pathologic Features

- Margins
  - High recurrence rate with positive margins

Pathologic Interpretation Pearls

- Proliferation of superficial &/or deep dilated vascular spaces lined by bland oval or flattened endothelial cells

SELECTED REFERENCES

1. Ozeki M et al: Clinical features and prognosis of generalized lymphatic anomaly, kaposiform lymphangiomatosis, and Gorham-Stout disease. Pediatr Blood Cancer. ePub, 2016
2. Chander B et al: Lymphangiomatosis: Two cases with unique presentations, salience of nomenclature, and diagnosis. J Cancer Res Ther. 11(3):652, 2015
3. Massa AF et al: Cutaneous Lymphangioma circumscriptum - dermoscopic features. An Bras Dermatol. 90(2):262-4, 2015
4. Núñez EC et al: Acquired vulvar lymphangioma: a case series with emphasis on expanding clinical contexts. Int J Gynecol Pathol. 33(3):235-40, 2014
5. Ji RC et al: Multiple expressions of lymphatic markers and morphological evolution of newly formed lymphatics in lymphangioma and lymph node lymphangiogenesis. Microvasc Res. 80(2):195-201, 2010
6. Chen EY et al: Similar histologic features and immunohistochemical staining in microcystic and macrocystic lymphatic malformations. Lymphat Res Biol. 7(2):75-80, 2009
7. Gedikbasi A et al: Multidisciplinary approach in cystic hygroma: prenatal diagnosis, outcome, and postnatal follow up. Pediatr Int. 51(5):670-7, 2009
8. Patel GA et al: Cutaneous lymphangioma circumscriptum: frog spawn on the skin. Int J Dermatol. 48(12):1290-5, 2009
9. Patel GA et al: Zosteriform lymphangioma circumscriptum. Acta Dermatovenerol Alp Panonica Adriat. 18(4):179-82, 2009
10. Richmond B et al: Adult presentation of giant retroperitoneal cystic lymphangioma: case report. Int J Surg. 7(6):559-60, 2009
11. Edwards JR et al: Lymphatics and bone. Hum Pathol. 39(1):49-55, 2008
12. François M et al: Sox18 induces development of the lymphatic vasculature in mice. Nature. 456(7222):643-7, 2008
13. Norgall S et al: Elevated expression of VEGFR-3 in lymphatic endothelial cells from lymphangiomas. BMC Cancer. 7:105, 2007
14. Wilting J et al: Embryonic development and malformation of lymphatic vessels. Novartis Found Symp. 283:220-7; discussion 227-9, 238-41, 2007
15. Wilting J et al: The transcription factor Prox1 is a marker for lymphatic endothelial cells in normal and diseased human tissues. FASEB J. 16(10):1271-3, 2002
16. Prevo R et al: Mouse LYVE-1 is an endocytic receptor for hyaluronan in lymphatic endothelium. J Biol Chem. 276(22):19420-30, 2001

Gross Specimen of Lymphangioma

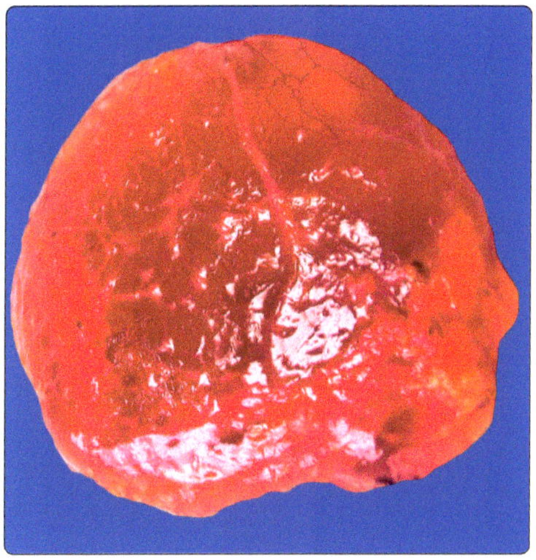

Superficial Lymphangioma

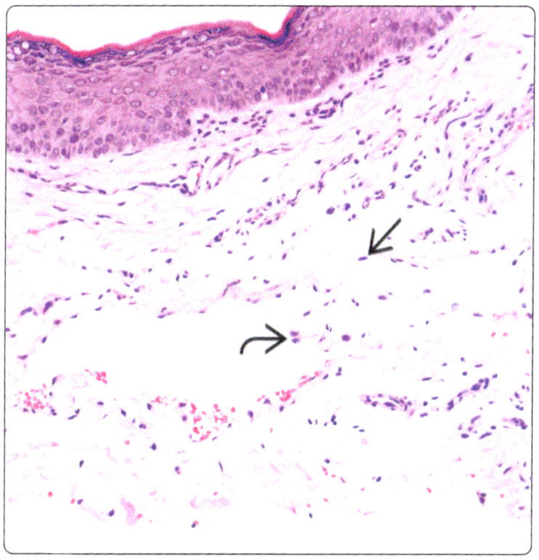

(Left) *Macroscopic view of a lymphangioma shows a reddish brown, translucent cystic mass. Small vessels are noted within the lining; the cyst was filled with clear, watery fluid.* **(Right)** *Examination of a superficial lymphangioma shows the dilated spaces lined by small, bland endothelial cells with uniform, hyperchromatic-staining oval ↗ to flattened → nuclei.*

Superficial Lymphangioma at Higher Magnification

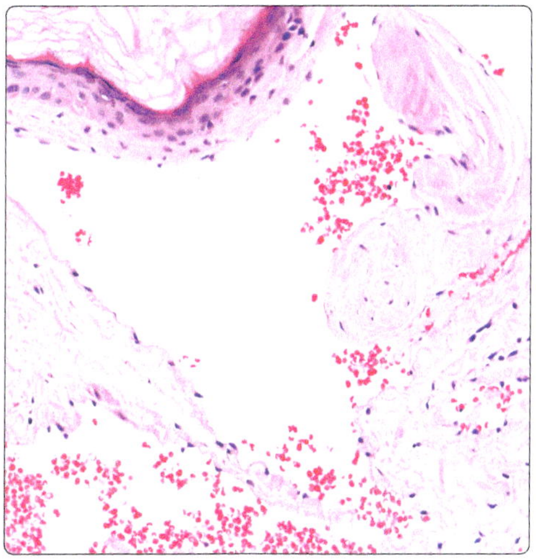

Deep Lymphangioma With Lymphoid Aggregates

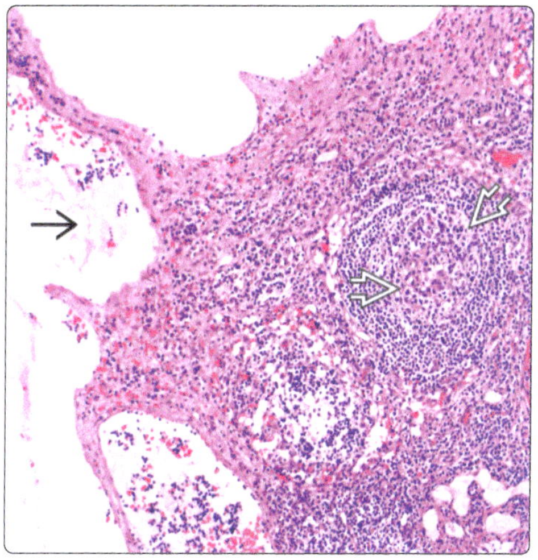

(Left) *Higher magnification examination of a superficial lymphangioma shows a large, irregularly dilated space lined by thin endothelial cells containing scattered red blood cells in the superficial dermis.* **(Right)** *Another deep lymphangioma shows a lumen lined by flattened endothelium and containing proteinaceous fluid →. There is a lymphocytic aggregate with a germinal center ➡ in the surrounding connective tissue.*

Differential Diagnosis: Progressive Lymphangioma

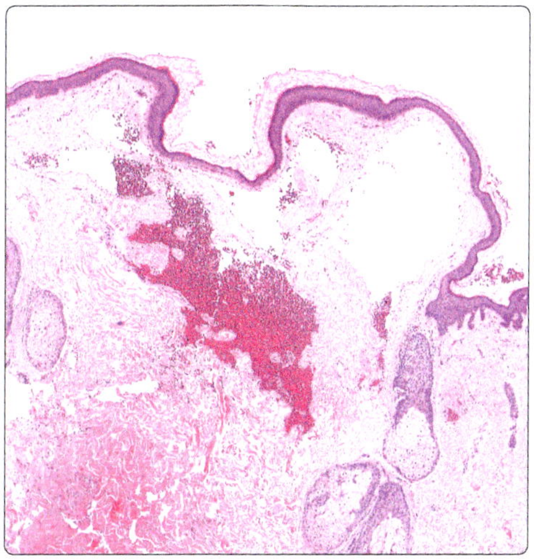

Differential Diagnosis: Atypical Vascular Lesion

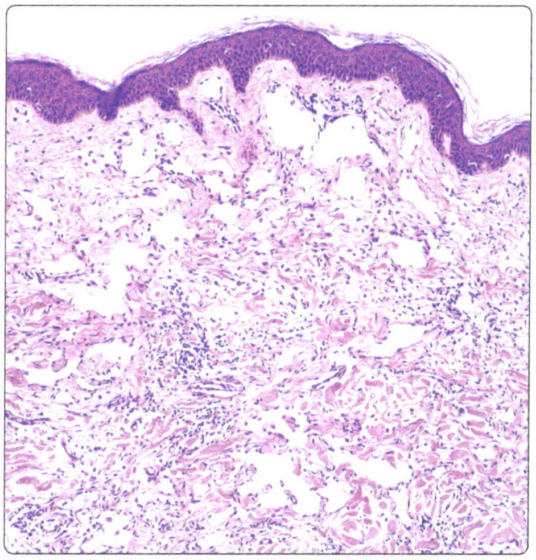

(Left) *Progressive lymphangioma shows similar histologic features but typically presents on the lower extremities of adults as slow-growing patches or plaques.* **(Right)** *Atypical vascular lesion shows a proliferation of irregularly shaped, thin-walled vessels in the superficial and deep dermis. Clinically, it typically presents as multiple small vesicles, most often in patients with a history of breast carcinoma and radiation therapy.*

KEY FACTS

TERMINOLOGY

- Benign, localized proliferation of lymphatic vessels
- a.k.a. acquired progressive lymphangioma and benign lymphangioendothelioma

ETIOLOGY/PATHOGENESIS

- May be related to trauma in some cases

CLINICAL ISSUES

- Usually presents on lower extremities but may occur anywhere
- Middle-aged or older adults
- Complete surgical excision is curative but not necessary
- Prognosis excellent; local recurrences rare, no metastases

MICROSCOPIC

- Dermal and subcutaneous proliferation of dilated vascular channels
- Spaces are often widely dilated superficially but become narrower with deep extension
- Endothelial-lined papillary projections with mild fibrosis may be present
- Endothelial cells may show mild hyperchromasia but no significant atypia

TOP DIFFERENTIAL DIAGNOSES

- Lymphangioma circumscriptum
  - Presents in infants or young children as multiple small vesicular lesions
- Lymphangiomatosis
  - Diffuse involvement of multiple organ systems, including skin, soft tissues, bone, and internal organs
- Atypical vascular lesion (radiotherapy-related)
  - Presents as multiple tiny vesicles in radiation field, usually on breast
- Lymphangioma-like Kaposi sarcoma
- Angiosarcoma

Progressive Lymphangioma

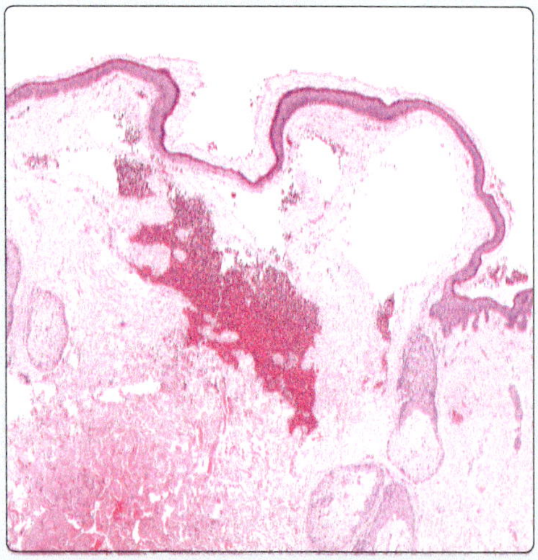

Progressive Lymphangioma at Higher Magnification

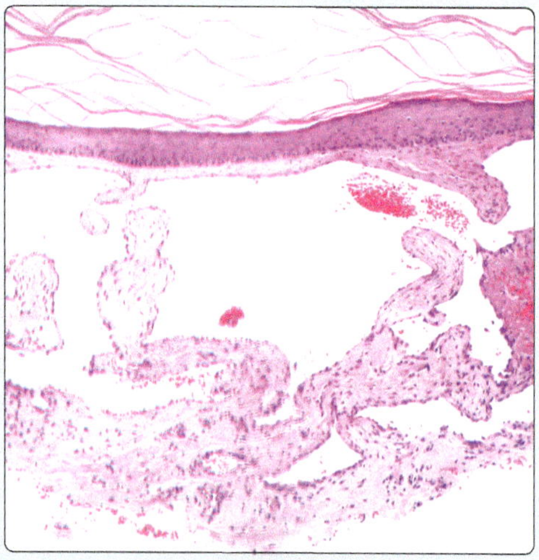

(Left) *Low-power examination of a progressive lymphangioma shows superficial, dermal-dilated, lymphatic spaces, some of which contain numerous red blood cells.* **(Right)** *Higher magnification examination of the superficial portion of a progressive lymphangioma shows widely dilated lymphatic spaces in the superficial dermis.*

Progressive Lymphangioma: High Magnification of Endothelial Cells

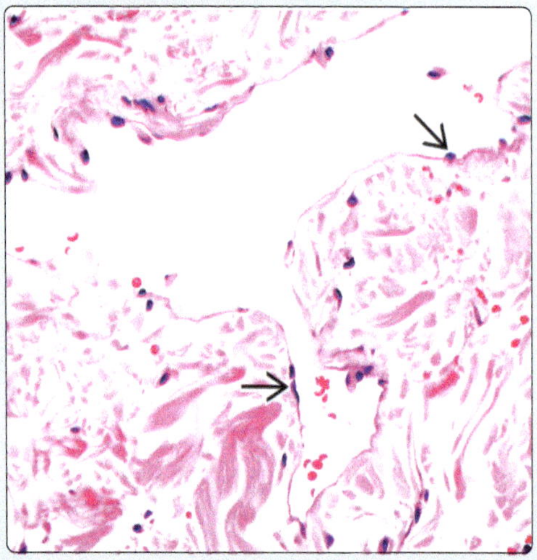

Progressive Lymphangioma: High Magnification of Papillary Projection

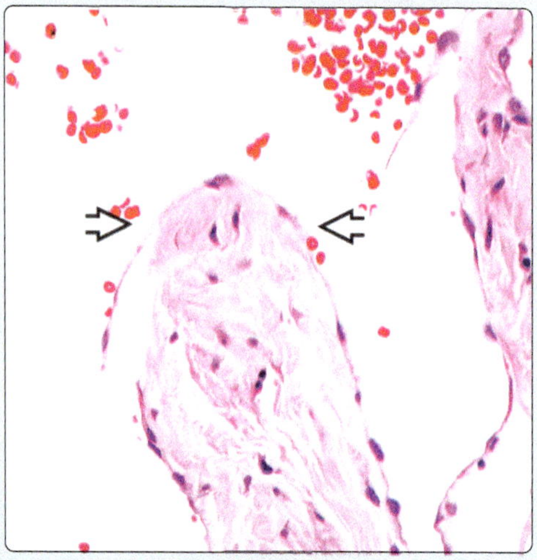

(Left) *High-power examination shows irregular contours of lymphatic spaces and small, bland-appearing, lining endothelial cells ➙.* **(Right)** *High-power examination of another section shows a large papillary projection ➙ protruding into the lymphatic space.*

TERMINOLOGY

Synonyms

- Acquired progressive lymphangioma
- Benign lymphangioendothelioma

Definitions

- Benign, localized proliferation of lymphatic vessels

ETIOLOGY/PATHOGENESIS

Unknown

- May be related to trauma in some cases

CLINICAL ISSUES

Epidemiology

- Age
  - Middle-aged or older adults
- Sex
  - No predilection

Site

- Usually presents on lower extremities but may occur anywhere

Presentation

- Slow-growing lesion
- Patches or plaques

Treatment

- Surgical approaches
  - Complete surgical excision is curative but not necessary given benign nature of this lesion
- Drugs
  - Corticosteroids have been reported to induce complete regression in some cases

Prognosis

- Excellent; local recurrences are rare, metastases do not occur

MACROSCOPIC

General Features

- Dermal-based mass lesion with cystic spaces and hemorrhage

Size

- May measure up to several centimeters

MICROSCOPIC

Histologic Features

- Dermal and subcutaneous proliferation of dilated vascular channels
- Spaces are often widely dilated superficially but become narrower with deep extension
  - Vascular channels are lined by monomorphous, bland-appearing endothelial cells
  - Endothelial cells may show mild hyperchromasia, but no significant atypia is present
- Endothelial-lined papillary projections with mild fibrosis may be present

ANCILLARY TESTS

Immunohistochemistry

- Usually not necessary for diagnosis
- Endothelial cells CD31, CD34, and podoplanin (D2-40) (+)

DIFFERENTIAL DIAGNOSIS

Lymphangioma Circumscriptum

- Presents at birth or in early childhood as multiple small vesicular lesions grouped together
- Superficial dermis is involved; may be deep dilated lymphatics as well

Lymphangiomatosis

- Clinically, very distinctive with diffuse involvement of many organ systems, including skin, soft tissues, bone, and internal organs

Atypical Vascular Lesion (Radiotherapy-Related)

- Clinically, presents as multiple tiny vesicles in radiation field, usually on breast
- Histologically, greater endothelial atypia in most cases, and lymphatic spaces are more widely dilated

Lymphangioma-Like Kaposi Sarcoma

- Usually shows more typical areas of Kaposi sarcoma and inflammatory infiltrate including plasma cells
- HHV8 immunohistochemistry (+)

Angiosarcoma

- Highly atypical vascular proliferation with dissection throughout dermis and subcutis in most cases
- Significant cytologic atypia, endothelial multilayering, and mitoses are present

DIAGNOSTIC CHECKLIST

Pathologic Interpretation Pearls

- Proliferation of dilated lymphatic channels lined by bland endothelial cells
- Widely dilated spaces superficially; narrower spaces with deep extension

SELECTED REFERENCES

1. Alkhalili E et al: Acquired progressive lymphangioma of the nipple. BMJ Case Rep. 2014, 2014
2. Zhu JW et al: Acquired progressive lymphangioma in the inguinal area mimicking giant condyloma acuminatum. Cutis. 93(6):316-9, 2014
3. Paik AS et al: Acquired progressive lymphangioma in an HIV-positive patient. J Cutan Pathol. 34(11):882-5, 2007
4. Hwang LY et al: Acquired progressive lymphangioma. J Am Acad Dermatol. 49(5 Suppl):S250-1, 2003
5. Guillou L et al: Benign lymphangioendothelioma (acquired progressive lymphangioma): a lesion not to be confused with well-differentiated angiosarcoma and patch stage Kaposi's sarcoma: clinicopathologic analysis of a series. Am J Surg Pathol. 24(8):1047-57, 2000
6. Cossu S et al: Lymphangioma-like variant of Kaposi's sarcoma: clinicopathologic study of seven cases with review of the literature. Am J Dermatopathol. 19(1):16-22, 1997
7. Rosso R et al: Acquired progressive lymphangioma of the skin following radiotherapy for breast carcinoma. J Cutan Pathol. 22(2):164-7, 1995
8. Meunier L et al: Acquired progressive lymphangioma. Br J Dermatol. 131(5):706-8, 1994

KEY FACTS

TERMINOLOGY

- Bacillary angiomatosis (BA)
- Reactive vascular proliferation associated with *Bartonella* infection

ETIOLOGY/PATHOGENESIS

- Caused by infection with *Bartonella* (gram-negative coccobacilli) species, usually *Bartonella henselae* or *Bartonella quintana*
- Most patients are immunosuppressed, especially HIV/AIDS
  - Also associated with organ transplantation, systemic steroids, and leukemia

CLINICAL ISSUES

- Occurs in both adults and children
- Can involve any cutaneous site; uncommonly involves mucosal sites, deep soft tissues
- Typically presents with multiple lesions, often pyogenic granuloma-like

MACROSCOPIC

- Reddish brown, dermal-based nodular, hemorrhagic lesion

MICROSCOPIC

- Nodular to dome-shaped/polypoid, dermal-based vascular proliferation
- May have overlying epidermal ulceration and collarette (similar to pyogenic granuloma)
- Vessels are arranged in loose lobular configuration
- Endothelial cells show mild enlargement and oval to epithelioid shape
- Background stroma shows fibrosis, edema, and mixed inflammatory infiltrate with many neutrophils

TOP DIFFERENTIAL DIAGNOSES

- Pyogenic granuloma
  - Ulceration and peripheral epidermal collarette are typically present but lack organisms of BA
- Kaposi sarcoma

Bacillary Angiomatosis

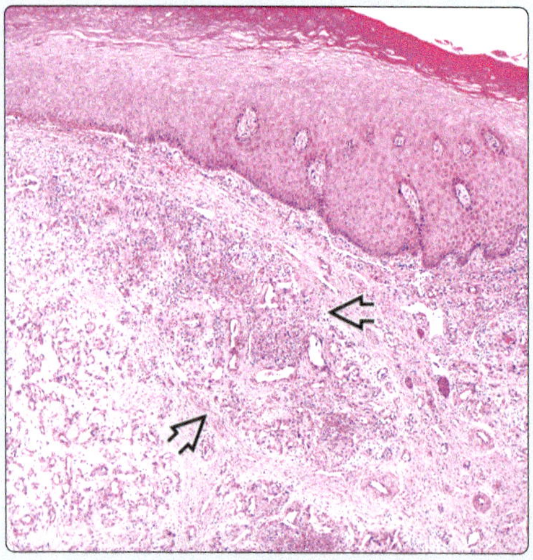

High Magnification of Bacillary Angiomatosis

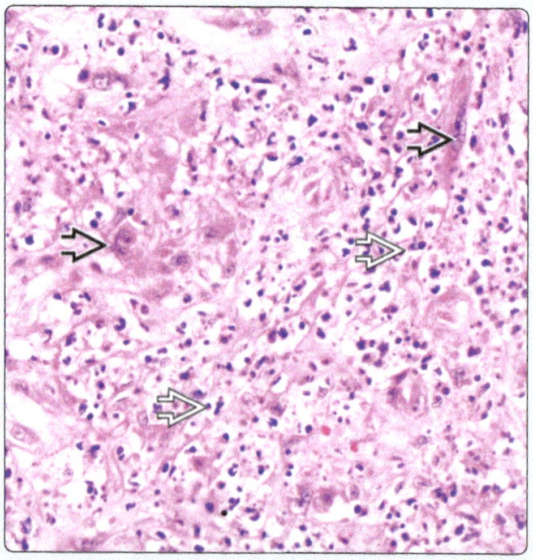

(Left) *Low-power examination of bacillary angiomatosis (BA) demonstrates a superficial dermal proliferation of blood vessels in a lobular configuration ➡ associated with edema and inflammation.* **(Right)** *High magnification of BA demonstrates a proliferation of small blood vessels with swollen endothelial cells ➡ surrounded by edema and inflammation ➡.*

Warthin-Starry Stain in Bacillary Angiomatosis

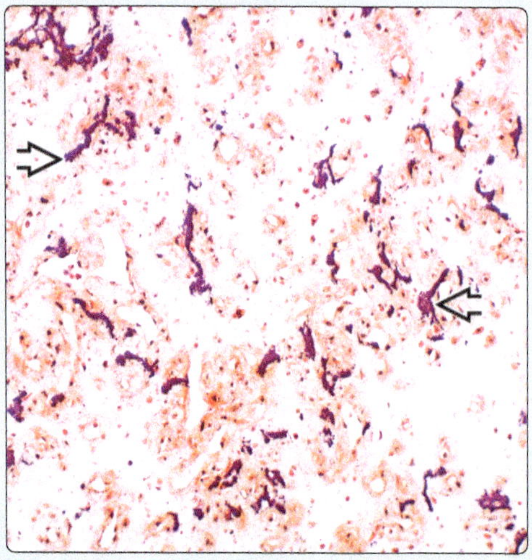

Warthin-Starry Stain at High Magnification

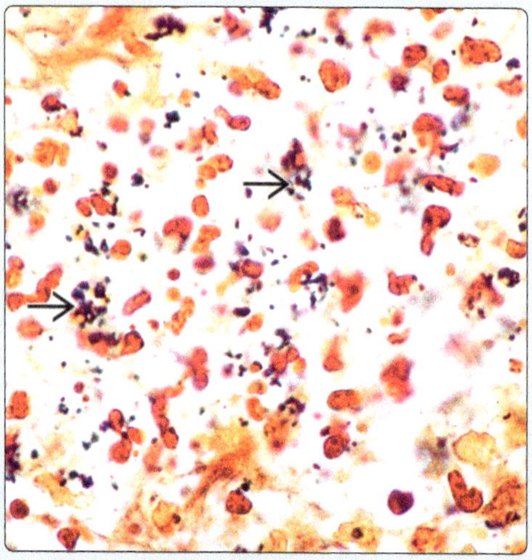

(Left) *Warthin-Starry silver stain preparation shows numerous clusters of bacterial organisms ➡ around blood vessels.* **(Right)** *Warthin-Starry stain demonstrates positive staining of numerous clusters ➡ and single bacterial organisms.*

TERMINOLOGY

Abbreviations

- Bacillary angiomatosis (BA)

Synonyms

- Epithelioid angiomatosis

Definitions

- Reactive vascular proliferation associated with *Bartonella* species bacterial infection

ETIOLOGY/PATHOGENESIS

Infectious Agents

- Caused by infection with *Bartonella* (gram-negative coccobacilli) species, usually *Bartonella henselae* or *Bartonella quintana*
  - Most patients have history of cat exposure (and may have preceding scratch or bite)
- Most patients are immunosuppressed, especially due to HIV/AIDS
  - Also associated with organ transplantation, systemic steroids, and leukemia

CLINICAL ISSUES

Epidemiology

- Age
  - May occur in adults and children

Site

- Can involve any cutaneous site; uncommonly may involve mucosal sites and deep soft tissues
  - Internal organ involvement rare, but may affect liver (peliosis hepatis)

Presentation

- Skin nodules or, less likely, plaques
  - Typically present with multiple lesions, often pyogenic granuloma-like

Treatment

- Drugs
  - Antibiotics typically lead to resolution of lesions

Prognosis

- Typically good, but depends on patient's immune status and sites involved

MACROSCOPIC

General Features

- Reddish brown, dermal-based nodular, hemorrhagic lesion

MICROSCOPIC

Histologic Features

- Typically nodular to dome-shaped/polypoid dermal-based vascular proliferation
  - May have overlying epidermal ulceration and collarette (similar to pyogenic granuloma)
- Vessels are arranged in loose lobular configuration
  - Endothelial cells show mild enlargement and oval to epithelioid shape
  - Deeper parts of lesion may show greater cellularity and crowding of vessels
  - No significant cytologic atypia or atypical mitotic activity
- Background stroma shows fibrosis, edema, and mixed inflammatory infiltrate
  - Infiltrate is rich in neutrophils with nuclear dust, macrophages, lymphocytes, and may show focal collections of basophilic granular material (clumps of bacteria)
    - Neutrophils are more plentiful in deeper lesions

ANCILLARY TESTS

Histochemistry

- Warthin-Starry (silver stain)
  - Highlights bacterial organisms
  - Staining pattern: Granular (coccobacillary organisms)
- Gram Stain
  - Organisms are gram negative

PCR

- PCR for *Bartonella* species may be ordered if organisms are not identified on histochemical stains

DIFFERENTIAL DIAGNOSIS

Pyogenic Granuloma

- Polypoid dermal-based lesion composed of lobular collection of capillary-type vessels
- Overlying ulceration and peripheral epidermal collarette are typically present, similar to BA
- No evidence of organisms identified on H&E or special stains (except for superficial colonies/impetiginization)

Kaposi Sarcoma

- Plaque-like or nodular collection of slit-like vessels lined by atypical spindle cells
- Inflammatory infiltrate is typically composed of lymphocytes and plasma cells, not neutrophils
- No bacterial organisms identified
- HHV8(+) is diagnostic

DIAGNOSTIC CHECKLIST

Clinically Relevant Pathologic Features

- Organ distribution

Pathologic Interpretation Pearls

- Proliferation of vessels associated with neutrophils and clumps of bacterial organisms

SELECTED REFERENCES

1. Orsag J et al: Cutaneous bacillary angiomatosis due to Bartonella quintana in a renal transplant recipient. Transpl Int. 28(5):626-31, 2015
2. Wanat KA et al: Tumoral bacillary angiomatosis in a child with human immunodeficiency virus. JAMA Dermatol. 150(9):1015-6, 2014
3. Amsbaugh S et al: Bacillary angiomatosis associated with pseudoepitheliomatous hyperplasia. Am J Dermatopathol. 28(1):32-5, 2006
4. Maurin M et al: Bartonella infections: diagnostic and management issues. Curr Opin Infect Dis. 11(2):189-93, 1998
5. LeBoit PE et al: Bacillary angiomatosis. The histopathology and differential diagnosis of a pseudoneoplastic infection in patients with human immunodeficiency virus disease. Am J Surg Pathol. 13(11):909-20, 1989

KEY FACTS

TERMINOLOGY

- Mesenchymal neoplasm composed of distinctive perivascular epithelioid cells (PEComa)
  - Includes angiomyolipoma (AML), clear cell sugar tumor of lung (CCST), lymphangioleiomyomatosis (LAM), clear cell myomelanocytic tumor of falciform ligament/ligamentum teres

ETIOLOGY/PATHOGENESIS

- Only AML, CCST, and LAM are associated with tuberous sclerosis, but not other types

CLINICAL ISSUES

- Most are benign, but rare malignant cases reported
- Rare tumors overall; very rare in skin

MICROSCOPIC

- PEC cell component consists of epithelioid to spindled cells arranged around vessels extending outward radially
- Clear to granular, lightly eosinophilic cytoplasm and round to oval nuclei with small nucleoli
- Myoid component with densely eosinophilic cytoplasm
- Adipose tissue component present in lesions termed AML
- Express smooth muscle markers and melanoma markers but lack S100 expression
- TFE3 rearrangements

TOP DIFFERENTIAL DIAGNOSES

- True smooth muscle tumors
- Renal cell carcinoma
- Clear cell sarcoma
- Melanoma
- Myoepithelioma
- Well-differentiated liposarcoma
- Metastatic gastrointestinal stromal tumor
- Metastatic hepatocellular carcinoma

PEComa at Scanning Magnification

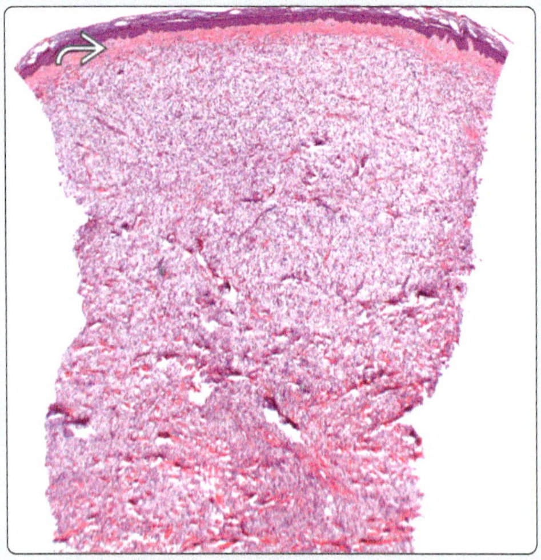

PEComa at High Magnification

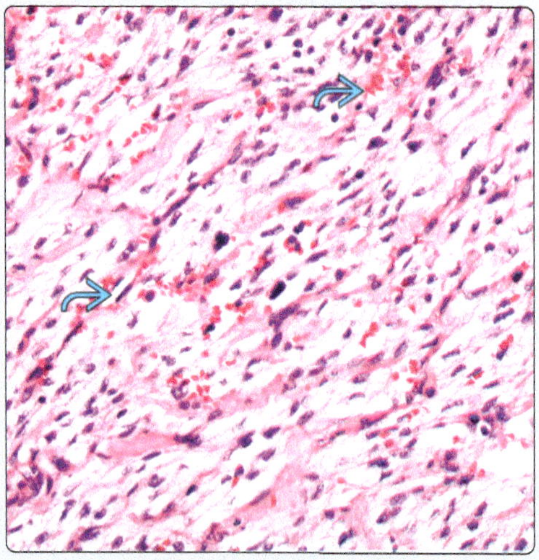

(Left) *This rare primary cutaneous PEComa shows a clear cell neoplasm diffusely involving the dermis and associated with many small blood vessels. There is a grenz zone separating the tumor from the overlying epidermis* ➡*.* **(Right)** *Higher magnification examination shows a clear cell tumor with numerous fibrovascular channels* ➡ *between the spindled and epithelioid clear cells.*

Cutaneous PEComa, SMA Labeling

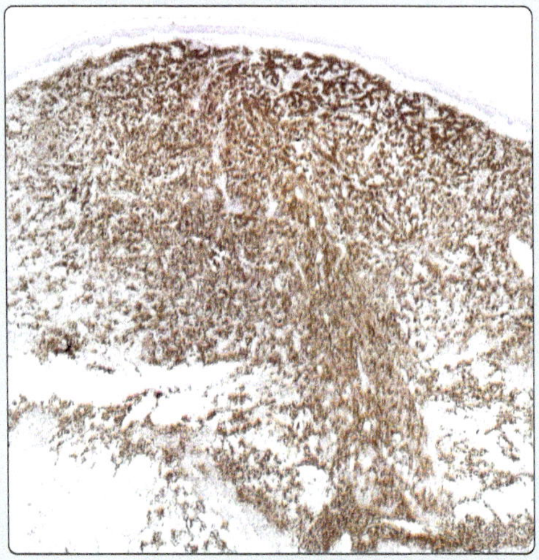

PEComa, HMB-45 Staining

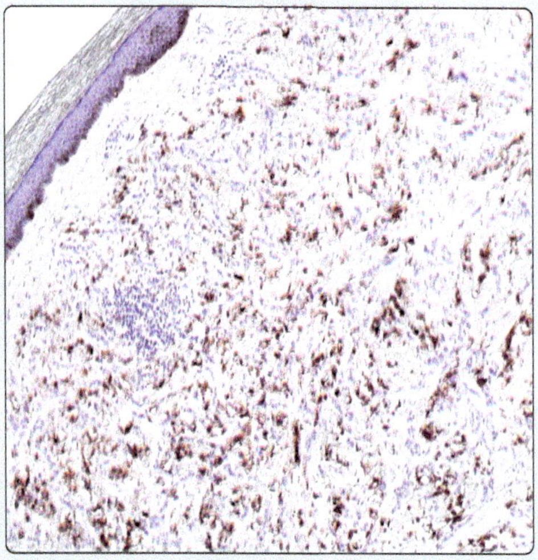

(Left) *SMA shows strong and diffuse cytoplasmic expression in this rare primary cutaneous PEComa.* **(Right)** *HMB-45 shows scattered, strong cytoplasmic expression in a primary cutaneous PEComa. These lesions also express other markers of melanocytic differentiation as well as CD117 and CD10, but typically lack S100 and keratin expression.*

TERMINOLOGY

Abbreviations

- Perivascular epithelioid cell (PEC)
  - Thus, neoplasms are termed PEComa

Synonyms

- Perivascular epithelioid cell tumor
- Extrapulmonary sugar tumor
- Monotypic epithelioid angiomyolipoma

Definitions

- Mesenchymal neoplasms composed of distinctive perivascular epithelioid cells; category includes
  - Angiomyolipoma (AML)
  - Clear cell sugar tumor of lung (CCST)
  - Lymphangioleiomyomatosis (LAM)
  - Clear cell myomelanocytic tumor of falciform ligament/ligamentum teres (CCMMT)
- In many respects, PEComas are simply angiomyolipomas without fat
- Subset displays overt histologic features of malignancy and malignant clinical behavior

ETIOLOGY/PATHOGENESIS

Association With Tuberous Sclerosis

- Genetic alterations of tuberous sclerosis complex (TSC), losses of *TSC1* (9q34) or *TSC2* (16p13.3) genes
- Autosomal dominant inheritance
- Benign tumors of brain (most common), kidneys, heart, eyes, lungs, and skin
  - Name comes from characteristic tuber or potato-like nodules in brain, which calcify with age and become hard or sclerotic
- AML, CCST, and LAM are associated with tuberous sclerosis but not other types

CLINICAL ISSUES

Epidemiology

- Incidence
  - AML, CCST, LAM are rare
    - Other PEComas extremely rare
- Age
  - CCMMT typically encountered in girls in late childhood
  - Most others seen in adults 50-60 yr old
  - AML detected in younger patients in setting of tuberous sclerosis
- Sex
  - Marked overall female predominance

Site

- Reported in multiple sites; rare in skin, but reported
  - Kidney, liver, falciform ligament, deep soft tissues of extremities, uterus, vulva, heart, gallbladder, gastrointestinal tract

Presentation

- CCMMT presents as painful abdominal mass
- Uterine examples manifest as uterine bleeding
- Most other categories of PEComas present as painless masses
- Brain tumors in patients with tuberous sclerosis present with seizures, developmental delay, behavioral problems

Treatment

- Surgical excision

Prognosis

- Most are benign
  - Rare documented examples of malignancy
    - Usually not in AML, LAM, or CCST types
    - Malignant examples behave as aggressive sarcomas

MICROSCOPIC

Histologic Features

- PEC cell component consists of epithelioid to spindled cells arranged around vessels extending outward radially
  - Clear to granular, lightly eosinophilic cytoplasm and round to oval nuclei with small nucleoli
  - Lesions are richly vascular
  - Small arching vessels divide tumor into packets (similar to pattern in renal cell carcinoma)
- Myoid component with densely eosinophilic cytoplasm
  - Nuclei less rounded than those of true smooth muscle
- Adipose tissue component present in lesions termed AML
- CCMMT is almost exclusively spindle cell lesion
  - Uniform moderate-sized cells set in elaborate lace-like vasculature

Rare Malignant Examples

- Criteria for malignancy
  - Infiltrative growth
  - Marked hypercellularity
  - Nuclear enlargement and hyperchromasia
  - Numerous &/or atypical mitotic figures
  - Necrosis

ANCILLARY TESTS

Immunolabeling

- Express smooth muscle markers, HMB-45, Melan-A/MART-1 and other melanoma markers, CD10, and cathepsin K

Genetics

- Most cases show rearrangements of *TFE3*

DIFFERENTIAL DIAGNOSIS

True Smooth Muscle Tumors

- Perpendicularly oriented fascicles of spindle cells with brightly eosinophilic cytoplasm and blunt-ended nuclei
  - Criteria for malignancy site specific and related to mitotic activity and nuclear atypia
- Intensely eosinophilic cytoplasm
- Usually lack adipose tissue component (exception is myolipoma)
- Lack PEC differentiation
  - Most smooth muscle tumors lack melanocytic antigens and express desmin
- Lack rich vascular pattern (although some leiomyosarcomas arise in association with vessels)
- Some examples are associated with Epstein-Barr virus

Renal Cell Carcinoma

- Clear epithelial cells and rich vascular pattern
  - Sarcomatoid examples overtly high-grade neoplasms
- Usually displays epithelial markers by immunohistochemistry
- Lacks adipose tissue component

Clear Cell Sarcoma

- Usually involves feet and hands of young adults
- Consists of highly uniform cells with clear cytoplasm and uniform nuclei with single large nucleolus
  - Packeted arrangement with groups of cells separated by slender connective tissue septa
- Most examples express S100
- Soft tissue examples express melanocytic markers
  - Subset of visceral examples only express S100 but not melanocytic markers
    - This relates to *EWS-CREB1* fusion in visceral examples (in contrast with *EWS-ATF1* fusion in other cases)
- Lack CD117 expression
- No adipose tissue component of myoid component
- Vessels inconspicuous

Melanoma

- Can be spindled to epithelioid
- Marked cytologic atypia with prominent nucleoli is rule
- Some cases display melanin pigment
- Large lesions highly aggressive clinically
- Label with S100
  - Melanocytic markers expressed in most classic examples, negative in spindled lesions
- Vessels inconspicuous

Well-Differentiated Liposarcoma

- Extremely rare in skin
- Shows fat punctuated by atypical nuclei
  - Fibrous septa containing enlarged hyperchromatic nuclei
  - Can have areas of dedifferentiation to high-grade sarcoma
    - Overt high-grade spindle cell sarcoma with numerous mitoses and atypical nuclei
- Most examples not richly vascular
- Show nuclear MDM2 or CDK4 immunolabeling
  - Negative melanocytic markers

Intramuscular Hemangioma

- Capillary or cavernous vascular lesion
- Often has abundant overgrowth of mature adipose tissue
- No spindle cell component
- No immunolabeling with melanocytic markers

Metastatic Gastrointestinal Stromal Tumor

- Epithelioid or spindle cell neoplasms usually involving muscularis propria of gastrointestinal tract
  - Cytoplasmic vacuoles common
  - Cytoplasm eosinophilic
  - Uniform nuclei
  - CD117 immunolabeling and *KIT* mutations in most cases
    - Variable immunolabeling with smooth muscle markers
    - Usually negative for melanocytic markers (some have focal MART-1/Melan-A)
- Lack adipose tissue component and clear cells
- Vessels inconspicuous

Metastatic Hepatocellular Carcinoma

- Large, atypical cells with opaque eosinophilic cytoplasm, rich vascularity
- Usually has marked nuclear pleomorphism
- Expresses epithelial markers (CAM5.2), sometimes Hep-Par1
  - Canalicular pattern on immunolabeling with CD10 or polyclonal CEA
- No adipose tissue component
- Some examples have cytoplasmic bile

Myoepithelioma

- Lobulated lesions
- Uniform epithelioid cells
- Variable colabeling with keratins, S100, and smooth muscle markers
- Some have *EWSR1* rearrangements

SELECTED REFERENCES

1. Cheng N et al: Clear cell proliferations of the skin. Adv Anat Pathol. 22(3):181-93, 2015
2. Rao Q et al: PSF/SFPQ is a very common gene fusion partner in TFE3 rearrangement-associated perivascular epithelioid cell tumors (PEComas) and melanotic Xp11 translocation renal cancers: clinicopathologic, immunohistochemical, and molecular characteristics suggesting classification as a distinct entity. Am J Surg Pathol. 39(9):1181-96, 2015
3. Charli-Joseph Y et al: Primary cutaneous perivascular epithelioid cell tumor: a clinicopathological and molecular reappraisal. J Am Acad Dermatol. 71(6):1127-36, 2014
4. Rao Q et al: Cathepsin K in the immunohistochemical diagnosis of melanocytic lesions. Int J Clin Exp Pathol. 7(3):1132-9, 2014
5. Shen Q et al: Perivascular epithelioid cell tumor (PEComa) with TFE3 gene rearrangement: clinicopathological, immunohistochemical, and molecular features. Virchows Arch. 465(5):607-13, 2014
6. Rao Q et al: Cathepsin K expression in a wide spectrum of perivascular epithelioid cell neoplasms (PEComas): a clinicopathological study emphasizing extrarenal PEComas. Histopathology. 62(4):642-50, 2013
7. Argani P et al: A distinctive subset of PEComas harbors TFE3 gene fusions. Am J Surg Pathol. 34(10):1395-406, 2010
8. Sukov WR et al: Perivascular epithelioid cell tumor (PEComa) of the urinary bladder: report of 3 cases and review of the literature. Am J Surg Pathol. 33(2):304-8, 2009
9. Hornick JL et al: Sclerosing PEComa: clinicopathologic analysis of a distinctive variant with a predilection for the retroperitoneum. Am J Surg Pathol. 32(4):493-501, 2008
10. Liegl B et al: Primary cutaneous PEComa: distinctive clear cell lesions of skin. Am J Surg Pathol. 32(4):608-14, 2008
11. Martignoni G et al: PEComas: the past, the present and the future. Virchows Arch. 452(2):119-32, 2008
12. Folpe AL et al: Perivascular epithelioid cell neoplasms of soft tissue and gynecologic origin: a clinicopathologic study of 26 cases and review of the literature. Am J Surg Pathol. 29(12):1558-75, 2005
13. Harris GC et al: Malignant perivascular epithelioid cell tumour ("PEComa") of soft tissue: a unique case. Am J Surg Pathol. 28(12):1655-8, 2004
14. Vang R et al: Perivascular epithelioid cell tumor ('PEComa') of the uterus: a subset of HMB-45-positive epithelioid mesenchymal neoplasms with an uncertain relationship to pure smooth muscle tumors. Am J Surg Pathol. 26(1):1-13, 2002
15. Folpe AL et al: Clear cell myomelanocytic tumor of the falciform ligament/ligamentum teres: a novel member of the perivascular epithelioid clear cell family of tumors with a predilection for children and young adults. Am J Surg Pathol. 24(9):1239-46, 2000
16. L'Hostis H et al: Renal angiomyolipoma: a clinicopathologic, immunohistochemical, and follow-up study of 46 cases. Am J Surg Pathol. 23(9):1011-20, 1999
17. Tsui WM et al: Hepatic angiomyolipoma: a clinicopathologic study of 30 cases and delineation of unusual morphologic variants. Am J Surg Pathol. 23(1):34-48, 1999

Cutaneous PEComa

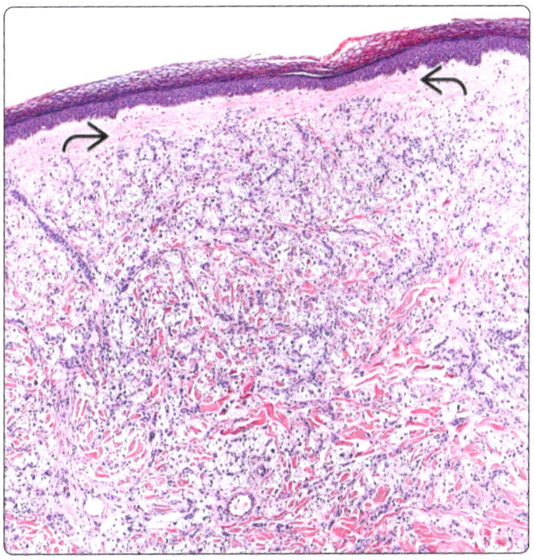

PEComa, Prominent Blood Vessels

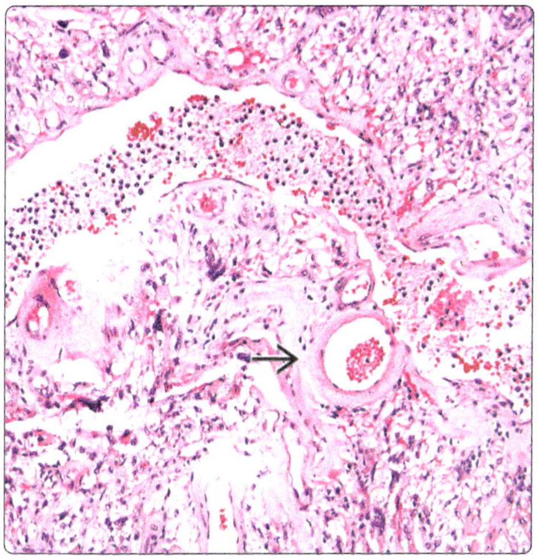

(Left) *Primary cutaneous PEComa shows a dermal-based clear cell neoplasm associated with numerous small blood vessels. This tumor diffusely involved the dermis and extended into the subcutaneous adipose tissue. Note the grenz zone separating the tumor from the overlying epidermis* ↗. **(Right)** *Higher magnification shows the lesional cells surrounding disorganized, medium-sized vessels* →.

PEComa, Nested Appearance

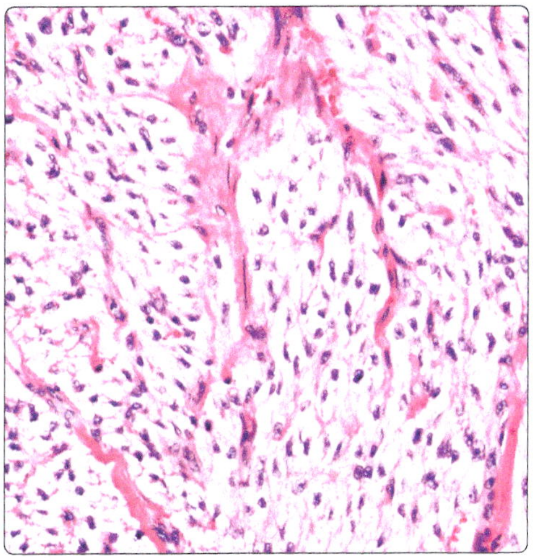

CD10 Staining in PEComa

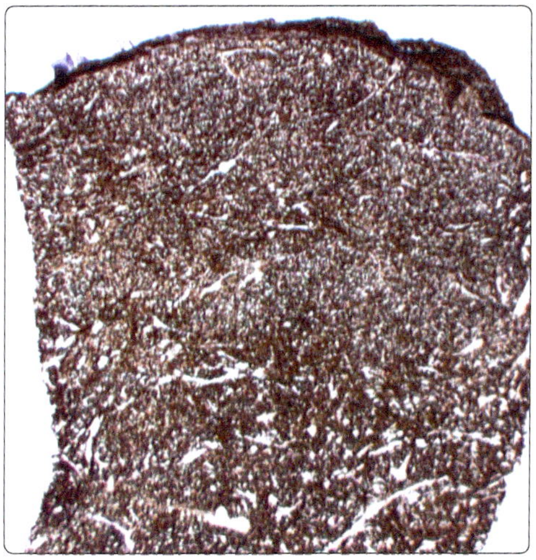

(Left) *PEComa often shows a packeted appearance formed by fibrovascular separations between bundles of proliferating cells. This pattern is reminiscent of that of renal cell carcinoma or clear cell sarcoma.* **(Right)** *CD10 is often strongly positive in PEComas, as illustrated in this case.*

HMB-45 Staining in PEComa

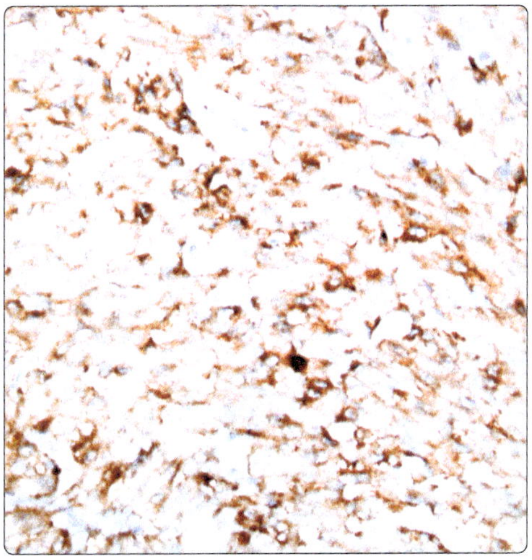

PEComa, Actin Labeling

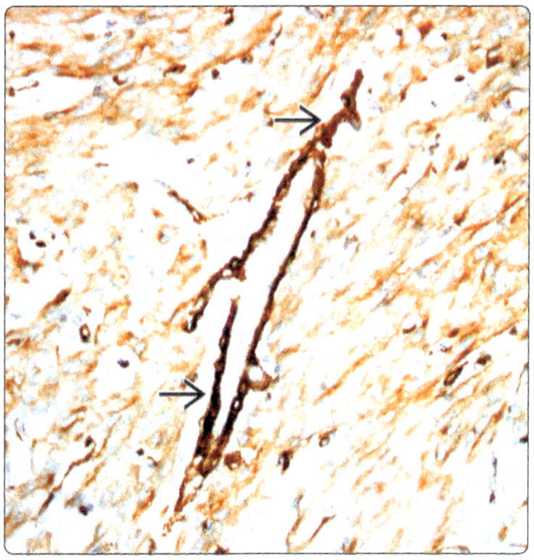

(Left) *HMB-45 typically shows cytoplasmic expression in PEComa. These lesions also express other markers of melanocytic differentiation such as MART-1/Melan-A and tyrosinase, but lack S100 and SOX10 expression.* **(Right)** *Actin-HHF-35 shows cytoplasmic labeling in a PEComa. Note that the internal control (vessel wall* →*) labels more intensely.*

PEComa, Cathepsin-K Immunolabeling

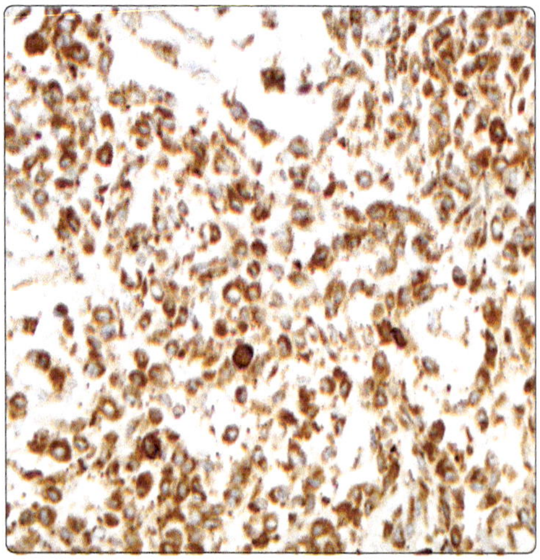

PEComa, Desmin Immunolabeling

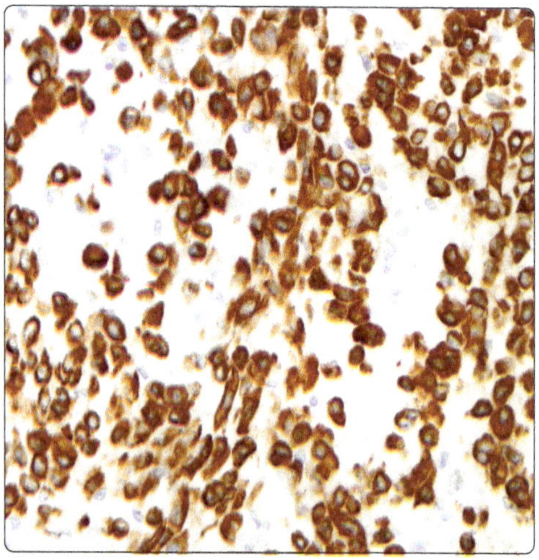

(Left) *Note the strong granular staining in this PEComa. This staining is characteristic of these tumors, but by no means specific. For example, melanomas often label with cathepsin-K (but they also express S100 and SOX10, which PEComas do not).* **(Right)** *Note the strong diffuse desmin expression in this PEComa.*

Malignant PEComa

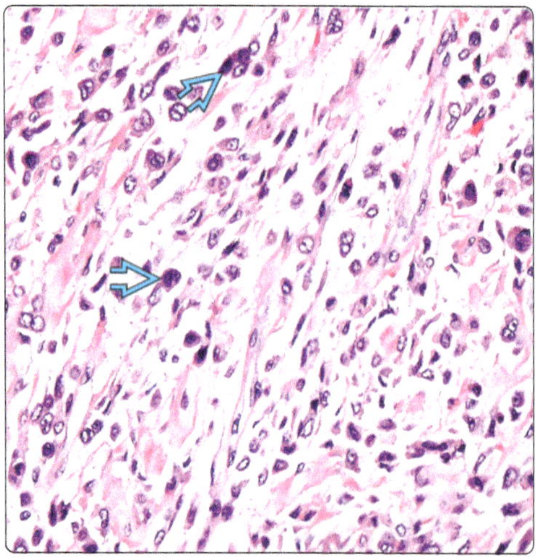

Malignant PEComa With Giant Cells

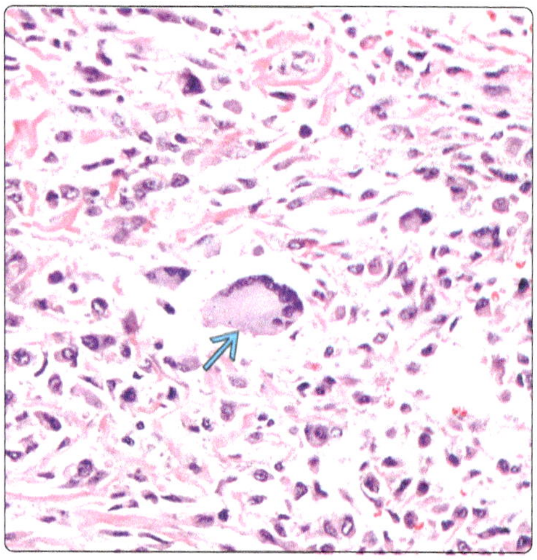

(Left) *This was a large intraabdominal mass with extensive necrosis and many mitoses. Note the prominent cytologic atypia and pleomorphism in this lesion.* **(Right)** *This lesion is spindled and epithelioid, and even features scattered giant cells. The epithelioid eosinophilic cytoplasm is not as brightly eosinophilic as that of smooth muscle neoplasms.*

Differential Diagnosis: Clear Cell Sarcoma

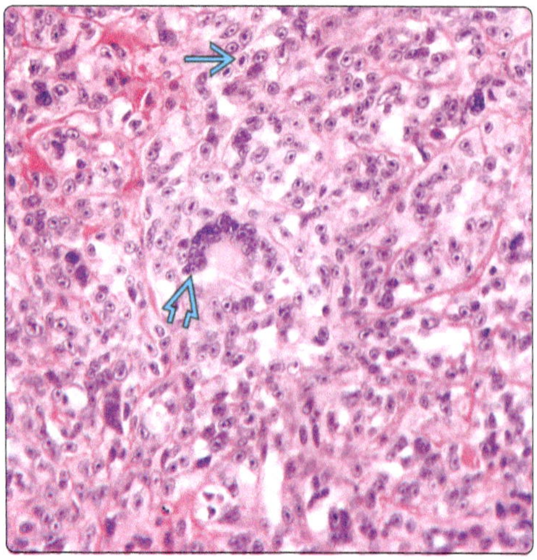

Clear Cell Sarcoma, Giant Cell

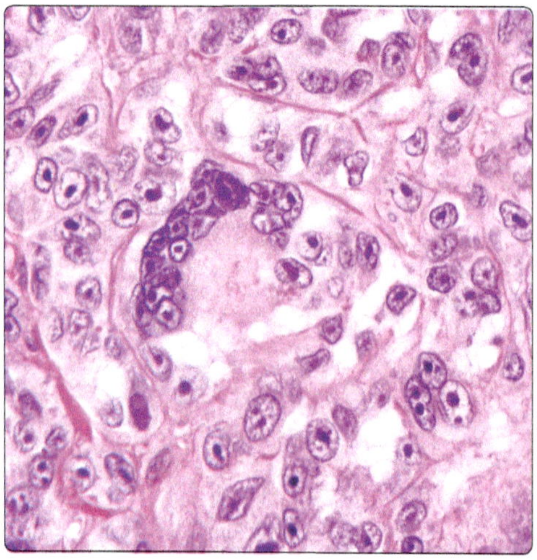

(Left) *In this example, note that each nucleus has a prominent nucleolus, even those in the wreath-like giant cell. Since clear cell sarcomas often arise in the distal extremities, the presence of the giant cells can result in a mistaken interpretation of tenosynovial giant cell tumor (giant cell tumor of tendon sheath).* **(Right)** *High magnification of this clear cell sarcoma shows the enlarged, atypical-appearing nuclei, each with a prominent red nucleolus, even those in the giant cell in the center of the field.*

Clear Cell Sarcoma, HMB-45 Staining

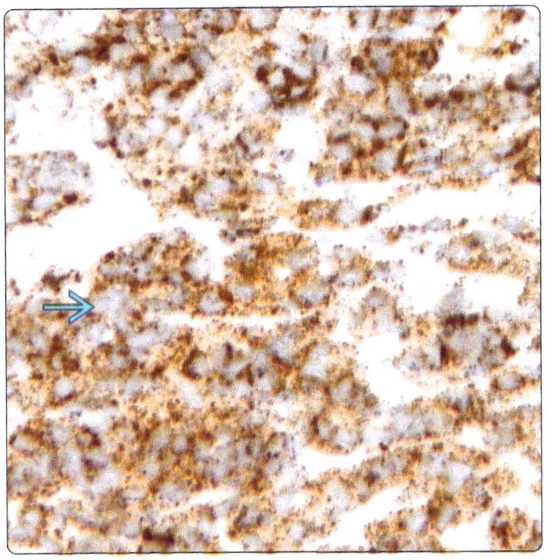

Clear Cell Sarcoma, S100 Staining

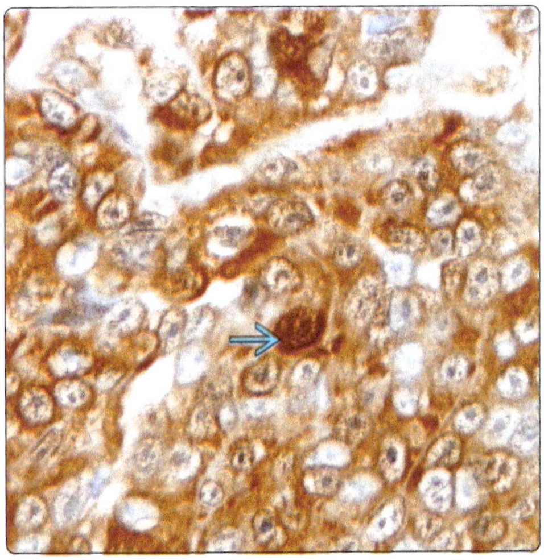

(**Left**) *Note the strong and diffuse (though granular) staining in this clear cell sarcoma. The labeling is more intense than that typically encountered in PEComas. The nuclei* → *do not stain.* (**Right**) *S100 immunolabeling shows both nuclear* → *and cytoplasmic expression in this clear cell sarcoma.*

Differential Diagnosis: Melanoma With Clear Cell Features

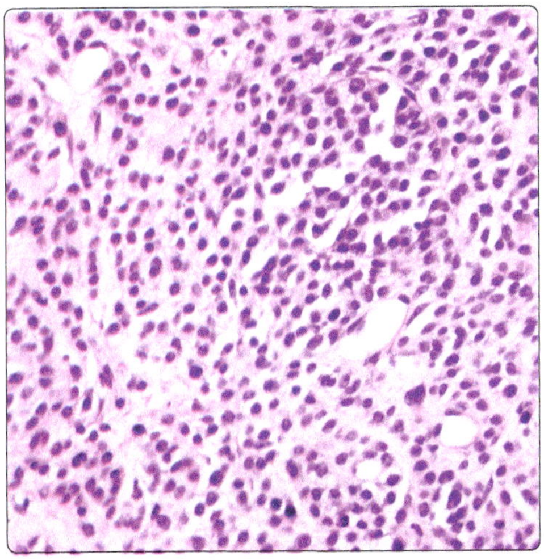

Melanoma With Clear Cell Features, Intranuclear Pseudoinclusion

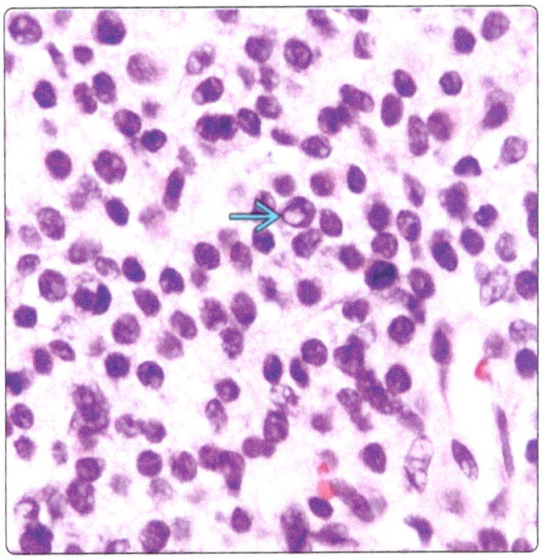

(**Left**) *Melanoma can assume a variety of appearances, including clear cell features in rare cases. This example also shows more bland-appearing cytologic features than most cases.* (**Right**) *Although this melanoma lacks the nuclear pleomorphism of many examples, it does contain an intranuclear cytoplasmic invagination (pseudoinclusion* →*), a characteristic feature.*

Melanoma, S100 Staining

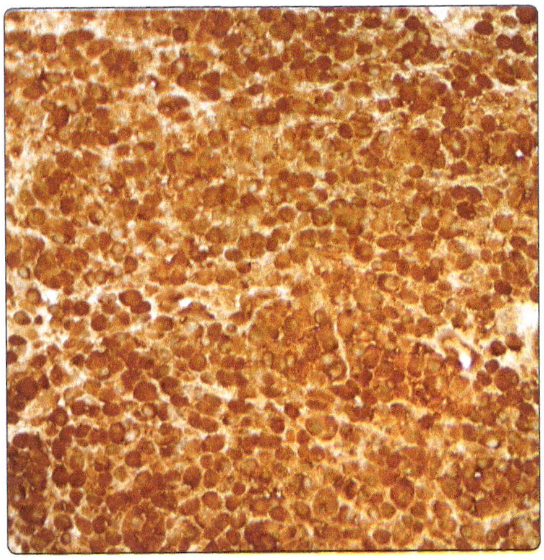

Differential Diagnosis: Myoepithelioma

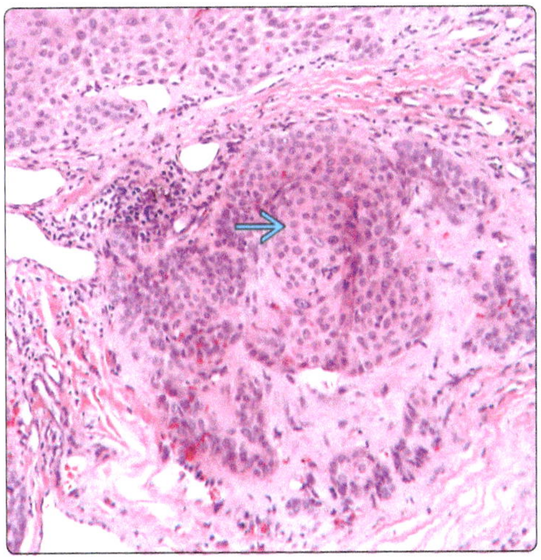

(**Left**) *This example shows very strong and diffuse nuclear and cytoplasmic S100 expression, a typical immunolabeling pattern for melanoma.* (**Right**) *This myoepithelioma shows lobulations and uniform nuclei* → *in the fashion of mesenchymal lesions associated with characteristic translocations and gene fusions. Myoepitheliomas often have rearrangements of EWSR1.*

Kaposi Sarcoma

KEY FACTS

TERMINOLOGY

- Vascular neoplasm (usually low grade) caused by HHV-8

CLINICAL ISSUES

- Sites: Skin (majority), mucosa, lymph nodes, organs
- Clinical variants
  - Classic: Lower legs/feet of elderly males; indolent
  - African/endemic: Children/adults in equatorial Africa
  - Iatrogenic: Immunosuppressed patients of any age
  - AIDS-associated: Aggressive (often disseminated)
- Many modalities for symptom control, but no cure

MICROSCOPIC

- Patch stage
  - Infiltrative interconnected vascular channels dissect dermal collagen; scattered plasma cells (useful clue)
- Plaque stage
  - Spindle cell proliferation infiltrating dermis and invading/destroying eccrine glands
- Tumor stage
  - Nodules with intersecting fascicles of spindle cells
  - Blood-filled slit/sieve-like spaces between spindle cells

ANCILLARY TESTS

- Positive HHV8 (LANA-1) in essentially 100% of cases

TOP DIFFERENTIAL DIAGNOSES

- Angiosarcoma
- Severe vascular stasis (acroangiodermatitis)
- Hobnail (targetoid hemosiderotic) hemangioma
- Microvenular hemangioma
- Spindle cell hemangioma
- Kaposiform hemangioendothelioma
- Acquired tufted angioma
- Progressive lymphangioma
- Cellular fibrous histiocytoma
- Leiomyosarcoma (cutaneous)

Classic KS

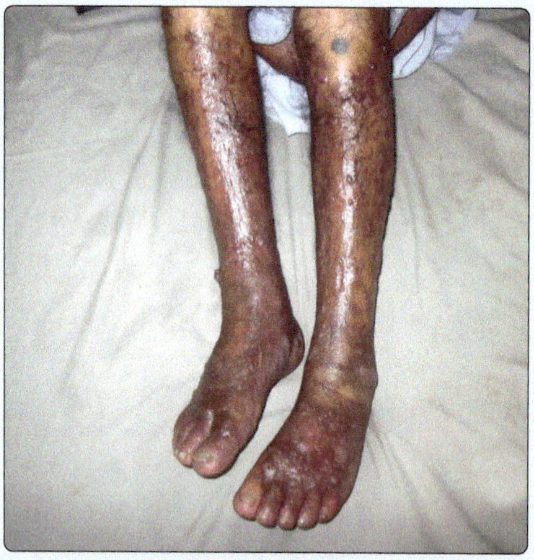

KS at Scanning Magnification

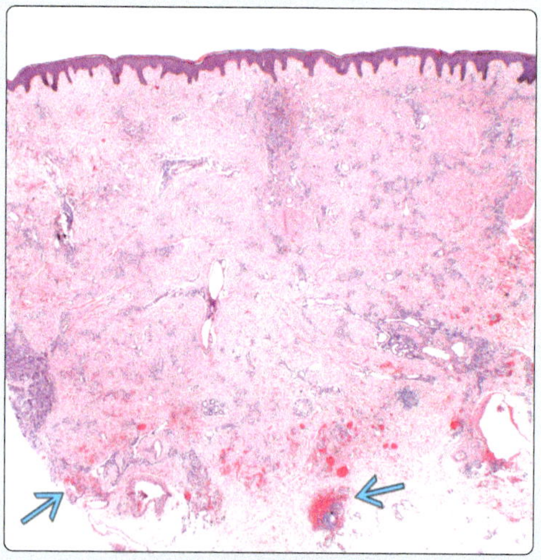

(Left) *Classic Kaposi sarcoma presents as diffuse erythematous and hyperpigmented plaques and nodules on the lower extremities of this elderly male. (Courtesy J. McMichael, MD.)* **(Right)** *Earlier lesions of KS display increased numbers of irregular vascular channels infiltrating the dermis. Hemorrhage is evident even from low power →.*

Infiltrative Growth Pattern in KS

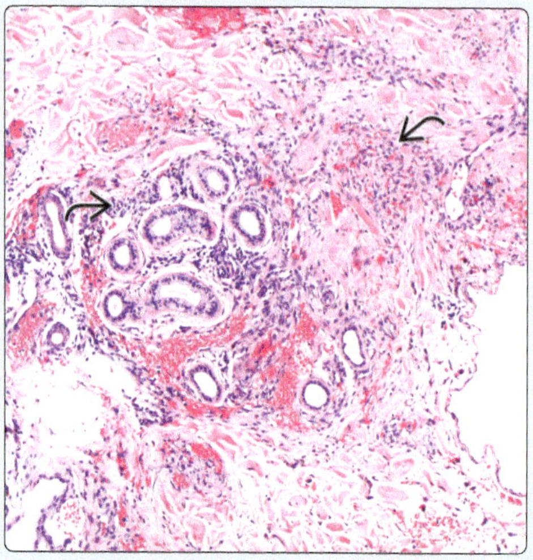

High Magnification Showing Slit- and Sieve-Like Spaces

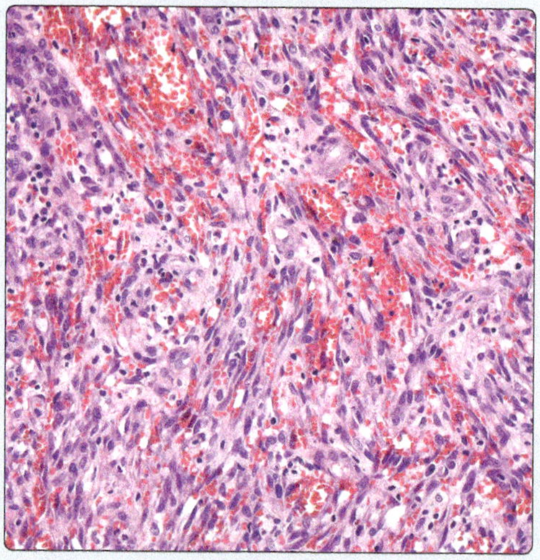

(Left) *In addition to vascular channels, infiltrative spindle cells → with hemorrhage are present in plaque stage KS. These have a tendency to infiltrate and destroy the eccrine sweat coils.* **(Right)** *In later stage lesions of KS, spindled endothelial cells form fascicles with intervening slit- and sieve-like vascular spaces containing numerous erythrocytes.*

TERMINOLOGY

Abbreviations

- Kaposi sarcoma (KS)

Definitions

- Locally aggressive vascular proliferation (usually low grade) caused by human herpesvirus 8 (HHV-8)

ETIOLOGY/PATHOGENESIS

Infectious Agents

- All forms of KS are caused by HHV-8
  - HHV-8 detectable in nearly 100% of KS
  - HHV-8 present in tumor cells & peripheral blood

CLINICAL ISSUES

Presentation

- Most cases involve skin
  - Also mucosa, lymph nodes, visceral organs
- Multiple lesions may arise in different sites simultaneously
  - Multifocality does not necessarily represent metastatic spread in classic sense
- 3 stages
  - Patch stage: Red or violaceous macules coalescing into patches
  - Plaque stage: Thickened red/blue/purple/brown plaques
  - Tumor stage: Larger nodules arise from plaques, may ulcerate and simulate pyogenic granuloma clinically
- These stages are same regardless of clinical variant of KS; stages may coexist with one another

Natural History

- Clinical variants of KS
  - Classic
    - Elderly men (90%), usually nodules/plaques on feet and lower legs
    - Most prevalent regions: Mediterranean, Eastern Europe, and central equatorial Africa
      - Rare in USA
    - Often associated with underlying malignancy, usually hematologic
    - Indolent behavior: Slow growth over years
      - Lymph node or organ involvement uncommon
  - African (endemic)
    - Young children & middle-aged adults in equatorial Africa
    - **Not** associated with HIV
    - Multiple skin nodules/tumors of lower legs, progressing over many years
    - Aggressive, often fatal disease if lymph node involvement (lymphadenopathic form)
  - Iatrogenic
    - Occurs in immunosuppressed patients of any age
    - Skin and mucosal involvement commonly; may be disseminated with organ involvement
    - Variable behavior
  - AIDS-associated
    - Occurs in patients coinfected by HIV-1 and HHV-8
      - Specific predilection for homosexual men and IV drug users with HIV
      - In Africa, has equal M:F incidence among HIV(+)
    - Usually patch stage at presentation with subsequent progression
    - Predilection for skin of face, genitals, lower extremities
    - Frequently disseminated with involvement of mucosa, lymph nodes, organs
    - Most aggressive type of KS

Treatment

- No cure for KS
- Wide variety of treatment options for symptom reduction, prevention of disease progression, &/or cosmesis
  - Surgical excision (only for individual more symptomatic lesions, not practical for all lesions)
  - External beam radiation
  - Cryo, laser, or photodynamic therapy
  - Topical or intralesional drugs
  - Systemic chemotherapy only in more severe scenarios
- In AIDS-associated KS, lesions may regress or flare with antiretroviral therapy
- In Iatrogenic KS, lesions may regress (sometimes entirely) once immunosuppression is removed

Prognosis

- Depends on epidemiological/clinical type of KS
- Strongly related to stage of disease
- Strongly related to coexisting infectious diseases

MICROSCOPIC

Histologic Features

- Histologic features differ by stage of disease but not by clinical/epidemiological type
- Distinction of stages not required of pathologist, but useful for recognition of varying histologic patterns in KS
- Patch stage
  - Increased jagged interconnected vascular channels in reticular dermis
    - Dissecting/wrapping around collagen bundles
    - Growing around adnexa
    - Growing into normal vessels (promontory sign: Characteristic but uncommon finding)
    - Lined by uniform endothelial cells with minimal atypia
  - Scattered plasma cells (very useful clue) and lymphocytes
  - Extravasated erythrocytes and hemosiderin deposits
- Plaque stage
  - More extensive vascular proliferation
  - Increased inflammatory infiltrate with plasma cells
  - Spindle cell proliferation infiltrating dermis and invading/destroying eccrine glands
- Tumor stage
  - Nodules of spindle cells arranged in intersecting fascicles
  - Blood-filled slit- and sieve-like spaces between spindle cells
    - When blood-filled spaces absent, may be difficult to recognize as vascular tumor
  - Mitoses often prominent, but nuclear atypia usually only mild to moderate
    - If severe atypia, consider spindled angiosarcoma
    - In AIDS, KS may have more atypical areas similar to angiosarcoma

- Intracytoplasmic hyaline globules in spindle cells
  - Some suggest these are degenerated erythrocytes
- Inflammatory infiltrate with plasma cells usually present
- Other unique histologic variants
  - Lymphangioma-like: Bulla-like clinical appearance, dilated lymphatic-like channels similar to lymphangioma
  - Hemangioma-like: Larger dilated blood-filled spaces similar to hemangioma
  - Poorly differentiated: Pleomorphism and numerous mitoses (more common in Africa)

ANCILLARY TESTS

Immunohistochemistry

- Positive for endothelial and lymphatic markers
  - CD31, CD34, ERG, podoplanin (D2-40), Prox1, Fli1
- Positive nuclear expression of HHV8 (LANA-1) in essentially 100% of cases
  - Often punctate or granular pattern of nuclear staining
  - Essentially all other vascular proliferations are HHV8 negative

DIFFERENTIAL DIAGNOSIS

Angiosarcoma

- Different clinical scenario
- Anastomosing infiltrating vascular channels lined by markedly atypical endothelium with multilayering
  - Negative for HHV8

Severe Vascular Stasis (Acroangiodermatitis)

- Very similar clinical and histologic appearance to KS
  - Violaceous plaques on lower extremities
  - Increased vascular channels & spindle cells in dermis
  - Extravasated RBCs & hemosiderin
- Dermal spindle cells are fibroblasts (not spindled endothelial cells as in KS)
  - Negative for vascular markers: CD31, CD34, ERG
- Negative for HHV8 (in vessels and spindle cells)

Hobnail Hemangioma (Targetoid Hemosiderotic Hemangioma)

- Solitary vascular lesion of skin
- Dilated lymphatic-like channels with bland hobnail endothelium in superficial dermis
- Compressed vessels involve underlying dermis
  - Apparently infiltrative thin vessels can mimic KS
- Negative for HHV8

Microvenular Hemangioma

- Solitary vascular lesion of skin
- Compressed vascular channels trickle between dermal collagen (similar to hobnail hemangioma)
  - Apparently infiltrative thin vessels can mimic KS
- Negative for HHV8

Spindle Cell Hemangioma

- Subcutaneous (or dermal) nodule, usually in leg
- Biphasic pattern
  - Cavernous zone: Similar to cavernous hemangioma
  - Cellular zone: Spindled endothelium & compressed vascular spaces can resemble KS
    - No mitoses, hemorrhage, plasma cells
    - Epithelioid endothelium with vacuoles resembling miniature adipocytes (not seen in KS)
- Negative for HHV8

Kaposiform Hemangioendothelioma

- Infants and young children (vast majority)
  - Very rare in adults
- Whorled nodules of spindled endothelium & slit-like vascular channels
  - No mitoses, hemorrhage, plasma cells
  - Whorled nodular pattern not seen in KS
- Negative for HHV8

Acquired Tufted Angioma

- Solitary skin lesion in adults
- Histologically identical to kaposiform hemangioendothelioma
- Negative for HHV8

Progressive Lymphangioma (Benign Lymphangioendothelioma)

- Slowly growing, solitary, patch or plaque
- Infiltrative channels with bland lymphatic endothelium
- No spindle cells, hemorrhage, plasma cells
- Negative for HHV8

Cellular Dermatofibroma (Fibrous Histiocytoma)

- Dermatofibroma with intersecting hypercellular fascicles
  - Similar fascicles in paucivascular tumor-stage KS
- Epidermal hyperplasia, peripheral collagen trapping, other features of dermatofibroma present
- Lacks infiltrative vascular channels
- Negative for HHV8 & vascular markers

Leiomyosarcoma (Superficial/Cutaneous)

- Intersecting fascicles of atypical smooth muscle cells
  - Similar fascicles in paucivascular tumor-stage KS
- SMA(+), desmin (+)
- Negative for HHV8 & vascular markers

SELECTED REFERENCES

1. Amerson E et al: Accuracy of clinical suspicion and pathologic diagnosis of Kaposi sarcoma in East Africa. J Acquir Immune Defic Syndr. ePub, 2015
2. Jackson CC et al: Kaposi Sarcoma of Childhood: Inborn or Acquired Immunodeficiency to Oncogenic HHV-8. Pediatr Blood Cancer. ePub, 2015
3. Schulz TF et al: Kaposi Sarcoma-associated Herpesvirus: mechanisms of oncogenesis. Curr Opin Virol. 14:116-28, 2015
4. Chadburn A et al: Molecular and immunohistochemical detection of Kaposi sarcoma herpesvirus/human herpesvirus-8. Methods Mol Biol. 999:245-56, 2013
5. Dittmer DP et al: Kaposi sarcoma associated herpesvirus pathogenesis (KSHV)--an update. Curr Opin Virol. 3(3):238-44, 2013
6. He M et al: Cancer angiogenesis induced by Kaposi sarcoma-associated herpesvirus is mediated by EZH2. Cancer Res. 2012 Jul 15;72(14):3582-92. Epub 2012 May 16. Erratum in: Cancer Res. 73(17):5603-5, 2013
7. Fatahzadeh M: Kaposi sarcoma: review and medical management update. Oral Surg Oral Med Oral Pathol Oral Radiol. 2012 Jan;113(1):2-16. Epub 2011 Sep 1. Review. Erratum in: Oral Surg Oral Med Oral Pathol Oral Radiol. 113(5):708, 2012
8. Rosado FG et al: Utility of immunohistochemical staining with FLI1, D2-40, CD31, and CD34 in the diagnosis of acquired immunodeficiency syndrome-related and non-acquired immunodeficiency syndrome-related Kaposi sarcoma. Arch Pathol Lab Med. 136(3):301-4, 2012
9. Dictor M: Kaposi's sarcoma. Origin and significance of lymphaticovenous connections. Virchows Arch A Pathol Anat Histopathol. 409(1):23-35, 1986

Nodules of Classic Kaposi Sarcoma

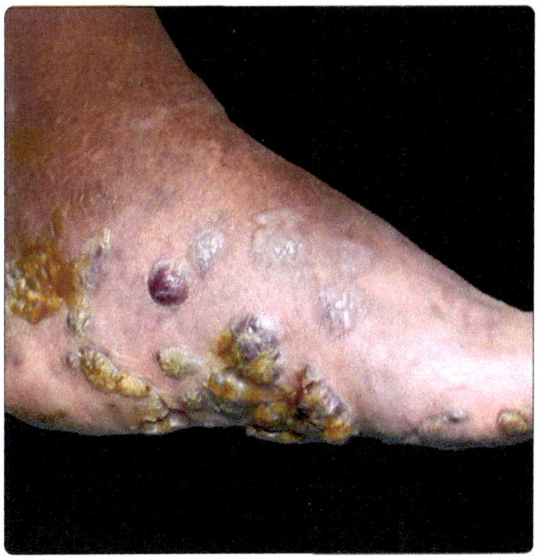

AIDS-Associated Kaposi Sarcoma

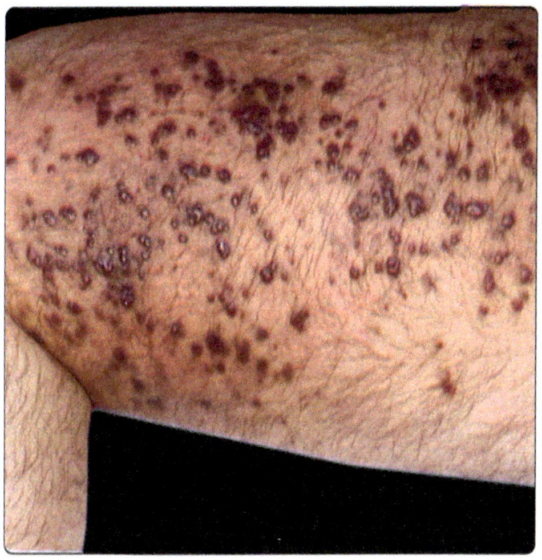

(Left) *Classic KS arose in an elderly man who presented with multiple violaceous and hyperkeratotic nodules on the foot.* **(Right)** *This image shows an HIV(+) patient exhibiting multiple erythematous to violaceous patches and coalescing papules on the thigh.*

Early Kaposi Sarcoma

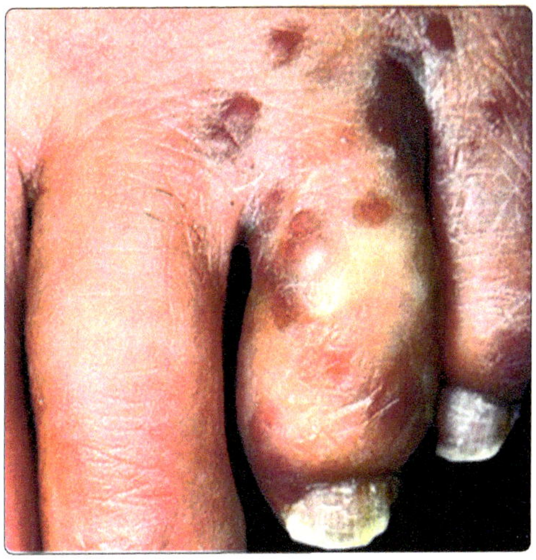

Patch-Stage Kaposi Sarcoma

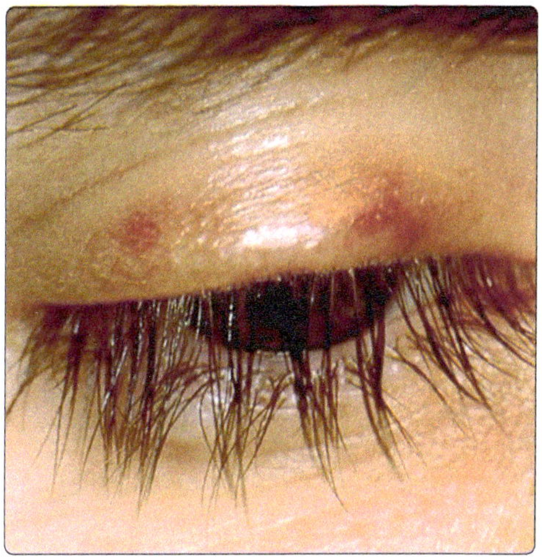

(Left) *Early forms of KS may be subtle and difficult to diagnose clinically. This elderly patient developed multiple erythematous macules and slightly elevated papules on the toe.* **(Right)** *Patients with AIDS-associated KS may present with lesions at unusual anatomic sites, as did this young patient who developed small erythematous patches on his upper eyelid.*

Classic Kaposi Sarcoma

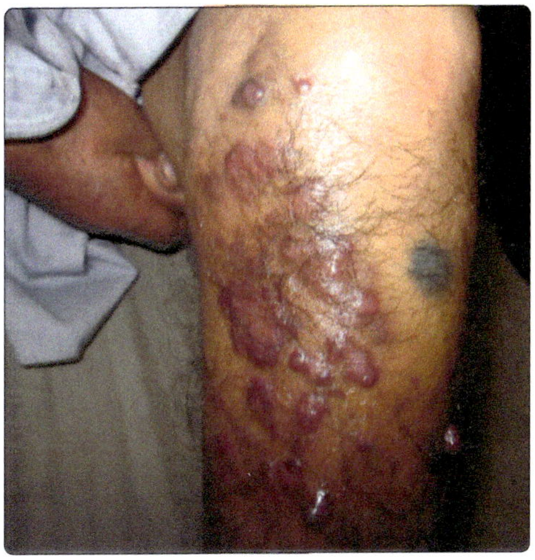

Patch Stage Kaposi Sarcoma

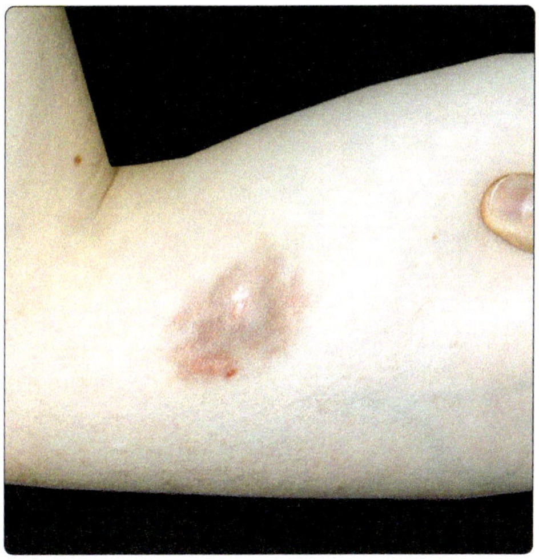

(Left) *This image shows multiple erythematous nodules and plaques of classic KS in an elderly man. (Courtesy J. McMichael, MD.)* **(Right)** *A 30-year-old man with HIV presented with an irregularly shaped erythematous to violaceous patch on the upper arm. The lesion proved to be KS.*

(Left) *Earlier lesions of KS display increased numbers of irregular vascular channels and spindle cells infiltrating the dermis. Hemorrhage is present. Some vessels protrude into the lumen of larger vascular channels (promontory sign)* . **(Right)** *Increased numbers of irregular vascular channels infiltrate the dermis. Mild associated inflammation is also present.*

Early KS With Increased Numbers of Vessels

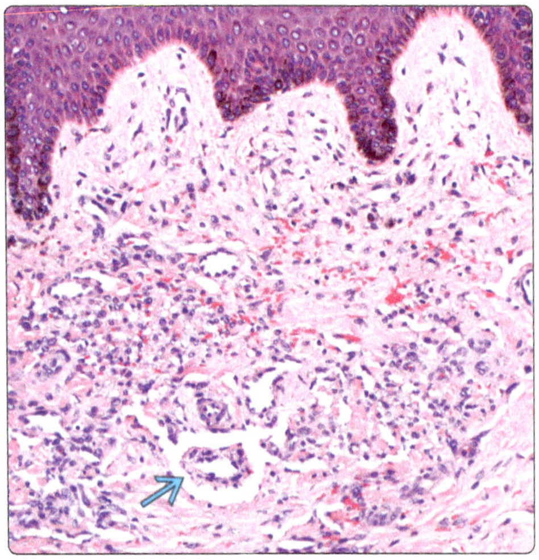

KS With Associated Inflammation

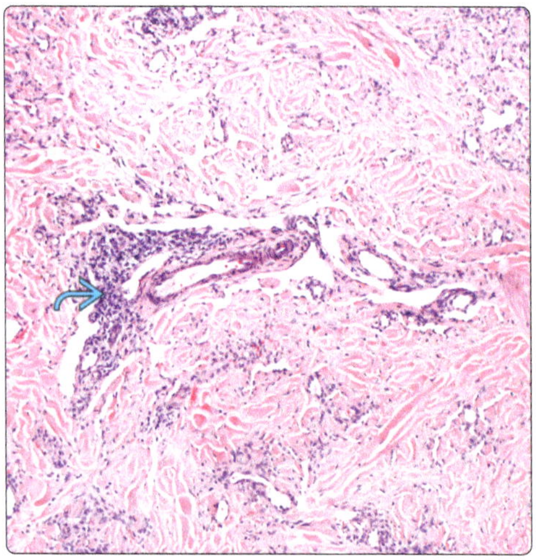

(Left) *Vessels protrude into the lumens of larger vascular channels (promontory sign), giving a vessel within a vessel appearance. This finding is characteristic of KS, although it is relatively uncommon.* **(Right)** *Bland spindle cells with associated hemorrhage infiltrate the dermis in plaque stage KS. Most of these are endothelial cells, not fibroblasts, and can be highlighted by CD31, CD34, and other vascular markers.*

Promontory Sign in KS

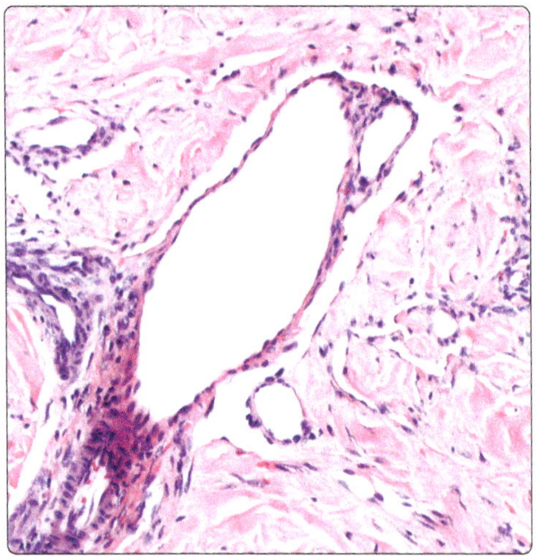

Infiltrative Spindle Cells

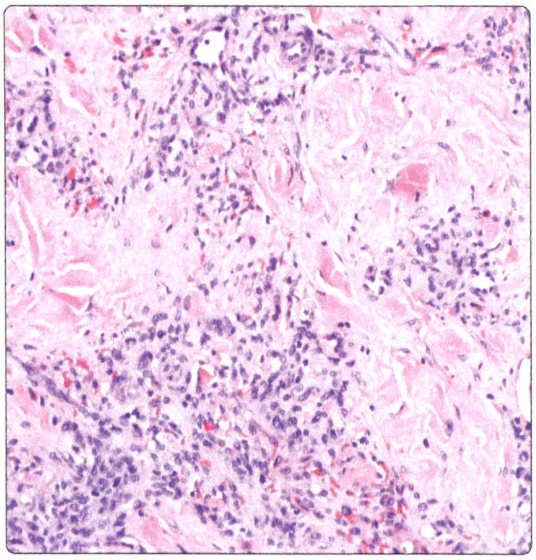

(Left) *Spindled endothelial cells often infiltrate and disrupt the eccrine coils , a very characteristic finding in KS.* **(Right)** *Bland spindled endothelial cells infiltrate and disrupt the eccrine coils in KS, intervening between individual eccrine ducts . Scattered extravasated erythrocytes are also present .*

Infiltration of Eccrine Coils by KS

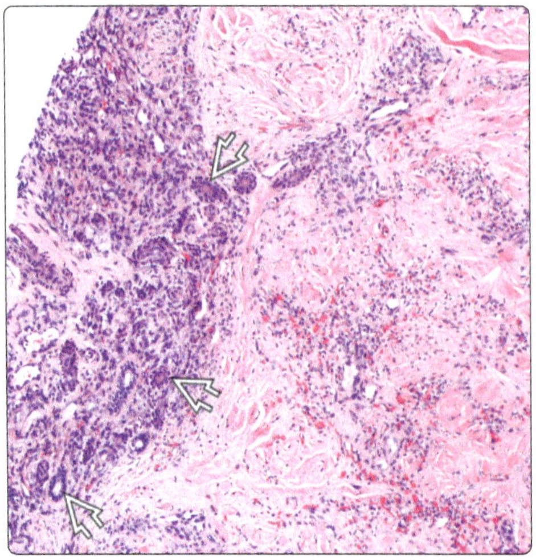

Disruption of Eccrine Coils

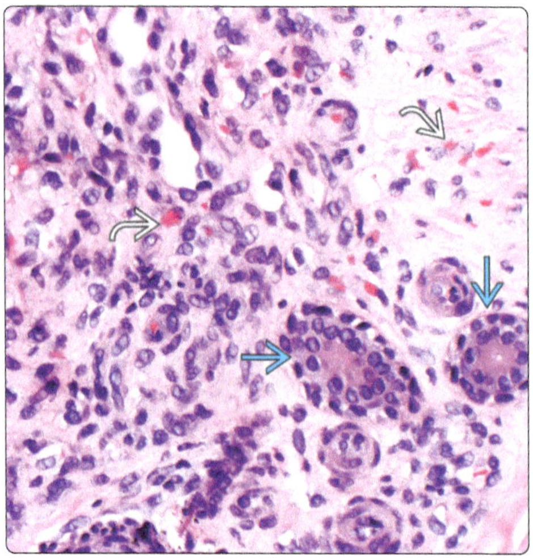

Early Kaposi Sarcoma in Superficial Dermis

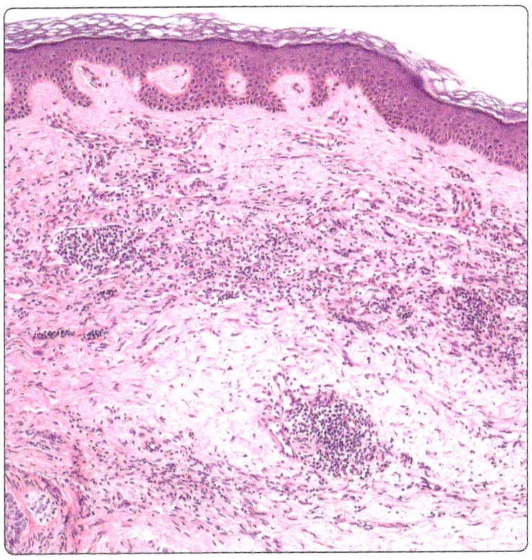

Spindle Cells and Inflammation

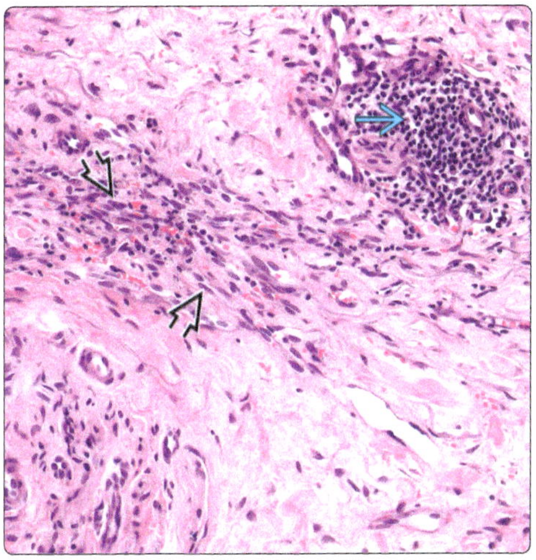

(Left) *Early KS displays infiltrating irregular thin-walled vascular channels, scattered spindle cells, and brisk inflammation.* **(Right)** *Spindle cells associated with small, slit-like spaces infiltrate the dermis. Extravasated erythrocytes are present, and there are also focal aggregates of lymphocytes and plasma cells.*

Mitotic Figure in KS

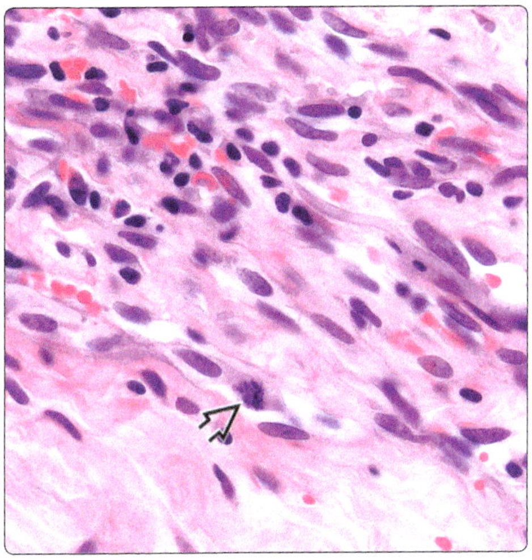

Plasma Cells in KS

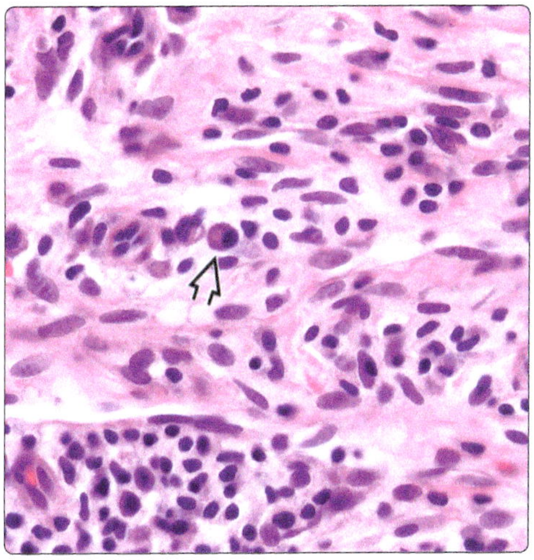

(Left) *At higher power, narrow vascular spaces and cytologically bland spindled cells are seen. Note the presence of inflammatory cells and scattered mitoses.* **(Right)** *The inflammatory infiltrate in KS usually contains at least a few plasma cells.*

Dilated Cavernous Channels in Superficial KS

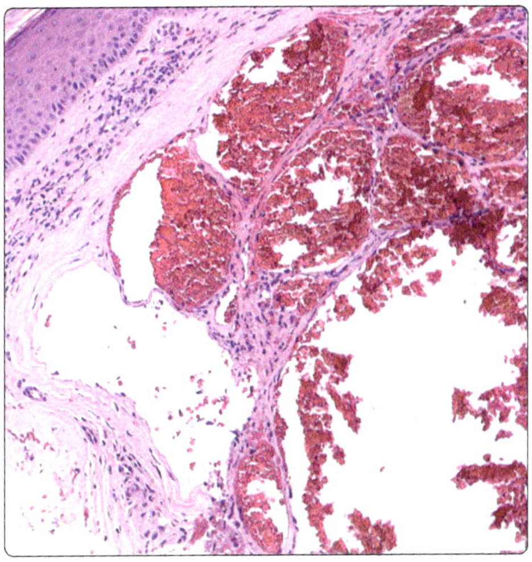

Dissection of Dermal Collagen in KS

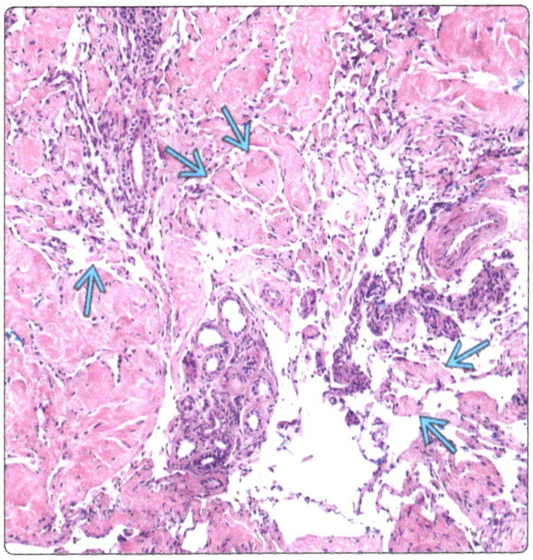

(Left) *Larger dilated blood-filled vessels may be present in some cases of KS, as depicted. These unique cases have been described as hemangioma-like variants of KS.* **(Right)** *Infiltrative dilated vascular channels dissect between deep dermal collagen. This may be so extensive that individual collagen bundles appear to be suspended within empty space.*

(Left) *Low-power view of tumor-stage KS shows an ulcerated, exophytic-appearing hypercellular dermal nodule with hemorrhage.* **(Right)** *Short fascicles of spindle cells intersect one another in tumor-stage KS. Abundant erythrocytes are present between tumor cells.*

Tumor-Stage Kaposi Sarcoma

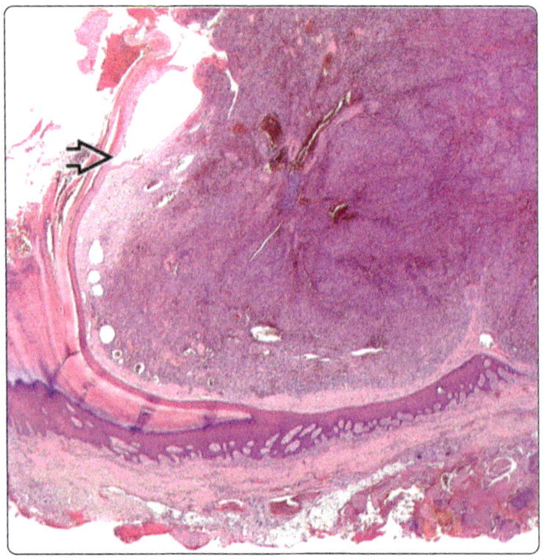

Intersecting Fascicles in Tumor-Stage KS

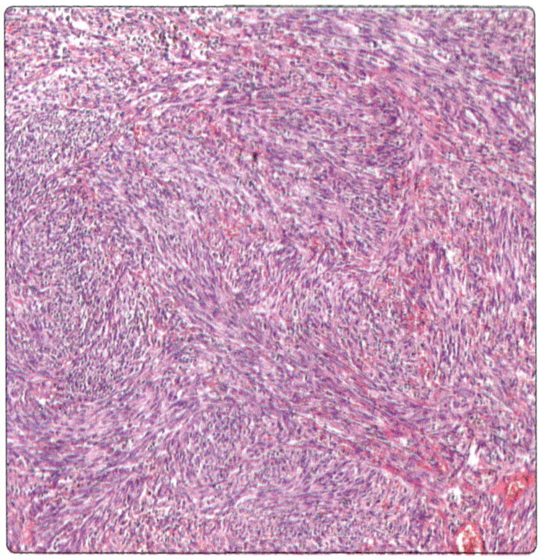

(Left) *Tumor-stage KS displays cellular fascicles of relatively uniform-appearing spindle cells with intervening slit- or sieve-like spaces filled with erythrocytes.* **(Right)** *KS displays tumor cells with relatively uniform spindled nuclei that typically have minimal nuclear atypia, but multiple mitoses can be seen. Small sieve-like spaces containing erythrocytes are seen between the spindled cells.*

Cellular Fascicles of Spindle Cells

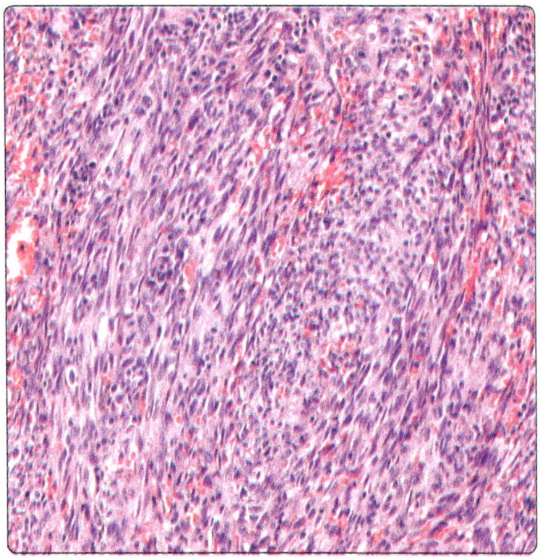

Mitoses but Minimal Nuclear Atypia

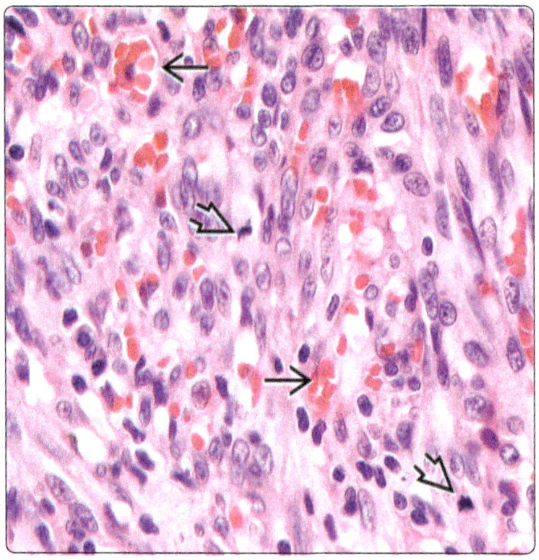

(Left) *Abundant erythrocyte extravasation is seen. Hemosiderin is also often present. Mitoses are readily identified.* **(Right)** *Tumor-stage KS sometimes has minimal or completely absent erythrocyte-filled spaces or hemorrhage. These cases may be easily confused with other fascicular-patterned spindle cell tumors.*

Hemorrhage and Hemosiderin

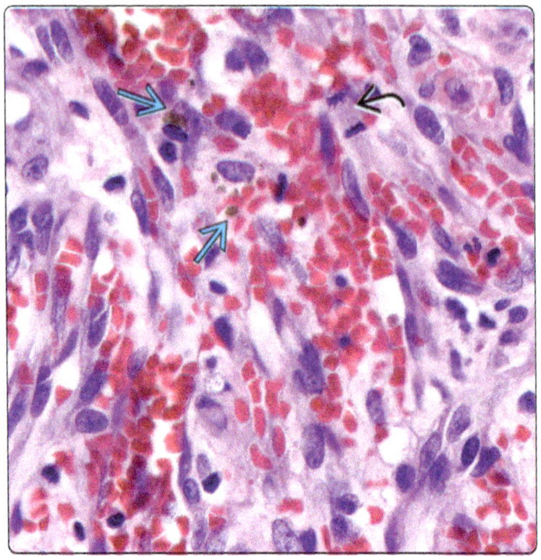

Tumor-Stage KS With Minimal Hemorrhage

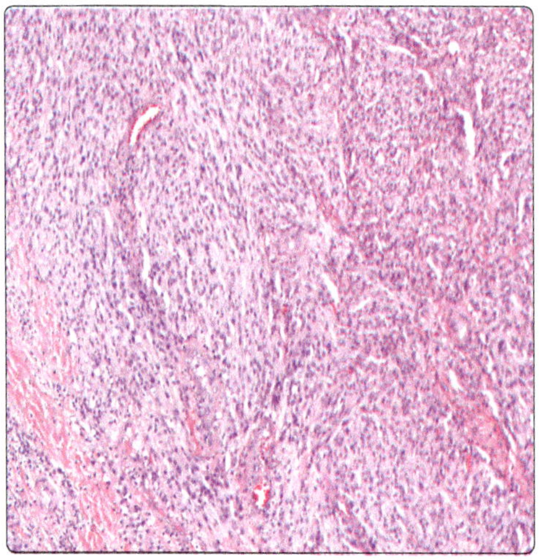

Fascicles Without Erythrocytes

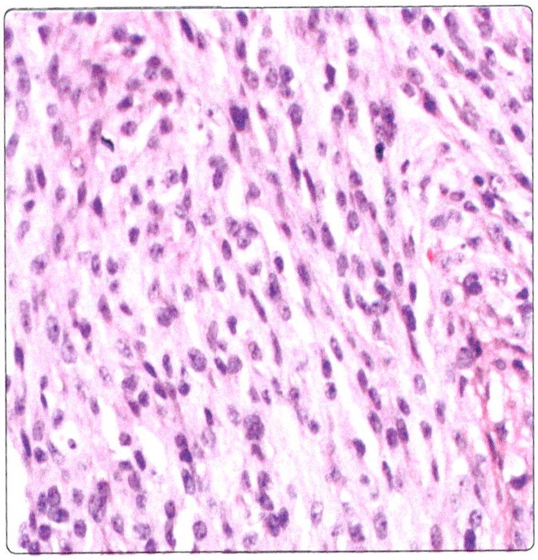

Characteristic Plasma Cells

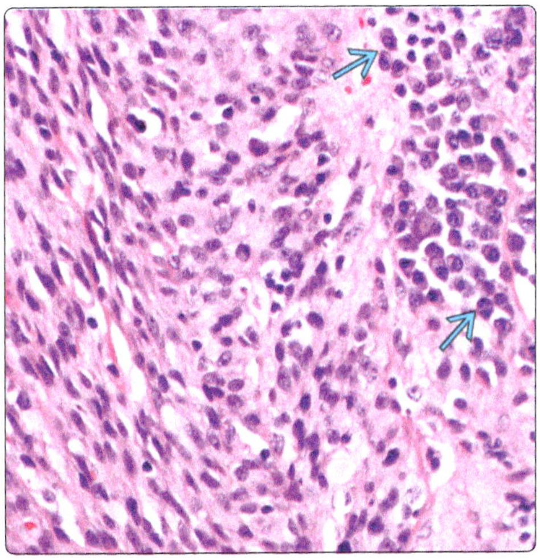

(Left) *Higher magnification shows tumor-stage KS composed of cellular fascicles of uniform spindle cells, devoid of erythrocytes. Recognizing the endothelial nature of these cells is very challenging in areas like this.* **(Right)** *In tumor-stage KS lacking erythrocytes, the presence of plasma cells* ➞ *may be a very important clue to the diagnosis.*

Nuclear HHV8 Expression in KS

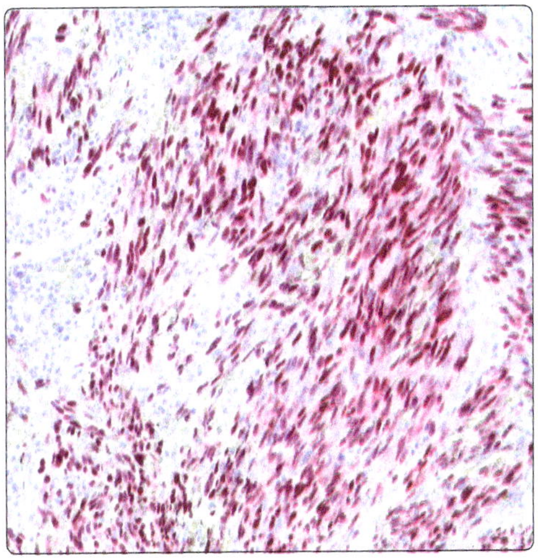

HHV8: Granular Nuclear Staining in KS

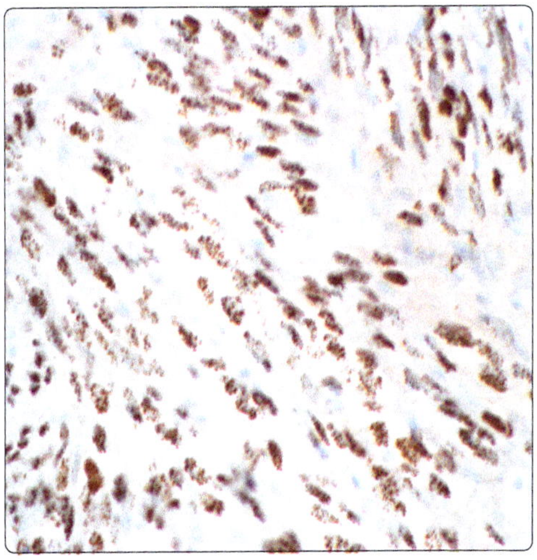

(Left) *Nuclear HHV8 expression is present in essentially 100% of KS but is absent in all other vascular proliferations.* **(Right)** *The HHV8 immunostain often displays a punctate granular nuclear staining pattern.*

CD34 Expression in KS

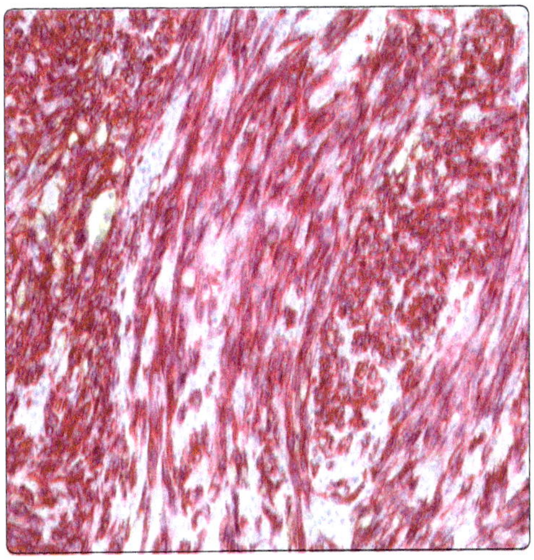

Podoplanin (D2-40) Expression in KS

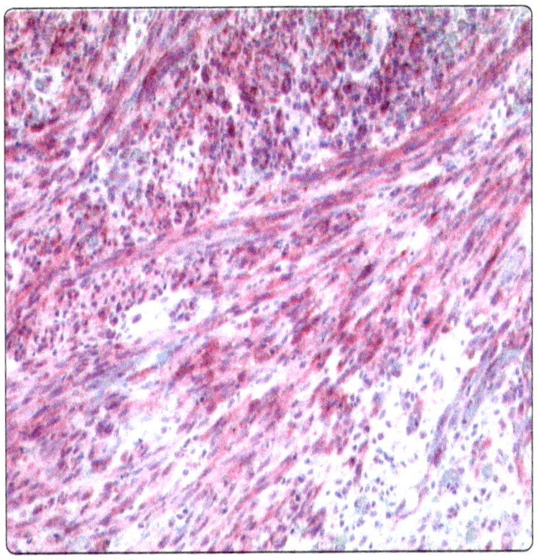

(Left) *Fascicles of spindle cells are diffusely positive for CD34 in this case of tumor-stage KS. CD31 is also typically expressed.* **(Right)** *Most cases of KS have a lymphatic endothelial phenotype, resulting in podoplanin expression (detected with D2-40 immunostaining).*

Kaposiform Hemangioendothelioma

KEY FACTS

CLINICAL ISSUES

- Presents in infants and young children
- Deep tumors, often multiple nodules
- Associated with Kasabach-Merritt phenomenon
  - Consumptive coagulopathy
  - Thrombocytopenia
  - Highest risk for coagulopathy in retroperitoneal and intrathoracic tumors, but also seen in association with large cutaneous tumors
- Rare regional lymph node metastases
- No distant metastases reported to date
- Mortality ~ 10%,usually related to Kasabach-Merritt phenomenon
- Chemotherapy often preferred treatment

MICROSCOPIC

- Spindled cell areas resembling Kaposi sarcoma
- Zones resembling capillary hemangiomas
- Minimal atypia
- Immunohistochemistry shows positive CD31, CD34, FLI-1, ERG, and podoplanin staining
- Negative for HHV8

TOP DIFFERENTIAL DIAGNOSES

- Tufted hemangioma (acquired tufted angioma)
  - Small cutaneous tumor
  - Histologically identical to kaposiform hemangioendothelioma, also occurs in children
  - Likely in same spectrum of tumors
- Kaposi sarcoma
  - Older and immunocompromised patients
  - Positive for HHV8
- Spindle cell hemangioma
  - Adults, usually distal extremities
  - Often partially intravascular
  - Spindled cells, blister cells, and ectatic vascular spaces

Kaposiform Hemangioendothelioma in Groin of Infant

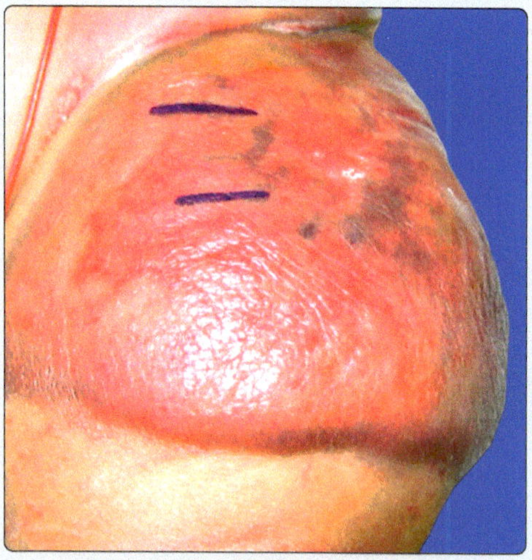

Kaposiform Hemangioendothelioma at Low Magnification

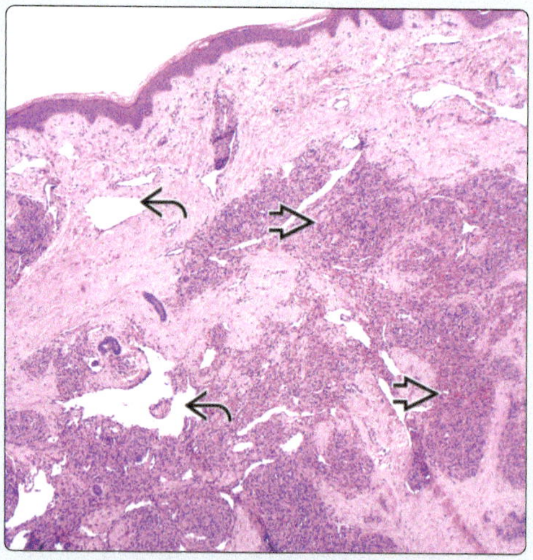

(Left) *Clinical photograph shows a large inguinal tumor in an infant. More superficial tumors typically present as an erythematous or violaceous mass.* **(Right)** *Histologic examination at low power of kaposiform hemangioendothelioma demonstrates irregular nodules ⇨ of spindled cells in the dermis as well as ectatic vessels at periphery of nodules of spindled cells ↶.*

Glomeruloid Area in Kaposiform Hemangioendothelioma

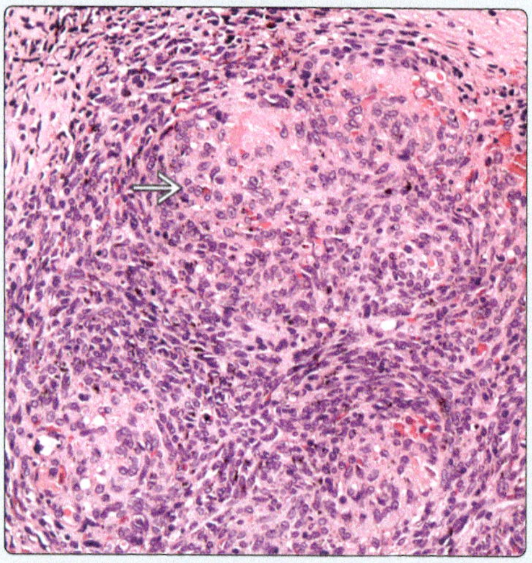

Kaposiform Hemangioendothelioma: Kaposi Sarcoma-Like Area

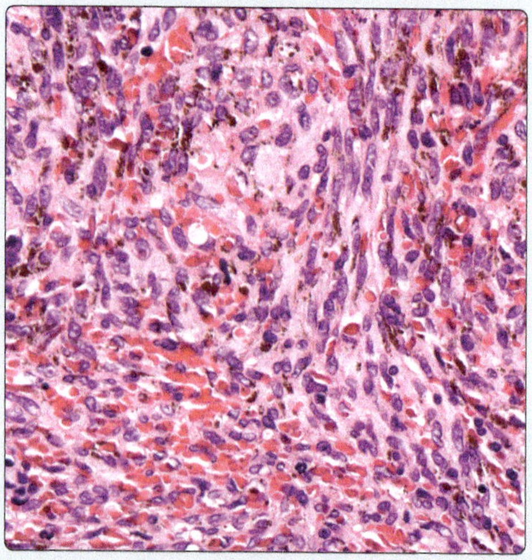

(Left) *In some areas, the spindled tumor cells can have a somewhat swirling growth pattern, imparting a glomeruloid ➡ appearance.* **(Right)** *The tumor cells have uniform hyperchromatic spindled nuclei and are arranged in short fascicles with slit-like vascular lumina.*

ETIOLOGY/PATHOGENESIS

Developmental Anomaly

- ~ 1/2 of kaposiform hemangioendothelioma cases present in 1st year of life

CLINICAL ISSUES

Epidemiology

- Age
  - Majority present in infancy to teenage years

Presentation

- Painful or painless mass
  - Presents as superficial or deep mass
  - Cutaneous lesions present as violaceous plaques
    - Cutaneous lesions most common
  - Deep tumors, often multiple nodules
    - Present in retroperitoneum and intrathoracic locations
- Systemic symptoms
  - Associated with Kasabach-Merritt phenomenon
    - Consumptive coagulopathy
    - Thrombocytopenia
    - Majority of all cases of Kasabach-Merritt phenomenon associated with kaposiform hemangioendothelioma
    - Retroperitoneal and intrathoracic tumors have highest risk of consumptive coagulopathy

Treatment

- Surgical approaches
  - Wide excision
- Drugs
  - Vincristine, cyclophosphamide, methotrexate, α-interferon, sirolimus
    - Patients may have dramatic responses to chemotherapy

Prognosis

- Rare regional lymph node metastasis
- No distant metastasis
- Mortality ~ 10%, usually related to coagulopathy

MICROSCOPIC

Histologic Features

- Multinodular growth pattern
- Spindled areas resembling Kaposi sarcoma
- Capillary hemangioma-like areas with telangiectatic vessels
- Mitoses present, but minimal atypia

ANCILLARY TESTS

Immunohistochemistry

- Positive for CD31, CD34, FLI-1, ERG, and podoplanin (especially in peripheral lymphatic component)
- Negative for GLUT1 (+ in juvenile hemangioma)

DIFFERENTIAL DIAGNOSIS

Tufted Hemangioma (Acquired Tufted Angioma)

- Clinical features
  - Similar demographics as kaposiform hemangioendothelioma
    - Most cases present in children
    - Occasional cases in adults
  - Often associated with Kasabach-Merritt phenomenon
- Microscopic features
  - Nodular proliferation of closely packed capillaries in dermis (cannonball pattern)
  - Bland oval to spindled endothelial cells
- Likely related to kaposiform hemangioendothelioma

Kaposi Sarcoma

- Clinical features
  - Immunocompromised and older patients
- Microscopic features
  - Early Kaposi sarcoma shows neoplastic spindle cells and slit-like vessels dissecting through dermal collagen
  - Later lesions show solid spindle cell areas
  - Lacks dilated vessel at periphery of spindle cell nodules
  - Positive for HHV8 nuclear antigen

Spindle Cell Hemangioma

- Clinical features
  - Occurs in adults
  - Distal extremities
- Microscopic features
  - Often partially intravascular
  - Ectatic vessels
  - Spindled cells
  - Vacuolated endothelial cells
    - So-called blister cells
  - May have areas of thrombosis or phleboliths

DIAGNOSTIC CHECKLIST

Clinically Relevant Pathologic Features

- Age distribution
  - Vast majority occur in children
- Symptom complex
  - Kasabach-Merritt phenomenon

SELECTED REFERENCES

1. Liu Q et al: Clinicopathological features of Kaposiform hemangioendothelioma. Int J Clin Exp Pathol. 8(10):13711-8, 2015
2. Vivas-Colmenares GV et al: The importance of early diagnosis and treatment of kaposiform hemangioendothelioma complicated by Kasabach-Merritt phenomenon. Dermatol Pract Concept. 5(1):91-3, 2015
3. Chan S et al: Rapidly enlarging "bruise" on the back of an infant. Kaposiform hemangioendothelioma complicated by Kasabach-Merritt syndrome. JAMA Dermatol. 149(11):1337-8, 2013
4. Croteau SE et al: Kaposiform hemangioendothelioma: atypical features and risks of Kasabach-Merritt phenomenon in 107 referrals. J Pediatr. 162(1):142-7, 2013
5. Debelenko LV et al: D2-40 immunohistochemical analysis of pediatric vascular tumors reveals positivity in kaposiform hemangioendothelioma. Mod Pathol. 18(11):1454-60, 2005
6. Lyons LL et al: Kaposiform hemangioendothelioma: a study of 33 cases emphasizing its pathologic, immunophenotypic, and biologic uniqueness from juvenile hemangioma. Am J Surg Pathol. 28(5):559-68, 2004
7. Mac-Moune Lai F et al: Kaposiform hemangioendothelioma: five patients with cutaneous lesion and long follow-up. Mod Pathol. 14(11):1087-92, 2001

Epithelioid Hemangioendothelioma

KEY FACTS

TERMINOLOGY

- Malignant angiocentric vascular neoplasm composed of epithelioid endothelial cells within characteristic myxohyaline stromal matrix

CLINICAL ISSUES

- Most common at 30-50 years of age
- Wide distribution in soft tissue
- Also visceral organs (particularly liver and lung)
- Solitary, often painful mass
  - Multicentricity at presentation likely represents locoregional metastases
- Treatment: Wide surgical excision with negative margins
- Indolent clinical course in majority of cases
- Metastases in 20-30%
- Overall mortality rate of 10-20%
  - High-risk EHE features size > 3 cm and > 3 mitoses/50 HPF
    - Associated with significant decrease in survival

MICROSCOPIC

- Infiltrative growth with absence of defined lobularity
- Epithelioid eosinophilic cells arranged in cords, nests
  - Intracytoplasmic vacuoles common (blister cells)
- Well-formed vascular channels typically absent
- Characteristic myxoid to hyaline stromal matrix
- Involvement of larger vessels common

ANCILLARY TESTS

- CD31(+), CD34(+), ERG(+), FLI-1(+)
- Nuclear TFE3(+) observed in distinctive genetic subset
- Keratin (+) in up to 35% of cases, often focal
- Molecular: t(1;3)(p36;q25) with *WWTR1-CAMTA1*
  - Distinctive subset contains *YAP1-TFE3* fusion

TOP DIFFERENTIAL DIAGNOSES

- Epithelioid hemangioma
- Epithelioid angiosarcoma
- Epithelioid sarcoma

Epithelioid Hemangioendothelioma: Clinical Photo

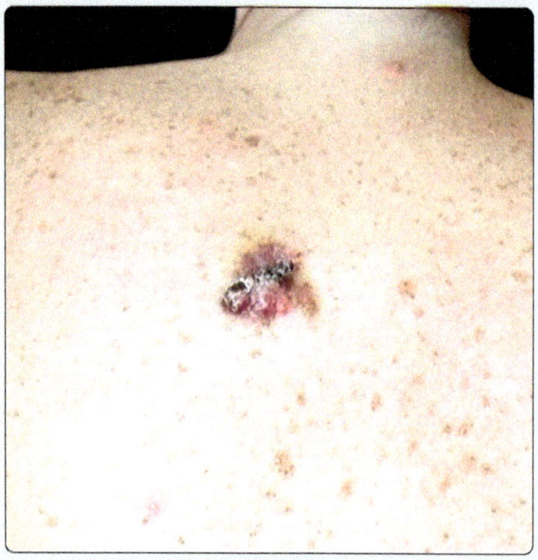

Epithelioid Hemangioendothelioma

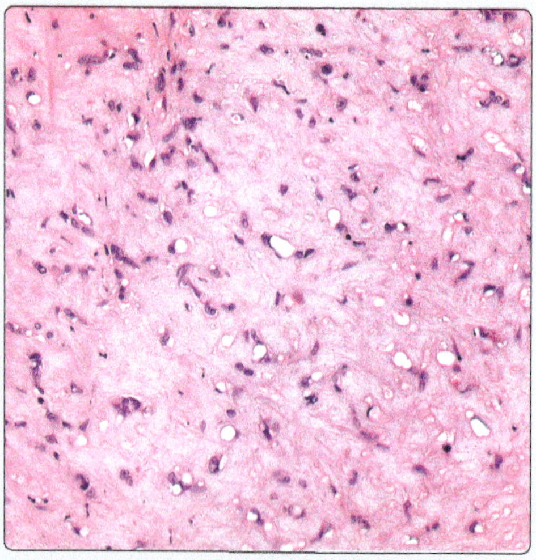

(Left) *Clinical photograph shows a rare cutaneous epithelioid hemangioendothelioma (EHE) presenting as an exophytic lesion.* **(Right)** *EHE is a distinctive malignant vascular neoplasm characterized predominantly by cords of epithelioid tumor cells within a characteristic myxoid to hyaline matrix.*

EHE With Involvement of Larger Vessel

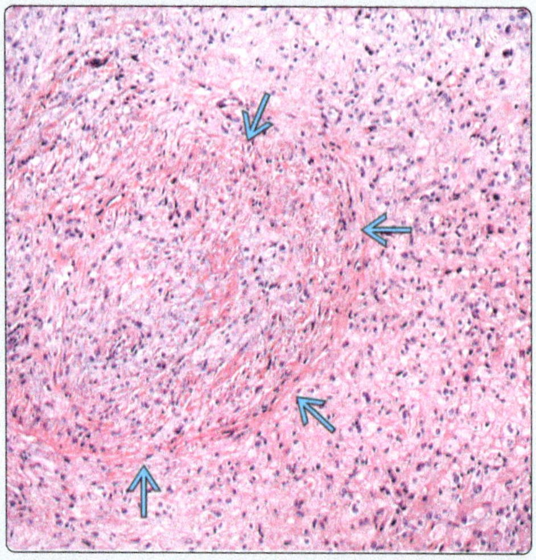

CD31 Expression by Immunohistochemistry

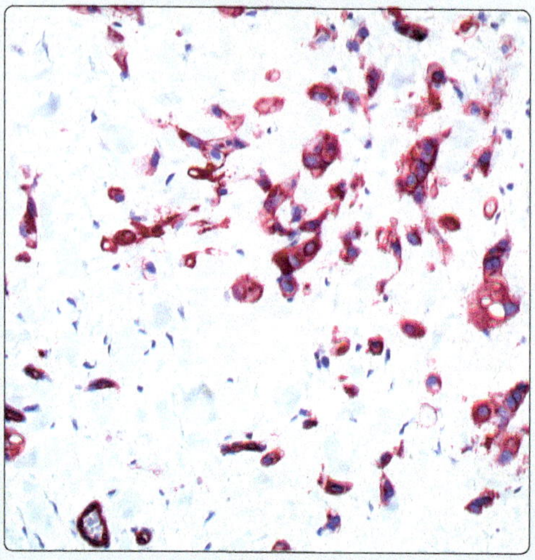

(Left) *EHE is an angiocentric neoplasm and evidence of origin from a larger vessel may be evident histologically. Note the residual smooth muscle wall ➡ in this image. Tumor cells often extend outward from the involved vessel into the surrounding tissues.* **(Right)** *EHE shows expression of endothelial markers, including CD31 (shown), CD34, ERG, and FLI-1. Focal keratin positivity is seen in up to 1/3 of cases.*

TERMINOLOGY

Abbreviations

- Epithelioid hemangioendothelioma (EHE)

Synonyms

- Intravascular bronchioloalveolar tumor (lung)

Definitions

- Malignant angiocentric vascular neoplasm composed of epithelioid endothelial cells within characteristic myxohyaline stromal matrix

CLINICAL ISSUES

Epidemiology

- Incidence
  - Rare tumors
- Age
  - Wide age range affected
    - Most common in 30- to 50-year-old patients
    - Rare in childhood
- Sex
  - Slight female predominance

Site

- Wide distribution in soft tissue
  - Extremities, head/neck region, others
- Visceral organs (particularly liver and lung)

Presentation

- Solitary, often painful mass
  - Superficial or deep
  - Rarely cutaneous
- Apparent multicentricity at time of presentation (up to 50% of cases)
  - Recent molecular data supports conclusion of locoregional metastases over multiple primary lesions
- Occlusion of vessels
  - 30-50% of cases arise in or are associated with preexisting vessel
  - May cause more profound vasoocclusive symptoms, including edema

Treatment

- Wide surgical excision with negative margins
- No proven role for adjuvant chemotherapy &/or radiotherapy

Prognosis

- Indolent clinical course in majority of cases
  - Local recurrence in 10-15%
- Metastases in 20-30%
  - Usually to liver, bone, lungs
  - Occasionally regional lymph nodes
- Overall mortality rate of 10-20%
- Proposed risk assessment
  - High-risk EHE features size > 3 cm and > 3 mitoses per 50 HPF
    - Significant decrease in survival in these cases

MACROSCOPIC

General Features

- Well-circumscribed nodular lesion
- Firm, tan-gray cut surface
- Intravascular tumors may simulate organizing thrombi

Size

- Wide size range
  - Mean: 2.5 cm in 1 large series

MICROSCOPIC

Histologic Features

- Infiltrative growth with absence of defined lobularity
- Epithelioid cells arranged in cords, singly, and in small aggregates or nests
  - Pale to densely eosinophilic cytoplasm
    - Intracytoplasmic vacuoles representing primitive vascular lumina (so-called blister cells)
      - May contain erythrocytes
  - Small, vesicular nuclei ± small nucleoli
    - Occasional tumors show marked nuclear pleomorphism and hyperchromasia
  - Mitotic rate usually low (< 3 figures per 50 HPF)
  - Occasional spindled cytomorphology
- Well-formed vascular channels typically absent
- Characteristic myxoid to hyaline stromal matrix
  - Contains sulfated acid mucopolysaccharides
- Involvement of larger vessels common
  - Obliteration of lumina
  - Outward growth of tumor cells into surrounding tissue
- Metaplastic calcification &/or ossification may be seen in minority of cases
- Necrosis infrequent
- Site-specific unique features (visceral EHE)
  - Lung
    - Characteristic alveolar-filling pattern
    - Central necrosis common
  - Liver
    - Distinct tumor nodules common
    - Entrapped hepatocytes and bile ducts common

Morphologic/Genetic Variant

- Epithelioid hemangioendothelioma with *YAP1-TFE3* fusion
  - Tumor cells often feature more abundant eosinophilic cytoplasm
  - Vasoformation more developed

ANCILLARY TESTS

Immunohistochemistry

- CD31(+), CD34(+), ERG(+), FLI-1(+)
- Nuclear TFE3(+) observed in distinctive genetic subset
- Keratin (+) in up to 35% of cases, often focal
- Nuclear CAMTA1 expression recently reported to be highly useful in distinguishing EHE from histologic mimics
- Negative for S100, SMA, desmin, CD117, EMA, HMB-45

Molecular Genetics

- Characteristic t(1;3)(p36;q25) in most cases (90%)
  - Results in *WWTR1-CAMTA1* fusion

- Distinctive subset contains *YAP1-TFE3* fusion

DIFFERENTIAL DIAGNOSIS

Epithelioid Hemangioma

- Lobular architecture
- Well-formed vascular channels present
- Complete rim of SMA(+) pericytes
- Characteristic mixed chronic inflammatory infiltrate, particularly eosinophils
- Lacks genetic signatures of EHE

Epithelioid Angiosarcoma

- Background of conventional angiosarcoma often present
- Large epithelioid tumor cells in nests or lining irregular vascular spaces
- Mitoses common, include atypical forms
- Frequent tumor necrosis

Epithelioid Sarcoma

- Most common in distal extremities of younger patients
- May show granuloma-like growth pattern with centralized necrosis
- Diffuse expression of keratins and EMA
- Negative for CD31; may be CD34(+)
- Loss of nuclear INI1 expression

Myoepithelioma of Soft Tissue

- Epithelial differentiation evidence in subset (mixed tumor)
- Lacks angiocentric growth
- Usually diffuse keratin (+)
- S100(+) in most cases
- Variable expression of SMA, GFAP, several other markers
- Negative for CD31, CD34, ERG

Pseudomyogenic Hemangioendothelioma

- Sheets and fascicles of predominantly plump spindled cells
- Neutrophilic infiltrate common
- Keratin (+), usually diffuse
- Negative for CD34

Extraskeletal Myxoid Chondrosarcoma

- Prominent lobular growth with fibrous septa
- Fibrous pseudocapsule common
- Small rounded to spindled tumor cells with uniform nuclei
- Prominent myxoid, hypovascular stroma
- Negative for keratins, CD31, CD34, ERG
- Fusions involving *NR4A3* (most commonly to *EWSR1*)

Metastatic Carcinoma

- Clinical history of primary tumor
- Usually higher degree of atypia
- Strong, diffuse keratins (+) in most cases
- Negative for CD31 and CD34

Chondroid Lipoma

- Lobular, often encapsulated
- Conspicuous lipogenic component (mature adipocytes, lipoblasts)
- Negative for CD31, CD34, keratins

DIAGNOSTIC CHECKLIST

Clinically Relevant Pathologic Features

- High-risk features include
  - Large size (> 3 cm)
  - Increased mitotic activity (> 3 mitoses/50 HPF)

Pathologic Interpretation Pearls

- Often arises from preexisting vessel
- Bland-appearing epithelioid endothelial cells with intracytoplasmic vacuoles
- Characteristic myxohyaline stroma
- Expression of endothelial immunohistochemical markers

SELECTED REFERENCES

1. Doyle LA et al: Nuclear expression of CAMTA1 distinguishes epithelioid hemangioendothelioma from histologic mimics. Am J Surg Pathol. ePub, 2015
2. Patel NR et al: Molecular characterization of epithelioid haemangioendotheliomas identifies novel WWTR1-CAMTA1 fusion variants. Histopathology. ePub, 2015
3. Puls F et al: YAP1-TFE3 epithelioid hemangioendothelioma: a case without vasoformation and a new transcript variant. Virchows Arch. 466(4):473-8, 2015
4. Flucke U et al: Epithelioid hemangioendothelioma: clinicopathologic, immunhistochemical, and molecular genetic analysis of 39 cases. Diagn Pathol. 9:131, 2014
5. Antonescu CR et al: Novel YAP1-TFE3 fusion defines a distinct subset of epithelioid hemangioendothelioma. Genes Chromosomes Cancer. 52(8):775-84, 2013
6. Chevreau C et al: Sorafenib in patients with progressive epithelioid hemangioendothelioma: a phase 2 study by the French Sarcoma Group (GSF/GETO). Cancer. 119(14):2639-44, 2013
7. Mistry AM et al: Diagnostic and therapeutic challenges in hepatic epithelioid hemangioendothelioma. J Gastrointest Cancer. 43(4):521-5, 2012
8. Wang LR et al: Clinical experience with primary hepatic epithelioid hemangioendothelioma: retrospective study of 33 patients. World J Surg. 36(11):2677-83, 2012
9. Murali R et al: Cytologic features of epithelioid hemangioendothelioma. Am J Clin Pathol. 136(5):739-46, 2011
10. Woelfel C et al: Molecular cytogenetic characterization of epithelioid hemangioendothelioma. Cancer Genet. 204(12):671-6, 2011
11. Emamaullee JA et al: Vascular endothelial growth factor expression in hepatic epithelioid hemangioendothelioma: Implications for treatment and surgical management. Liver Transpl. 16(2):191-7, 2010
12. Gill R et al: Utility of immunohistochemistry for endothelial markers in distinguishing epithelioid hemangioendothelioma from carcinoma metastatic to bone. Arch Pathol Lab Med. 133(6):967-72, 2009
13. Clarke LE et al: Cutaneous epithelioid hemangioendothelioma. J Cutan Pathol. 35(2):236-40, 2008
14. Deyrup AT et al: Epithelioid hemangioendothelioma of soft tissue: a proposal for risk stratification based on 49 cases. Am J Surg Pathol. 32(6):924-7, 2008
15. Bagan P et al: Prognostic factors and surgical indications of pulmonary epithelioid hemangioendothelioma: a review of the literature. Ann Thorac Surg. 82(6):2010-3, 2006
16. Tsarouha H et al: Chromosome analysis and molecular cytogenetic investigations of an epithelioid hemangioendothelioma. Cancer Genet Cytogenet. 169(2):164-8, 2006
17. Leowardi C et al: Malignant vascular tumors: clinical presentation, surgical therapy, and long-term prognosis. Ann Surg Oncol. 12(12):1090-101, 2005
18. Mendlick MR et al: Translocation t(1;3)(p36.3;q25) is a nonrandom aberration in epithelioid hemangioendothelioma. Am J Surg Pathol. 25(5):684-7, 2001
19. Quante M et al: Epithelioid hemangioendothelioma presenting in the skin: a clinicopathologic study of eight cases. Am J Dermatopathol. 20(6):541-6, 1998
20. Mentzel T et al: Epithelioid hemangioendothelioma of skin and soft tissues: clinicopathologic and immunohistochemical study of 30 cases. Am J Surg Pathol. 21(4):363-74, 1997
21. Tsang WY et al: The family of epithelioid vascular tumors. Histol Histopathol. 8(1):187-212, 1993
22. Weiss SW et al: Epithelioid hemangioendothelioma: a vascular tumor often mistaken for a carcinoma. Cancer. 50(5):970-81, 1982

EHE Growing in Nests and Cords

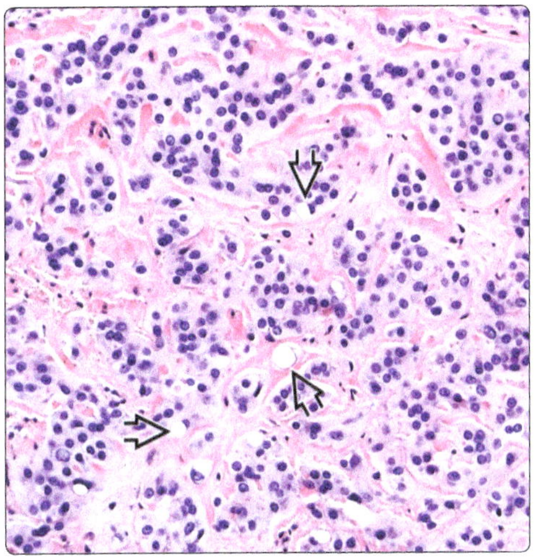

Occasional Spindled Tumor Cells and Atypia

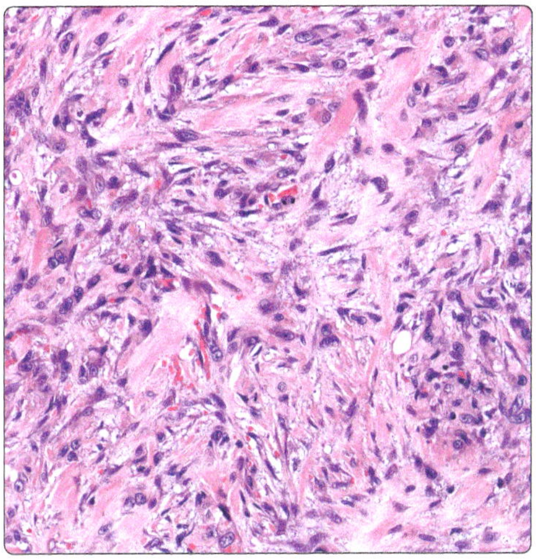

(Left) *In addition to growth in cords and chains, tumor cells in EHE may also be arranged in small aggregates and nests, as depicted. Note the intracytoplasmic vacuoles. The stroma is more hyaline than myxoid in this image.* **(Right)** *Spindling of tumor cells is seen in a minor proportion of cases of EHE. Areas of more conventional epithelioid morphology are usually also present. Nuclear atypia may be seen but does not correlate well with more aggressive behavior (which is related to increased size and mitoses).*

Intracytoplasmic Vacuoles Are Characteristic Finding

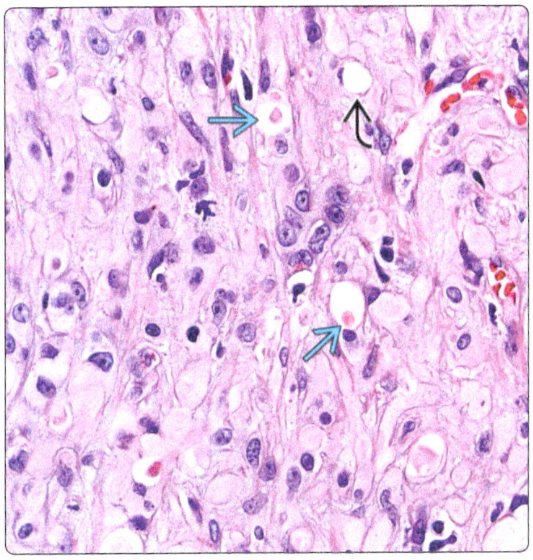

Increased Cellularity Present in Some Tumors

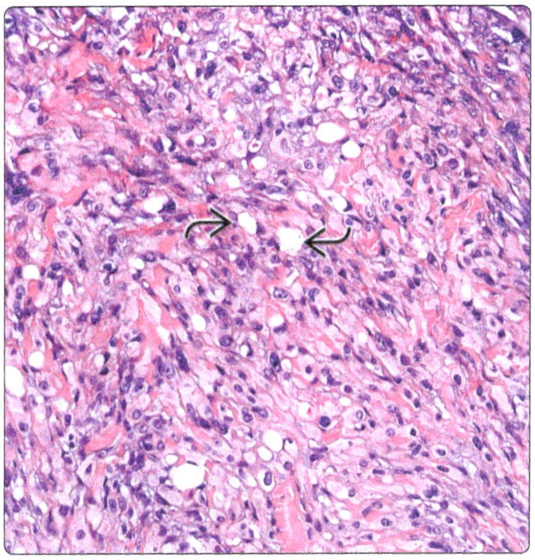

(Left) *Another characteristic finding in EHE is the presence of intracytoplasmic vacuoles. Despite their resemblance to fat cells, these spaces actually represent immature vascular lumina and may at times contain erythrocytes.* **(Right)** *Some cases of EHE feature areas of increased cellularity, as depicted. Note also that some tumor cells can appear to contain multiple intracytoplasmic vacuoles, mimicking true lipoblastic cells.*

Metaplastic Bone Formation Is Rare Finding

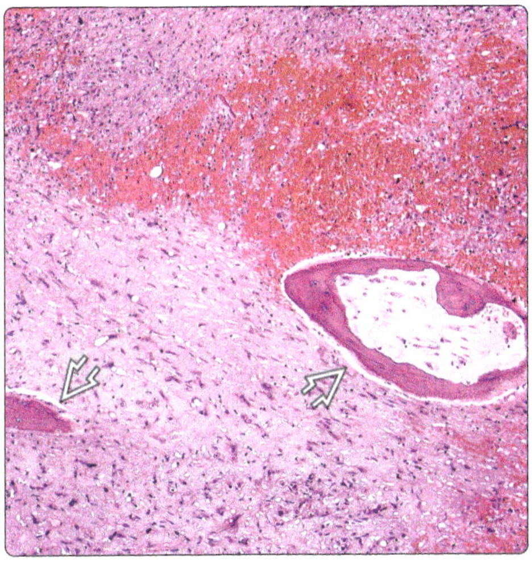

EHE Arising in Liver

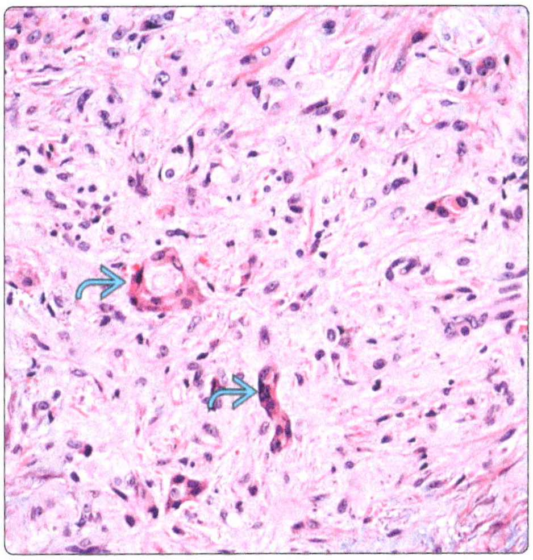

(Left) *Foci of metaplastic ossification may be seen in up to 10% of EHE.* **(Right)** *Hepatic EHE shows a similar morphology to soft tissue EHE; however, entrapped hepatocytes and reactive bile ducts are often present. Growth as multiple distinct nodules is also more common in this site.*

Retiform Hemangioendothelioma

KEY FACTS

TERMINOLOGY

- Retiform hemangioendothelioma (RHE)
- Low-grade malignant vascular tumor composed of elongated vessels resembling rete testes

ETIOLOGY/PATHOGENESIS

- Rare cases associated with lymphedema or preceding radiation

CLINICAL ISSUES

- Typically middle-aged adults but may occur in children
- Locally aggressive, very rarely metastasizing (although lymph node metastases reported)
- Trunk or extremities
- Locally aggressive, rarely metastasizing (although lymph node metastases reported in several cases)

MICROSCOPIC

- Distinctive elongated, arborizing blood vessels resembling rete testis
- Often show papillary-like intraluminal projections, some of which may have hyaline core
- Vascular spaces are lined by endothelial cells with characteristic hobnail morphology
- Some cases show significant overlap with Dabska tumor
- Hobnail cells with oval nuclei with mild hyperchromasia

ANCILLARY TESTS

- Tumor cells react with vascular endothelial markers CD31, CD34, and FVIIIRAg

TOP DIFFERENTIAL DIAGNOSES

- Papillary intralymphatic angioendothelioma (Dabska tumor)
  - More common in children
- Composite hemangioendothelioma (HE)
  - Composed of at least 2 distinct HE types
- Kaposi sarcoma
- Angiosarcoma

Retiform Hemangioendothelioma at Low Magnification

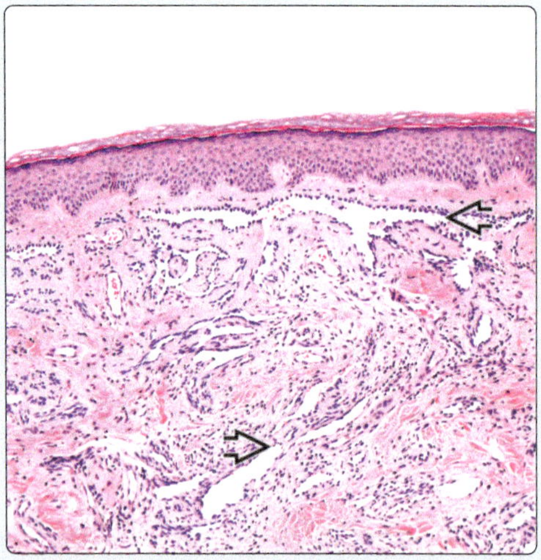

Retiform Hemangioendothelioma at Higher Magnification

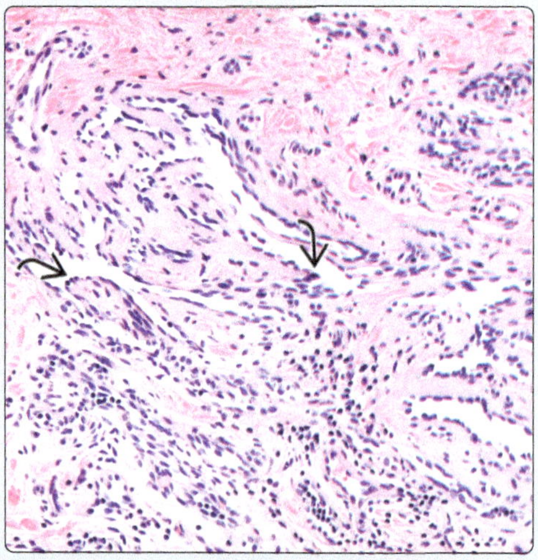

(Left) *Low-magnification examination of a retiform hemangioendothelioma (RHE) shows superficial dermal involvement by irregular, elongated, branching vascular spaces.* **(Right)** *Higher magnification view shows a proliferation of elongated vessels lined by hyperchromatic-staining hobnailed endothelial cells. The surrounding stroma shows fibrosis and scattered lymphocytes.*

Retiform Hemangioendothelioma With Dense Lymphoid Aggregates

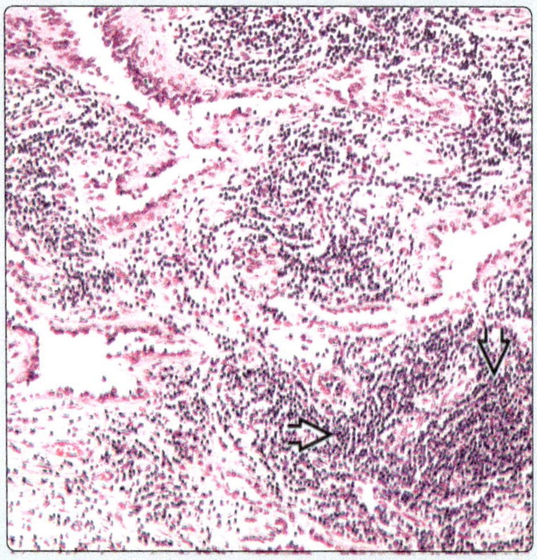

Retiform Hemangioendothelioma: Cytologic Features

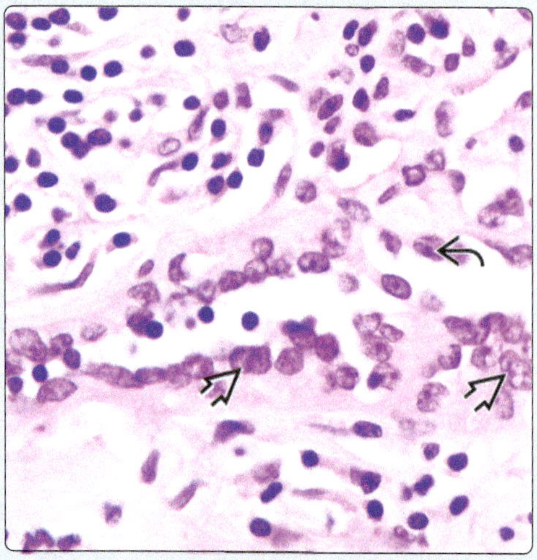

(Left) *A deep area of an RHE shows elongated vascular spaces surrounded by prominent lymphoid aggregates.* **(Right)** *High-magnification view shows hyperchromatic endothelial cells with hobnail features, nuclear crowding, and focally enlarged nucleoli.*

TERMINOLOGY

Abbreviations

- Retiform hemangioendothelioma (RHE)

Synonyms

- Hobnail hemangioendothelioma (HE)

Definitions

- Low-grade malignant vascular tumor composed of elongated vessels resembling rete testis

ETIOLOGY/PATHOGENESIS

Unknown

- Rare cases associated with lymphedema or preceding radiation
- 1 case reported to be positive for HHV8

CLINICAL ISSUES

Epidemiology

- Incidence
  - Rare vascular tumor
- Age
  - Typically middle-aged adults but may occur in children
- Sex
  - More common in females

Site

- Trunk or extremities

Presentation

- Large nodular to plaque-like lesion

Treatment

- Surgical approaches
  - Complete excision is necessary to prevent recurrence

Prognosis

- Locally aggressive, rarely metastasizing (although lymph node metastases reported in several cases)

MACROSCOPIC

General Features

- Typically poorly circumscribed dermal &/or subcutaneous tumor

Size

- May be large tumors (up to 12 cm)

MICROSCOPIC

Histologic Features

- Dermal-based infiltrative proliferation of distinctive elongated, arborizing blood vessels resembling rete testis
- Vascular spaces are lined by endothelial cells with characteristic hobnail morphology
  - Endothelial cells show hyperchromasia but typically do not show prominent cytologic atypia
  - Mitotic figures may be present but are usually rare
- Very prominent lymphocytic infiltrate in most cases
- May show invasion of subcutaneous tissues
- Some cases show significant overlap with Dabska tumor (both have hobnailed cells), with prominent papillary structures and hyaline cores

Cytologic Features

- Hobnail cells with oval nuclei with mild hyperchromasia

ANCILLARY TESTS

Immunohistochemistry

- Tumor cells react with vascular endothelial markers CD31, CD34, and FVIIIRAg
- Most cases negative with lymphatic markers D2-40 and VEGFR-3 but rare positive cases

DIFFERENTIAL DIAGNOSIS

Papillary Intralymphatic Angioendothelioma (Dabska Tumor)

- More common in children but some cases in young adults reported
- Papillary structures more common
- Typically do not show prominent rete-like elongated vessels of RHE
- Some cases show significant overlap with RHE (both have hobnailed cells)
- Most cases positive for lymphatic markers (D2-40, VEGFR-3)

Composite Hemangioendothelioma

- By definition, composed of at least 2 distinct HE types
  - Predominant histologic components usually are epithelioid HE and RHE

Kaposi Sarcoma

- Much more common, associated with HIV/AIDS
- Proliferation of small, slit-like vascular spaces lined by spindle cells, lacking rete-like pattern of RHE
- HHV8 positive (only 1 case of RHE reported to be positive)

Angiosarcoma

- Typically occurs in older adults or post mastectomy
- Proliferation of atypical spindled or epithelioid endothelial cells, often forming anastomosing vascular spaces and showing infiltrative features

DIAGNOSTIC CHECKLIST

Pathologic Interpretation Pearls

- Proliferation of distinctive elongated blood vessels (lined by hobnail cells) resembling rete testis

SELECTED REFERENCES

1. Tamhankar AS et al: Retiform hemangioendothelioma over forehead: A rare tumor treated with chemoradiation and a review of literature. J Cancer Res Ther. 11(3):657, 2015
2. Zheng LQ et al: Cutaneous retiform hemangioendothelioma on the right foot with an unusual clinicopathological feature. Am J Dermatopathol. 36(9):757-9, 2014
3. Mota A et al: Clinical, dermoscopic and histopathologic findings of retiform hemangioendothelioma. Dermatol Pract Concept. 3(4):11-4, 2013
4. Emberger M et al: Retiform hemangioendothelioma: presentation of a case expressing D2-40. J Cutan Pathol. 36(9):987-90, 2009
5. Tan D et al: Retiform hemangioendothelioma: a case report and review of the literature. J Cutan Pathol. 32(9):634-7, 2005
6. Calonje E et al: Retiform hemangioendothelioma. A distinctive form of low-grade angiosarcoma delineated in a series of 15 cases. Am J Surg Pathol. 18(2):115-25, 1994

Papillary Intralymphatic Angioendothelioma (Dabska Tumor)

KEY FACTS

TERMINOLOGY

- Dabska tumor
- Endovascular papillary angioendothelioma

CLINICAL ISSUES

- Rare tumors
- Typically occur in children (minority in adults)
- Distal extremities most common but may occur in other sites
- High rate of local recurrence, rare metastasis

MICROSCOPIC

- Dermal proliferation of vessels with papillary projections lined by enlarged, cuboidal endothelial cells
- Endothelial cells show prominent hobnail features with plump, rounded profiles protruding into lumina
- Typically associated with surrounding lymphoid infiltrate and sclerotic collagen
- Hobnail cells show high nuclear:cytoplasmic ratio, nuclei may show grooves
- Cytoplasmic vacuolation may be seen

ANCILLARY TESTS

- Typically positive for vascular markers including CD31 and CD34

TOP DIFFERENTIAL DIAGNOSES

- Retiform hemangioendothelioma
  - Most cases occur in adults but some occur in children
  - May show significant overlap with Dabska tumor, with prominent papillary structures
- Composite hemangioendothelioma
  - Composed of at least 2 distinct HE types
- Kaposi sarcoma
  - Proliferation of small, slit-like vascular spaces lined by HHV8(+) spindle cells
- Angiosarcoma

Scanning Magnification of Dabska Tumor

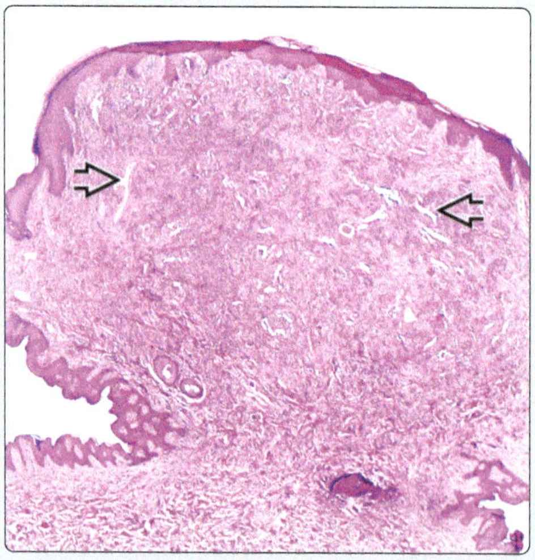

Low Magnification of Dabska Tumor

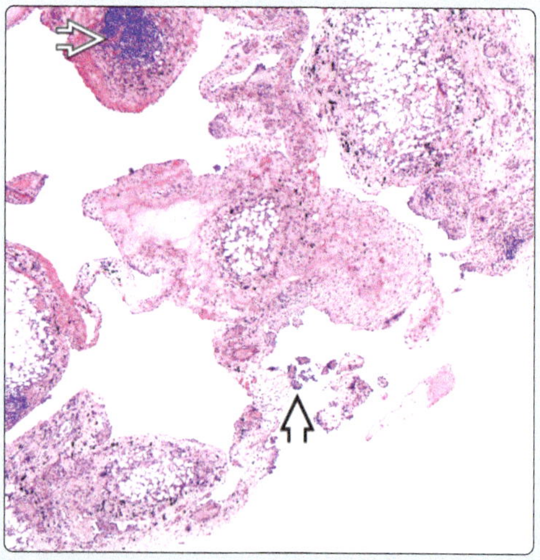

(Left) *Scanning magnification view of a papillary intralymphatic angioendothelioma (Dabska tumor) shows a polypoid lesion in the dermis with irregularly dilated vascular spaces* ⇨. **(Right)** *Low magnification shows a background of lymphangioma-like areas with scattered lymphoid aggregates* ➡. *Note the focal intraluminal papillary projections* ⇨.

High Magnification Showing Cytologic Details

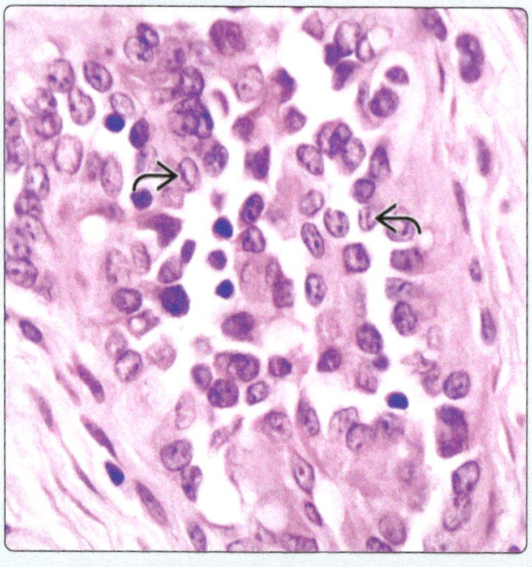

Papillae Lined by Plump Endothelial Cells

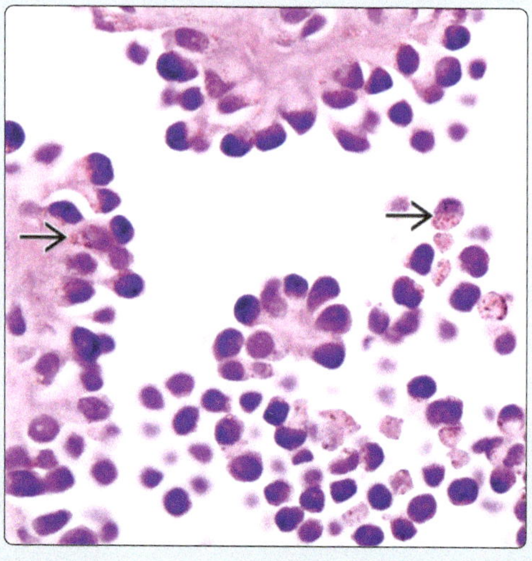

(Left) *High power shows papillae lined by mildly enlarged hobnailed cells projecting into the vascular lumina. The cells show vesicular chromatin, small nucleoli, and occasional grooves* ↷. **(Right)** *Multiple prominent intralymphatic projections of papillary structures with hyaline cores are lined by plump, hyperchromatic-staining endothelial cells, some of which contain cytoplasmic hemosiderin pigment* →.

TERMINOLOGY

Synonyms

- Dabska tumor

Definitions

- Low-grade malignant vascular tumor composed of hobnailed endothelial cells

ETIOLOGY/PATHOGENESIS

Unknown

- May be associated with vascular or lymphatic tumor/malformation

CLINICAL ISSUES

Epidemiology

- Incidence
  - Rare tumors
- Age
  - Typically occur in children (minority in adults)
- Sex
  - Slight female predominance

Site

- Distal extremities most common but may occur in other sites

Presentation

- Plaque-like lesion of dermis and subcutis
  - May show overlying violaceous skin discoloration

Treatment

- Surgical approaches
  - Complete surgical excision recommended to prevent metastasis (rare) or recurrence

Prognosis

- High rate of local recurrence but only rare metastasis

MACROSCOPIC

General Features

- Dermal-based, infiltrative tumor

Size

- Can be quite large (average: 7 cm)

MICROSCOPIC

Histologic Features

- Dermal proliferation of vessels lined by enlarged, cuboidal endothelial cells
  - Intravascular papillary projections with hyaline cores
  - Endothelial cells show prominent hobnail features with plump, rounded profiles protruding into lumina
  - Cytoplasmic vacuolation may be seen
  - Mitotic figures absent or rare
- Typically associated with surrounding lymphoid infiltrate and sclerotic collagen
- Vessels often extend into subcutaneous tissues
- Associated lymphatic or vascular tumor or malformation in some cases

Cytologic Features

- Hobnail cells show high nuclear:cytoplasmic ratio; nuclei may show grooves

ANCILLARY TESTS

Immunohistochemistry

- Typically positive for vascular markers including CD31, CD34, and FVIIIRAg
- Most cases also positive for lymphatic markers D2-40 and VEGFR-3

DIFFERENTIAL DIAGNOSIS

Retiform Hemangioendothelioma

- Most cases occur in adults but some present in children
- Proliferation of vessels forming distinct, elongated, rete-like structures lined by hobnail cells
- Some cases of retiform hemangioendothelioma (RHE) show significant overlap with Dabska tumor, with prominent papillary structures
- Most cases negative with lymphatic markers D2-40 and VEGFR-3; rare positive cases

Composite Hemangioendothelioma

- By definition, composed of at least 2 distinct composite hemangioendothelioma (HE) types
  - Predominant histologic components usually are epithelioid HE and RHE

Kaposi Sarcoma

- Much more common; associated with HIV infection and AIDS in most cases
- Proliferation of small, slit-like vascular spaces lined by spindle cells, lacking papillary pattern of Dabska
- HHV8(+)

Angiosarcoma

- Typically occurs in older adults or post mastectomy
- Proliferation of atypical spindled or epithelioid endothelial cells, forming anastomosing vascular spaces and showing infiltrative features

DIAGNOSTIC CHECKLIST

Pathologic Interpretation Pearls

- Dermal proliferation of vessels with papillary projections lined by enlarged, cuboidal endothelial cells

SELECTED REFERENCES

1. Kugler A et al: Papillary intralymphatic angioendothelioma (PILA), also referred to as Dabska tumour, in an 83-year-old woman. J Eur Acad Dermatol Venereol. ePub, 2015
2. Llamas-Velasco M et al: Hemangioma with dabskoid features: a rare histopathologic variant of acquired hemangioma. J Cutan Pathol. ePub, 2015
3. Neves RI et al: Endovascular papillary angioendothelioma (Dabska tumor): underrecognized malignant tumor in childhood. J Pediatr Surg. 46(1):e25-8, 2011
4. Emanuel PO et al: Dabska tumor arising in lymphangioma circumscriptum. J Cutan Pathol. 35(1):65-9, 2008
5. Fanburg-Smith JC et al: Papillary intralymphatic angioendothelioma (PILA): a report of twelve cases of a distinctive vascular tumor with phenotypic features of lymphatic vessels. Am J Surg Pathol. 23(9):1004-10, 1999
6. Dabska M: Malignant endovascular papillary angioendothelioma of the skin in childhood. Clinicopathologic study of 6 cases. Cancer. 24(3):503-10, 1969

Atypical Vascular Lesion

KEY FACTS

TERMINOLOGY

- Synonym: Atypical vascular proliferation
- Benign cutaneous vascular lesion presenting as small papule or patch in radiated skin, composed of thin-walled lymphatic vessels, usually limited to dermis

ETIOLOGY/PATHOGENESIS

- Median latency 3 years post radiotherapy

CLINICAL ISSUES

- Wide age range; median in late 50s
- Skin of breast or chest wall most common following radiotherapy for breast cancer
- Small, flesh-colored papule or erythematous patch
- Solitary or multiple
- Most lesions pursue benign course
- New lesions frequently appear
- Few reports of transformation to angiosarcoma
- Complete excision of all lesions recommended

MICROSCOPIC

- Dermal-based, small, symmetrical, often wedge-shaped
- Usually confined to superficial dermis
- Thin-walled lymphatic capillary vessels
- Dilated or jagged, anastomosing vascular structures
- Dissects preexisting dermal collagen
- Rarely extends into subcutis
- Lacks endothelial multilayering and significant atypia
- Mitoses rarely present
- No amplification of *MYC*

TOP DIFFERENTIAL DIAGNOSES

- Well-differentiated angiosarcoma
  - Endothelial multilayering and nuclear atypia
- Hobnail hemangioma
- Lymphangioma circumscriptum
- Progressive lymphangioma (benign lymphangioendothelioma)

Clinical Appearance as Small Papules and Patches

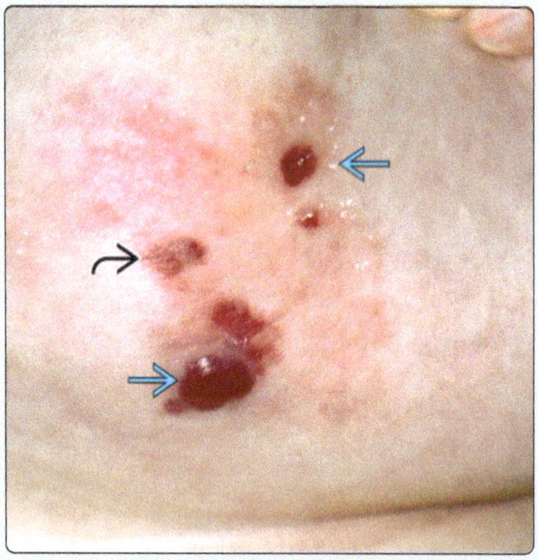

Atypical Vascular Lesion in Superficial Dermis

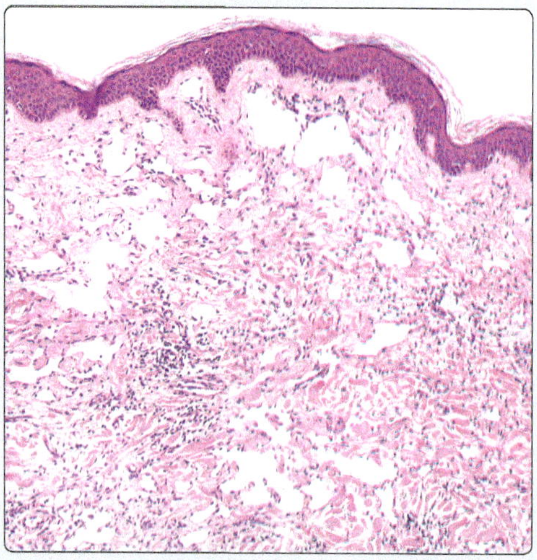

(Left) *An atypical vascular lesion (AVL) typically presents as small papules ➡ and patches ➡ in radiated skin at a median time of 3 years post radiotherapy. The breast or chest wall are most common sites. The lesions can be solitary or multiple.* **(Right)** *Low-magnification view shows a superficially located, lymphangioma-like vascular lesion composed of dilated vascular structures lined by cytologically bland endothelial cells.*

Higher Magnification of Superficial Atypical Vascular Lesion

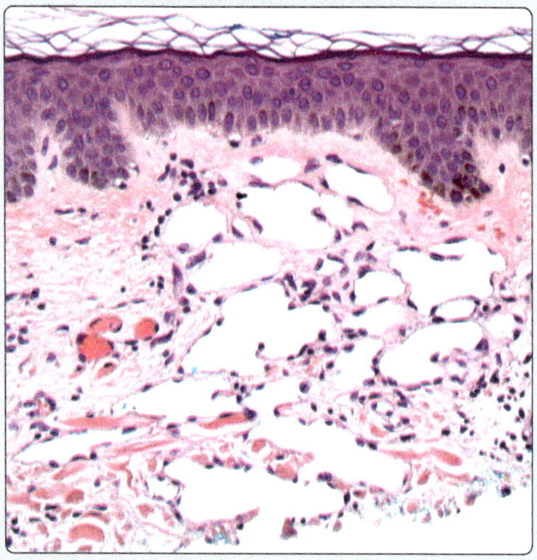

Dissecting Growth Pattern Is Typically Present

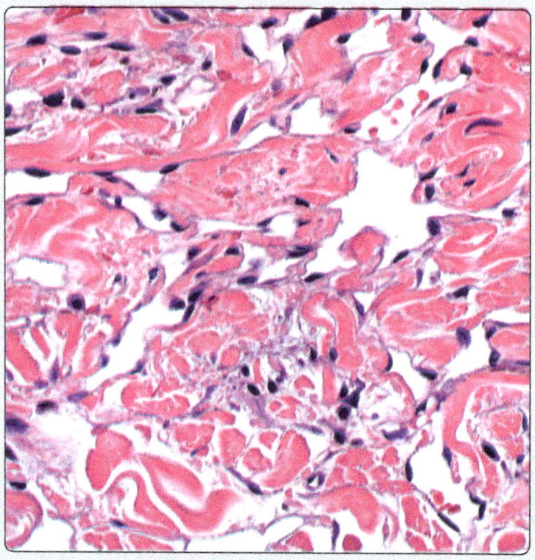

(Left) *Higher magnification of this superficial dermal AVL shows a proliferation of dilated vascular channels lined by small, relatively bland-appearing endothelial cells.* **(Right)** *AVLs often have a dissecting growth pattern consisting of jagged, anastomosing channels that infiltrate dermal collagen; a pattern that mimics well-differentiated angiosarcoma. Unlike angiosarcoma, however, there is no significant nuclear atypia, no multilayering of cells, and rarely any mitotic activity.*

TERMINOLOGY

Abbreviations

- Atypical vascular lesion (AVL)

Synonyms

- Atypical vascular proliferation

Definitions

- Benign cutaneous vascular lesion presenting as small papule or patch in radiated skin, composed of thin-walled lymphatic vessels, usually limited to dermis

ETIOLOGY/PATHOGENESIS

Environmental Exposure

- Radiation (40-60 Gy)
- Median latency: 3 years post radiotherapy

CLINICAL ISSUES

Epidemiology

- Incidence
  - Exact incidence unknown
- Age
  - Wide age range; median in late 50s
  - Usually 1 decade earlier than radiation-associated cutaneous angiosarcoma

Site

- Skin of breast or chest wall most common site, following radiotherapy for breast cancer
- Less frequent in radiation fields associated with gynecological and other malignancies

Presentation

- Small, flesh-colored papule or erythematous patch
- Solitary or multiple

Treatment

- Complete excision of all lesions recommended

Prognosis

- Most lesions pursue benign course
- New lesions frequently appear
- Few reports of transformation to angiosarcoma
  - Usually following multiple recurrences

MICROSCOPIC

Histologic Features

- Dermal-based, small, symmetrical, often wedge-shaped vascular proliferation
- Usually confined to superficial dermis
  - Rarely extends into subcutis
- Thin-walled lymphatic-type vessels
- Dilated or jagged, anastomosing vascular structures
- Dissects preexisting dermal collagen
- Single layer of slightly enlarged endothelial cells
- Lacks endothelial multilayering and significant cytologic atypia in most cases
- Mitoses rarely present

DIFFERENTIAL DIAGNOSIS

Well-Differentiated Angiosarcoma

- Clinical: Large, erythematous plaque (median: 7 cm)
- Anastomosing and infiltrating vascular structures
- Endothelial multilayering and nuclear atypia
- Mitotic figures often present
- Often show *MYC* amplification by FISH or immunohistochemistry

Hobnail Hemangioma

- Solitary papule or nodule
- Biphasic pattern (dilated superficial vessels; narrow deep vessels)
- Hobnail endothelial cells
- Stromal fibrosis, hemosiderin deposits

Lymphangioma Circumscriptum

- Clinically, groups of small vesicles containing clear fluid
- Small and superficially located lesion
- Large, ectatic lymphatic channels
- Represents developmental malformation (infants, adults)
- Similar lesion seen in radiated skin

Progressive Lymphangioma (Benign Lymphangioendothelioma)

- Presents clinically as large, slowly increasing, pink to red-brown plaque
- Infiltrating, dissecting lymphatic channels
- Lymphatics orientated horizontally in dermis
- Similar lesion seen in radiated skin

DIAGNOSTIC CHECKLIST

Clinically Relevant Pathologic Features

- Symptom time frame
- Gross appearance

SELECTED REFERENCES

1. Fraga-Guedes C et al: Angiosarcoma and atypical vascular lesions of the breast: diagnostic and prognostic role of MYC gene amplification and protein expression. Breast Cancer Res Treat. 151(1):131-40, 2015
2. Fernandez AP et al: FISH for MYC amplification and anti-MYC immunohistochemistry: useful diagnostic tools in the assessment of secondary angiosarcoma and atypical vascular proliferations. J Cutan Pathol. 39(2):234-42, 2012
3. Manner J et al: MYC high level gene amplification is a distinctive feature of angiosarcomas after irradiation or chronic lymphedema. Am J Pathol. 176(1):34-9, 2010
4. Lucas DR: Angiosarcoma, radiation-associated angiosarcoma, and atypical vascular lesion. Arch Pathol Lab Med. 133(11):1804-9, 2009
5. Patton KT et al: Atypical vascular lesions after surgery and radiation of the breast: a clinicopathologic study of 32 cases analyzing histologic heterogeneity and association with angiosarcoma. Am J Surg Pathol. 32(6):943-50, 2008
6. Gengler C et al: Vascular proliferations of the skin after radiation therapy for breast cancer: clinicopathologic analysis of a series in favor of a benign process: a study from the French Sarcoma Group. Cancer. 109(8):1584-98, 2007
7. Brenn T et al: Radiation-associated cutaneous atypical vascular lesions and angiosarcoma: clinicopathologic analysis of 42 cases. Am J Surg Pathol. 29(8):983-96, 2005
8. Requena L et al: Benign vascular proliferations in irradiated skin. Am J Surg Pathol. 26(3):328-37, 2002
9. Fineberg S et al: Cutaneous angiosarcoma and atypical vascular lesions of the skin and breast after radiation therapy for breast carcinoma. Am J Clin Pathol. 102(6):757-63, 1994

Angiosarcoma

KEY FACTS

TERMINOLOGY

- Malignant neoplasm showing morphologic &/or immunophenotypic evidence of vascular/endothelial differentiation

ETIOLOGY/PATHOGENESIS

- Subsets associated with prior radiotherapy, chronic lymphedema, exposure to certain chemicals, certain syndromes

CLINICAL ISSUES

- Wide age range overall (more common in adults)
- Various clinical features depending upon subset
  - Cutaneous scalp/face in elderly, cutaneous breast with history of radiotherapy or chronic lymphedema, parenchymal breast in young women
  - Deep soft tissue forms most common in lower extremity
- Treatment: Aggressive surgical resection with widely negative margins
- Poor prognosis (overall survival rate: 30%)
  - Epithelioid angiosarcoma is often more aggressive

MICROSCOPIC

- Infiltrative tumors
  - Dissecting growth of fat and collagen characteristic
- Histologic appearance depends upon degree of vasoformation
- Lesional endothelial cells show variable nuclear atypia; often multilayering
- Morphologic variant: Epithelioid angiosarcoma

ANCILLARY TESTS

- CD31(+), CD34(+), ERG(+), FLI-1(+)
- Keratin (+) in significant subset of epithelioid angiosarcoma

TOP DIFFERENTIAL DIAGNOSES

- Hemangioma
- Atypical vascular lesion
- Metastatic carcinoma

(Left) *Angiosarcoma is an aggressive vascular malignancy that occurs most commonly in adults. It is most common in cutaneous sites (particularly the scalp and face), but can also involve the breast, deep soft tissues, bone, and visceral organs.* **(Right)** *The lesion is composed of atypical, infiltrative vessels with hyperchromatic endothelial cell nuclei ⇒. Stromal inflammatory cells may be seen in angiosarcoma, particularly in cutaneous forms. When extensive, they may obscure the underlying neoplasm.*

Scanning Magnification of Primary Cutaneous Angiosarcoma

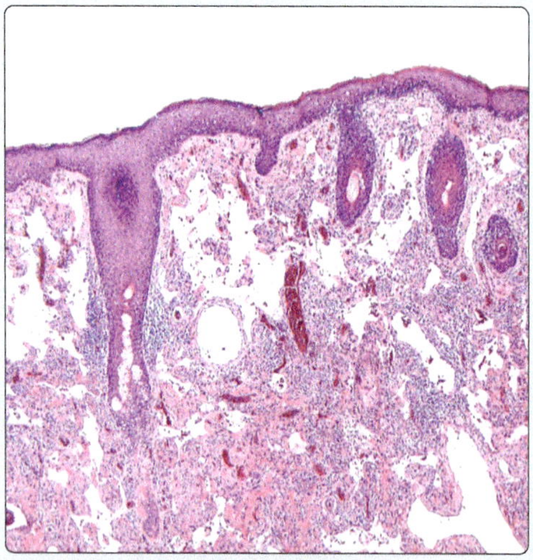

High Magnification of Atypical Vascular Channels With Inflammation

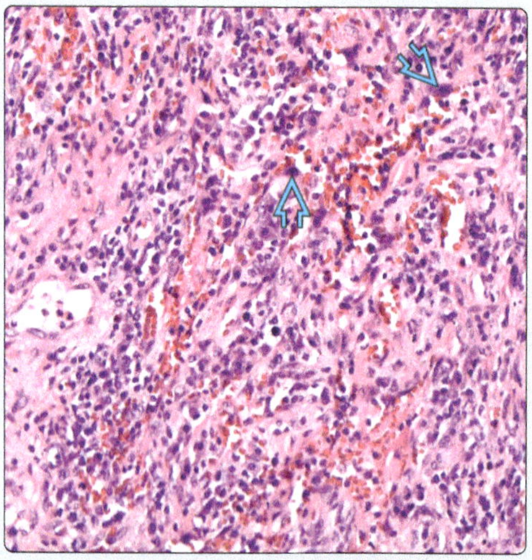

(Left) *Epithelioid angiosarcoma may mimic a variety of epithelioid neoplasms, including carcinoma, melanoma, and epithelioid sarcoma. Immunohistochemistry is often necessary to confirm the diagnosis in such cases.* **(Right)** *FLI-1 immunohistochemical stain shows strong nuclear expression in most cases of angiosarcoma.*

Epithelioid Angiosarcoma With Marked Atypia

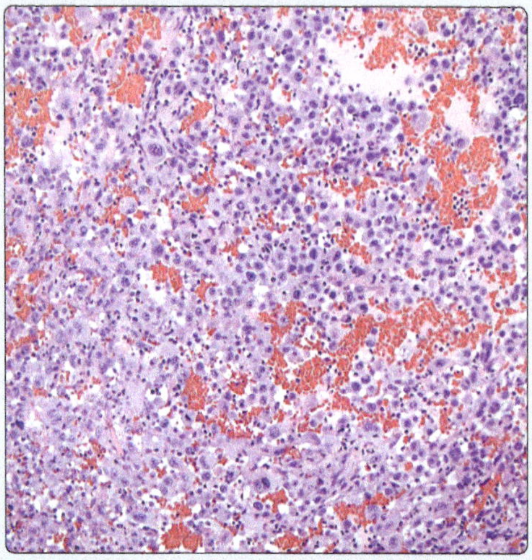

Nuclear FLI-1 Expression in Angiosarcoma

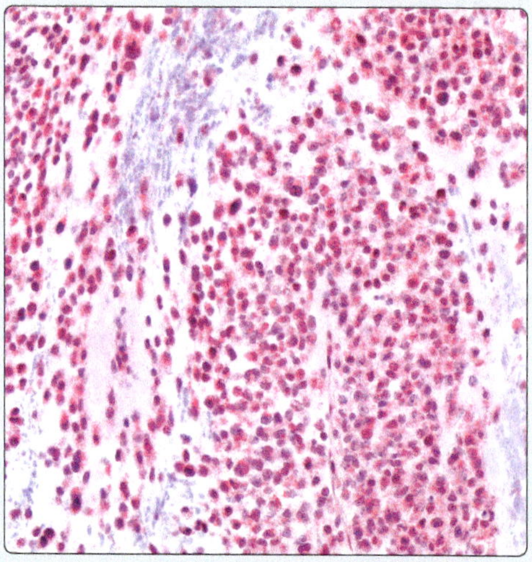

TERMINOLOGY

Synonyms

- Hemangiosarcoma
- Malignant hemangioendothelioma

Definitions

- Malignant neoplasm showing morphologic &/or immunophenotypic evidence of vascular/endothelial differentiation
- Many clinicopathologic subsets (cutaneous, deep soft tissue, radiation- or lymphedema-associated, breast parenchymal, others)

ETIOLOGY/PATHOGENESIS

Developmental Anomaly

- Develops rarely in association with genetic syndromes
  - Klippel-Trenaunay, Maffucci syndrome, neurofibromatosis
  - Often deep soft tissue angiosarcoma

Environmental Exposure

- Associated with exposure to radiation or certain chemicals (e.g., polyvinyl chloride)
- Can arise within setting of chronic lymphedema
- Rarely develops adjacent to foreign material or synthetic vascular grafts

Tumor Associations

- May rarely arise in benign nerve sheath tumors, malignant nerve sheath tumors, germ cell tumors, others

CLINICAL ISSUES

Epidemiology

- Incidence
  - Rare (< 1-2% of all sarcomas)
    - Cutaneous angiosarcoma is more common than other forms
- Age
  - Wide age range overall
    - Cutaneous: 60-80 years most common
    - Breast parenchymal: 30-40 years most common
  - Rare in childhood
- Sex
  - Male predominance in nonbreast cutaneous and deep soft tissue
  - Female predominance in breast (cutaneous and parenchymal)

Site

- Most common site overall is scalp and face (cutaneous type)
  - Superficial cutaneous tumors may also arise elsewhere, including breast and lower extremity
- Deep soft tissue tumors are most common in deep muscles of lower extremity
  - Also retroperitoneum, abdominal cavity, mesentery
- Also arises in breast parenchyma, spleen, liver, heart, bone, other viscera

Presentation

- Cutaneous
  - Dark red or purple nodules, plaques, or bruise-like areas
  - May be multifocal
- Breast
  - May be cutaneous or parenchymal
    - Cutaneous
      - Macroscopically similar to other cutaneous forms
      - Often history of irradiation to breast or chest wall area (short latency, usually < 7 years)
      - Occurrence in setting of postsurgical lymphedema (Stewart-Treves syndrome)
    - Parenchymal
      - Solitary or multiple breast masses
      - May show purple discoloration of overlying skin
- Deep soft tissue
  - Slow-growing, often large, painful mass
  - Hematologic abnormalities (e.g., coagulopathy) in up to 1/3 of cases
  - May also arise within field of previous irradiation

Treatment

- Aggressive surgical resection with widely negative margins
- Chemotherapy

Prognosis

- Overall poor prognosis (overall survival rate: 30%) for all forms
  - Local recurrences and distant metastases common
    - Cutaneous disease is often more extensive than clinically/macroscopically apparent
    - Metastases to lung, brain, bone, soft tissue sites, others
  - High mortality rate
- In general, prognosis unrelated to histologic grade
  - Possible exception: Breast parenchymal tumors
- Adverse prognostic factors for deep soft tissue cases: Older age, larger size, high proliferation rate, retroperitoneal origin
- Tumors with prominent epithelioid morphology (epithelioid angiosarcoma) are often more clinically aggressive than conventional forms

MACROSCOPIC

General Features

- Poorly demarcated or nodular
- Red, brown hemorrhagic cut surface

Size

- Highly variable, but often large

MICROSCOPIC

Histologic Features

- Often highly infiltrative, poorly circumscribed tumor
  - Poorly differentiated areas are often more nodular and better demarcated
- Apparent multifocality within same tissue section is common
- Morphologic appearance depends upon degree of vasoformation
  - Formation of irregular, anastomosing vascular channels in well-differentiated areas

- Vessels characteristically appear to "dissect" through collagen, fat, and other soft tissues
  - May entrap fragments of collagen and form intraluminal papillary structures
- Endothelial cell lining may show multilayering or intraluminal tufting
  - Nuclear atypia varies, but hyperchromasia, enlargement, and irregularity often present
  - Mitotic activity variable, often conspicuous
  - Intracytoplasmic lumina may be present focally
- Back-to-back vascular channels may appear sieve-like
- Solid growth in more poorly differentiated areas
  - Cells may be spindled, epithelioid, or pleomorphic
- Intraluminal erythrocytes and hemorrhage common
- Stromal lymphoid infiltrate may be present (particularly cutaneous forms)
- Pericytes usually absent
- Rare findings: Solid spindle cell, granular, inflammatory morphologies

Morphologic Variants

- Epithelioid angiosarcoma
  - More frequent in deep soft tissues
  - Predominantly large epithelioid cells in nests and sheets
    - Abundant eosinophilic cytoplasm
    - Large vesicular nuclei with prominent macronucleoli
  - Irregular vascular spaces lined by protuberant epithelioid cells may also be seen
  - Mitoses often numerous
  - Necrosis common

ANCILLARY TESTS

Immunohistochemistry

- Endothelial differentiation
  - CD31(+), CD34(+), ERG(+), FLI-1(+)
    - Multistain panel recommended, as sensitivity varies
  - Variable D2-40 (podoplanin)
- Keratin (+) in significant subset of epithelioid angiosarcoma
- Negative for SMA, desmin, HHV8
- Retention of nuclear INI1 expression

Molecular Genetics

- High-level *MYC* (8q24) amplification in radiation/lymphedema-associated (secondary) tumors
- *FLT4* (*VEGFR3*) (5q35) amplification in 25% of secondary tumors

DIFFERENTIAL DIAGNOSIS

Hemangioma

- Well-defined lobular architecture
  - No peripheral infiltrative or dissecting growth
- Well-formed vascular channels lined by bland endothelial cells
  - No endothelial multilayering and tufting

Atypical Vascular Lesion

- Distinction from angiosarcoma can be challenging on small biopsy
- Small, solitary, or multiple lesion(s) in previously irradiated skin
  - Small size (median 0.5 cm) of atypical vascular lesion is helpful feature
- Histologically resemble lymphangioma
  - Rare cases appear as lobular capillary proliferations (vascular type)
- Usually no multilayering or significant nuclear atypia

Kaposi Sarcoma

- Predominantly spindled cellular morphology
- Vasoformation generally less developed than in angiosarcoma
- Characteristically HHV8(+)

Atypical Fibroxanthoma

- Usually smaller, more superficial lesions
- Variety of morphology patterns
  - Lacks vasoformation
- Negative for CD31, CD34, ERG expression
  - CD31 stains histiocytes

Epithelioid Sarcoma (Proximal Type)

- Can resemble epithelioid angiosarcoma
- Diffuse keratin(+); CD34(+) in 50% of cases
- May express ERG
- Negative for CD31
- Loss of nuclear INI1 expression

Metastatic Carcinoma

- Can resemble epithelioid angiosarcoma
- Lacks vasoformation
- Diffuse keratin (+)
  - Often focal and less impressive in epithelioid angiosarcoma
- Negative for CD31, CD34

Metastatic Melanoma

- Can resemble epithelioid angiosarcoma
- Lacks vasoformation
- S100(+), CD31(-), CD34(-)
- Expression of melanocytic markers

SELECTED REFERENCES

1. Patel SH et al: Angiosarcoma of the scalp and face: the Mayo Clinic experience. JAMA Otolaryngol Head Neck Surg. 141(4):335-4, 2015
2. Ginter PS et al: Diagnostic utility of MYC amplification and anti-MYC immunohistochemistry in atypical vascular lesions, primary or radiation-induced mammary angiosarcomas, and primary angiosarcomas of other sites. Hum Pathol. 45(4):709-16, 2014
3. Deyrup AT et al: Pediatric cutaneous angiosarcomas: a clinicopathologic study of 10 cases. Am J Surg Pathol. 35(1):70-5, 2011
4. Guo T et al: Consistent MYC and FLT4 gene amplification in radiation-induced angiosarcoma but not in other radiation-associated atypical vascular lesions. Genes Chromosomes Cancer. 50(1):25-33, 2011
5. Suchak R et al: Primary cutaneous epithelioid angiosarcoma: a clinicopathologic study of 13 cases of a rare neoplasm occurring outside the setting of conventional angiosarcomas and with predilection for the limbs. Am J Surg Pathol. 35(1):60-9, 2011
6. Lucas DR: Angiosarcoma, radiation-associated angiosarcoma, and atypical vascular lesion. Arch Pathol Lab Med. 133(11):1804-9, 2009
7. Nascimento AF et al: Primary angiosarcoma of the breast: clinicopathologic analysis of 49 cases, suggesting that grade is not prognostic. Am J Surg Pathol. 32(12):1896-904, 2008
8. Fayette J et al: Angiosarcomas, a heterogeneous group of sarcomas with specific behavior depending on primary site: a retrospective study of 161 cases. Ann Oncol. 18(12):2030-6, 2007
9. Meis-Kindblom JM et al: Angiosarcoma of soft tissue: a study of 80 cases. Am J Surg Pathol. 22(6):683-97, 1998

Variable Degrees of Vasoformation in Angiosarcoma

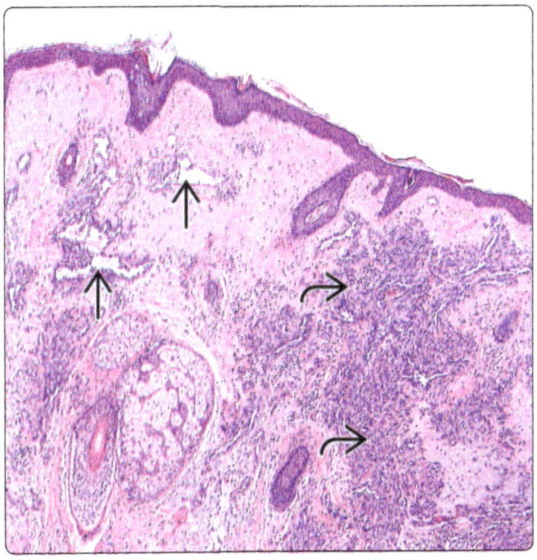

Angiosarcoma With Very Focal/Subtle Cutaneous Involvement

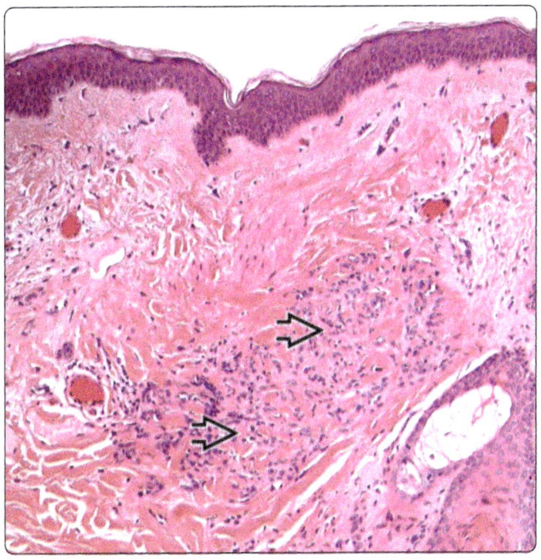

(Left) *Depending upon the degree of vasoformation in a given case, some areas of angiosarcoma may appear more clearly vascular (with luminal spaces →), and others may appear more solid/less well differentiated ↪.* **(Right)** *Conspicuous vascular lumina are not present in all areas of angiosarcoma, and identification of subtle tumor foci ⇨ can be challenging. This appearance can be problematic when evaluating margins by frozen section at the time of surgery.*

Infiltrating, Dissecting Growth is Common

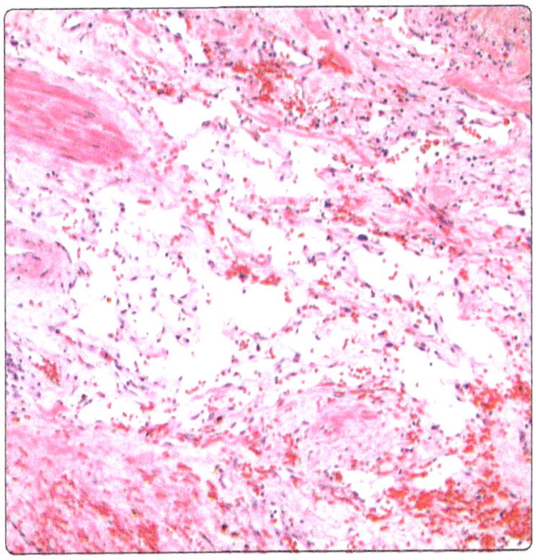

Nuclear Atypia Can be Subtle in Angiosarcoma

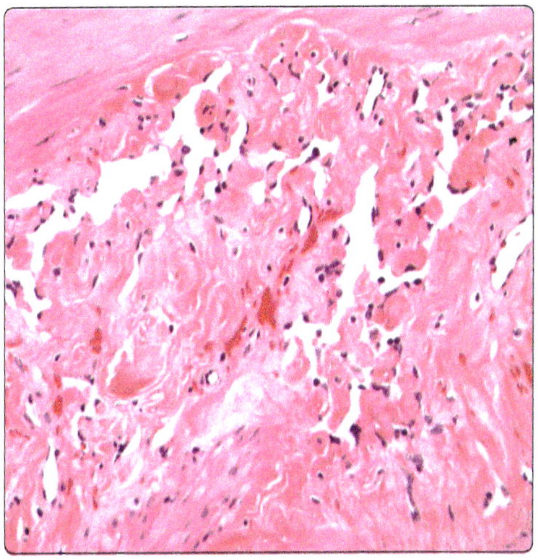

(Left) *Infiltrative and dissecting growth through collagenous connective tissue by irregularly shaped and anastomosing vascular channels is a characteristic feature of angiosarcoma. The depth and extent of infiltration can be striking.* **(Right)** *In well-differentiated areas of angiosarcoma, the lesional endothelial cells may show very little atypia; however, the irregular and dissecting growth pattern can help establish the diagnosis.*

Angiosarcoma With Variable Infiltration of Adipose Tissue

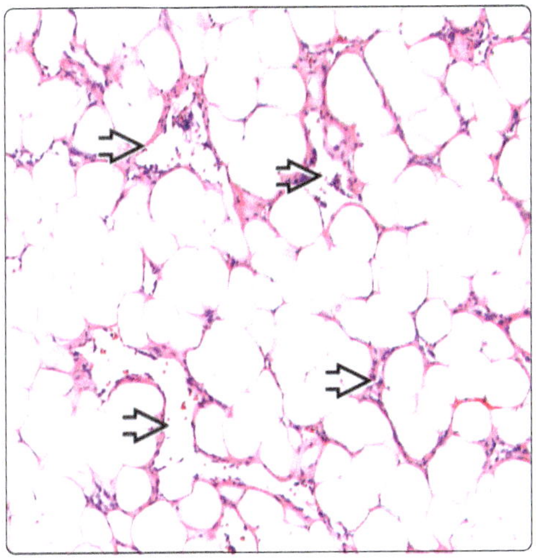

Prominent Fat Infiltration in Angiosarcoma

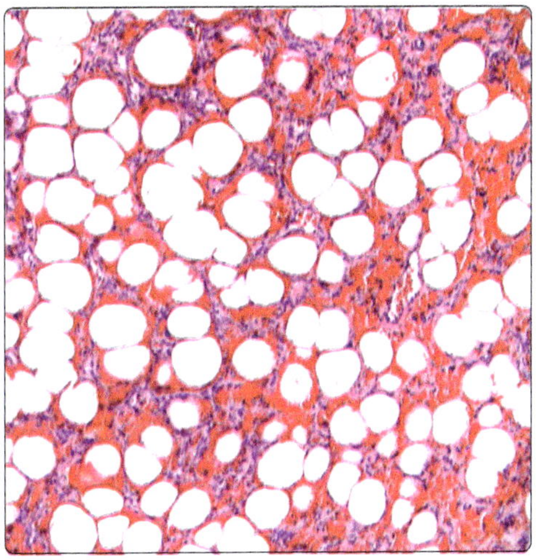

(Left) *Angiosarcoma can infiltrate normal subcutaneous adipose tissue, and may show extensive or subtle involvement. Note the irregular, infiltrating vascular channels ⇨.* **(Right)** *This case of angiosarcoma shows a highly infiltrative tumor in the adipose tissue, with extensive hemorrhage, somewhat obscuring the malignant tumor cells.*

Prominent Nuclear Atypia in Angiosarcoma

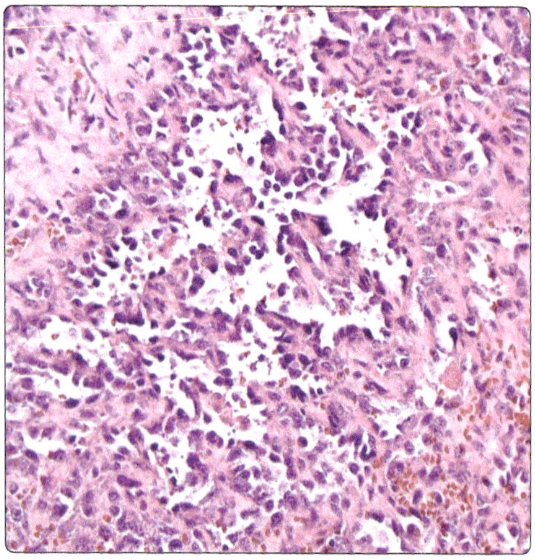

Marked Nuclear Pleomorphism in Angiosarcoma

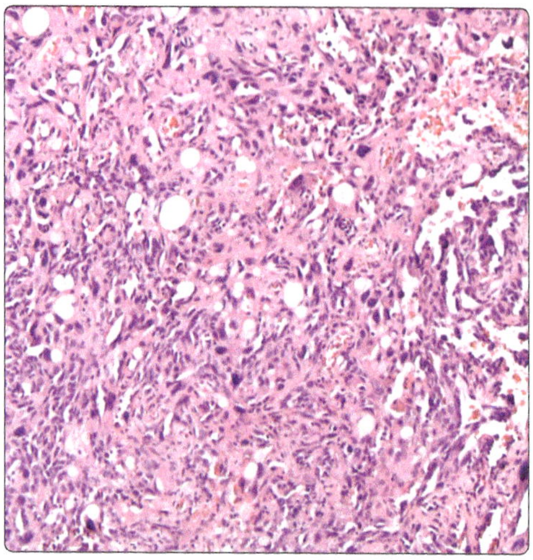

(Left) *In some cases of angiosarcoma, the lesional endothelial cells show a much greater degree of nuclear enlargement and hyperchromasia.* **(Right)** *In occasional cases, there is marked nuclear pleomorphism in angiosarcoma. This may lead to consideration of other malignant entities in solid areas in a small biopsy.*

Degree of Vasoformation Varies in Angiosarcoma

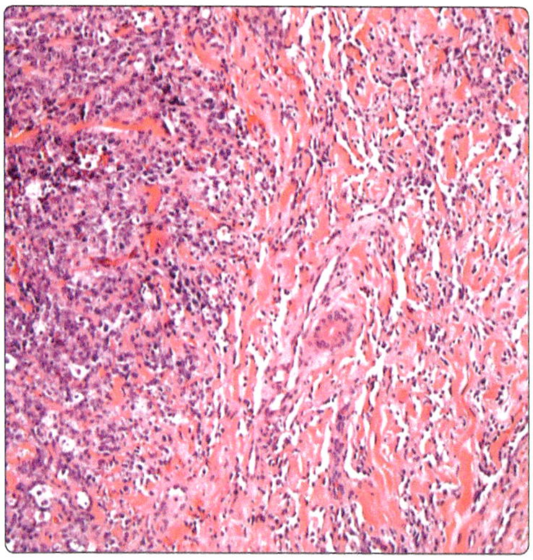

Solid Growth in Poorly Differentiated Areas of Angiosarcoma

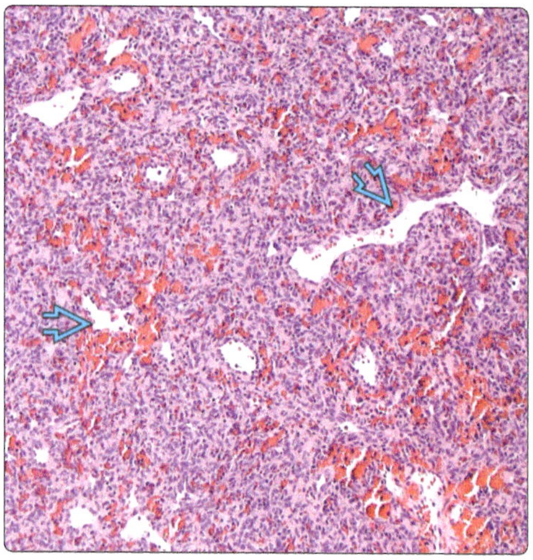

(Left) *A variable degree of vasoformation is a common occurrence in angiosarcoma. Note the more well-differentiated vasoformative areas (right) and less-differentiated, more solid areas (left).* **(Right)** *Poorly differentiated areas of angiosarcoma often show a greater degree of solid growth; however, vasoformation ➡ is still evident, at least focally.*

Occasional Sieve-Like Pattern in Angiosarcoma

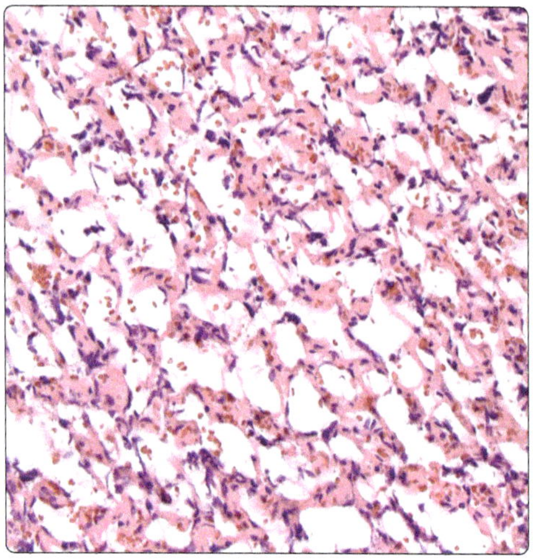

Angiosarcoma With Extensive Hemorrhage

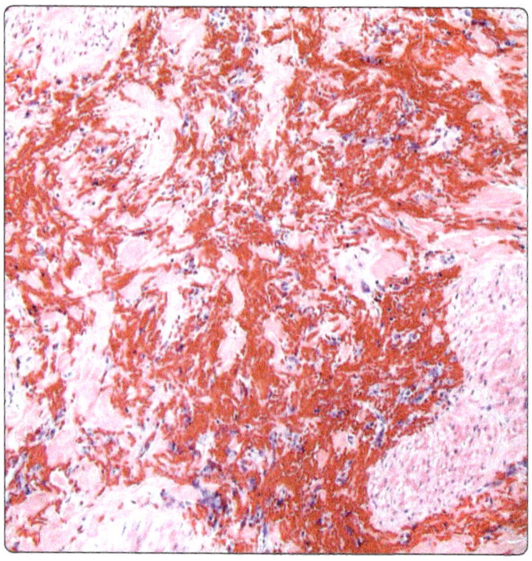

(Left) *A sieve-like or lattice-like growth pattern may be seen in some areas of angiosarcoma. These back-to-back channels may also contain abundant erythrocytes.* **(Right)** *Hemorrhage is not uncommon in angiosarcoma and may be prominent in some cases. It can occasionally be so extensive that the neoplastic cells are obscured and underrecognized.*

Papillary-Like Structures Are Common in Angiosarcoma

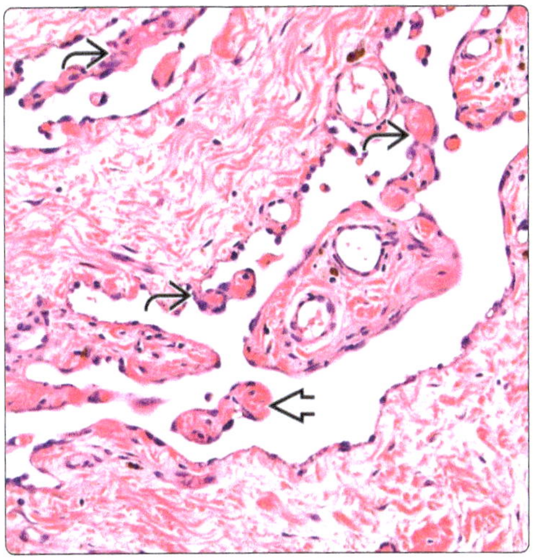

Papillary Structures May Resemble Papillary Endothelial Hyperplasia

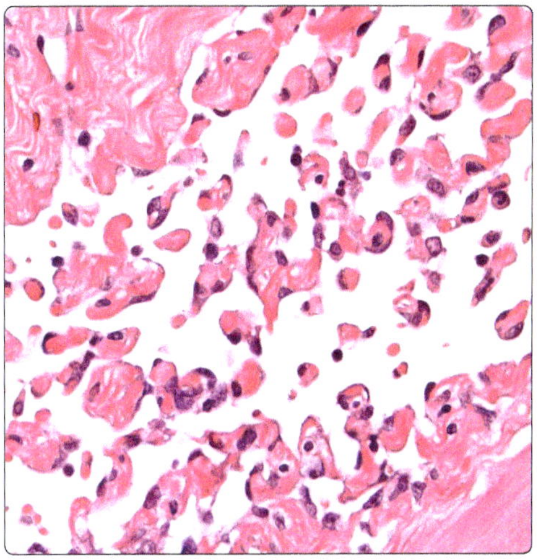

(Left) *A frequent finding in angiosarcoma is variably sized papillary-like structures ➩ composed of collagen lined by lesional endothelial cells. These structures can also appear to float freely ➩ within the open vascular spaces.* **(Right)** *In some areas, the papillary-like structures may be abundant and resemble papillary endothelial hyperplasia (Masson tumor/change).*

Spindled Morphology in Angiosarcoma

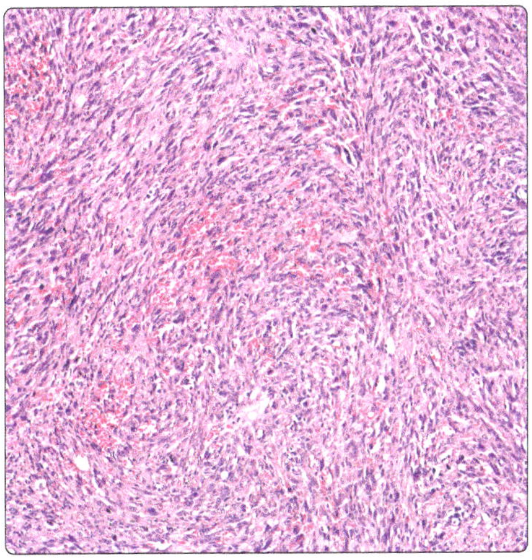

Epithelioid Angiosarcoma

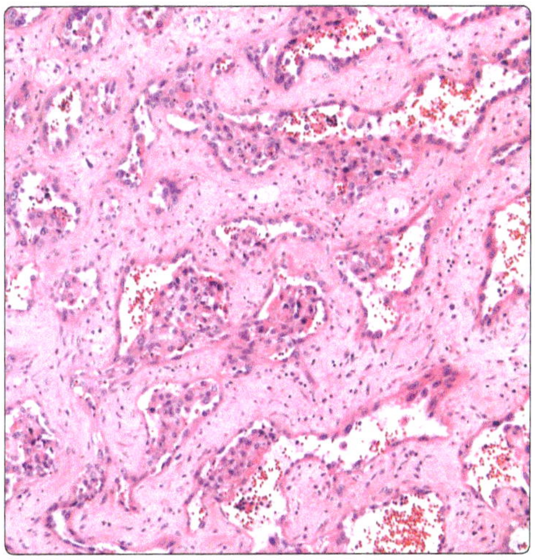

(Left) *A solid, cellular tumor with spindled morphology may be seen in some poorly differentiated areas of angiosarcoma. It can also be the dominant pattern in rare tumors.* **(Right)** *The lesional endothelial cells of angiosarcoma may show an epithelioid morphology in some cases, rarely is it a predominant feature of the tumor. In the latter scenario, the term epithelioid angiosarcoma is often utilized.*

Prominent Nucleoli in Epithelioid Angiosarcoma

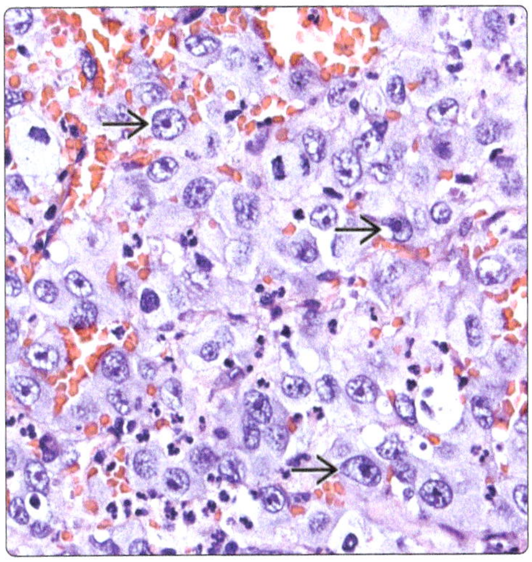

CD31 Expression in Angiosarcoma

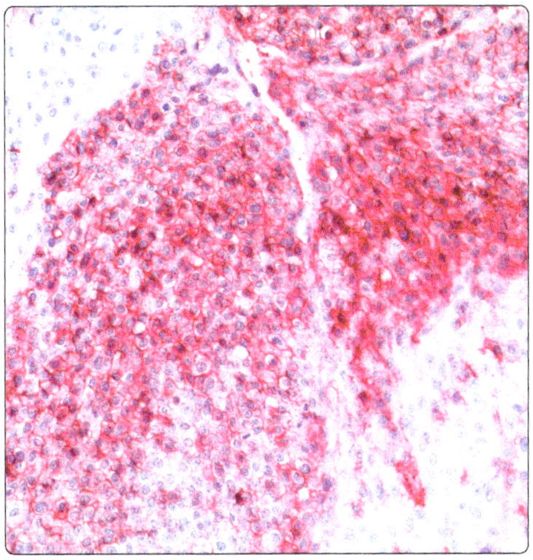

(Left) *A characteristic finding in epithelioid angiosarcoma is the presence of enlarged vesicular nuclei with prominent macronucleoli ➞.* **(Right)** *This image shows relatively strong expression of CD31 in the atypical epithelioid tumor cells in epithelioid angiosarcoma.*

PART I
SECTION 9

Tumors and Tumor-Like Conditions With Neural, Nerve Sheath, and Neuroendocrine Differentiation

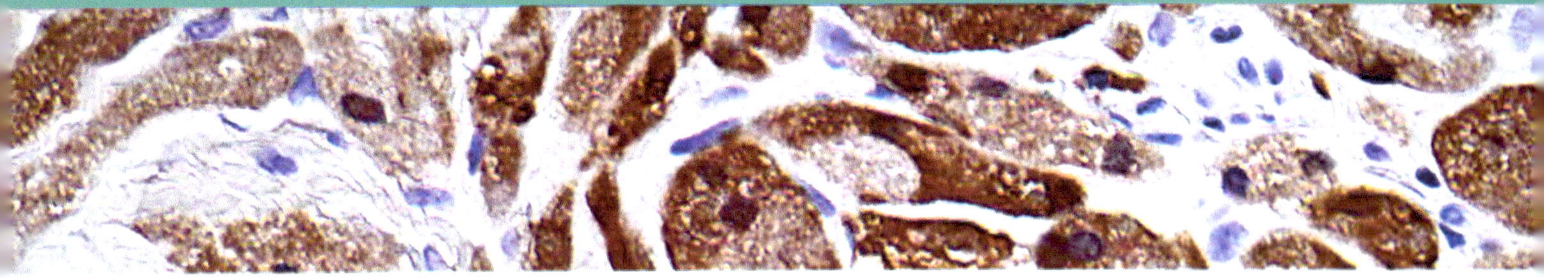

Neuromas

KEY FACTS

TERMINOLOGY

- Proliferation of peripheral nerve fibers in which ratio of axons to Schwann cell fascicles is close to 1:1
  - Solitary circumscribed neuroma ("palisaded encapsulated neuroma") represents spontaneous proliferation of peripheral nerve fibers
  - Multiple mucosal neuromas associated with multiple endocrine neoplasia syndrome (type 2B) represents rare autosomal dominant condition
  - Traumatic neuroma represents posttraumatic proliferation of peripheral nerve fibers
  - Morton neuroma represents degenerative neural change with reactive fibrosis on foot
  - Pacinian neuroma represents painful hyperplasia of Pacinian bodies on finger
  - Epithelial sheath neuroma represents proliferation of enlarged dermal nerves ensheathed by squamous epithelium

CLINICAL ISSUES

- Solitary circumscribed neuroma most common on face
- Morton neuroma occurs in distal parts of peripheral nerves of 3rd and 4th metatarsals

MICROSCOPIC

- Spindled Schwann cells &/or peripheral nerve fibers
- Clefts in solitary circumscribed neuroma
- Perineural fibrosis in traumatic neuroma
- No cytologic atypia

ANCILLARY TESTS

- Strong S100(+) in Schwann cells and nerve fibers
- Negative for SMA, desmin, melanocytic markers

TOP DIFFERENTIAL DIAGNOSES

- Benign nerve sheath tumors
- Superficial (pilar) leiomyoma
- Dermatofibroma

Solitary Circumscribed Neuroma

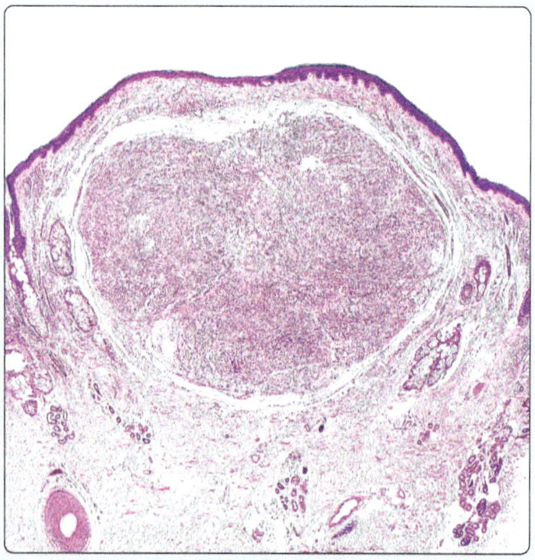

PEN With Characteristic Clefts

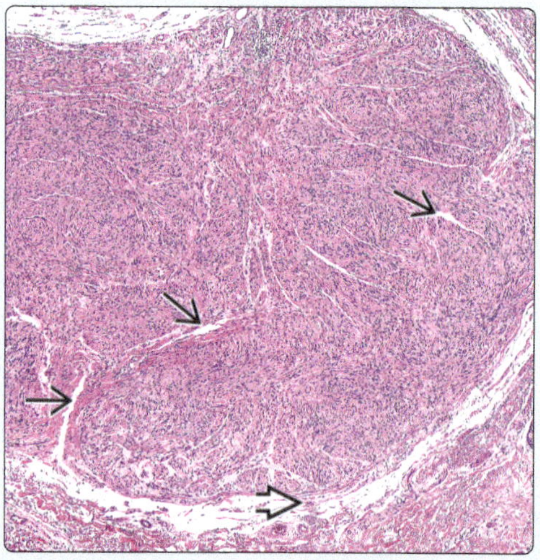

(Left) *Solitary circumscribed neuroma ["palisaded encapsulated neuroma" (PEN)] represents a well-circumscribed, partially encapsulated, dermal-based neural neoplasm. Note the absence of overlying epidermal hyperplasia.* **(Right)** *Solitary circumscribed neuroma is a circumscribed, sometimes partly encapsulated dermal lesion composed of Schwann cells and associated axons. Characteristic clefts ⇨ and a small, preexisting nerve at the base of the lesion ⇨ can be seen.*

Bland Spindled Schwann Cells in PEN

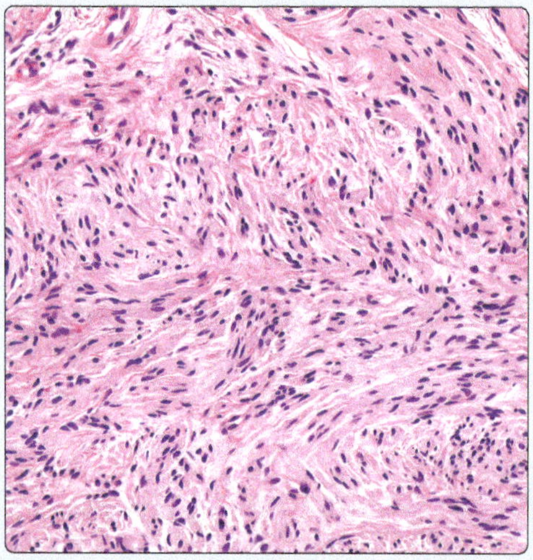

PEN Tumor Cells Positive for S100

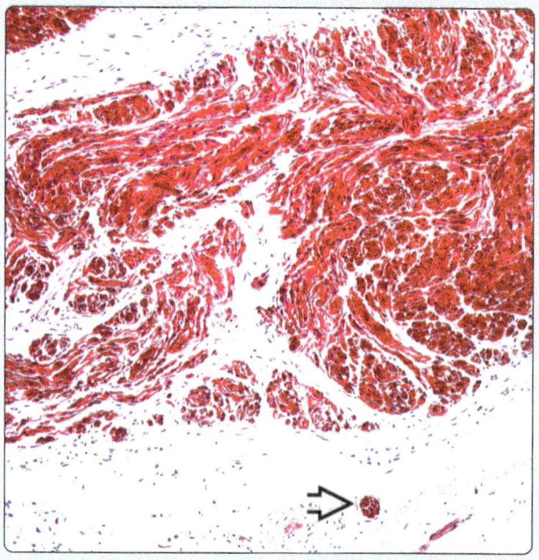

(Left) *The neoplastic Schwann cells contain ill-defined, pale, eosinophilic cytoplasm and cytologically bland spindled nuclei with evenly distributed chromatin. No prominent cytologic atypia and no increased mitoses are present.* **(Right)** *Solitary circumscribed neuroma is composed mainly of S100-positive Schwann cells. Preexisting peripheral nerves ⇨ can often be seen at the base of these lesions.*

TERMINOLOGY

Definitions

- Proliferation of peripheral nerve fibers in which ratio of axons to Schwann cell fascicles is in nearly equal proportions
  - Solitary circumscribed neuroma ["palisaded encapsulated neuroma" (PEN)] is spontaneous proliferation of peripheral nerve fibers
  - Multiple mucosal neuromas associated with multiple endocrine neoplasia (MEN) syndrome (type 2B), rare autosomal dominant condition
  - Traumatic neuroma represents posttraumatic proliferation of peripheral nerve fibers
  - Morton neuroma is due to degenerative neural changes with reactive fibrosis on foot
  - Pacinian neuroma represents painful hyperplasia of pacinian bodies on finger
  - Epithelial sheath neuroma is proliferation of nerves ensheathed by squamous epithelium

ETIOLOGY/PATHOGENESIS

Developmental Anomaly

- Multiple mucosal neuromas in MEN 2B syndrome
  - Represents rare autosomal dominant condition
  - Also includes medullary carcinoma of thyroid, pheochromocytoma, and somatic abnormalities
  - Mucosal neuromas have been rarely reported without any other systemic features of syndrome

Environmental Exposure

- Traumatic neuroma
  - Amputation neuroma is painful, reactive proliferation of nerve fibers after amputation
  - Proliferation of nonencapsulated nerve fibers after intrauterine or perinatal amputation of supernumerary digits
  - Can occur on penis after circumcision
- Morton neuroma
  - Degenerative damage of peripheral nerves

CLINICAL ISSUES

Epidemiology

- Age
  - Solitary circumscribed neuroma most common in 5th and 7th decades
- Sex
  - Solitary circumscribed neuroma occurs in equal ratio in both genders

Site

- Solitary circumscribed neuroma
  - Majority (90%) located on face
  - Rare in other anatomic locations
  - Mucosal involvement has been reported rarely
- Mucosal neuroma
  - Lips, tongue, eyelids
  - Upper GI tract
- Morton neuroma
  - Sole of foot
  - Usually in distal parts of peripheral nerves of 3rd and 4th metatarsals
- Pacinian neuroma
  - Usually on fingers
- Epithelial sheath neuroma
  - Usually on back
  - In superficial dermis

Presentation

- Painful or painless mass
  - Traumatic neuroma typically painful
- Slow growing

Treatment

- Simple excision is curative

Prognosis

- Biologically benign

MACROSCOPIC

General Features

- Raised dermal, papular, or nodular lesions

MICROSCOPIC

Histologic Features

- Solitary circumscribed neuroma PEN
  - Single dermal nodule
  - Multinodular &/or plexiform growth are very uncommon
  - Well-developed fascicles of Schwann cells
  - Numerous associated axons
  - Characteristic clefts present
  - Superficial part is rather loosely arranged
  - Capsule-like fibroblasts and perineurial cells are seen in deeper parts
  - Small nerves can grow into lesion from below
  - Epithelioid cytomorphology is seen very rarely
  - Vascular variant has been reported rarely
- Multiple mucosal neuromas associated with MEN syndrome
  - Morphology resembles that of solitary circumscribed neuroma
- Traumatic neuroma
  - Irregular arrangement of proliferating nerve fascicles embedded in fibrous scar tissue
  - Perineural fibrosis
  - Perineurial cells surround each small nerve fascicle
- Morton neuroma
  - Enlargement of plantar digital nerves
  - Edema of nerve
  - Perineural fibrosis
- Pacinian neuroma
  - Hyperplasia of Pacinian bodies
- Epithelial sheath neuroma
  - Large hyperplastic peripheral nerves in upper parts of dermis
  - Nerve fibers are surrounded by mature squamous epithelium
  - Associated fibroplasia and scattered inflammatory cells
  - Can simulate appearance of epithelial tumor invading nerve

Cytologic Features

- Elongated, spindled Schwann cells
- Ill-defined, pale eosinophilic cytoplasm
- Bland, elongated fusiform nuclei
- No cytologic atypia

ANCILLARY TESTS

Immunohistochemistry

- Strong S100(+) in Schwann cells and nerve fibers
- Neurofilament protein (NFP) highlights axons
- EMA(+) perineurial cells
- Epithelial structures in epithelial sheath neuroma are keratin (+)
- Negative for SMA, desmin, melanocytic markers

DIFFERENTIAL DIAGNOSIS

Schwannoma

- Encapsulated neoplasm composed almost exclusively of Schwann cells
- Antoni A (hypocellular) and Antoni B (hypercellular) growth patterns
- Usually no NFP(+) axons
- Hyalinized blood vessels common

Neurofibroma

- Often poorly circumscribed dermal-based lesions
- Typically shows myxoid stroma and mast cells
- No proliferation of peripheral nerve fibers

Perineurioma

- Composed of EMA(+) perineurial cells
- Spindled tumor cells with elongated nuclei and long, thin cytoplasmic processes
- No S100(+) Schwann cells
- No NFP(+) axons

Superficial (Pilar) Leiomyoma

- Ill-defined dermal neoplasms
- Composed of spindled eosinophilic tumor cells
- Negative for S100
- SMA(+), MSA(+), desmin (+)

Dermatofibroma

- Ill-defined dermal spindle cell lesion
- Admixed lymphocytes, foamy histiocytes common
- Negative for CD34 and S100

Dermatomyofibroma

- Plaque-like dermal lesion similar to dermatofibroma, but with myofibroblastic differentiation
- Composed of spindled myofibroblasts
- SMA(+); negative for S100

Dermal Melanocytic Nevus

- Epithelioid-appearing nevus cells, usually present in nests
- Often at least focal presence of melanin pigment superficially
- Expression of melanocytic antigens HMB-45, MART-1/Melan-A

Sclerotic Fibroma (Storiform Collagenoma)

- Collagenous stroma with lamellar clefts
- CD34(+); negative for S100

Dermatofibrosarcoma Protuberans

- Characteristic storiform growth pattern
- Diffuse infiltrative growth into subcutaneous fat
- CD34(+) spindled cells
- Negative for S100

Superficial (Acral) Fibromyxoma

- Fascicles of spindled tumor cells
- Collagenous and myxoid stroma
- Negative for S100
- Often focal expression of EMA &/or CD34

DIAGNOSTIC CHECKLIST

Clinically Relevant Pathologic Features

- Multiple mucosal neuromas associated with MEN syndrome

Pathologic Interpretation Pearls

- Proliferation of peripheral nerve fibers with relatively equal number of axons and Schwann cell fascicles

SELECTED REFERENCES

1. Vandergriff TW et al: Multifocal epithelial sheath neuroma. Am J Dermatopathol. 37(2):176-7, 2015
2. Salcedo E et al: Traumatic neuromas of the penis: a clinical, histopathological and immunohistochemical study of 17 cases. J Cutan Pathol. 36(2):229-33, 2009
3. Misago N et al: Unusual benign myxoid nerve sheath lesion: myxoid palisaded encapsulated neuroma (PEN) or nerve sheath myxoma with PEN/PEN-like features? Am J Dermatopathol. 29(2):160-4, 2007
4. Lin TY et al: Epithelial sheath neuroma: a case report and discussion of the literature. Am J Dermatopathol. 28(3):216-9, 2006
5. Lombardi T et al: [Solitary circumscribed neuroma (palisaded encapsulated neuroma) of the oral mucosa.] Ann Dermatol Venereol. 129(2):229-32, 2002
6. Dubovy SR et al: Palisaded encapsulated neuroma (solitary circumscribed neuroma of skin) of the eyelid: report of two cases and review of the literature. Br J Ophthalmol. 85(8):949-51, 2001
7. Navarro M et al: Palisaded encapsulated neuroma (solitary circumscribed neuroma) of the glans penis. Br J Dermatol. 142(5):1061-2, 2000
8. Requena L et al: Epithelial sheath neuroma: a new entity. Am J Surg Pathol. 24(2):190-6, 2000
9. Magnusson B: Palisaded encapsulated neuroma (solitary circumscribed neuroma) of the oral mucosa. Oral Surg Oral Med Oral Pathol Oral Radiol Endod. 82(3):302-4, 1996
10. Bennett GL et al: Morton's interdigital neuroma: a comprehensive treatment protocol. Foot Ankle Int. 16(12):760-3, 1995
11. Megahed M: Palisaded encapsulated neuroma (solitary circumscribed neuroma). A clinicopathologic and immunohistochemical study. Am J Dermatopathol. 16(2):120-5, 1994
12. Argenyi ZB et al: Plexiform and other unusual variants of palisaded encapsulated neuroma. J Cutan Pathol. 20(1):34-9, 1993
13. Argenyi ZB et al: Vascular variant of palisaded encapsulated neuroma. J Cutan Pathol. 20(1):92-3, 1993
14. Dakin MC et al: The palisaded, encapsulated neuroma (solitary circumscribed neuroma). Histopathology. 20(5):405-10, 1992
15. Tsang WY et al: Epithelioid variant of solitary circumscribed neuroma of the skin. Histopathology. 20(5):439-41, 1992
16. Butterworth DM et al: Solitary circumscribed neuroma of the skin. Histopathology. 19(6):577-9, 1991
17. Fletcher CD et al: Digital pacinian neuroma: a distinctive hyperplastic lesion. Histopathology. 15(3):249-56, 1989
18. Reed RJ et al: Palisaded, encapsulated neuromas of the skin. Arch Dermatol. 106(6):865-70, 1972

Traumatic Penile Neuroma

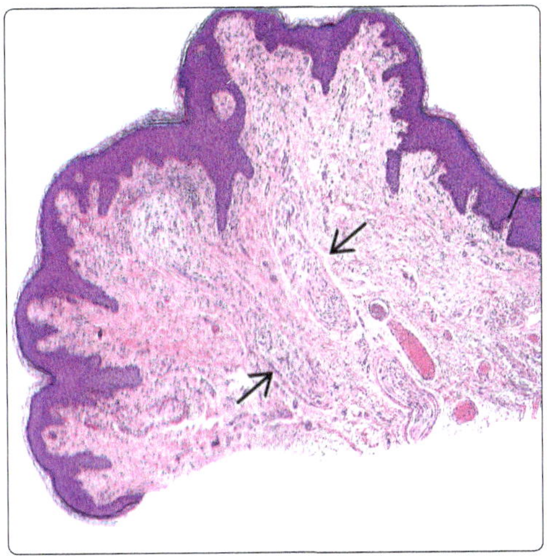

Nerve Fibers Surrounded by Fibrosis in Traumatic Neuroma

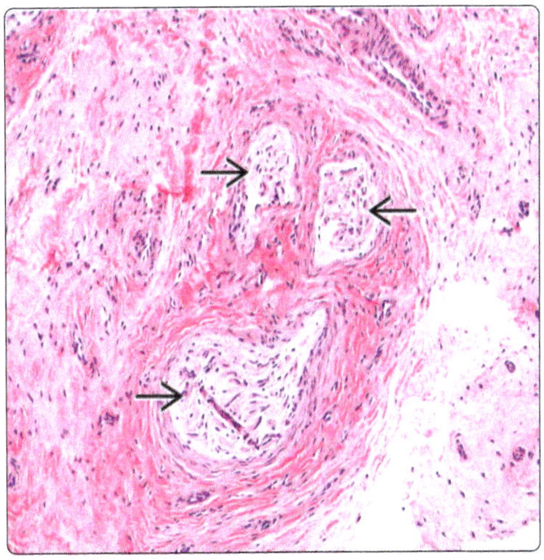

(Left) *Traumatic neuroma of the penis after circumcision has hyperplastic nerve fibers ⇒ with mild perineural fibrosis. This lesion can clinically mimic a condyloma, but the clinical history and the demonstration of excess nerves lead to the correct diagnosis.* **(Right)** *Nerve fibers ⇒ in traumatic neuroma are often separated from one another by abundant fibrous scar tissue.*

Fibrosis and Perineurial Cell Hyperplasia

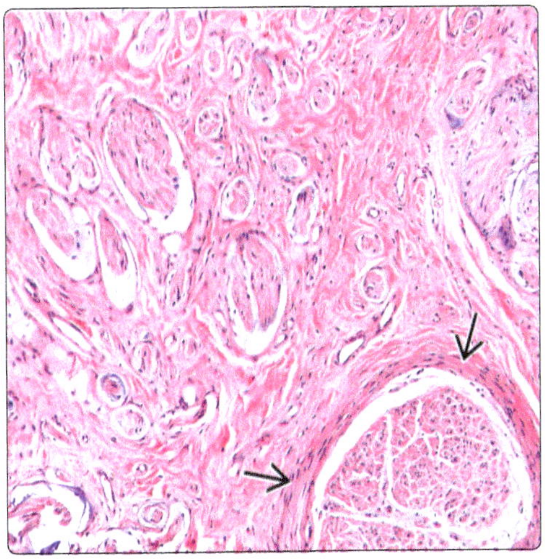

Epithelial Sheath Neuroma

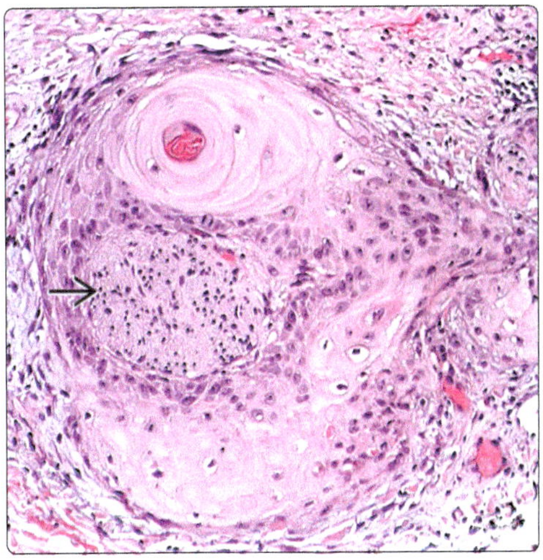

(Left) *A rim of hyperplastic perineurial cells ⇒ can often be identified around some of the nerve fibers in a traumatic neuroma. Note also the scattered small nerve fibers within abundant fibrosis in this image (top left).* **(Right)** *Epithelial sheath neuroma is a rare benign superficial dermal lesion. An enlarged nerve bundle ⇒ is surrounded by keratinizing squamous epithelium. (Courtesy C. Cockerell, MD and C. Etufugh, MD.)*

Pacinian Neuroma

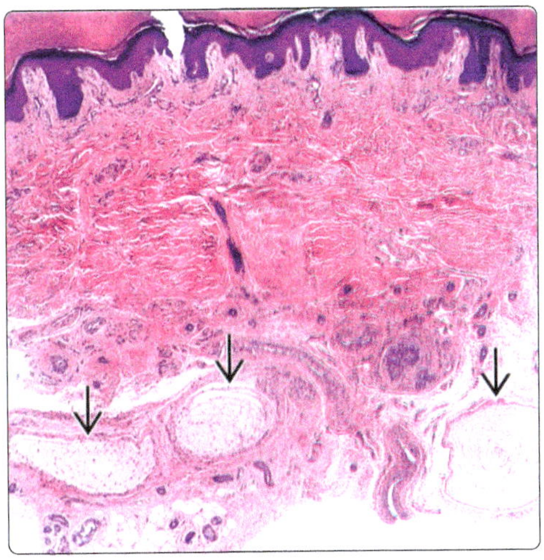

Perineurial Cells in Concentric Lamellae in Pacinian Neuroma

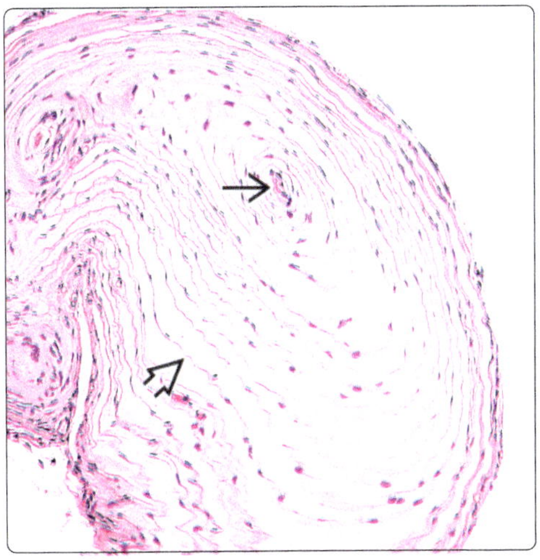

(Left) *Pacinian neuroma is comprised of round or oval nodules with multiple cell layers ⇒, resembling normal Pacinian corpuscles. This occurs mainly in the digits in subcutaneous tissue and can be painful. (Courtesy C. Cockerell, MD and C. Etufugh, MD.)* **(Right)** *The corpuscles comprise concentric lamellae ⇒ of perineurial cells with elongated, slender processes. These are immunoreactive for epithelial membrane antigen. In the center is an axon ⇒, which is positive for neurofilaments.*

KEY FACTS

TERMINOLOGY

- Benign peripheral nerve sheath tumor composed of Schwann cells, fibroblasts, perineurial-like cells, and residual nerve axons within extracellular matrix

CLINICAL ISSUES

- Most common peripheral nerve sheath tumor
  - 3 main types: Localized (cutaneous or intraneural), diffuse, and plexiform
    - Plexiform type is essentially pathognomonic for neurofibromatosis type 1 (NF1)
- Wide age range
  - Diffuse and plexiform types most common in young
- Most (90%) of neurofibromas are sporadic
- Benign; very rare local recurrence
- Malignant transformation usually occurs in setting of NF1 (up to 10% of patients)

MICROSCOPIC

- Loosely arranged spindle cells in haphazard arrangement
  - Small, hyperchromatic, wavy or buckled nuclei
  - Variable myxoid to collagenous matrix
- Diffuse type: Ill-defined, dermal and subcutaneous proliferation that entraps adnexa
  - Pseudomeissnerian bodies are characteristic
- Plexiform: Multinodular/serpentine growth pattern
- Malignant transformation: Combination of increased cellularity, nuclear atypia, mitotic activity, &/or necrosis

ANCILLARY TESTS

- Mixture of S100(+), CD34(+), and EMA(+) cells

TOP DIFFERENTIAL DIAGNOSES

- Malignant peripheral nerve sheath tumor
- Dermatofibrosarcoma protuberans
- Schwannoma
- Perineurioma

Neurofibroma Gross Image

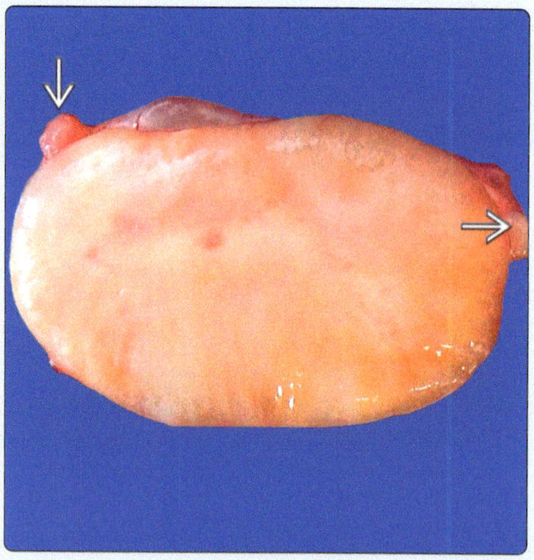

Localized Neurofibroma at Low Power

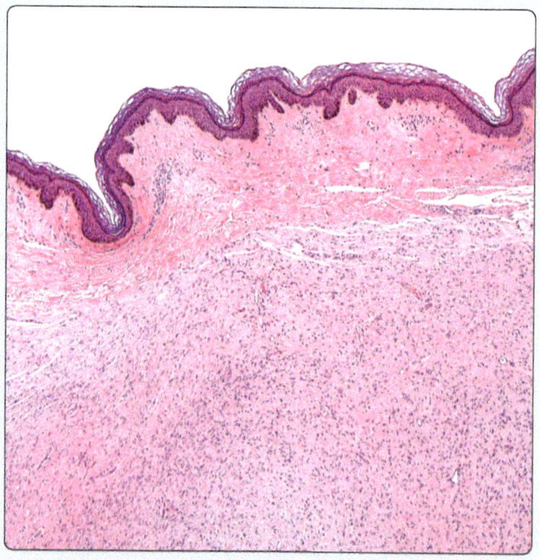

(Left) *Grossly, neurofibroma often appears as an ovoid or fusiform mass and usually shows a pale, wavy to gelatinous cut surface. The gross degenerative changes often seen in schwannomas are seldom present in neurofibroma. Note the transected nerve fibers ➔ at both ends of the mass.* **(Right)** *Localized cutaneous neurofibroma forms a well-circumscribed, but unencapsulated, dermal proliferation. This lesion may also occur in the nerve (intraneural localized neurofibroma).*

Small Elongated Spindle Cells in Neurofibroma

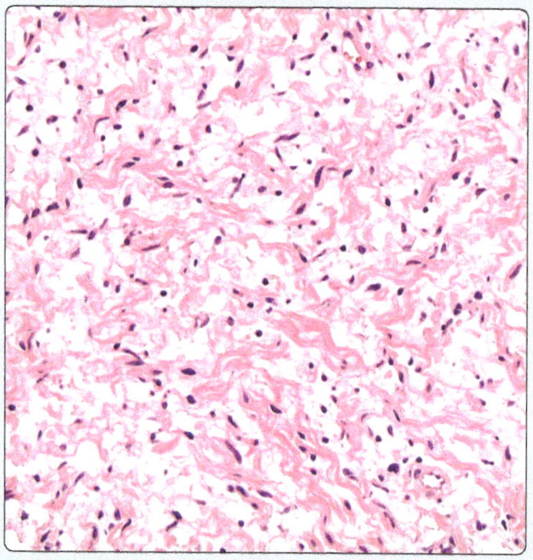

S100 Expression in Schwann Cells

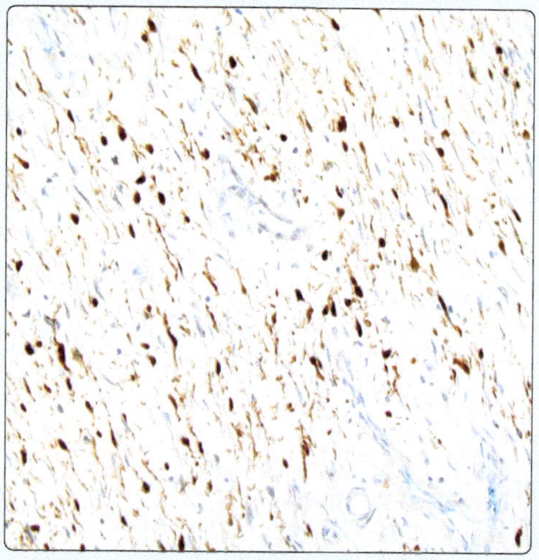

(Left) *All forms of neurofibroma are cytologically similar and are characterized by small, elongated, spindled cells in a variably collagenous background stroma. Rare tumors show epithelioid features (not shown).* **(Right)** *Consistent S100 expression is seen in all forms of neurofibroma; however, it is usually less impressive than that seen in schwannoma due to the lower overall cellularity and mixture of cell types in the former (e.g., fibroblasts, perineurial-like cells).*

TERMINOLOGY

Definitions

- Benign peripheral nerve sheath tumor composed of Schwann cells, fibroblasts, perineurial-like cells, and residual nerve axons within extracellular matrix
  - 3 major types: Localized (cutaneous or intraneural), diffuse, and plexiform
    - Plexiform neurofibroma is essentially pathognomonic of neurofibromatosis type 1 (NF1)

ETIOLOGY/PATHOGENESIS

Histogenesis

- Sporadic in ~ 90% of cases; others are syndromic in association with NF1
  - NF1 results from germline mutation in *NF1* gene on chromosome 17q11.2
    - *NF1* gene encodes for neurofibromin protein, which is GTPase-activating protein
  - Sporadic tumors arise from somatic mutations in *NF1*

CLINICAL ISSUES

Epidemiology

- Incidence
  - Most common peripheral nerve sheath tumor
    - Localized type most common among neurofibromas
- Age
  - Wide range (most common in young to middle-aged adults)
    - Plexiform and diffuse variants occur more often in younger age groups, including children
- Sex
  - M = F

Site

- Localized
  - Usually skin of trunk, head/neck, extremities
  - Less common in deeply situated nerves, nerve plexi, major nerve trunks, viscera
- Diffuse
  - Skin &/or subcutaneous tissue of head/neck
- Plexiform
  - Superficial or deep soft tissues, large nerve trunks
  - Head/neck, trunk, extremities

Presentation

- Most (90%) neurofibromas are sporadic and unassociated with NF1
- Usually slow-growing masses overall
  - Rapid growth in preexisting neurofibroma is worrisome for malignant transformation
- Localized
  - Usually small, sporadic, solitary mass
    - Deep lesions may be large
  - Rarely associated with NF1
    - Numerous localized neurofibromas; however, usually indicate NF1
  - Intraneural tumors present as fusiform swellings
    - Often cause sensory or motor disturbances related to affected nerve
- Diffuse type
  - Poorly defined, plaque-like growth, often large
  - 10% of cases associated with NF1
- Plexiform
  - Considered pathognomonic for NF1
    - Occurs in up to 40% of NF1 patients
  - Irregular, nodular mass with bag-of-worms appearance
  - Entire extremity may be involved (elephantiasis neuromatosa)
- Rare, massive soft tissue neurofibromas may result in large, pendulous folds of neurofibromatous tissue ("localized gigantism")

Treatment

- Complete surgical excision

Prognosis

- Benign
  - All forms (including atypical/bizarre neurofibroma)
- Local recurrence very rare
- Malignant transformation
  - Usually occurs in setting of NF1 (rare in sporadic tumors)
    - Seen in 5-10% of NF1 patients
  - Plexiform and localized intraneural types are most frequent precursors to malignant peripheral nerve sheath tumor (MPNST)
    - Essentially no risk for localized cutaneous type
    - Very low risk for diffuse type

MACROSCOPIC

General Features

- Most are well circumscribed or well demarcated
  - Diffuse type is ill defined, plaque-like, cutaneous growth
- Unencapsulated
- Gray-tan firm/fibrous to gelatinous cut surface
- Generally lack degenerative changes (hemorrhage, cystic change)

Size

- Wide range
  - Localized cutaneous types usually small (< 2 cm)
  - Diffuse type often large
  - Rare tumors may be massive

MICROSCOPIC

Histologic Features

- Localized type
  - Well-circumscribed, unencapsulated; grenz zone in skin
    - Intraneural tumors may have peripheral rim of perineurium or thickened epineurium
  - Usually low or moderate cellularity
  - Loosely arranged spindle cells in haphazard arrangement
    - Poorly defined cytoplasmic borders/processes
    - Small, hyperchromatic, wavy or buckled nuclei
    - Scattered nuclei may show degenerative changes (pleomorphic, hyperchromatic, "smudgy" nuclei)
      - Described as atypical (or bizarre) neurofibroma
  - Variable myxoid to collagenous matrix
    - Coarse collagen bundles often described as having shredded carrot appearance

- Mast cells are common
- Rarely contain small nerve twigs
- Many rare variants described: Cellular, epithelioid, granular cell, dendritic cell, others
- Diffuse type
  - Ill-defined, expansive dermal and subcutaneous proliferation
    - Proliferates around cutaneous adnexal structures, entrapping them
      - Entrapped nerve twigs are often hypertrophic or edematous
    - Extends into subcutaneous tissue along connective tissue septa and infiltrates fat
  - Loosely arranged spindle cells in haphazard arrangement
    - Small, hyperchromatic, wavy or buckled nuclei
    - Some cases have epithelioid cytomorphology, at least focally
  - Evenly distributed, fibrillar collagenous stroma
    - May be myxoid
  - Pseudomeissnerian bodies are characteristic
    - Individual or aggregates of whorled eosinophilic fibrillary clusters
    - Vary in number and distribution
  - Rare cases show scattered dendritic cells containing melanin pigment
- Plexiform
  - Defined by growth pattern
    - Multiple, irregularly arranged structures resembling hypertrophic nerve fascicles
      - Imparts mixed multinodular and serpentine appearance
      - Usually markedly myxoid or edematous with abundant collagen bundles
  - May also show areas indistinguishable from diffuse-type neurofibroma
  - May show scattered nuclear atypia (degenerative) without increased mitoses or necrosis
- Hybrid neurofibroma/schwannoma
  - Schwannoma-like nodules within otherwise typical neurofibroma
  - Identified in some patients with NF1, per recent reports
- Malignant transformation (MPNST)
  - Many cases are clear-cut, with increased cellularity, generalized nuclear pleomorphism and hyperchromasia, mitotic activity, &/or necrosis
    - Some cases are extremely challenging to prognosticate
      - No clear criteria currently exist to apply to all cases
  - Subtle/early low-grade transformation is generally heralded by combination of markedly increased cellularity and more than rare mitoses
    - Generalized nuclear atypia may or may not be present
  - Nuclear atypia in isolation (atypical/bizarre neurofibroma) does not qualify
  - Mitotic figures in isolation (rare) do not qualify

ANCILLARY TESTS

Immunohistochemistry

- S100(+) in ~ 50% of total cells (Schwann cells)
- CD34(+) admixed spindled fibroblasts
- EMA(+) admixed perineurial cells
- Neurofilament protein highlights intratumoral axons

DIFFERENTIAL DIAGNOSIS

Malignant Peripheral Nerve Sheath Tumor

- Usually large, deep tumors
- Variable combination of high cellularity with nuclear atypia, mitotic figures, &/or necrosis
- Perivascular tumor cell accentuation
- May contain peripheral component of preexisting neurofibroma

Dermatofibrosarcoma Protuberans

- Cellular, highly infiltrative tumor with honeycomb infiltration of subcutaneous fat
- Usually prominent storiform architecture
- Diffuse CD34(+), S100(-)

Schwannoma

- Biphasic, encapsulated tumor with Antoni A and Antoni B areas
- Verocay body formation, perivascular hyalinization
- Diffuse, uniform S100(+)
- Cellular plexiform schwannoma may be mistaken for MPNST arising in plexiform neurofibroma

Perineurioma

- Usually prominent storiform, whorling, or lamellar architecture
- EMA(+), claudin-1(+), GLUT1(+)
  - Expression is often more diffuse than in neurofibroma (focal, patchy)
- S100(-), CD34(+/-)

Ganglioneuroma

- Most common in posterior mediastinum and retroperitoneum
- Contains enlarged, irregularly scattered ganglion cells
- Predominant neural component may resemble neurofibroma

SELECTED REFERENCES

1. Thareja S et al: Glomus-like bodies within a neurofibroma: a novel neoplasm arising in neurofibromatosis type 1 or a coincidence? J Cutan Pathol. 42(4):285-8, 2015
2. Harder A et al: Hybrid neurofibroma/schwannoma is overrepresented among schwannomatosis and neurofibromatosis patients. Am J Surg Pathol. 36(5):702-9, 2012
3. Jokinen CH et al: Atypical neurofibroma of the skin and subcutaneous tissue: clinicopathologic analysis of 11 cases. J Cutan Pathol. 37(1):35-42, 2010
4. Magro G et al: Multinucleated floret-like giant cells in sporadic and NF1-associated neurofibromas: a clinicopathologic study of 94 cases. Virchows Arch. 456(1):71-6, 2010
5. Spurlock G et al: Molecular evolution of a neurofibroma to malignant peripheral nerve sheath tumor (MPNST) in an NF1 patient: correlation between histopathological, clinical and molecular findings. J Cancer Res Clin Oncol. 136(12):1869-80, 2010
6. Val-Bernal JF et al: Cutaneous lipomatous neurofibroma: characterization and frequency. J Cutan Pathol. 32(4):274-9, 2005
7. Fetsch JF et al: Pigmented (melanotic) neurofibroma: a clinicopathologic and immunohistochemical analysis of 19 lesions from 17 patients. Am J Surg Pathol. 24(3):331-43, 2000

Classic Neural Cytologic Features

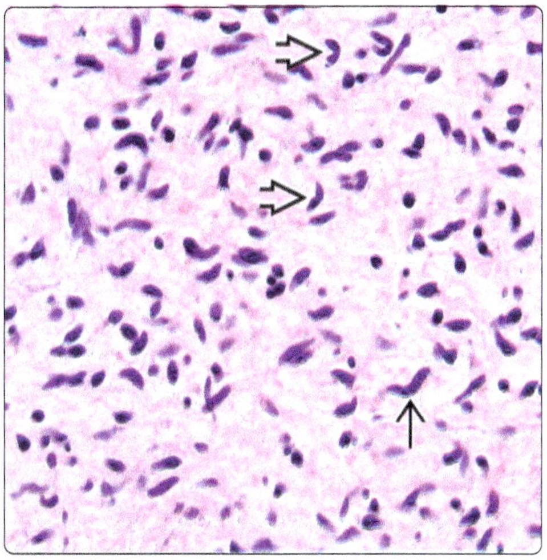

Mast Cells in Neurofibroma

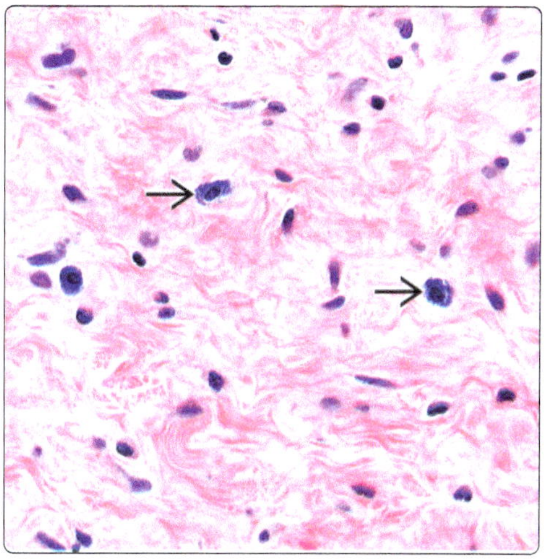

(Left) *The lesional Schwann cell nuclei of neurofibroma are generally elongated with pointed or tapered ends and often appear wavy → or buckled (comma-shaped ⇨). Mitotic activity is essentially nonexistent.* **(Right)** *Mast cells → are commonly identified in neurofibromas, particularly localized and diffuse forms. They may be sparse or relatively abundant.*

Low to Moderate Cellularity in Neurofibroma

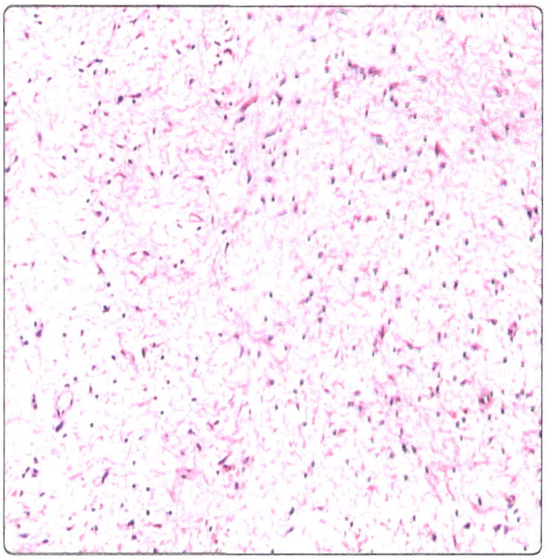

Myxoid Stromal Change in Neurofibroma

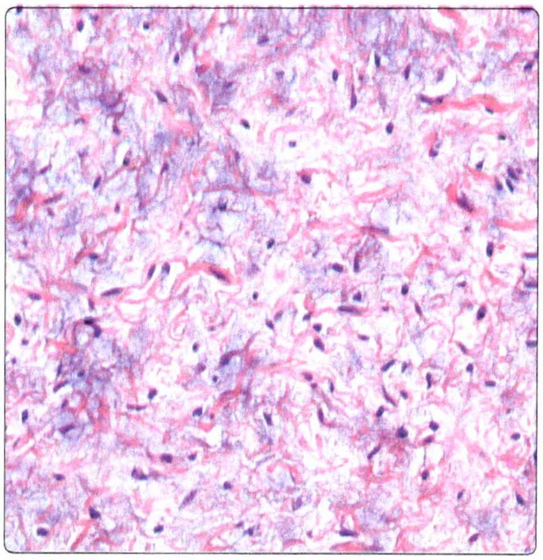

(Left) *Neurofibroma is generally a low to moderately cellular neoplasm. Some cases are heavily edematous (shown). Even at low power, the characteristic wavy nuclei are apparent.* **(Right)** *Myxoid stromal change is not uncommon in neurofibroma. Note the numerous separated pink collagen fibers, which somewhat resemble shredded carrots. Examples in which myxoid change is extensive may show morphologic overlap with myxoma or spindle cell lipoma.*

Rare, Multinucleated, Floret-Like Giant Cells

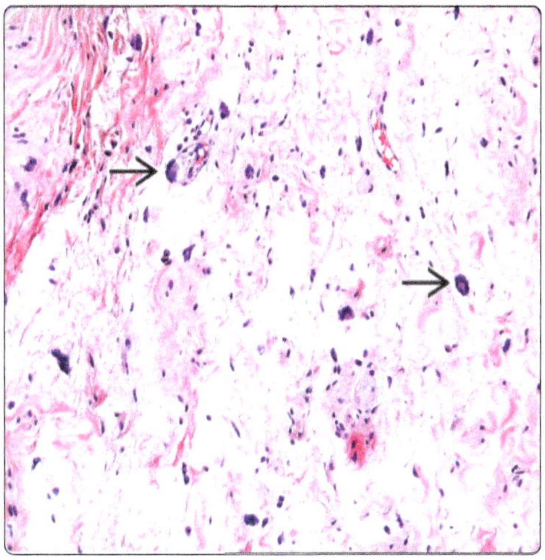

Rare Tumor With Increased Cellularity

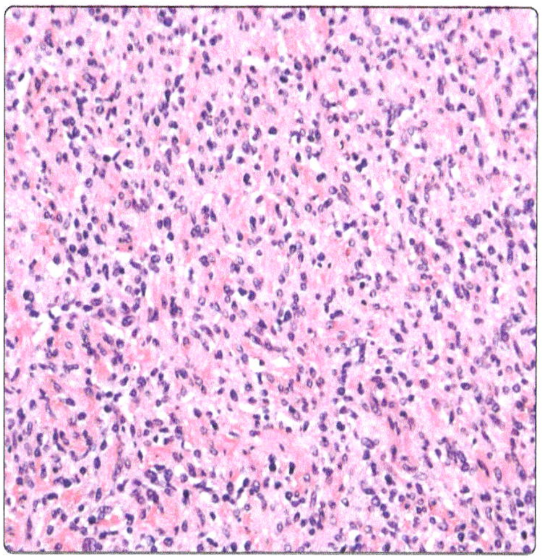

(Left) *Multinucleated, floret-like giant cells →, similar to those seen in pleomorphic lipoma, are occasionally encountered in neurofibroma. They are seen in both sporadic tumors and those associated with neurofibromatosis type 1 (NF1), and are typically CD34(+) and S100(-).* **(Right)** *Rare cases of neurofibroma show increased cellularity. Importantly, mitotic activity and high-grade cytologic atypia are absent.*

(Left) *Diffuse-type neurofibroma usually presents as an ill-defined, cutaneous plaque in the head and neck. It is characteristically highly infiltrative and grows around normal anatomic structures.* **(Right)** *Intralesional adipose tissue may rarely be identified within localized cutaneous neurofibroma; however, it is far more common in diffuse-type neurofibroma (due to peripheral infiltration of subcutaneous fat).*

Diffuse-Type Neurofibroma

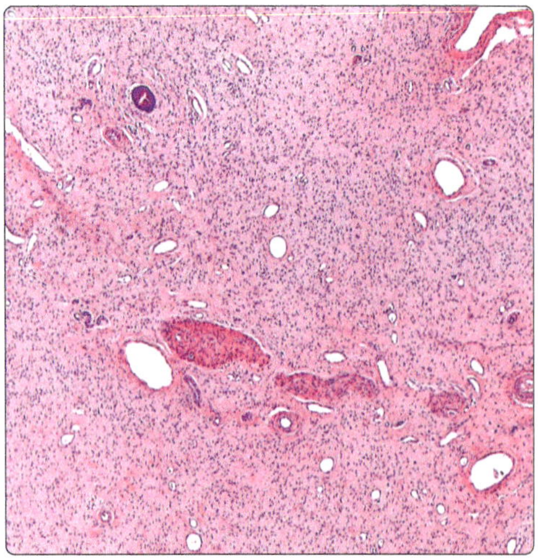

Intralesional Adipose Tissue

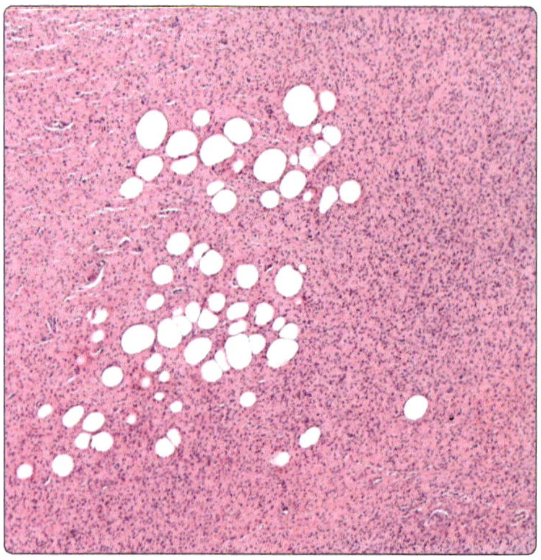

(Left) *The lesional tissue of diffuse-type neurofibroma characteristically grows around and entraps cutaneous adnexa, such as hair follicles and eccrine structures (shown). Note that there is no destruction of these normal structures.* **(Right)** *Infiltration of peripheral soft tissues, including fat and skeletal muscle, is commonly seen in diffuse-type neurofibroma.*

Entrapment of Cutaneous Adnexa in Diffuse Neurofibroma

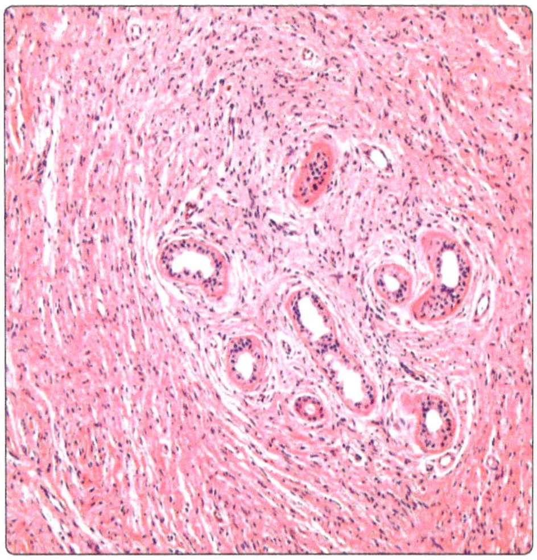

Infiltration of Fat and Muscle in Diffuse Neurofibroma

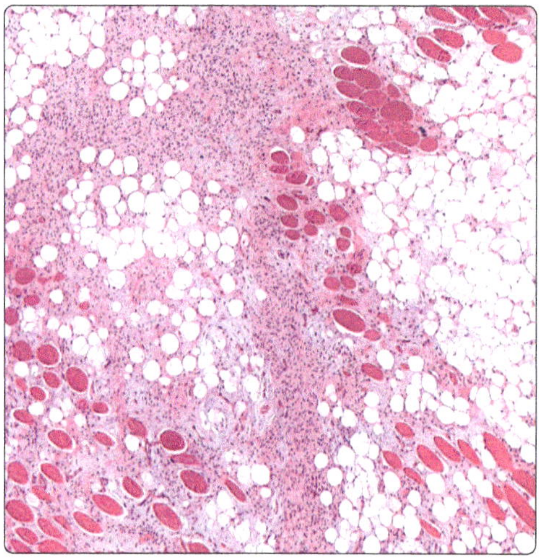

(Left) *Some cases of diffuse-type neurofibroma grow as thin rays ➡ of lesional tissue within abundant fat, resembling fibrous septa. This morphology can mimic lipofibromatosis or fibrolipoma.* **(Right)** *The nuclei of Schwann cells in diffuse-type neurofibroma are identical to those of other forms. Note the admixed non-Schwannian nuclei, which are larger ➡ and paler.*

Infiltration of Fat in Diffuse Neurofibroma

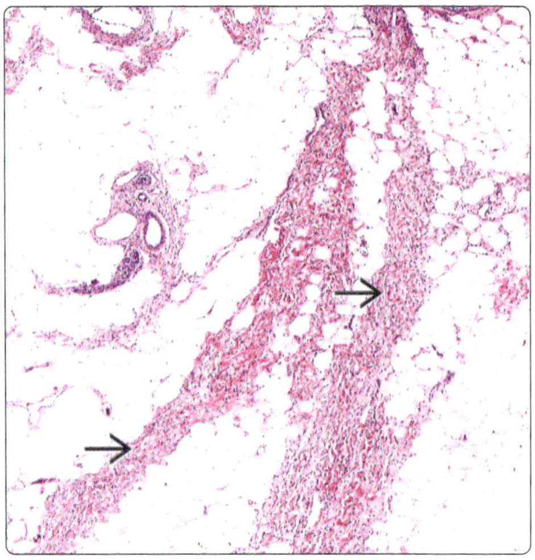

Diffuse-Type Neurofibroma Cytology

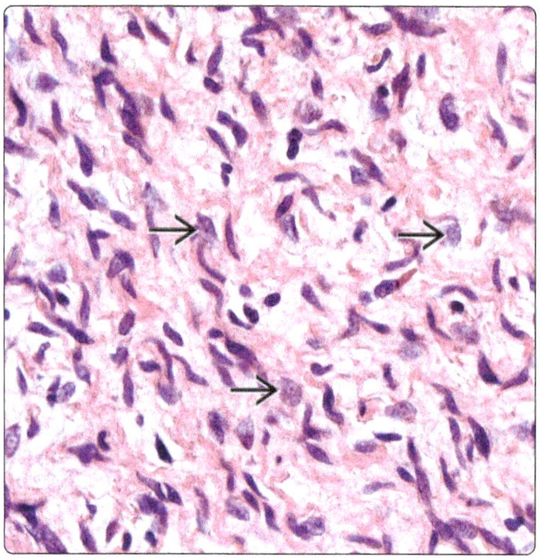

Rounded Nuclei in Diffuse Neurofibroma

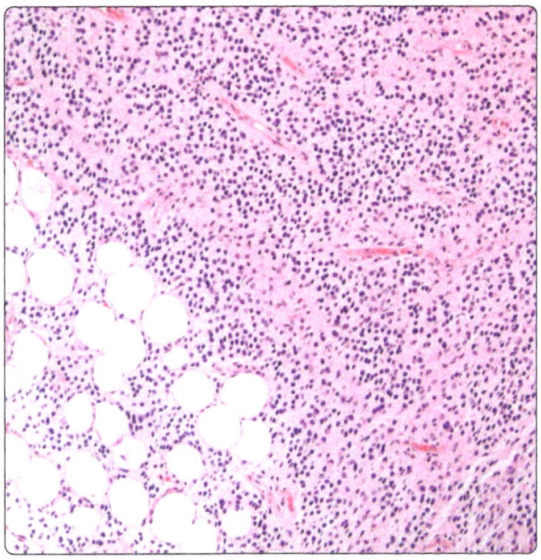

Very Rare Nuclear Palisading in Diffuse Neurofibroma

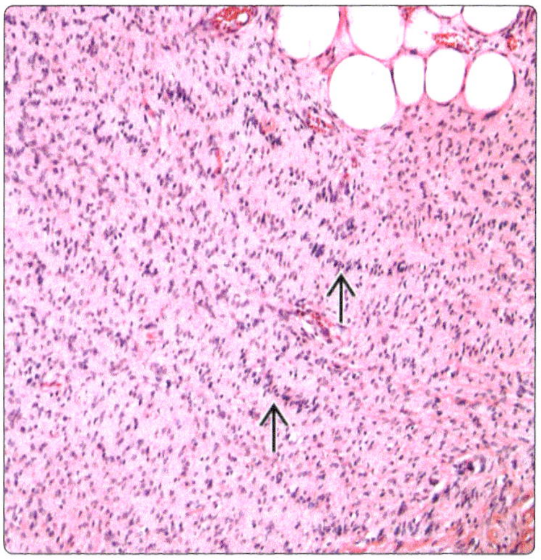

(Left) *Lesional Schwann cells with a rounded nuclear profile may be seen in some cases of diffuse-type neurofibroma. This appearance is more common in this subtype than in the others.* **(Right)** *Nuclear palisading is very uncommon in neurofibroma. This unusual case of otherwise typical diffuse-type neurofibroma had focal areas of increased cellularity with vague palisading ➡.*

Wagner-Meissner Bodies Characteristic of Diffuse-Type Neurofibroma

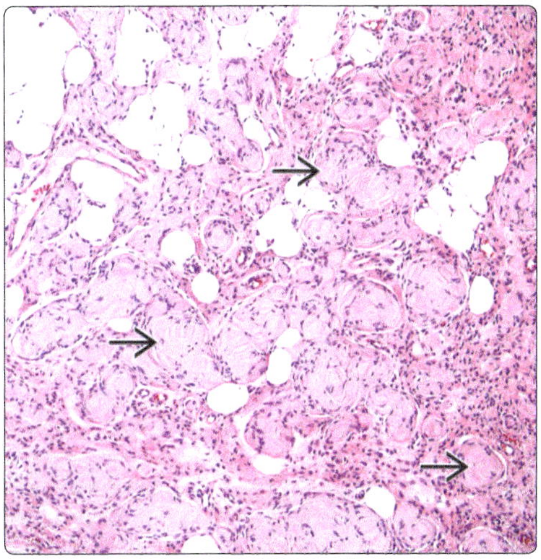

Morphology of Wagner-Meissner Bodies

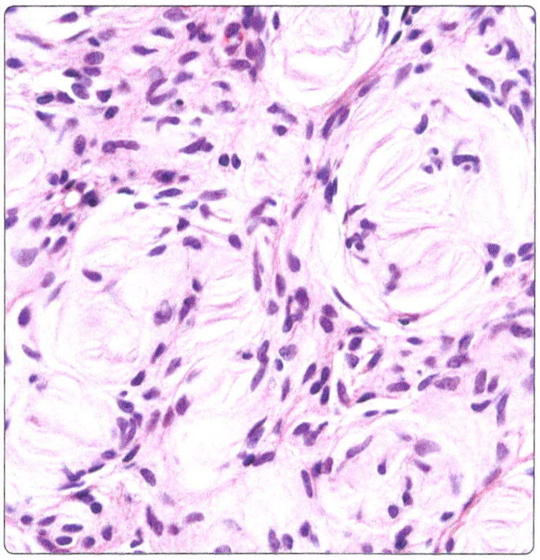

(Left) *Wagner-Meissner (pseudomeissnerian) bodies ➡ are very characteristic of diffuse-type neurofibroma and may arrange in small aggregates, linear arrays, or larger sheets.* **(Right)** *Wagner-Meissner (pseudomeissnerian) bodies are composed of spherical, layered clusters of thin and elongated, spindled cells with long delicate cytoplasmic processes. They resemble Meissner corpuscles.*

Scattered Wagner-Meissner Bodies

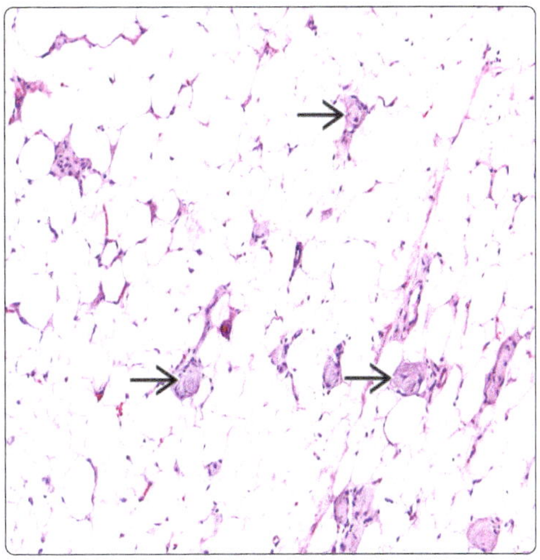

Pigmented Neurofibroma

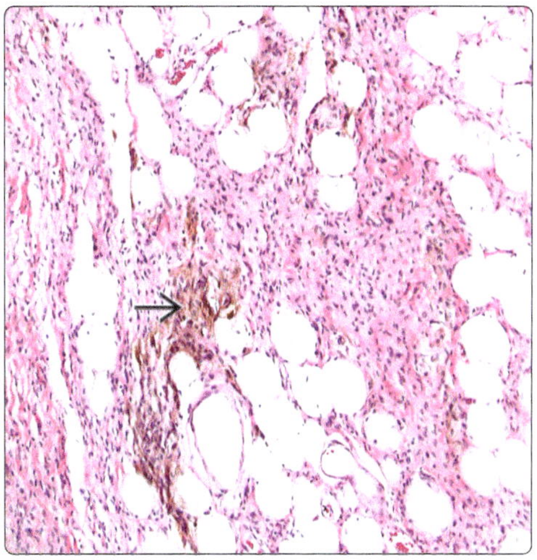

(Left) *Diffuse-type neurofibroma may contain large zones of predominantly mature adipose tissue with scattered small Wagner-Meissner bodies ➡. This finding may be the only clue to the diagnosis in a small biopsy.* **(Right)** *Rare cases of diffuse-type neurofibroma contain collections of pigmented Schwann cells ➡ with intracytoplasmic melanin. Most of these tumors occur in the setting of NF1, and some may also show a plexiform morphology.*

(Left) *Plexiform neurofibroma is identified by a characteristic irregular, multinodular, and serpentine growth pattern of expanded nerves. This variant usually first arises in childhood and is virtually diagnostic of NF1.* **(Right)** *Many of the expanded nerves in plexiform neurofibroma contain a centralized core → of residual nerve within otherwise typical neurofibromatous tissue.*

Plexiform Neurofibroma

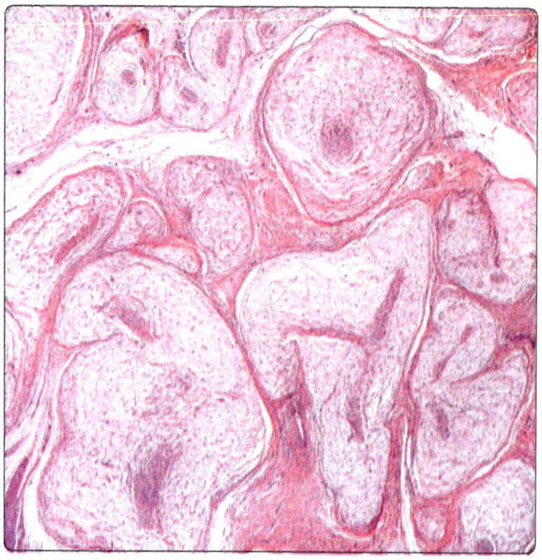

Expanded Nerves in Plexiform Neurofibroma

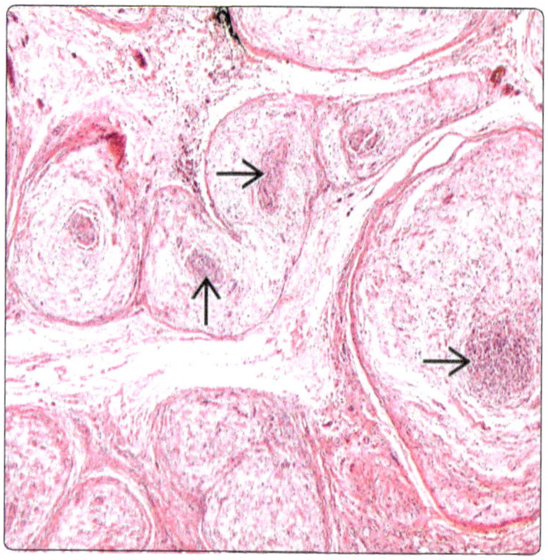

(Left) *Myxoid change is common in plexiform neurofibroma, and collagen fibers are typically splayed apart throughout each expanded nerve, reminiscent of shredded carrots. This morphology is similar to other forms of neurofibroma.* **(Right)** *Collagen fibers may be thicker in some foci of plexiform neurofibroma. Note the small core → of centralized residual nerve.*

Myxoid Change in Plexiform Neurofibroma

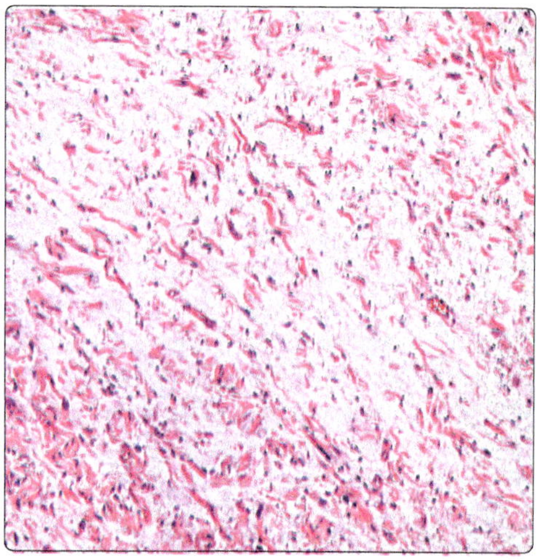

Collagen Fibers in Plexiform Neurofibroma

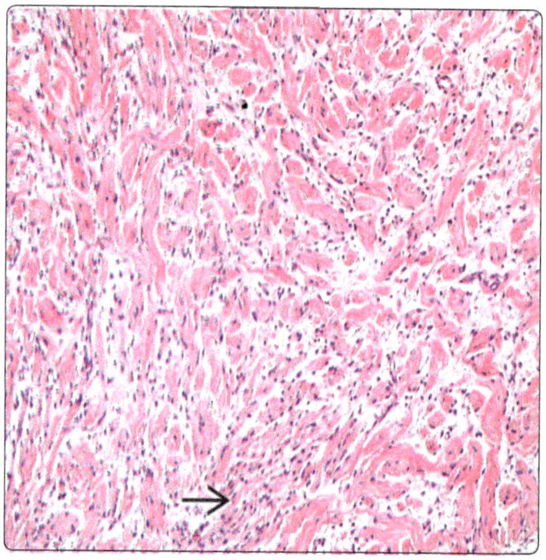

(Left) *This example of plexiform neurofibroma shows foci with extensive bundled collagen between clusters of lesional spindled cells.* **(Right)** *Many cases of plexiform neurofibroma show extension → of lesional tissue out of the expanded nerves → in plexiform areas and into the surrounding tissue. The morphology of this extraneural tissue is indistinguishable from diffuse-type neurofibroma.*

Prominent Collagen in Plexiform Neurofibroma

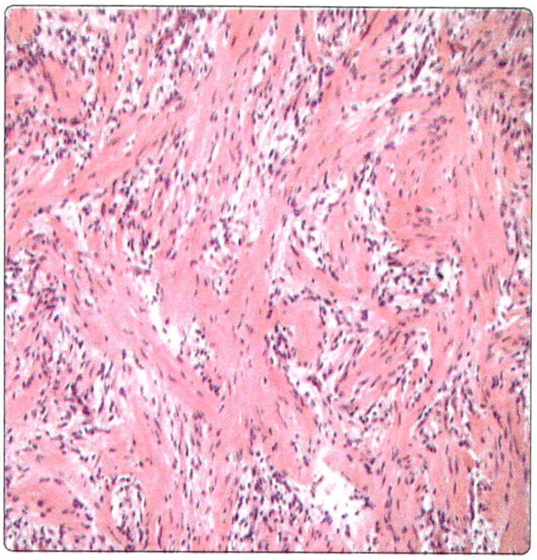

Combined Diffuse and Plexiform Morphologies

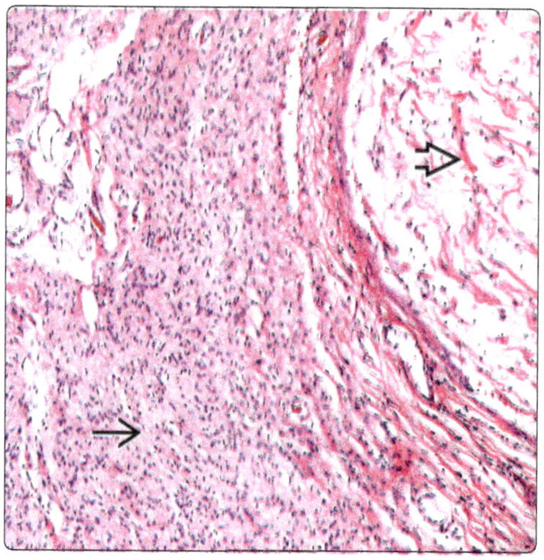

Degenerative Nuclear Atypia

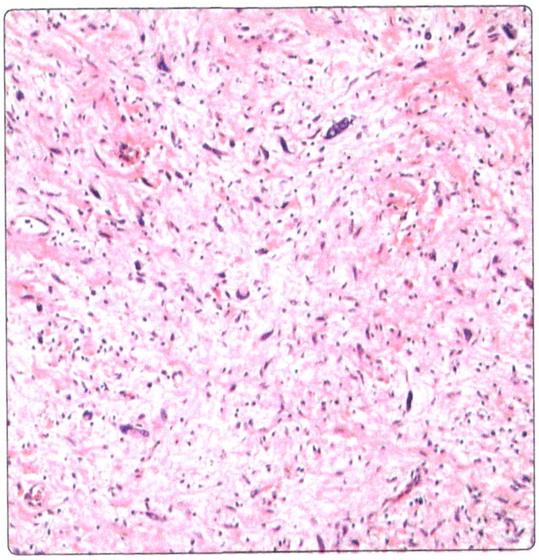

Degenerative Changes Include Foamy Histiocytes

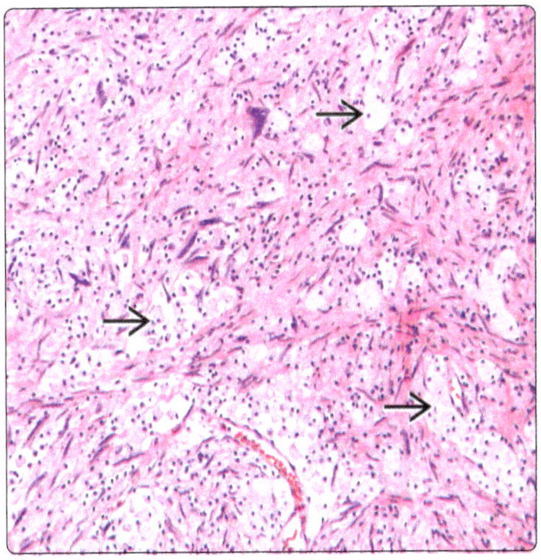

(Left) *Degenerative nuclear atypia, identical to the "ancient change" seen in schwannoma, may be seen in localized or plexiform neurofibroma. The nuclei generally show "smudgy" chromatin and commonly contain pseudoinclusions. When this change is prominent, these tumors may be referred to as atypical (or bizarre) neurofibroma.* **(Right)** *Collections of foamy histiocytes ⇨ may also be seen in degenerative (atypical/bizarre) neurofibromas.*

Central Cellularity in Atypical Neurofibroma

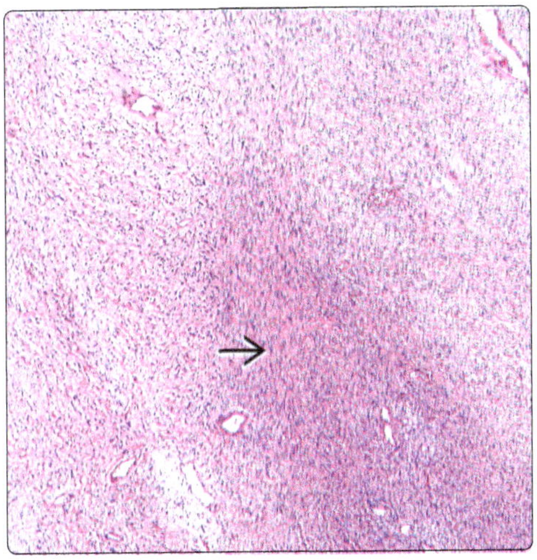

Increased Cellularity in Atypical Neurofibroma

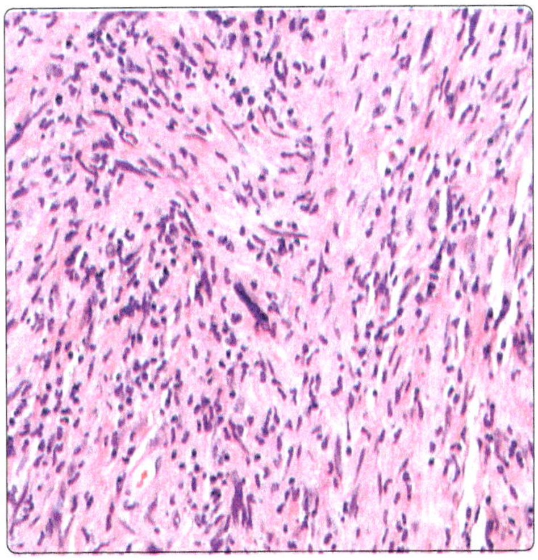

(Left) *Large examples of localized soft tissue neurofibroma may show centralized increases in cellularity ⇨. These areas should be evaluated at higher power for other features that might indicate possible malignant transformation.* **(Right)** *Increased cellularity in atypical (bizarre) neurofibroma does not necessarily imply malignant transformation. However, marked cellularity with generalized nuclear atypia and more than rare mitoses suggests transformation into an MPNST.*

Malignant Transformation in Neurofibroma

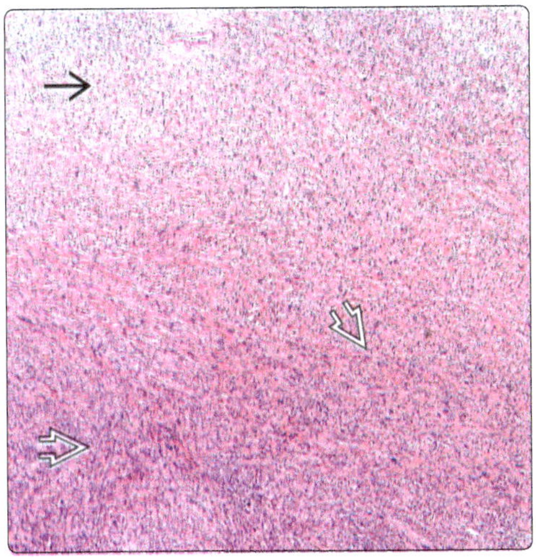

MPNST Arising in Neurofibroma

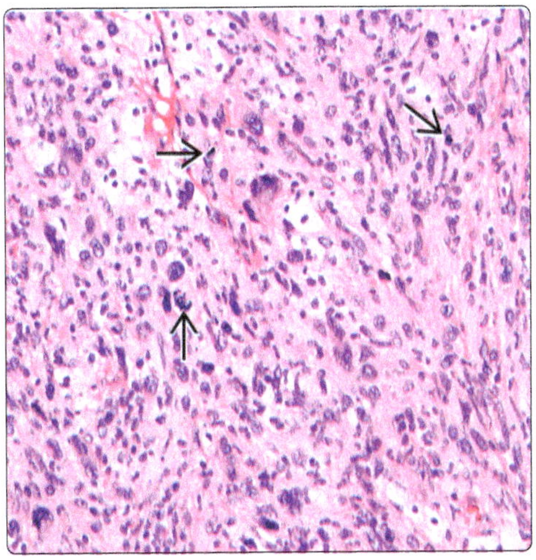

(Left) *This image shows transformation of a localized soft tissue neurofibroma ⇨ into an malignant peripheral nerve sheath tumor (MPNST) ➡. Note the marked increase in cellularity from benign to malignant zones.* **(Right)** *This image shows the MPNST portion of a neurofibroma with malignant transformation, as evidence by the significant nuclear atypia and several mitotic figures ⇨ in 1 field. Necrosis may or may not be present (not shown).*

Schwannoma

KEY FACTS

TERMINOLOGY

- Encapsulated, benign peripheral nerve sheath tumor composed predominantly of Schwann cells

CLINICAL ISSUES

- Any age
  - Most common: 20-50 years
- Most occur in superficial soft tissues of head/neck and upper or lower extremities
  - Also retroperitoneum, posterior mediastinum, and viscera (GI tract, kidney, etc.)
- Surgical excision is generally curative and recurrences are rare

MICROSCOPIC

- Well-circumscribed, nodular mass with fibrous capsule
- Hallmark: Variable amounts of hypercellular Antoni A and hypocellular Antoni B areas
- Morphologic variants: Ancient, cellular, plexiform, epithelioid, pseudoglandular, neuroblastoma-like, microcystic/reticular
- Schwannomas in neurofibromatosis type 2 (NF2) and schwannomatosis
  - Similar morphologically to sporadic tumors

ANCILLARY TESTS

- Diffuse, strong S100 positivity is characteristic of all schwannoma variants
- Type IV collagen is present around individual cells and small groups of cells
- Cytokeratin AE1/AE3 and GFAP expression common in tumors of retroperitoneum, posterior mediastinum, and GI tract

TOP DIFFERENTIAL DIAGNOSES

- Neurofibroma
- Malignant peripheral nerve sheath tumor
- Pleomorphic hyalinizing angiectatic tumor

Schwannoma at Low Magnification

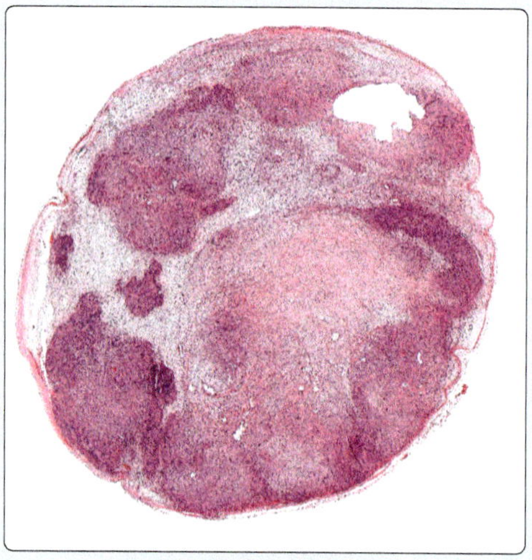

Encapsulation Common

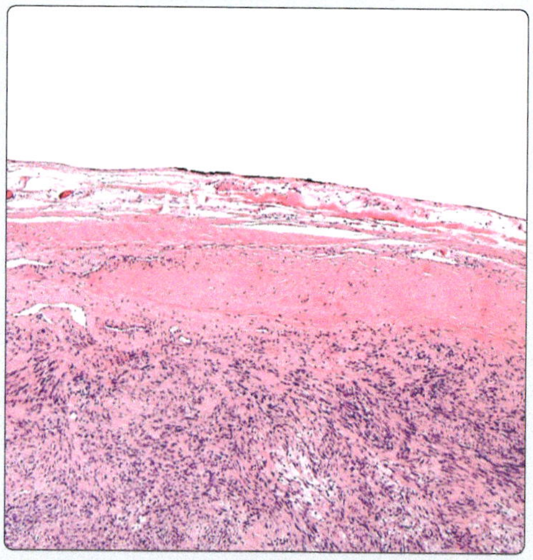

(Left) *Schwannoma is a well-circumscribed, encapsulated peripheral nerve sheath tumor that, in its conventional form, shows a variable admixture of zones of high and low cellularity, imparting a somewhat marbled appearance at low magnification.* **(Right)** *Most schwannomas are surrounded by a thick or thin fibrous capsule that contains epineurium and residual nerve fibers.*

Classic Alternating Cellularity

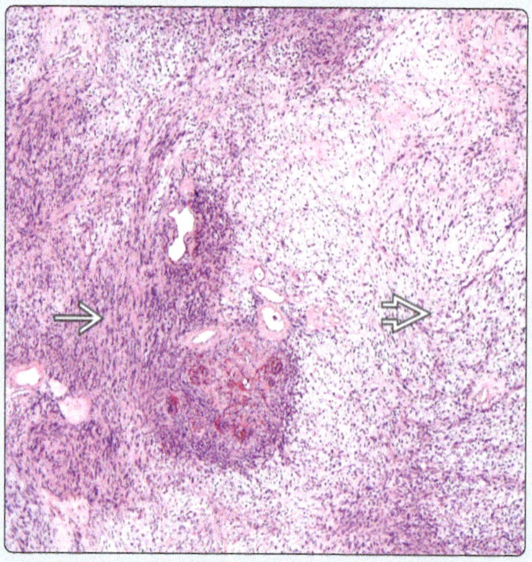

Antoni A and Antoni B Zones

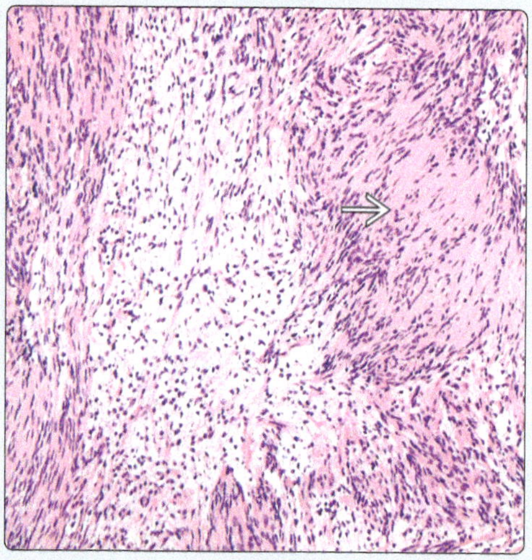

(Left) *The classic marbled appearance of schwannoma is created by interfaces between the cellular Antoni A zones* ➡ *and the loose edematous or myxoid Antoni B zones* ⇨*. This interface may be discretely abrupt or a gradual transition.* **(Right)** *Antoni A zones* ➡ *are more cellular and organized than Antoni B zones. Most schwannomas show a complex admixture of these 2 types of zones, but occasional cases are composed predominantly of either Antoni A or B.*

TERMINOLOGY

Synonyms

- Neurilemmoma

Definitions

- Encapsulated, benign peripheral nerve sheath tumor composed predominantly of Schwann cells

ETIOLOGY/PATHOGENESIS

Molecular Aberrations

- Somatic *NF2* gene mutations present in most tumors
- Bilateral vestibular schwannomas occur in setting of germline *NF2* gene mutations

Associated Syndromes

- Neurofibromatosis type 2 (NF2)
  - Inactivating germline mutations of *NF2* gene on chromosome 22
  - Autosomal dominant condition
    - Incidence around 1:30,000-40,000
  - Bilateral vestibular schwannomas are characteristic and diagnostic
    - Schwannomas involving other cranial nerves may be present
  - CNS tumors like meningioma, ependymoma, and gliomas are also part of disease spectrum
  - Schwannomas in NF2 resemble their sporadic counterparts
    - Of note, plexiform schwannomas are **not** diagnostic of NF2
- Schwannomatosis
  - Rare sporadic or familial (autosomal dominant) condition characterized by formation of multiple peripheral schwannomas
    - Familial cases that follow autosomal-dominant inheritance with reduced penetrance occur but are less common
    - Schwannomatosis locus identified on chromosome 22 proximal to *NF2* gene
    - Not associated with germline mutations in *NF1* or *NF2* genes
    - Some cases of inherited and sporadic schwannomatosis may be associated with germline *SMARCB1* mutations
  - By definition, patients do not have bilateral vestibular schwannomas and lack other criteria for NF2
  - Morphology similar to sporadic schwannomas

CLINICAL ISSUES

Epidemiology

- Incidence
  - 90% are sporadic
  - 10% are syndromic
    - ~ 3% with NF2
    - 2% with schwannomatosis
    - 5% with multiple meningiomas
    - Very rarely in association with NF1
- Age
  - All ages
    - Common between 20 and 50 years
- Sex
  - Affects male and female patients equally

Site

- Most occur in superficial soft tissues of head/neck and upper or lower extremities
  - Deep-seated soft tissue tumors much less common
- Retroperitoneum and mediastinum (often large)
- May also be seen in GI tract and parenchymal organs (kidney, pancreas, etc.)
- May involve cranial nerve VIII in setting of NF2 (vestibular/acoustic neuroma)

Presentation

- Slow-growing, painless mass
  - Large tumors may be painful
- Cystic tumors may show fluctuation in size
- Examples that occur in neck often confused clinically for lymph nodes

Treatment

- Surgical excision, often nerve sparing

Prognosis

- Benign
- Excision is generally curative and recurrences are rare (usually deep-seated tumors)

MACROSCOPIC

General Features

- Surrounded by true capsule consisting of epineurium
- Eccentric growth off of large nerve, or less likely, as nodular or fusiform mass seemingly unassociated with nerve
  - Dumbbell-shaped tumors occur in vertebral canal, usually in posterior mediastinum
- Variable size (often < 5 cm)
- Cut surface is gray-tan-white to yellow
- Large tumors may show cystic change, hemorrhage, or calcification on cut section

MICROSCOPIC

Histologic Features

- Well-circumscribed, nodular mass with fibrous capsule
- Hallmark: Variable amounts of admixed cellular Antoni A and hypocellular Antoni B areas
  - Antoni A
    - Spindle cells in short or interconnecting fascicles, loosely or tightly formed
    - Generally indistinct cytoplasmic borders
    - Nuclear palisading or whorling is common
      - Verocay bodies: Compact rows of palisaded nuclei separated by fibrillary processes
    - May contain lymphocytic infiltrate
  - Antoni B
    - Less orderly than Antoni A
    - Spindle or ovoid cells with indistinct cytoplasmic borders
    - Loose edematous or myxoid matrix with cystic change and inflammatory cells, particularly lymphocytes and histiocytes

- ◻ Presence of scattered collagen bundles may impart resemblance to neurofibroma
  - Large vessels with thick hyalinized walls and luminal thrombi, ± hemosiderin deposition
- Nuclei are either thin and elongated with buckled or carrot-like shape or plump and ovoid
  - Intranuclear inclusions may be seen
- Mitotic rate is generally low to absent with no atypical forms
  - Cellular schwannomas may show more conspicuous mitotic activity
- Longstanding lesions often show degenerative changes
  - Nuclear atypia (ancient change) but without increase in mitotic activity
  - Cystic change may be focal or widespread with abundant hemorrhage
  - Stromal hyalinization or marked hypocellularity
  - Calcification ± metaplastic bone formation
  - Infarct-type necrosis may be present
    - True coagulative necrosis is rarely seen cellular schwannoma (usually focal)
- Malignant transformation in schwannomas extremely rare
  - Usually epithelioid malignant peripheral nerve sheath tumor (MPNST), also epithelioid angiosarcoma

Morphologic Variants

- **Ancient schwannoma**
  - Demonstrates marked nuclear atypia of degenerative type (often "smudgy")
  - Lacks mitotic activity
  - Cystic change, hemorrhage, calcification, and hyalinization present
  - Usually seen in tumors of long duration (particularly deep-seated cases)
- **Cellular schwannoma**
  - By definition, composed almost exclusively of hypercellular Antoni A areas, which lack Verocay bodies
  - Encapsulated tumors; some may be multinodular or plexiform in architecture
    - Many show subcapsular &/or intratumoral lymphoid aggregates
  - Short to long sweeping fascicles of spindle-shaped cells
    - Cells may appear round/ovoid in fascicles that are cut in cross section
  - Mitotic activity is low (< 4/10 HPF)
  - Small foci of necrosis may be present
  - More common in mediastinum, retroperitoneum, and GI tract
- **Plexiform schwannoma**
  - Encapsulated tumors with striking multinodular or plexiform architecture
  - Often more cellular than ordinary schwannoma
    - Highly cellular examples reported in infants and children (cellular plexiform schwannoma)
  - Usually occur in skin or superficial soft tissues
  - Most common in head and neck region; infrequent in deeper locations
  - Association with NF syndromes is weak (unlike plexiform neurofibroma)
- **Epithelioid schwannoma**
  - Epithelioid or polygonal Schwann cells with sharp cell borders and variable amount of eosinophilic cytoplasm
  - Arranged in clusters, cords, or as single cells in variably myxoid or collagenous stroma
  - Foci of conventional schwannoma may be present
  - Small, bland nuclei
    - Degenerative nuclear atypia may be seen
  - Lacks mitotic activity
- **Pseudoglandular schwannoma**
  - Contains cystic spaces that are lined by small round tumor cells, resembling epithelial surfaces
    - Cells may show "apical" cytoplasm
      - ◻ May mimic glandular or ductal epithelium
  - Often contains areas of conventional schwannoma
- **Neuroblastoma-like schwannoma**
  - Contains rosette-like structures composed of round to ovoid Schwann cells around acellular collagen cores
    - Collagen cores may lack peripheral cells
    - Structures may be centered around small vessels
  - Mimics rosettes seen in neuroblastoma
- **Microcystic/reticular schwannoma**
  - Anastomosing strands of eosinophilic spindle cells in myxoid, fibrillary, or collagenous matrix
  - Predilection for visceral locations, particularly GI tract
  - Foci of conventional schwannoma or other schwannoma variants may be present

ANCILLARY TESTS

Immunohistochemistry

- Diffuse, strong S100 expression is characteristic
  - Applies to all morphologic variants
  - SOX10 shows similar diffuse expression in nuclei
- Type IV collagen is present around individual cells and small groups of cells
- Neurofilament protein expression is often limited to entrapped axons at periphery of tumor but may be also seen within tumor in some cases
- Cytokeratin AE1/AE3 and GFAP expression common in tumors of retroperitoneum, posterior mediastinum, and GI tract
  - In peripheral sites, GFAP expression is rare, and CK AE1/AE3 has not been reported
  - CK AE1/AE3 expression due to cross-reactivity with GFAP
- Negative for CD34, EMA, claudin-1, GLUT1
  - Mixed expression of S100 with 1 or more of these markers may indicate hybrid peripheral nerve sheath tumor

DIFFERENTIAL DIAGNOSIS

Neurofibroma

- Unencapsulated and lacks Antoni A areas
  - Antoni B areas of schwannoma can look very similar to neurofibroma
- Composed of mixture of Schwann cells, fibroblasts, and perineurial cells
- S100 is diffusely positive but less striking overall compared to schwannoma (due to lower cellularity)
- CD34 is commonly positive in admixed population of fibroblasts

Malignant Peripheral Nerve Sheath Tumor

- Often larger and more deep-seated than schwannoma
- Cytology varies from monomorphic to highly pleomorphic, and mitotic activity is generally high and conspicuous
- Tumor necrosis common
- S100 expression is characteristically negative or at most focal
  - Lower grade MPNST may show more extensive S100 positivity
  - Very rare cases of high-grade MPNST are diffusely S100 positive
- Most likely to be confused with cellular, plexiform, and ancient schwannoma variants
  - Cellular examples of plexiform schwannoma may be mistaken for MPNST arising in plexiform neurofibroma
- Epithelioid MPNST is larger and more cellular than epithelioid schwannoma and contains larger nuclei with prominent macronucleoli

Malignant/Metastatic Melanoma

- Always consider in dermal tumors and in patients with history of melanoma
- Lack admixed Antoni A and Antoni B zones
- Primary melanoma often contains cutaneous junctional component
- Spindle cell melanoma may be relatively bland but often shows at least focal nuclear atypia and mitotic activity
- Epithelioid melanoma cells are often cytologically malignant with prominent, eosinophilic, cherry red nucleoli
- Strong expression of S100 and SOX10; often diffuse
- Variable expression of melanocytic markers (HMB-45, MART-1/Melan-A, MITF, tyrosinase)
  - Focal expression of HMB-45 and MART-1/Melan-A can be easily missed
  - Desmoplastic melanomas are characteristically negative for HMB-45 and MART-1

Pleomorphic Hyalinizing Angiectatic Tumor

- Can show markedly similar appearance to ancient schwannoma
- S100(-); CD34(+) (~ 50% of cases)
- Predilection for foot, ankle, and leg
- Significant risk of local recurrence with simple excision

Leiomyoma

- Generally very pink microscopic appearance
- Lack admixed Antoni A and Antoni B zones
- Composed of fascicles of plump eosinophilic spindle cells with cigar-shaped nuclei
  - May show epithelioid morphology
- SMA, caldesmon, and desmin expression
- S100(-)

SELECTED REFERENCES

1. Luzar B et al: Cutaneous microcystic/reticular schwannoma: a poorly recognized entity. J Cutan Pathol. 43(2):93-100, 2016
2. Zong S et al: Treatment results in the differential surgery of intradural extramedullary schwannoma of 110 cases. PLoS One. 8(5):e63867, 2013
3. Blakeley J: Development of drug treatments for neurofibromatosis type 2-associated vestibular schwannoma. Curr Opin Otolaryngol Head Neck Surg. 20(5):372-9, 2012
4. Carter JM et al: Epithelioid malignant peripheral nerve sheath tumor arising in a schwannoma, in a patient with "neuroblastoma-like" schwannomatosis and a novel germline SMARCB1 mutation. Am J Surg Pathol. 36(1):154-60, 2012
5. Harder A et al: Hybrid neurofibroma/schwannoma is overrepresented among schwannomatosis and neurofibromatosis patients. Am J Surg Pathol. 36(5):702-9, 2012
6. Rezanko T et al: Epithelioid schwannoma of soft tissue: unusual morphological variant causing a diagnostic dilemma. Ann Diagn Pathol. 16(6):521-6, 2012
7. Voltaggio L et al: Gastric schwannoma: a clinicopathologic study of 51 cases and critical review of the literature. Hum Pathol. 43(5):650-9, 2012
8. Chetty R: Reticular and microcystic schwannoma: a distinctive tumor of the gastrointestinal tract. Ann Diagn Pathol. 15(3):198-201, 2011
9. Gaudi S et al: Intravascular schwannoma. Am J Dermatopathol. 33(8):850-4, 2011
10. Ida CM et al: Primary schwannoma of the bone: a clinicopathologic and radiologic study of 17 cases. Am J Surg Pathol. 35(7):989-97, 2011
11. Agaimy A et al: Peripheral nerve sheath tumors of the gastrointestinal tract: a multicenter study of 58 patients including NF1-associated gastric schwannoma and unusual morphologic variants. Virchows Arch. 456(4):411-22, 2010
12. Küsters-Vandevelde HV et al: Improved discrimination of melanotic schwannoma from melanocytic lesions by combined morphological and GNAQ mutational analysis. Acta Neuropathol. 120(6):755-64, 2010
13. Santos PP et al: Clinicopathologic analysis of 7 cases of oral schwannoma and review of the literature. Ann Diagn Pathol. 14(4):235-9, 2010
14. Trufant JW et al: Melanotic schwannoma arising in association with nevus of Ota: 2 cases suggesting a shared mechanism. Am J Dermatopathol. 31(8):808-13, 2009
15. Liegl B et al: Microcystic/reticular schwannoma: a distinct variant with predilection for visceral locations. Am J Surg Pathol. 32(7):1080-7, 2008
16. Fanburg-Smith JC et al: Keratin expression in schwannoma; a study of 115 retroperitoneal and 22 peripheral schwannomas. Mod Pathol. 19(1):115-21, 2006
17. MacCollin M et al: Diagnostic criteria for schwannomatosis. Neurology. 64(11):1838-45, 2005
18. Woodruff JM et al: Congenital and childhood plexiform (multinodular) cellular schwannoma: a troublesome mimic of malignant peripheral nerve sheath tumor. Am J Surg Pathol. 27(10):1321-9, 2003
19. McMenamin ME et al: Expanding the spectrum of malignant change in schwannomas: epithelioid malignant change, epithelioid malignant peripheral nerve sheath tumor, and epithelioid angiosarcoma: a study of 17 cases. Am J Surg Pathol. 25(1):13-25, 2001
20. Antinheimo J et al: Population-based analysis of sporadic and type 2 neurofibromatosis-associated meningiomas and schwannomas. Neurology. 54(1):71-6, 2000
21. Kindblom LG et al: Benign epithelioid schwannoma. Am J Surg Pathol. 22(6):762-70, 1998
22. Chan JK et al: Pseudoglandular schwannoma. Histopathology. 29(5):481-3, 1996
23. Goldblum JR et al: Neuroblastoma-like neurilemoma. Am J Surg Pathol. 18(3):266-73, 1994
24. Brooks JJ et al: Benign glandular schwannoma. Arch Pathol Lab Med. 116(2):192-5, 1992
25. Carney JA: Psammomatous melanotic schwannoma. A distinctive, heritable tumor with special associations, including cardiac myxoma and the Cushing syndrome. Am J Surg Pathol. 14(3):206-22, 1990
26. Fletcher CD et al: Cellular schwannoma: a distinct pseudosarcomatous entity. Histopathology. 11(1):21-35, 1987
27. Fletcher CD et al: Benign plexiform (multinodular) schwannoma: a rare tumour unassociated with neurofibromatosis. Histopathology. 10(9):971-80, 1986

Antoni A Cellular Areas

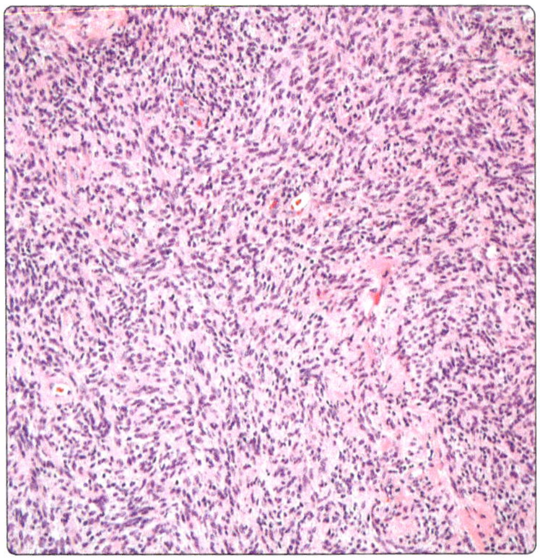

Antoni A Cytologic Features

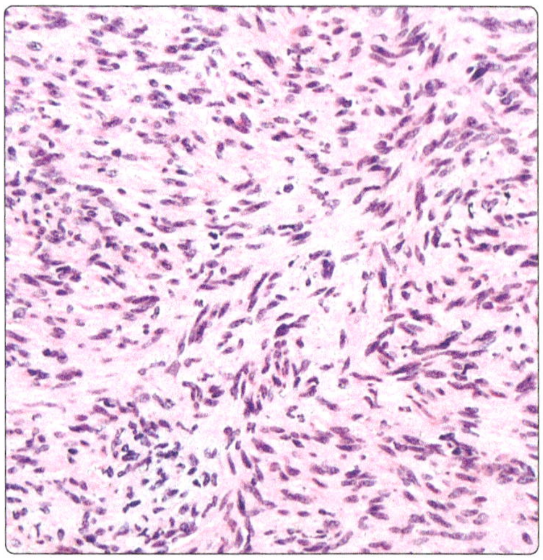

(Left) *Antoni A zones of schwannoma are cellular and relatively organized. Not all Antoni A zones exhibit nuclear palisading, Verocay body formation, or whorling.* **(Right)** *The spindle cells in Antoni A zones of schwannoma typically show indistinct cytoplasmic borders and elongated, buckled, wavy, or twisted nuclei. The matrix is fine, fibrillary, and eosinophilic.*

Nuclear Palisading in Antoni A

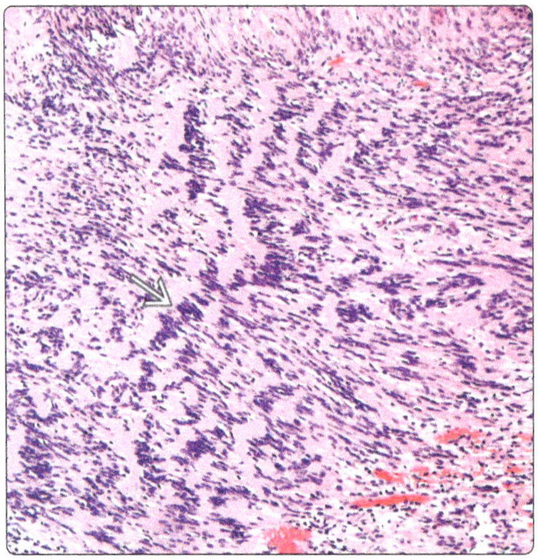

Morphology of Verocay Bodies

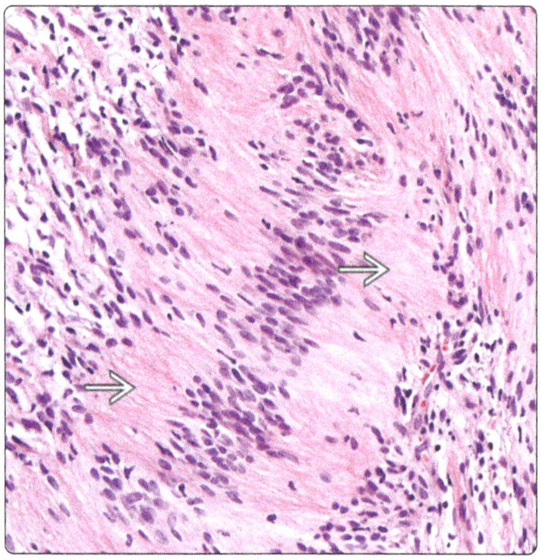

(Left) *A characteristic finding in some Antoni A zones of schwannoma is the presence of focal to prominent nuclear palisading* ➡*. This finding is not pathognomonic, however, as other unrelated tumors can show similar morphology.* **(Right)** *In schwannoma, the term Verocay body is used to describe the finding of eosinophilic fibrillary cell processes* ➡ *between 2 rows of palisading Schwann cell nuclei.*

Whorling Architecture in Some Cases

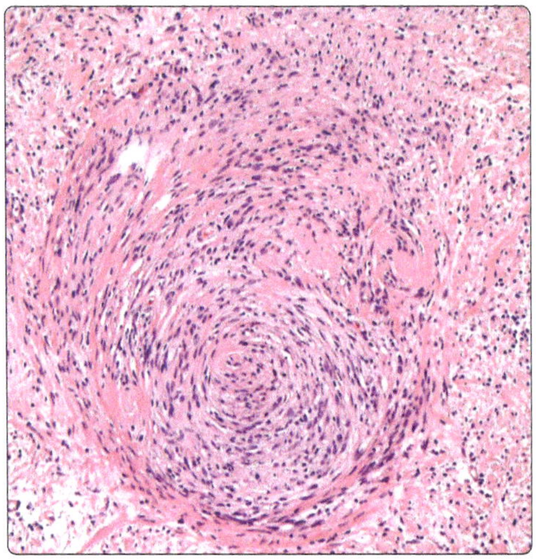

Schwann Cell Nuclear Features

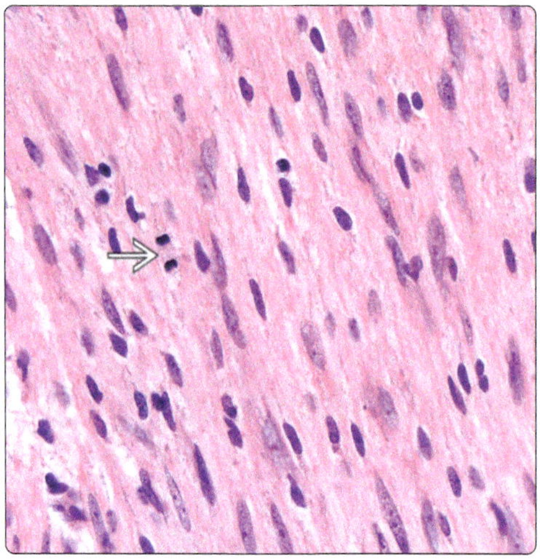

(Left) *In addition to nuclear palisading, a whorling architecture may be identified within Antoni A zones of schwannoma.* **(Right)** *Cytologically, most Schwann cell nuclei are bland, elongated, and often tapered at 1 or both ends. Nucleoli are inconspicuous. Clear nuclear pseudoinclusions (not pictured) are also seen in some cases. Mitotic figures* ➡ *are rarely identified in schwannoma and, if present, are never atypical.*

Stromal Inflammation Common

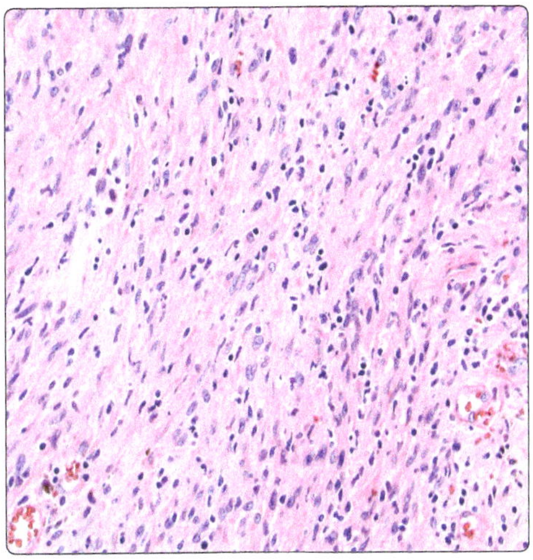

Variable Stromal Collagen

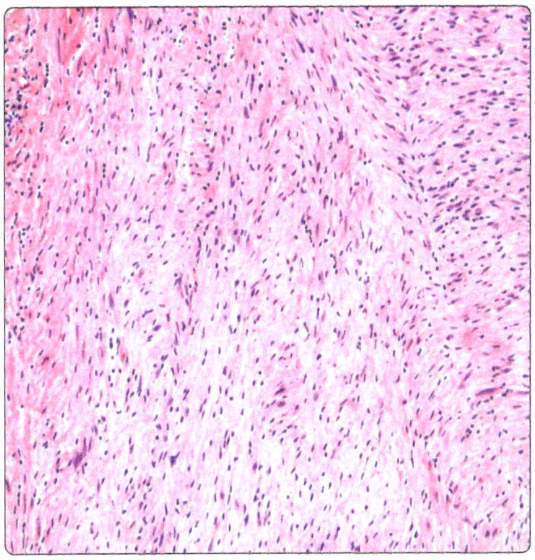

(Left) *A chronic inflammatory infiltrate is not uncommon in schwannoma and usually consists of predominantly reactive lymphocytes. This finding varies in prominence and may be seen in both Antoni A and Antoni B zones.* **(Right)** *Some areas in a schwannoma may show a typical loose fascicular growth of Antoni A but with increased stromal collagen. This finding is a feature of some cellular schwannomas.*

Antoni B Zones

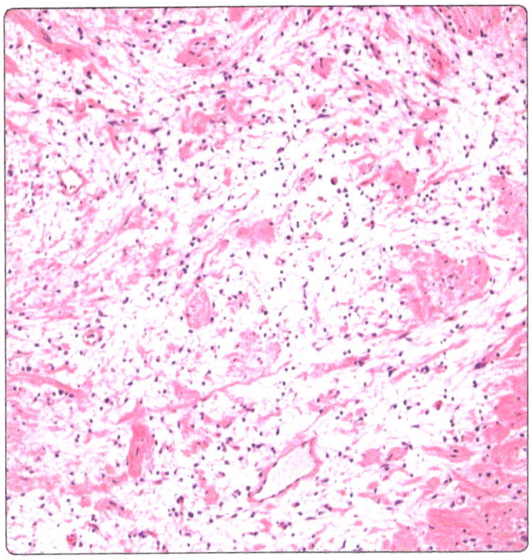

Antoni B Collagen Distribution

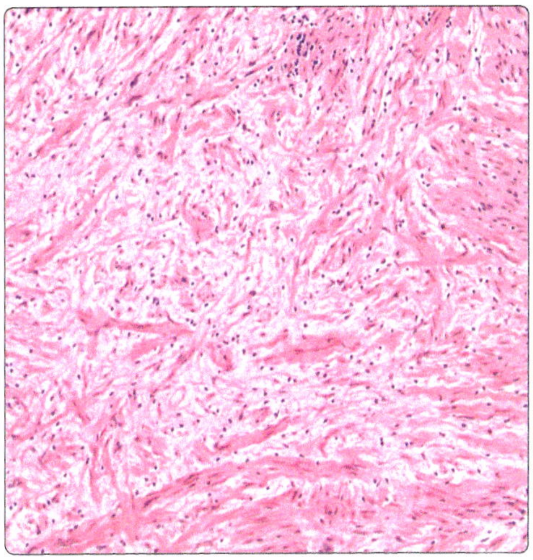

(Left) *Antoni B zones in schwannoma are distinctly less cellular than Antoni A zones and demonstrate a loose edematous or myxoid matrix with scattered collagen fibers.* **(Right)** *In some areas of schwannoma, the distribution of collagen fibers in Antoni B zones may closely resemble that of a neurofibroma, particularly the plexiform type; however, the characteristic multinodular growth pattern of the latter is generally absent.*

Hypocellularity or Myxoid Change in Antoni B

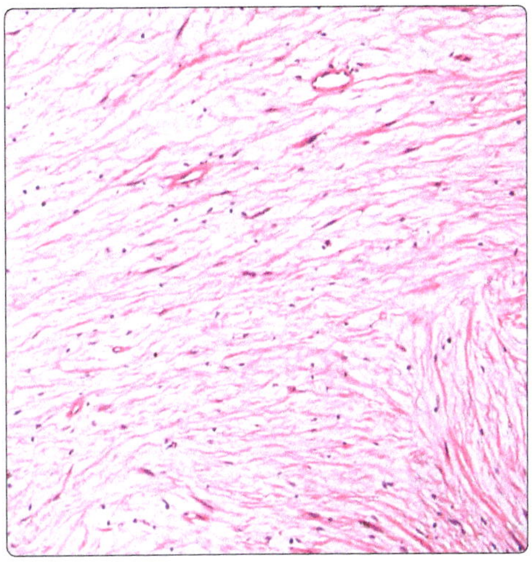

Strong and Diffuse S100 Expression

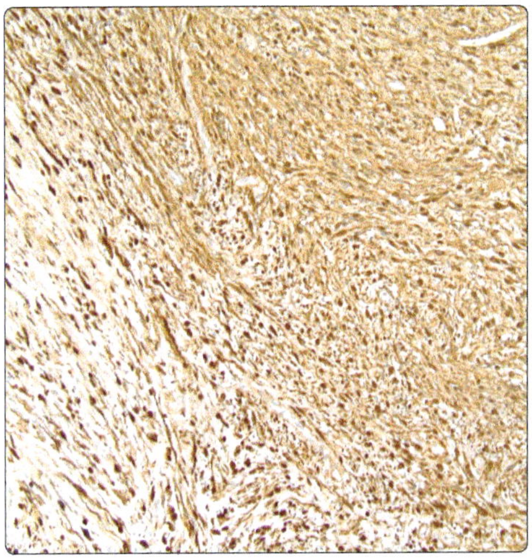

(Left) *Antoni B zones in schwannoma may be significantly myxoid and hypocellular and be easily confused with a variety of other low-grade myxoid neoplasms, such as myxoma or neurofibroma.* **(Right)** *S100 expression is essentially always strong and diffuse in schwannoma and is characteristic of all variants. The staining pattern is typically both nuclear and cytoplasmic.*

(Left) *An often conspicuous and characteristic finding in schwannoma is the presence of single or clusters of irregular vascular channels with hyalinized walls. These vessels predominate in Antoni B zones but may occasionally be identified in cellular Antoni A zones.* **(Right)** *A variety of benign vascular changes may be identified in the vessels of schwannoma, including papillary endothelial hyperplasia and thrombosis.*

Hyalinized Vessels Characteristic

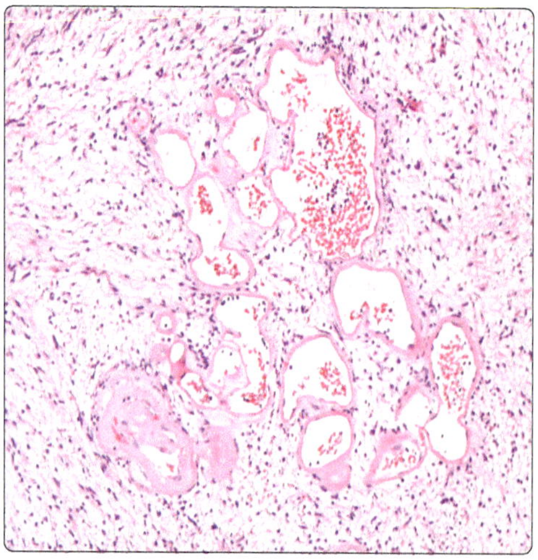

Hyperplastic Vascular Changes in Some Tumors

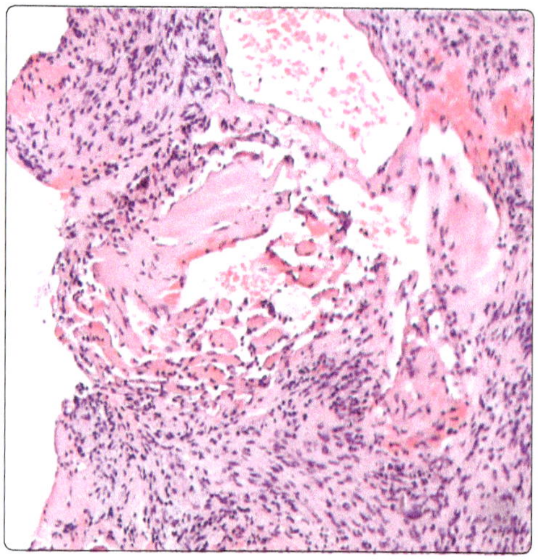

(Left) *Occasional vessels in schwannoma may show fibrinoid change in the wall ± thrombosis. This finding is most commonly seen in ancient schwannoma. Similar vascular changes can be seen in other tumors, particularly pleomorphic hyalinizing angiectatic tumor.* **(Right)** *Some examples of schwannoma show an interesting morphologic arrangement of relatively eosinophilic Antoni A zones and highly myxoid Antoni B. The overall marbled pattern is characteristic of most cases of conventional schwannoma.*

Occasional Vessels With Fibrinoid Changes

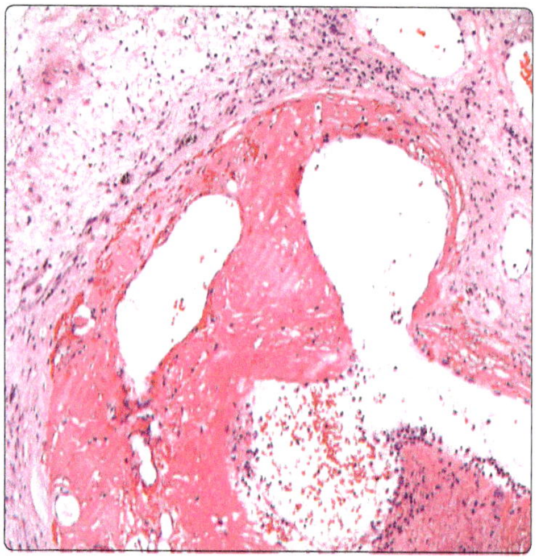

Myxoid Areas in Schwannoma

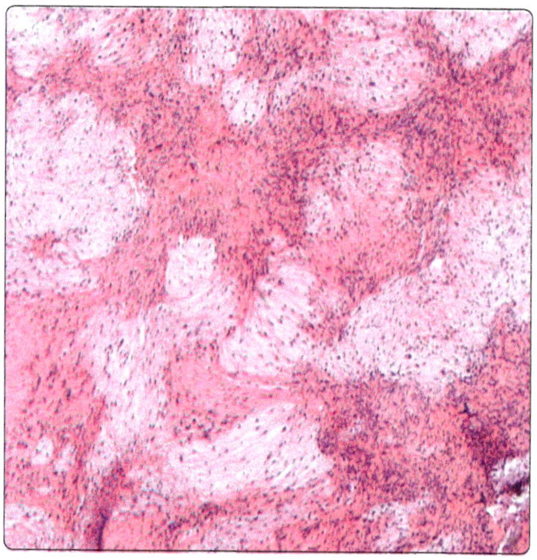

(Left) *This particular case of schwannoma shows large areas of myxoid matrix, resembling other low-grade myxoid neoplasms. S100 positivity was helpful in supporting the diagnosis of schwannoma.* **(Right)** *Antoni B zones in schwannoma may be markedly hyalinized and hypocellular, particularly longstanding tumors or those with abundant other degenerative features.*

Rare, Prominent Myxoid Stroma

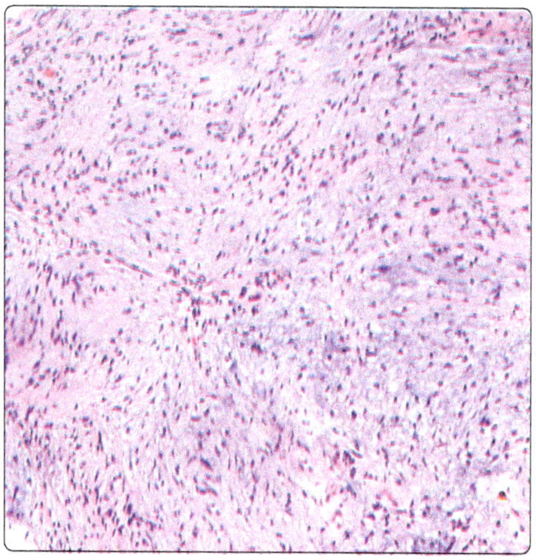

Stromal Hyalinization in Antoni B

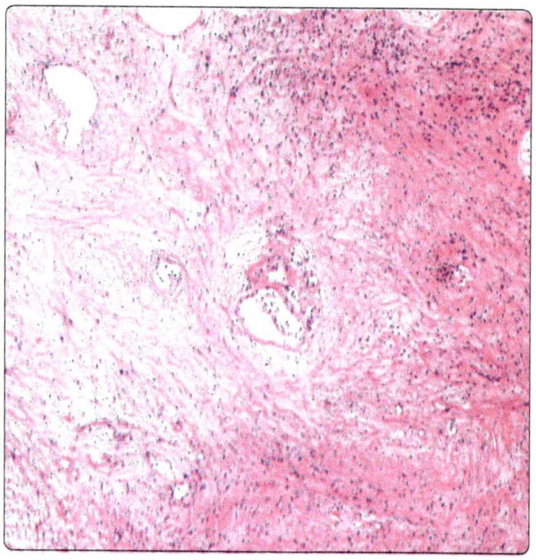

Diffuse Stromal Sclerosis in Older Tumors

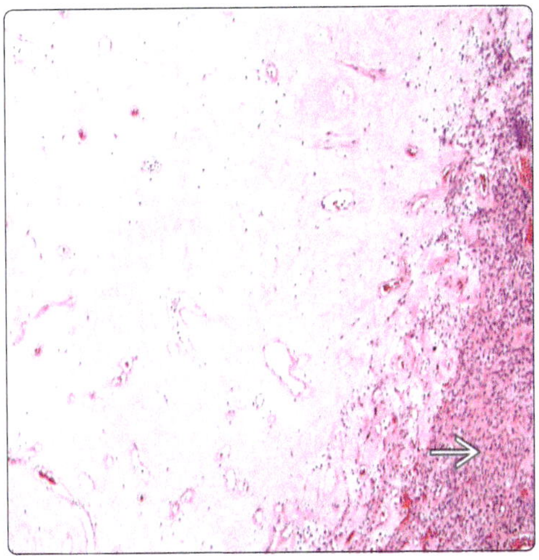

Calcification in Degenerative Schwannoma

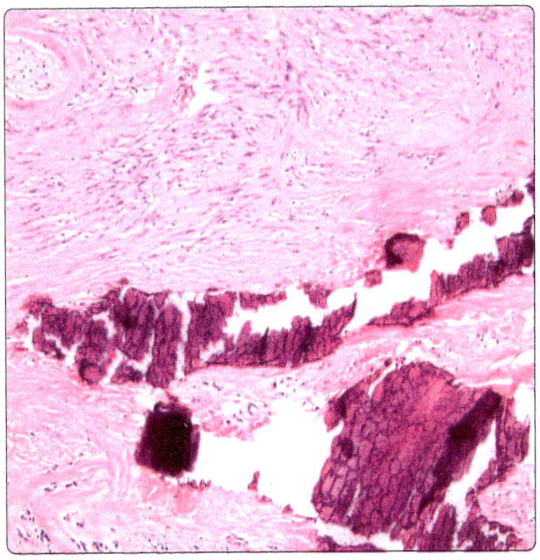

(Left) *Diffuse stromal hyalinization or sclerosis may be seen in degenerative schwannoma, and areas of conventional morphology* ➡ *may be focal or absent altogether.* **(Right)** *Calcification is not uncommon in schwannoma and is often associated with other degenerative changes, including vascular hyalinization, stromal sclerosis, cystic change, and hemosiderin deposition.*

Metaplastic Bone Formation Uncommon

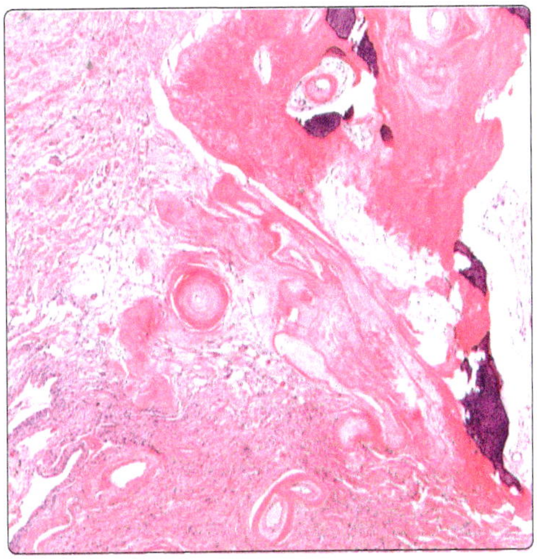

Foamy Histiocytes

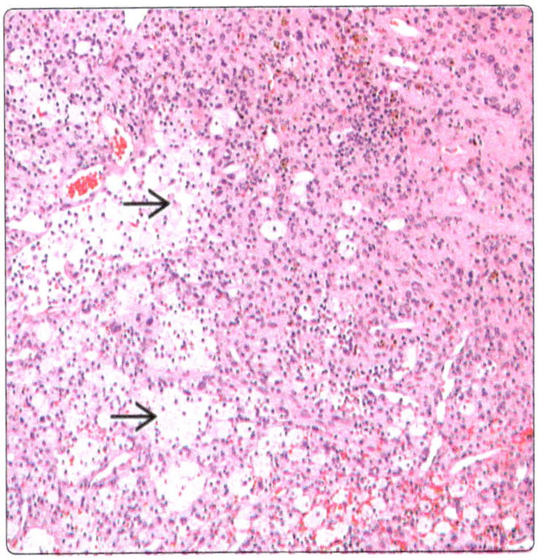

(Left) *Metaplastic bone formation is an uncommon event in schwannoma but is more likely to be seen in longstanding cases.* **(Right)** *Foamy histiocytes* ⇨ *may be identified in some cases of schwannoma, particularly cellular variants. They can also be seen as a component of Antoni B zones.*

Cystic Change in Degenerative Schwannoma

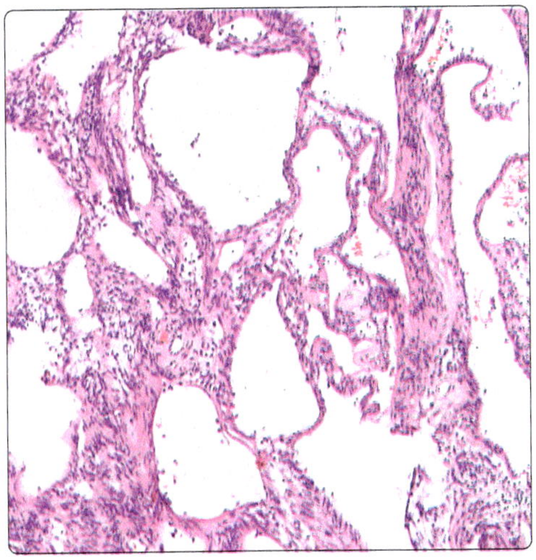

Rare Prominent Cystic Change

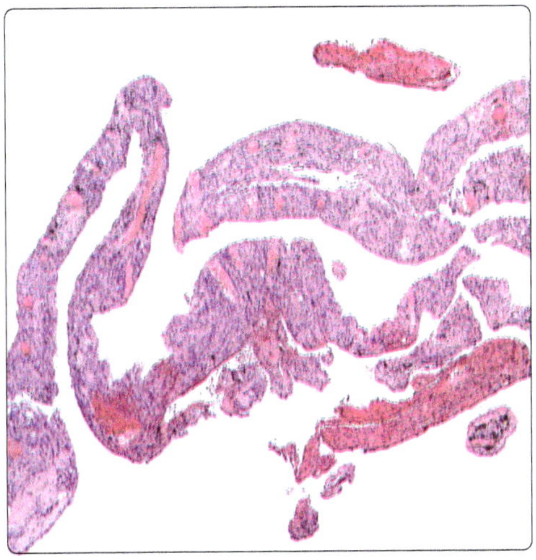

(Left) *Cystic change is not uncommon in schwannoma but is more frequently encountered in ancient/degenerative tumors. Clinically, larger schwannomas are more likely to have central cystic hemorrhage.* **(Right)** *Rare cases of schwannoma are predominantly or exclusively cystic and may be challenging to diagnose. This type of schwannoma is usually very hemorrhagic intraoperatively, clinically suggesting a vascular neoplasm.*

Hemosiderin Deposition Common

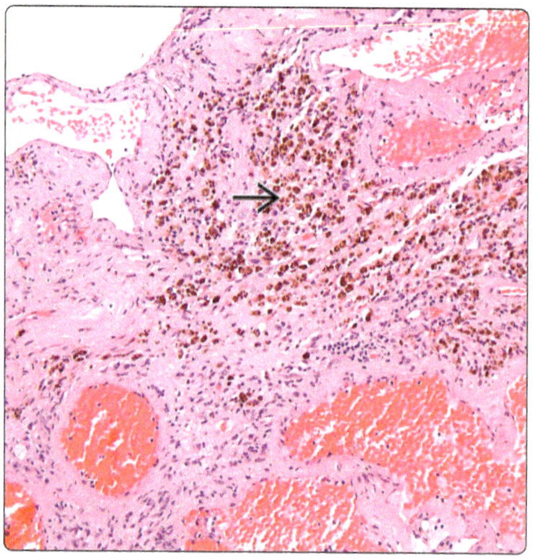

Degenerative Microcystic Stromal Change

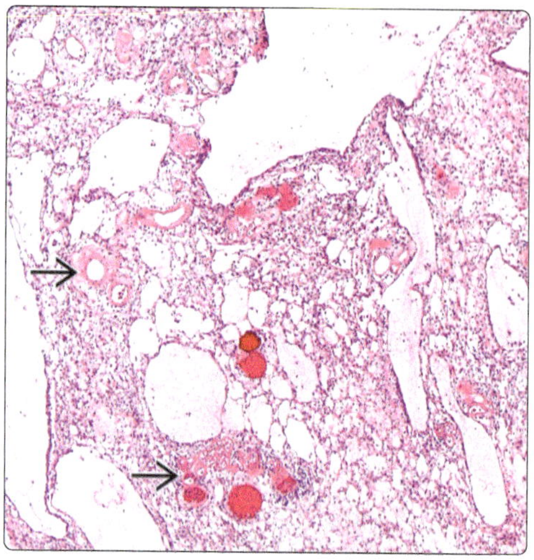

(Left) *Hemosiderin deposition is common in schwannoma, particularly cases with intratumoral hemorrhage. Rare cases show abundant hemosiderin and blood, simulating a hematoma or vascular neoplasm.* **(Right)** *Microcystic stromal changes may be seen in some cases of schwannoma. The microcysts vary in size and are often more prominent around large cystic spaces. Note the hyalinized vessels.*

Microcystic Stromal Change Associated With Inflammation

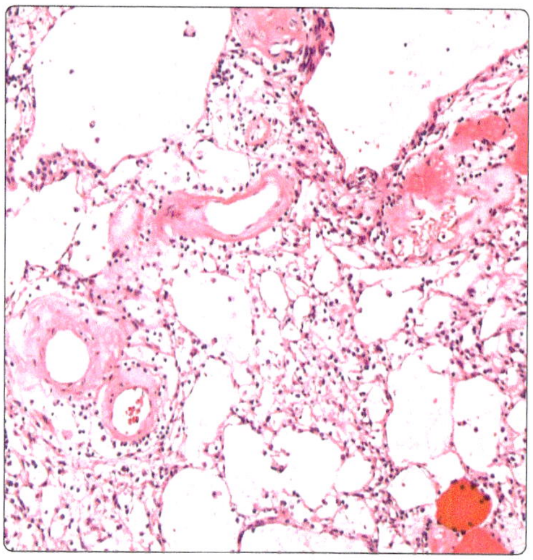

"Smudgy" Degenerative Nuclear Changes

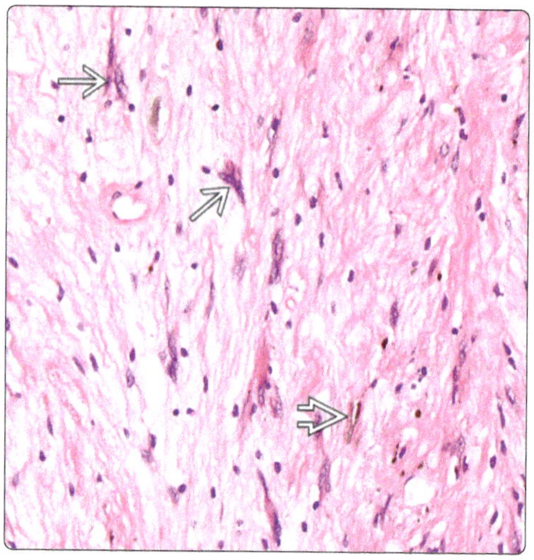

(Left) *Microcystic stromal change in degenerative schwannomas may be associated with a brisk chronic inflammatory infiltrate, as well as hyalinized vessels and histiocytes.* **(Right)** *A common finding in many schwannomas is the presence of scattered enlarged cells with hyperchromatic, "smudgy" nuclei, termed ancient change. Another common finding in these cases is lipofuscin pigment.*

Ancient Schwannoma Variant

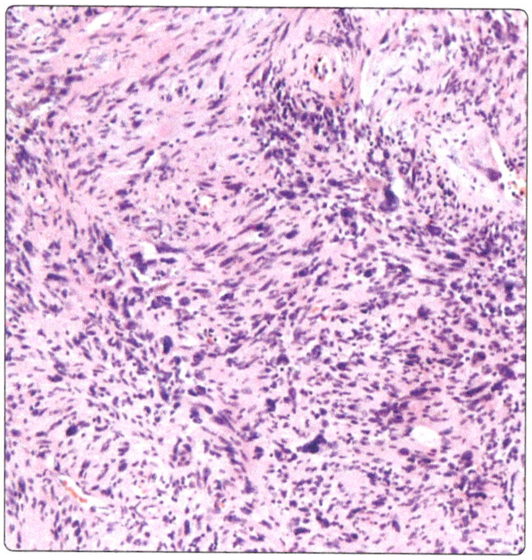

Atypical, "Smudgy" Nuclei in Schwannoma

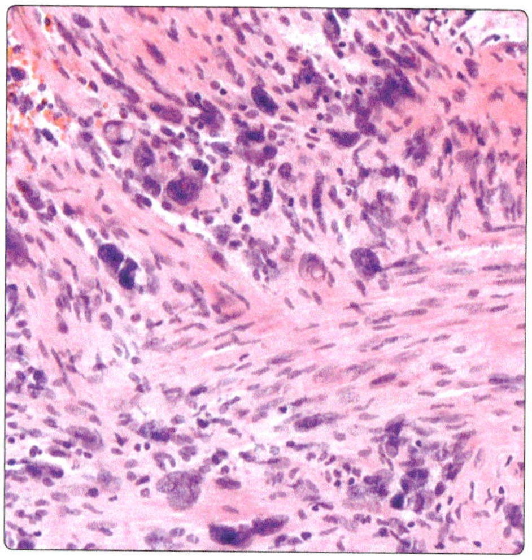

(Left) *Ancient change in a schwannoma may be very prominent in some cases, mostly in Antoni B areas but even in Antoni A zones. This finding may lead one to suspect malignancy; however, mitoses are discrepantly rare, and there is no tumor necrosis.* **(Right)** *At high magnification, the degenerative nuclei are often hyperchromatic and irregular with "smudgy" contours and may show nuclear vacuolization. Mitoses are inconspicuous or absent.*

Cellular Schwannoma Variant

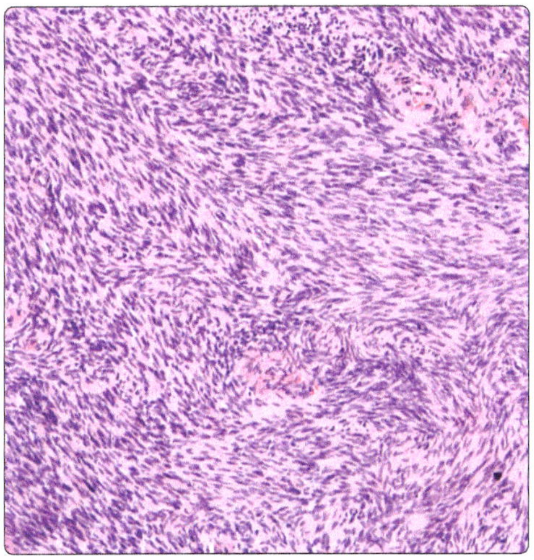

Short Fascicles and Whorls

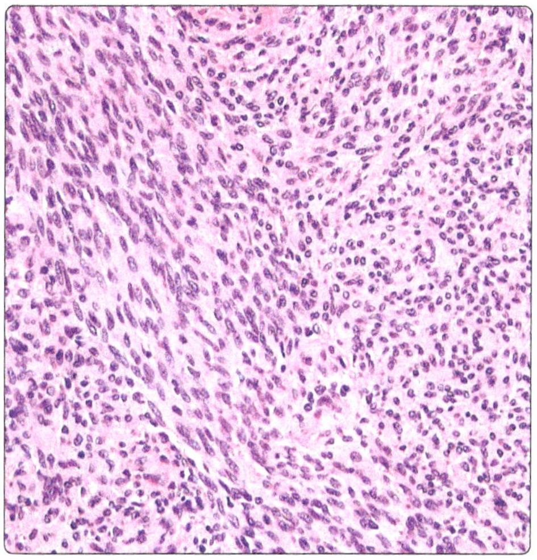

(Left) *The cellular variant of schwannoma is defined as being composed exclusively or predominantly of Antoni A zones. Focal Antoni B zones may be identified but usually do not comprise > 10% of the tumor.* **(Right)** *Cellular schwannoma often shows the formation of short fascicular or vague whorling architectures. Mitoses are more likely to be identified in this variant; however, they are generally not numerous.*

Stromal Collagen in Cellular Schwannoma

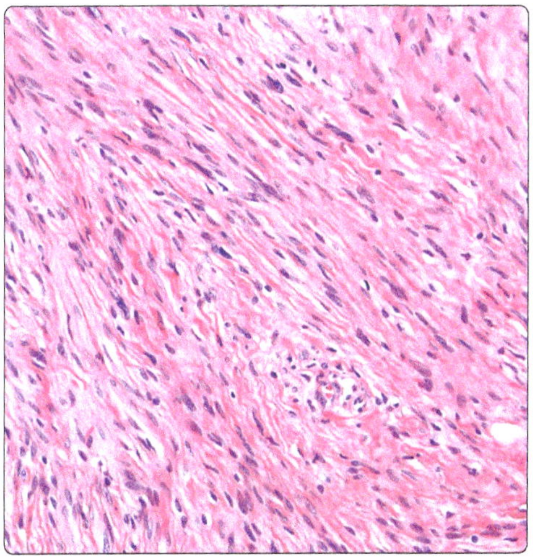

Rare Nuclear Palisading in Cellular Tumors

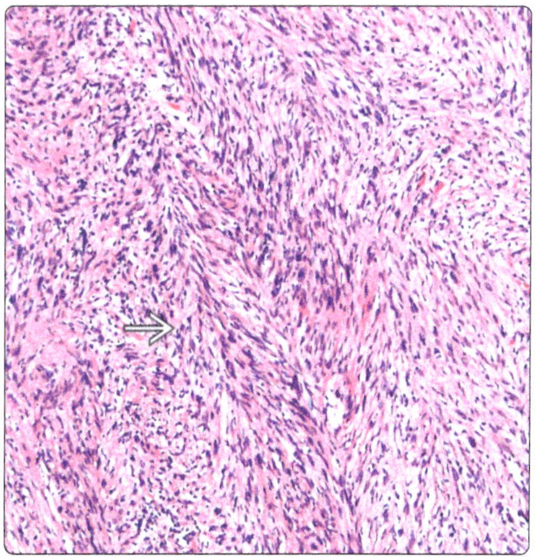

(Left) *Some examples of cellular schwannoma show increased stromal collagen and are overall more eosinophilic in appearance. Gastrointestinal schwannomas in particular routinely show this morphology.* **(Right)** *In contrast to Antoni A zones in conventional schwannoma, those of cellular schwannoma often lack distinct nuclear palisading and Verocay body formation. Rare herringbone fascicular architecture ➔ may be identified in some cases.*

Microtrabecular Pattern in Cellular Schwannoma

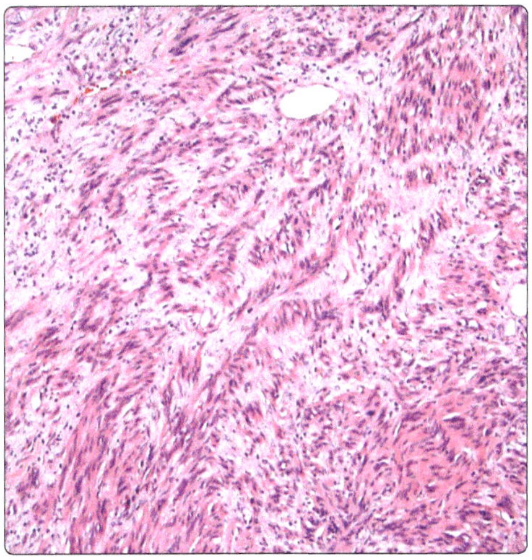

Collections of Foamy Histiocytes

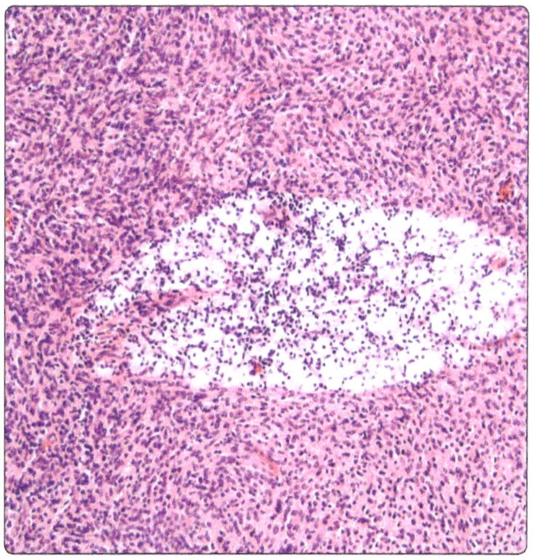

(Left) *A microtrabecular architecture is another interesting and recurrent pattern that can be seen in cellular schwannoma. It is characterized by discrete, small clusters or rows of spindled Schwann cells.* **(Right)** *Collections or aggregates of foamy histiocytes are a common finding in cellular schwannoma and can be diagnostically helpful in identifying this particular variant.*

Lymphoid Aggregates Common

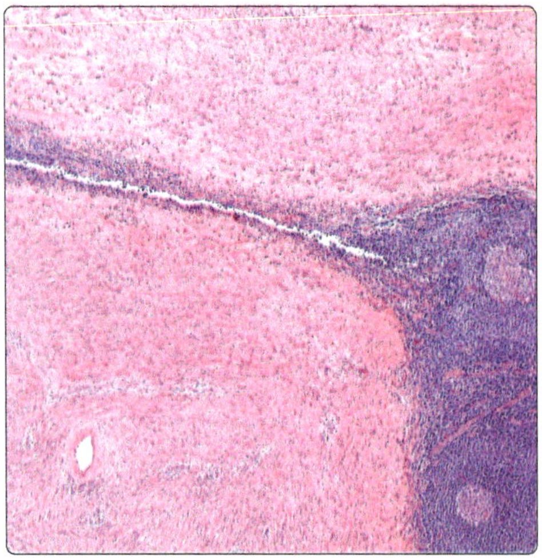

Plexiform Schwannoma Variant

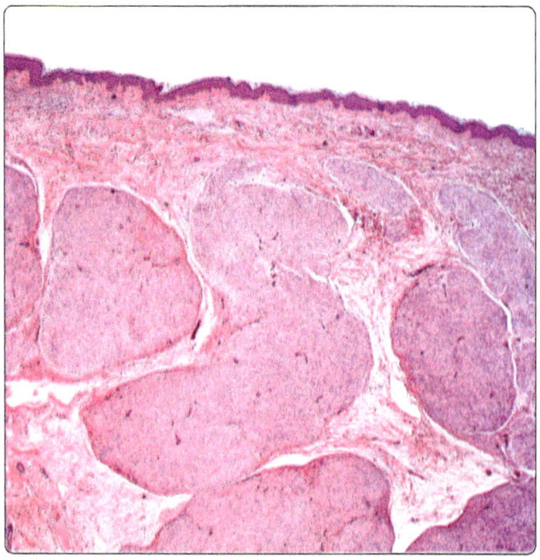

(Left) *Lymphoid aggregates are a very common and characteristic feature of most cellular schwannomas. These aggregates are often subcapsular, pericapsular, or intratumoral and may show reactive germinal center formation.* **(Right)** *The plexiform variant of schwannoma has a distinct multinodular or serpentine growth pattern. It shows a predilection for the skin and is rarely at deep sites. Unlike plexiform neurofibroma, plexiform schwannoma is not diagnostic of neurofibromatosis type 1.*

Plexiform Schwannoma With Palisading

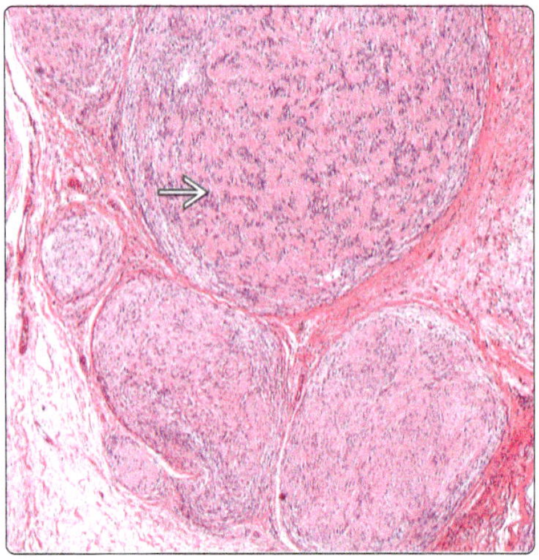

Plexiform Schwannoma Without Palisading

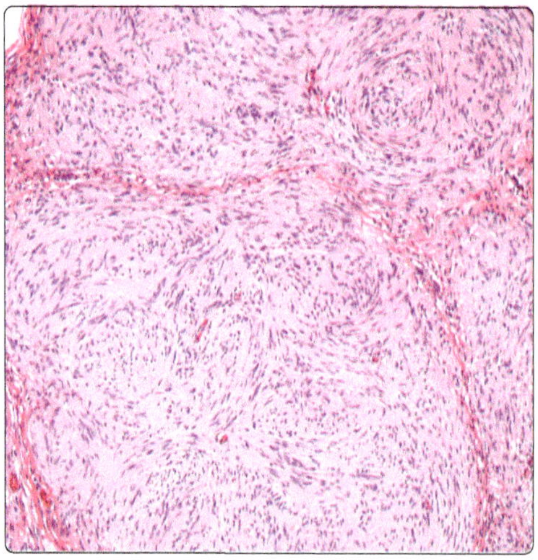

(Left) *Plexiform schwannoma generally contains minimal Antoni B and therefore has an overall cellular appearance. Typical features of Antoni A, including nuclear palisading* ➡*, may be seen.* **(Right)** *Some examples of plexiform schwannoma may show diffuse cellularity without nuclear palisading. In the context of a plexiform growth pattern, this appearance may lead to misdiagnosis of malignant peripheral nerve sheath tumor in a plexiform neurofibroma; however, mitotic activity is low and there is no tumor necrosis.*

Epithelioid Schwannoma Variant

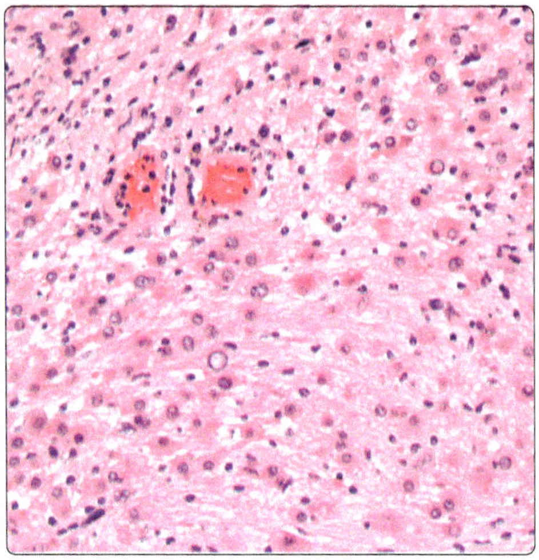

Epithelioid Schwannoma With Clusters of Small Cells

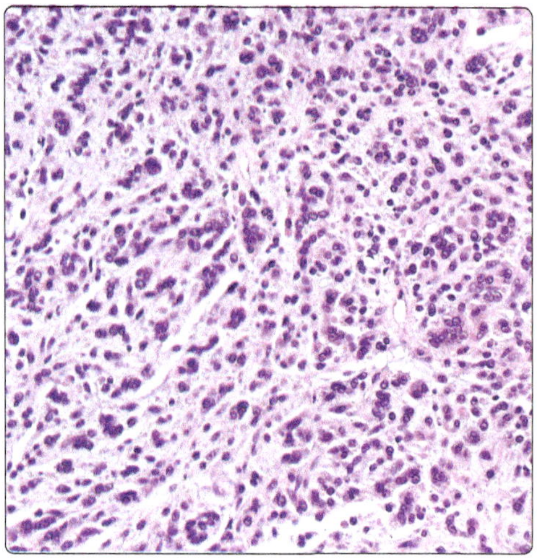

(Left) *Epithelioid cellular change in a schwannoma is seen focally in many cases. Rarely, this morphology may be diffuse and warrant classification as an epithelioid schwannoma.* **(Right)** *Epithelioid schwannoma may show clusters of small, bland tumor cells in small clusters or linear arrays within a myxoid matrix. Mitotic figures are rare or absent.*

Bland Nuclei in Epithelioid Tumors

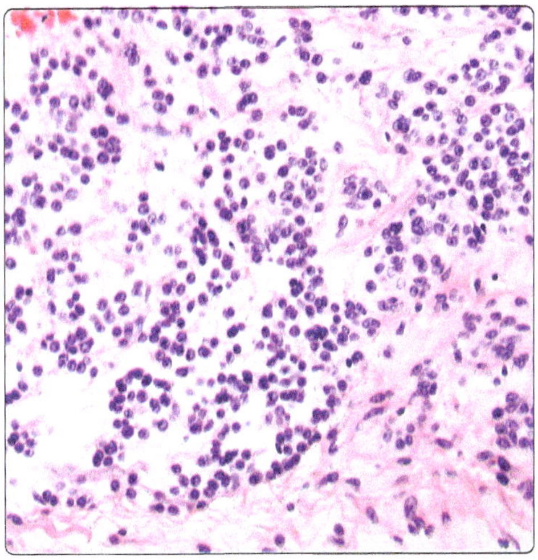

Mixed Epithelioid and Spindled Cells

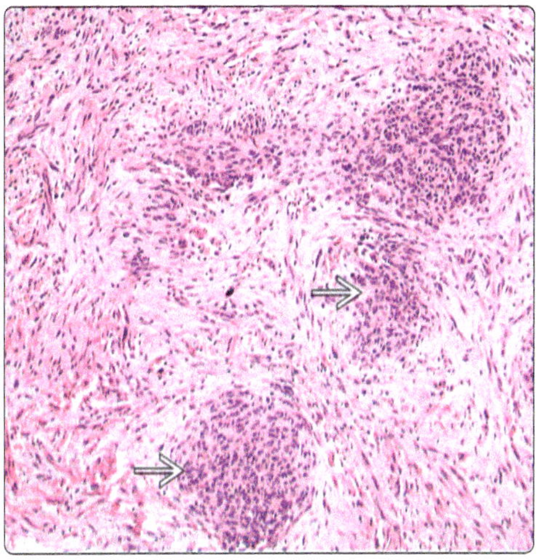

(Left) *Cytologically, the cells of epithelioid schwannoma are generally small and show bland nuclei. Features of epithelioid malignant peripheral nerve sheath tumor, including enlarged nuclei with prominent macronucleoli and conspicuous mitoses, are not seen.* **(Right)** *Foci of epithelioid Schwann cells* ➡ *may be seen in the background of an otherwise typical spindle cell schwannoma.*

Pseudoglandular Spaces in Schwannoma

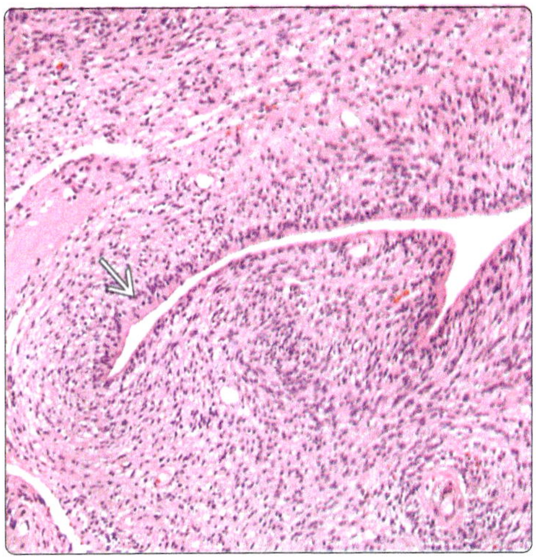

Schwann Cell Lining Resembles Gland Formation

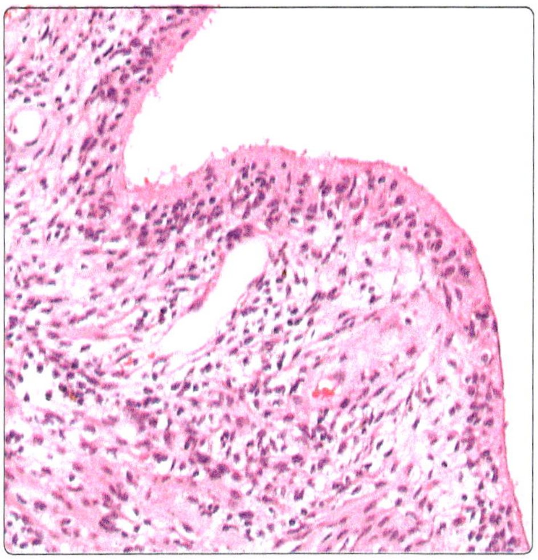

(Left) *Schwannomas with cystic change may show a lining* ➡ *that is very reminiscent of glandular epithelium. This lining is clearly schwannian, as evidenced by strong S100 expression and negative keratin staining. Also, there is an absence of intracytoplasmic mucin.* **(Right)** *The basal polarity of the Schwann cell nuclei lining the cystic spaces helps impart a pseudoglandular appearance.*

Pseudoglandular Schwannoma Variant

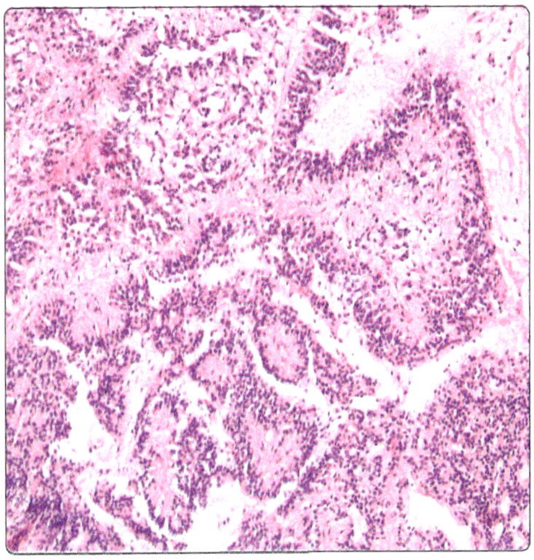

Neuroblastoma-Like Schwannoma Variant

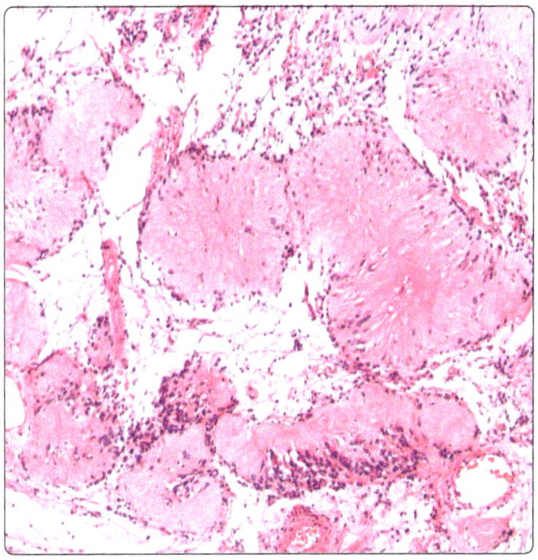

(Left) *In some rare cases of schwannoma, the pseudoglandular change is extensive or predominant, warranting classification as a pseudoglandular schwannoma. Other areas of more typical schwannoma are often present.* **(Right)** *Variably sized, hyalinized, rosette-like structures lined by peripheral Schwann cell nuclei are a rare finding in schwannoma and may be numerous.*

(Left) *The neuroblastoma-like rosettes seen in rare cases of schwannoma are formed by rounded Schwann cells radially oriented around a collagen core. The nuclei of these cells are cytologically banal.* **(Right)** *In some cases of neuroblastoma-like schwannoma, the rosette structures are formed around what appear to be tiny vascular channels* ⇒.

Radial Cellular Arrangement in Rosettes

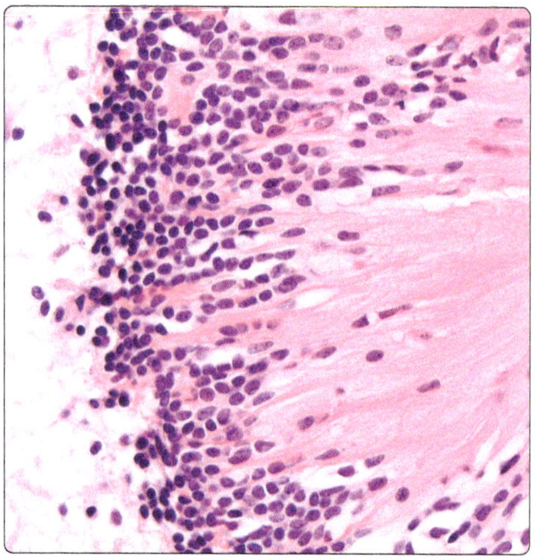

Focal Perivascular Arrangement

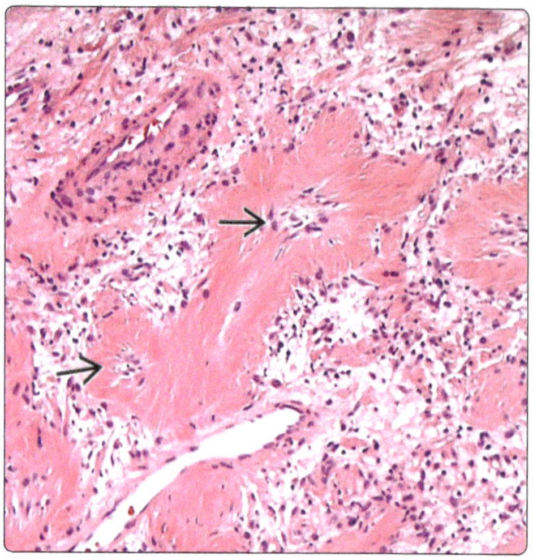

(Left) *The radially oriented cells of neuroblastoma-like schwannoma may rarely be spindled rather than epithelioid, warranting consideration of low-grade fibromyxoid sarcoma (hyalinizing spindle cell tumor with giant rosette morphology).* **(Right)** *Rare cases of schwannoma show a striking reticular growth pattern in a myxoid to hyalinized stroma. This morphology may be predominant or associated with areas of more conventional schwannoma morphology.*

Rosettes With Spindled Cells in Schwannoma

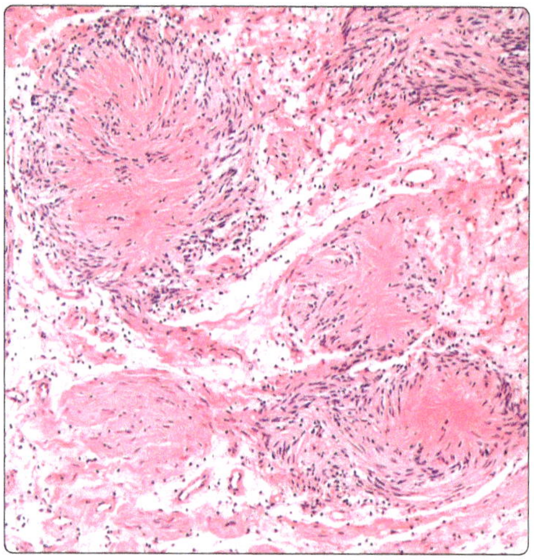

Microcystic/Reticular Schwannoma Variant

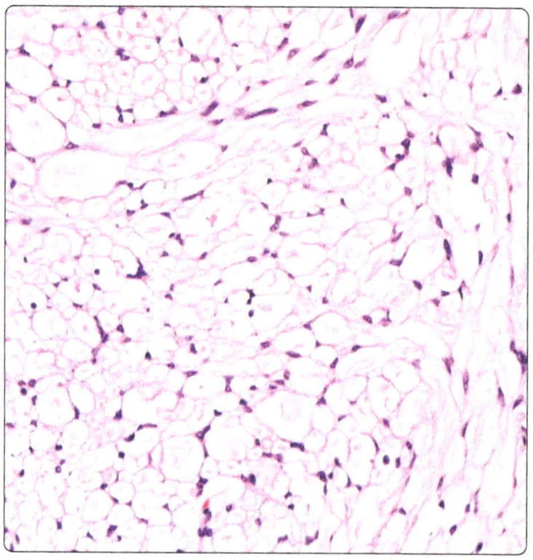

(Left) *The cytoplasmic eosinophilia is more conspicuous in this example of microcystic/reticular schwannoma.* **(Right)** *Microcyst formation* ⇒ *may also be identified in association with the reticular morphology in some schwannomas. Similar to other forms of schwannoma, this morphologic variant strongly and diffusely expresses S100.*

Cytoplasmic Eosinophilia in Reticular Schwannoma

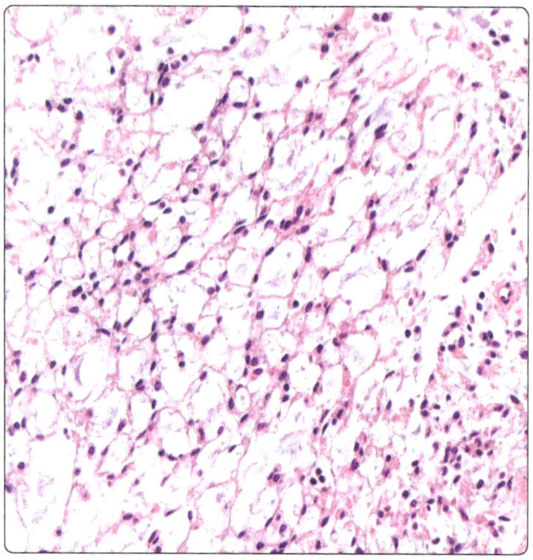

Microcyst Formation

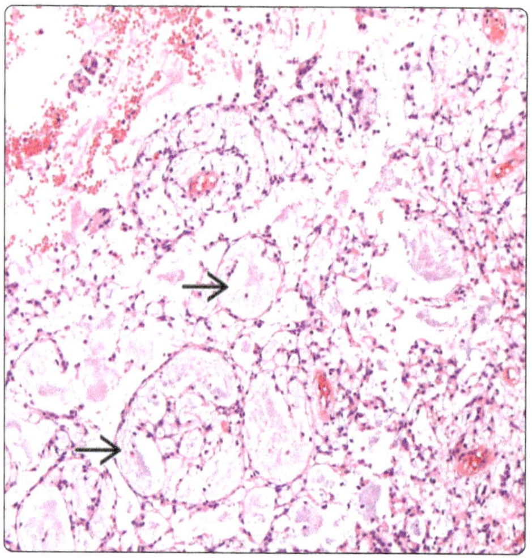

Focal Microcystic/Reticular Change in Otherwise Typical Schwannoma

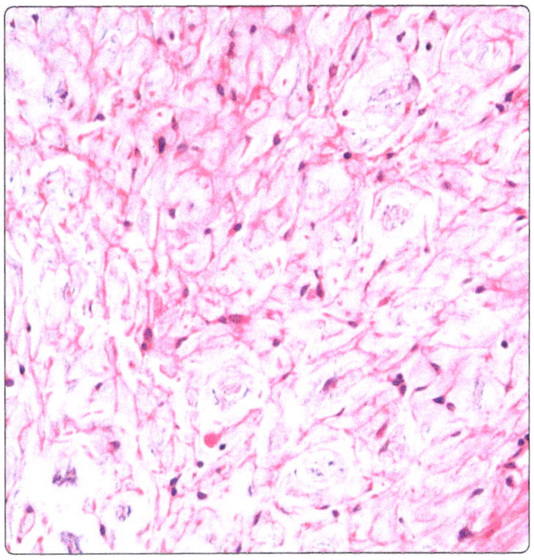

Rare Presence of Eosinophilic Granular Bodies

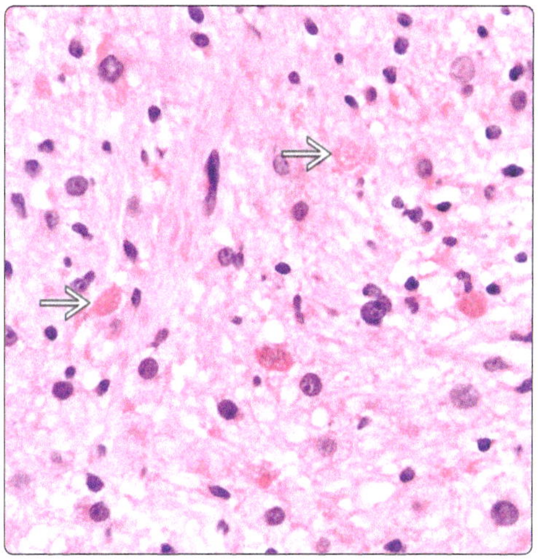

(Left) *This case of schwannoma shows small focal areas demonstrating reticulated growth within a myxoid stroma intermixed with areas of more conventional schwannoma.* **(Right)** *Eosinophilic, granular body-like structures ➡ are a rare finding in schwannoma but appear to be more prevalent in schwannomas of the vestibulocochlear nerve (acoustic schwannoma), along with Rosenthal fibers.*

Unusual Case of Schwannoma With Hemangioma

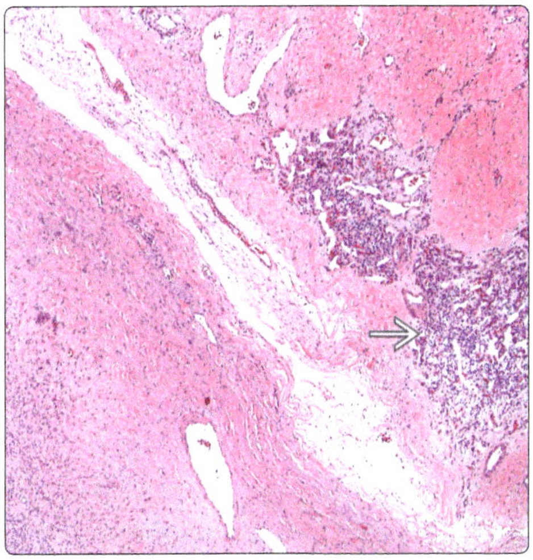

Direct Association With Nerve

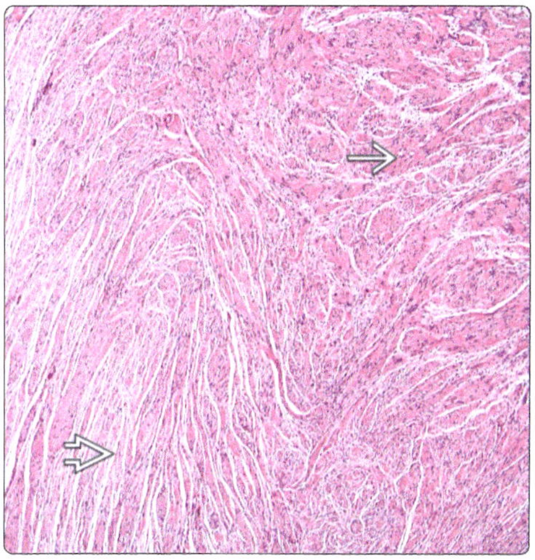

(Left) *This unusual case of schwannoma was associated with an adjacent benign capillary hemangioma ➡ that arose in the epineurium of an adjacent nerve.* **(Right)** *Occasionally, a small or incipient schwannoma may be detected intraoperatively as a small nodule growing on an otherwise unremarkable nerve. This image shows the tumor ➡ arising in a background of peripheral nerve ⇨.*

Adjacent Ganglion in Schwannoma Mimicking Ganglioneuroma

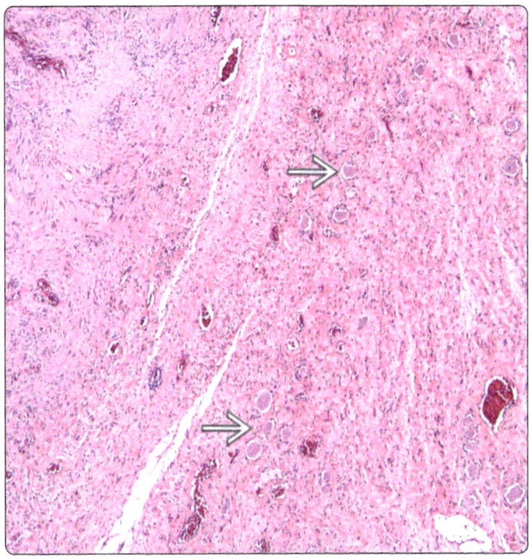

Very Rare Malignant Change in Schwannoma

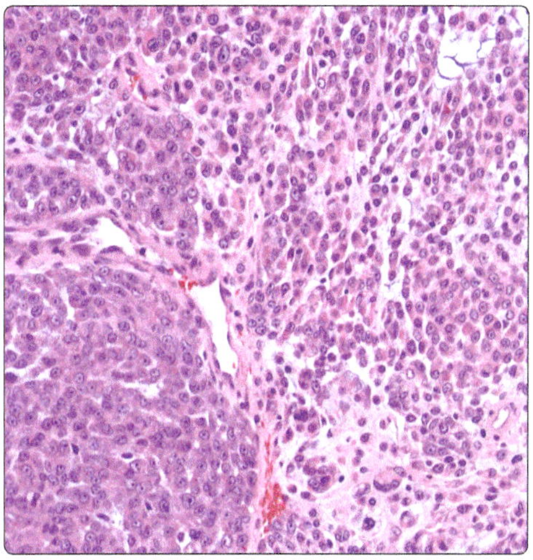

(Left) *Schwannomas that arise in the immediate vicinity of a ganglion will often show scattered collections of benign ganglion cells ➡ in or adjacent to the peripheral capsule. This pattern differs from a true ganglioneuroma, in which ganglion cells are widely scattered throughout the tumor.* **(Right)** *Malignant change in schwannoma is an extremely rare event. Most well-documented cases of this transformation are in the form of an epithelioid malignant peripheral nerve sheath tumor (pictured) or epithelioid angiosarcoma.*

Cellular Neurothekeoma

KEY FACTS

TERMINOLOGY

- Rare dermal tumor of uncertain histogenesis composed of epithelioid cells in multiple nests divided by fibrous septa
- Unrelated to dermal nerve sheath myxoma (conventional neurothekeoma)

CLINICAL ISSUES

- Children & young adults (mean age: 25 years)
- Head/neck & upper extremity (most on face & shoulder)
- Benign (even if atypical histologic features)

MICROSCOPIC

- Epithelioid to spindled cells with abundant pale eosinophilic cytoplasm arranged in nests divided by dense fibrous septa
- Myxoid change common (30%)
- Multinucleated giant cells (osteoclastic or Touton)
- Nuclear atypia/pleomorphism in 25%
- Mitotic activity common (mean: 3/10 HPF, range: 0-22)
    - Subset have brisk mitotic activity (> 5/10 HPF in 20%; > 10/10 HPF in 5%)
    - Atypical mitotic figures may be seen

ANCILLARY TESTS

- Often positive for variety of nonspecific markers, including NKI/C3, NSE, PGP9.5
    - No specific positive IHC marker
- Negative for S100 & SOX10
    - Most important IHC; essentially excludes melanocytic tumor

TOP DIFFERENTIAL DIAGNOSES

- Spitz nevus or spitzoid melanoma
- Dermal nerve sheath myxoma (conventional neurothekeoma)
- Plexiform fibrohistiocytic tumor
- Epithelioid cutaneous fibrous histiocytoma

Cellular Neurothekeoma

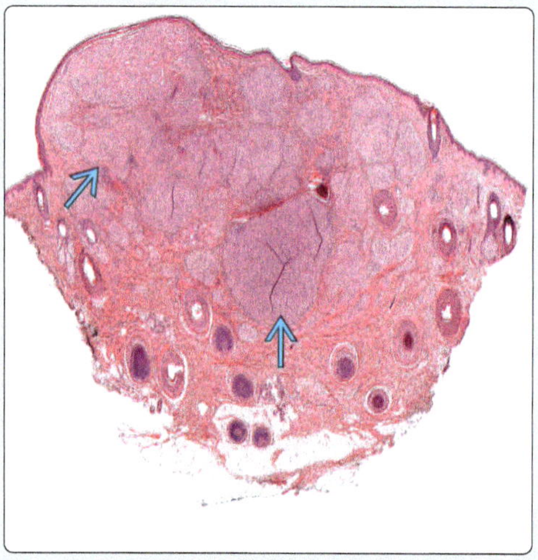

Nests and Aggregates of Tumor Cells

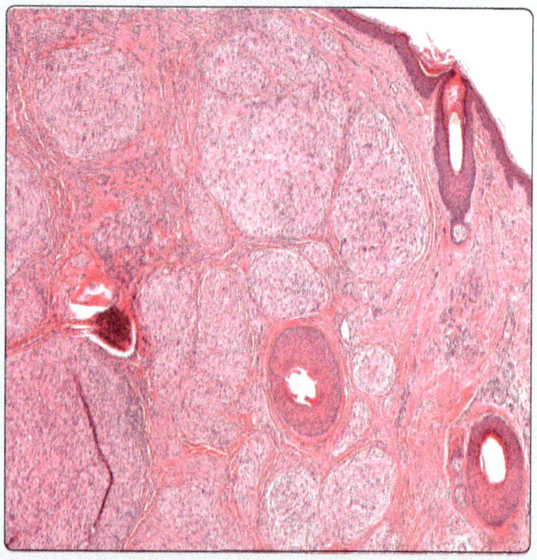

(Left) *Cellular neurothekeoma is a benign tumor of uncertain histogenesis that typically presents as a multilobular tumor ➡ centered in the dermis.* **(Right)** *Cellular neurothekeoma is generally characterized by multiple nests or aggregates of histiocytoid tumor cells divided by intervening fibrous bands.*

Bland Histiocytoid Cells in Cellular Neurothekeoma

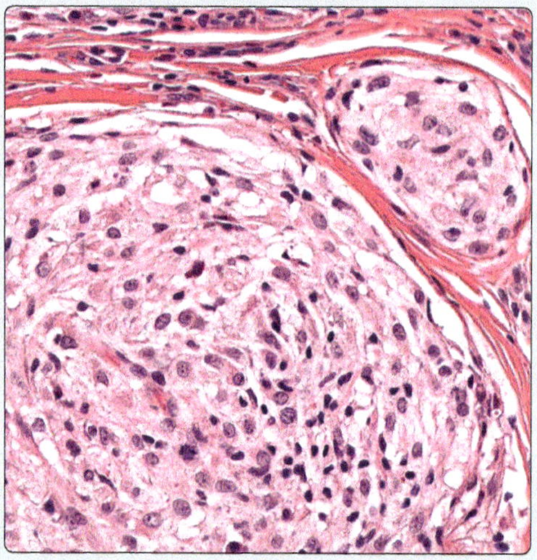

Atypia and Mitotic Activity in Cellular Neurothekeoma

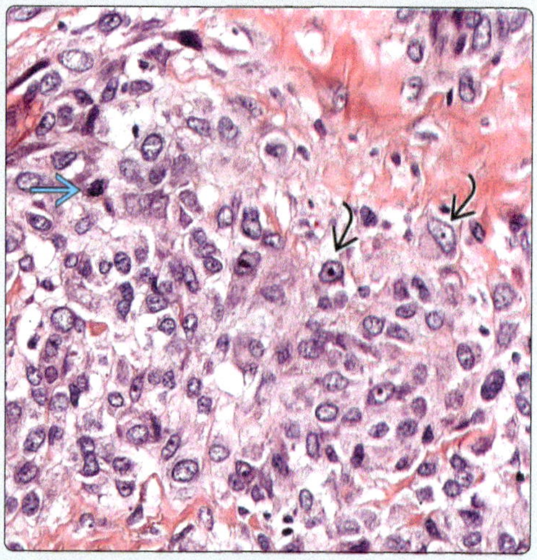

(Left) *The nests are composed of histiocytoid cells with abundant pale cytoplasm and uniform-appearing, round nuclei.* **(Right)** *Nuclear atypia ➔ and pleomorphism are seen in 25% of cellular neurothekeoma and do not indicate aggressive behavior. Mitotic activity ➡ is common and may even be brisk.*

TERMINOLOGY

Definitions

- Rare dermal tumor of uncertain histogenesis composed of epithelioid cells in nests divided by fibrous septa
- Unrelated to dermal nerve sheath myxoma (conventional neurothekeoma)

CLINICAL ISSUES

Site

- Head/neck & upper extremity (most on face & shoulder)

Presentation

- Children & young adults (mean: 25 years; most < 40 years)
- Painless solitary skin nodule, often present > 1 year
  - Rarely agminated (cluster of multiple lesions in 1 site)

Treatment

- Simple but complete excision

Prognosis

- Benign (even if atypical histologic features)
- Small subset recur, especially if incompletely excised

MACROSCOPIC

General Features

- Rounded or dome-shaped skin lesion, usually > 2 cm

MICROSCOPIC

Histologic Features

- Micronodular or lobulated dermal tumor
  - No epidermal involvement
  - Usually has infiltrative borders
  - 50% also involve subcutis
- Epithelioid to spindled cells with abundant pale, eosinophilic cytoplasm, arranged in nests divided by dense fibrous septa
- Plexiform or focally sheet-like growth pattern sometimes
- Myxoid change common (30%)
  - Spindling more prominent in myxoid areas; may resemble pattern of dermal nerve sheath myxoma
- Multinucleated giant cells (osteoclastic or Touton) in some cases
- Nuclear atypia/pleomorphism in 25%
  - Atypical multinucleated tumor giant cells may be seen
- Mitotic activity common (mean: 3 mitoses/10 HPF; range: 0-22 mitoses)
  - Subset have brisk mitotic activity (> 5/10 HPF in 20%; > 10/10 HPF in 5% of cases)
  - Atypical mitotic figures may be seen
- Lymphovascular or perineural invasion rarely seen
- Necrosis also rarely seen

ANCILLARY TESTS

Immunohistochemistry

- Often positive for variety of nonspecific markers
  - NKI/C3, NSE, MITF, PGP9.5 (most cases)
  - SMA, p63 (~ 1/2 of cases)
  - Lack of specificity limits utility of these stains
- No specific positive IHC marker
- Negative for S100 & SOX10
  - Most important IHC; essentially excludes melanocytic
- Also negative: MART-1, HMB-45, desmin, keratin

DIFFERENTIAL DIAGNOSIS

Spitz Nevus or Spitzoid Melanoma

- Small skin nodule, sometimes nonpigmented, on face or extremity of young patients
- Nests of epithelioid to spindled cells with abundant eosinophilic cytoplasm
- Often have intraepidermal component
- S100(+), SOX10(+), MART-1(+), HMB-45(+)
- Cellular neurothekeoma should always be in differential of **intradermal** atypical spitzoid lesion, especially on face of child or young adult
  - Atypical spitzoid lesions often treated with wider excision ± sentinel lymph node biopsy; sometimes behave aggressively
  - S100 & Melan-A/MART-1 can easily distinguish

Dermal Nerve Sheath Myxoma (Conventional Neurothekeoma)

- Skin nodule of middle-aged adults
- Vast majority on distal extremities (especially fingers)
- Circumscribed, multilobulated dermal tumor
- Hypocellular myxoid nodules with strands of spindle cells
- Nodules divided by fibrous septa
- S100(+) in 100% of cases

Plexiform Fibrohistiocytic Tumor

- Skin nodule on extremities of children & young adults
- Plexiform pattern of multiple small nodules infiltrating deep dermis & subcutis
- Nodules composed of round histiocytoid cells ± multinucleated giant cells
  - Similar to nested pattern of cellular neurothekeoma
- Usually has fascicles of spindled fibroblasts
- Usually lacks dense collagen septa

Epithelioid Cell Histiocytoma

- Often polypoid nodule with epidermal collarette
- Epithelioid histiocytoid cells arranged in sheet (not nests)
- Overlying epidermal hyperplasia
- Usually negative for MITF

SELECTED REFERENCES

1. Navarrete-Dechent C et al: Cellular neurothekeoma: case report and its (un) relation with nerve sheath myxoma. An Bras Dermatol. 90(3 Suppl 1):156-9, 2015
2. Fried I et al: SOX-10 and MiTF expression in cellular and 'mixed' neurothekeoma. J Cutan Pathol. 41(8):640-5, 2014
3. Linos K et al: Benign cutaneous biphasic hybrid tumor of perineurioma and cellular neurothekeoma: a case report expanding the clinical and histopathologic features of a recently described entity. Am J Dermatopathol. 37(4):319-22, 2015
4. Yun SJ et al: Myxoid cellular neurothekeoma: a new entity of S100-negative, CD68-positive myxoid neurothekeoma. Ann Dermatol. 26(4):510-3, 2014
5. Stratton J et al: Cellular neurothekeoma: analysis of 37 cases emphasizing atypical histologic features. Mod Pathol. Epub ahead of print, 2013
6. Cardoso J et al: Cellular neurothekeoma with perineural extension: a potential diagnostic pitfall. J Cutan Pathol. 39(6):662-4, 2012
7. Hornick JL et al: Cellular neurothekeoma: detailed characterization in a series of 133 cases. Am J Surg Pathol. 31(3):329-40, 2007

Cellular Neurothekeoma at Low Magnification Showing Dome-Shaped Nodule

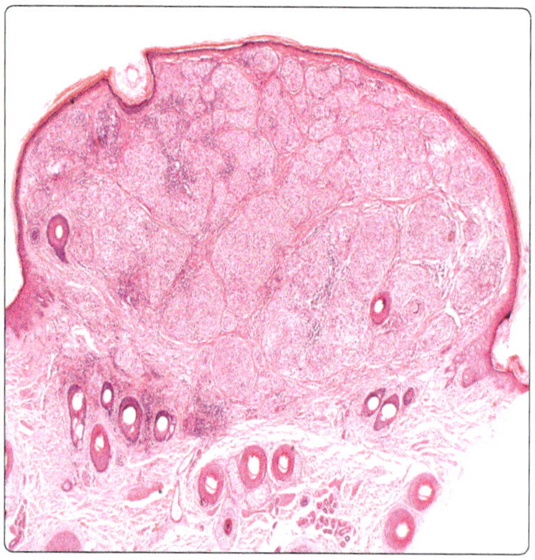

Higher Magnification Showing Nested Growth Pattern

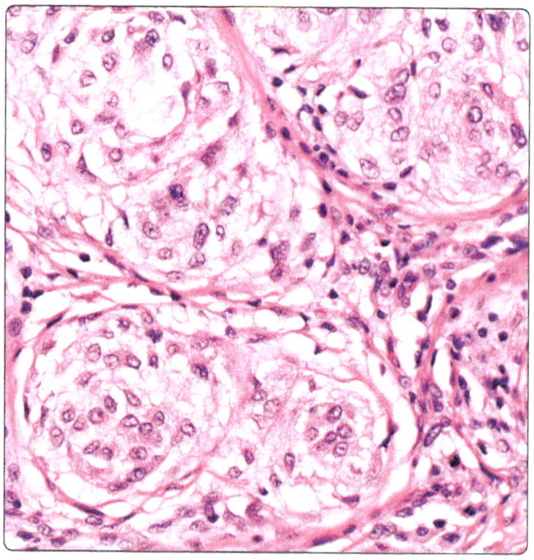

(Left) *Nests of tumor cells fill the dermis forming a dome-shaped nodule in this low-power image of cellular neurothekeoma.* **(Right)** *Nests of histiocytoid cells are separated by thin fibrous septa. The cells have uniform nuclei, moderate amounts of cytoplasm, and variably distinct cell margins in this case.*

Myxoid Change in Cellular Neurothekeoma

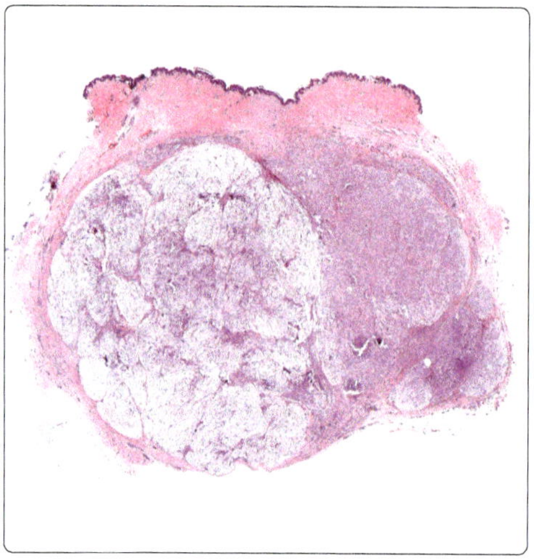

Myxoid Areas Mimicking Nerve Sheath Myxoma

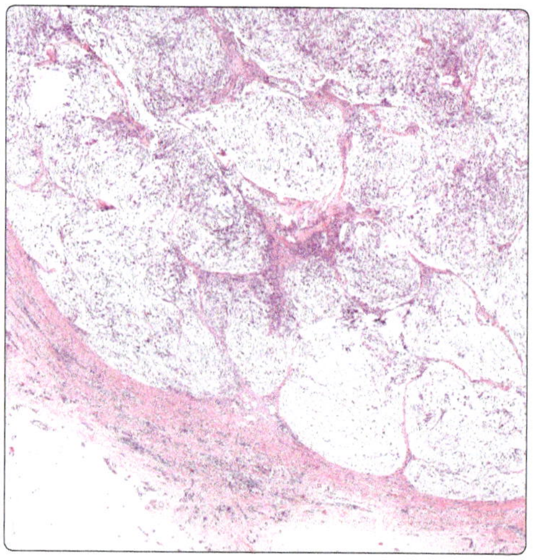

(Left) *Myxoid change is present in ~ 30% of cases of cellular neurothekeoma and may be prominent, as seen here.* **(Right)** *Areas of myxoid change in cellular neurothekeoma may be arranged into myxoid nodules with intervening fibrous septa, an appearance very similar to that of dermal nerve sheath myxoma (conventional neurothekeoma), which is an unrelated entity.*

Myxoid and Nonmyxoid Zones

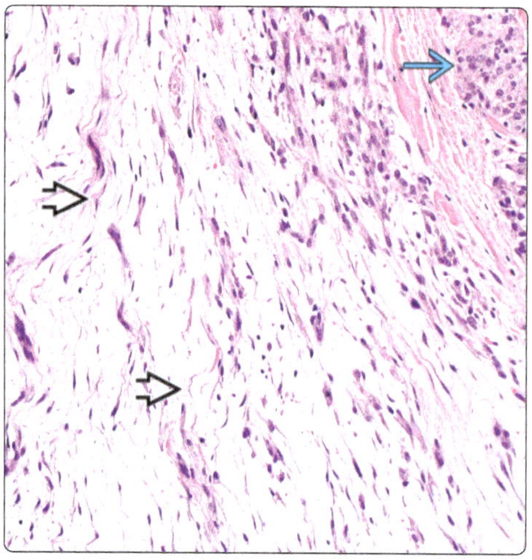

Multinucleated Tumor Giant Cells

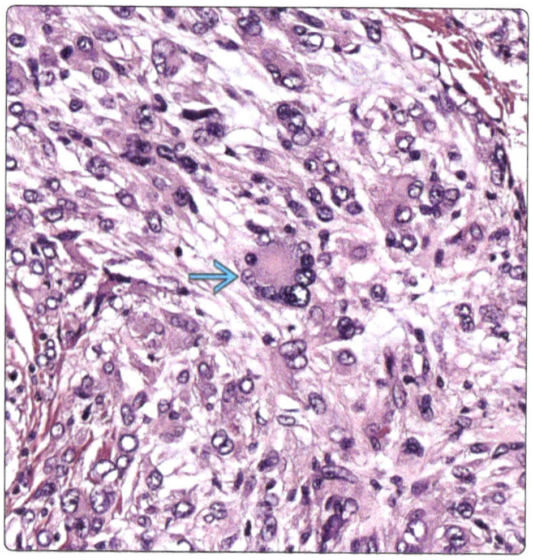

(Left) *Nests of typical nonmyxoid cellular neurothekeoma → transition to myxoid spindled zones resembling nerve sheath myxoma ⇨ in this case.* **(Right)** *Atypical multinucleated tumor giant cells may be present → in cellular neurothekeoma. This is a benign finding not indicative of aggressive behavior. Classic Touton or osteoclastic giant cells may also be seen.*

Atypia in Cellular Neurothekeoma

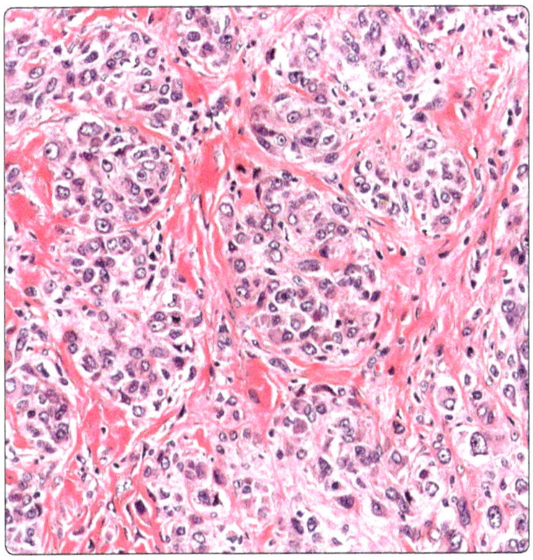

Mitotic Activity Common in Cellular Neurothekeoma

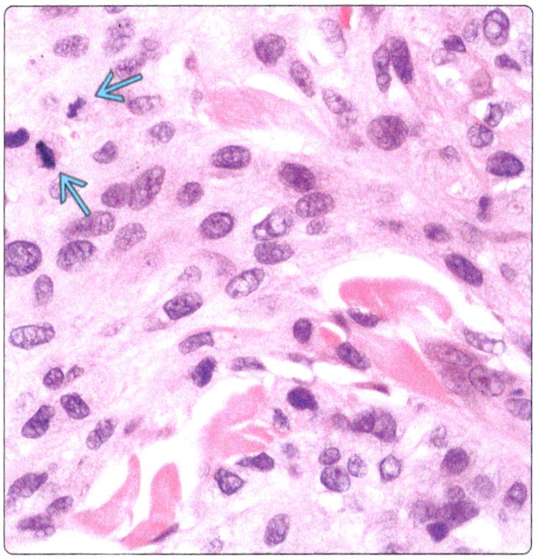

(Left) *This image shows a case of cellular neurothekeoma that has typical nests of tumor cells but with the additional feature of cellular atypia. This finding has no clinical significance.* **(Right)** *Mitotic activity ⇨ is common in cellular neurothekeoma and may be brisk (up to or greater than 10 figures/10 HPF).*

Nuclear Pleomorphism in Cellular Neurothekeoma

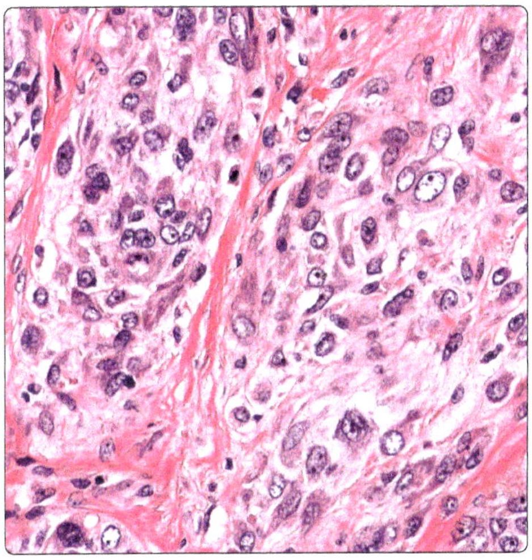

Subcutaneous Involvement in Cellular Neurothekeoma

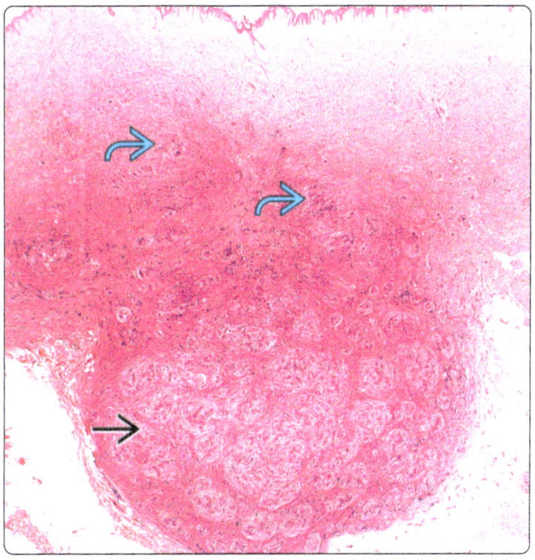

(Left) *Nuclear pleomorphism is a relatively common finding in cellular neurothekeoma and does not appear to alter the benign behavior of the lesion.* **(Right)** *Subcutaneous involvement ⇨ is present in 50% of cases of cellular neurothekeoma. Note the several small, discrete nests ⇨ of tumor cells in the overlying dermis.*

Sheet-Like Growth Pattern

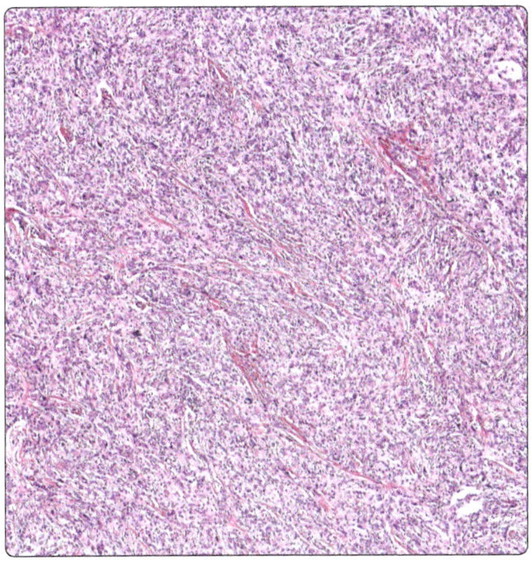

Spindle Cell Areas

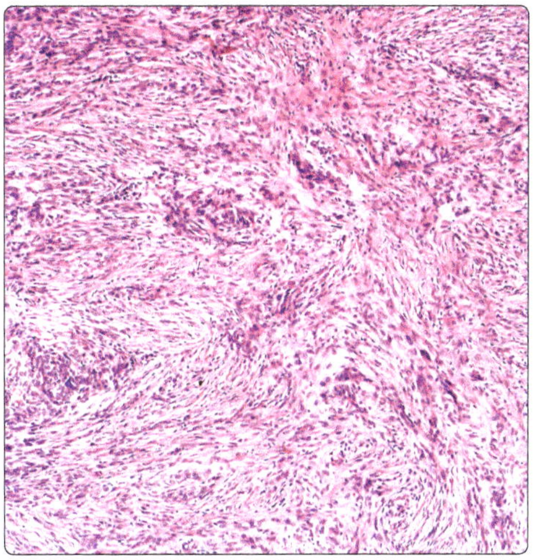

(Left) *Areas of cellular sheet-like growth without nesting may be seen in occasional cases of cellular neurothekeoma, as depicted here. More conventional nested or nodular areas are typically seen elsewhere.* **(Right)** *Sheets or fascicles of more spindled tumor cells are occasionally encountered in cellular neurothekeoma.*

KEY FACTS

TERMINOLOGY

- Benign cutaneous nerve sheath tumor with Schwann cell differentiation, abundant myxoid matrix, and well-defined lobular architecture

CLINICAL ISSUES

- Fingers and hand most common sites
  - Pretibial skin also common
  - Uncommon on face
- Benign but up to 50% recur
- Rare intraoral, orbital, intradural, and paraspinal cases

MICROSCOPIC

- Multiple lobules with abundant myxoid matrix
- Well-defined lobular architecture and dense fibrous septa
- Usually limited to dermis and subcutis
- Spindle-shaped and epithelioid cells
- Interconnecting cords, networks, syncytial nests, ring-like structures
- Stellate and vacuolated cells common
- No atypia, very low mitotic rate

ANCILLARY TESTS

- Diffuse S100(+)
- GFAP(+) in most
- SMA, desmin, CD68, HMB-45, synaptophysin, chromogranin-A, CD31 (-)

TOP DIFFERENTIAL DIAGNOSES

- Neurothekeoma
- Superficial angiomyxoma
- Digital mucoid cyst
- Myxoid neurofibroma
- Superficial acral fibromyxoma
- Myxoid dermatofibrosarcoma protuberans
- Myxofibrosarcoma (low grade)

Dermal Papule

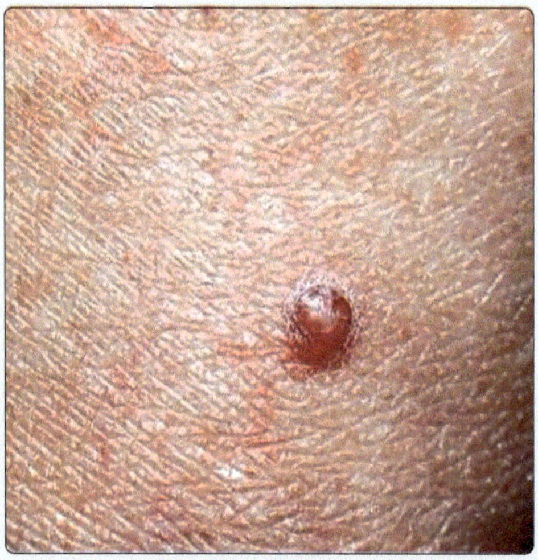

Dermal Nerve Sheath Myxoma

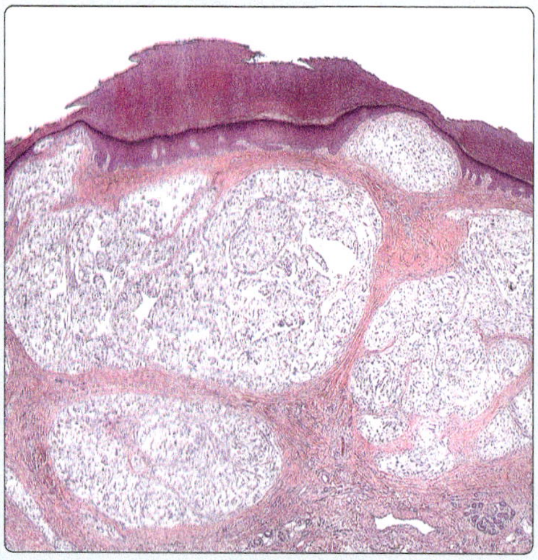

(Left) *Dermal nerve sheath myxoma typically presents as a firm papule that varies from 0.5-4.5 cm in size. It usually occurs in adults. Common locations are the finger, hand, and pretibial skin.* **(Right)** *Dermal nerve sheath myxoma has a very distinctive architecture, consisting of well-defined myxoid lobules. It is typically centered within the dermis and can involve the underlying subcutis as well.*

Composed of Schwann Cells

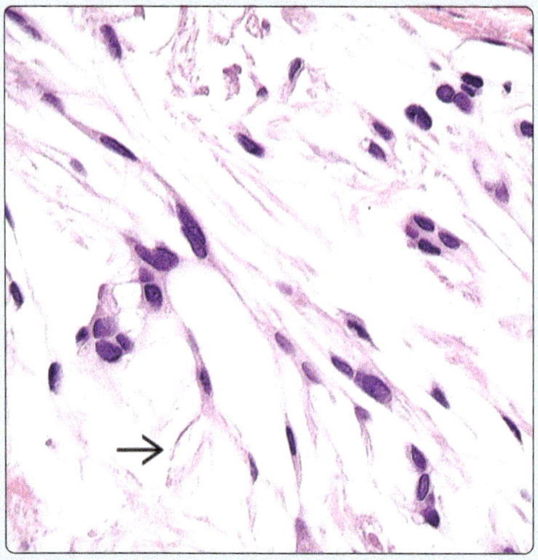

Strong, Diffuse S100 Expression

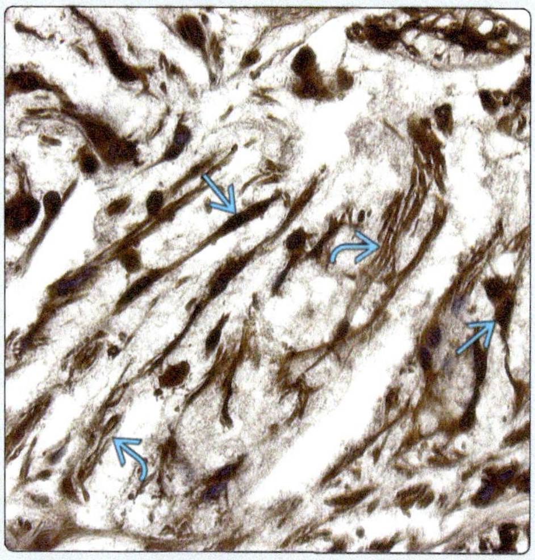

(Left) *The cells in dermal nerve sheath myxoma have schwannian differentiation. They have uniform spindle-shaped or oval nuclei, evenly distributed chromatin, and long fibrillary cytoplasmic processes ➔ forming bipolar and stellate configurations.* **(Right)** *Dermal nerve sheath myxomas are strongly S100(+) consonant with Schwann cell differentiation. This immunohistochemically stained section depicts diffuse and intense nuclear ➔ and cytoplasmic ↗ reactivity.*

TERMINOLOGY

Definitions

- Benign cutaneous nerve sheath tumor with Schwann cell differentiation, abundant myxoid matrix, and well-defined lobular architecture

CLINICAL ISSUES

Epidemiology

- Incidence
  - Rare; fewer than 100 reports
- Age
  - Mostly adults; median age: 34 years

Site

- Extremities
  - Fingers and hand most common
  - Pretibial skin common
- Rare intraoral, orbital, intradural, and paraspinal cases
- Uncommon on face

Presentation

- Slowly growing, painless mass

Prognosis

- Benign and nonaggressive but often excised with positive margins
  - Up to 50% recur

MACROSCOPIC

Size

- 0.5-4.5 cm

MICROSCOPIC

Histologic Features

- Multiple myxoid lobules
  - Well-defined borders separated by dense fibrous septa
- Usually limited to dermis and subcutis
- Paucicellular proliferation of bland spindle cells
  - Interconnecting cords, networks, syncytial nests, ring-like structures, Verocay-like bodies

Cytologic Features

- Spindle-shaped and epithelioid Schwann cells
- Stellate and vacuolated cells
- No atypia, very low mitotic rate

ANCILLARY TESTS

Immunohistochemistry

- Diffuse S100(+) in 100% of tumors
- GFAP(+) in most
- SMA, desmin, CD68, HMB-45, synaptophysin, chromogranin-A, CD31 (-)

DIFFERENTIAL DIAGNOSIS

Neurothekeoma

- Multinodular but less myxoid matrix and less-defined border
- Whorling pattern common
- Spindle and large plump epithelioid cells, ill-defined cytoplasm
- Lacks cords, syncytial aggregates, vacuolated cells
- S100(-)
- Predilection for face

Superficial Angiomyxoma

- Poorly circumscribed, extends into adjacent tissue
- Fibroblastic cells, often bi- or multinucleated
- Prominent vascularity; small, thin-walled, curvilinear, congested vessels
- Sparse dispersed inflammation, often neutrophils
- S100(-)

Cutaneous Myxoma in Carney Complex

- Indistinguishable from superficial angiomyxoma
- Predilection for ear, eyelid, nipple
- Spotty pigmentation, endocrine overactivity, psammomatous melanotic schwannoma

Digital Mucoid Cyst

- Extruded myxoid material, possibly from underlying joint
- Limited to fingers over dorsal aspect of distal interphalangeal joints

Myxoid Neurofibroma

- Small spindle cells with buckled, wavy nuclei and ill-defined cytoplasm
- Lacks lobular architecture; may be plexiform or diffuse
- Collagen bundles within myxoid stroma

Superficial Acral Fibromyxoma

- Variable fibrous and myxoid areas
- Lacks well-defined lobules
- CD34(+); S100(-)
- Acral extremities, often periungual

Myxoid Dermatofibrosarcoma Protuberans

- Storiform or fascicular, lacks lobular architecture
- Infiltrates subcutis, classic honeycomb pattern
- Plexiform vascular pattern
- CD34(+); S100(-)

Myxofibrosarcoma (Low Grade)

- Variable lobular architecture
- Infiltrative growth into dermis and subcutis
- Pleomorphism and mitotic figures in most cases
- S100(-)

SELECTED REFERENCES

1. Rozza-de-Menezes RE et al: Intraoral nerve sheath myxoma: case report and systematic review of the literature. Head Neck. 35(12):E397-404, 2013
2. Sheth S et al: Differential gene expression profiles of neurothekeomas and nerve sheath myxomas by microarray analysis. Mod Pathol. 24(3):343-54, 2011
3. Nishioka M et al: Nerve sheath myxoma (neurothekeoma) arising in the oral cavity: histological and immunohistochemical features of 3 cases. Oral Surg Oral Med Oral Pathol Oral Radiol Endod. 107(5):e28-33, 2009
4. Fetsch JF et al: Nerve sheath myxoma: a clinicopathologic and immunohistochemical analysis of 57 morphologically distinctive, S-100 protein- and GFAP-positive, myxoid peripheral nerve sheath tumors with a predilection for the extremities and a high local recurrence rate. Am J Surg Pathol. 29(12):1615-24, 2005

(Left) *This scanning-power micrograph of a dermal nerve sheath myxoma illustrates its well-defined lobular architecture composed of rounded lobules containing copious, pale blue myxoid matrix.* **(Right)** *The lobular architecture in dermal nerve sheath myxoma is defined by thick fibrous septa* [→]*, which separate the myxoid lobules* [↪].

Well-Defined Lobular Architecture

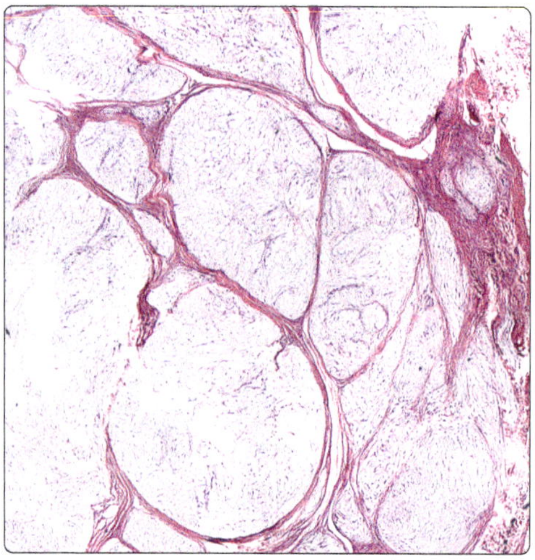

Lobules Divided by Fibrous Septa

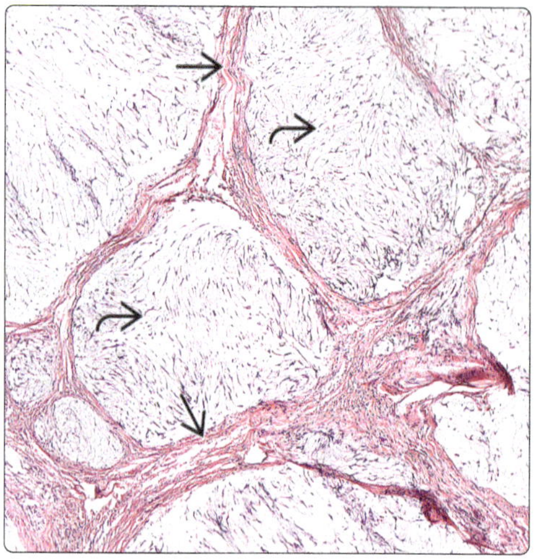

(Left) *This medium-power view of a dermal nerve sheath myxoma depicts a thick fibrous septum composed of dense, mature collagen* [→] *in between myxoid lobules.* **(Right)** *Verocay-like bodies consist of parallel arrays of spindle cells* [→] *surrounding a fine fibrillary matrix* [↪]*. Although rarely seen in dermal nerve sheath myxomas, they provide additional evidence of schwannian differentiation.*

Thick Fibrous Septa

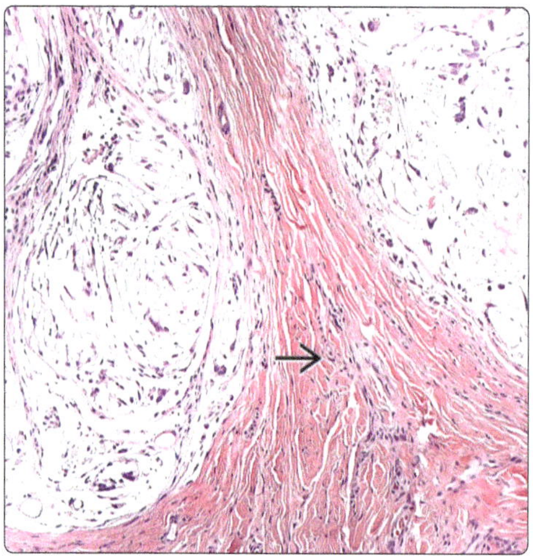

Verocay-Like Body Formed by Schwann Cells

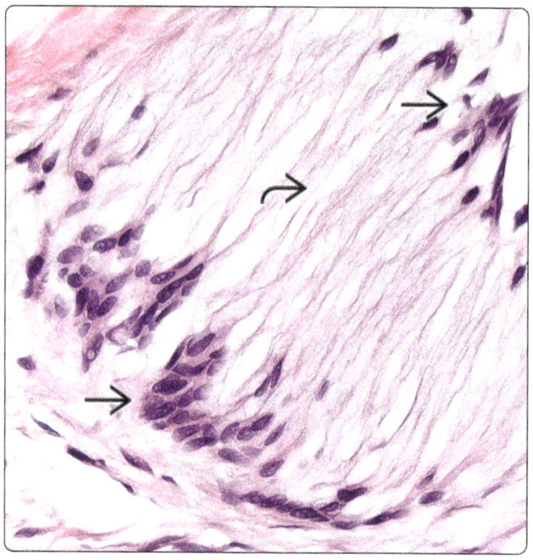

(Left) *The neoplastic cells of nerve sheath myxoma consist of spindle and epithelioid cells with uniform, bland, oval, and elongated nuclei and abundant eosinophilic cytoplasm. They are frequently arranged in syncytial nests and often have intracytoplasmic vacuoles* [→] *as depicted.* **(Right)** *The spindle cells may interconnect via elongated cytoplasmic processes to form ring-like structures* [→].

Syncytial Nests and Vacuoles

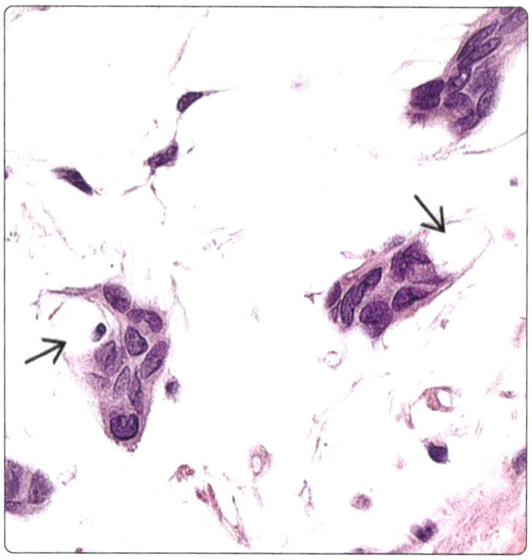

Ring-Like Cellular Structures

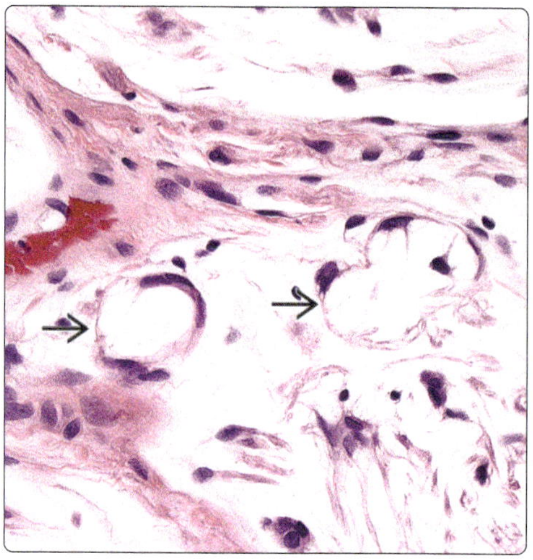

Nerve Sheath Myxoma at Low Power

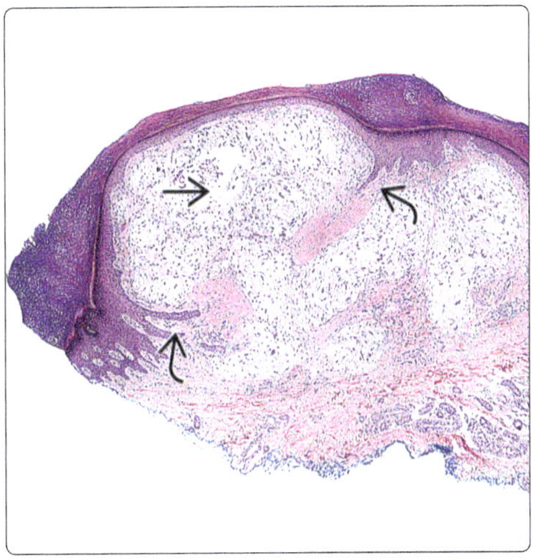

Cohesive Structures Within Myxoid Matrix

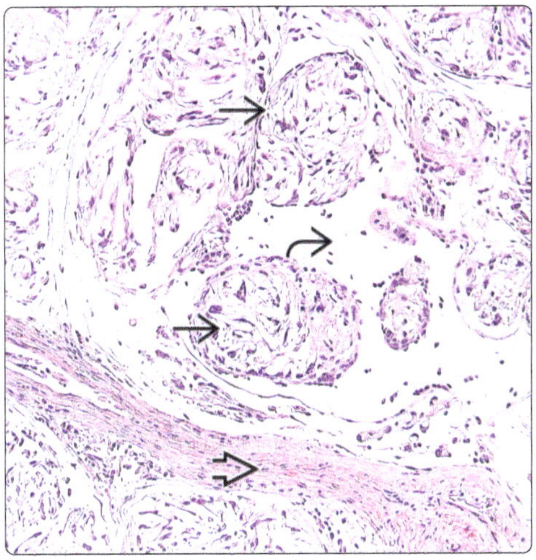

(Left) *This scanning-power micrograph depicts a dermal nerve sheath myxoma with a raised, exophytic pattern due to an expansile myxoid lobule* → *in the superficial dermis. Clinically, it presented as a papule. Note the peripheral epidermal collarette* ↷. **(Right)** *Dermal nerve sheath myxomas often form cohesive structures* → *floating within a myxoid matrix* ↷. *Note the thick fibrous septum at the bottom, which divides adjacent lobules* ⇨.

Reticulated Pattern

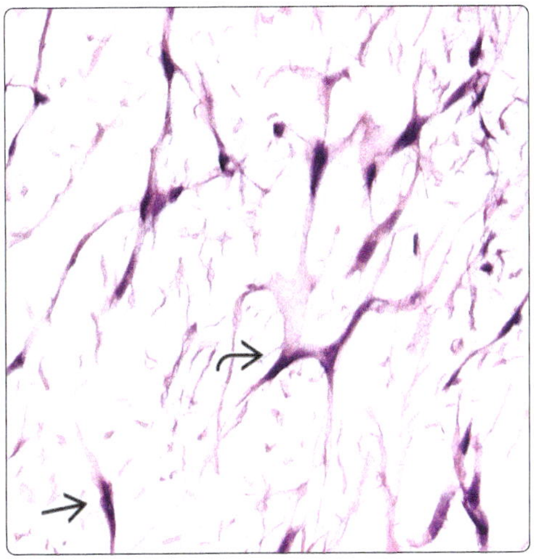

Multilobular and Plexiform Architecture

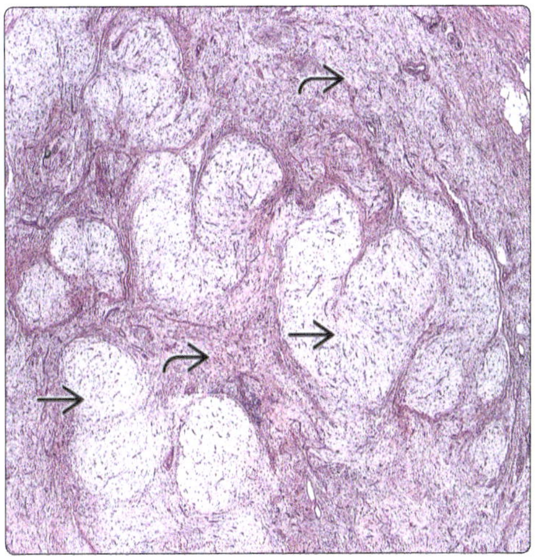

(Left) *This micrograph shows bipolar* → *and stellate* ↷ *spindle cells in a dermal nerve sheath myxoma, with abundant eosinophilic cytoplasm and long, interconnecting cell processes, forming a reticulated or network pattern.* **(Right)** *This low-power micrograph highlights a multilobular and plexiform pattern in a dermal nerve sheath myxoma, consisting of sharply demarcated, serpiginous myxoid lobules* → *situated within dense fibroconnective tissue* ↷.

S100 Expression in Nerve Sheath Myxoma

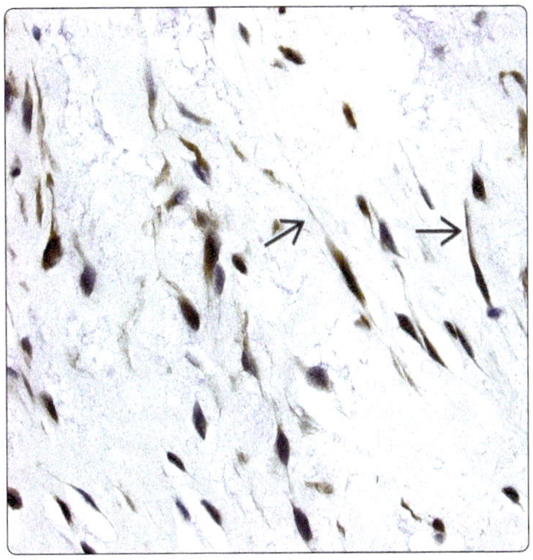

CD34(+) Fibroblasts

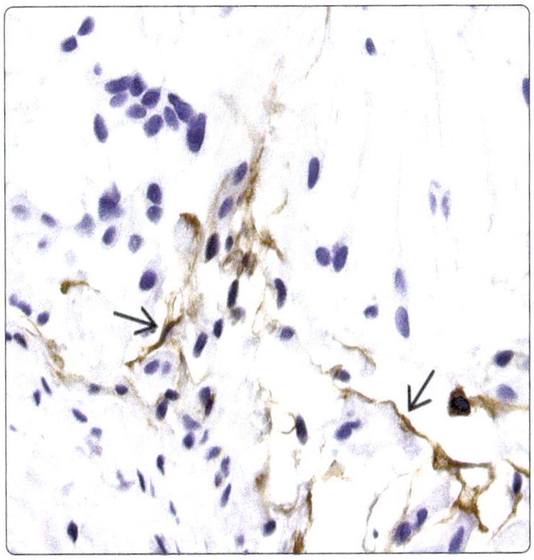

(Left) *S100 immunostain in a dermal nerve sheath myxoma shows diffuse nuclear and cytoplasmic staining, which highlights its long, delicate cytoplasmic processes* →. **(Right)** *Immunohistochemical stain for CD34 highlights the long, slender cell processes* → *of intraneural fibroblasts, which are frequently detected in dermal nerve sheath myxoma. In addition, EMA(+) perineurial cells (not depicted) are also detected in most tumors.*

Granular Cell Tumor

KEY FACTS

TERMINOLOGY

- Benign tumor of putative schwannian origin composed of cells with abundant granular cytoplasm

CLINICAL ISSUES

- Wide age range (peak: 40-60 years)
  - Female predilection
  - More prevalent in African Americans
- Wide anatomic distribution, usually arises in skin and subcutaneous tissue
  - Head and neck region common (tongue, oral cavity)
- Usually solitary, painless nodule, plaque, or mass
  - Multicentricity in 10% of cases
- Excellent prognosis for benign lesions
- Malignant granular cell tumor (GrCT) (very rare) metastasizes in up to 50% of cases

MACROSCOPIC

- Usually small (mean: 1-2 cm)

MICROSCOPIC

- Nonencapsulated, usually with irregular borders
- Overlying pseudoepitheliomatous hyperplasia in 30%
- Sheets, nests, and cords of plump, polygonal cells with abundant eosinophilic granular cytoplasm
- Typically prominent collagenous stroma
- Malignant GrCT shows ≥ 3 atypical features (pleomorphism, prominent nucleoli, increased mitoses, etc.)

ANCILLARY TESTS

- PAS(+), diastase-resistant cytoplasmic granules
- Strong, diffuse S100(+), SOX10(+)
- Nuclear TFE3(+) in majority

TOP DIFFERENTIAL DIAGNOSES

- Congenital granular cell epulis
- Nonneural GrCT
- Hibernoma
- Melanoma

(Left) *Granular cell tumor (GrCT) is a benign tumor of putative Schwann cell origin that occurs in a variety of anatomic sites but shows a predilection for the head and neck region, especially the tongue. This case presented as a dermal nodule on the chest wall, which was clinically suspicious for breast carcinoma.* **(Right)** *This tumor is composed of sheets, nests, and cords of plump, polygonal cells with abundant eosinophilic granular cytoplasm within a collagenous stroma.*

Granular Cell Tumor at Low Magnification

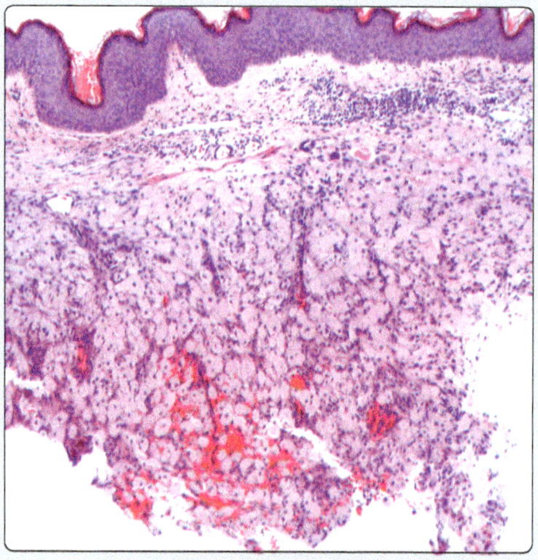

Sheets, Nests, and Cords of Tumor Cells

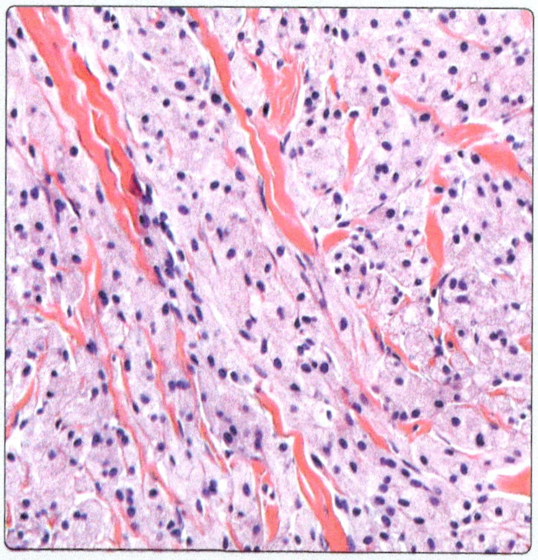

(Left) *Cytologically, the cells of GrCT show prominent, granular cytoplasm, which represents numerous lysosomal structures. Nuclei are generally small and may be dark with dense chromatin or vesicular with a small nucleolus. Occasional scattered larger nuclei and nucleoli ➚ may be seen in otherwise benign GrCT.* **(Right)** *Strong, diffuse S100 expression is characteristic of GrCT and can help to distinguish it from most entities in its differential diagnosis.*

Prominent Granular Cytoplasm

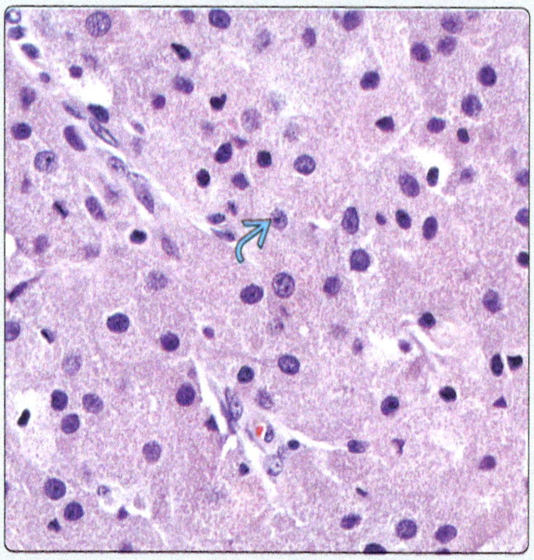

S100 Immunohistochemistry

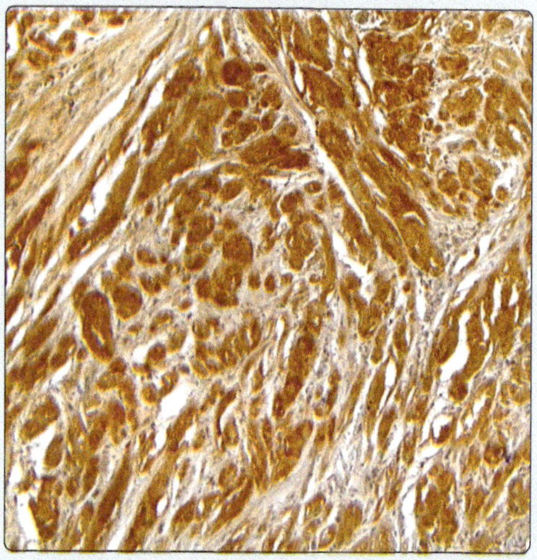

TERMINOLOGY

Abbreviations

- Granular cell tumor (GrCT)

Synonyms

- Granular cell myoblastoma
- Abrikossoff tumor
- Granular cell schwannoma

Definitions

- Benign tumor of putative schwannian origin composed of cells with abundant granular cytoplasm

CLINICAL ISSUES

Epidemiology

- Incidence
  - Benign GrCT not uncommon
    - Malignant GrCT extremely rare
- Age
  - Any (peak: 40-60 years)
- Sex
  - Female predilection
- Ethnicity
  - More prevalent in African Americans

Site

- Wide distribution, usually arises in skin and subcutaneous tissue
  - Rarely in deep soft tissue sites
- Head and neck region common
  - Particularly tongue and oral cavity
- Also breast, bronchus, larynx, neurohypophysis, other viscera
- Rarely in nerves, lymph nodes

Presentation

- Usually solitary, slowly growing, painless nodule, plaque, or mass
  - Multicentric in ~ 10% of cases
    - May appear synchronously or metachronously
    - May rarely arise in association with Noonan syndrome or LEOPARD syndrome
- Oral cavity/tongue lesions may show concurrent candidiasis

Treatment

- Complete surgical excision

Prognosis

- Overall excellent prognosis for benign lesions
  - Local recurrence in < 10% of cases
- Multicentric tumors usually benign
- Malignant GrCT
  - Up to 30% recur
  - Up to 50% metastasize
  - Adverse prognostic factors
    - Local recurrence, metastasis
    - Tumor size (> 5 cm), older patient age (> 50 years)

MACROSCOPIC

General Features

- Cutaneous lesions may show hyperplastic/verrucous appearance
- Cut surface firm, pale yellow, or cream colored

Size

- Usually small (mean: 1-2 cm)
  - Deep lesions often larger (5-6 cm)

MICROSCOPIC

Histologic Features

- Nonencapsulated, usually with irregular borders
  - May appear to infiltrate adjacent tissues (dermal collagen, adipose tissue, skeletal muscle)
    - Tumor cells often appear to entrap small nerves
  - Can extend directly up to surface epithelium
    - May incite overlying pseudoepitheliomatous hyperplasia (30% of cases)
      - Can mimic invasive squamous cell carcinoma in superficial biopsies
  - Rare, plexiform growth pattern in dermis
- Sheets, nests, and cords of plump, polygonal cells
  - Abundant granular, eosinophilic cytoplasm
    - Enlarged granules with halos (phagolysosomes) frequent (referred to as pustulo-ovoid bodies of Milian)
    - Cell membrane often indistinct; appears syncytial
  - Central small nuclei with variable dense to vesicular nuclei
    - Small, subtle nucleoli may be present
    - Mitoses absent
- Typically prominent collagenous stroma
  - May be fibrotic or desmoplastic in longstanding lesions
- Intratumoral lymphoid aggregates in some cases
- Necrosis absent
- Atypical features
  - Pleomorphism, prominent nucleoli, high nuclear:cytoplasmic ratio, spindling of cells
    - Should be prominent in tumor, not focal
  - Mitoses > 2 per 10 HPF
  - Necrosis
- Malignant GrCT shows ≥ 3 atypical features
  - Tumors with 1 or 2 prominent atypical features may be regarded as atypical GrCT

ANCILLARY TESTS

Histochemistry

- PAS(+), diastase-resistant cytoplasmic granules
  - Diffuse, chunky staining

Immunohistochemistry

- Strong, diffuse S100(+) and nuclear SOX10(+)
- Calretinin (+), CD68(+), inhibin (+), nestin (+)
- Nuclear TFE3(+) in majority of cases
- Type IV collagen (+) around nests of cells
- SMA, desmin, myogenin, GFAP, HMB-45, neurofilament (-)

Electron Microscopy

- Continuous external lamina around cell nests
- Pleomorphic secondary lysosomes
  - Autophagosomes
  - Myelin-like figures
  - Angulate lysosomes

DIFFERENTIAL DIAGNOSIS

Congenital Granular Cell Epulis

- Can be histologically indistinguishable from GrCT
- Arises in gingiva of newborns (congenital)
- S100(-)

Nonneural Granular Cell Tumor

- Cutaneous lesion, often polypoid with epidermal collarette
- Sheet-like growth of spindled to epithelioid cells with abundant granular, eosinophilic cytoplasm
- Variable nuclear atypia and mitotic activity
- S100(-)

Hibernoma

- Sheets and lobules of multivacuolated brown fat cells
  - Often contains areas of white fat cells
- Most common in subcutis (not cutaneous)
- Cells lack intracytoplasmic phagolysosomes

Malignant Melanoma

- Granular cell change rare
- Junctional component usually present
- HMB-45(+), MART-1(+) in most cases

Invasive Squamous Cell Carcinoma

- Absence of underlying GrCT (key finding)
- Desmoplastic stroma

Leiomyoma

- Rare granular cell change
- Areas of conventional smooth muscle cytology
- SMA(+) and desmin (+)
- S100(-)

Alveolar Soft Part Sarcoma

- Deep, usually large mass
- Compartmentalized growth; pseudoalveolar pattern common
- Rare granular cell change
- Majority of cases show PAS(+), diastase resistant, intracytoplasmic, rod-like crystals
- S100, SOX10, and nestin (-)
- Nuclear TFE3(+)

Reactive Granular Cell Change

- Collections of granular histiocytes
- Occurs at sites of trauma or prior surgical procedures
- Lack diffuse S100 expression

Adult-Type Rhabdomyoma

- Sheets of polygonal cells with homogeneous, eosinophilic cytoplasm
- Desmin (+), myogenin (+)
- S100(-)

Granular Cell Dermatofibroma (Fibrous Histiocytoma)

- Other typical features of dermatofibroma
- Lacks prominent overlying pseudoepitheliomatous hyperplasia
- S100(-)

DIAGNOSTIC CHECKLIST

Pathologic Interpretation Pearls

- Large granular cells
- Pseudoepitheliomatous hyperplasia of overlying epithelium is common
- Diffuse S100 positivity

SELECTED REFERENCES

1. Machado I et al: Solitary, multiple, benign, atypical, or malignant: the "Granular Cell Tumor" puzzle. Virchows Arch. 468(5):527-38, 2016
2. Pérez-González YC et al: Primary cutaneous malignant granular cell tumor: an immunohistochemical study and review of the literature. Am J Dermatopathol. 37(4):334-40, 2015
3. Battistella M et al: Vascular invasion and other invasive features in granular cell tumours of the skin: a multicentre study of 119 cases. J Clin Pathol. 67(1):19-25, 2014
4. Chamberlain BK et al: Alveolar soft part sarcoma and granular cell tumor: an immunohistochemical comparison study. Hum Pathol. 45(5):1039-44, 2014
5. Gomes CC et al: Evidence for loss of heterozygosity (LOH) at chromosomes 9p and 17p in oral granular cell tumors: a pilot study. Oral Surg Oral Med Oral Pathol Oral Radiol. 115(2):249-53, 2013
6. Izquierdo F et al: Perineurial cells in granular cell tumors and neoplasms with perineural invasion: an immunohistochemical study. Am J Dermatopathol. 34(8):800-9, 2012
7. Nasser H et al: Malignant granular cell tumor: a look into the diagnostic criteria. Pathol Res Pract. 207(3):164-8, 2011
8. Papalas JA et al: Recurrence risk and margin status in granular cell tumors of the breast: a clinicopathologic study of 13 patients. Arch Pathol Lab Med. 135(7):890-5, 2011
9. Rejas RA et al: The neural histogenetic origin of the oral granular cell tumor: an immunohistochemical evidence. Med Oral Patol Oral Cir Bucal. 16(1):e6-10, 2011
10. Shintaku M: Immunohistochemical localization of autophagosomal membrane-associated protein LC3 in granular cell tumor and schwannoma. Virchows Arch. 459(3):315-9, 2011
11. Papalas JA et al: Isolated and synchronous vulvar granular cell tumors: a clinicopathologic study of 17 cases in 13 patients. Int J Gynecol Pathol. 29(2):173-80, 2010
12. Aldabagh B et al: Plexiform pattern in cutaneous granular cell tumors. J Cutan Pathol. 36(11):1174-6, 2009
13. Rose B et al: Granular cell tumours: a rare entity in the musculoskeletal system. Sarcoma. 2009:765927, 2009
14. Vered M et al: Granular cell tumor of the oral cavity: updated immunohistochemical profile. J Oral Pathol Med. 38(1):150-9, 2009
15. Bhattacharyya I et al: Granular cell leiomyoma of the oral cavity. Oral Surg Oral Med Oral Pathol Oral Radiol Endod. 102(3):353-9, 2006
16. Zarovnaya E et al: Distinguishing pseudoepitheliomatous hyperplasia from squamous cell carcinoma in mucosal biopsy specimens from the head and neck. Arch Pathol Lab Med. 129(8):1032-6, 2005
17. Chrysomali E et al: Immunohistochemical evaluation of cell proliferation antigen Ki-67 and apoptosis-related proteins Bcl-2 and caspase-3 in oral granular cell tumor. Oral Surg Oral Med Oral Pathol Oral Radiol Endod. 96(5):566-72, 2003
18. van der Meij EH et al: Granular cells in oral lichen planus. Oral Dis. 7(2):116-8, 2001
19. Fanburg-Smith JC et al: Malignant granular cell tumor of soft tissue: diagnostic criteria and clinicopathologic correlation. Am J Surg Pathol. 22(7):779-94, 1998
20. Junquera LM et al: Granular-cell tumours: an immunohistochemical study. Br J Oral Maxillofac Surg. 35(3):180-4, 1997
21. Collins BM et al: Multiple granular cell tumors of the oral cavity: report of a case and review of the literature. J Oral Maxillofac Surg. 53(6):707-11, 1995

Granular Cell Tumor in Superficial Dermis

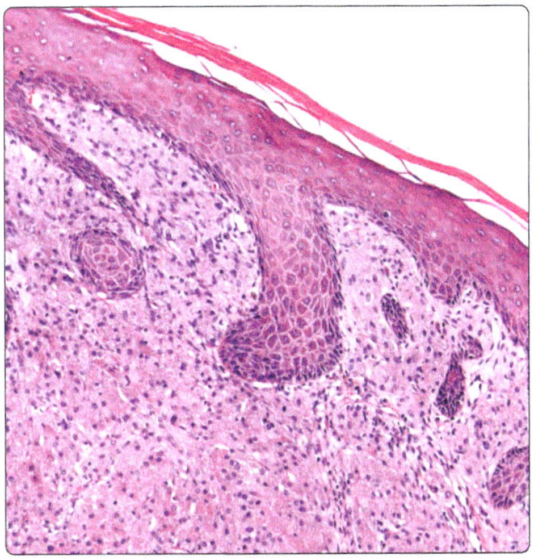

Occasional Pale Granular Cells

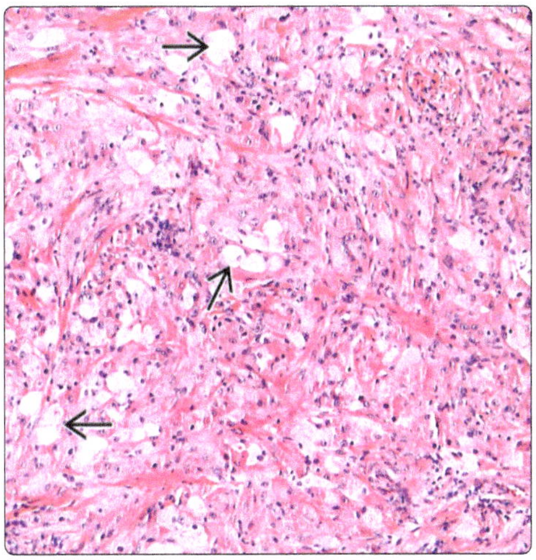

(Left) *Most cases of GrCT are dermal or subcutaneous, but some may extend directly up under the overlying epidermis, as in this case.* **(Right)** *Occasional cases of GrCT contain scattered tumor cells with abundant pale/foamy-appearing cytoplasm →, resembling foamy histiocytes.*

Abundant Intracytoplasmic Granules

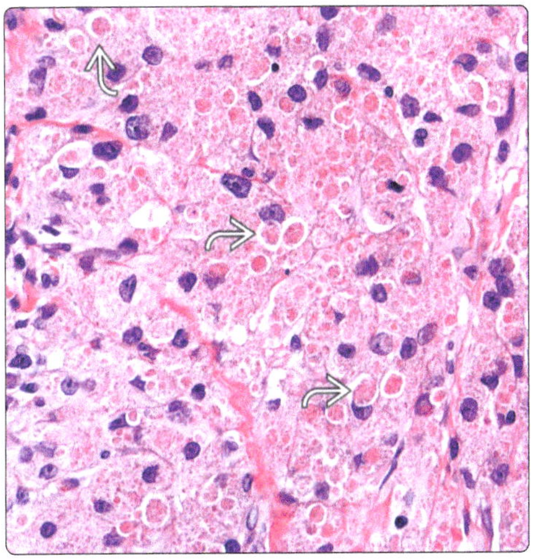

High Magnification of Intracytoplasmic Granules

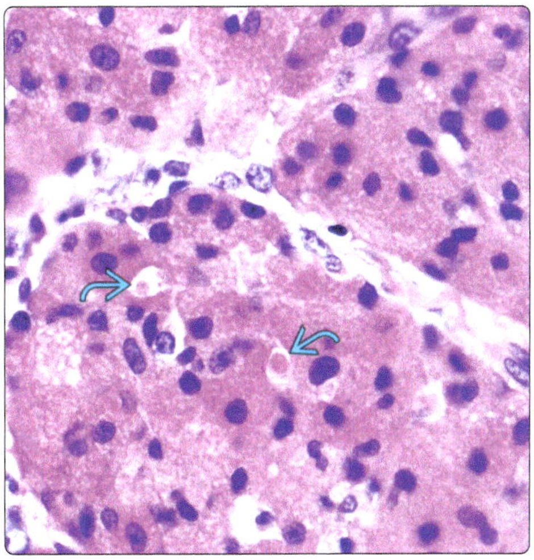

(Left) *Large, intracytoplasmic, granular structures (pustulo-ovoid bodies of Milian) ➔ are common in GrCT but vary widely in number from case to case. In some tumors, such as this one, they can be quite abundant.* **(Right)** *This is another case with a few large, intracytoplasmic granules (pustulo-ovoid bodies) ↪.*

Entrapment of Nerve Fibers

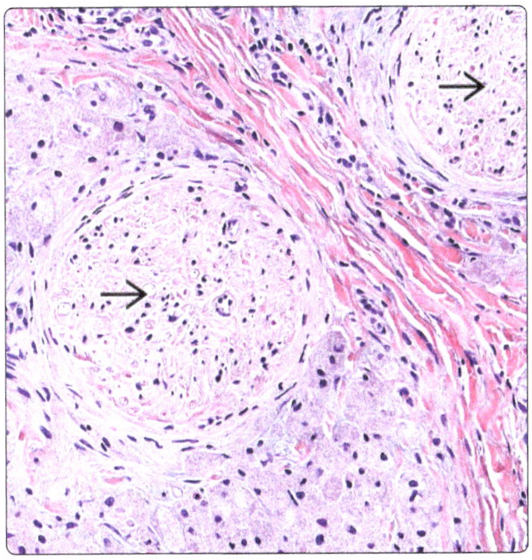

Entrapment of Nerve Fibers

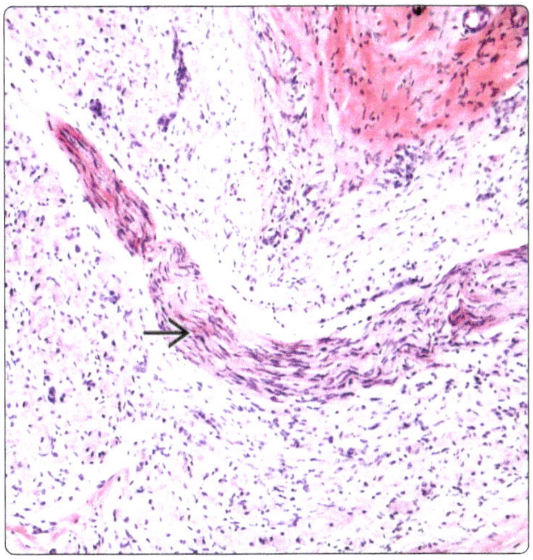

(Left) *In keeping with the likely schwannian origin of this lesion, entrapped nerve fibers → are commonly identified in GrCT, both within the tumor and around the periphery. However, to the unwary, this finding may suggest perineural invasion by a malignant process.* **(Right)** *This H&E of GrCT shows almost complete entrapment of a nerve fiber → by the lesional tumor cells, which is not a concerning feature in these tumors.*

(Left) *In ~ 1/3 of cases of cutaneous GrCT, the overlying squamous epithelium shows marked hyperplasia and may simulate the appearance of an invasive well-differentiated squamous cell carcinoma. Detection of the GrCT component is critical on a superficial biopsy.* **(Right)** *Note the irregular, small nests of keratinizing squamous epithelial cells → that, out of the context of GrCT, would be highly suspicious for invasive carcinoma.*

Pseudoepitheliomatous Hyperplasia Mimicking Invasive Carcinoma

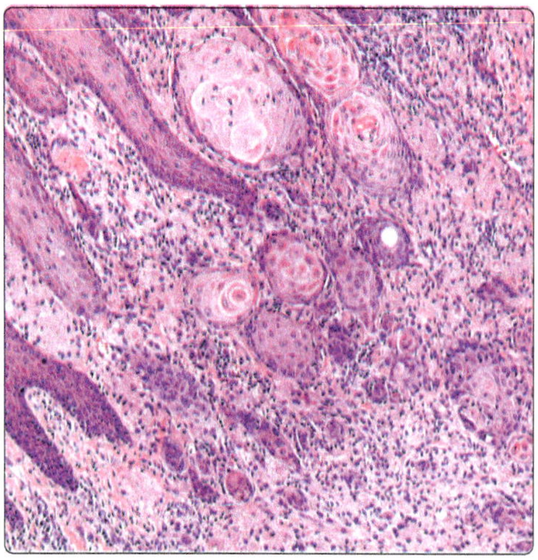

Pseudoepitheliomatous Hyperplasia

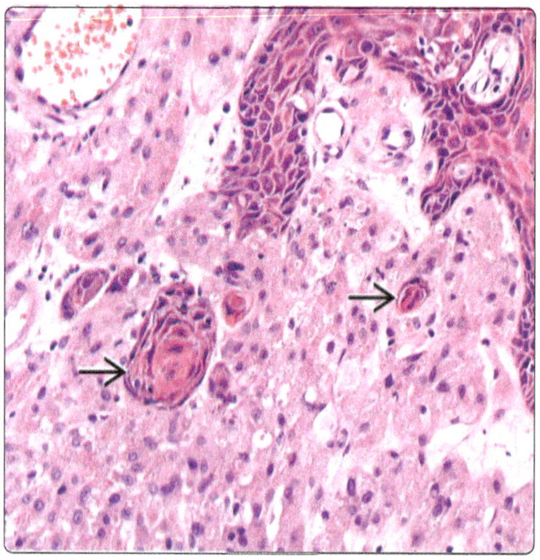

(Left) *Occasional cases of GrCT may show surface ulceration and inflammation, which may obscure the actual diagnosis. Note the subtle eosinophilic granular cells → underlying the ulceration.* **(Right)** *Some cases of dermal GrCT can show a multinodular growth pattern with satellite nodules. Rarely, an apparent plexiform pattern is seen (as shown here).*

Surface Ulceration With Inflammation

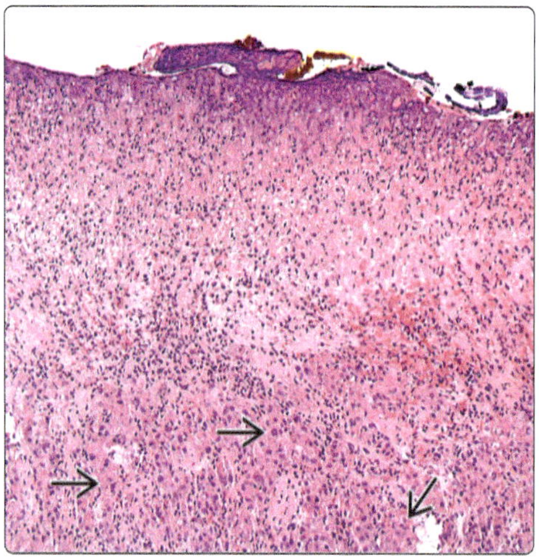

Rare Plexiform Growth Pattern

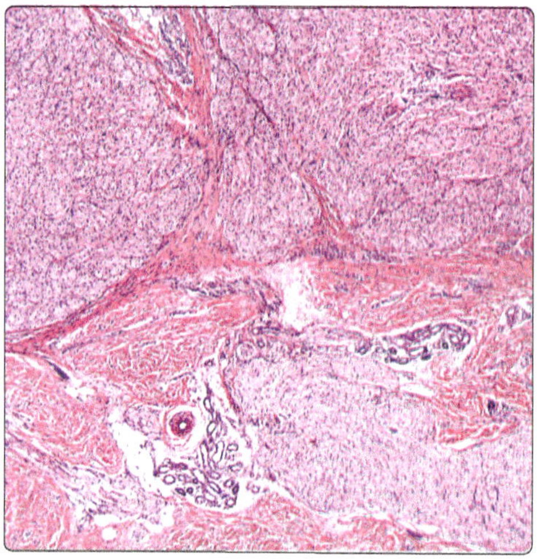

(Left) *Most cases of GrCT are characterized by an ill-defined proliferation of tumor cells that appear to infiltrate adjacent tissues, including dermal collagen, adipose tissue, and skeletal muscle (shown here). This finding should not be equated with malignancy.* **(Right)** *Scattered intratumoral lymphoid aggregates may be seen in occasional cases of GrCT, similar to what is seen in some examples of schwannoma.*

Infiltrative Appearance Common

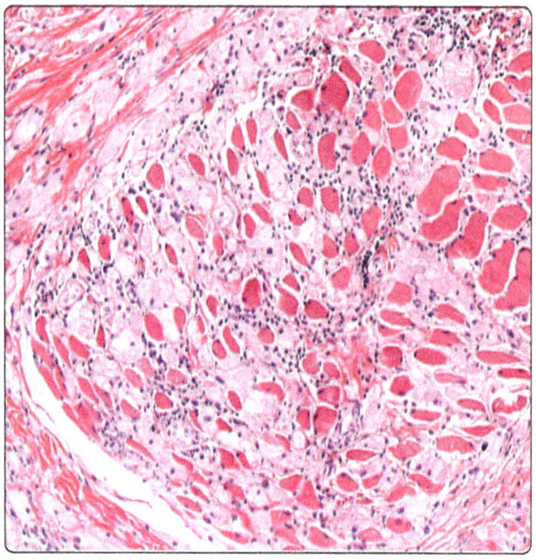

Intratumoral Lymphoid Aggregates

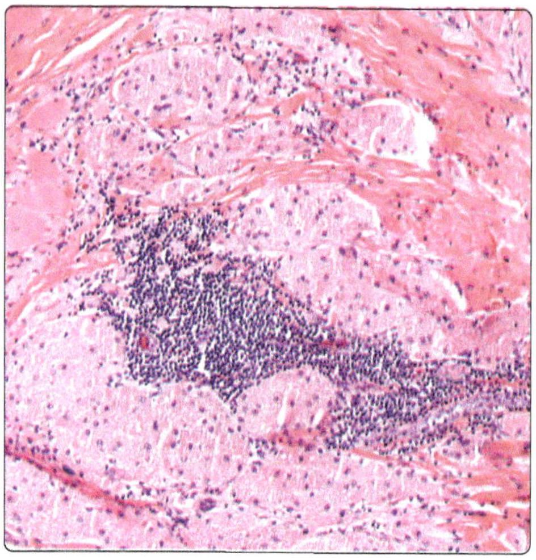

Histologically Subtle Longstanding Lesions

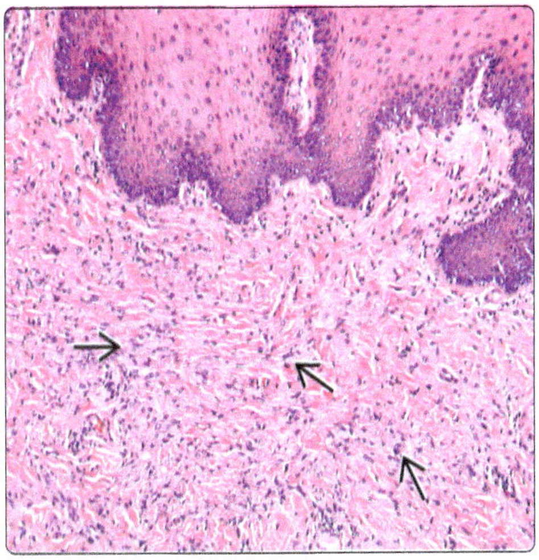

Sclerosis in Longstanding Lesions

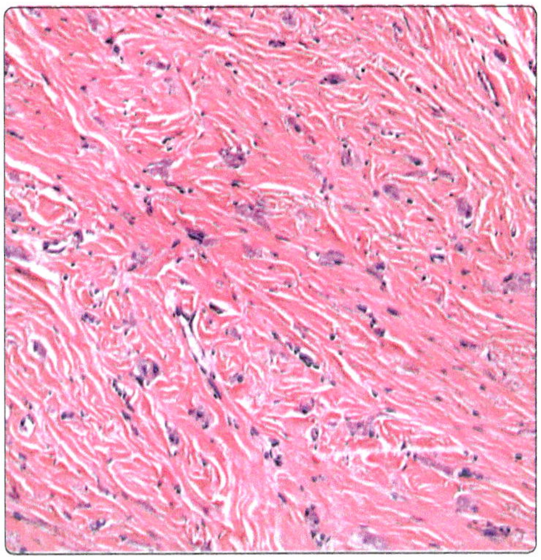

(Left) *Longstanding cases of GrCT may show subtle diagnostic findings that can be overlooked. This image shows a hypocellular tumor in the dermis, with relatively few granular cells → infiltrating collagen bundles, findings that can mimic a dermatofibroma.* **(Right)** *The stroma in GrCT is characterized in most cases by prominent, dense collagen. In older lesions, this stroma may appear even more fibrotic, or even desmoplastic, and lesional cells may be identified singly &/or in scattered small aggregates or cords.*

Degenerative Nuclear Atypia

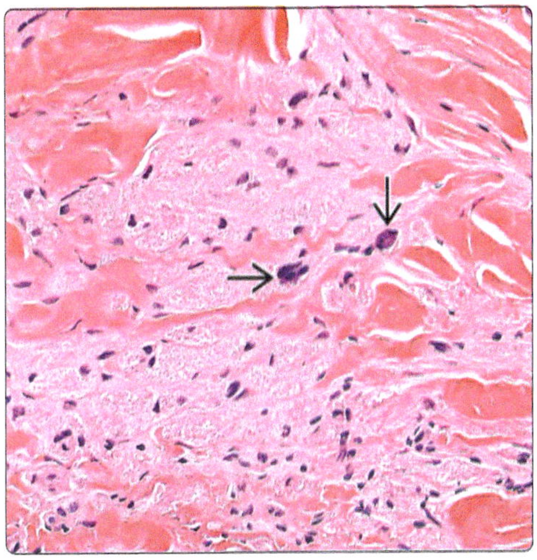

Focal Cellular Spindling

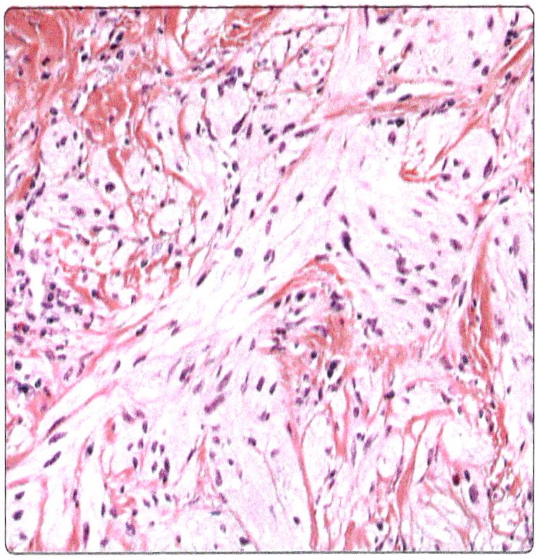

(Left) *Degenerative nuclear atypia → may be seen in occasional cases of GrCT and is rarely prominent. This finding is similar to that seen in other nerve sheath tumors.* **(Right)** *Although most cases of GrCT are composed of polygonal tumor cells, occasional tumors show focal cellular spindling. This finding, when focal and in isolation, is of no prognostic significance. Of note, spindling is not uncommon in GI tract GrCT.*

Malignant Granular Cell Tumor

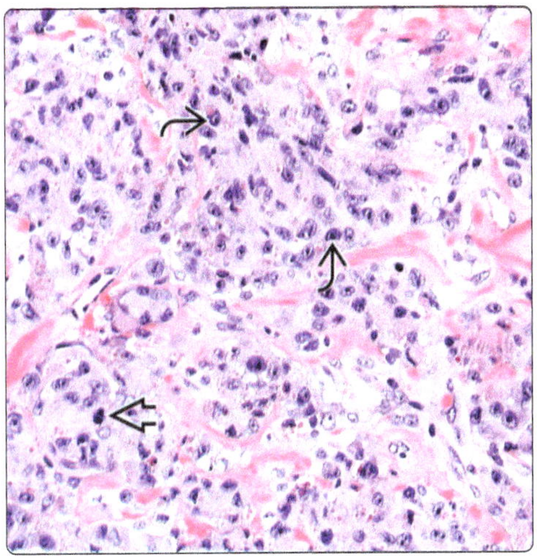

Malignant Granular Cell Tumor

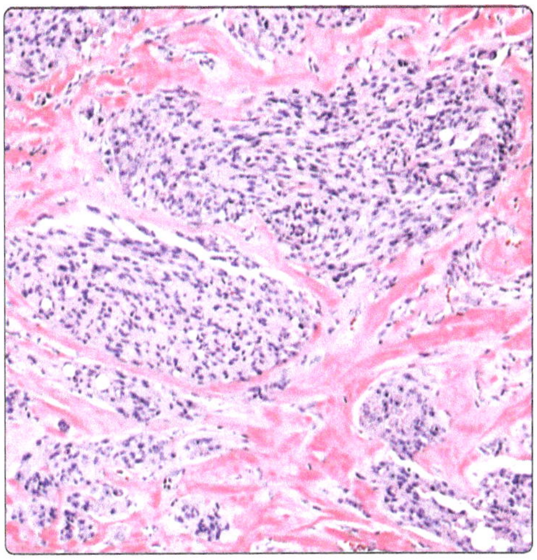

(Left) *Malignant examples of GrCT are extremely rare and usually show atypical features, such as large, vesicular nuclei with prominent nucleoli ↷, high nuclear:cytoplasmic ratio, pleomorphism, and increased mitoses ⇨ (> 2 figures/10 HPF). Necrosis, both single cell and geographic types, is also common.* **(Right)** *Areas of prominent spindling, increased cellularity, and an overall sarcomatoid appearance are common features of malignant GrCT.*

Lipomatosis of Nerve

KEY FACTS

TERMINOLOGY

- Increased fibrofatty tissue infiltrating and surrounding nerves
- Synonym: Fibrolipomatous hamartoma of nerve

CLINICAL ISSUES

- Predominantly in children, often congenital
  - Some in young adults up to 30 yr; rare in older adults
- Median nerve and digital branches most common (80%)
  - Symptoms often similar to compression neuropathy or carpal tunnel syndrome
- Slowly progressive swelling/mass of palm (if median nerve affected)
- Macrodactyly present in 30%
- Biopsy not needed if classic MR findings
  - Complete excision usually contraindicated because of potential nerve damage
- Good prognosis when conservatively managed

IMAGING

- Coaxial cable-like (axial view) and spaghetti-like (coronal view) appearances due to linear nerve bundles encased in fat

MACROSCOPIC

- Sausage-shaped mass
- Yellow-white fibroadipose tissue surrounds and distends nerve

MICROSCOPIC

- Mature adipose and fibrous tissue infiltrate nerve
  - Individual nerve bundles separated and encased by fat
- Marked epineurial and perineurial fibrous thickening
- Concentric hyperplasia of perineurium

TOP DIFFERENTIAL DIAGNOSES

- Lipoma of nerve
- Neuroma

Lipomatosis of Nerve

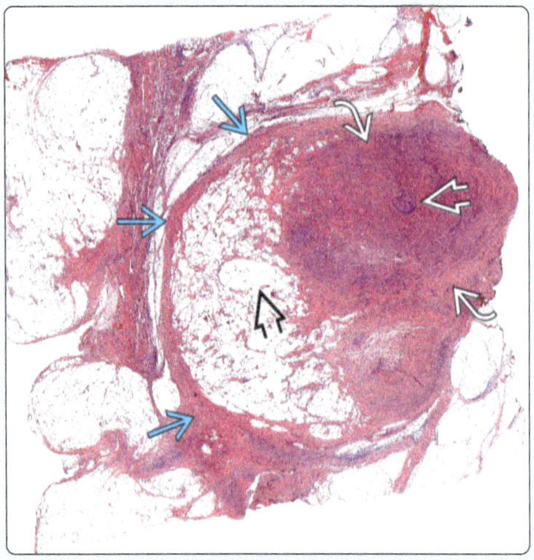

Nerve Bundles Separated by Fibrofatty Tissue

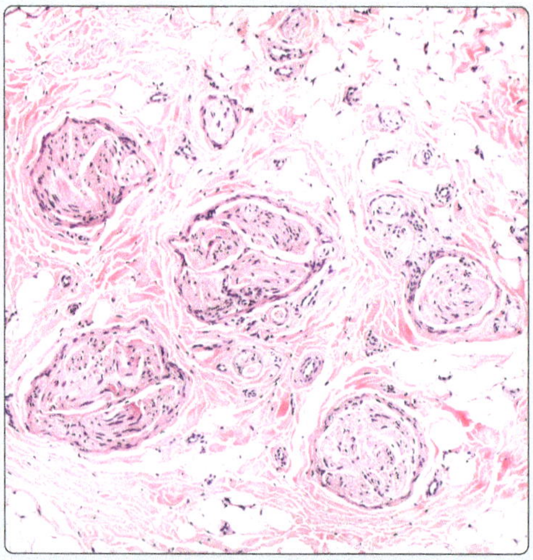

(Left) *In this image of lipomatosis of nerve (fibrolipomatous hamartoma), a small, solitary nerve bundle* ➡ *is surrounded by concentric layers of dense fibrosis* ➡*, mature adipose tissue* ➡*, and a thick layer of epineurial fibrosis* ➡*.* **(Right)** *At higher magnification, nerve bundles with perineurial hyperplasia are separated from one another by fibrous tissue and mature fat.*

Frequent Involvement of Median Nerve

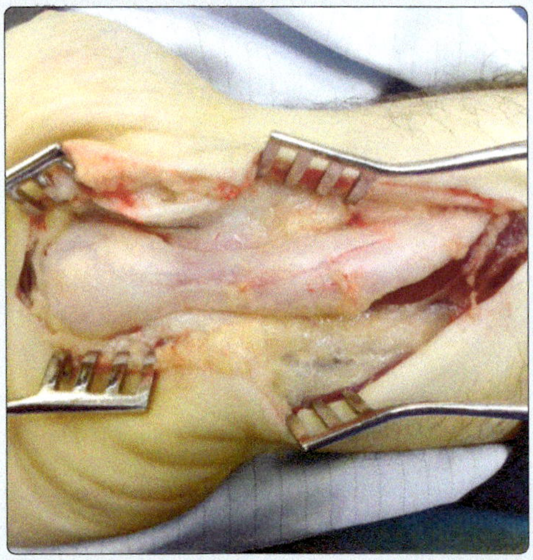

Appearance on Axial MR

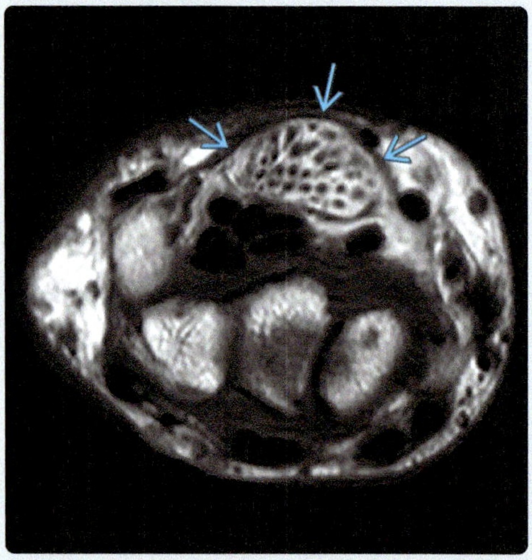

(Left) *In this gross photo of lipomatosis of nerve, the median nerve is markedly enlarged and distended by pale yellow-white adipose tissue. (Courtesy T. Al-Jabri, MD.)* **(Right)** *The median nerve* ➡ *is massively enlarged on this axial T1 MR and has an appearance likened to cross section of coaxial cable. Multiple individual nerve bundles (dark) are divided from one another by intervening fibroadipose tissue (light). (Courtesy A. Lawson, MBBCh.)*

TERMINOLOGY

Synonyms

- Fibrolipomatous hamartoma of nerve
- Neural fibrolipoma, neurolipomatosis
- Fatty infiltration of median nerve

Definitions

- Increased fibrofatty tissue infiltrating and surrounding nerves

CLINICAL ISSUES

Epidemiology

- Age
  - Predominantly in children, often congenital
  - Some in young adults up to 30 years; rare in older adults

Site

- Median nerve and digital branches most common (80%)
  - Affects palmar surface of hand, wrist, forearm, digits
- Rarely ulnar, radial, sciatic, peroneal, or cranial nerve; any nerve can be involved
- Vast majority are unilateral

Presentation

- Slowly progressive swelling/mass of palm (if median nerve affected)
- Paresthesia and dysesthesia
  - Symptoms often similar to compression neuropathy or carpal tunnel syndrome
- Macrodactyly (digital gigantism, macrodystrophia lipomatosa) in 30%
  - Can be congenital and progressive
  - Increased growth of bone and soft tissue of affected digit

Treatment

- Biopsy not needed if classic MR findings
- Complete excision usually contraindicated because of potential nerve damage
- Surgical decompression (e.g., carpal tunnel release) or debulking may reduce symptoms
- For macrodactyly, may remove deformed digit

Prognosis

- Good prognosis when conservatively managed

IMAGING

MR Findings

- Fusiform enlargement of affected nerve segment
- Coaxial cable-like (axial view) and spaghetti-like (coronal view) appearances due to linear nerve bundles encased in fat

MACROSCOPIC

General Features

- Sausage-shaped mass
- Yellow-white fibroadipose tissue surrounds and distends nerve

Size

- Variable, up to 10-cm length of nerve may be involved

MICROSCOPIC

Histologic Features

- Mature adipose and fibrous tissue infiltrate nerve
  - Individual nerve bundles separated and encased by fat
- Marked epineurial and perineurial fibrous thickening
- Concentric hyperplasia of perineurium
- Nerves can become atrophic in longstanding cases
- Rare metaplastic bone formation

DIFFERENTIAL DIAGNOSIS

Lipoma of Nerve

- Circumscribed and confined within nerve
- Fat does not entrap and separate individual nerve bundles

Traumatic Neuroma

- Increased number of nerve bundles
- No fatty component

Lipomatosis

- Histologically similar
- May have secondary nerve involvement, but is primarily lesion of skin/subcutis or muscle

Neurofibromatosis Type 1

- Also may cause macrodactyly
- Expanded nerve in neurofibromatosis type 1 (NF1) may grossly resemble lipomatosis of nerve
  - Histologically easy to distinguish by typical features of neurofibroma and lack of fat
- Other distinct clinical features of NF1 not usually seen in lipomatosis of nerve

SELECTED REFERENCES

1. Mahan MA et al: Long-term progression of lipomatosis of nerve. World Neurosurg. 82(3-4):492-9, 2014
2. Chiaradia G et al: Precalcaneal congenital fibrolipomatous hamartoma: report of 2 cases. J Pediatr Surg. 46(3):e11-2, 2011
3. Yang JH et al: Precalcaneal congenital fibrolipomatous hamartoma. Ann Dermatol. 23(1):92-4, 2011
4. Al-Jabri T et al: Lipofibromatous hamartoma of the median nerve. J Orthop Surg Res. 5:71, 2010
5. Chiang CL et al: MRI diagnosis of fibrolipomatous hamartoma of the median nerve and associated macrodystrophia lipomatosa. J Chin Med Assoc. 73(9):499-502, 2010
6. Flann S et al: Precalcaneal congenital fibrolipomatous hamartoma. Clin Exp Dermatol. 34(4):495-6, 2009
7. Bisceglia M et al: Neural lipofibromatous hamartoma: a report of two cases and review of the literature. Adv Anat Pathol. 14(1):46-52, 2007
8. Jain TP et al: Fibrolipomatous hamartoma of median nerve. Australas Radiol. 51 Spec No.:B98-B100, 2007
9. Razzaghi A et al: Lipofibromatous hamartoma: review of early diagnosis and treatment. Can J Surg. 48(5):394-9, 2005
10. Al-Qattan MM: Lipofibromatous hamartoma of the median nerve and its associated conditions. J Hand Surg [Br]. 26(4):368-72, 2001
11. Marom EM et al: Fibrolipomatous hamartoma: pathognomonic on MR imaging. Skeletal Radiol. 28(5):260-4, 1999
12. Berti E et al: Fibrolipomatous hamartoma of a cranial nerve. Histopathology. 24(4):391-2, 1994
13. Amadio PC et al: Lipofibromatous hamartoma of nerve. J Hand Surg [Am]. 13(1):67-75, 1988
14. Silverman TA et al: Fibrolipomatous hamartoma of nerve. A clinicopathologic analysis of 26 cases. Am J Surg Pathol. 9(1):7-14, 1985

Perineurioma

KEY FACTS

TERMINOLOGY

- Benign peripheral nerve sheath tumor, specifically of perineurial cell derivation that surrounds endoneurial connective tissue space of nerve fibers

CLINICAL ISSUES

- Wide age range: 2-85 years; mean: 45 years
- Superficial subcutaneous soft tissues of head and neck
- Local recurrence is uncommon (< 5% of cases)

MACROSCOPIC

- Usually discrete, solitary, well circumscribed, but without easily detected capsule
- Range: 0.3-20.0 cm; mean: ~ 3 cm

MICROSCOPIC

- Well circumscribed, focally showing changes suggesting collagenous capsule
- Spindled tumor cells organized in many patterns
- Fascicles, storiform or pinwheel
- Whorled to concentrically stratified
- Bipolar, bland, plump spindled cells with pale, eosinophilic long and thin cytoplasmic processes
- Nuclei vary: Oval, tapered, elongate, triangular, curved, or wavy with finely distributed chromatin
- Background stroma is collagenous, myxoid, or mixture
- Sclerosing, reticular (retiform), granular and epithelioid subtypes recognized

ANCILLARY TESTS

- EMA: Strong and diffuse
- Claudin-1: Distinctly particulate pattern along cell membrane
- GLUT1: Usually membranous to stippled

TOP DIFFERENTIAL DIAGNOSES

- Neurofibroma, schwannoma, solitary fibrous tumor, myoepithelioma, meningioma, desmoid fibromatosis

Submucosal Spindle Cell Proliferation

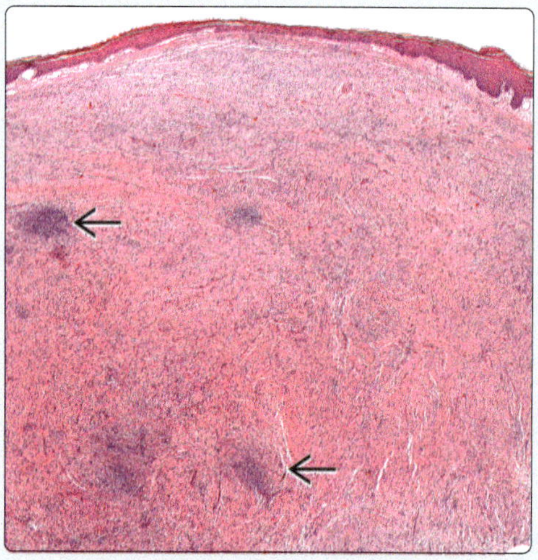

Syncytial Appearance to Spindled Cells

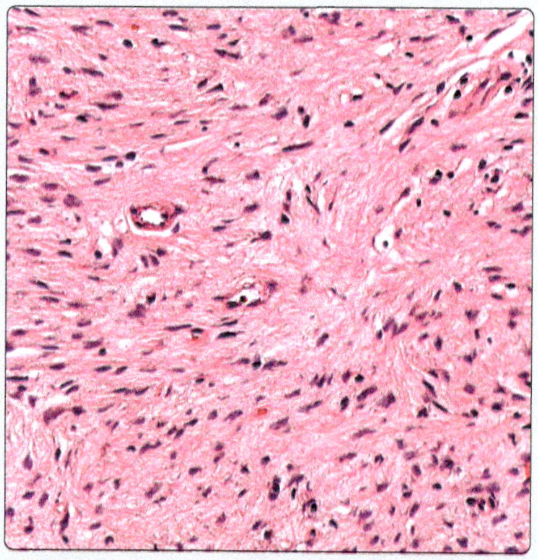

(Left) *H&E shows an intact surface epithelium overlying a proliferation of spindled cells arranged in a vaguely storiform pattern with focal small whorls. Collections of inflammatory cells are present* ⇨. **(Right)** *H&E shows a haphazard spindle cell proliferation showing a syncytial appearance. The cells show slightly spindled nuclei with cytoplasmic processes. The background stroma is slightly loose to myxoid.*

Epithelioid Cells in Sclerosing Perineurioma

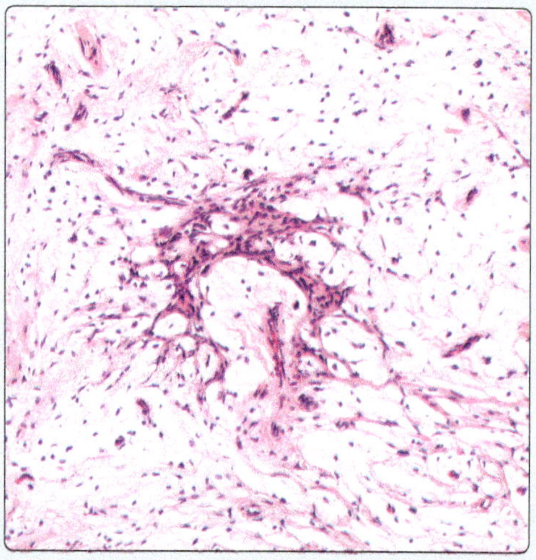

Haphazard Storiform Proliferation

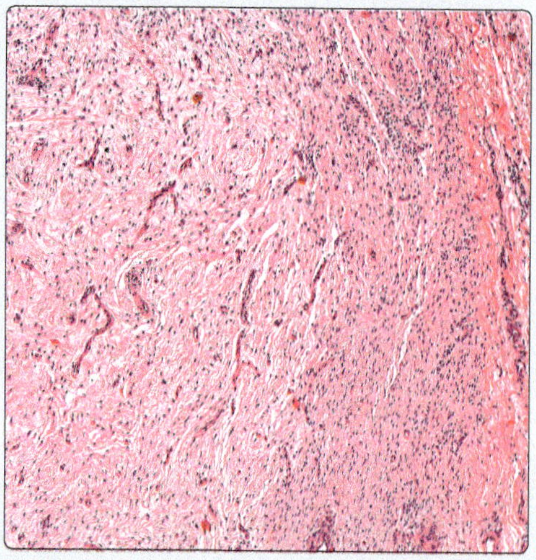

(Left) *Epithelioid and spindle cells in a trabecular or whorled pattern are shown within a background of myxoid to fibrotic stroma.* **(Right)** *The proliferation blends at the periphery with the densely collagenized stroma. There is a haphazard storiform appearance to the proliferation. The stroma is myxoid to edematous, perhaps having a vaguely tissue culture-like appearance.*

TERMINOLOGY

Abbreviations

- Soft tissue perineurioma (STP)

Synonyms

- Sclerosing perineurioma

Definitions

- Benign peripheral nerve sheath tumor, specifically of perineurial cell derivation that surrounds endoneurial connective tissue space of nerve fibers
  - Tumors are traditionally separated into intraneural, sclerosing, and soft tissue perineurioma
  - Perineurial cells can be seen in other tumors, such as neurofibroma and schwannoma

ETIOLOGY/PATHOGENESIS

Pathogenesis

- May be related to Schwann cells, fibroblasts, or arachnoid cap cells

CLINICAL ISSUES

Epidemiology

- Incidence
  - Exceedingly rare
  - Represents < 0.5% of peripheral nerve sheath tumors
- Age
  - Wide range: 2-85 years; mean: 45 years
    - Majority: 2nd-5th decades
- Sex
  - Slight female predilection (for extraneural tumors)

Site

- Superficial subcutaneous soft tissues of head and neck
  - ~ 15% of all perineuriomas affect head and neck sites
  - May rarely affect gnathic bones (mandible)
- Oral cavity is affected ~ 4% of time

Presentation

- Most patients present with solitary, painless mass
  - Sclerosing type usually affects superficial dermis
- May have syndrome/familial association
  - Neurofibromatosis type 2 (NF2): Only for intraneural type tumors
  - Nevoid basal cell carcinoma (Gorlin) syndrome
  - Interestingly, both have meningioma in common
    - Perineurium may be derived from arachnoid cap cells

Treatment

- Complete, wide excision to prevent recurrence

Prognosis

- Local recurrence is uncommon (< 5% of cases)
  - May develop late, and only if incompletely excised
- Pleomorphic cells and infiltrative margins do not affect clinical outcome

MACROSCOPIC

General Features

- Usually discrete, solitary, well circumscribed, but without easily detected capsule

Size

- Range: 0.3-20.0 cm; mean: ~ 3 cm

MICROSCOPIC

Histologic Features

- Superficial subcutaneous or dermal site
- Well circumscribed, focally showing changes suggesting collagenous capsule
  - Infiltrating borders can be seen, but not significant invasion
- Spindled tumor cells organized in many patterns
  - Fascicles, storiform or pinwheel
  - Whorled to concentrically stratified
  - Lamellar architecture
- Tumors are hypo- or hypercellular, with alternating zones
- Bipolar, bland, plump spindled cells with pale, eosinophilic long and thin cytoplasmic processes
- Nuclei vary: Oval, tapered, elongate, triangular, curved, compressed, twisted, or wavy with finely distributed chromatin
  - Intranuclear pseudoinclusions are rare
- Isolated pleomorphic cells (ancient change) are unusual
- Background stroma is collagenous, myxoid, or mixture
  - Sclerotic, round to elliptical collagen deposits may be present
  - Pericellular cracking or clefting between collagen and cells
- Mitoses are sparse to absent
- Degeneration and hemorrhage may be present
- Calcifications (calcospherites or metaplastic bone) are exceptional
- Chronic inflammation is uncommon
- Peripheral nerve association is unique, usually "twigs" of nerves
- Vessel hyalinization is not present
- Sclerosing, reticular (retiform), granular and epithelioid subtypes are recognized, although very rare in head and neck
  - Reticular: Lace-like growth pattern of anastomosing cords of spindle cells
  - Sclerosing: Epithelioid and spindle cells in trabecular or whorled pattern within markedly dense sclerotic stroma
  - Intraneural: Perineurial cells form concentric layers around nerve fibers (pseudo-onion bulb)

ANCILLARY TESTS

Cytology

- Cellular smears with sheets and clusters of spindle-shaped tumor cells
- Cells are bipolar with cytoplasmic extensions
- May have signet ring appearance
- Prominent myxoid background

Immunohistochemistry

Antibody	Reactivity	Staining Pattern	Comment
EMA	Positive	Cytoplasmic	Strong and diffuse in all cases
Claudin-1	Positive	Cell membrane	Distinctly particulate pattern along cell membrane in nearly all cases
GLUT1	Positive	Cell membrane and cytoplasm	Usually membranous to stippled
CD34	Positive	Cytoplasmic	Seen in up to 65% of cases
Collagen IV	Positive	Stromal matrix	Strong membranous staining of cells
Actin-sm	Positive	Cytoplasmic	Up to 20% of cases
S100	Positive	Nuclear & cytoplasmic	Only in up to 5% of cases
CK-PAN	Negative		
GFAP	Negative		
NFP	Negative		Axons adjacent to tumor may be highlighted
Desmin	Negative		
TLE1	Equivocal	Nuclear	Present in normal perineurial cells

Immunohistochemistry

- Variably positive with perineurial markers
  - EMA: Strong and diffuse in all cases
  - Claudin-1: Distinctly particulate pattern along cell membrane in nearly all cases
  - GLUT1: Usually membranous to stippled
  - CD34: Up to 65% of tumors may be positive
  - May have smooth muscle actin (~ 20%) and S100 (~ 5%)
- Strong membranous staining with collagen IV

Genetic Testing

- Monosomy of chromosome 22 in conventional STP
- Chromosome 10 aberrations seen in sclerosing variants
  - Deletion of 10q; t(2;10)(p23;q24); monosomy 10

Electron Microscopy

- Long, thin, cytoplasmic processes with incomplete basal lamina (basement membrane) and pinocytotic vesicles, and well-formed tight junctions
- Axons absent

DIFFERENTIAL DIAGNOSIS

Neurofibroma and Schwannoma

- Benign peripheral nerve sheath tumors include neurofibromas, schwannomas, and perineuriomas
  - Hybrid combinations of schwannoma/neurofibroma and perineurioma are known
  - Show alternating layers of S100 and EMA positive cells layered adjacent to one another
- Schwannoma are encapsulated tumors, which may be associated with nerve in many cases
- Perivascular hyalinization is usually found
- **Positive**: S100, SOX10; CD34 in neurofibroma

Solitary Fibrous Tumor

- Cellular tumors with spindled cells, vascular pattern, and much more heavily collagenized stroma
- **Positive**: CD34, Bcl-2, STAT6; **negative**: S100, SOX10

Myoepithelioma

- Epithelial neoplasm arranged in nests, cords, and clusters, sometimes with ductal differentiation but usually spindled to plasmacytoid cells
- **Positive**: CK-PAN, CK7, S100, p63, GFAP, SMA, MSA, calponin

Meningioma

- Central nervous system association is usual, but ectopic tumors may be seen
- Whorled architecture with psammoma bodies
- Lacks collagen IV immunoreactivity
- **Positive**: EMA
  - Perineurial and arachnoidal cells may be related

Desmoid Fibromatosis

- Ill-defined, infiltrative lesions with bland, purposefully directed spindled cells parallel to vessels
- **Positive**: Nuclear β-catenin

SELECTED REFERENCES

1. Folpe AL: Selected topics in the pathology of epithelioid soft tissue tumors. Mod Pathol. 27 Suppl 1:S64-79, 2014
2. Xiao WL et al: Soft tissue perineurioma of the tongue: report of a case and review of the literature. World J Surg Oncol. 12:11, 2014
3. Rodriguez FJ et al: Pathology of peripheral nerve sheath tumors: diagnostic overview and update on selected diagnostic problems. Acta Neuropathol. 123(3):295-319, 2012
4. Koutlas IG et al: Intraoral perineurioma, soft tissue type: report of five cases, including 3 intraosseous examples, and review of the literature. Head Neck Pathol. 4(2):113-20, 2010
5. Fang WS et al: An unusual sinonasal tumor: soft tissue perineurioma. AJNR Am J Neuroradiol. 30(2):437-9, 2009
6. Hornick JL et al: Hybrid schwannoma/perineurioma: clinicopathologic analysis of 42 distinctive benign nerve sheath tumors. Am J Surg Pathol. 33(10):1554-61, 2009
7. Ahrens WA et al: GLUT-1 expression in mesenchymal tumors: an immunohistochemical study of 247 soft tissue and bone neoplasms. Hum Pathol. 39(10):1519-26, 2008
8. Hornick JL et al: Soft tissue perineurioma: clinicopathologic analysis of 81 cases including those with atypical histologic features. Am J Surg Pathol. 29(7):845-58, 2005
9. Housini I et al: Fine needle aspiration cytology of perineurioma. Report of a case with histologic, immunohistochemical and ultrastructural studies. Acta Cytol. 34(3):420-4, 1990

Epithelioid Nests Within Stroma

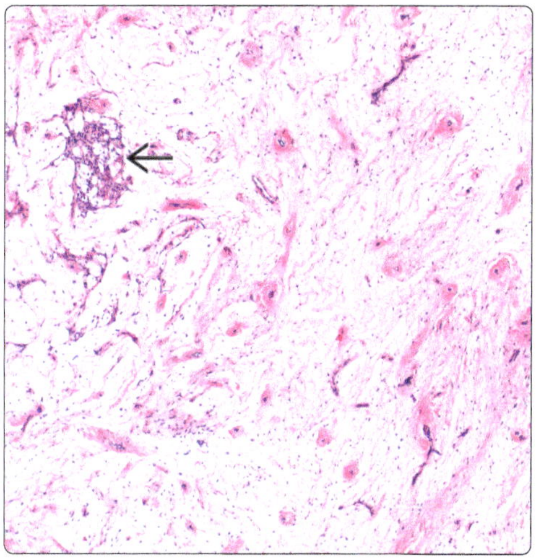

Syncytium of Spindled Cells

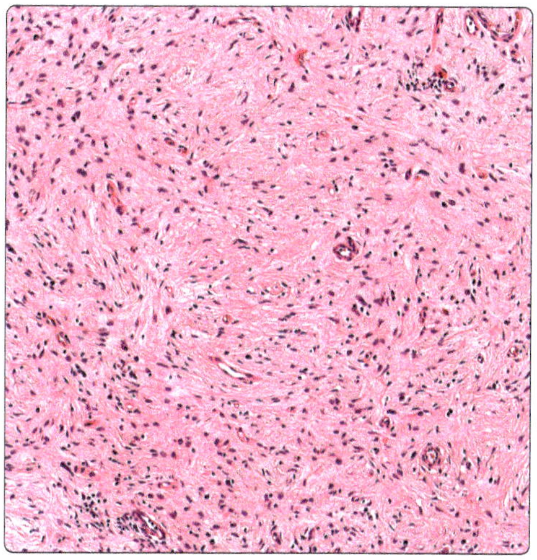

(Left) *H&E shows an epithelioid nest → set within an otherwise storiform to spindled cell population.* **(Right)** *H&E shows the cells are arranged in a syncytial pattern, although the spindle cells are easily identified. There are vessels within the proliferation, but they do not show hyalinized walls.*

Prominent Vessels in Perineurioma

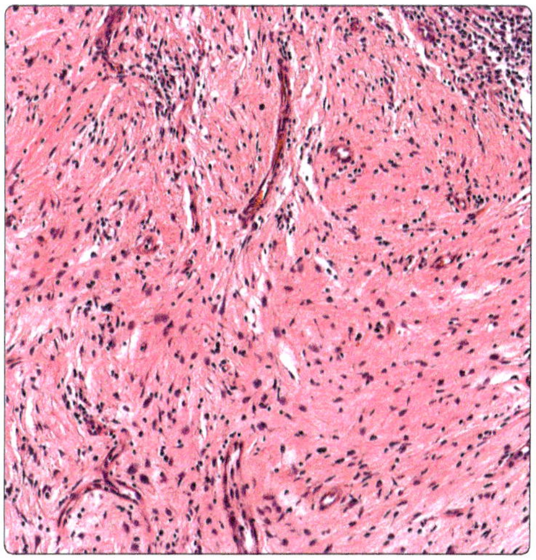

GLUT1 Highlights Spindled Cells

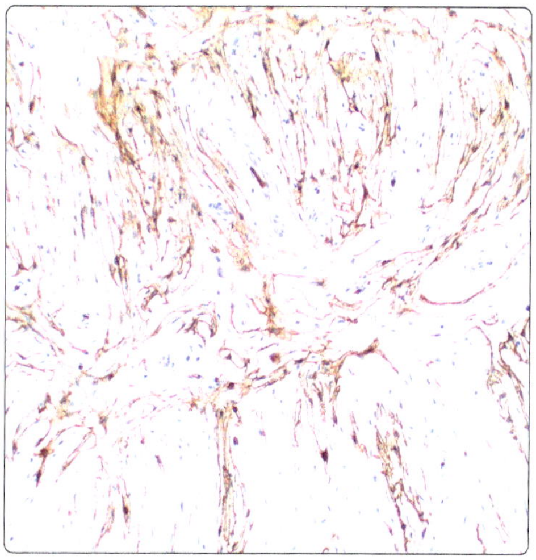

(Left) *The proliferation is less cellular in this field, although the vessels are more prominent. There is still a lack of perivascular hyalinization. The nuclei are small and spindled. There is a lack of cytologic atypia and mitoses.* **(Right)** *The neoplastic spindle cells seen here are highlighted by GLUT1, giving a slightly stippled to granular appearance. The wisps of cytoplasm are stained, creating a feathery appearance to the cells.*

Claudin-1: Perineural Marker

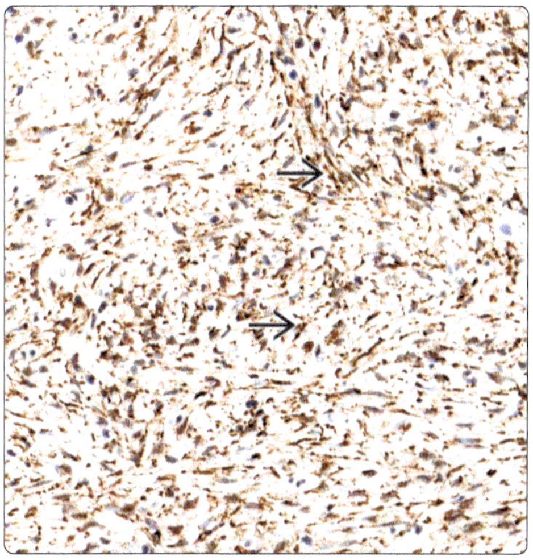

EMA Stains Epithelioid Cells

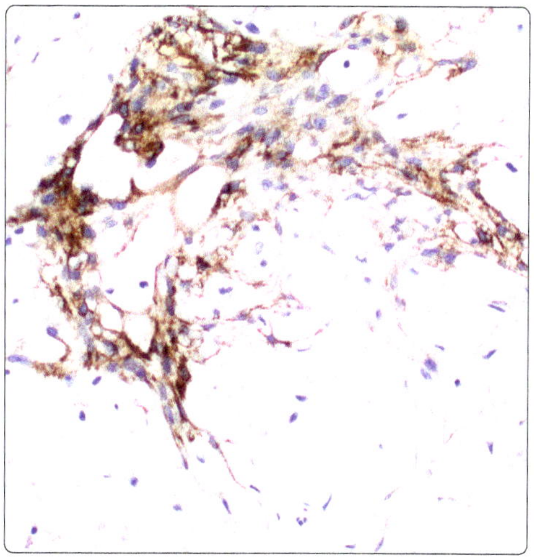

(Left) *Claudin-1 will frequently display a stippled, beaded, or granular staining →, while also highlighting the cell membranes. This staining pattern is quite unique to this tumor.* **(Right)** *The cell membranes and cytoplasm show a variably strong reaction in the cells of a perineurioma. However, it is important to know the staining can be quite weak.*

Nasal Glial Heterotopia

KEY FACTS

TERMINOLOGY

- Nasal glial heterotopia are congenital malformations of displaced normal, mature glial tissue (choristomas)
- Encephalocele represents herniation of brain tissue and leptomeninges through bony defect of skull

CLINICAL ISSUES

- NGH usually presents during infancy
- Separated into 2 types, based on location
- Extranasal (60%): Subcutaneous bridge of nose
- Intranasal (30%): Superior nasal cavity
- Firm, subcutaneous nodule at bridge of nose
- Obstruction, nasal polyps, chronic rhinosinusitis, nasal drainage
- Radiographs are prerequisite to avoid postbiopsy complications, including meningitis and CSF rhinorrhea
- Excellent outcome with surgery, although recurrences occur (up to 30%) if incompletely excised

MICROSCOPIC

- Skin or surface mucosa is intact
- Fibrous connective tissue blended with glial tissue
- Fibrosis frequently obliterates or obscures glial tissue; special stains required to confirm
- Prominent glial fibrillar network
- Gemistocytes may be noted

ANCILLARY TESTS

- Trichrome: Glial tissue is bright red; fibrosis is blue
- Glial tissue is highlighted with S100 and GFAP (latter more sensitive)

TOP DIFFERENTIAL DIAGNOSES

- Fibrosed nasal polyp: Lacks glial tissue, contains mucoserous glands, and usually has greater amount of inflammation

Glial Tissue Blended With Fibrosis

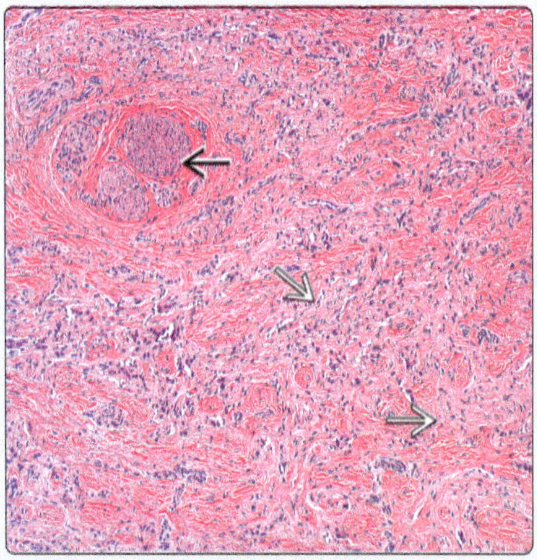

Glial Tissue in Fibrosis

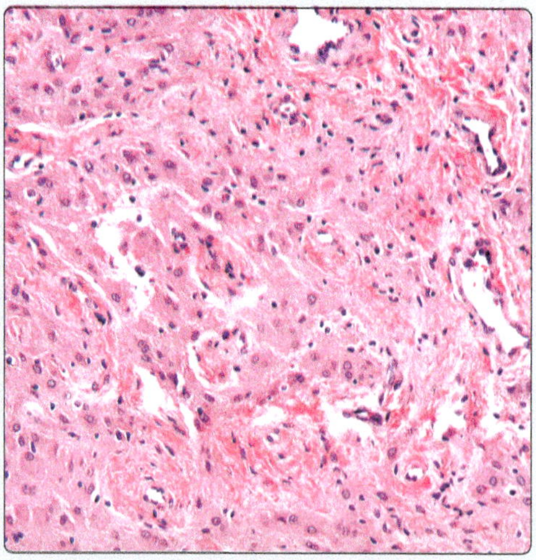

(Left) *The glial tissue ➡ identified as part of nasal glial heterotopia can be very challenging to separate from the adjacent fibrous connective tissue that is a common component of the lesion. Note the peripheral nerve ➡ intermixed with the proliferation.* **(Right)** *Hematoxylin & eosin shows the intermingling of glial elements with fibrosis. This is a very subtle finding, highlighting the reason for performing special studies in many cases.*

Gemistocytic-Like Glial Cells in Fibrosis

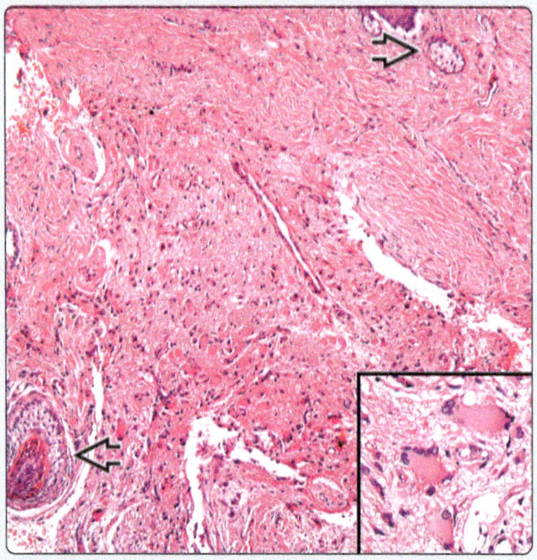

GFAP Strongly Highlights Neural Tissue

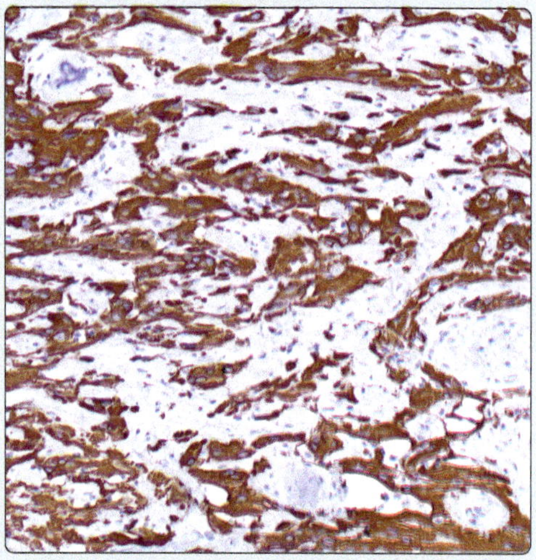

(Left) *Hematoxylin & eosin shows pilosebaceous units ➡, with a gemistocytic-like glial proliferation within the fibrous connective tissue. The tissue often extends into the dermis or subcutaneous tissue. The inset shows higher power magnification of the gemistocytes.* **(Right)** *GFAP strongly and diffusely highlights the neural tissue in this example of nasal glial heterotopia. The fibrous connective tissue is negative.*

TERMINOLOGY

Abbreviations

- Nasal glial heterotopia (NGH)

Synonyms

- Glioma: Implies tumor and is to be discouraged

Definitions

- Nasal glial heterotopia are congenital malformations of displaced normal, mature glial tissue (choristomas)
- Encephalocele represents herniation of brain tissue and leptomeninges through bony defect of skull

ETIOLOGY/PATHOGENESIS

Developmental Anomaly

- Congenital malformation of displaced normal and mature glial tissue

Iatrogenic

- Encephalocele is herniation of brain tissue through bony defect
  - Often secondary to infections, trauma, or surgery

CLINICAL ISSUES

Epidemiology

- Incidence
  - NGH is rare, while encephalocele is uncommon
- Age
  - NGH usually presents during infancy
  - Encephalocele may present in older children and adults
- Sex
  - Equal gender distribution

Site

- Separated into 2 types, based on location
  - Extranasal (60%): Subcutaneous bridge of nose
  - Intranasal (30%): Superior nasal cavity
  - Mixed (10%)

Presentation

- Firm, subcutaneous nodule at bridge of nose
- Polypoid mass within superior nasal cavity
- Obstruction, nasal polyps, chronic rhinosinusitis, nasal drainage
- Chronic otitis media
- CSF rhinorrhea represents encephalocele

Treatment

- Excision must be adequate

Prognosis

- Excellent, with recurrences (up to 30%) if incompletely excised

IMAGING

Radiographic Findings

- Radiographs are prerequisite to avoid postbiopsy complications, including meningitis and CSF rhinorrhea
- Sharply demarcated, expansile mass
- Need to document continuity with central nervous system
- Intracranial extension (tract or cribriform plate defect) must be excluded
  - Especially difficult to document with CT or MR if defect is small

MACROSCOPIC

General Features

- Smooth, homogeneous glistening cut surface, similar to brain tissue
- Sometimes fibrous connective tissue dominates, making it firm

Size

- Usually < 2 cm

MICROSCOPIC

Histologic Features

- Skin or surface mucosa is intact
- Glial tissue appears similar to gliosis
- Fibrous connective tissue blended with glial tissue
  - Fibrosis frequently obliterates or obscures glial tissue; special stains required to confirm
- Nests and sheets of fibrillar neuroglial tissue
- Prominent glial fibrillar network
- Gemistocytes may be noted, while neurons are uncommon
- Choroid plexus, ependyma, and retinal pigmented cells are exceedingly rare
- Encephalocele shows glial degeneration but requires radiographic/clinical correlation

ANCILLARY TESTS

Histochemistry

- Trichrome: Glial tissue is bright red; fibrosis is blue

Immunohistochemistry

- Glial tissue **positive** with S100 and GFAP (latter more sensitive)

DIFFERENTIAL DIAGNOSIS

Fibrosed Nasal Polyp

- Lacks glial tissue, contains mucoserous glands, and usually has greater amount of inflammation

SELECTED REFERENCES

1. Kau T et al: Transsphenoidal extension of heterotopic glioneuronal tissue: pathoanatomic considerations in symptomatic neonates. Childs Nerv Syst. 27(5):771-8, 2011
2. Meoded A et al: Pre- and postnatal ultrasound and magnetic resonance imaging of intracranial extra-axial glioneuronal heterotopia. Fetal Diagn Ther. 30(4):314-6, 2011
3. Kadom N et al: Radiological reasoning: pediatric midline nasofrontal mass. AJR Am J Roentgenol. 194(3 Suppl):WS10-3, 2010
4. Pereyra-Rodríguez JJ et al: Nasal glial heterotopia (nasal glioma). J Pediatr. 156(4):688-688.e1, 2010
5. Yorgancılar E et al: Ganglioglioma in the nasal cavity: a case report. Kulak Burun Bogaz Ihtis Derg. 20(5):267-70, 2010
6. Penner CR et al: Nasal glial heterotopia. Ear Nose Throat J. 83(2):92-3, 2004
7. Penner CR et al: Nasal glial heterotopia: a clinicopathologic and immunophenotypic analysis of 10 cases with a review of the literature. Ann Diagn Pathol. 7(6):354-9, 2003
8. Kardon DE: Nasal glial heterotopia. Arch Pathol Lab Med. 124(12):1849, 2000

Ectopic Meningioma

KEY FACTS

TERMINOLOGY

- Meningothelial neoplasm occurring outside of cranial vault and spinal column
  - Soft tissue extension from intracranial or intraspinal tumor are excluded from definition

CLINICAL ISSUES

- Rare tumors
- Most common in children and young adults
- Usually occur in head and neck region
  - Skin and subcutis of scalp
  - Sinonasal tract
- Treatment: Complete surgical excision, if possible
- Overall prognosis depends upon grade of tumor and completeness of resection
  - Similar to CNS meningiomas
- Meningothelial hamartoma is benign; recurrences rare

MICROSCOPIC

- Often infiltrative into surrounding tissues
- Morphologic spectrum similar to CNS tumors
  - Meningothelial, fibrous, psammomatous, transitional
- Meningothelial hamartoma variant: Slit-like pseudovascular spaces lined by meningothelial cells; variable meningothelial nodules

ANCILLARY TESTS

- Positive for EMA, progesterone receptor
- Variable for claudin-1, S100, p63
- Negative for chromogranin, synaptophysin, CD31, SMA

TOP DIFFERENTIAL DIAGNOSES

- Primary meningioma of CNS
- Cellular neurothekeoma
- Squamous cell carcinoma
- Plexiform fibrohistiocytic tumor

Ectopic (Cutaneous) Meningioma

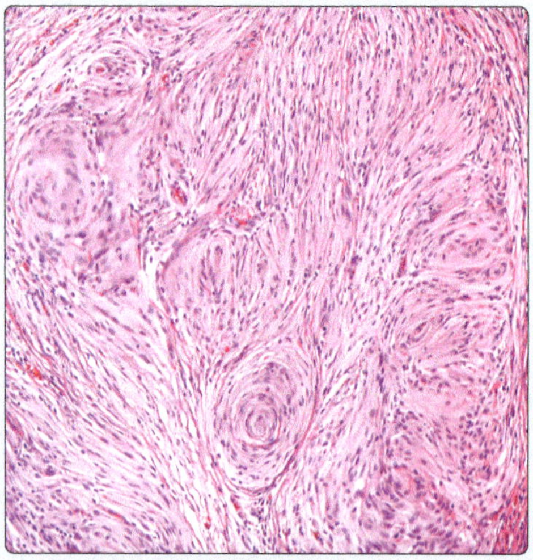

Cells Forming Whorls and Nodules

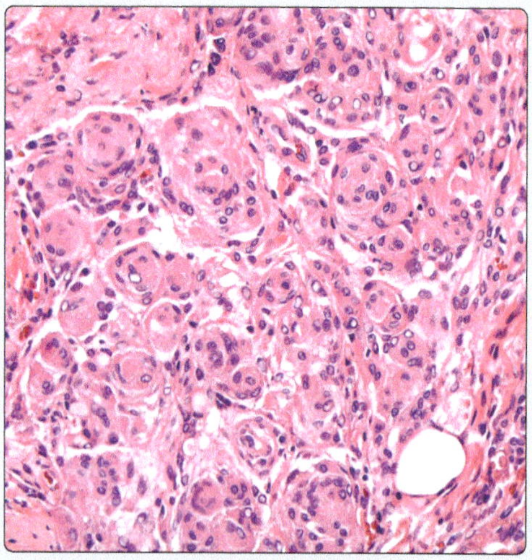

(Left) *Ectopic meningioma shows a similar morphologic spectrum to intracranial/ intraspinal tumors. The meningiothelial or transitional form is most common. Foci of whorling and small nest/nodule formation are characteristic.* **(Right)** *Extensive nested features may mimic a cellular neurothekeomam or even paraganglioma, depending on the site. Immunohistochemistry is valuable in the distinction.*

Infiltrative Growth Pattern

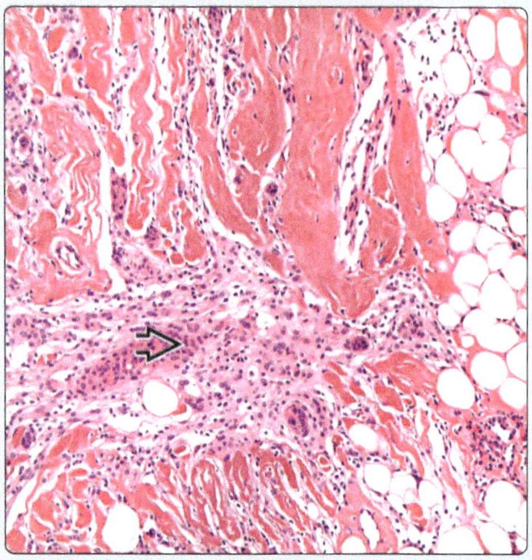

Meningothelial Hamartoma Variant

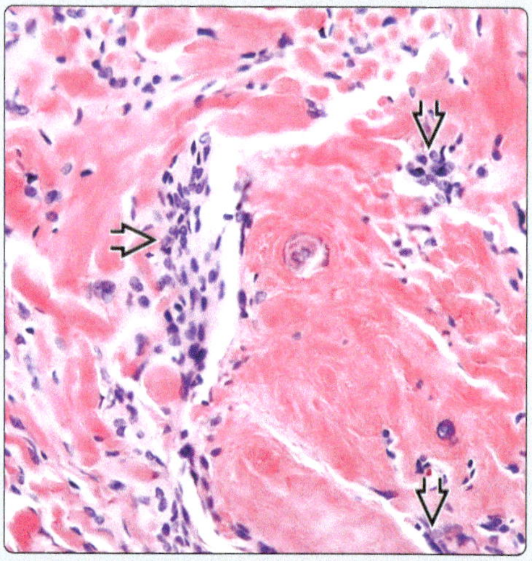

(Left) *Ectopic meningioma ➡ typically shows infiltrative growth within the surrounding soft tissues, as evidenced in this image by the admixed collagen bundles and mature adipose tissue.* **(Right)** *Meningothelial hamartoma is a variant of ectopic meningioma that classically occurs in infants around the posterior scalp. Histologically, it shows collagenous stroma with slit-like pseudovascular spaces lined by meningothelial cells ➡.*

TERMINOLOGY

Synonyms

- Cutaneous meningioma, meningothelial choristoma, extracranial meningioma

Definitions

- Meningothelial proliferation or neoplasm occurring outside of cranial vault and interior spinal column (a.k.a. classic or type 2 lesion)
  - Meningothelial hamartoma (a.k.a. type 1 lesion) is distinctive, benign clinical variant
  - Soft tissue extension from intracranial or intraspinal tumor (a.k.a. type 3 lesion) are not included in definition

ETIOLOGY/PATHOGENESIS

Unknown

- Various hypotheses, including ectopic arachnoid cap cells, displaced meningothelial cells, others

CLINICAL ISSUES

Epidemiology

- Incidence
  - Rare tumors
- Age
  - Wide range reported (most common in children and young adults)
    - Meningothelial hamartoma usually in neonates/infants

Site

- Most common in head and neck region
  - Skin and subcutis of scalp, paravertebral areas
    - Meningothelial hamartoma most common in posterior scalp
  - Sinonasal tract
  - Rarely in other sites, including orbit (unassociated with optic nerve dural sheath), skull, facial bones, oropharynx

Presentation

- Varies widely depending upon site of origin
  - Skin/subcutis
    - Often painless, slow-growing mass
    - May be mistaken for skin tag or epidermal cyst
  - Sinonasal tract
    - Nasal obstruction, discharge, epistaxis

Treatment

- Complete surgical excision

Prognosis

- Similar to CNS tumors
  - Overall prognosis depends upon grade of tumor and completeness of resection
    - Recurrences not uncommon
    - Distant metastases in rare malignant (anaplastic) meningiomas
- Meningothelial hamartoma is benign and recurrences are rare

MACROSCOPIC

General Features

- Usually tan-white-gray, rubbery mass
- May infiltrate bone

Size

- Range: 1-8 cm (mean: 3.5 cm)

MICROSCOPIC

Histologic Features

- Often infiltrative into surrounding tissues
- Morphologic spectrum similar to CNS tumors
  - Meningothelial (most common)
    - Syncytial lobules of cells without distinct borders
    - Whorled architecture
    - Round, regular nuclei with even nuclear chromatin and small nucleoli
    - Pale intranuclear cytoplasmic inclusions
  - Variant morphologies: Transitional, fibroblastic, psammomatoid, atypical, others
- Meningothelial hamartoma (type 1) variant
  - Pseudovascular spaces lined by meningothelial cells
  - Small to large clusters of meningothelial cells

ANCILLARY TESTS

Immunohistochemistry

- Positive for EMA, progesterone receptor
- Variable for claudin-1, S100, p63
- Negative for chromogranin, synaptophysin, CD31, SMA

DIFFERENTIAL DIAGNOSIS

Primary Meningioma of CNS

- May grow out into (or metastasize to) extracranial/extraspinal soft tissues
  - Must always be excluded through imaging

Cellular Neurothekeoma

- May show morphological overlap with meningioma
- Head, neck, upper extremity of young adults
- Prominent micronodular growth
- CD63(+); MiTF(+); EMA(-); S100(-)

Squamous Cell Carcinoma

- Cytologic atypia and keratin formation
- Cytokeratin (+)
- Overlying squamous dysplasia

Plexiform Fibrohistiocytic Tumor

- Usually mixture of spindled fibroblastic cells and histiocytoid nodules
  - Multinucleated giant cells common
- Plexiform growth pattern
- SMA(+), EMA(-)

SELECTED REFERENCES

1. Miedema JR et al: Cutaneous meningioma. Arch Pathol Lab Med. 136(2):208-11, 2012
2. Thompson LD et al: Extracranial sinonasal tract meningiomas: a clinicopathologic study of 30 cases with a review of the literature. Am J Surg Pathol. 24(5):640-50, 2000

Superficial Malignant Peripheral Nerve Sheath Tumor

KEY FACTS

TERMINOLOGY

- Superficial sarcoma arising from cutaneous nerve or benign nerve sheath tumor, or showing nerve sheath differentiation

ETIOLOGY/PATHOGENESIS

- 40% associated with NF1

CLINICAL ISSUES

- Very rare
- Mostly adults but wide age range (4-79 years)
- Most arise in dermis &/or subcutis of head/neck
- Similar reported rates of recurrence and metastasis as deep-seated tumors
  - But may have better overall prognosis (limited data)

MICROSCOPIC

- Mostly intermediate- and high-grade sarcomas
- Spindle cell pattern most common
  - Long fascicles of hyperchromatic spindle cells
  - Wavy nuclei with tapered ends
  - Variable nuclear pleomorphism
  - Extensive necrosis with perivascular preservation
- Epithelioid MPNST
  - Sheets and nodules of epithelioid cells with prominent nucleoli
- Heterologous differentiation in subset
  - Rhabdomyoblastic, osseous, chondroid, others

ANCILLARY TESTS

- S100 positive in ~ 60% of cases, usually focal
  - Diffuse expression in epithelioid MPNST

TOP DIFFERENTIAL DIAGNOSES

- Malignant melanoma
- Atypical neurofibroma
- Dermatofibrosarcoma protuberans
- Clear cell sarcoma

Superficial MPNST

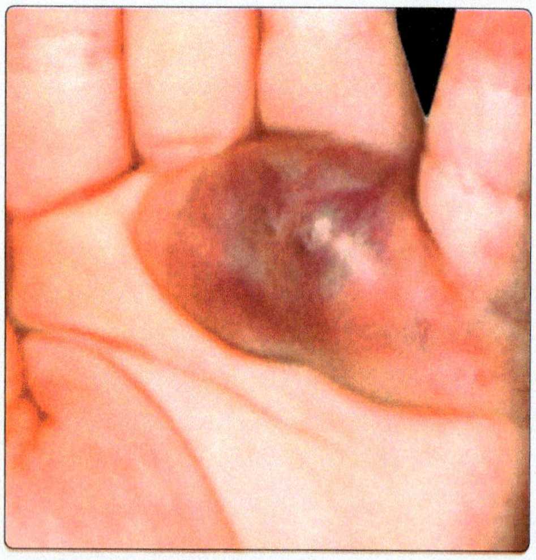

MPNST With Origin in Dermis

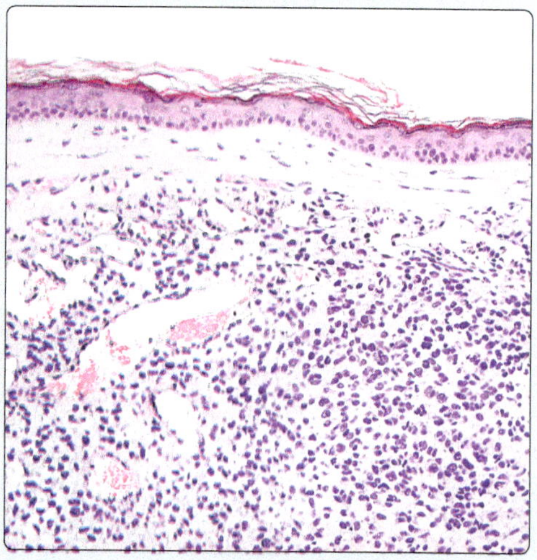

(Left) *Superficial malignant peripheral nerve sheath tumor (MPNST) presents as a cutaneous or soft tissue tumor, as seen in this hand tumor. Average size is around 3 cm. However, massive tumors up to 16 cm have been reported.* **(Right)** *MPNST can rarely present as a primary skin tumor, such as this scalp tumor excised from a 90-year-old woman. Superficial MPNST typically occurs in the mid to deep dermis or as a subcutaneous primary.*

Epithelioid MPNST

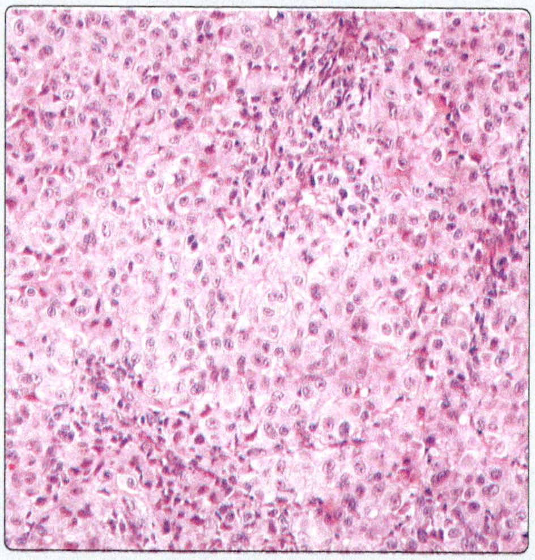

Focal S100 Expression

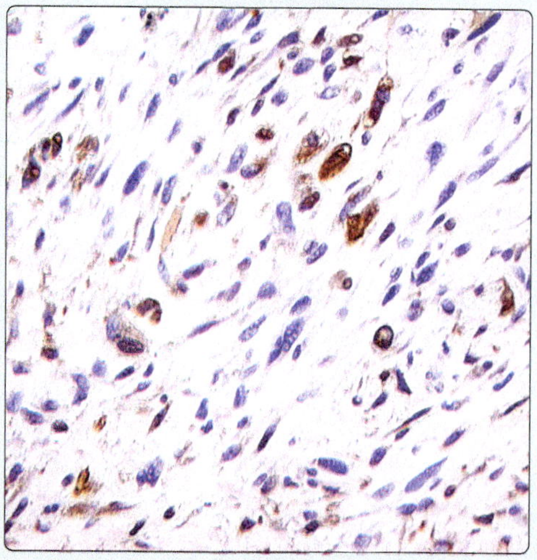

(Left) *Epithelioid MPNST may occur as a primary cutaneous tumor. It is characterized by sheets of epithelioid cells with abundant eosinophilic cytoplasm in a vaguely nodular pattern.* **(Right)** *Only around 60% of superficial MPNSTs are positive for S100 immunohistochemically, and, in most cases, the staining reaction is focal, as shown here. Well-differentiated tumors can show more diffuse staining.*

TERMINOLOGY

Abbreviations

- Malignant peripheral nerve sheath tumor (MPNST)

Synonyms

- Neurofibrosarcoma, malignant schwannoma (older, obsolete terms)

Definitions

- Superficial sarcoma arising from cutaneous nerve or benign nerve sheath tumor, or showing evidence of nerve sheath differentiation
  - Diagnostic criteria
    - Arises from nerve or benign nerve sheath tumor
      - Or shows histological evidence of nerve sheath differentiation in neurofibromatosis type 1 (NF1) patient
      - Or shows histological plus immunohistochemical evidence of nerve sheath differentiation in non-NF1 patient

ETIOLOGY/PATHOGENESIS

Genetic Predisposition

- 40% associated with NF1
  - Lifetime incidence: 2-16%

Molecular Pathogenesis

- NF1 caused by germline mutation of *NF1* tumor suppressor gene
  - Somatic loss of 2nd *NF1* allele required for tumorigenesis
- Malignant transformation in both NF1-associated and sporadic MPNST often involves *CDKN2A* (INK4A) and *TP53* (P53) and their downstream pathways

CLINICAL ISSUES

Epidemiology

- Incidence
  - MPNST accounts for 5-10% of soft tissue sarcomas
    - Superficial MPNST very rare
- Age
  - Mostly adults (20-50 years)
    - Average: 40 years
    - Wide range: 4-79 years
- Sex
  - M = F

Site

- Head and neck (60%), trunk, upper and lower extremities
- Dermis &/or subcutis
  - Mid- or deep dermis in most cases
  - May invade deeper structures

Presentation

- Painful or painless mass

Treatment

- Wide surgical excision/resection
- Radiation
- Response to chemotherapy generally poor

Prognosis

- Similar rates of recurrence and metastasis as deep-seated tumors
  - But may have better overall prognosis (limited data)

IMAGING

General Features

- Morphology
  - Cutaneous nodule
  - Superficial soft tissue mass

MACROSCOPIC

General Features

- Epidermal alterations absent
- Coexisting neurofibroma in some cases

Size

- Average: 3 cm (range: 2-16 cm)

MICROSCOPIC

Histologic Features

- Wide spectrum of cytoarchitectural patterns
  - Mostly intermediate- or high-grade sarcomas
    - High mitotic rate and necrosis
    - Only ~ 15% are low grade
  - Nerve sheath differentiation
    - Nuclear palisading uncommon, usually focal
    - Tactoid differentiation with whorling or Wagner-Meissner body-like features
  - Intraneural tumors
    - Plexiform architecture
    - Microscopic extension within nerve fascicle
  - Tumors arising from preexisting benign nerve sheath tumor
    - Neurofibroma most common, transitional areas, usually in NF1 patients
  - Diffuse infiltrative sarcomatous proliferation without evidence of nerve or nerve sheath tumor origin
- **Spindle cell MPNST (most common pattern)**
  - Long fascicles of uniform, closely spaced, hyperchromatic spindle cells
  - Alternating cellular fascicles and hypocellular areas (tapestry or marbled pattern)
  - Myxoid matrix, focal
  - Storiform arrays
  - Wavy nuclei with tapered ends
  - Small round blue cells
  - Pleomorphic cells
    - Multinucleated giant cells
  - Extensive necrosis with perivascular preservation
- **Epithelioid MPNST**
  - Multinodular architecture
  - Cords and clusters in some
  - Large epithelioid cells
    - Abundant eosinophilic cytoplasm
    - Large vesicular nuclei with macronucleoli
    - Clear cytoplasm in some
  - Often mixed with spindle cells

- **Heterologous differentiation (15% of MPNSTs)**
  - Osseous and osteosarcomatous
  - Chondroid and chondrosarcomatous
  - Rhabdomyosarcomatous (malignant Triton tumor)
  - Angiosarcomatous
  - Glandular

Cytologic Features

- Spindle cells
  - Ill-defined cytoplasm
  - Hyperchromatic nucleus with dispersed coarse chromatin
  - Tapered and wavy nuclei in well-differentiated tumors
  - Very brisk mitotic activity in high-grade tumors
- Epithelioid cells
  - Abundant eosinophilic or clear cytoplasm
  - Vesicular nucleus with prominent inclusion-like nucleolus

ANCILLARY TESTS

Immunohistochemistry

- S100(+) in ~ 60% of cases of spindle cell MPNST, usually focal
  - Diffuse expression in epithelioid MPNST

Genetic Testing

- Complex structural and numeric chromosomal abnormalities
  - Frequent loss of *NF1* at 17q11
  - Frequent loss of *TP53* at 17q13

DIFFERENTIAL DIAGNOSIS

Malignant Melanoma

- Spindle cell/desmoplastic melanoma
  - Often have overlying melanoma in situ (> 70% of cases), usually lentigo maligna type
  - May have clustered or thèque-like areas
  - Diffusely and strongly positive for S100 and SOX10
    - MPNST often shows only weak/focal staining
  - Usually negative for HMB-45, tyrosinase, and MART-1/Melan-A
- Epithelioid melanoma
  - Almost always have overlying melanoma in situ (unless metastatic)
  - Amelanotic melanoma may be indistinguishable from epithelioid MPNST
  - Diffusely S100(+)
    - Epithelioid MPNST often diffusely S100 (+) as well
  - Usually positive for HMB-45, tyrosinase, SOX10, and MART-1/Melan-A
    - MPNST negative for these markers

Atypical Neurofibroma

- Large, hyperchromatic-staining spindle cells
- Degenerated (smudged) chromatin
- Low mitotic rate
- Lacks necrosis
- Usually retains cytoarchitectural features of neurofibroma
  - Edematous fibrillary or myxoid matrix with collagen bundles (shredded carrots pattern)

Dermatofibrosarcoma Protuberans

- Dermal-based tumor composed of uniform spindle cells with tapered nuclei and indistinct cytoplasm
- Well-defined storiform architecture usually prominent
- Broadly infiltrates subcutis and entraps adipocytes in honeycomb pattern
- CD34(+), FXIIIA(-), S100(-)
- t(17;22)(q22;q13) by cytogenetics
- *COL1A1-PDGFRB* by FISH or RT-PCR

Clear Cell Sarcoma

- Predilection for acral extremities
- Usually deep soft tissue tumor but can invade skin in some cases
  - Rare cutaneous primary tumors
- Multinodular, packeted or nested architecture
  - Nests often surrounded by fibrous tissue bands
- Uniform epithelioid and spindle cells
- Vesicular chromatin with prominent nucleoli
- Diffuse S100, HMB-45, and MART-1/Melan-A staining in most cases
- t(12:22) by cytogenetics
- *EWSR1* break apart by FISH
- *EWSR1-ATF1* or *EWSR1-CREB1* by RT-PCR

SELECTED REFERENCES

1. Luzar B et al: Cutaneous epithelioid malignant peripheral nerve sheath tumour: a clinicopathological analysis of 11 cases. Histopathology. 68(2):286-96, 2016
2. Inoue T et al: Superficial malignant peripheral nerve sheath tumor arising from diffuse neurofibroma in a neurofibromatosis type 1 patient. J Dermatol. 41(7):631-3, 2014
3. Salgado R et al: Molecular diagnosis of dermatofibrosarcoma protuberans: A comparison between reverse transcriptase-polymerase chain reaction and fluorescence in situ hybridization methodologies. Genes Chromosomes Cancer. 50(7):510-7, 2011
4. Gottfried ON et al: Neurofibromatosis type 1 and tumorigenesis: molecular mechanisms and therapeutic implications. Neurosurg Focus. 28(1):E8, 2010
5. Hantschke M et al: Cutaneous clear cell sarcoma: a clinicopathologic, immunohistochemical, and molecular analysis of 12 cases emphasizing its distinction from dermal melanoma. Am J Surg Pathol. 34(2):216-22, 2010
6. Jokinen CH et al: Atypical neurofibroma of the skin and subcutaneous tissue: clinicopathologic analysis of 11 cases. J Cutan Pathol. 37(1):35-42, 2010
7. Tanas MR et al: Utilization of fluorescence in situ hybridization in the diagnosis of 230 mesenchymal neoplasms: an institutional experience. Arch Pathol Lab Med. 134(12):1797-803, 2010
8. Jagdis A et al: Prospective evaluation of TLE1 as a diagnostic immunohistochemical marker in synovial sarcoma. Am J Surg Pathol. 33(12):1743-51, 2009
9. Olsen SH et al: Cluster analysis of immunohistochemical profiles in synovial sarcoma, malignant peripheral nerve sheath tumor, and Ewing sarcoma. Mod Pathol. 19(5):659-68, 2006
10. Allison KH et al: Superficial malignant peripheral nerve sheath tumor: a rare and challenging diagnosis. Am J Clin Pathol. 124(5):685-92, 2005
11. Birindelli S et al: Rb and TP53 pathway alterations in sporadic and NF1-related malignant peripheral nerve sheath tumors. Lab Invest. 81(6):833-44, 2001
12. Lucas DR et al: Clear cell sarcoma of soft tissues. Mayo Clinic experience with 35 cases. Am J Surg Pathol. 16(12):1197-204, 1992
13. Dabski C et al: Neurofibrosarcoma of skin and subcutaneous tissues. Mayo Clin Proc. 65(2):164-72, 1990
14. Hruban RH et al: Malignant peripheral nerve sheath tumors of the buttock and lower extremity. A study of 43 cases. Cancer. 66(6):1253-65, 1990
15. George E et al: Malignant peripheral nerve sheath tumors of the skin. Am J Dermatopathol. 11(3):213-21, 1989
16. Ducatman BS et al: Malignant peripheral nerve sheath tumors. A clinicopathologic study of 120 cases. Cancer. 57(10):2006-21, 1986

Spindle Cell Pattern in MPNST

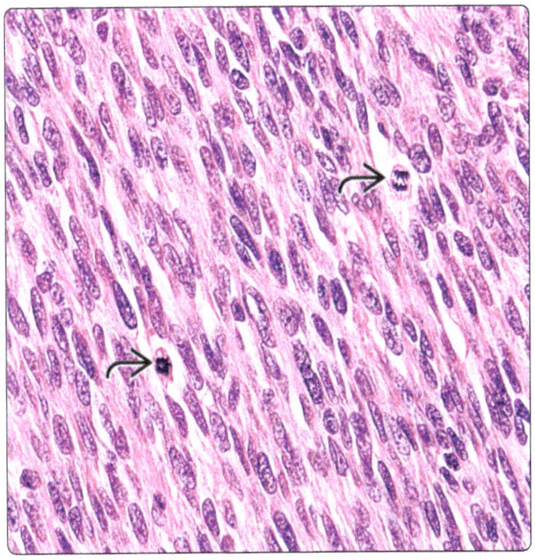

Marbled Growth Pattern in MPNST

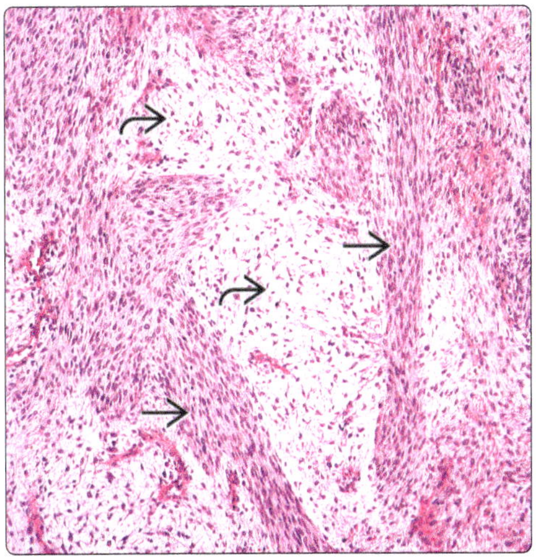

(Left) *The most common pattern of MPNST is a high-grade spindle cell sarcoma composed of long fascicles of closely spaced, uniform spindle cells with ill-defined cytoplasmic borders, coarse nuclear hyperchromasia, and brisk mitotic activity ⮫.* **(Right)** *A distinctive pattern seen in spindle cell MPNST consists of alternating hypercellular fascicles ➙ and less cellular myxedematous regions ⮫, sometimes referred to as a tapestry or marbled pattern.*

Origin from Nerve or Benign Nerve Sheath Tumor

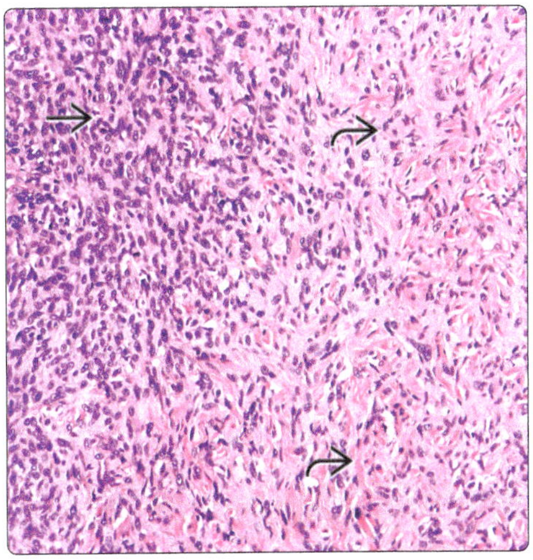

Prominent Nucleoli in Epithelioid MPNST

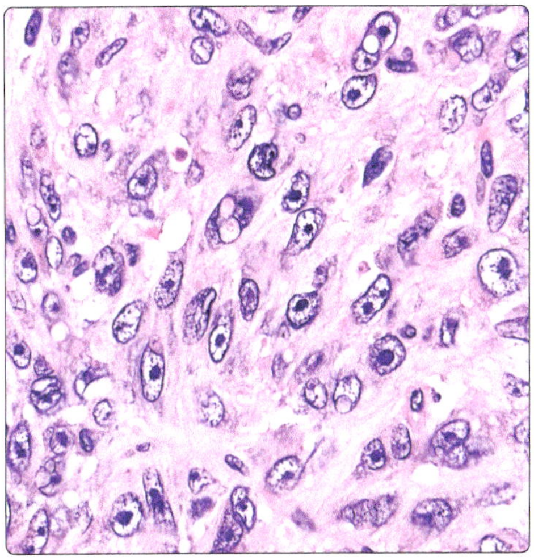

(Left) *Superficial MPNSTs may arise from either cutaneous nerves or from benign nerve sheath tumors. This spindle cell MPNST ➙ arose from a neurofibroma ⮫ in the neck of a 46-year-old woman with type 1 neurofibromatosis.* **(Right)** *Epithelioid MPNST is characterized by large polygonal cells with abundant eosinophilic cytoplasm and vesicular nuclei with prominent large nucleoli. It is usually diffusely S100(+) but HMB-45 and MART-1/Melan-A (-), which distinguishes it from melanoma.*

Corded Growth in MPNST

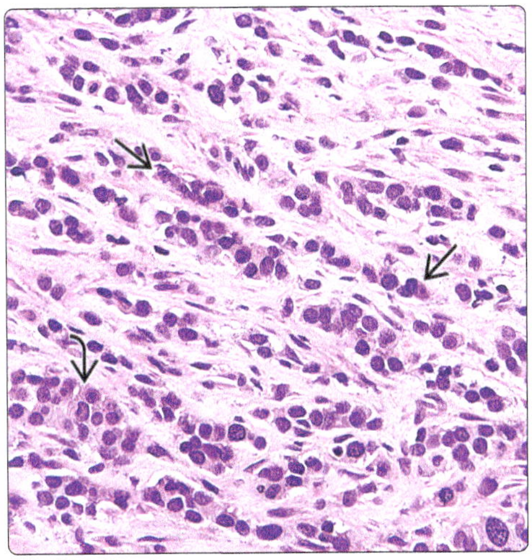

Heterologous Elements in MPNST

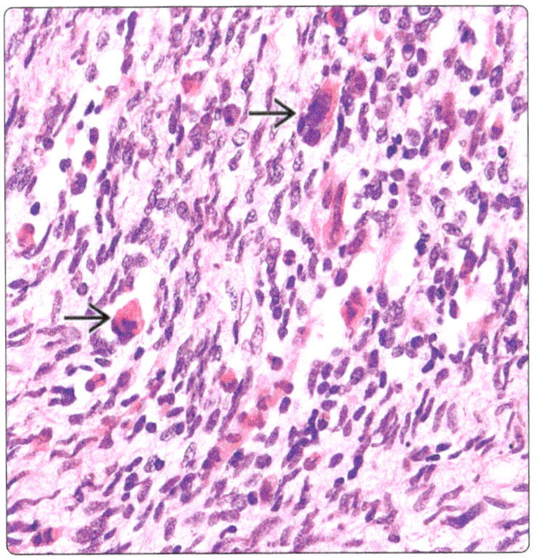

(Left) *In some epithelioid MPNSTs, the cells are arranged in single file cords ➙ and small clusters ⮫, mimicking carcinoma. However, immunostaining for cytokeratins is negative.* **(Right)** *Heterologous differentiation is present in around 15% of MPNSTs. Rhabdomyosarcomatous differentiation (so-called Triton tumor) has been reported in superficial MPNST. Note the malignant rhabdomyoblasts with brightly eosinophilic cytoplasm ➙ in this spindle cell MPNST.*

KEY FACTS

TERMINOLOGY

- Primary malignant small round blue cell tumor of dermis and superficial subcutis
  - Variable evidence of neuroectodermal differentiation

CLINICAL ISSUES

- Very rare
- Most common in teenagers and young adults
- More common in women
- Extremities, trunk, head/neck, other sites
- Complete surgical resection
- Chemotherapy &/or radiation
- Cutaneous ES/PNET appears to have improved prognosis

MACROSCOPIC

- Most < 2.5 cm

MICROSCOPIC

- Localized to dermis or dermis/subcutis
- Resembles conventional deep forms of ES/PNET
  - Sheets &/or vague lobules
  - Monomorphic small round tumor cells
  - Fine chromatin with small or absent nucleoli
- Mitotic figures and necrosis common
- Intercellular rosettes may be present (PNET morphology)

ANCILLARY TESTS

- Diffuse, strong CD99(+) in membranous pattern
- Negative for lymphoid, myoid, and melanocytic markers
- Characteristic t(11;22)(q24;q12) in 90% of cases
  - *EWSR1-FLI1* gene fusion

TOP DIFFERENTIAL DIAGNOSES

- Metastatic ES/PNET
- Merkel cell carcinoma
- Alveolar rhabdomyosarcoma
- Lymphoblastic lymphoma

(Left) *Superficial cutaneous forms of ES/PNET are morphologically, immunophenotypically, and genetically identical to conventional, deep forms of ES/PNET. The superficial types differ, however, by having a better prognosis. For this to apply, a cutaneous metastasis from a deep ES/PNET must be completely excluded.* **(Right)** *ES/PNET has the overall appearance of a typical small round blue cell tumor. That is, sheets &/or lobules of small monomorphic cells with minimal cytoplasm.*

Superficial ES/PNET

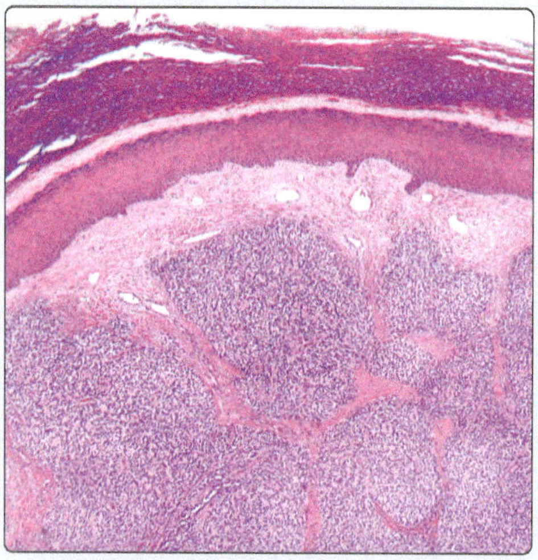

ES/PNET With Sheets of Monomorphic Tumor Cells

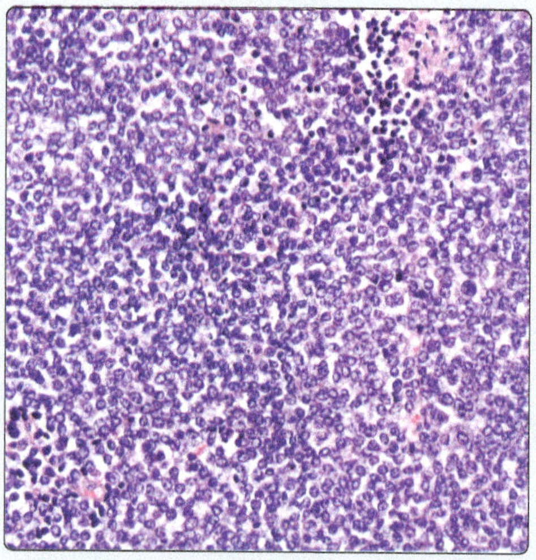

(Left) *The cytologic features of ES/PNET include rounded nuclei with fine chromatin and small to absent nucleoli. Rare variants feature scattered nuclear atypia and pleomorphism.* **(Right)** *Immunohistochemical stain for CD99 in ES/PNET typically shows strong membranous immunoreactivity in the tumor cells. Of note, this finding, although helpful, is not entirely specific for the diagnosis.*

High Magnification Showing Nuclear Features

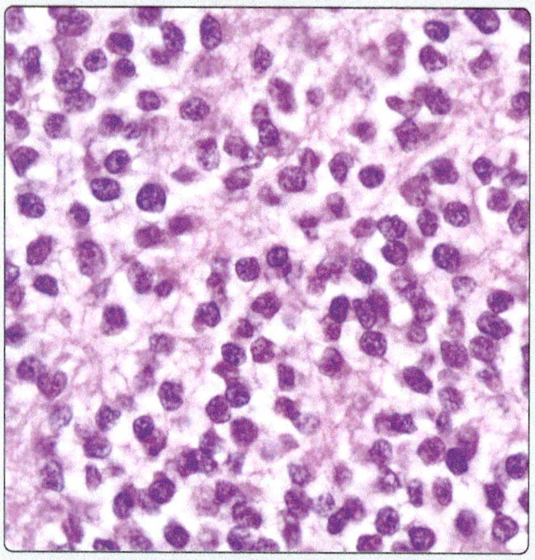

Strong, Membranous CD99 Expression

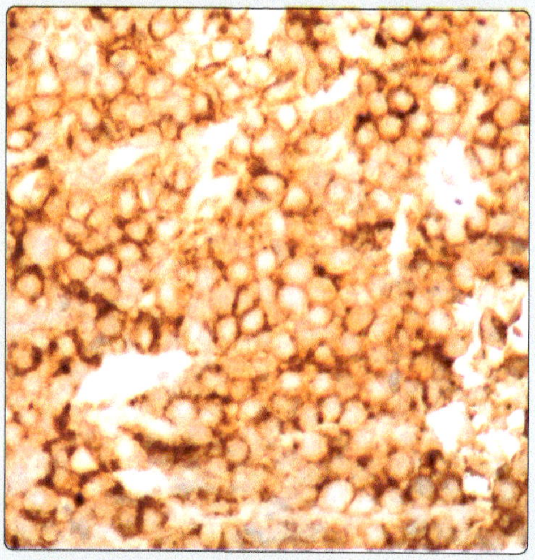

TERMINOLOGY

Abbreviations

- Ewing sarcoma (ES)
- Primitive neuroectodermal tumor (PNET)

Synonyms

- Cutaneous ES/PNET
- Ewing sarcoma family of tumors
- Primitive neuroepithelioma

Definitions

- Primary malignant small round blue cell tumor of dermis and superficial subcutis
  - Variable evidence of neuroectodermal differentiation (morphologic, ultrastructural, immunohistochemical)
  - Essentially, cutaneous/superficial variant of conventional ES/PNET
- Cutaneous metastasis of deep ES/PNET must always be excluded

ETIOLOGY/PATHOGENESIS

Genetics

- Characteristic t(11;22)(q24;q12) in most cases
  - *EWSR1-FLI1* gene fusion

CLINICAL ISSUES

Epidemiology

- Incidence
  - Very rare
    - < 100 cases reported
- Age
  - Most common in teenagers and young adults
- Sex
  - F > M

Site

- Extremities most common
- Trunk
- Head and neck
- Groin

Presentation

- Small nodule, often present for < 1 yr
- Can be painful
- May be clinically misdiagnosed as benign tumor or cyst

Treatment

- Complete surgical resection
- Chemotherapy
- Radiation

Prognosis

- Cutaneous metastasis from deep ES/PNET must be rigorously excluded
- True cutaneous ES/PNET appears to have improved prognosis
  - Lower rate of recurrence and metastasis

MACROSCOPIC

General Features

- Nodular
- May be polypoid/pedunculated

Size

- Most < 2.5 cm

MICROSCOPIC

Histologic Features

- Localized to dermis or dermis/subcutis
  - Well demarcated or mildly infiltrative
  - May appear encapsulated
- Resembles conventional deep forms of ES/PNET
  - Monomorphic small round tumor cells
    - Fine chromatin
    - Small or absent nucleoli
    - Limited or scant, pale eosinophilic cytoplasm
  - Sheets &/or vague lobules
  - Delicate fibrovascular stroma
- Mitotic figures often abundant
- Necrosis is common
  - Can be single cell or geographic type
- Intercellular rosettes may be present (PNET morphology), but are often not well formed
  - Homer Wright rosettes with central neuropil
- Rare variants
  - Large cell (atypical), adamantinoma-like, spindle cell, sclerosing

ANCILLARY TESTS

Immunohistochemistry

- Diffuse, strong CD99 (membranous staining)
- Nuclear FLI-1(+) and ERG(+)
- Focal low molecular weight keratin expression in up to 25% of cases
- Very limited expression (if any) of S100, synaptophysin, chromogranin, CD56
- Negative for lymphoid, myoid, and melanocytic markers

Electron Microscopy

- Elongated, interdigitating cytoplasmic processes
- Rudimentary intercellular junctions, rarely desmosomes, intermediate filaments, microtubules
- Membrane-bound dense core neurosecretory granules

Molecular Genetics

- Characteristic t(11;22)(q24;q12)
  - Results in *EWSR1-FLI1* gene fusion
  - 90% of cases
- t(21;22)(q22;q12)
  - *EWSR1-ERG* gene fusion
  - < 5% of cases
- Other genetic variants very rare (< 1%)
  - Usually involve *EWSR1*; very rarely *FUS*

DIFFERENTIAL DIAGNOSIS

Metastatic ES/PNET

- Critical to exclude metastasis from deep ES/PNET
  - Requires clinical and radiologic correlation
- Morphologically, immunohistochemically, and genetically identical

Merkel Cell Carcinoma

- Usually older/elderly adults
- EMA(+), keratins (+)
  - CK20(+)
    - Characteristic perinuclear dot-like expression
- Synaptophysin (+), chromogranin (+), NSE(+)
- Negative for CD99
- Lacks *EWSR1* translocations

Alveolar Rhabdomyosarcoma

- Greater degree of nuclear variability
- May contain wreath cells or rhabdomyoblasts
- Desmin (+)
- Nuclear myogenin (+), MYOD1(+)
- CD99(+) common
- Features *FOXO1* translocations
- Lacks *EWSR1* translocations

Lymphoblastic Lymphoma

- Most common in children
- Can show histologic and immunohistochemical overlap with ES/PNET
- Often strongly CD99(+)
- Also FLI-1(+)
- TdT(+), CD43(+)
- Negative for CD45
- Lacks *EWSR1* translocations

Small Cell Melanoma

- Overlying melanoma in situ usually present
- Can be S100(-)
- HMB-45(+)
- Negative for CD99
- Lacks *EWRS1* translocations

Metastatic Small Cell Carcinoma

- Usually older adults
- Presence of primary tumor in lung or elsewhere
- Keratin (+), EMA(+)
- Synaptophysin (+), CD56(+)
- Negative for CD99
- Lacks *EWSR1* translocations

Metastatic Neuroblastoma

- Difficult to distinguish histologically
- Usually in young children
- Shows adrenergic expression, metabolic excretion
  - Catecholamines and metabolites
- May contain mature neural elements
  - Ganglion cells
  - Neuropil (fibrillary intercellular network)
- NB84(+)
- Negative for CD99
- Lacks *EWSR1* translocations

Synovial Sarcoma (Poorly Differentiated)

- Often contain areas of more conventional monophasic spindled or biphasic morphology
- Keratin (+)
- Nuclear TLE-1(+)
- CD99(+) common
- Negative for FLI-1 and ERG
- Characteristic *SS18(SYT)* rearrangement
- Lacks *EWSR1* translocations

DIAGNOSTIC CHECKLIST

Clinically Relevant Pathologic Features

- Must exclude possibility of cutaneous metastasis from deep ES/PNET
- Most common in teens and young adults
- More common in women
- Better prognosis than conventional ES/PNET

Pathologic Interpretation Pearls

- Strong, diffuse CD99(+) with membranous reactivity
  - Not completely specific for ES/PNET
- Characteristic t(11;22)(q24;q12) in vast majority of cases
  - *EWSR1-FLI1* gene fusion

SELECTED REFERENCES

1. Hung YP et al: Evaluation of NKX2-2 expression in round cell sarcomas and other tumors with EWSR1 rearrangement: imperfect specificity for Ewing sarcoma. Mod Pathol. 29(4):370-80, 2016
2. Renard C et al: [Ewing/PNET sarcoma family of tumors: towards a new paradigm?.] Ann Pathol. 35(1):86-97, 2015
3. Boland JM et al: Cutaneous neoplasms showing EWSR1 rearrangement. Adv Anat Pathol. 20(2):75-85, 2013
4. Fernandez-Flores A et al: Study of EWS/FLI-1 rearrangement in 18 cases of CK20+/CM2B4+ Merkel cell carcinoma using FISH and correlation to the differential diagnosis of Ewing sarcoma/peripheral neuroectodermal tumor. Appl Immunohistochem Mol Morphol. 21(5):379-85, 2013
5. Machado I et al: Superficial small round-cell tumors with special reference to the Ewing's sarcoma family of tumors and the spectrum of differential diagnosis. Semin Diagn Pathol. 30(1):85-94, 2013
6. Delaplace M et al: Primary cutaneous Ewing sarcoma: a systematic review focused on treatment and outcome. Br J Dermatol. 166(4):721-6, 2012
7. Machado I et al: Superficial Ewing's sarcoma family of tumors: a clinicopathological study with differential diagnoses. J Cutan Pathol. 38(8):636-43, 2011
8. Vural C et al: The evaluation of CD99 immunoreactivity and EWS/FLI1 translocation by fluorescence in situ hybridization in central PNETs and Ewing's sarcoma family of tumors. Pathol Oncol Res. 17(3):619-25, 2011
9. Shingde MV et al: Primary cutaneous Ewing sarcoma/primitive neuroectodermal tumour: a clinicopathological analysis of seven cases highlighting diagnostic pitfalls and the role of FISH testing in diagnosis. J Clin Pathol. 62(10):915-9, 2009
10. Terrier-Lacombe MJ et al: Superficial primitive Ewing's sarcoma: a clinicopathologic and molecular cytogenetic analysis of 14 cases. Mod Pathol. 22(1):87-94, 2009
11. Ehrig T et al: Superficial primitive neuroectodermal tumor/Ewing sarcoma (PN/ES): same tumor as deep PN/ES or new entity? Ann Diagn Pathol. 11(3):153-9, 2007
12. Sangueza OP et al: Multiple primitive neuroectodermal tumors. J Am Acad Dermatol. 31(2 Pt 2):356-61, 1994
13. Van Nguyen A et al: Cutaneous neuroblastoma. Peripheral neuroblastoma. Am J Dermatopathol. 15(1):7-14, 1993
14. Gorman PA et al: Cytogenetic analysis of primitive neuroectodermal tumors. Absence of the t(11;22) in two of three cases and a review of the literature. Cancer Genet Cytogenet. 51(1):13-22, 1991
15. Jacinto CM et al: Malignant primitive neuroectodermal tumor presenting as a scalp nodule. Am J Dermatopathol. 13(1):63-70, 1991
16. Klapman MH et al: Cutaneous and subcutaneous neuroblastoma in children and adults: case reports and population study. J Am Acad Dermatol. 24(6 Pt 1):1025-7, 1991

Sheets of Tumor Cells in ES/PNET

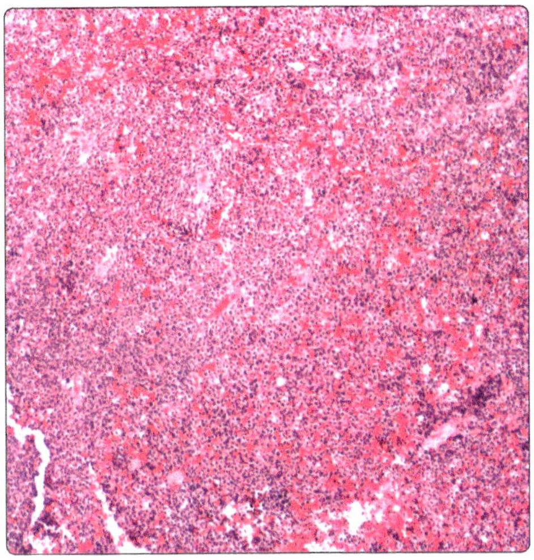

Tumor Cells With Clear Cytoplasm

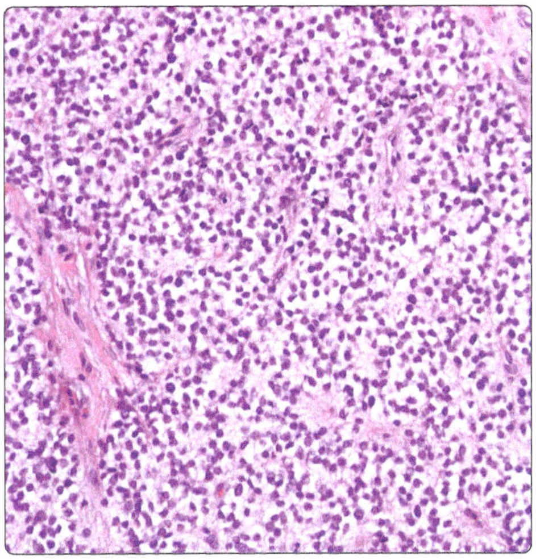

(Left) *Low-power view shows ES/PNET with the classic appearance of patternless, hypercellular lobules to sheets of undifferentiated, small round blue cells.* **(Right)** *The cytoplasm in tumor cells of ES/PNET varies from pale eosinophilic to clear as seen here. The cytoplasmic clearing is due to the presence of intracytoplasmic glycogen.*

Formation of Vague Rosettes

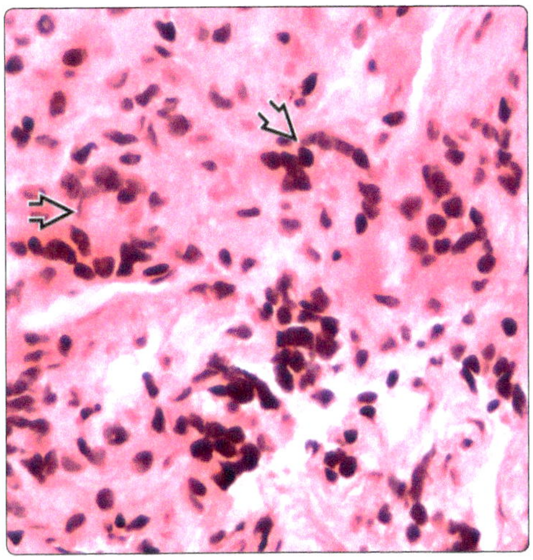

Primitive, Poorly Differentiated Tumor Cells

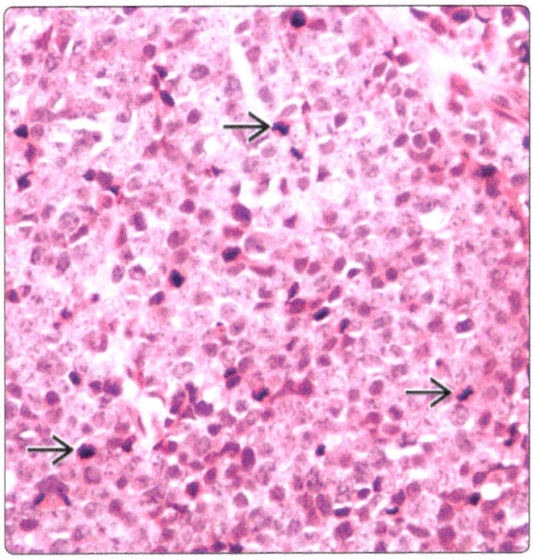

(Left) *High magnification shows an ES/PNET with vague arrangement of cells into rosettes* ⇨, *reminiscent of Homer Wright rosettes with central neuropil.* **(Right)** *High-power view shows ES/PNET with sheet-like areas of dense cellularity composed of monotonous, poorly differentiated tumor cells with little cytoplasm and numerous mitoses* →.

High Proliferation Index Common

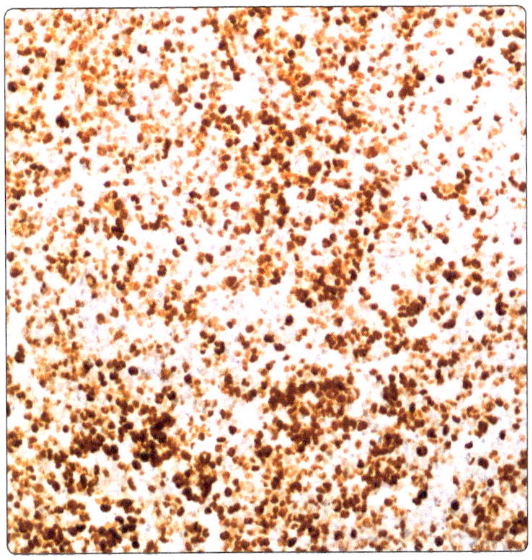

Focal Synaptophysin Expression

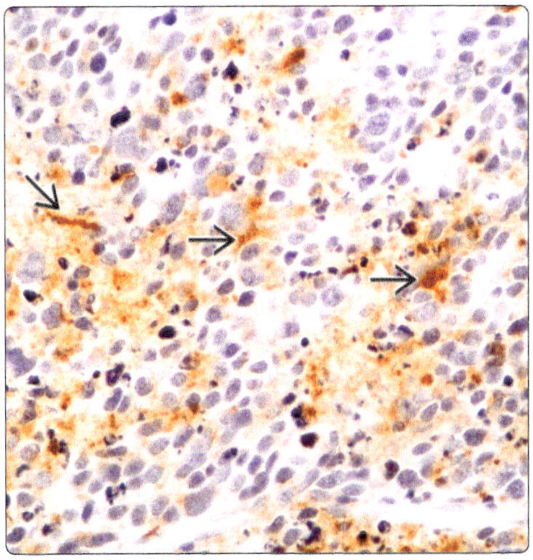

(Left) *Immunohistochemical stain for Ki-67 (MIB-1) shows an ES/PNET with a very high proliferation index, approaching 80-90%.* **(Right)** *Immunohistochemical stain for synaptophysin shows an ES/PNET with highlighted areas of neuronal differentiation* →, *characterized by nuclei-free fibrillar zones with tumor cells radially arranged around them, akin to neuroblastic Homer Wright rosettes. Extensive synaptophysin expression is not seen in ES/PNET.*

Primary Neuroendocrine (Merkel Cell) Carcinoma

KEY FACTS

TERMINOLOGY

- Merkel cell carcinoma (MCC)

ETIOLOGY/PATHOGENESIS

- Recent studies have shown strong link to infection with polyomavirus
- Associated with immunosuppression

CLINICAL ISSUES

- Highly aggressive tumors with greater metastatic potential than melanoma
- Rare (~ 470 cases/yr in USA)
- Typically occur in sun-damaged skin of elderly
- More common in males

MICROSCOPIC

- Highly atypical basaloid neoplasm composed of infiltrative cords, trabeculae, nodular and sheet-like areas
- Typically dermal based, but may show epidermal (pagetoid) involvement in up to 20% of cases
- Numerous mitoses and apoptotic bodies
- Nuclear crush artifact and streaming may be seen, similar to small cell carcinomas
- Basaloid cells with high nuclear:cytoplasmic ratio, scant cytoplasm, large nuclei, granular to clear chromatin, and indistinct nucleoli

ANCILLARY TESTS

- Immunohistochemistry is important in confirming diagnosis and excluding metastatic carcinoma
- MCC is typically positive for keratins, including CK20, with perinuclear dot-like staining

TOP DIFFERENTIAL DIAGNOSES

- Basal cell carcinoma
- Metastatic small cell carcinoma (especially pulmonary origin)
  - Especially lung, which are TTF-1(+), CK20(-)
- Small cell melanoma
- Lymphoma

Clinical Photograph of MCC

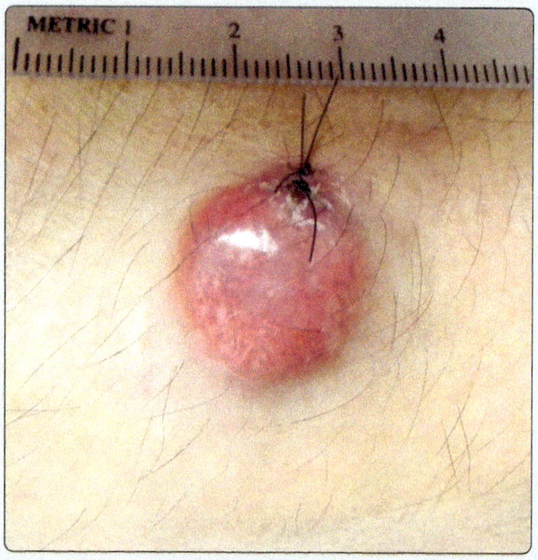

MCC Involving Superficial Dermis

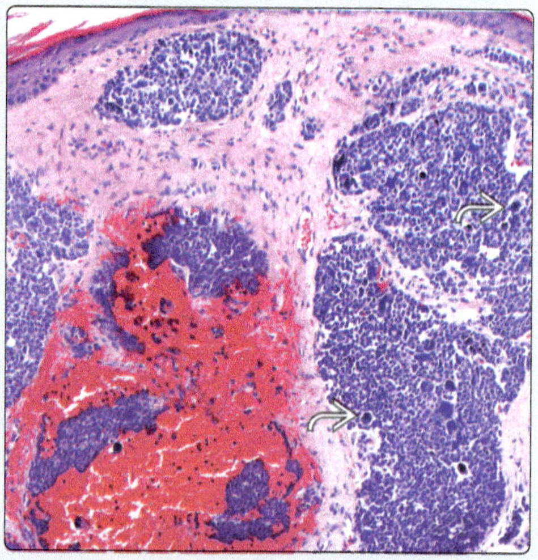

(Left) *Clinical photograph of Merkel cell carcinoma (MCC) shows a well-circumscribed, erythematous dermal nodule. (Courtesy J. Wu, MD.)* **(Right)** *The superficial dermal portion of this tumor shows enlarged, crowded and markedly atypical-appearing basaloid cells with several large, atypical mitotic figures ➡ easily identified.*

Higher Magnification of MCC With Lymphatic Invasion

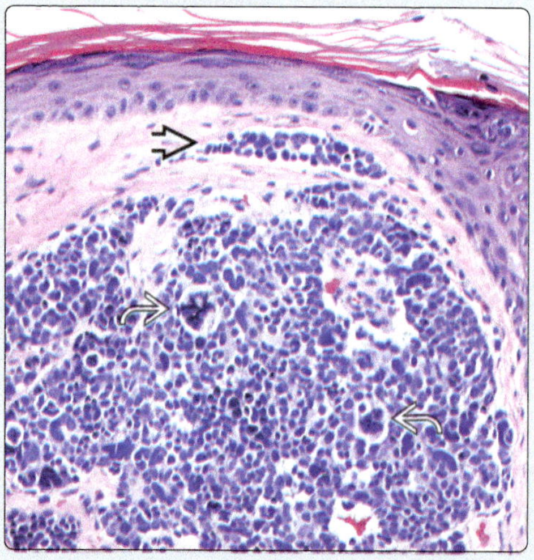

High Magnification of MCC

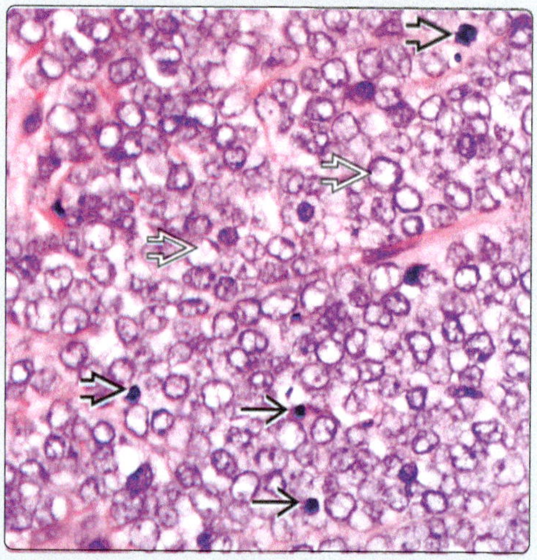

(Left) *High magnification of the superficial dermal portion of this tumor shows enlarged, atypical basaloid cells with several frankly atypical mitotic figures ➡. Invasion of a superficial lymphatic vessel is also seen →.* **(Right)** *Nuclear clearing ➡ is often seen in MCC, a feature not seen in basal cell carcinoma or most other small round blue cell tumors. Note the numerous apoptotic bodies → and mitotic figures →.*

TERMINOLOGY

Abbreviations

- Merkel cell carcinoma (MCC)

Synonyms

- Cutaneous neuroendocrine carcinoma

Definitions

- Malignant proliferation of cutaneous neuroendocrine cells

ETIOLOGY/PATHOGENESIS

Infectious Agents

- Recent studies have shown strong link to infection with polyomavirus
  - Merkel cell polyoma virus infection is found in > 90% of cases by PCR studies
- Associated with immunosuppression
  - Organ transplant and HIV(+) patients have much higher incidence

Cell of Origin

- Postulated to represent malignant transformation of cutaneous neuroendocrine (Merkel) cells or pluripotent stem cells, but this remains speculative

CLINICAL ISSUES

Epidemiology

- Incidence
  - Rare
    - < 500 cases/yr in USA
- Age
  - Typically in elderly patients (> 65 yr old)
- Sex
  - M > F (2.5:1)
- Ethnicity
  - Caucasians much more commonly affected than other races

Site

- Sun-damaged skin
- Usually head and neck or extremities

Presentation

- Dermal nodular or plaque-like mass lesion
- Rapidly enlarging dermal mass lesion
  - May be ulcerated &/or hemorrhagic

Natural History

- Aggressive tumors with high incidence of local recurrence, lymph node, and distant metastasis
- Clinical staging should include imaging studies, especially chest and abdominal CT scans

Treatment

- Surgical approaches
  - Complete and wide excision to ensure complete local removal
  - Consideration may be given to sentinel lymph node (SLN) biopsy
    - However, SLN positivity does not seem to be very sensitive for regional lymph node involvement, as many patients progress to distant metastases
- Adjuvant therapy
  - Radiotherapy is generally used and may lead to remission in some cases
  - Chemotherapy is less effective and does not prolong overall survival

Prognosis

- High incidence of recurrence (up to 30%) and metastasis (up to 75%)
- Overall prognosis is poor
  - Death due to disease is high, even with treatment
  - Worse prognosis associated with advanced age, head and neck location, large size, and immunosuppression

MACROSCOPIC

General Features

- Nodular tumor with blue or red appearance

Size

- Typically < 2 cm

MICROSCOPIC

Histologic Features

- Highly atypical invasive basaloid neoplasm
  - Composed of infiltrative cords, trabeculae, nests, nodular and sheet-like areas
    - Associated dermal desmoplasia may be present
  - Enlarged, hyperchromatic basaloid tumor cells with scant cytoplasm, large nuclei, granular to vesicular chromatin, and indistinct nucleoli
  - Nuclear clearing is distinctive feature often seen
    - This finding is not present in basal cell carcinoma (BCC)
  - Mitotic figures are abundant
  - Numerous apoptotic bodies
  - Areas of geographic necrosis often present, especially in larger tumors
  - Nuclear crush artifact and streaming may be seen, similar to small cell carcinomas
  - Angiolymphatic invasion identified in significant percentage of cases, often at periphery of tumor
  - Partial tumor regression may be present
- Typically dermal based
  - May show epidermal (pagetoid) involvement in up to 20% of cases
  - Purely pagetoid (in situ) cases have been reported
- Areas of squamoid or adnexal (including follicular, ductal, or glandular) differentiation may be present in minority of cases
  - Rarely, melanocytic differentiation may be present
  - These findings suggest that MCC may arise from primitive pluripotential (stem) cell that can differentiate along multiple different lines, rather than specific neuroendocrine cell
- Rarely, spindle cell/sarcomatoid differentiation mimicking atypical fibroxanthoma, leiomyosarcoma, osteosarcoma, or rhabdomyosarcoma may be seen

Immunohistochemistry

Antibody	Reactivity	Staining Pattern	Comment
CK-PAN	Positive	Dot positivity	May or may not show dot-like positivity but will be positive
CK20	Positive	Dot positivity	Rare cases may be negative
CK8/18/CAM5.2	Positive	Dot positivity	Most cases show dot reactivity
NFP	Positive	Cytoplasmic	Most cases are positive [often positive in CK20(-) cases]
Chromogranin-A	Positive	Cytoplasmic	Most cases are positive
Synaptophysin	Positive	Cytoplasmic	Most cases are positive
CK7	Negative	Dot positivity	Isolated cases may be CK7 positive when CK20 negative
S100	Negative		
Melan-A103	Negative		
HMB-45	Negative		
TTF-1	Negative		

Cytologic Features

- Basaloid cells with high nuclear:cytoplasmic ratio, scant cytoplasm, large nuclei, granular to clear chromatin, and indistinct nucleoli

ANCILLARY TESTS

Immunohistochemistry

- IHC is important in confirming diagnosis and excluding metastatic neuroendocrine carcinoma
  - MCC is typically positive for keratins (CK-PAN, CK20, CK8/18/CAM5.2), often with perinuclear dot-like staining
  - Positive for neuroendocrine markers including chromogranin, synaptophysin, and NFP [may be useful in CK20(-) cases]
  - Negative staining for TTF-1, melanocytic markers, and lymphoid markers

Genetic Testing

- Trisomy 6 is identified in many cases of MCC, up to 50% in some studies

DIFFERENTIAL DIAGNOSIS

Basal Cell Carcinoma

- Less atypia and mitotic activity
- Most cases show areas of peripheral palisading, mucinous stroma, and tumor-stromal retraction artifact
- MCC should always be considered in high-grade/pleomorphic-appearing cases of BCC
- Almost always positive for EpCAM/BER-EP4/CD326, but negative for CK20, chromogranin, and synaptophysin

Metastatic Small Cell Carcinoma

- Especially pulmonary origin, which are positive for TTF-1, negative for CK20
- Small cell carcinomas from other sites are TTF-1(-)
- Clinical history and complete examination important to exclude metastasis

Small Cell Melanoma

- Rare variant of melanoma; typically see areas of associated junctional nesting and overlying pagetoid spread
- Cells show more abundant cytoplasm, prominent nucleoli, and may see cytoplasmic pigmentation and intranuclear pseudoinclusions
- S100, HMB-45, MART-1/Melan-A typically positive; negative for cytokeratins, CK20, and neuroendocrine markers

Lymphoma

- Lymphomas are dyscohesive, lacking cord-like and trabecular growth pattern of MCC
- Various lymphoid markers including CD45, and CD3 or CD20 should be positive

Small Round Blue Cell Tumors

- These tumors include neuroblastoma, Ewing/primitive neuroectodermal tumor, rhabdomyosarcoma
- Very rare in skin (typically metastatic from other sites); most cases occur in children

DIAGNOSTIC CHECKLIST

Pathologic Interpretation Pearls

- High-grade tumor with neuroendocrine features
- Composed of infiltrative cords, trabeculae, nests, and sheet-like areas

SELECTED REFERENCES

1. Mauzo SH et al: Molecular characteristics and potential therapeutic targets in Merkel cell carcinoma. J Clin Pathol. 69(5):382-90, 2016
2. Servy A et al: Merkel cell carcinoma: value of sentinel lymph-node status and adjuvant radiation therapy. Ann Oncol. 27(5):914-9, 2016
3. Grundhoff A et al: Merkel cell polyomavirus, a highly prevalent virus with tumorigenic potential. Curr Opin Virol. 14:129-37, 2015
4. Saini AT et al: Merkel cell carcinoma of the head and neck: pathogenesis, current and emerging treatment options. Onco Targets Ther. 8:2157-67, 2015
5. Feng H et al: Clonal integration of a polyomavirus in human Merkel cell carcinoma. Science. 319(5866):1096-100, 2008
6. Calder KB et al: A case series and immunophenotypic analysis of CK20-/CK7+ primary neuroendocrine carcinoma of the skin. J Cutan Pathol. 34(12):918-23, 2007
7. Sandel HD 4th et al: Merkel cell carcinoma: does tumor size or depth of invasion correlate with recurrence, metastasis, or patient survival? Laryngoscope. 116(5):791-5, 2006
8. Gancberg D et al: Trisomy 6 in Merkel cell carcinoma: a recurrent chromosomal aberration. Histopathology. 37(5):445-51, 2000
9. Yanguas I et al: Spontaneous regression of Merkel cell carcinoma of the skin. Br J Dermatol. 137(2):296-8, 1997

Low Magnification of MCC

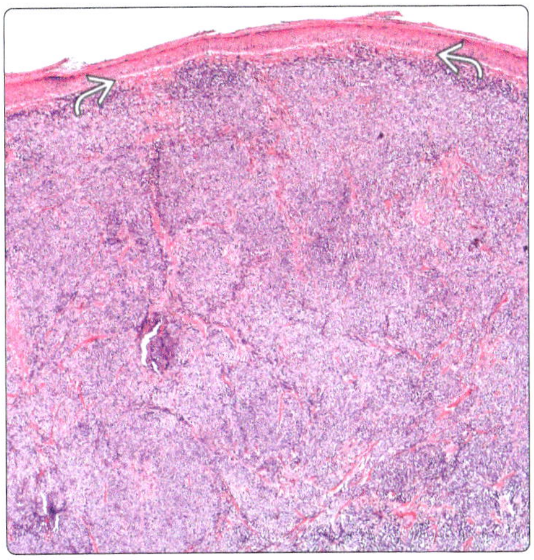

MCC With Pagetoid Carcinoma in Situ

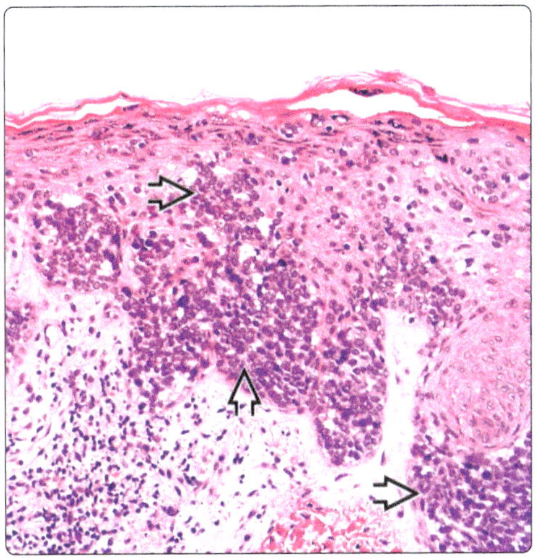

(Left) *Low magnification of MCC shows diffuse dermal involvement by sheets and nodules of atypical basophilic cells. There is a thin grenz zone separating the tumor from the epidermis* ➡. **(Right)** *Pagetoid intraepidermal spread of MCC* ⇨ *is seen in a minority of cases (< 20%). No dermal component is present in this image.*

High Magnification of Pagetoid MCC in Situ

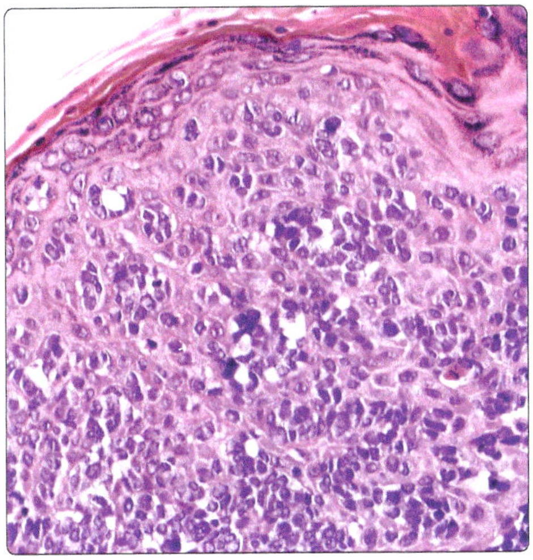

High Magnification of MCC

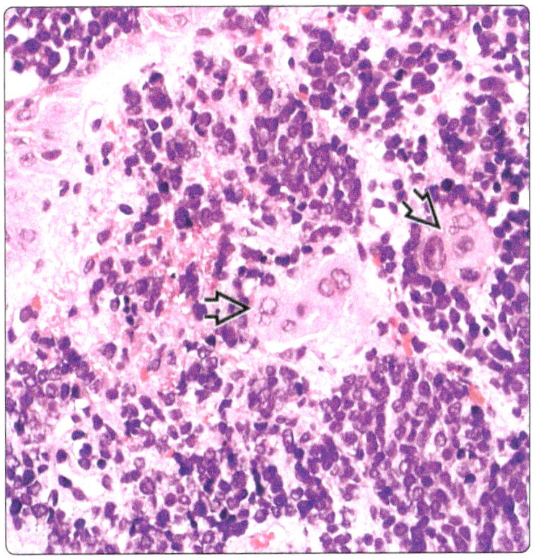

(Left) *High magnification of the same case of pagetoid MCC shows prominent full-thickness, intraepidermal spread of atypical hyperchromatic-staining cells.* **(Right)** *High magnification of another case of MCC shows that the neoplastic cells are predominantly basophilic with a high nuclear:cytoplasmic ratio. The nuclear chromatin is dense, and nucleoli are not appreciated. Focal squamous differentiation* ⇨ *is seen in this example.*

PANCK Immunohistochemistry in MCC

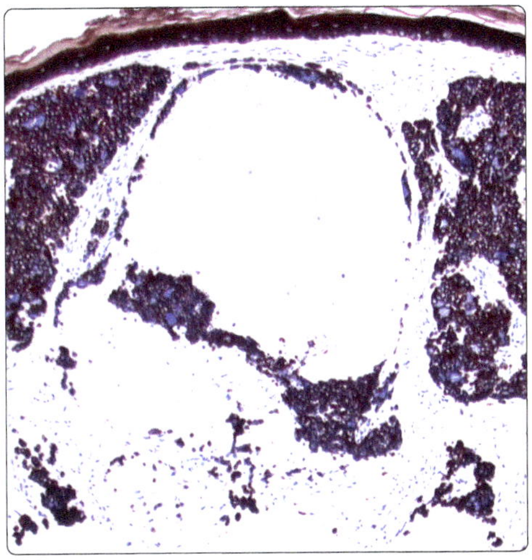

CK20 Immunohistochemistry in MCC

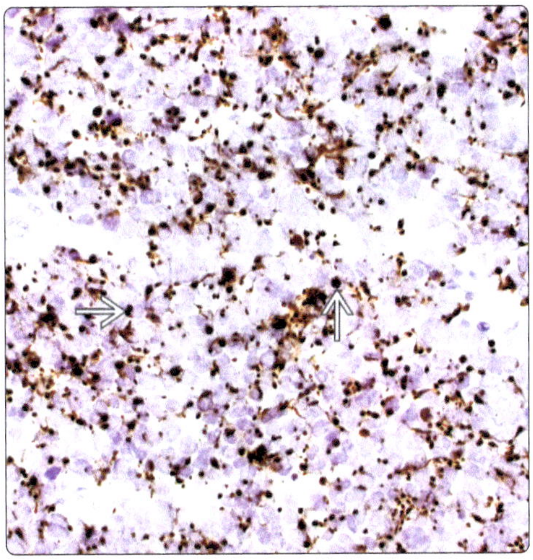

(Left) *Pancytokeratin immunohistochemical stain is strongly and diffusely positive in MCC. A perinuclear dot-like pattern may be seen in some cases. Neuroendocrine markers are also typically positive and TTF-1 negative.* **(Right)** *CK20 immunohistochemistry shows cytoplasmic and perinuclear dot-like* ➡ *positivity. This pattern is not a feature identified in other basaloid tumors, helping to confirm the diagnosis.*

PART I
SECTION 10

Tumors of Muscle, Fat, Cartilage, and Bone

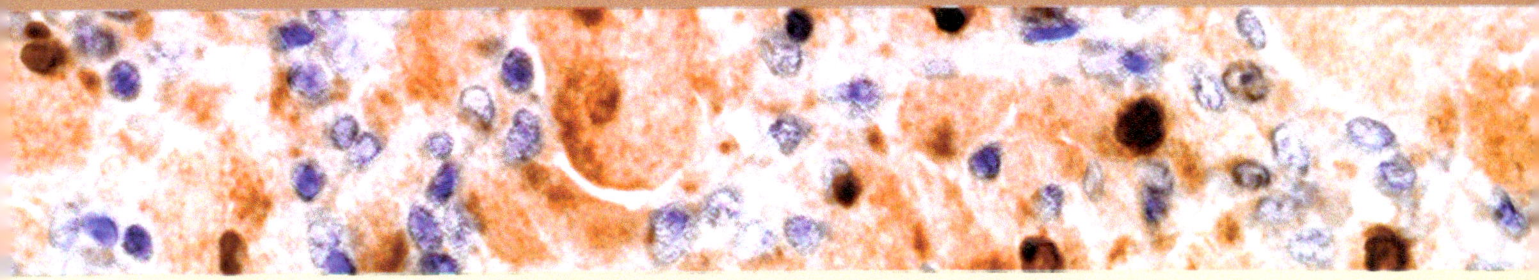

Congenital Smooth Muscle Hamartoma

KEY FACTS

TERMINOLOGY

- Smooth muscle hamartoma
- Rare lesion presenting in infants, characterized by disorganized proliferation of benign smooth muscle bundles in dermis, often involving subcutis

CLINICAL ISSUES

- Infants
- Most common in lumbosacral area
- Macule or plaque
- Often hyperpigmented, may have coarse hairs

MICROSCOPIC

- Benign smooth muscle bundles
  - Haphazard arrangement
  - Thin fascicles rather than solid growth pattern
  - No atypia
  - No mitoses
  - No necrosis
  - Immunohistochemistry (+) for muscle markers

TOP DIFFERENTIAL DIAGNOSES

- Cutaneous leiomyoma (pilar leiomyoma)
  - Occurs in adults
  - Different anatomic distribution
  - Lobules of mature smooth muscle
- Leiomyosarcoma
  - Adults
  - Deeply infiltrative dermal and subcutaneous tumor
  - Cytologic atypia
  - Mitotic activity
- Neurofibroma
  - Wavy nuclei
  - Myxocollagenous stroma
  - S100(+)
- Normal skin from special sites
  - Nipple and genital skin

Smooth Muscle Hamartoma: Low Power

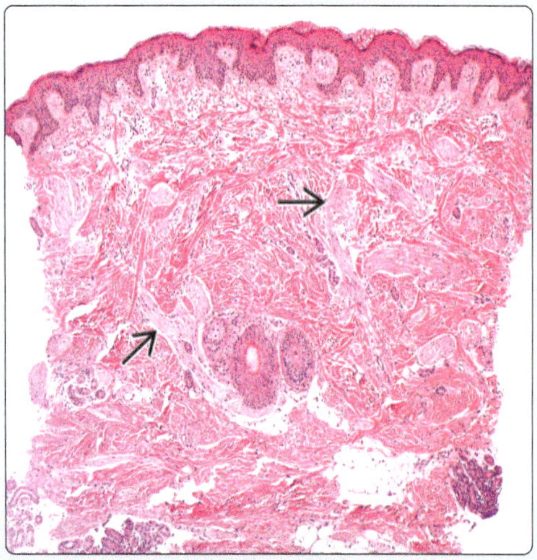

Smooth Muscle Hamartoma: Medium Power

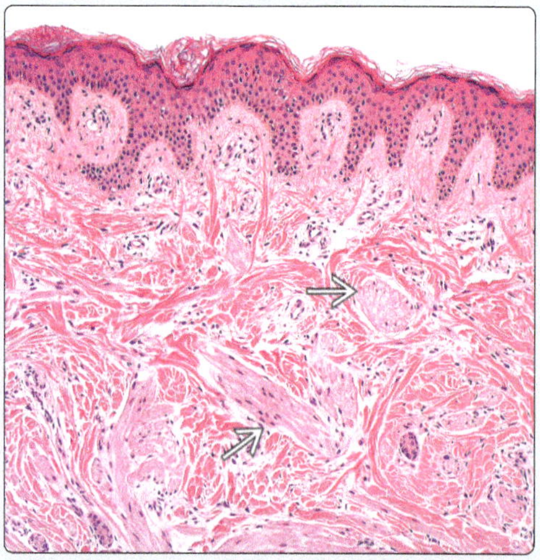

(Left) *Congenital smooth muscle hamartoma shows a haphazard arrangement of smooth muscle bundles* → *present throughout the dermis.* **(Right)** *Medium-power view of congenital smooth muscle hamartoma shows a disorganized proliferation of smooth muscle bundles* ➡ *present in the dermis.*

Smooth Muscle Hamartoma Surrounding Adnexal Structures

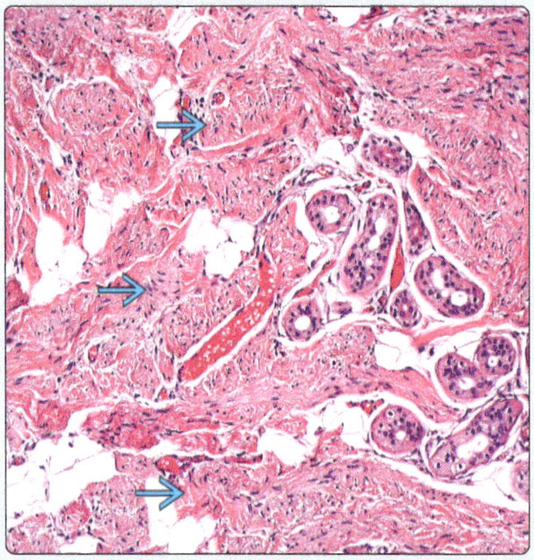

Smooth Muscle Hamartoma: High Magnification of Smooth Muscle Bundles

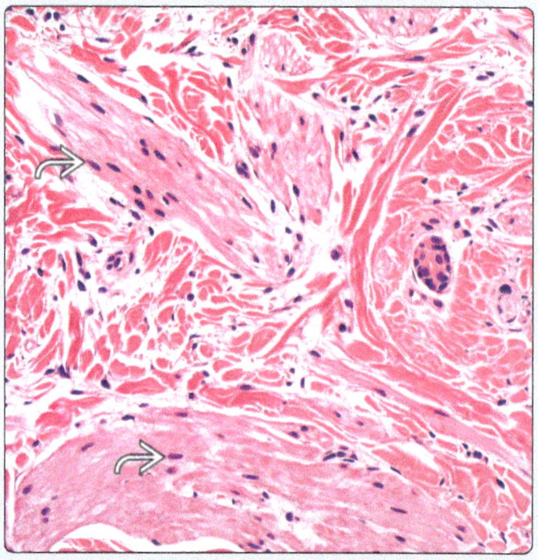

(Left) *Higher magnification shows the numerous bundles of smooth muscle. The smooth muscle bundles resemble arrector pili muscles but are present in a greater density than normal arrector pili muscles* →*. In this case, they infiltrate around eccrine units.* **(Right)** *High magnification shows a fascicular arrangement of smooth muscle with characteristic elongated, spindle-shaped to blunt-ended nuclei* ↷*.*

TERMINOLOGY

Synonyms

- Smooth muscle hamartoma

Definitions

- Rare, benign smooth muscle tumor presenting in infants
- Characterized by disorganized proliferation of smooth muscle bundles

CLINICAL ISSUES

Epidemiology

- Age
  - Infants

Site

- Lumbosacral area and proximal extremities

Presentation

- Macule or plaque
  - Indurated
  - Often hyperpigmented
  - May have coarse hairs
- Pseudo-Darier sign
  - Piloerection induced by mechanical stimulation
- Occasionally presents as multiple lesions
- Rare familial cases

Treatment

- Surgical approaches
  - Simple excision

Prognosis

- Excellent

MACROSCOPIC

General Features

- Ill-defined dermal thickening

Size

- Usually < 2 cm in diameter

MICROSCOPIC

Histologic Features

- Haphazard arrangement of benign smooth muscle bundles
  - Resembles arrector pili muscle
  - Spindled cells arranged in fascicles
  - Elongated, spindled to blunt-ended nuclei
  - Eosinophilic cytoplasm
  - No pleomorphism
  - No significant mitotic activity
  - No areas of necrosis

Predominant Pattern/Injury Type

- Fascicular

Predominant Cell/Compartment Type

- Mesenchymal, muscle, smooth

DIFFERENTIAL DIAGNOSIS

Cutaneous Leiomyoma (Pilar Leiomyoma)

- Presents in young adults
- May be multiple
- Lobules rather than haphazard fascicles

Becker Nevus

- Dermal proliferation of smooth muscle bundles may be similar to smooth muscle hamartoma
- However, clinically hyperpigmented and shows growth of coarse hair
- Epidermal acanthosis with basal hyperpigmentation also present

Normal Skin From Special Sites

- Skin from nipple, vulva, and scrotum has high concentration of normal smooth muscle bundles

Schwannoma

- Circumscribed, deep dermal or subcutaneous lesion
- Often encapsulated
- Strongly S100(+)
- EMA/MUC1(+) rim of perineurial cells

Neurofibroma

- Wavy spindle cells in myxoid to collagenous stroma
- Meissner bodies in diffuse neurofibroma
- S100(+)

Fetal Rhabdomyoma

- Skeletal muscle differentiation
  - Striations present
  - Myogenin, MYOD1(+)

Leiomyosarcoma

- Diffuse or nodular atypical spindle cell tumor
- Often deeply invasive throughout dermis and into subcutis
- Mitotic activity
- Nuclear atypia

DIAGNOSTIC CHECKLIST

Pathologic Interpretation Pearls

- Confined to dermis
- No atypical features
- Lumbosacral region of infants/young children most common site

SELECTED REFERENCES

1. Bilgiç Ö et al: Pseudo Darier sign: a distinctive finding for congenital smooth muscle hamartoma. J Pediatr. 169:318, 2016
2. Guarneri C et al: A case of hypertrichotic smooth muscle hamartoma: is it an amelanotic Becker naevus? Clin Exp Dermatol. 40(5):577-9, 2015
3. Fernandez-Flores A et al: Combined cutaneous smooth muscle hamartoma and nevus flammeus. J Cutan Pathol. 41(7):612-6, 2014
4. Nuñez D et al: Congenital smooth muscle hamartoma at unusual location. Indian J Dermatol. 59(4):409-10, 2014
5. Tzu J et al: Combined blue nevus-smooth muscle hamartoma: a series of 12 cases. J Cutan Pathol. 40(10):879-83, 2013
6. Gualandri L et al: Multiple familial smooth muscle hamartomas. Pediatr Dermatol. 18(1):17-20, 2001
7. Gagné EJ et al: Congenital smooth muscle hamartoma of the skin. Pediatr Dermatol. 10(2):142-5, 1993
8. Zvulunov A et al: Congenital smooth muscle hamartoma. Prevalence, clinical findings, and follow-up in 15 patients. Am J Dis Child. 144(7):782-4, 1990

KEY FACTS

TERMINOLOGY

- Benign dermal smooth muscle neoplasm
  - Pilar type (piloleiomyoma) arises from arrector pili
  - Genital type arises from specialized genital smooth muscle

ETIOLOGY/PATHOGENESIS

- Hereditary leiomyomatosis and renal cell cancer syndrome
  - Multiple leiomyomas of skin and uterus
  - Subset develop renal cell carcinoma
  - Mutations in fumarate hydratase (*FH*) gene (autosomal dominant)

CLINICAL ISSUES

- Pilar leiomyoma: Multiple painful, pink/brown papules/nodules, most < 2 cm
- Genital leiomyoma: Solitary painless nodule on scrotum, penis, vulva, or nipple of adults

MICROSCOPIC

- Pilar leiomyoma
  - Ill-defined, dermal nodule composed of haphazardly arranged smooth muscle bundles/fascicles
  - Bland, blunt-ended spindled nuclei
  - Abundant fibrillary eosinophilic cytoplasm
  - Focal atypia and occasional mitoses (up to 1/10 HPF) acceptable
  - Fascicles often dissect between dermal collagen
- Genital leiomyoma
  - Usually more circumscribed, cellular, and histologically heterogeneous (e.g., myxoid change, hyalinization, epithelioid cells) than pilar leiomyoma

TOP DIFFERENTIAL DIAGNOSES

- Superficial leiomyosarcoma
- Congenital smooth muscle hamartoma
- Angioleiomyoma
- Dermatomyofibroma

Cutaneous Leiomyomas and HLRCC

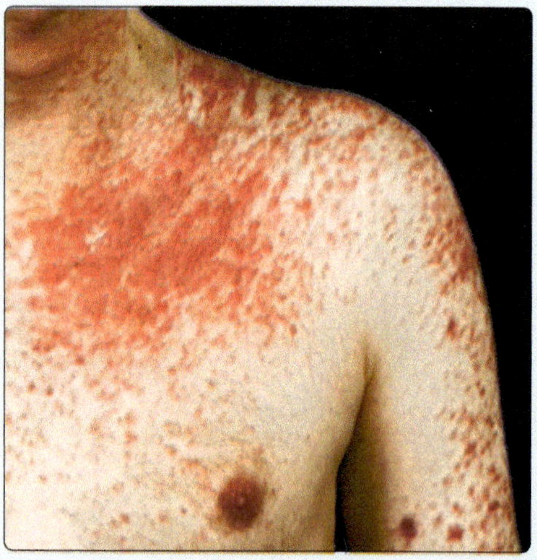

Pilar Leiomyoma at Low Magnification

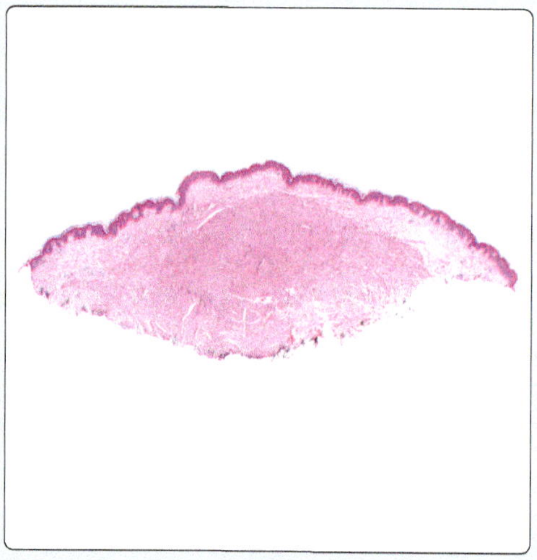

(Left) *This clinical photo shows cutaneous leiomyomas in a patient with hereditary leiomyomatosis and renal cell cancer (HLRCC). Numerous red/brown papules coalescing into plaques are present on the chest, lower neck, shoulder, and upper arm.* **(Right)** *The pilar type of superficial leiomyoma is an ill-defined dermal nodule composed of multiple eosinophilic smooth muscle bundles.*

Resemblance to Arrector Pili Muscles

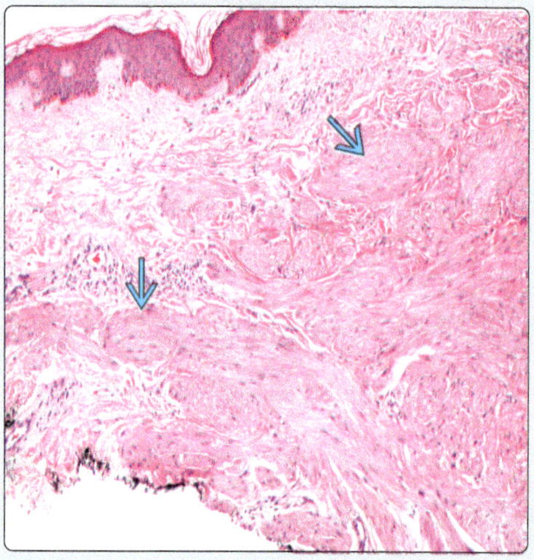

Well-Differentiated Smooth Muscle Cells

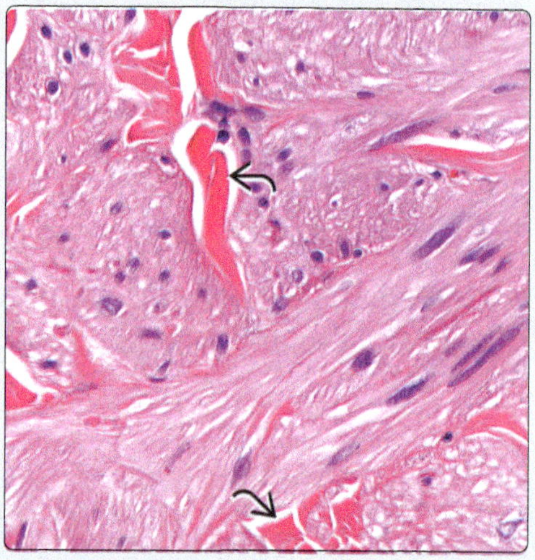

(Left) *The individual eosinophilic smooth muscle bundles* ➔ *of pilar leiomyoma resemble normal arrector pili muscles.* **(Right)** *The smooth muscle fascicles/bundles of pilar leiomyoma consist of elongated spindled cells with abundant fibrillary eosinophilic cytoplasm. Nuclei are oval with blunt ends (cigar shaped) and show little cytologic atypia or mitotic activity. Note the characteristic pattern of fascicles dissecting between dermal collagen bundles* ➔.

TERMINOLOGY

Synonyms

- Superficial/cutaneous leiomyoma, leiomyoma cutis

Definitions

- Benign dermal smooth muscle neoplasm
  - Pilar type (piloleiomyoma) arises from arrector pili
  - Genital type arises from specialized genital smooth muscle

ETIOLOGY/PATHOGENESIS

Hereditary Leiomyomatosis and Renal Cell Cancer Syndrome

- Synonyms: Multiple cutaneous and uterine leiomyomatosis syndrome, Reed syndrome
- Multiple leiomyomas of skin and uterus, risk of renal cell carcinoma (RCC)
- Familial autosomal dominant germline loss of function mutations in fumarate hydratase (*FH*) gene
  - Most with multiple cutaneous leiomyomas have *FH* mutation
  - Most women with *FH* mutation have uterine leiomyomas
- Features of uterine leiomyomas in hereditary leiomyomatosis and renal cell cancer syndrome (HLRCC)
  - Multiple; 1-8 cm; presenting at young age
  - Increased cellularity and nuclear atypia
  - Unique prominent eosinophilic inclusion-like nucleoli surrounded by clear halo
    - Similar distinct nucleoli seen in RCC occurring in HLRCC
    - These nucleoli not present in cutaneous leiomyomas of HLRCC
- Subset of HLRCC patients develop RCC
  - Often more aggressive; usually papillary, tubulopapillary, or collecting duct types
  - Distinct large eosinophilic nucleoli with clear halo

CLINICAL ISSUES

Presentation

- Pilar leiomyoma
  - Most arise in adolescents or young adults
  - Multiple painful pink/brown papules/nodules, most < 2 cm
    - Rare cases are solitary and painless
  - Papules may coalesce into nodules/plaques
  - Extensor surfaces of extremities, trunk, head, and neck
    - Often 2 or more body sites affected
- Genital leiomyoma
  - Solitary painless nodule on scrotum, penis, vulva, or nipple of adults

Treatment

- Depends on number of lesions and symptomatology
- Excision for localized or symptomatic lesions
- Conservative management for extensive lesions
- Imaging of kidneys and uterus if multiple skin lesions
- Cryotherapy and laser ablation: Mixed results

Prognosis

- Benign; does not undergo malignant transformation
- Excised lesions may recur (or new lesions may develop)

MICROSCOPIC

Histologic Features

- Pilar leiomyoma
  - Ill-defined, dermal nodule composed of haphazardly arranged smooth muscle bundles/fascicles
  - Bland, blunt-ended, spindled nuclei
  - Abundant fibrillary eosinophilic cytoplasm
  - Focal atypia and occasional mitoses (up to 1 figure per 10 HPF) acceptable
    - Numerous mitoses, diffuse/marked atypia, necrosis: Leiomyosarcoma
  - Fascicles often dissect between dermal collagen
  - Rare cases are circumscribed
- Genital leiomyoma: Usually more circumscribed, cellular, and histologically heterogeneous (e.g., myxoid change, hyalinization, epithelioid cells) than pilar leiomyoma

ANCILLARY TESTS

Immunohistochemistry

- Strong, diffuse SMA(+), MSA(+), desmin (+)
- Leiomyoma in HLRCC often fumarate hydratase (-) by IHC (not 100% sensitive or specific)

DIFFERENTIAL DIAGNOSIS

Superficial Leiomyosarcoma

- Usually solitary; marked atypia and mitotic activity

Congenital Smooth Muscle Hamartoma

- Usually solitary lumbosacral plaque in child, often with increased hair and pigmentation
- Horizontal, band-like, dermal proliferation of haphazard smooth muscle bundles

Angioleiomyoma

- Solitary painful subcutaneous nodule, usually in lower extremity of middle-aged women
- Sharply circumscribed; smooth muscle intimately admixed with thick-walled vessels; usually lacks discrete bundles; no dermal involvement

Dermatomyofibroma

- Solitary plaque on shoulder/trunk of young adult
- Fascicles of spindled myofibroblasts arranged parallel to epidermis
- Lacks well-formed smooth muscle bundles; most desmin (-)

SELECTED REFERENCES

1. Llamas-Velasco M et al: Fumarate hydratase immunohistochemical staining may help to identify patients with multiple cutaneous and uterine leiomyomatosis (MCUL) and hereditary leiomyomatosis and renal cell cancer (HLRCC) syndrome. J Cutan Pathol. 41(11):859-65, 2014
2. Idriss MH et al: Phosphohistone-H3 and Ki-67 immunostaining in cutaneous pilar leiomyoma and leiomyosarcoma (atypical intradermal smooth muscle neoplasm). J Cutan Pathol. 40(6):557-63, 2013
3. Sanz-Ortega J, Vocke C, Stratton P, Linehan WM, Merino MJ. Morphologic and molecular characteristics of uterine leiomyomas in hereditary leiomyomatosis and renal cancer (HLRCC) syndrome. Am J Surg Pathol. 37(1):74-80, 2013

Multiple Pilar Leiomyomas

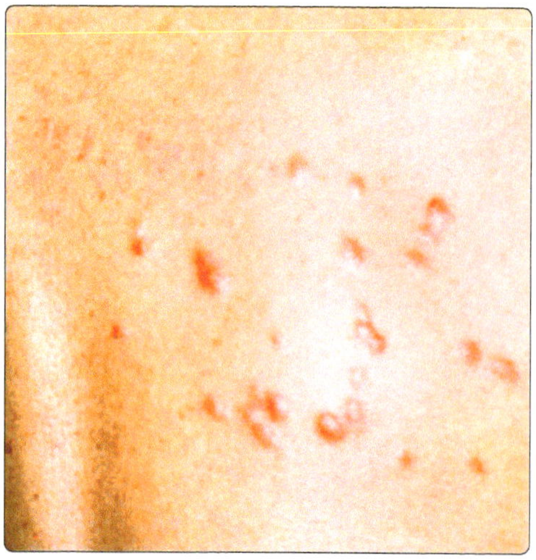

Ill-Defined Dermal Nodule

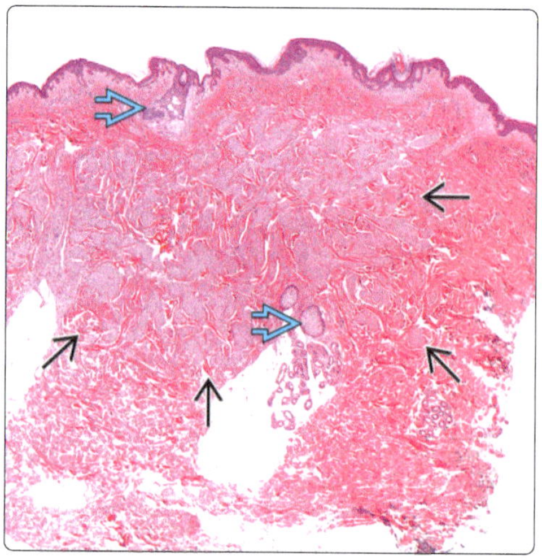

(Left) *Superficial leiomyomas (pilar type) are usually < 2 cm and appear as multiple pink or brown papules or nodules. Clinically, they tend to elicit pain and are often distributed in a dermatomal fashion.* **(Right)** *This low-power H&E shows a superficial (pilar type) leiomyoma involving the majority of the dermis. The lesion is unencapsulated and vaguely circumscribed but does have an irregular border with displacement of dermal appendages.*

Collagen Bundles in Leiomyoma

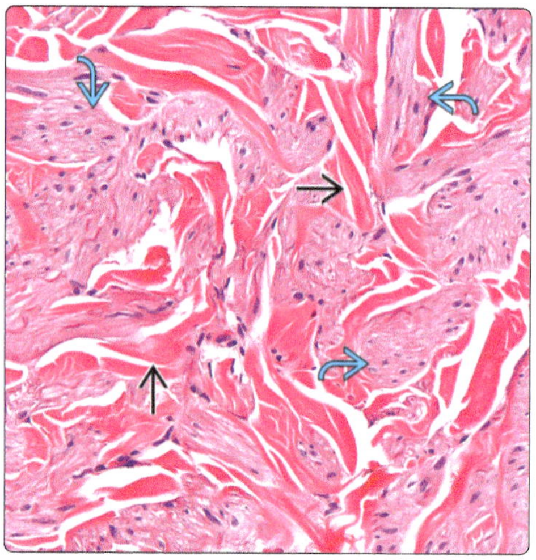

Grenz Zone in Leiomyoma

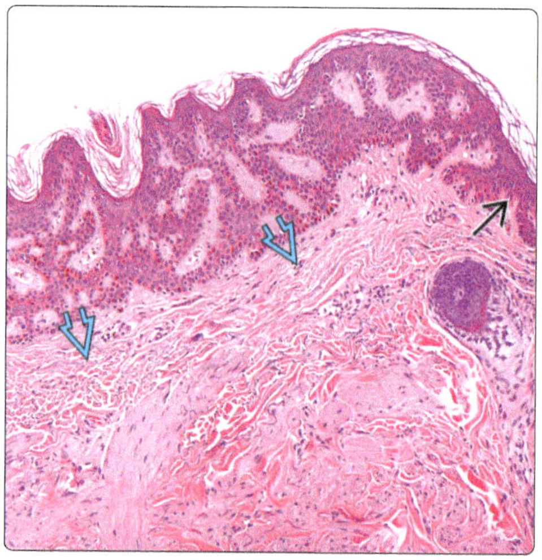

(Left) *At higher power, cutaneous leiomyomas consist of short fascicles or bundles of smooth muscle haphazardly arranged within the dermis and tend to dissect between dermal collagen bundles.* **(Right)** *Many superficial leiomyomas have a grenz zone and epidermal hyperplasia with elongated rete pegs adjacent to normal epidermis.*

Incipient Pilar Leiomyoma

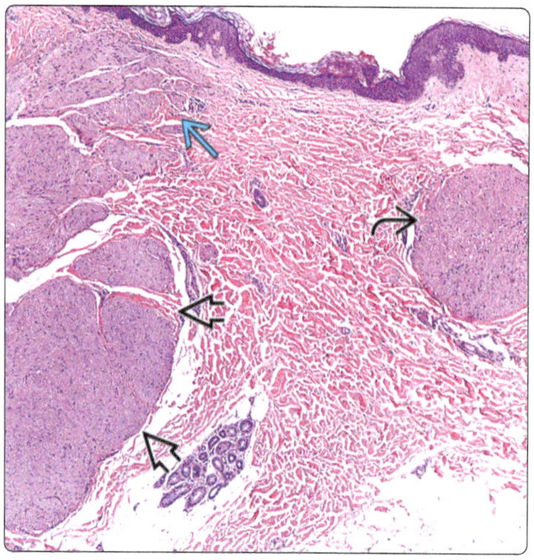

Rare Sharp Circumscription

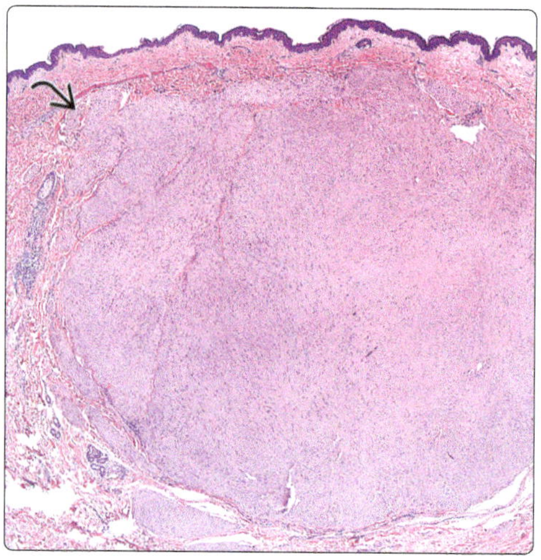

(Left) *Surgical specimens often reveal incipient pilar leiomyomas adjacent to the primary tumor. The primary tumor in this example does show areas of circumscription, but other areas have the more typical infiltrative pattern.* **(Right)** *Rare examples of superficial leiomyoma are well circumscribed, such as this solitary lesion, which shows only focal areas with an irregular border. Solitary lesions, such as the example shown, often present without pain symptoms.*

Solitary, Circumscribed Leiomyoma

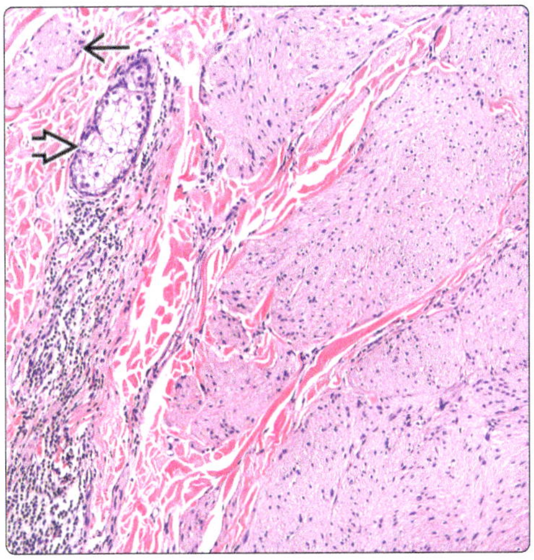

Solitary Leiomyoma

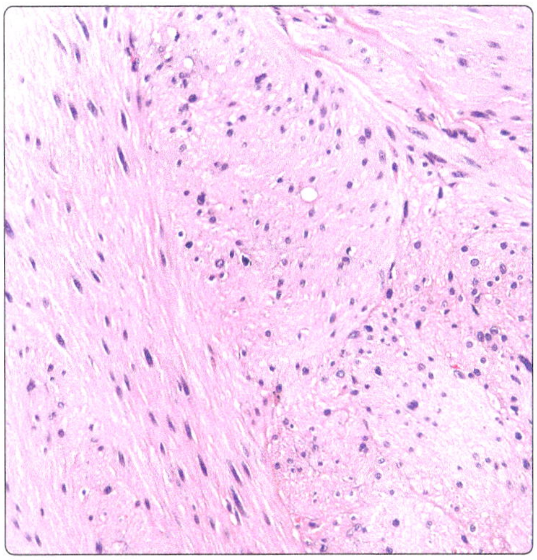

(Left) *Solitary and circumscribed cutaneous leiomyomas can arise from the pilar smooth muscle. This solitary and circumscribed tumor was located adjacent to a sebaceous gland* ⇨ *and pilar smooth muscle bundle* ➡, *indicating likely origin from this pilosebaceous unit.* **(Right)** *Compared to typical pilar leiomyomas, solitary superficial leiomyomas are more often solid and less often characterized by small smooth muscle fascicles intersecting between dermal collagen.*

DDx: Angioleiomyoma

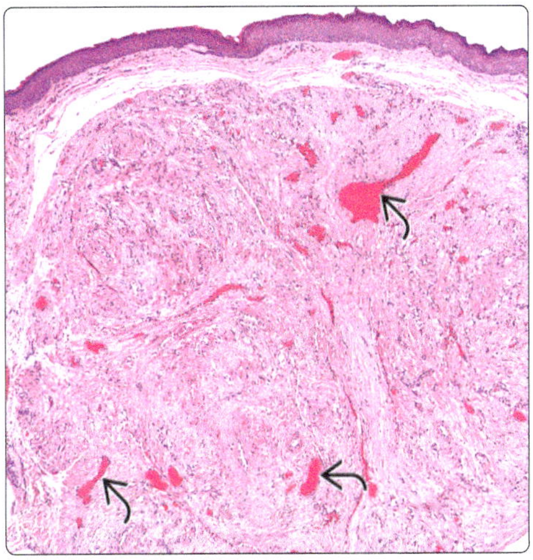

Vessels in Angioleiomyoma

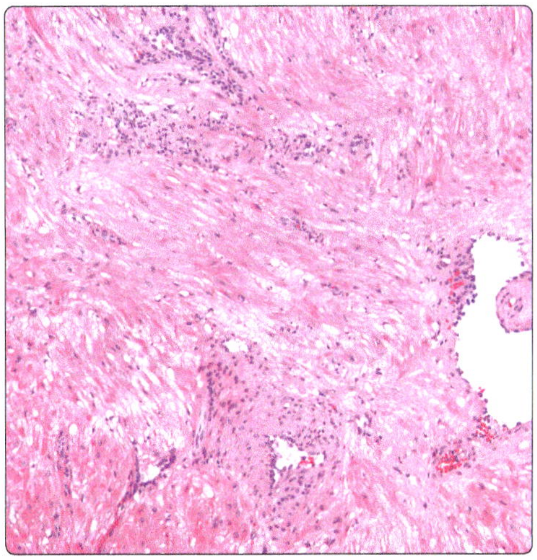

(Left) *In contrast to superficial leiomyoma, angioleiomyoma is usually circumscribed and contains numerous variably sized vascular channels that stand out at low power* ↪. *In addition, it is usually solitary and located in the lower extremity.* **(Right)** *Sheets of smooth muscle cells with abundant fibrillary eosinophilic cytoplasm intimately associated with thick-walled, often slit-like vascular channels characterize angioleiomyoma at higher power.*

DDx: Superficial Leiomyosarcoma

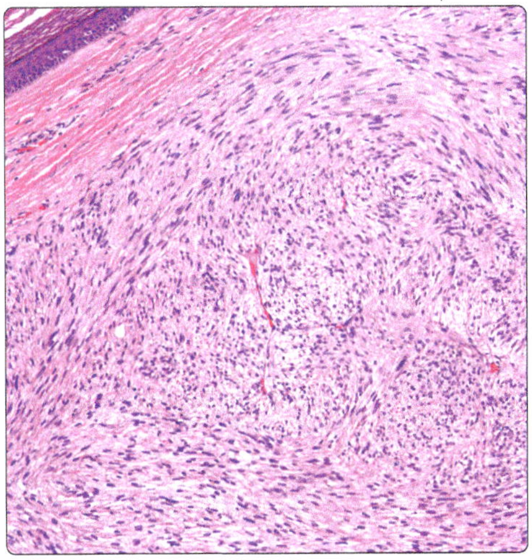

Atypia and Mitoses in Leiomyosarcoma

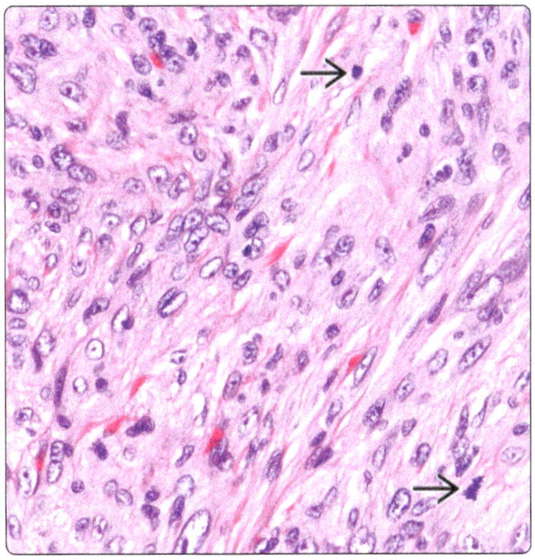

(Left) *Superficial (or cutaneous) leiomyosarcoma also consists of fascicles of cells with abundant fibrillary eosinophilic cytoplasm with blunt-ended oval nuclei. However, this tumor is more cellular and demonstrates less dissection of dermal collagen. It is also usually larger than superficial leiomyoma.* **(Right)** *At higher power, superficial leiomyosarcoma usually features moderate to marked nuclear atypia with a higher nuclear:cytoplasmic ratio than leiomyoma. Mitotic figures* ➡ *are also generally more frequent.*

Angioleiomyoma

KEY FACTS

TERMINOLOGY

- Benign, well-circumscribed neoplasm composed of mature smooth muscle cells arranged around prominent blood vessels
- Synonyms: Vascular leiomyoma, angiomyoma

CLINICAL ISSUES

- Wide range (most common: 40-70 years)
- Upper and lower extremities (most common in lower leg)
- Usually small, solitary, subcutaneous nodule
  - > 50% are painful
- Treatment: Simple, conservative excision
- Excellent prognosis; very rarely recurs

MACROSCOPIC

- Usually < 2 cm

MICROSCOPIC

- Sharp circumscription
- 3 types described: Solid (most common), venous, and cavernous
- Well-differentiated smooth muscle component
- Prominent component of medium- to large-sized blood vessels with dilated or compressed lumina
  - Smooth muscle cells can show concentric, perivascular accentuation in some cases
- No significant nuclear atypia or mitotic activity
- Mature adipose tissue, stromal hyalinization, myxoid changes, or calcification may be present

ANCILLARY TESTS

- Strong, diffuse SMA(+) and h-caldesmon (+)
- Desmin (+) but varies in extent

TOP DIFFERENTIAL DIAGNOSES

- Myopericytoma
- Hemangioma
- PEComa

Angioleiomyoma

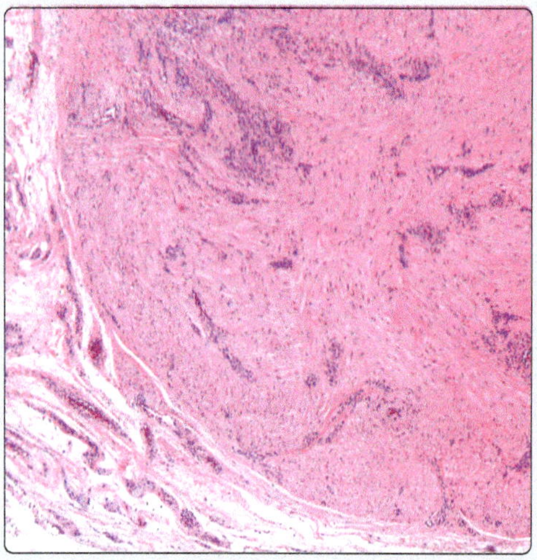

Perivascular Growth by Smooth Muscle Cells

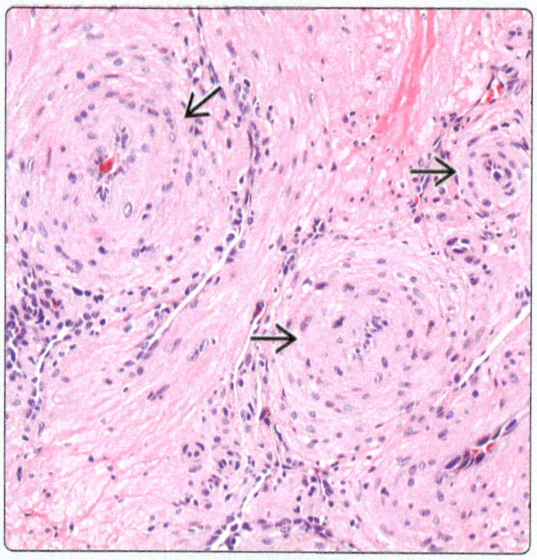

(Left) *Angioleiomyoma is a small, sharply circumscribed smooth muscle neoplasm containing a prominent component of stromal blood vessels. These vessels vary in size and may be compressed (solid variant, shown) or markedly dilated/ectatic (venous and cavernous variants).* **(Right)** *Perivascular arrangement ➔ of the lesional smooth muscle cells is a common finding in angioleiomyoma and creates morphologic overlap with myopericytoma. This finding, however, may be focal or absent in some cases.*

Mature Smooth Muscle Cells

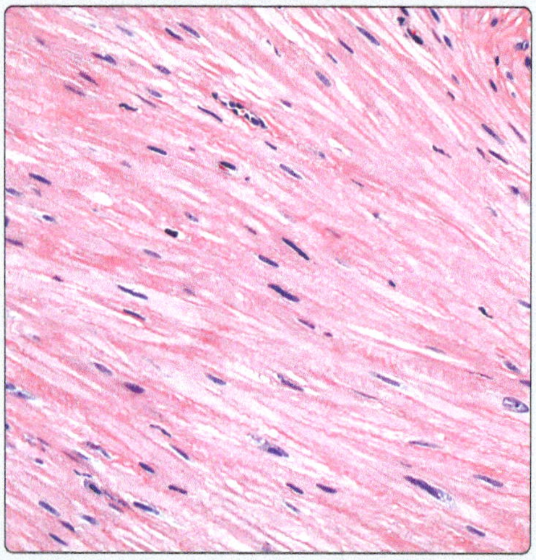

Cavernous Morphology

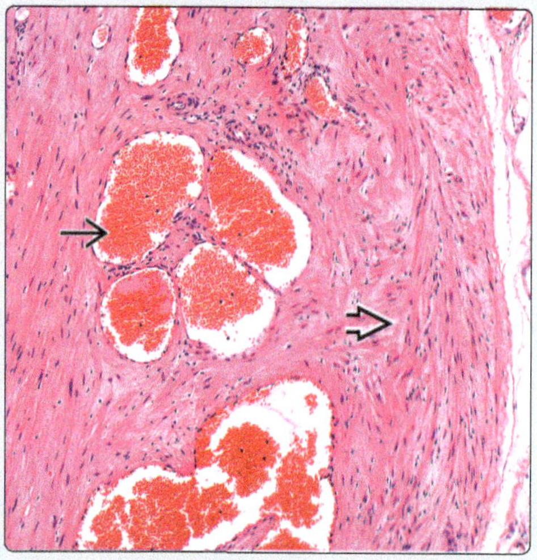

(Left) *The well-differentiated smooth muscle cells of angioleiomyoma show classic cytologic features including prominent eosinophilic cytoplasm and elongated, blunt, cigar-shaped nuclei. They are also typically arranged in bundles and fascicles, as seen in other smooth muscle neoplasms.* **(Right)** *The cavernous type of angioleiomyoma has thin-walled, dilated vascular channels ➔ arranged in small clusters within a stroma composed of smooth muscle fibers ➩ that form branching fascicles.*

TERMINOLOGY

Synonyms

- Vascular leiomyoma
- Angiomyoma

Definitions

- Benign, well-circumscribed neoplasm composed of mature smooth muscle cells arranged around prominent blood vessels
  - Now classified as tumor of pericytic (perivascular) origin (2013 WHO classification)
  - Considered to exist on morphologic spectrum with myopericytoma

CLINICAL ISSUES

Epidemiology

- Age
  - Wide range (most common: 40-70 years)
- Sex
  - Male predominance in upper extremity
  - Female predominance in lower extremity

Site

- Upper and lower extremities (most common in lower leg)
- Head and neck (particularly oral cavity, lip, palate)
- Rare on trunk

Presentation

- Usually small, solitary, subcutaneous nodule
- Often slow growing
- > 50% are painful
  - May be exacerbated by pregnancy, menses, or change in temperature

Treatment

- Simple, conservative excision

Prognosis

- Excellent
- Recurrences very rare

MACROSCOPIC

General Features

- Small, well circumscribed
- White, rubbery cut surface
  - Calcified examples may be gritty

Size

- Usually < 2 cm

MICROSCOPIC

Histologic Features

- Sharp circumscription
- 3 morphologic forms described
  - Solid type (most common)
    - Bundles and fascicles of spindled, well-differentiated smooth muscle cells
    - Intervening compressed, slit-like vessels
  - Venous type
    - Mature smooth muscle arranged around dilated, thick-walled vascular channels
      - Smooth muscle cells often show concentric, perivascular accentuation
  - Cavernous type (least common)
    - Resembles cavernous hemangioma
    - Intervascular septa contain smooth muscle cells
- Occasional cases show some morphologic overlap with myopericytoma
- No significant nuclear atypia or mitotic activity
  - Focal (likely degenerative) atypia may be present in older lesions
- Mature adipose tissue, stromal hyalinization, or myxoid changes may be present
- Calcification is more common in older lesions
- Small nerve twigs are occasionally identifiable within or at periphery of lesion

ANCILLARY TESTS

Immunohistochemistry

- Strong, diffuse SMA(+) and h-caldesmon (+)
- Desmin (+) but varies in extent
- HMB-45(-)

DIFFERENTIAL DIAGNOSIS

Myopericytoma

- May show morphologic overlap with angioleiomyoma
- Prominent perivascular growth
- Lesional cells lack mature smooth muscle cytomorphology
- SMA(+), desmin (-)

Hemangioma

- Vascular (capillary or cavernous) channels are numerous
- Lacks prominent intervascular smooth muscle cell proliferation

PEComa (Perivascular Epithelioid Cell Tumor)

- Tumor cell cytoplasm varies from eosinophilic to clear
- Variably sclerotic stroma
- May contain fat (angiomyolipoma)
- Most coexpress SMA and melanocytic marker (HMB-45, MART-1, etc.)

SELECTED REFERENCES

1. Agaimy A et al: Angioleiomyoma of the sinonasal tract: analysis of 16 cases and review of the literature. Head Neck Pathol. 9(4):463-73, 2015
2. Liu Y et al: Angioleiomyomas in the head and neck: A retrospective clinical and immunohistochemical analysis. Oncol Lett. 8(1):241-247, 2014
3. Christopher DM et al: WHO Classification of Tumours of Soft Tissue and Bone. 4th ed. Lyon: IARC Press, 2013
4. Houdek MT et al: Angioleiomyoma of the upper extremity. J Hand Surg Am. 38(8):1579-83, 2013
5. Matsuyama A et al: Angioleiomyoma: a clinicopathologic and immunohistochemical reappraisal with special reference to the correlation with myopericytoma. Hum Pathol. 38(4):645-51, 2007
6. Nishio J et al: Chromosomal imbalances in angioleiomyomas by comparative genomic hybridization. Int J Mol Med. 13(1):13-6, 2004
7. Fox SB et al: Angioleiomyomas: an immunohistological study. Histopathology. 16(5):495-6, 1990
8. Hachisuga T et al: Angioleiomyoma. A clinicopathologic reappraisal of 562 cases. Cancer. 54(1):126-30, 1984

Leiomyosarcoma

KEY FACTS

TERMINOLOGY

- Malignant neoplasm composed of cells exhibiting smooth muscle differentiation

ETIOLOGY/PATHOGENESIS

- Epstein-Barr virus associated in immunosuppressed patients

CLINICAL ISSUES

- Uncommon: 10-15% of extremity sarcomas
- Most common sarcoma type if uterine examples are included
- Cutaneous lesions present as superficial or deep soft tissue mass, often asymptomatic, in extremities
- Retroperitoneum most common site overall
- Treatment is complete surgical excision
- Prognosis is site and stage dependent, as with other sarcoma types
  - Lesions restricted to cutis only rarely metastasize

MICROSCOPIC

- Perpendicularly oriented fascicles of spindle cells
- Brightly eosinophilic cytoplasm
- Blunt-ended nuclei
- Nuclear atypia and mitoses

ANCILLARY TESTS

- Labels as per smooth muscle: Desmin, actin, calponin, caldesmon
  - Some cases stain with keratins

TOP DIFFERENTIAL DIAGNOSES

- Sarcomatoid squamous cell carcinoma
- Atypical fibroxanthoma
- Leiomyoma
- Dermatofibroma/fibrous histiocytoma
- Nodular fasciitis
- Inflammatory myofibroblastic tumor

Cutaneous Leiomyosarcoma (Atypical Smooth Muscle Tumor)

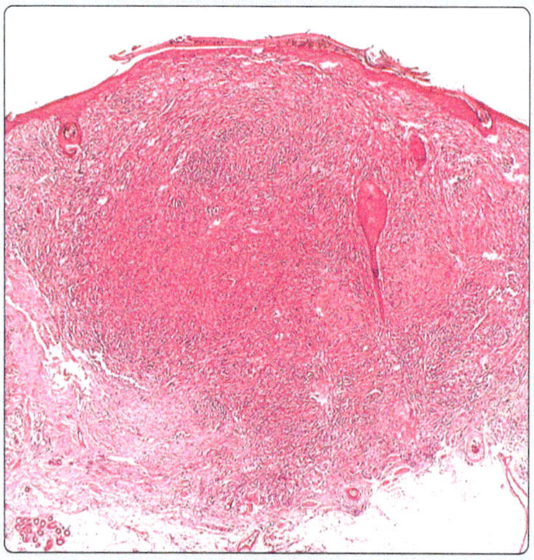

Superficial Area of Cutaneous Leiomyosarcoma

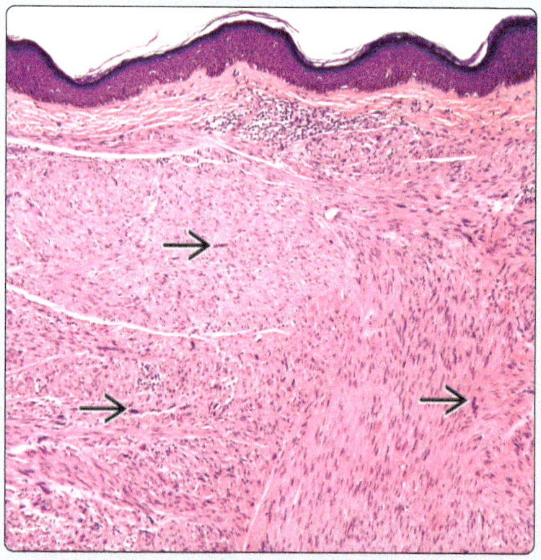

(Left) *Based on the lack of involvement of the subcutaneous adipose tissue, a favorable prognosis would be anticipated for this lesion. In fact, some observers have suggested diagnosing such superficial cutaneous lesions as atypical smooth muscle tumors.* **(Right)** *This leiomyosarcoma (LMS) extended into the subcutis. It is composed of perpendicularly oriented fascicles of brightly eosinophilic cells. Even at scanning magnification, atypical nuclei stand out ➔.*

Leiomyosarcoma at High Magnification

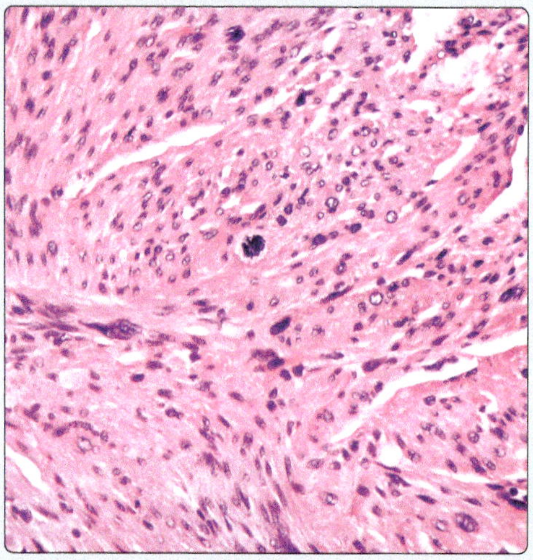

Leiomyosarcoma With Anaphase Bridge

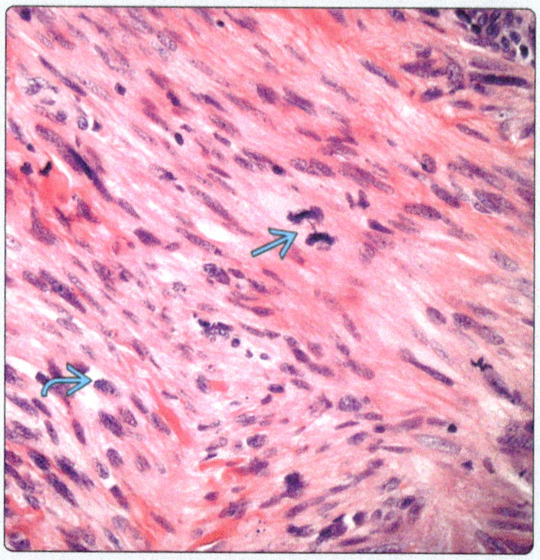

(Left) *Mitotic figures are usually easily found in LMS. There is no need to search for numerous mitoses, although mitotic counts assist in assigning a sarcoma grade. Note the bright pink color of the tumor cells' cytoplasm.* **(Right)** *LMSs do not show a characteristic translocation and have chromosome instability, as indicated by the presence of anaphase bridges ➔, long cords of chromatin that remain as cells separate in anaphase. Note the blunt-ended nuclei ➔.*

TERMINOLOGY

Abbreviations

- Leiomyosarcoma (LMS)

Definitions

- Malignant neoplasm composed of cells exhibiting smooth muscle differentiation

ETIOLOGY/PATHOGENESIS

Infectious Agents

- Epstein-Barr virus (EBV) smooth muscle tumors (SMT) in immunosuppressed patients
- Occasional examples are radiation associated

CLINICAL ISSUES

Epidemiology

- Incidence
  - Uncommon: 10-15% of extremity sarcomas
  - Most common overall sarcoma type if uterine and visceral examples are included
- Age
  - Middle-aged adults
- Sex
  - No gender preference overall

Presentation

- Cutaneous LMS presents as single nodule or plaque-like tumor
  - May be ulcerated or show serum crusting/hemorrhage
- Deep soft tissue tumors present as mass, often asymptomatic, in extremities
  - Retroperitoneum most common site
  - Vena cava examples often symptomatic
- Uterine examples considered separately with unique diagnostic criteria

Treatment

- Surgical excision
  - Radiation
  - Chemotherapy for metastatic tumors

Prognosis

- Outcome site and stage dependent as with other sarcoma types
  - Lesions restricted to cutis only rarely metastasize
    - Some observers have advocated diagnosing them as atypical SMTs
  - Subcutaneous lesions
    - Up to 40% of tumors metastasize
    - Over 30% of patients with subcutaneous tumors die of disease
  - Retroperitoneum: About 80% of patients die of disease, typically with metastases
  - Bone: Metastases in up to 1/2 of patients
  - Vena cava: 5- and 10-yr survival 50% and 30%, respectively
  - Head and neck: Over 1/2 metastasize

MICROSCOPIC

Histologic Features

- Perpendicularly oriented fascicles of spindle cells
- Cells show brightly eosinophilic cytoplasm
- Blunt-ended nuclei with nuclear atypia
- Some examples are epithelioid-appearing
- Any number of mitoses sufficient in subcutis, scrotal lesions, or deep soft tissue if nuclear atypia is present
- In vulva, some observers offered > 5 mitosis per 10 HPF as cutoff, but recurrences reported in lesions with any mitotic activity

Predominant Pattern/Injury Type

- Fascicular

Predominant Cell/Compartment Type

- Mesenchymal, smooth muscle

Variant and Special Forms

- **Epithelioid leiomyosarcoma**
  - Literature confounded because many epithelioid gastrointestinal stromal tumors (GIST) were termed epithelioid LMS in past
  - Found anywhere in body
  - Distinct epithelioid morphology, but more nuclear atypia than GISTs
  - Older studies reported smooth muscle actin (SMA) and muscle specific actin (MSA)-positive, desmin-negative immunophenotype, but desmin labels most lesions using modern methods
    - Possible reflection of misdiagnosed GISTs
    - Less sensitive desmin antibodies used in past
- **Myxoid leiomyosarcoma**
  - Grossly gelatinous
  - Extensive myxoid change, but zones of typical leiomyosarcoma allow for diagnosis
    - Express desmin and actin
    - Subset labels with keratin antibodies
  - Tend to be low grade
  - Clinicopathologic features otherwise same as typical leiomyosarcoma
- **Inflammatory leiomyosarcoma**
  - Characterized by dense inflammation that masks underlying lesion
    - Histiocytes, xanthoma cells, lymphocytes, neutrophils
  - Areas of more typical morphology must be sought
  - Clinicopathologic features otherwise as per typical leiomyosarcoma
- **Pleomorphic leiomyosarcoma**
  - Defined as pleomorphic areas in > 2/3 of tumor
    - Ordinary leiomyosarcomatous fascicular area covers < 1/3
  - More aggressive since higher grade
    - In one series, 65% of patients died of disease
  - Subset features osteoclast-like giant cells
- **Epstein-Barr virus-associated**
  - a.k.a. EBV-associated SMT (EBV-SMT)
    - Classified as leiomyoma and leiomyosarcoma, but term EBV-SMT may be more appropriate
    - Appearances are somewhat unique

- Found in immunosuppressed patients
- Frequently multifocal
- No clear-cut metastases reported
- Histologic features
  - Monomorphic, spindled, smooth muscle cells arranged in short, intersecting fascicles
  - Subpopulation of more primitive round cells are either admixed with spindled cells or form discrete nodules
  - Variable lymphocytic infiltrate composed primarily of T cells
  - Mitotic activity variable (0-18 per 10 HPF)
  - Necrosis and myxoid change in some cases
  - All are EBV-encoded RNA (EBER) positive
  - All express SMA; desmin in ~ 1/2
- Reducing immunosuppression in transplant patients should be key treatment
  - Rapid tumor reduction following reduced immunosuppression reported, but some lesions persist
  - About 5% die of disease
- Treatment is primarily surgical
- Sirolimus (inhibitor of mTOR-associated protein pathway) effective in some lesions

- **Leiomyosarcoma with osteoclast-like giant cells**
  - Same demographics as conventional LMS
  - Areas with same histology as typical LMS
    - Reactive with smooth muscle markers: Actins and desmin
  - Areas with osteoclast-like giant cells
    - Some giant cells appear bland (likely histiocytes), but others cytologically malignant
    - Benign-appearing osteoclast-like giant cells label with CD68, but not muscle markers
    - Cytologically malignant giant cells label with smooth muscle markers
  - No osteoid/matrix formation seen

ANCILLARY TESTS

Immunohistochemistry

- Label as SMT: (+) for desmin, actin, calponin, caldesmon
  - Some cases stain with keratins (usually focal)

Genetic Testing

- Complex variable karyotypes
- No characteristic translocation, mutation, or fusion product known

DIFFERENTIAL DIAGNOSIS

Based on Anatomic Site

- **Skin and subcutaneous fat/fascia**
  - **Sarcomatoid squamous cell carcinoma**
    - May have overlying in situ component
    - Expresses HMWCKs (CK5/6, CK903) and p63, in contrast to LMS
  - **Atypical fibroxanthoma**
    - Occurs in heavily sun-damaged skin of elderly
    - Composed of population of atypical to bizarre and pleomorphic-appearing spindled and epithelioid cells
    - Typically negative for muscle markers including desmin and MSA (although SMA can be focally positive in some cases); positive for nonspecific markers (CD10, CD68, CD99)
  - **Leiomyoma**
    - Bland cytology
    - Mitoses infrequent
  - **Dermatofibroma/fibrous histiocytoma**
    - Uniform, bland-appearing histiocytoid and fibroblastic cells
    - Collagen trapping pattern at periphery
    - Often has secondary inflammatory constituents (lymphoplasmacytic cells, foamy histiocytes, hemosiderin)
    - Typically lacks desmin; FXIIIA and CD10 positive
  - **Nodular fasciitis**
    - Bland nuclei
    - Loose storiform rather than fascicular pattern
    - Backdrop of lymphocytes and extravasated erythrocytes, often osteoclast-like giant cells
    - Immunoreactive for actin or calponin, but not desmin or caldesmon
  - **Inflammatory myofibroblastic tumor**
    - Inflammatory backdrop
    - Myofibroblastic differentiation (stellate cytoplasm)
    - About 60% of cases show ALK expression and *ALK* rearrangements
    - High-grade form overtly sarcomatous
      - Subset termed epithelioid inflammatory myofibroblastic sarcoma is typically intraabdominal

DIAGNOSTIC CHECKLIST

Pathologic Interpretation Pearls

- Attention to depth of involvement important in evaluating SMTs of skin
  - Lesions restricted to cutis essentially never metastasize; subcutaneous tumors have significant metastatic potential

SELECTED REFERENCES

1. Aneiros-Fernandez J et al: Primary cutaneous and subcutaneous leiomyosarcomas: review of their evolution and prognostic factors. Eur J Dermatol. 26(1):9-12, 2016
2. Winchester DS et al: Skin metastases of leiomyosarcoma (LMS): a retrospective review of 21 cases. J Am Acad Dermatol. 72(5):910-2, 2015
3. Cantile M et al: A cutaneous inflammatory myofibroblastic tumour with ALK rearrangement in the upper extremity. Pathology. 46(6):575-6, 2014
4. Mariño-Enríquez A et al: Epithelioid inflammatory myofibroblastic sarcoma: An aggressive intra-abdominal variant of inflammatory myofibroblastic tumor with nuclear membrane or perinuclear ALK. Am J Surg Pathol. 35(1):135-44, 2011
5. Oda Y et al: Pleomorphic leiomyosarcoma: clinicopathologic and immunohistochemical study with special emphasis on its distinction from ordinary leiomyosarcoma and malignant fibrous histiocytoma. Am J Surg Pathol. 25(8):1030-8, 2001
6. de Saint Aubain Somerhausen N et al: Leiomyosarcoma of soft tissue in children: clinicopathologic analysis of 20 cases. Am J Surg Pathol. 23(7):755-63, 1999
7. Kaddu S et al: Cutaneous leiomyosarcoma. Am J Surg Pathol. 21(9):979-87, 1997
8. Mentzel T et al: Leiomyosarcoma with prominent osteoclast-like giant cells. Analysis of eight cases closely mimicking the so-called giant cell variant of malignant fibrous histiocytoma. Am J Surg Pathol. 18(3):258-65, 1994
9. Suster S: Epithelioid leiomyosarcoma of the skin and subcutaneous tissue. Clinicopathologic, immunohistochemical, and ultrastructural study of five cases. Am J Surg Pathol. 18(3):232-40, 1994

Leiomyosarcoma, Paranuclear Vacuoles

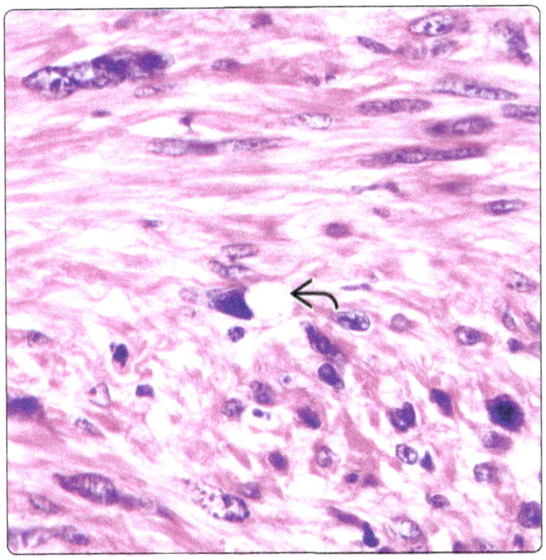

Leiomyosarcoma, Paranuclear Vacuole at High Magnification

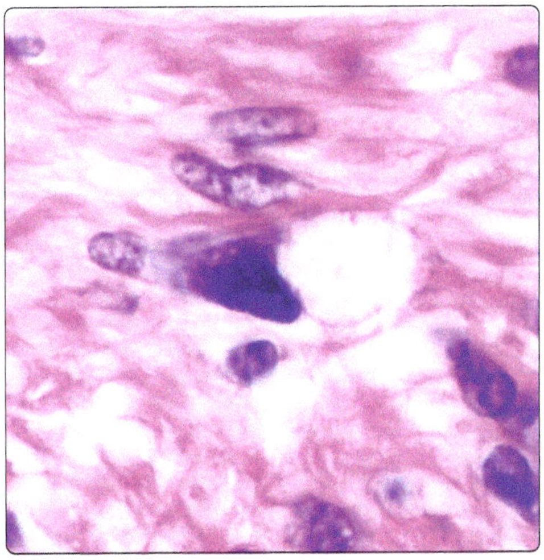

(Left) *High magnification shows a classic appearance of leiomyosarcoma. The proliferating cells contain blunt-ended nuclei and fibrillary eosinophilic cytoplasm. A paranuclear large vacuole is in the center of the field ⮊.* **(Right)** *High magnification shows a large paranuclear vacuole in a leiomyosarcoma. The cells above the vacuolated one have blunt-ended nuclei.*

Leiomyosarcoma, Perpendicularly Oriented Fascicles

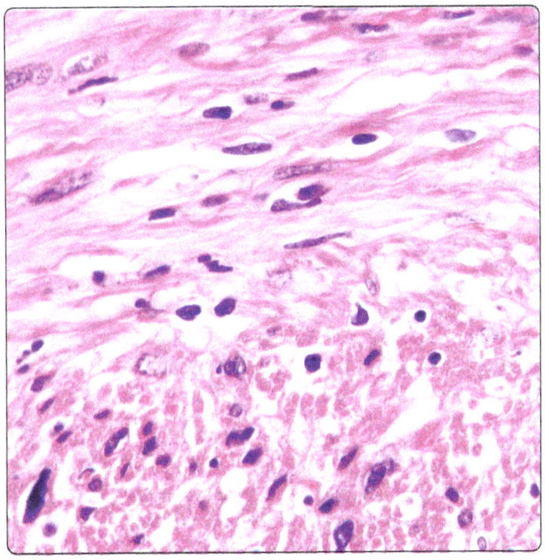

Leiomyosarcoma With Mitoses

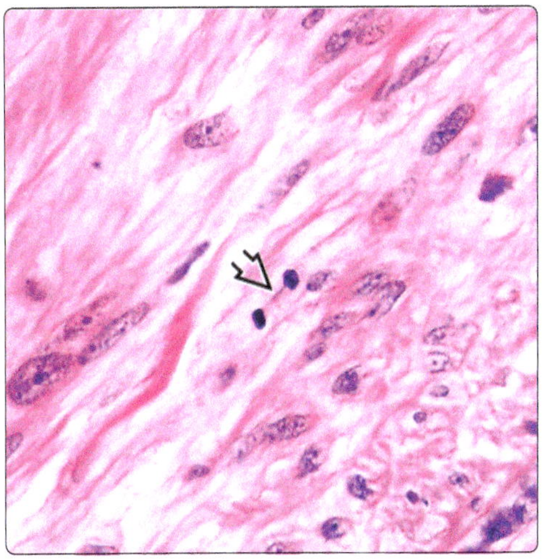

(Left) *High magnification shows perpendicularly oriented fascicles. The cells in the upper part of the field are in a fascicular arrangement, whereas the ones at the bottom of the field are mostly aligned en face.* **(Right)** *This image shows an anaphase bridge ⮊ in the center of the field, an indication that this neoplasm has chromosome instability rather than a characteristic translocation or gene rearrangement.*

Leiomyosarcoma, Trichrome Stain

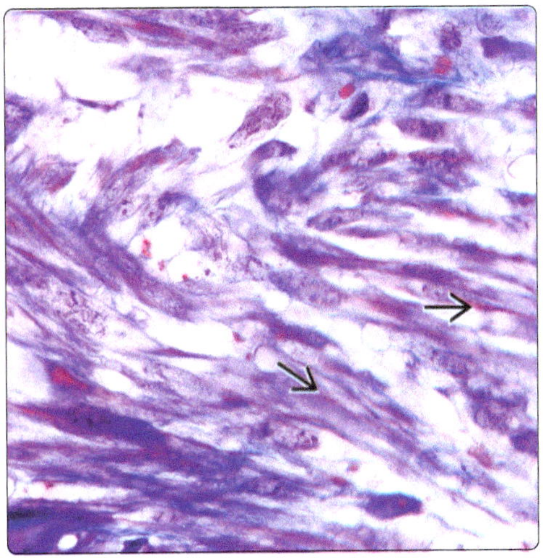

Leiomyosarcoma, Desmin Immunostaining

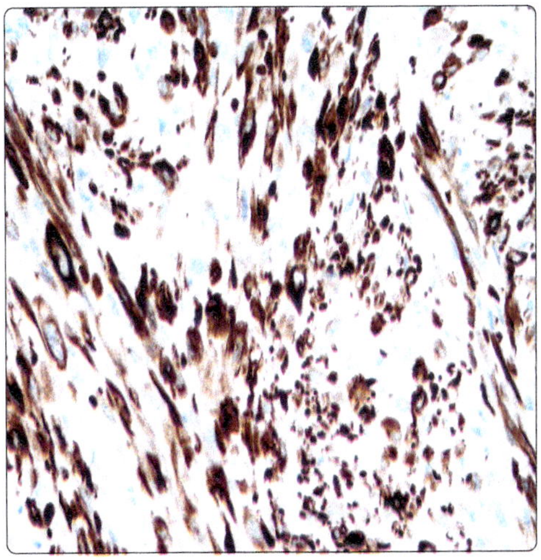

(Left) *Masson trichrome stain highlights delicate red cytoplasmic filaments ⮊ in this well-differentiated leiomyosarcoma.* **(Right)** *Desmin shows striking cytoplasmic labeling in this leiomyosarcoma. In contrast to myofibroblastic lesions such as nodular fasciitis (which show smooth muscle actin staining), leiomyosarcomas express desmin and caldesmon, whereas nodular fasciitis usually lacks these markers or shows only focal expression.*

(Left) *The lesional cells in this inflammatory leiomyosarcoma show blunt-ended nuclei and brightly eosinophilic cytoplasm, although obscuring inflammation masks the typical fascicular pattern. This tumor was strongly reactive with desmin and lacked ALK expression.* **(Right)** *This leiomyosarcoma displays prominent osteoclast-like giant cells ➢. In the past, such lesions were sometimes mistaken for undifferentiated pleomorphic sarcomas (or malignant fibrous histiocytomas).*

Inflammatory Leiomyosarcoma

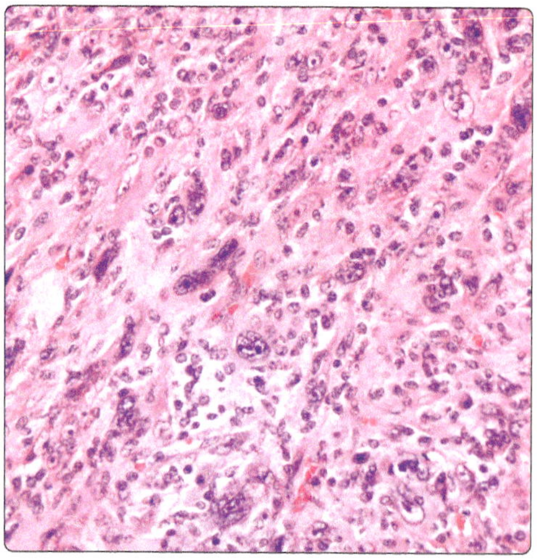

Leiomyosarcoma, Giant Cells

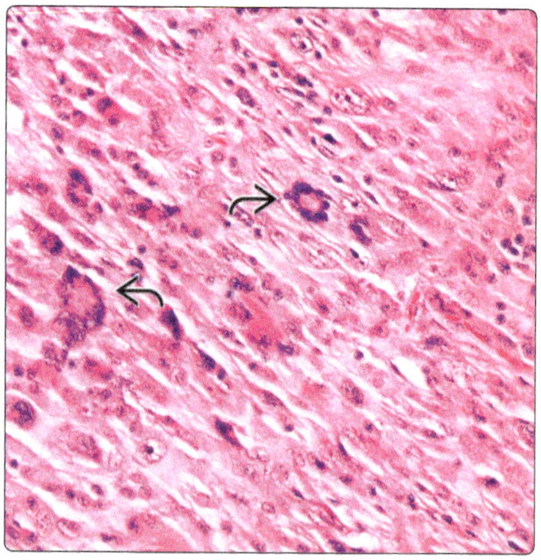

(Left) *This oil immersion image shows an anaphase bridge ➢. Blunt-ended (cigar-shaped) nuclei ➢ are also present in this field. Note also the delicate longitudinally oriented fibrillary cytoplasm ➢.* **(Right)** *Note the nuclear palisading in this cutaneous leiomyosarcoma case. Although this pattern could suggest a nerve sheath tumor, the perpendicular arrangement of the fascicles supports the interpretation of leiomyosarcoma.*

Leiomyosarcoma, Anaphase Bridge at High Magnification

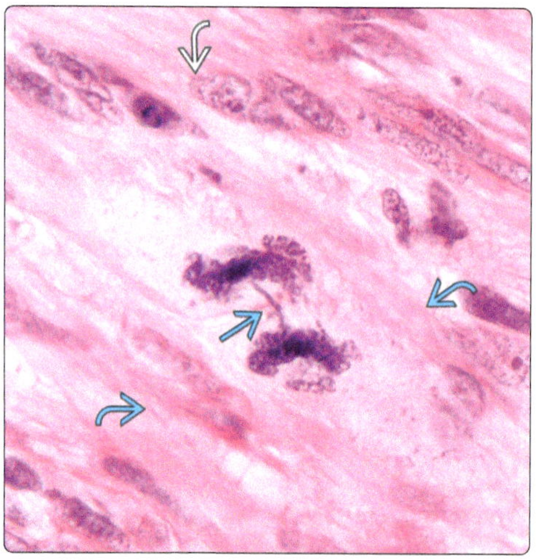

Leiomyosarcoma With Nuclear Palisading

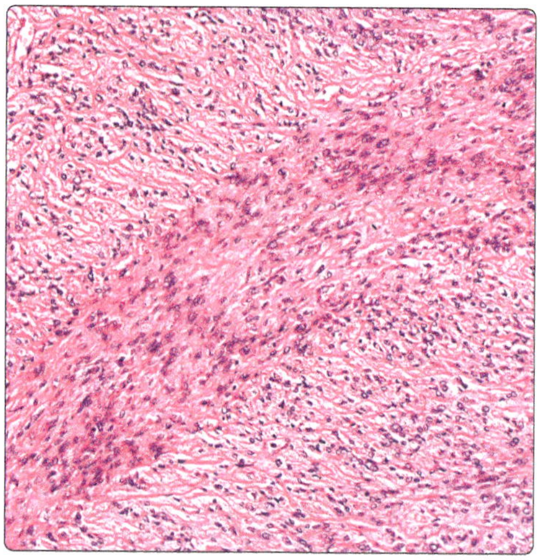

(Left) *Histologic examination of a myxoid leiomyosarcoma is shown. The bottom of the field shows typical leiomyosarcoma features, whereas the top is myxoid with a pleomorphic cell ➢. A predominance of pleomorphic zones would qualify a tumor as a pleomorphic leiomyosarcoma.* **(Right)** *This cell, found in the myxoid zone of the myxoid leiomyosarcoma, shows blunt-ended nuclear contours. Note the delicate eosinophilic filaments ➢ in the cytoplasm.*

Myxoid Leiomyosarcoma

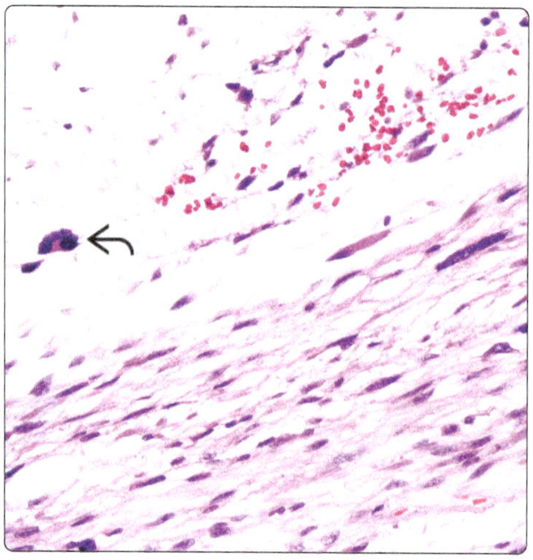

Leiomyosarcoma, Fibrillary Longitudinal Striations

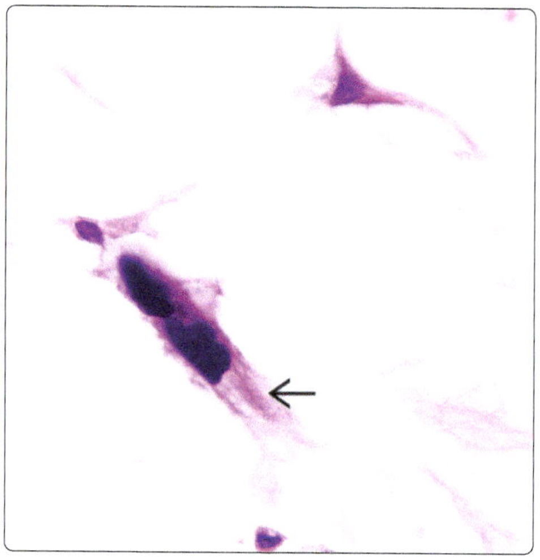

Leiomyosarcoma With Nuclear Pleomorphism

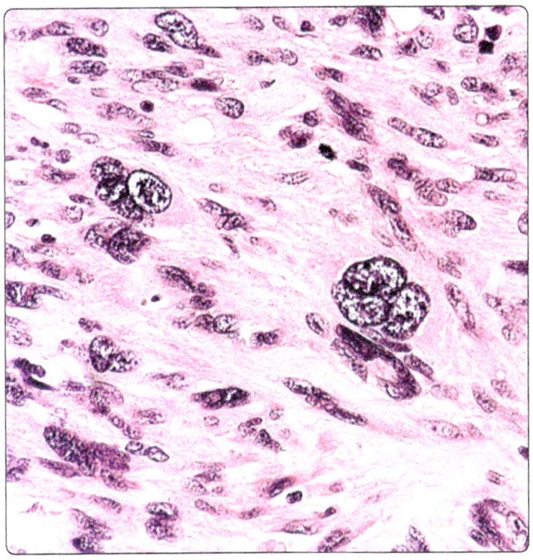

Epithelioid Leiomyosarcoma With Marked Atypia

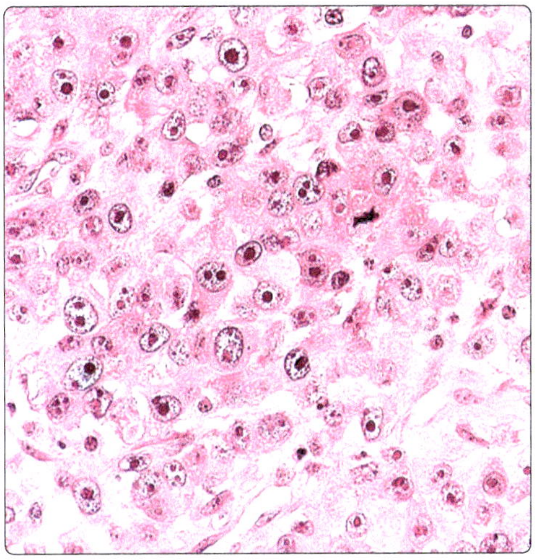

(Left) *This leiomyosarcoma displays striking nuclear pleomorphism. When this feature is the overriding one, such tumors have been classified as pleomorphic leiomyosarcoma and behave more aggressively.* **(Right)** *Epithelioid leiomyosarcoma shows abundant eosinophilic cytoplasm and cytologically malignant nuclei. The diagnosis in such cases often requires use of immunohistochemistry to exclude melanoma and poorly differentiated carcinomas.*

Epstein-Barr Virus-Associated Smooth Muscle Tumor

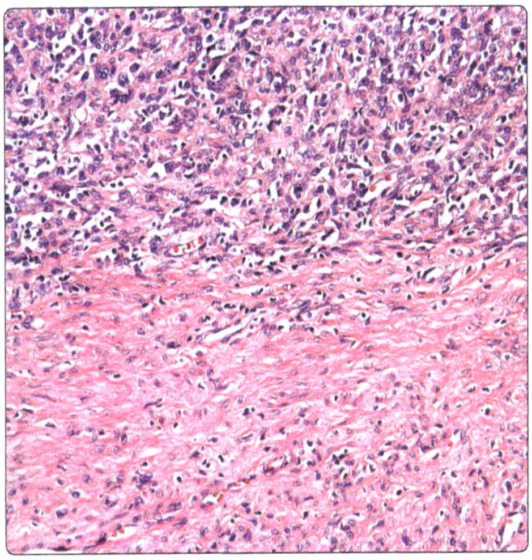

Epstein-Barr Virus In Situ Hybridization

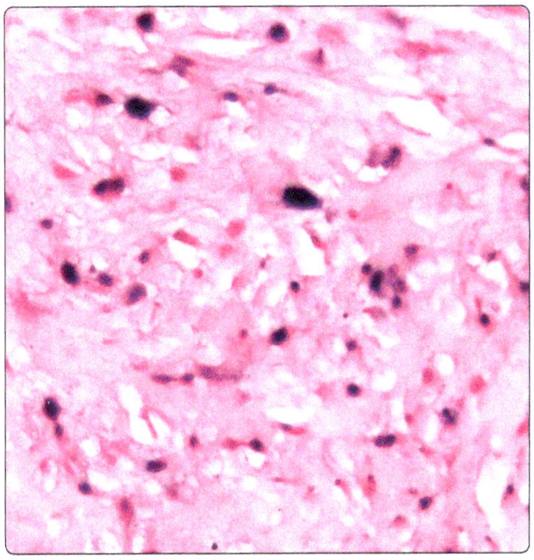

(Left) *Epstein-Barr virus (EBV)-associated smooth muscle tumor manifests a dual population of fascicular eosinophilic cells and smaller darker cells at the top of the field. (Courtesy A. Deyrup, MD.)* **(Right)** *This EBV in situ hybridization study shows strong nuclear labeling in an EBV-associated smooth muscle tumor.*

Inflammatory Leiomyosarcoma

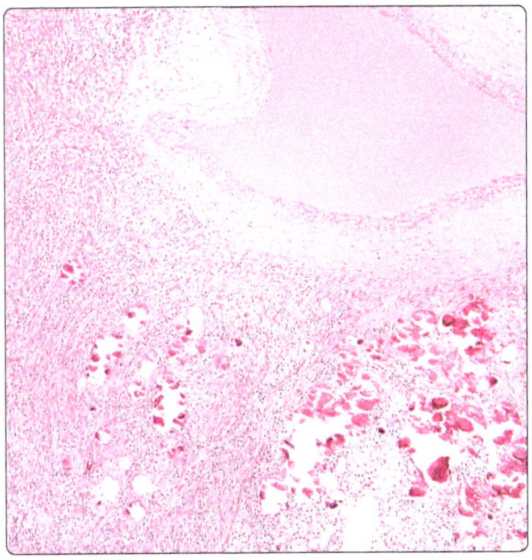

Inflammatory Leiomyosarcoma

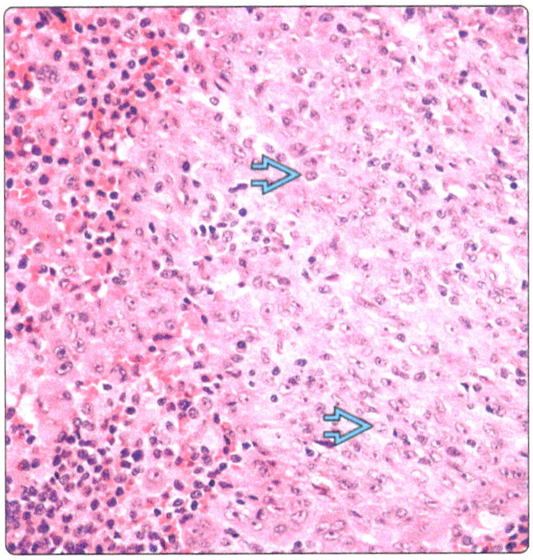

(Left) *An inflammatory leiomyosarcoma associated with a large vein and microcalcifications is depicted here.* **(Right)** *At a higher magnification of an inflammatory leiomyosarcoma, the proliferating cells show epithelioid features ⇨. The inflammatory component is primarily lymphoplasmacytic.*

KEY FACTS

TERMINOLOGY

- Benign tumor with skeletal muscle differentiation
  - Adult, fetal, and genital types

ETIOLOGY/PATHOGENESIS

- No association with tuberous sclerosis (unlike cardiac type)
- Some fetal rhabdomyomas associated with nevoid basal cell carcinoma syndrome (Gorlin syndrome)

CLINICAL ISSUES

- Fetal type: Usually infants and children
- Adult and genital types: Most common in adults
- Genital type shows strong female predilection
- Adult and fetal types most common in head and neck region
- Excellent prognosis after complete excision

MICROSCOPIC

- No significant atypia or necrosis; mitoses usually absent
- Fetal rhabdomyoma
  - Classic (immature) type: Bland spindle cells in abundant myxoid stroma
  - Intermediate (juvenile) type: Increased cellularity with more skeletal muscle differentiation
- Adult rhabdomyoma
  - Large polygonal cells with eosinophilic cytoplasm
  - Intracytoplasmic cross striations or rod-like inclusions
- Genital rhabdomyoma
  - Hypocellular proliferation of bland spindle cells and mature rhabdomyoblastic elements

ANCILLARY TESTS

- Desmin (+), myogenin (+), MYOD1(+)

TOP DIFFERENTIAL DIAGNOSES

- Carcinoma or melanoma
- Granular cell tumor
- Hibernoma

Adult Rhabdomyoma | Fetal Rhabdomyoma

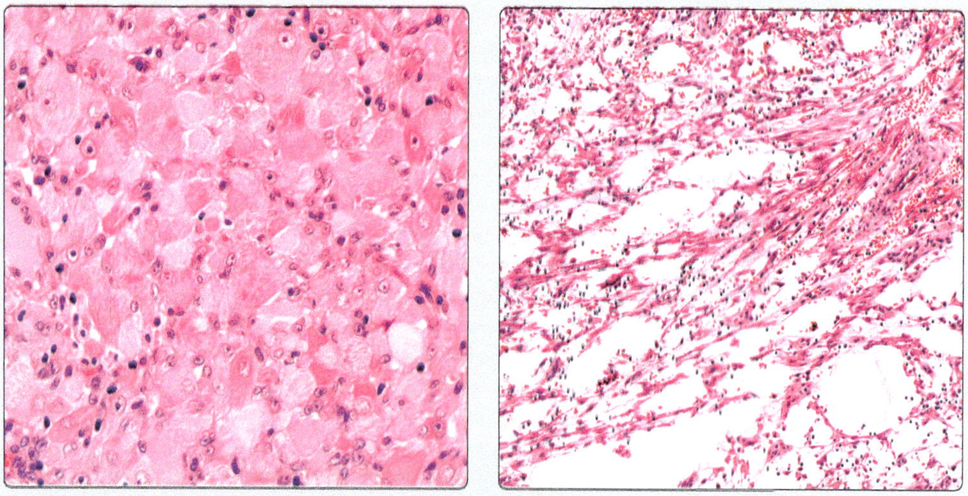

(Left) *High magnification shows adult rhabdomyoma composed of large polygonal cells with copious eosinophilic cytoplasm (varying in staining intensity) and small round nuclei with uniform nucleoli.* **(Right)** *Intermediate magnification shows fetal rhabdomyoma of classic (immature) type. Slender spindle cells form loosely organized fascicles in myxoid stroma. Note the absence of pleomorphism and necrosis.*

Desmin Expression in Rhabdomyoma | Myogenin Expression in Rhabdomyoma

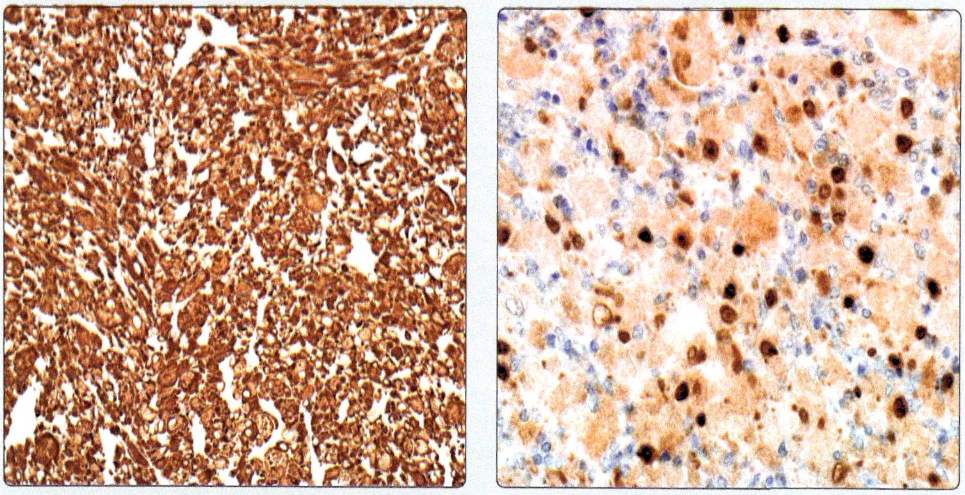

(Left) *Desmin stain in an adult rhabdomyoma shows strong, diffuse positivity throughout the lesion. This is a typical finding in rhabdomyoma and can also highlight cross striations.* **(Right)** *Positive myogenin in an adult rhabdomyoma shows immunoreactivity in the nuclei of many of the lesional cells. This is diagnostic of skeletal muscle differentiation. Cytoplasmic staining is sometimes seen, but it is nonspecific. MYOD1 is also useful, although less sensitive.*

TERMINOLOGY

Definitions

- Benign tumor with skeletal muscle differentiation
- Extracardiac rhabdomyoma includes adult, fetal, and genital types

ETIOLOGY/PATHOGENESIS

Developmental Anomaly

- No association with tuberous sclerosis (unlike cardiac type)
- Some fetal rhabdomyomas associated with nevoid basal cell carcinoma syndrome (Gorlin syndrome)
  - *PTCH1* gene mutations

CLINICAL ISSUES

Epidemiology

- Incidence
  - Rare
- Age
  - Fetal type
    - Infants and children (particularly in 1st year of life)
  - Adult and genital types
    - Most common in adults (mean: 50 years)
- Sex
  - Adult and fetal types: Male predilection
  - Genital type: Strong female predilection

Site

- Rarely cutaneous lesion
- Adult and fetal types are most common in head and neck region
  - Larynx, oropharynx, mouth, neck
- Genital lesions are subepithelial
  - Mostly in vagina, occasionally in vulva or cervix

Presentation

- Slowly growing, painless mass
- Often solitary
  - Subset of adult and fetal types can be multifocal

Treatment

- Complete surgical excision

Prognosis

- Excellent after complete excision
- Adult type may recur
- No metastatic potential

MACROSCOPIC

General Features

- Well circumscribed; may be pedunculated/polypoid

MICROSCOPIC

Key Microscopic Features

- Fetal rhabdomyoma, classic (immature)
  - Solitary circumscribed lesion, can be polypoid
  - Spindle cells with eosinophilic cytoplasm, occasional cross striations
  - No atypia or necrosis, mitoses usually absent
  - Prominent myxoid stroma
- Fetal rhabdomyoma, intermediate (juvenile)
  - Greater cellularity and mitotic activity than classic type
  - Myxoid stroma less prominent
  - Greater degree of rhabdomyoblastic differentiation
  - No significant nuclear atypia or atypical mitotic figures
- Adult rhabdomyoma
  - Sheets of large polygonal cells with abundant finely granular, eosinophilic cytoplasm
  - Cross striations and rod-like crystalline cytoplasmic inclusions occasionally seen
  - Small bland nuclei, some with prominent nucleoli
  - Occasional vacuolated ("spider") cells
- Genital rhabdomyoma
  - Polypoid subepithelial lesion in women
  - Hypocellular proliferation of bland spindle cells with eosinophilic cytoplasm and mature rhabdomyoblastic elements
  - No atypia, mitoses, or necrosis
  - Sclerosing variant features abundant dense collagenous stroma

ANCILLARY TESTS

Immunohistochemistry

- Desmin (+), myogenin (+), MYOD1(+)

DIFFERENTIAL DIAGNOSIS

Fetal and Genital Rhabdomyomas

- Embryonal rhabdomyosarcoma
  - Infiltrative growth
  - Mitoses, nuclear pleomorphism, necrosis
  - Cellular cambium layer in submucosal tumors

Adult Rhabdomyoma

- Granular cell tumor
  - Lacks cytoplasmic vacuolizations
  - S100(+); desmin and myogenin (-)
- Hibernoma
  - Eosinophilic cells containing numerous tiny intracytoplasmic vacuoles
  - Usually shows obvious component of adipocytic differentiation
  - Myogenic markers (-)
- Carcinoma or melanoma
  - In situ components
  - Mitoses, pleomorphism
  - Prior history and immunohistochemistry helpful
- Alveolar soft part sarcoma
  - Mitoses, pleomorphism, necrosis, vascular invasion
  - Nuclear TFE3 (+); desmin and myogenin (-)

SELECTED REFERENCES

1. Diociaiuti A et al: Naevoid basal cell carcinoma syndrome in a 22-month-old child presenting with multiple basal cell carcinomas and a fetal rhabdomyoma. Acta Derm Venereol. 95(2):243-4, 2015
2. Yang SH et al: Supraorbital cutaneous fetal rhabdomyoma of intermediate type: a case report. Am J Dermatopathol. 36(5):e93-6, 2014
3. Walsh SN et al: Cutaneous fetal rhabdomyoma: a case report and historical review of the literature. Am J Surg Pathol. 32(3):485-91, 2008

(Left) *Low magnification shows an adult rhabdomyoma of the larynx. The tumor is separated from the epithelium by a narrow clear zone and forms a solid sheet of cells. Laryngeal rhabdomyomas are most commonly of the adult type, although examples of fetal rhabdomyoma also occur.* **(Right)** *Intermediate-power examination shows an adult rhabdomyoma. The large, rounded, uniform cells have abundant eosinophilic cytoplasm. They are arranged in confluent sheets with interspersed inflammatory cells.*

Adult Rhabdomyoma at Low Power

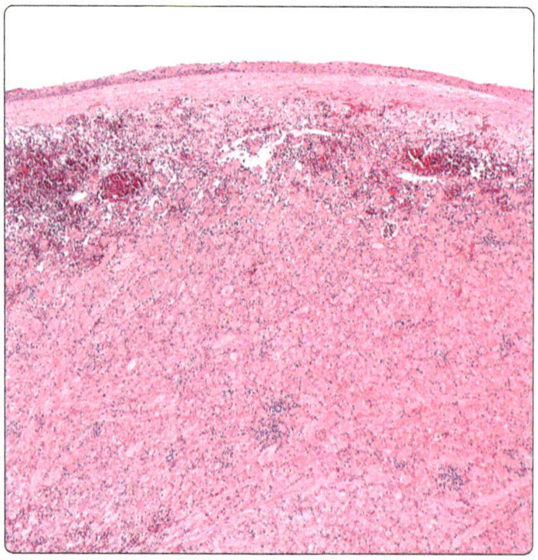

Adult Rhabdomyoma With Sheets of Eosinophilic Cells

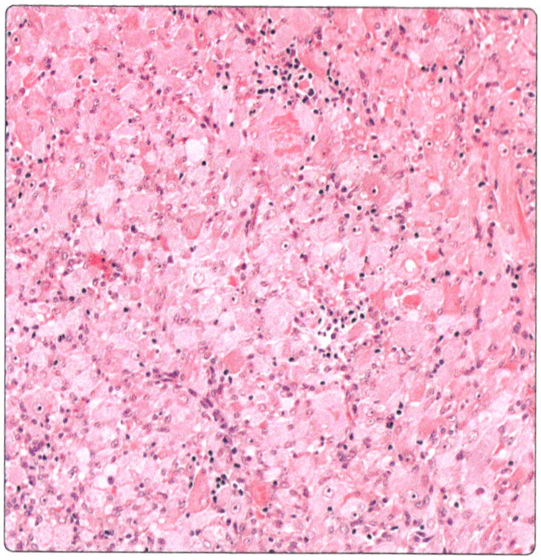

(Left) *High magnification shows an adult rhabdomyoma with vacuolated cells, some with strands of cytoplasm extending to the cell's periphery ("spider" cell) ⇨. These cells are generally more prominent in cardiac rhabdomyoma.* **(Right)** *Adult rhabdomyoma is shown with a large lesional cell containing crystalline, rod-shaped intracytoplasmic inclusions ⇨. With electron microscopy, these are seen to be composed of hypertrophic Z-band structures.*

Occasional "Spider" Cells

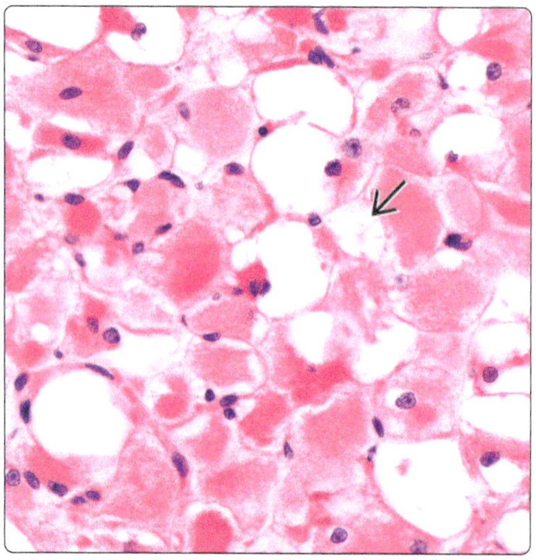

Intracytoplasmic Inclusions

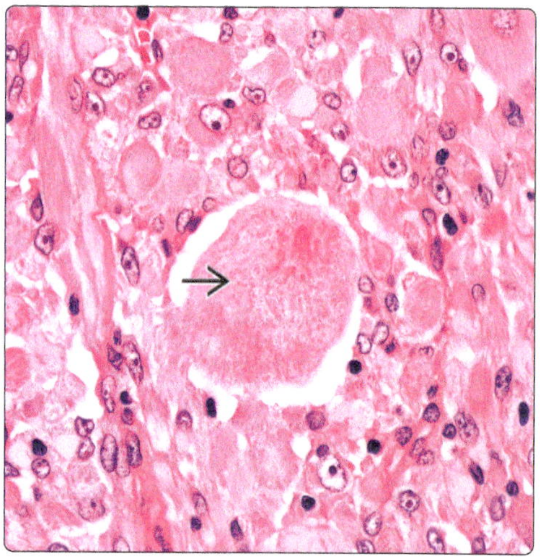

(Left) *Classic (immature) type of fetal rhabdomyoma features bland spindle cells arranged in loose bundles and fascicles in a prominent myxoid stroma. Pleomorphism and necrosis are absent.* **(Right)** *Fetal rhabdomyoma (intermediate type) is shown. Cells show varying stages of skeletal muscle maturation, including rhabdomyoblast-like cells. As in other types of rhabdomyoma, mitotic figures, pleomorphism, and necrosis are absent, which help to exclude embryonal rhabdomyosarcoma.*

Classic Fetal Rhabdomyoma With Myxoid Stroma

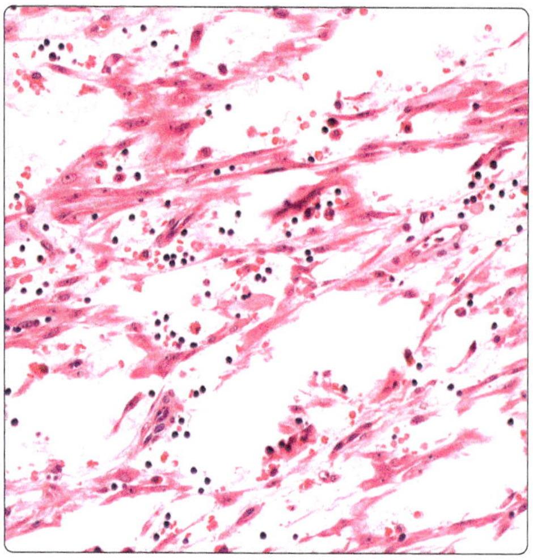

Intermediate-Type Fetal Rhabdomyoma With Increased Cellularity

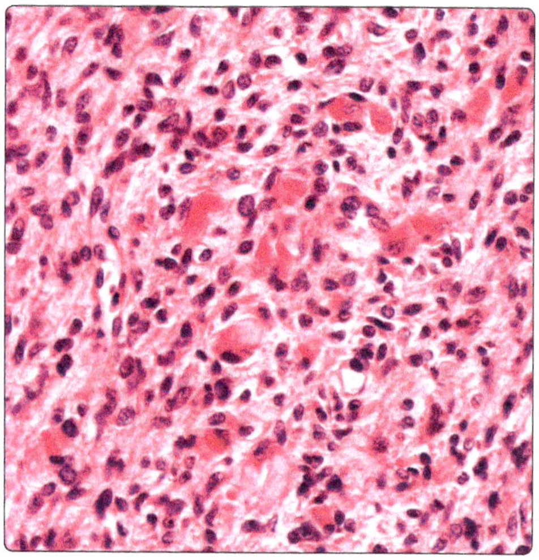

Cellular Proliferation of Uniform Spindle Cells

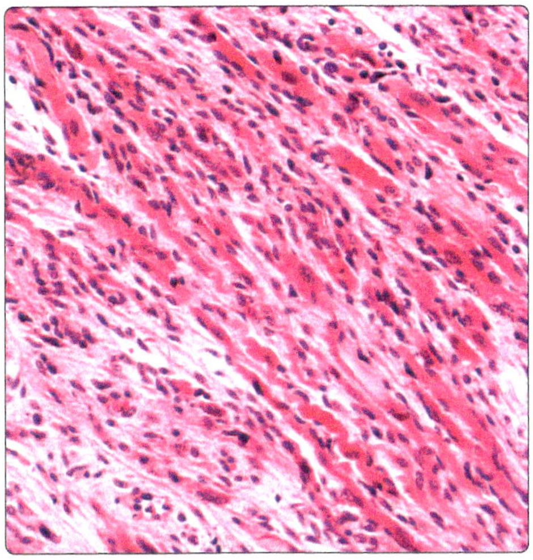

Evidence of Rhabdomyoblastic Differentiation

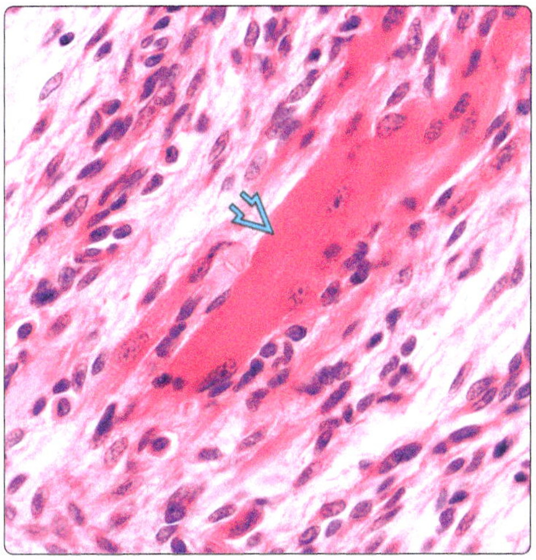

(Left) *Intermediate-type fetal rhabdomyoma manifesting relatively uniform spindle cells with differentiation resembling late-stage embryonic skeletal muscle development is shown. Nuclei are uniform, and no mitotic activity is seen.* **(Right)** *Intermediate-type fetal rhabdomyoma at higher magnification is shown. Note the variation in cell type. Typical cross striations ⇨, characteristic of skeletal muscle differentiation, are apparent in the cytoplasm.*

Desmin in Fetal Rhabdomyoma

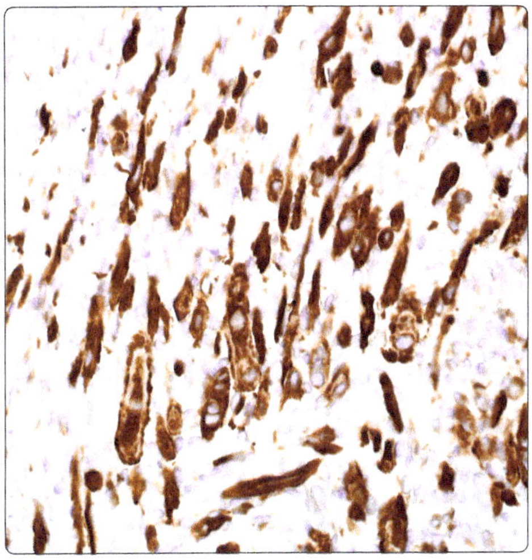

Genital Rhabdomyoma

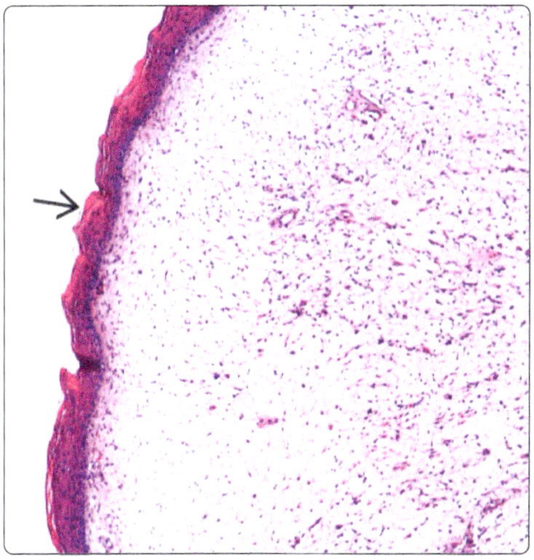

(Left) *Desmin expression in intermediate-type fetal rhabdomyoma highlights the more differentiated rhabdomyoblastic elements.* **(Right)** *Genital rhabdomyoma is the rarest form of rhabdomyoma and most often arises in women in the vagina. Lesions are generally polypoid and show overlying squamous epithelium →. Note the absence of a cellular, subepithelial cambium layer.*

Hypocellular Proliferation of Bland Spindle Cells

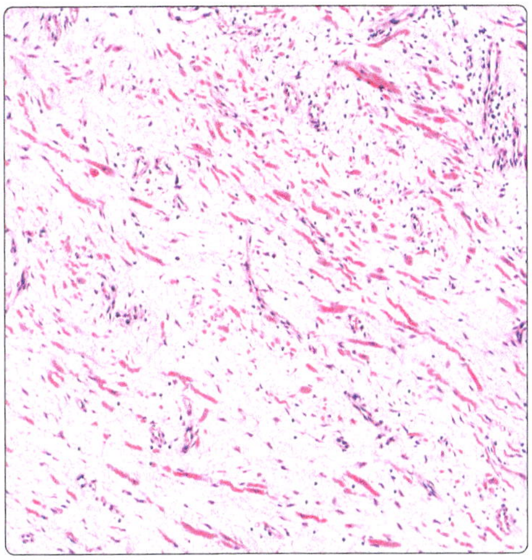

Mature Rhabdomyoblastic Elements

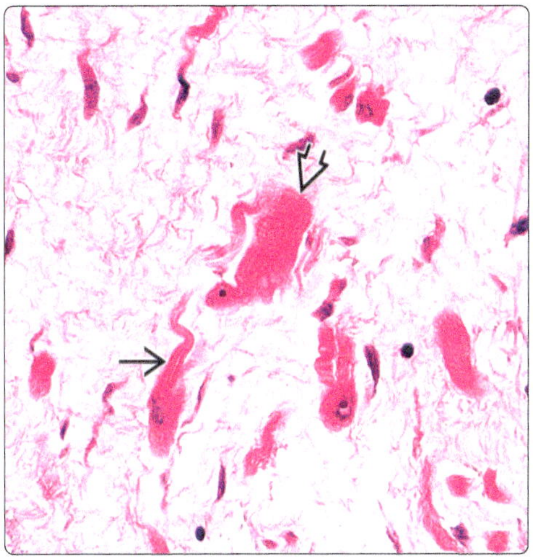

(Left) *Genital rhabdomyoma shows widely separated cords of cells with eosinophilic cytoplasm in a fibrous and myxoid stroma.* **(Right)** *Higher magnification shows spindle cells that vary in shape and size. Some are slender and wavy, others are tadpole-like →, and occasional cells are strap-shaped ⇨, with cross striations evident in this example. As with most rhabdomyomas, no mitoses are seen.*

Cutaneous Rhabdomyosarcoma

KEY FACTS

TERMINOLOGY

- Malignant mesenchymal neoplasm arising in dermis &/or subcutis and showing variable differentiation toward skeletal muscle

CLINICAL ISSUES

- Very rare
  - Cutaneous metastases or secondary involvement of skin by deep primary must be thoroughly excluded
- Bimodal age distribution
  - Children and young adults: Embryonal and alveolar types
  - Older adults: Pleomorphic and epithelioid types
- Limited data available regarding treatment and prognosis
  - However, recurrences and metastases reported

MICROSCOPIC

- Confined to dermis &/or subcutaneous tissue
- Embryonal rhabdomyosarcoma (RMS)
  - Variably cellular sheets of spindle and ovoid cells
- Alveolar RMS
  - Nests of small round cells with fibrous septa
- Pleomorphic RMS
  - Sheets of markedly pleomorphic, atypical cells
- Epithelioid RMS
  - Sheets of uniform epithelioid cells with abundant eosinophilic cytoplasm
  - Eccentric nuclei with prominent nucleoli

ANCILLARY TESTS

- Desmin (+), myogenin (+), MYOD1(+)
- Negative for S100, SOX10, p63, CD31, melanocytic markers

TOP DIFFERENTIAL DIAGNOSES

- Superficial Ewing sarcoma/PNET
- Carcinoma, melanoma
- Merkel cell carcinoma
- Atypical fibroxanthoma

(Left) *This cutaneous rhabdomyosarcoma (RMS) from the ear is a polypoid tumor with extensive infiltration of the dermis by hypercellular sheets of fairly uniform, small, hyperchromatic, ovoid cells.* **(Right)** *High magnification of a cutaneous RMS shows a nodular dermal proliferation of medium-sized, blue-staining, ovoid cells. A grenz zone separates the tumor from overlying epidermis.*

Cutaneous Rhabdomyosarcoma

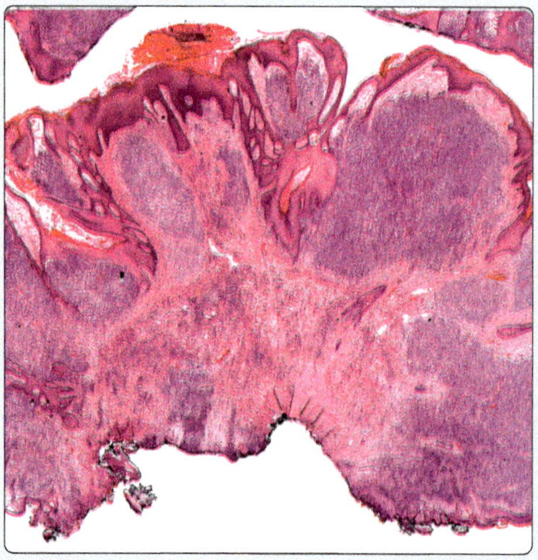

Cutaneous Rhabdomyosarcoma at High Power

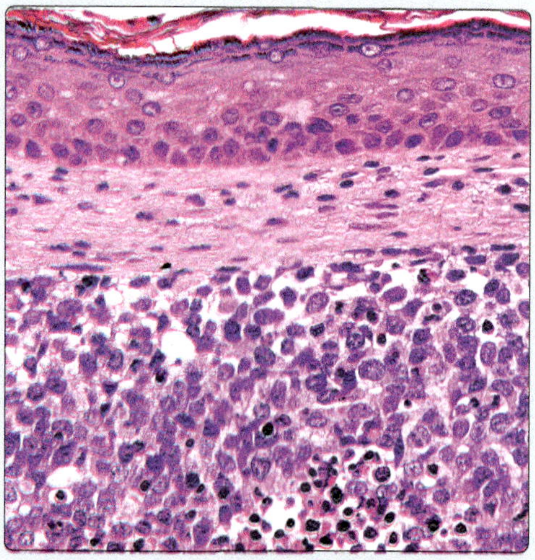

(Left) *Desmin expression in RMS is typically diffuse and strong in the cytoplasm of the neoplastic cells. Cross striations may be highlighted.* **(Right)** *Immunostaining for myogenin shows well-defined nuclear localization (→). The proportion of nuclei expressing this marker varies. It is most widespread in alveolar RMS, with lesser degrees in embryonal and pleomorphic subtypes. Cytoplasmic staining is nonspecific and seen in many tumor types.*

Desmin Expression in Rhabdomyosarcoma

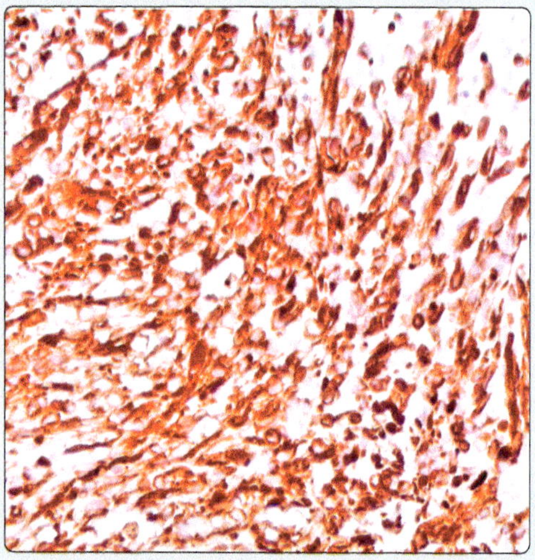

Myogenin Expression in Rhabdomyosarcoma

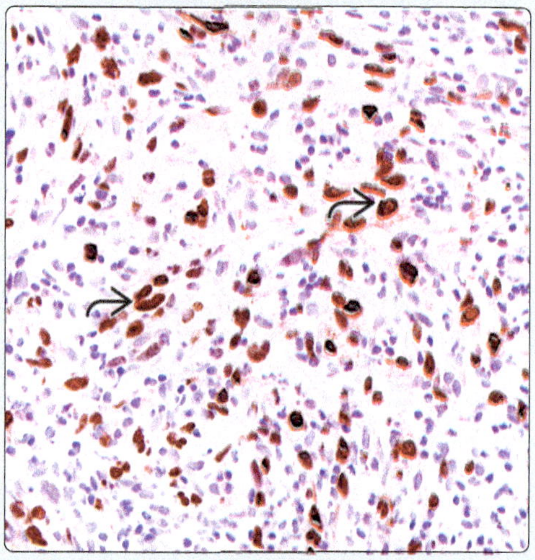

TERMINOLOGY

Abbreviations

- Rhabdomyosarcoma (RMS)

Definitions

- Malignant mesenchymal neoplasm arising in dermis &/or subcutis and showing variable differentiation toward skeletal muscle
  - Cutaneous metastases or secondary involvement by deep primary tumor must be excluded
  - Embryonal, alveolar, pleomorphic, and epithelioid types of RMS have been described as primary cutaneous tumors

CLINICAL ISSUES

Epidemiology

- Incidence
  - However, primary cutaneous RMS is very rare
    - Cutaneous metastases or secondary involvement of skin must be thoroughly excluded
- Age
  - Bimodal age distribution
    - Children and young adults
      - Embryonal and alveolar types most common
    - Older adults
      - Pleomorphic and epithelioid types most common
- Sex
  - M = F

Site

- May occur at any cutaneous site
  - Including head and neck, trunk, extremities

Presentation

- Often presents as asymptomatic papule or nodule
  - May cause pain
- Nonspecific clinical features
  - Diagnosis may therefore be delayed

Treatment

- Complete surgical excision
- Chemotherapy &/or radiation

Prognosis

- Data limited due to small number of cases reported
- However, documented cutaneous cases prone to repeated recurrences and metastases (including to lymph nodes and lung)
- Overall mortality rate 36% in one small series

MACROSCOPIC

Size

- Usually 1-4 cm

MICROSCOPIC

Histologic Features

- May be confined to dermis, subcutis, or involve both dermis and subcutis
- May show ulceration of overlying skin
- Rhabdomyoblasts
  - Cells with eccentric nuclei and variable amounts of eosinophilic cytoplasm
  - Cytoplasmic cross striations may be visible
  - Variable numbers and stages of differentiation
  - Can be found in all RMS subtypes
- Embryonal RMS
  - Alternating regions of cellularity
  - Spindled, stellate, and ovoid cells
    - Ovoid and elongated, hyperchromatic or vesicular nuclei
    - Varying stages of myogenic differentiation
  - Myxoid stroma common
  - Mitoses and necrosis
- Alveolar RMS
  - Nests of small to medium-sized ovoid cells divided by fibrous septa
    - Alveolar-like spaces formed by central loss of cohesion
    - Central cells poorly preserved and necrotic
  - Solid variant lacks alveolar pattern
  - Multinucleated tumor giant cells ("wreath cells" may be present)
- Pleomorphic RMS
  - Sheet-like growth of markedly pleomorphic cells with abundant eosinophilic cytoplasm
    - Resembles undifferentiated pleomorphic sarcoma and other pleomorphic sarcomas
  - Can have prominent rhabdoid morphology
  - Abundant mitoses, often atypical
  - Necrosis common
- Epithelioid RMS
  - Sheets of uniform epithelioid cells with abundant eosinophilic cytoplasm
  - Eccentric nuclei with prominent nucleoli
    - Absence of significant pleomorphism
  - Mitoses common, including abnormal forms
  - Stroma may be myxoid
  - Necrosis
- RMS, not otherwise specific
  - Contains indistinct or unexplained morphologies for RMS
  - Diagnosis of exclusion

ANCILLARY TESTS

Immunohistochemistry

- Strongly desmin (+)
  - Often diffuse in alveolar RMS
  - Can be patchy/focal in embryonal and pleomorphic RMS
- Nuclear myogenin (+) and MYOD1(+)
  - May be focal or diffuse
    - Often diffuse in alveolar RMS
  - Very rare cases may be negative for one of these markers
- Variable SMA(+)
- Focal keratin (+) reported in several reported cases
- Retained nuclear SNF5 (INI1)
- Negative for CD99 and synaptophysin (but both can be focally expressed in alveolar RMS)
- Negative for S100, SOX10, melanocytic markers
- Negative for CK5/6, p63

- Negative for CD31, CD34, ERG

Genetic Testing

- Limited testing in reported cutaneous RMS
- Alveolar RMS
  - t(2;13)(q35;q14)
    - *PAX3-FOXO1* gene fusion
    - Most common
  - t(1;13)(p36;q14) (10-15% of alveolar RMS)
    - *PAX7-FOXO1* gene fusion
- Embryonal RMS
  - Complex karyotypes
    - Often gains of chromosomes 2, 8, 12, and 13
    - LOH at 11p15.5 considered hallmark of embryonal RMS
    - Genes located in 11p15.5 region include some that encode proteins involved in growth regulation
- Pleomorphic RMS
  - Complex karyotypes

DIFFERENTIAL DIAGNOSIS

Superficial Ewing Sarcoma/Primitive Neuroectodermal Tumor

- Nests and sheets of uniform small cells
- Strong membranous CD99(+)
- Very rare focal desmin (+)
- Negative for myogenin and MYOD1
- Characteristic translocations involving *EWSR1*

Neuroendocrine Carcinoma

- Includes Merkel cell carcinoma (MCC) and metastatic small cell carcinoma
- Older adults
- Primary tumor site may be identifiable (small cell carcinoma)
- Cells often show nuclear modling
- Keratin (+), chromogranin and synaptophysin (+)
  - Cytoplasmic dot-like expression of CK20 in MCC
- Merkel cell polyomavirus (+) in MCC
- Negative for desmin, myogenin, MYOD1
  - Rare cases reported of heterologous rhabdomyoblastic elements in MCC

Sarcomatoid Squamous Cell Carcinoma

- Overlying in situ component may be present
  - May be inapparent in ulcerated cases
- May contain well-differentiated areas with obvious keratin formation
- Keratin (+), p63(+)
- Negative for desmin, myogenin, MYOD1

Malignant Melanoma

- Junctional component often present
- S100(+), SOX10(+)
- Expression of melanocytic markers

Atypical Fibroxanthoma

- Should be considered diagnosis of exclusion
- Usually arises in sun-damaged skin of elderly adults
- Small lesion confined to dermis
- Lacks necrosis
- Can show SMA(+), but is usually focal/weak
- Negative for myogenin, MYOD1

Cutaneous Leiomyosarcoma

- Intersecting fascicular architecture
- Typical cytological features of smooth muscle, e.g., blunt-ended nuclei
- Strong SMA(+), HCAD(+)
- Variable desmin(+)
- Negative for myogenin and MYOD1

Pleomorphic Dermal Sarcoma

- Also known as superficial undifferentiated pleomorphic sarcoma
- Diagnosis of exclusion (similar to atypical fibroxanthoma)
- Negative for desmin, myogenin, MYOD1

Epithelioid Angiosarcoma

- Sheets of epithelioid cells with prominent nucleoli
- May contain areas of obvious vasoformation
- CD31(+), CD34(+), ERG(+)
- Negative for desmin, myogenin, MYOD1

Myoepithelial Carcinoma

- Often rhabdoid or plasmacytoid morphology
- Usually keratin (+), S100(+), SOX10(+)
- Variable expression of calponin, SMA, desmin, p63
- Negative for myogenin and MYOD1

Epithelioid Sarcoma

- Nests of epithelioid to ovoid cells with eosinophilic cytoplasm
- Centralized granuloma-like necrosis can be seen
- Keratin (+)
- CD34(+) in 50% of cases
- Loss of nuclear INI1
- Negative for desmin, myogenin, MYOD1

Rhabdomyomatous Mesenchymal Hamartoma

- Congenital or in infants
- Dermal and subcutaneous
- Mature skeletal muscle, fat, nerves, and adnexa
- No mitoses, necrosis, or atypia

Lymphoma/Leukemia

- Often systemic involvement by disease
- Architecture dispersed and sheet-like, rather than nested
- Expression of broad spectrum hematolymphoid markers
- Negative for desmin, myogenin, MYOD1

SELECTED REFERENCES

1. Li JJ et al: Cutaneous pleomorphic rhabdomyosarcoma occurring on sun-damaged skin: a case report. Am J Dermatopathol. 37(8):653-7, 2015
2. Feasel PC et al: Primary cutaneous epithelioid rhabdomyosarcoma: a rare, recently described entity with review of the literature. J Cutan Pathol. 41(7):588-91, 2014
3. Sabater-Marco V et al: Postradiation cutaneous pleomorphic rhabdomyosarcoma with extracellular collagen deposits reminiscent of so-called amianthoid fibers. J Cutan Pathol. 41(3):316-21, 2014
4. Marburger TB et al: Primary cutaneous rhabdomyosarcoma: a clinicopathologic review of 11 cases. J Cutan Pathol. 39(11):987-95, 2012
5. Kuroiwa M et al: Manifestation of alveolar rhabdomyosarcoma as primary cutaneous lesions in a neonate with Beckwith-Wiedemann syndrome. J Pediatr Surg. 44(3):e31-5, 2009
6. Gong Y et al: Primary cutaneous alveolar rhabdomyosarcoma of the perineum. Arch Pathol Lab Med. 126(8):982-4, 2002

Cutaneous Embryonal Rhabdomyosarcoma

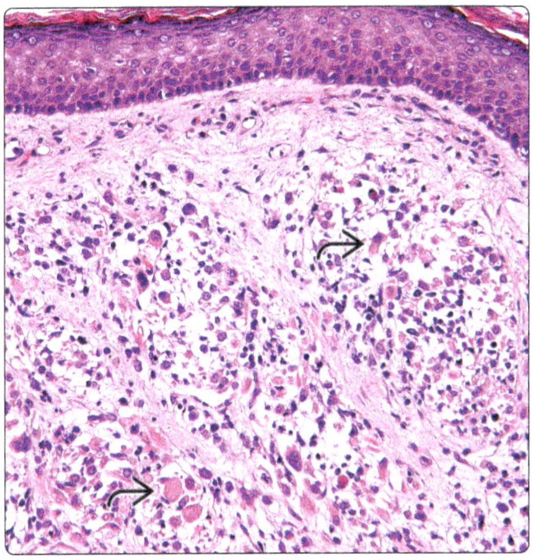

Undifferentiated Ovoid Cells With Scattered Rhabdomyoblasts

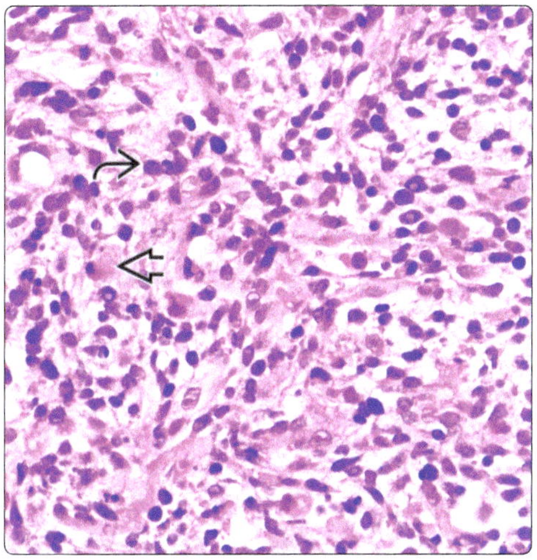

(Left) *This embryonal subtype of cutaneous RMS shows extensive dermal invasion by collections of primitive cells with ovoid nuclei within myxoid stroma. Note numerous intermixed rhabdomyoblasts.* **(Right)** *In this embryonal RMS, the cells show a range of appearances, with relatively undifferentiated ovoid cells with hyperchromatic nuclei and a few rhabdomyoblasts with large amounts of eosinophilic cytoplasm and eccentric nuclei.*

Cutaneous Alveolar Rhabdomyosarcoma

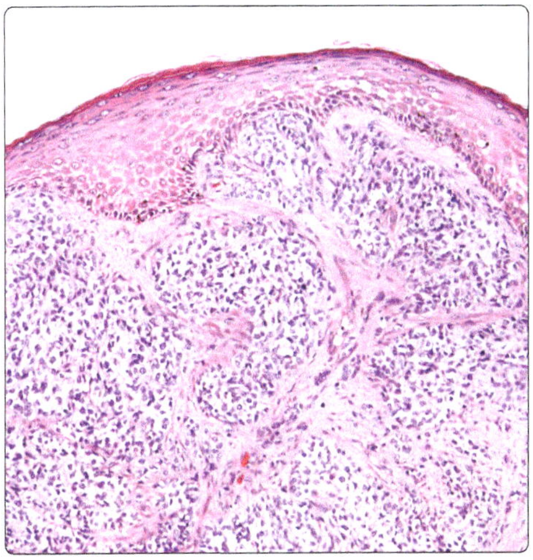

Pseudoalveolar Spaces in Alveolar Rhabdomyosarcoma

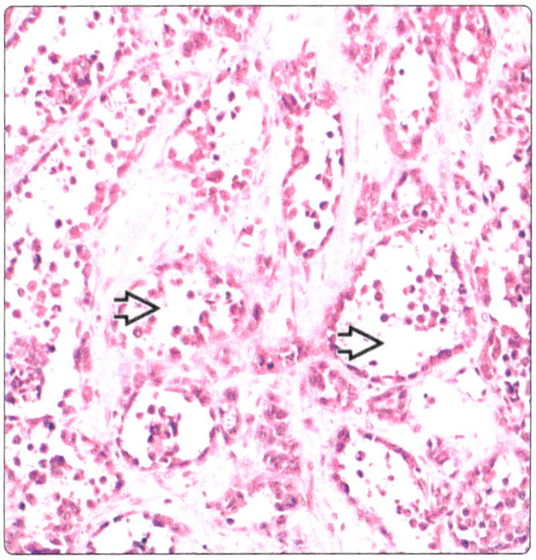

(Left) *Alveolar RMS may rarely present as a primary lesion in the skin; however, the more likely situation is secondary involvement of the skin by a larger underlying tumor or metastatic disease.* **(Right)** *This example of alveolar RMS is composed of nests of round cells separated by fibrous septa. In the nests, there is peripheral cellular preservation but central dyscohesion and necrosis, somewhat resembling the appearance of pulmonary alveoli.*

Pleomorphic Rhabdomyosarcoma

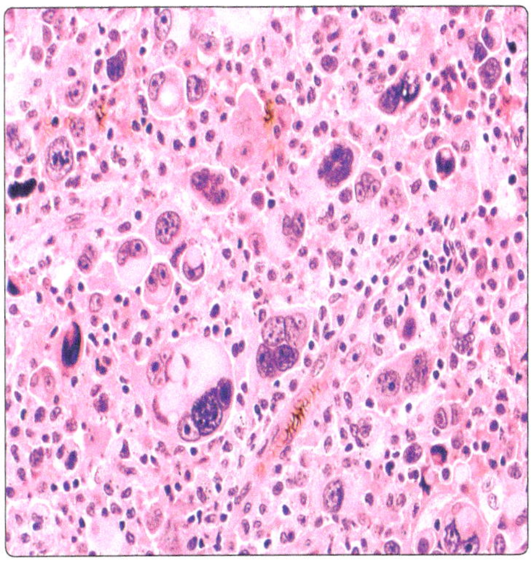

Epithelioid Rhabdomyosarcoma

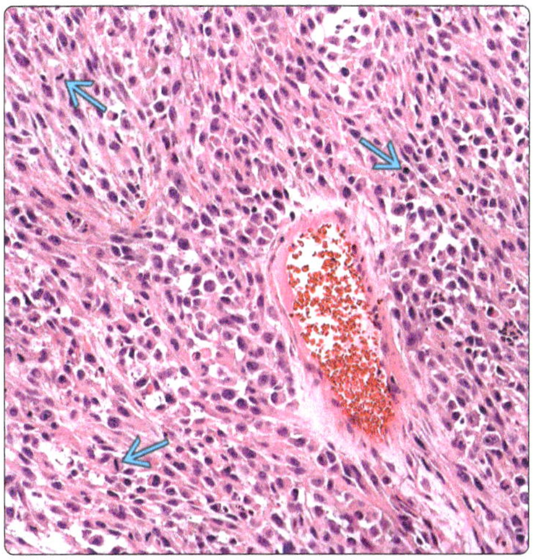

(Left) *This pleomorphic RMS is composed of sheets of large, polygonal, often bizarre-appearing cells with abundant eosinophilic-staining cytoplasm. Some examples feature a prominent rhabdoid morphology.* **(Right)** *Epithelioid RMS is composed of sheets of uniform epithelioid cells with abundant eosinophilic-staining cytoplasm and eccentric nuclei with prominent nucleoli. Mitoses are often easily identified.*

Lipoma

KEY FACTS

TERMINOLOGY

- Benign neoplasm of mature adipocytes (white fat)

CLINICAL ISSUES

- Very common (most common soft tissue tumor overall)
- Wide range (most between 40-60 yr old)
- Present as painless mass
- Superficial lipomas are most common in upper back, shoulder, neck, and abdomen
  - Rarely may be multiple
- Surgical excision is generally curative
  - Intramuscular lipoma can recur (15% rate)
- Lipomatosis: Diffuse &/or regional overgrowth of mature adipose tissue

MACROSCOPIC

- Well circumscribed, often lobulated, with thin capsule
- Yellow, greasy cut surface with very thin to no fibrous septa
- Usually 2-10 cm in size

MICROSCOPIC

- Lobules and sheets of mature adipocytes with minimal size variation and no nuclear atypia
- May show fat necrosis, myxoid changes, or other degenerative features
- Variants: Fibrolipoma, myxolipoma, intramuscular lipoma, lipoma with osseous or cartilaginous metaplasia

ANCILLARY TESTS

- Aberrations involving locus at 12q13-15 are most common
- No amplification of MDM2

TOP DIFFERENTIAL DIAGNOSES

- Atypical lipomatous tumor/well-differentiated liposarcoma
- Spindle cell lipoma
- Myxoid liposarcoma
- Hibernoma
- Lipomatosis of nerve

Lipoma Gross Specimen

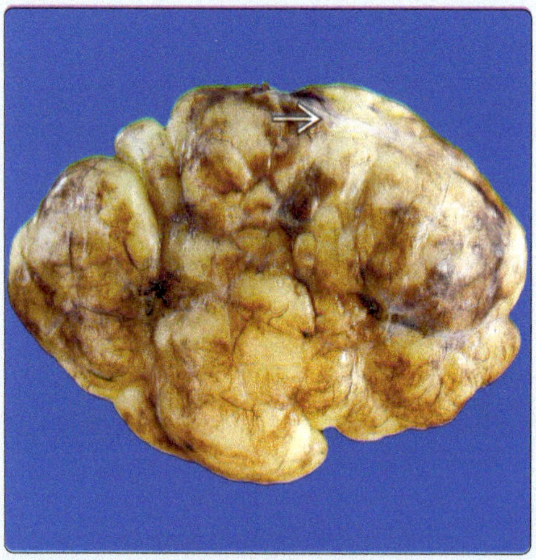

Lipoma, Cut Surface

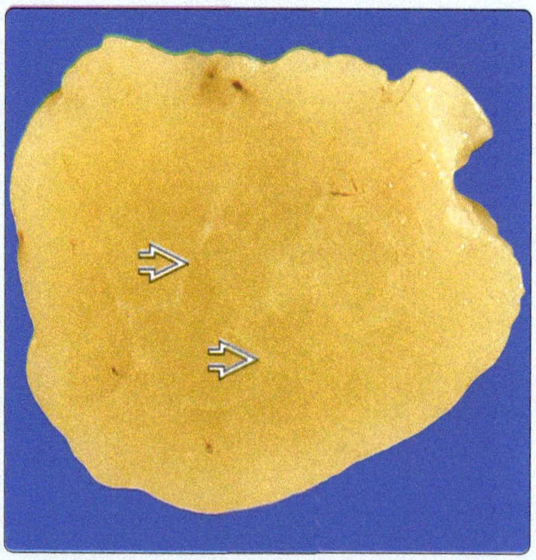

(Left) *This lipoma is surrounded by a thin, delicate, and transparent capsule ➡, and is highly lobulated. It is often taken out by the surgeon piecemeal.* **(Right)** *The cut surface of a lipoma is yellow, homogeneous, and greasy. Note the thin, delicate fibrous septa ➡, which separate the tumor into lobules. Some variants may show myxoid areas or small foci of hemorrhage.*

Lipoma Showing Abundant Mature Adipose Tissue

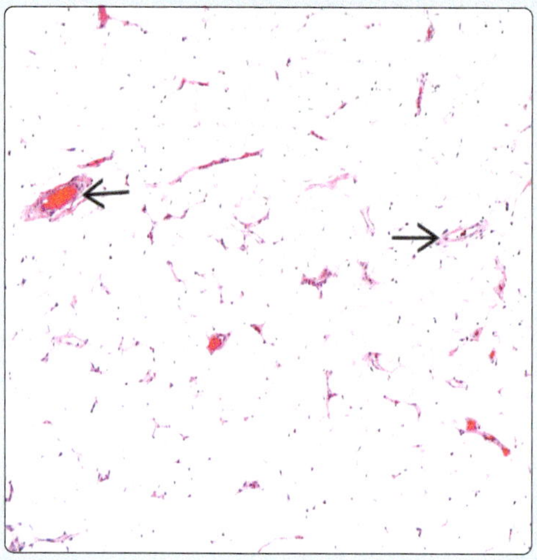

Mature Adipose Tissue

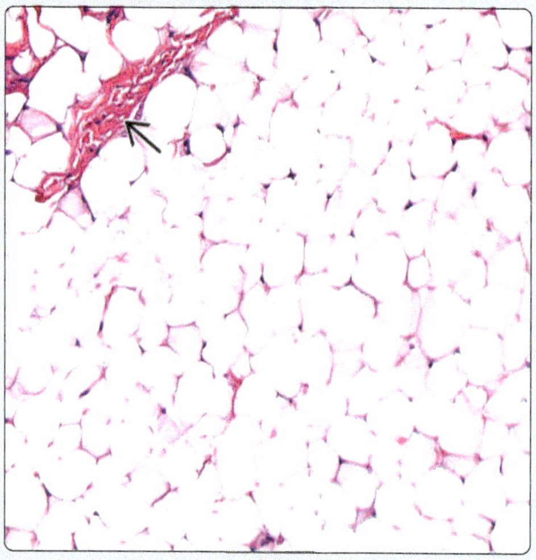

(Left) *A conventional lipoma is composed of lobules and sheets of mature adipocytes (white fat). Small- to medium-sized vessels ➡ are often scattered in the background but are usually not prominent.* **(Right)** *The mature adipocytes of a lipoma usually vary little in size from one another. Thin fibrous septa ➡ are commonly seen separating the lobules; however, thicker, more fibrotic septa may be present along with fat necrosis in traumatized tumors.*

TERMINOLOGY

Definitions

- Benign neoplasm of mature adipocytes (white fat)

CLINICAL ISSUES

Epidemiology

- Incidence
  - Very common (most common soft tissue tumor overall)
  - More common in obese people
- Age
  - Wide range (40-60 yr most common)
  - Rare in patients < 20 yr old

Site

- Superficial lipomas are most common in upper back, shoulder, neck, and abdomen
  - Rare in hands, feet, lower legs, and face
- Deep lipomas may arise in deep soft tissues as well as thorax, mediastinum, pelvis, and, rarely, retroperitoneum
  - May also occur near bone (periosteal/parosteal lipoma)
- Intramuscular lipoma is most common within large muscles of thigh, upper arm, and shoulder
- Mature adipose tissue proliferation within synovium of large joint (synovial lipoma or lipoma arborescens) may clinically simulate diffuse-type tenosynovial giant cell tumor/pigmented villonodular synovitis

Presentation

- Painless mass
  - Larger lesions may be painful
- May be multiple (5% of cases)
  - Range in number from several to hundreds
  - Predilection for upper arm, shoulder, and back in older men
  - May be hereditary in 30% of cases (familial multiple lipomas)
  - Multiple lipomas can occur in various syndromes including Cowden, Proteus, and Fröhlich

Treatment

- Surgical excision is curative

Prognosis

- Recurrences are rare
- Higher recurrence rate in intramuscular lipoma (15%)

Clinical Variants

- Lipomatosis
  - Diffuse &/or regional overgrowth of mature adipose tissue
    - Not the same as multiple discrete lipomas
  - Subtypes: Diffuse, symmetric, pelvic, steroid, and HIV-associated lipodystrophy
  - Adipose tissue proliferation is poorly marginated, lending tendency toward recurrence
  - Significant growth may lead to obstruction of regional structures (larynx, ureter, bowel, etc.)
  - Cytologically and morphologically similar to conventional lipoma, except may show infiltration of muscle or regional structures

MACROSCOPIC

General Features

- Well circumscribed, often lobulated
- Thin, delicate capsule
- Yellow, greasy cut surface
- Myxoid change, focal hemorrhages, bone, or cartilage may be evident
- Infiltrative margins may be present in intramuscular cases

Size

- Usually 2-10 cm
- Deep and intramuscular lipomas are often larger

MICROSCOPIC

Histologic Features

- Lobules and sheets of mature adipocytes
  - In small samples, adipocytes are often indistinguishable from normal, nonlesional fat
- Minimal variation in adipocyte size
- Bland nuclei are small and often peripherally flattened
  - May appear absent
  - May show small intranuclear vacuoles (Lockhern change)
- Small- to medium-sized vessels sparsely distributed throughout tumor
  - May be more prominent in atrophic lipomas
- Thin, discontinuous fibrous bands with collagen may be present, particularly in larger lesions
- Degenerative changes including foci of fat necrosis, myxoid change, or hemorrhage are not uncommon
  - Fat necrosis may be extensive in some cases
- Ischemic changes, infarction, and cystic degeneration may be present, particularly in traumatized lipomas

Morphologic Variants

- **Fibrolipoma**
  - Contains variably prominent fibrous tissue and septa with abundant collagen
  - Extensively fibrous examples (sclerotic lipoma) have predilection for hands and scalp of young men
- **Myxolipoma**
  - Prominent/diffuse stromal myxoid change in otherwise conventional lipoma
  - May also show prominent vascular component (so-called angiomyxolipoma)
- **Lipoma with cartilaginous metaplasia (chondrolipoma)**
  - Additional component of mature cartilage
- **Lipoma with osseous metaplasia (osteolipoma)**
  - Additional component of mature bone
- **Intramuscular lipoma**
  - Often much larger than subcutaneous forms
  - Variable amounts of admixed mature skeletal muscle fibers, most prominent at periphery
    - Imparts checkerboard appearance at low magnification
    - Often infiltrative margins
  - Atrophic skeletal muscle fibers, if present, often mimic atypical stromal cells (smudge cells) of atypical lipomatous tumor/well-differentiated liposarcoma

ANCILLARY TESTS

Immunohistochemistry

- Mature adipocytes express S100
- MDM2(-), CDK4(-)

Genetic Testing

- Majority of lipomas have abnormal karyotype
  - Aberrations involving 12q13-15 (most cases)
    - t(3;12)(q27-28;q13-15) most common translocation
  - Also aberrations involving 6p21-23, 13q11-12, and 12q22-24
- No amplification of *MDM2*

DIFFERENTIAL DIAGNOSIS

Atypical Lipomatous Tumor (ALT)/Well-Differentiated Liposarcoma

- Often larger and more deeply seated than lipoma, but may occur in subcutaneous tissue (ALT)
- Contain variably thickened fibrous septa containing atypical stromal cells (smudge cells)
  - Atypical stromal cells may be extremely focal
- Lipoblasts may or may not be present and are not required for diagnosis
- May arise intramuscularly and show similar myoinfiltrative checkerboard pattern as in intramuscular lipoma
- *MDM2* amplification by FISH
- In retroperitoneum, well-differentiated liposarcoma is far more common than lipoma

Spindle Cell Lipoma

- Predilection for upper arms, shoulders, and posterior neck of older males
- Classically contains ropey collagen and population of bland, spindled fibroblastic cells [CD34(+)]
- Myxoid stroma is common and may be extensive
- Mast cells common

Myxoid Liposarcoma

- Plexiform chicken wire capillary vascular pattern
- Variable numbers of early lipoblasts and maturing adipocytes
- Generally more cellular than myxolipoma
- Most show chromosomal translocations involving *DDIT3* (*CHOP*)

Hibernoma

- Often occurs in younger patients than conventional lipoma
- Most common in thigh, but can occur in variety of sites
- Contains multivacuolated brown fat cells
  - May be very focal (lipoma-like hibernoma)
- Karyotypic aberrations involving 11q13-21

Lipomatosis of Nerve

- Predominantly in hands, wrists, and forearms of children and young adults
- May be associated with macrodactyly
- Mature adipose tissue infiltrating around and between nerve branches and along perineurium

Diffuse-Type Neurofibroma

- Infiltrative growth within connective and adipose tissues
- Neural element may be sparse compared to adipocytic component
- S100(+) spindle cells
- Often show pseudomeissnerian bodies

Intramuscular Hemangioma

- May contain abundant mature adipose tissue, mimicking intramuscular lipoma
- Most patients < 30 yr of age
- Contain prominent capillary or large vessel vascular component
- Significant recurrence rate (~ 50%)

Chondroid Lipoma

- Contains regions of myxoid or sclerotic lipoblastic differentiation that superficially resemble cartilage
- Lacks mature cartilage and contains numerous lipoblasts
- May contain large zones of relatively unremarkable-appearing mature adipose tissue

DIAGNOSTIC CHECKLIST

Pathologic Interpretation Pearls

- Most examples are clinically superficial/subcutaneous
- Homogeneous yellow cut surface and lacking prominent, thick fibrous septations
- Adipocytes are mature and nuclei lack enlargement, irregularity, and hyperchromasia
- Fat necrosis and atrophic skeletal muscle fibers may mimic atypical stromal cells of well-differentiated liposarcoma/atypical lipomatous tumor

SELECTED REFERENCES

1. Nodelman LO et al: Neural fibrolipoma of the ankle: a case report and review of the literature. J Foot Ankle Surg. ePub, 2016
2. Clay MR et al: MDM2 amplification in problematic lipomatous tumors: analysis of FISH testing criteria. Am J Surg Pathol. 39(10):1433-9, 2015
3. Wang SY et al: Pedunculated subcutaneous lipoma in the popliteal fossa causing eczema. Med J Malaysia. 70(1):33-5, 2015
4. Manor E et al: Oral lipoma: analysis of 58 new cases and review of the literature. Ann Diagn Pathol. 15(4):257-61, 2011
5. Zhang H et al: Molecular testing for lipomatous tumors: critical analysis and test recommendations based on the analysis of 405 extremity-based tumors. Am J Surg Pathol. 34(9):1304-11, 2010
6. Macarenco RS et al: Retroperitoneal lipomatous tumors without cytologic atypia: are they lipomas? A clinicopathologic and molecular study of 19 cases. Am J Surg Pathol. 33(10):1470-6, 2009
7. Ida CM et al: Primary retroperitoneal lipoma: a soft tissue pathology heresy?: report of a case with classic histologic, cytogenetics, and molecular genetic features. Am J Surg Pathol. 32(6):951-4, 2008
8. Sakurai H et al: Intrathoracic lipomas: their clinicopathological behaviors are not as straightforward as expected. Ann Thorac Surg. 86(1):261-5, 2008
9. Laskin WB et al: Sclerotic (fibroma-like) lipoma: a distinctive lipoma variant with a predilection for the distal extremities. Am J Dermatopathol. 28(4):308-16, 2006
10. Gaskin CM et al: Lipomas, lipoma variants, and well-differentiated liposarcomas (atypical lipomas): results of MRI evaluations of 126 consecutive fatty masses. AJR Am J Roentgenol. 182(3):733-9, 2004
11. Tardío JC et al: Angiomyxolipoma (vascular myxolipoma) of subcutaneous tissue. Am J Dermatopathol. 26(3):222-4, 2004
12. Willén H et al: Comparison of chromosomal patterns with clinical features in 165 lipomas: a report of the CHAMP study group. Cancer Genet Cytogenet. 102(1):46-9, 1998
13. Zelger BG et al: Sclerotic lipoma: lipomas simulating sclerotic fibroma. Histopathology. 31(2):174-81, 1997
14. Fletcher CD et al: Intramuscular and intermuscular lipoma: neglected diagnoses. Histopathology. 12(3):275-87, 1988

Mature Adipocytes Without Atypia

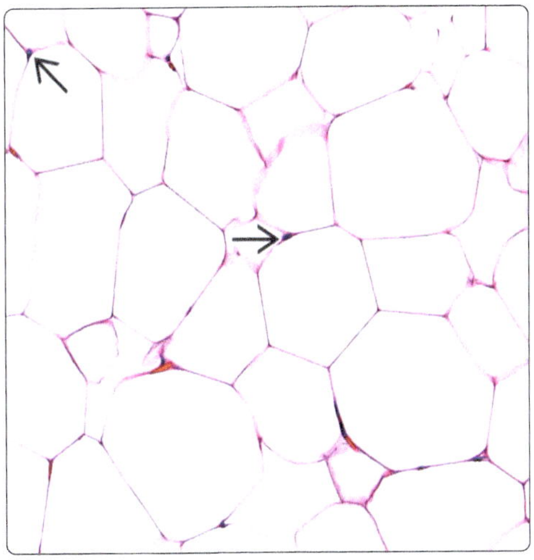

Lockhern Nuclear Change

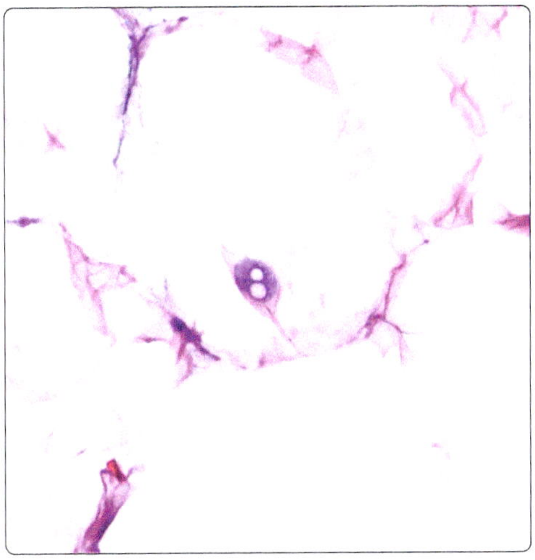

(Left) *A lipoma is composed entirely of mature white fat. The adipocyte nucleus* → *is bland, small, and typically compressed against the periphery of the cell by the large fat vacuole. Of note, most adipocytes appear to lack a nucleus as a result of 2D tissue sectioning.* **(Right)** *Adipocytes showing nuclear vacuolization are relatively common and may be mistaken for multivacuolated lipoblasts. However, the vacuoles (usually 1 or 2) are not external to the nucleus, as would be seen in lipoblasts.*

Myxoid Stromal Change

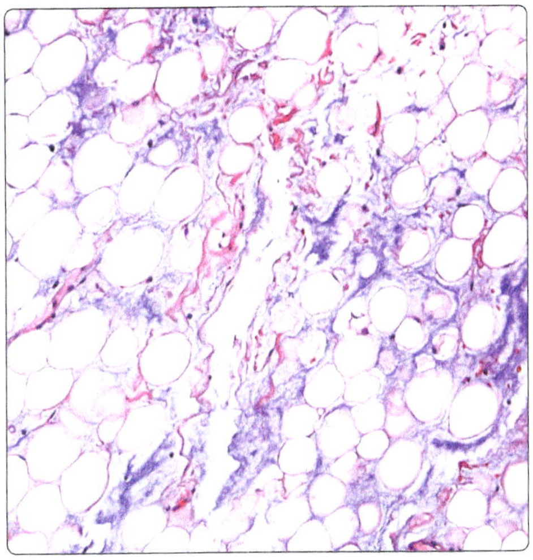

Fat Necrosis in Traumatized Lipoma

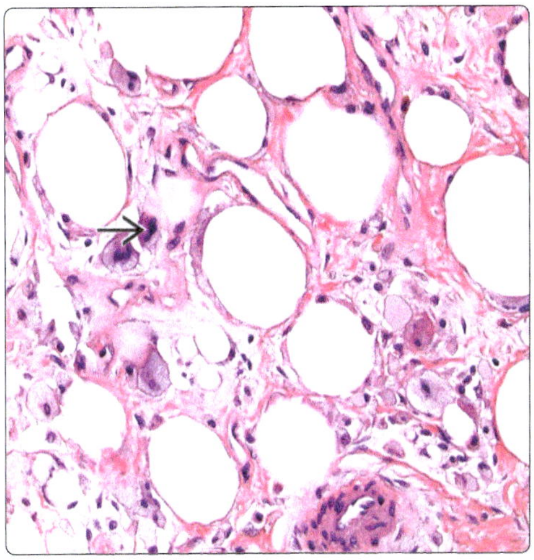

(Left) *Focal myxoid stromal change is a common finding in lipomas, particularly ones that have been traumatized. Fat necrosis is also often present elsewhere.* **(Right)** *Fat necrosis is represented by foamy histiocytes surrounding and reacting to damaged adipocytes. Not uncommonly, the histiocytes are multinucleated, and the apparent hyperchromasia caused by nuclear overlap* → *may raise concern for an atypical lipomatous tumor/well-differentiated liposarcoma.*

Focal Fat Necrosis

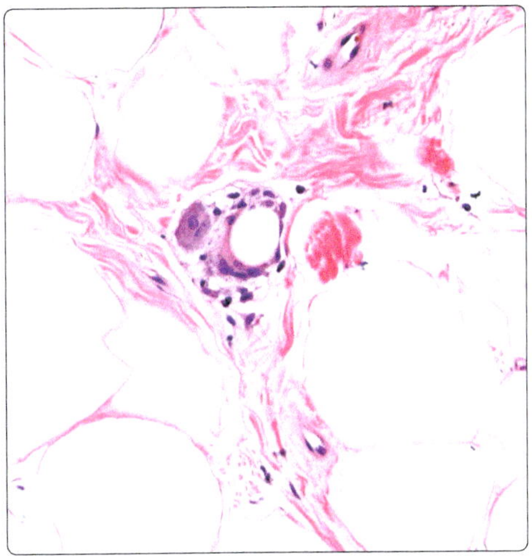

Fibrous Variant of Lipoma

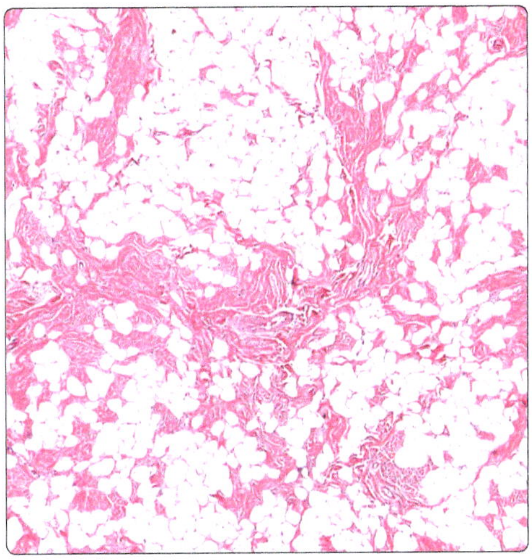

(Left) *Fat necrosis presents in a wide variety of histologic patterns, and the constituent histiocytes are commonly misidentified as lipoblasts or atypical cells suggestive of an atypical lipomatous tumor/well-differentiated liposarcoma, particularly when focal and isolated.* **(Right)** *A lipoma containing abundant fibrous tissue and collagen is appropriately designated as a fibrolipoma. Examples with extensive fibrosis have also been referred to as sclerotic lipomas.*

(Left) *Fibrolipomas often contain an abundance of dense collagen in the form of apparent septa or ill-defined aggregates. The exact amount of collagen varies from case to case.* **(Right)** *Some cases of fibrolipoma show well-demarcated bundles of collagen* → *cut in cross section. This morphology may be easily confused with the smooth muscle bundles of a myolipoma when diffuse or even neural elements when focal.*

Fibrolipoma With Dense Collagen

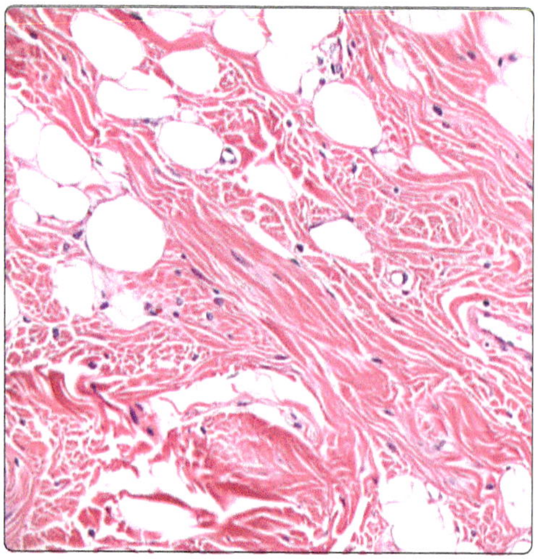

Fibrolipoma With Collagen Bundles

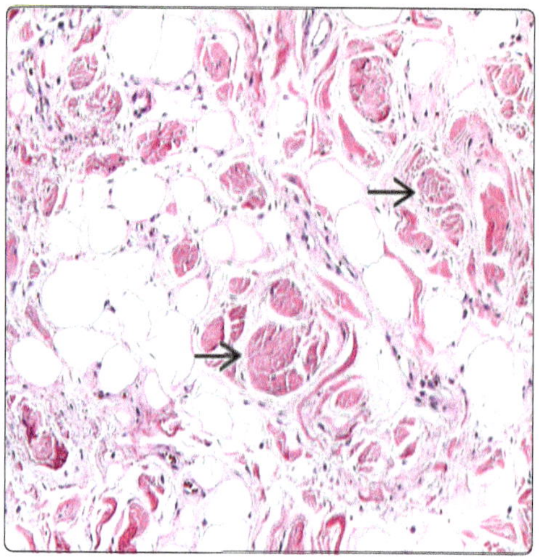

(Left) *This example of an otherwise conventional fibrolipoma contained foci of ropey collagen bundles such as those typically seen in spindle cell lipoma. The distinction in such cases is largely academic.* **(Right)** *A lipoma that demonstrates extensive and diffuse stromal myxoid change is appropriately classified as a myxolipoma. If a component of bland spindle cells is also present, a diagnosis of spindle cell lipoma is more appropriate.*

Fibrolipoma With Ropey Collagen

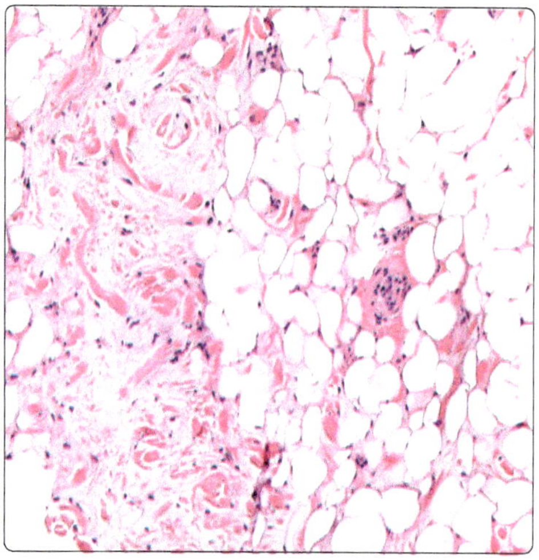

Myxoid Variant of Lipoma (Myxolipoma)

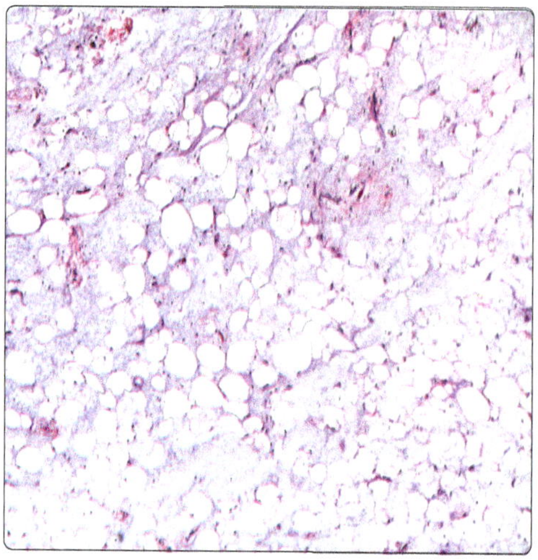

(Left) *Compared to a myxoid spindle cell lipoma, myxolipoma lacks a component of bland spindle cells as well as the ropey collagen bundles. The myxoid stroma is largely acellular. Although not seen in this image, prominent vessels may also be seen (so-called angiomyxolipoma).* **(Right)** *Metaplastic bone formation in a lipoma may be focal or extensive and is often first evident at the time of gross examination.*

Myxolipoma at Higher Magnification

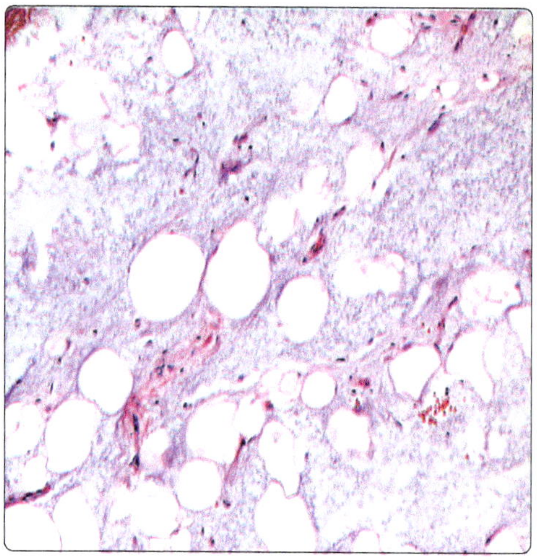

Osseous Metaplasia in Lipoma

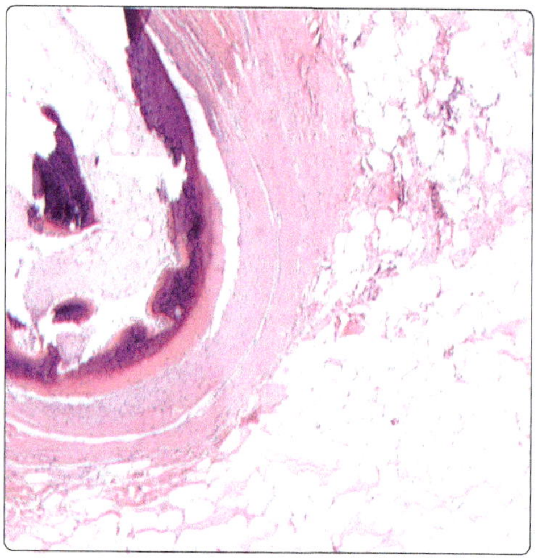

Cartilaginous Metaplasia in Lipoma

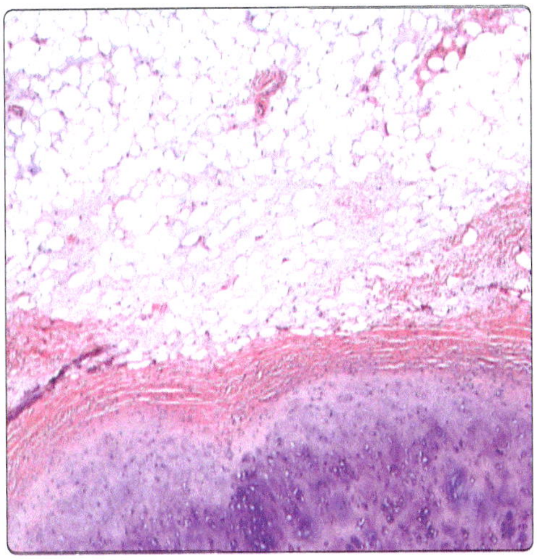

Intramuscular Lipoma

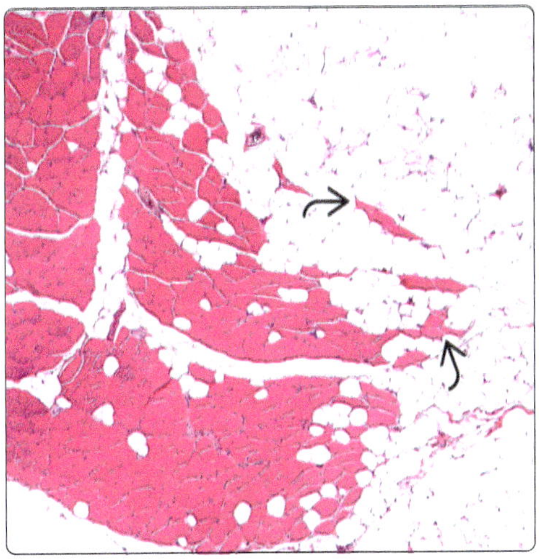

(Left) *Cartilaginous metaplasia in a lipoma may be isolated or associated with foci of metaplastic bone. Not uncommonly, the background adipose tissue shows increased fibrosis and collagen or myxoid stromal change.* **(Right)** *Intramuscular or intermuscular lipomas typically show bundles of mature skeletal muscle ➔ intermixed to some degree with the elements of mature adipose tissue.*

Intramuscular Lipoma With Checkerboard Pattern

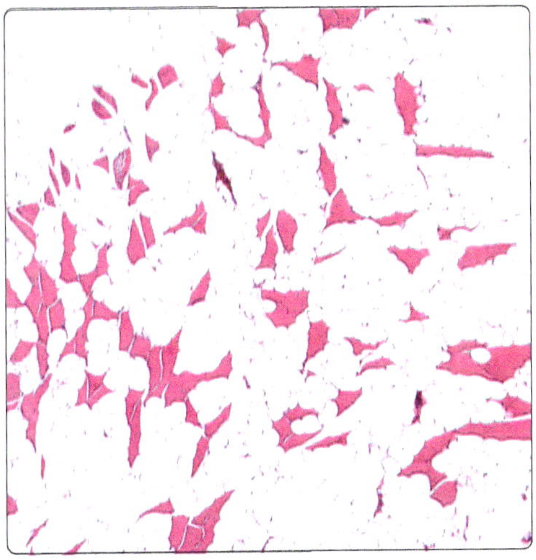

Mature Myocytes in Intramuscular Lipoma

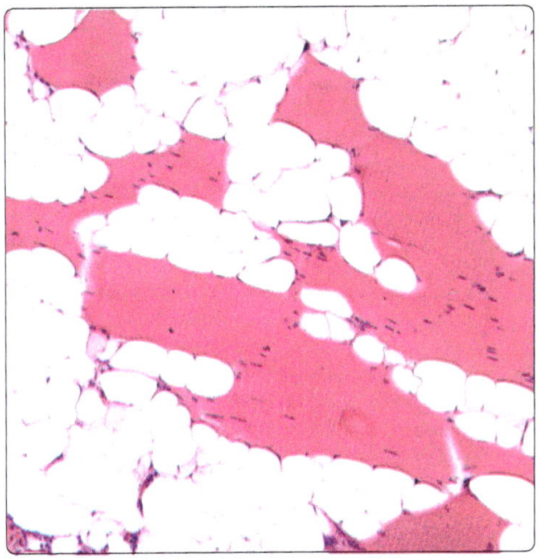

(Left) *The adipose tissue component of intramuscular lipoma is often highly intermixed with the skeletal muscle bundles, demonstrating the classic alternating checkerboard appearance.* **(Right)** *The skeletal muscle bundles in an intramuscular lipoma are composed of mature myocytes. They may be present focally in some tumors and extensively in others.*

Atrophic Skeletal Muscle

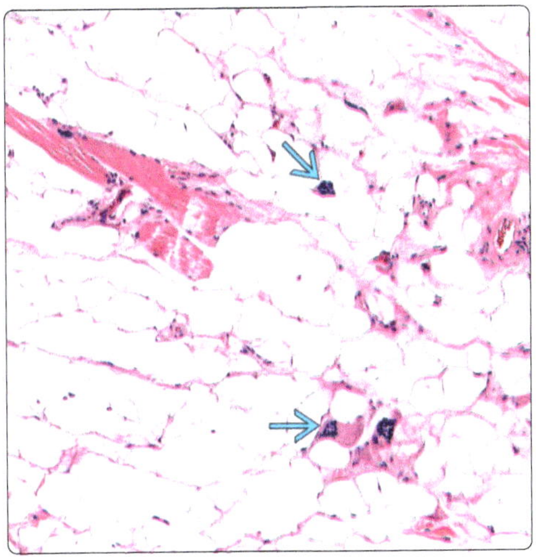

Atrophic Skeletal Muscle Cytologic Features

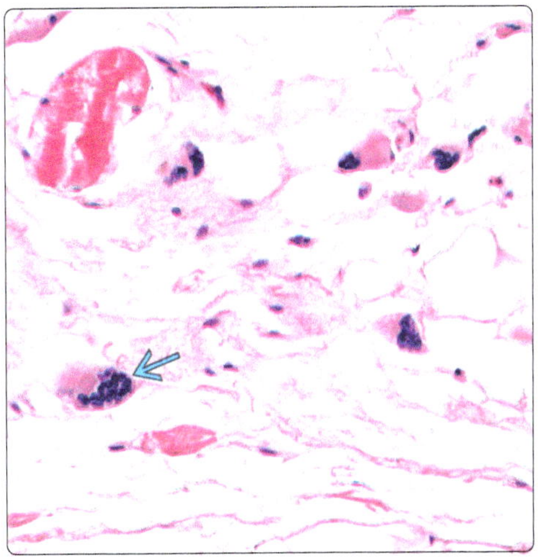

(Left) *Atrophic skeletal muscle fibers ➔ are commonly identified in cases of intramuscular lipoma, although the extent of this finding may be very focal. This finding is not specific to lipomas and may be seen in other intramuscular tumors.* **(Right)** *Atrophic myocytes characteristically contain bright pink cytoplasm and numerous small, overlapping nuclei in a cluster-of-grapes configuration ➔. It is important to not confuse these cells with the atypical stromal cells (smudge cells) of liposarcoma.*

KEY FACTS

TERMINOLOGY

- Benign tumor consisting of mature adipocytes and thin-walled blood vessels with intraluminal fibrin thrombi

ETIOLOGY/PATHOGENESIS

- Majority are sporadic; rare familial cases

CLINICAL ISSUES

- Commonly in young adults
  - Male predominance
- Forearm, trunk, and upper arm most common sites
- Painful tender subcutaneous nodules
  - Often multiple
- Treatment: Simple surgical excision
- Excellent prognosis
  - Local recurrence very rare
  - No risk of malignant transformation

MACROSCOPIC

- Circumscribed, yellow-red nodule
- Typically < 2 cm in size

MICROSCOPIC

- Admixture of mature adipocytes and capillary-sized blood vessels
  - Hallmark: Fibrin thrombi within vessels
- Vascularity often more prominent in periphery
- No nuclear atypia in adipocytic or endothelial components
- Morphologic variant: Cellular angiolipoma

TOP DIFFERENTIAL DIAGNOSES

- Lipoma
- Intramuscular hemangioma
- Kaposi sarcoma
- Spindle cell hemangioma
- Angiomyolipoma

(Left) *Angiolipoma is composed of both vascular ➡ and mature adipocytic ⇨ components admixed together in varying proportions. They are often small, circumscribed lesions, as seen here.* **(Right)** *This angiolipoma is predominantly composed of adipose tissue. The focal vascular component is present as clusters of small vessels near the periphery ➡ and around the thin, fibrous septa ➡.*

Angiolipoma at Low Magnification

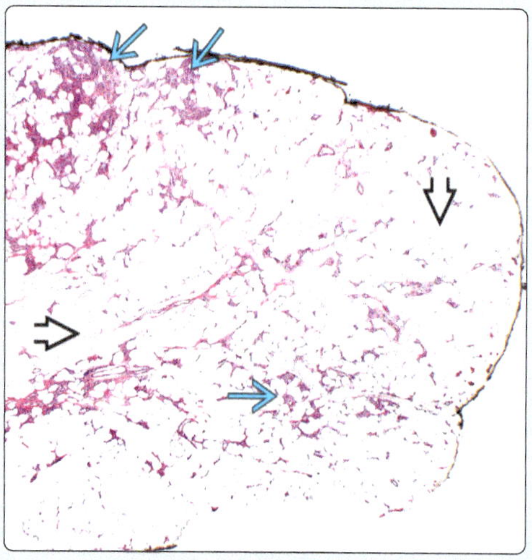

Prominent Adipose Tissue Component

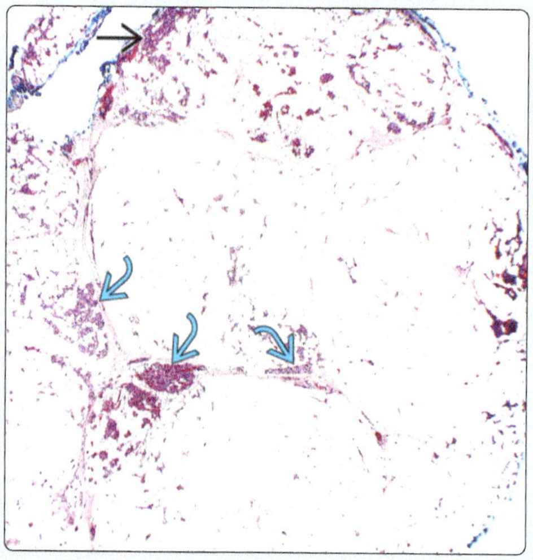

(Left) *The focal vascular component of angiolipoma is present as clusters of small vessels near the periphery of the lesion ➡. The remainder of the tumor is composed of mature adipocytes ➡.* **(Right)** *Bright pink fibrin thrombi ➡ are present in small clustered capillary vessels. This is the hallmark feature of angiolipoma.*

Peripheral Vascular Component

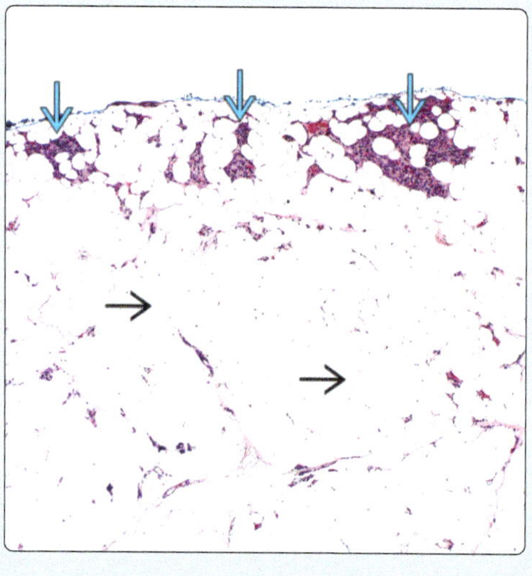

Characteristic Fibrin Thrombi

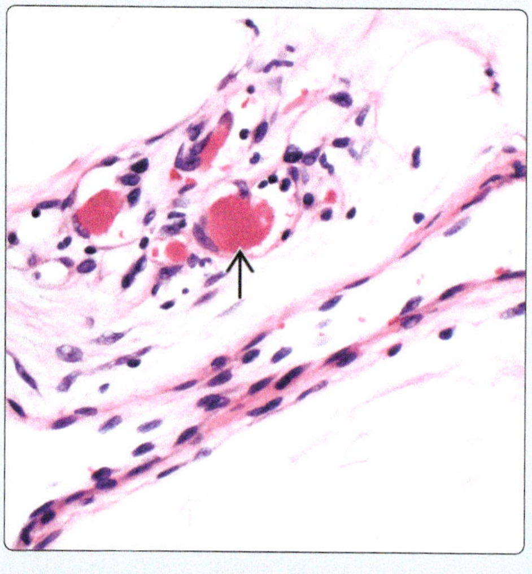

TERMINOLOGY

Definitions

- Benign tumor composed of mature adipocytes and clustered small blood vessels with intraluminal fibrin thrombi

ETIOLOGY/PATHOGENESIS

Unknown

- Majority are sporadic
- Rare familial predilection (5%)

CLINICAL ISSUES

Epidemiology

- Age
  - Most common in young adults
  - Rare in children or in adults > 50 years
- Sex
  - Male predominance

Site

- Forearm, trunk, and upper arm most common sites
- Rare on scalp or face

Presentation

- Painful subcutaneous nodule, often multiple (in 2/3 of cases)

Treatment

- Simple surgical excision

Prognosis

- Excellent: Benign
  - Very low risk of local recurrence
  - No known risk of malignant transformation

MACROSCOPIC

Gross Features

- Well circumscribed
- Yellow-red nodules
- Typically < 2 cm in size

MICROSCOPIC

Histologic Features

- 2 components present in varying proportions
  - Mature adipocytes
  - Clustered capillary-sized vessels with fibrinoid thrombi
    - Vascularity often more prominent in periphery
- No nuclear atypia in adipocytic or endothelial components

Morphologic Variant

- Cellular angiolipoma
  - Vascular component predominates
  - Can be spindled, raising concern for Kaposi sarcoma

ANCILLARY TESTS

Immunohistochemistry

- Immunostains not useful for diagnosis

DIFFERENTIAL DIAGNOSIS

Lipoma

- Mass composed of mature adipose tissue
  - May have increased single vessels but lacks clustered vessels and fibrinoid thrombi
- Lipomas possess various translocations of chromosome 12q or 6p
- Fat-predominant angiolipoma may mimic lipoma

Intramuscular Hemangioma

- Previously known as infiltrating angiolipoma
- Large infiltrative lesion in deep muscle (not in subcutis)
- Often has adipose tissue and large thick-walled vessels
  - Lacks clustered small vessels with luminal thrombi

Kaposi Sarcoma

- More spindled and fascicular endothelial proliferation
- Blood-filled, slit-like spaces and extravasated RBCs
- PAS(+) hyaline globules but no fibrinoid thrombi
- HHV8(+) endothelial cells

Angiomyolipoma

- Spindle cells in angiomyolipoma are HMB-45(+) smooth muscle cells
- Vessels are larger caliber and thick walled
- Vanishingly rare in subcutis and peripheral soft tissue

Spindle Cell Hemangioma

- Painful multiple subcutaneous nodules in extremities
- Unlike cellular angiolipoma, spindle cell hemangioma has
  - Large, cavernous vascular spaces
  - Cellular zones of spindled and epithelioid endothelial cells and clustered endothelial vacuoles resembling miniature adipocytes
  - Large calcified thrombi (phleboliths) but lacks clustered vessels with small thrombi

DIAGNOSTIC CHECKLIST

Pathologic Interpretation Pearls

- Mature adipocytes
- Clusters of capillary-sized vessels
- Fibrinoid microthrombi in vessels

SELECTED REFERENCES

1. Mayooran N et al: Infiltrating angiolipoma of the chest wall: a rare clinical entity. J Surg Case Rep. 2016(1), 2016
2. Roncati L et al: Subcutaneous cavernous angiolipoma: a new soft-tissue entity. Acta Dermatovenerol Croat. 23(2):144-5, 2015
3. Shahi AK et al: Cellular infiltrative angiolipoma of cheek in an infant. Natl J Maxillofac Surg. 5(2):202-5, 2014
4. Sheng W et al: Cellular angiolipoma: a clinicopathological and immunohistochemical study of 12 cases. Am J Dermatopathol. 35(2):220-5, 2013
5. Sciot R et al: Cytogenetic analysis of subcutaneous angiolipoma: further evidence supporting its difference from ordinary pure lipomas: a report of the CHAMP Study Group. Am J Surg Pathol. 21(4):441-4, 1997
6. Fletcher CD et al: Correlation between clinicopathological features and karyotype in lipomatous tumors. A report of 178 cases from the Chromosomes and Morphology (CHAMP) Collaborative Study Group. Am J Pathol. 148(2):623-30, 1996
7. Kanik AB et al: Cellular angiolipoma. Am J Dermatopathol. 17(3):312-5, 1995
8. Dixon AY et al: Angiolipomas: an ultrastructural and clinicopathological study. Hum Pathol. 12(8):739-47, 1981

(Left) *Fibrin thrombi within capillary lumina are pink and amorphous.* **(Right)** *The capillaries in angiolipoma often have a lobular arrangement and may appear reminiscent of a hemangioma in some cases; however, pink fibrin thrombi are present in many of the lumina in angiolipoma.*

Pink and Amorphous Fibrin Thrombi

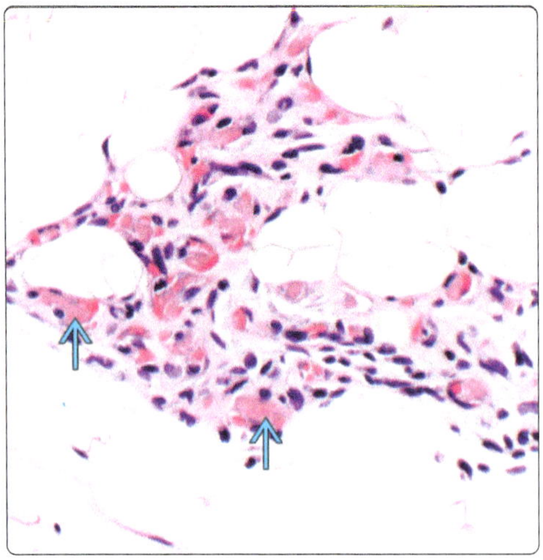

Abundant Fibrin Thrombi

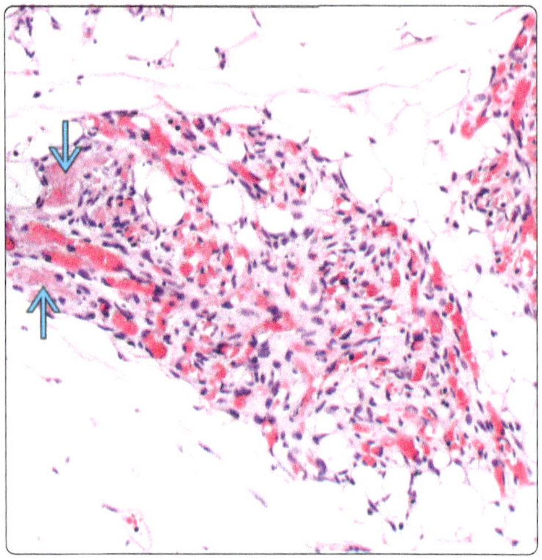

(Left) *More cellular vascular areas are admixed with mature adipose tissue in this angiolipoma. The vascularity is still enhanced at the peripheral aspect of the mass.* **(Right)** *Spindled endothelial cells and pericytes appear to infiltrate into mature adipose tissue. This more cellular and spindled pattern can mimic Kaposi sarcoma; however, note the characteristic fibrin thrombi.*

Angiolipoma With Moderate Cellularity

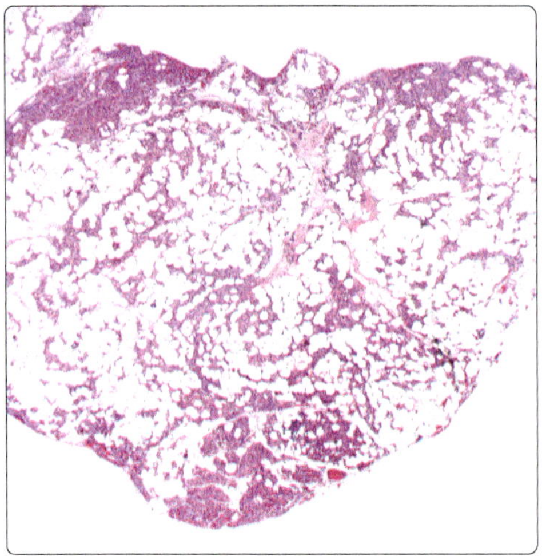

Kaposi Sarcoma-Like Morphology

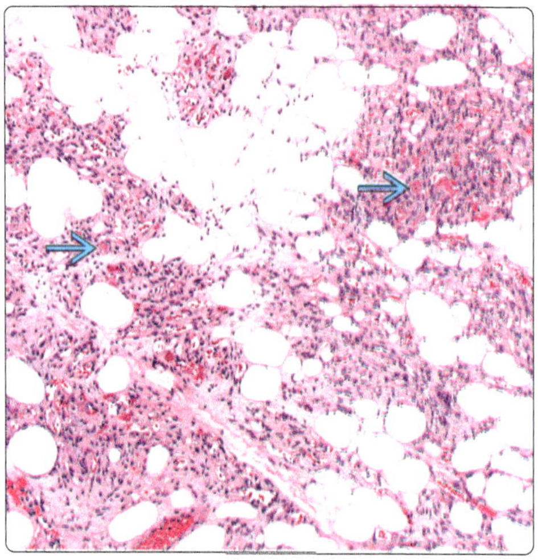

(Left) *Capillary lumina with bland endothelial cells can be appreciated at high power in the cellular zones. Fibrin thrombi are present, unlike in Kaposi sarcoma.* **(Right)** *Angiolipoma may have spindled cellular foci, but there are still small, well-formed vessels. The spindled cells are endothelial and pericytic (perivascular modified smooth muscle cells). Both cell types are bland and lack nuclear atypia or significant mitotic activity in angiolipoma.*

Moderate Cellularity With Fibrin Thrombi

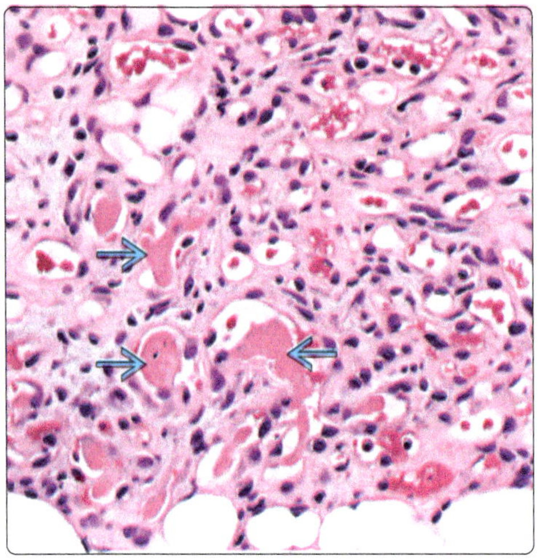

Focal Spindled Morphology

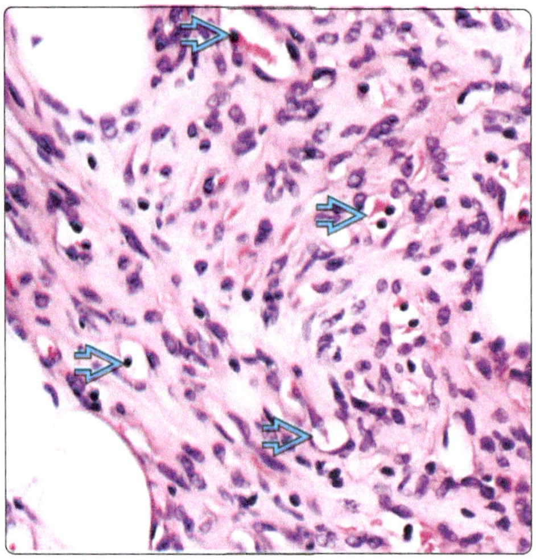

Cellular Foci in Angiolipoma

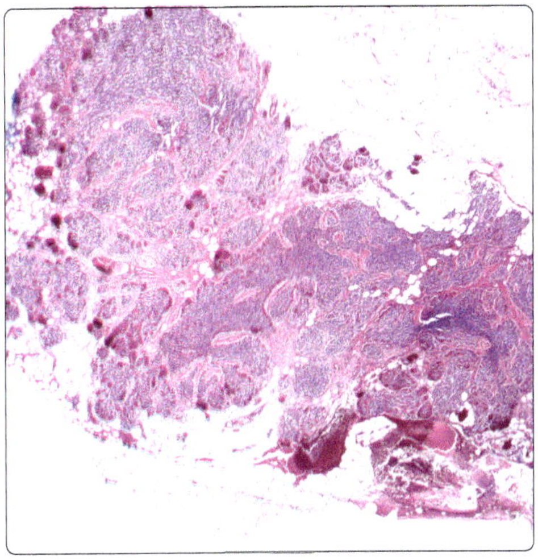

Cellular Angiolipoma

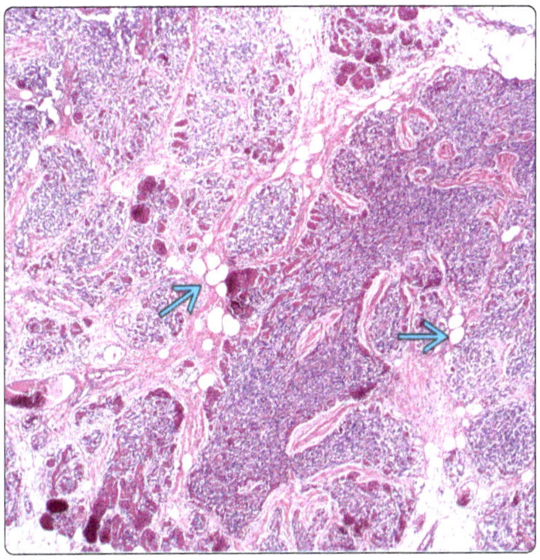

(Left) *The cellular variant of angiolipoma is composed almost entirely of densely packed small blood vessels. There is very little adipose component within the mass.* **(Right)** *There is often a lobular arrangement of vessels in cellular angiolipoma. Focal adipocytes ➡ appear to be entrapped between the vascular lobules, which may give the false impression of an infiltrative growth pattern.*

Cellular Angiolipoma With Tightly Packed Capillaries

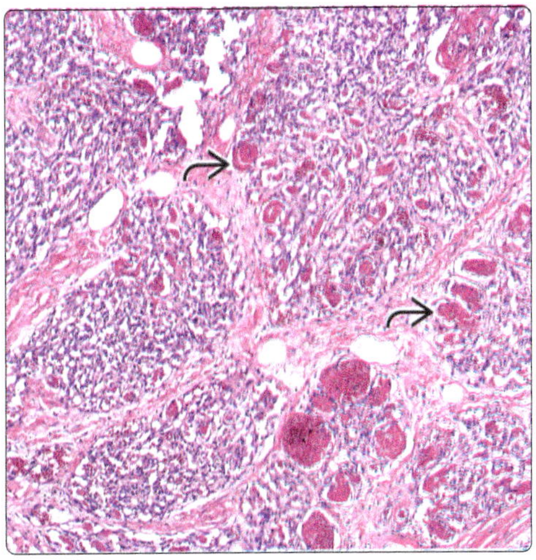

Fibrin Thrombi in Cellular Angiolipoma

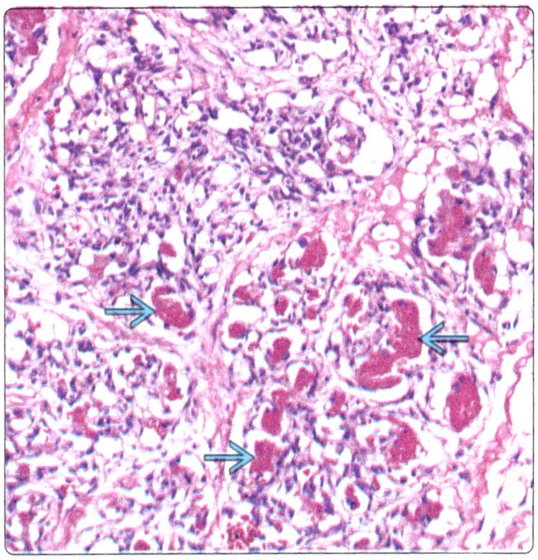

(Left) *Vascular zones in cellular angiolipoma are composed of tightly packed, well-formed small vessels, similar to a lobular capillary hemangioma. However, the characteristic fibrin thrombi ↗ are prominent in this case.* **(Right)** *Numerous fibrin thrombi ➡ are present within the lumina of the vessels, helping to establish the diagnosis of angiolipoma.*

Bland Capillary Channels in Cellular Angiolipoma

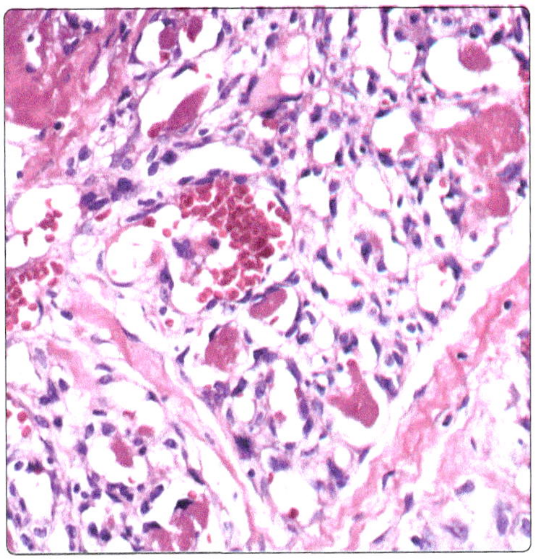

Uniform Cytologic Features

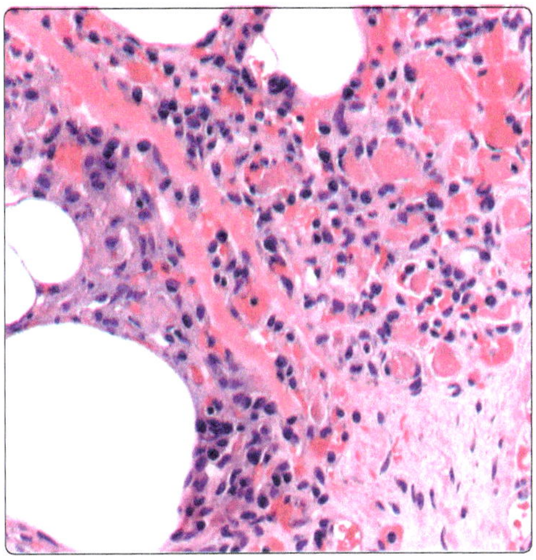

(Left) *High magnification shows that the vessels in a cellular angiolipoma are well formed and lined by bland endothelial cells.* **(Right)** *The endothelial cells are bland and uniform-appearing. The presence of intraluminal fibrin thrombi in cellular angiolipoma is helpful in distinguishing it from Kaposi sarcoma. Immunohistochemistry for HHV8 can also be utilized, if necessary.*

Spindle Cell/Pleomorphic Lipoma

KEY FACTS

CLASSIFICATION

- Benign adipocytic tumor with variable admixture of spindle cells, ropey collagen, mature adipose tissue, and multinucleate tumor giant cells
- Spindle cell lipoma (SCL) and pleomorphic lipoma (PL) are morphologic variations of same neoplasm

CLINICAL ISSUES

- Most common in older (> 50 years) men
- Typically arise in shoulder, posterior neck, or back
- Benign; conservative surgical excision only treatment needed

MACROSCOPIC

- Well-circumscribed subcutaneous (or less commonly dermal) mass
- Yellow-tan cut surface with variable gray-white &/or myxoid foci

MICROSCOPIC

- Tumors may show morphology of SCL exclusively, PL exclusively, or admixed SCL/PL
- SCL
  - Variable admixture of bland spindle cells, ropey collagen, mature adipose tissue, myxoid stroma, and mast cells
- PL contains multinucleated tumor cells
- Morphologic variants: Fat-free, fat-poor, angiomatous

ANCILLARY TESTS

- CD34(+); loss of nuclear retinoblastoma (Rb) expression
- Molecular: Deletion of *RB1* (13q14)

TOP DIFFERENTIAL DIAGNOSES

- Atypical lipomatous tumor
- Neurofibroma
- Myxoid liposarcoma
- Solitary fibrous tumor

Spindle Cell Lipoma, Gross Specimen

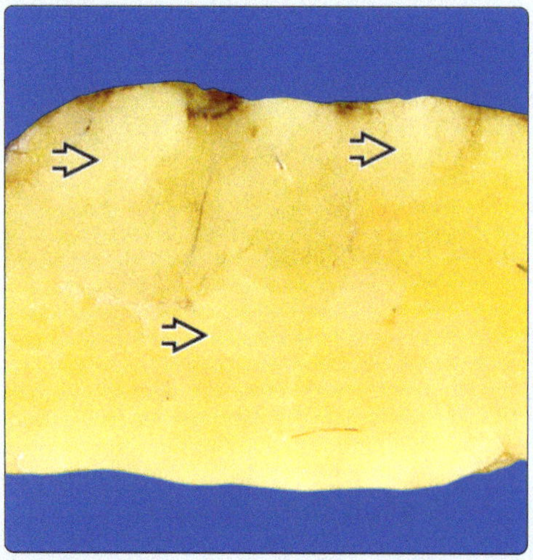

Spindle Cell Lipoma at Low Magnification

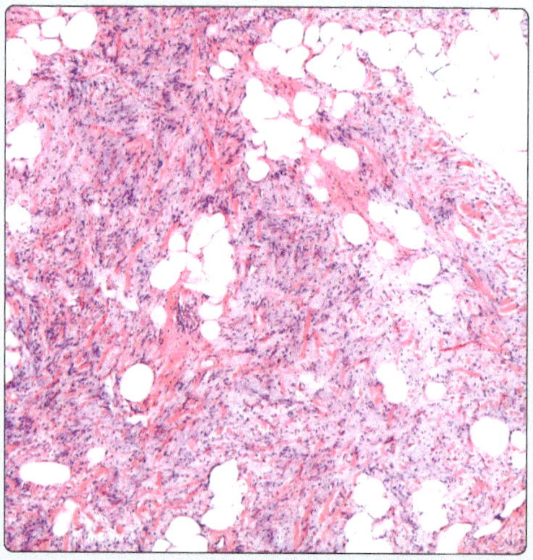

(Left) *Like conventional lipomas, spindle cell (SCL) and pleomorphic lipomas (PL) have a homogeneous yellow cut surface. Both tumors also often show subtle gray-white foci ➩ that are firm in consistency and correlate histologically with spindle cell areas containing ropey collagenous matrix.* **(Right)** *At low power, SCL is composed of a mixture of adipose tissue and a variable myxoid to collagenous stroma containing bland spindle cells.*

Ropey Collagen and Mast Cells

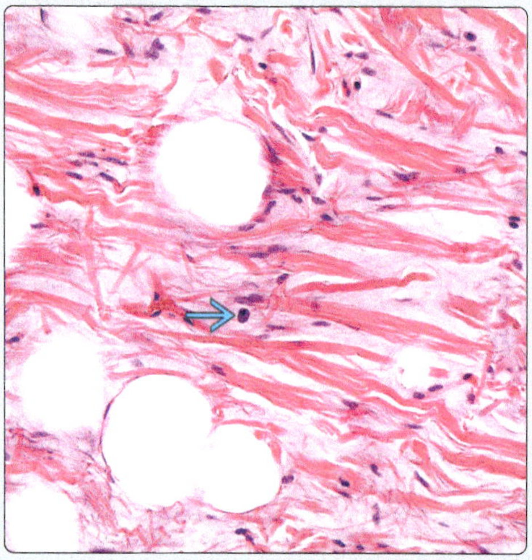

Bland Spindle Cells in Spindle Cell Lipoma

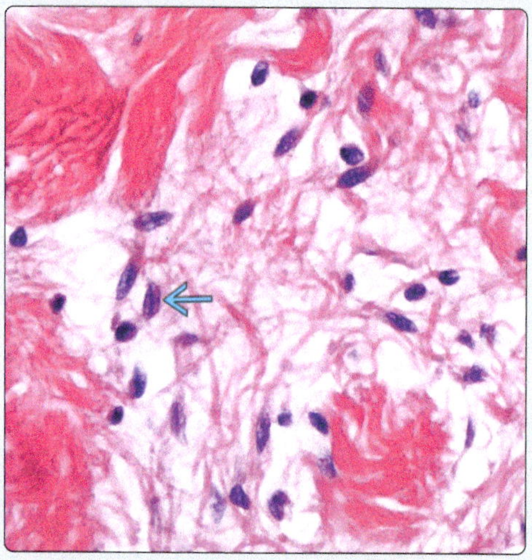

(Left) *Thickened bundles and strips of collagen are a consistent finding in SCL/PL and a helpful diagnostic feature. Mast cells ➙ are also very commonly identified.* **(Right)** *The lesional cells of SCL are cytologically bland and show bipolar or stellate cytoplasmic processes. Nuclear grooves may be identified in some cases ➙. Mitoses are rare.*

TERMINOLOGY

Abbreviations

- Spindle cell lipoma (SCL)/pleomorphic lipoma (PL)

Definitions

- Benign adipocytic tumor with variable admixture of spindle cells, ropey collagen, and mature adipose tissue
  - PL additionally contains multinucleated tumor giant cells
- SCL and PL are considered morphologic variations on same entity

CLINICAL ISSUES

Epidemiology

- Age
  - Typically in older age group (> 50 years old)
  - Very rare in patients < 20 years old
- Sex
  - Strong male predilection
    - Dermal SCL may be more common in females

Site

- Most occur superficially in subcutaneous tissue or dermis
  - Exceptionally rare in deep soft tissues
- Shoulder, posterior neck, and back most common (80% of cases)
  - Also face, oral cavity, trunk, extremities

Presentation

- Very similar to conventional lipoma
  - Painless, slow-growing mass
  - Often present for long duration
- Rarely arise in multiple sites (synchronous or metachronous)
  - May be familial

Treatment

- Conservative surgical excision

Prognosis

- Benign
- Local recurrence is very rare
  - Atypical findings in PL, such as lipoblasts and rare atypical mitoses, do not appear to affect behavior

MACROSCOPIC

General Features

- Well circumscribed
  - Dermal tumors usually less circumscribed
- Yellow-tan cut surface
- Subtle gray-white foci correlate with spindle cell foci
- May show focal myxoid areas or be extensively gelatinous
- Very rare multinodular, plexiform growth pattern

Size

- Usually 3-5 cm (rarely > 10 cm)

MICROSCOPIC

Histologic Features

- SCL and PL exist as 2 ends of single morphologic spectrum
  - Some tumors show morphology of SCL exclusively and some show morphology of PL exclusively
  - Tumors demonstrating intermixed features or discrete areas of both SCL and PL are common
- SCL
  - Variable admixture of 3 components
    - Uniform, bland spindle cell proliferation
      - Bipolar to stellate cytoplasmic projections
      - May cluster together akin to schools of fish or show nuclear palisading
      - May show nuclear grooves
      - Mitotic figures rare to absent
    - Mature adipocytes
    - Bundles of ropey (thickened) collagen fibers
  - Myxoid stroma is common and may be extensive
  - Mast cells are very common and nearly constant finding
  - Thick-walled vessels may show perivascular hyalinization or fibrosis or grow in focal ectatic staghorn pattern
- PL
  - Characterized by variable numbers of multinucleated giant cells with dense eosinophilic cytoplasm and peripherally arranged nuclei (floret cells)
    - Also cells with "smudgy" nuclei &/or nuclear pseudoinclusions
  - Bland spindled cells, ropey collagen, mast cells, and adipose tissue also usually present
  - May rarely contain multivacuolated lipoblasts
  - Mitotic figures rare to absent (may be atypical)

Morphologic Variants

- Fat-free or low-fat SCL
  - Minimal to no mature adipose tissue component
  - May show abundant collagen, abundant myxoid stroma, or predominantly spindle cells
  - Fat-free and low-fat forms of PL also exist
- Angiomatous SCL
  - Also described as pseudoangiomatous SCL
  - Contains prominent slit-like to ectatic vascular spaces lined by endothelial cells
  - Nodules or lobules of tumor may appear to float in empty space
  - May also show prominent myxoid stroma or minimal mature adipose tissue

ANCILLARY TESTS

Immunohistochemistry

- Strong, diffuse CD34(+)
- Loss of nuclear retinoblastoma (Rb) expression
- S100, smooth muscle actin, and desmin (-)

Molecular Genetics

- Characteristic deletion (monoallelic or biallelic) of *RB1* on 13q14
  - Identical deletion present in mammary-type myofibroblastoma and cellular angiofibroma

DIFFERENTIAL DIAGNOSIS

Atypical Lipomatous Tumor/Well-Differentiated Liposarcoma

- Usually large tumors

- Commonly arise in deep locations (especially retroperitoneum in well-differentiated liposarcoma)
- Ropey collagen bundles and mast cells are not typical features
- MDM2(+), CDK4(+) by IHC
  - Rare cases of SCL show focal expression
- Amplification of *MDM2* by FISH in most cases

Neurofibroma

- Presence of bland spindle cells with intermixed adipose tissue in SCL may suggest diffuse-type neurofibroma
- Ropey collagen bundles in myxoid background in SCL may suggest plexiform neurofibroma
- S100(+) in most spindle cells
- CD34(+) component of admixed fibroblastic cells

Cellular Angiofibroma

- Most cases occur in lower external genital tract in women
  - May also occur in men in same general region
- Can show morphologic overlap with SCL
  - Hyalinized vessels common in cellular angiofibroma
- Strong CD34(+)
- Loss of nuclear Rb expression
- Deletion of *RB1* on 13q14

Mammary-Type Myofibroblastoma

- Histologically identical to myofibroblastoma of breast
- Short fascicles of monomorphic spindle cells in collagenous stroma
- Can show morphologic overlap with SCL
  - Thickened, coarse collagen bundles are characteristic feature of myofibroblastoma
- Strong CD34(+), desmin (+)
- Loss of nuclear Rb expression
- Deletion of *RB1* on 13q14

Solitary Fibrous Tumor

- Prominent ectatic "staghorn" vascular network in most cases
- Ropey collagen bundles are not feature
- Diffusely CD34(+) in vast majority of cases
- May also show intratumoral adipose tissue (lipomatous solitary fibrous tumor)

Myxoid Liposarcoma

- Usually affects younger age group than SCL/PL
- Often strikingly lobular growth pattern
- Usually shows prominent delicate plexiform capillary vascular pattern
- Uni- and multivacuolated lipoblasts are common
- May contain cellular ("round cell") foci
- CD34(-)
- Characteristic t(12;16) in most cases

Spindle Cell Liposarcoma

- Currently controversial entity; may be related to SCL
- Spindle cells arranged in loose fascicles with admixed lipoblasts
- Lacks ropey collagen bundles
- Strong CD34(+)
- Deletion of *RB1* on 13q14

Dermatofibrosarcoma Protuberans

- Usually occurs in younger individuals than SCL/PL
- Monomorphic spindle cells arranged in broad or tight storiform pattern
- May be focally or extensively myxoid
- Prominent infiltration of peripheral adipose tissue or skeletal muscle (honeycomb infiltration)
- Mast cells uncommon
- Diffuse CD34(+) in vast majority of cases
- t(17;22) with *COL1A1-PDGFRB* fusion

Schwannoma

- Usually contains discrete Antoni A and B areas
- Intratumoral fat uncommon
- Strong diffuse S100(+); CD34(-)
- Nuclear palisading in SCL may suggest schwannoma

Giant Cell Fibroblastoma

- Most common in children < 6 years
- Multinucleated stromal giant cells lining pseudovascular spaces/clefts
  - Tumors with inconspicuous pseudovascular spaces can resemble PL
- CD34(+)
- t(17;22) with *COL1A1-PDGFRB* fusion

SELECTED REFERENCES

1. Cheah A et al: Spindle cell/pleomorphic lipomas of the face: an under-recognized diagnosis. Histopathology. 66(3):430-7, 2015
2. Forcucci JA et al: "Low-fat" pseudoangiomatous spindle cell lipoma: a rare variant with loss of 13q14 region. Am J Dermatopathol. 37(12):920-3, 2015
3. Creytens D et al: Atypical spindle cell lipoma: a clinicopathologic, immunohistochemical, and molecular study emphasizing its relationship to classical spindle cell lipoma. Virchows Arch. 465(1):97, 2014
4. Chen BJ et al: Loss of retinoblastoma protein expression in spindle cell/pleomorphic lipomas and cytogenetically related tumors: an immunohistochemical study with diagnostic implications. Am J Surg Pathol. 36(8):1119-28, 2012
5. Wood L et al: Cutaneous CD34+ spindle cell neoplasms: Histopathologic features distinguish spindle cell lipoma, solitary fibrous tumor, and dermatofibrosarcoma protuberans. Am J Dermatopathol. 32(8):764-8, 2010
6. Sachdeva MP et al: Low-fat and fat-free pleomorphic lipomas: a diagnostic challenge. Am J Dermatopathol. 31(5):423-6, 2009
7. Billings SD et al: Diagnostically challenging spindle cell lipomas: a report of 34 "low-fat" and "fat-free" variants. Am J Dermatopathol. 29(5):437-42, 2007
8. Fanburg-Smith JC et al: Multiple spindle cell lipomas: a report of 7 familial and 11 nonfamilial cases. Am J Surg Pathol. 22(1):40-8, 1998
9. Dal Cin P et al: Lesions of 13q may occur independently of deletion of 16q in spindle cell/pleomorphic lipomas. Histopathology. 31(3):222-5, 1997
10. Hawley IC et al: Spindle cell lipoma--a pseudoangiomatous variant. Histopathology. 24(6):565-9, 1994
11. Shmookler BM et al: Pleomorphic lipoma: a benign tumor simulating liposarcoma. A clinicopathologic analysis of 48 cases. Cancer. 47(1):126-33, 1981
12. Enzinger FM et al: Spindle cell lipoma. Cancer. 36(5):1852-9, 1975

Classic Ropey Collagen Bundles in Spindle Cell Lipoma

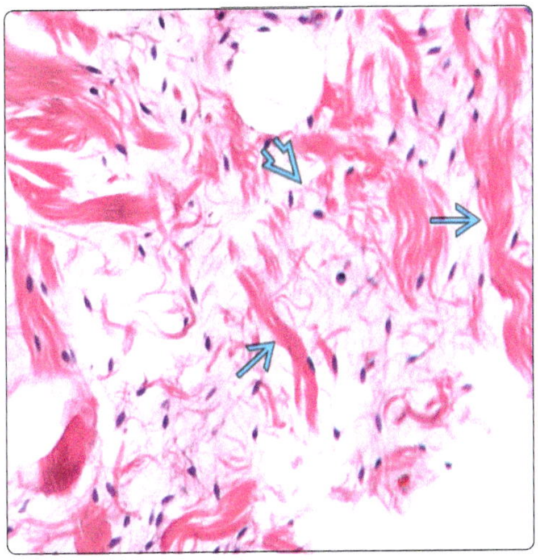

Thicker Collagen Bundles

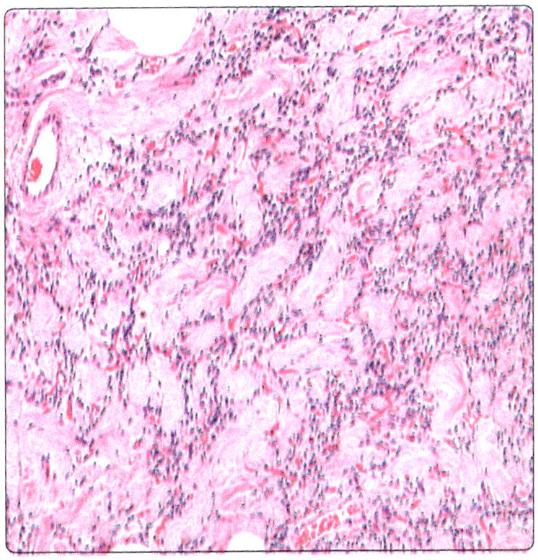

(Left) *The characteristic ropey collagen bundles ➡ of SCL/PL vary widely in extent and distribution. Thin, wispy fibers ➡ are often present as well and may be the predominant form of collagen in some cases.* **(Right)** *In some cases of SCL, the collagen fibers have a thickened and organized appearance reminiscent of mammary-type myofibroblastoma, a tumor that appears to be histogenetically related to SCL.*

Haphazard Cellular Components

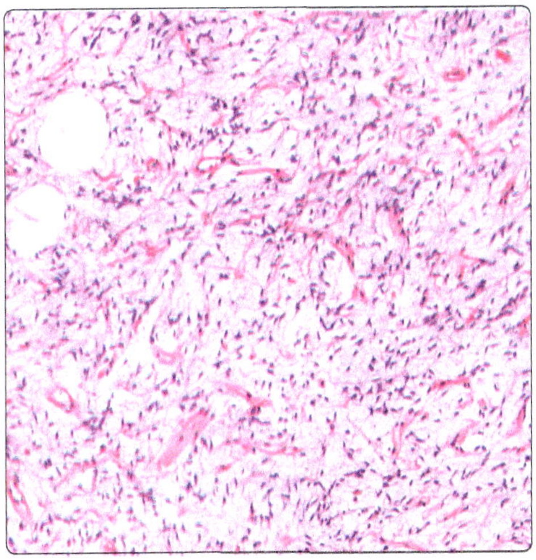

Occasional Nuclear Palisading

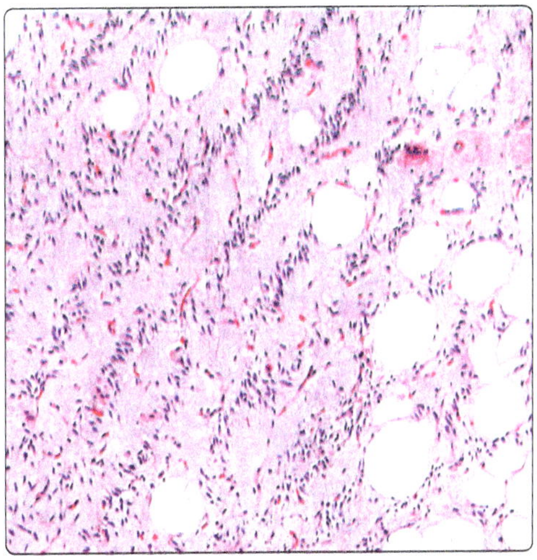

(Left) *Some cases of SCL show a haphazard, disorganized distribution of bipolar and stellate spindle cells with ropey or wispy collagen. This morphology may lead to consideration of a peripheral nerve sheath tumor.* **(Right)** *Nuclear palisading is not an uncommon finding in myxoid SCL, but it is usually not extensive. Many cases, however, show small clusters or linear arrangements of tumor cells, akin to schools of fish.*

Prominent Myxoid Stroma

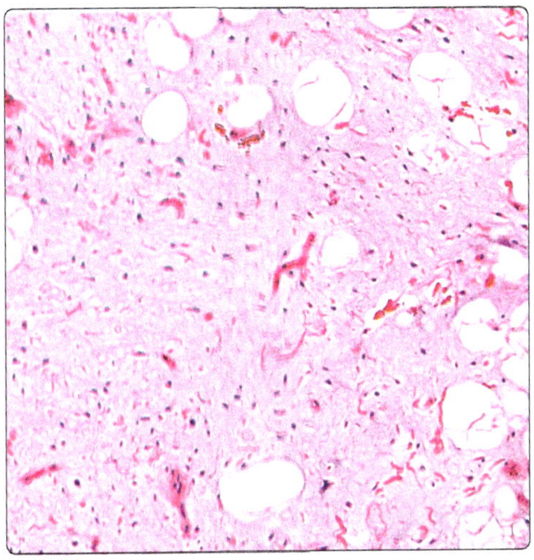

Spindled and Stellate Cells Within Myxoid Stroma

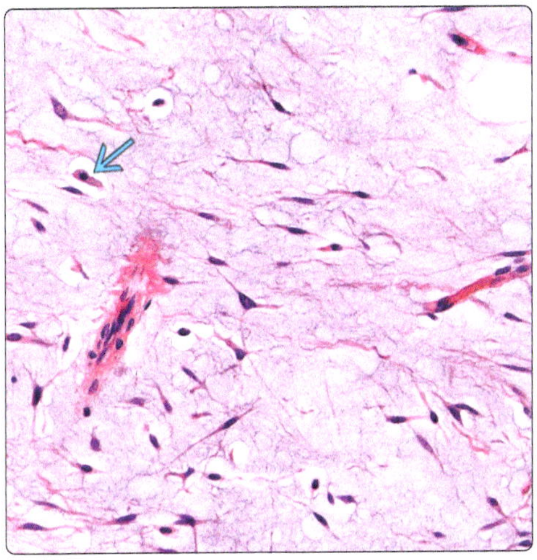

(Left) *SCL may show a markedly abundant myxoid stroma and overall striking hypocellularity that is suggestive of a myxoma or myxolipoma. Identification of a discrete component of scattered bland spindle cells is helpful, as are foci of ropey collagen.* **(Right)** *As in other cases of SCL, the lesional spindle cells in myxoid variants show bipolar to stellate cytoplasmic processes. Note the mast cell ➡.*

(Left) *In some cases of SCL, there is little to no mature adipose tissue. These cases can be very challenging to diagnose; however, the characteristic spindle cells and collagen bundles are helpful clues, as is possibly the clinical presentation.* **(Right)** *The cellularity of fat-poor and fat-free SCL may be strikingly increased in some cases, resulting in the lesion looking nothing like an adipocytic tumor.*

Fat-Free and Low-Fat Variants of Spindle Cell Lipoma

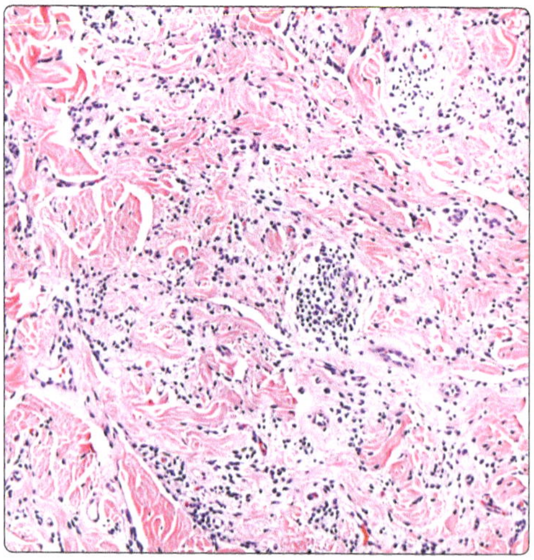

Fat-Free Variant of Spindle Cell Lipoma

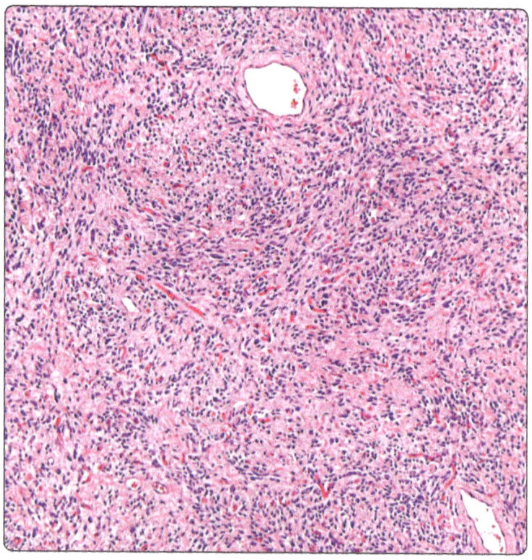

(Left) *Despite the cellularity, the cytologic features of this fat-free variant of SCL are not worrisome for malignancy, and mitotic figures are inconspicuous or absent. Note the mast cell →.* **(Right)** *Some cases of the angiomatous SCL variant show nodules of tumor "floating" in relatively empty spaces, as depicted. Red blood cells may also be seen in these spaces. This particular example was highly myxoid as well.*

Cytologic Features of Fat-Free Spindle Cell Lipoma

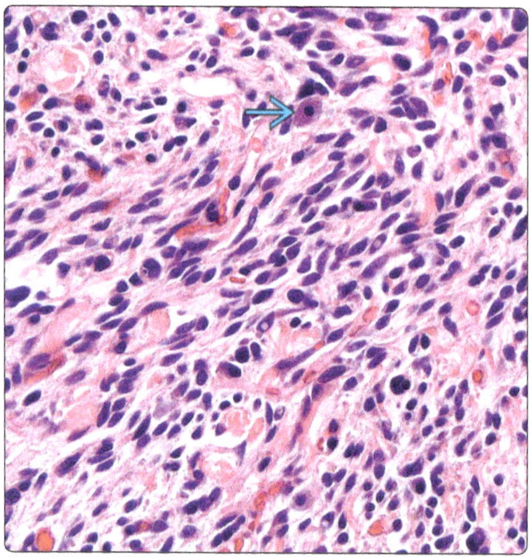

Angiomatous Variant of Spindle Cell Lipoma

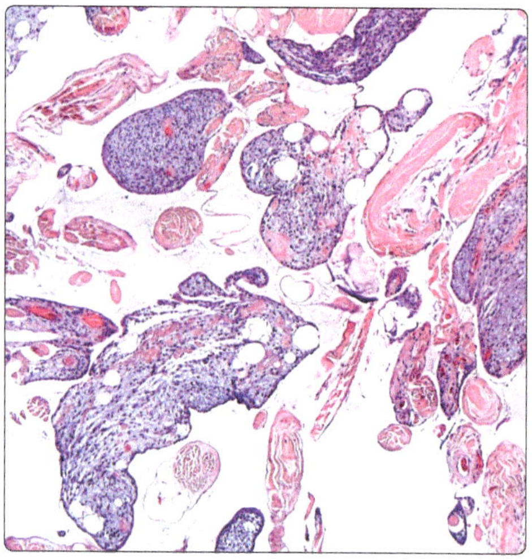

(Left) *The unusual angiomatous variant of SCL demonstrates slit-like to markedly dilated endothelial-lined channels associated with the otherwise characteristic features of SCL.* **(Right)** *Although originally considered to be pseudoangiomatous, a conspicuous endothelial lining → can often be identified in this variant of SCL. A CD31 immunostain will highlight the endothelial cells.*

Angiomatous Variant of Spindle Cell Lipoma

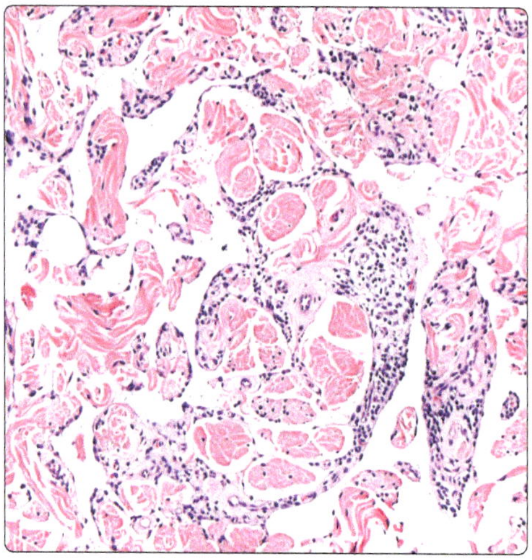

Angiomatous Variant Shows Endothelial Lining

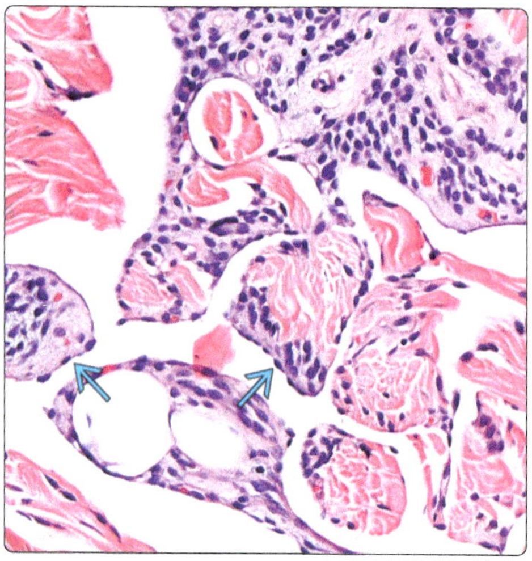

Focal Hyalinized Vessels

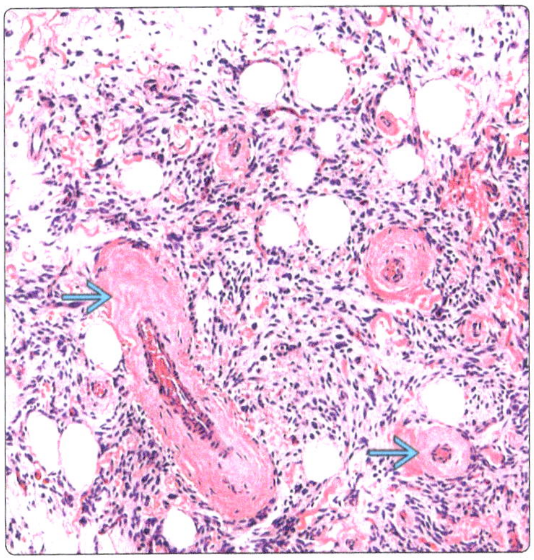

Spindle Cell and Pleomorphic Lipoma

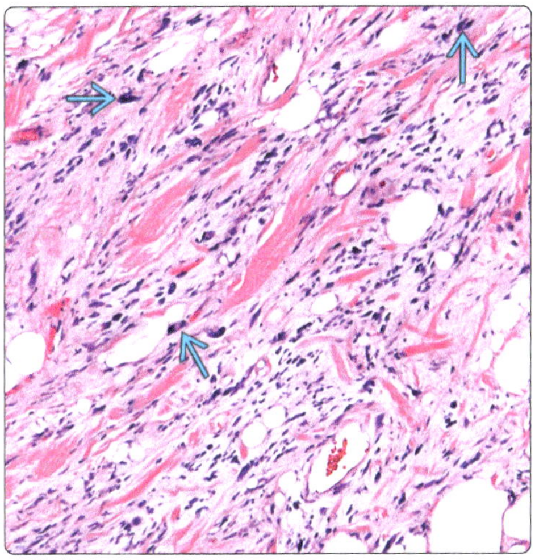

(Left) *Rare cases of SCL contain foci of vessels showing perivascular hyalinization* → *or even concentric onion-skinning fibrosis. This finding may impart an overall appearance to cellular angiofibroma.* **(Right)** *PL is essentially the same neoplasm as SCL. Accordingly, many features of SCL are often present in PL, including bland spindle cells and ropey collagen bundles. Notably, there is also a variably prominent population of multinucleated tumor giant cells, termed floret cells* →.

Pleomorphic Lipoma at Low Magnification

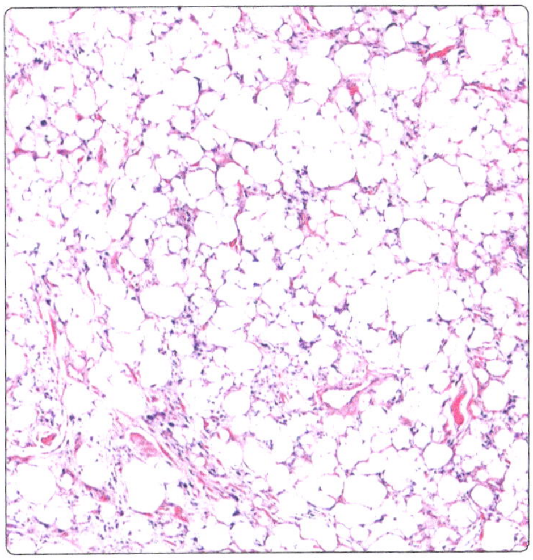

Characteristic Floret Tumor Cells at High Magnification

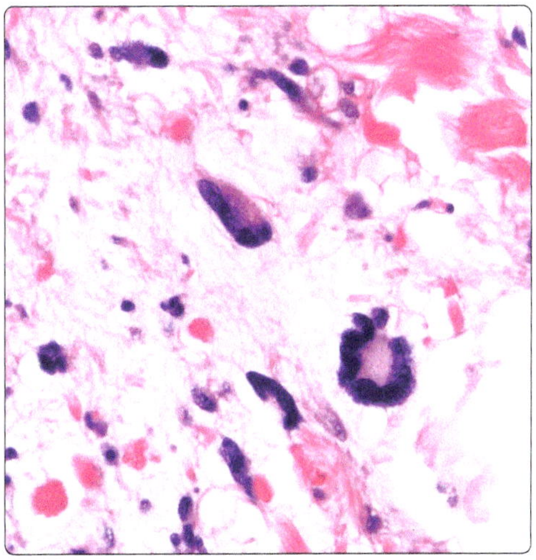

(Left) *Some cases of PL are mostly adipocytic, with scattered foci of myxoid stroma containing the diagnostic findings. Examples such as these may at first resemble a myxolipoma or liposarcoma. Occasional cases of PL are also low-fat or fat-free.* **(Right)** *The floret cell defines the morphology of PL. These cells have eosinophilic cytoplasm and contain multiple hyperchromatic nuclei often arranged in a peripheral distribution, resembling that of a floral arrangement.*

Rare Multivacuolated Lipoblasts in Pleomorphic Lipoma

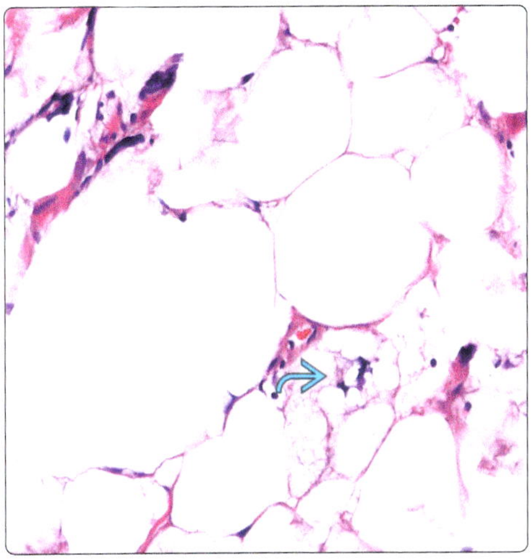

Diffuse CD34 Expression in Spindle Cell Lipoma/Pleomorphic Lipoma

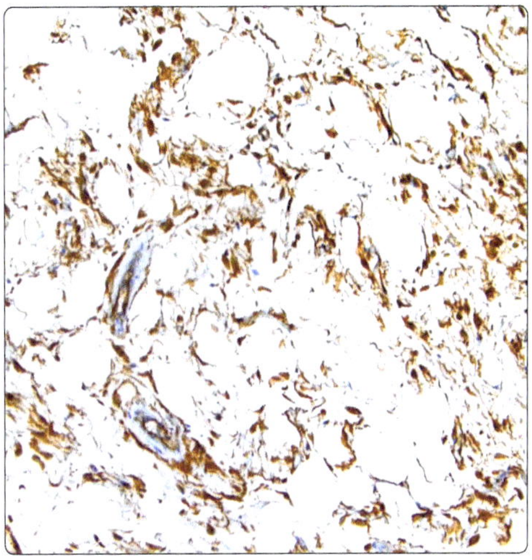

(Left) *Multivacuolated lipoblasts* ↪ *may be rarely encountered in otherwise typical cases of PL. Similarly, a scattered atypical mitotic figure may also rarely be identified. Neither of these findings appear to alter the usual benign clinical course of these neoplasms.* **(Right)** *CD34 expression is strong, diffuse, and consistent in both SCL and PL and stains both the spindle cells and the multinucleated floret cells. S100 is expressed in adipocytes but is generally negative in the lesional cells.*

Chondroid Lipoma

KEY FACTS

TERMINOLOGY

- Benign mesenchymal neoplasm composed of lipoblastic cells and mature adipocytes within myxochondroid matrix

CLINICAL ISSUES

- Very rare
- Adults (20-40 years most common)
- Strong female predilection (4:1)
- Slow-growing, painless mass
- Most common in proximal limbs and limb girdles
  - Also trunk, head and neck
- Occurs in both superficial and deep tissues
- Simple complete excision is curative

MICROSCOPIC

- Well circumscribed, often encapsulated
- Nests, sheets, and cords of uni- and multivacuolated round cells
  - Some nonvacuolated tumor cells have granular eosinophilic cytoplasm
  - Classic multivacuolated lipoblasts common
- Myxochondroid to hyalinized matrix
- Variable mature adipose tissue component
- Interspersed thick- and thin-walled vessels with variable hemorrhage and hemosiderin deposition

ANCILLARY TESTS

- Variable S100(+) in lipoblast-like cells
- Characteristic chromosomal translocation
  - t(11;16)(q13;p12-13) (*C11orf95-MKL2*)

TOP DIFFERENTIAL DIAGNOSES

- Atypical lipomatous tumor/well-differentiated liposarcoma
- Myxoid liposarcoma
- Extraskeletal myxoid chondrosarcoma
- Soft tissue chondroma
- Myoepithelioma of soft tissue

(Left) *Chondroid lipoma is classically a very well-circumscribed lesion with a multilobulated and yellow to tan cut surface. As in other forms of lipoma, foci of hemorrhage may be identified.* **(Right)** *Chondroid lipoma is usually sharply delineated from adjacent tissues and may or may not be encapsulated. It can occur in both superficial and deep soft tissues, the latter evidenced in this case by the presence of surrounding mature skeletal muscle* ➡*.*

Chondroid Lipoma: Gross Specimen

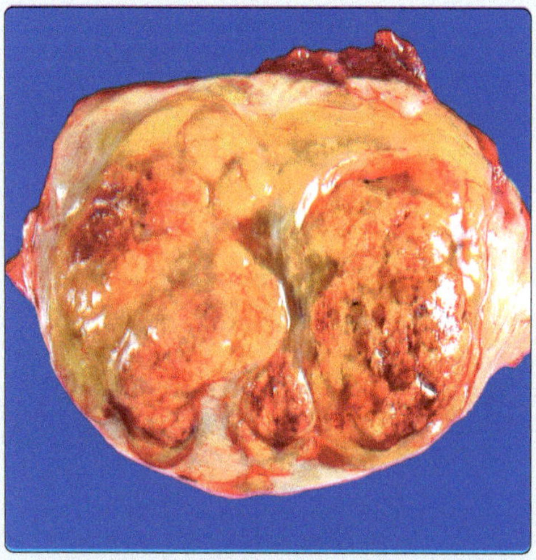

Chondroid Lipoma With Sharp Circumscription

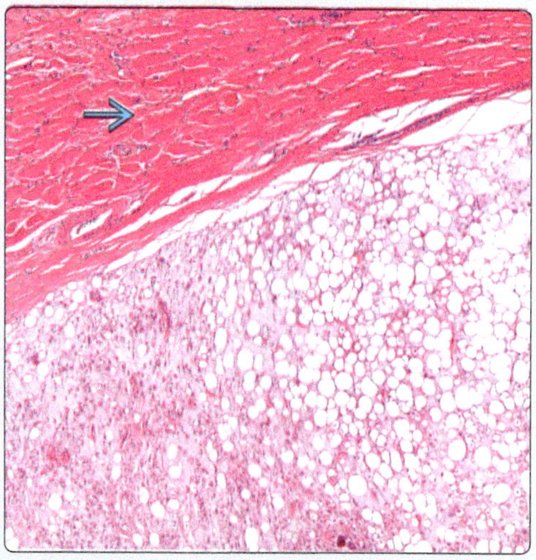

(Left) *Most cases of chondroid lipoma show a multilobulated growth pattern, with each lobule delineated by a thin or thick fibrous septa. Dilated blood vessels* ➡ *are also abundant and conspicuous in this tumor.* **(Right)** *The classic image of chondroid lipoma shows a mixture of rounded eosinophilic cells with 1 to several intracytoplasmic vacuoles deposited in a myxochondroid matrix. Some cells, however, are not vacuolated.*

Chondroid Lipoma With Multilobulated Growth

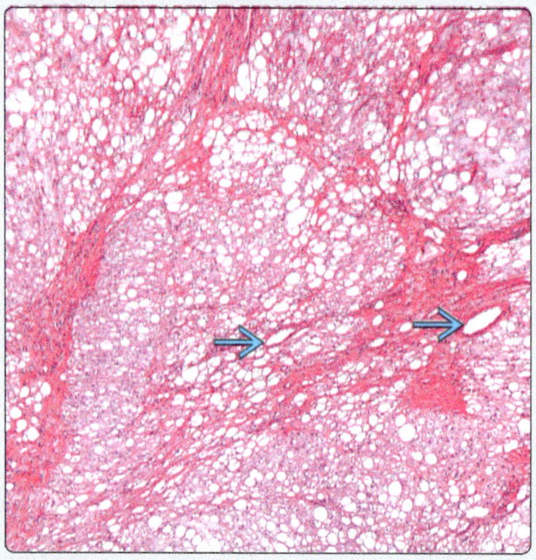

Classic Appearance of Chondroid Lipoma

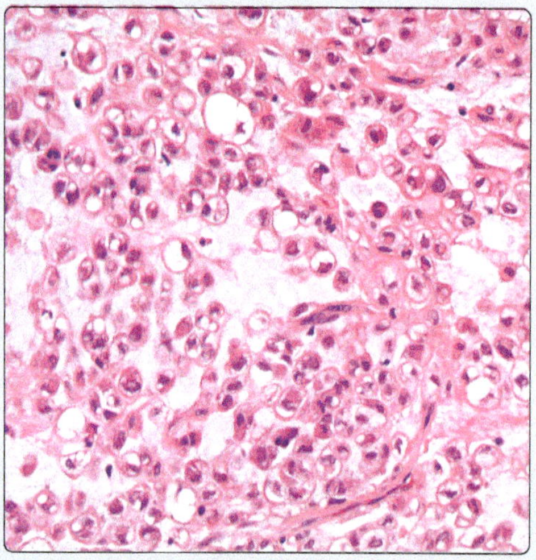

TERMINOLOGY

Definitions

- Benign mesenchymal neoplasm composed of lipoblastic cells and mature adipocytes within myxochondroid matrix

CLINICAL ISSUES

Epidemiology

- Incidence
  - Very rare
- Age
  - Adults (20-40 years most common)
- Sex
  - Strong female predilection (4:1)

Site

- Predominantly proximal limbs and limb girdles
- Also trunk, head and neck (particularly oral cavity)
- Occurs in both superficial and deep soft tissue

Presentation

- Painless, slowly enlarging mass
  - History of recent enlargement in half of cases

Treatment

- Simple complete excision

Prognosis

- Benign
- Does not recur or metastasize

MACROSCOPIC

General Features

- Well circumscribed and frequently encapsulated
- Tan-yellow cut surface; occasionally with hemorrhagic foci

Size

- 1.5-11 cm (median: 4 cm)

MICROSCOPIC

Histologic Features

- Well circumscribed
- Often lobulated with fibrous septa
- Nests, sheets, and cords of uni- and multivacuolated epithelioid cells
  - Cells may appear to be in lacunar spaces (chondrocyte-like)
  - Some nonvacuolated tumor cells have granular eosinophilic cytoplasm
  - No significant nuclear atypia or mitotic activity
- Classic multivacuolated lipoblasts common
- Myxochondroid matrix
  - May be hyalinized
- Variable mature adipose tissue component
- Interspersed thick- and thin-walled vessels with variable hemorrhage and hemosiderin deposition
- Can show fibrosis, calcification, metaplastic bone

ANCILLARY TESTS

Immunohistochemistry

- Variable S100(+) in lipoblast-like cells
- Rarely focal keratin (+)
- Negative for smooth muscle actin, HMB-45, EMA

Genetic Testing

- Characteristic chromosomal translocation
  - t(11;16)(q13;p12-13) (*C11orf95-MKL2*)
- No amplification of *MDM2* or *CDK4*

DIFFERENTIAL DIAGNOSIS

Atypical Lipomatous Tumor/Well-Differentiated Liposarcoma

- Often large, slowly growing
- Lobules of atypical fat separated by thick fibrous septa containing atypical "smudgy" stromal cells
- Multivacuolated lipoblasts may be few, absent, or numerous
- May show prominent myxoid stroma
- *MDM2* amplification

Myxoid Liposarcoma

- Bland spindle cell component
- Plexiform capillary vascular pattern (staghorn vessels)
- Cellular (round cell) myxoid liposarcoma has larger, ovoid cells with monomorphic nuclei
- Characteristic translocations t(12;16), t(12;22)

Extraskeletal Myxoid Chondrosarcoma

- Often larger, slowly growing, and infiltrative
- Anastomosing cords of spindled to stellate cells in prominent myxoid stroma
- No adipose tissue or lipoblasts
- Characteristic translocations t(9;17), t(9:22)

Soft Tissue Chondroma

- Occurs in fingers, toes, hands, feet
- Contains true hyaline cartilage
- Lacks adipocytic component

Myoepithelioma of Soft Tissue

- Lacks lipoblasts
- Most cases show diffuse keratin (+) &/or S100(+)
- Variable expression of SMA, EMA, calponin, GFAP, desmin

SELECTED REFERENCES

1. Flucke U et al: Presence of C11orf95-MKL2 fusion is a consistent finding in chondroid lipomas: a study of eight cases. Histopathology. 62(6):925-30, 2013
2. Thway K et al: Chondroid lipoma: an update and review. Ann Diagn Pathol. 16(3):230-4, 2012
3. de Vreeze RS et al: Delineation of chondroid lipoma: an immunohistochemical and molecular biological analysis. Sarcoma. 2011:638403, 2011
4. Ballaux F et al: Chondroid lipoma is characterized by t(11;16)(q13;p12-13). Virchows Arch. 444(2):208-10, 2004
5. Kindblom LG et al: Chondroid lipoma: an ultrastructural and immunohistochemical analysis with further observations regarding its differentiation. Hum Pathol. 26(7):706-15, 1995
6. Meis JM et al: Chondroid lipoma. A unique tumor simulating liposarcoma and myxoid chondrosarcoma. Am J Surg Pathol. 17(11):1103-12, 1993

(Left) *The constituent cell of chondroid lipoma is small and round, contains abundant eosinophilic cytoplasm, and has a small, bland nucleus with irregular contours. Focal enlargement* → *may be seen, but significant nuclear pleomorphism is not typically a feature.* **(Right)** *Chondroid lipoma resembles a cartilaginous tumor in part due to the presence of cells* → *with cytoplasmic vacuoles surrounding the nucleus that create a compressed peripheral rim of eosinophilic cytoplasm, simulating a chondrocyte within a lacuna.*

Round Cells With Eosinophilic Cytoplasm

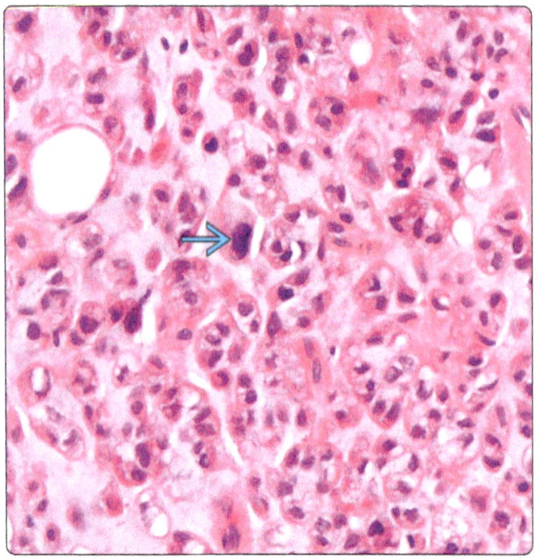

Chondroid Cytomorphology

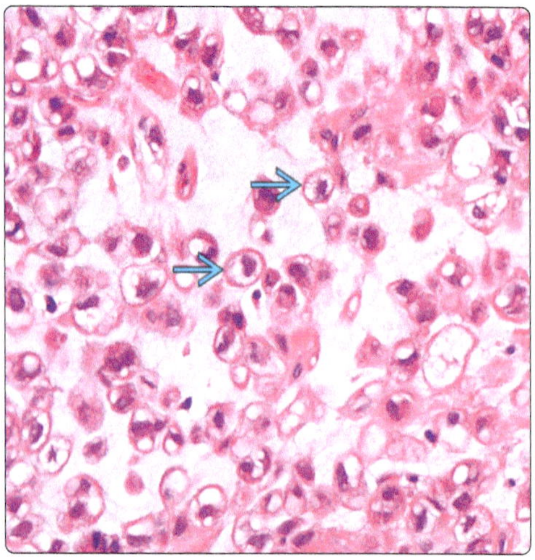

(Left) *Most cells of chondroid lipoma contain at least 1 cytoplasmic vacuole. In those cells that contain only 1* →*, the nucleus may be compressed at the periphery, reminiscent of a signet ring cell. When prominent, this morphology may be confused with carcinoma.* **(Right)** *Vague spindling of tumor cells is a very rare finding in chondroid lipoma and is often focal.*

Univacuolated Tumor Cells

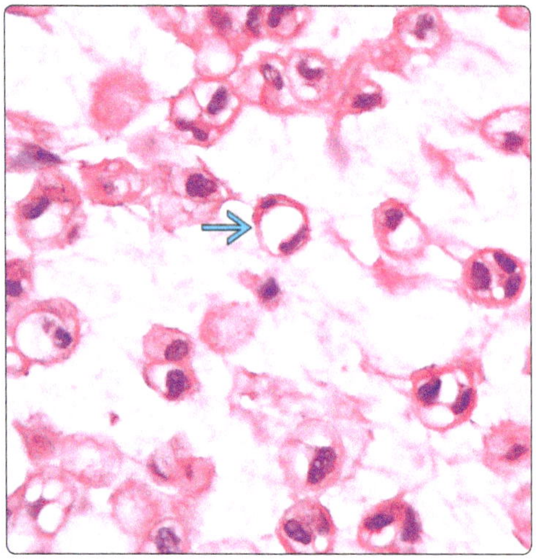

Focal Spindled Cellular Morphology

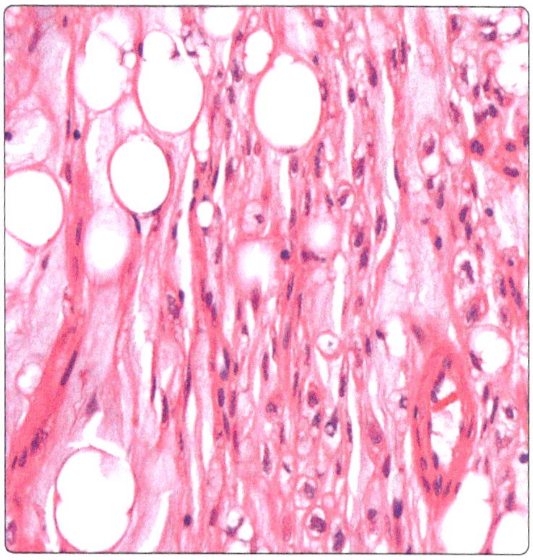

(Left) *Some of the multivacuolated tumor cells of chondroid lipoma are morphologically indistinguishable from the classic multivacuolated lipoblasts encountered in liposarcoma. They vary in number from sparse to numerous but are usually quite abundant.* **(Right)** *A component of mature adipose tissue is almost always identified in chondroid lipoma, but the distribution varies from focal to extensive. In the latter setting, limited sampling may lead to diagnostic error.*

Multivacuolated Lipoblasts

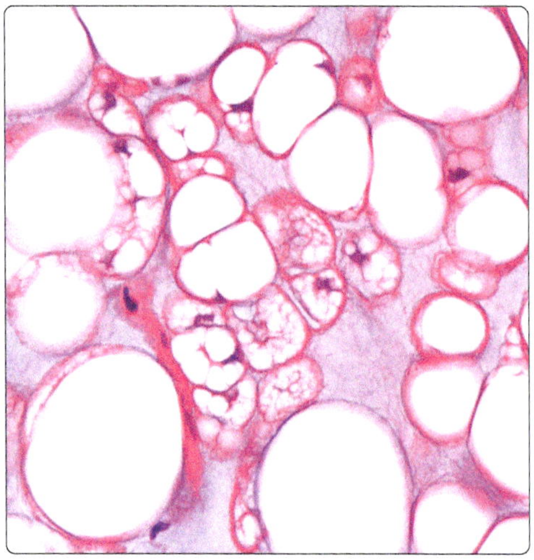

Mature Adipose Tissue Component

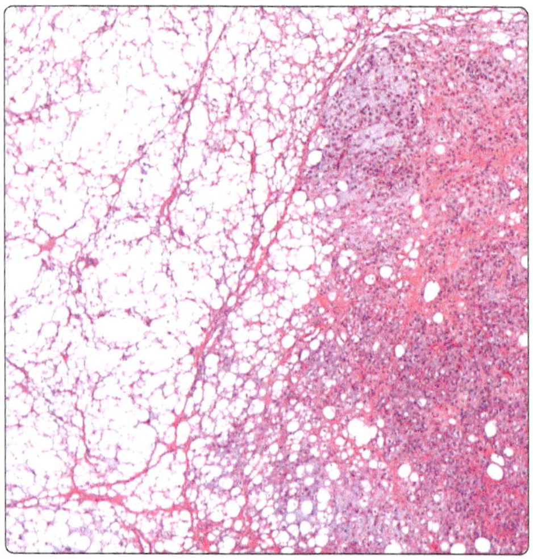

Abundant Mature Adipose Tissue

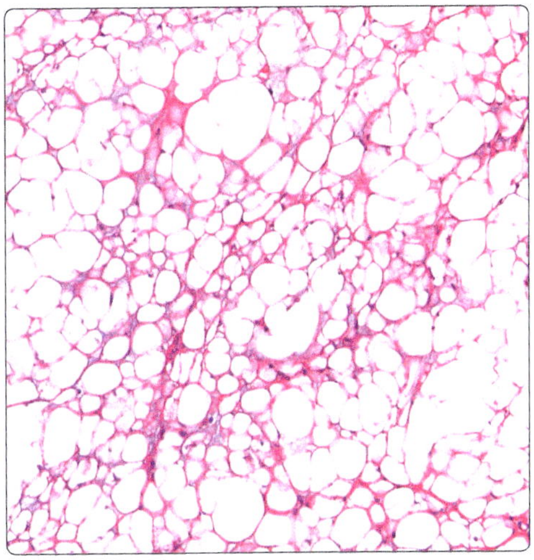

Aggregates of Tumor Cells Within Mature Adipose Tissue

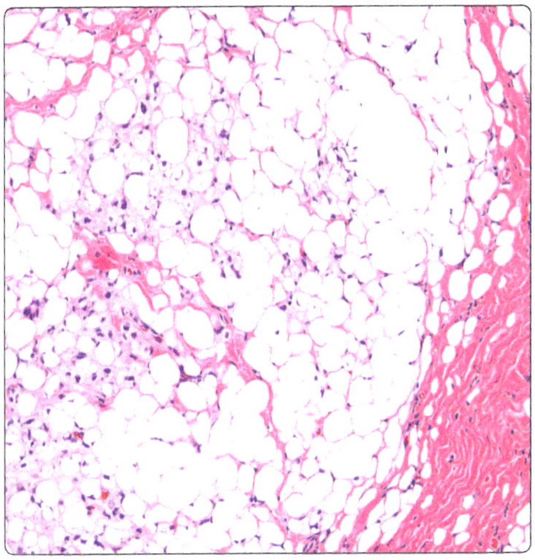

(Left) *In areas of chondroid lipoma that show abundant mature adipose tissue, it is not uncommon to see mild myxoid stromal change or scattered multivacuolated tumor cells. This pattern may lead to serious consideration of a liposarcoma if other, more conventional areas of chondroid lipoma are not identified.* **(Right)** *In some cases of chondroid lipoma, the constituent tumor cells form small aggregates or nests within a background of abundant mature adipose tissue.*

Myxoid Stroma Common

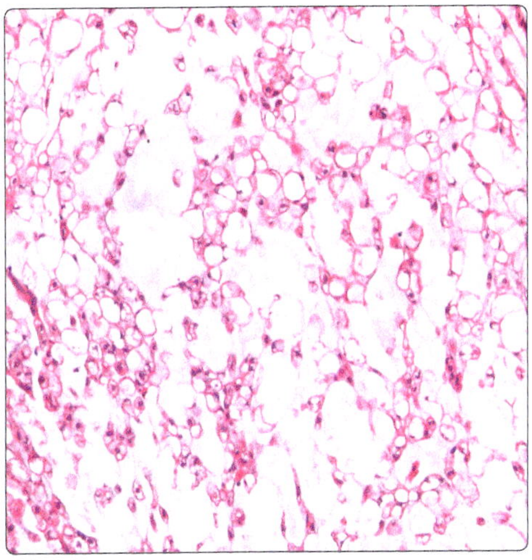

Abundant Myxoid Stroma

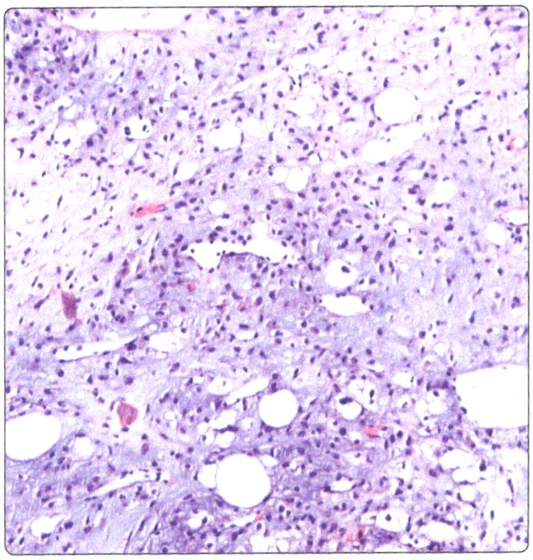

(Left) *Myxoid stroma is a common and relatively consistent feature of chondroid lipoma.* **(Right)** *In some heavily myxoid cases of chondroid lipoma, the overall appearance of scattered small, bland tumor cells associated with adipose tissue and multivacuolated lipoblast-like cells may closely resemble a myxoid liposarcoma. However, chondroid lipoma does not demonstrate a delicate, plexiform vascular network.*

Focally Hyalinized Stroma

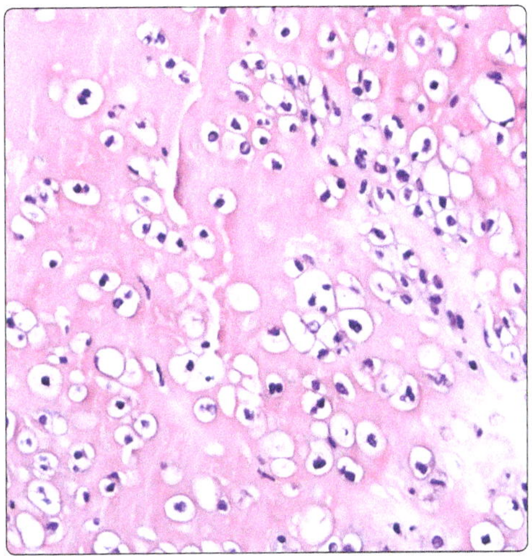

Conspicuous Vasculature

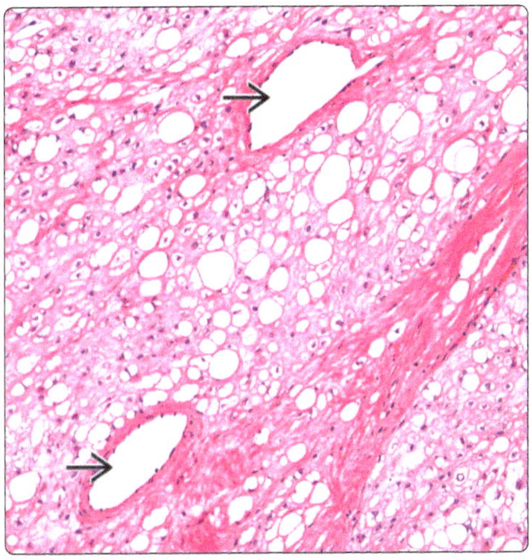

(Left) *Foci of hyalinization are often intermingled with myxoid zones in chondroid lipoma; however, they are usually not prominent. In rare cases, the stroma is almost entirely hyalinized.* **(Right)** *Thin- to thick-walled dilated blood vessels → are a common finding in chondroid lipoma and are usually easily identified. They may be associated with stromal hemorrhage, as well as hemosiderin deposition and fibrosis.*

Nevus Lipomatosus

KEY FACTS

TERMINOLOGY

- Nevus lipomatosus superficialis
- a.k.a. pedunculated lipofibroma
- Connective tissue nevus characterized by mature adipose tissue in reticular dermis

CLINICAL ISSUES

- Solitary or multiple grouped papules or polypoid lesions
- Rarely diffuse
- Classic form: Children and young adults
- Solitary form: Adults
- Posterior surfaces
  - Buttocks and upper thighs, lower back
- Excellent prognosis

MICROSCOPIC

- Mature adipose tissue in reticular dermis
- Absence of adnexal structures associated with adipose tissue
- Increased numbers of small blood vessels
- No increased cellularity or cytologic atypia

TOP DIFFERENTIAL DIAGNOSES

- Acrochordon (skin tag)
  - Lacks mature adipose tissue
- Lipoma
  - Arises in subcutis not dermis
- Fibrolipoma
  - Arises in subcutis not dermis
  - Also used to refer to skin tag with adipose tissue
- Spindle cell lipoma
  - Usually arises in subcutis
  - Associated with proliferation of bland spindle cells
  - Ropey collagen
- Focal dermal hypoplasia
  - Clinically different: Widespread, depressed, atrophic lesions
  - Loss of normal dermis

Nevus Lipomatosus at Scanning Magnification

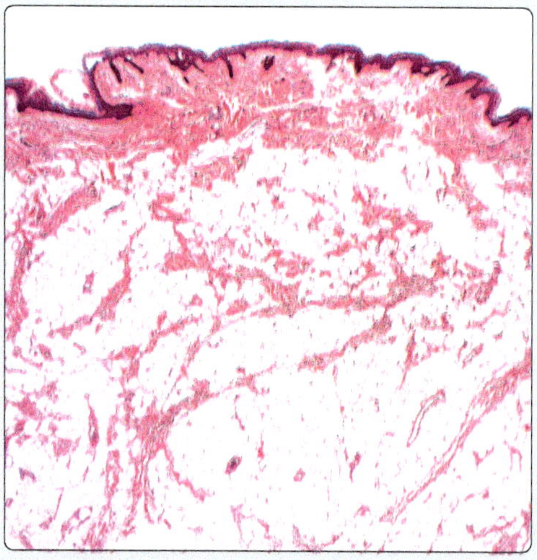

Nevus Lipomatosus With Polypoid Architecture

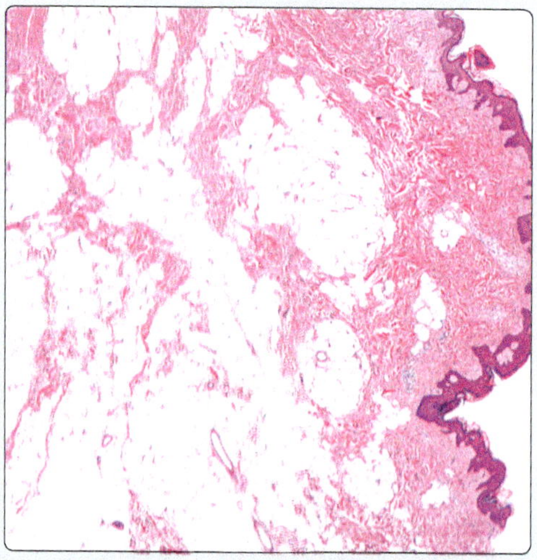

(Left) *In this case of nevus lipomatosus superficialis, the mature adipose tissue is quite prominent and diffusely present throughout the dermis.* **(Right)** *Nevus lipomatosus often appears polypoid, as in this case, and consists of mature fat within the dermis.*

Nevus Lipomatosus: Mature Adipose Tissue Within Reticular Dermis

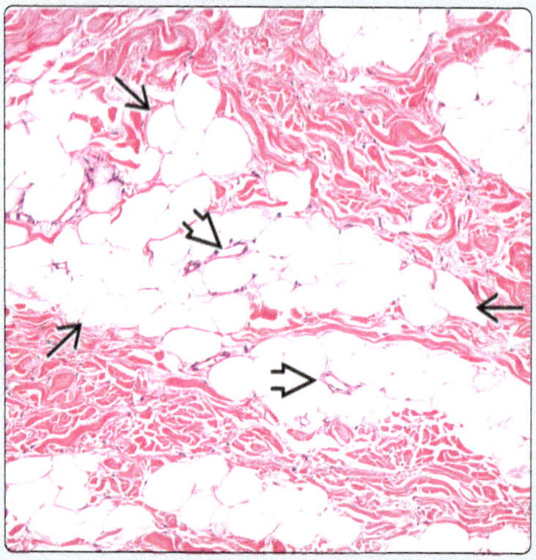

Nevus Lipomatosus at High Power

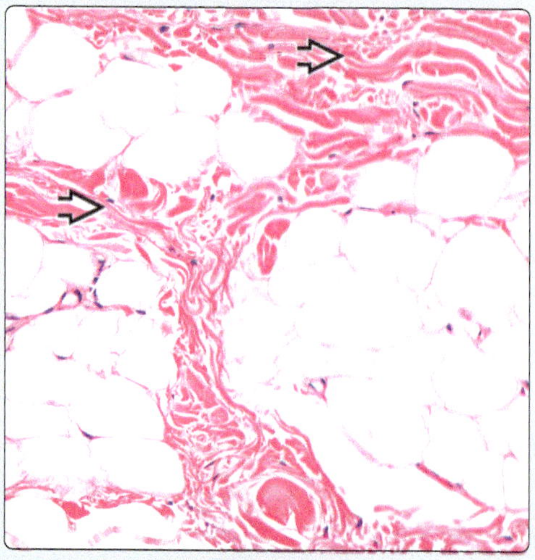

(Left) *The aggregates of mature adipose tissue → are often found around small dermal blood vessels ⇒.* **(Right)** *Note that the collagen otherwise resembles normal reticular dermis ⇒, with the characteristic spaces between bands of eosinophilic-staining collagen.*

TERMINOLOGY

Synonyms

- Nevus lipomatosus superficialis
- Pedunculated lipofibroma

Definitions

- Connective tissue nevus/hamartoma characterized by mature adipose tissue in reticular dermis

ETIOLOGY/PATHOGENESIS

Unknown

- Most cases are idiopathic

Genetic

- Single case described with 2p24 deletion
  - Importance in pathogenesis remains unclear

CLINICAL ISSUES

Epidemiology

- Incidence
  - Uncommon
- Age
  - Classic form: Children and young adults
  - Solitary form: Adults
- Sex
  - M = F

Site

- Posterior surfaces
  - Buttocks
  - Upper thigh
  - Lower back

Presentation

- Classic form
  - Multiple, grouped papules, polypoid lesions, or plaques
  - Rarely diffuse
  - Rarely associated with
    - Lipedematous scalp
    - Dermoid cysts
    - Folliculosebaceous cystic hamartoma
    - Angiokeratoma
- Solitary form
  - Locations similar to classic form
  - May also occur in areas where acrochordons present

Treatment

- Surgical approaches
  - Simple excision is curative
  - Laser removal also reported

Prognosis

- Excellent: Benign lesions
  - Primarily cosmetic issue

MACROSCOPIC

General Features

- Papule, plaque, or nodule with smooth or wrinkled surface
- Skin-colored to yellow appearance

MICROSCOPIC

Histologic Features

- Polypoid silhouette at low magnification
- Mature adipose tissue in upper dermis
  - Often clustered around dermal blood vessels
  - Few small, immature-appearing lipocytes may be present
- Increased numbers of small blood vessels
- Absence of adnexal structures
- No increased cellularity or cytologic atypia
- Rare cases with pagetoid adipocytes along dermoepidermal junction

DIFFERENTIAL DIAGNOSIS

Acrochordon/Fibroepithelial Polyp (Skin Tag)

- Similar clinical/gross appearance
  - However, acrochordons typically show thin stalk
- Acrochordons usually lack mature adipose tissue

Lipoma

- Presents deep to dermis
- Well-circumscribed nodule of mature adipose tissue
- Lacks admixed reticular dermal collagen

Fibrolipoma

- Typically presents deep to dermis
- Collagen bands represent fibrotic areas within lipoma, not reticular dermal collagen
- Term is also commonly used for acrochordons with adipose tissue

Spindle Cell Lipoma

- Presents on upper back and head and neck
- Usually tumor of subcutis
- Short fascicles of bland CD34(+) spindled cells
- Ropey collagen and myxoid stroma
- Frequent mast cells

Focal Dermal Hypoplasia (Goltz Syndrome)

- Histologically appears similar
  - But reticular dermis diminished
- Clinically different
  - Widespread, depressed, atrophic lesions
  - May have polypoid lesions from herniation of fat through atrophic dermis
  - Associated with skeletal abnormalities

SELECTED REFERENCES

1. Fatah S et al: Successful CO2 laser treatment of naevus lipomatosus cutaneous superficialis. Clin Exp Dermatol. 35(5):559-60, 2010
2. Cardot-Leccia N et al: Naevus lipomatosus superficialis: a case report with a 2p24 deletion. Br J Dermatol. 156(2):380-1, 2007
3. Kang H et al: Nevus lipomatosus cutaneous superficialis with folliculosebaceous cystic hamartoma. J Am Acad Dermatol. 56(2 Suppl):S55-7, 2007
4. Mansur AT et al: Colocalization of lipedematous scalp and nevus lipomatosus superficialis: a case report. J Cutan Pathol. 34(4):342-5, 2007
5. Orteu CH et al: Naevus lipomatosus cutaneous superficialis: overlap with connective tissue naevi. Acta Derm Venereol. 76(3):243-5, 1996
6. Eyre SP et al: Rubbery zosteriform nodules on the back. Nevus lipomatosus cutaneous superficialis (Hoffmann-Zurhelle). Arch Dermatol. 128(10):1395, 1398, 1992

Hibernoma

KEY FACTS

TERMINOLOGY

- Benign lipomatous tumor composed of lobules of cells resembling brown fat

CLINICAL ISSUES

- Age: 20-40 years most common
- Painless, slow-growing mass
- Most common in thigh, upper trunk, and neck
  - Subcutaneous (most common) or intramuscular
- Treatment: Simple surgical excision
- Benign; very rare recurrences

MACROSCOPIC

- Circumscribed, lobulated lesion
- Mean size: 9.3 cm

MICROSCOPIC

- Lobulated tumor composed of mixture of cell types in varying proportions
  - Polygonal cells with granular eosinophilic cytoplasm, multivacuolated cells, univacuolated adipocytes
- Small, bland, central nuclei ± nucleoli
- Medium-sized stromal vessels are common and may be prominent
- Morphologic variants: Lipoma-like, myxoid, spindle cell

ANCILLARY TESTS

- Variable S100(+)
- Molecular: Rearrangements of 11q13-21 common and characteristic

TOP DIFFERENTIAL DIAGNOSES

- Normal brown fat
- Lipoma (conventional)
- Lipoblastoma
- Atypical lipomatous tumor/well-differentiated liposarcoma
- Granular cell tumor

Hibernoma With Classic Findings

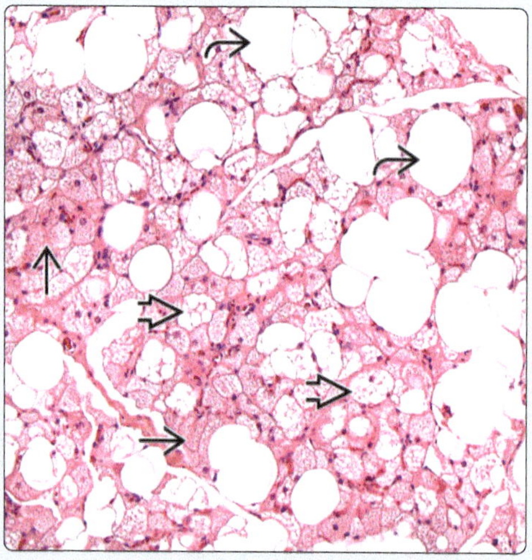

Multivacuolated Cells Containing Lipid

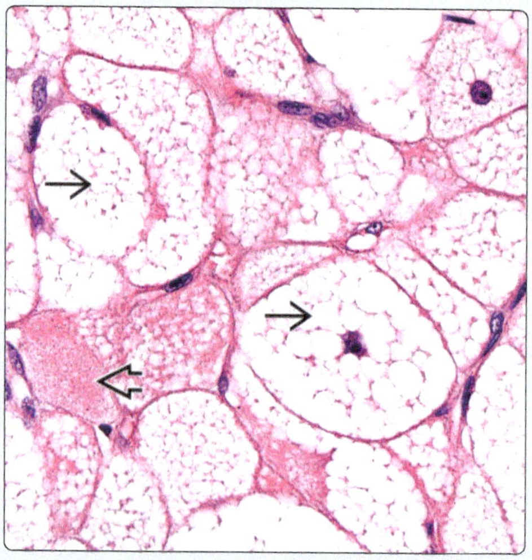

(Left) *Hibernoma is a benign lipomatous neoplasm composed of cells resembling brown fat. This classic case shows a mixture of granular eosinophilic cells →, multivacuolated cells ⇨, and scattered univacuolated mature adipocytes ↷.* **(Right)** *The multivacuolated cells → usually contain innumerable lipid droplets and resemble multivacuolated lipoblasts; however, the latter have enlarged, hyperchromatic, and scalloped nuclei. The eosinophilic cells ⇨ derive their coloration from numerous mitochondria.*

Lipoma-Like Variant of Hibernoma

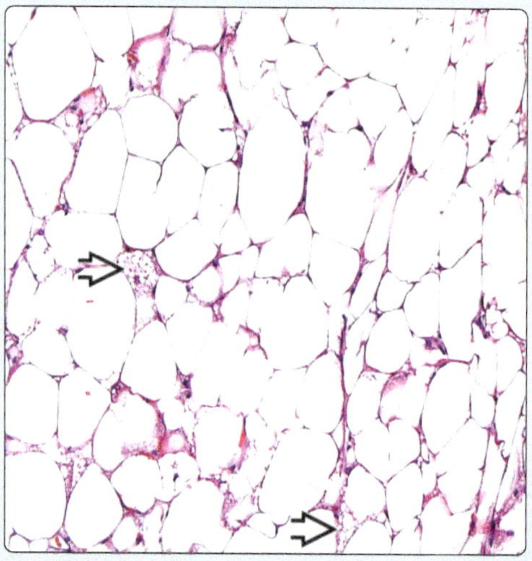

Myxoid Variant of Hibernoma

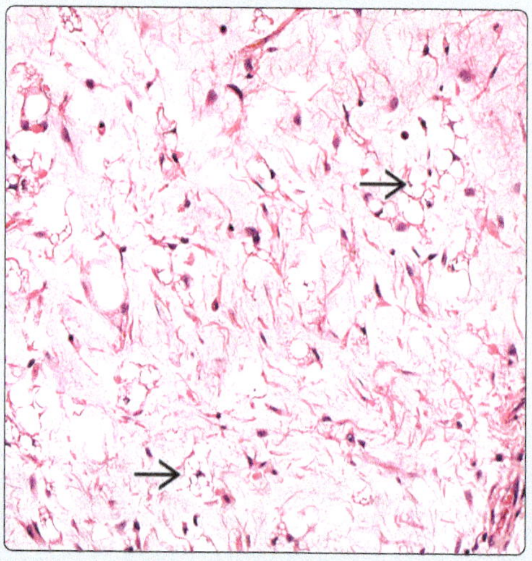

(Left) *Occasional cases of hibernoma show predominantly univacuolated white fat cells with only scattered multivacuolated ⇨ and eosinophilic granular cells. These tumors may be easily misclassified as conventional lipoma.* **(Right)** *Rare cases of hibernoma show myxoid stromal change, which may be diffuse. Scattered multivacuolated cells → and mature adipocytes can be identified. Identification of other more typical areas of hibernoma is helpful.*

TERMINOLOGY

Synonyms

- Fetal lipoma
- Lipoma of embryonic fat

Definitions

- Benign lipomatous tumor composed of lobules of cells resembling brown fat

CLINICAL ISSUES

Epidemiology

- Incidence
  - Rare
- Age
  - 20-40 years most common
  - Rare in children and elderly > 60 years of age

Site

- Subcutaneous (most common) or intramuscular
- Most common in thigh
- Also neck, arm, trunk, back, shoulder, and retroperitoneum
  - Rarely breast, kidney, or mediastinum

Presentation

- Painless, slow-growing mass

Treatment

- Simple surgical excision

Prognosis

- Benign
- Recurrences are very rare

MACROSCOPIC

General Features

- Circumscribed, lobulated lesions
- Tan-yellow to yellow-brown, greasy cut surface

Size

- Range: 1-24 cm (mean: 9.3 cm)

MICROSCOPIC

Histologic Features

- Lobulated tumor composed of mixture of cell types in varying proportions
  - Polygonal cells with granular eosinophilic cytoplasm
  - Multivacuolated cells with numerous lipid droplets
  - Univacuolated adipocytes
- Medium-sized stromal vessels are common and may be prominent
- Small, bland, central nuclei ± nucleoli
- Mitotic figures are rare

Morphologic Variants

- Lipoma-like hibernoma
  - Mostly univacuolated adipocytes
  - Eosinophilic granular and multivacuolated cells are sparse
  - Most common in thigh
- Myxoid variant
  - Predominantly occurs in males and in head and neck region
  - Constituent cells separated by acellular myxoid stroma
- Spindle cell variant
  - Rare; found in posterior neck or scalp
  - Hibernoma cells, thick collagen bundles, mast cells, mature fat

ANCILLARY TESTS

Immunohistochemistry

- Variable S100(+)
- Spindle cell variant is often CD34(+)

Electron Microscopy

- Numerous intracytoplasmic mitochondria
- Also lipid droplets, lysosomes

Molecular Genetics

- Rearrangements of 11q13-21 common and characteristic
- Concomitant deletions of tumor suppressor genes *AIP* and *MEN1*
- No amplification of *MDM2*

DIFFERENTIAL DIAGNOSIS

Normal Brown Fat

- More abundant in children and young adults than older adults
- Usually found in neck, axilla, mediastinum, and paraspinal regions
- No discrete mass lesion

Lipoma (Conventional)

- Lacks multivacuolated cells

Lipoblastoma

- May contain brown fat cells
- Usually occurs in infants (< 3 years of age)
- Prominent lobularity with myxoid stroma and lipoblasts

Atypical Lipomatous Tumor/Well-Differentiated Liposarcoma

- Atypical "smudge" cells in thickened fibrous septa
- True lipoblasts with hyperchromatic scalloped nuclei may be present
- *MDM2* amplification by FISH

Granular Cell Tumor

- Diffuse cytoplasmic granularity
- No multivacuolated cells
- Diffuse S100(+)

SELECTED REFERENCES

1. Vassos N et al: Deep-seated huge hibernoma of soft tissue: a rare differential diagnosis of atypical lipomatous tumor/well differentiated liposarcoma. Int J Clin Exp Pathol. 6(10):2178-84, 2013
2. Moretti VM et al: Spindle-cell hibernoma: a clinicopathologic comparison of this new variant. Orthopedics. 33(1):52-5, 2010
3. Chirieac LR et al: Characterization of the myxoid variant of hibernoma. Ann Diagn Pathol. 10(2):104-6, 2006
4. Furlong MA et al: The morphologic spectrum of hibernoma: a clinicopathologic study of 170 cases. Am J Surg Pathol. 25(6):809-14, 2001
5. Mertens F et al: Hibernomas are characterized by rearrangements of chromosome bands 11q13-21. Int J Cancer. 58(4):503-5, 1994

Atypical Lipomatous Tumor and Liposarcoma

KEY FACTS

TERMINOLOGY

- Intermediate (locally aggressive, nonmetastasizing) lipogenic neoplasm composed of atypical adipocytes
- Atypical lipomatous tumor (ALT)
- Well-differentiated liposarcoma

CLINICAL ISSUES

- Accounts for 40-45% of all liposarcomas
- Occurs most frequently in deep soft tissues of limbs followed by retroperitoneum, abdominal cavity, paratesticular region, and mediastinum
- Usually presents as deep-seated, painless, and slowly enlarging tumor mass
- Lesions located in surgically amenable soft tissues recur only rarely after complete excision
- Variable risk of dedifferentiation in extremities (< 2%) and retroperitoneum (> 25%)
- May also arise in subcutaneous tissue and very rarely in skin
- Middle-aged to elderly adults
- Intermediate (locally aggressive but nonmetastasizing) malignant mesenchymal tumor

MICROSCOPIC

- Atypical adipocytes, atypical stromal cells, lipoblasts
  - Adipocytes show striking variations in size and shape
  - Typically show enlarged hyperchromatic-staining nuclei
  - Hyperchromatic and multinucleated stromal cells
  - Lipoblasts may be seen, but are not essential for diagnosis
- Lipoma-like subtype
- Sclerosing subtype
- Inflammatory subtype
- Spindle cell subtype

TOP DIFFERENTIAL DIAGNOSES

- Spindle cell and pleomorphic lipoma
- Massive localized lymphedema in morbidly obese
- Lipoma

ALT: Clinical Image

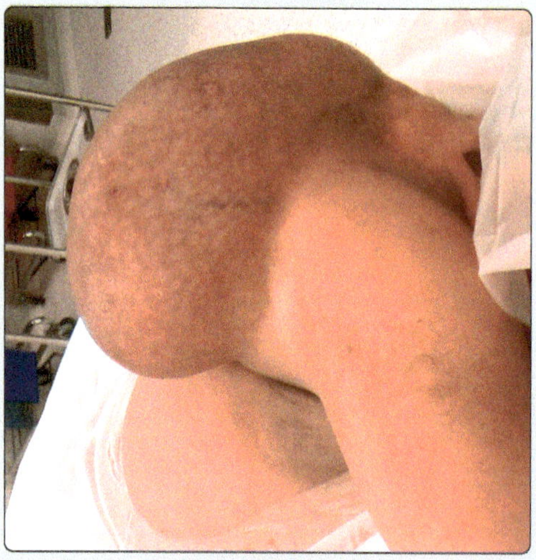

ALT: Gross Image

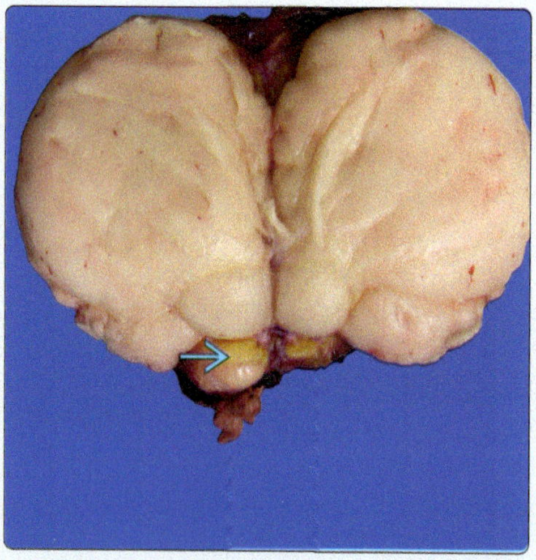

(Left) *A large lipomatous tumor on the shoulder of an adult male patient is shown.* **(Right)** *Note that the neoplasm has appearances that are somewhat different from that of normal adipose tissue. The lesion appears firmer and more whitish than the surrounding nonneoplastic adipose tissue ➡.*

ALT: Fibrous Septa

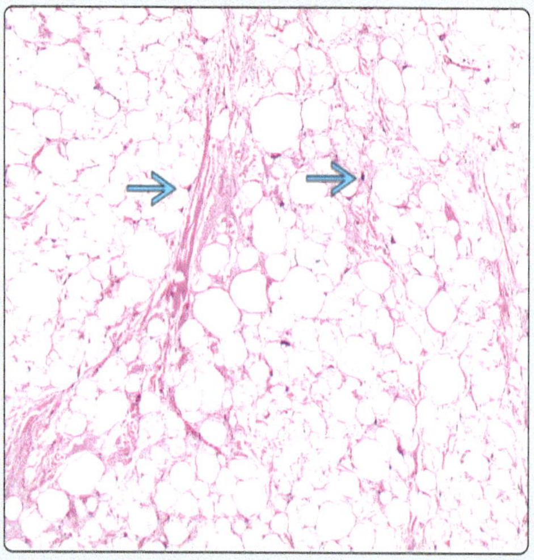

ALT: Atypical Adipocytic Nuclei

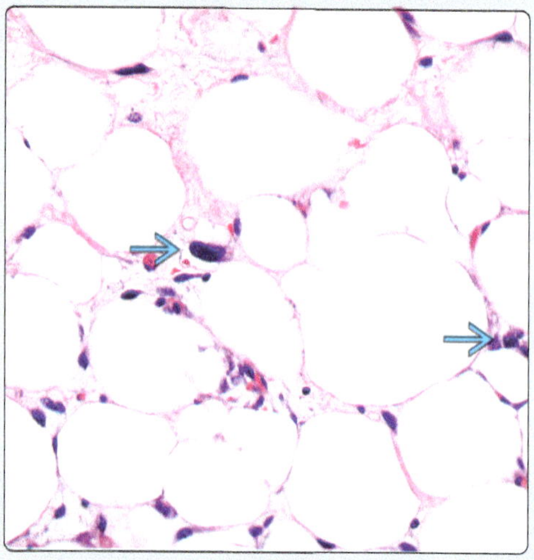

(Left) *Histologic examination of atypical lipomatous tumor (ALT) shows striking variations in size and shape of lipogenic cells, as well as scattered enlarged cells with enlarged hyperchromatic nuclei. The atypical cells ➡ are found along the fibrous connective tissue septa.* **(Right)** *Note the deeply hyperchromatic appearance of the lesional cell nuclei ➡. This is the key diagnostic clue, rather than the detection of lipoblasts, which are often absent in such neoplasms.*

TERMINOLOGY

Abbreviations

- Atypical lipomatous tumor (ALT)

Synonyms

- Well-differentiated liposarcoma

Definitions

- Intermediate (locally aggressive, nonmetastasizing) lipogenic neoplasm composed of atypical adipocytes

CLINICAL ISSUES

Epidemiology

- Incidence
  - Accounts for 40-45% of all liposarcomas
  - Most frequently in deep soft tissues
    - Retroperitoneum, abdominal cavity, paratesticular region, mediastinum
    - Limbs
  - May also arise in subcutaneous tissue and very rarely in skin
- Age
  - Middle-aged to elderly adults
  - Extremely rare in childhood
- Sex
  - M = F

Presentation

- Deep-seated, painless, slowly enlarging tumor mass

Treatment

- Complete surgical excision

Prognosis

- In surgically amenable sites
  - Recur only rarely after complete excision
- Intraabdominal, retroperitoneal, mediastinal, or paratesticular lesions
  - Often recur locally and may be fatal
- Variable risk of dedifferentiation in extremities (< 2%) and in retroperitoneum (> 20%)

IMAGING

General Features

- Best diagnostic clue
  - Circumscribed, lobular mass
- Location
  - Deep soft tissues
- Size
  - Variable
  - Usually > 5 cm
- Morphology
  - Circumscribed, lipomatous lesion

MACROSCOPIC

General Features

- Well-circumscribed lobular neoplasms
- Color varies from yellow to white
- Fat necrosis may be seen in large lesions

Sections to Be Submitted

- Sample margins and representative sections of tumor
- Look for indurated, firm areas

Size

- May attain very large size

MICROSCOPIC

Histologic Features

- **Lipoma-like subtype**
  - Adipocytes show significant variation in size and shape
  - Enlarged, hyperchromatic-staining nuclei
  - Hyperchromatic and multinucleated stromal cells
  - Lipoblasts may be seen, but are not essential for diagnosis
  - Involvement of large vessel walls by atypical tumor cells
  - Prominent myxoid stromal changes may be present
  - Rare chondroid stromal changes
- **Sclerosing subtype**
  - Scattered bizarre stromal cells with hyperchromatic nuclei
  - Rare atypical lipogenic cells and multivacuolated lipoblasts
  - Fibrillary, collagenous stroma
- **Inflammatory subtype**
  - Prominent inflammatory infiltrate (lymphocytes, plasma cells)
  - Scattered atypical lipogenic cells/lipoblasts
  - Often edematous stroma
- **Spindle cell subtype (controversial; may be related to spindle cell lipoma)**
  - Atypical lipogenic cells
  - Slightly atypical neuroid spindle cells
  - Fibrous, fibromyxoid stroma
  - Alternate term: Fibrosarcoma-like lipomatous neoplasm
- **Heterologous differentiation rarely seen**
  - Smooth or striated muscle
  - Cartilage, bone

Grade

- Intermediate (locally aggressive but nonmetastasizing in absence of dedifferentiation) mesenchymal tumor

ANCILLARY TESTS

In Situ Hybridization

- *MDM2* and *CDK4* amplification can be identified by FISH
  - Immunolabeling can also be used

Genetic Testing

- Supernumerary ring and giant marker chromosomes
  - Contain amplified sequences originating from 12q14-15 region
  - *MDM2*, *CDK4*, *TSPAN31*, *HMGA2* are amplified

DIFFERENTIAL DIAGNOSIS

Lipoma

- Lobular growth pattern
- No or only slight atypia of adipocytes

- Lack increased number of enlarged and hyperchromatic nuclei
- No lipoblasts should be identifiable
- No amplification of *MDM2* &/or *CDK4*
- Hibernoma can be considered form in younger adults, which shows brown fat differentiation

Spindle Cell and Pleomorphic Lipoma

- Usually occurs in elderly male patients
- Arises usually in subcutaneous tissues of neck, shoulder, or upper back
- No or only slight atypia of adipocytes
- Bland CD34(+) spindled &/or multinucleated giant cells (floret-like giant cells)
- Rope-like collagen bundles
- Often myxoid stromal changes and cleft-like spaces
- Scattered mast cells
- No amplification of *MDM2* &/or *CDK4*

Sclerosing Lipoma

- Dermal-based neoplasms
- Typically present on scalp or hands of young adult males
- No atypical lipogenic tumor cells

Angiolipoma

- Subcutaneous nodules in young adults
- Often multiple lesions
- Often tender to painful clinically
- Forearm represents most common site
- Mature fat separated by small blood vessels
- Vascular channels typically contain fibrin thrombi

Angiomyolipoma

- Myogenic tumor cells expressing myogenic and melanocytic markers [HMB-45(+)]
- Currently considered type of PEComa
- Often associated with tuberous sclerosis
- Thick-walled blood vessels
- Predominantly renal/perirenal tissues

Pseudolipoblastic Granulomatous Foreign Body Reaction

- Multivacuolated, CD68(+) histiocytes
- No atypical lipogenic cells

Inflammatory Myofibroblastic Tumor

- Fascicles of myofibroblastic spindled cells in mixed inflammatory cell background
- No atypical lipogenic tumor component
- Expression of ALK1 protein in many cases (especially in children and adolescents) and *ACVRL1* (ALK1) rearrangements by FISH

Dedifferentiated Liposarcoma

- Abrupt or gradual transition from atypical lipomatous tissue to higher grade nonlipogenic component
- Atypical nonlipogenic tumor component with variable morphologic features, but typically high-grade spindle cell tumor
- Strong expression of MDM2 and CDK4

Massive Localized Lymphedema in Morbidly Obese

- Very large lesions (mean: 31 cm) in obese patients (mean weight ~ 400 lbs)
- Most involve thigh, some in calf, pedunculated lesions
- Overlying thickened with cobblestone appearance
- Striking dermal fibrosis, expansion of fibrous septa between fat lobules with reactive fibroblasts, numerous dilated lymphatic spaces, especially towards surface

DIAGNOSTIC CHECKLIST

Clinically Relevant Pathologic Features

- Gross appearance
- Organ distribution
- Age distribution

Pathologic Interpretation Pearls

- Atypical lipogenic cells
- Atypical stromal cells
- Often focal nuclear expression of MDM2 &/or CDK4
- Amplification of *MDM2* and *CDK4* detected by FISH analysis

SELECTED REFERENCES

1. Deyrup AT et al: Fibrosarcoma-like lipomatous neoplasm: a reappraisal of so-called spindle cell liposarcoma defining a unique lipomatous tumor unrelated to other liposarcomas. Am J Surg Pathol. 37(9):1373-8, 2013
2. Shon W et al: Cutaneous angiosarcoma arising in massive localized lymphedema of the morbidly obese: a report of five cases and review of the literature. J Cutan Pathol. 38(7):560-4, 2011
3. Manduch M et al: Massive localised lymphoedema: a clinicopathological study of 22 cases and review of the literature. J Clin Pathol. 62(9):808-11, 2009
4. Evans HL: Atypical lipomatous tumor, its variants, and its combined forms: a study of 61 cases, with a minimum follow-up of 10 years. Am J Surg Pathol. 31(1):1-14, 2007
5. Folpe AL et al: Lipoleiomyosarcoma (well-differentiated liposarcoma with leiomyosarcomatous differentiation): a clinicopathologic study of nine cases including one with dedifferentiation. Am J Surg Pathol. 26(6):742-9, 2002
6. Dei Tos AP et al: Primary liposarcoma of the skin: a rare neoplasm with unusual high grade features. Am J Dermatopathol. 20(4):332-8, 1998
7. Farshid G et al: Massive localized lymphedema in the morbidly obese: a histologically distinct reactive lesion simulating liposarcoma. Am J Surg Pathol. 22(10):1277-83, 1998
8. Kraus MD et al: Well-differentiated inflammatory liposarcoma: an uncommon and easily overlooked variant of a common sarcoma. Am J Surg Pathol. 21(5):518-27, 1997
9. Mentzel T et al: Lipomatous tumours of soft tissues: an update. Virchows Arch. 427(4):353-63, 1995
10. Nilbert M et al: Characterization of the 12q13-15 amplicon in soft tissue tumors. Cancer Genet Cytogenet. 83(1):32-6, 1995
11. Dal Cin P et al: Cytogenetic and fluorescence in situ hybridization investigation of ring chromosomes characterizing a specific pathologic subgroup of adipose tissue tumors. Cancer Genet Cytogenet. 68(2):85-90, 1993
12. Weiss SW et al: Well-differentiated liposarcoma (atypical lipoma) of deep soft tissue of the extremities, retroperitoneum, and miscellaneous sites. A follow-up study of 92 cases with analysis of the incidence of "dedifferentiation". Am J Surg Pathol. 16(11):1051-8, 1992
13. Azumi N et al: Atypical and malignant neoplasms showing lipomatous differentiation. A study of 111 cases. Am J Surg Pathol. 11(3):161-83, 1987
14. Bolen JW et al: Liposarcomas. A histogenetic approach to the classification of adipose tissue neoplasms. Am J Surg Pathol. 8(1):3-17, 1984
15. Kindblom LG et al: Atypical lipoma. Acta Pathol Microbiol Immunol Scand [A]. 90(1):27-36, 1982
16. Evans HL et al: Atypical lipoma, atypical intramuscular lipoma, and well differentiated retroperitoneal liposarcoma: a reappraisal of 30 cases formerly classified as well differentiated liposarcoma. Cancer. 43(2):574-84, 1979

ALT: Gross Specimen

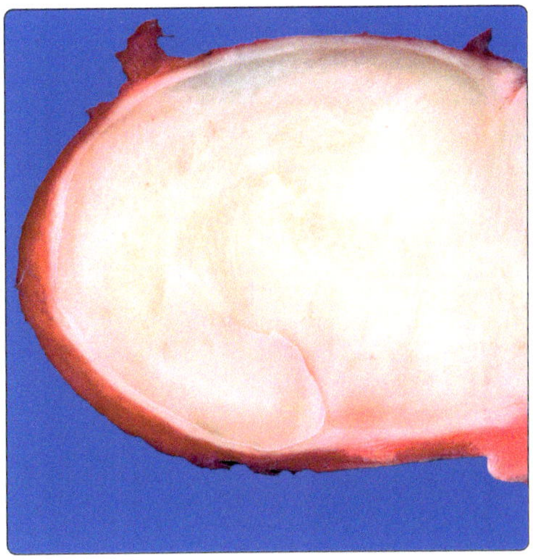

ALT: Atypical Nuclei

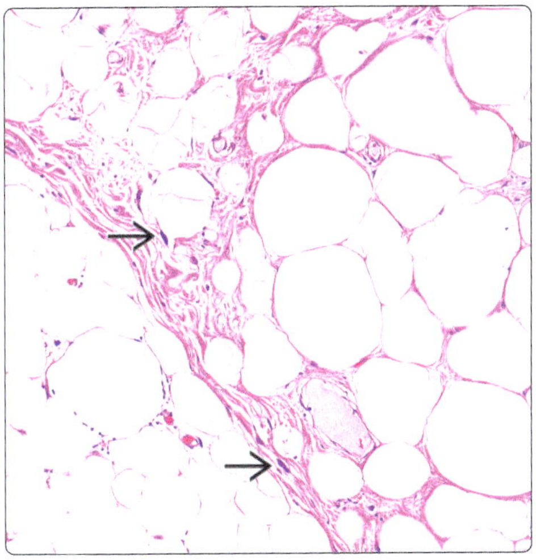

(Left) *Gross photograph shows an indurated, gray-white cut surface in this example of an ALT, in contrast to the surrounding nonneoplastic fatty tissue.* **(Right)** *Histologic examination shows the lipoma-like subtype of an atypical lipomatous tumor with variation in size and shape of the lipogenic tumor cells and scattered cells with enlarged, hyperchromatic-staining nuclei* ⇒.

ALT: Fibrous Septa

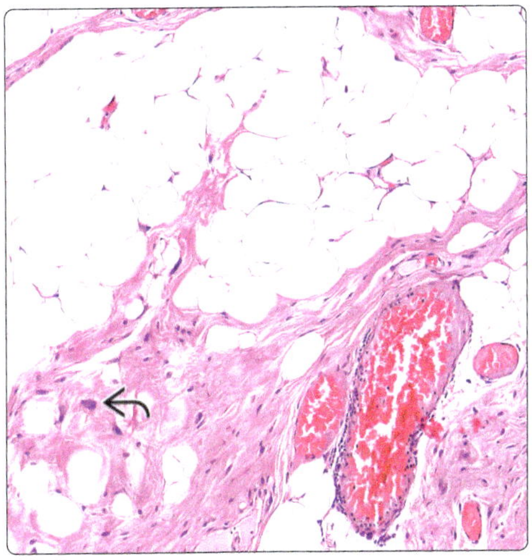

ALT: Lipoblasts

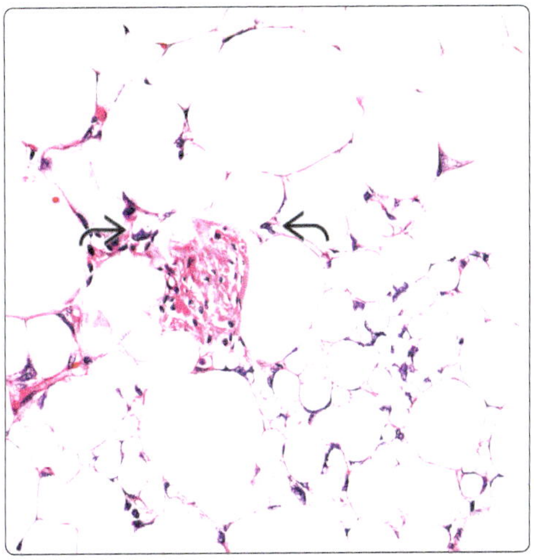

(Left) *Low magnification of ALT shows fibrous septa with enlarged cells containing irregularly shaped, hyperchromatic-staining nuclei* ⇒. **(Right)** *Examination of another example of ALT shows scattered lipoblasts* ⇒ *in a perivascular location.*

ALT: Lipoblasts

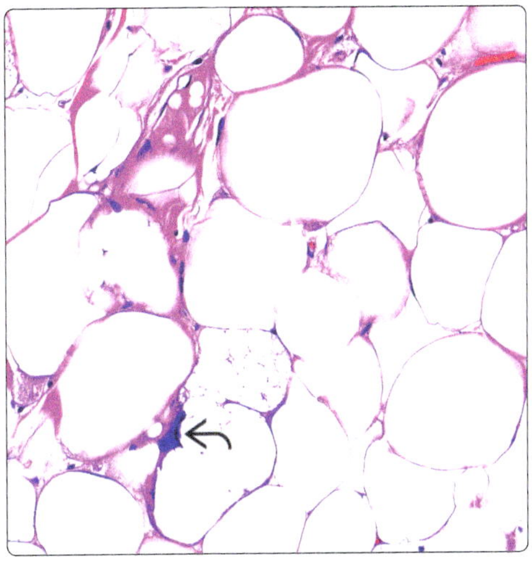

ALT: Lipoma-Like With Myxoid Stroma

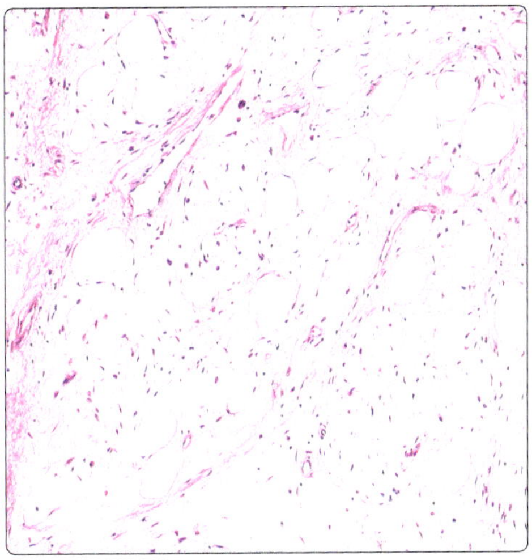

(Left) *Higher magnification shows multivacuolated lipoblasts containing hyperchromatic nuclei* ⇒. *Note the indentation of the hyperchromatic nuclei.* **(Right)** *Low magnification shows the lipoma-like subtype of an atypical lipomatous tumor with myxoid stromal changes.*

(Left) *Low magnification shows the lipoma-like subtype of an ALT with a focus of chondroid metaplasia. The cartilaginous tissue appears histologically benign.* **(Right)** *S100 immunostaining shows lipogenic cells of variable size and shape and multivacuolated lipoblasts.*

ALT: Chondroid Metaplasia

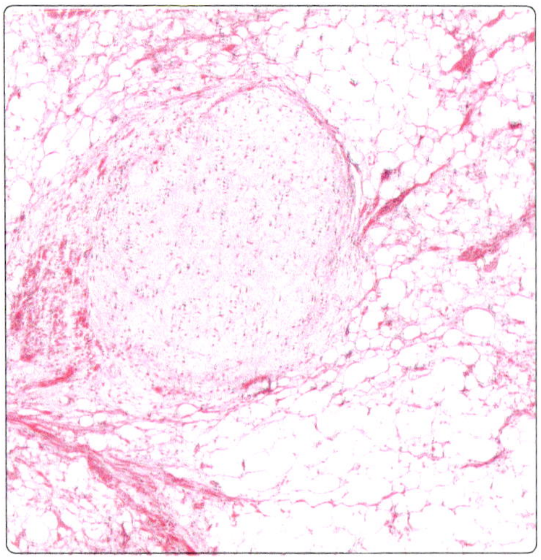

ALT: S100 Immunohistochemical Stain

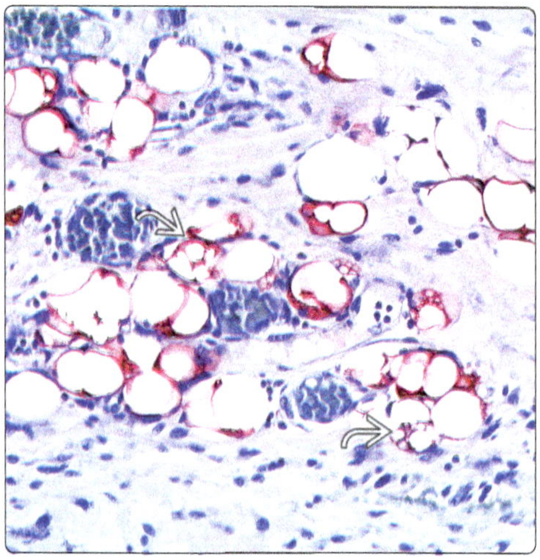

(Left) *MDM2 immunostaining shows nuclear expression in the atypical cells.* **(Right)** *CDK4 immunostaining shows focal nuclear expression in this atypical lipomatous tumor.*

ALT: MDM2 Immunolabeling

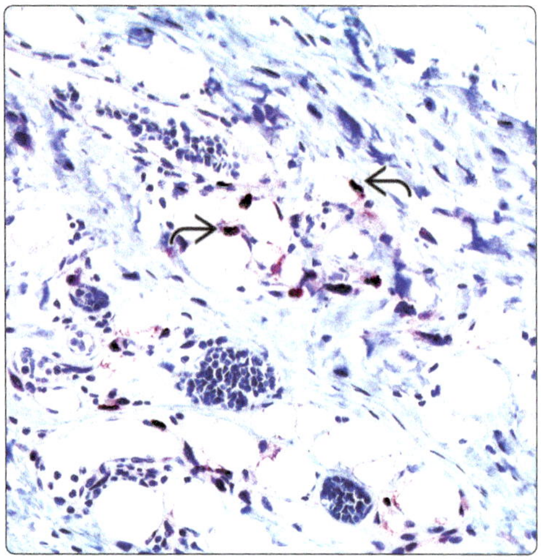

ALT: CDK4 Immunolabeling

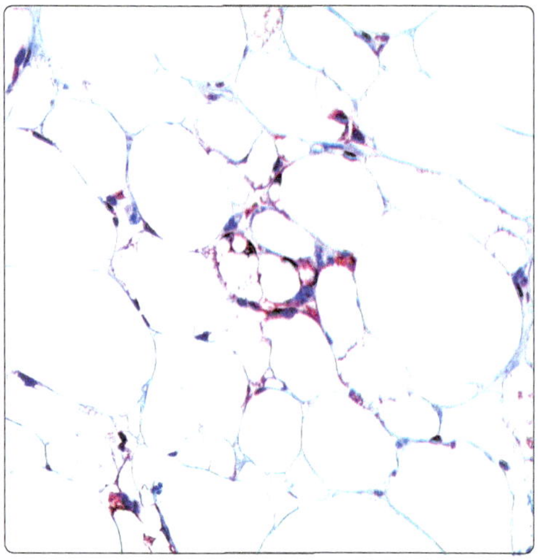

(Left) *Histologic examination shows scattered lipogenic cells including bivacuolated lipoblasts set in a prominent collagenous stroma in this example of the sclerosing subtype of ALT.* **(Right)** *Low magnification shows an example of the inflammatory subtype of ALT, with a prominent inflammatory infiltrate, edematous stroma, and only scattered atypical lipogenic tumor cells.*

ALT: Sclerosing Type

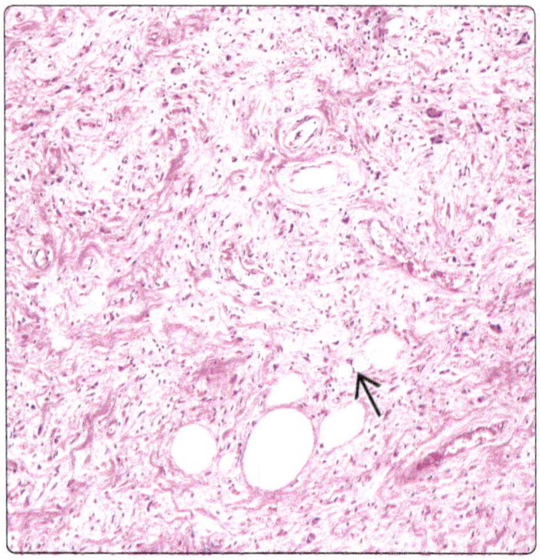

ALT: Inflammatory Type

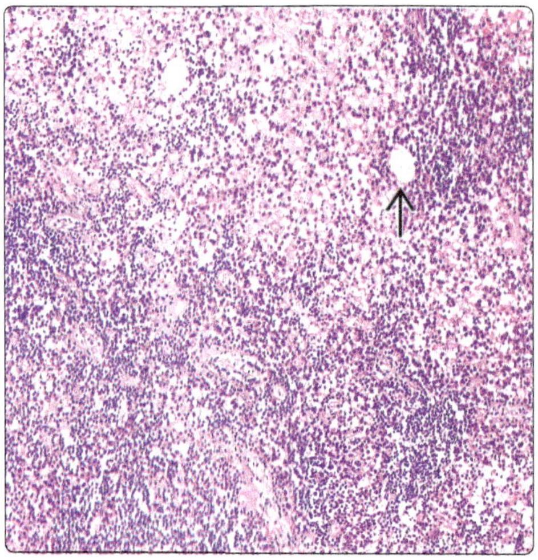

ALT Spindle Cell Type: Fibrosarcoma-Like Lipomatous Neoplasm

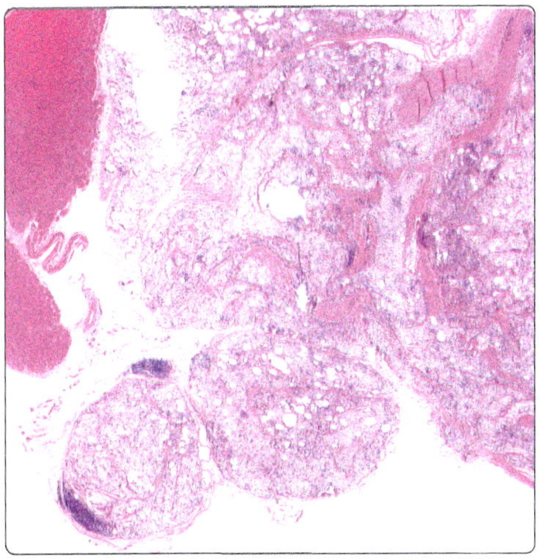

ALT Spindle Cell Type: Fibrosarcoma-Like Lipomatous Neoplasm

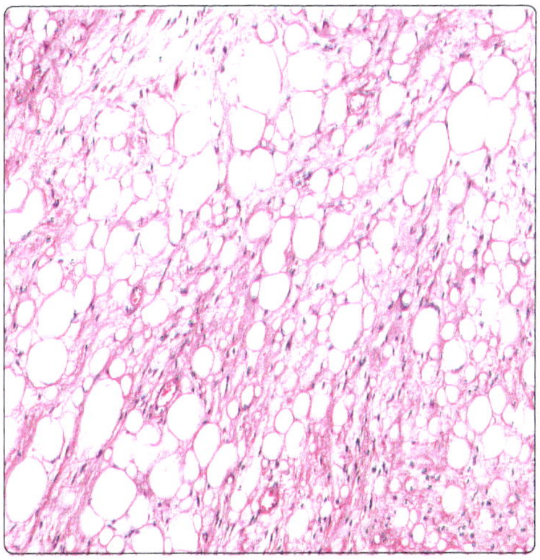

(Left) *Low-magnification examination of this spindle cell subtype of ALT shows a deep-seated lobular neoplasm. These may be more closely related to spindle cell lipoma and have also been termed fibrosarcoma-like lipomatous neoplasm.* **(Right)** *Higher magnification shows an ALT of the spindle cell subtype with atypical lipogenic cells admixed with slightly enlarged spindled tumor cells.*

ALT Spindle Cell Type: Fibrosarcoma-Like Lipomatous Neoplasm

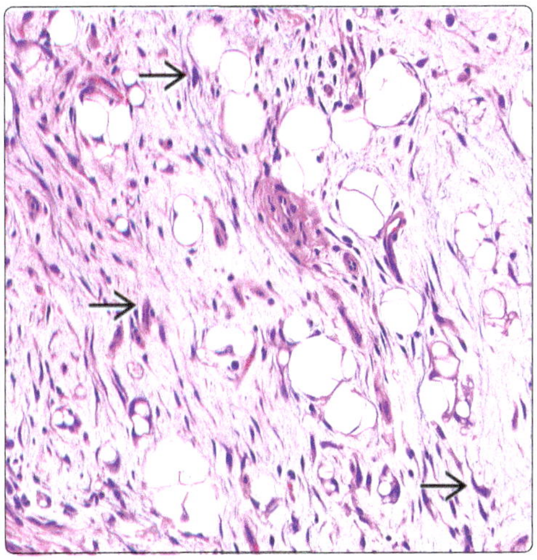

ALT Spindle Cell Type: Cutaneous

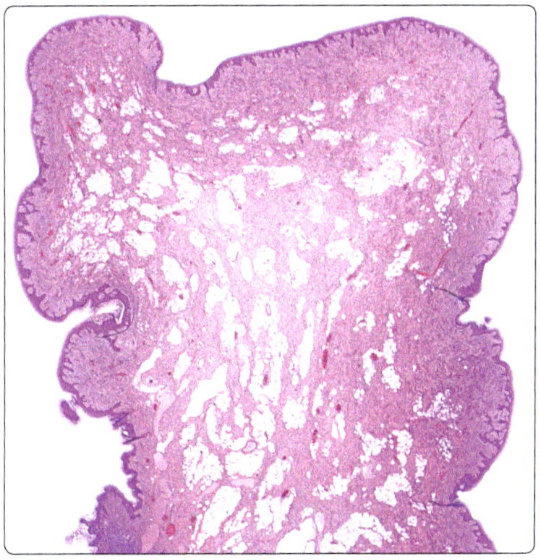

(Left) *High-power examination shows a neoplasm composed of atypical lipogenic and spindled tumor cells ⇒ with enlarged and hyperchromatic nuclei.* **(Right)** *Histologic examination shows a low-power view of a rare cutaneous ALT with a polypoid configuration mimicking a fibroepithelial polyp.*

ALT Spindle Cell Type: Cutaneous

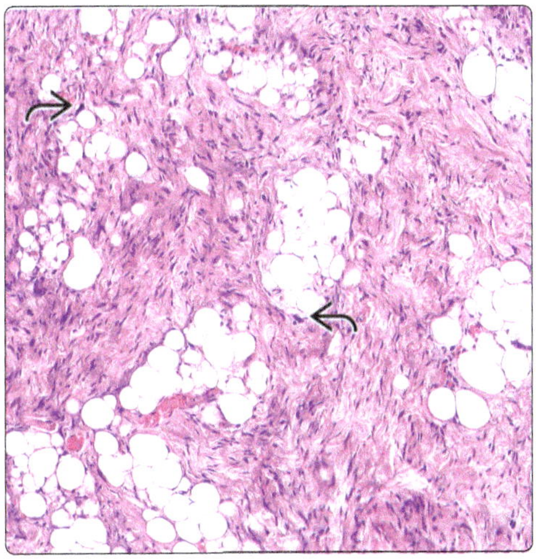

ALT Spindle Cell Type: MDM2 Amplification

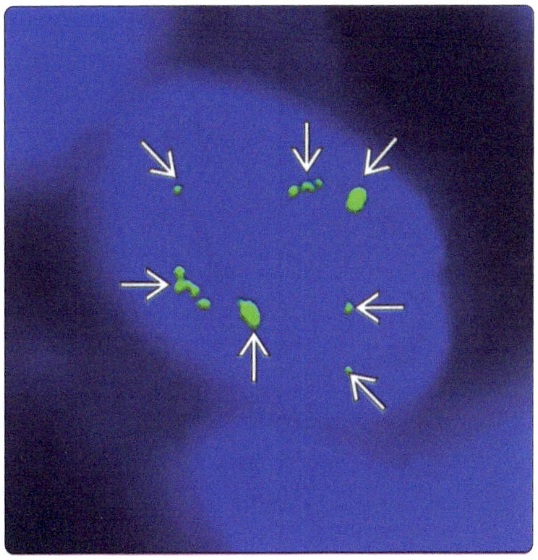

(Left) *Higher power examination shows a cutaneous ALT as an ill-defined dermal neoplasm composed of atypical lipogenic cells with enlarged and hyperchromatic-staining nuclei ↷.* **(Right)** *In situ hybridization FISH analysis shows MDM2 amplification. Note numerous signals ⇒ in an analyzed tumor cell nucleus.*

(Left) *This superficial lesion was well marginated, but its cut surface appears whitish rather than yellowish.* **(Right)** *The lesion consists of fat , cleft-like spaces , and well-aligned spindle cells with hyperchromatic-staining nuclei .*

Differential Diagnosis: Spindle Cell Lipoma, Gross Sample

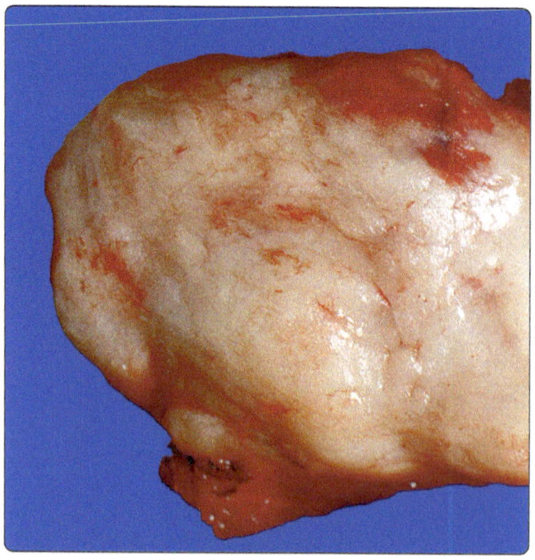

Spindle Cell Lipoma: Cleft-Like Spaces and Spindle Cells

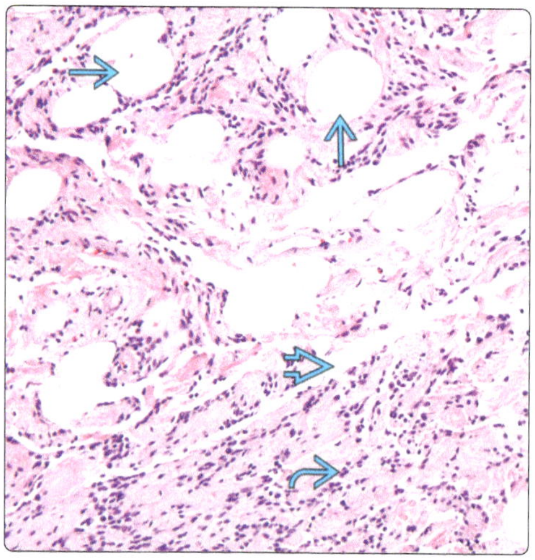

(Left) *The wiry collagen found in both spindle cell and pleomorphic lipomas is a diagnostic clue. Mast cells are often abundant in these tumors.* **(Right)** *Mast cells are very common in spindle cell lipomas and are identified by their metachromatic cytoplasm.*

Spindle Cell Lipoma: Wiry Collagen and Mast Cells

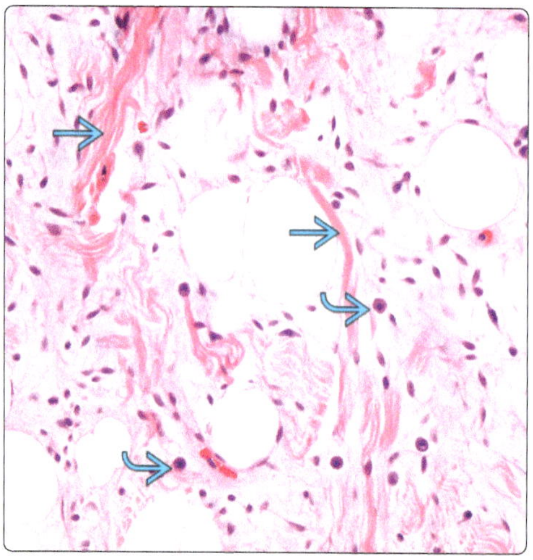

Spindle Cell Lipoma: Mast Cells

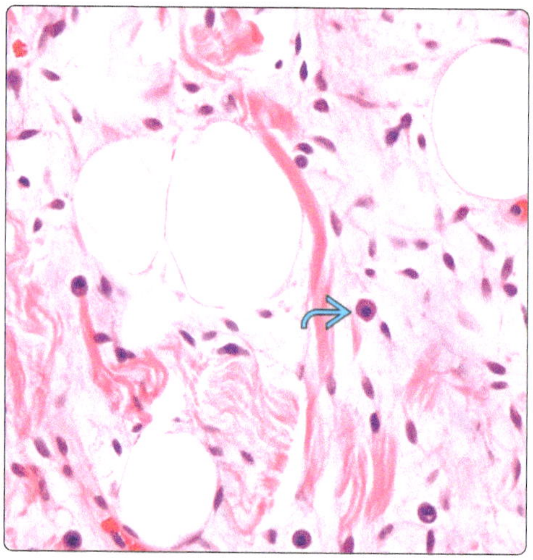

(Left) *In this image, this obese patient's right thigh is present at the left of the field and a massive lesion that originated from his right thigh, hiding his scrotum, is shown. Note the appearance of the skin overlying the process.* **(Right)** *Note the edematous appearance of the dermis and subcutis as well as the lymphangiectasia .*

Differential Diagnosis: Massive Localized Lymphedema in Morbidly Obese

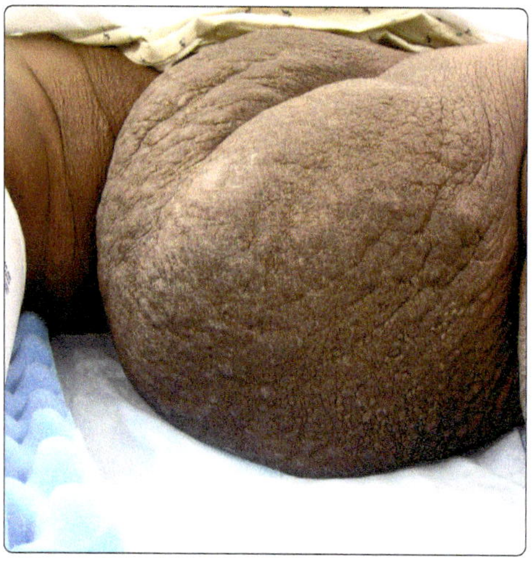

Differential Diagnosis: Massive Localized Lymphedema

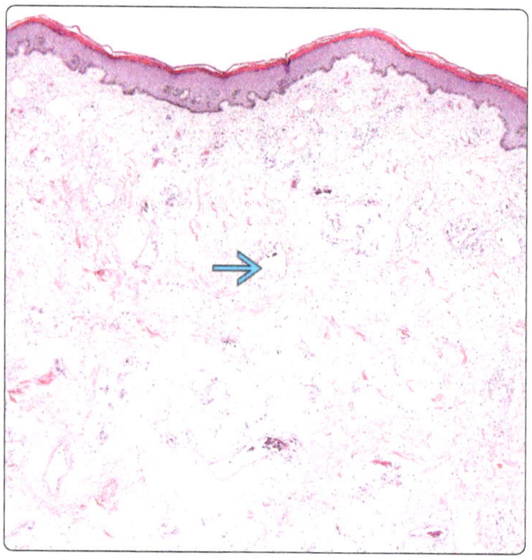

Differential Diagnosis: Massive Localized Lymphedema, Reactive Fibroblast

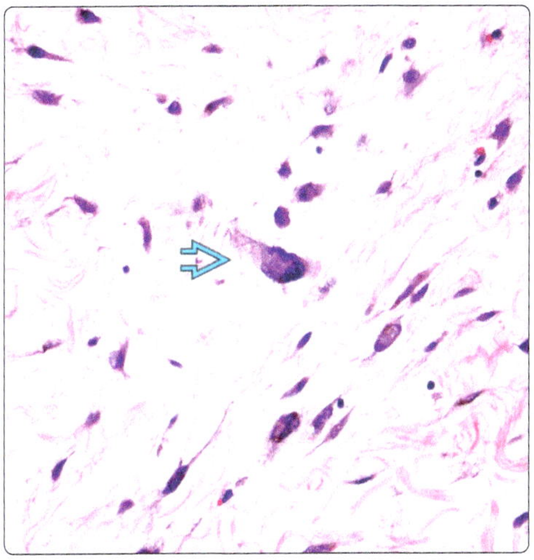

Massive Localized Lymphedema: MDM2 Immunolabeling

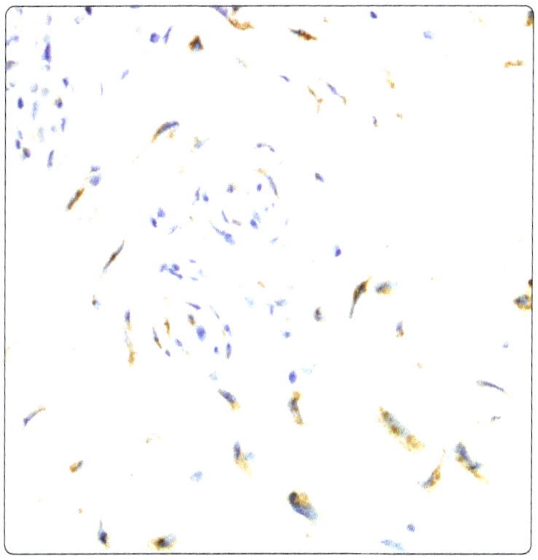

(Left) *The presence of reactive fibroblasts ⇨ in the stroma of massive localized lymphedema can raise concern for an ALT. However, the nuclei of these cells are less hyperchromatic than those of atypical lipomatous tumors.* **(Right)** *A lack of nuclear MDM2 labeling can be reassuring in the evaluation of massive localized lymphedema in the morbidly obese.*

Differential Diagnosis: Hibernoma

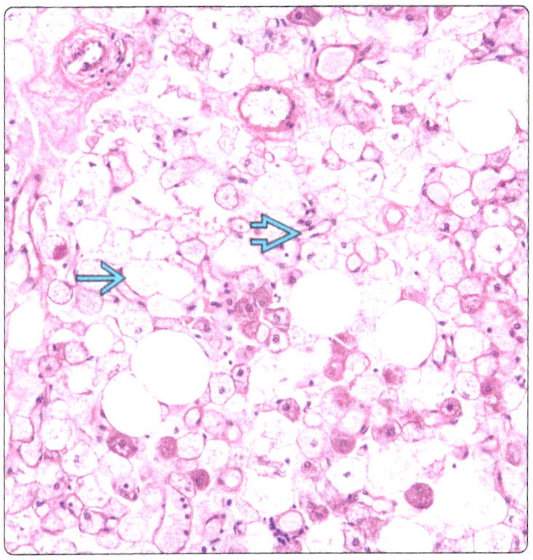

Hibernoma: White and Brown Fat

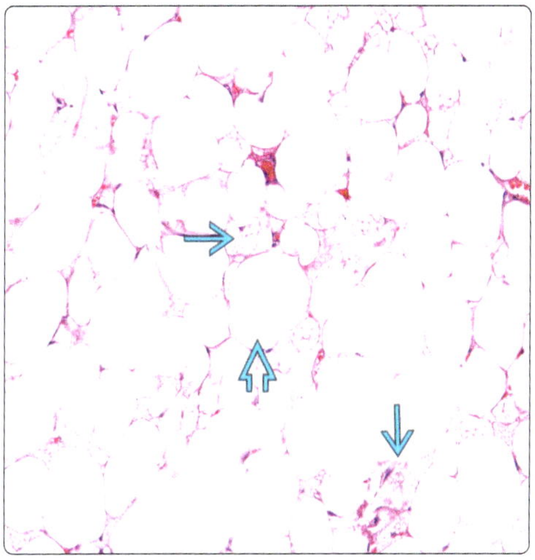

(Left) *These are essentially lipomas of young adults (arising in younger persons than usual lipomas). They are lesions with brown fat differentiation; the cells have microvacuoles → that contain lipid, and an associated capillary network ⇨.* **(Right)** *This example has a prominent white fat component ⇨ as well as the brown fat component →.*

Hibernoma: Numerous Capillaries

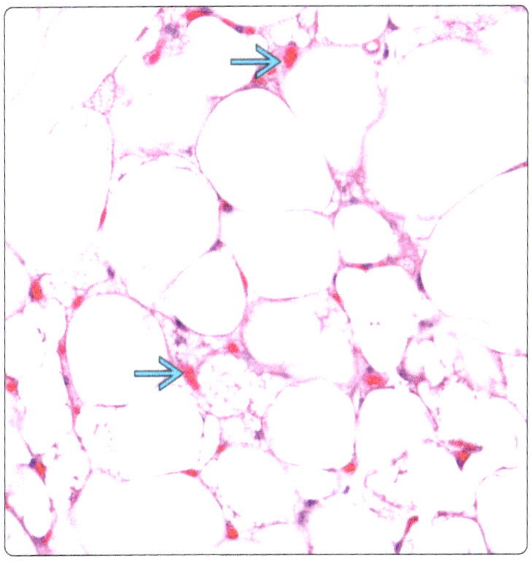

Hibernoma: High Magnification

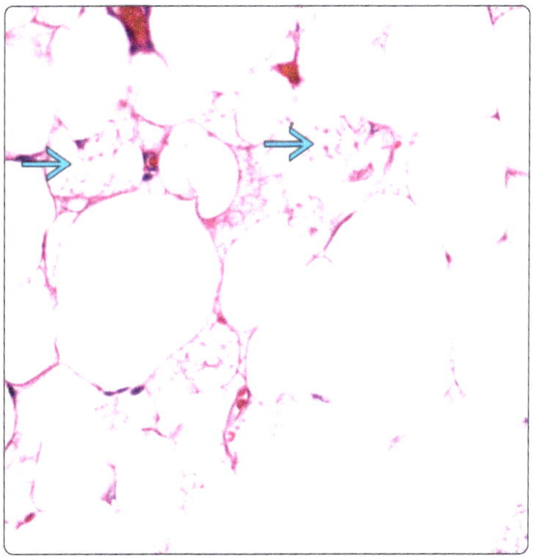

(Left) *Note the prominent capillaries → in this hibernoma, analagous to the rich vascularity in brown fat.* **(Right)** *Note the delicate microvesicular lipid vaculoes → seen in some cells in this hibernoma example.*

Soft Tissue Chondroma

KEY FACTS

TERMINOLOGY

- Benign hyaline cartilage neoplasm of soft tissue with predilection for hands and feet

CLINICAL ISSUES

- Low recurrence rate (15-20%)
- Recurrences controlled by reexcision

IMAGING

- Small, well demarcated
- Mineralized soft tissue mass
- Most common in acral extremities

MACROSCOPIC

- Median size: 1.6 cm
  - Range: 0.3-6.5 cm

MICROSCOPIC

- Well circumscribed and lobulated
- Mostly composed of mature hyaline cartilage
- Variable amounts of calcification
- Ossification common
- Granulomatous inflammation in 15% of cases
- Rare tumors with extensive xanthogranulomatous inflammation
- Myxoid matrix common (myxochondroma)
- Rare tumors with extensive stromal fibrosis (fibrochondroma)
- Morphologic variant: Chondroblastoma-like chondroma

TOP DIFFERENTIAL DIAGNOSES

- Synovial chondromatosis
- Tophaceous pseudogout
- Tumoral calcinosis
- Extraskeletal myxoid chondrosarcoma
- Calcifying aponeurotic fibroma
- Myxochondroid metaplasia of plantar foot
- Cutaneous mixed tumor with chondroid metaplasia
- Tenosynovial giant cell tumor

CT Scan of Soft Tissue Chondroma

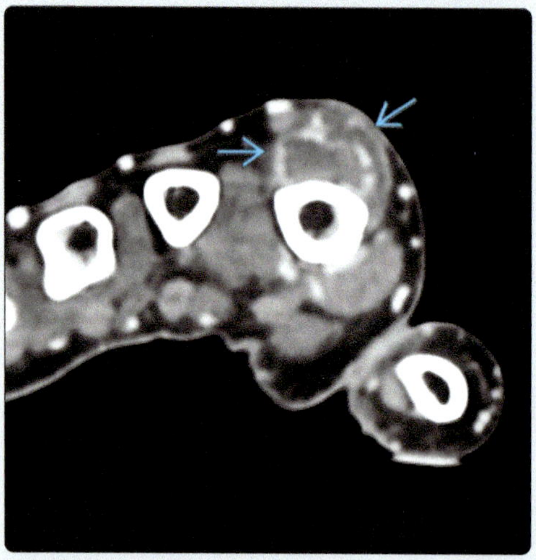

Lobular Architecture of Chondroma

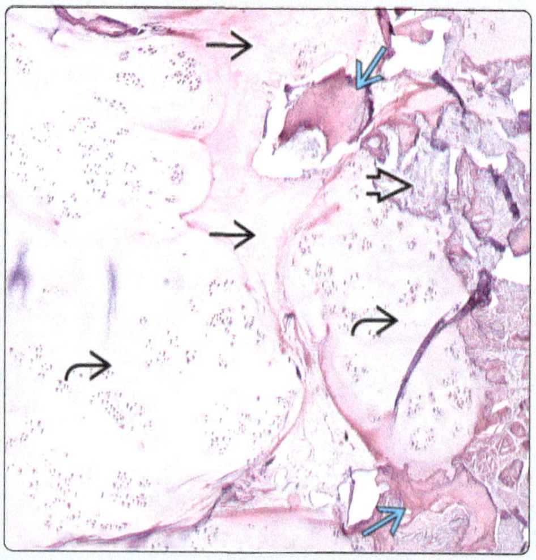

(Left) *Soft tissue chondroma typically occurs in the digits of the hands and feet. It presents as a painless, well-demarcated mineralized mass, as demonstrated in this CT of a dorsal index finger lesion. Note the peripheral distribution of mineralization.* **(Right)** *Soft tissue chondroma typically has a lobular architecture with islands of hyaline cartilage separated by fibrous bands. Matrix calcification and ossification are common.*

Cytological Features of Chondroma

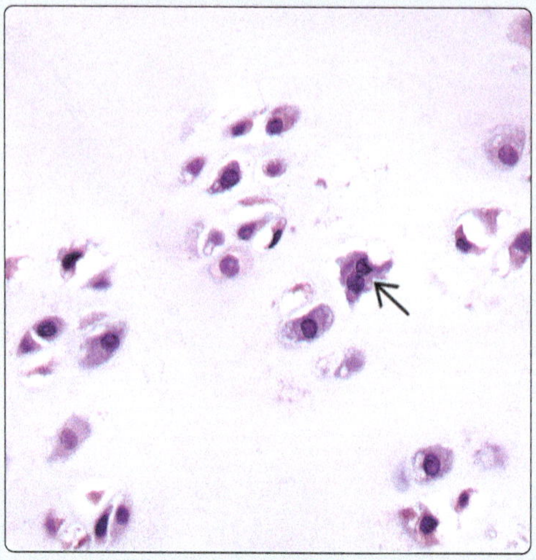

Calcified Hyaline Cartilage

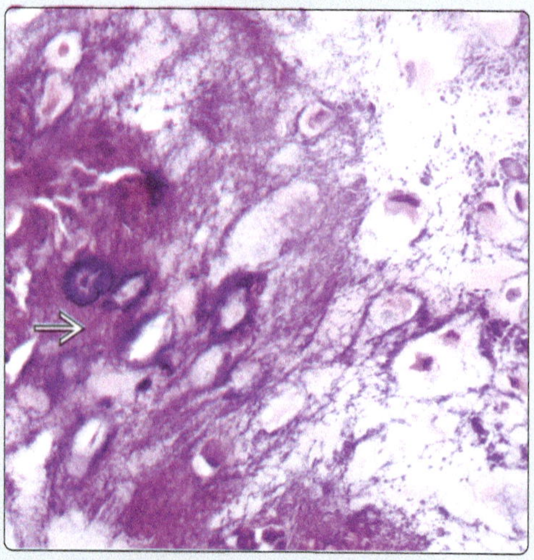

(Left) *High-power micrograph illustrates typical cytological features of soft tissue chondroma. The chondrocytes are often arranged in clusters, situated in lacunar spaces within a pale blue hyaline matrix, and have uniform round nuclei and abundant eosinophilic cytoplasm. Rare binucleated cells can be seen. Mitoses are rare.* **(Right)** *Areas of very dense calcification are common, illustrated by heavy basophilic staining of the cartilage matrix.*

TERMINOLOGY

Synonyms

- Extraskeletal chondroma
- Chondroma of soft parts
- Fibrochondroma
- Osteochondroma
- Myxochondroma
- Chondroblastoma-like chondroma

Definitions

- Benign hyaline cartilage neoplasm of soft tissue with predilection for hands and feet

ETIOLOGY/PATHOGENESIS

Neoplasm With Genetic Abnormalities

- Rearrangement of 12q13-15
- Trisomy 5
- Aberrations of chromosome 11
- *HMGA2* abnormalities

CLINICAL ISSUES

Epidemiology

- Incidence
  - Uncommon
    - Exact incidence unknown
- Age
  - Median: 4th decade
    - Range: Infancy to 9th decade
- Sex
  - F = M

Presentation

- Painless mass
- Most common in hands and feet (60-95%)
  - Especially in fingers (40-50%)
- Rare sites
  - Proximal extremities, trunk, head and neck, oral cavity, ear, upper aerodigestive tract, dura/extradural, skin, fallopian tube

Treatment

- Simple surgical excision

Prognosis

- Low recurrence rate (15-20%)
  - Recurrences controlled by reexcision
- No reports of malignant degeneration

IMAGING

General Features

- Best diagnostic clue
  - Small, well-demarcated lesion
  - Mineralized soft tissue mass
  - Acral extremity
- Location
  - Hands and feet
  - Often in vicinity of joint or tendon
  - No intraarticular or subperiosteal localization by definition
- Morphology
  - Most are calcified or ossified
  - Sometimes erode and deform underlying bone

MACROSCOPIC

General Features

- Well demarcated and bosselated
- Spherical or oval
- Rubbery or hard
- Sometimes soft, friable, gelatinous, or cystic

Size

- Median: 1.6 cm
  - Range: 0.3-6.5 cm

MICROSCOPIC

Histologic Features

- Well-circumscribed and lobulated subcutaneous tumor
- Mostly composed of mature hyaline cartilage
- Chondrocytes located in lacunae
  - Arranged diffusely or in small clusters
  - Some have enlarged nuclei and moderate pleomorphism
  - Very low mitotic rate
- Variable amounts of calcification
  - Granular stippled calcification that surrounds chondrocytes in lace-like pattern
  - Some with extensive calcification
    - Deep basophilia of cartilage
- Ossification common
- Granulomatous inflammation in 15% of cases
  - Epithelioid macrophages and osteoclastic giant cells
  - Most pronounced in heavily calcified tumors
- Myxoid areas and cystic degeneration in some
- Rare tumors with extensive xanthogranulomatous inflammation
  - Mimics xanthoma, tenosynovial giant cell tumor, or lipidized fibrous histiocytoma
- Rare tumors with extensive stromal fibrosis (fibrochondroma)

Morphologic Variant

- Chondroblastoma-like chondroma
  - Abundant myxoid matrix
  - Immature chondrocytes
    - Resemble cells of chondroblastoma of bone
      - Polygonal or elongated cells
      - Abundant eosinophilic or vacuolated cytoplasm
      - Eccentrically located, grooved or reniform nuclei

ANCILLARY TESTS

Immunohistochemistry

- S100(+) and ERG(+)
- Keratin (-) and SMA(-)

DIFFERENTIAL DIAGNOSIS

Tophaceous Pseudogout

- Wide distribution, including acral extremities
  - Predilection for temporomandibular joint

- Heavily calcified lesions with metaplastic cartilage formation
- Rhomboid-shaped calcium pyrophosphate dihydrate crystals
  - Positive birefringence under polarized light

Tumoral Calcinosis

- Predilection for large joints
- Calcium hydroxyapatite crystals (psammomatous)
- Histiocytic giant cells with intracytoplasmic calcifications
- Familial and nonfamilial cases

Calcifying Aponeurotic Fibroma

- Hands and feet
  - Especially palms of children
- Geographic areas of calcification surrounded by chondroid cells
- Fibromatous areas

Myxochondroid Metaplasia of Plantar Foot

- All reports from plantar foot, including toes
- Fibromyxoid background
- Areas with distinct stromal basophilia and chondroid appearance
- Cystic change common
- Reactive, nonneoplastic

Cutaneous Mixed Tumor With Chondroid Metaplasia

- Massive chondroid metaplasia in some cases
- Epithelial glandular structures should be present

Synovial Chondromatosis

- Larger tumors
- Most often in synovium of large joints, especially knee
  - Also found in tenosynovium of acral extremities
- More discrete lobular architecture and chondrocyte clusters
- Intrarticular loose bodies

Tenosynovial Giant Cell Tumor

- Localized forms also referred to as giant cell tumor of tendon sheath
- Similar location, most common in fingers
- Calcified soft tissue chondromas can have extensive granulomatous inflammation
- Osteoclastic giant cells
- Xanthoma cells

Extraskeletal Myxoid Chondrosarcoma

- Large, lobulated soft tissue mass
- Abundant myxoid matrix
- Thick fibrous septa
- Interconnecting cords of neoplastic cells
- Lacks true cartilage
- Necrosis

DIAGNOSTIC CHECKLIST

Clinically Relevant Pathologic Features

- Predilection for acral extremities

Pathologic Interpretation Pearls

- Features that can lead to misdiagnosis
  - Chondrocyte atypia
  - Increased cellularity
  - Extensive calcification and ossification
  - Granulomatous or xanthogranulomatous reaction
  - Fibrous and myxoid areas
  - Chondroblastoma-like features

SELECTED REFERENCES

1. Cho SJ et al: Chondro-osseous lesions of soft tissue. Surg Pathol Clin. 8(3):419-44, 2015
2. Sugiura Y et al: Convexity dural chondroma: a case report with pathological and molecular analysis. Clin Neuropathol. 34(1):13-18, 2015
3. Pace J et al: Extradural chondroma presenting as lumbar mass with compressive neuropathy. J Craniovertebr Junction Spine. 5(3):131-3, 2014
4. Shon W et al: ERG expression in chondrogenic bone and soft tissue tumours. J Clin Pathol. 68(2):125-9, 2014
5. Vescovi P et al: Soft tissue chondroma of the oral cavity: an extremely rare tumour localized on the hard palate. Case Rep Med. 2014:414861, 2014
6. Choi Y et al: A case of auricular chondroma. Korean J Audiol. 17(3):156-8, 2013
7. Choi Y et al: Extraskeletal chondroma of the scalp: an atypical location. Indian J Dermatol Venereol Leprol. 79(3):435-6, 2013
8. Raparia K et al: Chondroblastoma-like chondroma of soft tissue: report of the first case in the base of skull. Ann Diagn Pathol. 17(3):298-301, 2013
9. Shon W et al: Myxochondroid metaplasia of the plantar foot: a distinctive pseudoneoplastic lesion resembling nuchal fibrocartilaginous pseudotumor and the equine digital cushion. Mod Pathol. 26(12):1561-7, 2013
10. Smith EJ et al: Case presentation of soft tissue parapharyngeal chondroma in a pediatric patient. Am J Otolaryngol. 34(6):720-3, 2013
11. Thompson J et al: Cutaneous mixed tumor with extensive chondroid metaplasia: a potential mimic of cutaneous chondroma. Dermatol Online J. 18(3):9, 2012
12. Kim HS et al: A true chondroma cutis. J Eur Acad Dermatol Venereol. 23(5):612-3, 2009
13. Khedhaier A et al: Soft tissues chondromas of the hand: a report of five cases. Acta Orthop Belg. 73(4):458-61, 2007
14. Hondar Wu HT et al: Imaging and pathological correlation of soft-tissue chondroma: a serial five-case study and literature review. Clin Imaging. 30(1):32-6, 2006
15. Dahlén A et al: Fusion, disruption, and expression of HMGA2 in bone and soft tissue chondromas. Mod Pathol. 16(11):1132-40, 2003
16. Fetsch JF et al: Tenosynovial (extraarticular) chondromatosis: an analysis of 37 cases of an underrecognized clinicopathologic entity with a strong predilection for the hands and feet and a high local recurrence rate. Am J Surg Pathol. 27(9):1260-8, 2003
17. Tallini G et al: Correlation between clinicopathological features and karyotype in 100 cartilaginous and chordoid tumours. A report from the Chromosomes and Morphology (CHAMP) Collaborative Study Group. J Pathol. 196(2):194-203, 2002
18. Cates JM et al: Chondroblastoma-like chondroma of soft tissue: an underrecognized variant and its differential diagnosis. Am J Surg Pathol. 25(5):661-6, 2001
19. Ishida T et al: Tophaceous pseudogout (tumoral calcium pyrophosphate dihydrate crystal deposition disease). Hum Pathol. 26(6):587-93, 1995
20. Pollock L et al: Childhood soft tissue chondroma: a case report. Pediatr Pathol Lab Med. 15(3):437-41, 1995
21. Bridge JA et al: Biologic and clinical significance of cytogenetic and molecular cytogenetic abnormalities in benign and malignant cartilaginous lesions. Cancer Genet Cytogenet. 69(2):79-90, 1993
22. Humphreys S et al: Soft tissue chondroma--a study of 15 tumours. Histopathology. 10(2):147-59, 1986
23. Chung EB et al: Chondroma of soft parts. Cancer. 41(4):1414-24, 1978
24. Dahlin DC et al: Cartilaginous tumors of the soft tissues of the hands and feet. Mayo Clin Proc. 49(10):721-6, 1974

Lobules of Hyaline Cartilage in Chondroma

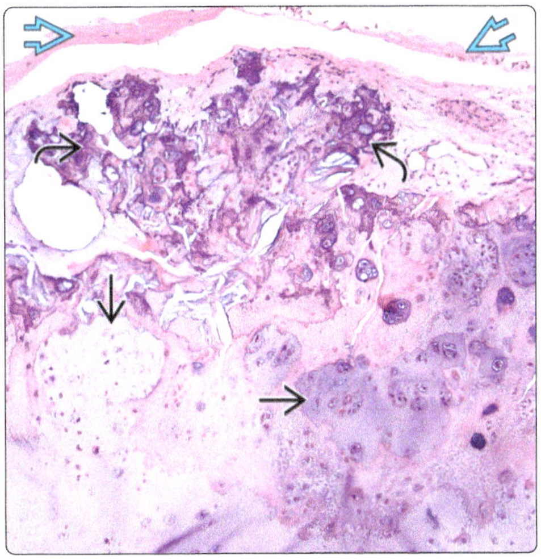

Calcification Is Common in Chondroma

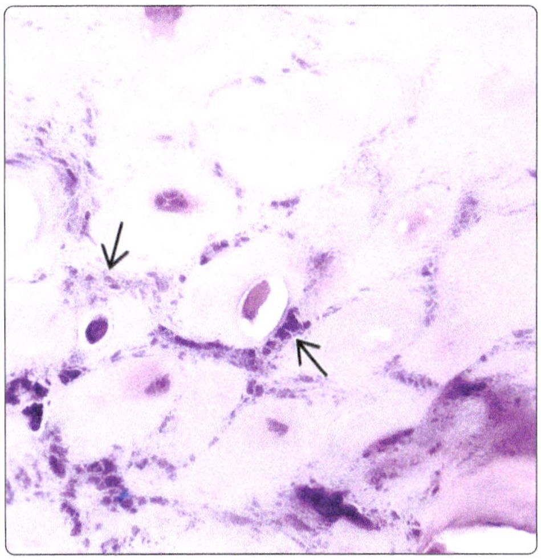

(Left) *Soft tissue chondroma is typically a well-circumscribed tumor composed of hyaline cartilage lobules* →*, with areas of calcification* ↷*, and sharp demarcation from adjacent soft tissue* ⇨*.* **(Right)** *Calcification is very common in soft tissue chondroma. It appears as granular basophilic stippling of the matrix, which often surrounds individual chondrocytes to form a reticular pattern* →*.*

Dense Calcifications

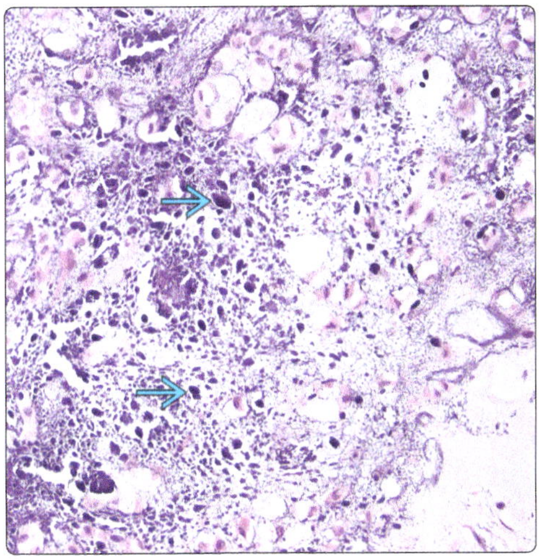

Granulomatous Inflammation and Giant Cells

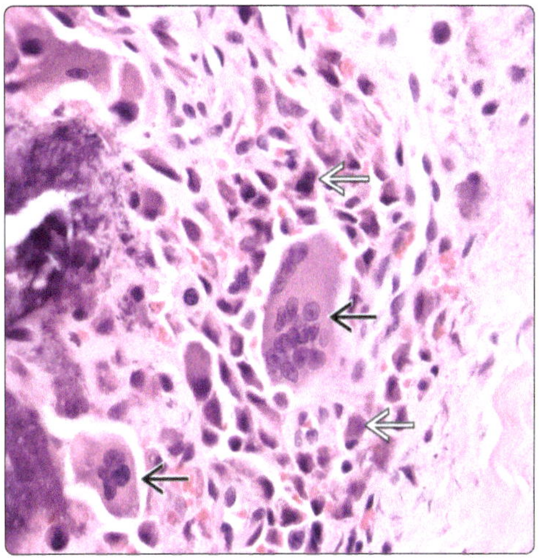

(Left) *This medium-power micrograph depicts very dense mineralization of the cartilage matrix consisting of coarse, basophilic particles of calcium* ⇨*.* **(Right)** *Granulomatous inflammation is often present in heavily calcified tumors. This micrograph illustrates epithelioid macrophages* ➡ *and osteoclastic giant cells* → *in a calcified tumor. When extensive, it mimics a tenosynovial giant cell tumor.*

Xanthogranulomatous Inflammation

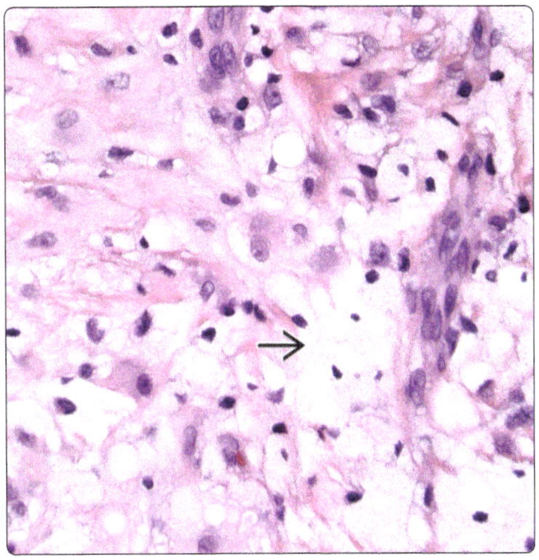

Ossification in Soft Tissue Chondroma

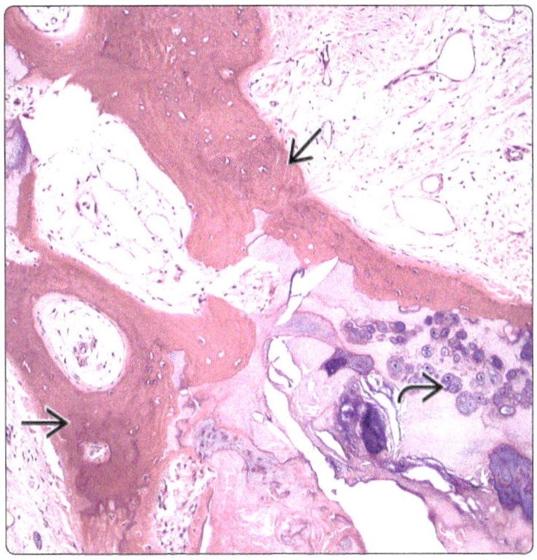

(Left) *Xanthogranulomatous inflammation can be present in soft tissue chondroma, consisting of sheets or clusters of foamy histiocytes* →*. When extensive, such a tumor can be mistaken for a xanthoma or tenosynovial giant cell tumor.* **(Right)** *Ossification* → *is common in soft tissue chondroma and can sometimes be extensive, as illustrated here. It can be located either at the center or periphery of the tumor and is formed via endochondral ossification of calcified cartilage matrix* ↷*.*

(Left) *This CT depicts a mineralized soft tissue chondroma involving the plantar soft tissue adjacent to the 4th metatarsal. Soft tissue chondroma has a predilection for the hands and feet, often near a joint or tendon.* **(Right)** *This low-power micrograph illustrates well-defined lobular architecture in a soft tissue chondroma consisting of cartilaginous lobules separated by fibrous bands. Note the deeply basophilic calcium deposits within the centers of the lobules.*

CT Scan of Soft Tissue Chondroma of Foot

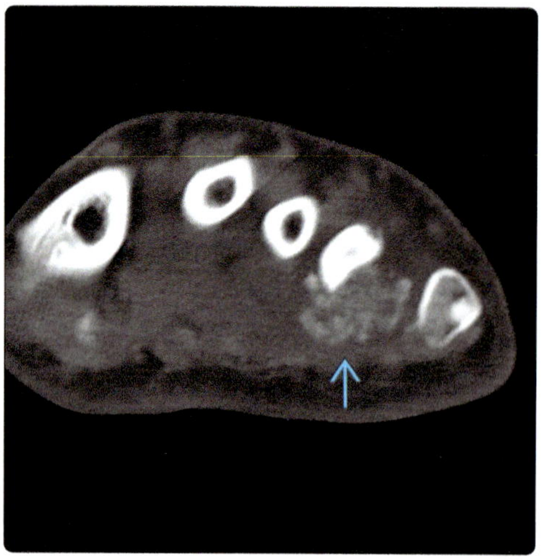

Lobular Architecture and Calcification

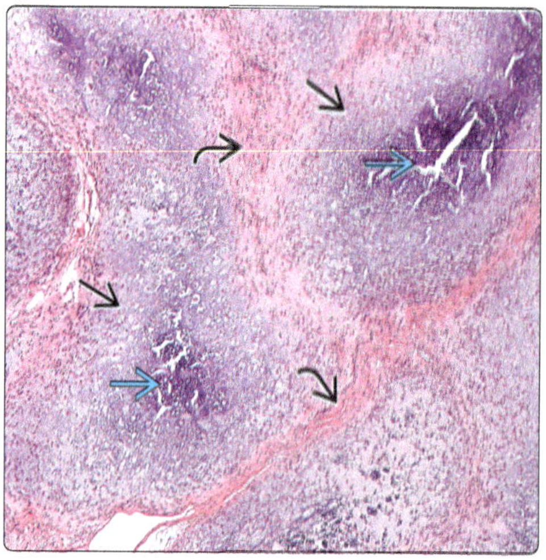

(Left) *This high-power micrograph of a densely calcified tumor depicts finely granular and coarse calcium deposits. The hyaline matrix is degenerated, and the chondrocytes are no longer contained within lacunae.* **(Right)** *Some tumors have an extensive myxoid matrix, where chondrocytes assume elongated and stellate configurations, sometimes interconnecting with each other to form a network, mimicking extraskeletal myxoid chondrosarcoma. Such tumors have been called myxochondromas.*

Calcified Cartilage Matrix

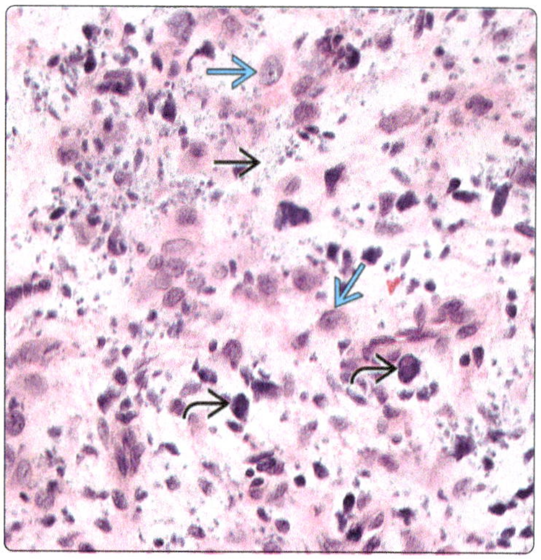

Extensive Myxoid Matrix

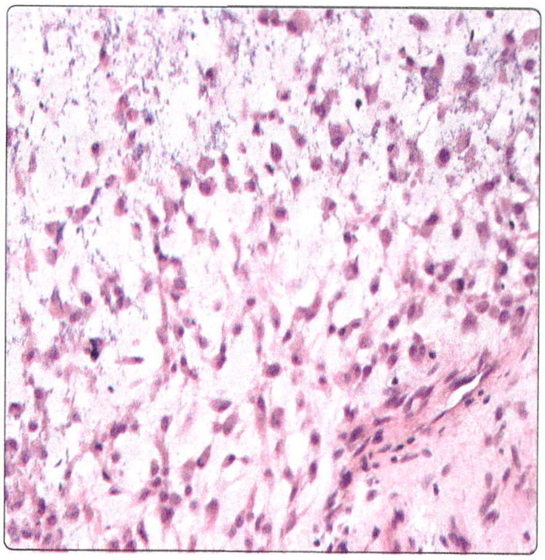

(Left) *In the myxoid areas, the chondrocytes lose their lacunae and assume stellate shapes. There are also rounded cells that resemble chondroblasts, with abundant eosinophilic cytoplasm and eccentric grooved or reniform nuclei.* **(Right)** *Soft tissue chondroma can have extensive fibrosis, as exemplified by the numerous collagen bundles traversing this tumor. Tumors with extensive fibrosis are sometimes referred to as fibrochondromas.*

Stellate and Chondroblastoma-Like Cells

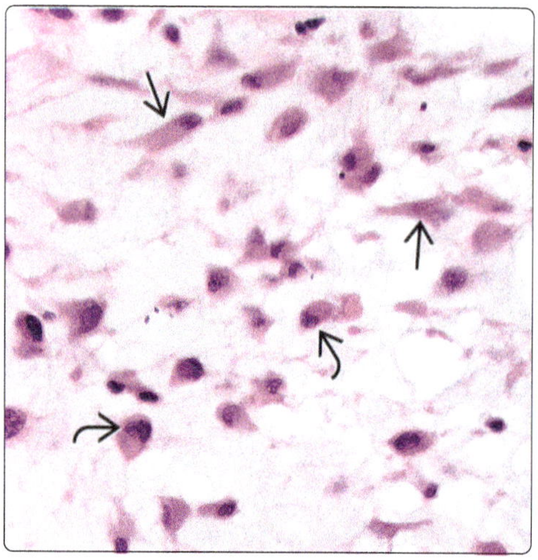

Fibrocollagenous Matrix

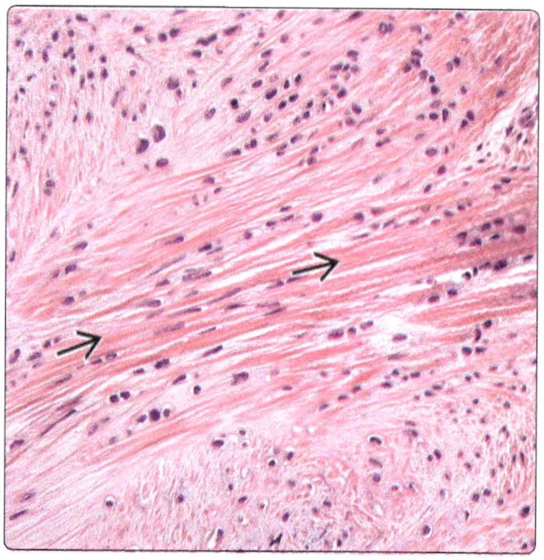

Circumscription and Lobular Architecture

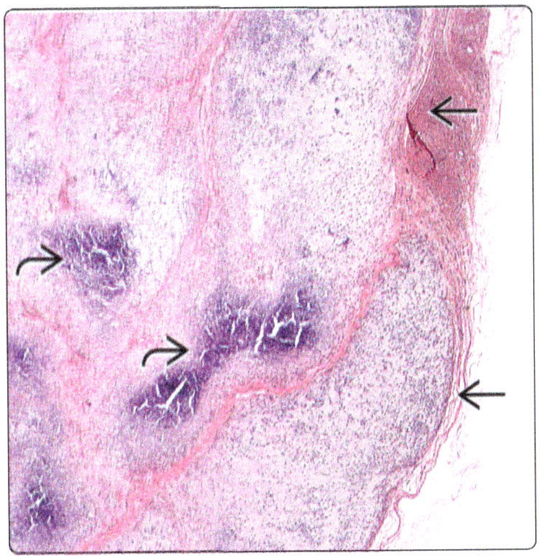

Calcification and Increased Cellularity

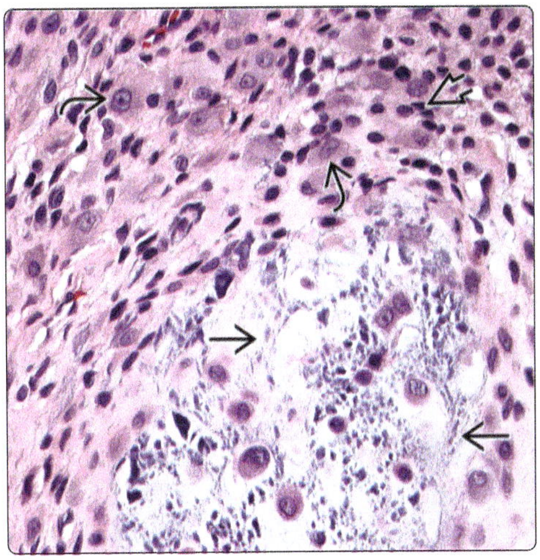

(Left) *Soft tissue chondroma is well circumscribed and well demarcated from adjacent soft tissues* ➡. *It typically has a multilobular architecture, as shown here, and zones of calcification* ↷. **(Right)** *This micrograph illustrates a zone of calcified matrix* ➡ *surrounded by an area of increased cellularity. The cellular area is comprised of a mixture of chondrocytes devoid of lacunae* ↷ *and mononuclear inflammatory cells* ⇨ *and resembles tenosynovial giant cell tumor.*

Areas of Increased Cellularity

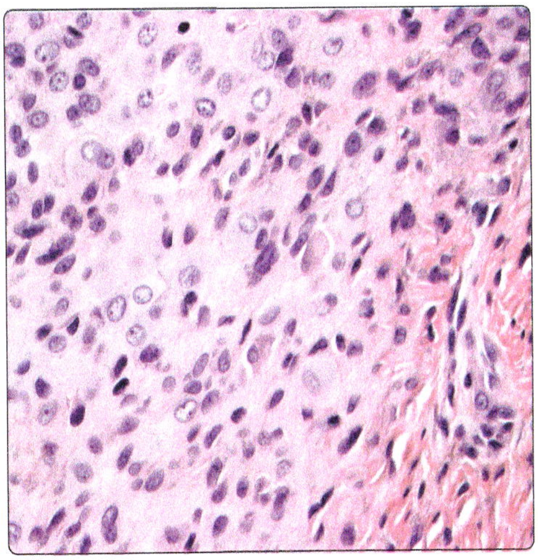

Degenerative Cytologic Atypia

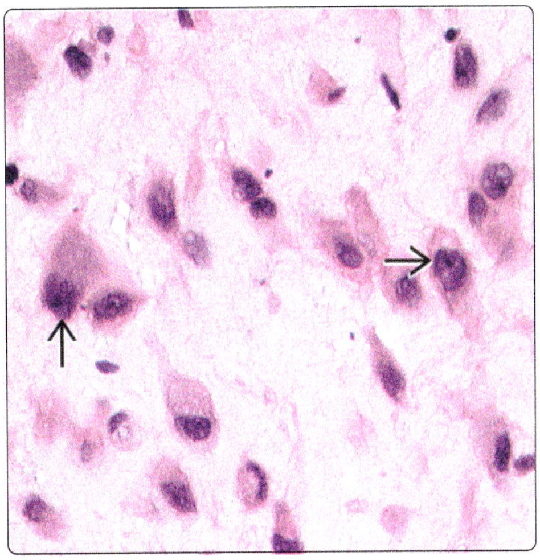

(Left) *Areas of increased cellularity can be present in soft tissue chondroma, as exemplified here, and do not portend a more aggressive behavior.* **(Right)** *Degenerative cytologic atypia is not uncommon in soft tissue chondroma. This high-power micrograph illustrates chondrocytes with nuclear enlargement* ➡ *and pleomorphism, which out of context would be suspicious for chondrosarcoma.*

Chondroblastoma-Like Features

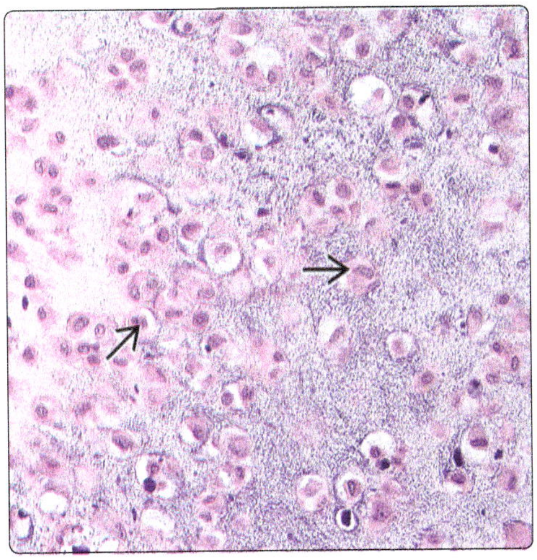

Cystic Degeneration of Matrix

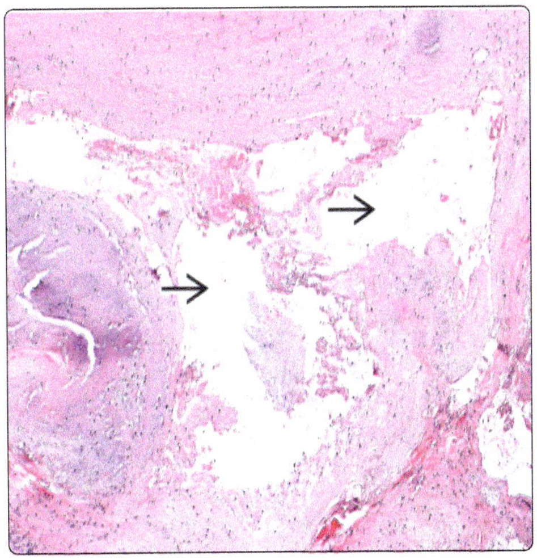

(Left) *This heavily calcified soft tissue chondroma contains cells with abundant eosinophilic cytoplasm and eccentric nuclei with reniform and grooved shapes* ➡, *resembling the cells of a chondroblastoma.* **(Right)** *Cystic degeneration can occur in some tumors, consisting of liquefaction of the hyaline cartilage matrix, as seen in this foot lesion* ➡.

KEY FACTS

TERMINOLOGY

- Primary cutaneous osteoma cutis
- Metaplastic (secondary) ossification

ETIOLOGY/PATHOGENESIS

- Primary: May be part of Albright hereditary osteodystrophy or other genetic syndromes
- Secondary: Associated with preexisting lesions, such as nevi, tumors, scars, and ruptured cysts

CLINICAL ISSUES

- Primary cases often present at birth or in early childhood; secondary cases in adults
- Dermal papule, plaque, or nodule
- Multiple lesions more common in primary types
- Excellent prognosis in vast majority of cases; no malignant potential
- Genetic cases may develop numerous debilitating lesions

MICROSCOPIC

- Appearance varies from small spicules to large masses of bone
- Mature-appearing bone, often with haversian systems and cement lines
- Osteoblastic activity may be present (especially in Albright syndrome), osteoclasts are less common
- Typically located in deep dermis &/or subcutaneous tissue
- Associated/precursor lesions often present in secondary ossification, including
    - Nevi, cysts, scars, pilomatrixomas, other tumors such as basal cell carcinoma

TOP DIFFERENTIAL DIAGNOSES

- Calcinosis cutis
- Chondroma
- Myositis ossificans
- Osteosarcoma

Osteoma Cutis Associated With Dermatofibroma

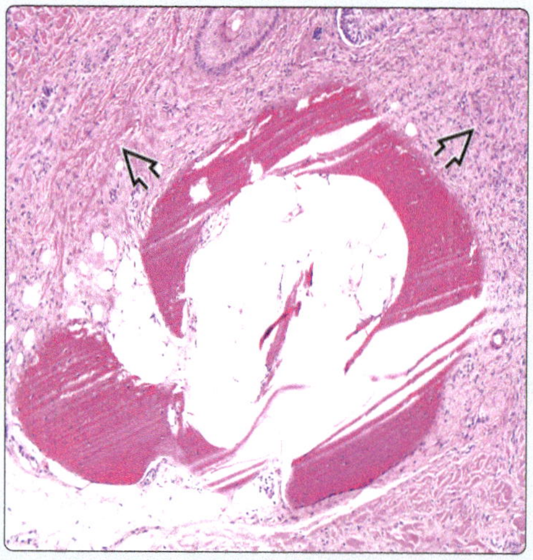

Osteoma Cutis Associated With Chondroid Syringoma

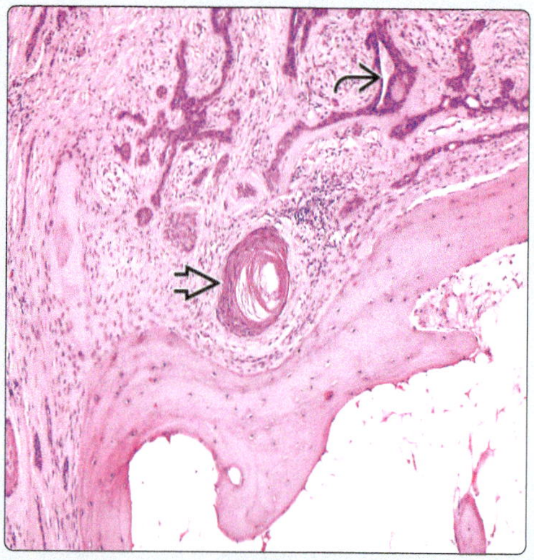

(Left) *Low-power view of an osteoma cutis arising in association with a dermatofibroma ⊡ shows a proliferation of mature osteoid surrounding large bland fat cells.* **(Right)** *Low magnification of an osteoma cutis associated with a chondroid syringoma (cutaneous mixed tumor) shows a proliferation of bland ductal ⊡ and folliculocystic structures ⊡ surrounding the bone.*

Osteoma Cutis With Chondroid Syringoma

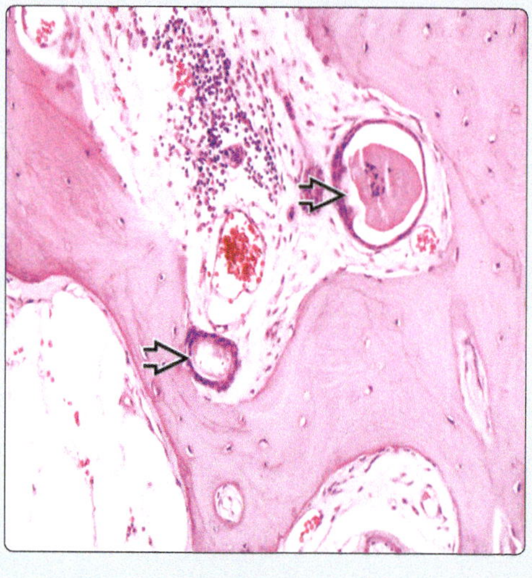

Osteoma Cutis With Mature Bone

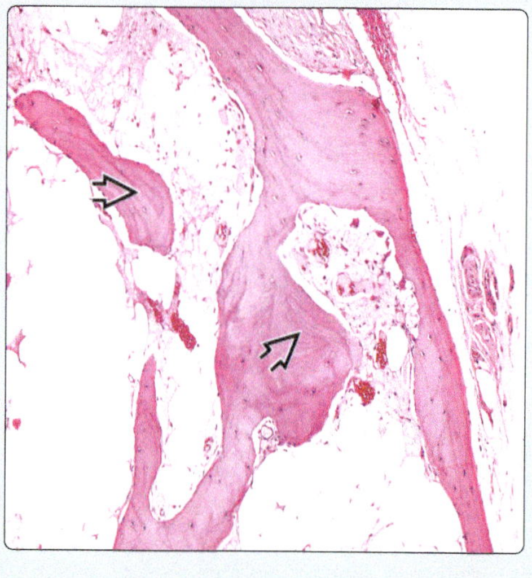

(Left) *Higher power examination of the same osteoma cutis shows a few bland adnexal ducts ⊡ trapped between the mature bony trabeculae.* **(Right)** *Low-magnification image of an osteoma cutis shows mature bone-forming trabeculae with cement lines ⊡ surrounding adipocytes and small blood vessels.*

TERMINOLOGY

Synonyms

- Primary cutaneous osteoma cutis
- Metaplastic (secondary) ossification
- Cutaneous ossification

Definitions

- Primary or secondary cutaneous mature bone formation

ETIOLOGY/PATHOGENESIS

Primary (Rare)

- Often genetic or developmental in origin; presents at early age
- May be part of Albright hereditary osteodystrophy or other genetic syndromes
  - Albright: X-linked dominant condition associated with characteristic facies, mental retardation, basal ganglia calcification, and cataracts
  - Other rare syndromes include congenital plaque-like osteomatosis, progressive osseous heteroplasia, and fibrodysplasia ossificans progressiva

Secondary (Common)

- Associated with preexisting lesions, such as nevi, benign tumors (including adnexal tumors, especially pilomatrixomas), basal cell carcinoma, scars, acne, and ruptured cysts

CLINICAL ISSUES

Epidemiology

- Age
  - Primary cases often present at birth or in early childhood
  - Secondary cases typically present in adulthood

Site

- Variable, but often involve extremities or face

Presentation

- Dermal papule, plaque, or nodule
  - Multiple lesions more common in primary types

Treatment

- Surgical approaches
  - Complete conservative excision is not necessary but curative

Prognosis

- Excellent in vast majority of cases; no malignant potential
- Genetic cases may develop numerous debilitating lesions

MACROSCOPIC

General Features

- Nodular, dermal-based solid bony lesion

MICROSCOPIC

Histologic Features

- Appearance varies from small spicules to large masses of bone
  - Typically located in deep dermis &/or subcutis
  - Mature-appearing bone, often with haversian systems and cement lines
  - Cartilaginous precursor usually absent
  - Osteoblastic activity may be present (especially in Albright syndrome); osteoclasts are less common
  - Stromal fat may be present
  - Hematopoietic cells occasionally present
- Transepidermal elimination may be seen, particularly in plaque-like osteomas
- Associated/precursor lesions often present in secondary ossification, including
  - Nevi (especially on face)
  - Pilomatrixomas (often ruptured lesions)
  - Basal cell carcinomas
  - Other tumors, including trichoepitheliomas, hemangiomas, schwannomas, lipomas, and dermatofibromas
  - Cysts, including epidermoid and pilar (tricholemmal) cysts, especially ruptured
  - Sites of trauma, scars, injections, and previous infection
- Pigmentation has been reported in patients treated with minocycline or tetracycline

Cytologic Features

- Osteocytes, osteoblasts, and osteoclasts show bland cytologic features without atypia

DIFFERENTIAL DIAGNOSIS

Calcinosis Cutis

- Nodules of dense basophilic material typically lacking well-formed bone
- Peripheral rim of secondary ossification may form

Chondroma

- Very rare dermal or subcutaneous tumor
- Cartilaginous tumor, which often lacks mature bone formation

Myositis Ossificans

- Subcutaneous tumor showing shell of reactive bone
- Central proliferation of fibroblastic cells with tissue-culture appearance (similar to nodular fasciitis)

Osteosarcoma

- Exceptionally rare in skin, most cases likely metastatic or from underlying bone tumor invading dermis
- Proliferation of highly atypical epithelioid, spindled, and multinucleated tumor giant cells

SELECTED REFERENCES

1. Kim BK et al: Acquired perforating osteoma cutis. Ann Dermatol. 27(4):452-3, 2015
2. Painsi C et al: Multiple miliary osteoma cutis of the scalp. J Dtsch Dermatol Ges. 13(11):1185-7, 2015
3. Chabra IS et al: Evaluation and management of multiple miliary osteoma cutis: case series of 11 patients and literature review. Dermatol Surg. 40(1):66-8, 2014
4. Haro R et al: Plaque-like osteoma cutis with transepidermal elimination. J Cutan Pathol. 36(5):591-3, 2009
5. Burford C: Pigmented osteoma cutis secondary to long-term tetracyclines. Australas J Dermatol. 48(2):134-6, 2007
6. Thielen AM et al: Multiple cutaneous osteomas of the face associated with chronic inflammatory acne. J Eur Acad Dermatol Venereol. 20(3):321-6, 2006
7. Cottoni F et al: Primary osteoma cutis. Clinical, morphological, and ultrastructural study. Am J Dermatopathol. 15(1):77-81, 1993

PART I
SECTION 11
Histiocytic Proliferations

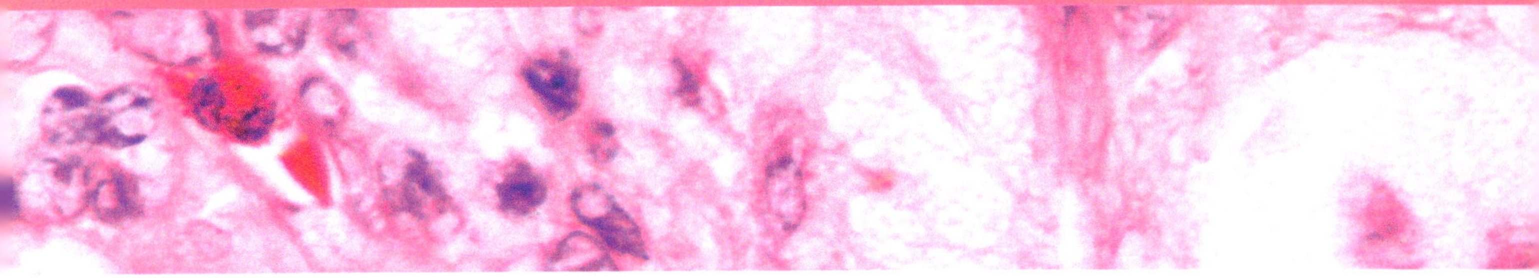

KEY FACTS

TERMINOLOGY

- Stable or regressing histiocytic lesion that usually occurs in childhood
- Form of non-Langerhans histiocytosis

CLINICAL ISSUES

- Majority in individuals under 3 years
- Visceral examples almost exclusively in infants and children
- Solitary cutaneous lesion in majority of cases
- Head and neck > trunk > extremities

MICROSCOPIC

- Mononuclear cells
- Multinucleated cells ± Touton features
- Variable lipid and foamy histiocytes
- Spindle cells
- Inflammatory cell background
- Eosinophils are frequent finding

ANCILLARY TESTS

- CD68(+)
- S100(-)
- CD1a(-)
- No *BRAF* mutations

TOP DIFFERENTIAL DIAGNOSES

- Langerhans cell histiocytosis
- Xanthoma
- Dermatofibroma/fibrous histiocytoma
- Reticulohistiocytoma
- Rosai-Dorfman disease/sinus histiocytosis with massive lymphadenopathy

DIAGNOSTIC CHECKLIST

- Multinucleated cells ± Touton features
- Mixed inflammatory background
- Negligible nuclear atypia

Juvenile Xanthogranuloma

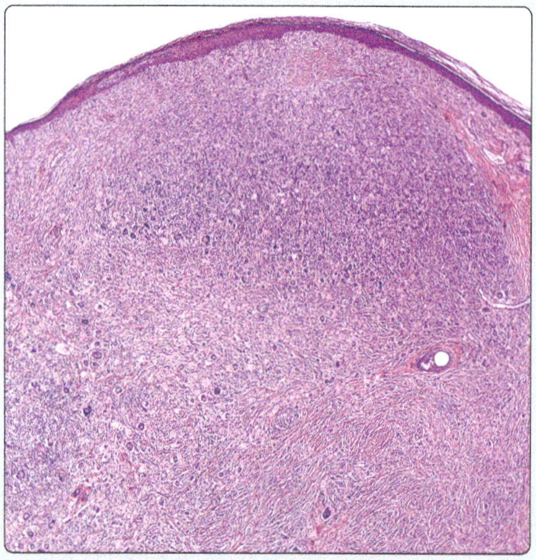

Juvenile Xanthogranuloma at High Magnification

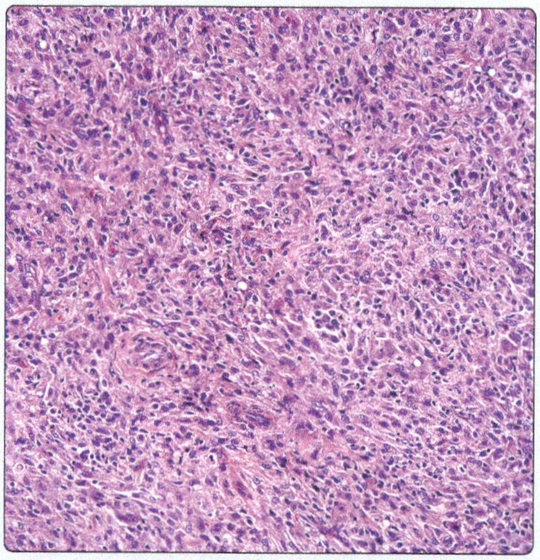

(Left) *This is a typical appearance of a juvenile xanthogranuloma removed from the face of a small boy. The lesion is uniform and cellular and proliferates in the dermis with no grenz zone.* **(Right)** *A cellular example at high magnification shows numerous mononucleated histiocytes associated with an inflammatory background composed mostly of mononuclear cells.*

Juvenile Xanthogranuloma: Touton Cells

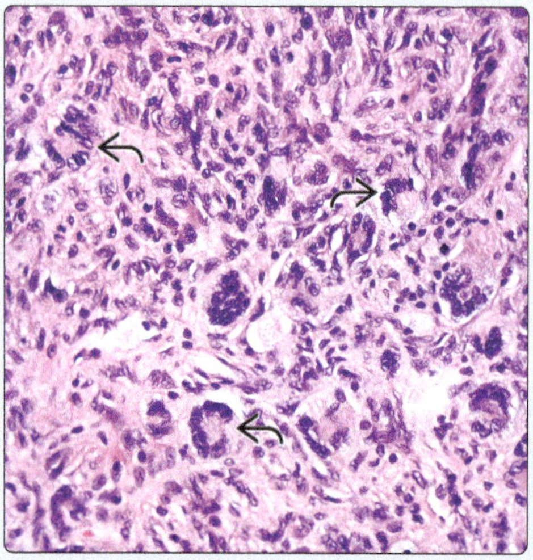

CD68 Staining in Juvenile Xanthogranuloma

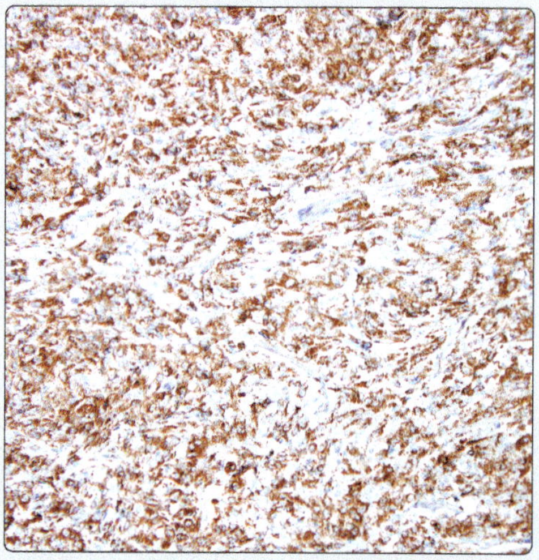

(Left) *Many Touton giant cells* ➩ *can be seen in this juvenile xanthogranuloma. The background cells are spindled to ovoid with eosinophilic cytoplasm, which shows only minimal lipid in this case.* **(Right)** *Essentially all examples of juvenile xanthogranuloma are reactive with CD68 (shown) and factor XIIIa by immunohistochemistry, but are negative for S100 and CD1a.*

TERMINOLOGY

Abbreviations

- Juvenile xanthogranuloma (JXG)

Synonyms

- Nevoxanthoendothelioma

Definitions

- Stable or regressing histiocytic lesion that usually occurs in childhood
  - Form of non-Langerhans histiocytosis

CLINICAL ISSUES

Epidemiology

- Incidence
  - Rare
- Age
  - Majority in individuals under 3 years
    - Visceral examples almost exclusively in infants and children
  - 13-30% in older children and adults
- Sex
  - Slight male predominance

Presentation

- Solitary cutaneous lesion in majority of cases
  - Head and neck > trunk > extremities
- Up to 10% of patients with multiple cutaneous lesions
- Up to 5% of patients with visceral-systemic disease

Treatment

- Simple excision
- Chemotherapy administered to rare patients with systemic disease

Prognosis

- Usually excellent
  - Most lesions regress or stabilize (including large visceral ones)
  - Rare deaths associated with multiorgan disease

MICROSCOPIC

Histologic Features

- Mononuclear cells typically predominate
- Multinucleated cells ± Touton features
- Spindle cells (typically minor component)
  - Variable finely vacuolated cytoplasm
  - Often lightly eosinophilic
- Variable lipid and foamy histiocytes
  - Minimal lipid in early lesions
- Inflammatory cell background
  - Acute and chronic inflammatory cells
    - Eosinophils are consistent finding
    - Neutrophils uncommon
- Negligible nuclear atypia
- Minimal mitotic activity

ANCILLARY TESTS

Immunohistochemistry

- CD68 expression; S100(-), CD1a(-)

DIFFERENTIAL DIAGNOSIS

Xanthoma

- Foamy histiocytes
- No Touton giant cells
- No background inflammation
- Can be associated with hyperlipidemia
  - Usually lesions of adults
- Benign

Dermatofibroma/Fibrous Histiocytoma

- Usually in adults
- Peripheral collagen trapping in cutaneous examples
- Overlying epidermal hyperplasia
- May show storiform pattern
- Eosinophils usually inconspicuous
- Intralesional hemorrhage, hemosiderin
- Benign
  - Rare metastases but no deaths associated with superficial lesions

Reticulohistiocytoma

- Benign histiocytic proliferation, which typically occurs in adults
- Brown-yellow papules at any site
- Nodules composed of brightly eosinophilic histiocytes, some multinucleated
- Nuclear atypia
- CD68(+), S100(-), CD1a(-)

Langerhans Cell Histiocytosis

- Usually presents as skeletal disease
- Atypical histiocytic cells with reniform nuclei
- Background of numerous eosinophils
- S100(+), CD1a(+), *BRAF* mutations

Rosai-Dorfman Disease/Sinus Histiocytosis With Massive Lymphadenopathy

- Usually involves lymph nodes but may present in skin and soft tissues
- Form of non-Langerhans histiocytosis
- Histiocytes and lymphoid aggregates
- Emperipolesis is key diagnostic feature
- Histiocytes are S100(+), CD1a(-), no *BRAF* mutations
- Most patients have good outcome

SELECTED REFERENCES

1. Salva KA et al: Possible association of cutaneous Rosai-Dorfman disease and chronic Crohn disease: a case series report. JAMA Dermatol. 150(2):177-81, 2014
2. Black J et al: Fibrohistiocytic tumors and related neoplasms in children and adolescents. Pediatr Dev Pathol. 15(1 Suppl):181-210, 2012
3. Janssen D et al: Clonality in juvenile xanthogranuloma. Am J Surg Pathol. 31(5):812-3, 2007
4. Dehner LP: Reawakening to the existence of juvenile xanthogranuloma. Am J Surg Pathol. 29(1):119-20, 2005

(Left) *The differential diagnosis can include Langerhans cell histiocytosis. Note the obscuring inflammation. The lesion is found in the paler areas.* **(Right)** *Note the ulceration. This is an excoriated lesion that present as a nodule in perianal skin. There is prominent chronic inflammation but a more eosinophilic zone.*

Langerhans Cell Histiocytosis, Dense Secondary Inflammation

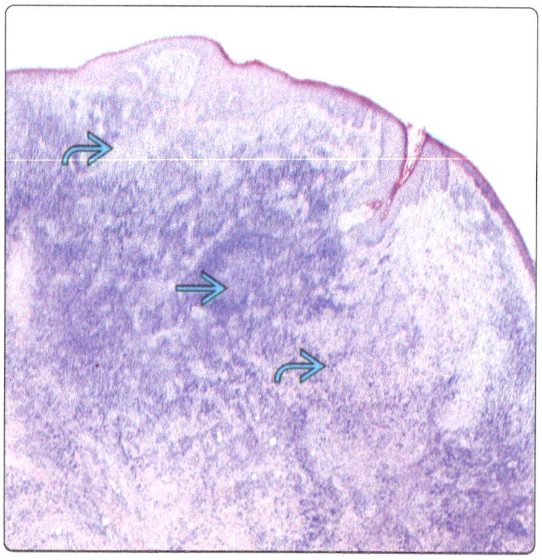

Langerhans Cell Histiocytosis

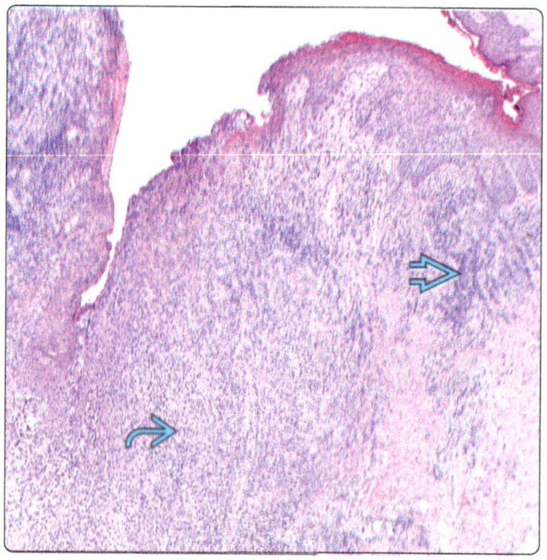

(Left) *This example lacks the classic backdrop of eosinophils, but the neoplastic histiocytic cells often display eosinophilic cytoplasm. These cells are known to harbor BRAF mutations, a feature they share with the histiocytes in Erdheim-Chester disease but not with the histiocytic cells in juvenile xanthogranuloma.* **(Right)** *The nuclei are enlarged and mildly atypical. Some of them have nuclear grooves. This field has a few plasma cells but not eosinophils.*

Langerhans Cell Histiocytosis, Eosinophilic Low-Magnification Appearance

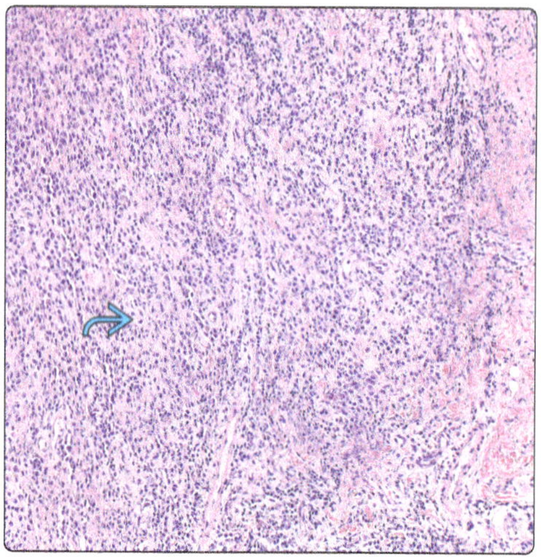

Langerhans Cell Histiocytosis, Cytologic Features

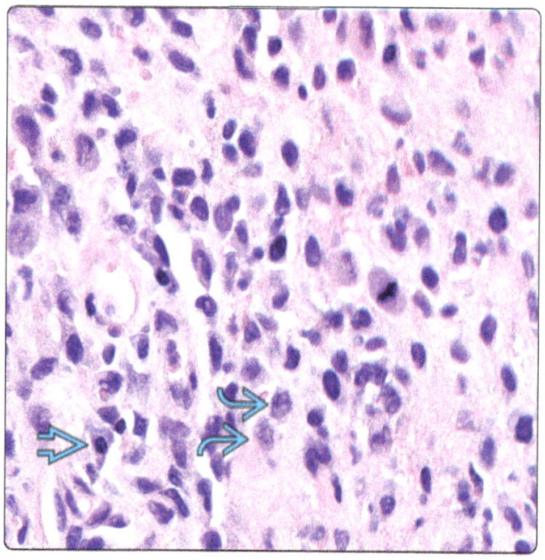

(Left) *There is both nuclear and cytoplasmic labeling with S100 in this example of Langerhans cell histiocytosis.* **(Right)** *CD1a is a cytoplasmic and membranous stain and is helpful in confirming the diagnosis. Another marker that has been promulgated to confirm a diagnosis of Langerhans cell histiocytosis is langerin.*

Langerhans Cell Histiocytosis, S100 Expression

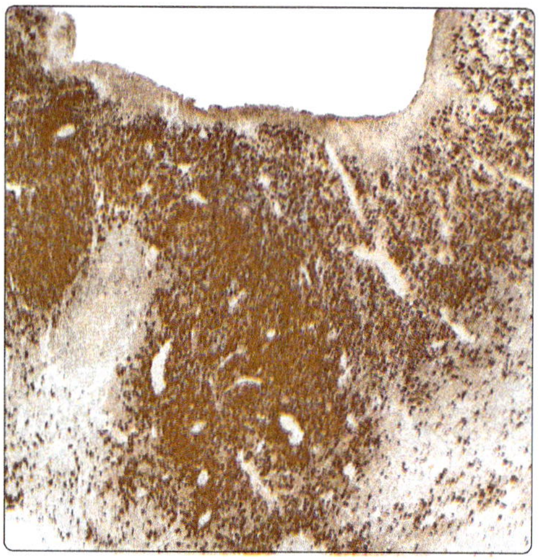

Langerhans Cell Histiocytosis, CD1a Labeling

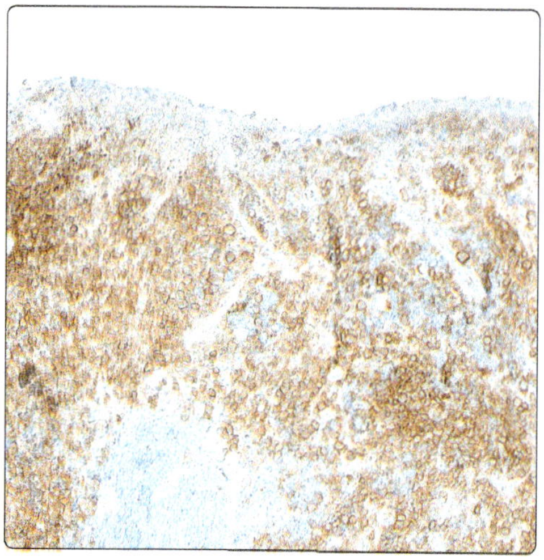

Rosai-Dorfman Disease, Needle Biopsy of Subcutaneous Mass

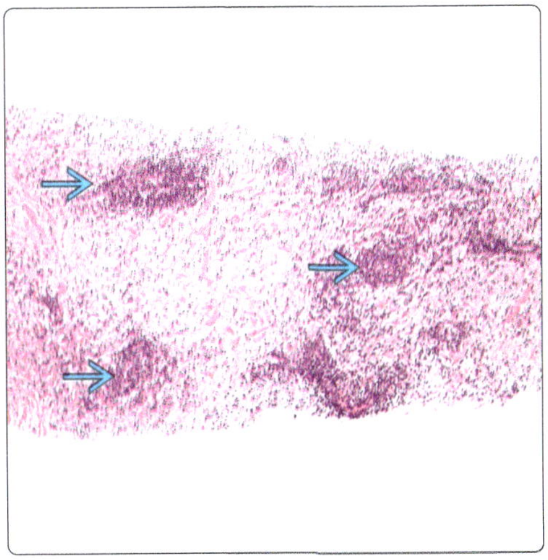

Rosai-Dorfman Disease, Atypical Cells

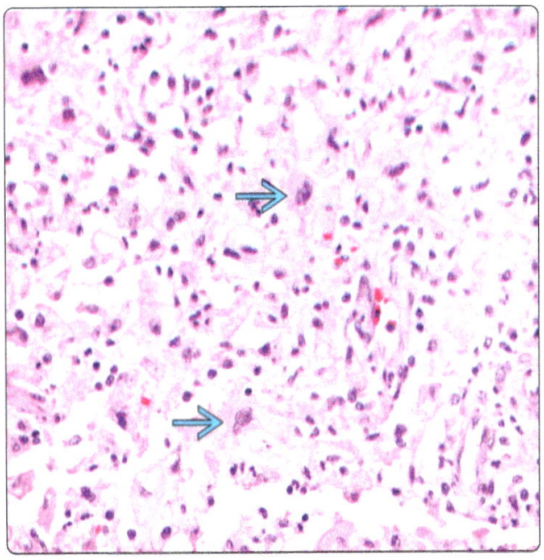

(Left) *The differential diagnosis can also include Rosai-Dorfman disease. Note the lymphoid aggregates ➔ spaced throughout the spindle cell lesion. This pattern is typical of extranodal disease.* **(Right)** *The presence of enlarged nuclei ➔ in the spindled areas of extranodal Rosai-Dorfman disease can lead to a mistaken impression of sarcoma.*

Rosai-Dorfman Disease, Enlarged Nuclei

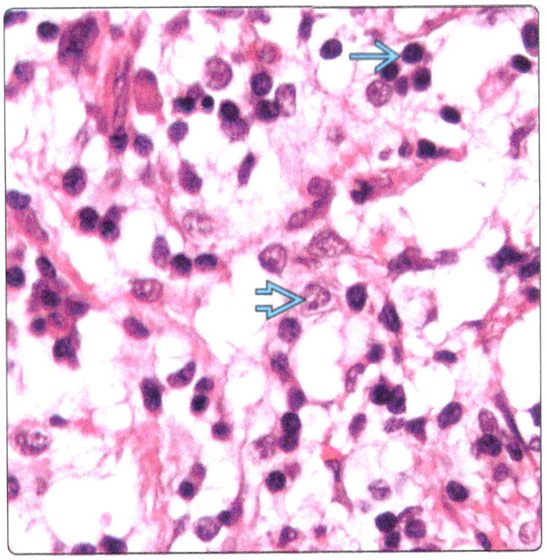

Rosai-Dorfman Disease, Emperipolesis

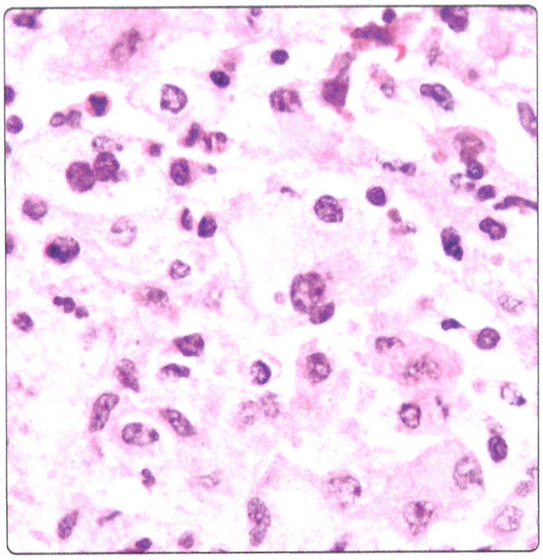

(Left) *In this field, enlarged nuclei ➔ are present in a background with many lymphocytes ➔. Rosai-Dorfman disease is a non-Langerhans cell histiocytosis that lacks BRAF mutations. It was classically described in lymph nodes.* **(Right)** *The abnormal histiocytic cells have engulfed lymphoid cells without destroying them.*

Rosai-Dorfman Disease, Emperipolesis

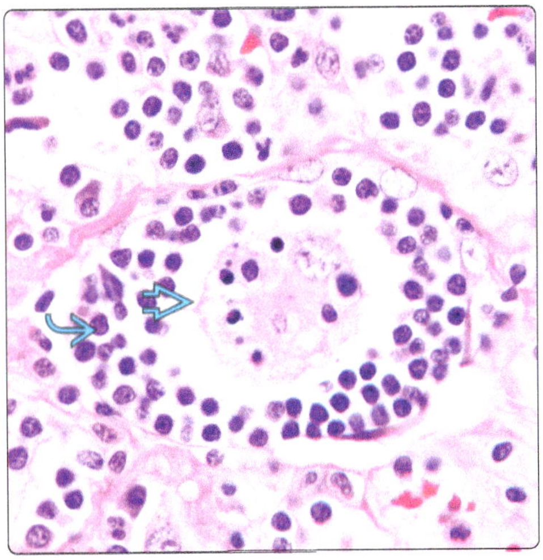

Rosai-Dorfman Disease, S100

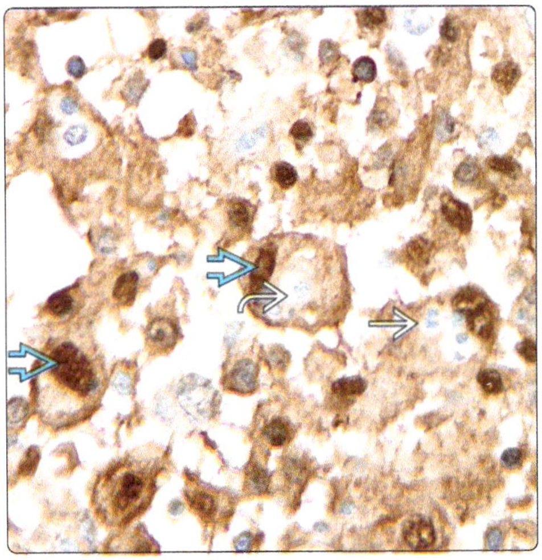

(Left) *This is a lymphatic space in a case of extranodal Rosai-Dorfman disease. It contains both lymphocytes ➔ as well as a lesional cell ➔ that has engulfed many lymphocytes without damaging them (emperipolesis).* **(Right)** *The abnormal histiocytes show nuclear expression of S100 ➔, whereas the engulfed lymphoid ➔ cells and neutrophils ➔ do not. The cytoplasm of the abnormal histiocytic cells is also reactive with S100, causing the nonlabeled emperipolesed cells to stand out on the S100 stain.*

Reticulohistiocytoma

KEY FACTS

TERMINOLOGY

- Proliferation of histiocytes with abundant dense, glassy-appearing eosinophilic cytoplasm

CLINICAL ISSUES

- Usually occurs in adults > 40 years old, but cases have been reported in adolescents
- Usually head and neck region, including mucosal sites, but may present at any cutaneous site
- Usually red-brown or yellow-brown appearing

MICROSCOPIC

- Dermal-based nodular proliferation of large mononuclear and multinucleated histiocytes
- Cells show characteristic abundant glassy/hyalinized-appearing eosinophilic cytoplasm
- Early lesions characterized by more mononuclear cells with lymphocytes
- Few Touton-type giant cells containing lipid may be present but not prominent
- Occasional atypical-appearing cells may be present but do not indicate malignancy

ANCILLARY TESTS

- Cells are typically positive for CD68, CD163, and lysozyme
- S100 negative in most cases; can be focally positive

TOP DIFFERENTIAL DIAGNOSES

- Multicentric reticulohistiocytosis and generalized cutaneous reticulohistiocytosis
    - Different clinical features: Multiple cutaneous lesions, may have joint &/or internal organ involvement in multicentric cutaneous reticulohistiocytosis
- Juvenile xanthogranuloma
- Langerhans cell histiocytosis
- Rosai-Dorfman disease (sinus histiocytosis with massive lymphadenopathy)

Solitary Reticulohistiocytoma at Low Magnification

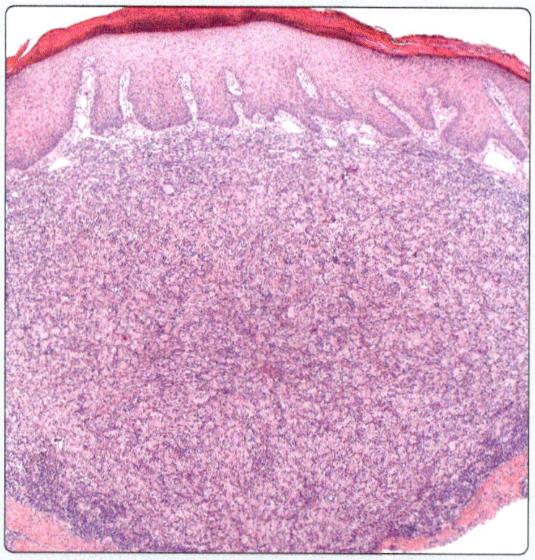

Solitary Reticulohistiocytoma

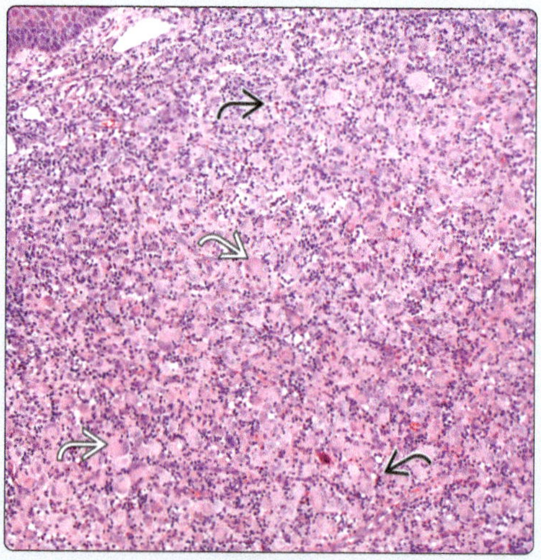

(Left) *Low magnification shows a nodular dermal infiltrate composed of large, eosinophilic-staining histiocytic cells, associated with mixed inflammatory infiltrate, including many lymphocytes and eosinophils.* **(Right)** *Higher magnification shows a population of large histiocytic-appearing cells with dense, eosinophilic-staining cytoplasm, associated with an infiltrate, including many lymphocytes and eosinophils.*

Solitary Reticulohistiocytoma at High Magnification

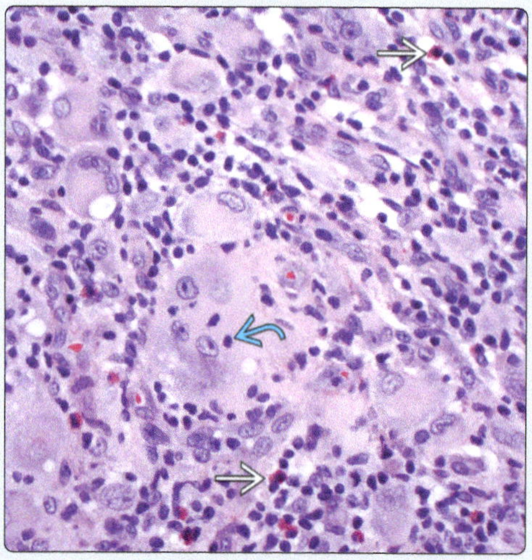

S100 Immunohistochemistry in Reticulohistiocytoma

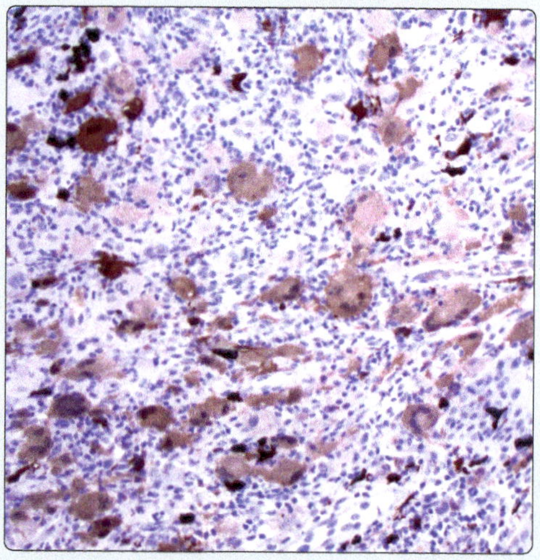

(Left) *High magnification shows the large, eosinophilic-staining histiocytic cells with dense, glassy cytoplasm and focal emperipolesis of lymphocytes. Note the mixed background inflammatory infiltrate, including many eosinophils.* **(Right)** *This case showed greater S100 staining than usual, although it is relatively weak and mostly cytoplasm. Entrapped dendritic cells show much stronger staining.*

TERMINOLOGY

Synonyms

- Solitary cutaneous reticulohistiocytoma
- Reticulohistiocytic granuloma
- Giant cell reticulohistiocytoma

Definitions

- Proliferation of histiocytes with abundant dense, glassy-appearing eosinophilic cytoplasm

ETIOLOGY/PATHOGENESIS

Environmental Exposure

- May be related to stimuli, such as insect bites, infection, trauma, or ruptured folliculitis or cyst in some cases

CLINICAL ISSUES

Epidemiology

- Incidence
  - Rare tumor
- Age
  - Usually occurs in adults > 40 years old
    - However, some cases have been reported in adolescents
- Sex
  - M:F = 1:1
- Ethnicity
  - Most cases occur in Caucasians

Site

- Usually head and neck region, including mucosal sites
  - However, may present at almost any cutaneous site

Presentation

- Skin papule or nodule
  - Usually single lesion, but several may be present in some cases
- Firm, rapidly growing lesion
- Usually appear as red-brown or yellow-brown
- May be preceded by trauma in some cases
- Lack of systemic symptoms, including fever, weight loss, or weakness (which may be seen in multicentric reticulohistiocytosis)

Treatment

- Surgical approaches
  - Complete conservative excision is curative
    - Usually not required, unless lesion is very large or fails to resolve

Prognosis

- Excellent; lesions often involute spontaneously
- No definite relationship with more aggressive multicentric reticulohistiocytosis
  - However, multiple skin lesions should suggest possibility of generalized cutaneous reticulohistiocytosis

MACROSCOPIC

General Features

- Dermal-based, nodular, well-circumscribed, but unencapsulated, lesion

Size

- Lesions typically range in size from 0.5-2.0 cm

MICROSCOPIC

Histologic Features

- Dermal-based nodular proliferation of large mononuclear and multinucleated histiocytes
  - Cells show characteristic abundant glassy/hyalinized-appearing eosinophilic cytoplasm
  - Some cells may show finely granular cytoplasm
  - Occasional Touton-type giant cells containing lipid may be present but not prominent
  - Cytologic atypia is usually minimal, and mitoses are few and nonatypical
  - No infiltrative features are present
- Overlying epidermis may show atrophy/thinning
  - Often grenz zone separating infiltrate from epidermis
- Early lesions characterized by background inflammatory infiltrate with many small mononuclear cells and lymphocytes
- Later lesions show greater numbers of large mononuclear and multinucleated cells, with background infiltrate including neutrophils and eosinophils
- Phagocytosis of inflammatory cells and collagen may be present (but not usually prominent, as in Rosai-Dorfman disease)
- Occasional bizarre-appearing cells may be present but do not indicate malignancy
- Rare cases may show deep subcutaneous, and even lymph node, involvement

Cytologic Features

- Large but cytologically bland-appearing cells that show characteristic abundant glassy/hyalinized-appearing eosinophilic cytoplasm

ANCILLARY TESTS

Histochemistry

- Periodic acid-Schiff with diastase digestion and Sudan black
  - Reactivity: Positive
  - Staining pattern: Cytoplasmic; highlights granules

Immunohistochemistry

- Cells are typically positive for CD68 (KP1), CD163, and lysozyme
- Variable positivity reported for FXIIIA, CD64, and α-1-antitrypsin
- S100 negative in most cases but has been reported to be rarely positive (usually weak/focal)
- Cells negative for CD1a, CD3, CD20, CD34, actin, desmin, HMB-45, MART-1/Melan-A

Electron Microscopy

- Large cells showing abundant granular cytoplasm containing numerous mitochondria, phagolysosomes, dense bodies, and myelin figures
- Also contain so-called pleomorphic cytoplasmic inclusions
  - Highly complex structures consisting mainly of unit membranes, which may surround vesicles
- Birbeck granules are absent

DIFFERENTIAL DIAGNOSIS

Multicentric and Generalized Cutaneous Reticulohistiocytosis

- These entities show different clinical features
  - Multicentric cutaneous reticulohistiocytosis (MCR) presents with multiple lesions involving skin, mucosal sites, joints, and occasionally internal organs
    - MCR may show aggressive course with destructive arthropathy and constitutional symptoms
  - Generalized cutaneous reticulohistiocytosis is characterized by eruption of multiple small cutaneous lesions
    - Some cases may progress to MCR
- Histologically, there is considerable overlap with solitary reticulohistiocytoma, but some differences have been described
  - Solitary lesions may be better circumscribed and show more multinucleated giant cells
  - Neutrophils and xanthomatized cells have been reported to be more common in solitary reticulohistiocytoma
  - FXIIIA expression may be lower in systemic cases

Juvenile Xanthogranuloma

- Typically occurs in children, but some cases occur in adults (adult-type xanthogranuloma)
- Multiple papules are common, and dozens of lesions have been reported in some cases
- Histologically, juvenile xanthogranuloma typically shows more foamy histiocytes and Touton-type giant cells with peripheral wreath-like arrangement of nuclei
  - Cells lack dense glassy eosinophilic cytoplasm of reticulohistiocytoma
- Cells positive by immunohistochemistry for CD68 and CD163 but negative for S100 and CD1a

Langerhans Cell Histiocytosis

- Includes Letterer-Siwe, Hand-Schüller Christian, eosinophilic granuloma, and congenital self-healing reticulohistiocytosis variants
- Predominantly occurs in children
  - Also 2nd peak in elderly adults (usually eosinophilic granuloma variant)
- Typically characterized by multiple skin lesions and systemic involvement (especially bone)
- Histologic examination shows proliferation of mononuclear cells in dermis and occasionally in epidermis
  - Cells show large, folded, or reniform vesicular nuclei and abundant eosinophilic cytoplasm
  - Cells lack dense eosinophilic cytoplasm of reticulohistiocytoma
  - Background infiltrate often contains numerous eosinophils and variable numbers of lymphocytes
- CD1a and S100 should be positive in vast majority of cases (both are typically negative in reticulohistiocytoma)

Rosai-Dorfman Disease

- a.k.a. sinus histiocytosis with massive lymphadenopathy
- Often shows concomitant lymphadenopathy and constitutional symptoms
- Lesions may be solitary or multiple
- Histology shows proliferation of large, pale-staining histiocytes with emperipolesis of lymphocytes, plasma cells, and erythrocytes (usually much more prominent than in reticulohistiocytoma)
  - Cells lack dense, glassy cytoplasm of reticulohistiocytoma
- Positive for S100 (typically negative in reticulohistiocytoma), CD68, and lysozyme; negative for CD1a

DIAGNOSTIC CHECKLIST

Pathologic Interpretation Pearls

- Nodular proliferation of large mononuclear and multinucleated histiocytes
  - Cells show characteristic abundant glassy-/hyalinized-appearing eosinophilic cytoplasm
  - Occasional Touton-type giant cells containing lipid may be present, but not prominent (as in JXG)
- Cells positive for CD68, CD163, and lysozyme
- Cells typically negative for S100, CD1a, CD3, CD20, and CD34

SELECTED REFERENCES

1. Shibuya R et al: A plaque-type solitary reticulohistiocytoma in a two-year-old boy. Case Rep Dermatol. 7(1):7-9, 2015
2. Cohen PR et al: Adult-onset reticulohistiocytoma presenting as a solitary asymptomatic red knee nodule: report and review of clinical presentations and immunohistochemistry staining features of reticulohistiocytosis. Dermatol Online J. 20(3), 2014
3. Caputo R et al: Unusual variants of non-Langerhans cell histiocytoses. J Am Acad Dermatol. 57(6):1031-45, 2007
4. Chen CH et al: Multicentric reticulohistiocytosis presenting with destructive polyarthritis, laryngopharyngeal dysfunction, and a huge reticulohistiocytoma. J Clin Rheumatol. 12(5):252-4, 2006
5. Miettinen M et al: Reticulohistiocytoma (solitary epithelioid histiocytoma): a clinicopathologic and immunohistochemical study of 44 cases. Am J Surg Pathol. 30(4):521-8, 2006
6. Wang KH et al: Cutaneous Rosai-Dorfman disease: clinicopathological profiles, spectrum and evolution of 21 lesions in six patients. Br J Dermatol. 154(2):277-86, 2006
7. Nguyen TT et al: Expression of CD163 (hemoglobin scavenger receptor) in normal tissues, lymphomas, carcinomas, and sarcomas is largely restricted to the monocyte/macrophage lineage. Am J Surg Pathol. 29(5):617-24, 2005
8. Bakri SJ et al: Recurrent solitary reticulohistiocytoma of the eyelid. Ophthal Plast Reconstr Surg. 19(2):162-4, 2003
9. Busam KJ et al: Immunohistochemical distinction of epithelioid histiocytic proliferations from epithelioid melanocytic nevi. Am J Dermatopathol. 22(3):237-41, 2000
10. Burgdorf WH et al: The non-Langerhans' cell histiocytoses in childhood. Cutis. 58(3):201-7, 1996
11. Suwabe H et al: Reticulohistiocytoma involving the skin, subcutaneous tissue and a regional lymph node. Pathol Int. 46(7):531-7, 1996
12. Hunt SJ et al: Solitary reticulohistiocytoma in pregnancy: immunohistochemical and ultrastructural study of a case with unusual immunophenotype. J Cutan Pathol. 22(2):177-81, 1995
13. Zelger B et al: Reticulohistiocytoma and multicentric reticulohistiocytosis. Histopathologic and immunophenotypic distinct entities. Am J Dermatopathol. 16(6):577-84, 1994
14. Davies BT et al: The so-called reticulohistiocytoma of the skin; a comparison of two distinct types. Br J Dermatol. 67(6):205-11, 1955

Solitary Reticulohistiocytoma at Low Magnification

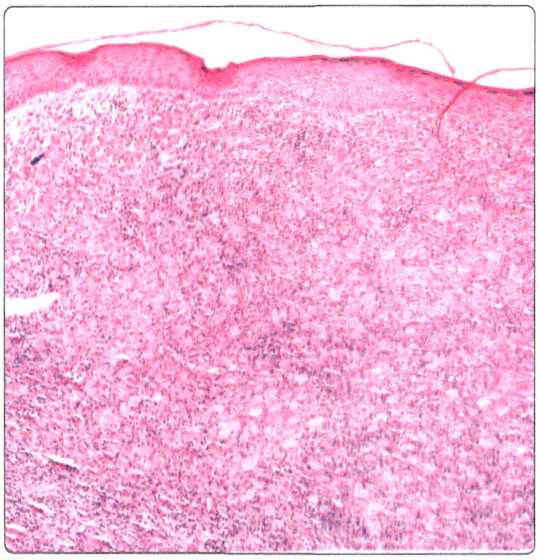

Reticulohistiocytoma With Associated Eosinophils

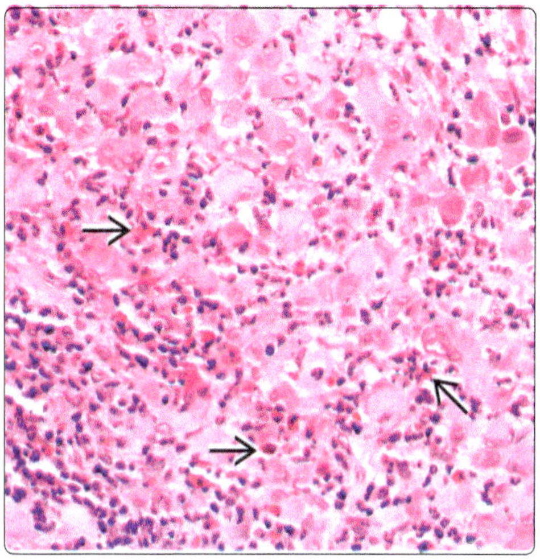

(Left) *Low-power examination shows a dense nodular to sheet-like collection of large histiocytic cells in the dermis, without any epidermal involvement.* **(Right)** *Higher magnification shows sheets of eosinophilic-staining histiocytic cells associated with an inflammatory infiltrate containing lymphocytes, neutrophils, and numerous eosinophils ⮕.*

High Magnification of Reticulohistiocytoma

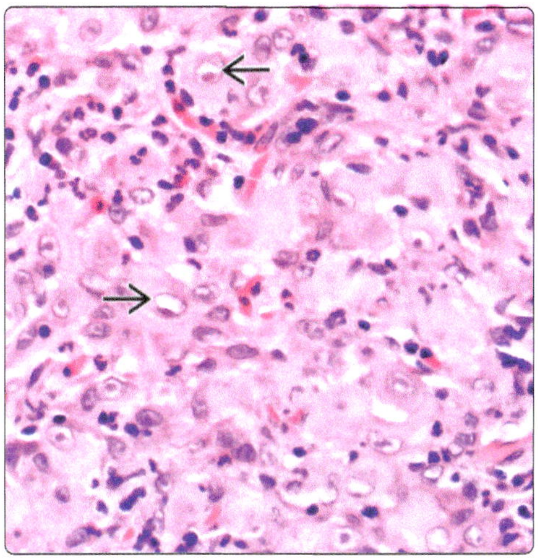

Hypocellular Reticulohistiocytoma

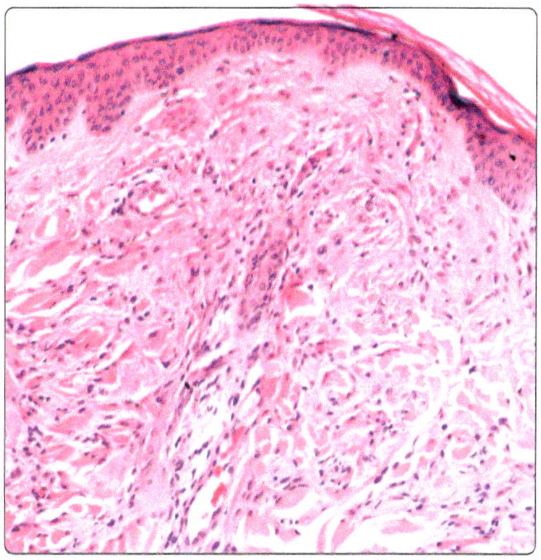

(Left) *Higher power examination shows the cytologic features of the cells, with abundant dense eosinophilic to glassy-appearing cytoplasm and vesicular nuclei ⮕ with prominent nucleoli.* **(Right)** *Low-power view of a hypocellular (possibly regressing) lesion shows only scattered large histiocytes in the superficial dermis.*

CD163 Immunohistochemical Stain in Reticulohistiocytoma

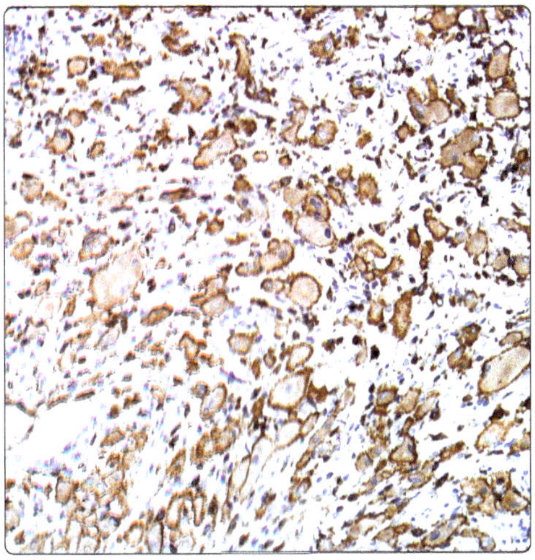

S100 Immunohistochemical Stain in Reticulohistiocytoma

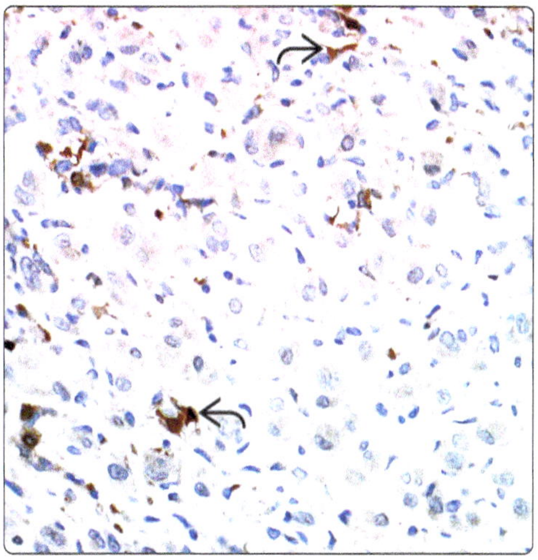

(Left) *CD163 immunohistochemical stain is strongly and diffusely positive, highlighting the histiocytic cell cytoplasm and membranes.* **(Right)** *S100 is essentially negative, with only very weak cytoplasmic, and no nuclear, staining. A few background dendritic cells are strongly positive ⮫.*

Multicentric Reticulohistiocytosis

KEY FACTS

TERMINOLOGY

- Giant cell reticulohistiocytosis

CLINICAL ISSUES

- Most cases occur in adults > 40 years
- Can affect multiple sites, including hands, face, juxtaarticular regions, oral, nasal/pharyngeal mucosa
- Prognosis is variable; some cutaneous lesions may regress
- Immunosuppressive medications typically used

MICROSCOPIC

- Dermal-based, nodular proliferation of large mononuclear & multinucleated histiocytes
- Often overlying epidermal atrophy
- Cells show characteristic abundant, glassy/hyalinized-appearing, eosinophilic cytoplasm
- Occasional Touton-type giant cells containing lipid may be present but not prominent
- Background of neutrophils & eosinophils
- Less well-circumscribed than solitary reticulohistiocytoma but no infiltrative features

ANCILLARY TESTS

- Typically positive for histiocytic markers, including CD68, lysozyme, & CD45
- Cells are usually negative for S100, CD1a, & MAC387

TOP DIFFERENTIAL DIAGNOSES

- Solitary cutaneous reticulohistiocytoma (SCR) & generalized cutaneous reticulohistiocytosis (GCR)
  - SCR presents as single papular or nodular cutaneous lesion
  - GCR is characterized by eruption of multiple small cutaneous lesions
- Juvenile xanthogranuloma
  - Typically single lesion occurring in children but can be multiple, & some cases occur in adults
- Langerhans cell histiocytosis
  - Strongly positive for S100 & CD1a

Low Magnification of Multicentric Reticulohistiocytosis

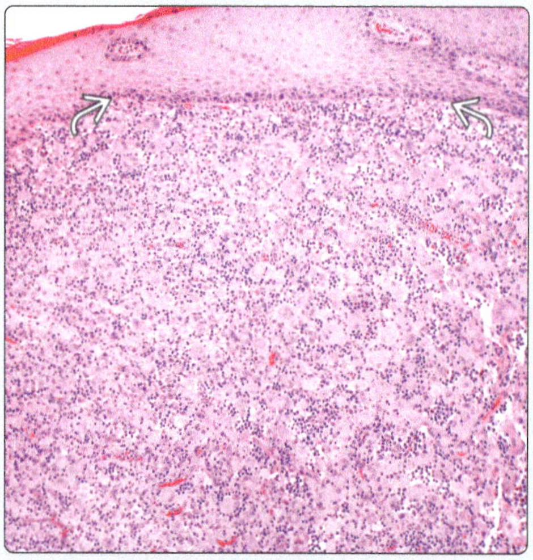

Higher Magnification of Multicentric reticulohistiocytosis

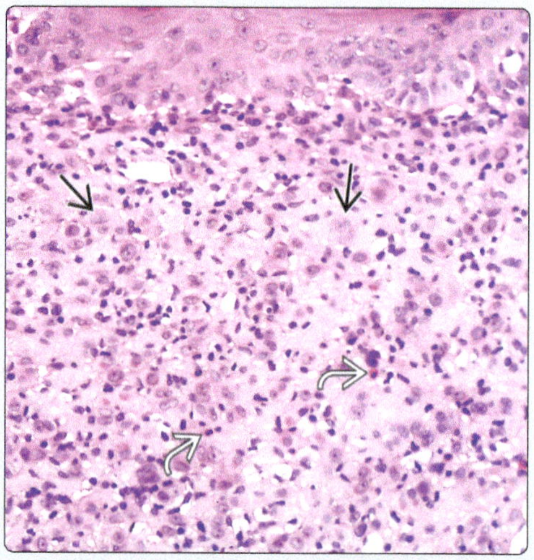

(Left) *Low magnification of multicentric reticulohistiocytosis (MCR) shows a nodular proliferation of enlarged histiocytic cells in the dermis. There is a very thin grenz zone, and the epidermis shows flattening of the rete ridges.* **(Right)** *Higher magnification of MCR shows a proliferation of numerous, enlarged, histiocytic-appearing cells associated with a background mixed inflammatory infiltrate containing scattered eosinophils.*

Multicentric Reticulohistiocytosis With Large Multinucleated Cell

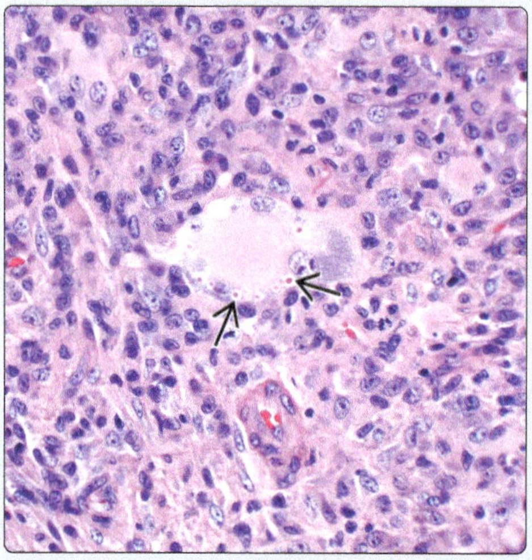

Hypocellular Variant of Multicentric Reticulohistiocytosis

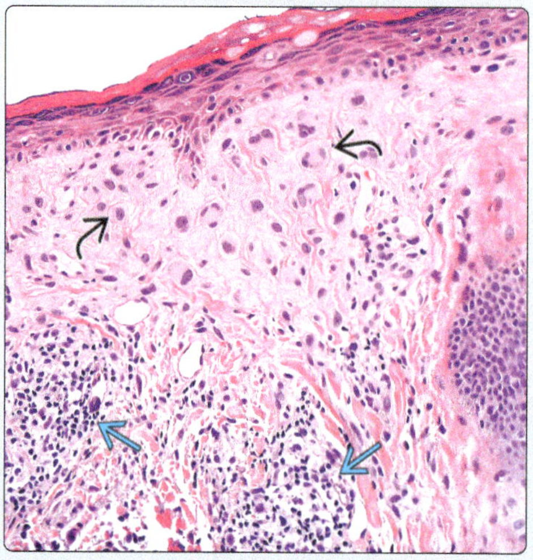

(Left) *High magnification of a cellular MCR shows a very large, central multinucleated cell containing fragments of phagocytosed erythrocytes.* **(Right)** *A hypocellular example of MCR shows a superficial, dermal-based proliferation of large epithelioid histiocytes, many of which are multinucleated, and a mild associated lymphocytic infiltrate.*

TERMINOLOGY

Abbreviations

- Multicentric reticulohistiocytosis (MCR)

Synonyms

- Giant cell reticulohistiocytosis
- Reticulohistiocytosis of skin & synovia

Definitions

- Proliferation of large histiocytes with dense eosinophilic cytoplasm involving multiple organs

ETIOLOGY/PATHOGENESIS

Associated Conditions

- Autoimmune disorders & internal malignancies

CLINICAL ISSUES

Epidemiology

- Age
  - Most cases occur in adults > 40 years

Site

- Can affect multiple sites, including hands, face, juxtaarticular regions, oral, nasal/pharyngeal mucosa

Presentation

- Multiple nodules & arthropathy
  - Most cases present with multiple cutaneous/mucocutaneous papulonodules & severe arthropathy, other visceral symptoms

Treatment

- Drugs
  - Immunosuppressive medications typically used
  - Underlying autoimmune disease or malignancy should be treated

Prognosis

- Variable; some cutaneous lesions may regress
- Osteoarticular involvement shows progressive course in ~ 50% of cases

MACROSCOPIC

General Features

- Dermal-based nodular, nonencapsulated lesion

Size

- Typically range from 2 mm to 2 cm in diameter

MICROSCOPIC

Histologic Features

- Dermal-based, nodular proliferation of large mononuclear & multinucleated histiocytes
  - Cells show characteristic abundant glassy/hyalinized-appearing eosinophilic cytoplasm
  - Some cells may show finely granular cytoplasm
  - Cytologic atypia is minimal; only few mitoses should be present
  - Less well circumscribed than solitary reticulohistiocytoma but no infiltrative features
- Overlying epidermis may show atrophy/thinning
- Early lesions characterized by background inflammatory infiltrate with many small mononuclear cells & lymphocytes
- Later lesions show greater numbers of large cells, neutrophils, & eosinophils

ANCILLARY TESTS

Immunohistochemistry

- Typically positive for histiocytic markers, including CD68, lysozyme, & CD45
- Cells are typically negative for S100 (may be focally positive in some cases), CD1a, & MAC387

DIFFERENTIAL DIAGNOSIS

Solitary Cutaneous Reticulohistiocytoma & Generalized Cutaneous Reticulohistiocytosis

- Solitary cutaneous reticulohistiocytoma presents as single papular or nodular cutaneous lesion
  - Histologically, there is considerable overlap with MCR, but some differences may be seen
    - May be better circumscribed & show more multinucleated giant cells & neutrophils
- Generalized cutaneous reticulohistiocytosis is characterized by eruption of multiple small cutaneous lesions
  - Some cases may progress to MCR

Juvenile Xanthogranuloma

- Typically, single lesion occurring in children but can be multiple, & some cases occur in adults
- Histologically, shows more foamy histiocytes & Touton-type giant cells with peripheral, wreath-like rim of nuclei & foamy cytoplasm

Langerhans Cell Histiocytosis

- Predominantly occurs in children but 2nd peak in elderly adults (usually eosinophilic granuloma variant)
- Characterized by multiple skin lesions & systemic involvement (especially bone)
- Cells show folded or reniform vesicular nuclei & abundant eosinophilic cytoplasm
- CD1a & S100 are strongly positive in vast majority

DIAGNOSTIC CHECKLIST

Pathologic Interpretation Pearls

- Nodular proliferation of large mononuclear & multinucleated histiocytes
  - Cells show characteristic abundant, glassy/hyalinized-appearing, eosinophilic cytoplasm

SELECTED REFERENCES

1. Chisolm SS et al: Adult xanthogranuloma, reticulohistiocytosis, and Rosai-Dorfman disease. Dermatol Clin. 33(3):465-72; discussion 473, 2015
2. Selmi C et al: Multicentric reticulohistiocytosis: a critical review. Curr Rheumatol Rep. 17(6):511, 2015
3. Islam AD et al: Multicentric reticulohistiocytosis: a rare yet challenging disease. Clin Rev Allergy Immunol. 45(2):281-9, 2013
4. Luz FB et al: Multicentric reticulohistiocytosis: a proliferation of macrophages with tropism for skin and joints, part I. Skinmed. 6(4):172-8, 2007
5. Baghestani S et al: Multicentric reticulohistiocytosis presenting with papulonodular skin eruption and polyarthritis. Eur J Dermatol. 15(3):196-200, 2005

Langerhans Cell Histiocytosis

KEY FACTS

TERMINOLOGY

- Langerhans cell histiocytosis is also known as
  - Histiocytosis X
  - Eosinophilic granuloma
- Defined as clonal proliferation of Langerhans cells

CLINICAL ISSUES

- Newborns and infants usually present with limited skin or bone lesions
- Erythematous, crusted, vesiculopustular rash
- Common sites include skin, bone and bone marrow, and lung
- M:F = 2:1
- **Eosinophilic granuloma** is restricted to bone
- **Hand-Schüller-Christian disease** has multiple organ involvement and diabetes insipidus
- **Letterer-Siwe disease** is aggressive with multisystem involvement

MICROSCOPIC

- Langerhans cells infiltrate dermis and subcutis and often extend throughout epidermis to stratum corneum
- Langerhans cells show
  - Abundant eosinophilic show cytoplasm
  - Coffee bean-shaped nucleus
- Large numbers of eosinophils and other inflammatory cells typically present
- Mitoses common, but usually not atypical

ANCILLARY TESTS

- CD1a and S100 immunostaining
- Birbeck granules seen on EM

TOP DIFFERENTIAL DIAGNOSES

- Granulomatous infiltrates
- Rosai-Dorfman disease
- Indeterminate cell histiocytosis
- Hodgkin and non-Hodgkin lymphoma

Clinical Photograph of Langerhans Cell Histiocytosis

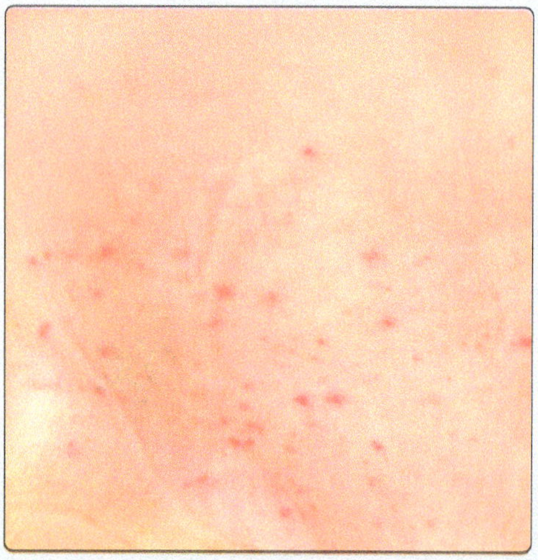

Dermal Involvement by Langerhans Cell Histiocytosis

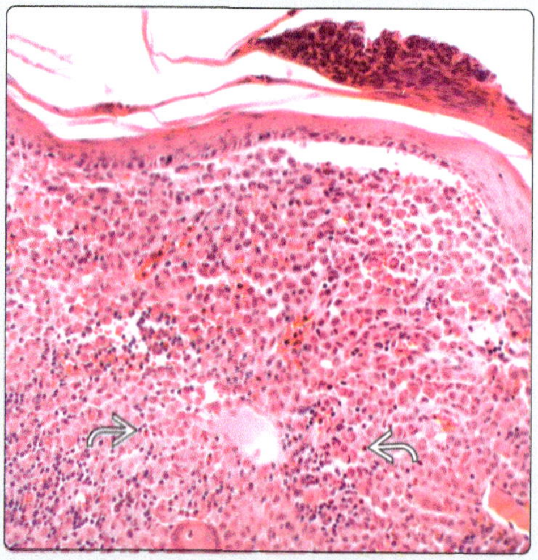

(Left) *This example of Langerhans cell histiocytosis (LCH) of the skin presented as a seborrheic-like erythematous rash with petechiae on the abdomen of a 23-month-old child. (Courtesy S. Vanderhooft, MD.)* **(Right)** *This example of LCH shows dense collections of histiocytic cells in the superficial dermis, with overlying epidermal atrophy and serum crust containing neutrophils. Scattered dermal eosinophils are also seen ➡.*

Higher Magnification of Langerhans Cell Histiocytosis

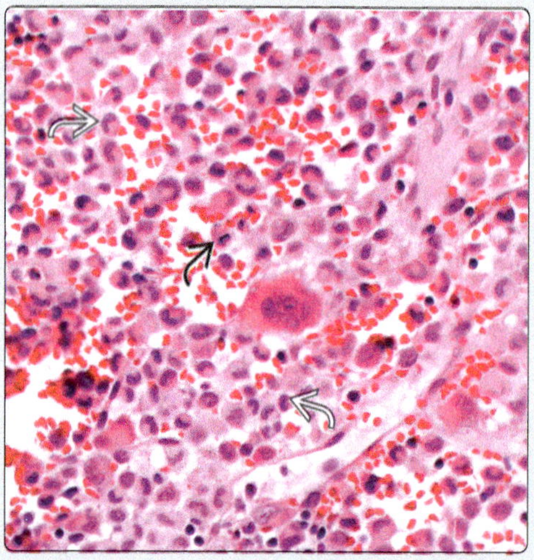

CD1a Immunohistochemistry in Langerhans Cell Histiocytosis

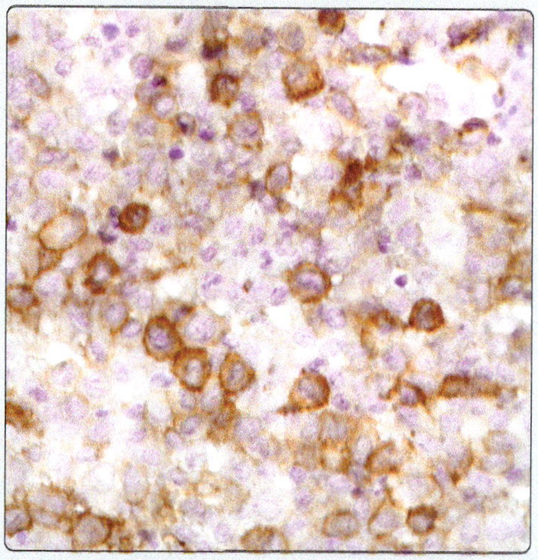

(Left) *Higher magnification shows the characteristic cytologic features, including folded or coffee bean-shaped nuclei ➡, and abundant eosinophilic-staining cytoplasm. This field also shows a mitosis ➡ and a few large multinucleated cells, which may seen in some cases.* **(Right)** *The Langerhans cells show positive cytoplasmic and membranous staining for CD1a.*

TERMINOLOGY

Abbreviations

- Langerhans cell histiocytosis (LCH)

Synonyms

- Histiocytosis X
- Eosinophilic granuloma

Definitions

- Clonal proliferation of Langerhans cells

CLINICAL ISSUES

Epidemiology

- Age
  - First 3 decades of life; rarely occurs in older adults
- Sex
  - M:F = 2:1

Site

- Skin
  - Erythematous, crusted, vesiculopustular rash, or salmon-colored macular-papular rash
- Bone and bone marrow
  - Skull, pelvis, long bones, vertebrae
- CNS
  - Primary in dura, leptomeninges, or parenchyma
  - May be secondary to skull or vertebral involvement
- Other organs that may be affected include lung, lymph nodes, liver, thymus, and GI tract

Presentation

- Newborns and infants usually present with limited skin or bone lesions
- Generalized disease is more common in young children
- **Eosinophilic granuloma**
  - Single or multiple lesions restricted to bone
- **Hand-Schüller-Christian disease**
  - Multiple organ involvement
  - Diabetes insipidus and exophthalmos
- **Letterer-Siwe disease**
  - Disseminated disease with skin, lymph node, visceral, and marrow involvement

Natural History

- May spontaneously resolve or progress

Treatment

- Surgical approaches
  - Local excision for limited disease
- Drugs
  - Chemotherapy for disseminated disease

Prognosis

- Poor prognosis associated with young age, hepatosplenomegaly, and thrombocytopenia

MICROSCOPIC

Histologic Features

- Langerhans cells infiltrate dermis and subcutis and often extend throughout epidermis
- Langerhans cells show
  - Abundant eosinophilic cytoplasm
  - Coffee bean-shaped nuclei or lobulated nucleus with central groove
  - Small nucleolus
- Large numbers of eosinophils frequently present
  - Other inflammatory cells also seen, including multinucleated giant cells
- Necrosis is common
- Mitoses common, but usually not atypical
- Lymph nodes
  - Architecture generally preserved
  - Sinuses are distended by Langerhans cells
- Disease passes through various stages
  - Necrosis and increasing fibrosis seen in older lesions

ANCILLARY TESTS

Immunohistochemistry

- CD1a is very specific for Langerhans cells
- Langerin is also specific for Langerhans cells
- S100 is not specific, but stains Langerhans cells

Electron Microscopy

- Birbeck granules
  - Tubular pentilaminar membrane-bound cytoplasmic bodies, often with terminal oval protrusion
  - Tennis racket shaped

DIFFERENTIAL DIAGNOSIS

Granulomatous Infiltrates

- Multinucleated, foreign body giant cells typically present
- Histiocytic cells are CD68(+), CD1a(-)

Rosai-Dorfman Disease

- LCH does not display emperipolesis
- Histiocytes are S100(+) but CD1a(-)

Indeterminate Cell Histiocytosis

- Histologic and immunohistochemical features essentially identical to LCH
- Lack Birbeck granules by ultrastructural examination

Hodgkin and Non-Hodgkin Lymphoma

- Cells lack characteristic nuclear features of LCH
- Neoplastic cells are usually CD15 and CD30 (+), CD1a(-)

SELECTED REFERENCES

1. Yasuda M et al: Langerhans cell histiocytosis masquerading as hidradenitis suppurativa. J Dermatol. ePub, 2016
2. Monsereenusorn C et al: Clinical characteristics and treatment of langerhans cell histiocytosis. Hematol Oncol Clin North Am. 29(5):853-73, 2015
3. Satpathy AT et al: Cellular morphology of BRAF V600E-positive Langerhans cell histiocytosis. Blood. 126(15):1857, 2015
4. Degar BA et al: Langerhans cell histiocytosis: malignancy or inflammatory disorder doing a great job of imitating one? Dis Model Mech. 2(9-10):436-9, 2009
5. Imashuku S et al: Langerhans cell histiocytosis with multifocal bone lesions: comparative clinical features between single and multi-systems. Int J Hematol. 90(4):506-12, 2009
6. Jaffe R: Is there a role for histopathology in predicting the clinical outcome in congenital and infant Langerhans cell disease? Pediatr Blood Cancer. 53(6):924-5, 2009

(Left) *Cutaneous involvement by LCH shows epidermal and dermal involvement, features that can mimic a melanocytic tumor. However, the correct diagnosis is easily made by identifying the characteristic nuclear features and using immunohistochemical stains.* **(Right)** *LCH in the skin shows numerous Langerhans cells infiltrating into the epidermis ➡. Usually, they are present as nests or small aggregates, as seen here.*

Langerhans Cell Histiocytosis Involving Epidermis and Dermis

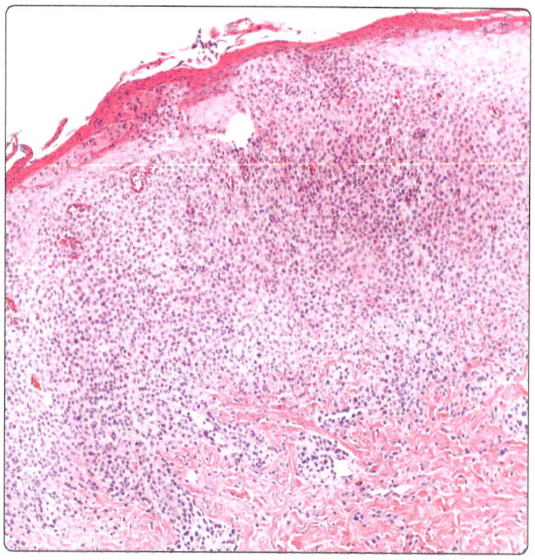

Langerhans Cell Histiocytosis Involving Epidermis

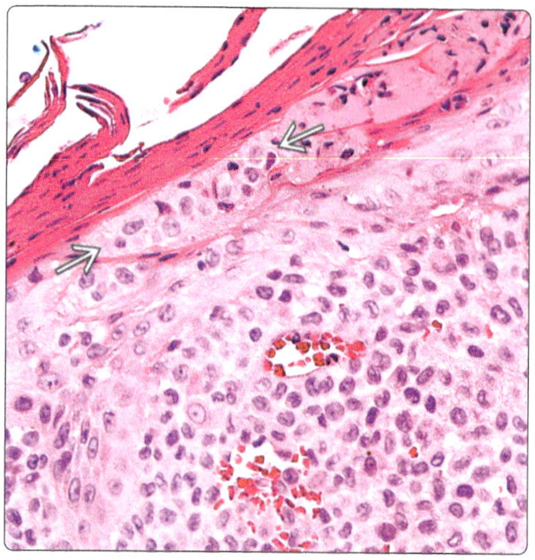

(Left) *Low-power view of LCH shows a collection of eosinophils → representing an eosinophilic granuloma. Eosinophilic granuloma is another term for LCH, which is used to describe nodules restricted to bone.* **(Right)** *High-power view highlights the typical nuclear features of Langerhans cells. The nuclei are folded, show long grooves ↪, and often resemble coffee beans. An eosinophil → is seen.*

Langerhans Cell Histiocytosis With Numerous Eosinophils

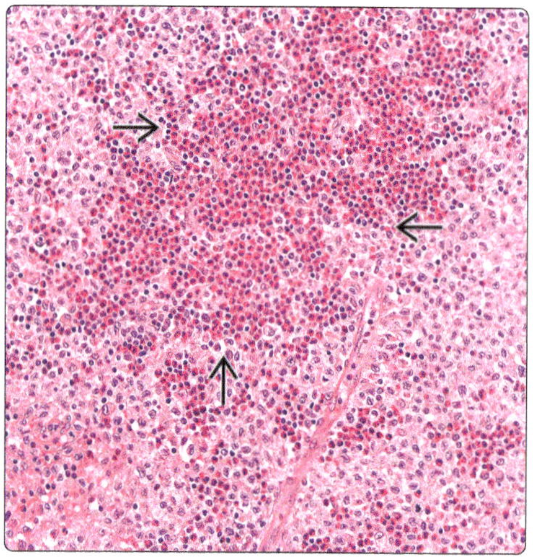

High Magnification of Langerhans Cell Histiocytosis

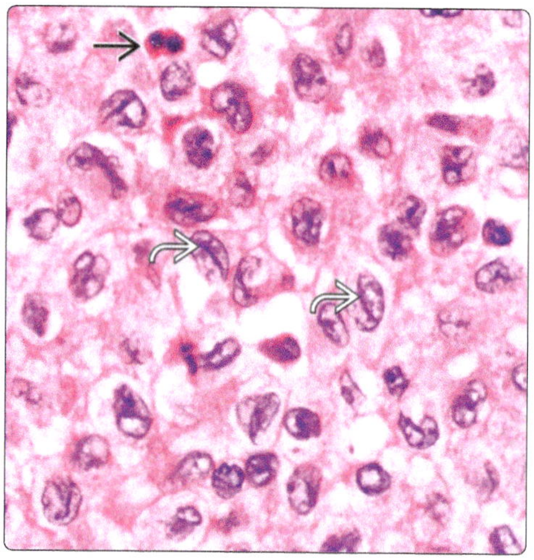

(Left) *Langerhans cells show positive nuclear and cytoplasmic immunoreactivity for S100. While S100 is not as specific as CD1a for Langerhans cells, it still can be quite useful as a confirmatory marker.* **(Right)** *Langerhans cells show positive membranous and cytoplasmic immunoreactivity for CD1a. Grooved nuclei → can be seen within the positive staining cells. CD1a is very specific for Langerhans cells and is very useful in cases where the cellularity is low.*

S100 Staining in Langerhans Cell Histiocytosis

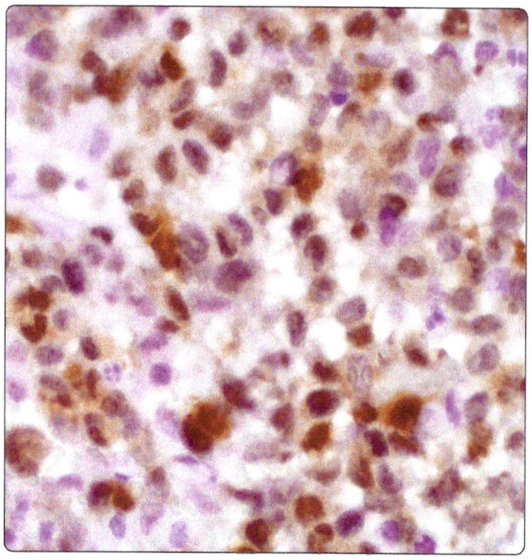

CD1a Staining in Langerhans Cell Histiocytosis

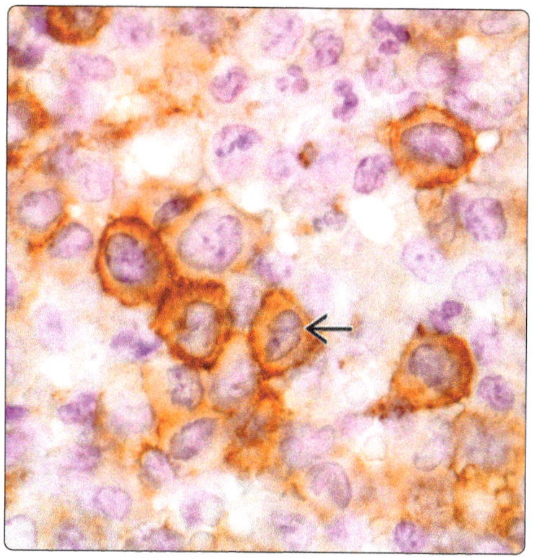

Langerhans Cell Histiocytosis Involving Skull Bones

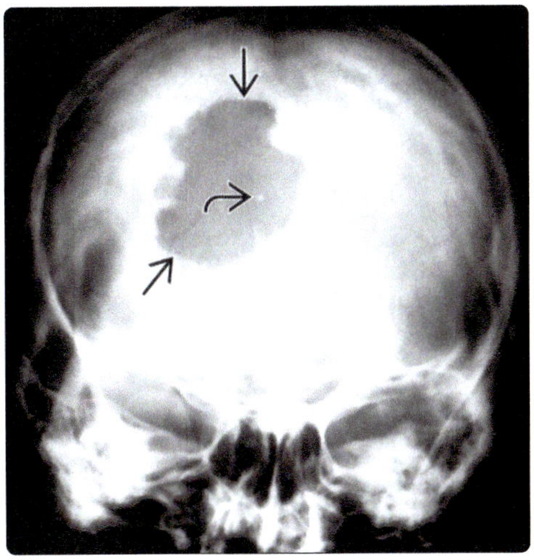

Langerhans Cell Histiocytosis of Skull Involving Bone

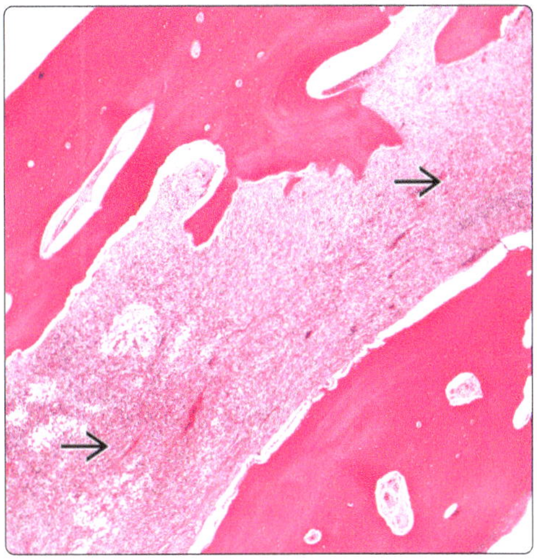

(Left) *This radiograph of the skull shows the typical appearance of LCH in bone. The lesion is lytic with scalloped edges and sharp borders, with a radiodense focus that is commonly seen in skull lesions.* **(Right)** *This low-power view of the skull shows LCH infiltrating through and replacing the marrow space. The skull is a common location for LCH to occur.*

Langerhans Cell Histiocytosis Involving Bone

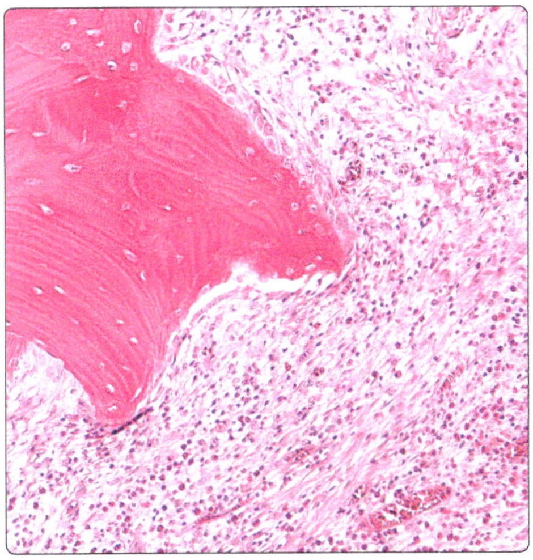

Langerhans Cell Histiocytosis Involving Liver

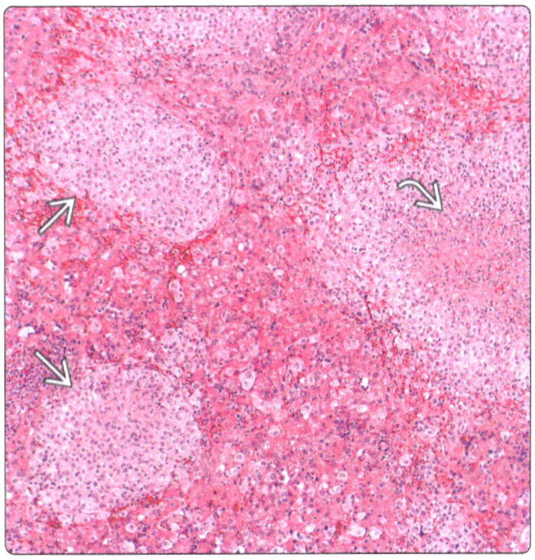

(Left) *The histology of LCH in bone can vary widely. In this example, there is fibrosis and less cellularity; Langerhans cells can be difficult to identify in some cases without the aid of immunostains.* **(Right)** *This low-power example of LCH in the liver shows multiple scattered nodules. The large nodule on the right has a necrotic center; necrosis is common in LCH.*

Touch Preparation of Langerhans Cell Histiocytosis

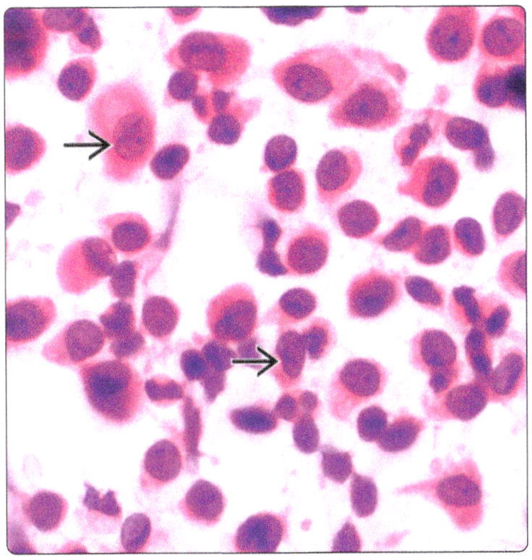

Langerhans Cell Sarcoma

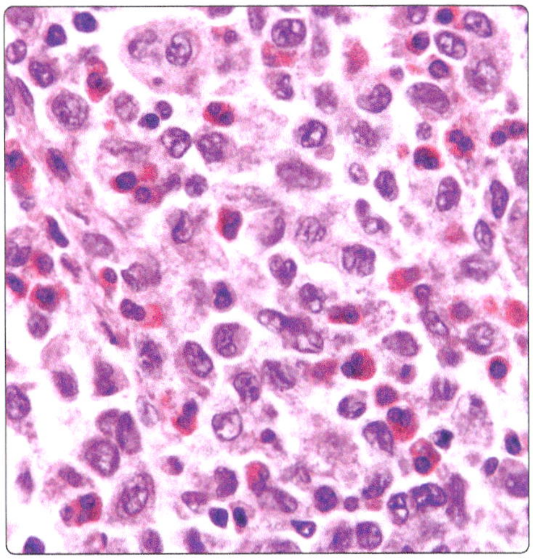

(Left) *Touch preparations made at the time of frozen section can be very helpful. The characteristic Langerhans cell features are easily identified, with grooved nuclei and abundant pink cytoplasm.* **(Right)** *This is an example of a higher grade Langerhans cell tumor, which shows more marked cytologic atypia and pleomorphism, features consistent with Langerhans cell sarcoma.*

KEY FACTS

TERMINOLOGY

- Wide range of histiocytic disorders that are not derived from Langerhans cells
  - Sometimes difficult to categorize because of overlapping morphologic and clinical findings

MICROSCOPIC

- Macrophages are large (15-80 µm in diameter) phagocytic cells with irregular shapes and pseudopodia

ANCILLARY TESTS

- Macrophages are CD14, CD68, CD163 (+)
- Dermal/interstitial dendritic cells are CD14, CD163, FXIIIA, fascin (+)

TOP DIFFERENTIAL DIAGNOSES

- Interdigitating dendritic cell sarcoma
  - Spindled to ovoid cells, usually forming fascicles or whorls, expressing S100, vimentin, and fascin (+)
- Follicular dendritic cell sarcoma
  - Neoplastic follicular dendritic cells showing spindled to ovoid cells forming fascicles, expressing follicular dendritic cell-associated markers CD21, CD23, and CD35
- Benign cephalic histiocytosis
  - Rare cutaneous condition in children characterized by skin lesions that initially present on head and consist of histiocytes
- Indeterminate cell histiocytosis
  - Features of macrophages, dendritic cells, and Langerhans cells; S100, CD68, CD1a (+)
- Progressive nodular histiocytosis
  - Part of xanthogranuloma family of disease but more clinically aggressive and disfiguring than others
- Atypical granuloma annulare
  - May be either clinically atypical (associated with malignancies) or histologically atypical (more cellular, pleomorphic, and mitoses)

Clinical Photograph of IDCS

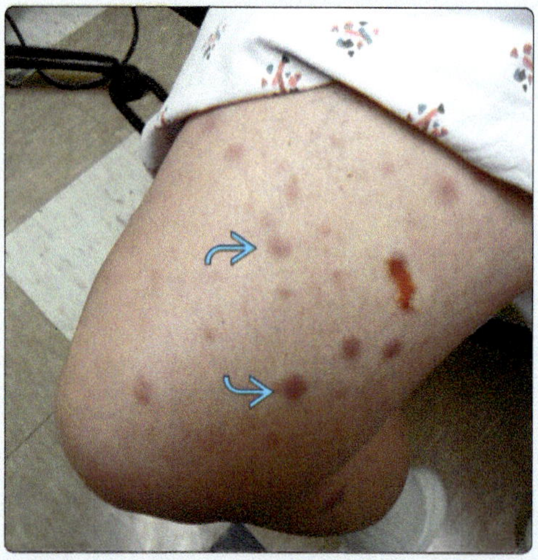

IDCS Morphology at Low Magnification

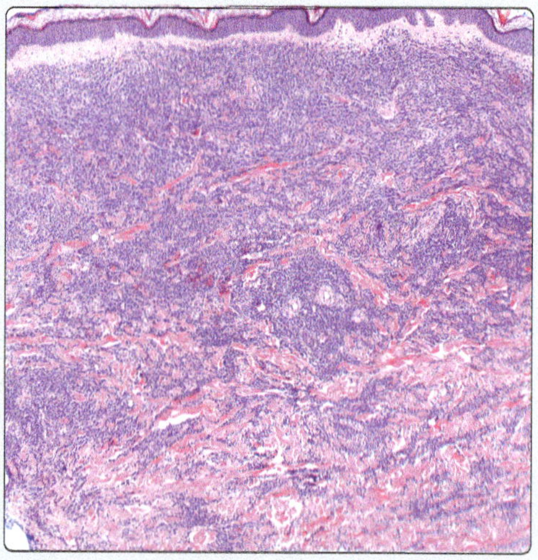

(Left) *This is a clinical photograph from a patient with interdigitating dendritic cell sarcoma (IDCS). There are multiple papules* ↷ *on his right leg.* **(Right)** *This IDCS is extensively involving the skin. The neoplastic cells involve the superficial and deep dermis, showing areas of dense storiforming patterns. Some of the cells are spindle-shaped.*

Lysozyme Immunohistochemistry in IDCS

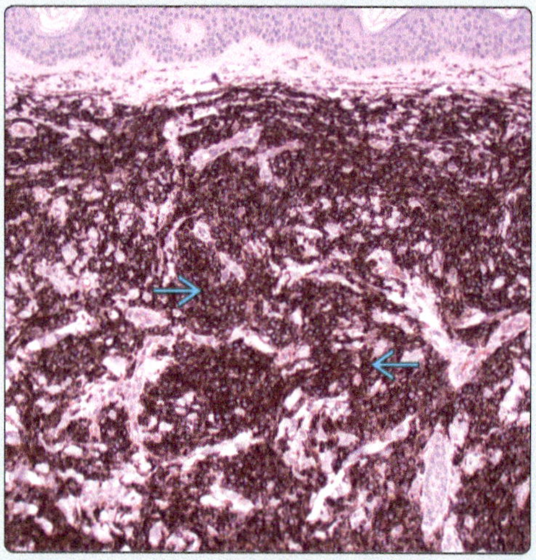

CD1a Immunohistochemistry in IDCS

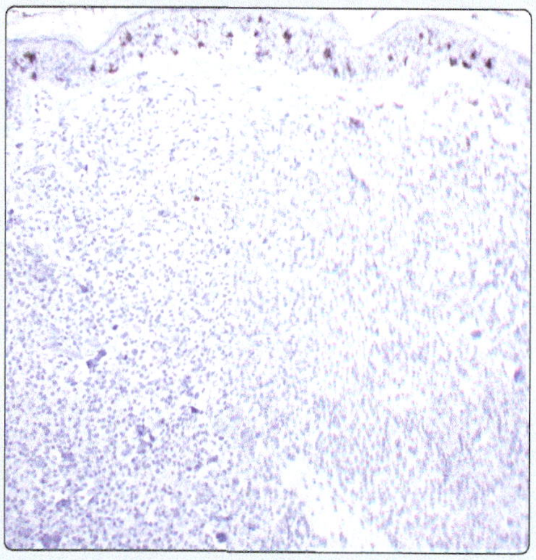

(Left) *This lysozyme stain is strongly positive* → *in a case of interdigitating dendritic cell sarcoma. S100 was also positive (not shown).* **(Right)** *This CD1a immunostain is negative in the same case of interdigitating dendritic cell sarcoma. CD1a negativity effectively excludes a Langerhans cell sarcoma. CD21, CD23, CD35, Langerin, and CD163 where also negative, excluding follicular dendritic cell sarcoma and other histiocytic lesions.*

TERMINOLOGY

Synonyms

- Non-X histiocytoses

Definitions

- Wide range of histiocytic disorders that are not derived from Langerhans cells
  - Sometimes difficult to categorize because of overlapping morphologic, immunohistochemical, and clinical findings
  - Includes juvenile xanthogranuloma, reticulohistiocytoma, and Rosai-Dorfman disease
- Histiocyte: Bone marrow-derived cell belonging to monocytes/macrophage &/or dendritic cell lineage and functional variants
  - Includes macrophages, Langerhans cells, interstitial dendritic cells, interdigitating dendritic cells, plasmacytoid dendritic cells, microglia, Kupffer cells, and alveolar macrophages

ETIOLOGY/PATHOGENESIS

Unknown

- Most cases are of undetermined etiology, although are likely genetic

CLINICAL ISSUES

Epidemiology

- Age
  - Depends on type of histiocytosis
    - Most benign histiocytoses

Treatment

- Benign tumors that do not require treatment in most cases

Prognosis

- Depends on type of histiocytosis

MICROSCOPIC

Histologic Features

- Macrophages are large (15-25 μm in diameter) phagocytic cells with irregular shapes and pseudopodia
  - Nucleus is round to oval but may be indented or reniform
  - Nuclear membrane is indistinct, and chromatin is fine
  - Cytoplasm is abundant and can be vacuolated or granulated
  - Phagocytosed material may be present
- Other features depend on type of histiocytosis

ANCILLARY TESTS

Immunohistochemistry

- Depends on type of histiocytosis
  - Macrophages are typically CD4, CD14, CD68, and CD163 (+)
  - Dermal/interstitial dendritic cells are FXIIIA, CD14, CD163, and fascin (+)
  - Indeterminate cells are S100, CD1a, and FXIIIA (+)

Electron Microscopy

- Non-Langerhans cell histiocytoses do not have Birbeck granules by ultrastructural studies, unlike Langerhans cell histiocytosis

DIFFERENTIAL DIAGNOSIS

Interdigitating Dendritic Cell Sarcoma

- Neoplastic proliferation of interdigitating dendritic cells
- Incidence is very rare
  - Patients mostly adults; mean age: 60 years
  - There is slight male predominance
- Most commonly involves single lymph node
  - Most frequently cervical, inguinal, or axillary lymph node
  - Usually presents as asymptomatic mass
  - B symptoms can occur in some cases
  - More rarely arising in patients with history of lymphoma
- Treatment typically involves surgical resection ± radiation for localized disease
  - Due to rarity of this disease, there is currently no standard treatment protocol
- Clinical course is variable, although ~ 50% of cases show disseminated disease
- Tumor usually forms fascicles, storiform pattern, and whorls of spindled to ovoid cells
- Cytology bland with infrequent mitoses
- Small lymphocytes and plasma cells may be interspersed with tumor cells
- Immunohistochemistry
  - S100(+), vimentin (+), fascin (+), CD68(+/-), lysozyme (+/-)
  - Melanoma markers, Langerhans cell markers (CD1a), B-cell markers, and T-cell markers (-)
  - FDC-associated markers (-)
    - CD21, CD23, and CD35
- Electron microscopy
  - Complex interdigitating cell processes but no well-formed desmosomes
    - No Birbeck granules

Follicular Dendritic Cell Sarcoma

- Neoplastic proliferation of follicular dendritic cells
- Follicular dendritic cells are found in B-cell areas
  - Form meshwork of cells in primary and secondary lymphoid follicles
  - Trap and present antigens to B cells involved in B-cell proliferation and differentiation
- Adults; median age: 40-50 years
- M:F = 1:1, except inflammatory pseudotumor-like variant, which is mostly in females
- Slow-growing, painless mass
- Most cases behave like low- to intermediate-grade soft tissue sarcoma
- Systemic symptoms uncommon in follicular dendritic cell sarcoma (FDCS), except in inflammatory pseudotumor-like variant
- Most patients are treated by complete surgical excision ± adjuvant radiotherapy or chemotherapy
- Local excision, frequent recurrence
- Subset of cases are clinically aggressive
- Inflammatory pseudotumor-like variant of FDCS is more indolent

- Spindled to ovoid cells forming fascicles, storiform arrays, whorls, diffuse sheets, or vague nodules
  - Small lymphocytes scattered throughout tumor commonly
  - Cytology may be low grade
- Morphologic variants include spindled/typical, epithelioid, and inflammatory pseudotumor-like variant
  - Epithelioid variant shows oval to round nuclei with moderate amount of cytoplasm
  - Inflammatory pseudotumor-like variant shows collections of lymphocytes, plasma cells, and histiocytes
- Immunohistochemistry is positive for 1 or more FDC-associated markers, such as CD21, CD23, CD35, CXCL13, clusterin, Ki-M4p, and CNA.42
  - Stains may be patchy and focally positive, especially in high-grade tumors and variant tumors
  - CD68(+/-), S100(+/-)
  - EBER(+) in inflammatory pseudotumor-like variant

Benign Cephalic Histiocytosis

- Rare histiocytosis characterized by asymptomatic, self-healing, reddish to brownish macules and papules on head, which spread later to trunk and arms
  - Begins in children ≤ 3 years old
- Morphology
  - Dermal histiocytes, fairly small with round nuclei
    - ± vacuolated cytoplasm
    - CD68, CD11a, and CD11c (+); S100 and CD1a (-)
  - Patterns include papillary dermal, lichenoid, and diffuse
    - Usually no epidermotropism
- Electron microscopy shows comma-shaped bodies, coated vesicles, and desmosome-like structures with absence of Birbeck granules

Generalized Eruptive Histiocytoma

- Rare benign histiocytosis characterized by crops of hundreds of blue-red papules, affecting mainly adults, and self-healing
  - Symmetrically distributed on trunk and extremities
    - May become hyperpigmented macules when they regress
- Clinical course
  - Usually self-limiting; may last from 1 month to over 12 years
    - May persist, may resolve, or may relapse
  - Sometimes associated with underlying tumors
    - Macules/papules may regress when underlying malignancy is treated
- Morphology
  - Histiocytes in upper dermis
    - Sometimes small and vacuolated cytoplasm
    - ± perivascular distribution
  - Usually no multinucleated giant cells
  - Older lesions may show fibrosis or giant cells
  - CD68(+), S100(-), CD1a(-)
- Electron microscopy shows dense bodies with myelin, but no Birbeck granules

Indeterminate Cell Histiocytosis

- Dendritic cells in dermis with features of histiocytes and Langerhans cells but no Birbeck granules
  - Only a few cases reported
- Presentation
  - Numerous red/brown papules
    - May coalesce
- Morphology
  - Monomorphous infiltrate of mononuclear histiocytes intermixed with clusters of lymphocytes
    - Rarely multinucleated cells
    - Often increased numbers of reactive T cells interspersed among histiocytic cells
    - Usually ample pale cytoplasm and clefted nuclei
    - Rare spindle cell variant has been described
    - Stroma can be myxoid
  - Immunohistochemistry
    - S100(+), CD68(+), CD1a(+), FXIIIA(±)
- Sometimes look like Langerhans cells with ample cytoplasm and grooves
  - But lack some Langerhans markers, such as Langerin and Birbeck granules

Progressive Nodular Histiocytosis

- Normolipemic non-Langerhans cells histiocytosis with multiple yellow-brown papules and nodules on skin and mucous membranes; part of xanthomatous family of lesions
  - Nodules mostly on trunk
  - Rarely systemic lesions
  - Disfiguring, much more aggressive than other xanthogranulomas
- CD68, CD163, and FXIIIA (+), but CD1a and S100 (-)
- Young adults present with numerous lesions

Erdheim-Chester Disease

- Rare infiltrative histocytic disorder characterized by symmetrical bone sclerosis involving long bones and systemic manifestations, mostly in lung, kidney, retroperitoneal, and heart with aggressive biology
  - ~ 30% involve skin
- Epidemiology
  - Mean age: 43 years (range: 7-84 years)
  - Slight male predominance
- Symptoms include fever, weight loss, dyspnea, diabetes insipidus, exophthalmos, periorbital xanthomas
  - Diaphyses of long bones show symmetrical osteosclerosis
- Morphology
  - Part of xanthogranuloma family of lesions
  - Collections of foamy histiocytes
    - Histiocytes have round to oval nuclei and moderate to abundant cytoplasm
    - May be multinucleated
    - Cytoplasm is usually eosinophilic and foamy
  - Varying degrees of fibrosis
  - Other inflammatory cells (lymphocytes, plasma cells, and eosinophils) may be present
  - Immunohistochemistry
    - Histiocytes CD68, factor XIIIa, ± S100 (+)
    - Histiocytes PAS, CD1a, CD45RB (-)
  - Ultrastructural studies show histiocytic cells with phagolysosomes containing lipid but no Birbeck granules
- Treatment and prognosis

- Systemic adult form, fatal in ~ 50% of patients after 5 years
- Attempted treatments include corticosteroids, chemotherapy, radiotherapy, surgery, and immunotherapy
- Differentiated from Langerhans cell histiocytosis because it lacks grooved nuclei and is CD1a(-)
- Lacks emperipolesis of Rosai-Dorfman disease

Atypical Granuloma Annulare

- Very rare histiocytic proliferation, whereas granuloma annulare is common
  - Usually affects older age than typical granuloma annulare
- Can either be clinically atypical or histologically atypical
  - Clinically atypical
    - Often associated with underlying malignancies, including lymphoma
    - Can be painful lesions on palms and soles
  - Histologically atypical
    - Often more cellular as compared to typical granuloma annulare
    - Histiocytes can have increased pleomorphism, including enlarged size, nuclear irregularity, and prominent nucleoli
    - Still areas of palisading, necrobiosis, and mucin
    - Can have increased mitotic figures as well as atypical mitoses, ≥ 1 mitoses per HPF
- Immunohistochemistry
  - Ki-67 shows fairly high proliferation rate
    - Up to 29% of histiocytes can be positive
- Need to exclude
  - Infections, which usually have true necrosis
  - Other histiocytic tumors, lymphomas, and epithelioid sarcoma
    - Recognition of atypical granuloma annulare is important to not overdiagnose as malignant condition

Hereditary Progressive Mucinous Histiocytosis

- Rare, often hereditary histiocytosis characterized by multiple persistent papules with prominent mucinosis
  - Reported primarily in female patients
  - Multiple small papules all over skin appearing in 1st decades of life and increasing gradually in number with age
- Histology
  - Unencapsulated dermal nodules composed of epithelioid histiocytes and abundant Alcian blue (+) mucin separating broad bundles of collagen
  - Histiocytes are CD68 and factor XIIIa (+), but S100, CD1a, and CD34 (-)
- Ultrastructural studies show histiocytes with cytoplasmic inclusions similar to zebra bodies and myelin bodies
- Genetic pattern remains unclear
  - Similar to autosomal dominant transmission but much more likely in women

SELECTED REFERENCES

1. Wu A et al: Follicular dendritic cell sarcoma. Arch Pathol Lab Med. 140(2):186-90, 2016
2. Lupato V et al: Head and neck extranodal interdigitating dendritic cell sarcoma: case report and review of the literature. Head Neck Pathol. 10(2):145-51, 2015
3. O'Malley DP et al: Evidence of BRAF V600E in indeterminate cell tumor and interdigitating dendritic cell sarcoma. Ann Diagn Pathol. 19(3):113-6, 2015
4. Pang J et al: Follicular dendritic cell sarcoma of the head and neck: case report, literature review, and pooled analysis of 97 cases. Head Neck. ePub, 2015
5. Dalia S et al: Clinicopathologic characteristics and outcomes of histiocytic and dendritic cell neoplasms: the moffitt cancer center experience over the last twenty five years. Cancers (Basel). 6(4):2275-95, 2014
6. Dalia S et al: Dendritic cell and histiocytic neoplasms: biology, diagnosis, and treatment. Cancer Control. 21(4):290-300, 2014
7. Go H et al: Frequent detection of BRAF(V600E) mutations in histiocytic and dendritic cell neoplasms. Histopathology. 65(2):261-72, 2014
8. Shan SJ et al: Primary cutaneous interdigitating dendritic cell sarcoma: a case report and review of the literature. Am J Dermatopathol. 37(8):639-42, 2014
9. Kim MS et al: Erdheim-chester disease. Ann Dermatol. 22(4):439-43, 2010
10. Kunimoto K et al: Progressive nodular histiocytosis. J Dermatol. 37(12):1071-3, 2010
11. Schlegel C et al: Hereditary progressive mucinous histiocytosis: first report in a male patient. Acta Derm Venereol. 90(1):65-7, 2010
12. Hasegawa S et al: Japanese case of benign cephalic histiocytosis. J Dermatol. 36(1):69-71, 2009
13. Watanabe T et al: Progressive nodular histiocytosis: a five-year follow up. Eur J Dermatol. 18(2):200-2, 2008
14. Stefanaki K et al: Histological and immunohistochemical study of granuloma annulare and subcutaneous granuloma annulare in children. J Cutan Pathol. 34(5):392-6, 2007
15. Kiliç A et al: Generalized eruptive histiocytoma: a pediatric case. Eur J Dermatol. 16(6):694-5, 2006
16. Shimizu S et al: Atypical generalized granuloma annulare associated with two visceral cancers. J Am Acad Dermatol. 54(5 Suppl):S236-8, 2006
17. Jih DM et al: Benign cephalic histiocytosis: a case report and review. J Am Acad Dermatol. 47(6):908-13, 2002
18. Rosenberg AS et al: Cutaneous indeterminate cell histiocytosis: a new spindle cell variant resembling dendritic cell sarcoma. J Cutan Pathol. 28(10):531-7, 2001
19. Gonzalez Ruíz A et al: Progressive nodular histiocytosis accompanied by systemic disorders. Br J Dermatol. 143(3):628-31, 2000
20. Sass U et al: A sporadic case of progressive mucinous histiocytosis. Br J Dermatol. 142(1):133-7, 2000
21. Matsushima Y et al: Generalized eruptive histiocytoma of childhood associated with rheumatic fever. Eur J Dermatol. 9(7):548-50, 1999
22. Manente L et al: Indeterminate cell histiocytosis: a rare histiocytic disorder. Am J Dermatopathol. 19(3):276-83, 1997
23. Trotter MJ et al: Mitotic granuloma annulare: a clinicopathologic study of 20 cases. J Cutan Pathol. 23(6):537-45, 1996

(Left) *This is a medium-powered image of follicular dendritic cell sarcoma (FDCS). Architecturally, FDCS typically shows a storiform or whorling growth pattern, at least focally. Other patterns include fascicular, nests, and sheet-like growth. (From DP: Soft Tissue, 2e.)* **(Right)** *This is a CD23 immunostain marking a case of FDCS. The neoplastic cells are strongly CD23(+). (From DP: Lymphomas.)*

Whorling Architecture FDCS

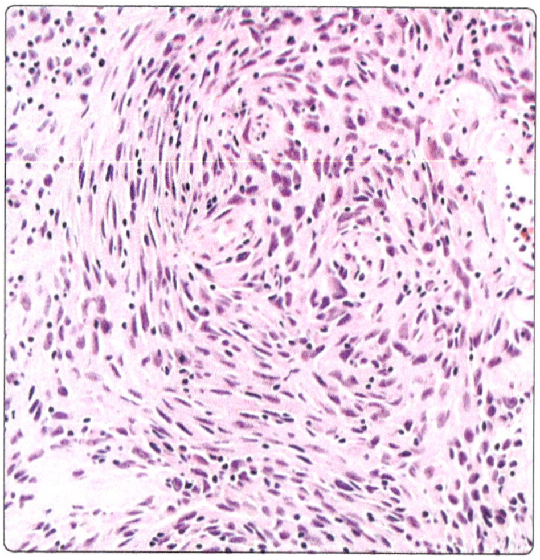

CD23 Immunohistochemistry in FDCS

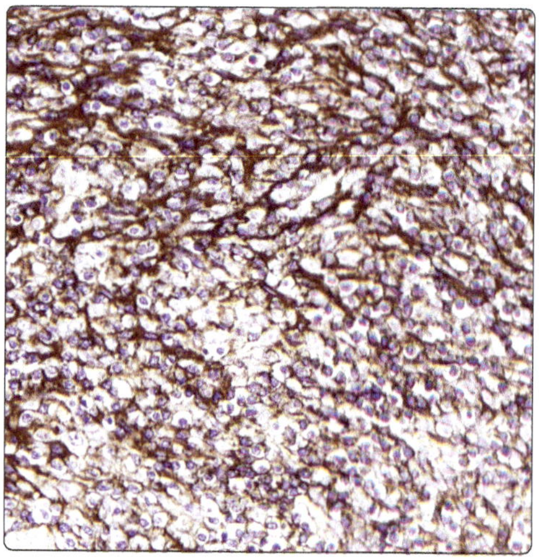

(Left) *This CD21 is strongly positive in a case of FDCS involving the lymph node. (From DP: Lymphomas.)* **(Right)** *This is another example of FDCS. The neoplastic cells are strongly CD35(+). CD21, CD23, and CD35 can be used to distinguish FDCS from IDCS. (From DP: Lymphomas.)*

CD21 Immunohistochemistry in FDCS

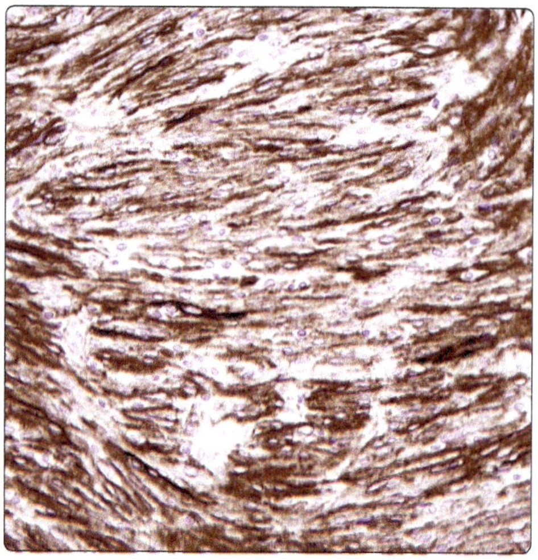

CD35 Immunohistochemistry in FDCS

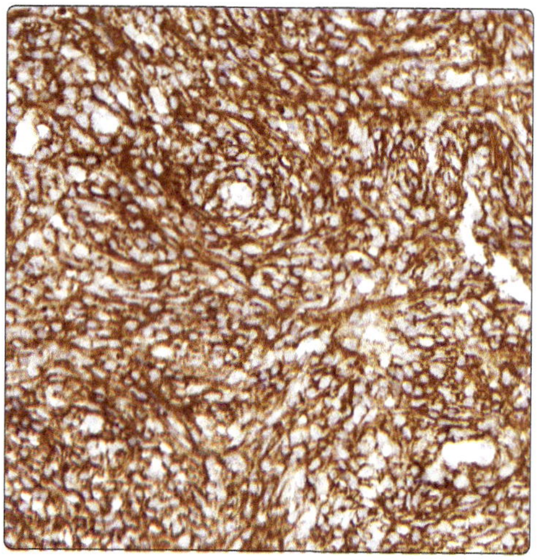

(Left) *Hereditary progressive mucinous histiocytosis shows a dermal proliferation composed of epithelioid histiocytes ➡ and mucin separating broad bundles of collagen ⇨.* **(Right)** *Indeterminate cell histiocytosis (ICH) is a very rare histiocytosis composed of cells with histologic and immunohistochemical similarities to Langerhans cells but lacking Birbeck granules by electron microscopy.*

Hereditary Progressive Mucinous Histiocytosis

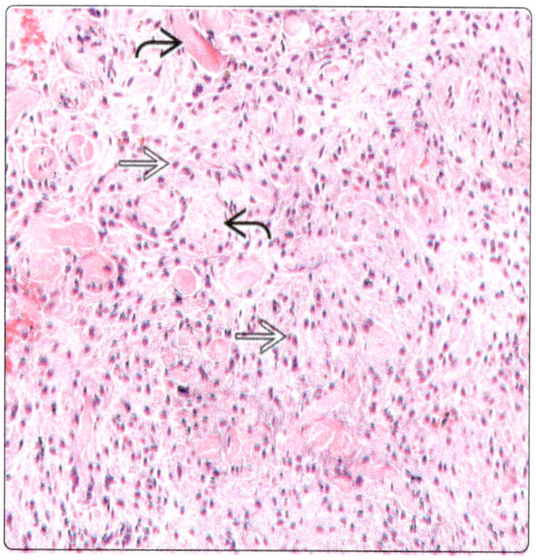

ICH

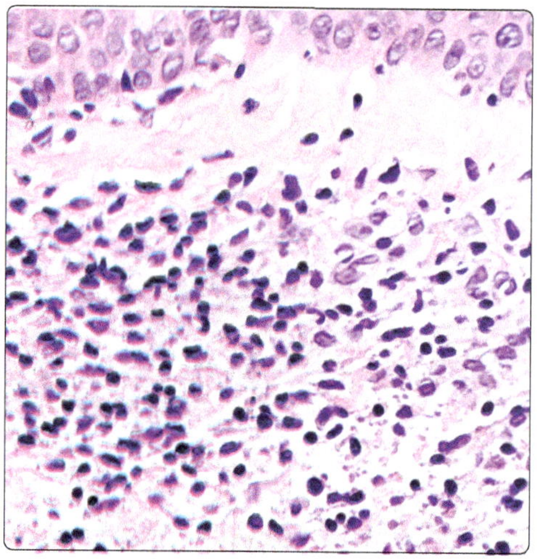

ICH

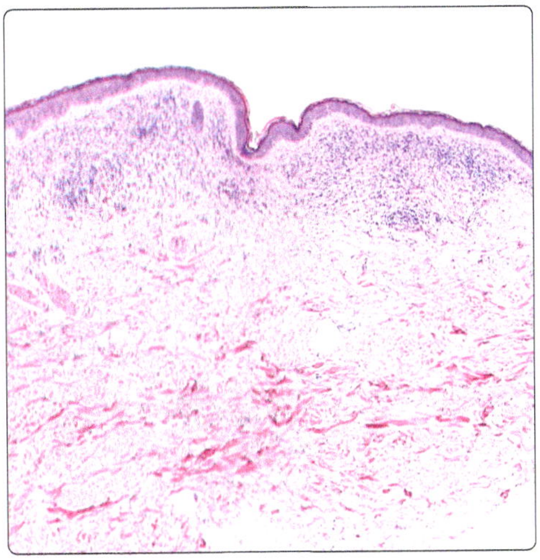

ICH, Higher Power

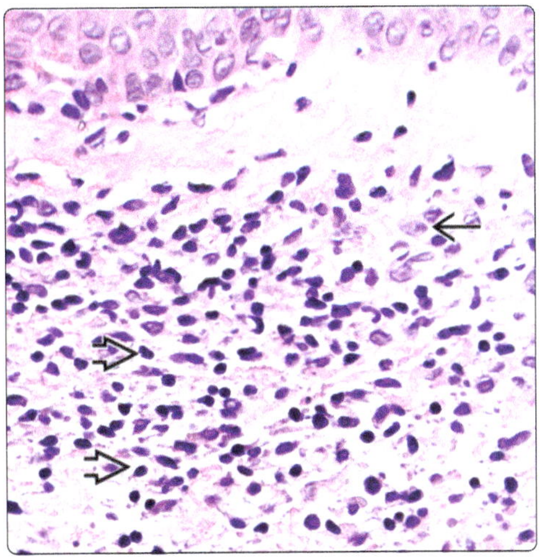

(Left) *In this case of ICH, the superficial dermis contains a histiocytic lesion intermixed with scattered lymphocytes. No epidermotropism is seen. The patient presented with numerous red/brown papules that were coalescing on his face.* **(Right)** *At higher power, 2 populations of cells are seen. The histiocyte-like cells appear with fine chromatin and clefted nuclei ⇨. There are also scattered small T cells with more coarse chromatin ⇨.*

CD1a Immunohistochemistry in ICH

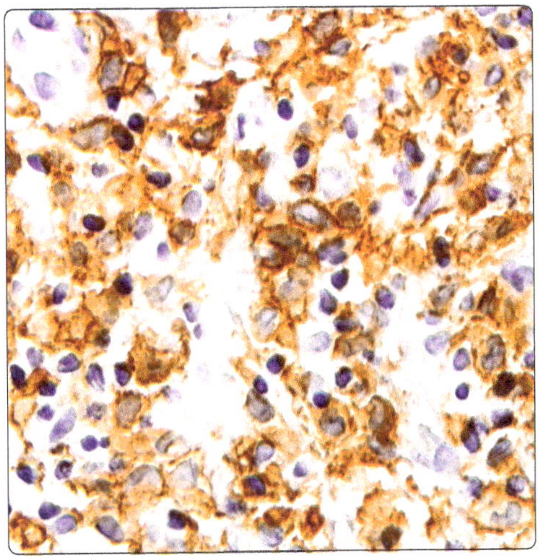

CD163 Immunohistochemistry in ICH

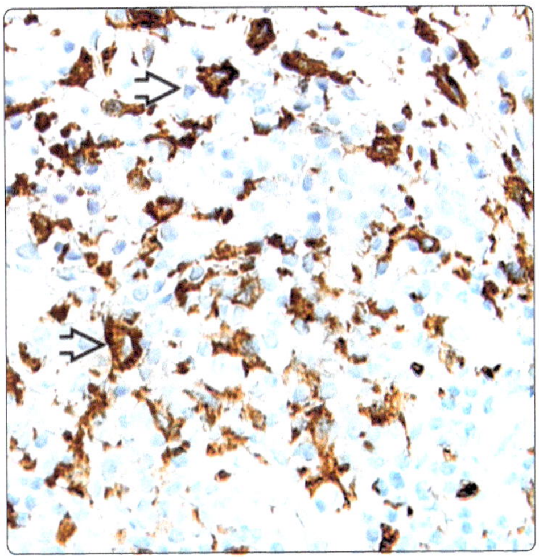

(Left) *ICH shows features of histiocytes and Langerhans cells. This is an image showing strong, diffuse positive CD1a in the cells of ICH. CD1a is often a marker of Langerhans cells.* **(Right)** *ICH shares phenotypic similarities with histiocytes, as the ICH cells are highlighted by CD163 ⇨, a macrophage marker. CD68 was also positive (not shown).*

S100 Immunohistochemistry in ICH

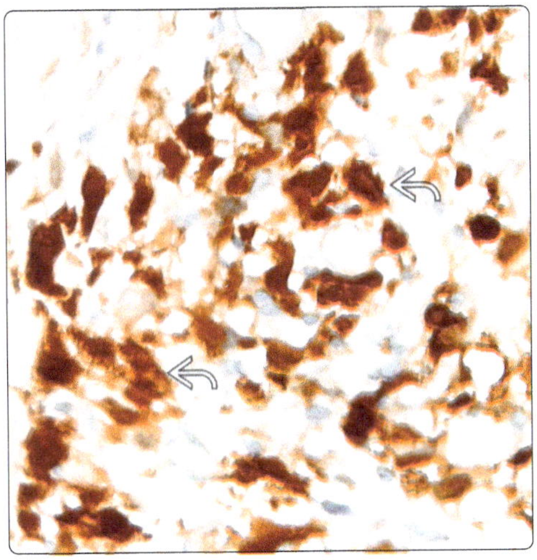

CD3 Immunohistochemistry in ICH

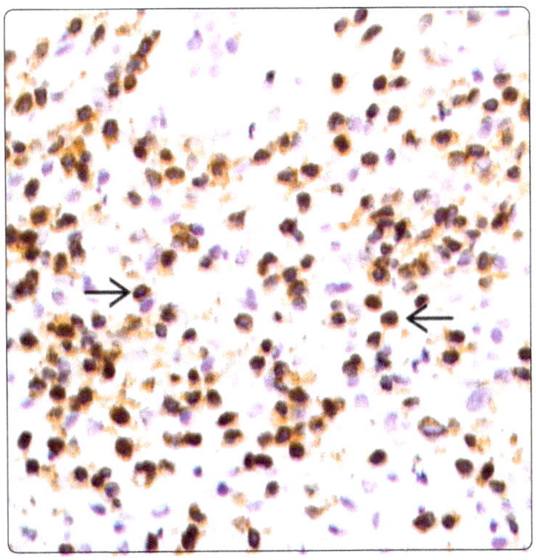

(Left) *In this case of ICH, the cells are immunoreactive for S100 ➡. The immunophenotype of histiocyte-like cells that are positive for CD1a, CD163, and S100 is unusual and points to the diagnosis of ICH instead of Langerhans cell histiocytosis (LCH). Langerin was negative, and no Birbeck granules were seen ultrastructurally, arguing against LCH.* **(Right)** *This CD3 immunostain shows increased numbers of small T cells ⇨ among the histiocyte-like cells.*

HPMH

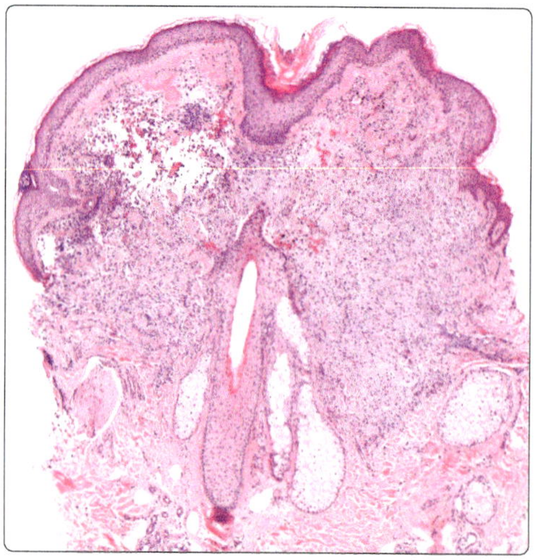

Higher Power of HPMH

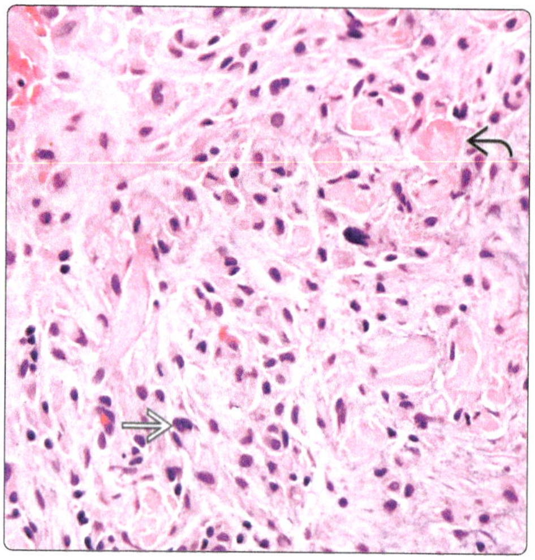

(Left) *This is a biopsy specimen from a 40-year-old woman with hereditary progressive mucinous histiocytosis (HPMH). She had multiple papules on her face, similar to those of her mother and daughter. HPMH has an autosomal dominant-like transmission mostly involving women. The dermal lesions consist of histiocytes and mucin.* **(Right)** *The dermal nodule is composed of epithelioid histiocytes ➡ and mucin separating broad bundles of collagen ⇨.*

CD68 Immunohistochemistry in HPMH

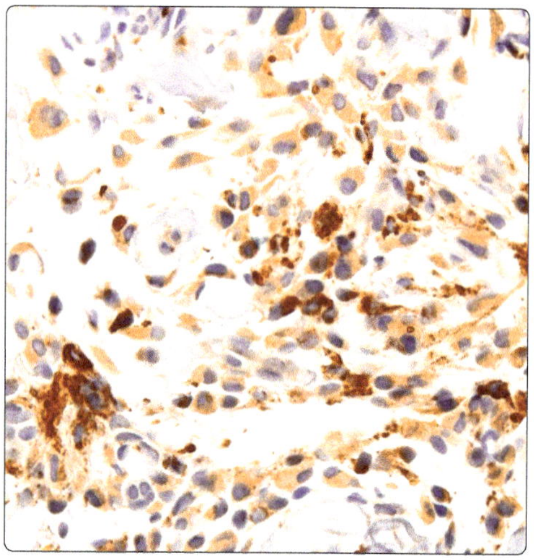

CD163 Immunohistochemistry in HPMH

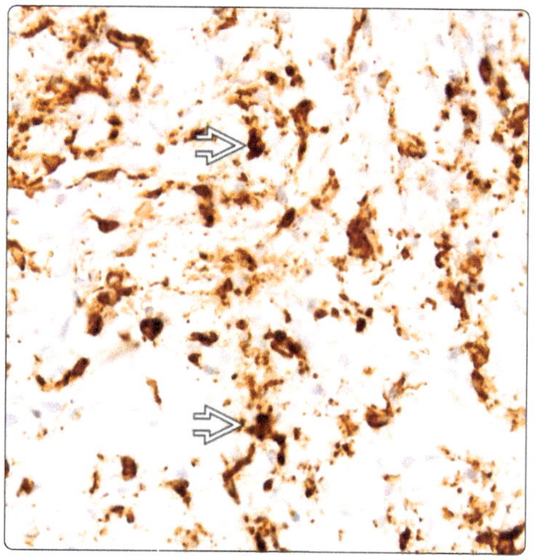

(Left) *In this case of HPMH, CD68 shows moderate to strong cytoplasmic staining.* **(Right)** *CD163, another macrophage marker, is also strongly positive ➡ in the histiocytes of HPMH. S100 and CD1a were negative (not shown). Ultrastructural studies showed myelin and zebra bodies.*

AGA

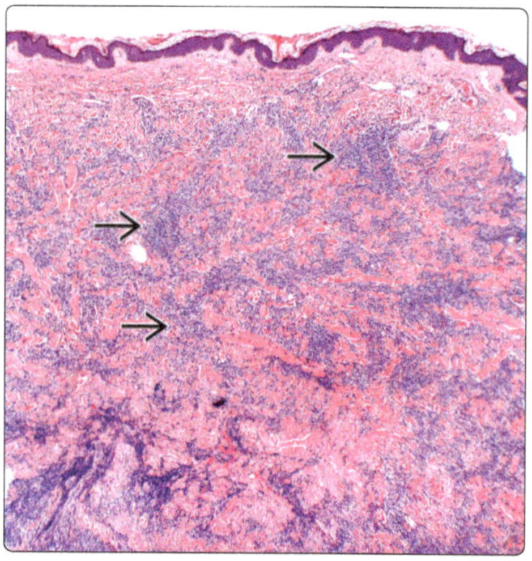

Mitotic Figures in AGA

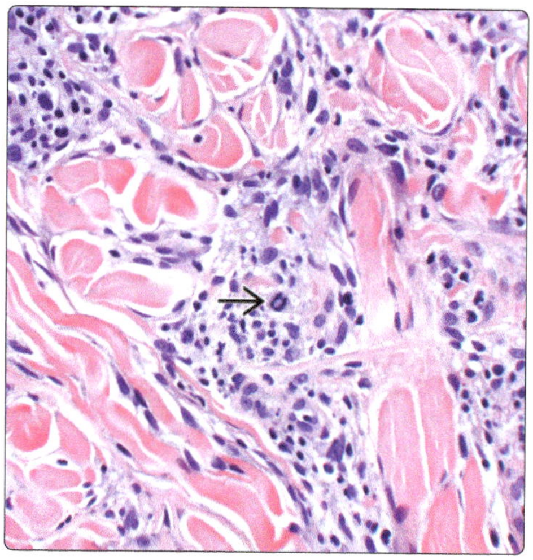

(Left) *Low-power magnification of a case of atypical granuloma annulare (AGA) shows that there are vaguely formed granulomas → with palisading though the collagen in the superficial and deep dermis. There is more cellularity than is seen in a typical granuloma annulare.* **(Right)** *High-power magnification of a case of AGA shows that there are more mitotic figures → than in a typical granuloma annulare. AGA usually has ≥ 1 mitotic figures per HPF.*

DDx: Dermatofibroma

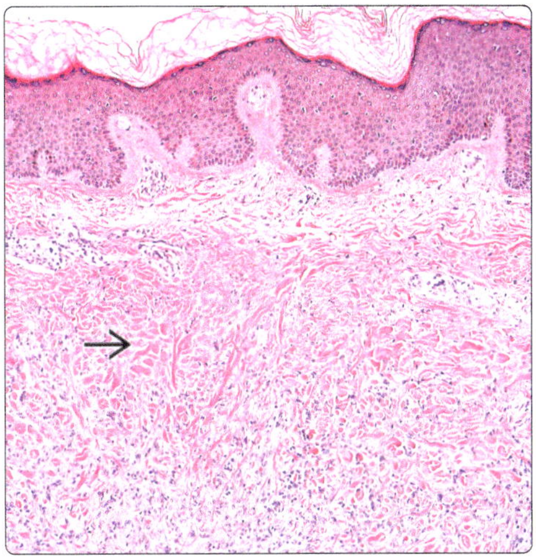

DDx: Juvenile Xanthogranuloma

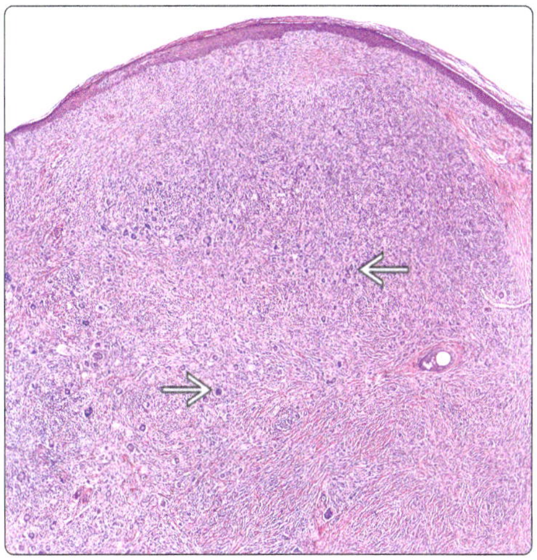

(Left) *This dermatofibroma shows bland spindled to histiocytoid-appearing cells in the dermis with overlying epidermal hyperplasia and basilar pigmentation. The spindled cells are entrapping numerous hyalinized balls of collagen* →. **(Right)** *This juvenile xanthogranuloma shows a uniform cellular lesion in the dermis with no grenz zone and scattered Touton giant cells* → *with a peripheral wreath-like arrangement of nuclei.*

DDx: Reticulohistiocytoma

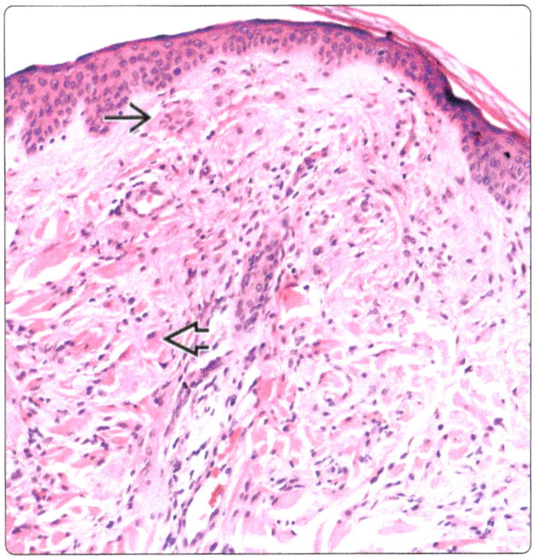

DDx: Rosai-Dorfman Disease

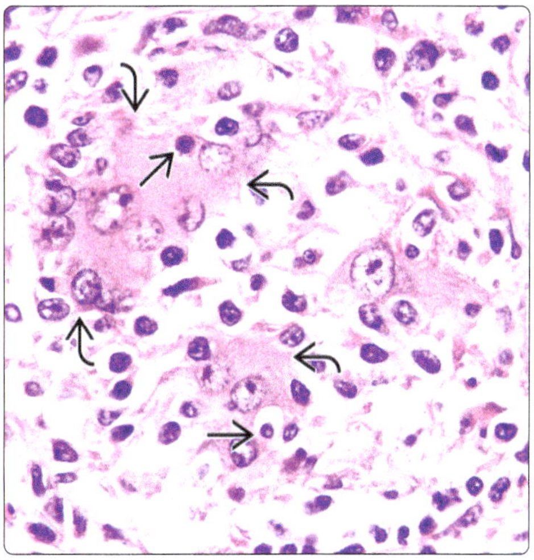

(Left) *This reticulohistiocytoma is seen as a hypocellular dermal lesion consisting of scattered large histiocytes with characteristic glassy cytoplasm* → *and rare multinucleated giant cells* →. **(Right)** *This example of Rosai-Dorfman disease shows striking emperipolesis by the proliferating histiocytes. Lymphocytes* → *are seen within the cytoplasm of histiocytes* →.

DDx: Histiocytic Sarcoma

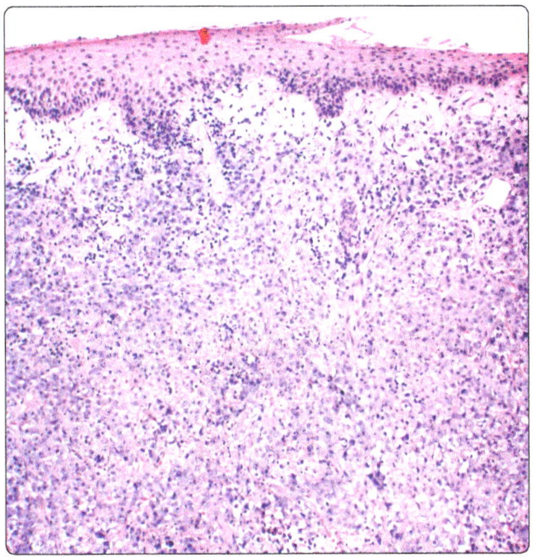

DDx: Cellular Atypia in Histiocytic Sarcoma

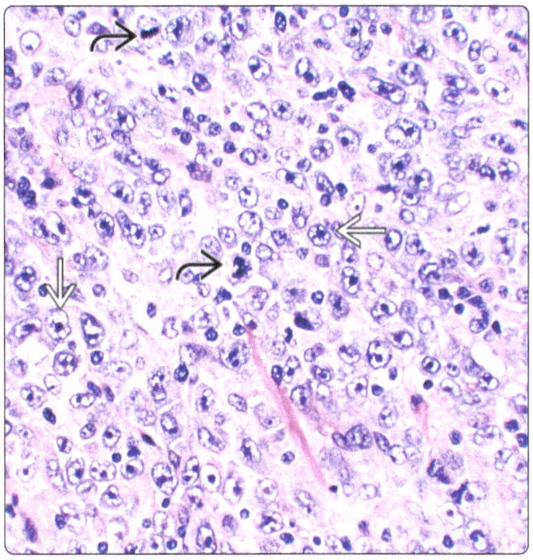

(Left) *This histiocytic sarcoma shows a diffuse, dermal-based, sheet-like proliferation of enlarged, undifferentiated-appearing cells at low-power magnification.* **(Right)** *High magnification of histiocytic sarcoma shows sheets of markedly enlarged and atypical cells* → *with abundant cytoplasm, enlarged nuclei with prominent nucleoli, and scattered mitotic figures* →.

Rosai-Dorfman Disease

KEY FACTS

TERMINOLOGY

- Rosai-Dorfman disease (RDD)
- Sinus histiocytosis with massive lymphadenopathy (term for disease involving lymph nodes)
- Lesional histiocytes contain variable numbers of intact inflammatory cells within their cytoplasm
  - Referred to as lymphophagocytosis or emperipolesis

CLINICAL ISSUES

- Painless lymphadenopathy most frequent presenting symptom
- Skin and soft tissue most common extranodal site
- Most patients have complete and spontaneous remission
  - Some may experience recurrent or persistent but stable lymphadenopathy
- Rarely, excision may be required for persistent/recurrent lesions
- Poor prognosis correlates with widespread dissemination
  - Involves kidneys, lower respiratory tract, liver, and immunologic abnormalities or anemia

MICROSCOPIC

- Skin and soft tissue cases have more subtle histologic features than lymph node counterparts
- Emperipolesis less conspicuous
- Proliferating histiocytes frequently spindled
- Majority of lesions label strongly with S100
- Vague storiform pattern
- Scattered lymphoplasmacytic aggregates

TOP DIFFERENTIAL DIAGNOSES

- Langerhans cell histiocytosis
- Juvenile xanthogranuloma
- Granulomatous inflammatory diseases
- Malakoplakia
- Sarcoidosis
- Histiocytic sarcoma (histiocytic lymphoma)

Cutaneous Rosai-Dorfman Disease, Clinical Image

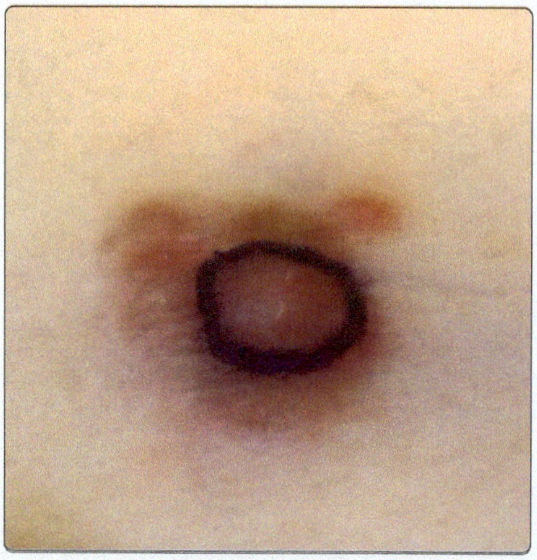

Rosai-Dorfman Disease, Low Magnification

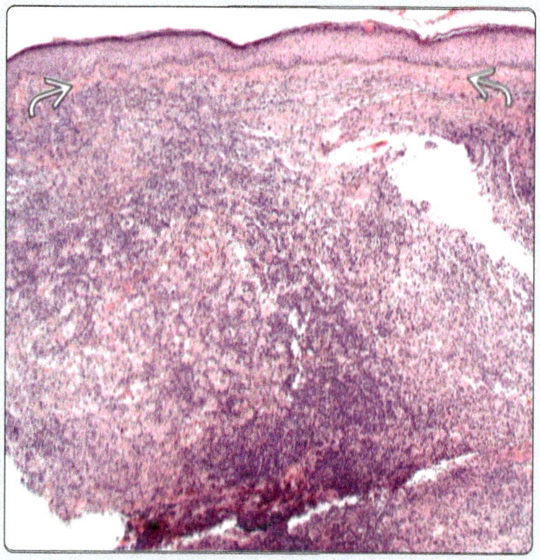

(Left) *The lesion consists of a poorly marginated process with a central nodule, marked in preparation for a punch biopsy.* **(Right)** *This case shows a lymphohistiocytic infiltrate diffusely involving the dermis and sparing the epidermis, with a grenz zone present. There is often a dense inflammatory background with many lymphoid aggregates.*

Rosai-Dorfman Disease, High Magnification Showing Emperipolesis

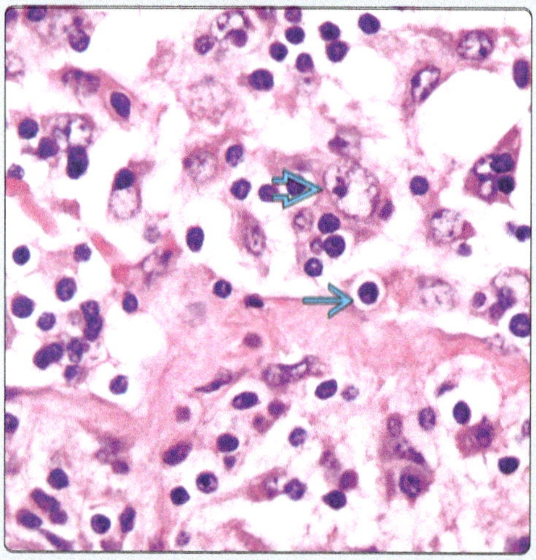

Rosai-Dorfman Disease, S100 Stain

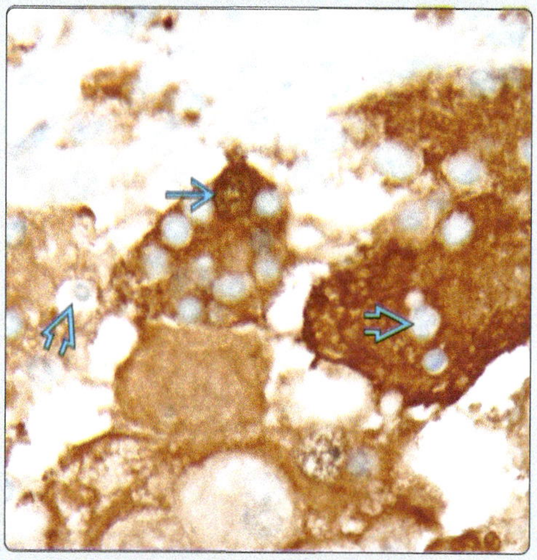

(Left) *In emperipolesis, cells are engulfed by the abnormal histiocytic cells, but they are not destroyed. Note the halos around the engulfed cells. The histiocytic nuclei are often quite large.* **(Right)** *In this high-magnification image, the emperipolesed cells are unlabeled, whereas the cytoplasm and nuclei of the abnormal histiocytic cells label strongly.*

TERMINOLOGY

Abbreviations

- Rosai-Dorfman disease (RDD)

Synonyms

- Sinus histiocytosis with massive lymphadenopathy (SHML)
  - Applies to disease involving lymph nodes
  - Primary skin cases lack lymphadenopathy

Definitions

- Rare, acquired, nonmalignant proliferation of distinctive histiocytes that presents with lymphadenopathy or extranodal disease
  - Lesional histiocytes contain variable numbers of inflammatory cells (usually lymphocytes) within cytoplasm
    - Phenomenon referred to as lymphophagocytosis or emperipolesis
  - Primarily in children and young adults

ETIOLOGY/PATHOGENESIS

Exuberant Hematopoietic Response to Undetermined Immunologic Trigger

- Association with autoimmune lymphoproliferative syndrome has been described
  - Inherited disorder of lymphocyte-programmed cell death with mutations in death receptor genes that specifically eliminate apoptosis in lymphocyte subsets
  - Occurs primarily in early childhood
  - May represent acquired disorder of deregulation of apoptotic signaling pathways
- Various infections associated with cases of RDD/SHML but none proven as etiologic infectious agent
  - Parvovirus
  - Epstein-Barr virus
  - HHV6
  - Polyoma virus

CLINICAL ISSUES

Presentation

- Varies with site
  - Painless lymphadenopathy is most frequent presenting symptom
    - Involves cervical region in up to 90% of patients
  - 30-45% of patients have at least 1 site of extranodal involvement as well as lymph node involvement
    - Hepatosplenomegaly uncommon
  - ~ 25% of patients have extranodal disease only
  - Skin and soft tissue most common extranodal sites; approximate frequency of extranodal sites
    - Skin and soft tissue (16%)
    - Nasal cavity and paranasal sinuses (16%)
    - Eye, orbit, and ocular adnexa (11%)
    - Bone (11%)
    - Salivary gland (7%)
    - Central nervous system (7%)
    - Oral cavity (4%)
    - Kidney and genitourinary tract (3%)
    - Respiratory tract (3%)
    - Liver (1%)
    - Tonsil (1%)
    - Breast (< 1%)
    - Gastrointestinal tract (< 1%)
    - Heart (< 1%)
  - Simultaneous involvement of multiple extranodal sites not unusual
  - Involvement of kidney, lower respiratory tract, and liver associated with worse clinical outcome (as is number of extranodal sites)

Treatment

- Most patients require little intervention
- Some require steroids to alleviate lesions
- Rarely, excision may be required for persistent/recurrent lesions

Prognosis

- Most patients have complete and spontaneous remission or are treated by excision
- Some may experience recurrent or persistent but stable lymphadenopathy
- In very few cases, disease follows aggressive course and may be fatal
  - Poor prognosis correlates with widespread dissemination, involvement of kidneys, lower respiratory tract, liver, and immunologic abnormalities or anemia

MACROSCOPIC

General Features

- In soft tissues and other extranodal sites
  - Firm, poorly marginated lesion
- In lymph nodes
  - Firm, massively enlarged lymph nodes

MICROSCOPIC

Histologic Features

- RDD of skin and soft tissue often has more subtle histologic features than its lymph node counterpart
  - Emperipolesis less conspicuous
  - Proliferating histiocytes frequently spindled
  - Abundant associated collagen deposition
  - Vague storiform pattern
  - Scattered lymphoplasmacytic aggregates
  - Mild cytologic atypia
- In lymph nodes (SHML)
  - Expanded sinuses contain histiocytic cells with abundant cytoplasm, sometimes multinucleated
  - Emperipolesis striking feature
- Majority of lesions label with S100
- Also positive for histiocytic markers, such as CD68, CD163, lysozyme

DIFFERENTIAL DIAGNOSIS

Langerhans Cell Histiocytosis

- Cells with nuclear grooves (coffee bean-shaped), background of eosinophils (often numerous)
- Expresses S100, CD1a, and langerin
- May harbor *BRAF* mutations

Juvenile Xanthogranuloma

- Non-Langerhans cell histiocytosis
- Cutaneous form most common
  - Nodules often develop shortly after birth
  - Most common site head and neck, followed by trunk and extremities
  - Many nodules regress spontaneously
- Rare deep cases
  - Skeletal muscle, parenchymal organs
- No association with lipid metabolism disorders
- Histiocytic cells with variable giant cells, lipid
- Background inflammatory cells, often many eosinophils
- CD68(+), CD31(+), S100(-), CD1a(-)

Granulomatous Inflammatory Diseases

- Mycobacterial infection
  - Granulomas composed of S100(-) histiocytes
  - No emperipolesis
  - Organisms can be detected by culture/special stains
- Chronic granulomatous disease (CGD)
  - Rare primary inherited immunodeficiency (incidence 1:200,000 in USA)
  - Affects phagocytes (neutrophils and macrophages) that contain nicotinamide adenine dinucleotide phosphate (reduced NADPH) oxidase enzyme
    - Generates superoxide required for killing microorganisms
  - Dysfunction of NADPH oxidase in CGD results in ineffective respiratory burst in phagocytes
    - Unable to kill and digest certain bacteria and fungi, predisposing patients to infections
  - Functional diagnosis of CGD
    - Demonstrates absence or marked reduction in phagocytic respiratory burst to form superoxides, using tests such as nitroblue tetrazolium (NBT) reduction
    - Neutrophils stimulated with phorbol myristate acetate and incubated with yellow dye NBT
    - Normal phagocytes reduce this to dark pigment formazan, with mixed NBT(+) and NBT(-) cells, denoting carrier status
  - Features loose collections of pigmented histiocytes typically in lung and GI tract with variable granuloma formation
  - S100(-)
- Malakoplakia
  - Acquired granulomatous disorder (1st described by Michaelis and Gutmann)
  - Believed to result from acquired bacteriocidal defect in macrophages
    - Occurring mostly in immunosuppressed patients or in setting of autoimmune disease
  - Usually in bladder or GI tract
  - Collections of histiocytes
    - S100(-)
  - Contain targetoid inclusions that stain with von Kossa stain
    - Believed to reflect concretions of phagocytosed bacteria

Sarcoidosis

- Well-formed granulomas with mild background infiltrate
- Histiocytes lack S100 labeling
- Emperipolesis not typical feature

Histiocytic Sarcoma (Histiocytic Lymphoma)

- Marked cytologic atypia
- Expresses multiple histiocytic markers but not S100
- Aggressive clinical course

Malignant Fibrous Histiocytoma (High-Grade Pleomorphic Undifferentiated Sarcoma)

- Composed of highly pleomorphic spindle cells
- S100 staining (-)
- Emperipolesis not typical feature

Follicular Dendritic Cell Tumor/Sarcoma

- Oval to spindle-shaped cells with eosinophilic cytoplasm in sheets and fascicles, focal storiform pattern and whorls (similar to those seen in meningioma)
- Oval or elongated nuclei with thin nuclear membranes, inconspicuous or small eosinophilic nucleoli, and clear or dispersed chromatin
- Tumor cells are intimately admixed with small lymphocytes, with prominent perivascular cuffing
- Multinucleate cells common
- Necrosis, marked cellular atypia, high mitotic rate, &/or abnormal mitoses common
- Express CD21, CD35, podoplanin (D2-40), S100

SELECTED REFERENCES

1. Alayed K et al: BRAF and MAP2K1 mutations in Langerhans cell histiocytosis: a study of 50 cases. Hum Pathol. ePub, 2016
2. Campochiaro C et al: BRAF mutations in Erdheim-Chester disease. Dermatol Clin. 34(1):xi-xii, 2016
3. Diamond EL et al: Diverse and targetable kinase alterations drive histiocytic neoplasms. Cancer Discov. 6(2):154-65, 2016
4. Hyman DM et al: Vemurafenib in multiple nonmelanoma cancers with BRAF V600 mutations. N Engl J Med. 373(8):726-36, 2015
5. Satpathy AT et al: Cellular morphology of BRAF V600E-positive Langerhans cell histiocytosis. Blood. 126(15):1857, 2015
6. Lin SK et al: Elusive diagnosis of left ear nodules. Cutaneous Rosai-Dorfman disease (RDD). JAMA Dermatol. 150(1):81-2, 2014
7. Al-Daraji W et al: Soft tissue Rosai-Dorfman disease: 29 new lesions in 18 patients, with detection of polyomavirus antigen in 3 abdominal cases. Ann Diagn Pathol. 14(5):309-16, 2010
8. Gaitonde S: Multifocal, extranodal sinus histiocytosis with massive lymphadenopathy: an overview. Arch Pathol Lab Med. 131(7):1117-21, 2007
9. Mehraein Y et al: Parvovirus B19 detected in Rosai-Dorfman disease in nodal and extranodal manifestations. J Clin Pathol. 59(12):1320-6, 2006
10. Wang KH et al: Cutaneous Rosai-Dorfman disease: clinicopathological profiles, spectrum and evolution of 21 lesions in six patients. Br J Dermatol. 154(2):277-86, 2006
11. Lauwers GY et al: The digestive system manifestations of Rosai-Dorfman disease (sinus histiocytosis with massive lymphadenopathy): review of 11 cases. Hum Pathol. 31(3):380-5, 2000
12. Levine PH et al: Detection of human herpesvirus 6 in tissues involved by sinus histiocytosis with massive lymphadenopathy (Rosai-Dorfman disease). J Infect Dis. 166(2):291-5, 1992
13. Montgomery EA et al: Rosai-Dorfman disease of soft tissue. Am J Surg Pathol. 16(2):122-9, 1992
14. Foucar E et al: Sinus histiocytosis with massive lymphadenopathy (Rosai-Dorfman disease): review of the entity. Semin Diagn Pathol. 7(1):19-73, 1990
15. Foucar E et al: Sinus histiocytosis with massive lymphadenopathy. An analysis of 14 deaths occurring in a patient registry. Cancer. 54(9):1834-40, 1984
16. Rosai J et al: Sinus histiocytosis with massive lymphadenopathy. A newly recognized benign clinicopathological entity. Arch Pathol. 87(1):63-70, 1969

Rosai-Dorfman Disease With Scattered Lymphoid Aggregates

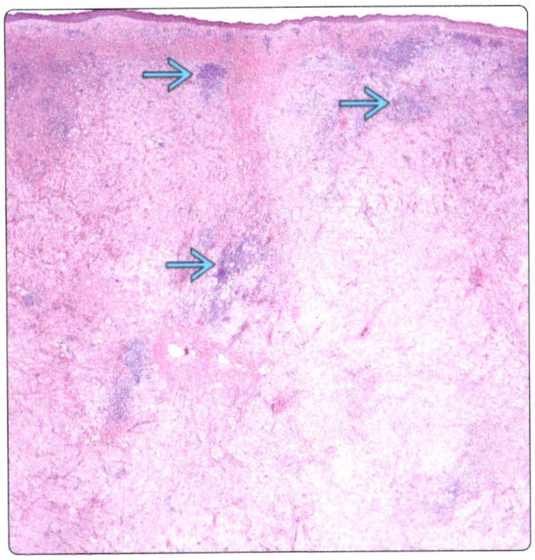

Rosai-Dorfman Disease With Lymphoid Aggregates

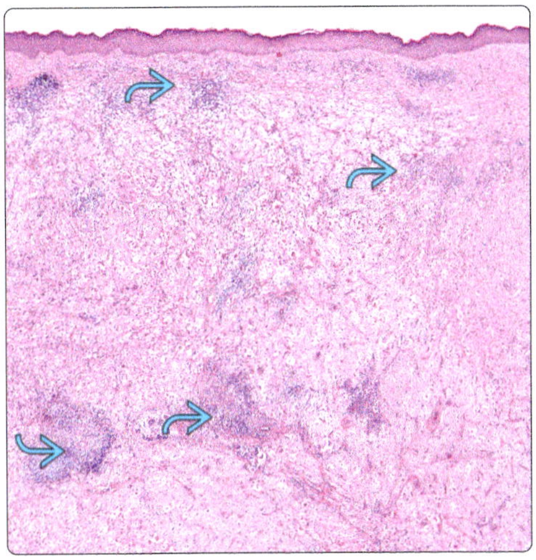

(Left) *Note the lymphoid aggregates in the dermis. They appear conspicuous against the pale background of sheets of abnormal histiocytic cells.* **(Right)** *Slightly higher magnification shows that the lesion is histiocyte rich but has scattered lymphoid aggregates as well. Their presence amongst the histiocytes is a diagnostic clue.*

Rosai-Dorfman Disease in Superficial Dermis

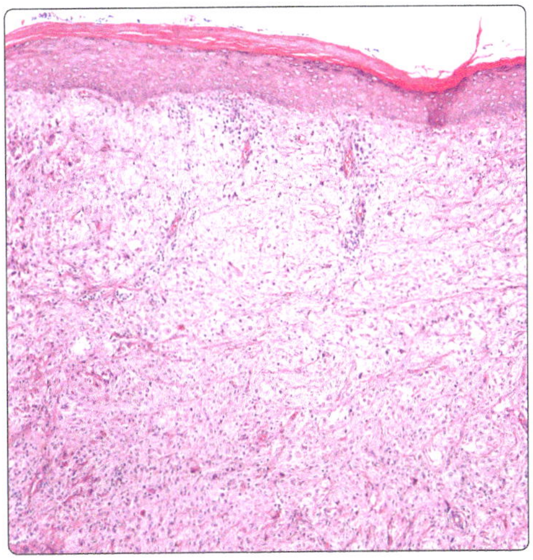

Rosai-Dorfman Disease, Higher Magnification

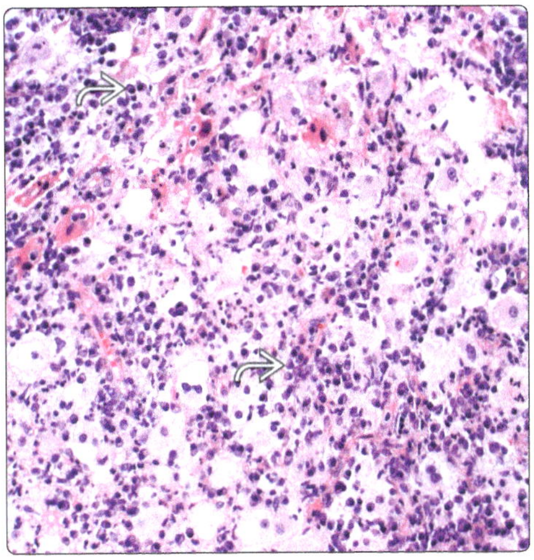

(Left) *There is a histiocyte-rich proliferation in the superficial dermis and closely abutting the epidermis. Some lesions show a dense inflammatory background, with many lymphoid aggregates and plasma cells.* **(Right)** *Higher magnification shows many large histiocytic cells, some of which contain inflammatory cells in their cytoplasm, including lymphocytes and plasma cells.*

Rosai-Dorfman Disease, High Magnification Showing Emperipolesis

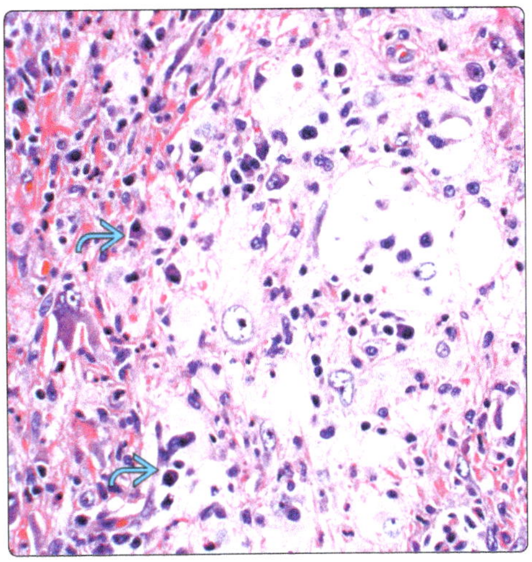

Rosai-Dorfman Disease, S100 Immunohistochemistry

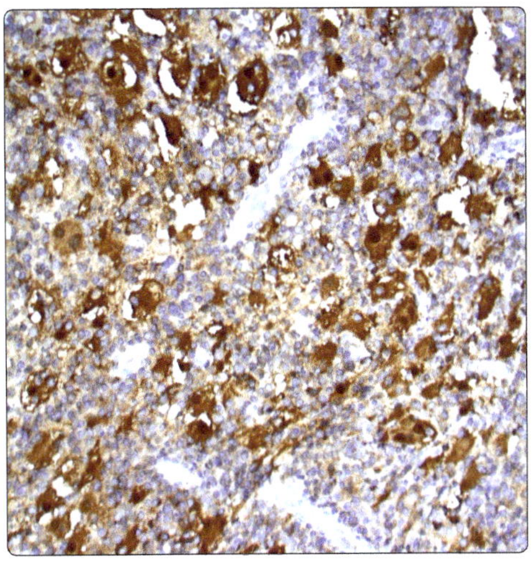

(Left) *Many large histiocytic-appearing cells with abundant cytoplasm and emperipolesis are seen in this field. Note the many plasma cells present.* **(Right)** *Usually Rosai-Dorfman disease displays strong S100 expression, with nuclear and cytoplasmic staining, as seen here.*

(Left) *In this case, the pattern of regularly spaced lymphoid aggregates amid the pale sea of histiocytic cells is reminiscent of the light and dark squares on a checkerboard.* **(Right)** *Many histiocytic cells in this image are participating in emperipolesis. Note their large nuclei. The cells are stuffed with lymphocytes, monocytes, and neutrophils.*

Rosai-Dorfman Disease, Low-Magnification Pattern

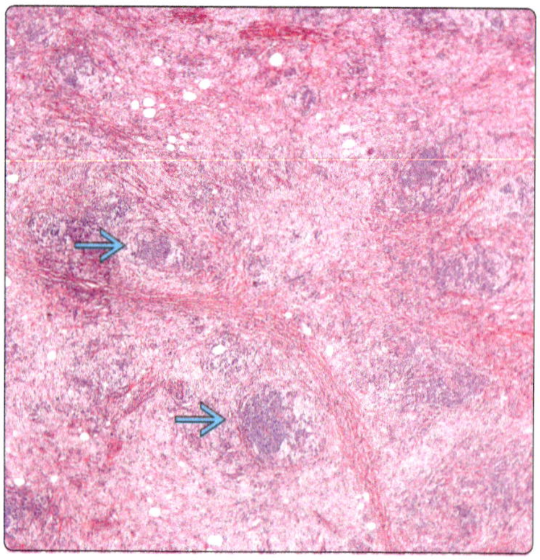

Rosai-Dorfman Disease, Emperipolesis

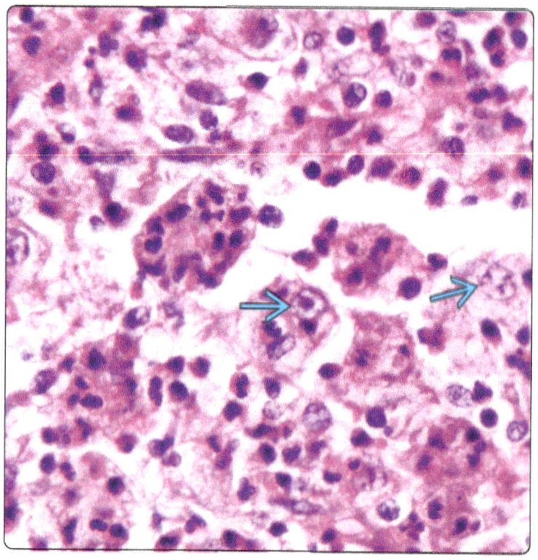

(Left) *This high magnification shows emperipolesis in Rosai Dorfman disease. Engulfed intact lymphocytes are present in a histiocytic cell with an enlarged nucleus.* **(Right)** *S100 shows nuclear and cytoplasmic labeling in the histiocytes. Note that the engulfed lymphocytes in the field do not express S100. They are undamaged and surrounded by a "halo". The S100 stain sometimes accentuates this emperipolesis.*

Rosai-Dorfman Disease, Emperipolesis

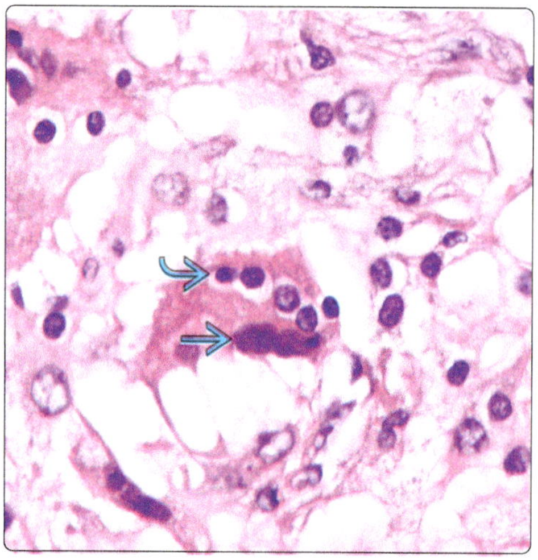

Rosai-Dorfman Disease, S100 Stain

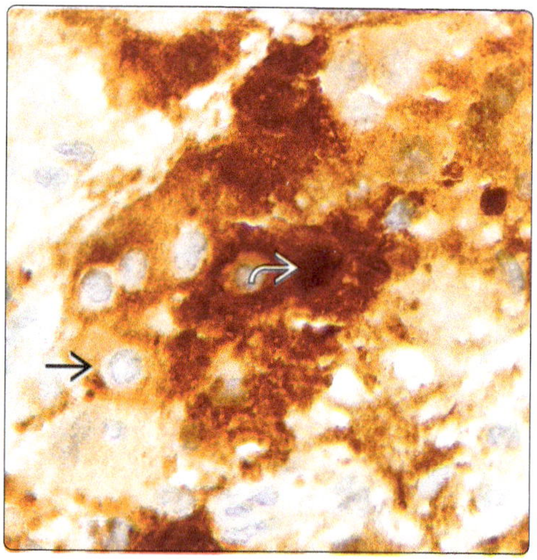

(Left) *This example shows overlying epidermal hyperplasia, a feature that is common to so-called fibrohistiocytic lesions (dermatofibroma/fibrous histiocytoma).* **(Right)** *There is a backdrop of mononuclear histiocytic cells punctuated in this case by multinucleated giant cells and many eosinophils. Most cases have varying amounts of each of these components.*

Differential Diagnosis, Juvenile Xanthogranuloma

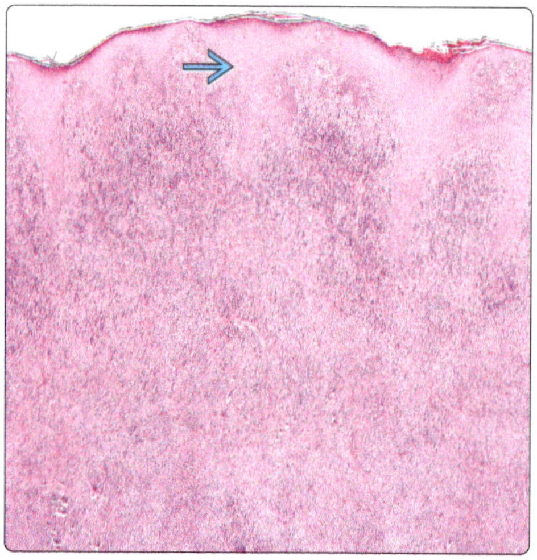

Differential Diagnosis, Juvenile Xanthogranuloma

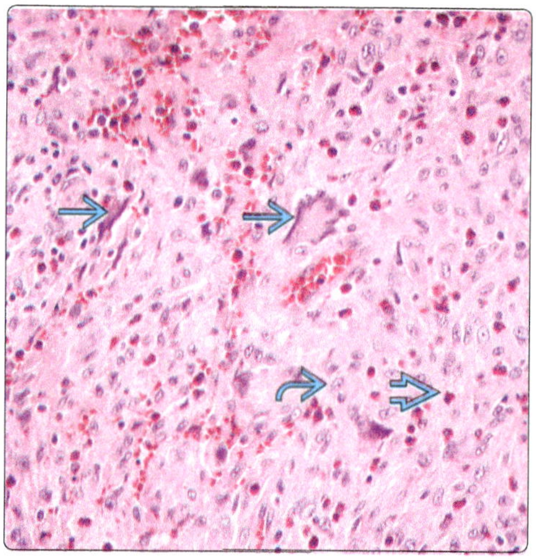

Differential Diagnosis, Langerhans Cell Histiocytosis

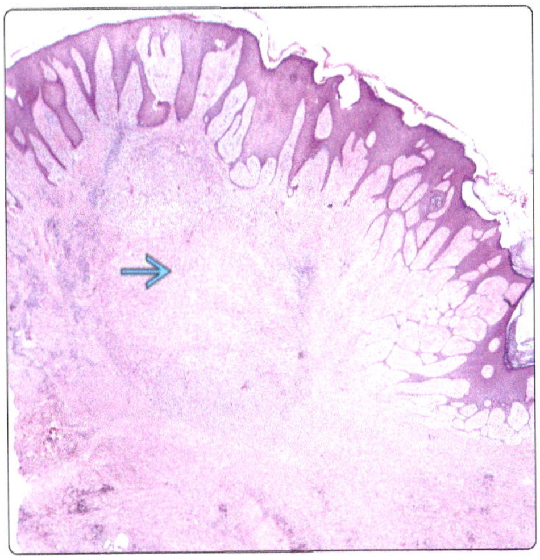

Langerhans Cell Histiocytosis, S100 Staining

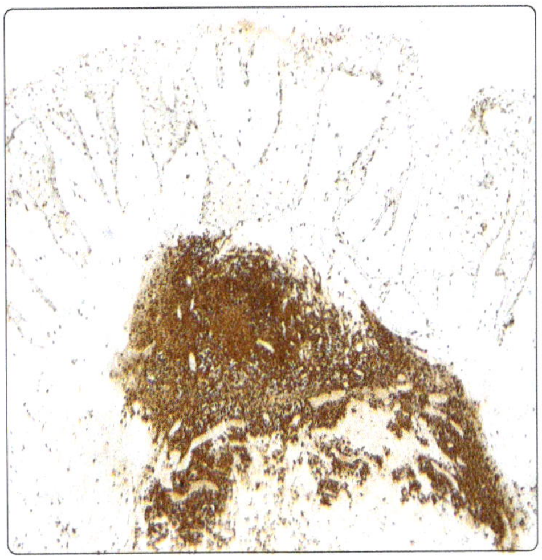

(Left) *The abnormal Langerhans cells are more eosinophilic-staining than Rosai-Dorfman cells. They also harbor BRAF mutations, which are absent in Rosai-Dorfman disease but shared with Erdheim-Chester disease (another form of histiocytosis characterized by deep tissue and bone involvement).* **(Right)** *Note the diffuse, strong S100 expression in Langerhans cell histiocytosis, a feature it shares with Rosai-Dorfman disease.*

Langerhans Cell Histiocytosis With Numerous Eosinophils

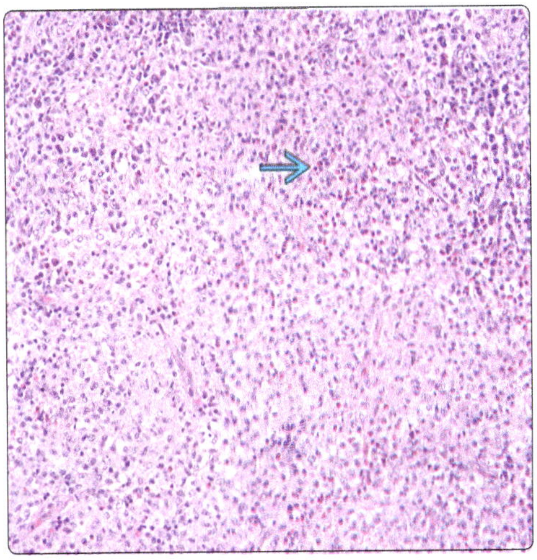

Langerhans Cell Histiocytosis, High Magnification Showing Nuclear Grooves

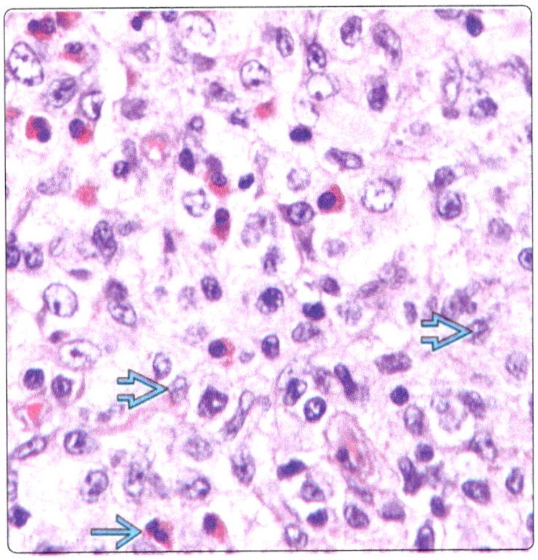

(Left) *Even at this magnification, eosinophils are readily noted. The lesional cells are eosinophilic-staining and have a higher nucleus:cytoplasmic ratio than the cells of Rosai-Dorfman disease.* **(Right)** *Coffee bean-shaped nuclei with nuclear grooves, and a background infiltrate including many eosinophils, are characteristically seen in Langerhans cell histiocytosis.*

Differential Diagnosis, Malakoplakia

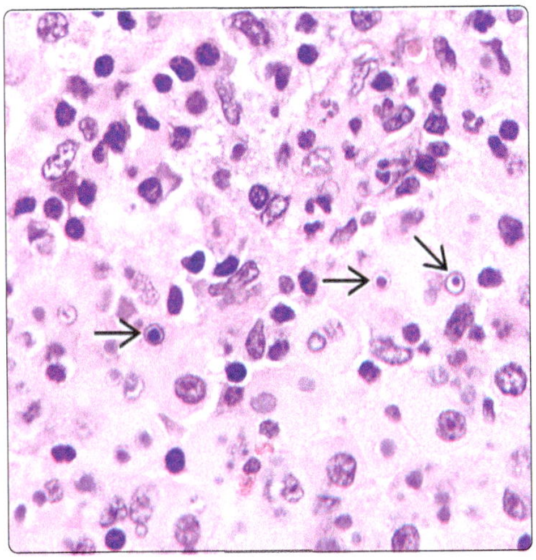

Malakoplakia, Von Kossa Stain

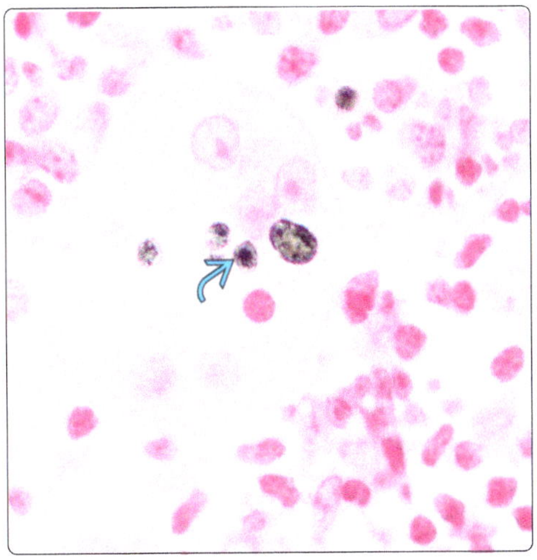

(Left) *Histologic examination shows an example of malakoplakia. There are several Michaelis-Gutmann bodies identified. These consist of incompletely eradicated engulfed bacteria.* **(Right)** *This von Kossa stain highlights the Michaelis-Gutmann bodies in malakoplakia that are within a histiocyte. One has a so-called targetoid appearance.*

KEY FACTS

TERMINOLOGY

- Malignancy with histologic and phenotypic evidence of histiocytic differentiation
- Neoplasm of mature malignant histiocytes

CLINICAL ISSUES

- Extremely rare tumor
- Usually rash or solitary mass on skin
- Some patients develop both histiocytic tumors and lymphoid tumors, known as transdifferentiation
- Complete surgical excision with subsequent chemotherapy &/or radiotherapy
- Poor prognosis but better for small localized tumors

MICROSCOPIC

- Dermal and subcutaneous infiltrate sparing epidermis
- Composed of large, noncohesive, atypical epithelioid tumor cells with abundant cytoplasm
- Histiocytes range from bland to pleomorphic

ANCILLARY TESTS

- Immunohistochemistry: CD163(+), CD68(+), lysozyme (+), CD4(+/-), S100(-)/focal(+)
- B-cell markers, melanoma markers, carcinoma markers, and myeloid markers (-)
- *BRAF* V600E mutations frequent
- *IGH*, *TRB*, or *TRG* can be monoclonal with transdifferentiation
    - And HS may have same clone as lymphoma

TOP DIFFERENTIAL DIAGNOSES

- Langerhans cell histiocytosis and Langerhans cell sarcoma
- Myeloid/monocytic sarcoma
- Diffuse large B-cell lymphoma
- Anaplastic large cell lymphoma
- Classic Hodgkin lymphoma
- Melanoma
- Carcinoma

Cutaneous HS at Low Magnification

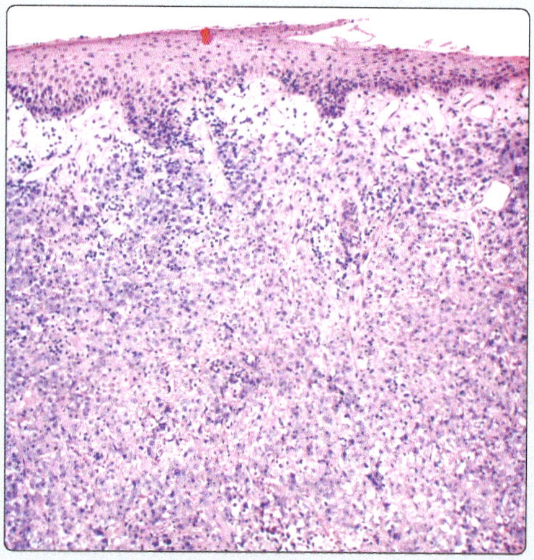

HS at High Magnification

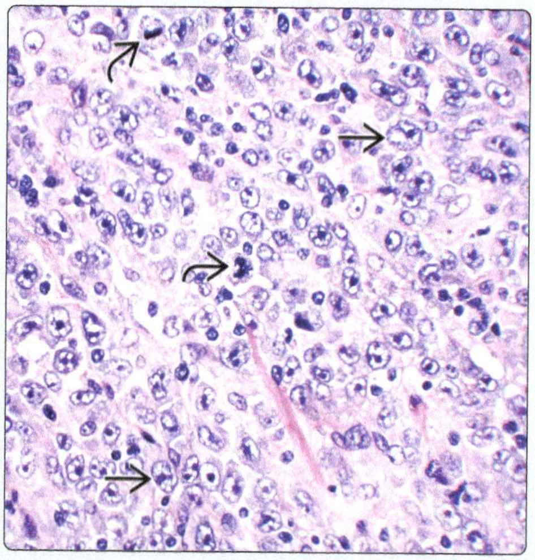

(Left) *Histiocytic sarcoma (HS) at low magnification shows a diffuse, dermal-based, sheet-like proliferation of enlarged, undifferentiated-appearing cells at this power.* **(Right)** *High magnification of HS shows sheets of markedly enlarged and atypical cells → with abundant cytoplasm, enlarged nuclei with prominent nucleoli, and scattered mitotic figures ↷.*

CD68 Immunohistochemistry in HS

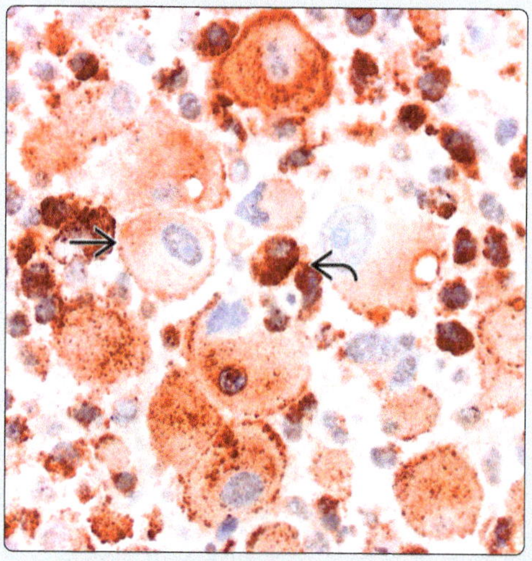

***BRAF* V600E in HS**

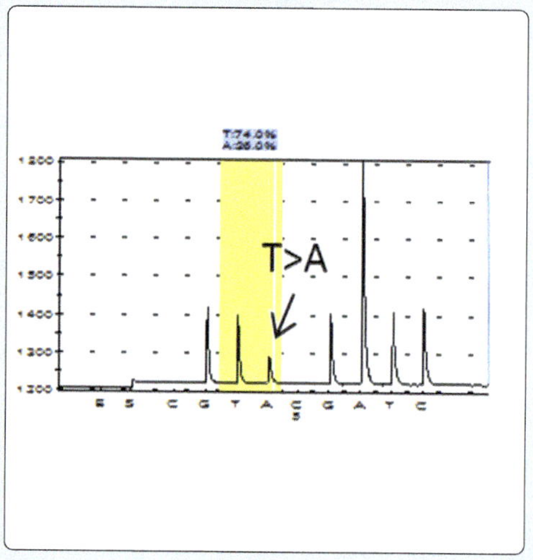

(Left) *CD68(+) HS is shown. CD68 immunohistochemistry highlights dim reactivity in large neoplastic cells → and strong reactivity in small nonneoplastic histiocytes ↷. (Courtesy R. Miranda, MD.)* **(Right)** *Graph shows a BRAF V600E mutation in histiocytic sarcoma with a substitution of nucleotide T for A →. The nucleotide substitution results in an amino acid substitution of valine for glutamic acid. BRAF mutations are often seen in HS. (From DP: Molecular Oncology.)*

TERMINOLOGY

Abbreviations

- Histiocytic sarcoma (HS)

Synonyms

- Extramedullary monocytic tumor, malignant histiocytosis, true histiocytic lymphoma

Definitions

- Malignant tumor of mature histiocytes
  - Neoplasms associated with acute monocytic leukemia are excluded
    - Now classified as monocytic sarcoma

ETIOLOGY/PATHOGENESIS

Etiology

- Idiopathic
  - Rarely associated with germ cell tumors
  - Also can be associated with lymphoma, leukemia, or myelodysplastic syndrome

CLINICAL ISSUES

Epidemiology

- Incidence
  - Extremely rare tumor
- Age
  - Mostly in adults
    - Median age: 52 years
    - Rare in children
- Sex
  - M:F = ~ 1:1
- Ethnicity
  - No known ethnic predilection

Site

- Most cases are extranodal
  - Skin, GI tract, and soft tissue most common
- Lymph node less common

Presentation

- Often single painless mass
  - B symptoms common
- Skin
  - Variable presentation
    - Can be seen as rash, single lesion, or multiple lesions (disseminated)

Laboratory Tests

- Cytopenias in some patients
  - Thrombocytopenia is most common

Natural History

- Some patients develop both histiocytic tumors and lymphoid tumors
  - Process known as transdifferentiation
  - Association with prior lymphoma suggests transdifferentiation

Treatment

- Surgical approaches
  - Surgical excision with wide margins
- Adjuvant therapy
  - Chemotherapy &/or radiation therapy
    - Non-Hodgkin lymphoma protocols (i.e., CHOP)
    - Acute leukemia protocols
  - BRAF inhibitors such as vemurafenib are promising treatments in cases with *BRAF* V600E mutations

Prognosis

- Low-stage (localized) lesions may be less clinically aggressive
- High-stage lesions (multiple lesions, systemic disease, recurrences) resistant to adjuvant therapy
  - 80% of patients die of disease
- HS with *BRAF* V600E mutations are not associated with worse outcomes

MACROSCOPIC

General Features

- Cutaneous papule or nodule
  - 1 or more firm lesions

MICROSCOPIC

Histologic Features

- Skin
  - Dermal and subcutaneous atypical histiocytic infiltrate with infiltrative borders
  - Spares epidermis, separated by grenz zone
- Lymph node
  - Usually diffuse effacement of lymph node architecture
  - Focal involvement is often in paracortex
  - Rarely tumor is seen in sinuses
- Hemophagocytosis, sometimes
  - Emperipolesis in some cases
- Mitotic figures and necrosis
- Inflammatory background
  - Often prominent
    - Reactive T cells, plasma cells, eosinophils
    - Especially in HS of central nervous system

Cytologic Features

- Range of bland to overtly malignant histiocytes
- Neoplastic cells, large and noncohesive
  - Nuclei
    - Usually round/epithelioid-shaped
    - Rarely spindle-shaped
    - Often highly pleomorphic cells, sometimes monomorphic
    - Vesicular chromatin
    - Nucleoli often prominent
    - Multinucleated cells can be seen
  - Cytoplasm is abundant
    - Eosinophilic
    - Cytoplasmic vacuoles in some cases
    - Xanthomatous appearance sometimes

ANCILLARY TESTS

Immunohistochemistry

- Histiocyte markers (+)

- CD163, CD68 (KP1, PGM1), lysozyme, CD4(+/-)
- Other (+) markers
  - LCA(+), HLA-DR(+), CD15[(+/-), weak], S100[(+/-), partial and weak], CD31(+)
- (-) for B cell, T cell, melanoma, carcinoma, myeloid, Langerhans cell, and follicular dendritic cell markers

PCR

- *BRAF* V600E exon 15 gene mutations are common
  - Found in ~ 60% of cases
- In cases of transdifferentiation, HS can show molecular alterations in lymphoma, including *IGH* gene rearrangement, *TRB* gene rearrangement, *TRG* gene rearrangement, and t(14;18)
  - *IGH* gene rearrangement does not exclude diagnosis
  - HS and lymphoma can show identical clones

Genetic Testing

- No specific chromosomal abnormalities
- Isochromosome 12p in cases with germ cell tumors
- In situ hybridization is (-) for EBER

Electron Microscopy

- Tumor cells with abundant cytoplasm and lysosomes

DIFFERENTIAL DIAGNOSIS

Langerhans Cell Histiocytosis and Langerhans Cell Sarcoma

- Similarities to HS
  - Histiocytic lineage
  - Often eosinophils in background
  - *BRAF* V600E mutations in ~ 40% of cases
- Differences from HS
  - Tumor cells have less atypia than HS
    - Grooved and twisted nuclei
  - Clusters of tumor cells often in epidermis, unlike HS
  - S100(+), CD1a(+), langerin (+)
  - Birbeck granules by electron microscopy

Rosai-Dorfman Disease

- Similarities to HS
  - Large histiocytes with abundant cytoplasm, bland cytologic features
  - Often plasma cells in background
- Differences from HS
  - Emperipolesis
  - Strongly S100(+)

Myeloid/Monocytic Sarcoma

- Often has monocytic, myelomonocytic, or monoblastic component
- Morphology and phenotype overlap with HS
- Differences from HS
  - Usually less atypia than HS
  - MPO(+/-) in myeloid sarcoma; (-) in HS
  - Immature markers, such as CD34, CD117, and rarely TdT, are (+)
- Bone marrow with patchy involvement (< 25% cellularity) may be classified as HS
- Bone marrow with extensive involvement (> 25% cellularity) classified as acute monocytic leukemia

Infection

- Granulomatous inflammation, special stains show organisms, &/or cultures are (+)

Juvenile Xanthogranuloma

- Also expresses CD14, CD68, and CD163
  - But FXIIIA(+), fascin (+), and LCA(-), contrary to HS
- Scattered Touton giant cells

Diffuse Large B-Cell Lymphoma

- Large cell proliferation that is often indistinguishable from HS by histology
- Different immunophenotype
  - B-cell markers expressed [CD20(+), CD79(+), pax-5(+)]
- Clonal *IGH* gene rearrangement
- Sometimes t(14;18)

Anaplastic Large Cell Lymphoma

- Similarities to HS
  - Large atypical dyscohesive cells
  - Sometimes sinusoidal infiltration pattern
  - CD68 may be dimly (+)
- Differences from HS
  - Hallmark cells with multiple nuclei in wreath-like or kidney-shaped pattern
  - Immunohistochemistry
    - T-cell antigens (+), CD30(+), ALK(+/-)
    - Histiocyte markers [CD163(-)], cytotoxic markers (+)
  - Molecular translocations involving *ALK* gene
    - More often in systemic ALK(+) cases, usually not in primary cutaneous anaplastic large cell lymphoma cases

Melanoma

- Nodular and metastatic melanomas often highly pleomorphic and may appear similar to HS
  - CD68 may be (+) in melanoma
  - Other histiocyte markers are usually (-)
- Melanoma markers should be (+)
  - S100, SOX10, HMB-45, Tyrosinase, MART-1/Melan-A, and KBA-62
- Look for past medical history of melanoma

Carcinoma

- Poorly differentiated carcinoma has overlapping morphology with HS
  - Immunophenotyping necessary to differentiate from HS
    - Cytokeratins, HMWCK, p63, and EMA(+) in most carcinomas
    - Histiocyte markers (-)

SELECTED REFERENCES

1. Bubolz AM et al: Potential clinical implications of BRAF mutations in histiocytic proliferations. Oncotarget. 5(12):4060-70, 2014
2. Dalia S et al: Dendritic cell and histiocytic neoplasms: biology, diagnosis, and treatment. Cancer Control. 21(4):290-300, 2014
3. Go H et al: Frequent detection of BRAF(V600E) mutations in histiocytic and dendritic cell neoplasms. Histopathology. 65(2):261-72, 2014
4. Feldman AL et al: Clonally related follicular lymphomas and histiocytic/dendritic cell sarcomas: evidence for transdifferentiation of the follicular lymphoma clone. Blood. 111(12):5433-9, 2008
5. Vos JA et al: Histiocytic sarcoma: a study of five cases including the histiocyte marker CD163. Mod Pathol. 18(5):693-704, 2005

Dermal Involvement in HS

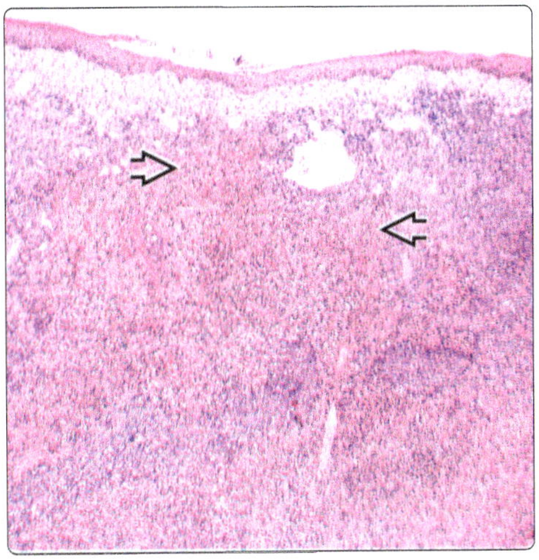

High-Power Magnification of HS

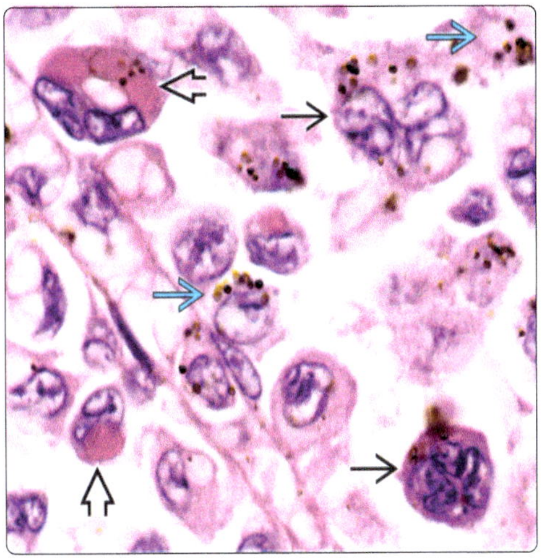

(Left) *HS at scanning magnification shows a diffuse, dermal-based, sheet-like proliferation of enlarged, undifferentiated-appearing cells with large areas of tumor necrosis* ⇨. **(Right)** *At high magnification, the malignant histiocytes are dyscohesive, atypical, and pleomorphic* →. *The malignant cells show erythrophagocytosis* ⇨ *and hemosiderin* →. *Nuclear irregularities are common. The spleen is a common site for HS. (From DP: Molecular Oncology.)*

HS of Palate

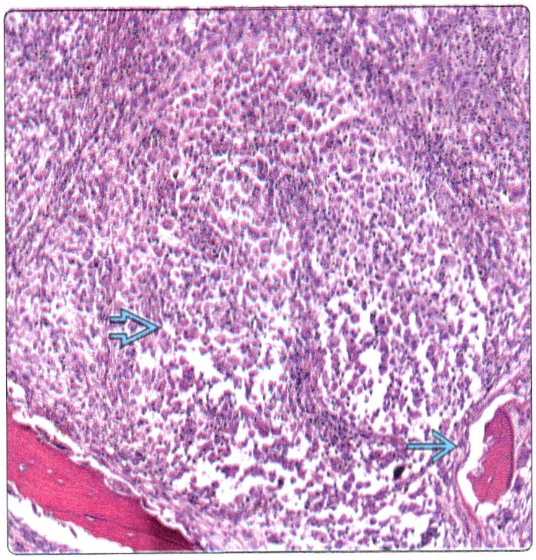

CD4 Immunohistochemistry in HS

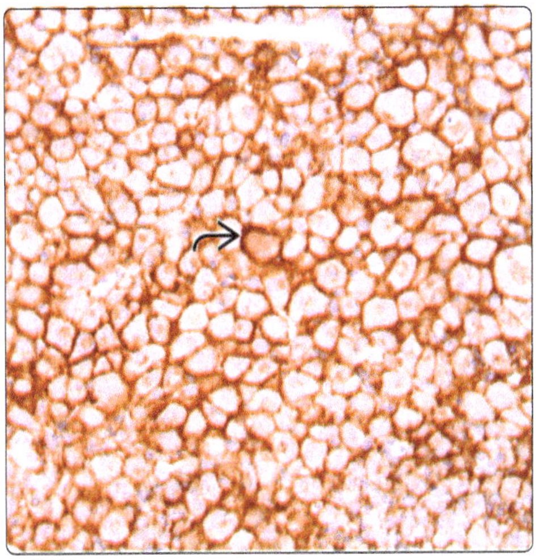

(Left) *This is a an example of HS of the palate showing dyscohesive sheets of large polygonal cells* ⇨. *The malignant cells are invading bone* →. *Benign histiocyte aggregates would not be expected to be this invasive. (From DP: Molecular Oncology.)* **(Right)** *CD4(+) histiocytic sarcoma is shown. CD4 immunohistochemistry highlights membrane reactivity in the large neoplastic cells* ↷. *(Courtesy R. Miranda, MD.)*

MPO Immunohistochemistry in HS

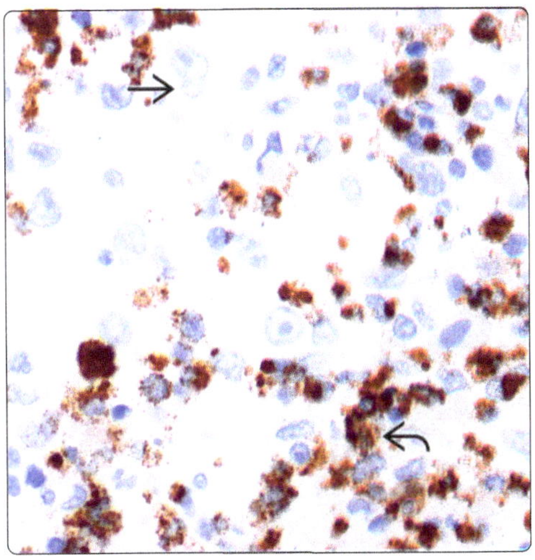

S100 Immunohistochemistry in HS

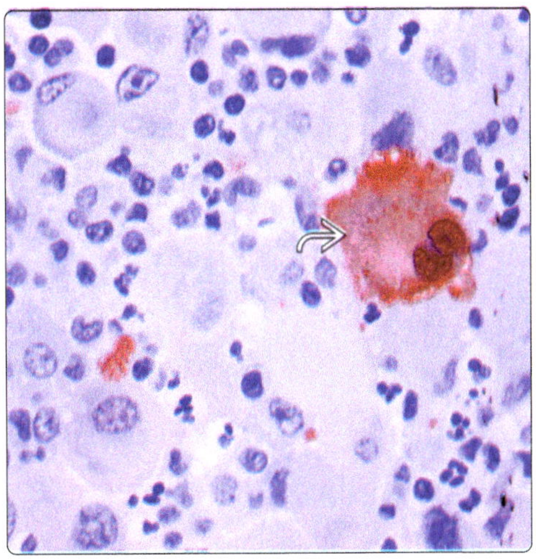

(Left) *Numerous reactive neutrophils are (+) for myeloperoxidase* ↶ *by immunohistochemistry in HS. Neoplastic histiocytes are (-)* →. *(Courtesy R. Miranda, MD.)* **(Right)** *A rare neoplastic cell is (+) for S100* ↷ *by immunohistochemistry, with staining of the nucleus and the cytoplasm. In certain cases of HS, a subset (< 25%) of neoplastic cells may express S100. (Courtesy R. Miranda, MD.)*

(Left) *Langerhans cell histiocytosis (LCH) is in the differential diagnosis of HS, especially in the skin. The dermis shows a diffuse infiltrate of ovoid histioid cells with relatively uniform, reniform-appearing nuclei and numerous eosinophils* ⇨. **(Right)** *At higher magnification, note that the histiocytes of LCH have longitudinal grooved* ➡ *&/or twisted* ➦ *nuclei. They also show relatively bland, fine chromatin. A mitotic figure* ⇨ *is also seen.*

Differential Diagnosis: Langerhans Cell Histiocytosis

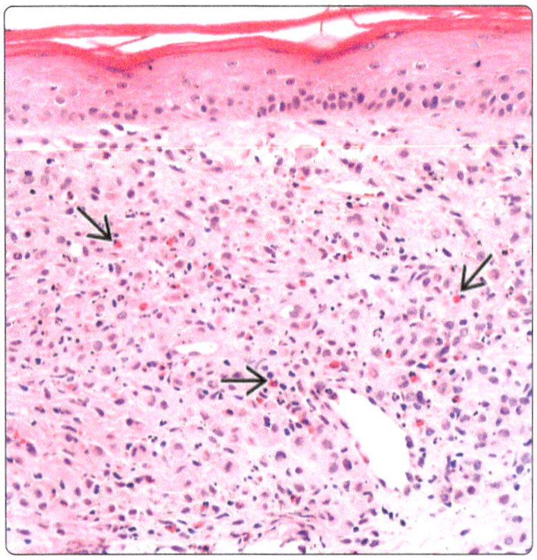

Langerhans Cell Morphology at High Magnification

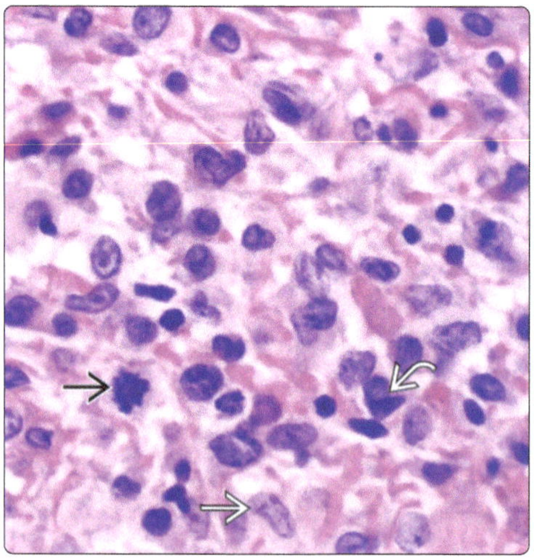

(Left) *This CD1a immunostain shows strong membrane (+) staining* ⇨ *of the Langerhans cells in LCH, which would be (-) in histiocytic sarcoma.* **(Right)** *Also in the differential is Rosai-Dorfman disease. The proliferating histiocytes are epithelioid-shaped and have abundant foamy cytoplasm. Lymphoid aggregates are present. The histiocytes show emperipolesis at high power, which can be seen on S100 immunostains (not shown).*

CD1a Immunohistochemistry in Langerhans Cell Histiocytosis

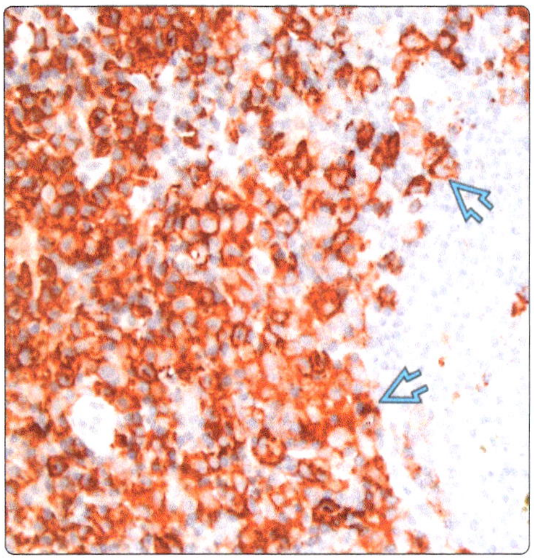

Differential Diagnosis: Rosai-Dorfman Disease

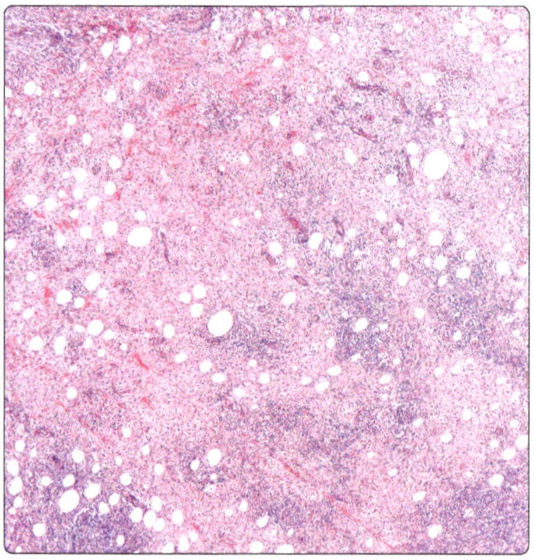

(Left) *Anaplastic large cell lymphoma (ALCL) can be mistaken for HS. There is epidermal ulceration over a diffuse dermal collection of large cells with irregular nuclei and abundant cytoplasm, similar to HS, with a background of mixed infiltrate, including neutrophils and eosinophils.* **(Right)** *The large malignant cells in ALCL show strong immunoexpression of CD30. The malignant cells of HS do not typically mark with CD30 but should be (+) for markers such as CD163.*

Differential Diagnosis: Anaplastic Large Cell Lymphoma

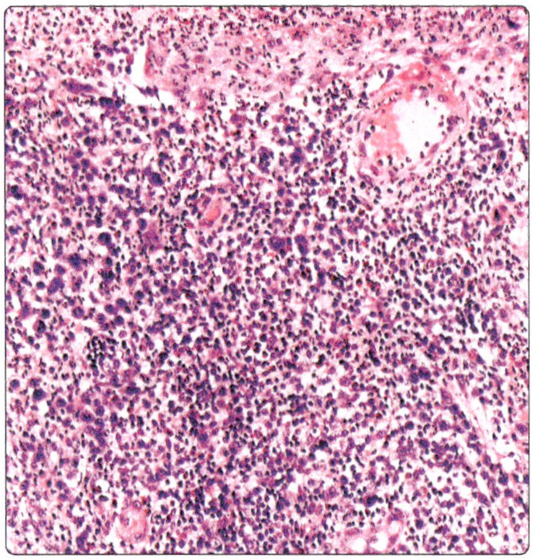

CD30 Immunohistochemistry in Anaplastic Large Cell Lymphoma

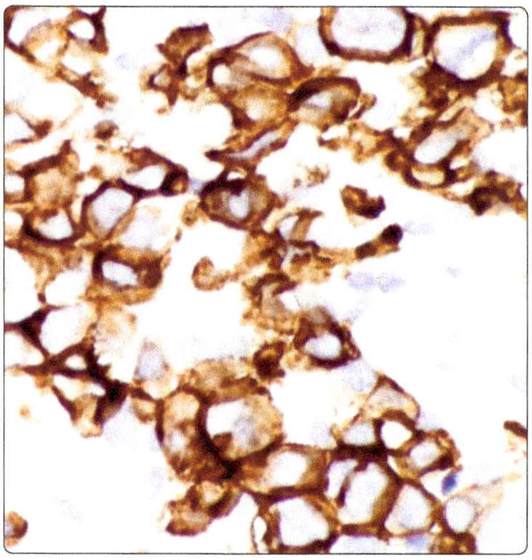

Differential Diagnosis: Diffuse Large B-Cell Lymphoma, Leg Type

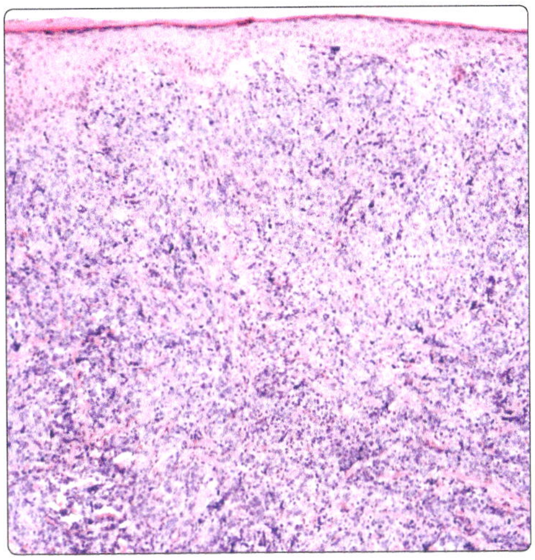

CD20 Immunohistochemistry in Diffuse Large B-Cell Lymphoma, Leg Type

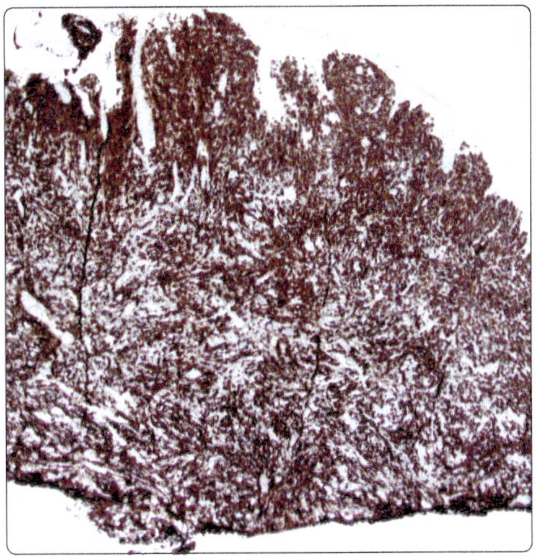

(Left) *This case of diffuse large B-cell lymphoma, leg type (DLBCL-L) may be indistinguishable from HS by histology, showing a large cell proliferation with nuclear hyperchromasia. However, DLBCL-L will express B-cell markers (e.g., CD20), and lack histiocyte markers.* **(Right)** *Strong and diffuse CD20 staining in DLBCL-L will typically express B-cell markers and lack histiocyte markers, such as CD68. With transdifferentiation, patients can rarely have both HS and B-cell lymphoma with the same clones.*

Differential Diagnosis: Myeloid Sarcoma

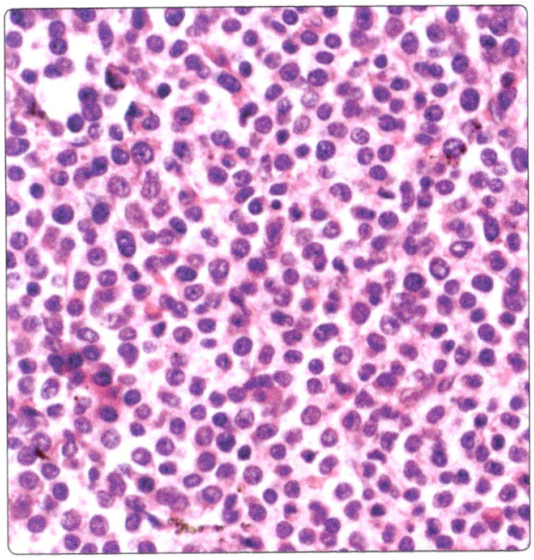

Myeloid Sarcoma: Myeloperoxidase Immunohistochemistry

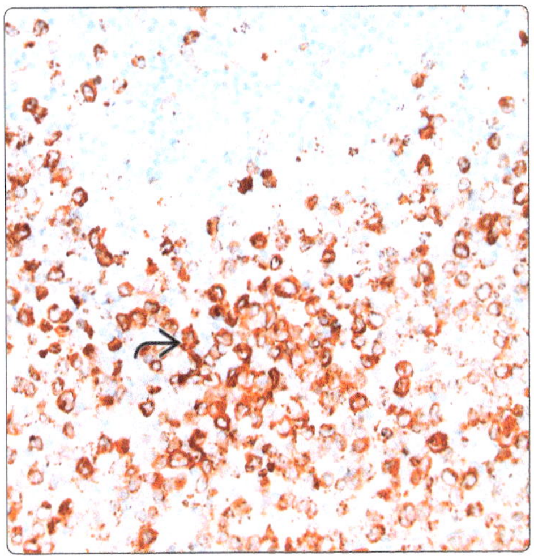

(Left) *This myeloid sarcoma (MS) shows an infiltrate composed of immature mononuclear cells, consistent with the blastic histologic subtype of MS. Some MS cases may show differentiation with components of maturing myeloid cells, including promyelocytes, myelocytes, and eosinophils. (From DP: Molecular Oncology.)* **(Right)** *This MS is (+) for MPO ➔. Immature markers, such as CD34 and CD117, as well as MPO, would help differentiate MS from HS. (Courtesy C. Bueso-Ramos, MD.)*

Histiocytic Sarcoma vs. Acute Monocytic Leukemia

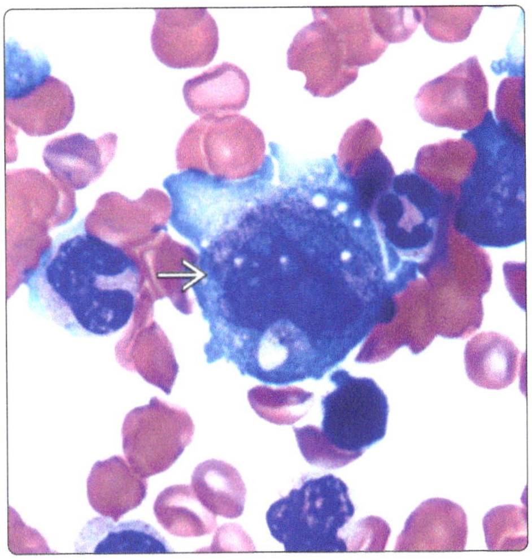

Differential Diagnosis: Acute Monocytic Leukemia

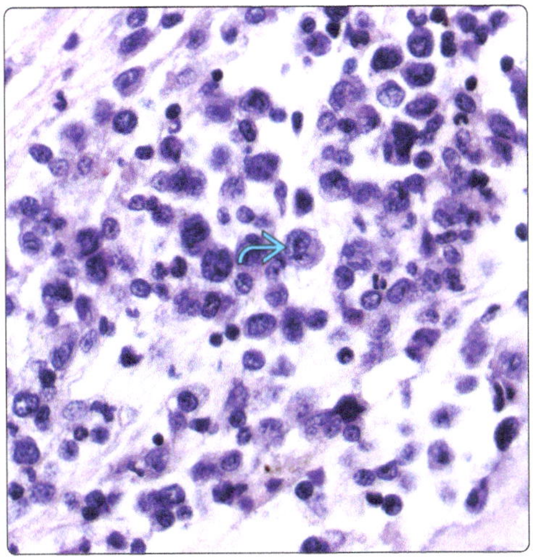

(Left) *This bone marrow aspirate shows a large cell ➔ with irregular nucleus and abundant cytoplasm. The WHO recommends classifying this case as acute monocytic leukemia (AMOL), but a diagnosis of HS can be suggested if these cells comprise < 25% of the tumor. (Courtesy R. Miranda, MD.)* **(Right)** *This is an AMOL in bone marrow. The neoplastic cells ➔ are similar to HS cells and represent ≥ 25% of bone marrow cellularity.*

Polyvinylpyrrolidone Storage Disease

KEY FACTS

ETIOLOGY/PATHOGENESIS

- Phagocytic foreign body-type reactive condition
- Found in aerosol hair sprays, adhesives, lithographic solutions, shaving products, plastics
- Used to improve clarity and stability of wine and fruit juice; used in oral medications and Betadine
- Presents as skin rash with nodules and macules, untreatable anemia due to bone marrow involvement

CLINICAL ISSUES

- Sites: Skin, bone marrow, lung
- Can lead to severe irreversible anemia when there is bone marrow involvement
- No effective treatment for removal of high-molecular-weight polyvinylpyrrolidone
  - Can only prevent additional administration

MICROSCOPIC

- Histiocytes with blue-gray, bubbly cytoplasm, in small groups or large sheets
- No nuclear atypia or mitotic activity
- Multinucleated giant cells may be present
- PAS, alcian blue, and Giemsa (-)
- Mucicarmine, Congo red, Sirius red, and colloidal iron (+)

ANCILLARY TESTS

- CD68(+), CD163(+)
- Keratin, S100, and CD1a (-)

TOP DIFFERENTIAL DIAGNOSES

- Sea-blue histiocytosis
- Signet ring cell adenocarcinoma
- Myxofibrosarcoma

Polyvinylpyrrolidone Storage Disease at Low Magnification

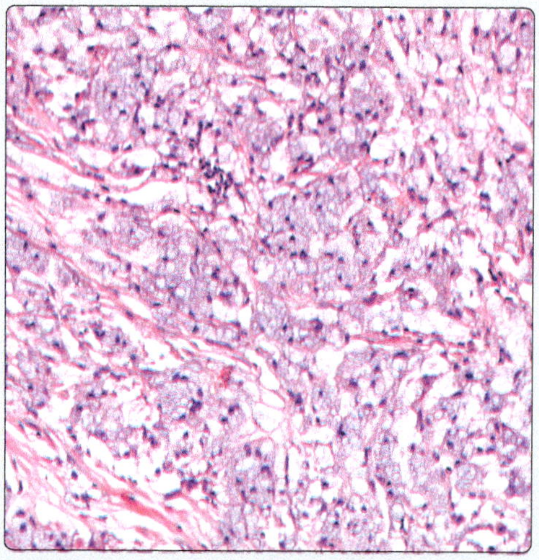

Histiocytes With Bubbly Cytoplasm

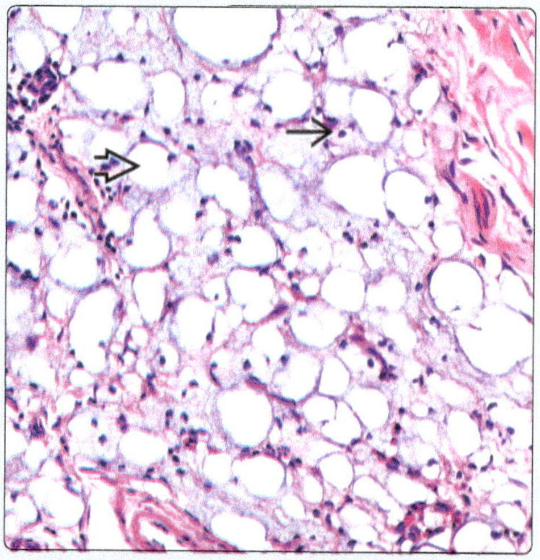

(Left) *Low-magnification H&E of polyvinylpyrrolidone (PVP) storage disease shows soft tissue infiltrated by sheets and nests of uniform macrophages containing basophilic material in their cytoplasm.* **(Right)** *Higher magnification shows histiocytic infiltrate with bubbly basophilic cytoplasm containing PVP and circular spaces. The nuclei are small and lack atypia and mitotic activity.*

Multinucleated Histiocytes Containing Material

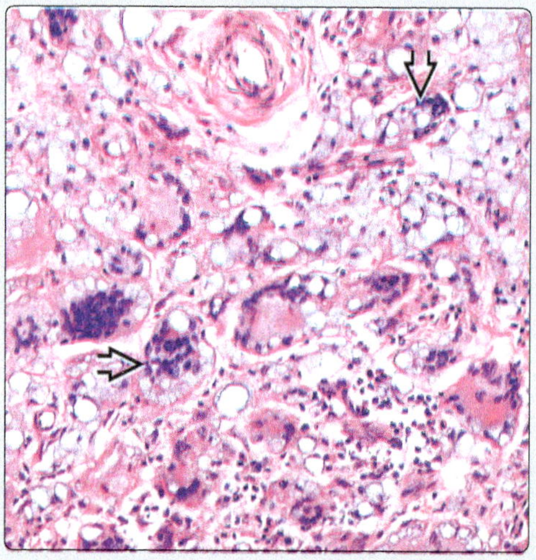

Polyvinylpyrrolidone Storage Disease Mimicking Myxoid Neoplasms

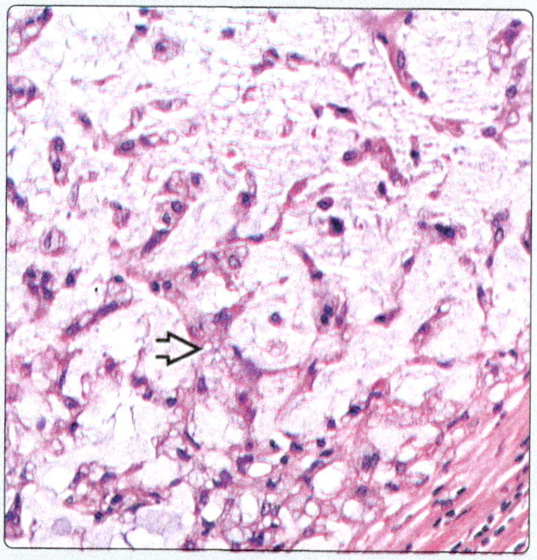

(Left) *High magnification of this case of PVP storage disease shows multinucleated histiocytes with abundant blue cytoplasm.* **(Right)** *Histologic examination shows basophilic bubbly material (PVP), largely extracellular but also within histiocytes, mimicking extraskeletal myxoid chondrosarcoma or myoepithelioma.*

TERMINOLOGY

Abbreviations

- Polyvinylpyrrolidone (PVP) storage disease

Synonyms

- Mucicarminophilic histiocytosis
- PVP granuloma

Definitions

- Phagocytic foreign body-type reactive condition in which PVP is deposited and retained in tissue

ETIOLOGY/PATHOGENESIS

Causes

- Synthesized during World War II, used intravenously as plasma expander
- PVP found in aerosol hair sprays, adhesives, lithographic solutions, and in cosmetics, including shaving products, plastics, and inks
- Used to improve clarity and stability of wine and fruit juice
- Used as component in oral medications and Betadine

CLINICAL ISSUES

Epidemiology

- Incidence
  - Associated with IV drug use

Site

- Skin, bone marrow, lung

Presentation

- Skin rash
  - Localized reactions may present as induration at injection site
  - Plaques, erythematous nodules, and purpuric to brown macules
  - Found during work-up for gastrointestinal bleeding in Munchausen syndrome
- Anemia
  - Due to marrow involvement, bony destruction

Treatment

- Prevent additional administration of high-molecular-weight PVP
- No effective treatment for removal of high-molecular-weight PVP

Prognosis

- Depending on amount of PVP accumulation, PVP storage disease may be incidental finding
- Can lead to severe irreversible anemia when there is bone marrow involvement
- Pulmonary angiothrombotic granulomatosis involving PVP (crospovidone) may lead to cor pulmonale and death

MICROSCOPIC

Histologic Features

- Microscopic
  - Blue-gray bubbly histiocyte with bubbly cytoplasmic contents, no pleomorphism
  - Multinucleated giant cells, foam cells, and granulomas may be present
  - Blue-gray material in extracellular pools, as well as within histiocyte cytoplasm
- Histochemistry
  - Mucicarmine red, Congo red, Sirius red, and colloidal iron (+)
  - PAS, alcian blue, and Giemsa (-)

ANCILLARY TESTS

Immunohistochemistry

- CD68(+), CD163(+)
- Keratin, S100, and CD1a (-)

DIFFERENTIAL DIAGNOSIS

Sea-Blue Histiocytosis

- Histiocytic proliferation
- Primary or secondary in hematologic/systemic disorders
- Blue with Giemsa; PAS(+)

Signet Ring Cell Adenocarcinoma

- Signet ring cells appear similar to PVP-containing histiocytes
- Mucicarmine and cytokeratin (+)
- PAS(-)

Myxofibrosarcoma

- Atypical spindle cells with presence of mitotic activity, cytologic activity, and prominent vasculature
- Alcian blue (+)

DIAGNOSTIC CHECKLIST

Clinically Relevant Pathologic Features

- May present as subcutaneous masses
- Material may be present at injection site
- Tissue distribution
  - Skin, bone marrow
  - Can be extensive

Pathologic Interpretation Pearls

- Histiocytes with blue-gray, bubbly cytoplasm, in small groups or large sheets, giant cells
- Nuclear pleomorphism, mitoses, necrosis are absent
- CD163(+); keratin (-)

SELECTED REFERENCES

1. Huang WC et al: Polyvinylpyrrolidone storage disease presenting as pathologic fracture and anemia: report of a case with imprint cytology. Diagn Cytopathol. 40(1):69-72, 2012
2. Chi CC et al: Localized cutaneous polyvinylpyrrolidone storage disease mimicking cheilitis granulomatosa. J Cutan Pathol. 33(6):454-7, 2006
3. Groisman GM et al: Mucicarminophilic histiocytosis (benign signet-ring cells) and hyperplastic mesothelial cells: two mimics of metastatic carcinoma within a single lymph node. Arch Pathol Lab Med. 122(3):282-4, 1998
4. Kuo TT et al: Cutaneous involvement in polyvinylpyrrolidone storage disease: a clinicopathologic study of five patients, including two patients with severe anemia. Am J Surg Pathol. 21(11):1361-7, 1997
5. Hizawa K et al: Subcutaneous pseudosarcomatous polyvinylpyrrolidone granuloma. Am J Surg Pathol. 8(5):393-8, 1984
6. Kuo TT et al: Mucicarminophilic histiocytosis. A polyvinylpyrrolidone (PVP) storage disease simulating signet-ring cell carcinoma. Am J Surg Pathol. 8(6):419-28, 1984

KEY FACTS

TERMINOLOGY

- Reactive mass-forming collection of lipidized macrophages, usually resulting from altered serum lipid levels
- Several forms
  - Xanthelasma, eruptive, tuberous, tendinous, planar, plexiform

ETIOLOGY/PATHOGENESIS

- Associated with hereditary lipoproteinemias and occasionally secondary lipoproteinemias
- May also occur in normolipemic patients
  - Particularly plexiform xanthoma

CLINICAL ISSUES

- Wide age range (children or adults)
- Usually occur in skin and subcutaneous tissue
- Occasionally arise in deep soft tissues (tendon, synovium, bone)
- Classified based on clinical features and gross appearance
- Treatment: Medical therapy or conservative excision
- Excellent prognosis

MICROSCOPIC

- Specific classification requires clinicopathologic correlation
- Sheets and aggregates of foamy macrophages
- Variable secondary changes including inflammation, giant cells, fibrosis, and cholesterol cleft formation
- Plexiform xanthoma features multinodular or plexiform growth pattern

TOP DIFFERENTIAL DIAGNOSES

- Localized-type tenosynovial giant cell tumor (giant cell tumor of tendon sheath)
- Solitary (juvenile) xanthogranuloma
- Lipidized-type dermatofibroma (fibrous histiocytoma)
- Verruciform xanthoma
- Plexiform fibrohistiocytic tumor

Xanthelasma

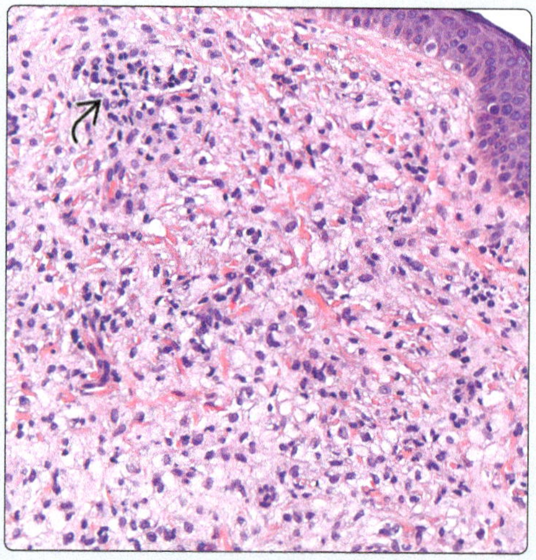

Eruptive Xanthoma

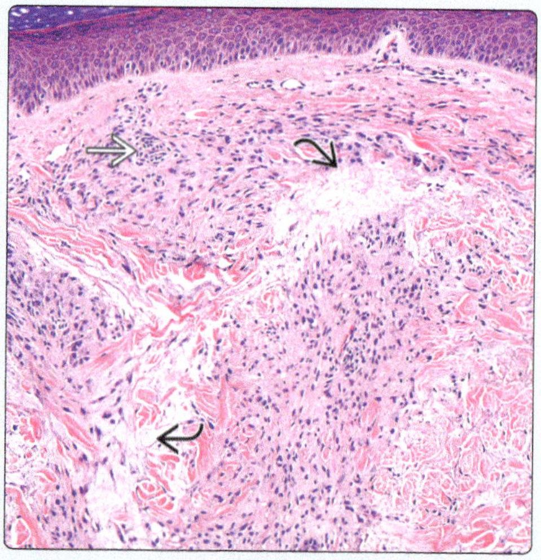

(Left) *Xanthelasmas (and planar xanthomas) consist of a sheet-like infiltrate of foamy macrophages involving the dermis and surrounding adnexal structures. Small areas of chronic inflammation ➚ may be present, but fibrosis and cholesterol clefts are not typical.* **(Right)** *Eruptive xanthoma is characterized by sheets of macrophages within the dermis. Extravascular lipid deposits with a blue-gray amorphous appearance are often seen ➚ between dermal collagen bundles. A sparse perivascular inflammatory infiltrate ➡ can also be seen.*

Early Eruptive Xanthoma

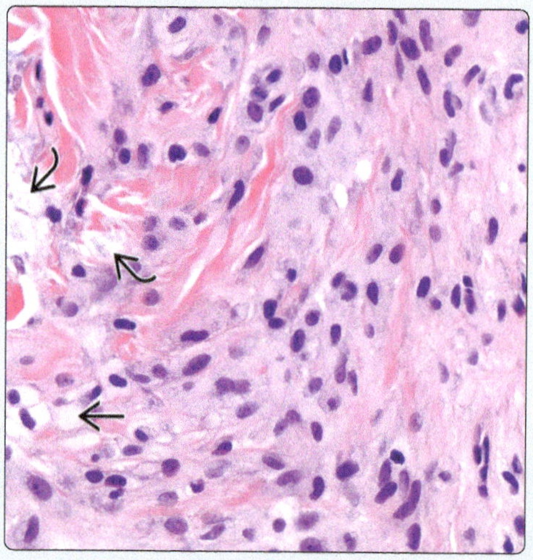

Older Eruptive Xanthoma

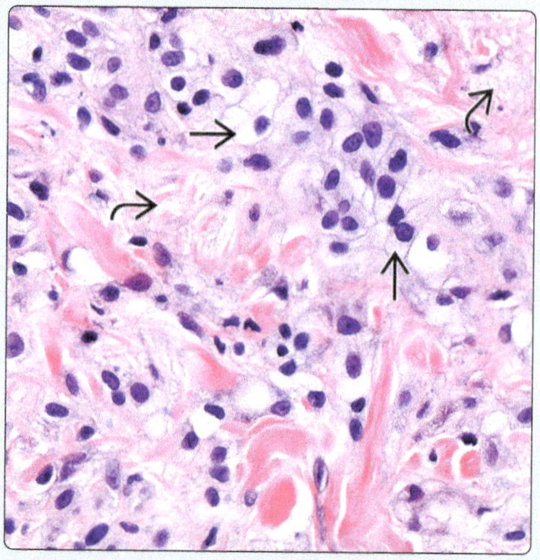

(Left) *In contrast to other forms of xanthoma, the cells in eruptive xanthoma are nonfoamy in early lesions. Note the rare foamy macrophages → and extravascular lipid ➚.* **(Right)** *Older eruptive xanthomas accumulate more foamy macrophages → and consist of a mixture of foamy and nonfoamy cells. Again, note areas of lace-like blue-gray extravascular lipid between the dermal collagen bundles ➚.*

TERMINOLOGY

Synonyms

- Plexiform xanthomatous tumor (for plexiform xanthoma)

Definitions

- Reactive mass-forming collection of lipidized macrophages, usually resulting from altered serum lipid levels
  - Several forms
    - Xanthelasma
    - Eruptive xanthoma
    - Tuberous xanthoma
    - Tendinous xanthoma
    - Planar xanthoma
    - Plexiform xanthoma

ETIOLOGY/PATHOGENESIS

Hereditary or Nonhereditary

- Associated with hereditary lipoproteinemias and occasionally secondary lipoproteinemias (e.g., diabetes, hypothyroidism, primary biliary cirrhosis)
- May also occur in normolipemic patients
  - Particularly plexiform xanthoma

CLINICAL ISSUES

Epidemiology

- Age
  - Wide age range (children or adults)

Presentation

- Usually occur in skin and subcutaneous tissue
- Occasionally arise in deep soft tissues (tendon, synovium, bone)
- Classified based on clinical features
  - **Xanthelasma**
    - Soft yellow plaques
    - Predilection for eyelids and periorbital skin; often bilateral
  - **Eruptive xanthoma**
    - Sudden onset of small, yellow papules with erythematous halo
    - Predilection for gluteal region, thigh, and shoulders
  - **Tuberous xanthoma**
    - Firm yellow subcutaneous nodules and plaques
    - Predilection for elbow, knee, gluteal region, and fingers
  - **Tendinous xanthoma**
    - Soft tissue mass associated with tendons, ligaments, &/or fascia; predilection for hands, feet, and Achilles tendon
    - May impair joint function but often asymptomatic
  - **Planar xanthoma**
    - Variably sized yellow macules; predilection for palmar creases
    - In normolipemic patients, consider underlying reticuloendothelial malignancy
  - **Plexiform xanthoma**
    - Dermal-based cutaneous nodule(s) occurring most often on extremities
      - Particularly extensor surfaces of elbow and knee regions
    - Usually in males
    - Patients usually normolipemic
  - **Cerebrotendinous xanthomatosis**
    - Rare autosomal recessive disease; sterol 27-hydroxylase gene (*CYP27A1*) mutation
    - Enzyme involved in bile acid synthesis; defect results in accumulation of cholestanol, which is deposited systemically
    - Bilateral Achilles tendon xanthomas and cataracts; CNS symptoms include ataxia, dementia, dysarthria, psychiatric disturbances, and seizures

Treatment

- May regress with medical therapy for hyperlipidemia or underlying cause if secondary
- Conservative excision can be employed for large or symptomatic lesions

Prognosis

- Excellent prognosis
- Surgically treated lesions may recur

MACROSCOPIC

General Features

- Diffuse or circumscribed
  - Plexiform xanthoma may appear grossly multinodular
- Variegated yellow, tan, and white appearance

Size

- Generally few millimeters to several centimeters depending on type
- Tendinous xanthomas can be quite large (up to 20 cm)

MICROSCOPIC

Histologic Features

- Specific classification requires clinicopathologic correlation
- Xanthelasma and planar xanthoma
  - Sheets of foamy macrophages
- Eruptive xanthomas
  - Sheets of mostly nonfoamy macrophages with some foamy macrophages
  - Later lesions contain more foamy macrophages
- Tuberous and tendinous xanthoma
  - Nodules of foamy macrophages
  - Chronic inflammation, fibrosis, and cholesterol clefts with giant cells common
- Plexiform xanthoma
  - Multinodular or plexiform growth of nodules of foamy histiocytes separated by fibrous or sclerotic stroma
  - Giant cells
  - Variable chronic inflammation, fibrosis, and cholesterol clefts

ANCILLARY TESTS

Immunohistochemistry

- CD68(+), CD163(+)
- S100(-)

Clinical Forms of Xanthoma

Feature	Xanthelasma	Eruptive	Tuberous	Tendinous	Planar	Plexiform
Lipoprotein association	None or IIa, III	I, III, V, secondary	IIa, III, secondary	IIa, secondary	None, III, secondary	Usually none
Characteristic location	Eyelids	Buttock	Elbow, knee, buttock, finger	Hand, foot, ankle (Achilles)	Palm creases	Elbow, knee, foot/hand
Foamy macrophages	Present	Present (absent in early lesions)	Present	Present	Present	Present
Characteristic histopathology	Foamy macrophages	Foamy and nonfoamy macrophages	Foamy macrophages, cholesterol clefts, giant cells, inflammation, fibrosis	Foamy macrophages, cholesterol clefts, giant cells, inflammation, fibrosis	Foamy macrophages	Plexiform nodules of foamy macrophages; giant cells

Hyperlipoproteinemia (Fredrickson) Classification

Feature	I	IIa	IIb	III	IV	V
Elevated lipoprotein	Chylomicrons	LDL	LDL, VLDL	Chylomicrons, VLDL remnants	VLDL	Chylomicrons, VLDL
Molecular defect	Lipoprotein lipase, apoC-II	LDL receptor, apoB-100	Unknown	ApoE	Unknown	Unknown

DIFFERENTIAL DIAGNOSIS

Localize-Type Tenosynovial Giant Cell Tumor

- Synonym: Giant cell tumor of tendon sheath
- Vast majority arise in digits
- Usually solitary; resembles tendinous xanthoma but contains multinucleated giant cells and hemosiderin
- Contains nonfoamy epithelioid, mononuclear stromal cells
- Osteoclast-like giant cells and hemosiderin common

Juvenile Xanthogranuloma

- Usually young children
- Touton giant cells often present
- Mixed inflammation including eosinophils and neutrophils

Lipidized-Type Dermatofibroma (Fibrous Histiocytoma)

- Usually lower leg (ankle predominant)
- Demonstrates dermal collagen entrapment

Verruciform Xanthoma

- Most are intraoral or anogenital
- Verrucous epithelium with parakeratin plugs and stromal foam cells

Plexiform Fibrohistiocytic Tumor

- In DDx for plexiform xanthoma
- Most common in children and adolescents
- Biphasic appearance
  - Fibromatosis-like fascicles of spindle cells
  - Nodules of epithelioid or histiocytoid cells ± multinucleated giant
- Xanthomatous change rare and usually limited in extent

Plexiform Schwannoma

- DDx for plexiform xanthoma
- Cellular nodules of spindled Schwann cells
- Nuclear palisading common
- Foamy histiocytes may be present but are not usually prominent
- S100(+)

SELECTED REFERENCES

1. Ghosh SK et al: Tuberous xanthoma as a presenting feature of familial homozygous hypercholesterolemia with aortic regurgitation. J Pediatr. 166(1):198, 2015
2. Blankenship DW et al: Verruciform xanthoma of the upper-extremity in the absence of chronic skin disease or syndrome: a case report and review of the literature. J Cutan Pathol. 40(8):745-52, 2013
3. Shahrabi Farahani S et al: Oral verruciform xanthoma associated with chronic graft-versus-host disease: a report of five cases and a review of the literature. Head Neck Pathol. 5(2):193-8, 2011
4. Reichwaldt I et al: Differential diagnosis of tendon tumors: xanthomas caused by hyperlipidemia in children. J Pediatr Surg. 45(10):e9-12, 2010
5. Oosterveer DM et al: 5-Lipoxygenase activating protein (ALOX5AP) gene variants associate with the presence of xanthomas in familial hypercholesterolemia. Atherosclerosis. 206(1):223-7, 2009
6. Chuang AY et al: Xanthoma of the prostate: a mimicker of high-grade prostate adenocarcinoma. Am J Surg Pathol. 31(8):1225-30, 2007
7. Tsouli SG et al: Pathogenesis, detection and treatment of Achilles tendon xanthomas. Eur J Clin Invest. 35(4):236-44, 2005
8. Moghadasian MH: Cerebrotendinous xanthomatosis: clinical course, genotypes and metabolic backgrounds. Clin Invest Med. 27(1):42-50, 2004
9. Michal M et al: Plexiform xanthomatous tumor: a report of 20 cases in 12 patients. Am J Surg Pathol. 26(10):1302-11, 2002
10. Michal M: Plexiform xanthomatous tumor. A report of three cases. Am J Dermatopathol. 16(5):532-6, 1994
11. Beham A et al: Plexiform xanthoma: an unusual variant. Histopathology. 19(6):565-7, 1991
12. Cruz PD Jr et al: Dermal, subcutaneous, and tendon xanthomas: diagnostic markers for specific lipoprotein disorders. J Am Acad Dermatol. 19(1 Pt 1):95-111, 1988
13. Parker F: Xanthomas and hyperlipidemias. J Am Acad Dermatol. 13(1):1-30, 1985

Tuberous Xanthoma

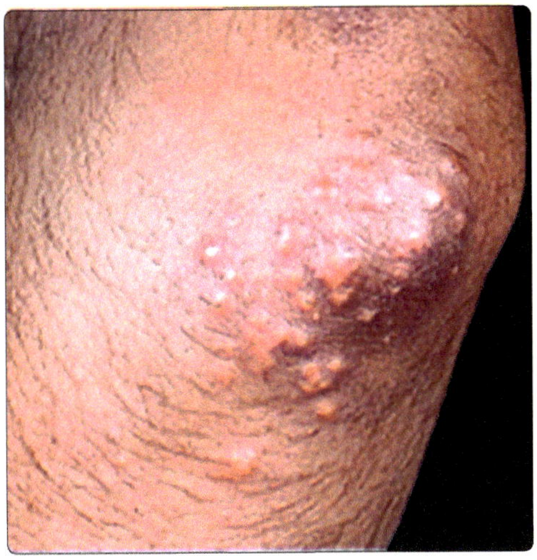

Tuberous Xanthoma

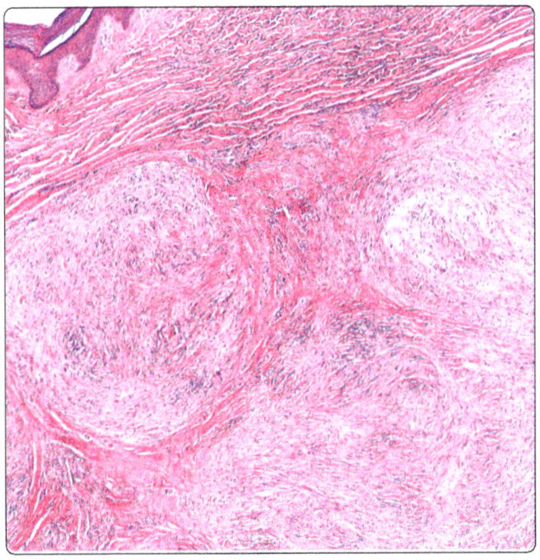

(Left) *Tuberous xanthoma is shown involving the knee. Tuberous xanthomas appear as firm yellow-red subcutaneous nodules and occur at pressure areas, such as the buttock and extensor surfaces of the knee and elbow. Smaller nodules often coalesce to form larger nodules or plaques.* **(Right)** *Tuberous xanthoma consists of a nodular infiltrate of foamy macrophages involving the dermis and may be uninodular or multinodular, as in this example.*

Cholesterol Clefts and Giant Cells

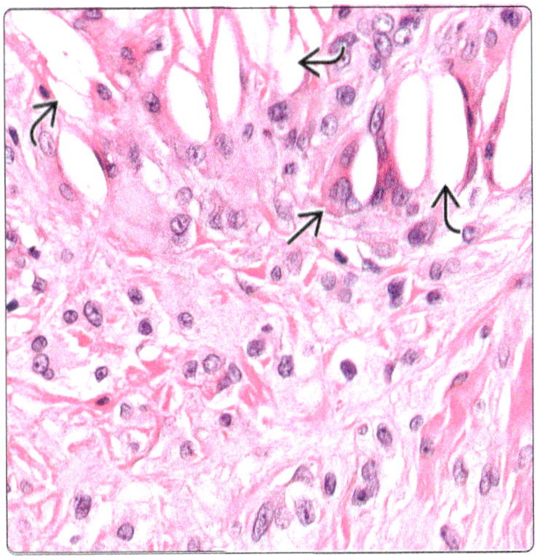

Fibrosis, Necrosis, and Cholesterol Clefts

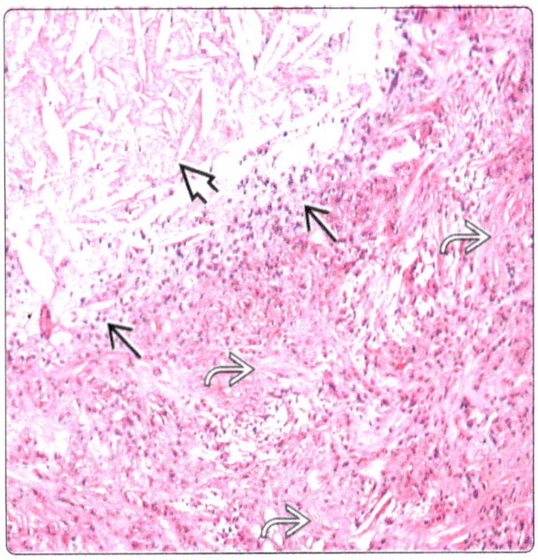

(Left) *Unlike the other forms of xanthoma, tuberous (and tendinous) xanthomas usually have secondary changes, including collections of extracellular cholesterol with cholesterol cleft formation* ↷ *and associated giant cells* →*.* **(Right)** *Other secondary changes in tuberous (and tendinous) xanthomas include varying degrees of fibrosis* ➔ *and foci of necrosis* ⇨ *containing amorphous eosinophilic debris with cholesterol clefts and a surrounding rim of foamy macrophages* →*.*

Tendinous Xanthoma

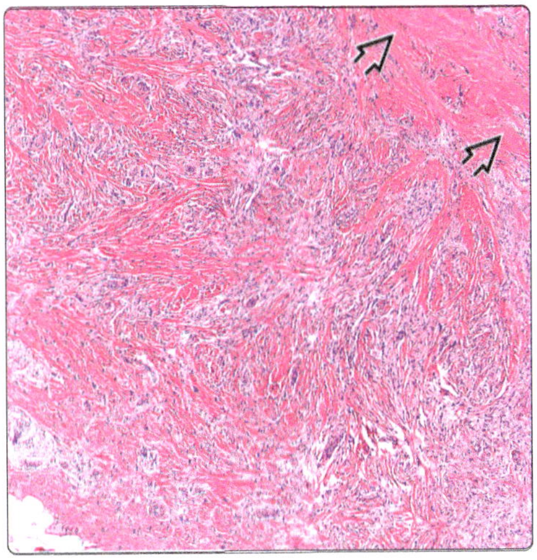

Plexiform Xanthoma

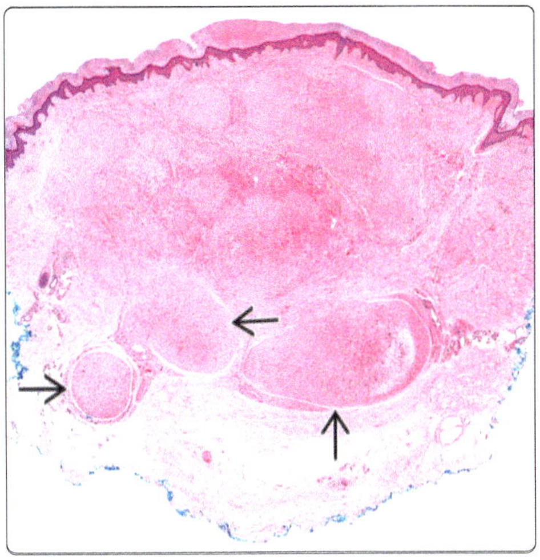

(Left) *Tendinous xanthomas are histologically identical to tuberous xanthomas except that they involve deeper structures, such as tendons* ⇨ *and ligaments.* **(Right)** *A multinodular proliferation with a plexiform architecture filling the dermis is typical of plexiform xanthoma. The deep nodules* → *tend to be more well developed than the superficial ones.*

Verruciform Xanthoma

KEY FACTS

TERMINOLOGY

- Verrucous epithelium/epidermis with foamy macrophages in lamina propria/dermis

CLINICAL ISSUES

- Usually occurs in oral cavity, but may occur in skin and other mucosal sites
- In oral cavity
  - Most commonly on palate, gingiva, or alveolar ridge mucosa
  - Usually single lesion, but on rare occasions, there may be multiple
  - Well-circumscribed, yellow, red, or gray plaque
  - Rough or granular surface
- In skin
  - Most commonly occur in anogenital area
  - Usually single lesion but may be multiple
  - Well-circumscribed, pink or grayish nodule or plaque
  - Rough or bosselated surface similar to warts
- No clear disease association

MICROSCOPIC

- Verrucous epithelial/epidermal hyperplasia
- Epidermal ridges extend downward but all extend to same depth
- Epidermal ridges are wide and bulbous
- Often keratinocyte necrosis
- Neutrophilic infiltrate is common
- Dermal pegs between elongated epidermal ridges are cellular
  - Vacuolated or foamy macrophages

TOP DIFFERENTIAL DIAGNOSES

- Condyloma acuminatum
- Verrucous carcinoma
- Granular cell tumor
- Verruca vulgaris
- Seborrheic keratosis

Verrucous Mucosa

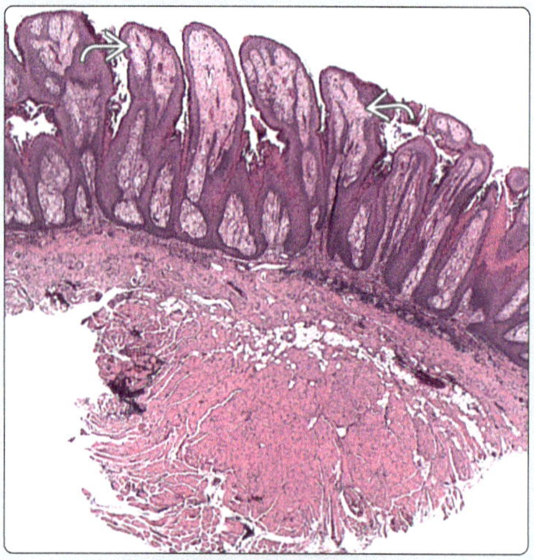

Pale Lamina Propria

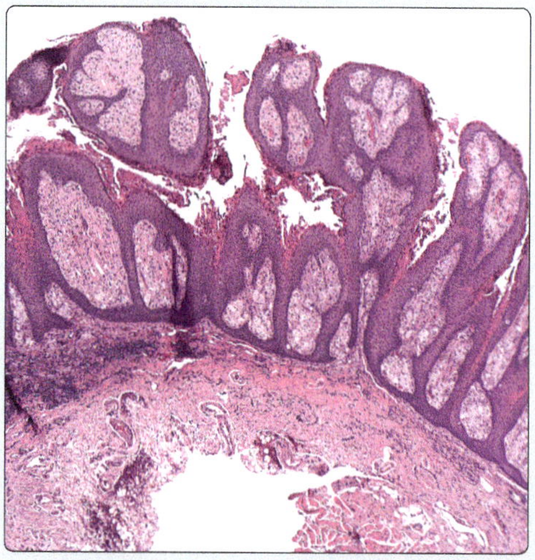

(Left) *Note the verrucous and papillomatous nature of the overlying mucosa. The lamina propria is abnormally pale ➡, indicative of the histiocytic infiltrate in those areas.* **(Right)** *At a slightly higher power, the pale nature of the superficial lamina propria is better appreciated when compared to the eosinophilic deeper soft tissue.*

Higher Magnification of Mucosa

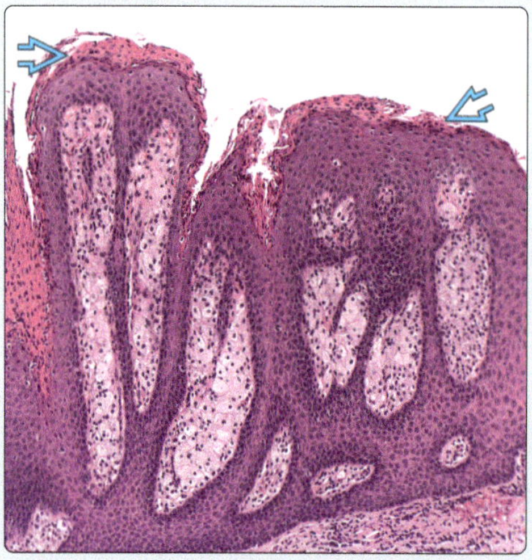

High Magnification Showing Foamy Histiocytes

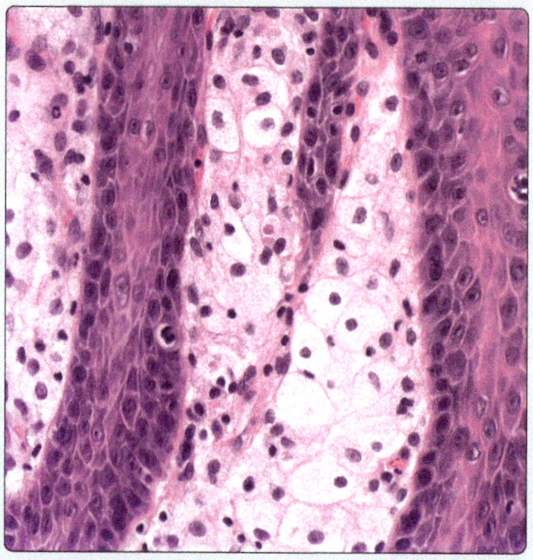

(Left) *Although the mucosa is verrucous and papillomatous, no keratinocytic atypia is present. Overlying parakeratosis ➡ with intracorneal neutrophils are seen. A mild lymphocytic infiltrate is seen in the lamina propria with some extension into the mucosa.* **(Right)** *High power clearly shows abundant foamy histiocytes in the superficial lamina propria. No atypia is present. Also, the cytoplasm is not granular as seen in granular cell tumors of the oropharynx.*

TERMINOLOGY

Definitions

- Verrucous epithelium/epidermis with foamy macrophages in lamina propria/dermis

CLINICAL ISSUES

Presentation

- Usually occurs in oral cavity, but may occur in skin and other mucosal sites
  - Anogenital region, ear, nose, digits
- In oral cavity
  - Most commonly on palate, gingiva, or alveolar ridge mucosa
  - Usually single lesion, but on rare occasions, there may be multiple
  - Well-circumscribed, yellow, red, or gray plaque
  - Rough or granular surface
  - May be raised or depressed
- In skin
  - Most commonly occur in anogenital area
  - Usually single lesion but may have multiple
  - Well-circumscribed, pink or grayish nodule or plaque
  - Rough or bosselated surface similar to warts
- No clear disease association
  - Reported in patients with chronic inflammation, various systemic diseases, metabolic diseases, and in normal patients

Treatment

- Surgical approaches
  - Surgical excision is usually curative

Prognosis

- If untreated, they will persist for months or years
  - Not locally aggressive or invasive
- If excised, then they typically do not recur

MICROSCOPIC

Histologic Features

- Similar features regardless of oral cavity or skin involvement
- Verrucous epithelial/epidermal hyperplasia
- Epidermal ridges extend downward but all extend to same depth
  - Epidermal ridges are wide and bulbous
- Often keratinocyte necrosis
- Neutrophilic infiltrate is common
- Dermal pegs between elongated epidermal ridges are cellular
  - Vacuolated or foamy macrophages
  - No multinucleated histiocytes (giant cells) or Touton giant cells
- May have underlying nonspecific lymphocytic infiltrate

ANCILLARY TESTS

Histochemistry

- Periodic acid-Schiff
  - Positive
- Periodic acid-Schiff diastase
  - Negative

Immunohistochemistry

- S100
  - Negative in foamy histiocytes
- CD68 and CD163
  - Positive in foamy histiocytes

DIFFERENTIAL DIAGNOSIS

Histopathological

- Granular cell tumor
  - Epidermis/epithelium may be acanthotic but often has more infiltrative growth pattern rather than bulbous
    - Does not appear as raised
  - Granular cells are larger without foamy cytoplasm
  - Granular cells are PAS(+) and S100(+)
- Verruca vulgaris
  - Keratohyaline clumping
  - Parakeratotic tiers above papillomatous tips
  - HPV viral effects (clear cytoplasm; hyperchromatic, wrinkled nuclei)
- Xanthoma/xanthelasma
  - Epidermis is normal in thickness
  - No acantholysis
  - No significant neutrophil infiltrate
  - Xanthelasma is more common around eyes rather than anogenital region
- Condyloma acuminatum
  - Acanthosis with undulating surface
    - May have papillomatosis
  - ± HPV viral change
  - No foamy histiocytes
- Seborrheic keratosis
  - Thickened epidermal ridges extending to same depth
  - No significant keratinocyte necrosis or neutrophils
  - No xanthoma cells in dermis
- Verrucous carcinoma
  - Bulbous epidermal downgrowths
  - May have mitotic activity
  - Minimal atypia
  - May have foci of squamous cell carcinoma

Clinical

- Condyloma acuminatum
  - Common in anogenital region
  - May be single or multiple
- Verrucous carcinoma
  - Usually larger (giant condyloma acuminatum of Buschke and Lowenstein)
    - Many view this as form of verrucous carcinoma
  - Usually single but may occasionally be multiple
  - May appear multinodular, bosselated, or filiform

SELECTED REFERENCES

1. Liu G et al: Verrucous Carcinoma of the vulva: a 20 year retrospective study and literature review. J Low Genit Tract Dis. 20(1):114-8, 2016
2. de Andrade BA et al: Oral verruciform xanthoma: a clinicopathologic and immunohistochemical study of 20 cases. J Cutan Pathol. 42(7):489-95, 2015
3. Hegde U et al: Verruciform xanthoma: a view on the concepts of its etiopathogenesis. J Oral Maxillofac Pathol. 17(3):392-6, 2013

PART I
SECTION 12

Lymphomas and Hematopoietic Proliferations

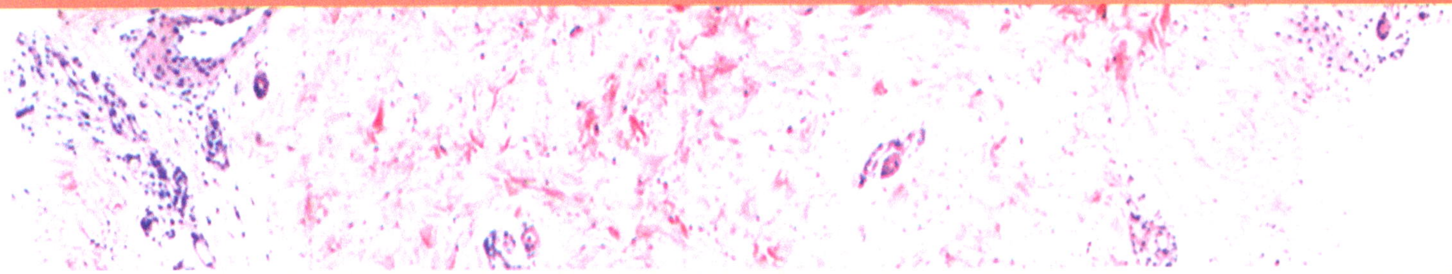

B-Cell Neoplasms

T-Cell and NK-Cell Neoplasms

Leukemic and Nonlymphoid Infiltrates

Cutaneous Plasmacytoma

KEY FACTS

TERMINOLOGY

- Extraosseous plasmacytoma of skin
- Neoplasm of monoclonal plasma cells
  - Must exclude cutaneous involvement in multiple myeloma and plasmacytoid B-cell lymphomas, such as primary cutaneous extranodal marginal zone lymphoma

ETIOLOGY/PATHOGENESIS

- Cell of origin is immunoglobulin-secreting, heavy-chain class-switched, terminally differentiated B cell

CLINICAL ISSUES

- Skin is rare site for plasmacytomas; most occur in respiratory tract
- Cutaneous lesions may be found anywhere on body
- Serum protein electrophoresis and urinary protein electrophoresis show low level of monoclonal gammopathy in 20%
- Usually local radiation or surgery
- Local recurrence may happen

MICROSCOPIC

- Diffuse or nodular collections of dermal plasma cells
- Oval-shaped plasma cells with eccentric nucleus, clock face or spoke wheel chromatin, without prominent nucleoli
- Increased pink cytoplasm with perinuclear hof
- Mature plasma cells, plasmablasts, and pleomorphic forms may be identified

ANCILLARY TESTS

- Immunohistochemistry shows CD38(+), CD138(+), CD45rb (-), CD20(-), pax-5(-), CD79a(+)
- Flow cytometry may underestimate number of plasma cells
- Plasmacytomas may show same molecular changes as seen in plasma cell myeloma

TOP DIFFERENTIAL DIAGNOSES

- Extranodal marginal zone lymphoma
- Reactive plasma cell infiltrates

Gross Image

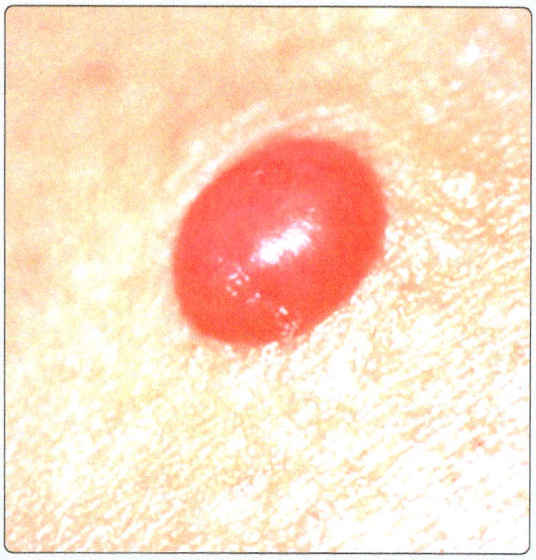

Low-Power of Cutaneous Plasmacytoma

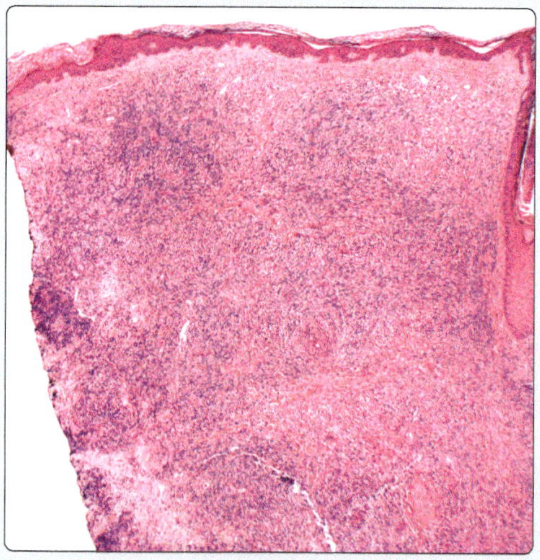

(Left) *A single red solitary plaque on the forearm is shown, which microscopically is a cutaneous plasmacytoma (CP).* **(Right)** *Low-magnification examination of a CP shows a diffuse, dermal-based lymphoid infiltrate with deep extension.*

Higher Magnification of Cutaneous Plasmacytoma

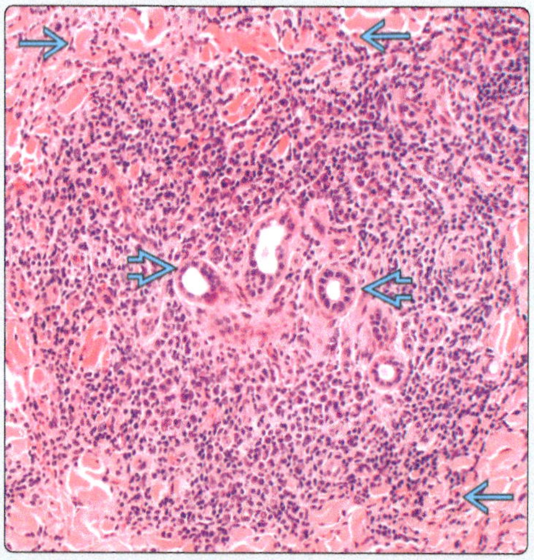

Plasma Cell Morphology

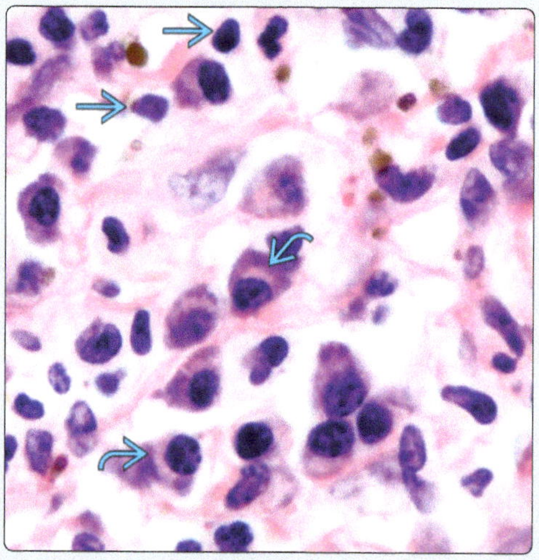

(Left) *This CP shows a prominent plasmacytoid infiltrate surrounding multiple adnexal ducts ⇨ and infiltrating between collagen bundles →.* **(Right)** *This CP shows multiple mature-appearing plasma cells with prominent perinuclear hofs ↷. Scattered small lymphocytes → are also present.*

TERMINOLOGY

Abbreviations

- Cutaneous plasmacytoma (CP)

Synonyms

- Extraosseous plasmacytoma of skin

Definitions

- Neoplasm of monoclonal plasma cells involving skin
  - Must exclude cutaneous involvement in multiple myeloma and plasmacytoid B-cell lymphomas, such as primary cutaneous extranodal marginal zone lymphoma
  - No clinical features of plasma cell myeloma and no evidence of bone marrow plasmacytosis

ETIOLOGY/PATHOGENESIS

Cell of Origin

- Clone of immunoglobulin-secreting, heavy-chain class-switched, terminally differentiated B cells that usually secrete single monoclonal immunoglobulin

CLINICAL ISSUES

Epidemiology

- Incidence
  - Extremely rare
    - Only 3-5% of all plasma cell neoplasms
    - Many cases previously reported as primary CPs would now be reclassified as extranodal marginal zone lymphomas
  - Rarely involve skin, more common in respiratory tract (80% of extraosseous plasmacytomas in oropharynx, nasopharynx, and nasal sinuses)
  - Rarely, may be seen as posttransplant lymphoproliferative disorder (PTLD)
    - Morphologically identical to other plasmacytomas, but PTLD plasmacytoma-like tumors are often EBV(+)
- Age
  - Median age: 55 years
- Sex
  - Mostly in men; M:F = 2:1

Site

- Skin (by definition)
- Lesions may occur anywhere on body

Presentation

- Usually single or rarely multiple lesions
  - Upper airway/nasal lesions may present with rhinorrhea, nasal obstruction, epistaxis

Laboratory Tests

- Serum protein electrophoresis
  - 20% reported to show monoclonal gammopathy
  - There is usually low level of M protein in serum &/or urine

Treatment

- Usually local radiation or surgery

Prognosis

- Local recurrence can occur
- Rare systemic dissemination
- Better prognosis if single lesion

MACROSCOPIC

General Features

- Patch, plaque, or tumor-like lesion of skin
- Tan to red in color

Size

- Usually varies from < 1 cm to several cm in diameter

MICROSCOPIC

Histologic Features

- Diffuse or nodular collections of plasma cells
- Usually located in deep dermis/subcutis
- Usually well differentiated; rarely, dysplastic with higher nuclear:cytoplasmic ratio and visible nucleoli
  - Mature plasma cells, plasmablasts, and pleomorphic forms may be identified
    - Mature plasma cells are small in size with eccentric nucleus and spoke wheel chromatin without nucleoli
    - Plasmablasts are more immature with delicate nuclear chromatin, higher nuclear:cytoplasmic ratio, and prominent nucleoli
    - Pleomorphic forms show irregular nuclear contours, more vesicular chromatin, and binucleation
- Cytoplasmic immunoglobulins may produce variety of morphologic findings
  - Russell bodies are eosinophilic, homogeneous cytoplasmic inclusions
  - Mott cells have grape-like clusters of cytoplasmic immunoglobulin inclusions
  - Crystalline rods are immunoglobulin-forming, rod-like structures
  - Gaucher-like cells have fibrillar-like inclusions
  - These inclusions are more likely to be seen in plasma cell myeloma than plasmacytoma
- May have scattered background lymphocytes
- No Castleman disease features

Cytologic Features

- Oval-shaped plasma cells
  - Eccentric nucleus with clock face or spoke wheel chromatin
  - Usually lacking prominent nucleoli
- Cytoplasm
  - Moderate to abundant, eosinophilic staining
  - Perinuclear hof representing Golgi apparatus

ANCILLARY TESTS

Immunohistochemistry

- Plasma cell and late B-cell markers are positive
  - CD38(+), CD138 (syndecan)(+), CD79a(+), MUM-1(+)
- Pan-B cell markers are usually negative
  - CD20 typically not reactive; rarely can aberrantly be expressed
- CD56(+) in malignant plasma cells; usually CD56(-) in reactive plasma cells
- CD45rb(-), unlike most types of non-Hodgkin B-cell lymphoma

- κ and λ monoclonality by immunohistochemistry
- Also can express CD117 and CD10
- Sometimes cyclin-D1 (+)

Flow Cytometry

- Underestimates number of plasma cells because of mechanical fragility
  - May need to defer to morphology and immunohistochemistry to evaluate plasma cells
- Strong CD138 expression with κ or λ monoclonality

Genetic Testing

- PCR
  - *IGH* gene rearrangement may or may not be detected
- Cytogenetics
  - Plasmacytomas may show same molecular changes as seen in plasma cell myeloma
    - However, this has not been specifically studied in CPs
    - Both numerical and structural chromosomal abnormalities are common
    - Translocations involving *IGH* on chromosome 14q32 are most common
  - Hyperdiploid subgroup
    - 48-74 chromosomes; gains of odd-numbered chromosomes
  - Hypodiploid subgroup
    - ≤ 44 chromosomes
  - Cyclin-D translocations: t(11;14)(q13;q32), t(6;14)(p21;q32), t(12;14)(p13;q32)
  - *WHSC1* (MMSET) translocation: t(4;14)(p16;q32)
  - *MAF* translocations: t(14;16)(q32;q23), t(14;20)(q32;q11), t(8;14)(q24;q32)
  - *TP53* deletion

DIFFERENTIAL DIAGNOSIS

Extranodal Marginal Zone Lymphoma With Plasmacytic Differentiation

- Can be difficult to exclude but usually express B-cell antigens (CD20, pax-5, CD79) and Bcl-2 and show reactive germinal centers
- Often have admixed mature B cells and show disrupted follicular dendritic cells on CD21

Reactive Plasma Cell Infiltrates

- Also well-differentiated plasma cells without dysplasia
- Often mixed infiltrate of plasma cells, lymphocytes, histiocytes, neutrophils, and eosinophils, whereas plasmacytoma is more homogenous population of plasma cells
- Often no mass lesion
- Polyclonal by κ/λ stains
- CD56(-) unlike most plasmacytomas
- Look for infectious organisms, such as spirochetes (i.e., syphilis)

IgG4-Related Disease

- Found in multiple organs, including skin, pancreas, and lymph nodes
- Morphology typically shows plasma cells with mixed background infiltrate and fibrosis
- Perform both IgG and IgG4 immunohistochemistry
  - IgG4:IgG > 0.4
    - Serum IgG4 levels may or may not be elevated in IgG4 disease
- Treatable in other organ systems with steroids

Castleman Disease

- Uncommon in skin
- Follicles with atretic germinal centers
- Occasionally > 1 germinal center per follicle
- Plasma cells found between secondary follicles
- Rarely light chain restricted, more λ restriction than κ restriction

Cutaneous Involvement by Plasma Cell Myeloma

- Increased plasma cells in bone marrow or peripheral blood, unlike plasmacytoma, which by definition spares bone marrow
- Clinical/laboratory findings: Lytic bone lesions, monoclonal gammopathy, anemia, hypercalcemia
- Both plasma cell myeloma and plasmacytoma are composed of monotypic plasma cells
- Similar molecular findings in both plasma cell myeloma and plasmacytoma

Plasmablastic Lymphoma

- Rare tumors characterized by larger plasmacytoid cells with more atypia
- Usually EBER or HHV8(+), unlike plasmacytoma; often in HIV-positive patients

Lymphoplasmacytic Lymphoma

- Associated with Waldenström macroglobulinemia
- Range of morphology from small lymphocytes to plasmacytoid lymphocytes to plasma cells
- Difficult to distinguish from marginal zone lymphoma

Solitary Plasmacytoma of Bone

- Localized malignant bone neoplasm consisting of monoclonal plasma cells
- Does not involve skin
- Typically has more aggressive clinical course than extraosseous plasmacytoma (plasmacytoma of skin)

SELECTED REFERENCES

1. Saidane O et al: Cutaneous and pleural involvement in a patient with multiple myeloma. BMJ Case Rep. 2015
2. Maejima H et al: Multiple primary cutaneous plasmacytoma. Acta Dermatovenerol Croat. 22(4):308-10, 2014
3. Tokura Y et al: IgG4-related skin disease. Br J Dermatol. 171(5):959-67, 2014
4. Uçmak D et al: Multiple primary cutaneous plasmacytomas: an unusual presentation. J Cutan Med Surg. 18(5):361-4, 2014
5. Wang E et al: Primary cutaneous giant cell plasmacytoma in an organ transplant recipient: a rare presentation of a posttransplant lymphoproliferative disorder. Am J Dermatopathol. 32(5):479-85, 2010
6. Rongioletti F et al: The histological and pathogenetic spectrum of cutaneous disease in monoclonal gammopathies. J Cutan Pathol. 35(8):705-21, 2008

Low Power of Cutaneous Plasmacytoma

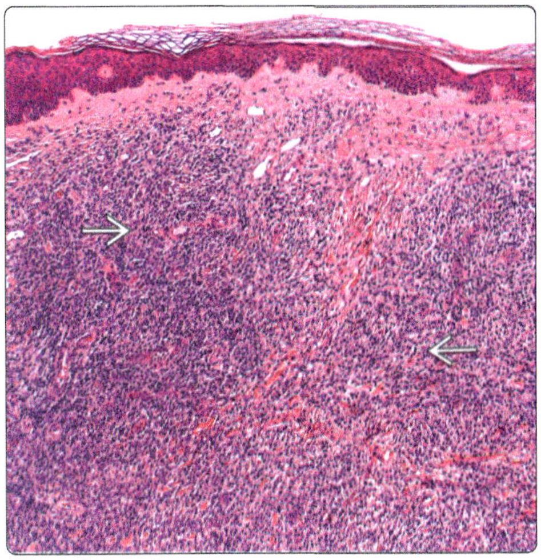

CD138 Immunohistochemistry

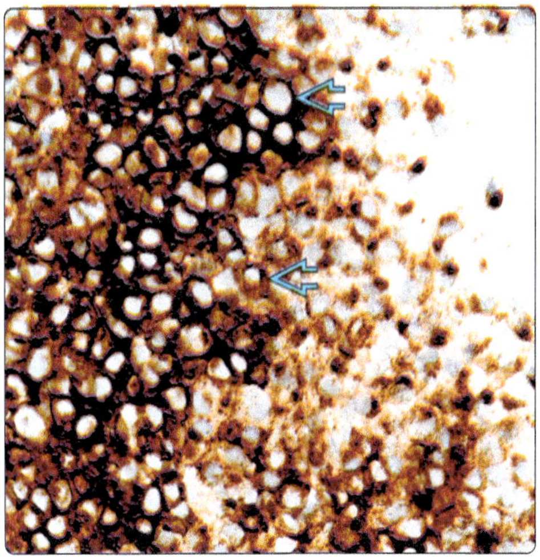

(Left) *This is a low-power image of a CP. There are sheet-like aggregates of plasma cells filling the superficial dermis* → *. A bone marrow biopsy did not show a plasma cell infiltrate, and the patient did not have evidence of a systemic B-cell lymphoma.* **(Right)** *This plasmacytoma is diffusely positive for CD138 by immunohistochemistry* → *. Benign and neoplastic plasma cells show membranous and cytoplasmic reactivity for CD138. Metastatic carcinomas may also express CD138. (From DP: Bone.)*

κ-Light Chain Immunohistochemistry

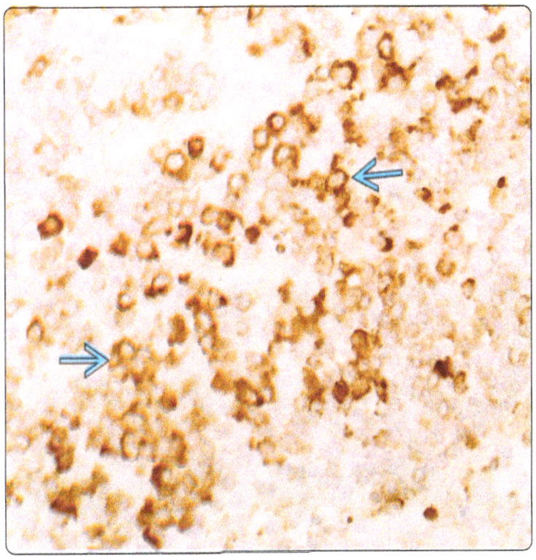

λ-Light Chain Immunohistochemistry

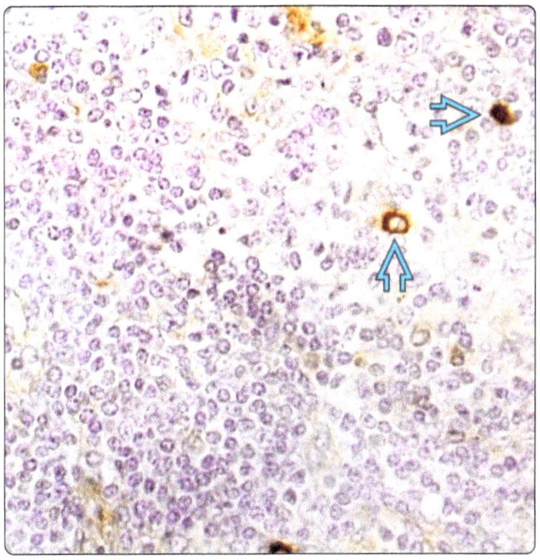

(Left) *This κ immunohistochemical stain is positive in the plasma cells* → *of this CP.* **(Right)** *The majority of plasma cells in this cutaneous plasmacytoma are negative for λ-light chain. Only rare reactive plasma cells are positive* → *. Monoclonality is demonstrated with the majority of cells positive for κ and negative for λ.*

Differential Diagnosis: Cutaneous Syphilis

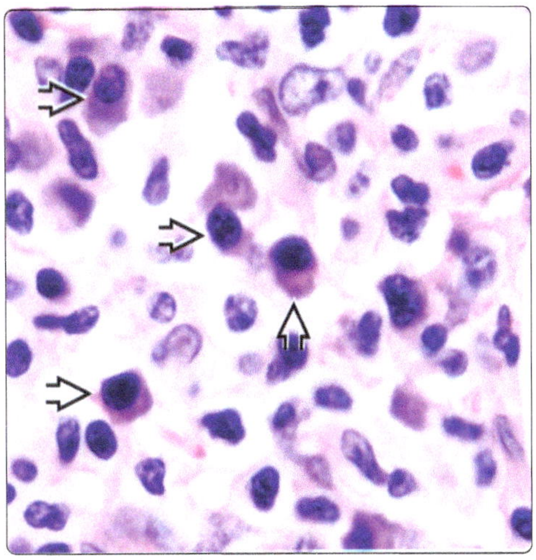

Spirochetal Antibody Stain Highlights Numerous Organisms in Syphilis

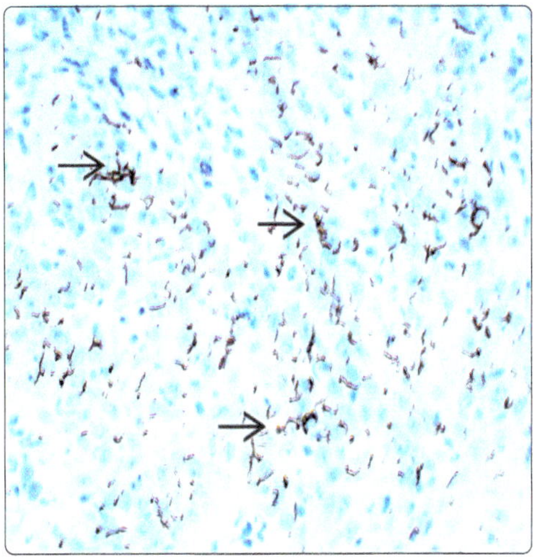

(Left) *This is a case of cutaneous syphilis. Numerous plasma cells* → *are seen, along with many lymphocytes. Spirochetal organisms were identified by Warthin-Starry and a spirochetal antibody stain.* **(Right)** *This is an example of secondary syphilis with numerous coiled organisms* → *easily identified by immunohistochemistry with an antispirochetal antibody.*

Primary Cutaneous Marginal Zone Lymphoma

KEY FACTS

TERMINOLOGY

- Non-Hodgkin small B-cell lymphoma of centrocyte-like marginal zone cells
- Malignant B cells often expanding marginal zones, surrounding reactive follicles and colonizing them

ETIOLOGY/PATHOGENESIS

- *Borrelia burgdorferi* in some cases (European)
- Associated with autoimmune disease and chronic antigen stimulation

CLINICAL ISSUES

- Excellent prognosis; 5-year survival: 90-100%
- Usually treated with excision or radiation

MICROSCOPIC

- Small B cells, monocytoid, plasmacytoid
- Colonized germinal centers
- Lymphoepithelial lesions rare
- ± Dutcher bodies

ANCILLARY TESTS

- B cells (+) for CD20, may coexpress CD43 and Bcl-2
- Germinal centers Bcl-6(+), CD10(+), Bcl-2(-)
- CD21(+) loose follicular dendric cell meshworks
- Usually IgG(+), often IgG4(+)
- Usually light chain restriction and clonally rearranged immunoglobulin genes
- No translocations involving *MALT1*, *BIRC3*, and *BCL10* genes
  - t(11;18)(q21;q21) negative
- No *MYD88* L265P mutations

TOP DIFFERENTIAL DIAGNOSES

- Primary cutaneous follicle center lymphoma
- Secondary involvement by systemic marginal zone lymphoma
  - Look for lymphoma at extracutaneous site
  - May be t(11;18)(q21;q21) positive

PCMZL

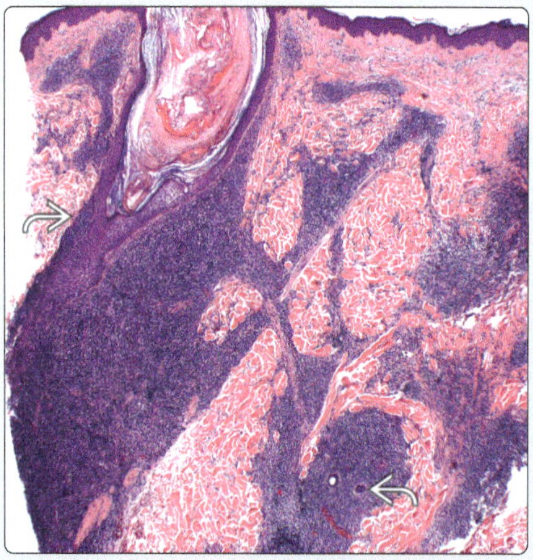

Higher Magnification of PCMZL

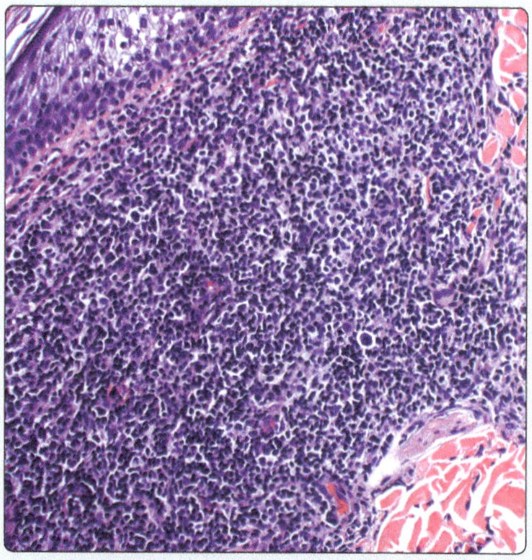

(Left) *Scanning magnification shows a primary cutaneous marginal zone lymphoma (PCMZL) involving the superficial and deep dermis. The infiltrate surrounds multiple blood vessels and adnexal structures.* **(Right)** *Higher magnification of the infiltrate shows a dense, nodular collection of crowded lymphocytes. The cells are small but show hyperchromatic-staining nuclei and scant mounts of pale eosinophilic-staining cytoplasm.*

CD20 Immunohistochemistry in PCMZL

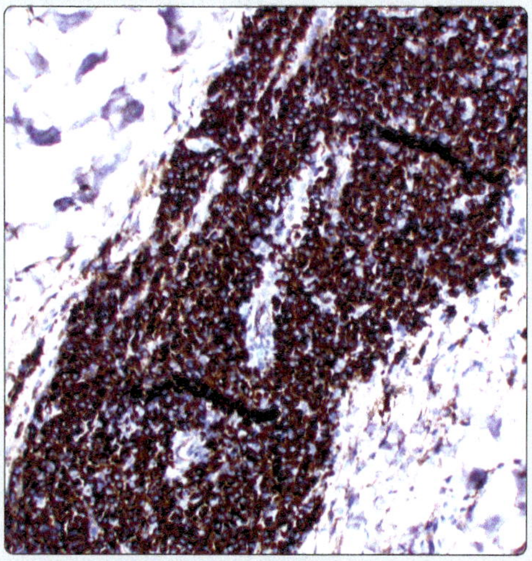

***BIRC3/MALT1* Dual Fusion Probes**

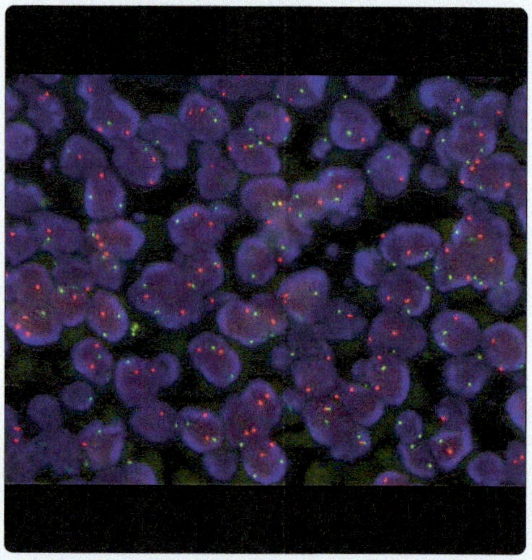

(Left) *CD20 strongly stains the majority of the lymphocytes, consistent with a B-cell lymphoma.* **(Right)** *This dual-color, dual-fusion FISH test probes the BIRC3 gene in green and the MALT1 gene in red. No translocation is identified since the green and red signals remain separate and no fusion (yellow signal) is present.*

TERMINOLOGY

Abbreviations

- Primary cutaneous marginal zone lymphoma (PCMZL)

Synonyms

- Primary cutaneous immunocytoma

Definitions

- Non-Hodgkin small B-cell lymphoma of centrocyte-like marginal zone cells with malignant B cells often expanding marginal zones, surrounding reactive follicles and colonizing them

ETIOLOGY/PATHOGENESIS

Infectious Agents

- *Borrelia burgdorferi* DNA found in skin in some European cases, but not in all other populations
  - Other infectious diseases noted in tissue other than skin

Autoimmune Diseases

- Marginal zone lymphoma has been associated with patients who have autoimmune diseases
  - Sjögren syndrome and parotid gland marginal zone lymphoma
  - Hashimoto thyroiditis and thyroid marginal zone lymphoma

Chronic Antigen Stimulation

- PCMZL cases have been related to tick bites, tattoo pigment, and antigen injection
- PCMZL recapitulates architecture of Peyer patches
  - Usually in sites without significant lymphoid tissue

CLINICAL ISSUES

Epidemiology

- Incidence
  - 2nd most common type of primary cutaneous B-cell lymphoma after primary cutaneous follicle center lymphoma
- Age
  - Usually adults > 40 years old, rare in children
- Sex
  - No gender predominance
- Ethnicity
  - No ethnic propensity

Site

- Mostly upper extremity and upper trunk
  - Also head and neck

Presentation

- 1 or more plaques or nodules
  - Rarely ulcerates
  - Multiple nodules often seen in systemic marginal zone lymphoma with secondary spread to dermis

Treatment

- Excision or radiation therapy
  - If solitary or only a few lesions
- Chemotherapy, including rituximab, considered for widespread disease, metastasis
- Antibiotics
  - Sometimes therapy for *Borrelia burgdorferi* infection

Prognosis

- Excellent
  - 5-year survival: 90-100%
  - But tendency to recur in skin
    - Rarely transforms to large B-cell lymphoma
    - Only rarely metastasize to extracutaneous sites

MACROSCOPIC

General Features

- 1 or more firm red nodules on skin

MICROSCOPIC

Histologic Features

- Nodular to diffuse dermal infiltrate
  - Spares epidermis with grenz zone
  - Rarely involves subcutis &/or epidermis
- Neoplastic cells
  - Small to medium-sized B cells with mild atypia, 1 or more inconspicuous nucleoli, and scant pale cytoplasm
  - Sometimes monocytoid with ample pale/clear cytoplasm
  - Sometimes plasmacytoid with eccentric nucleus and pink cytoplasm
  - Variable numbers of plasma cells, neutrophils, and eosinophils
  - Mostly small in size with coarse chromatin and mild atypia
- Dutcher bodies (intranuclear inclusions)
  - Sometimes present
  - More often in marginal zone lymphoma than plasmacytoma
  - Russell bodies are cytoplasmic inclusions that may also be seen, but are less specific
- Reactive germinal centers
  - Colonized by neoplastic marginal zone B cells
  - Still contain tingible body macrophages
  - If tissue is small, may not see follicles
- Follicular dendric cell meshworks
  - Often disrupted/loosened in colonized germinal centers
- Lymphoepithelial lesions
  - 3 or more lymphocytes entering epithelial structure (usually gland) and destroying it
  - Very rarely seen in skin
- May be difficult to diagnose because of nonspecificity of many morphologic features, absence of 1 or more classic features, and nature of small biopsies

ANCILLARY TESTS

Immunohistochemistry

- Neoplastic B cells
  - Express B-cell markers
    - Positive for CD19, CD20, CD22
    - Sheets of B cells with few T cells are concerning for B-cell lymphoma over reactive infiltrate
    - If there is a mix of B and T cells, then look for other features (IHC, clonality) to diagnose lymphoma

- B-cell coexpression of T-cell markers is feature of malignancy
  - B cells may coexpress CD43 or Bcl-2
  - Bcl-2 is normally expressed on reactive mantle zone cells and marginal zone cells
- Neoplastic B cells usually do not express
  - CD5, CD10, Bcl-6, CD21, or CD23
- Light chain restriction
  - Usually in plasma cells &/or lymphoplasmacytic cells
- Plasma cells express CD138 and CD79a

- Reactive germinal centers
  - Positive markers
    - Bcl-6(+), CD10(+)
  - Negative markers
    - Bcl-2(-)
- Lymphoepithelial lesions
  - B-cell markers (+) in B cells in gland
  - Cytokeratin stains can highlight disrupted glands
- Follicular dendritic cell meshworks
  - Highlighted by CD21 and CD23
  - Show expanded or loose pattern
- Immunoglobulins
  - Most are IgG(+) and to lesser extent for IgA
    - IgG4 in ~ 40%, but no evidence of IgG4-related disease
    - IgG4(+) in skin usually represents PCMZL
  - Few cases are IgM(+)
    - These cases are also CXCR3(+)
    - These cases can show extracutaneous extension
- PD1 is usually (-) in neoplastic B cells, but can be (+) in reactive T cells

Flow Cytometry

- Strong CD19 and CD20 co-expression with κ or λ restriction and lack of CD5 or CD10

In Situ Hybridization

- No translocations involving *MALT1*, *BIRC3*, and *BCL10* genes
  - Including no t(11;18)(q21;q21)
  - These translocations are detected at various rates in noncutaneous marginal zone lymphomas
    - t(11;18) in 25-50% gastric marginal zone lymphoma
- t(14;18)(q32;q21) almost always negative
  - Rarely positive; present in 1 series

Genetic Testing

- Clonal *IGH* gene rearrangement
- No *MYD88* L265P mutations in PCMZL
- *FAS* gene mutations are rarely found

DIFFERENTIAL DIAGNOSIS

Follicular Hyperplasia

- Contains reactive germinal centers, similar to PCMZL
  - But germinal centers are not colonized in follicular hyperplasia
- Lacks expanded/confluent neoplastic marginal zones
- Lacks light chain restriction
- Polyclonal *IGH* gene rearrangement

Primary Cutaneous Follicle Center Lymphoma

- Follicles are neoplastic, not reactive as in PCMZL
  - Monomorphic follicle center cells
  - Lack tingible body macrophages
  - Attenuated mantle zones
- Nodular or diffuse growth pattern
- Immunohistochemistry
  - Bcl-6(+)
  - CD10(+/-)
    - Often negative in diffuse areas
  - No coexpression of CD43
  - Bcl-2(-/+)
    - Often negative in diffuse areas
    - More common in nodal follicular lymphoma

Plasmacytoma

- Sheets of plasma cells
  - Not plasmacytoid B cells
- Must exclude cutaneous marginal zone lymphoma
  - Marginal zone lymphoma should have at least small population of malignant small B cells
- Must exclude plasmacytoid variants of other small B-cell lymphomas and plasma cell myeloma

Secondary Involvement by Systemic Marginal Zone Lymphoma

- Immunohistochemistry and morphology identical to PCMZL
  - Secondary involvement favors head and neck regions and is limited to older patients
  - t(11;18) may be positive
  - Often IgM and IgD(+), unlike PCMZL

Subcutaneous Panniculitis-Like T-Cell Lymphoma and Primary Cutaneous γδ T-Cell Lymphoma

- Within DDx of PCMZL involving subcutis
- Subcutaneous panniculitis-like T-cell lymphoma has cytotoxic T cells and are CD8(+)
- Primary cutaneous γδ T-cell lymphoma is CD56(+), CD4(-), CD8(-)

SELECTED REFERENCES

1. Brenner I et al: Lack of myeloid differentiation primary response protein MyD88 L265P mutation in primary cutaneous marginal zone lymphoma. Br J Dermatol. 173(6):1527-8, 2015
2. Chui MH et al: Primary marginal zone lymphoma of the subcutis associated with panniculitis and fat necrosis. Am J Clin Pathol. 144(2):341-6, 2015
3. Goyal A et al: PD-1, S-100 and CD1a expression in pseudolymphomatous folliculitis, primary cutaneous marginal zone B-cell lymphoma (MALT lymphoma) and cutaneous lymphoid hyperplasia. J Cutan Pathol. 42(1):6-15, 2015
4. Guitart J: Rethinking primary cutaneous marginal zone lymphoma: shifting the focus to the cause of the infiltrate. J Cutan Pathol. 42(9):600-3, 2015
5. Guitart J et al: High incidence of gastrointestinal tract disorders and autoimmunity in primary cutaneous marginal zone B-cell lymphomas. JAMA Dermatol. 150(4):412-8, 2014
6. Servitje O et al: Primary cutaneous marginal zone B-cell lymphoma: response to treatment and disease-free survival in a series of 137 patients. J Am Acad Dermatol. 69(3):357-65, 2013
7. Takino H et al: Primary cutaneous marginal zone B-cell lymphoma: a molecular and clinicopathological study of cases from Asia, Germany, and the United States. Mod Pathol. 21(12):1517-26, 2008
8. Mandekou-Lefaki I et al: Primary cutaneous MALT-type lymphoma and Helicobacter pylori: a possible relationship. J Eur Acad Dermatol Venereol. 20(5):606-8, 2006
9. Hoefnagel JJ et al: Primary cutaneous marginal zone B-cell lymphoma: clinical and therapeutic features in 50 cases. Arch Dermatol. 141(9):1139-45, 2005
10. Baldassano MF et al: Cutaneous lymphoid hyperplasia and cutaneous marginal zone lymphoma: comparison of morphologic and immunophenotypic features. Am J Surg Pathol. 23(1):88-96, 1999

Low Magnification of PCMZL

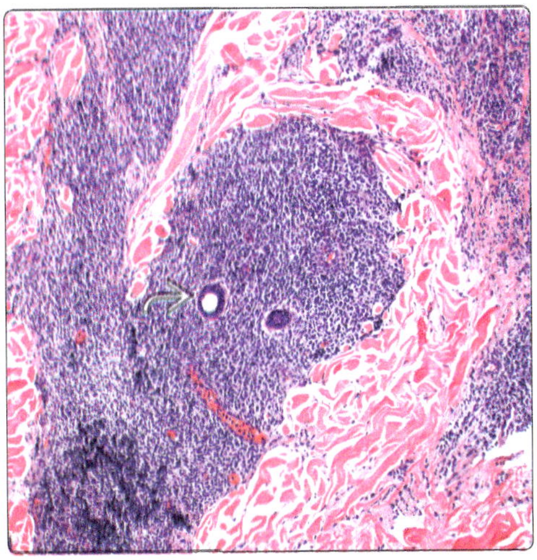

Higher Magnification of PCMZL

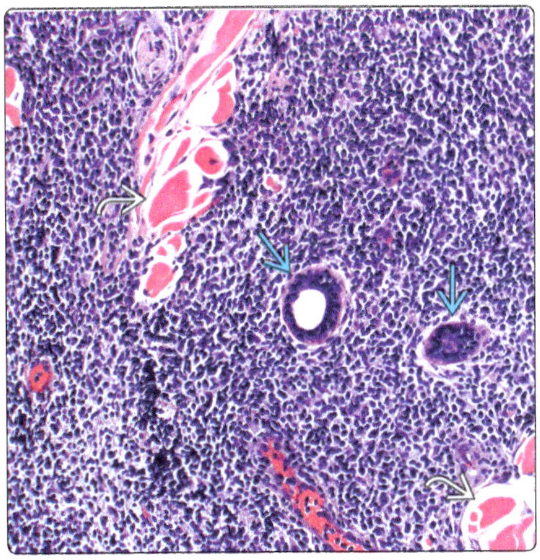

(Left) *Low magnification of a PCMZL involving the mid to deep dermis. Note the dense infiltrate surrounding multiple blood vessels and adnexal structures* . **(Right)** *Higher magnification shows the dense infiltrate of lymphocytes and plasma cells surrounding and entrapping collagen bundles and several adnexal structures* .

Monocytoid Cells in PCMZL

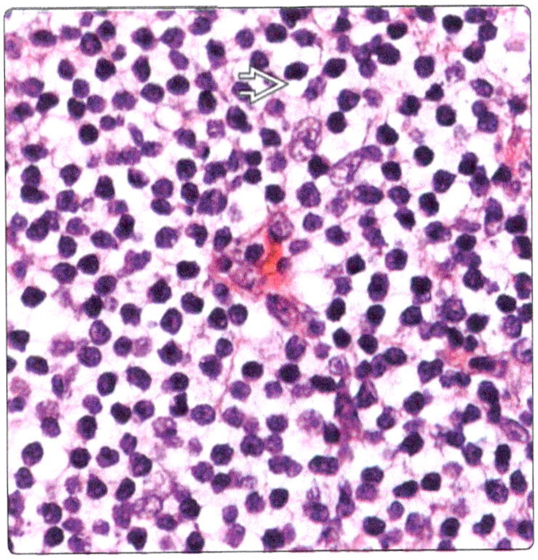

Dutcher Bodies in PCMZL

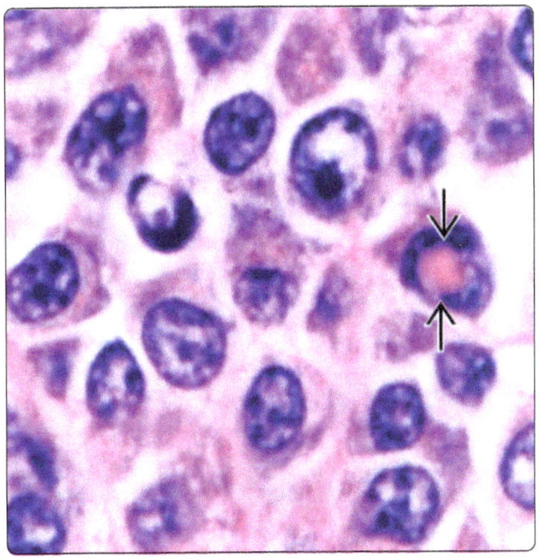

(Left) *In many cases of PCMZL, the tumor cells have a monocytoid appearance. In this image, the monocytoid cells have increased amounts of clear cytoplasm* . **(Right)** *There is a Dutcher body in this case of PCMZL. Dutcher bodies are intranuclear inclusions that have a round pink appearance.*

Reactive Germinal Centers in PCMZL

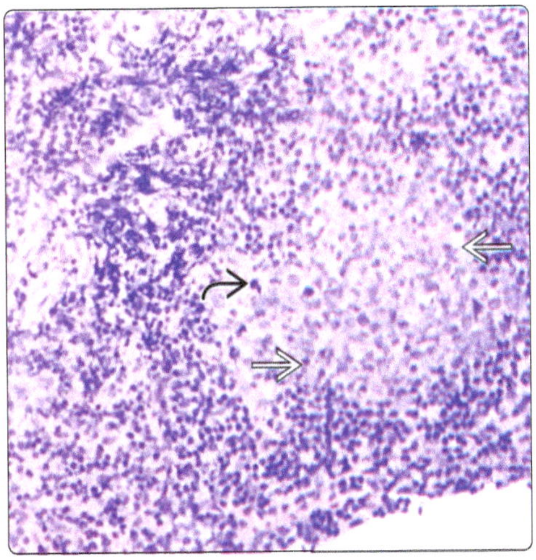

Lymphoepithelial Lesions in PCMZL

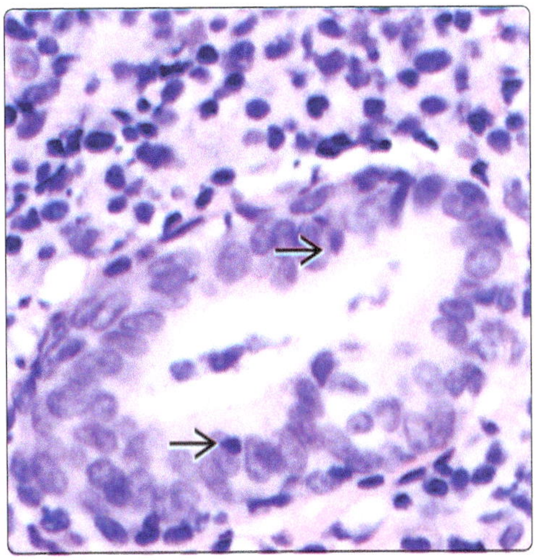

(Left) *As in this image, most cases of PCMZL have reactive germinal centers . However, the germinal centers are colonized or infiltrated by lymphoma. There are small cleaved neoplastic B cells penetrating this reactive germinal center.* **(Right)** *Lymphoepithelial lesions are common in systemic marginal zone lymphoma, although rarely seen in cutaneous marginal zone lymphoma. This gland has a few lymphocytes penetrating it.*

(Left) *This is a CD20(+) marginal zone lymphoma. CD20 is strongly positive in the neoplastic B cells. Other B-cell markers, such as CD79a and pax-5, are also positive.* **(Right)** *This CD3 immunostain is negative in the neoplastic B cells ⮕, but there are numerous reactive-appearing T cells ⮕ that are positive for CD3. Compared to CD20 staining, there is much less CD3 staining.*

CD20 Immunohistochemistry in PCMZL

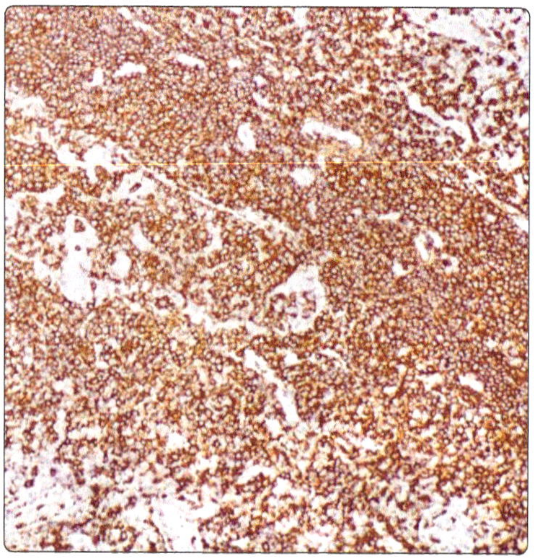

CD3 Immunohistochemistry in PCMZL

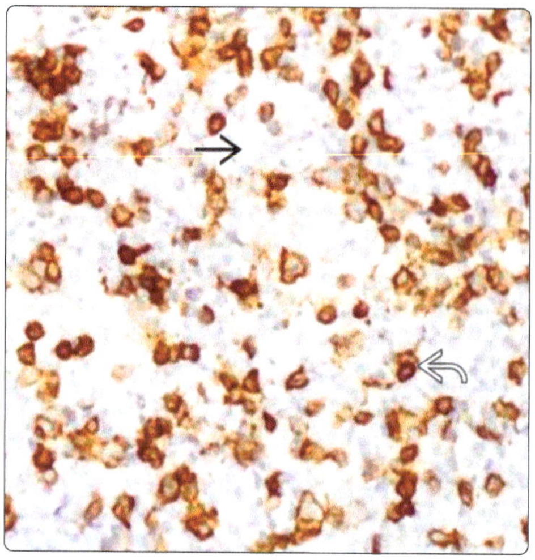

(Left) *κ light chain stain highlights the vast majority of the plasmacytoid cells ⮕ in a case of PCMZL (κ:λ ratio > 50:1).* **(Right)** *λ light chain stain highlights only a few plasmacytoid cells in the same case of PCMZL (κ:λ ratio > 50:1).*

Immunohistochemistry for κ Light Chain

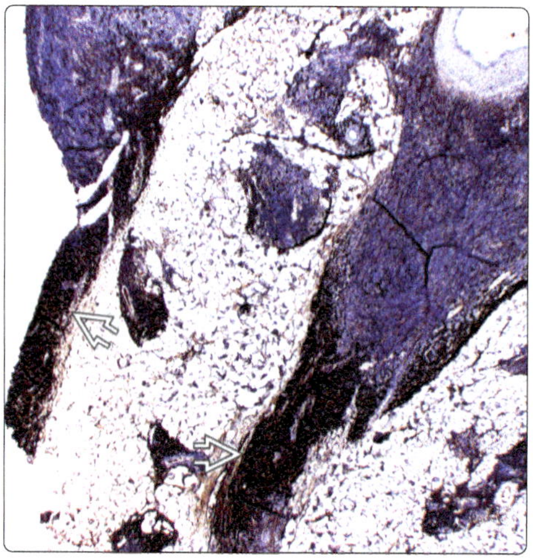

Immunohistochemistry for λ Light Chain

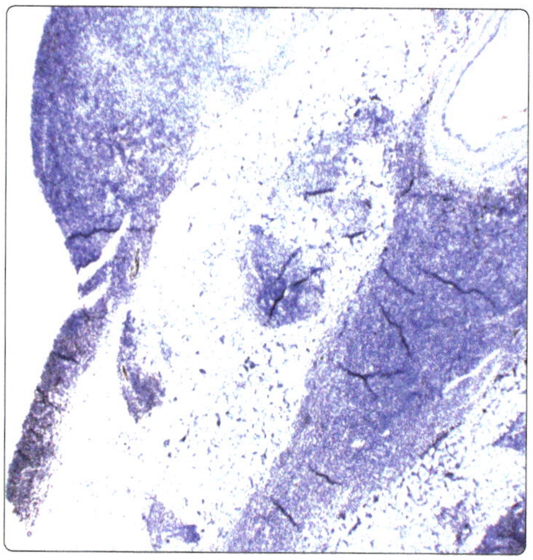

(Left) *This image shows CD21 expressed on follicular dendritic cells (FDCs) ⮕, but it is negative in the neoplastic cells in PCMZL. Because the germinal centers are colonized by malignant B cells, the FDCs show a loose/disrupted pattern as seen here.* **(Right)** *CD20 can be used to highlight the neoplastic B cells in lymphoepithelial lesions. In this case, there are large numbers of small B cells ⮕ in a glandular structure ⮕.*

CD21 Immunohistochemistry in PCMZL

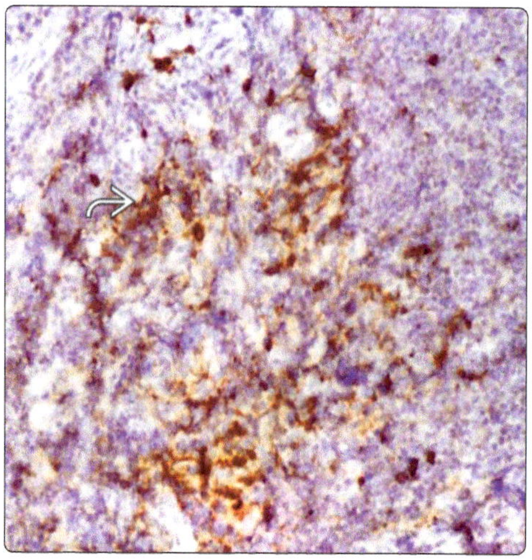

CD20(+) Lymphoepithelial Lesions in PCMZL

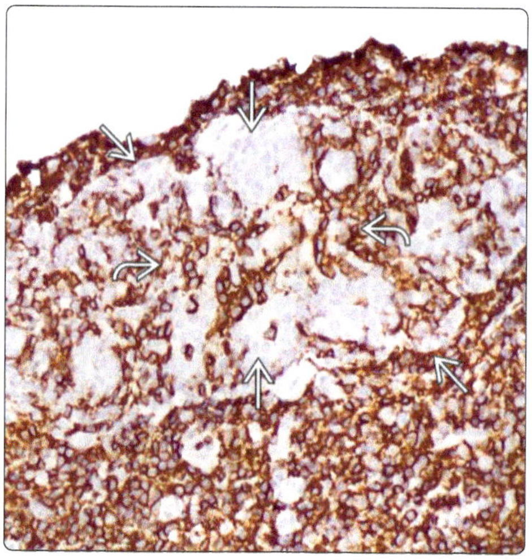

DDx: PCFCL

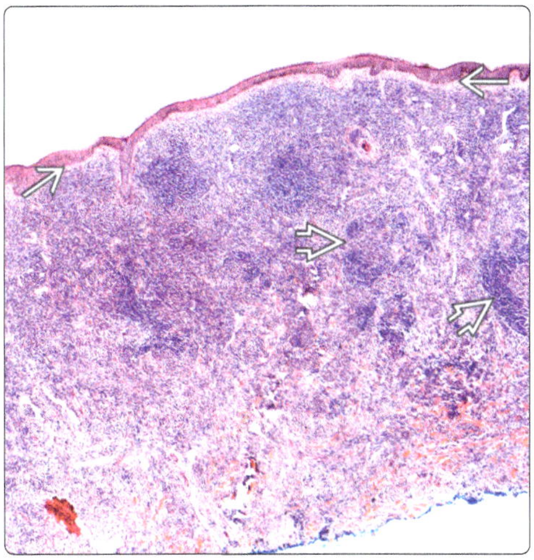

DDx: PCFCL at Higher Power Magnification

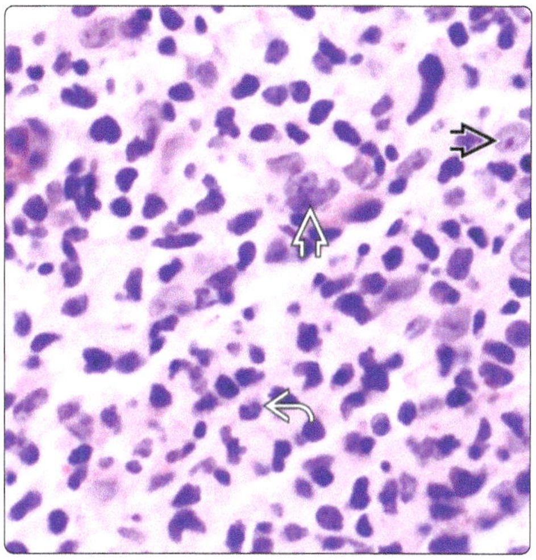

(Left) *Primary cutaneous follicle center lymphoma (PCFCL) displays a dense lymphocytic infiltrate in the dermis, sparing the subepidermal layer (grenz zone* ➡*). The neoplasm contains ill-defined follicles* ➡*. (Courtesy R. Miranda, MD.)* **(Right)** *PCFCL shows a mix of centrocytes* ➡*, centroblasts* ⇨*, and rare follicular dendritic cells* ➡*. Monocytoid change, plasmacytoid change, and Dutcher bodies typical to marginal zone lymphoma are not usually seen in follicle center lymphoma.*

DDx: Plasmacytoma

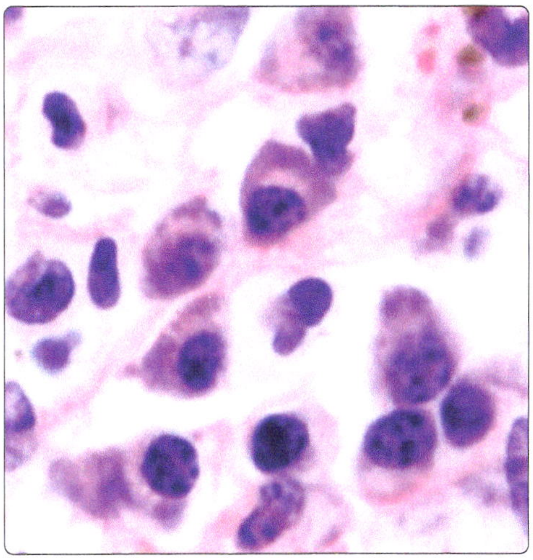

DDx: Small Lymphocytic Lymphoma/Chronic Lymphocytic Leukemia

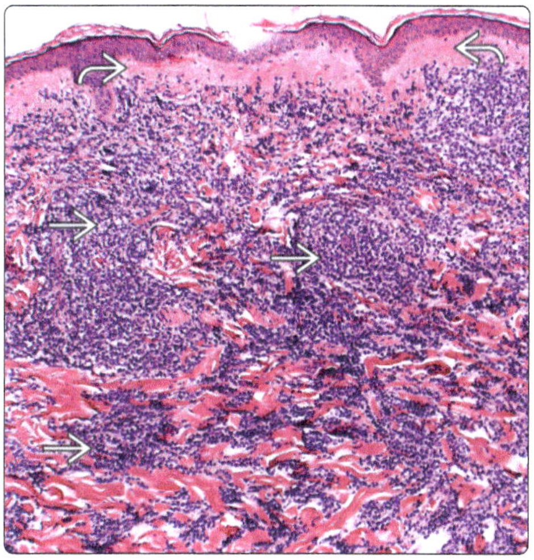

(Left) *Cutaneous plasmacytoma is very rare, and most would be reclassified as PCMZL today. These are collections of plasma cells, not plasmacytoid B cells, as in PCMZL.* **(Right)** *This image is of small lymphocytic lymphoma/chronic lymphocytic leukemia (SLL/CLL) of the skin. Atypical lymphocytes* ➡ *are seen in superficial and deep dermis with an infiltrative growth pattern. the epidermis is uninvolved and separated from the proliferation by a grenz zone* ➡*.*

CD20 Immunohistochemistry in SLL/CLL

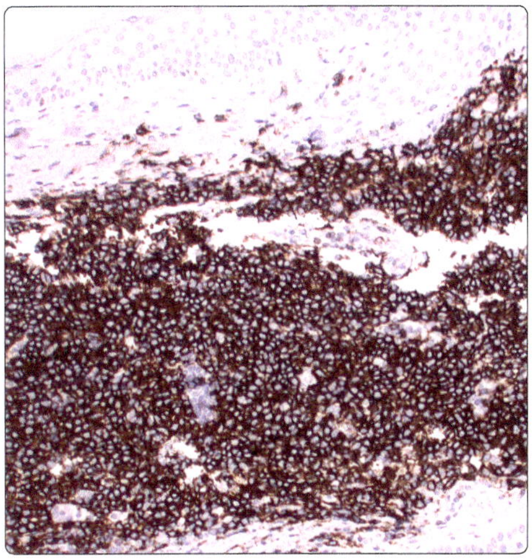

CD5 Immunohistochemistry in SLL/CLL

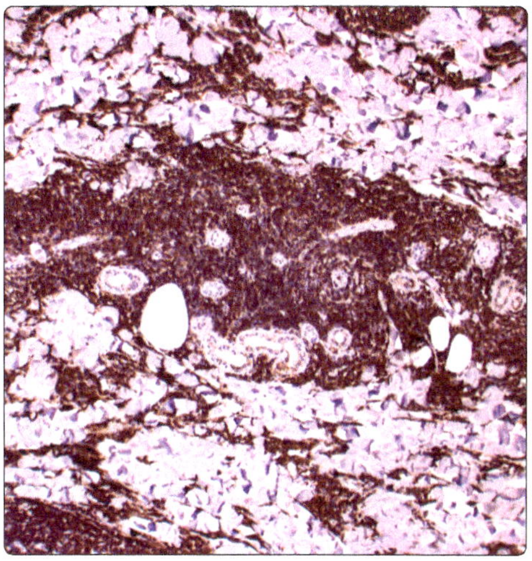

(Left) *CD20 immunohistochemical stain in SLL/CLL shows that the cells are strongly and diffusely CD20(+).* **(Right)** *A CD5 immunohistochemical stain in SLL/CLL shows that the cells are strongly CD5(+). CLL is typically CD5 and CD23(+). With PCMZL, CD5 is expressed by reactive T cells and not by the tumor B cells.*

KEY FACTS

TERMINOLOGY

- Primary cutaneous follicle center lymphoma (PCFCL)
- Mature B-cell lymphoma of follicle center cells, primary to skin and not originating in another anatomic site

CLINICAL ISSUES

- Mostly single lesion on scalp; trunk 2nd most common site
- > 95% 5-year survival with local recurrences

MICROSCOPIC

- Nodular, diffuse, and nodular/diffuse growth patterns
- Lack of mantle zones, lack tingible body macrophages

ANCILLARY TESTS

- CD20(+), Bcl-6(+)
- CD10(+/-) (often negative in diffuse variant)
- Bcl-2(+/-) and MUM1/IRF4 (-)
- CD23, CD21, and CD35 (+) in follicular dendritic cell meshworks
- Usually CD43(-), unlike other B-cell lymphomas
- CD5(-), Bcl-1(-)
- Clonal Ig heavy chain (*IgH*) gene rearrangement
- t(14;18), often not detected
- Gene expression profiling findings akin to germinal center-like large B-cell lymphoma

TOP DIFFERENTIAL DIAGNOSES

- Reactive follicular hyperplasia
  - Usually top heavy infiltrate, whereas PCFCL is often bottom heavy infiltrate
- Primary cutaneous marginal zone lymphoma
  - Has reactive germinal centers, which can be confused with PCFCL
- Secondary skin involvement of follicular lymphoma
  - Clinically and genetically different from systemic follicle center lymphoma
- Primary cutaneous diffuse large B-cell lymphoma, leg type

Clinical Presentation of Primary Cutaneous Follicle Center Lymphoma

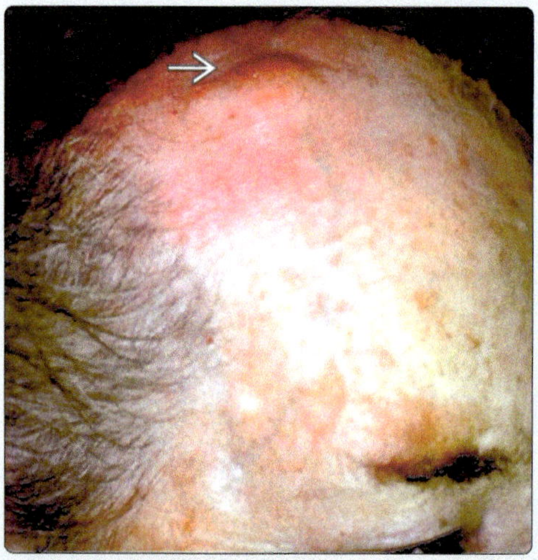

Primary Cutaneous Follicle Center Lymphoma Nodular Pattern, Low Magnification

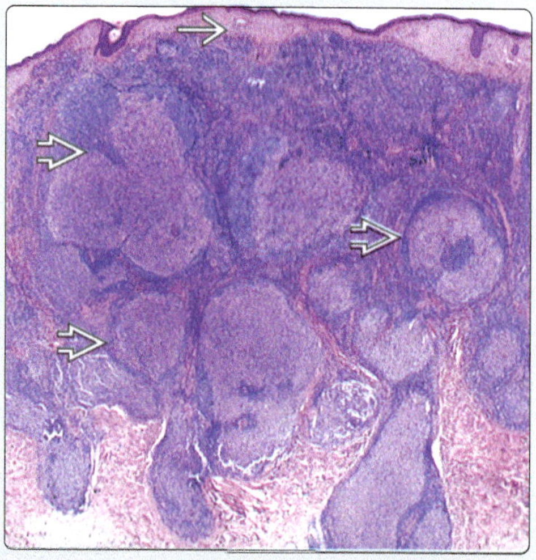

(Left) *This patient presented with a single large raised red nodule ➡ on the scalp, 5 cm in largest dimension. (Courtesy M. Tomaszewski, MD.)* **(Right)** *Low-power magnification shows primary cutaneous follicle center lymphoma (PCFCL) with a multinodular ➡ dermal infiltrate that is separated from the epidermis by a grenz zone ➡. (Courtesy M. Tomaszewski, MD.)*

FISH Showing t(14;18) Negative in Primary Cutaneous Follicle Center Lymphoma

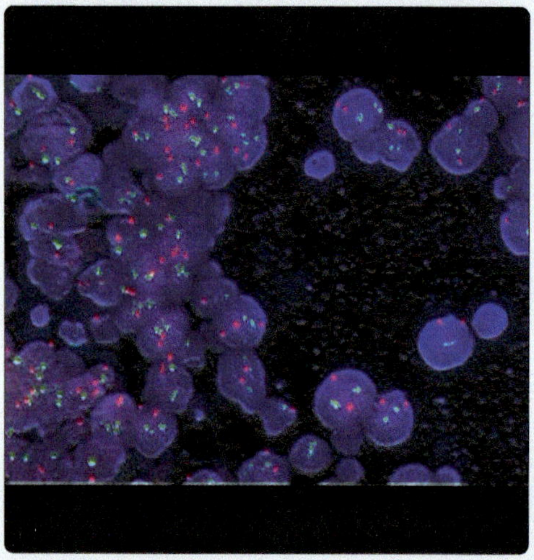

FISH Showing Positive t(14;18) in Systemic Follicular Lymphoma

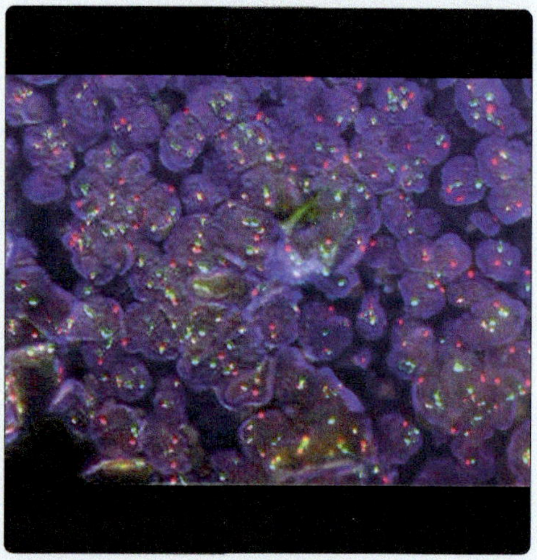

(Left) *This is an example of a FISH dual fusion probe for BCL2/IGH representing t(14;18). Numerous separate green and red signals are seen without fusion (yellow) signals, indicating that t(14;18) is not present. The t(14;18) is typically absent in PCFCL.* **(Right)** *This is an example of a FISH dual-fusion probe for BCL2/IGH representing t(14;18). Numerous fusion (yellow) signals are present, indicating that there is t(14;18) in this case of systemic follicle center/follicular lymphoma.*

TERMINOLOGY

Abbreviations

- Primary cutaneous follicle center lymphoma (PCFCL)

Synonyms

- Follicular lymphoma of skin
- Crosti disease (reticulohistiocytoma of dorsum)
  - Plaques/tumors surrounded by erythematous macules/papules
- Centroblastic/centrocytic lymphoma

Definitions

- Mature B-cell lymphoma of follicle center cells, arising in skin
  - Disease must be limited to skin for 6 months after diagnosis

ETIOLOGY/PATHOGENESIS

Classification

- Distinct disease from systemic/nodal follicular lymphoma (FL)
  - Different clinical findings
    - Indolent, less dissemination
  - Different genetic findings
    - Less common *BCL2* rearrangements than systemic follicular lymphoma

CLINICAL ISSUES

Epidemiology

- Incidence
  - 0.1-0.2 cases per 100,000 people per year
  - Most common primary cutaneous B-cell lymphoma
    - ~ 20% of all skin lymphomas
    - ~ 60% of all B-cell skin lymphomas
  - 2nd most common extranodal lymphoma after gastric MALT lymphomas
- Age
  - Usually adults
    - Median age: 60 years
- Sex
  - More common in males (M:F = 1.5:1)

Site

- Usually head and neck, especially scalp, forehead, and upper trunk

Presentation

- Usually single papule/nodule or grouped lesions
  - ~ 15% multifocal
- Papules, plaques, nodules, or tumors of differing sizes
  - From < 1 cm to > 40 cm in greatest dimension
  - Slowly enlarge
- Rarely ulcerate
- Rare variants
  - Miliary and agminated type: Multiple, firm, erythematous papules grouped together in small clusters
  - Anetodermic form: Lesions regress leaving anetoderma

Natural History

- Slow increase in size of untreated lesions
- Extracutaneous dissemination in only ~ 10% of cases
- ~ 35% recur, typically proximal to primary lesion

Treatment

- Observation, surgical removal, or local radiation
- Rituximab, if extensive skin involvement
- Chemotherapy in rare extensive disease or extracutaneous spread

Prognosis

- Good: ~ 95% 5-year survival
  - Much better than systemic follicular lymphoma
- Not affected by
  - Grade or growth pattern
  - Bcl-2 expression or t(14;18) status
- Worse prognosis associated with
  - PCFCL arising legs
  - Expression of FOXP1

MACROSCOPIC

Gross Pathology

- Dermal-based papule, plaque, or tumor, usually solitary

MICROSCOPIC

Histologic Features

- Dermal B-cell infiltrate, often extends into subcutis (~ 75% of cases)
  - No overlying epidermotropism
- Growth pattern
  - Nodular, diffuse, or nodular and diffuse
  - May be classified as follicular (> 75% follicular architecture), follicular and diffuse (25-75% follicular architecture), or diffuse (< 25% follicular architecture) growth pattern
    - Diffuse growth pattern does not represent tumor progression from follicular to diffuse pattern
    - Can initially present as diffuse
- Follicles
  - Often not well defined
  - Usually seen in small lesions
  - Lack mantle zones
  - Lack tingible body macrophages, unlike pseudolymphoma and primary cutaneous marginal zone lymphoma
  - Contain follicular dendritic cells
- Tumor cells
  - Mostly centrocytes (small to medium sized, cleaved) derived from germinal center B cells
  - Variable numbers of centroblasts (larger in size)
- Cases with ↑ numbers of centroblasts
  - Diagnose as PCFCL if nodular or nodular and diffuse growth pattern
  - Diagnose as diffuse pattern PCFCL if large cells and only diffuse growth pattern
- Grading of follicular lymphoma
  - Not necessary or of prognostic value for PCFCL
  - Necessary for systemic FL
    - Grade 1: < 5 centroblasts per HPF; grade 2: 6-15 centroblasts per HPF; grade 3: > 15 centroblasts per HPF

- Grades 1 and 2 show minimal differences in long-term outcome.
- Thus, 2008 WHO classification lumps cases with few centroblasts as "follicular lymphoma grade 1-2 (low grade)" in systemic follicular lymphoma, and does not advise grading of PCFCL
- Variable fibrosis and sclerosis
- Rare cases have shown Reed-Sternberg-like cells &/or follicular mucinosis

Cytologic Features

- Small cleaved cells with coarse chromatin and 1 or more indistinct nucleoli on peripheral smear

ANCILLARY TESTS

Immunohistochemistry

- B-cell markers (+)
  - CD20, CD19, CD79a, pax-5
  - Mostly MUM1/IRF4 or FOXP1 (-), unlike primary cutaneous diffuse large B-cell lymphoma, leg type
- Follicle center markers (+)
  - Bcl-6(+); CD10(+/-)
    - Bcl-6 more consistently (+)
    - CD10 usually (-) in diffuse areas
  - HGCAL (human germinal center-associated lymphoma), E2A, and AID can be (+) in PCFCL
- Bcl-2(+/-)
  - (+) in 20-40% of cases, often weak if (+)
  - Usually (+) in nodular cases and (-) in diffuse cases
- Usually CD43(-), unlike other B-cell lymphomas
- CD23, CD21, and CD35(+) in follicular dendritic cell meshworks
  - Remnants of meshworks are usually observed in diffuse growth pattern
- Express surface immunoglobulins IgM, IgD, IgG, and rarely IgA
- Kappa and lambda can show restriction ~ 1-20% of cases
- Scattered proliferating markers (Ki-67 and MIB-1) in entire infiltrate, unlike in pseudolymphoma where high activity is restricted at the germinal centers

Flow Cytometry

- Light chain restriction, CD20(+), CD10(+), CD19(+ dim), FMC-7(+)

In Situ Hybridization

- t(14;18)(*IGH/BCL2*) only seen in ~ 30% of cases
  - More common in systemic (lymph node) follicular lymphoma
  - Usually in cases with CD10 and Bcl-2(+) immunohistochemistry
- *BCL2* break apart detected in a subset of cases
- 1p36 detected in rare cases

Genetic Testing

- Clonal *IGH* gene rearrangement in ~ 45% by PCR
- 10% p15 inactivation and 30% p16 inactivation by promoter hypermethylation
- Rare inactivation of *CDKN2A* and *CDKN2B*

Gene Expression Profiling

- Findings akin to germinal center-like large B-cell lymphoma
  - Often *REL* gene amplification

DIFFERENTIAL DIAGNOSIS

Primary Cutaneous Marginal Zone Lymphoma

- Malignancy of marginal zone cells (postgerminal center cells), and not malignant follicles
- Clinical differences
  - More often multifocal than PCFCL
  - Associated with *Borrelia burgdorferi* in some European studies
- Often monocytoid B cells ± plasmacytoid cells
- Germinal centers often small/reactive and not as larger/irregular-appearing as in PCFCL
  - Colonization of germinal centers by marginal zone lymphoma
- Immunohistochemistry
  - CD21 shows expanded follicular dendritic cell meshwork, contrary to tight follicular dendritic cell meshwork in PCFCL
  - More often Bcl-2(+) than PCFCL
  - Clusters of CD123(+) plasmacytoid cells
  - CD10(+)/Bcl-6(+) residual germinal centers
- > 95% 5-year survival

Reactive Lymphoid Hyperplasia (Cutaneous "Pseudolymphoma")

- Can be caused by drugs, arthropod bites, infections, or folliculitis, but often idiopathic
- Reactive follicles
  - Well defined with polarization
  - Tingible body macrophages present
  - Well-formed mantle zones
  - Often in superficial to middermis, not in deeper tissue
- Germinal centers CD10(+), Bcl-6(+), Bcl-2(-)
- Often mixed infiltrate, including histiocytes, eosinophils, and plasma cells
- Polyclonal plasma cells and no clonal *IGH* gene rearrangement
- Negative for t(14;18)

Secondary Skin Involvement by Systemic Follicular Lymphoma

- Similar morphology and phenotype to PCFCL
- Follicular lymphoma present in other anatomic site, such as lymph node or bone marrow
- CD10(+), Bcl-2(+), unlike many PCFCL cases
  - Secondary skin involvement by systemic follicular lymphoma is suspected when tumor cells express Bcl-2 protein, reflecting *BCL2* translocation
  - However, Bcl-2 expression may be difficult to assess because of numerous Bcl-2 reactive T cells
- t(14;18)(q32;q21) more common in secondary follicular lymphoma
  - Present in ~ 80-90% of secondary follicular lymphoma cases
- More commonly treated with chemotherapy than PCFCL
- Worse overall prognosis as compared to PCFCL

Primary Cutaneous Diffuse Large B-Cell Lymphoma, Leg Type

- Clinical differences

- Usually female, older median age, worse prognosis with only 50% 5-year survival
- More commonly treated with chemotherapy than PCFCL
- Usually on leg
  - Cases of PCFCL on leg have similar prognosis to primary cutaneous diffuse large B-cell lymphoma, leg type (PCDLBCL-LT)
- Morphology
  - Diffuse growth pattern, unlike PCFCL, which usually has follicular pattern
  - Large malignant B cells, unlike PCFCL, which has mix of large centroblasts and smaller centrocytes
  - Lacks meshwork of follicular dendritic cells, unlike PCFCL
- Immunohistochemistry
  - High expression of Bcl-2, but t(14;18) can be (-)
  - MUM1/IRF4 (+), FOXP1(+) in PCDLBCL-LT and MUM1/IRF4 (-), FOXP1(-) in PCFCL
  - More often expresses cytoplasmic staining for IgM, which may be an additional tool for differentiating this lymphoma from PCFCL in clinical practice
  - Rarely (+) for PD1, which is (-) in PCFCL
  - Deletions in 9p21.3 may lead to deletions of *CDKN2A* and *CDKN2B*

Primary Cutaneous Diffuse Large B-Cell Lymphoma, Not Otherwise Specified

- Needs to be differentiated from PCFCL with diffuse growth pattern and large cells
  - Diagnose as PCFCL if there is at least partial nodular architecture or if there are fewer centroblasts
  - Diagnose as primary cutaneous diffuse large B-cell lymphoma (PCDLBCL) if there are all large cells and only diffuse growth pattern
- Bcl-2(+/-), Bcl-6(+/-)
- Need to exclude PCDLBCL-LT
- Need to exclude systemic DLBCL

Small Lymphocytic Lymphoma/Chronic Lymphocytic Leukemia

- Common peripheral blood involvement, unlike follicular lymphoma
- Mostly diffuse architecture
- Pseudofollicles identified
- Different immunophenotype: CD23(+), CD5(+), CD10(-), Bcl-6(-)
- t(14;18) negative

B-Cell Lymphoblastic Lymphoma

- Lymphoblasts with sparse cytoplasm, finely stippled chromatin, and inconspicuous nucleoli
- TdT(+), variably CD34(+), CD19(+), CD10(+), variable CD20

Mantle Cell Lymphoma

- Only very rarely involves skin, usually in patients with known history of mantle cell lymphoma
- Bcl-1/cyclin-D1(+) (nuclear), CD5(+), which are (-) in PCFCL and primary cutaneous marginal zone lymphoma
- CD10(-), Bcl-6(-)
- t(11;14)(+)

DIAGNOSTIC CHECKLIST

Pathologic Interpretation Pearls

- Nodules to sheet-like collections of B cells, back-to-back, lacking tingible body macrophages, showing attenuated mantle zones
- Similar features to systemic follicle center lymphoma, but often lacks Bcl-2 staining and t(14;18)
- Must exclude primary cutaneous diffuse large B-cell lymphoma, leg type, which has worse prognosis and expresses MUM1/IRF4 and Bcl-2

SELECTED REFERENCES

1. Akhtari M et al: Primary cutaneous B-cell lymphoma (non-leg type) has excellent outcomes even after very low dose radiation as single-modality therapy. Leuk Lymphoma. 57(1):34-8, 2016
2. O'Suoji C et al: Rare pediatric non-Hodgkin lymphomas: a report from Children's Oncology Group Study ANHL 04B1. Pediatr Blood Cancer. 63(5):794-800, 2016
3. Szablewski V et al: Primary cutaneous follicle center lymphomas expressing BCL2 protein frequently harbor BCL2 gene break and may present 1p36 deletion: a study of 20 cases. Am J Surg Pathol. 40(1):127-36, 2016
4. Haverkos B et al: Primary cutaneous B-cell lymphoma: management and patterns of recurrence at the multimodality cutaneous lymphoma clinic of The Ohio State University. Oncologist. 20(10):1161-6, 2015
5. Lima M: Cutaneous primary B-cell lymphomas: from diagnosis to treatment. An Bras Dermatol. 90(5):687-706, 2015
6. Palacios-Álvarez I et al: Cutaneous annular lesions as the first sign of transformation of follicular lymphoma into diffuse large B-cell lymphoma. Indian J Dermatol Venereol Leprol. 81(5):495-7, 2015
7. Pinter-Brown LC: Diagnosis and management of cutaneous B-cell lymphoma. Dermatol Clin. 33(4):835-40, 2015
8. Subramaniyam S et al: Primary cutaneous follicle center lymphoma associated with an extracutaneous dissemination: a cytogenetic finding of potential prognostic value. Am J Clin Pathol. 144(5):805-10, 2015
9. Sutton AM et al: Clinical practice guidelines for cutaneous lymphomas. Mo Med. 112(4):292-5, 2015
10. Wilcox RA: Cutaneous B-cell lymphomas: 2015 update on diagnosis, risk-stratification, and management. Am J Hematol. 90(1):73-6, 2015
11. Kempf W et al: Cutaneous lymphomas: an update. Part 2: B-cell lymphomas and related conditions. Am J Dermatopathol. 36(3):197-208; quiz 209-10, 2014
12. Marie D et al: Primary cutaneous follicle center lymphoma with Hodgkin and Reed-Sternberg-like cells: a new histopathologic variant. J Cutan Pathol. 41(10):797-801, 2014
13. Çetinözman F et al: Programmed death-1 expression in cutaneous B-cell lymphoma. J Cutan Pathol. 41(1):14-21, 2014
14. Koens L et al: MicroRNA profiling of primary cutaneous large B-cell lymphomas. PLoS One. 8(12):e82471, 2013
15. Swerdlow SH et al: Cutaneous B-cell lymphoproliferative disorders: report of the 2011 Society for Hematopathology/European Association for Haematopathology workshop. Am J Clin Pathol. 139(4):515-35, 2013
16. Sokol L et al: Primary cutaneous B-cell lymphomas: recent advances in diagnosis and management. Cancer Control. 19(3):236-44, 2012
17. Massone C et al: Miliary and agminated-type primary cutaneous follicle center lymphoma: report of 18 cases. J Am Acad Dermatol. 65(4):749-55, 2011
18. Senff NJ et al: Reclassification of 300 primary cutaneous B-Cell lymphomas according to the new WHO-EORTC classification for cutaneous lymphomas: comparison with previous classifications and identification of prognostic markers. J Clin Oncol. 25(12):1581-7, 2007
19. Zinzani PL et al: Prognostic factors in primary cutaneous B-cell lymphoma: the Italian Study Group for Cutaneous Lymphomas. J Clin Oncol. 24(9):1376-82, 2006
20. Hoefnagel JJ et al: Distinct types of primary cutaneous large B-cell lymphoma identified by gene expression profiling. Blood. 105(9):3671-8, 2005
21. Kim BK et al: Clinicopathologic, immunophenotypic, and molecular cytogenetic fluorescence in situ hybridization analysis of primary and secondary cutaneous follicular lymphomas. Am J Surg Pathol. 29(1):69-82, 2005
22. Willemze R et al: WHO-EORTC classification for cutaneous lymphomas. Blood. 105(10):3768-85, 2005

(Left) *PCFCL displays a dense, multinodular-appearing lymphocytic infiltrate in the dermis, sparing the subepidermal layer (grenz zone ➡). The neoplasm exhibits a few ill-defined follicles ➡. (Courtesy R. Miranda, MD.)* **(Right)** *This example of PCFCL shows a mostly diffuse growth pattern ➡, with only a few vaguely follicular-appearing areas ➡.*

Primary Cutaneous Follicle Center Lymphoma at Low Magnification

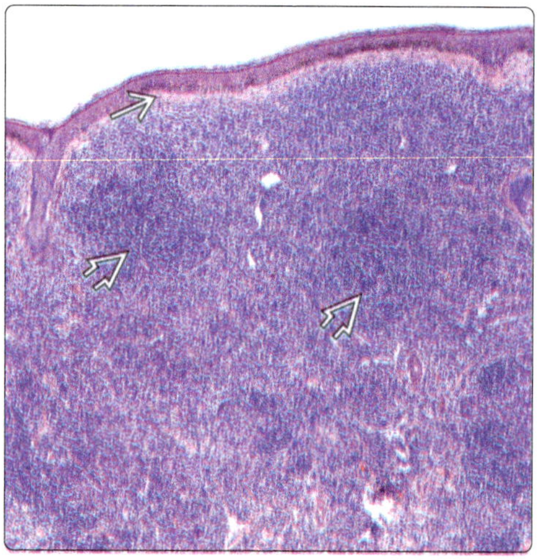

Primary Cutaneous Follicle Center Lymphoma Diffuse Pattern

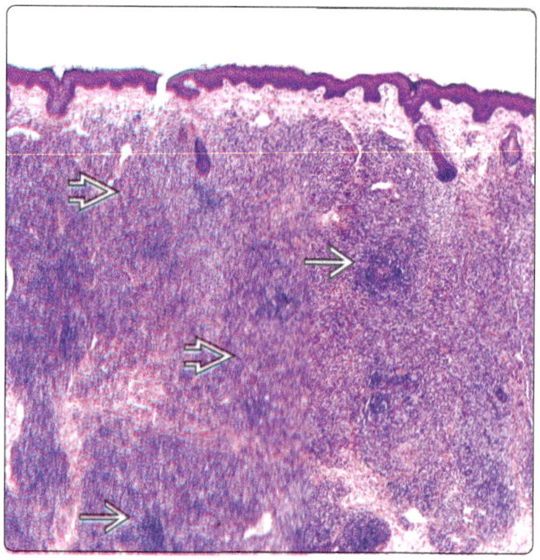

(Left) *In most cases of PCFCL, there is a mixture of small cleaved centrocytes ➡ and larger centroblasts. Centroblasts ➡ are bigger cells and usually have 1 or more nucleoli near the edge of the nuclear membrane.* **(Right)** *Within the follicles of a PCFCL, there is loss of the normal tingible body macrophages that are typically seen in reactive follicles.*

Mixture of Centrocytes and Centroblasts

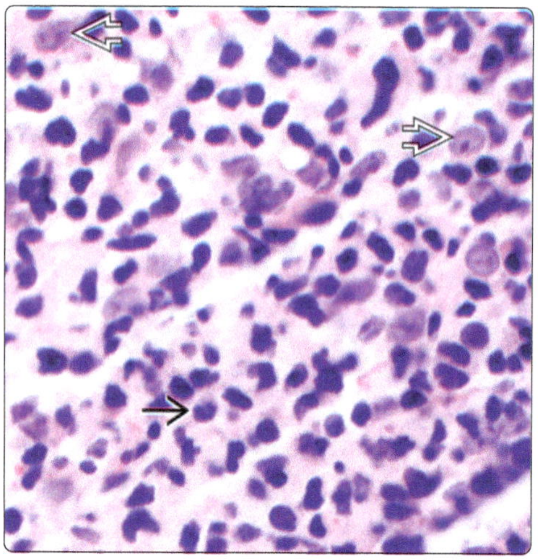

Primary Cutaneous Follicle Center Lymphoma, High Magnification

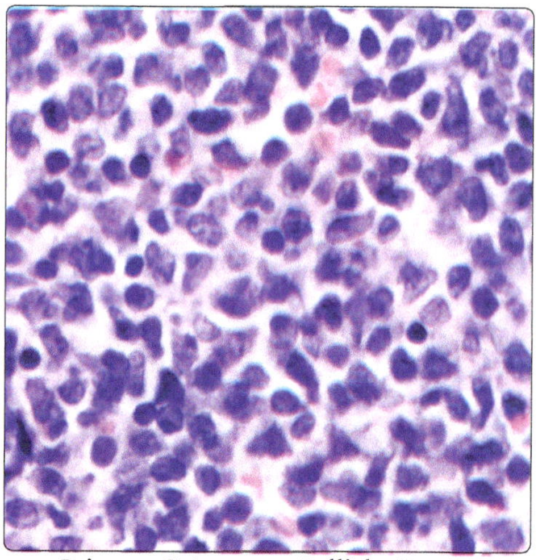

(Left) *This is a PCFCL with a diffuse pattern, composed of sheets of markedly enlarged and atypical-appearing cells, many of which have large nucleoli ➡.* **(Right)** *This diffuse type PCFCL is composed of sheets of markedly enlarged and atypical-appearing cells with large nucleoli. Although histologically very concerning, such cases show similar clinical behavior to nodular type PCFCL.*

Primary Cutaneous Follicle Center Lymphoma Diffuse Pattern, High Power

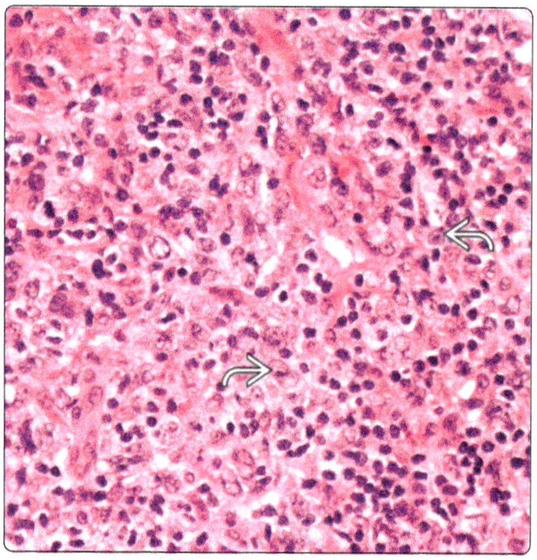

Primary Cutaneous Follicle Center Lymphoma, Diffuse Pattern, With Marked Atypia

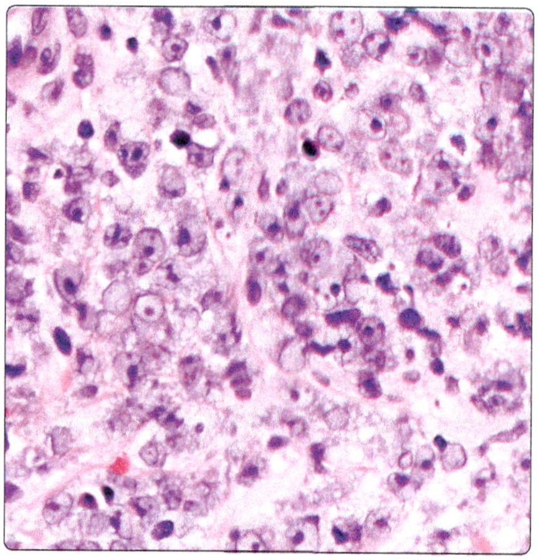

CD20 Immunohistochemistry in Primary Cutaneous Follicle Center Lymphoma

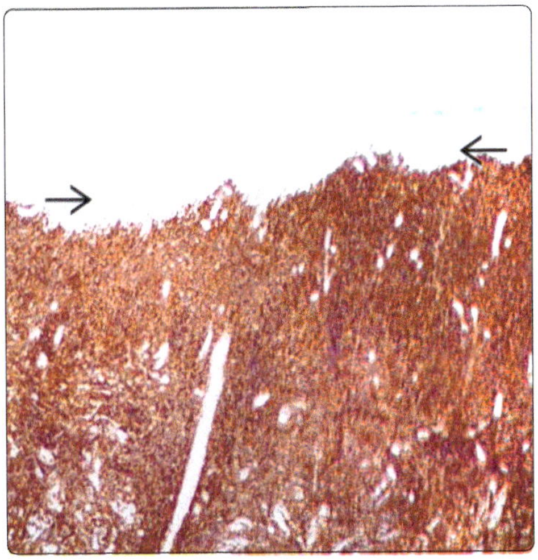

CD20 in Another Case of Primary Cutaneous Follicle Center Lymphoma

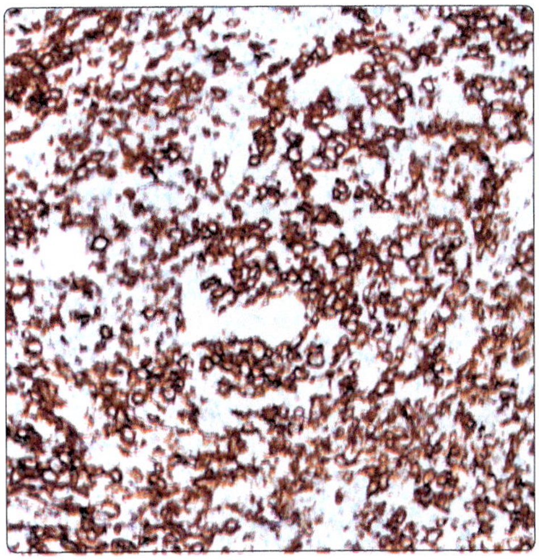

(Left) *CD20 is strongly expressed in the B cells throughout the dermal infiltrate. Note that the epidermis is uninvolved, with a grenz zone separating the infiltrate from the epidermis* ⇨. *Other B-cell markers, such as CD79a and pax-5 (not shown), are also immunoreactive in the malignant cells.* **(Right)** *Higher magnification in another case shows that CD20 is very strongly expressed in the B cells throughout the dermal infiltrate.*

Bcl-6 Immunohistochemistry in Primary Cutaneous Follicle Center Lymphoma

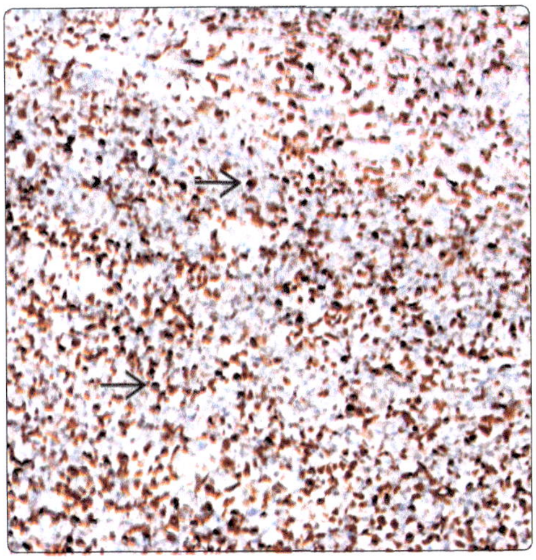

Bcl-2 Immunohistochemistry in Primary Cutaneous Follicle Center Lymphoma

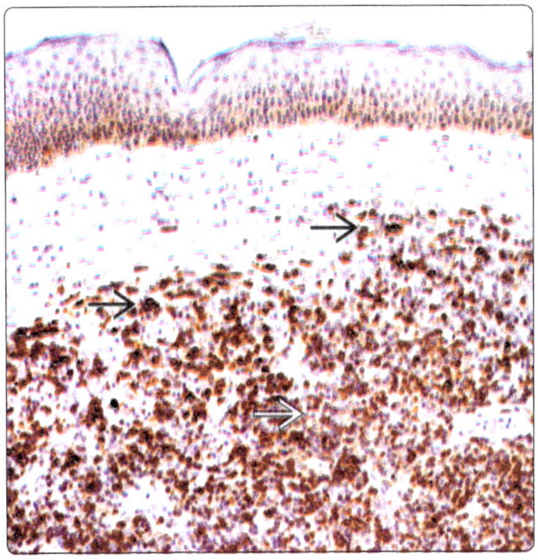

(Left) *Bcl-6 is positive in the vast majority of cases of PCFCL. The neoplastic lymphocytes express Bcl-6 even in diffuse areas, as is shown here, with strong and diffuse nuclear staining* ⇨. **(Right)** *Bcl-2 can be positive or negative in the neoplastic cells in PCFCL. In this case, there is weak to moderate Bcl-2 staining in the tumor cells* ➡, *with stronger staining of background T cells* ⇨. *Bcl-2 tends to be positive in follicular areas but negative in diffuse areas. (Courtesy R. Miranda, MD.)*

CD10 Negativity in Diffuse Type Primary Cutaneous Follicle Center Lymphoma

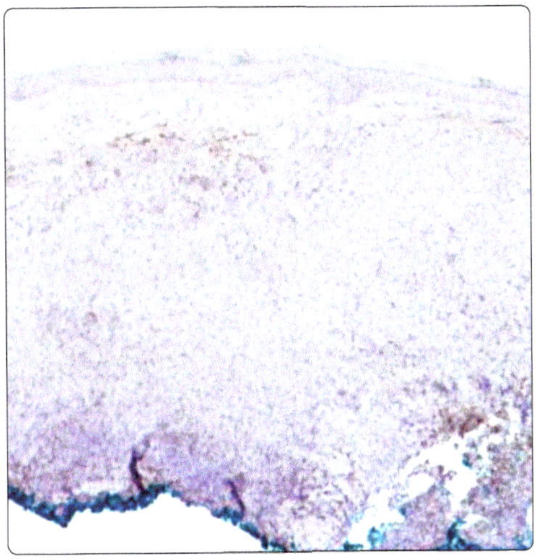

CD10 Positivity in Nodular Type Primary Cutaneous Follicle Center Lymphoma

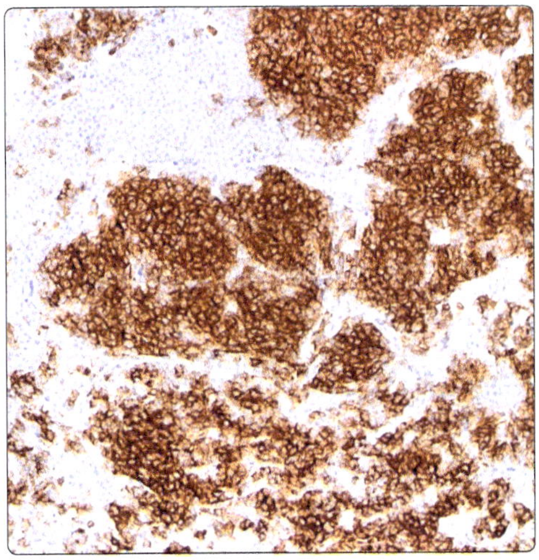

(Left) *This case of PCFCL is negative for CD10 in the neoplastic cells. CD10 is often negative in the diffuse areas of PCFCL, whereas it is more commonly positive in the follicular/nodular areas.* **(Right)** *Anti-CD10 strongly highlights the follicular pattern in this nodular PCFCL case. CD10 is usually reactive in PCFCL with a follicular pattern and tends to be negative in diffuse areas. (Courtesy R. Miranda, MD.)*

KEY FACTS

TERMINOLOGY

- Primary cutaneous diffuse large B-cell lymphoma (DLBCL) composed exclusively of large transformed cells

CLINICAL ISSUES

- 20% of primary cutaneous B-cell lymphomas
- Most cases arise in skin of lower leg(s)
  - ~ 85% of all cases
- Subset of cases arise in skin of other sites (trunk, arms, head and neck)
  - ~ 15% of cases
- Single or multiple lesions at time of presentation
- Relapse is common; 50% 5-year survival
- Treated with systemic chemotherapy plus rituximab

MICROSCOPIC

- Diffuse pattern of involvement in dermis
- Monotonous sheets of large, atypical-appearing immunoblasts or centroblasts
- Few small reactive T cells in background
- No centrocytes (or small B cells) present
- No epidermotropism

ANCILLARY TESTS

- Pan-B-cell antigens (+), Bcl-2(+), Bcl-6(+)
- MUM1(+), FOXP1(+), IgM(+), CD10(-)
- FISH often shows rearrangements of *MYC*, *BCL6*, or *IGH* genes
- Monoclonal *IGH* gene rearrangements

TOP DIFFERENTIAL DIAGNOSES

- Primary cutaneous follicle center lymphoma (PCFCL)
  - PCFCL cases with diffuse pattern and predominance of large centrocytes or centroblasts are challenging
  - CD10(+), Bcl-6(+); Bcl-2 often (-); if positive, often weak and focal
- Systemic DLBCL involving skin
- EBV(+) DLBCL of elderly

Morphologic Features of PCDLBCL-LT

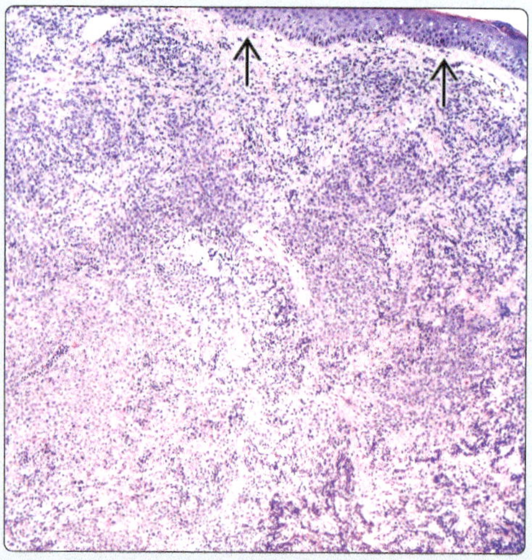

Morphologic Features of PCDLBCL-LT

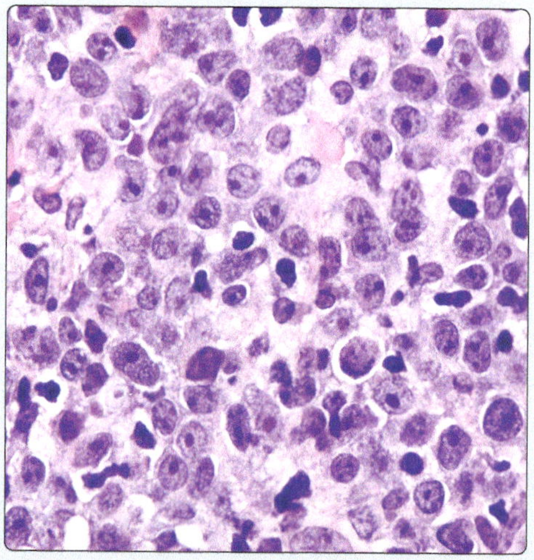

(Left) *Primary cutaneous diffuse large B-cell lymphoma, leg type (PCDLBCL-LT) shows a diffuse infiltrate replacing the dermis with sparing of the epidermis* ➡. **(Right)** *The lymphoma cells in PCDLBCL-LT are large and strikingly round with centrally located nucleoli (immunoblasts).*

CD20 IHC in PCDLBCL-LT

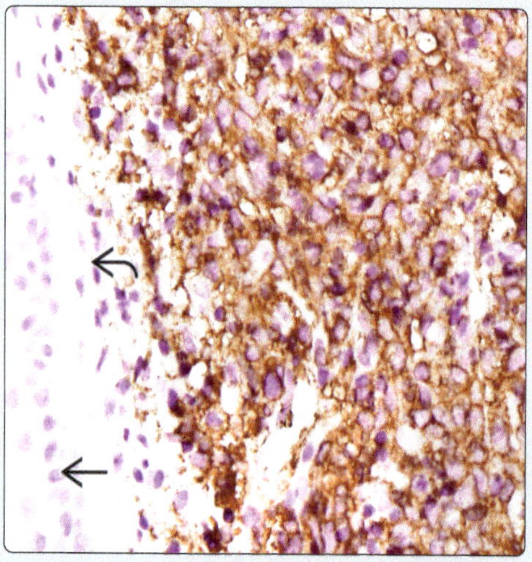

Bcl-2 Staining in PCDLBCL-LT

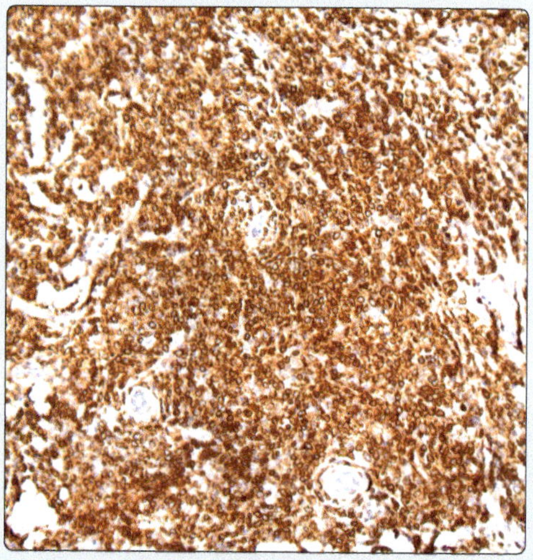

(Left) *In this case of PCDLBCL-LT, the lymphoma cells are strongly CD20(+) and form cohesive-appearing sheets. The epidermis* ➡ *is not involved, and a thin grenz zone is present* ↩. **(Right)** *Most cases of PCDLBCL-LT are strongly and diffusely Bcl-2(+), as shown in this case.*

TERMINOLOGY

Abbreviations

- Primary cutaneous diffuse large B-cell lymphoma, leg type (PCDLBCL-LT)

Synonyms

- Primary cutaneous large B-cell lymphoma, leg type
- Primary cutaneous diffuse large B-cell lymphoma

Definitions

- Primary cutaneous diffuse large B-cell lymphoma composed exclusively of large transformed B cells
  - Often occurs in lower leg(s) but can arise at other sites

ETIOLOGY/PATHOGENESIS

Cell of Origin

- Peripheral B cell of postgerminal center cell origin
  - Immunophenotype: IRF-4/MUM1(+), FOXP1(+)
  - High frequency of somatic mutations of *IGH* variable (V)-region genes

Possible Role of Antigen Selection

- Preferential use of certain *IGH* (IGHV) gene segments
  - Suggests that antigen stimulation may be involved in pathogenesis

Role of Molecular Abnormalities

- Number of genetic rearrangements and deletions reported
- No abnormality consistently present

CLINICAL ISSUES

Epidemiology

- Incidence
  - Rare
    - 4% of all cutaneous lymphomas
    - 20% of primary cutaneous B-cell lymphomas
- Age
  - Elderly patients; median age: 7th decade
- Sex
  - More common in women
    - M:F ratio: 1:1.6; as high as 1:4 in some studies

Site

- Most cases arise in skin of lower leg(s): 1 or both legs may be involved
  - ~ 85% of all cases
- Subset of cases arise in skin of other sites (trunk, arms, head and neck)
  - ~ 15% of cases
  - Similar morphologic and immunophenotypic characteristics
- Single or multiple lesions at time of presentation
  - Some patients have dissemination at initial diagnosis

Presentation

- Red or blue-red cutaneous lesions
  - Plaque, verrucous plaques, or deep plaques
  - Nodular, tumoral lesions
  - Often associated with ulceration
  - Multiple lesions are common
- B symptoms in 10-20% of patients

Treatment

- Anthracycline-containing systemic chemotherapy plus rituximab
- Radiotherapy has role for localized lesions in elderly patients

Prognosis

- Relapse is common
- 40-50% 5-year survival rate
  - Factors adversely correlated with prognosis
    - Older age
    - Multiple lesions at presentation
    - Inactivation of *CDKN2A*
  - Factors not correlated with prognosis
    - Duration of lesions before diagnosis
    - Gender, B symptoms, performance status, or serum lactate dehydrogenase level
    - Bcl-2 or IRF-4/MUM1 expression

MICROSCOPIC

Histologic Features

- Diffuse pattern of involvement of dermis
  - Infiltrate can be deep, often extending into superficial subcutaneous adipose tissue
- Cohesive, monotonous sheets of atypical-appearing large cells
  - Centroblasts or immunoblasts
  - Often very round nuclei; can also be oval
- Mitotic figures numerous
- Few small reactive T cells in background
- No centrocytes (or small B cells) present
- No epidermotropism

ANCILLARY TESTS

Immunohistochemistry

- Pan-B-cell antigens (+)
- Cytoplasmic IgM(+), IgD(+/-)
- Bcl-2(+), IRF-4/MUM1(+), FOXP1(+)
- Bcl-6(+), CD10(-)
- No follicular dendritic cell (FDC) meshworks
  - CD21(-), CD23(-), CD35(-)
- T-cell antigens (-), LMP1(-), HHV8(-)

In Situ Hybridization

- FISH often shows rearrangements of *MYC*, *BCL6*, or *IGH* genes
  - No evidence of *IGH-BCL2*/t(14;18) or *BCL2* rearrangements
- EBER(-)

Genetic Testing

- Monoclonal *IGH* gene rearrangements
- No evidence of *IGH-BCL2*/t(14;18)

Array Comparative Genomic Hybridization

- Amplification of 18q21.31-33 involving *BCL2* and *MALT1* genes

Gene Expression Profiling

- Profile is consistent with activated B-cell phenotype

DIFFERENTIAL DIAGNOSIS

Primary Cutaneous Follicle Center Cell Lymphoma

- Most primary cutaneous follicle center cell lymphoma (PCFCL) have follicular pattern and can therefore be distinguished from PCDLBCL-LT
- PCFCL cases with diffuse pattern and predominance of large centrocytes or centroblasts are challenging
  - Used to be designated as diffuse large B-cell lymphoma (DLBCL)
    - However, clinically they are confined to skin, and prognosis is good
    - Could lead to over-treatment with multiagent chemotherapy
- Sites of skin involvement
  - Mostly in head and neck, trunk, back, arms
  - Some cases of PCFCL can present on leg
    - Patients with PCFCL on leg often have worse prognosis than patients with PCFCL at other sites
    - Prognosis of PCFCL of leg is similar to, or slightly better than, PCDLBCL-LT
- Histologic features of PCFCL
  - Areas of follicular pattern can be predominant, focal, or absent
  - Often, perivascular &/or periadnexal pattern in dermis is present
  - Mixture of centrocytes and centroblasts
    - Cells can be polylobated or spindle-shaped
  - Stromal reaction with fibrosis and sclerosis is common
- Immunophenotype
  - CD10(+), Bcl-6(+); Bcl-2 often (-); if positive, often weak and focal
  - FDC meshwork is present
    - CD21, CD23, CD35, or other markers
  - IRF-4/MUM1(-), FOXP1(-)
  - Small B cells/centrocytes (+) (absent in PCDLBCL-LT)
  - CD3(+) reactive T cells relatively numerous (compared with PCDLBCL-LT)
  - Cases of PCFCL with diffuse pattern
    - CD10 often (-) in areas of diffuse pattern
    - Residual FDC meshwork usually can be identified

Systemic DLBCL Involving Skin

- Can be difficult to distinguish from PCDLBCL-LT based on morphology and immunophenotype
- Clinical history of systemic disease is key for differential diagnosis
- If patient has systemic and skin involvement at time of initial presentation
  - Can be difficult to distinguish systemic DLBCL from PCDLBCL-LT
  - Large tumors on lower leg(s) support PCDLBCL-LT

Plasmablastic Lymphoma Involving Skin

- Most patients have high-stage disease at time of presentation
  - Mucosal involvement is common
- Any skin site can be involved; leg uncommon
- Histologic features
  - Cohesive sheets of monomorphic plasmablasts can closely mimic PCDLBCL-LT
  - Some cases may show plasmacytic differentiation
- Immunophenotype
  - CD138(+), CD38(+)
  - Cytoplasmic monotypic Ig light chain (+)
  - EBER(+)

EBV(+) Diffuse Large B-Cell Lymphoma of Elderly

- Cutaneous involvement can be initial presentation
- Histologic features
  - Tumor cells are often more polymorphic than PCDLBCL-LT
    - Plasmacytoid or plasmacytic differentiation (+)
    - Large transformed cells, Reed-Sternberg-like cells
    - Background often has small lymphocytes, neutrophils, plasma cells, and histiocytes
  - Necrosis is common
- Immunophenotype is similar to PCDLBCL-LT; EBER(+)

Monomorphic Posttransplant Lymphoproliferative Disorder

- Monomorphic monomorphic posttransplant lymphoproliferative disorder can involve skin
- Histologic features
  - Tumor cells are often more polymorphic than PCDLBCL-LT
    - Plasmacytoid or plasmacytic differentiation (+)
    - Large transformed cells, Reed-Sternberg-like cells
  - Necrosis is common, often with geographic pattern
- Immunophenotype is similar to PCDLBCL-LT; EBER(+)
- Clinical history of organ transplantation

DIAGNOSTIC CHECKLIST

Clinically Relevant Pathologic Features

- PCDLBCL-LT usually involves lower leg(s); can present at other sites
  - Leg location is adverse prognostic factor

Pathologic Interpretation Pearls

- Diffuse involvement of dermis by sheets of round immunoblasts or centroblasts
  - Very few or absent small B cells
  - Relatively few reactive T cells (compared with PCFCL)
- Immunophenotype
  - Bcl-2(+), Bcl-6(+), MUM1(+), FOXP1(+), IgM(+)

SELECTED REFERENCES

1. Demirkesen C et al: The expression of IgM is helpful in the differentiation of primary cutaneous diffuse large B cell lymphoma and follicle center lymphoma. Leuk Res. 35(9):1269-72, 2011
2. Guyot A et al: Combined treatment with rituximab and anthracycline-containing chemotherapy for primary cutaneous large B-cell lymphomas, leg type, in elderly patients. Arch Dermatol. 146(1):89-91, 2010
3. Grange F et al: Primary cutaneous diffuse large B-cell lymphoma, leg type: clinicopathologic features and prognostic analysis in 60 cases. Arch Dermatol. 143(9):1144-50, 2007
4. Senff NJ et al: Reclassification of 300 primary cutaneous B-Cell lymphomas according to the new WHO-EORTC classification for cutaneous lymphomas: comparison with previous classifications and identification of prognostic markers. J Clin Oncol. 25(12):1581-7, 2007

Comparison of PCDLBCL-LT With PCFCL With Diffuse Pattern and Increased Large Cells

Parameter	PCDLBCL-LT	PCFCL With Diffuse Pattern and Increased Large Cells
Demographic Information		
Age	Older, 7th decade	6th decade
Gender	Female preponderance	Slight male preponderance
Sites of Involvement		
Location	Leg, 1 or both	Head and neck most frequent, followed by trunk or arms
	15% involving other sites, e.g., trunk, arm, head and neck	Rarely on leg, which has worse prognosis than PCFCL on other sites
	Multiple lesions common, some with deep plaques	Multiple sites of involvement are common
Risk for developing extracutaneous disease	~ 50%	~ 10%
Disseminated	~ 30%	~ 10%
Morphologic Features		
	Cohesive sheets of centroblasts or immunoblasts	Diffuse growth pattern with predominance of large centrocytes or centroblasts
	Cells often have strikingly round nuclei with many mitoses	Often cleaved, polylobated, irregular, or spindle-shaped
	No centrocytes (or small B cells) present	Often have admixed small centrocytes
Small reactive T cells	Very few, often in perivascular areas	Less pronounced but more than PCDLBCL-LT
Epidermotropism	Not present	Not present
Perivascular/periadnexal	Not present	Often
Follicular dendritic cell (FDC) meshwork	Not present	Small broken clusters of FDC may be present
Immunohistochemistry		
Bcl-6	Mostly positive	Positive
Bcl-2	Positive ~ 90%	Often negative; if positive, often weak or focal
CD10	Negative	Often negative in diffuse areas; often positive in follicular areas
MUM1	Positive, 50-80%	Negative
FOXP1	Positive	Negative
IgM &/or IgD	Positive	Negative
Molecular Genetics		
	Similar to systemic DLBCL	Different from nodal follicular lymphoma
MYC, *BCL6*, and *IGH* rearrangement by FISH	Can be present	Often absent
Amplification of *BCL2* and *MALT1* genes	Can be present	Absent
Deletions of chromosome 9p21.3 (containing *CDKN2a* and *CDKN2b*)	Reported in 67% of cases	Absent
t(14;18)(q32;q21)	Absent	Reported in 10-40% of cases
Treatment		
	Anthracycline-containing chemotherapy plus rituximab	If single lesion, radiation therapy or surgical excision
	Radiation therapy for localized lesion in elderly	If multiple lesions, systemic chemotherapy may be used
Prognosis		
Relapse	Yes, frequent	Yes, ~ 30% of patients
5-year survival rate	50%	85-100%

(Left) *This case of PCDLBCL-LT almost completely fills the dermis. The neoplasm has a diffuse pattern with a grenz zone → between the neoplasm and the uninvolved epidermis.* **(Right)** *PCDLBCL-LT often appears confluent at low-power magnification. Small reactive T cells can be seen in 1 corner ↪ of the field, but relatively few are admixed with the lymphoma cells.*

Morphologic Features of PCDLBCL-LT

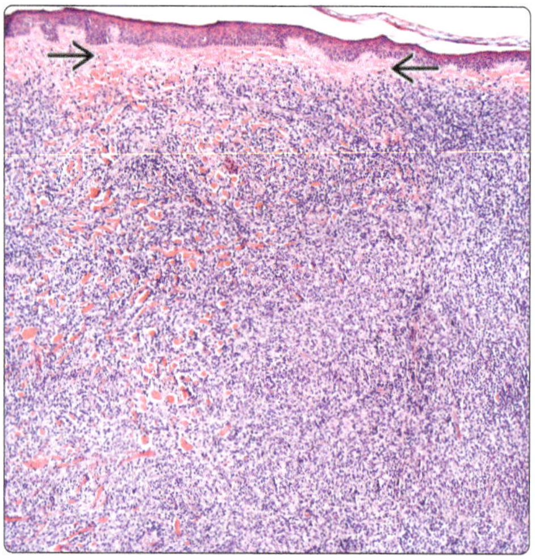

Morphologic Features of PCDLBCL-LT

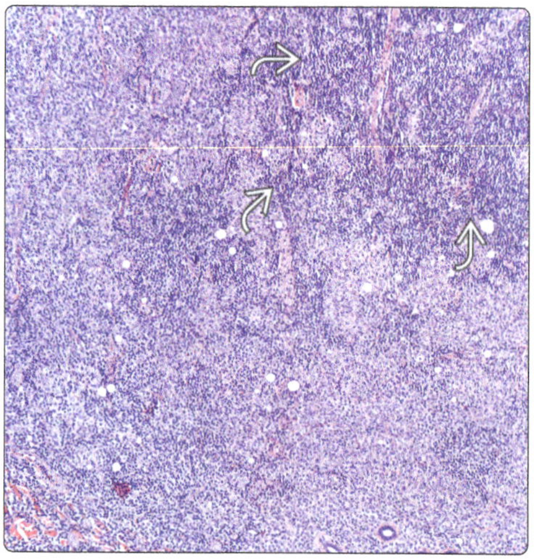

(Left) *In PCDLBCL-LT, the lymphoma cells often have a strikingly round cell morphology and grow in sheets that appear cohesive. The cells surround a central vessel in this field.* **(Right)** *In this case of PCDLBCL-LT, the lymphoma cells are centroblasts that appear very similar to each other, imparting a monotonous appearance.*

Morphologic Features of PCDLBCL-LT

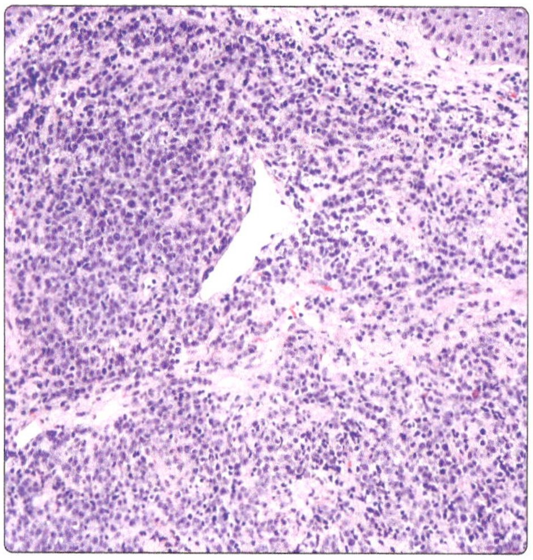

Morphologic Features of PCDLBCL-LT

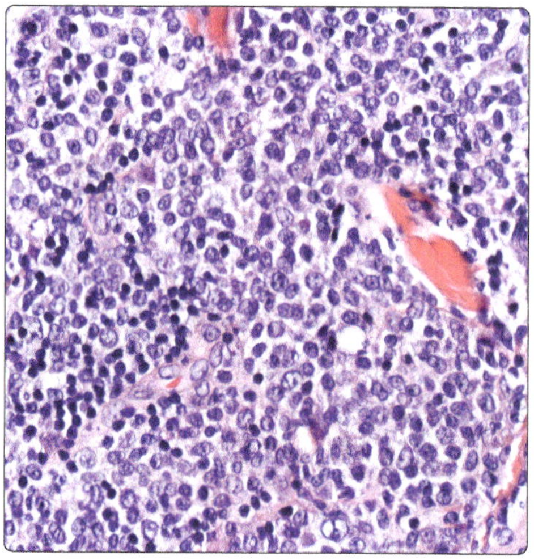

(Left) *CD20 is strongly expressed in this case of PCDLBCL-LT. The lymphoma cells form cohesive-appearing sheets.* **(Right)** *Strong Bcl-2 expression is observed in this case of PCDLBCL-LT. Bcl-2 expression is observed in most cases.*

CD20 Positivity in PCDLBCL-LT

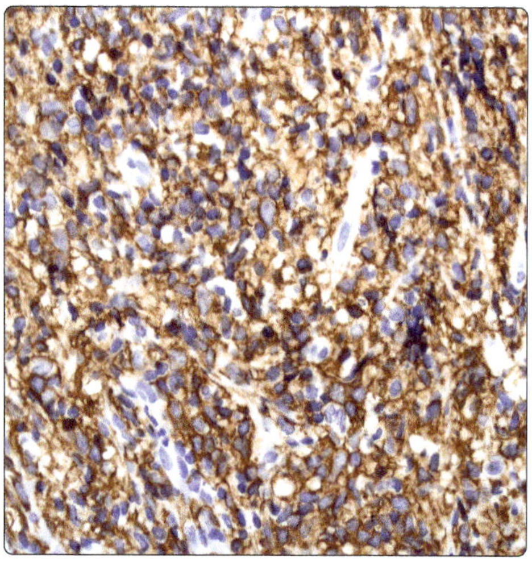

Strong Bcl-2 Staining in PCDLBCL-LT

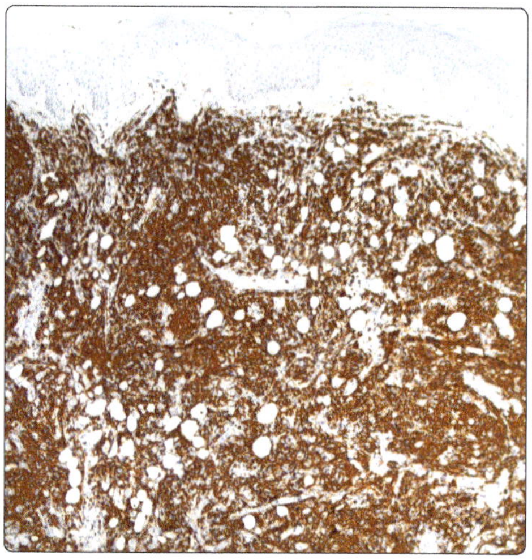

CD10 Staining in PCDLBCL-LT

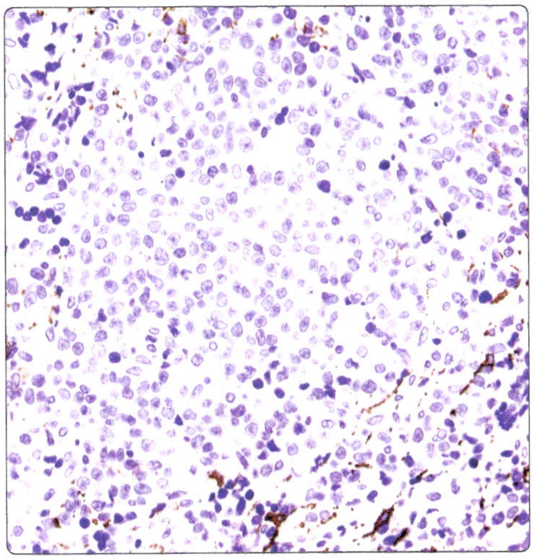

Bcl-6 Staining in PCDLBCL-LT

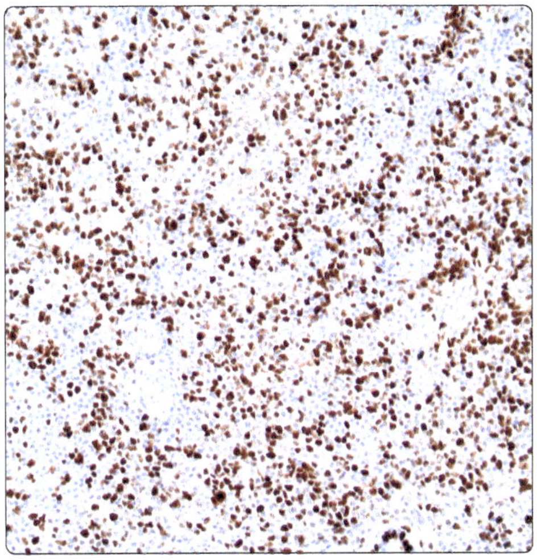

(Left) *In PCDLBCL-LT, the lymphoma cells are usually CD10(-), consistent with a postgerminal center origin of lymphoma cells.* **(Right)** *In PCDLBCL-LT, the lymphoma cells are often at least partially Bcl-6(+).*

IRF-4/MUM1 Staining in PCDLBCL-LT

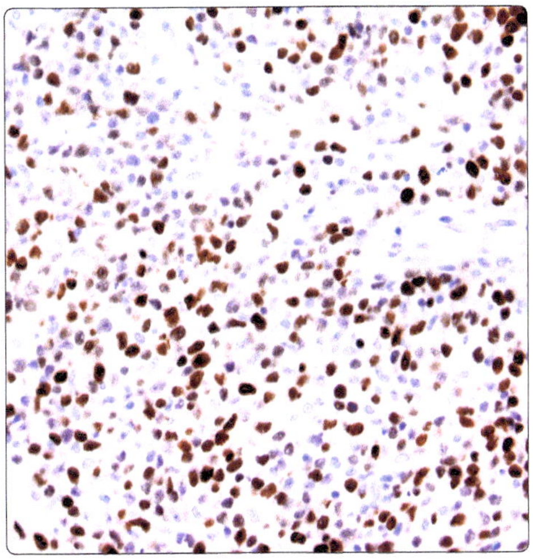

Ki-67 Staining in PCDLBCL-LT

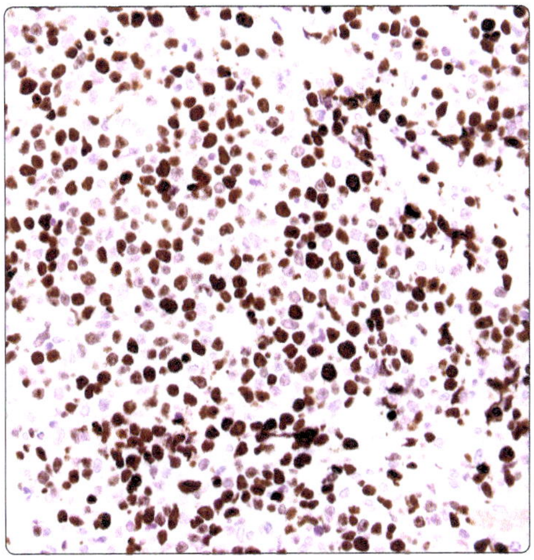

(Left) *Approximately 50-80% of cases of PCDLBCL-LT are IRF-4/MUM1(+), a marker associated with more aggressive lymphomas and indicating a postgerminal center origin.* **(Right)** *In PCDLBCL-LT, Ki-67 shows a high proliferation fraction in the lymphoid cells.*

CD23 Staining in PCDLBCL-LT

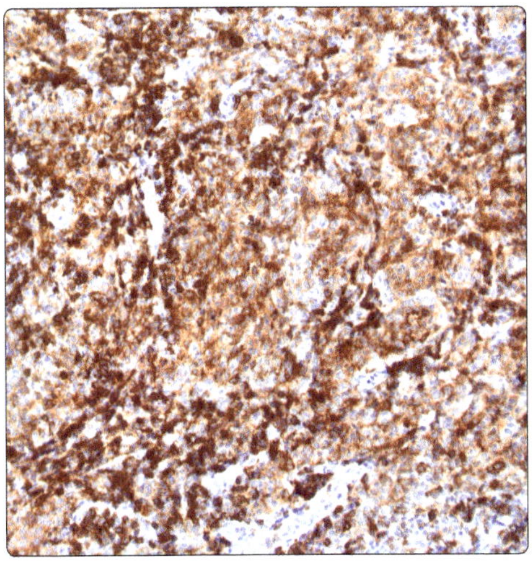

CD21 Staining in PCDLBCL-LT

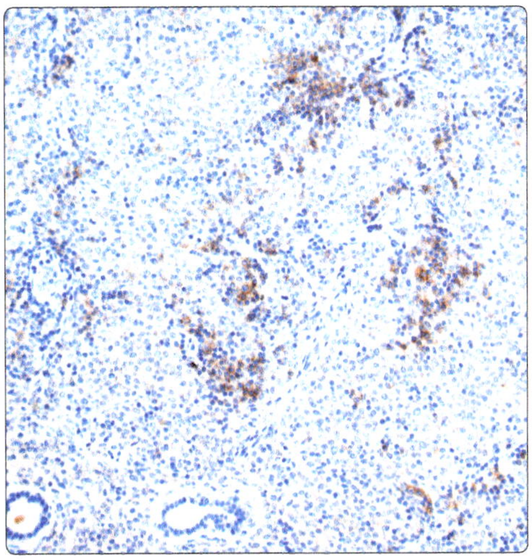

(Left) *This case of PCDLBCL-LT is strongly CD23(+). A subset of these tumors are CD23(+), unlike primary cutaneous follicle center lymphoma (PCFCL). Also note that no CD23(+) follicular dendritic cells are present, confirming the presence of a diffuse growth pattern.* **(Right)** *In this case of PCDLBCL-LT, a CD21 immunostain does not highlight any follicular dendritic cells, supporting a diffuse growth pattern. A small subset of lymphoma cells are CD21(+) in this field.*

(Left) *PCFCL with a diffuse pattern is shown. As with PCDLBCL-LT, the lymphoma cells spare the epidermis, leaving a grenz zone* ⇨*.* **(Right)** *This case of PCFCL also shows a predominance of large cells. In contrast with PCDLBCL-LT, the tumor cells are cleaved, polylobated, irregular, spindle-shaped (large centrocytes and centroblasts), and admixed with many small lymphocytes.*

Differential Diagnosis: Primary Cutaneous Follicular Center Lymphoma

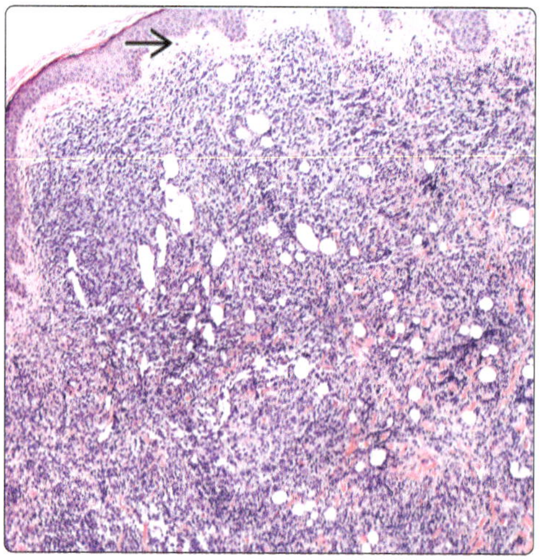

Differential Diagnosis: Primary Cutaneous Follicular Center Lymphoma

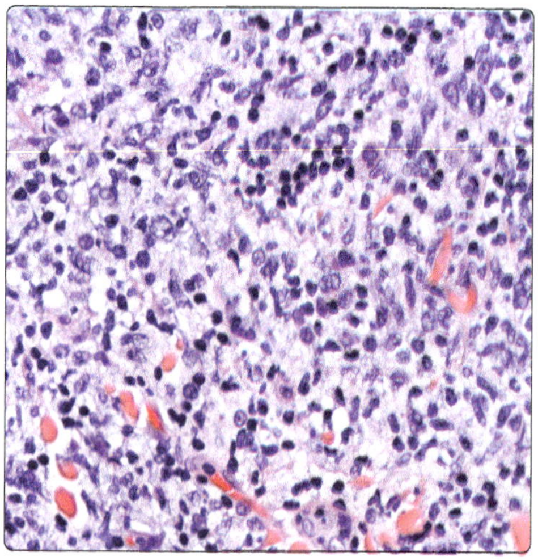

(Left) *PCFCL with a predominance of large cells is shown. The infiltrate appears to be noncohesive and is associated with a fibrotic stromal reaction, unlike cases of PCDLBCL-LT.* **(Right)** *PCFCL often shows vascular invasion or has a perivascular pattern of infiltration. These features are uncommon in PCDLBCL-LT.*

Differential Diagnosis: Primary Cutaneous Follicular Center Lymphoma

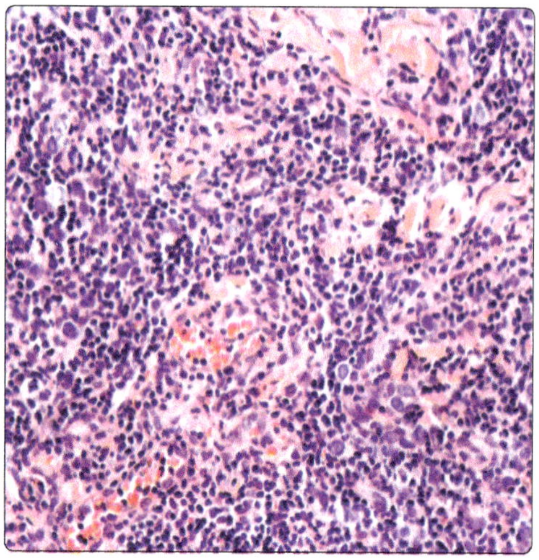

Differential Diagnosis: Primary Cutaneous Follicular Center Lymphoma

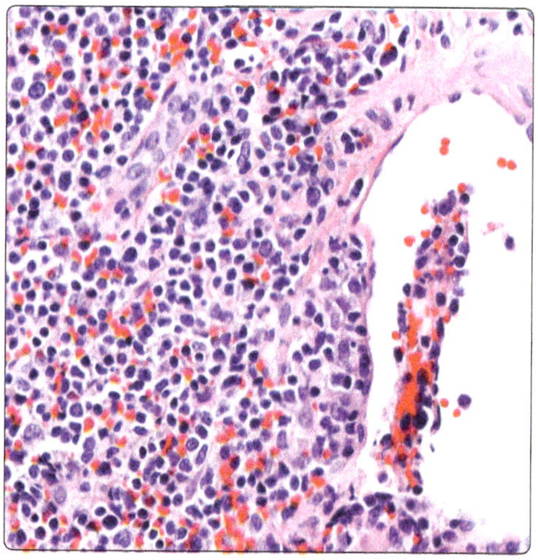

(Left) *This case of PCFCL with a diffuse pattern was CD10(-). It should be remembered that CD10 is commonly expressed in follicular areas but is often negative in diffuse areas of PCFCL.* **(Right)** *Many cases of PCFCL are negative for Bcl-2. In some cases of PCFCL, the lymphoma cells can be Bcl-2(+), but expression is often weak or present in only a subset of cells* ➡*, as shown in this field. Small reactive T cells are strongly Bcl-2(+).*

CD10 Staining in PCFCL

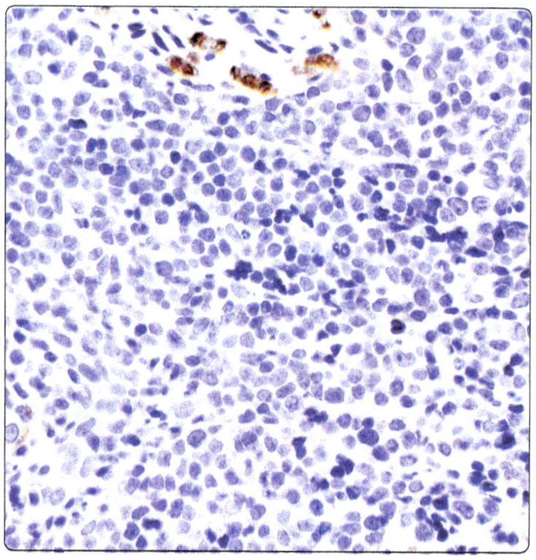

Bcl-2 Staining in PCFCL

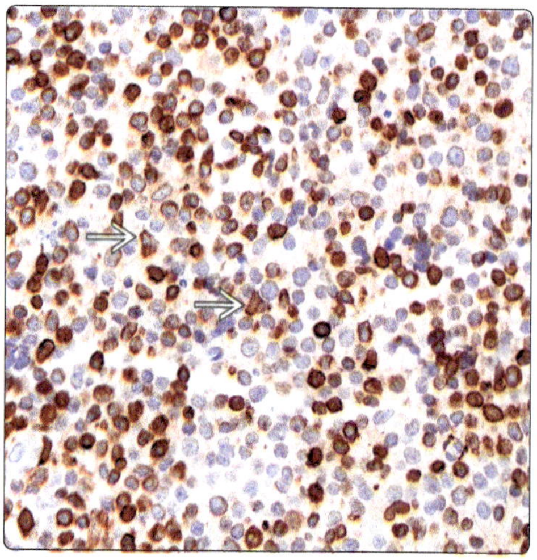

Differential Diagnosis: Primary Mediastinal Large B-Cell Lymphoma

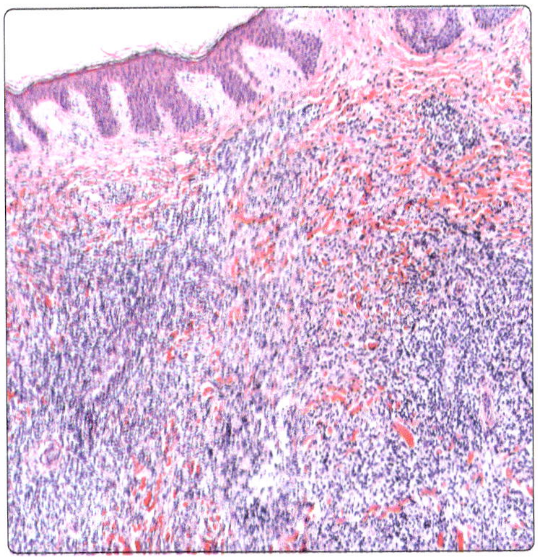

Differential Diagnosis: Primary Mediastinal Large B-Cell Lymphoma

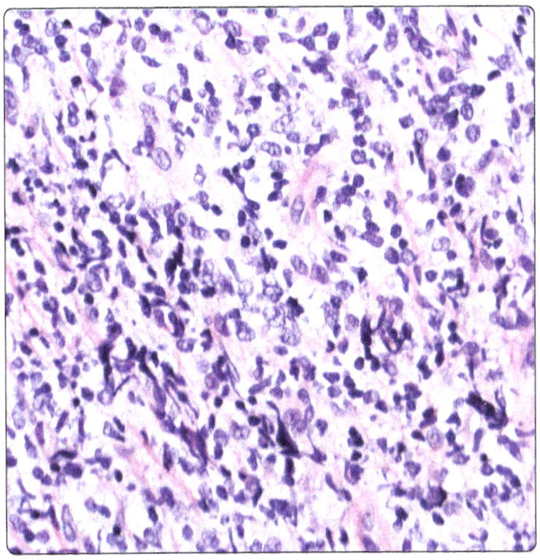

(Left) *A case of primary mediastinal (thymic) large B-cell lymphoma disseminated to skin is shown. The pattern of infiltration mimics primary cutaneous lymphoma at low-power magnification.* **(Right)** *High magnification of a primary mediastinal (thymic) large B-cell lymphoma disseminated to skin is shown. The lymphoma cells are polylobated and spindle-shaped.*

Differential Diagnosis: Systemic Diffuse Large B-Cell Lymphoma

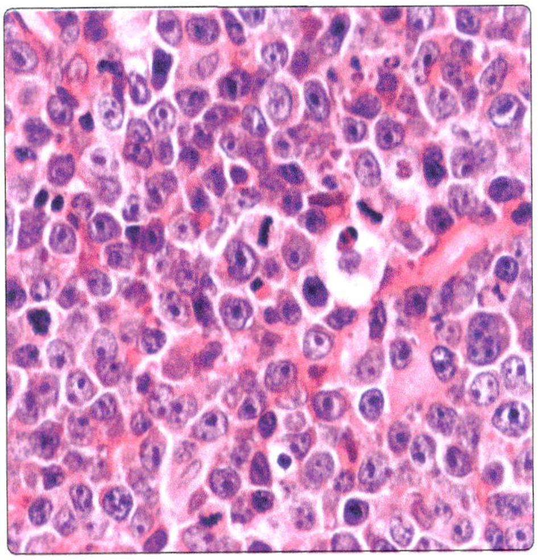

Differential Diagnosis: EBV(+) Diffuse Large B-Cell Lymphoma

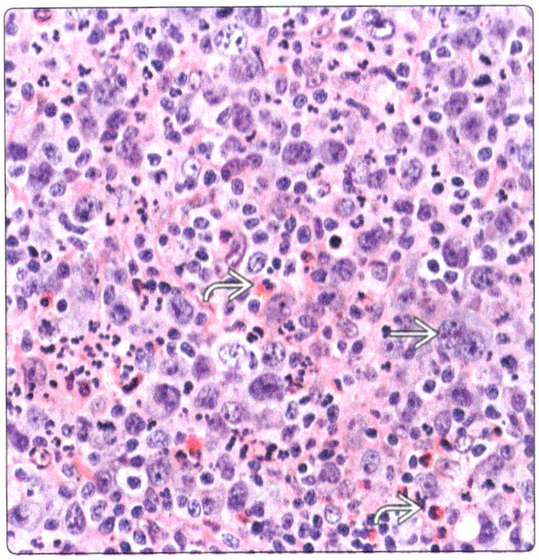

(Left) *A case of systemic diffuse large B-cell lymphoma, immunoblastic variant, involving the skin is shown. The lymphoma cells resemble the immunoblasts observed in some cases of PCDLBCL-LT.* **(Right)** *EBV(+) diffuse large B-cell lymphoma of the elderly involving skin is shown. The lymphoma cells are large and polymorphous, with Reed-Sternberg-like cells ➔ and plasmacytoid cells present. Many neutrophils, as well as eosinophils ➔, are also present in the background.*

Differential Diagnosis: Plasmablastic Lymphoma

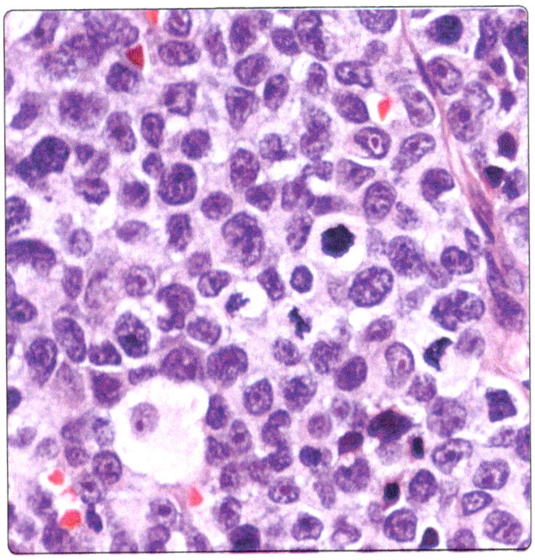

EBER Staining in Plasmablastic Lymphoma

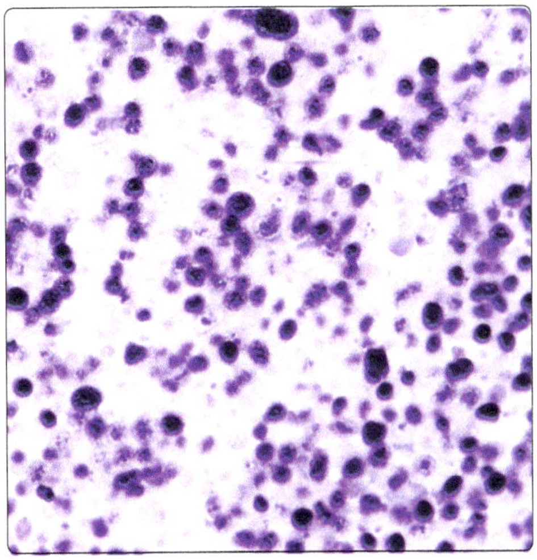

(Left) *Plasmablastic lymphoma involving the skin is shown. Plasmablastic lymphoma usually shows a cohesive proliferation of plasmablasts or immunoblasts, and these features overlap with PCDLBCL-LT.* **(Right)** *Plasmablastic lymphoma involving the skin is shown. In situ hybridization for Epstein-Barr virus small-encoded RNA is usually positive in plasmablastic lymphoma, unlike in PCDLBCL-LT.*

KEY FACTS

TERMINOLOGY

- Angiocentric and angioinvasive Epstein-Barr virus (EBV)-associated mature B-cell lymphoproliferative disorder

CLINICAL ISSUES

- Most common site is lung
- Skin is most common extrapulmonary site
- Cases with larger number of atypical B cells expressing EBV have worse prognosis
- Grading can be inconsistent and poorly reproducible among observers
- Grade 1 and grade 2 may be treated with interferon α
- Grade 3 lesions show some response to aggressive chemotherapy

MICROSCOPIC

- B cells in subcutis and sometimes dermis are scattered showing angiocentric distribution

ANCILLARY TESTS

- CD20(+), pax-5(+), EBV(+) (less in skin than lung), CD30(+/-), CD15(-)
- Clonal *IGH* gene rearrangement
- Mixed population of T cells, but most express CD4

TOP DIFFERENTIAL DIAGNOSES

- NK-/T-cell lymphoma: Also angiocentric & EBV(+), but tumor cells are NK or T cells [CD56(+) &/or CD3(+) & CD4(+)]
- EBV(+) diffuse large B-cell lymphoma of elderly
  - Diffuse growth pattern, not scattered cells of lymphomatoid granulomatosis (LYG)
  - Not angiocentric, usually no necrosis, and no mixed background infiltrate
- Vasculitis
  - Can show similar histologic features to LYG with inflammation of blood vessels and involvement of multiple organ systems
  - Usually not EBV(+), vasculitis has nonmonoclonal B cells

LYG at Low Power

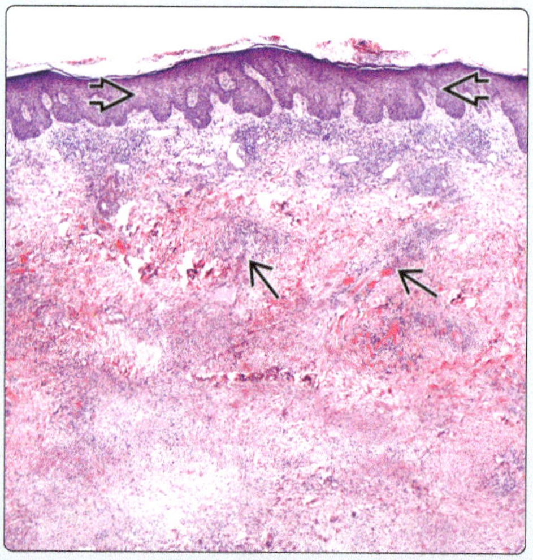

LYG Involving Subcutis

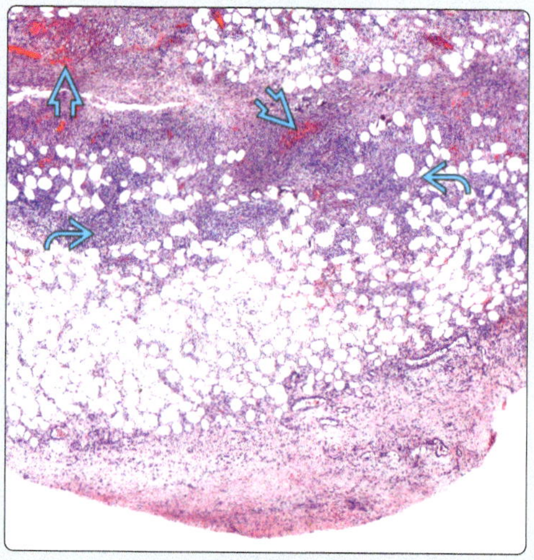

(Left) *Low-power view of cutaneous lymphomatoid granulomatosis (LYG) shows an extensive B-cell infiltrate with a perivascular angiodestructive distribution →. The epidermis ⇨ is not involved. (Courtesy M. Royer, MD.)* **(Right)** *LYG diffusely infiltrating into the fat ↗ can mimic a reactive panniculitis. There is angiocentric involvement with tumor cells surrounding and infiltrating blood vessels ⇨.*

Epstein-Barr Virus Encoded Receptor in LYG

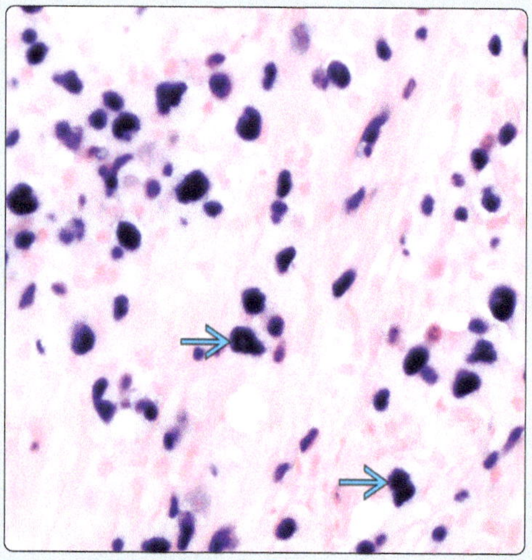

***IGH* Gene Rearrangement in LYG**

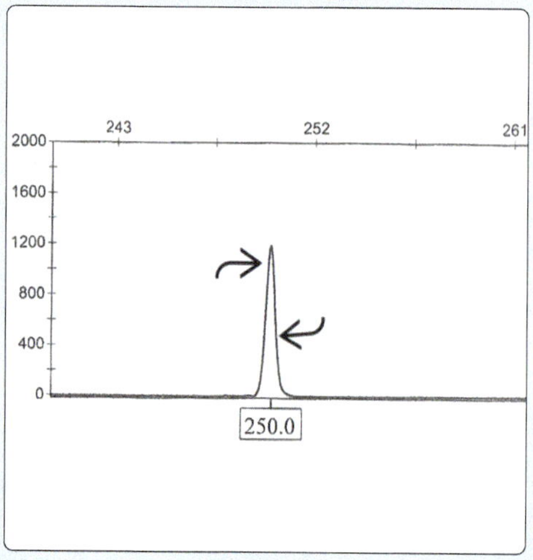

(Left) *A higher power magnification of the same lesion shows that many of the Epstein-Barr virus (EBV)-encoded receptor (EBER)(+) cells are large in size → and show some nuclear irregularity. The smaller reactive T cells are EBER(-).* **(Right)** *PCR test for IGH gene rearrangements shows a dominant monoclonal peak at position 250 ↗. IGH gene rearrangements are often detected in LYG since it is a B-cell lymphoma.*

TERMINOLOGY

Abbreviations

- Lymphomatoid granulomatosis (LYG)

Synonyms

- Angiocentric immunoproliferative lesion

Definitions

- Extranodal Epstein-Barr virus (EBV)-driven mature B-cell lymphoma that is angiocentric
  - It is uncertain whether LYG represents unique disease or is part of spectrum of EBV-associated B-cell lymphoproliferative disorders

ETIOLOGY/PATHOGENESIS

Epstein-Barr Virus

- Due to dysregulated immune surveillance of EBV-infected B cells, particularly by CD8(+) T cells
- Type III latency pattern, LMP and EBNA2(+)

Immunodeficiency

- Most have no clearly defined underlying immunodeficiency
- However, some patients have had allogeneic organ transplant, HIV infection, X-linked lymphoproliferative disorder, and Wiskott-Aldrich syndrome

CLINICAL ISSUES

Epidemiology

- Age
  - Mostly adults, commonly in 6th decade
  - Children with immunodeficiency syndromes
- Sex
  - M:F > 2.0:1.0

Site

- Most common site is lung; skin is most frequent extrapulmonary site
  - For skin lesions, often trunk or limbs, cutaneous nodules often develop after pulmonary disease
  - May show any anatomic distribution, but usually spares bone marrow, lymph nodes, and spleen

Presentation

- Most commonly as erythematous subcutaneous and dermal nodules
- Pulmonary symptoms (cough and dyspnea)

Treatment

- Grade 1 and grade 2 may be treated more conservatively
  - Interferon α has been used
- Grade 3 lesions show some response to aggressive chemotherapy + rituximab

Prognosis

- Variable, but often related to grading
  - Most patients have aggressive disease, survival < 2 years
  - Grading based on number of EBV(+) B cells
    - Grade 1: < 5 EBV-encoded receptor (EBER)(+) cells per high-power field, large atypical B cells are rare, polymorphous background infiltrate, focal or no necrosis
    - Grade 2: 5-20 EBER(+) cells per high-power field, small clusters of B cells, more necrosis
    - Grade 3: > 20 EBER(+) cells per high-power field, large atypical B cells, larger B-cell aggregates, often Reed-Sternberg-like cells, more necrosis
    - Grading can be inconsistent and poorly reproducible among observers
    - As areas of necrosis are always negative for EBER, this can greatly underestimate number of EBER(+) cells, especially when necrosis is extensive, as in high-grade lesions

MICROSCOPIC

Histologic Features

- Dense, atypical lymphoid infiltrate usually in subcutis and sometimes in dermis
  - B cells scattered and may not form sheets
    - May be immunoblasts, multinucleated, and Reed-Sternberg-like cells
  - Often numerous reactive T cells, ↑ plasma cells and histiocytes, usually normal neutrophils and eosinophils, rarely granulomatous inflammation in subcutis
    - Originally was considered T-cell lymphoma due to increased numbers of T cells
- Tumor cells angiocentric, angiodestructive with lymphocytic vasculitis and fibrinoid necrosis of injured blood vessels
- Commonly shows subcutaneous panniculitis, with frequent nonnecrotizing granulomas

Cytologic Features

- Medium to large atypical lymphocytes, sometimes with 1 or more prominent nucleoli

ANCILLARY TESTS

Immunohistochemistry

- Malignant cells are positive for B-cell markers [CD20(+), CD19(+), pax-5(+)], CD30(+/-), CD15(-)
- Mixed population of T cells, but most express CD4
- Maybe increased number of CXCL13(+) T-regulatory cells, especially in higher grade lesions

Genetic Testing

- Clonal Ig heavy chain (*IGH*) gene rearrangement more often detected in higher grade lesions
- Polyclonal for T-cell receptor gene rearrangement studies
- EBER in situ hybridization
  - Less commonly positive in skin than in lung

DIFFERENTIAL DIAGNOSIS

NK-/T-Cell Lymphoma

- Also angiocentric with necrosis and EBV(+), but tumor cells are NK or T cells [CD56(+) &/or CD3(+) and CD4(+)]

SELECTED REFERENCES

1. Piña-Oviedo S et al: Primary pulmonary lymphomas. Adv Anat Pathol. 22(6):355-75, 2015
2. Rysgaard CD et al: Lymphomatoid granulomatosis presenting with cutaneous involvement: a case report and review of the literature. J Cutan Pathol. 42(3):188-93, 2015

High Power of Atypical Cells in LYG

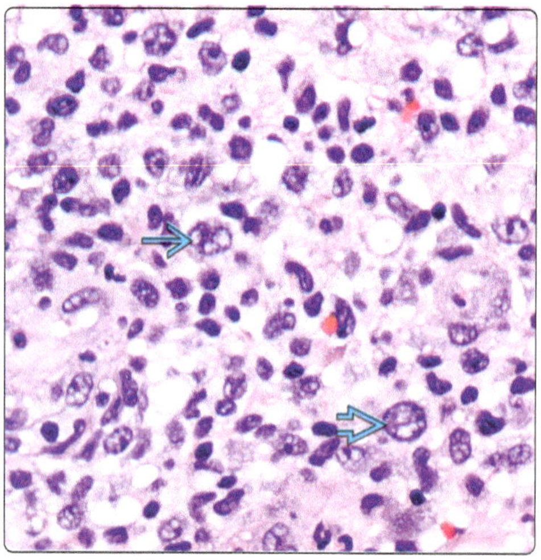

Angioinvasion in LYG

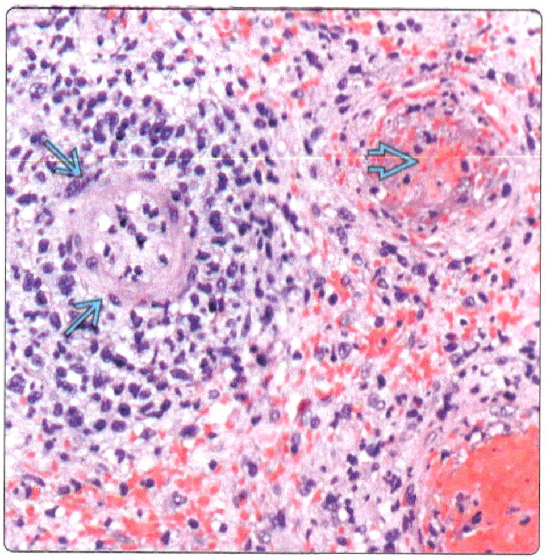

(Left) *High-power magnification of LYG shows that some of the malignant B cells have considerable atypia, including irregular nuclear shapes, enlarged nuclei, and vesicular chromatin. There were also rare multinucleated cells and Reed-Sternberg-like cells. Note that the malignant cells are scattered and not forming large aggregates.* **(Right)** *Lymphocytes cuff blood vessels and penetrate the vessel walls, causing prominent fibrinoid necrosis of injured vessels.*

Epstein-Barr Virus-Encoded Receptor in LYG

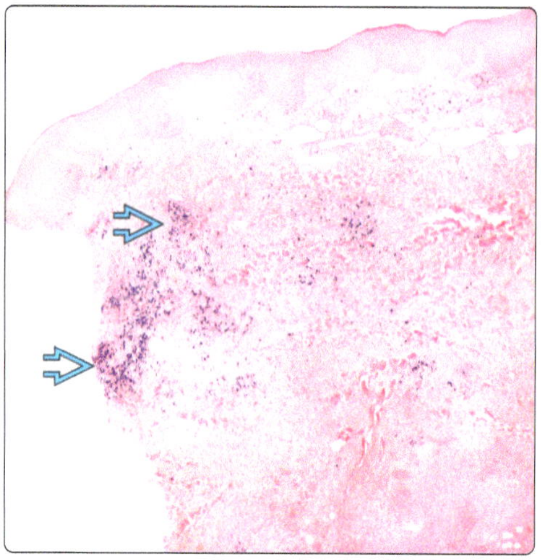

CD20 Staining in LYG

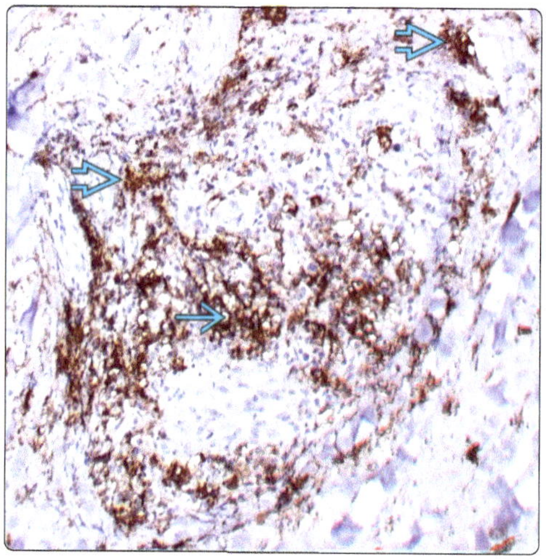

(Left) *Low-power image of in situ hybridization for EBER in a case of cutaneous LYG shows clusters of EBER(+) cells (blue) within the dermis in a perivascular distribution. There are no EBER(+) cells in the epidermis.* **(Right)** *This CD20 immunohistochemical (IHC) stain reveals that the mononuclear cells in the blood vessel in the center of the slide are B cells. CD20 also highlights increased numbers of lymphocytes outside of the vessel.*

CD3 Staining in LYG

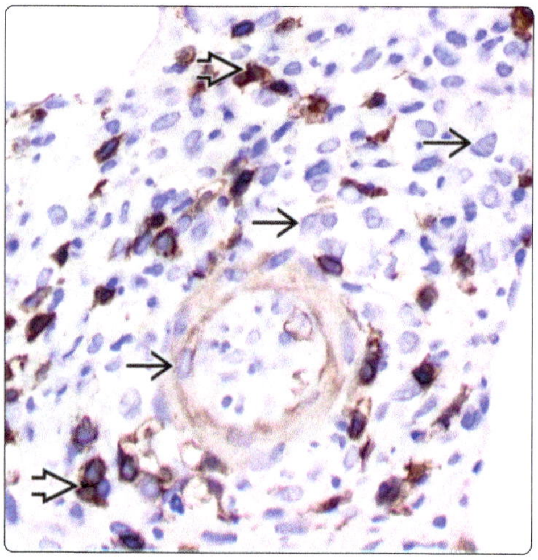

CD7 Staining in LYG

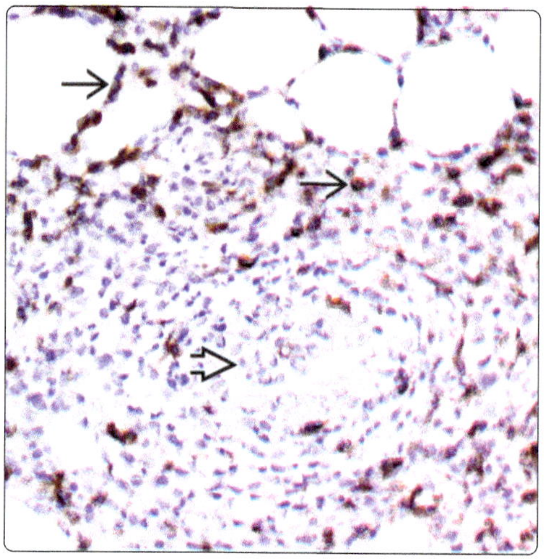

(Left) *A CD3 IHC is not reactive in the larger, malignant B cells within and surrounding the blood vessel in the center. The CD3 immunostain marks increased numbers of scattered, reactive T cells, which are commonly seen in LYG.* **(Right)** *A CD7 IHC is mostly negative in the lymphocytes penetrating the blood vessel in the center of the image. Reactive T cells are seen surrounding the fat cells at the top of the image. (Courtesy M. Royer, MD.)*

Vascular Involvement in LYG

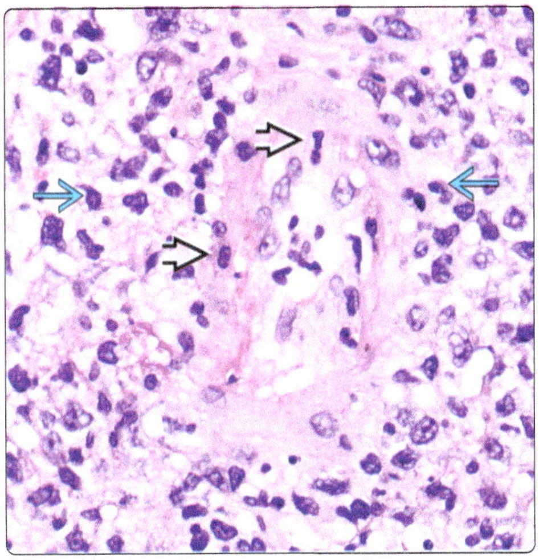

EBER Staining in LYG

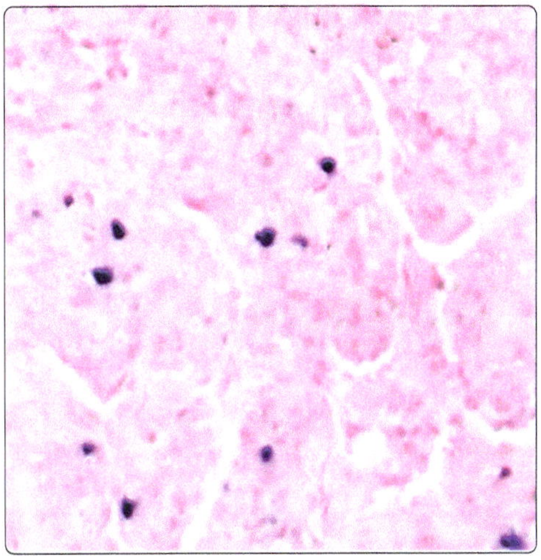

(Left) *In a high-power field, mononuclear cells ⇨ penetrate the wall of the blood vessel, and many lymphocytes are seen surrounding the blood vessel →. Mononuclear cells continue to invade the blood vessel until the vessel is destroyed.* **(Right)** *There are scattered EBER(+) cells in this case of cutaneous LYG.*

DDx: ENNK/TCL, Nasal Type

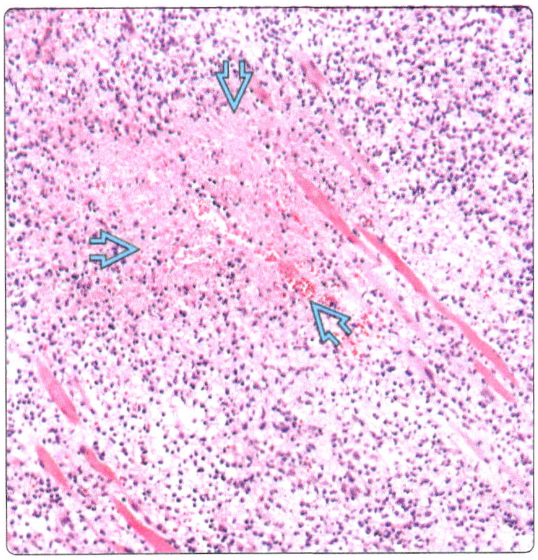

DDx: High-Power ENNK/TCL, Nasal Type

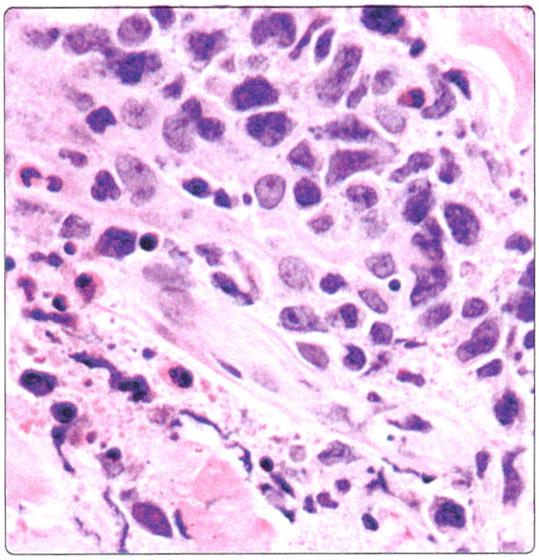

(Left) *The differential diagnosis of LYG includes extranodal NK-/T-cell lymphoma (ENNK/TCL), nasal type, a case of which is shown here involving the deep soft tissue of the cheek. Necrosis is present ⇨ surrounding a vessel. (Courtesy L. J. Medeiros, MD.)* **(Right)** *H&E shows high magnification of a nasal-type ENNK/TCL of NK cell lineage. The neoplastic cells are large and atypical and were positive for CD3, CD56, cytotoxic proteins, and EBER. (Courtesy L. J. Medeiros, MD.)*

CD56 Immunohistochemical in ENNK/TCL

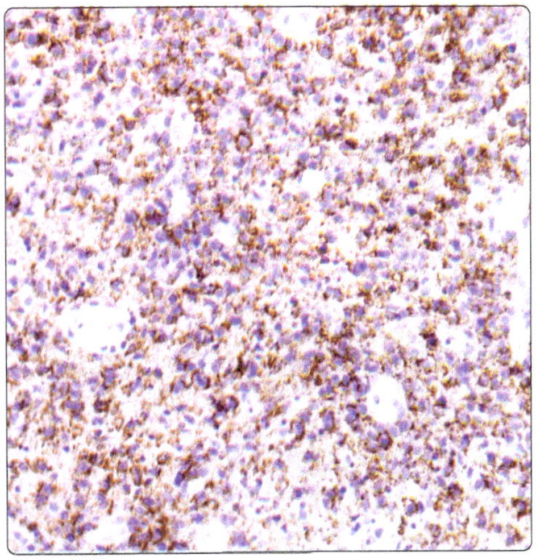

CD3 Staining in ENNK/TCL

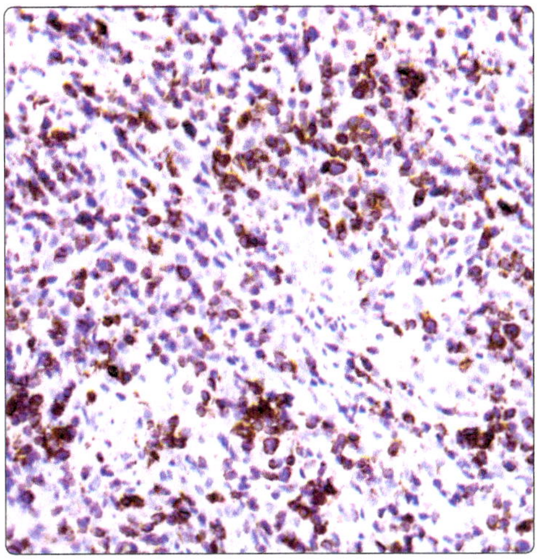

(Left) *CD56 IHC stain shows many positive neoplastic cells in ENNK/TCL, nasal type, and is highly suggestive of, but not specific for, NK-cell lineage. CD56 would be negative in LYG. (Courtesy L. J. Medeiros, MD.)* **(Right)** *CD3 IHC stain shows that the neoplastic cells are positive in ENNK/TCL. This antibody detects the epsilon chain of CD3 within the cell cytoplasm. Expression of CD3 epsilon chain is seen in both T cells and NK cells. (Courtesy L. J. Medeiros, MD.)*

KEY FACTS

TERMINOLOGY

- B-cell lymphoma that has spread to skin as secondary site of disease

CLINICAL ISSUES

- Systemic B-cell lymphoma more often involves skin, compared to systemic T-cell lymphoma
- Single or multiple lesions, usually tumors or nodules
- May present at diagnosis or develop during disease progression
- Often requires aggressive chemotherapy
- **Hodgkin lymphoma**
  - Direct extension to chest by tumor cells in patients with mediastinal disease
  - Reed-Sternberg cells CD30(+), CD15(+), pax-5(+), EBER(+)
- **Mantle cell lymphoma**
  - CD5(+), cyclin-D1(+), CD43(+), Bcl-2(+), t(11;14)(+)
- **Burkitt lymphoma**
  - CD10(+), Bcl-6(+), Bcl-2(-), t(8;14)(+)
- **SLL/CLL**
  - CD5(+), CD23(+), cyclin-D1(-)
  - CD200(+), CD10(-), FMC7(-)
  - ZAP70(+) (> 30% of cells) has worse prognosis than ZAP70(-)
  - Multiprobe FISH testing and cytogenetics detect changes on several chromosomes
- **Follicular lymphoma**
  - CD10(+), Bcl-6(+)
  - Often Bcl-2(+), unlike primary cutaneous follicle center lymphoma
  - Often t(14;18)(+), unlike primary cutaneous follicle center lymphoma

TOP DIFFERENTIAL DIAGNOSES

- B-cell lymphomas primary to skin
  - Higher stage than primary cutaneous lymphomas
  - Generally, much worse prognosis than primary cutaneous lymphoma

Clinical Photograph of Hodgkin Lymphoma

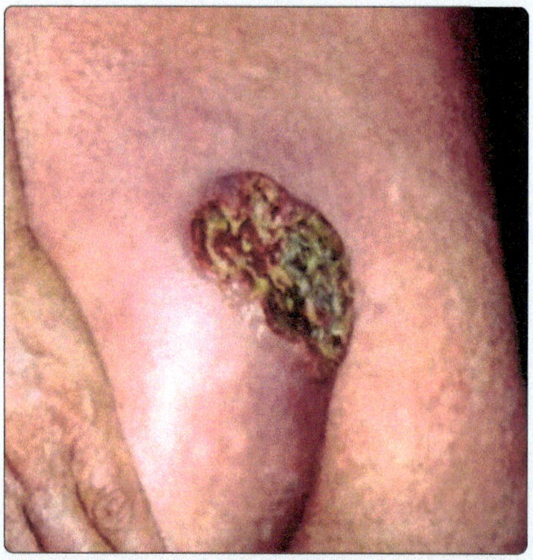

Classic Hodgkin Lymphoma Histology

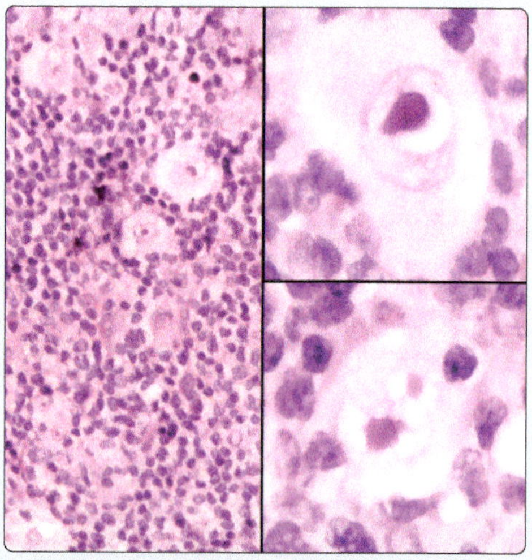

(Left) *This clinical photograph of cutaneous Hodgkin lymphoma shows a solitary ulcerating skin lesion. The lesion in the left gluteal area enlarged from 2 to 10 cm over several months. (Courtesy C. Hsai, MD.)* **(Right)** *Examination of the gluteal lesion shows Reed-Sternberg cells in the deep dermis, which expressed CD30 and CD15. Note the mixed inflammatory background with many eosinophils. (Courtesy C. Hsai, MD.)*

FISH for *CCND1-IGH* in Mantle Cell Lymphoma

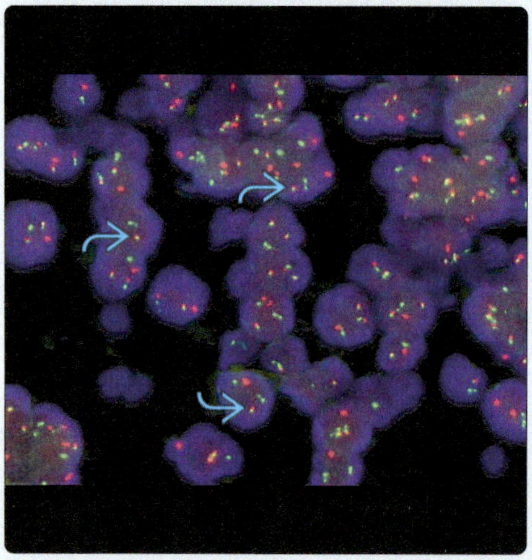

***MYC* FISH Break-Apart Probe in Burkitt Lymphoma**

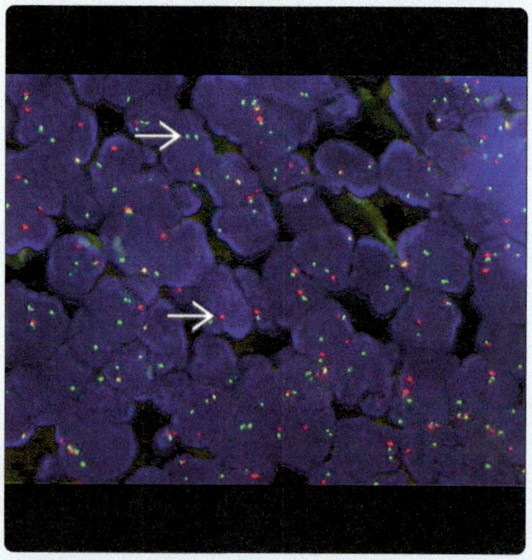

(Left) *This is a dual fusion FISH test for t(11;14), which is positive in a case of mantle cell lymphoma. This translocation is identified by the presence of numerous fused (yellow) signals ➔.* **(Right)** *This is a break-apart FISH test for the MYC gene, which is positive in a case of Burkitt lymphoma. The MYC gene translocation is identified by the presence of multiple green and red signals ➔.*

TERMINOLOGY

Synonyms

- Secondary cutaneous B-cell lymphoma

Definitions

- B-cell lymphoma that has spread to skin as secondary site of disease

ETIOLOGY/PATHOGENESIS

Infectious Agents

- Epstein-Barr virus infection in some types of lymphomas

Radiation

- Can be therapy related

CLINICAL ISSUES

Epidemiology

- Incidence
  - Systemic B-cell lymphoma more often involves skin, compared to systemic T-cell lymphoma
  - 25% of systemic peripheral T-cell lymphomas also have skin lesions
- Age
  - Any age but mostly adults
- Sex
  - Occurs in both males and females

Presentation

- Single or multiple lesions, usually tumors or nodules
  - Any cutaneous site; no site of predilection
- Skin involvement may present at diagnosis or develop later
- **Classic Hodgkin lymphoma**
  - Single or multiple dermal or subcutaneous nodules
  - Usually direct extension to skin (chest) by tumor cells in patients with mediastinal disease
    - Rare primary skin cases
  - Sometimes pruritus, hyperpigmentation, or urticaria, may be due to paraneoplastic syndrome, and not tumor
- **Mantle cell lymphoma (MCL)**
  - Often multiple macules, papules, plaques, or nodules on trunk or extremities
  - Involves skin ≤ 2% of cases
    - Primary to skin, extremely rare
- **Burkitt lymphoma**
  - Often in Africa (jaw tumors), in immunosuppressed, and in gastrointestinal tract
  - Often infection with Epstein-Barr virus
  - 12% of Burkitt lymphoma at autopsy have skin lesions
    - Sometimes direct invasion from underlying lesion
    - Can relapse with cutaneous lesions
- **Small lymphocytic lymphoma/chronic lymphocytic leukemia (SLL/CLL)**
  - Cutaneous lesion frequently follows initial diagnostic lesion
  - May develop at previous sites of viral infection
  - May occur at same site as other tumors
  - Cases with plasmacytoid differentiation are usually single nodule on trunk or extremity
  - 2% show skin lesions, usually already peripheral blood involvement
    - No apparent worse prognosis with skin involvement
- **Follicular lymphoma**
  - Secondary skin involvement is uncommon
- **Plasmablastic lymphoma**
  - Aggressive course and associated with HIV infection
  - Often arises in mucosa of oral cavity

Treatment

- Adjuvant therapy
  - Frequently aggressive chemotherapy, unlike most primary cutaneous B-cell lymphomas

Prognosis

- Higher stage than primary cutaneous lymphoma
- Usually much worse prognosis than primary cutaneous lymphoma

MICROSCOPIC

Histologic Features

- Depend on type of lymphoma
- Morphology and immunophenotype often identical to systemic disease
- **Classic Hodgkin lymphoma**
  - Scattered Reed-Sternberg cells with multinucleated giant cells, enlarged nuclei, and > 1 nucleoli sitting within lacunae
  - Many small lymphocytes, eosinophils, and plasma cells
  - Sometimes collagen bands
  - Most common subtype is nodular sclerosing Hodgkin lymphoma
    - Lymphocyte predominant Hodgkin lymphoma not reported in skin
  - Rare skin involvement, unlike non-Hodgkin B-cell lymphoma
    - Skin lesion in < 5% of cases and < 1% at presentation, more common in immunosuppressed
    - Extremely poor prognosis
- **MCL**
  - Nodular, diffuse, mantle zone or follicular growth pattern
  - B cells in dermis with grenz zone, often perivascular, sometimes surrounds reactive germinal center
  - Irregular nuclear contours, inconspicuous nucleoli
  - Scattered single epithelioid histiocytes
  - Blastoid variant may be more common in skin; has cells with dispersed chromatin, resembling lymphoblasts, or more atypia, similar to diffuse large B-cell lymphoma
- **Burkitt lymphoma**
  - Patchy dermal and subcutaneous infiltrate with grenz zone
  - Medium- to large-sized B cells with squared-off borders (i.e., cobblestone or jigsaw puzzle)
  - Dispersed chromatin with multiple medium-sized nucleoli
  - Can have basophilic cytoplasm, especially on touch preparation
  - ↑ mitosis and apoptosis
  - Tingible body macrophages creates starry-sky appearance

- **SLL/CLL**
  - Nodular or diffuse dermal B-cell infiltrate with small lymphocytes and minimal atypia
  - Sometimes patchy, sometimes perivascular
  - Small B cells with indistinct nucleoli and coarse chromatin
  - Rarely see proliferation centers in skin
  - Rare cases contain large cells (i.e., Richter syndrome) and may have worse prognosis
- **Follicular lymphoma**
  - Nodular or diffuse dermal infiltrate, usually with grenz zone
  - Germinal centers with decreased tingible body macrophages
  - Attenuated mantle zones
- **Plasmablastic lymphoma**
  - Diffuse neoplasm with immunoblastic or plasmablastic features and plasma cell immunophenotype
  - Starry-sky pattern frequent and high mitotic rates
  - Pan-B-cell antigens (CD20, pax-5) are weak or absent

ANCILLARY TESTS

Immunohistochemistry

- **Classical Hodgkin lymphoma**
  - Reed-Sternberg cells CD15, CD30, pax-5, LMP, CD20 (weak), and EBER (+)
  - Rarely T-cell antigens (+) and show T-cell receptor gene rearrangement
  - Must differentiate from anaplastic large cell lymphoma, which is CD30(+), CD15(-), pax-5(-), LMP(-), EBER(-)
- **MCL**
  - B-cell marker (+), CD5(+), cyclin-D1(+), SOX11(+/-), CD23(-), CD43(+), Bcl-2(+)
- **Burkitt lymphoma**
  - B-cell markers, including CD20(+), CD10(+), Bcl-6(+), Bcl-2(-) (usually), Ki-67 ~ 100%
- **SLL/CLL**
  - B-cell markers (+)
  - Usually CD5(+), CD23(+), LFE1(+), and cyclin-D1(-) (unlike MCL)
    - CD23 can differentiate SLL/CLL from MCL
    - Although some cases of CLL may only be weakly or partially CD23(+), and some cases of MCL can be dimly CD23(+)
    - CD200(+), CD10(-), FMC7(-)
    - ZAP70(+) (> 30% of cells) has worse prognosis than ZAP70(-) SLL/CLL
- **Follicular lymphoma**
  - B-cell antigens (+), CD10(+), Bcl-6(+)
  - Often Bcl-2(+), unlike primary cutaneous follicle center lymphoma
- **Plasmablastic lymphoma**
  - Plasma cell markers, such as CD138(+)
    - EBER(+), HHV8(-)

Genetic Testing

- **MCL**
  - t(11;14)(q13;q32) by cytogenetics or *CCND1-IGH* by FISH
- **Burkitt lymphoma**
  - *MYC* translocations are driving genetic change
  - *MYC* partners are *IGH* at 14q32, *IGK* at 2p11, and *IGL* at 22q11
  - t(8;14)(q24:q32) in ~ 80% of cases, t(8;22)(q24;q11) in ~ 15% of cases, t(2;8)(p11;q24) in ~ 5% of cases
- **SLL/CLL**
  - ~ 50% of cases have abnormal karyotypes
  - Trisomy 12 reported in 1/3 of cases portends more aggressive clinical course
  - 13q abnormalities in ~ 25% of cases; associated with longer survival
  - 11q23 abnormalities are detected in small subset of cases and are associated with aggressive course
  - Deletions of 6q21 in 5% of cases
  - Deletions of 17p13 (*TP53*) in 10% of cases have worse prognosis
- **Follicular lymphoma**
  - Often t(14;18)(*IGH-BCL2*)(+), unlike primary cutaneous follicle center lymphoma
  - *BCL6* alterations in only small percentage of cases

DIFFERENTIAL DIAGNOSIS

B-Cell Lymphomas Primary to Skin

- Usually more indolent clinically
- Usually treated less aggressive

SELECTED REFERENCES

1. Fabbri G et al: The molecular pathogenesis of chronic lymphocytic leukaemia. Nat Rev Cancer. 16(3):145-62, 2016
2. Fedoriw Y et al: The expanding spectrum of follicular lymphoma. Surg Pathol Clin. 9(1):29-40, 2016
3. Kluk MJ et al: MYC immunohistochemistry to identify MYC-driven B-cell lymphomas in clinical practice. Am J Clin Pathol. 145(2):166-79, 2016
4. Narurkar R et al: SOX11 is a biomarker for cyclin D1-negative mantle cell lymphoma. Biomark Res. 4:6, 2016
5. Park D et al: Novel insights into the early histopathogenesis of immunodeficiency-associated Burkitt lymphoma: A case report of Burkitt microlymphoma arising within HIV lymphadenitis. Histopathology. ePub, 2016
6. Ansell SM: Hodgkin lymphoma: diagnosis and treatment. Mayo Clin Proc. 90(11):1574-83, 2015
7. Elyamany G et al: Plasmablastic lymphoma: a review of current knowledge and future directions. Adv Hematol. 2015:315289, 2015
8. Pettey AA et al: Cutaneous involvement with Burkitt-like lymphoma. Am J Dermatopathol. 29(2):184-6, 2007
9. Jacobson MA et al: Cutaneous involvement by Burkitt lymphoma. J Am Acad Dermatol. 54(6):1111-3, 2006
10. Fullen DR et al: Granuloma annulare-like infiltrates with concomitant cutaneous involvement by B-cell non-Hodgkin's lymphoma: report of a case. Am J Dermatopathol. 25(1):57-61, 2003
11. Kim BK et al: Primary and secondary cutaneous diffuse large B-cell lymphomas: a multiparameter analysis of 25 cases including fluorescence in situ hybridization for t(14;18) translocation. Am J Surg Pathol. 27(3):356-64, 2003
12. Cerroni L et al: Specific cutaneous infiltrates of B-cell chronic lymphocytic leukemia (B-CLL) at sites typical for Borrelia burgdorferi infection. J Cutan Pathol. 29(3):142-7, 2002
13. Dubus P et al: Value of interphase FISH for the diagnosis of t(11:14)(q13;q32) on skin lesions of mantle cell lymphoma. Am J Clin Pathol. 118(6):832-41, 2002
14. Sen F et al: Mantle cell lymphoma involving skin: cutaneous lesions may be the first manifestation of disease and tumors often have blastoid cytologic features. Am J Surg Pathol. 26(10):1312-8, 2002
15. Starz H et al: Secondary lymph node involvement from primary cutaneous large B-cell lymphoma of the leg: sentinel lymph nodectomy as a new strategy for staging circumscribed cutaneous lymphomas. Cancer. 85(1):199-207, 1999

Clinical Image of Burkitt Lymphoma

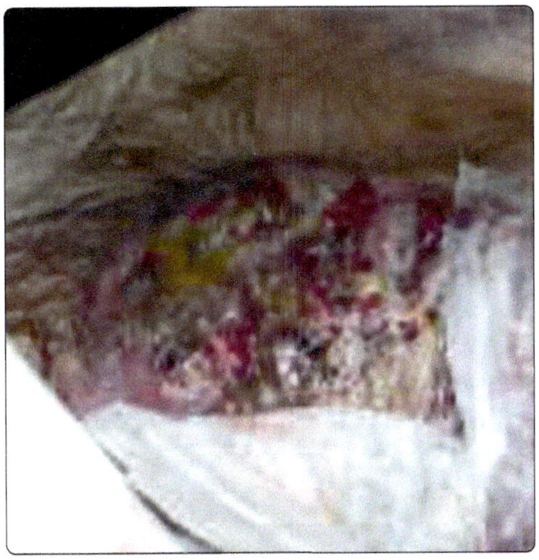

Burkitt Lymphoma Histology

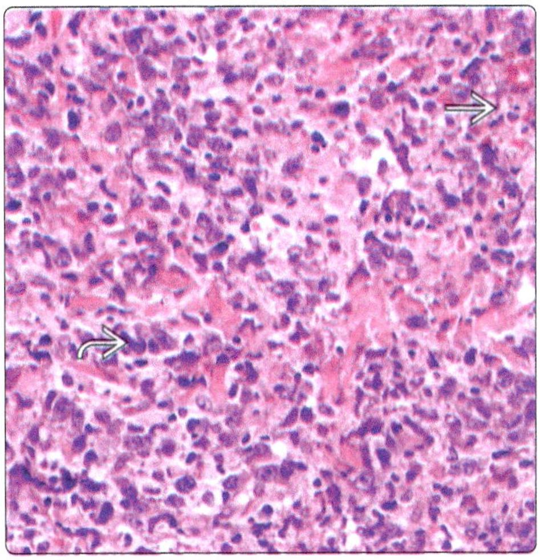

(Left) *This clinical photograph of Burkitt lymphoma involving the skin shows a large erythematous, slightly indurated verrucous plaque along the left chest and abdomen with erosions and bullae. (Courtesy D. Berke, MD.)* **(Right)** *This is a cutaneous Burkitt lymphoma with atypical B cells → [CD10(+), Bcl-2(-), t(8;14)(+) by FISH] in the dermis and rare tingible body macrophages →. The patient was also diagnosed with cecal Burkitt lymphoma.*

Lymphomatoid Granulomatosis

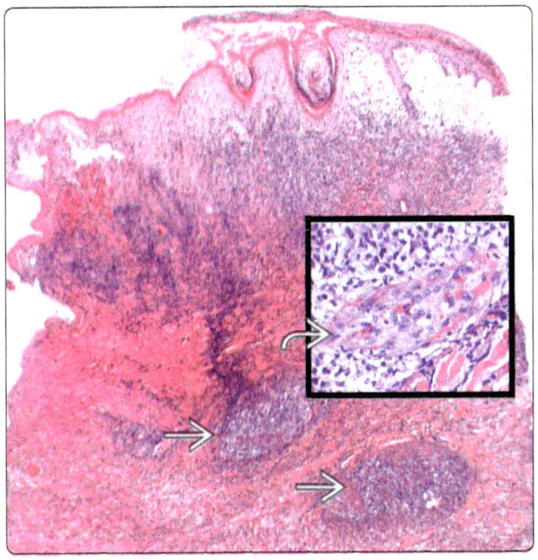

Lymphomatoid Granulomatosis Phenotype

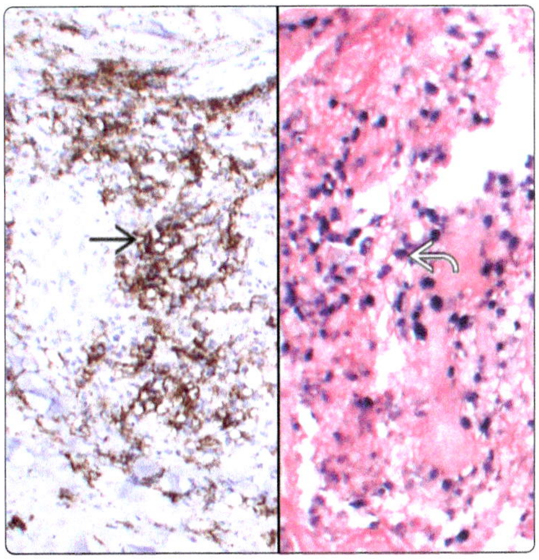

(Left) *This is lymphomatoid granulomatosis, and the patient had documented pulmonary lymphomatoid granulomatosis. The skin shows an angiocentric lymphoid infiltrate →. In the inset, there are medium-sized atypical lymphocytes in the wall of the blood vessel →.* **(Right)** *Ancillary testing on the same skin biopsy with lymphomatoid granulomatosis shows CD20(+) → on the left and EBER(+) → on the right, a phenotype consistent with lymphomatoid granulomatosis.*

Follicular Lymphoma Clinical Image

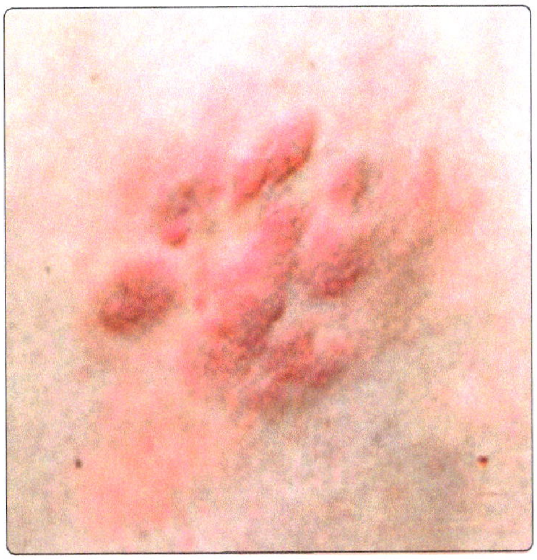

Follicular Lymphoma Morphology

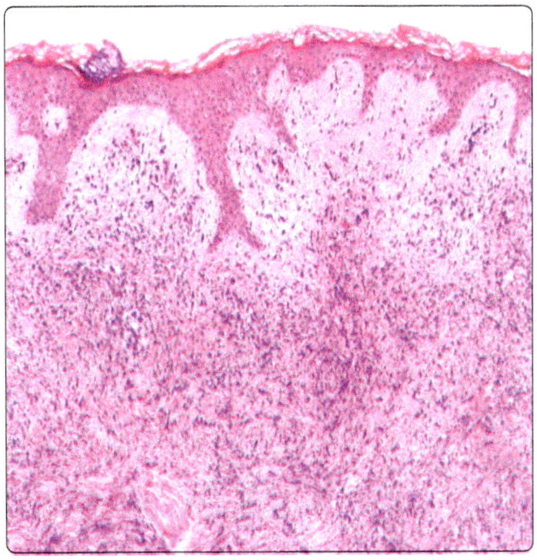

(Left) *This is a clinical photograph of systemic follicular lymphoma presenting in the skin, which shows nodules on the lower back in a grouped/zosteriform pattern. The patient was diagnosed with follicular lymphoma in the left axilla 10 months earlier. (Courtesy E. Moreira, MD.)* **(Right)** *This is skin involved with follicular lymphoma. The patient also has follicular lymphoma in lymph nodes. The malignant B cells have a mostly diffuse and vaguely nodular pattern [and were CD10(+), Bcl-6(+), Bcl-2(+)].*

(Left) *This is skin with small lymphocytic lymphoma/chronic lymphocytic leukemia, and the B cells ➡ are in the superficial and deep dermis with a sheet-like growth pattern. The epidermis is uninvolved and separated from the malignant B cells by a thin grenz zone ⇨. No germinal centers are present.* **(Right)** *A CD20 immunohistochemical stain shows that the chronic lymphocytic leukemia consists of aggregates of B cells. Pax-5 (not shown) marked the same population of B cells.*

Small Lymphocytic Lymphoma/Chronic Lymphocytic Leukemia

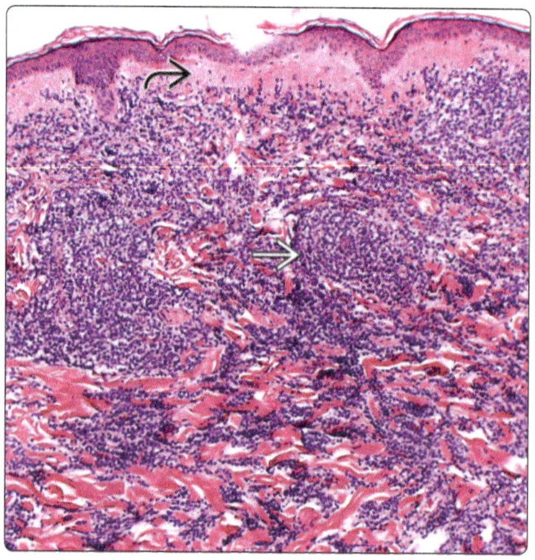

CD20(+) Small Lymphocytic Lymphoma/Chronic Lymphocytic Leukemia

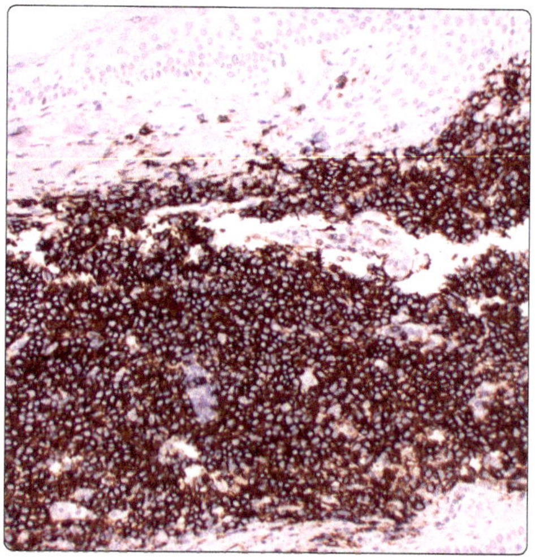

(Left) *CD5 immunohistochemical stain shows that the chronic lymphocytic leukemia is CD5(+). With reactive lymphocytes, CD5 is expressed in T cells and not B cells, but in CLL, CD5 is usually immunoreactive in the malignant B cells.* **(Right)** *CD23 immunohistochemical stain shows that the CD20(+) and CD5(+) B cells also are positive for CD23. Chronic lymphocytic leukemia is typically CD20(+), CD5(+), and CD23(+), although a subset of cases do not express CD5 or CD23.*

CD20(+) Small Lymphocytic Lymphoma/Chronic Lymphocytic Leukemia

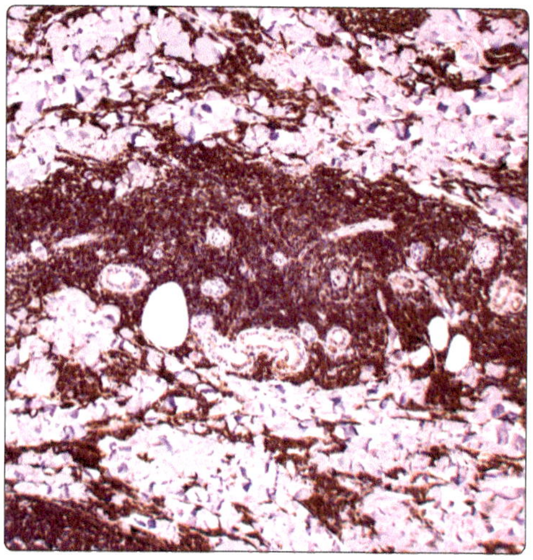

CD23(+) Small Lymphocytic Lymphoma/Chronic Lymphocytic Leukemia

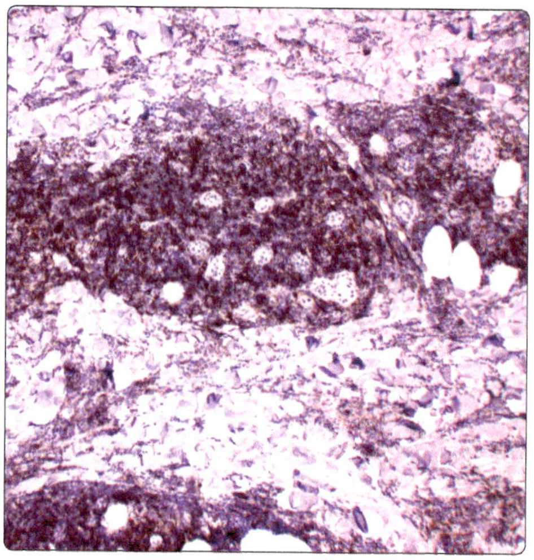

(Left) *This peripheral blood with chronic lymphocytic leukemia shows B cells ⇨ that are small and round with minimal atypia and coarse chromatin. Numerous smudge cells ➡ are usually identified.* **(Right)** *Flow cytometry shows a population of cells with coexpression CD19 and CD5, typical of chronic lymphocytic leukemia. These cells also expressed CD23, CD43, and Bcl-2 (not shown).*

Small Lymphocytic Lymphoma/Chronic Lymphocytic Leukemia Peripheral Blood

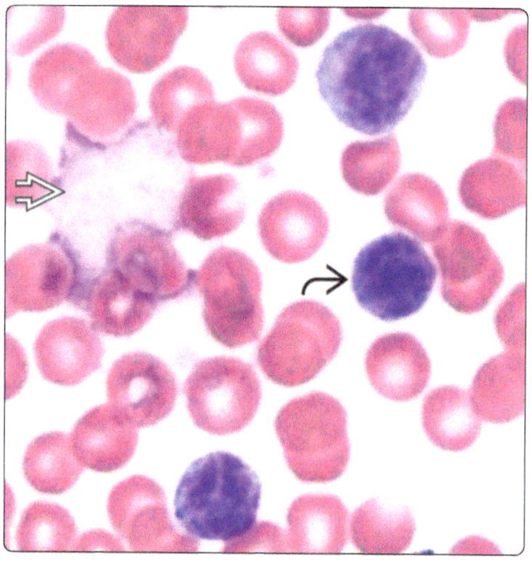

Flow Cytometry Small Lymphocytic Lymphoma/Chronic Lymphocytic Leukemia

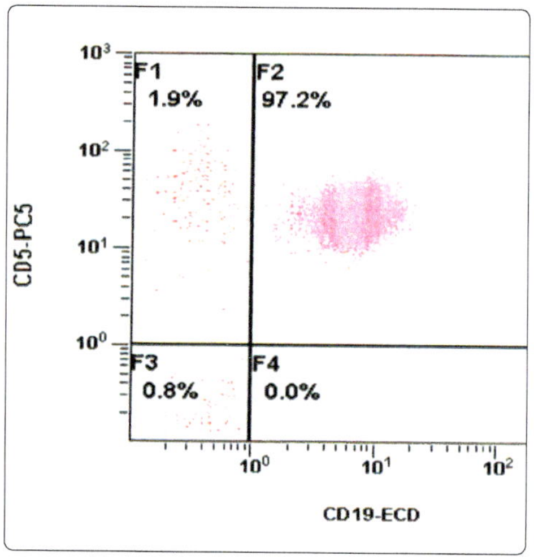

Mantle Cell Lymphoma

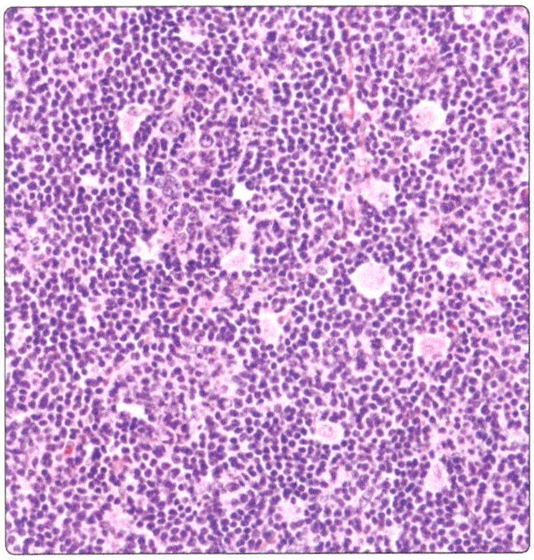

Cyclin-D1(+) Mantle Cell Lymphoma

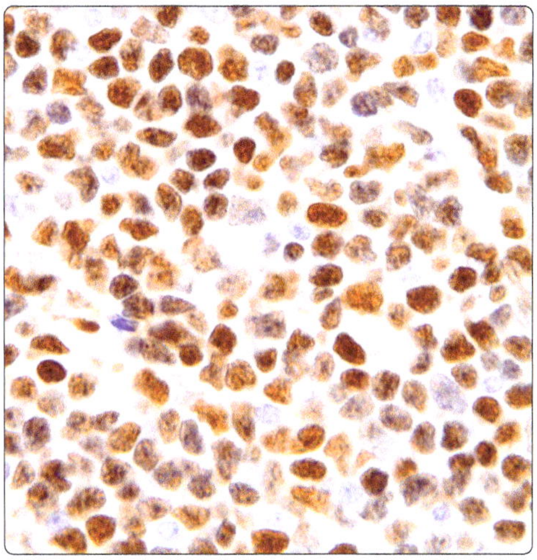

(Left) *A case of mantle cell lymphoma (MCL) shows small lymphocytes and many benign histiocytes with eosinophilic cytoplasm (so-called pink histiocytes). Pink histiocytes are a helpful clue for the diagnosis of MCL but are not specific. MCL is uncommon in the skin. (Courtesy C. Yin, MD.)* **(Right)** *Cyclin-D1 immunostain shows nuclear expression in the cells of MCL. PRAD1 and Bcl-1 are different names for cyclin-D1. (Courtesy C. Yin, MD.)*

Plasmablastic Lymphoma

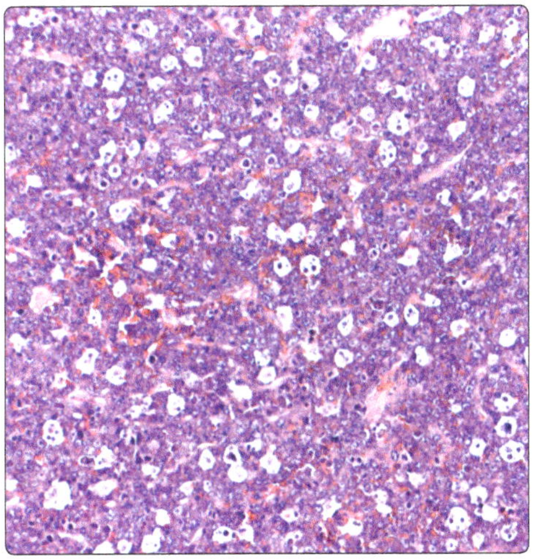

CD138(+) Plasmablastic Lymphoma

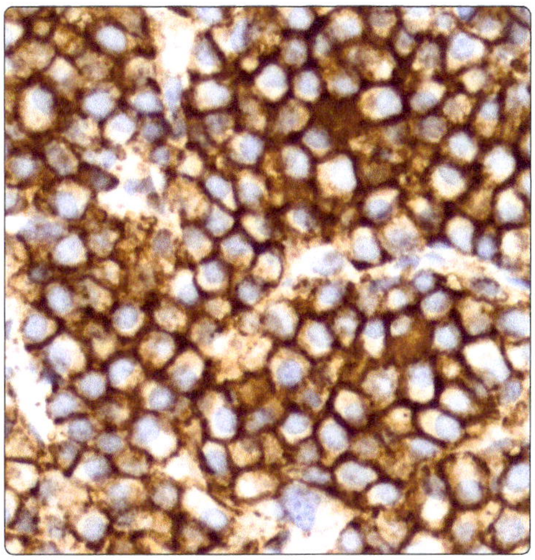

(Left) *This case of plasmablastic lymphoma (PBL) is characterized by a diffuse infiltrate of large atypical lymphoid cells with a starry-sky pattern. (Courtesy F. Vega, MD.)* **(Right)** *In PBL, the neoplastic cells show strong expression of CD138/syndecan (shown). Other plasma cell-associated antigens that are usually strongly expressed in PBL cases include IRF-4/MUM1, Vs38/p63, and CD38.*

Pax-5(-) Plasmablastic Lymphoma

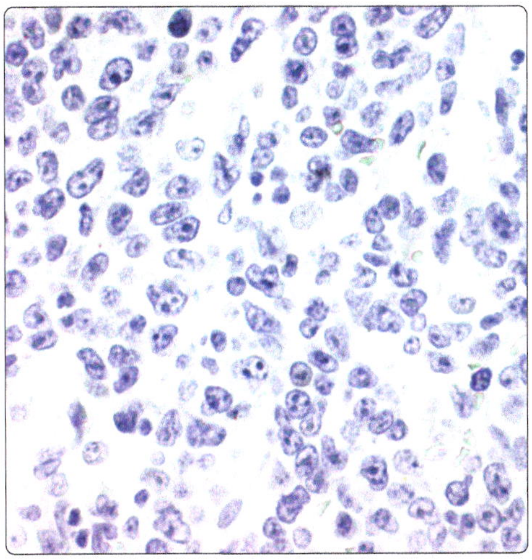

EBER(+) Plasmablastic Lymphoma

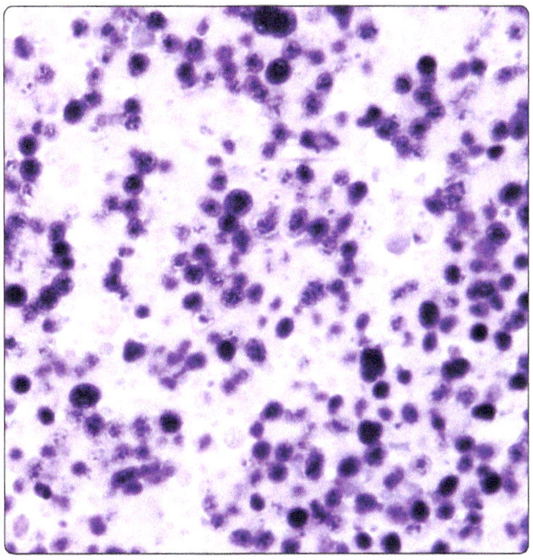

(Left) *The tumor cells in PBL are negative for pax-5. Strong expression of B-cell markers supports the diagnosis of diffuse large B-cell lymphoma over PBL. (Courtesy F. Vega, MD.)* **(Right)** *In situ hybridization for Epstein-Barr virus small-encoded RNA (EBER) is usually positive in PBL. (Courtesy F. Vega, MD.)*

Intravascular Large B-Cell Lymphoma

KEY FACTS

TERMINOLOGY

- Rare large B-cell lymphoma characterized by selective intravascular growth

CLINICAL ISSUES

- Heterogeneous clinical signs: Nodules/plaques (49%), macules (23%), telangiectatic patches (20%)
- Absence of marked lymphadenopathy
- Middle-aged or elderly patients
- Neurologic and dermatologic manifestations common
- Patients from Asia often show hemophagocytic syndrome
- Cutaneous variant
  - Most frequent in females, usually younger patients
  - Better prognosis (3-year survival rate of 56%, systemic variant: 22%)

MICROSCOPIC

- IVLBCL cells are large, with vesicular nuclear chromatin, distinct nucleoli, and frequent mitoses
- Lymphoma cells are mainly located in lumina of small vessels
- Mitoses are frequent
- Fibrin thrombi, hemorrhage, and necrosis often seen
- Circulating lymphoma cells can be occasionally seen in peripheral blood

ANCILLARY TESTS

- Pan-B-cell markers (+), Bcl-2(+), MUM1(+)
- Bcl-2(+) (90%), MUM1(+) (95%)
- CD5(+) (30%); other T-cell markers (-)
- Ki-67 high

TOP DIFFERENTIAL DIAGNOSES

- Peripheral T- or NK-cell lymphomas with intravascular pattern
- Hepatosplenic T-cell lymphoma
- T-cell large granular lymphocytic leukemia
- Diffuse large B-cell lymphoma, not otherwise specified

(Left) *Intravascular large B-cell lymphoma (IVLBCL) involving skin is shown. Note that the infiltration by neoplastic cells is difficult to recognize at this low magnification.* **(Right)** *IVLBCL involving the skin is shown. At high power, atypical lymphoid cells are seen inside of small dermal vessels ➡.*

Morphologic Features of IVLBCL

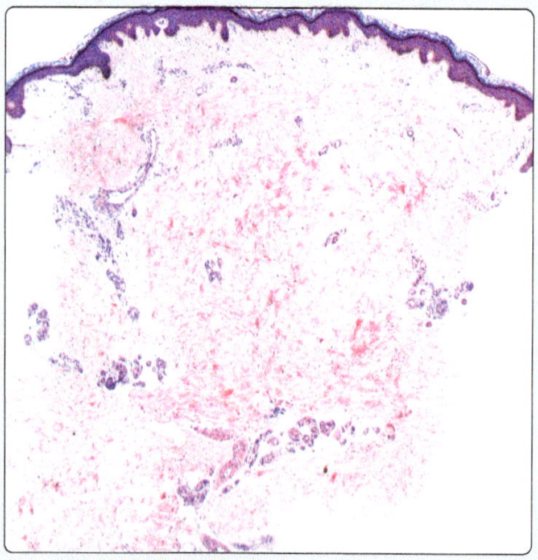

Morphologic Features of IVLBCL

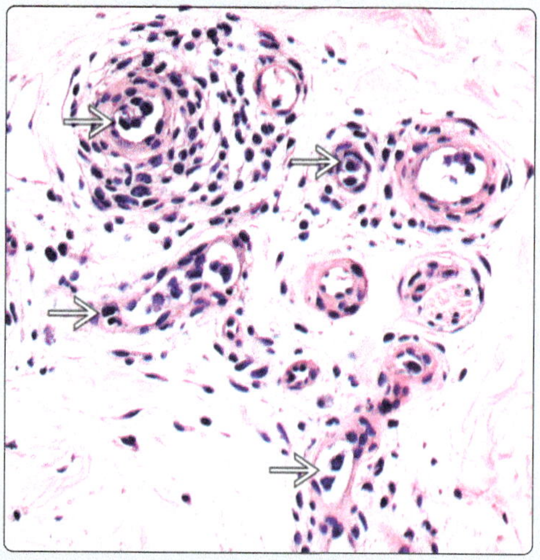

(Left) *Subcutaneous adipose tissue shows involvement by IVLBCL. Small blood vessels are filled with large atypical neoplastic cells.* **(Right)** *CD20 highlights the intravascular large neoplastic cells, supporting B-cell lineage and the diagnosis of IVLBCL involving subcutaneous adipose tissue.*

Morphologic Features of IVLBCL

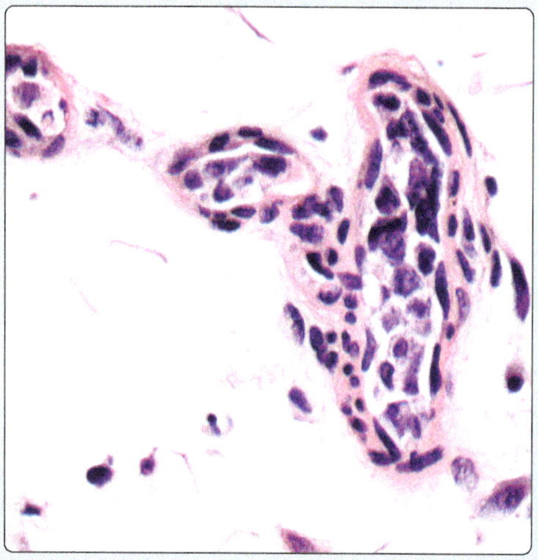

Ancillary Studies (CD20)

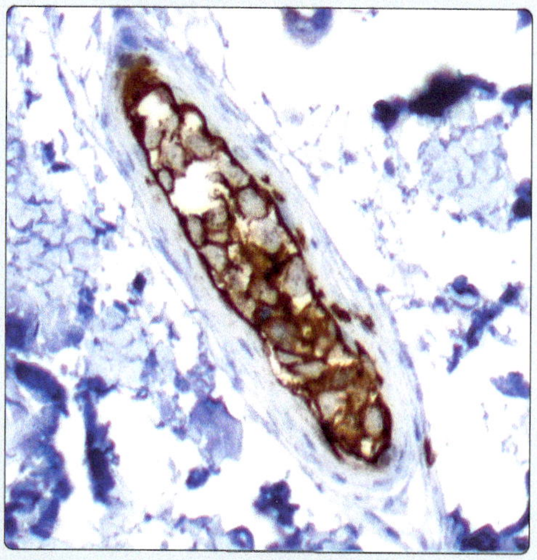

TERMINOLOGY

Abbreviations

- Intravascular large B-cell lymphoma (IVLBCL)

Synonyms

- Angiotropic large cell lymphoma
- Angioendotheliotropic (intravascular) lymphoma
- Intravascular lymphomatosis

Definitions

- Large B-cell lymphoma characterized by selective intravascular growth
- Preferential intravascular growth is condition sine qua non for diagnosing IVLBCL
  - Concomitant and minimal extravascular location of neoplastic cells, usually surrounding involved vessels, can be seen

CLINICAL ISSUES

Site

- Selective tumor growth within lumina of small blood vessels, particularly capillaries
- Widely disseminated
- Any organ can be involved
- Absence of marked lymphadenopathy
- Mechanisms responsible for selective growth of neoplastic cells within blood vessel lumina are unknown; possible explanations include
  - Chemokine-chemokine receptor interactions
    - e.g., CXCL9 (expressed in endothelium) and CXCR3 (expressed in IVLBCL)
  - Decreased expression of adhesion molecules on surface of IVLBCL cells
    - e.g., CD29 and CD54

Presentation

- Middle-aged or elderly patients; median: 67 years
- M:F ratio = 1.3:1
- IVLBCL can involve any organ with heterogeneous, often nonspecific symptoms
  - Fever of unknown origin
  - General fatigue
  - Deterioration in performance status
- Diagnosis can be clinically difficult and some cases are diagnosed postmortem
- 2 major patterns of clinical presentation
  - Western IVLBCL
    - Predominant neurologic and dermatologic manifestations
    - Central nervous system is involved in most patients
  - Asian IVLBCL
    - Hemophagocytic syndrome
    - Fever and B symptoms
    - Pancytopenia and bone marrow infiltration
    - Skin and central nervous system involvement are uncommon
- Skin
  - Heterogeneous clinical presentation
    - Nodules/plaques (49%)
    - Macules (22.5%)
    - Telangiectatic patches (20%)
    - Cellulitis
    - Ulcerated nodules
  - Waxing and waning lesions (16%)
  - Lower and upper extremities, trunk and lower abdomen
  - Skin involvement is sometimes detected by random skin biopsy of grossly unremarkable skin
  - Cutaneous variant
    - Most frequent in females
    - Younger than other IVLBCL patients
    - Usually not associated with leucopenia or thrombocytopenia
    - Better prognosis (3-year survival rate of 56%, systemic variant: 22%)
- Kidney
  - Increased creatinine
  - Proteinuria
  - Renal insufficiency
- Liver
  - Hepatomegaly
  - Increased bilirubin and liver enzymes
- Central nervous system
  - Alteration of consciousness
  - Motor and sensory deficits
  - Seizures
- Lungs
  - Dyspnea and hypoxia
- Hematopoietic system
  - Splenomegaly
  - Hemophagocytosis
  - Anemia, thrombocytopenia, and leukopenia
- Other
  - Increased LDH
  - Endocrine dysfunction (hypopituitarism)
  - Multiorgan failure

Treatment

- Rituximab-containing chemotherapy plus central nervous system-oriented therapy
  - R-CHOP plus high-dose methotrexate

Prognosis

- Aggressive behavior and often fatal course
- Predictive factors that are useful for risk stratification are not established

MICROSCOPIC

Histologic Features

- Large, atypical cells mainly located in lumina of small vessels in reticular dermis and subcutis
- Minimal extravascular location of tumor cells can be seen
  - Usually surrounding involved vessels
- Fibrin thrombi, hemorrhage, and necrosis often present
- Overlying telangiectases can be prominent
- Mitoses are frequently seen
- No criteria enable distinction between lesions restricted to skin and skin lesions concurrent with IVLBCL in other organs
- Sinusoidal involvement of liver, spleen, and bone marrow
- Spleen: Red pulp involvement

- Kidney: Neoplastic cells within glomerular capillaries and peritubular capillaries
- Circulating lymphoma cells can be occasionally seen in peripheral blood

Cytologic Features

- Usually tumor cells are large, with vesicular nuclear chromatin with prominent nucleoli
- In some cases, tumor cells have coarse nuclear chromatin and irregular or indented nuclei
- IVLBCL cell size may be smaller than usual in some cases

ANCILLARY TESTS

Immunohistochemistry

- Pan-B-cell markers typically (+)
  - CD19, CD20, CD22, CD79a, and pax-5
- Bcl-2(+) (90%), MUM1(+) (95%)
- Less frequently: CD5(+) (30%), CD10(+) (10%), Bcl-6(+) (25%)
- Ki-67: High proliferative activity
- T-cell markers (-)
  - CD2(-), CD3(-), CD4(-), CD8(-)

Genetic Testing

- Monoclonal rearrangements of *IGH* gene can be detected by PCR
- *TCR* genes in germline configuration
- Pathognomonic cytogenetic abnormalities have not been reported

DIFFERENTIAL DIAGNOSIS

Peripheral T- or NK-Cell Lymphomas With Intravascular Pattern

- Rare cases of T-cell lymphoma or NK-cell lymphoma can be purely intravascular
- (+) for T-cell or NK-cell markers
- These rare lymphomas do not have diagnostic category in 2008 WHO classification

Hepatosplenic T-Cell Lymphoma

- Some reported cases of intravascular T-cell lymphomas are probably γ-δ T-cell lymphoma or hepatosplenic T-cell lymphoma
- More frequent in young men
- Splenomegaly and hepatomegaly
- Bone marrow biopsy
  - Early stage disease: Small to intermediate in size lymphoma cells; intrasinusoidal pattern
  - Late stage disease: Large blastic lymphoma cells; interstitial or diffuse pattern
- T-cell markers: CD2(+), CD3(+), and cytotoxic markers TIA(+), GZM-B(+)
- Isochromosome 7q is consistent abnormality

T-Cell Large Granular Lymphocytic Leukemia

- Indolent clinical course with long survival
- Peripheral blood: Increased large granular lymphocytes
- Bone marrow, usually interstitial pattern, but sinusoidal pattern can be seen
- CD8(+), GZM-B(+), perforin(+), CD16(+), CD57(+), CD5(+) (dim)

Aggressive NK-Cell Leukemia/Lymphoma

- Leukemic cells can have cytoplasmic azurophilic granules
- NK-cell markers (+), GZM-B(+), perforin(+), EBV(+/-)
- Surface CD3(-), CD5(-)
- No *TCR* gene rearrangements

Splenic B-Cell Marginal Zone Lymphoma

- Patients often present with cytopenias
- Small neoplastic cells with abundant pale cytoplasm
- Pan-B-cell markers (+), CD3(-), CD10(-)
- Allelic loss of chromosome 7q22-36 (40%)

Diffuse Large B-Cell Lymphoma, Not Otherwise Specified

- Tumor cells are cytologically (and can be immunophenotypically) identical
  - IVLBCL does not present with lymphadenopathy or mass, unlike most cases of systemic diffuse large B-cell lymphoma (DLBCL)
- Cases of nodal DLBCL can relapse with appearance of IVLBCL
- Rare cases of IVLBCL may have derived from low-grade B-cell lymphomas
  - Identical *IGH* gene rearrangements in low-grade B-cell lymphoma and IVLBCL (in some cases)

DIAGNOSTIC CHECKLIST

Pathologic Interpretation Pearls

- Large lymphoid cells in intravascular spaces
  - B-cell immunophenotype (CD19, CD20, CD22, CD79a, and pax-5)

SELECTED REFERENCES

1. Pongpudpunth M et al: Usefulness of random skin biopsy as a diagnostic tool of intravascular lymphoma presenting with fever of unknown origin. Am J Dermatopathol. 37(9):686-90, 2015
2. Shimada K: Current understanding and future prospects for intravascular large B-cell lymphoma. Rinsho Ketsueki. 56(8):1032-7, 2015
3. Tanaka Y et al: Intravascular large B-cell lymphoma secondary to lymphoplasmacytic lymphoma: a case report and review of literature with clonality analysis. Int J Clin Exp Pathol. 8(3):3339-43, 2015
4. Kempf W et al: Cutaneous lymphomas: an update. Part 2: B-cell lymphomas and related conditions. Am J Dermatopathol. 36(3):197-208; quiz 209-10, 2014
5. Orwat DE et al: Intravascular large B-cell lymphoma. Arch Pathol Lab Med. 136(3):333-8, 2012
6. Kong YY et al: Intravascular large B-cell lymphoma with cutaneous manifestations: a clinicopathologic, immunophenotypic and molecular study of three cases. J Cutan Pathol. 36(8):865-70, 2009
7. Shimada K et al: Presentation and management of intravascular large B-cell lymphoma. Lancet Oncol. 10(9):895-902, 2009
8. Gleason BC et al: Intravascular cytotoxic T-cell lymphoma: a case report and review of the literature. J Am Acad Dermatol. 58(2):290-4, 2008
9. Ponzoni M et al: Definition, diagnosis, and management of intravascular large B-cell lymphoma: proposals and perspectives from an international consensus meeting. J Clin Oncol. 25(21):3168-73, 2007
10. Röglin J et al: Skin manifestations of intravascular lymphoma mimic inflammatory diseases of the skin. Br J Dermatol. 157(1):16-25, 2007
11. Shimizu I et al: Asian variant of intravascular lymphoma: aspects of diagnosis and the role of rituximab. Intern Med. 46(17):1381-6, 2007
12. Ferreri AJ et al: Intravascular lymphoma: clinical presentation, natural history, management and prognostic factors in a series of 38 cases, with special emphasis on the 'cutaneous variant'. Br J Haematol. 127(2):173-83, 2004

Morphologic Features of IVLBCL

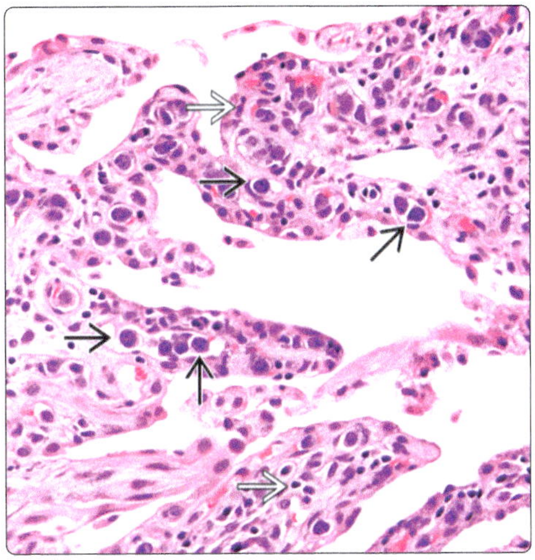

Morphologic Features of IVLBCL

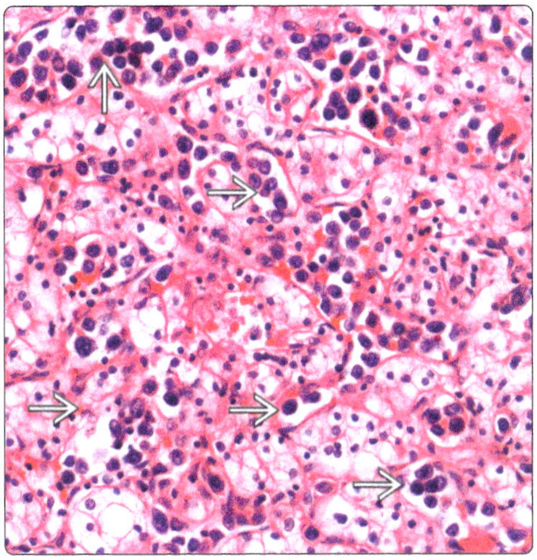

(Left) *IVLBCL involving a lung biopsy specimen is shown. The tumor cells are large and located within the alveolar capillaries. Some of the tumor cells are highlighted ⇒. Note the size of the neoplastic cells compared with that of small reactive lymphocytes ➡.* **(Right)** *IVLBCL in nephrectomy specimen of a patient with renal clear cell carcinoma is seen here. Large atypical lymphoid cells are seen inside of small sinusoid-like vessels ➡.*

Morphologic Features of IVLBCL

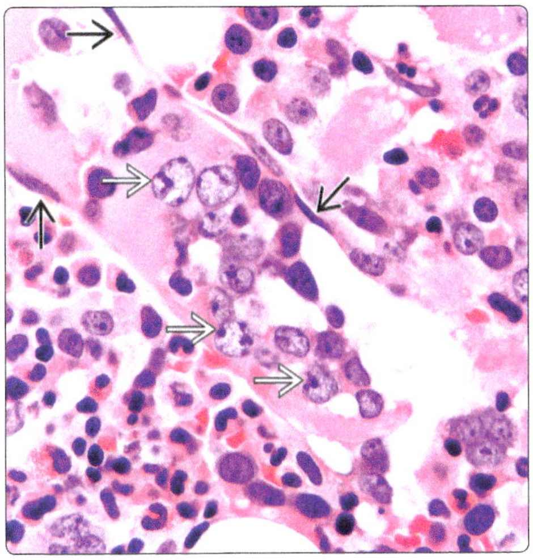

Morphologic Features of IVLBCL

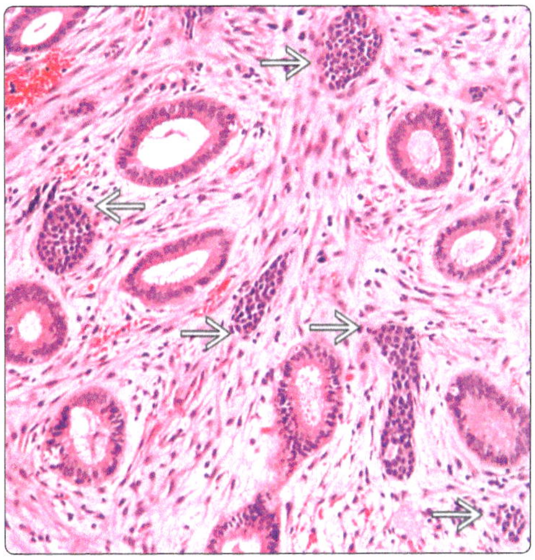

(Left) *IVLBCL involving bone marrow is shown. Note the presence of large atypical lymphoid cells inside this small blood vessel. The neoplastic cells characteristically have open nuclear chromatin, distinct nucleoli ➡, and are larger than adjacent endothelial cells ⇒.* **(Right)** *Endometrium shows involvement by IVLBCL with classical morphologic features. Small blood vessels in the endometrial mucosa are filled with large atypical neoplastic cells ➡. The endometrial glands are unremarkable.*

Ancillary Studies (CD20)

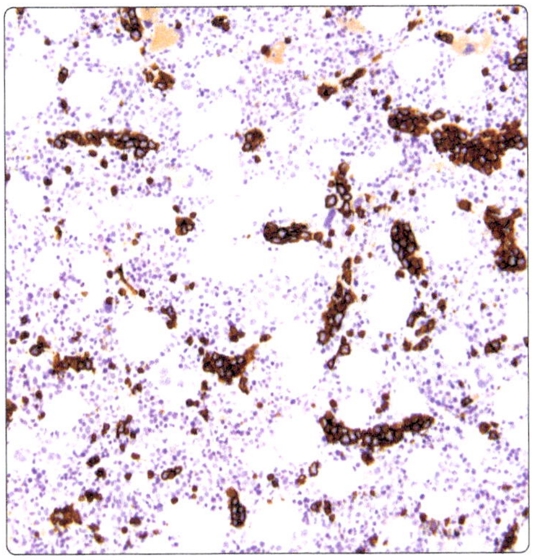

Ancillary Studies (Ki-67)

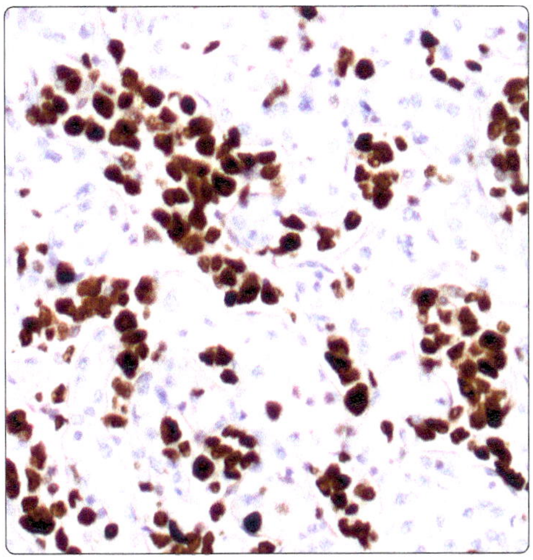

(Left) *CD20(+) IVLBCL involving bone marrow is shown. The intrasinusoidal infiltrate is easily recognized using immunostains specific for B-cell markers, such as CD20.* **(Right)** *IVLBCL is usually characterized by a high proliferation rate as shown by reactivity with the Ki-67 (MIB-1) antibody in this field.*

KEY FACTS

TERMINOLOGY

- Mycosis fungoides (MF)
- Primary cutaneous T-cell lymphoma characterized by
  - Epidermotropism
  - Clinical course showing stepwise evolution of patches, plaques, and tumors

CLINICAL ISSUES

- 50% of all cases of primary cutaneous lymphoma
- Typically presents in adults, 5th-6th decades
- Overall, indolent clinical course
- Clinical stage is most important predictor of prognosis
- **Pagetoid reticulosis (localized)**
  - a.k.a. Woringer-Kolopp disease
- **Folliculotropic (pilotropic) and syringotropic MF**
  - Closely related variants; often more aggressive course
  - Follicular papules (often grouped), alopecia, and acneiform lesions

MICROSCOPIC

- Superficial band-like or lichenoid infiltrate in patch and thin plaque stage
- Dense, band-like infiltrate in thick plaque stage
- Nodular dermal infiltrate in tumor stage
- Neoplastic lymphocytes are small, slightly cerebriform, and some have halos
- Large cell transformation: Large cells comprise ≥ 25% of infiltrate

ANCILLARY TESTS

- Immunophenotype
  - CD3(+), TCR-αβ/βF1(+)
  - CD4(+), CD8(-), CD5(+/-), CD7(-), CD26(-)

TOP DIFFERENTIAL DIAGNOSES

- Drug reactions, inflammatory dermatoses
- Primary cutaneous CD30(+) T-cell lymphoproliferative disorders (LyP and ALCL)

Clinical Presentation of Mycosis Fungoides

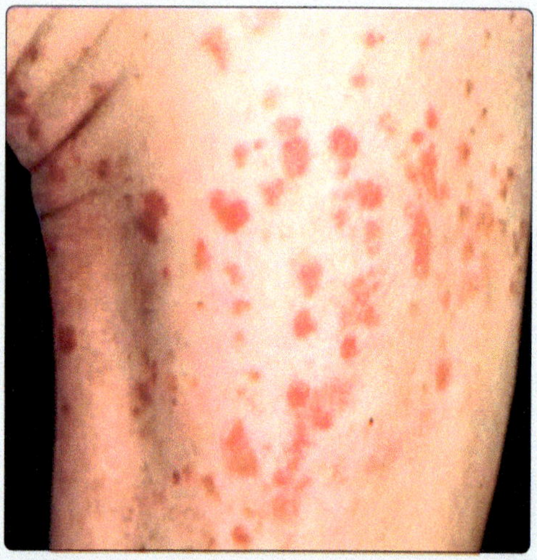

Plaque Stage Mycosis Fungoides

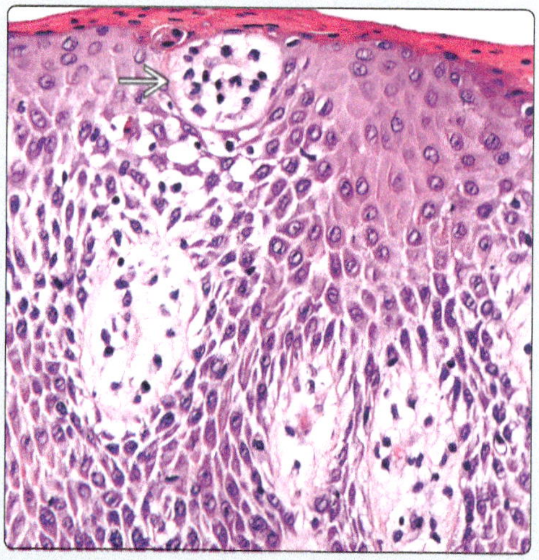

(Left) *The plaque stage of mycosis fungoides (MF) shows the presence of multiple red plaques on much of the body surface of this patient.* **(Right)** *The plaque stage of MF often shows the presence of Pautrier microabscesses ➡ containing small atypical tumor cells.*

Patch Stage Mycosis Fungoides

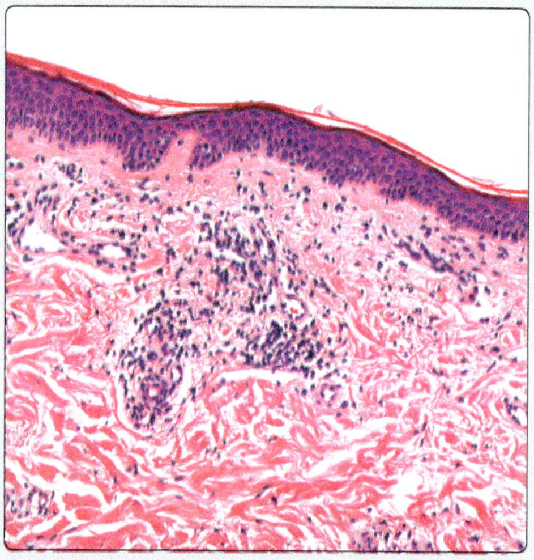

Patch Stage at High Magnification

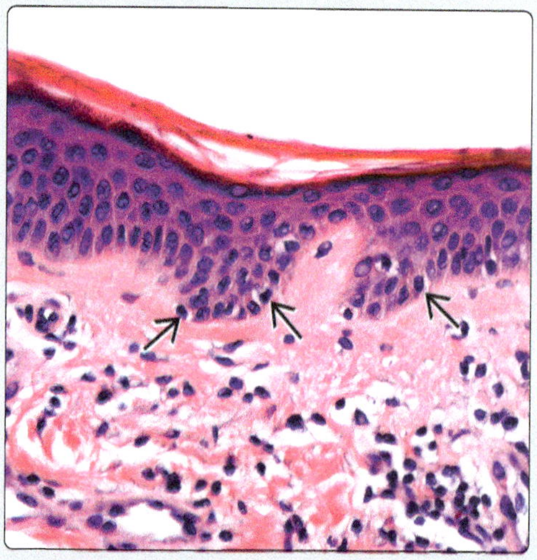

(Left) *This biopsy shows an early patch stage lesion of MF. Changes in the early patch stage are often very subtle. This specimen shows a mild perivascular lymphocytic infiltrate consisting of small lymphocytes and minimal epidermotropism.* **(Right)** *This higher power view of patch stage MF reveals epidermotropism of lymphocytes into the epidermal basal layer ➡. The tumor cells are small but hyperchromatic staining and have irregular nuclear contours.*

TERMINOLOGY

Abbreviations

- Mycosis fungoides (MF)

Definitions

- Primary cutaneous T-cell lymphoma characterized by
  - Epidermotropism
  - Clinical course showing stepwise evolution of patches, plaques, and tumors

ETIOLOGY/PATHOGENESIS

Unknown

- Chronic antigenic stimulation, possibly due to infectious agent, may play role
- Genetic abnormalities are likely involved

CLINICAL ISSUES

Epidemiology

- Incidence
  - 0.6/100,000 people per year
  - 50% of all cases of primary cutaneous lymphoma
- Age
  - Adults; 5th-6th decades
  - Can be seen in patients < 35 years, especially hypo- and hyperpigmented variants
- Sex
  - M:F = 2:1
- Ethnicity
  - Incidence is 1.7x higher in African Americans than in Caucasians

Presentation

- Premycotic period
  - Nonspecific skin lesions; often slight scaling, pruritus
    - Lesions can wax and wane for years; may never progress to MF
    - Skin biopsy findings are nondiagnostic
- Stepwise evolution of disease with development of patches, plaques, and tumors
  - Patches
    - Mostly on trunk but can arise anywhere on body, including palms and toes
    - Can be associated with alopecia
  - Plaques
    - Palpable lesions rise above skin surface
    - Can be associated with patch lesions
  - Tumors
    - Usually manifest as skin nodule(s)
    - Can coexist with patches and plaques
- MF variants
  - **Pagetoid reticulosis (localized)**
    - Also referred to as Woringer-Kolopp disease
    - Solitary, slow-growing, psoriasiform, crusty or hyperkeratotic patch or plaque
    - Often arises on distal limb
  - **Folliculotropic (pilotropic) MF**
    - Often involves head and neck area
    - Follicular papules (often grouped), alopecia, and acneiform lesions
    - Clinically more aggressive than other MF types; responds less well to skin-directed therapy
  - **Syringotropic MF**
    - Solitary, well-circumscribed, red-brown plaque, often associated with alopecia
    - Skin-directed therapy may be inadequate (similar to folliculotropic MF)
  - **Granulomatous slack skin**
    - Circumscribed areas of pendulous folds of lax skin in intertriginous areas (axillae, groin)
    - May coexist with classic MF lesions or classic Hodgkin lymphoma

Laboratory Tests

- Morphologic assessment of peripheral blood for Sézary cells
  - Insensitive
- Flow cytometry immunophenotypic analysis
  - Aberrant T-cell immunophenotypes support involvement by MF
- Assessment of T-cell clonality by PCR
- Serum lactate dehydrogenase &/or β-2-microglobulin
  - High levels associated with poorer prognosis

Natural History

- Evolution from patches to plaques to tumors over time
- Some patients develop visceral involvement by MF
  - Most common sites: Lungs, liver, spleen

Treatment

- Early-stage disease (stages I and IIA): Direct skin therapy
  - Topical chemotherapy with nitrogen mustard or carmustine
  - Topical corticosteroids and retinoids
  - Phototherapy; local radiation (radiograph or electron beam)
- Advanced-stage disease (stages IIB-IV)
  - Extracorporeal photopheresis
  - Single-agent chemotherapy
    - Methotrexate, pegylated liposomal doxorubicin (Doxil), purine analogs (fludarabine, 2-deoxycoformycin), others
  - Combination chemotherapy: Many regimens have been used
    - Cyclophosphamide, doxorubicin, vincristine, and prednisone
    - Cyclophosphamide, vincristine, and prednisone (CVP)
  - Hematopoietic stem cell transplantation

Prognosis

- Indolent clinical course overall
- Disease prognosis depends on clinical stage
- Clinical significance of T-cell receptor (*TCR*) gene rearrangements in MF staging is controversial
  - Monoclonal *TCR* gene rearrangement in blood is extremely common in early-stage disease
    - Not synonymous with blood involvement by MF in absence of morphologic or immunophenotypic evidence of disease
  - Monoclonal *TCR* gene rearrangement in lymph nodes is common finding
    - Not prognostically significant in multivariate analysis

MACROSCOPIC

General Features

- Patches
  - Circumscribed lesions with discoloration of variable size, color, and shape
  - Little scaling, not palpable
- Plaques
  - Palpable infiltrate of variable stage (thin and thick)
- Tumors
  - Often exophytic and ulcerated (hence, term fungoides)

MICROSCOPIC

Histologic Features of Skin

- Premycotic stage
  - Biopsy findings are typically nondiagnostic
  - Mild lymphocytic infiltrate
    - Mainly in upper dermis, not in subepidermal zone
    - Lacks obvious epidermotropism
- Patch and early (thin) plaque stage
  - Superficial band-like or lichenoid infiltrate of lymphocytes and histiocytes
    - Atypical lymphocytes often line up along basilar layer, especially at tips of rete ridges
    - Epidermotropism by single cells
    - Neoplastic lymphocytes are small, slightly cerebriform, some with perinuclear halos
  - Other changes
    - Mild acanthosis, hyperkeratosis; basal layer damage
    - Edema and fibrosis, increased postcapillary venules
  - In some early lesions, biopsy findings may be nondiagnostic
- Thick plaque stage
  - Dense, subepidermal, band-like infiltrate with many cerebriform lymphocytes
  - Epidermotropism is more prominent
    - Intraepidermal clusters and Pautrier microabscesses
    - Confluent Pautrier microabscesses that can result in subcorneal and subepidermal bullae
- Tumor stage
  - Dermal infiltrate becomes more diffuse and prominent
    - Tumor cells range in size from small to large
  - Epidermotropism may be lost
  - Large cell transformation
    - Often occurs in tumor stage
    - Large cells comprise ≥ 25% of tumor
    - CD30 often positive (but not necessary for diagnosis); high proliferation rate (by Ki-67)
- **MF variants**
  - **Pagetoid reticulosis**
    - Marked intraepidermal proliferation of T cells
    - Sponge-like disaggregation of epidermis
    - Atypical cells have medium- or large-sized, hyperchromatic, and cerebriform nuclei
    - Often CD8(+) but may be CD4(+) in some cases
    - Often CD30(+); Ki-67 > 30%
  - **Folliculotropic MF (pilotropic MF)**
    - Atypical lymphocyte infiltrating epithelium of hair follicles
    - Infiltrate often spares epidermis
    - Often (but not always) associated with mucinosis (follicular mucinosis)
    - Often many eosinophils present
  - **Syringotropic MF**
    - Hyperplastic eccrine ducts and glands infiltrated by atypical lymphocytes
    - Often abundant eosinophils present
    - Often seen in combination with folliculotropic MF
  - **Granulomatous slack skin**
    - Dense granulomatous dermal infiltrate containing atypical T cells, macrophages, and often many multinucleated giant cells
    - Infiltrate often shows destruction of elastic tissue; ± epidermotropism
    - CD4(+), CD8(-)
  - **Hypopigmented and hyperpigmented MF**
    - Similar to conventional MF but with postinflammatory pigment incontinence
    - Typically CD8(+), CD4(-)

Histologic Features of Lymph Nodes

- Best to biopsy lymph nodes draining area of involved skin or node with highest standardized uptake value on FDG PET scan
- Early involvement by MF (N1 and N2)
  - LN architecture is well maintained
  - Dermatopathic changes common
  - Cerebriform lymphocytes are either absent, singly scattered, or in small clusters or aggregates
    - Often difficult to identify morphologically
- Ancillary testing is important to demonstrate involvement by MF
  - Flow cytometric immunophenotyping
  - Assessment for *TCR* gene rearrangement
- Extensive involvement by MF (N3)
  - Overt involvement or complete effacement of architecture
  - May show large cell transformation

Cytologic Features

- Small- to medium-sized lymphocytes (unless large cell transformation)
- Cerebriform nuclear contours and hyperchromatic nuclei

ANCILLARY TESTS

Immunohistochemistry

- CD4(+), CD8(-)
  - Some cases can be CD4(-)/CD8(+); rarely CD4(+)/CD8(+) or CD4(-)/CD8(-)
- CD2(+), CD3(+), CD5(+/-), βF1(+)
- Often shows CD7 loss (all disease stages)
- CD45/LCA(+), CLA(+), CD25(-/+)
- CD30(+/-), usually expressed by large cells
- Ig(-), B-cell antigens (-)

Flow Cytometry

- Can be performed on skin, peripheral blood, lymph nodes, and other tissue specimens
- Flow panel should include
  - CD2, CD3, CD4, CD5, CD7

- CD8, CD25, CD26, TCR-αβ, TCR-γδ
- CD4:CD8 ratio is often increased
- Typical immunophenotype: CD3(+), CD4(+), CD8(-), CD5(+), TCR-αβ(+)
- Frequent immunophenotypic aberrancies
  - CD26(-), loss of CD7
  - Dim expression of CD2, CD3, CD4, or CD5

Genetic Testing

- Monoclonal *TCR* gene rearrangements
- Inactivation of *CDKN2A* (P16) or *PTEN* in subsets of cases

DIFFERENTIAL DIAGNOSIS

Drug Reactions, Inflammatory Dermatoses

- Exocytosis of lymphocytes can simulate MF, but there is often background of spongiosis &/or interface changes
- Perivascular lymphocytic infiltrate
- Often increased numbers of eosinophils in dermis
- Dyskeratotic keratinocytes and parakeratosis may or may not be present

Lymphomatoid Papulosis, Type B

- Recurrent, self-healing, waxing and waning lesions
  - Papular, papulonecrotic, &/or nodular skin lesions at different stages of development
- Morphological features
  - Often wedge-shaped infiltrate in dermis
  - Epidermotropic infiltrate of small atypical cells with cerebriform nuclei similar to MF
- Immunophenotype: T-cell antigens (+), TCR-αβ(+), TCL1(+); CD30 often negative
- Differential diagnosis in some cases can only be made by obtaining complete clinical information

Cutaneous Anaplastic Large Cell Lymphoma

- Cases of MF with large cell transformation can be uniformly CD30(+), similar to cutaneous anaplastic large cell lymphoma (C-ALCL)
- Clinical findings are different: Usually single nodule in C-ALCL, patches/plaques in MF

Primary Cutaneous γ/δ T-Cell Lymphoma

- Clinical presentation
  - Patients often present with generalized skin lesions, preferentially affecting extremities
  - Disease may be predominantly epidermotropic and present with patches/plaques that simulate MF
- Morphologic features
  - Can be epidermotropic, dermal, or subcutaneous infiltrate
  - Medium to large atypical lymphoid cells with coarse chromatin
  - Apoptosis and necrosis are common
- Immunophenotype
  - CD2(+), CD3(+), CD7(+/-), CD56(+), TCR-γδ(+)
  - Cytotoxic proteins(+), CD30(-/+)
  - CD4(-), CD5(-), CD8(-), TCR-αβ/βF1(-)

Primary Cutaneous Aggressive Epidermotropic CD8(+) Cytotoxic T-Cell Lymphoma

- Clinical presentation
  - Generalized skin lesions
  - Eruptive papules, nodules, and tumors with central ulceration and necrosis
  - May disseminate to other visceral sites but often spares lymph nodes
- Morphological features
  - Variable, ranging from lichenoid pattern to marked, pagetoid epidermotropism and subepidermal to deeper nodular infiltrates
  - Epidermis may show necrosis, ulceration, and blister formation
  - Tumor cells are small to medium in size
  - Angiocentricity and angioinvasion may be present, and tissue destruction is often present
- Immunophenotype
  - CD3(+), CD8(+), βF1(+)
  - Cytotoxic proteins (+), CD45RA(+/-), CD2(-/+), CD7(+/-)
  - CD4(-), CD5(-), CD45RO(-)

Primary Cutaneous Small/Medium Pleomorphic T-Cell Lymphoma

- Clinically indolent
  - Most cases present with solitary skin lesion; no evidence of patches and plaques typical of MF
    - Commonly on face, neck, or upper trunk
- Morphological features
  - Dense, diffuse, or nodular infiltrates within dermis with tendency to infiltrate subcutis
  - Epidermotropism may be present focally, but if conspicuous, more likely to be MF
  - Small-/medium-sized pleomorphic T cells
- Immunophenotype
  - CD3(+), CD4(+), CD8(-), βF1(+)

T-Cell Prolymphocytic Leukemia Involving Skin

- T-cell prolymphocytic leukemia (T-PLL) can involve skin, usually with dermal involvement, but epidermotropism can be seen
- Clinical history is helpful, as patients usually have history of T-PLL with
  - High peripheral blood leukocyte count; bone marrow involvement
- Immunophenotype: T-cell antigens (+), TCR-αβ(+), TCL1(+)

SELECTED REFERENCES

1. Desai M et al: Clinical characteristics, prognostic factors, and survival of 393 patients with mycosis fungoides and Sézary syndrome in the southeastern United States: A single-institution cohort. J Am Acad Dermatol. 72(2):276-85, 2015
2. Ahn CS et al: Mycosis fungoides: an updated review of clinicopathologic variants. Am J Dermatopathol. 36(12):933-48; quiz 949-51, 2014
3. Ally MS et al: A review of the solitary cutaneous T-cell lymphomas. J Cutan Pathol. 41(9):703-14, 2014
4. Feng B et al: Flow cytometric detection of peripheral blood involvement by mycosis fungoides and Sézary syndrome using T-cell receptor Vbeta chain antibodies and its application in blood staging. Mod Pathol. 23(2):284-95, 2010
5. Nikolaou VA et al: Clinical characteristics and course of CD8+ cytotoxic variant of mycosis fungoides: a case series of seven patients. Br J Dermatol. 161(4):826-30, 2009
6. Gerami P et al: The spectrum of histopathologic and immunohistochemical findings in folliculotropic mycosis fungoides. Am J Surg Pathol. 31(9):1430-8, 2007

TNMB Staging of Mycosis Fungoides

Tumor Stage (T)	
T1	Limited patches, papules, &/or plaques covering < 10% of skin surface; may further stratify into T1a (patch only) vs. T1b (plaque ± patch)
T2	Patches, papules, or plaques covering ≥ 10% of skin surface; may further stratify into T2a (patch only) vs. T2b (plaque ± patch)
T3	≥ 1 tumors (1-cm diameter)
T4	Confluence of erythema covering 80% of body surface area
Lymph Node Stage* (Lymph Nodes > 1.5 cm in Greatest Dimension) (N)	
N0	No clinically abnormal peripheral lymph nodes; biopsy not required
N1	Dermatopathic lymphadenopathy; none or few scattered atypical cerebriform mononuclear cells with nuclei > 7.5 μm
N2	Dermatopathic lymphadenopathy; aggregates or clusters of atypical cerebriform mononuclear cells with nuclei > 7.5 μm; architecture is preserved
N3	Partial or complete effacement of architecture with many atypical lymphocytes
Extracutaneous Disease (Visceral Involvement) (M)	
M0	No visceral organ involvement
M1	Visceral involvement (must have pathologic confirmation)
	Bone marrow involvement has not been considered as visceral involvement by ISCL/EORTC
Blood Stage (B)	
B0	Absence of significant blood involvement: 5% of peripheral blood lymphocytes are atypical (Sézary) cells
B1	Low blood tumor burden: > 5% of peripheral blood lymphocytes are atypical (Sézary) cells, but < 1,000/μL, or > 1,000/μL atypical cells with no clonality
B2	High blood tumor burden: ≥ 1,000/μL Sézary cells with positive clonality studies

**Central adenopathy may be secondary to a 2nd malignancy (especially lymphoma), infection, or a reactive process. The ISCL/EORTC recommends that central enlarged nodes be excluded from the determination of "N" status, except in cases where an excisional biopsy of a central node has proven lymphomatous (N3) involvement with MF.*

Clinical Staging of Patients With Mycosis Fungoides (ISCL/EORTC)*

Stage	T	N	M	B	Clinical Presentation
Stage I					
IA	T1	N0	M0	B0 or B1	Disease confined to skin with patches/papules/plaques < 10% of skin surface; no clinically abnormal lymph nodes
IB	T2	N0	M0	B0 or B1	Disease confined to skin with patches/papules/plaques > 10% of skin surface; no clinically abnormal lymph nodes
Stage II					
IIA	T1 or T2	N1 or N2	M0	B0 or B1	Skin involvement with patches/papules/plaques associated with no or early lymph node involvement
IIB	T3	N0 to N2	M0	B0 or B1	Skin involvement with patches/papules/plaques and with ≥ 1 or more tumors (> 1 cm) associated with no or early lymph node involvement
Stage III					
IIIA	T4	N0 to N2	M0	B0	Skin involvement with erythroderma, no or early lymph node involvement, and absent blood tumor burden (< 5% Sézary cells)
IIIB	T4	N0 to N2	M0	B0	Skin involvement with erythroderma, no or early (N1-N2) lymph node involvement, and low blood tumor burden (> 5% but < 1,000/μL circulating Sézary cells)
Stage IV					
IVA1	T1 to T4	N0 to N2	M0	B2	High blood tumor burden (> 1,000/μL circulating Sézary cells) with no or early lymph node involvement and no visceral involvement
IVA2	T1 to T4	N3	M0	B0 to B2	High blood tumor burden (> 1,000/μL circulating Sézary cells) with extensive lymph node involvement and no visceral involvement
IVB	T1 to T4	N0 to N3	M1	B0 to B2	High blood tumor burden (> 1,000/μL circulating Sézary cells) ± extensive lymph node involvement and positive for visceral involvement

**ISCL and the Cutaneous Lymphoma Task Force of the EORTC.*

Mycosis Fungoides With Prominent Epidermotropism

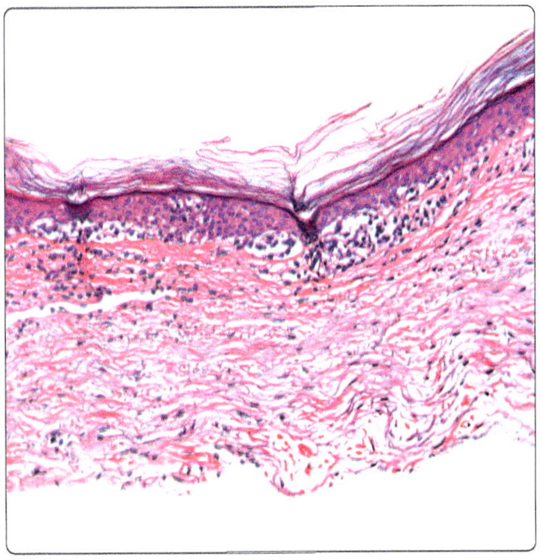

CD4 Immunohistochemistry in Mycosis Fungoides

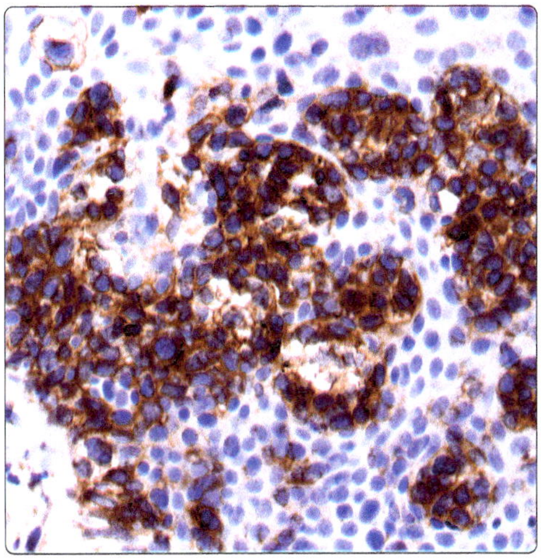

(Left) *Later patch stage and early plaque stage of MF shows intraepidermal clusters of atypical lymphocytes. There is only a mild superficial dermal infiltrate.* **(Right)** *Immunohistochemistry in the plaque stage of MF shows that the intraepidermal atypical lymphocytes within Pautrier microabscesses are CD4(+).*

Clinical Photograph of Tumor Stage Mycosis Fungoides

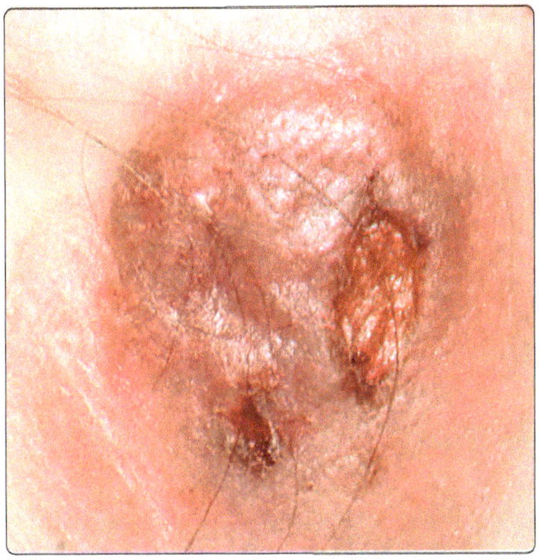

Tumor Stage Mycosis Fungoides

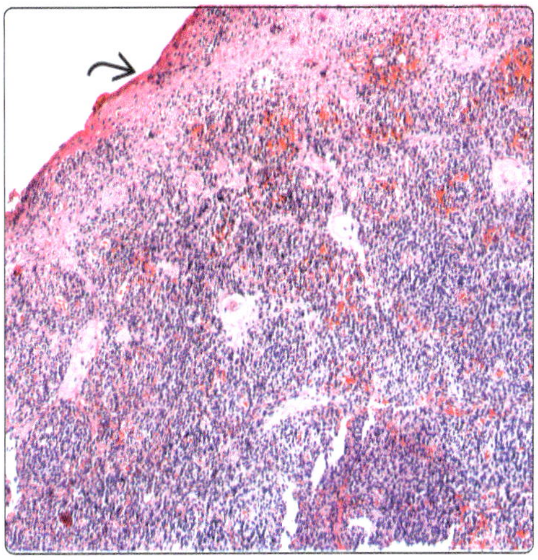

(Left) *Clinical photograph of the tumor stage is shown in a patient with MF.* **(Right)** *The tumor stage of MF shows a diffuse and prominent dermal infiltrate. Also present is dermal hemorrhage and focal overlying epidermal erosion* ➔.

Tumor Stage Mycosis Fungoides at High Magnification

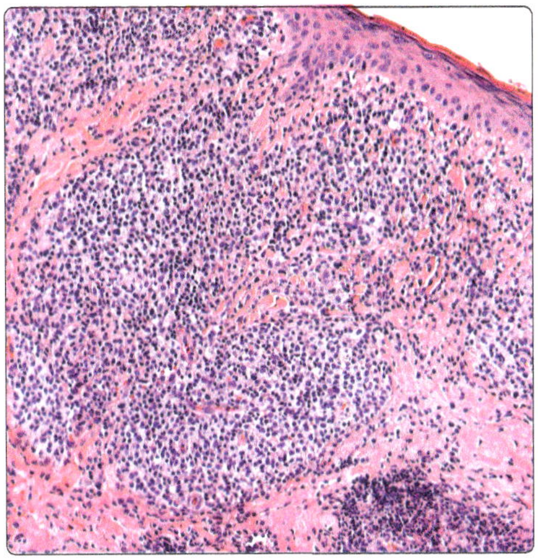

Large Cell Transformation in Mycosis Fungoides

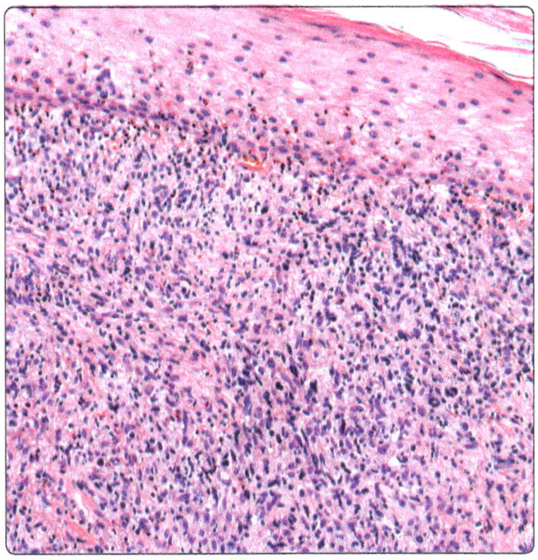

(Left) *Higher power view of the tumor stage of MF with large cell transformation shows no significant epidermotropism but a proliferation of large, atypical cells growing in sheets in the dermis.* **(Right)** *Another case of MF with large cell transformation shows a diffuse dermal infiltrate with increased numbers of large cells. There is no significant epidermotropism.*

(Left) *This is an example of MF with large cell transformation at high magnification. The tumor cells are large and pleomorphic-appearing, with angulated nuclei and nuclear hyperchromasia* ➡*.* **(Right)** *Immunohistochemistry in MF with large cell transformation shows that the large tumor cells are strongly CD3(+).*

Large Cell Transformation in Mycosis Fungoides at High Magnification

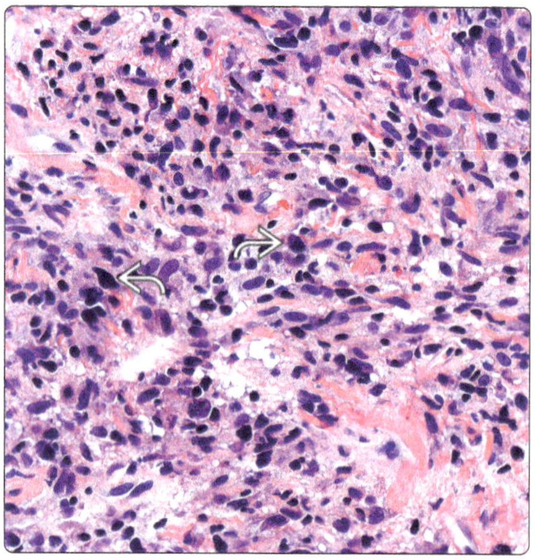

CD3 Immunohistochemistry in Mycosis Fungoides With Large Cell Transformation

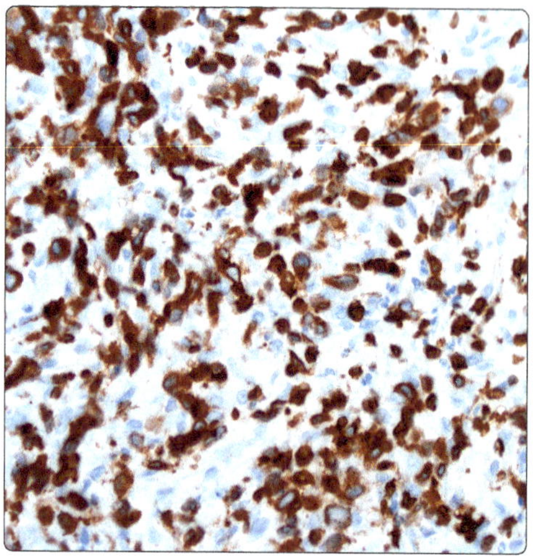

(Left) *In MF with large cell transformation, the large tumor cells are CD7(-), with only small reactive T cells staining.* **(Right)** *The large tumor cells are strongly CD30(+) in MF with large cell transformation; the lesional cells in large cell transformation often, but not always, show CD30 expression.*

CD7 Immunohistochemistry in Mycosis Fungoides With Large Cell Transformation

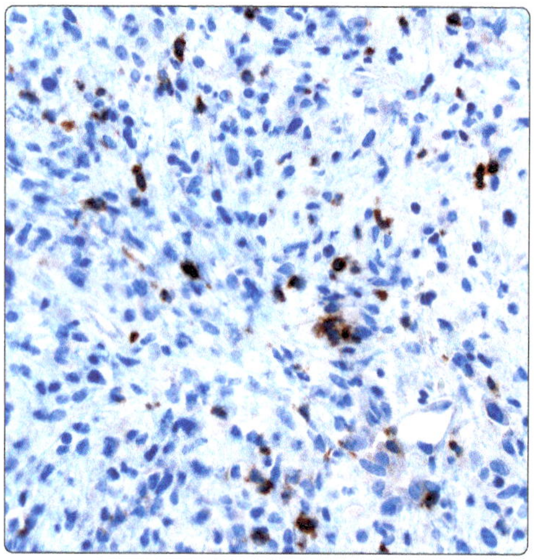

CD30 Immunohistochemistry in Mycosis Fungoides With Large Cell Transformation

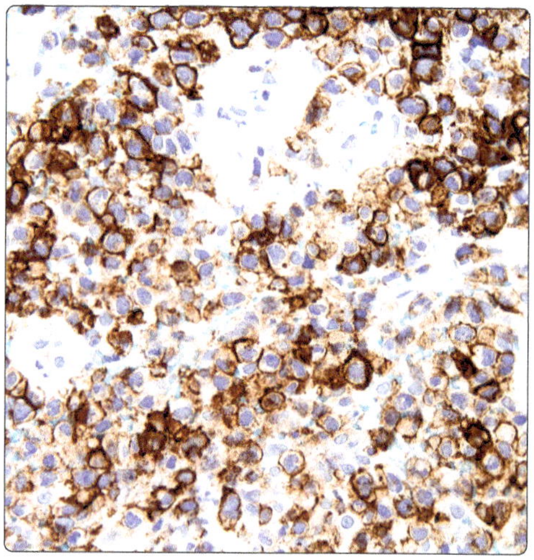

(Left) *In MF with large cell transformation, the large tumor cells are often CD25(+).* **(Right)** *A case of folliculotropic MF (pilotropic mycosis fungoides) shows a lymphocytic infiltrate predominantly in and around the hair follicles* ➡*, with relative sparing of the interfollicular skin* ➡*.*

CD25 Immunohistochemistry in Mycosis Fungoides With Large Cell Transformation

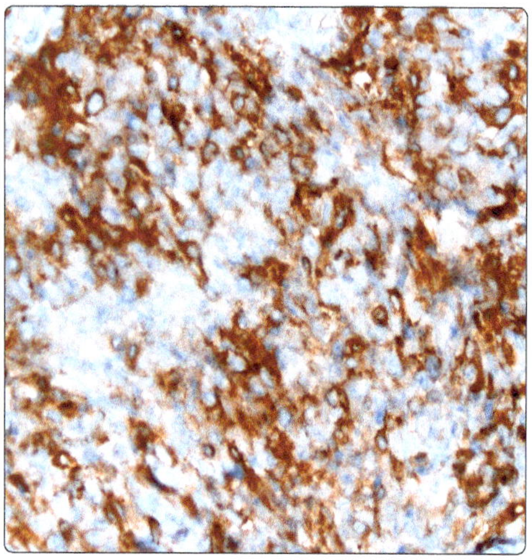

Folliculotropic Mycosis Fungoides

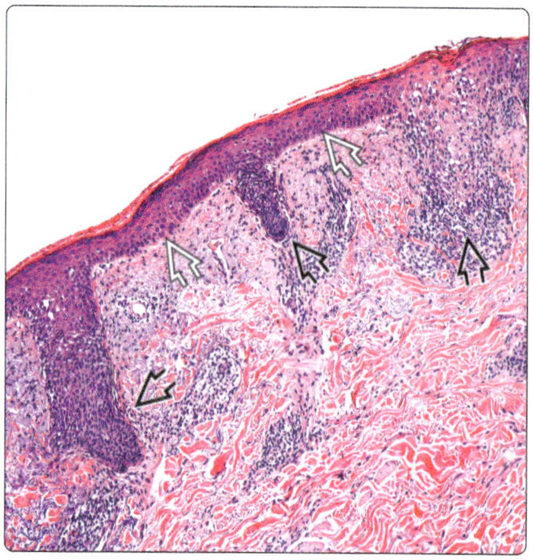

Folliculotropic Mycosis Fungoides With Prominent Folliculotropism

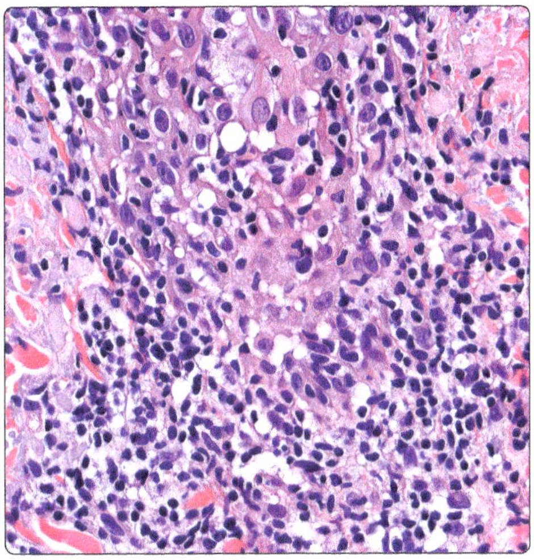

Folliculotropic Mycosis Fungoides at High Magnification

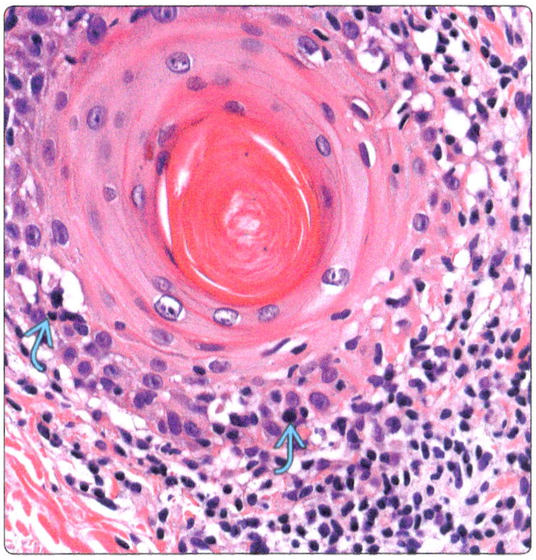

(Left) *Folliculotropic MF shows atypical lymphocytes within and surrounding the follicular epithelium.* **(Right)** *A cornified hair follicle is infiltrated by atypical lymphocytes ➜ in folliculotropic MF on high-power examination.*

Syringotropic Mycosis Fungoides

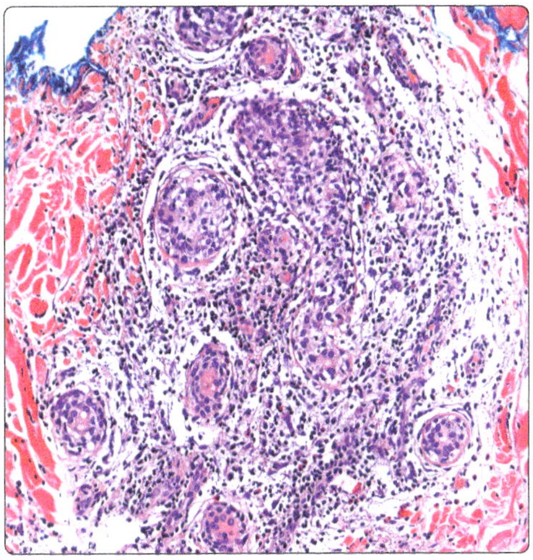

Syringotropic Mycosis Fungoides at High Magnification

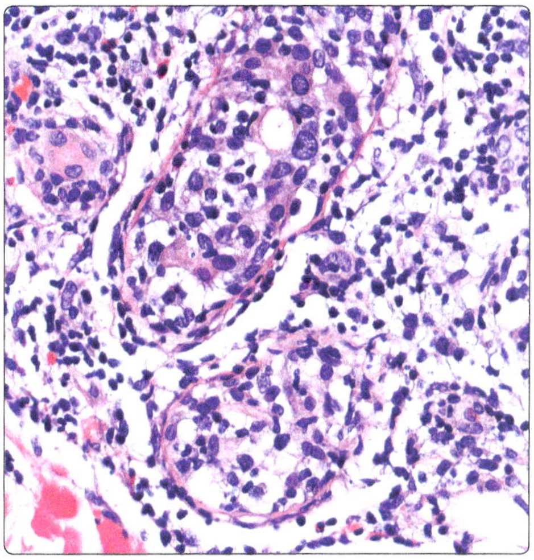

(Left) *This case of the syringotropic variant of MF shows a lymphocytic infiltrate predominantly surrounding and infiltrating eccrine sweat glands.* **(Right)** *Higher magnification of the syringotropic type of MF shows atypical small cerebriform lymphocytes involving and surrounding eccrine glands.*

Granulomatous Slack Skin Variant of Mycosis Fungoides

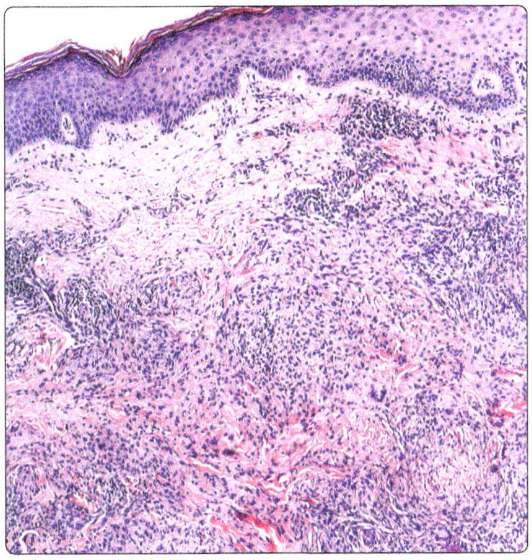

Granulomatous Slack Skin

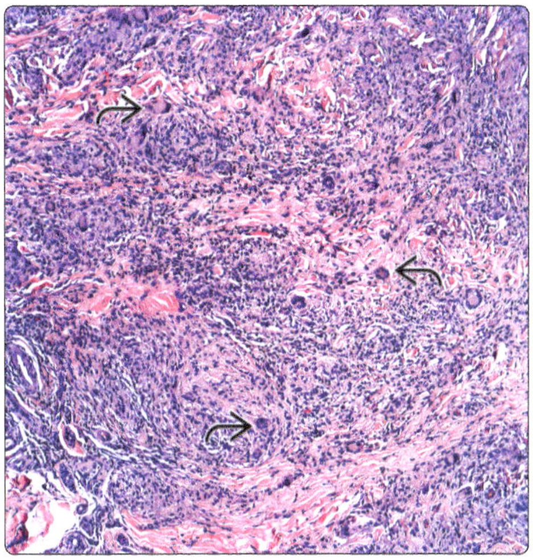

(Left) *Granulomatous slack skin disease is a rare variant of MF. This is an advanced-stage lesion and shows a dense lymphohistiocytic infiltrate in the dermis.* **(Right)** *Granulomatous slack skin disease shows a dense lymphohistiocytic infiltrate extending to the deep dermis, with many giant cells ➜ easily identified.*

(Left) *Granulomatous slack skin disease often shows giant cells containing 20-30 nuclei. Some of the giant cells have nuclei localized in the periphery of the cytoplasm. Focal elastophagocytosis is present ⇗. The lymphocytes between the giant cells are small without pronounced cytological atypia.* **(Right)** *Immunohistochemistry in granulomatous slack skin variant of MF shows that the infiltrating lymphocytes are strongly CD3(+); the giant cells are negative.*

Giant Cells in Granulomatous Slack Skin

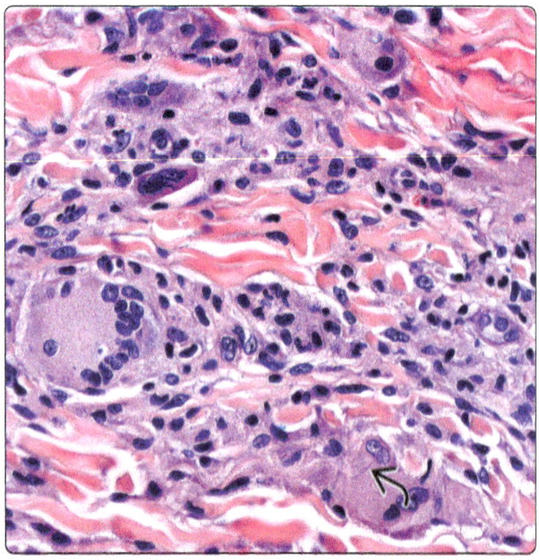

CD3 Immunohistochemistry in Granulomatous Slack Skin

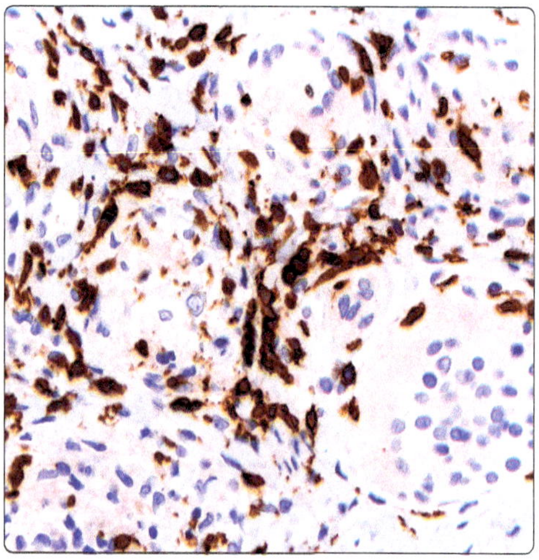

(Left) *Pagetoid reticulosis is a slow-growing, psoriasiform, crusty patch or plaque typically found on the distal limb. Note the hyperkeratotic and parakeratotic epithelium with marked exocytosis of numerous lymphocytes.* **(Right)** *High magnification of pagetoid reticulosis shows that the infiltrating lymphocytes are atypical-appearing and small to medium in size, with perinuclear halos.*

Pagetoid Reticulosis Variant of Mycosis Fungoides

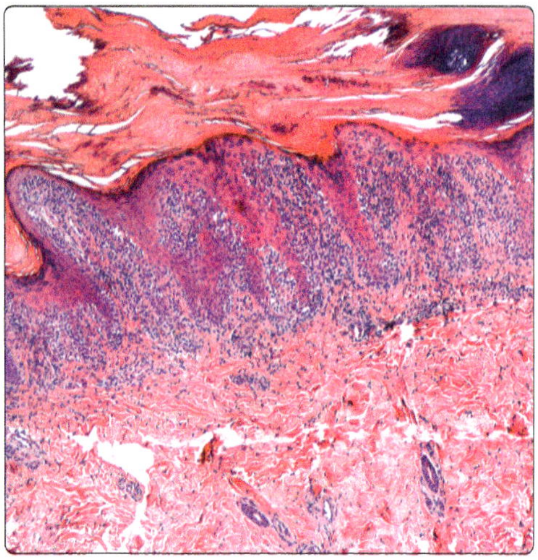

Pagetoid Reticulosis at High Magnification

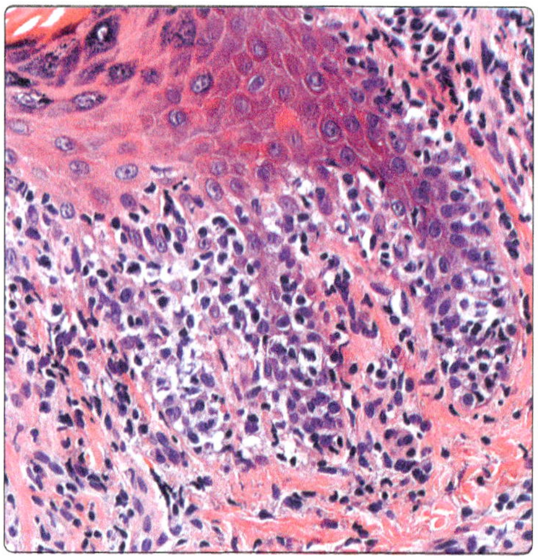

(Left) *As in this case, the lymphocytes in pagetoid reticulosis are typically CD3(+) and CD8(+) (not shown); however, CD8(-) pagetoid reticulosis is not uncommon.* **(Right)** *The atypical epidermotropic lymphocytes in pagetoid reticulosis are strongly and diffusely CD8(+).*

CD3 Immunohistochemistry in Pagetoid Reticulosis

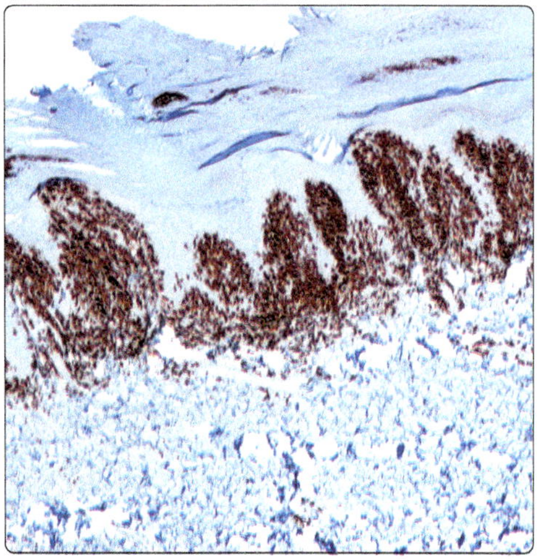

CD8 Immunohistochemistry in Pagetoid Reticulosis

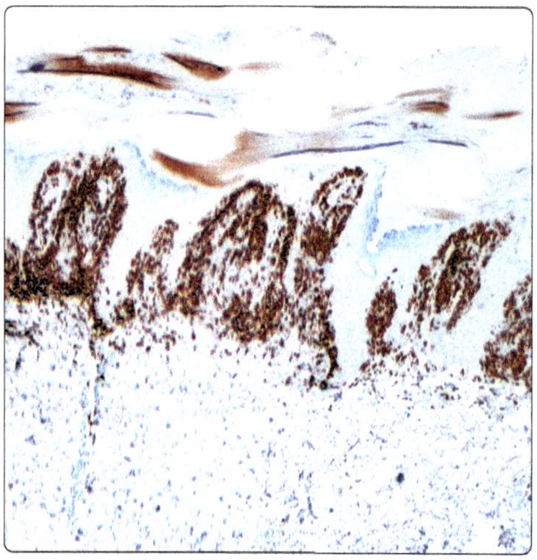

Mycosis Fungoides With CD8 Positivity

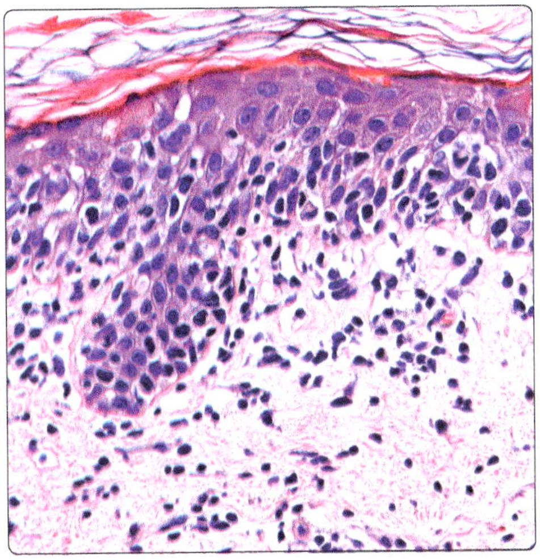

CD8 Staining in Mycosis Fungoides With CD8 Positivity

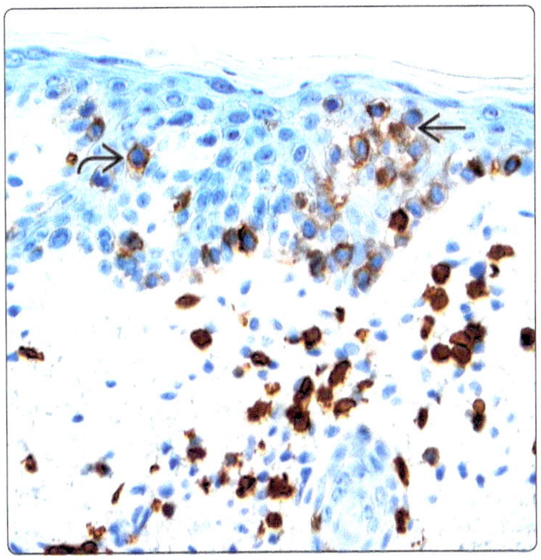

(Left) *This case of otherwise typical-appearing MF was CD8(+). The histologic features are identical to conventional CD4(+) MF, and they differ from pagetoid reticulosis and primary cutaneous aggressive epidermotropic CD8(+) cytotoxic T-cell lymphoma.* **(Right)** *This case of otherwise typical MF is CD8(+). The CD8 immunostain highlights the neoplastic intraepidermal T cells that express CD8 ⮳ more dimly than reactive CD8(+) T cells ⇨ in this field.*

Lymph Node With Dermatopathic Changes in Mycosis Fungoides

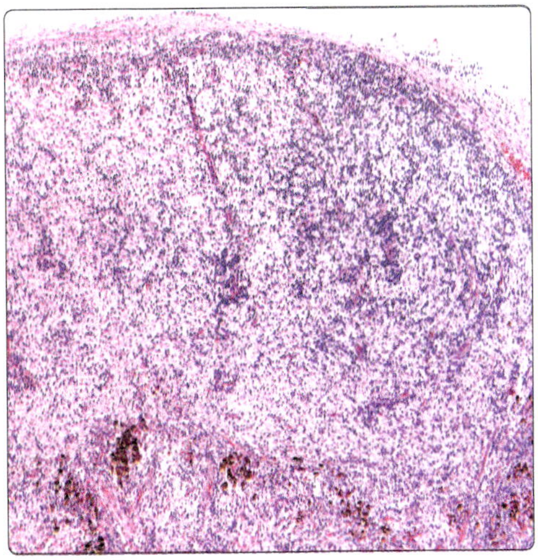

Lymph Node Changes in Mycosis Fungoides

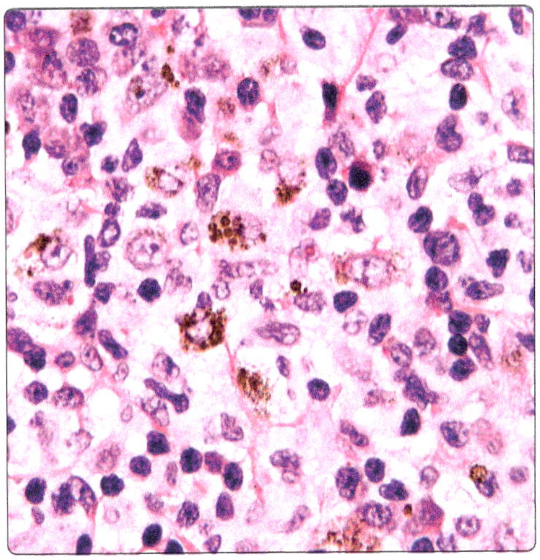

(Left) *This lymph node biopsy specimen from a patient with MF shows marked dermatopathic changes and maintained nodal architecture.* **(Right)** *Lymph node biopsy specimen from a patient with MF shows many interdigitating dendritic cells, Langerhans cells, and melanin-containing macrophages. The lymphocytes are not atypical. This would be interpreted as no histologic evidence of mycosis fungoides (N1).*

Lymph Node Involvement in Mycosis Fungoides

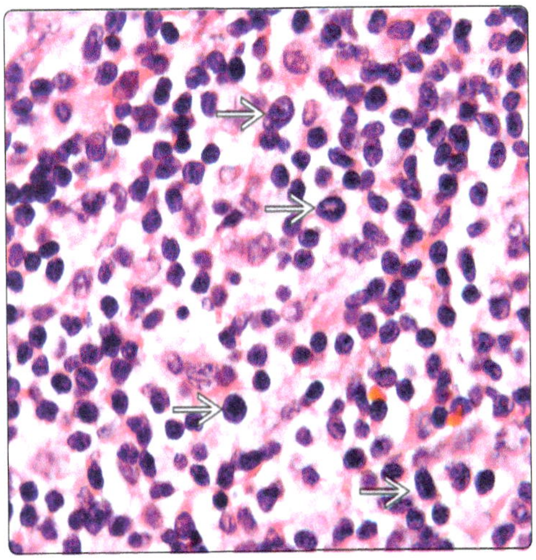

Lymph Node Involvement in Mycosis Fungoides

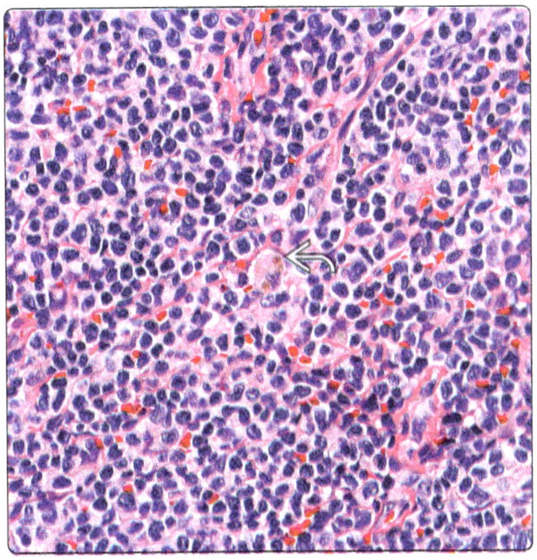

(Left) *Lymph node biopsy specimen from a patient with MF shows a few scattered, larger, atypical cells ➡. The histological grading of this involvement is still N1.* **(Right)** *Lymph node biopsy specimen from a patient with MF shows sheets of tumor cells present (N3). Macrophages containing melanin pigment ➡ are also present focally.*

Bone Marrow Involvement in Mycosis Fungoides

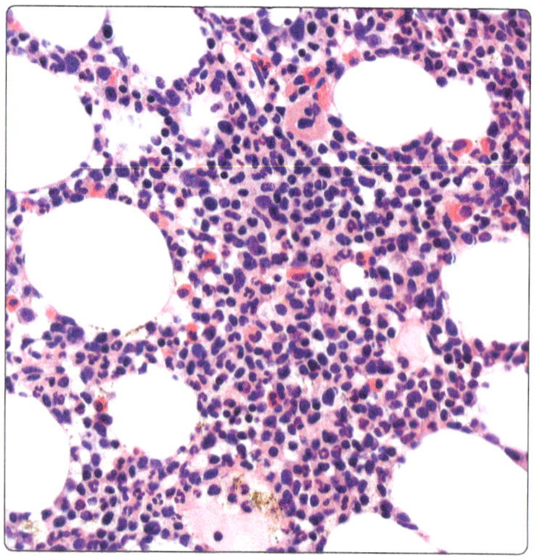

Bone Marrow Involvement in Mycosis Fungoides

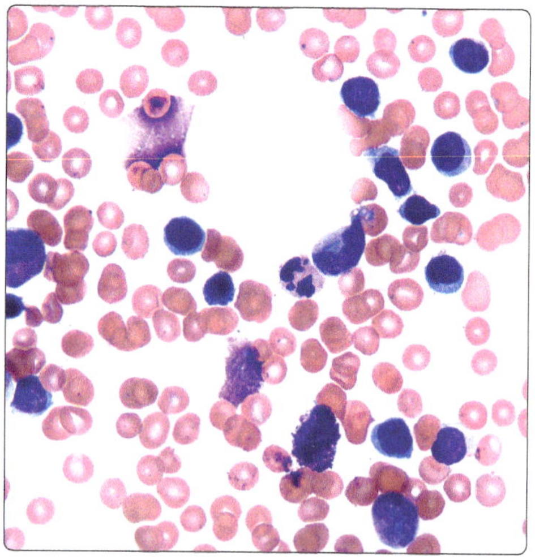

(Left) *Bone marrow involvement by MF is uncommon. When the bone marrow is involved, there often is an interstitial pattern of infiltration.* **(Right)** *Bone marrow aspirate smear reveals many atypical small- to medium-sized lymphocytes, consistent with involvement by MF.*

Sézary Cells in Peripheral Blood

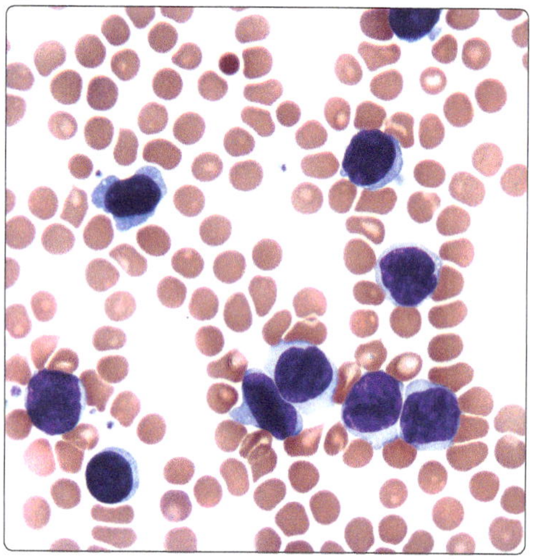

Peripheral Blood Lymphocytosis in Mycosis Fungoides

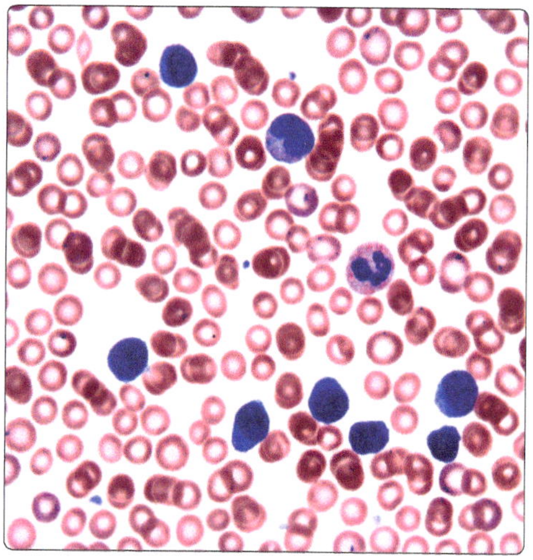

(Left) *Peripheral blood smear shows many large cerebriform (Sézary) cells, consistent with MF in the leukemic phase (so-called secondary Sézary syndrome).* **(Right)** *Peripheral blood smear in a case of MF shows lymphocytosis. The lymphocytes are small with round nuclei and lack typical Sézary cell morphology. However, flow cytometry and molecular studies confirmed the lymphocytes to be neoplastic T cells.*

Differential Diagnosis: CD8(+) Cytotoxic T-Cell Lymphoma

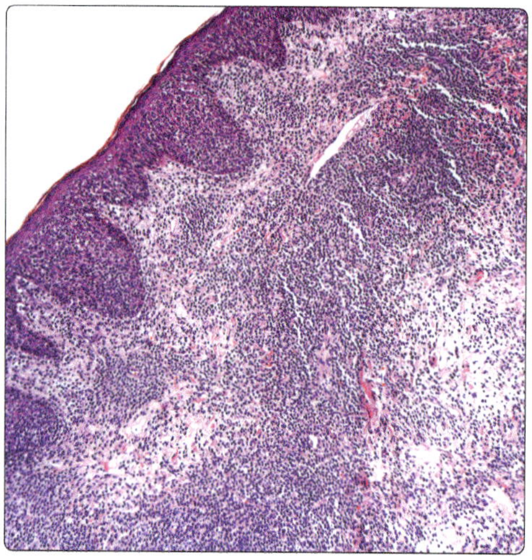

Differential Diagnosis: CD8(+) Cytotoxic T-Cell Lymphoma

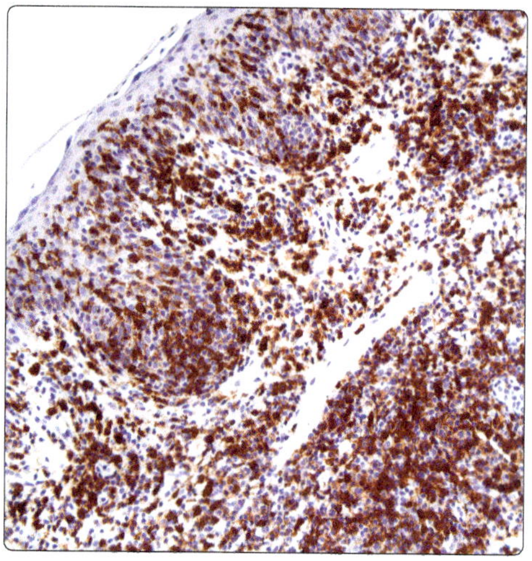

(Left) *Primary cutaneous aggressive epidermotropic CD8(+) cytotoxic T-cell lymphoma shows a pronounced epidermal and dermal infiltrate.* **(Right)** *Immunohistochemistry in primary cutaneous aggressive epidermotropic CD8(+) cytotoxic T-cell lymphoma shows that the lymphoma cells are very strongly CD8(+).*

CD8(+) Cytotoxic T-Cell Lymphoma

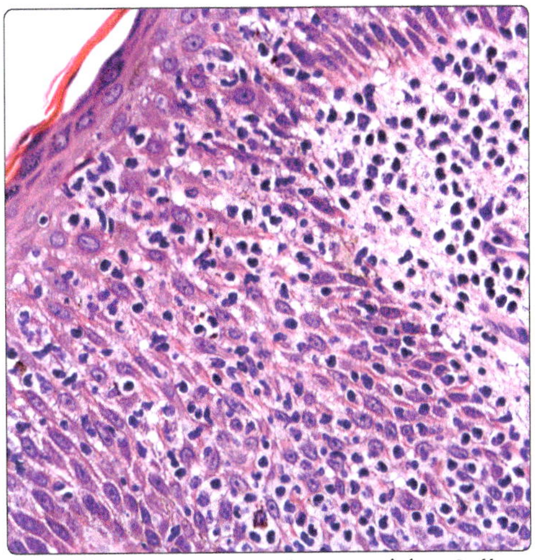

CD8(+) Cytotoxic T-Cell Lymphoma in Dermis

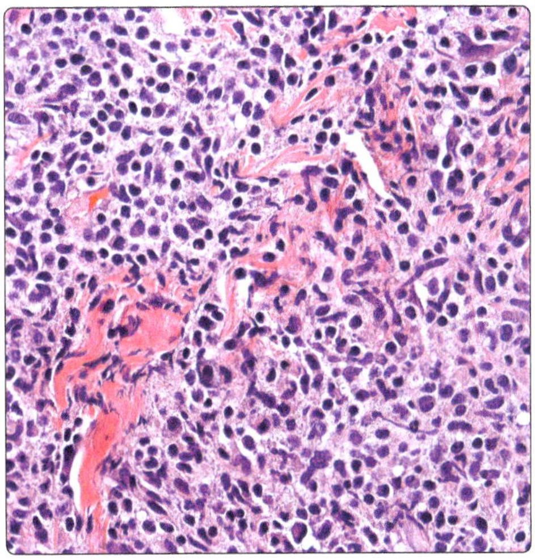

(Left) *Primary cutaneous aggressive epidermotropic CD8(+) cytotoxic T-cell lymphoma shows atypical epidermotropic lymphoid cells, which are small- to medium-sized, with irregular nuclear contours, and diffusely infiltrate the epidermis.* **(Right)** *The atypical lymphoid cells also diffusely infiltrate the dermis. Morphologically, the cells are medium-sized, angulated, and show nuclear atypia and pleomorphism.*

Differential Diagnosis: CD30(+) T-Cell Lymphoproliferative Disorder (Lymphomatoid Papulosis)

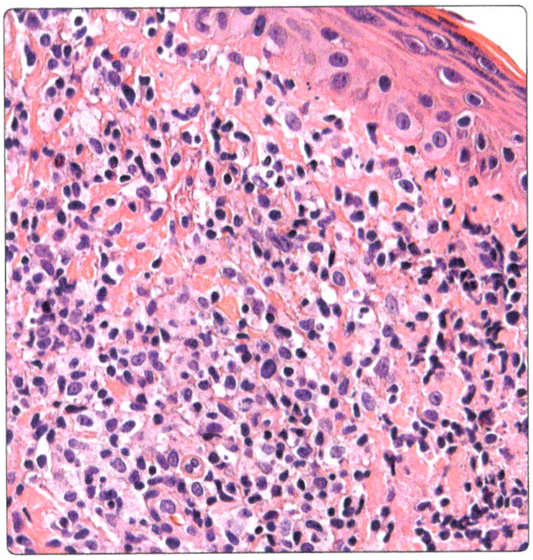

CD30 Immunohistochemistry in Lymphomatoid Papulosis

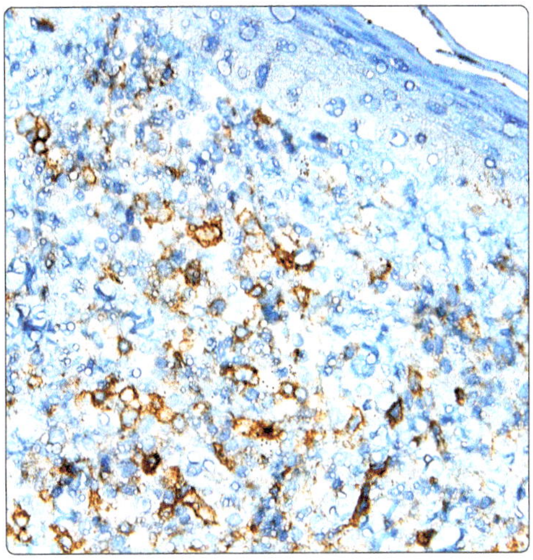

(Left) *This is an example of a primary cutaneous CD30(+) T-cell lymphoproliferative disorder, consistent with lymphomatoid papulosis (LyP), type A. The dermal infiltrate consists of a mixture of small lymphocytes, histiocytes, and scattered large cells.* **(Right)** *In this primary cutaneous CD30(+) T-cell lymphoproliferative disorder (consistent with LyP, type A), CD30 highlights scattered large cells.*

CD30(+) Lymphoproliferative Disorder (Anaplastic Large Cell Lymphoma)

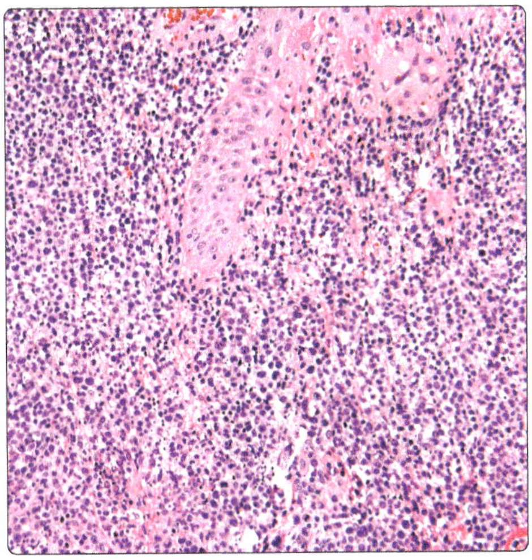

CD30 Immunohistochemistry in Anaplastic Large Cell Lymphoma

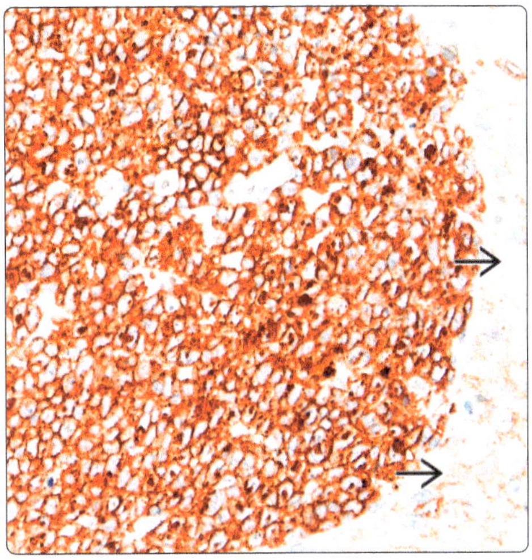

(Left) *This is an example of a cutaneous anaplastic large cell lymphoma (C-ALCL). Some cases of MF with large cell transformation can be uniformly CD30(+) and mimic C-ALCL. History of MF or evidence of MF elsewhere in the patient, or at the margins of the lesion in the biopsy, is helpful in this differential diagnosis.* **(Right)** *The neoplastic cells in C-ALCL are strongly and uniformly CD30(+); note the epidermis present at the right* ⇒.

Adult T-Cell Leukemia/Lymphoma

KEY FACTS

ETIOLOGY/PATHOGENESIS

- Long latency period between HTLV-I infection & tumor development
- Small risk of adult T-cell leukemia/lymphoma (ATLL) in human T-cell leukemia virus type I (HTLV-I) infected people
- Tax viral oncoprotein linked to tumorigenesis

CLINICAL ISSUES

- 4 clinical presentations: Acute, chronic, lymphomatous, & smoldering
- Skin lesions are mostly in acute & lymphomatous subtypes

MICROSCOPIC

- Atypical T-cell infiltrate in epidermis, dermis, &/or subcutis
  - Epidermotropism &/or Pautrier microabscesses
- Peripheral blood with multilobated "flower cells"
- Lymph nodes with effaced architecture & diffuse infiltrate

ANCILLARY TESTS

- Confirmation of HTLV-I infection by serology
- Immunophenotype
  - Regulatory T cells CD3(+), CD4(+), CD25(+), FOXP3(+), CD194(+)
  - Often lose CD7 expression
  - Cytotoxic markers (-)
- Clonal T-cell receptor gene rearrangement

TOP DIFFERENTIAL DIAGNOSES

- Mycosis fungoides
  - Similar clinical picture with epidermotropism & peripheral blood lymphocytosis
  - Also CD4(+), CD8(-) T cells, but CD25(-), FOXP3(-), & CD30(-)
- Anaplastic large cell lymphoma
  - FOXP3(-), CD194(-); ALK1 & EMA(+/-), unlike ATLL

Clinical Photograph of Adult T-Cell Leukemia/Lymphoma

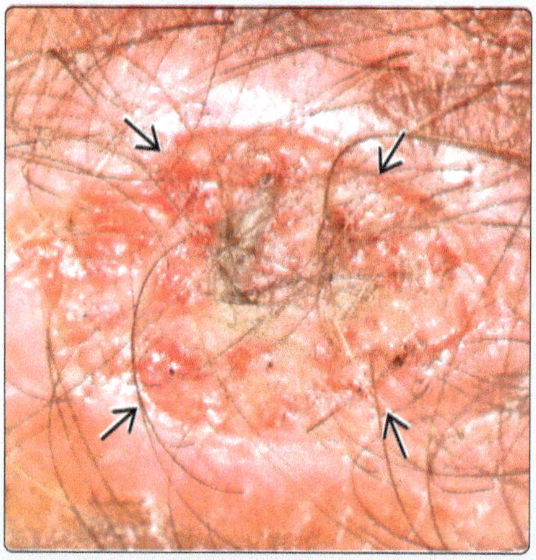

Epithelial Involvement in Adult T-Cell Leukemia/Lymphoma

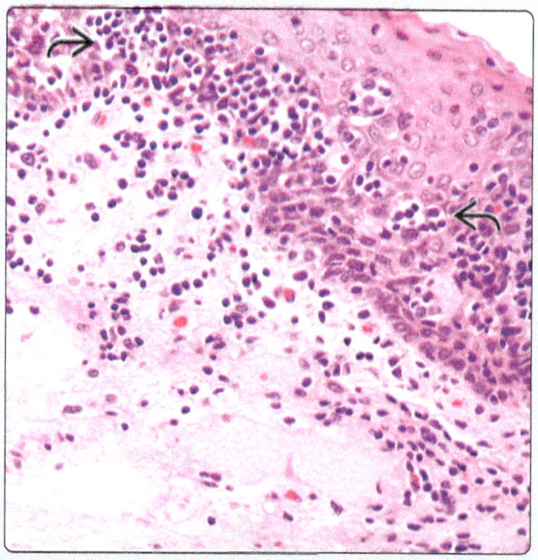

(Left) *This clinical photograph shows an ulcerating lesion, which is 2.5 cm in the greatest dimension, from the foot of a person from the Caribbean region who was human T-cell leukemia virus type I (HTLV-I) (+).* **(Right)** *This adult T-cell leukemia/lymphoma (ATLL) involves the mucosal epithelium. Note the small lymphocytes with irregular hyperchromatic nuclei infiltrating the squamous mucosa, forming Pautrier-like microabscesses. (Courtesy C. Bueso-Ramos, MD.)*

Adult T-Cell Leukemia/Lymphoma at High Magnification

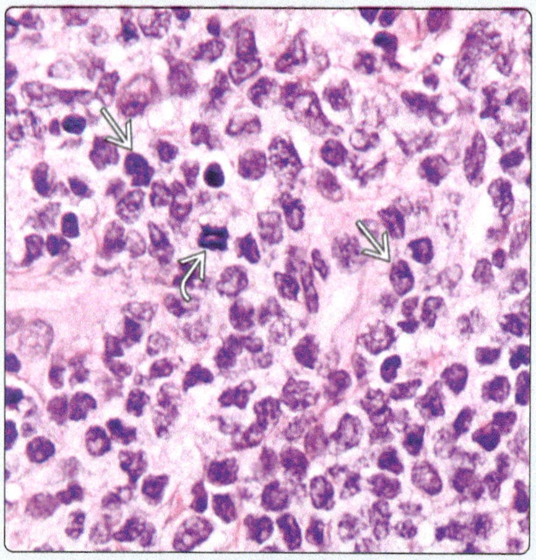

Lack of *ALK* Gene Rearrangements

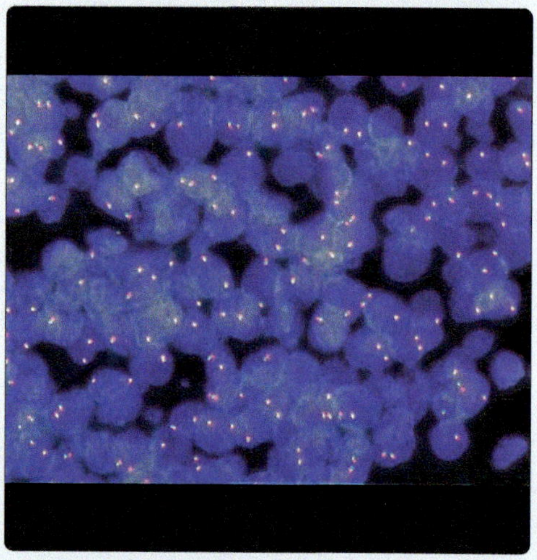

(Left) *High magnification of ATLL shows a population of medium-sized, atypical, and pleomorphic-appearing cells with hyperchromasia, atypical nuclear contours, focally prominent nucleoli, and vesicular chromatin. Mitotic figures are also seen.* **(Right)** *This is a break-apart FISH test for the ALK gene, which shows fused (yellow) signals. This indicates that the lesion does not have ALK gene rearrangements. Unlike systemic anaplastic large cell lymphoma, ATLL does not show ALK gene rearrangements.*

TERMINOLOGY

Abbreviations

- Adult T-cell leukemia/lymphoma (ATLL)

Synonyms

- Adult T-cell leukemia

Definitions

- T-cell lymphoma/leukemia of regulatory T cells [CD4(+), CD25(+), FOXP3(+)] caused by human T-cell leukemia virus type I (HTLV-I)

ETIOLOGY/PATHOGENESIS

Infectious Agents

- HTLV-I
  - Type C retrovirus, composed of single-stranded RNA, which is converted into double-strand DNA during infection
  - Virus is monoclonally integrated into host genome
  - Progresses to leukemia/lymphoma in < 5% of infected individuals
  - Long latency period
    - Most exposed as infants/children
    - Tumor often develops after 20 years of viral exposure
  - Transmitted through blood, sexual intercourse, or breast milk
  - HLA alleles A26, B4002, B4006, & B4801 may be predisposed to developing ATLL
  - Inflammatory diseases related to HTLV-I include tropical spastic paraparesis, HTLV-I-associated myelopathy, HTLV-I-associated uveitis, & infective dermatitis
  - Encodes tax (viral oncoprotein)
    - Activates transcription factors for T-cell proliferation genes

CLINICAL ISSUES

Epidemiology

- Age
  - Adults; most commonly in 6th or 7th decades
- Sex
  - M:F = 1.5:1.0
- Ethnicity
  - Endemic to Southwest Japan, Caribbean, South America, Australia, & Central Africa

Presentation

- Skin lesions
  - Develop in 50% of ATLL patients
  - Usually multiple nodules/tumors, papules, plaques, or macules
    - Papules may cover large segments of body
  - Rarely, erythroderma, purpura, prurigo, or erythema multiforme
- Other sites of disease include lymph nodes, peripheral blood, bone, spleen & sometimes lung, liver, & CNS
  - Most patients have generalized lymphadenopathy
  - Hypercalcemia from increased osteoclast bone resorption
- 4 clinical subtypes of ATLL
  - Acute subtype
    - Most common subtype, 60%, often in children
    - Severe peripheral blood lymphocytosis, ↑ WBC, ↑ lactate dehydrogenase (LDH), skin lesions, lymphadenopathy
    - Hypercalcemia, lytic bone lesions, renal dysfunction, neuropsychiatric problems
    - Immunodeficiency leads to other opportunistic infections
  - Chronic subtype
    - Lymphocytosis but ↓ WBC than acute subtype
    - No hypercalcemia, exfoliative skin rash
  - Lymphomatous subtype
    - ↑ lymphadenopathy; usually no peripheral blood involvement
    - Less hypercalcemia than acute subtype; skin often involved
  - Smoldering subtype
    - > 5% tumor cells in peripheral blood, even though normal WBC count
    - Tumor cells small with less pleomorphism & lobation
    - No hypercalcemia or lymphadenopathy
- Skin lesions are mostly in acute & lymphomatous subtypes

Treatment

- There is no standard modality of treatment
  - Prevention of HTLV-I transmission prevents ATLL
- Indolent subtypes
  - Antiviral therapy (zidovudine & interferon-α) or watch & wait
- Aggressive forms
  - Multiagent chemotherapy allogeneic
  - Hematopoietic stem cell transplantation
  - Valproic acid (histone deacetylase inhibitor)
  - Anti-CD194 monoclonal antibody, mogamulizumab

Prognosis

- Better in chronic & smoldering variants than acute & lymphomatous variants
  - < 10% 5-year survival for acute & lymphomatous variants
  - 1/4 of chronic & smoldering variants transform to acute & lymphomatous variants
- Favorable prognostic markers include only superficial skin infiltrates
- Primary skin disease without systemic involvement has better prognosis than secondary skin involvement
- Poor prognostic indicators
  - Hypercalcemia, ↑ LDH, tumors as compared to papules, age > 40, high serum CD25, high proviral HTLV-I load

IMAGING

Radiographic Findings

- Osteolytic bone lesions

MICROSCOPIC

Histologic Features

- Skin
  - Atypical lymphoid infiltrate in epidermis, dermis, &/or subcutis

    - Frequent epidermotropism &/or Pautrier microabscesses
    - Nodular, perivascular, & diffuse patterns
    - Follicular mucinosis in some cases
    - Lymphohistiocytic infiltrates may be precursor to lymphoma
  - Eosinophils present (usually absent in mycosis fungoides)

Cytologic Features

- Usually medium- to large-sized pleomorphic T cells with marked atypia, coarse clumped chromatin, & small/absent nucleoli
  - "Flower cells" (a.k.a. cauliflower cells) are multilobated atypical T cells
    - More easily seen in peripheral blood

Lymph Nodes

- Effaced architecture with heterogeneous infiltrate & paracortical distribution

Bone Marrow

- Diffuse, interstitial, or sinusoidal collections of tumor cells, osteoclasts may be increased
- Variably involved with subtle & patchy infiltrates

ANCILLARY TESTS

Immunohistochemistry

- T-cell antigens (+) (CD3, CD5)
  - CD7 is often lost
- Usually CD4(+)/CD8(-)
  - Rarely CD4(-)/CD8(+) or CD4(+)/CD8(+)
- Regulatory T-cell markers, CD25(+), FOXP3(+), CD194(+)
- CD30 often stains scattered large cells but they are ALK1(-)
- Cytotoxic markers (TIA1 & granzyme-B) (-)
- HTLV-I/HTLV-II antigen (+)
- CD62 (L-selectin) (+), PD1(-)

PCR

- Clonal T-cell receptor gene rearrangement
- Quantitative HTLV-I levels

Genetic Testing

- Cytogenetics
  - Numerous complex chromosomal abnormalities especially in acute & lymphomatous variants
  - No single consistent cytogenetic abnormality
- *RHOA* mutations detected in ~ 15% of cases
- Array CGH shows gains of 1q, 2p, 4q, 7p, 7q & losses of 10p, 13q, 16q, & 18p
- Gene expression profiles have shown some signatures, which show clinical response to zidovudine & α-interferon

Serologic Testing

- Diagnosis requires confirmation of HTLV-I infection

DIFFERENTIAL DIAGNOSIS

Mycosis Fungoides/Sézary Syndrome

- Less acute clinical presentation
- Skin lesions with epidermotropism & Pautrier microabscesses, similar to ATLL
- Circulating atypical lymphocytes, as in ATLL
  - Cerebriform nuclei of mycosis fungoides fold inward, whereas "flower cells" of ATLL have outward nuclear projections
- Immunophenotypic CD4(+), CD8(-) T cells, like ATLL
  - But usually not CD25(+), FOXP3(+), or CD30(+)
  - Patients not infected with HTLV-I

Anaplastic Large Cell Lymphoma

- CD30(+) T-cell lymphoma with large cells like ATLL
- FOXP3(-), CD194(-); ALK1 & EMA(+/-), unlike ATLL

Hodgkin Lymphoma

- ATLL with Hodgkin-like cells shows Reed-Sternberg-like cells that are CD30(+)
- Usually no aggregates of malignant T cells in Hodgkin lymphoma
- Lacks malignant cells in peripheral blood, skin lesions, & hypercalcemia

Angioimmunoblastic-Like T-Cell Lymphoma

- ↑ high endothelial venules, plasma cells, & eosinophils
- Tumor cells are CD10(+), Bcl-6(+), & CXCL13(+), unlike ATLL
- ↑ follicular dendritic cells expressing CD21

T-Cell Large Granular Lymphocytic Leukemia

- Also peripheral blood involved with variable absolute lymphocyte count & large granular lymphocytes in blood
- Large granular lymphocytes
  - Different morphology from ATLL T cells, with increased pale cytoplasm & prominent azurophilic granules
  - Mild nuclear indenting but no polylobated nuclei as in ATLL
- Immunohistochemistry differs from ATLL
  - T-cell large granular lymphocytic leukemia is CD8(+), CD16(+), CD57(+)

T-Cell Prolymphocytic Leukemia

- Involves blood at presentation with ↑ WBC
- Some nuclear irregularity, but no "flower cell" morphology as in ATLL

Infection

- HTLV-I infection can also cause nonneoplastic lymphohistiocytic lesions
- Usually less atypia & no T-cell gene receptor γ chain rearrangements

SELECTED REFERENCES

1. Arango M: Adult T-cell leukemia/lymphoma. Blood. 126(20):2343, 2015
2. Bailey NG et al: Mature T-cell leukemias: molecular and clinical aspects. Curr Hematol Malig Rep. 10(4):421-8, 2015
3. Kato K et al: Recent advances in therapeutic approaches for adult T-cell leukemia/lymphoma. Viruses. 7(12):6604-12, 2015
4. Sawada Y et al: Type of skin eruption is an independent prognostic indicator for adult T-cell leukemia/lymphoma. Blood. 117(15):3961-7, 2011
5. Bittencourt AL et al: Adult T-cell leukemia/lymphoma (ATL) presenting in the skin: clinical, histological and immunohistochemical features of 52 cases. Acta Oncol. 48(4):598-604, 2009

Adult T-Cell Leukemia/Lymphoma

Dermal Infiltrate in Adult T-Cell Leukemia/Lymphoma

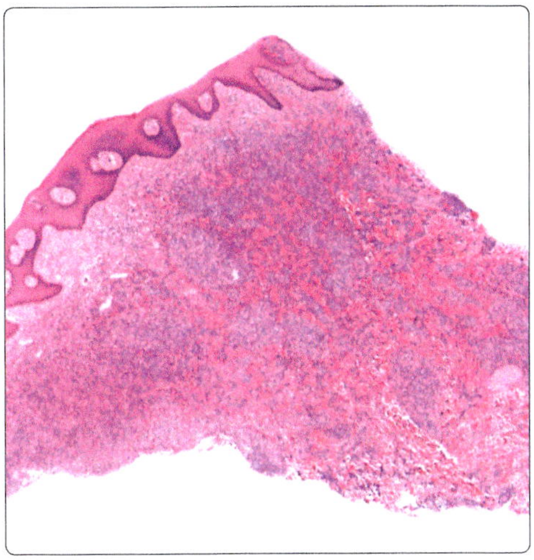

Pautrier-Like Microabscess

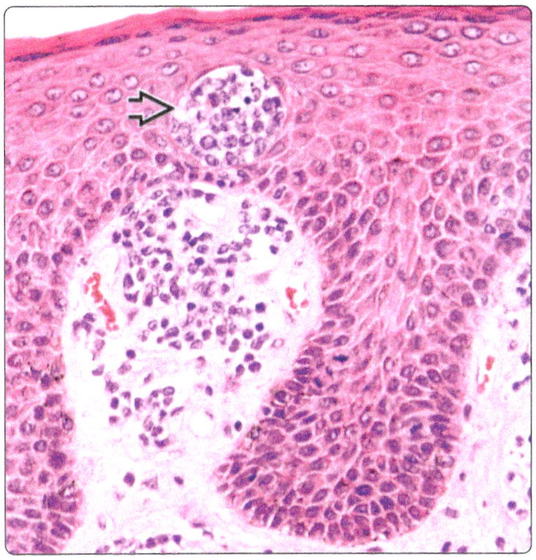

(Left) *ATLL involving the skin shows diffuse multinodular lymphoid aggregates present throughout the dermis. (Courtesy C. Bueso-Ramos, MD.)* **(Right)** *High magnification of ATLL shows atypical cells in the epidermis forming a well-circumscribed, Pautrier-like microabscess ⇨. Smaller and less cellular aggregates are more characteristic of mycosis fungoides, although sometimes the distinction is not possible. (Courtesy C. Bueso-Ramos, MD.)*

Cellular Atypia in Adult T-Cell Leukemia/Lymphoma

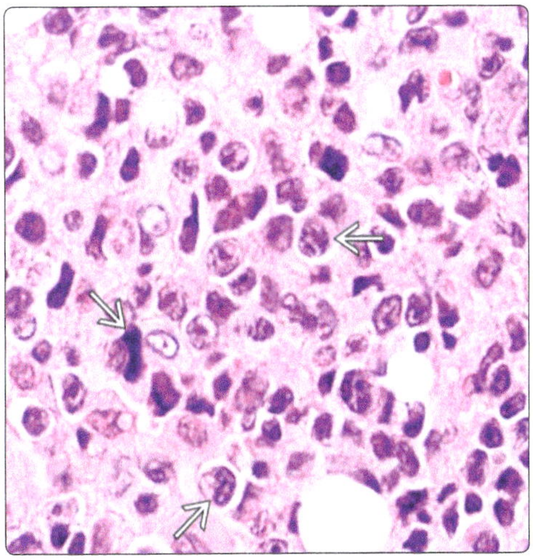

CD25 Immunohistochemistry

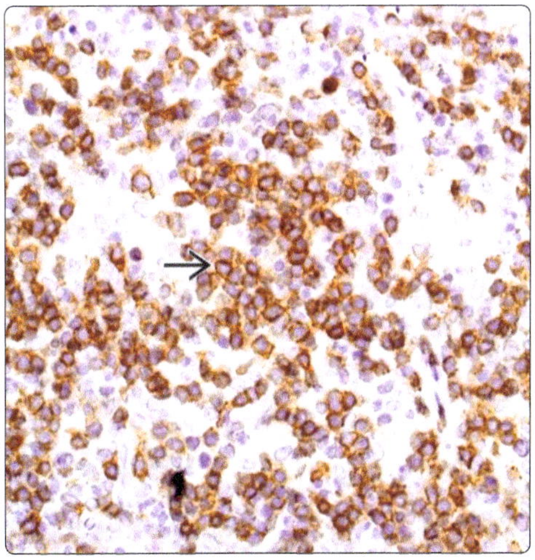

(Left) *In this high magnification of ATLL, there is a diffuse infiltrate of medium-sized, pleomorphic-appearing cells ➡ with hyperchromasia, atypical nuclear contours, focally prominent nucleoli, and vesicular chromatin.* **(Right)** *The malignant T cells are strongly positive for CD25 in a membranous/cytoplasmic distribution pattern ⇨. FOXP3 and HTLV-I antibodies are also immunoreactive (not shown).*

Bone Marrow Involvement in Adult T-Cell Leukemia/Lymphoma

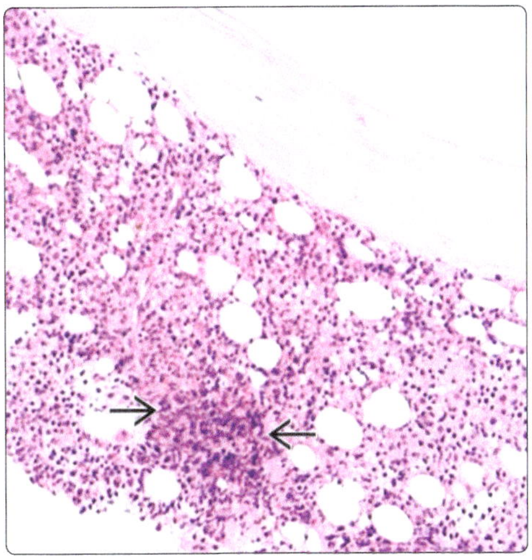

Flower Cells of Adult T-Cell Leukemia/Lymphoma in Peripheral Blood

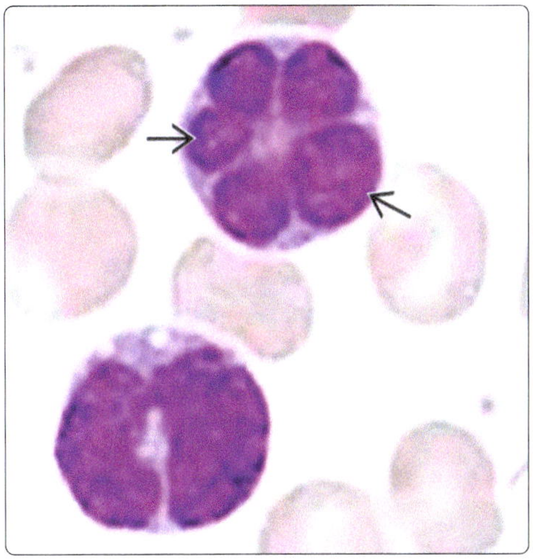

(Left) *This image shows malignant T cells in the bone marrow of a patient with ATLL. There is a patchy distribution pattern with malignant T cells in clusters ⇨. The T cells are CD25(+) and FOXP3(+) (not shown). The acute subtype shows the most severe bone marrow involvement.* **(Right)** *High-magnification image (oil) of peripheral blood shows large lymphocytes with irregular nuclei. These cells are called "flower cells" because of the multiple nuclear lobules or convolutions ⇨.*

KEY FACTS

TERMINOLOGY

- T-cell lymphoma of αβ cells usually involving subcutaneous tissue with prominent karyorrhexis and CD8(+) phenotype

CLINICAL ISSUES

- 20% hemophagocytic syndrome
- Excellent prognosis
- < 1% of all non-Hodgkin lymphoma
- Extremities and trunk most common
- Median: ~ 35 years (range: 5 months to 84 years)

MICROSCOPIC

- Atypical lobular panniculitic T-cell infiltrate confined to subcutis
- Malignant T cells rim around adipocytes
- Prominent necrosis/apoptosis
- Vacuolated histiocytes
- Erythrophagocytosis or cytophagocytosis (beanbag cells)
- Usually lacks plasma cells, eosinophils, or neutrophils

ANCILLARY TESTS

- Immunohistochemistry
  - CD8(+), CD4(-)
  - TCR-βF1(+), TCR-δ(-), CD56(-), EBER(-)
  - (+) for cytotoxic markers
- T-cell receptor gene rearrangements
- No diagnostic translocations

TOP DIFFERENTIAL DIAGNOSES

- Cutaneous γ/δ T-cell lymphoma
  - Panniculitis but also in dermis &/or epidermis often with ulceration; TCR-βF1(-), TCR-δ(+)
  - Worse prognosis than SPTCL
- Lupus profundus panniculitis
  - Similar inflammation in subcutis in panniculitic pattern
  - Lobular panniculitis but shows plasma cells and germinal centers unlike SPTCL
- Atypical lymphocytic lobular panniculitis

Clinical Image of SPTCL

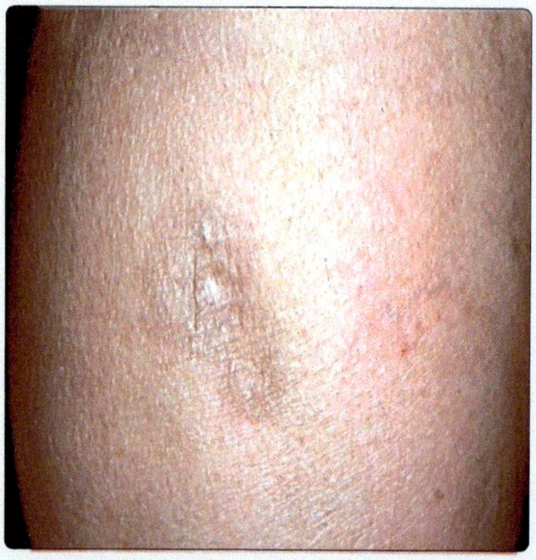

Scanning Magnification of SPTCL

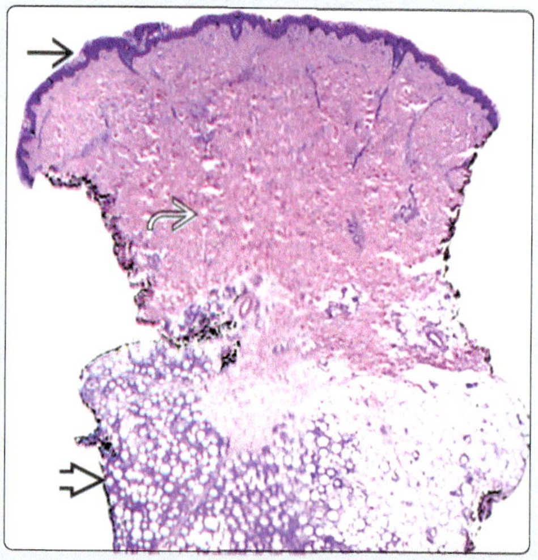

(Left) *This clinical photograph shows a single nonulcerated subcutaneous nodule on the arm of a 35-year-old patient. Upon excision, the nodule was diagnosed as subcutaneous panniculitis-like T-cell lymphoma (SPTCL). (Courtesy M. Tomaszewsky, MD.)* **(Right)** *Low-power view of SPTCL shows malignant T cells confined to the subcutaneous tissue ⇨. The dermis ➡ and epidermis → are both spared and are morphologically unremarkable-appearing at this power. (Courtesy M. Tomaszewsky, MD.)*

Higher Magnification of SPTCL

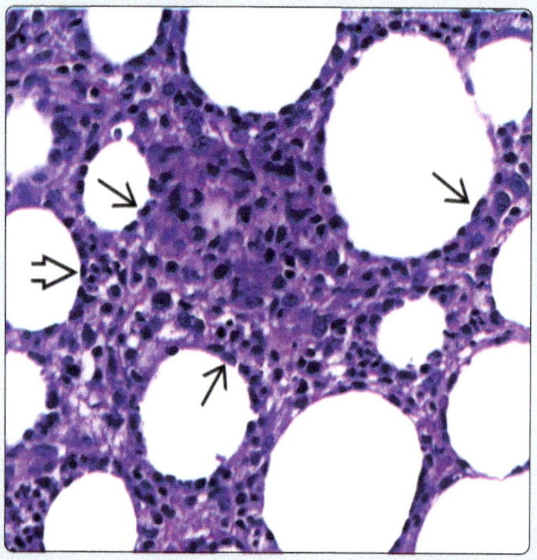

High Magnification of SPTCL With Fat Rimming

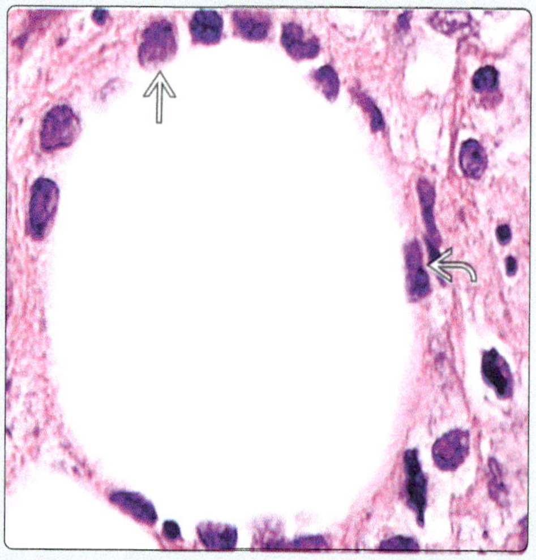

(Left) *Higher power shows a lobular pattern of atypical T cells rimming adipocytes →. There are also numerous histiocytes containing apoptotic debris (bean bag cells) ⇨ and markedly atypical lymphocytes present between the fat cells.* **(Right)** *This fat cell is surrounded by T cells that are medium to large in size ➡ and that show some nuclear irregularities ➡. This degree of atypia is not typically seen in reactive lesions with panniculitis.*

TERMINOLOGY

Abbreviations

- Subcutaneous panniculitis-like T-cell lymphoma (SPTCL)

Definitions

- T-cell lymphoma of αβ cells involving subcutaneous tissue with prominent karyorrhexis and cytotoxic phenotype
  - Cases composed of γδ cells are reclassified as cutaneous γ/δ T-cell lymphoma in WHO classification of hematopoietic and lymphoid tumors

ETIOLOGY/PATHOGENESIS

Autoimmune Disease

- Autoimmune disease present in ~ 20% of patients
  - Systemic lupus erythematosus (SLE) most common

Viral Infection

- Rarely, SPTCL is seen with Epstein-Barr virus infection
  - May be due to immunosuppression

CLINICAL ISSUES

Epidemiology

- Incidence
  - < 1% of all non-Hodgkin lymphoma
    - Presents sporadically without familial involvement
- Age
  - Median: ~ 35 years (range: 5 months to 84 years)
- Sex
  - M = F
- Ethnicity
  - No ethnic predisposition

Site

- Extremities and trunk most common
- Uncommonly disseminates
  - Can involve lymph nodes but not at initial diagnosis

Presentation

- Single or multiple erythematous subcutaneous nodules or plaques
  - Painless mass, rarely ulcerates
  - Symptoms due to mass effects
- B symptoms in up to 50%
  - Diagnosis often not discovered until months to years after onset of symptoms
- Hemophagocytic syndrome (HPS) in up to 20%
  - Related to release of cytotoxic molecules
  - May occur up to 5 years after presenting diagnosis

Laboratory Tests

- Cytopenias (anemia, leukopenia, thrombocytopenia)

Treatment

- Surgery
  - Sometimes excision of single lesion with no further recurrence
- Immunosuppressive agents
  - Often given, at least initially
  - High-dose systemic corticosteroids
- Chemotherapy
  - Recurrence or resistant cases treated with CHOP or CHOP-like therapy
- Radiation
  - Sometimes for localized disease
- Stem cell transplant
  - Can be considered for refractory/recurrent disease

Prognosis

- Indolent disease
  - 5-year overall survival ~ 80%
  - Mostly stage I (confined to skin)
  - Rare systemic spread
  - May be more aggressive in children
- HPS poor prognostic indicator
  - Medium survival ~ 2 years

IMAGING

CT Findings

- Enhancing nodules in subcutaneous tissue

MICROSCOPIC

Histologic Features

- Atypical T-cell infiltrate of subcutaneous fat lobules
  - Involves lobules, usually spares septa
    - Uncommon septal pattern represents spilling of T cells from lobules
    - Typically, no tumor in overlying dermis or epidermis
  - Malignant T cells rim individual adipocytes
    - Characteristic, but not specific for SPTCL
  - Neoplastic cells
    - Small to large in size
    - Mild to marked atypia with irregular nuclear contours
    - Hyperchromatic nuclei
    - Pale, clear cytoplasm
- Karyorrhexis (apoptosis) and fat necrosis characteristic
  - Necrosis from released cytotoxic molecules
- Initial biopsy commonly shows minimal T-cell atypia
  - Later biopsies show more atypia
- Angioinvasion in some cases
  - Poor prognostic indicator
- Reactive inflammatory cells
  - Histiocytes
    - Vacuolated foamy cytoplasm from imbibed material/lipid
    - Erythrophagocytosis or cytophagocytosis (so-called beanbag cells)
    - Sometimes poorly formed granulomas with multinucleated giant cells
  - Usually lacks plasma cells, eosinophils, or neutrophils
  - Plasma cells may be conspicuous in pediatric cases
- Bone marrow may be involved and shows similar morphology as in skin

ANCILLARY TESTS

Immunohistochemistry

- T-cell antigens (+) (CD2, CD3, CD5, CD7)
  - May lose 1 or more T-cell antigens
- CD8(+)/CD4(-) in > 95% of cases

- CD4(-)/CD8(-) and CD4(+)/CD8(-) rarely
- TCR-βF1(+), TCR-δ-1(-) (alpha-beta T cells)
- Cytotoxic markers (+) (perforin, TIA1, and granzyme)
  - But GZM-M(-), unlike other T-cell lymphomas
- CD56(-), CD30(-), Bcl-2(-)

In Situ Hybridization

- Epstein-Barr encoded receptor (EBER) usually (-)
  - Rare EBER(+) cases associated with immunocompromised and Asian patients

Genetic Testing

- Monoclonal T-cell receptor gene rearrangement
- No specific cytogenetic abnormalities
- Upregulated genes include
  - *IDO1*, immunotolerance-inducing enzyme
  - Th1-specific cytokines, known to be associated with autoimmune inflammation, including *IFNG*, *CXCR3*, *CXCL9*, *CXCL10*, *CXCL11*, and *CCL5*
- Neuron navigator 3 (*NAV3*) gene deletions have been identified
  - *NAV3* deletion has also been seen in mycosis fungoides and Sézary syndrome

DIFFERENTIAL DIAGNOSIS

Cutaneous γ/δ T-Cell Lymphoma

- Panniculitic pattern of involvement, like SPTCL
  - Dermal and epidermal involvement, unlike SPTCL
  - Ulcerated epidermis, contrary to SPTCL
- γδ cells, not αβ cells of SPTCL
  - Immunophenotype
    - TCR-βF1(-), TCR-δ-1(+), CD56(+), unlike SPTCL
    - Usually CD4(-), CD8(-) (double negative)
- Clinical features compared to SPTCL
  - Older median age of diagnosis (~ 60 years)
  - Generalized lesions
  - More B symptoms
  - More often HPS ~ 50% (of patients)
  - Worse prognosis than SPTCL ~ 10% 5-year survival
  - More often given multiagent chemotherapy; systemic corticosteroids often given in SPTCL

Other Hematopoietic Neoplasms

- Usually involve epidermis or dermis, contrary to SPTCL
  - **Anaplastic large cell lymphoma**
    - Superficial nodules, rarely panniculitic, diffusely CD30(+)
  - **Blastic plasmacytoid dendritic cell neoplasm**
    - Different phenotype than SPTCL, with CD4(+), CD56(+), CD123(+), cytotoxic markers negative
  - **Enteropathy-associated T-cell lymphoma**
    - Can have subcutaneous involvement
    - But will typically present with gastrointestinal mass, &/or other features of celiac disease
  - **Diffuse large B-cell lymphoma**
    - Can have subcutaneous involvement
    - But will have B-cell phenotype and Ig heavy chain immunoglobulin gene rearrangement

Reactive Panniculitis

- **Lupus profundus panniculitis**
  - Difficult to differentiate from SPTCL in some cases
    - Patients can have both lupus profundus panniculitis and SPTCL
  - Similarities to SPTCL
    - Inflammation in subcutis in panniculitic pattern
    - No/minimal lymphocyte atypia, like early lesions of SPTCL
    - Self-heal and improve with steroids, similar to many SPTCL cases
  - Differences from SPTCL
    - Plasma cells and germinal centers
    - Mixed inflammatory infiltrate with histiocytes, eosinophils, and neutrophils
    - Less T-cell atypia, minimal rimming of fat cells
    - B-cell aggregates
    - Mix of CD4(+) and CD8(+) T cells
    - T cells (-) for cytotoxic markers
    - Vacuolar epidermal change (some cases) and interstitial mucin
    - Usually polyclonal *TCR* rearrangement, but rarely oligoclonal T-cell populations are present
  - Other features of lupus
    - History of SLE
    - Laboratory tests: ANA(+), antidouble stranded DNA antibodies, rheumatoid factor(+), ↓ C4 levels
    - Superficial epidermal and dermal findings, including interface inflammation and perivascular and periadnexal infiltrates
- **Atypical lymphocytic lobular panniculitis**
  - Clonal lymphoid infiltrate without histologic criteria for lymphoma
  - Chronic condition that usually spontaneously regresses
  - Lobular T-cell infiltrate of small- to medium-sized cells without atypia
    - Less rimming of fat cells
    - No karyorrhexis
    - Can have CD4(+) cells
  - ↑ numbers of histiocytes
  - May develop into SPTCL
- **Histiocytic cytophagic panniculitis (HCP)**
  - Most cases are reclassified as SPTCL
    - Few HCP cases still remain
    - Rarely if ever progresses to SPTCL
  - ↑ histiocytes
  - No clonal T-cell receptor gene rearrangement

SELECTED REFERENCES

1. Brown NA et al: Subcutaneous panniculitis-like T-cell lymphoma with bone marrow involvement. Am J Clin Pathol. 143(2):265-73, 2015
2. Hu ZL et al: Subcutaneous panniculitis-like T-cell lymphoma in children: a review of the literature. Pediatr Dermatol. 32(4):526-32, 2015
3. Acree SC et al: Subcutaneous panniculitis-like T-cell lymphoma in two pediatric patients: an HIV-positive adolescent and a 4-month-old infant. Fetal Pediatr Pathol. 32(3):175-83, 2013
4. Huppmann AR et al: Subcutaneous panniculitis-like T-cell lymphoma in the pediatric age group: a lymphoma of low malignant potential. Pediatr Blood Cancer. 60(7):1165-70, 2013
5. Pincus LB et al: Subcutaneous panniculitis-like T-cell lymphoma with overlapping clinicopathologic features of lupus erythematosus: coexistence of 2 entities? Am J Dermatopathol. 31(6):520-6, 2009
6. Willemze R et al: Subcutaneous panniculitis-like T-cell lymphoma: definition, classification, and prognostic factors: an EORTC Cutaneous Lymphoma Group Study of 83 cases. Blood. 111(2):838-45, 2008

Septal Sparring in SPTCL

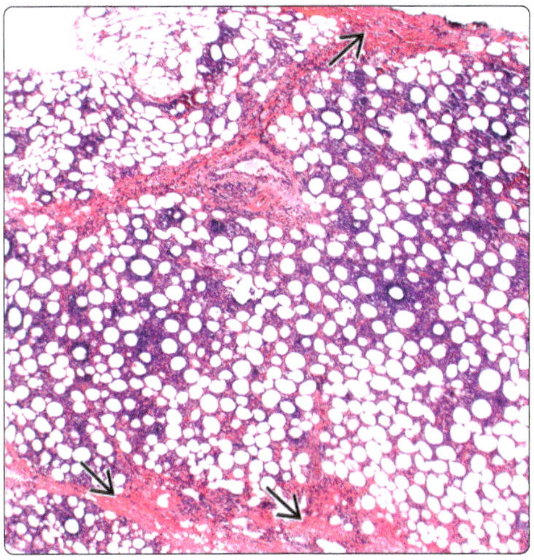

Karyorrhexis in SPTCL

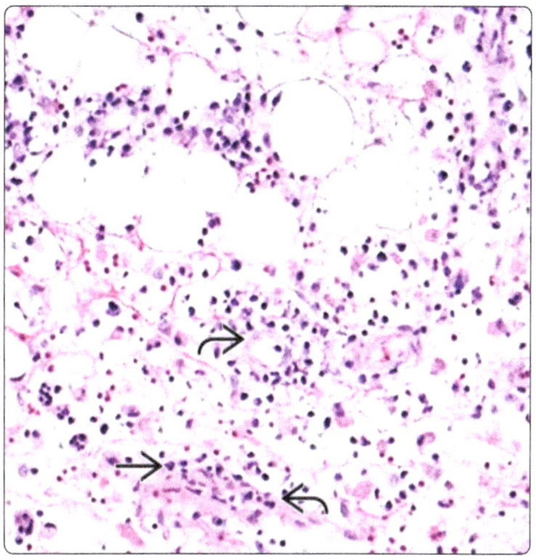

(Left) *Even at low-power examination, this SPTCL shows infiltration of the fat lobules by atypical lymphoid cells. However, the septa are relatively uninvolved.* **(Right)** *This SPTCL shows prominent karyorrhexis and angiocentricity. There is prominent karyorrhexis and focal necrosis in this tumor. The malignant cells also appear to surround and involve small blood vessels.*

Apoptosis and Mitoses in SPTCL

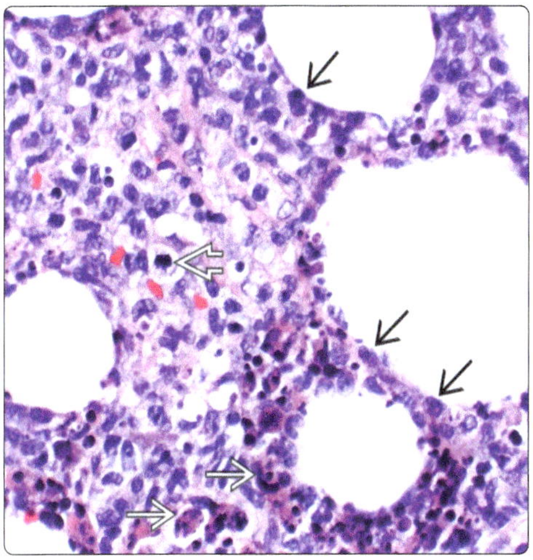

SPTCL With Histiocytes

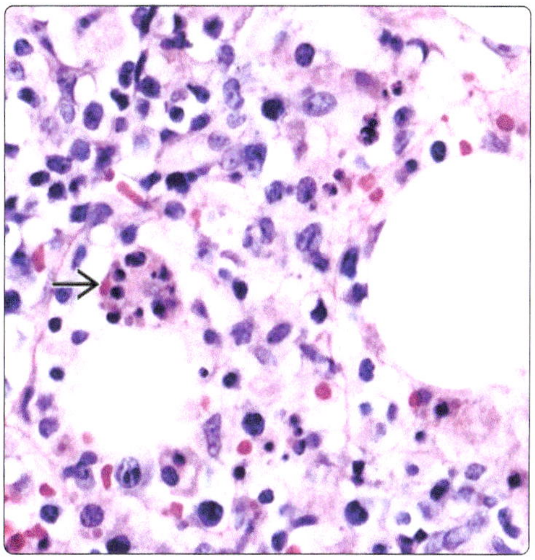

(Left) *Higher power shows a lobular pattern of atypical T cells rimming fat cells. There are also numerous histiocytes containing apoptotic debris (so-called beanbag cells) and markedly atypical lymphocytes present between the fat cells, with a mitotic figure.* **(Right)** *In this high-power view of SPTCL, there are abundant histiocytes containing apoptotic cellular debris (beanbag cells), a finding typical of SPTCL. Sometimes these histiocytes have a vacuolated appearance.*

SPTCL With Septal Involvement

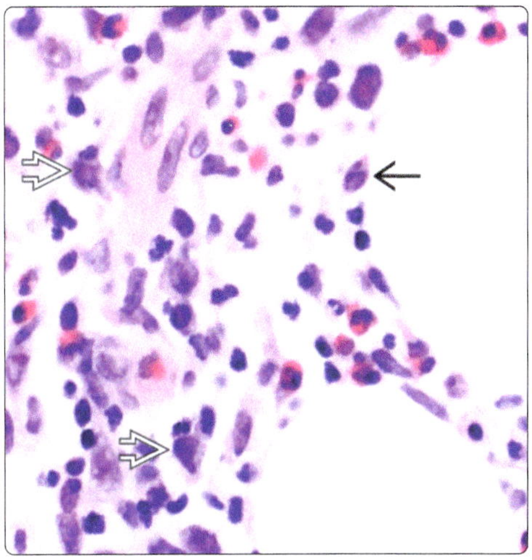

SPTCL With Many Eosinophils

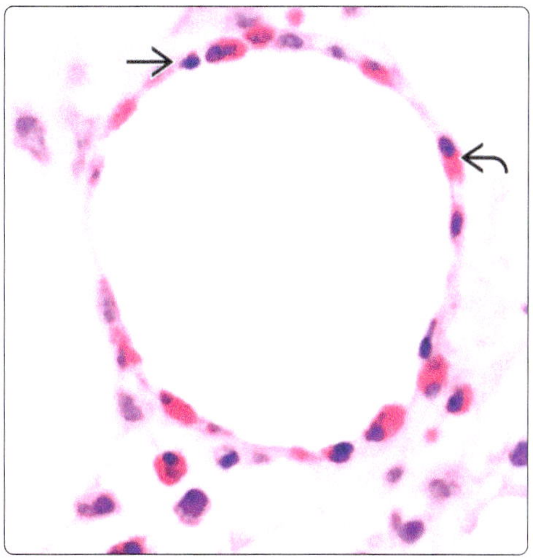

(Left) *Higher power showing a lobular pattern with atypical T cells rimming fat. There is also spillage of neoplastic lymphocytes into the septa.* **(Right)** *This is an unusual case of SPTCL with many eosinophils. A few atypical T cells rim the fat. It is unusual that eosinophils also surround this fat lobule, since eosinophils, plasma cells, and neutrophils are more common in reactive panniculitis than SPTCL.*

CD3 Immunohistochemical Stain

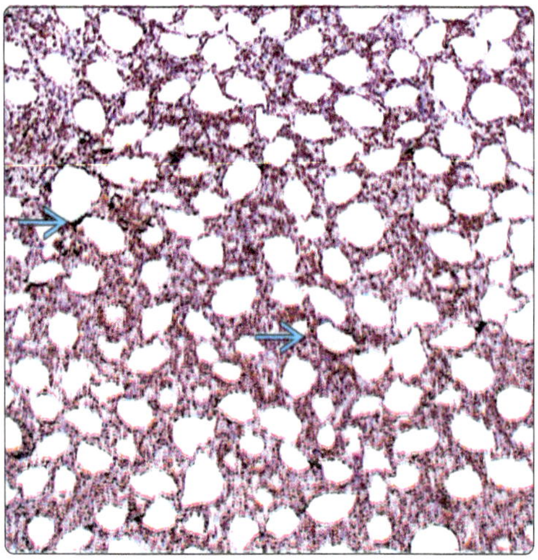

CD4 and CD8 in SPTCL

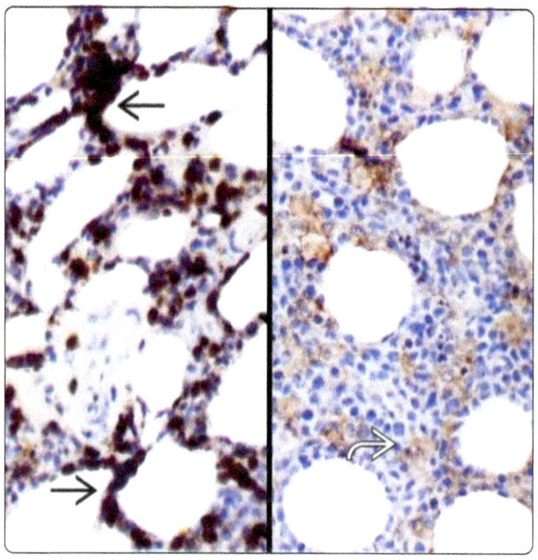

(Left) *In this CD3(+) SPTCL, the CD3 immunostain strongly highlights the numerous malignant T cells diffusely infiltrating and rimming the fat cells →.* **(Right)** *This image is a composite picture with a CD8 stain on the left and a CD4 stain on the right. In this case of SPTCL, the malignant T cells strongly express CD8 → but are nonimmunoreactive for CD4 → [only scattered histiocytes and reactive T cells are CD4(+)].*

TCR-β-F1 Immunohistochemical Stain

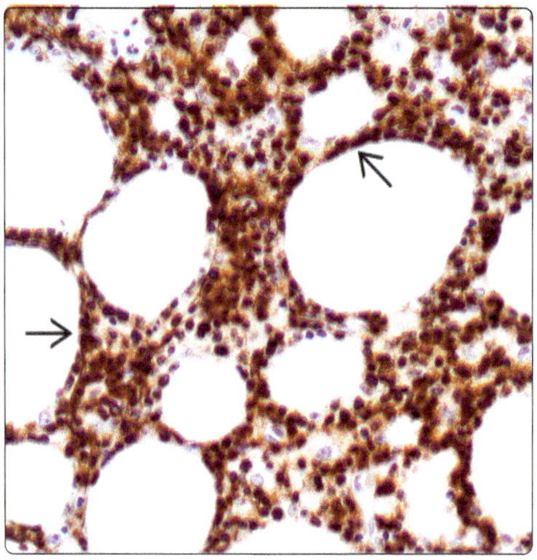

Granzyme-B Immunohistochemical Stain

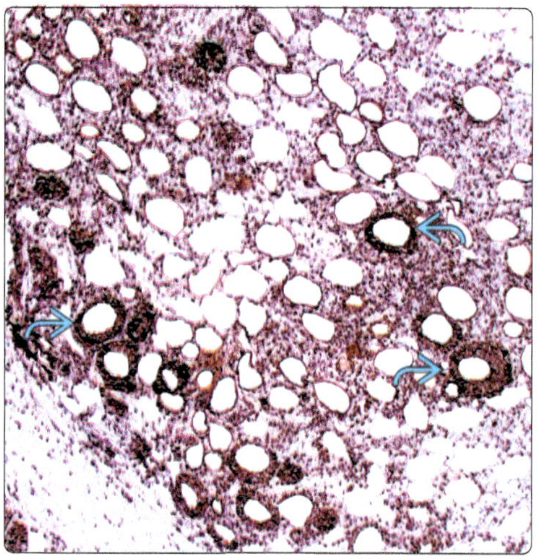

(Left) *TCR-β-F1 immunohistochemical stain is expressed in the malignant T cells rimming the fat →, similar to the CD3 and CD8 stains. This is evidence that the cells in SPTCL are αβ T cells and not γδ T cells. (Courtesy T. Muzzafar, MD.)* **(Right)** *Granzyme-B is a cytotoxic marker that is typically strongly and diffusely positive in SPTCL. Note the staining of areas of fat rimming →. These cells were also positive for other cytotoxic markers, including TIA-1 and perforin (not shown).*

CD56 Immunohistochemical Stain

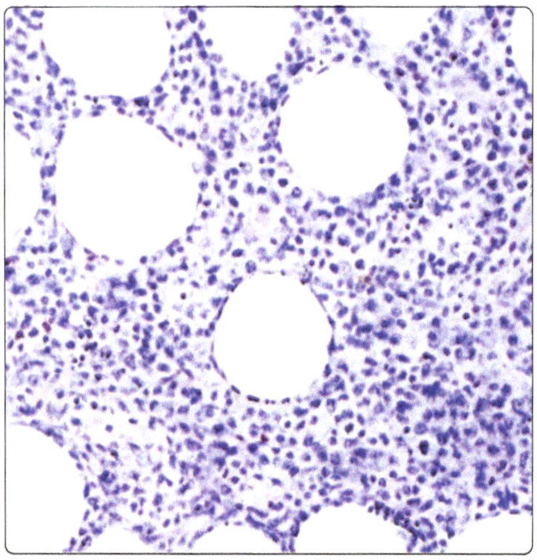

T-Cell Receptor Beta Gene Rearrangement

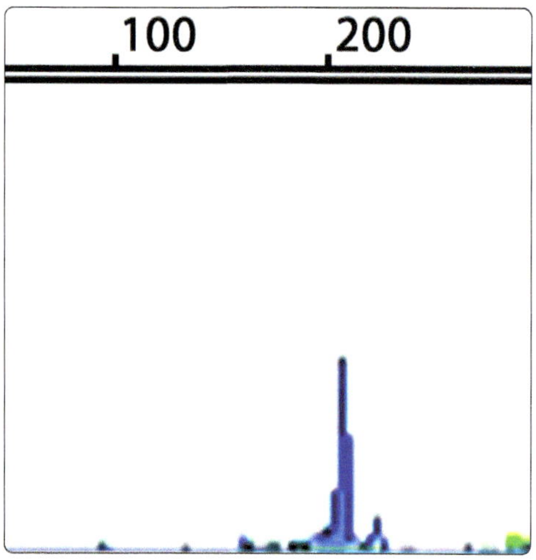

(Left) *CD56 immunohistochemical stain is typically negative in the malignant cells of SPTCL. In cases of cutaneous γδ T-cell lymphoma, CD56 is typically positive.* **(Right)** *This test is a PCR T-cell receptor beta gene rearrangement performed on a case of SPTCL. The appearance of a blue peak between 180 and 280 base pairs in size is suggestive of a clonal T-cell rearrangement, as is commonly seen in this tumor.*

Differential Diagnosis: Primary Cutaneous γδ T-Cell Lymphoma

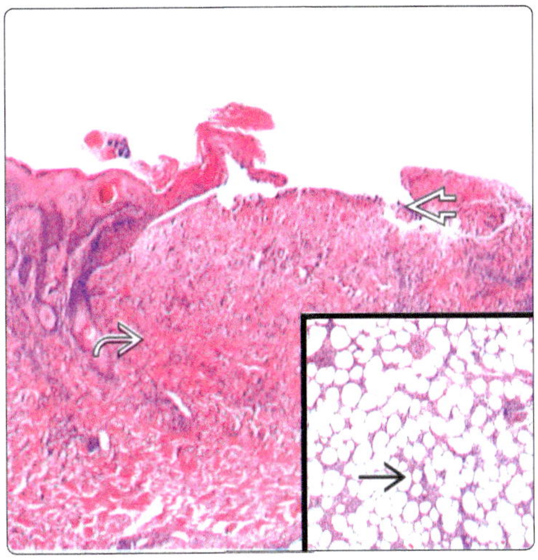

Atypia in PCGDTCL

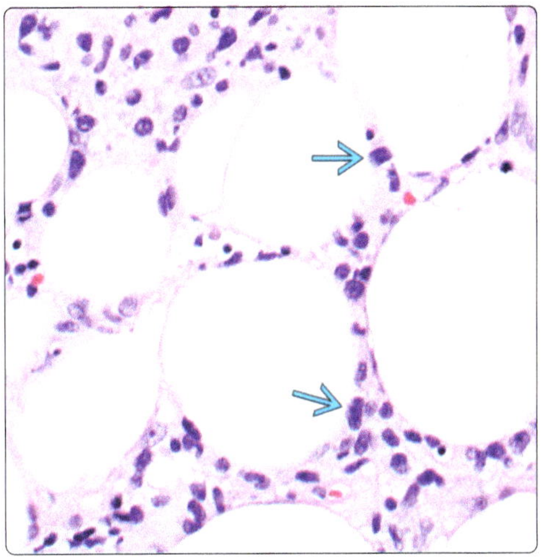

(Left) *Primary cutaneous γδ T-cell lymphoma (PCGDTCL) is the main differential diagnosis of SPTCL. In this cutaneous γδ T-cell lymphoma, T cells rim fat (lower right inset →), similar to SPTCL. However, there is an overlying ulcer → and dermal infiltrate →, unlike SPTCL.* **(Right)** *In this PCGDTCL, the neoplastic cells exhibit greater cytologic atypia → than those of SPTCL and rim the adipocytes.*

βF1 Immunohistochemical Stain in PCGDTCL

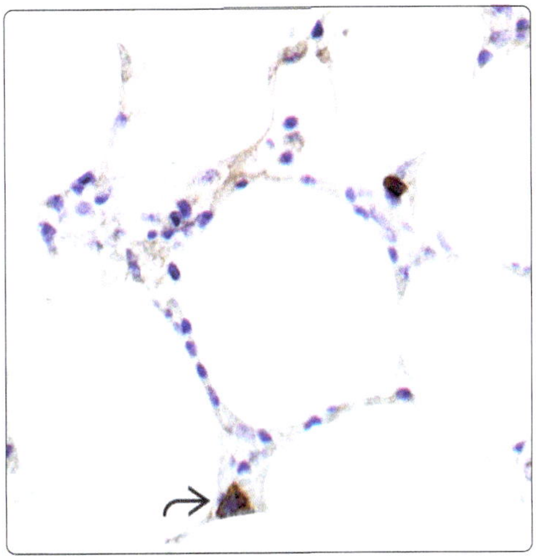

Differential Diagnosis: Lupus Profundus

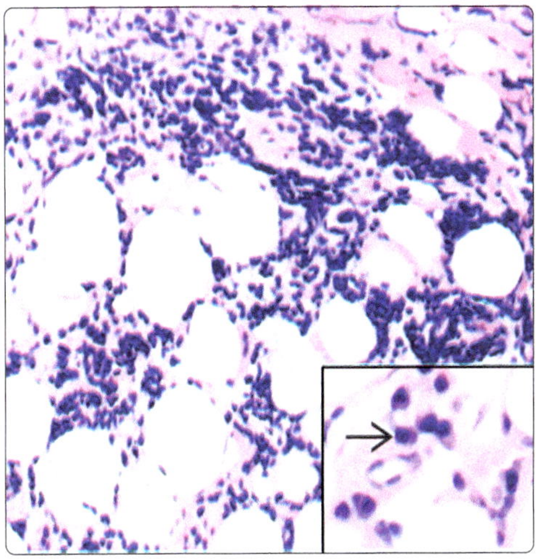

(Left) *This is a βF1 stain done on a PCGDTCL. The neoplastic T cells are negative for TCR-βF1, although a few scattered reactive T cells are positive →. Many believe that absence of TCR-βF1 is presumptive evidence that the neoplastic cells express the TCR-γδ.* **(Right)** *This case of lupus profundus shows a lobular panniculitis. Scattered plasma cells are seen →. Plasma cells are a component of lupus profundus but are not commonly seen in SPTCL.*

CD20(+) Immunohistochemical Stain in Lupus

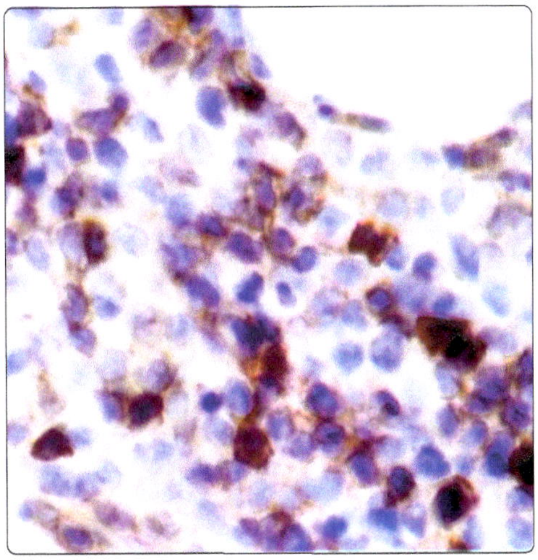

CD4/CD8 Immunohistochemical Stains in Lupus

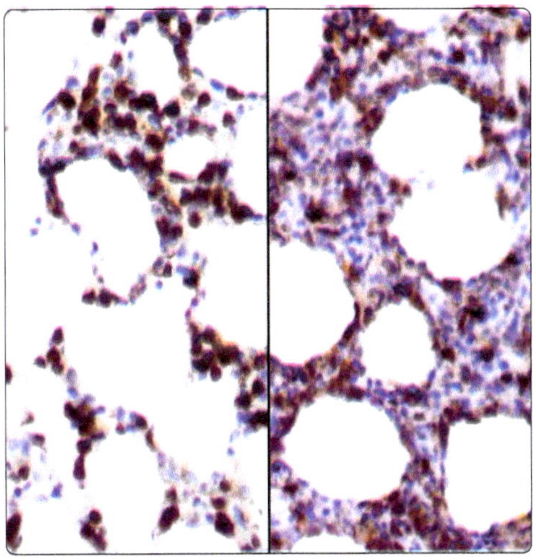

(Left) *This is a case of lupus profundus with CD20(+) B cells. This CD20 immunohistochemical stain shows several clusters of B cells. This finding favors lupus profundus over SPTCL, which usually does not show B-cell aggregates.* **(Right)** *Unlike SPTCL, which consists of CD8(+) T cells, lupus profundus (as seen here) usually has a mixture of CD4(+) and CD8(+) cells. In this image, the CD4 stain (left) and the CD8 stain (right) both show clusters of positive cells in the subcutis.*

Extranodal NK-/T-Cell Lymphoma, Nasal Type

KEY FACTS

TERMINOLOGY

- Tumor of NK cells or T cells, with necrosis, Epstein-Barr virus infection, and angioinvasion

ETIOLOGY/PATHOGENESIS

- Epstein-Barr virus

CLINICAL ISSUES

- Common in adults in South America, Central America, and Asia
- Nasopharynx most common site, skin is 2nd

MICROSCOPIC

- Diffuse dermal/subcutaneous infiltrate of variably sized tumor cells, angiocentric with necrosis
- Dense chromatin, can be vesicular in large cells
- Coagulative necrosis in most cases

ANCILLARY TESTS

- Epstein-Barr virus antigen (+) and cytotoxic markers (+)
- Mostly NK-cell markers phenotype
    - **βF1(-)**, CD2(+), cytoplasmic CD3-ε(+), **CD56(+/-)**
- Less often T-cell marker phenotype
    - **βF1(+)**, CD2(+), cytoplasmic CD3-ε(+), **CD56(+/-)**
- Mutation in *FAS, P53, β-catenin, KRAS, KIT* reported, but not specific
- Gains of 1q, 7q, and 17p detected in skin lesions
- NF-κB and JAK-STAT pathways preferentially activated
- Isochromosome 7q has been detected in rare cases

TOP DIFFERENTIAL DIAGNOSES

- Wegener granulomatosis
- Infections
- B-cell lymphomas (DLBCL, lymphomatoid granulomatosis)
- PTCL-NOS, NK-cell leukemia
- Hydroa vacciniforme-like lymphoma
- Anaplastic large cell lymphoma
- Primary cutaneous CD4(+) small/medium pleomorphic T-cell lymphoma

Nasal-Type Extranodal NK-/T-Cell Lymphoma

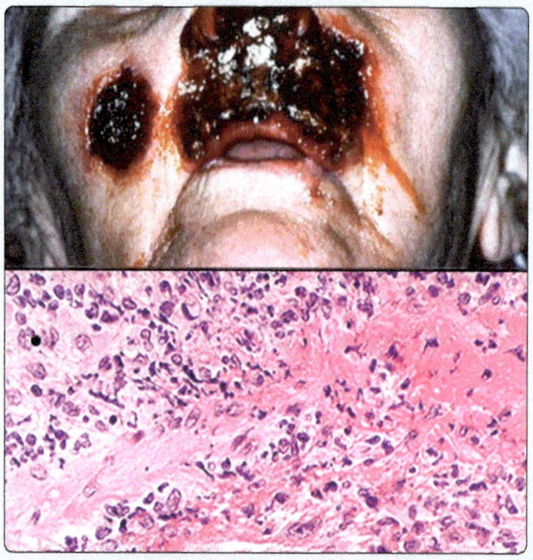

ENNKTCL Involving Dermis

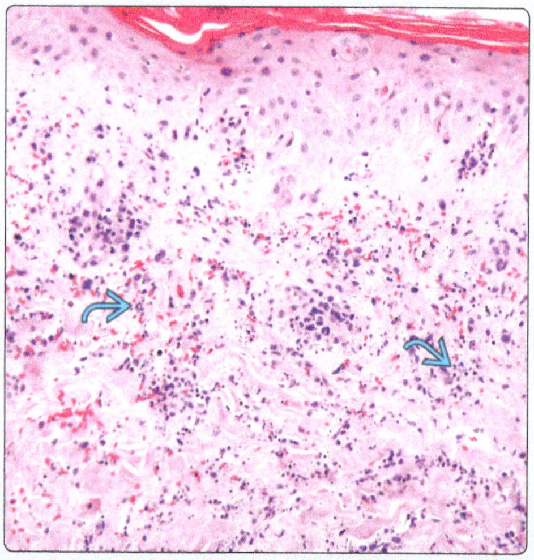

(Left) *Clinical photograph of nasal-type extranodal NK-/T-cell lymphoma (ENNKTCL) shows extensive destruction of the nasolabial region (above). High magnification of this lesion shows an atypical lymphoid infiltrate with vascular destruction.* **(Right)** *This is a nasal-type ENNKTCL of NK-cell lineage involving the skin. The neoplastic cells are enlarged, show nuclear hyperchromasia, and there are areas of necrosis ↷. (Courtesy L. J. Medeiros, MD.)*

High Magnification of ENNKTCL

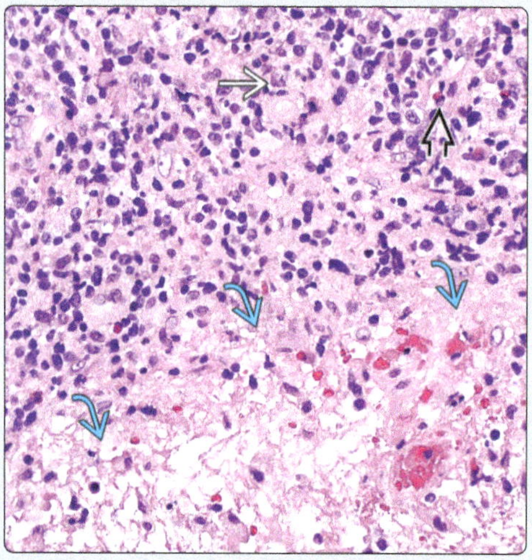

EBV In Situ Hybridization

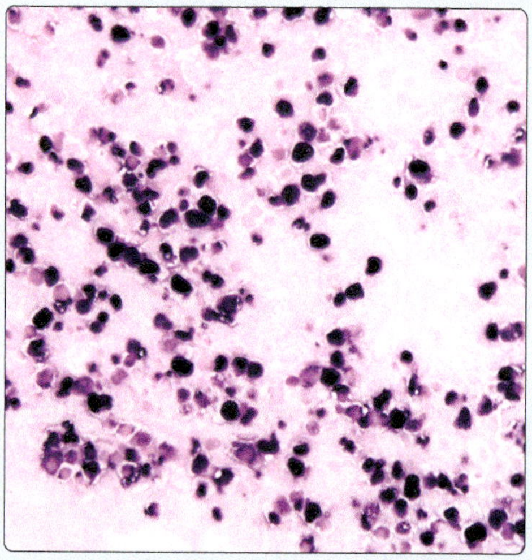

(Left) *This is a high-powered image of ENNKTCL, nasal type, which shows a proliferation of medium- to large-sized lymphoid cells, → some with pale to clear cytoplasm. Eosinophils → are also present, as is necrosis ↷, which is often associated with this lymphoma.* **(Right)** *This in situ hybridization test for Epstein-Barr virus small-encoded RNA (EBER) is strongly positive. EBV infection is an invariable feature of ENNKTCL, nasal type. (Courtesy L. J. Medeiros, MD.)*

TERMINOLOGY

Abbreviations

- Extranodal NK-/T-cell lymphoma (ENNKTCL), nasal type

Synonyms

- Angiocentric T-cell lymphoma, malignant midline reticulosis, lethal midline granuloma, polymorphic reticulosis

Definitions

- Lymphoma composed of natural killer (NK) cells or T cells that is characterized by necrosis, Epstein-Barr virus (EBV) infection, angioinvasion, and is usually extranodal

ETIOLOGY/PATHOGENESIS

Infectious Agents

- EBV
  - EBV antigens, usually type A, are identified by immunohistochemistry and in situ hybridization

CLINICAL ISSUES

Epidemiology

- Incidence
  - Rare in United States; more common in South America, Central America, and Asia
- Age
  - Usually adults

Site

- Nasal
  - Most common location of disease
  - Anywhere in upper aerodigestive tract
    - Includes nasal cavity, nasopharynx, sinuses, and palate
- Extranasal
  - Skin
    - Most common extranasal site
    - Skin can be primary disease or secondary to disease elsewhere
    - Often extremities or torso
  - Other sites include gastrointestinal tract, lymph nodes (rare but cases have been published), and testes

Presentation

- Skin
  - Nodules &/or plaques on skin, often ulcerated
- Nasal obstruction or epistaxis
- Gastrointestinal tract, mass, or perforation
- B symptoms, including fever &/or weight loss
- Hemophagocytic syndrome in some cases

Laboratory Tests

- EBV DNA can be assessed to check disease activity

Natural History

- Can spread to regional lymph nodes
  - Tumor only in lymph nodes and not other anatomic sites is uncommon
  - Primary lymph node involvement is very rare
- Can involve bone marrow

Treatment

- Chemotherapy and radiation therapy

Prognosis

- Median survival < 15 months
- Poor prognostic indicators
  - High stage of disease
  - Bone marrow with EBV(+) cells
  - High International or Korean Prognostic Index
    - B symptoms, serum LDH, regional lymph nodes, stage
  - Increased EBV DNA
  - ↑ C-reactive protein, thrombocytopenia
  - Ki-67 > 50%
- More favorable prognostic indicators
  - Nasal disease is better than extranasal
  - High absolute lymphocyte count
  - CD56(+), CD30(+) coexpression has been reported

IMAGING

General Features

- Mass lesion that can destroy bone, especially in nasal tumors

MACROSCOPIC

General Features

- 1 or more firm nodules

MICROSCOPIC

Histologic Features

- Skin/mucosa
  - Diffuse pattern of infiltration
    - Mostly dermal infiltrate, sometimes subcutis
    - Rare foci of epidermotropism in 30%
  - Tumor cells can be small, medium, or large
    - Irregular nuclear shapes
    - Dense chromatin, can be vesicular in large cells
    - Sometimes ↑ amounts of clear cytoplasm
  - Coagulative necrosis in most cases
  - Tumor cells are angiocentric and angiodestructive
  - Overlying epithelium/mucosa
    - ± ulceration
    - Often shows pseudoepitheliomatous hyperplasia
  - Increased mitoses
  - Erythrophagocytosis is sometimes seen
- Lymph node
  - Tumor tends to involve paracortical areas

Cytologic Features

- Rarely, diagnosis can be made by fine-needle aspirate
  - Azurophilic granules in some tumor cells

ANCILLARY TESTS

In Situ Hybridization

- In situ hybridization for EBV small-encoded RNA (EBER) is (+) in both T and NK subtypes

Immunohistochemistry

- EBV antigens (+)

- Immunohistochemistry for latent membrane protein (LMP)
  - LMP is less sensitive than EBER
- EBV antigens can be found in patients before tumor develops

- NK-cell markers (75% of cases)
  - **βF1(-)**, CD2(+), cytoplasmic CD3-ε(+), surface CD3(-), CD4(-), CD5(-), CD8(-), **CD56(+/-)**, cytotoxic markers (+), CD94(+)
- T-cell markers (25% of cases)
  - **βF1(+)**, CD2(+), cytoplasmic CD3-ε(+), CD5(+), CD8(+/-), CD43(+), **CD56(+/-)**, cytotoxic markers (+)
- CD56(-) cases should be EBER(+) or cytotoxic markers(+)
- CMYC is (+) in 60%, and is not specific for Burkitt lymphoma

PCR

- T-cell receptor gene rearrangements (*TRB* and *TRG*)
  - In T-cell tumors but not in NK-cell tumors

Genetic Testing

- Gene mutation analysis
  - Mutations in *FAS*, *P53*, *β-catenin*, *KRAS*, *KIT* reported, but not specific
  - Platelet-derived growth factor α is overexpressed; *HACE1* is deregulated
- Cytogenetics
  - Isochromosome 7q has been detected in rare cases of ENNKTCL
  - Partial trisomy chromosome 13, del(6)(q21q25) and i(6)(p10) have also been reported
- Array CGH
  - Gains of 1q, 7q, and 17p detected in skin lesions
- Gene expression profiles
  - Overexpression of angiogenesis genes
  - NF-κB and JAK-STAT pathways preferentially activated

Electron Microscopy

- Electron-dense membrane-bound granules

DIFFERENTIAL DIAGNOSIS

Wegener Granulomatosis

- Morphology classically shows triad of necrosis, vasculitis, and granulomas
  - All 3 components only seen in < 25% of cases
- Usually more of mixed inflammatory infiltrate than ENNKTCL
  - Neutrophils, eosinophils, lymphocytes, plasma cells, histiocytes

Infections

- Similarities to ENNKTCL
  - Common in upper airways and may involve skin
  - Pools of necrosis on H&E
- Differences from ENNKTCL
  - No large atypical tumor cells
  - More mixed inflammatory infiltrate with neutrophils
  - Lack of *TRB* or *TRG* gene rearrangements
  - No EBER or LMP
  - Organisms can be identified
- Infectious mononucleosis
  - Also EBV(+) but usually no mass lesion, no clonality and no metastasis, good prognosis

T-Cell or Other NK-Cell Neoplasms

- Peripheral T-cell lymphoma, NOS
  - Overlapping histologic features with ENNKTCL
    - Both can have necrosis and angioinvasion
  - Different immunophenotype
    - Often CD56(-) and EBV(-)
- Hydroa vacciniforme-like lymphoma
  - Also, EBER(+), cytotoxic markers(+), T cells &/or NK cells
  - Also, necrosis and angioinvasion
  - Usually in children, unlike ENNKTCL
  - Patients present with papulovesicular eruption on sun-exposed areas
- NK-cell leukemia
  - Presents more as leukemia with primary involvement of bone marrow and peripheral blood
    - Also EBV(+) and can have skin lesions
- Posttransplant lymphoproliferative disorder, ENNKTCL, nasal type
  - Rarely, tumors can develop post transplant that morphologically and phenotypically mimic ENNKTCL
  - Necrosis and angioinvasion
  - EBER(+), CD56(+), CD3(+), cytotoxic markers (+)
- Anaplastic large cell lymphoma (ALCL)
  - Both ALCL and ENNKTCL can be CD30(+), CD56(+)
    - ALCL is usually not necrotic or angiocentric
    - ALCL has much better clinical course
    - *ALK* gene rearrangement, often in ALCL
- Primary cutaneous CD4(+) small/medium pleomorphic T-cell lymphoma (SMPTCL)
  - Both can present with dermal T-cell infiltrate
  - SMPTCL is EBER(-), CD4(+), CD8(-)
    - Less necrosis and angioinvasion than ENNKTCL
- Angioimmunoblastic T-cell lymphoma
  - Also presents as a dermal T-cell infiltrate and is EBER(+)
  - Less necrosis and angioinvasion than ENNKTCL
  - Increased follicular dendritic cells, unlike ENNKTCL
  - PD1(+), Bcl-6(+), CXCL13(+), unlike ENNKTCL

SELECTED REFERENCES

1. Chang D et al: Evaluation of the 2008 World Health Organization classification for non-mycosis fungoides, non-Sezary syndrome T/NK-cell lymphomas with primary cutaneous involvement. J Cutan Pathol. ePub, 2015
2. Lima M: Extranodal NK/T cell lymphoma and aggressive NK cell leukaemia: evidence for their origin on CD56+bright CD16-/+dim NK cells. Pathology. 47(6):503-14, 2015
3. Takata K et al: Primary cutaneous NK/T-cell lymphoma, nasal type and CD56-positive peripheral T-cell lymphoma: a cellular lineage and clinicopathologic study of 60 patients from Asia. Am J Surg Pathol. 39(1):1-12, 2015
4. Suzuki R: Pathogenesis and treatment of extranodal natural killer/T-cell lymphoma. Semin Hematol. 51(1):42-51, 2014
5. Berti E et al: Cutaneous extranodal NK/T-cell lymphoma: a clinicopathologic study of 5 patients with array-based comparative genomic hybridization. Blood. 116(2):165-70, 2010
6. Choi YL et al: Extranodal NK/T-cell lymphoma with cutaneous involvement: 'nasal' vs. 'nasal-type' subgroups--a retrospective study of 18 patients. Br J Dermatol. 160(2):333-7, 2009
7. Chan JK et al: Nonnasal lymphoma expressing the natural killer cell marker CD56: a clinicopathologic study of 49 cases of an uncommon aggressive neoplasm. Blood. 89(12):4501-13, 1997

CT Scan of ENNKTCL

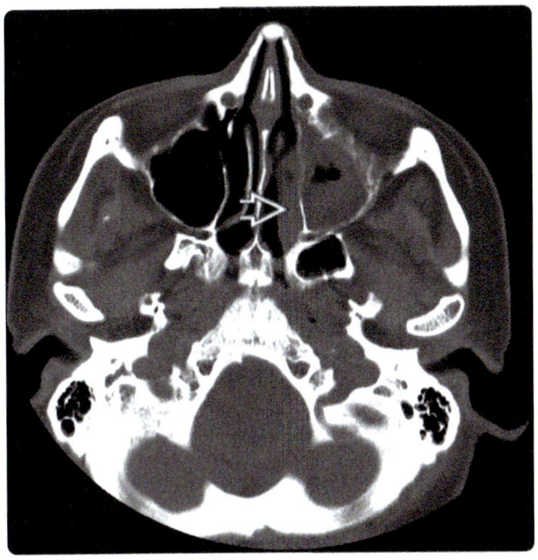

ENNKTCL With Overlying Ulceration

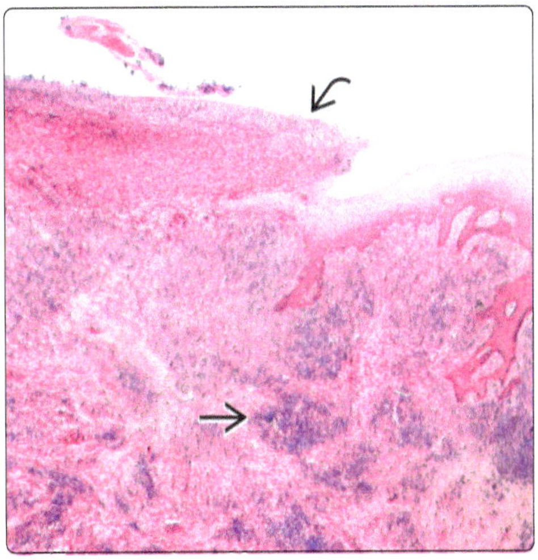

(Left) *This is a CT scan of ENNKTCL, nasal type, that shows an almost completely opacified maxillary sinus and thickening of mucosa in the nasopharynx . (Courtesy L. J. Medeiros, MD.)* **(Right)** *The surface of this example of ENNKTCL is extensively ulcerated . Beneath the ulcerated surface, the tumor replaces the normal dermal architecture.*

Higher Magnification Showing Perivascular Infiltrate

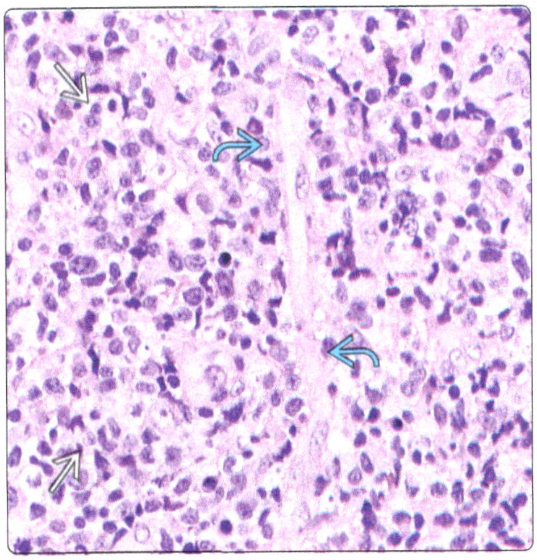

ENNKTCL With Necrosis

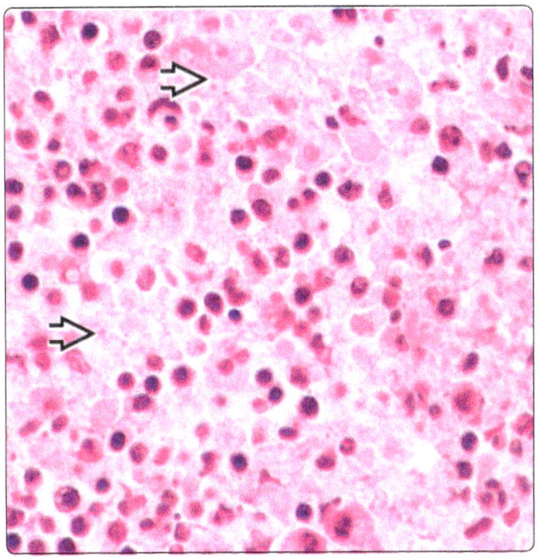

(Left) *At high-power examination, the lymphoid infiltrate consists of large atypical T cells , which are surrounding a blood vessel .* **(Right)** *There is extensive coagulative necrosis in this case of ENNKTCL. Necrosis is a classic morphologic feature in these tumors.*

ENNKTCL With Atypical Cells

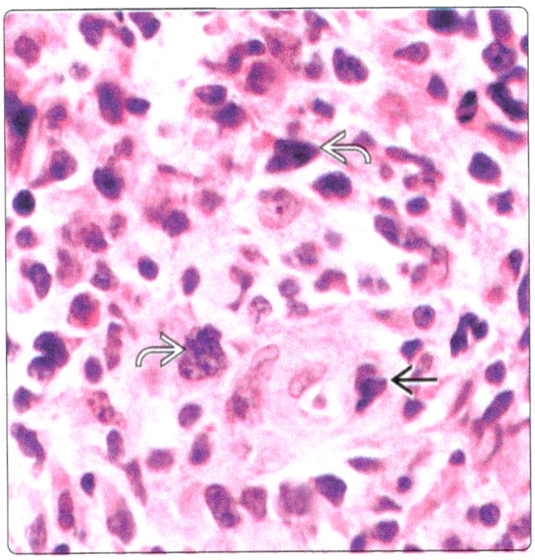

Nasopharynx With ENNKTCL

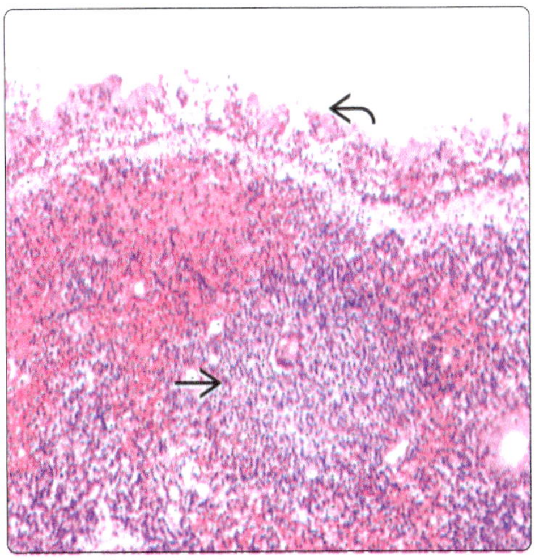

(Left) *The tumor cells in ENNKTCL tend to be angiocentric and angioinvasive. The blood vessel is surrounded by frankly atypical tumor cells and shows malignant cells invading its wall .* **(Right)** *The nasopharynx is the most common site of presentation for ENNKTCL. In this case, there is a diffuse/nodular infiltrate deep to the mucosal surface .*

CD3 Immunohistochemistry in ENNKTCL

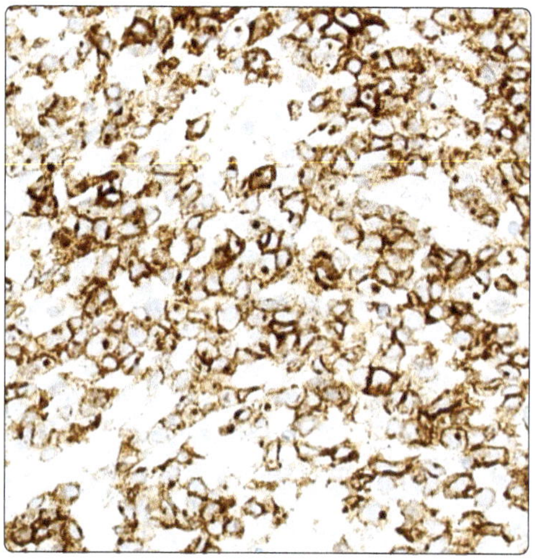

CD56 Immunohistochemistry in ENNKTCL

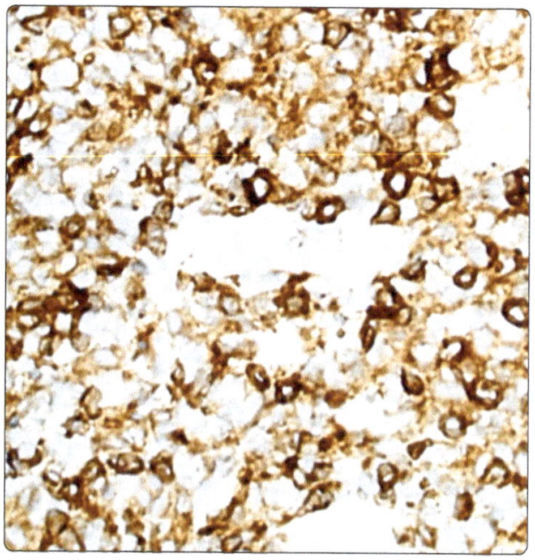

(Left) *This is a CD3(+) stain in a case of ENNKTCL. This antibody detects the epsilon chain of CD3 within the cell cytoplasm. Expression of CD3-ε chain is positive in both T cells and NK cells.* **(Right)** *CD56 shows many positive neoplastic cells in ENNKTCL. CD56 is commonly (but not invariably) expressed, and CD56 is highly suggestive of, but not specific for, NK cell lineage.*

TIA1 Staining in ENNKTCL

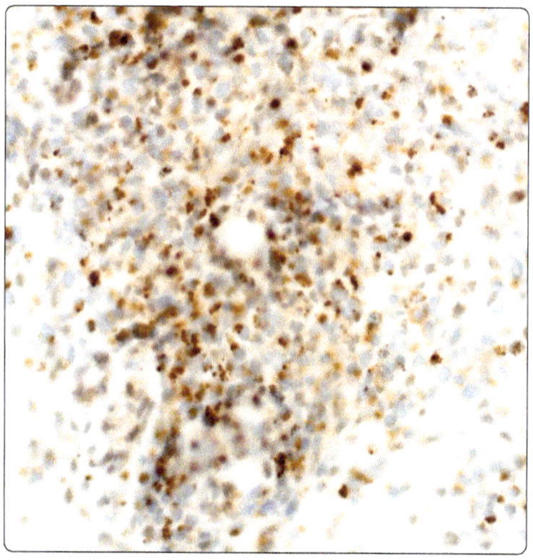

Granzyme-B Staining in ENNKTCL

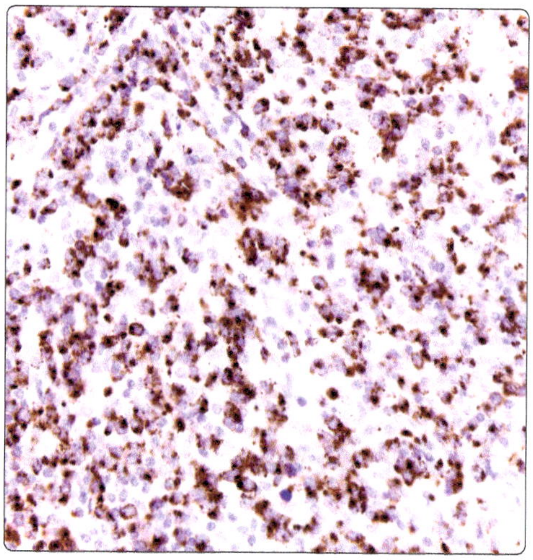

(Left) *TIA-1 immunohistochemical stain shows that many of the neoplastic cells in ENNKTCL are strongly positive. TIA, as well as granzyme-B and perforin, are cytotoxic markers that are usually expressed in ENNKTCL.* **(Right)** *Granzyme-B immunohistochemical stain highlights numerous neoplastic cells supporting cytotoxic lineage in ENNKTCL. (Courtesy L. J. Medeiros, MD.)*

CD8 Staining in ENNKTCL

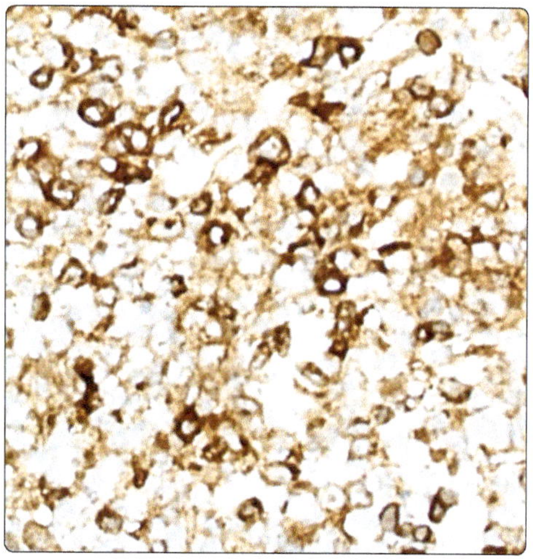

EBV-Encoded Small RNA

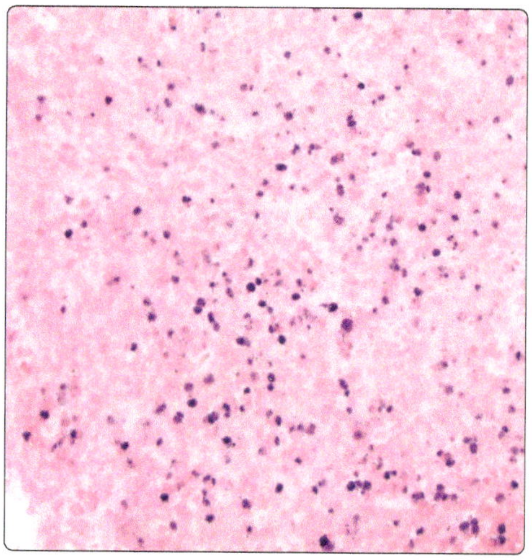

(Left) *This CD8 immunohistochemical stain shows that the neoplastic cells are CD8(+), supporting T-cell lineage.* **(Right)** *This in situ hybridization test for Epstein-Barr virus small-encoded RNA (EBER) is strongly positive. EBV infection is an invariable feature of ENNKTCL, nasal type.*

DDx: Herpes Infection

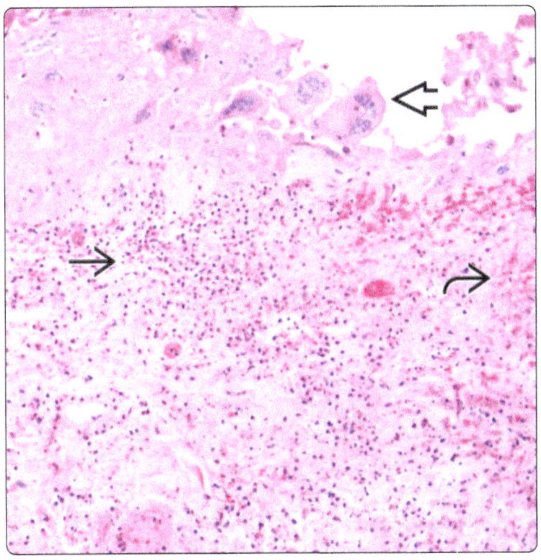

DDx: Anaplastic Large Cell Lymphoma

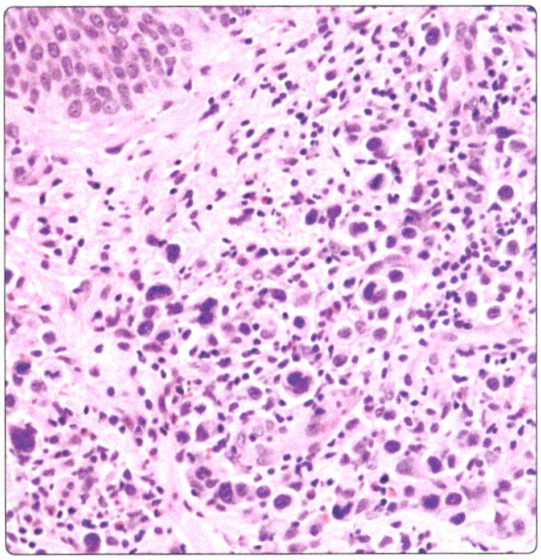

(Left) *Herpes infection can mimic ENNKTCL. Many infections involve the nasal region. This herpes infection shows necrosis →, like ENNKTCL, but has more acute inflammation →, and virus-infected cells with multinucleation, chromatin margination, and moulding are identified →.* **(Right)** *Histologic section from a patient with cutaneous anaplastic large cell lymphoma shows large anaplastic cells with abundant cytoplasm and irregular multilobated nuclei, admixed with inflammatory cells.*

DDx: Lymphomatoid Granulomatosis

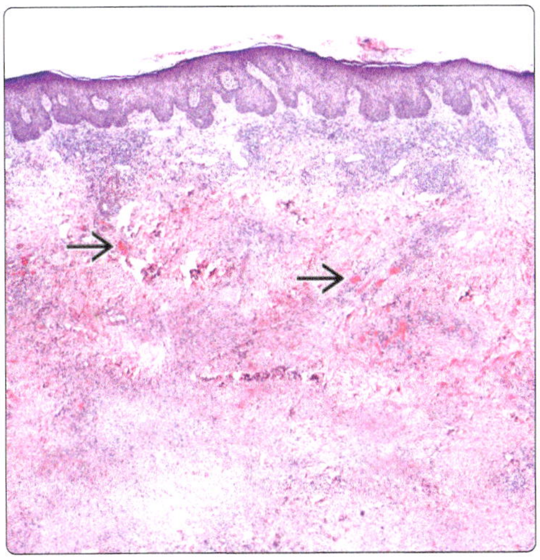

DDx: Diffuse Large B-Cell Lymphoma

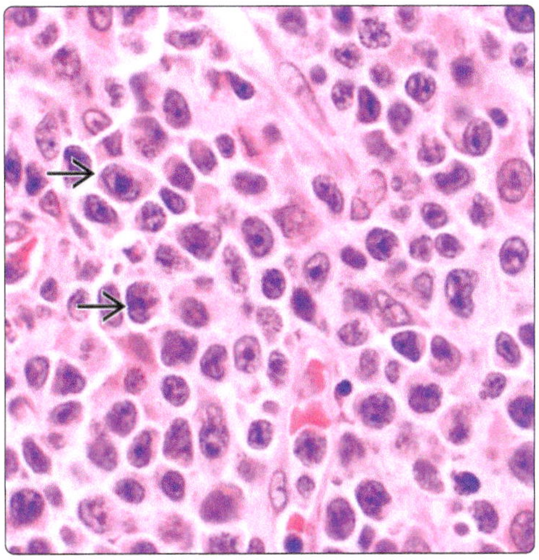

(Left) *Lymphomatoid granulomatosis of skin is angiocentric →, angiodestructive, and EBER(+), like ENNKTCL. However, this is a B-cell neoplasm and expresses multiple B-cell antigens.* **(Right)** *Diffuse large B-cell lymphoma (DLBCL) can also involve the upper airways like ENNKTCL. This DLBCL involves the maxillary sinuses. The tumor cells → are large and morphologically indistinguishable from ENNKTCL but are CD20(+), CD19(+), and pax-5(+).*

DDx: Posttransplant Lymphoproliferative Disorder

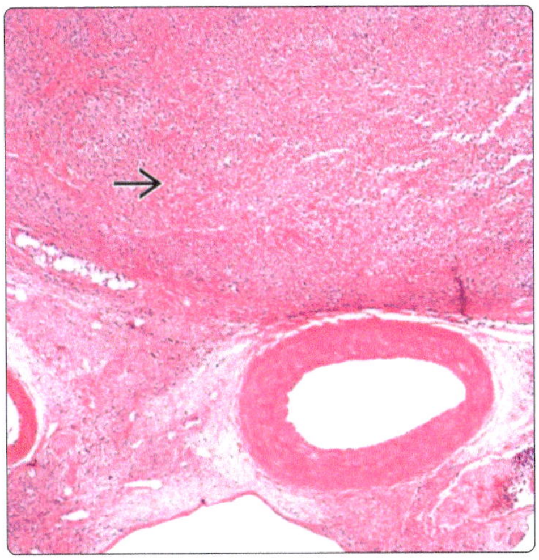

DDx: Posttransplant Lymphoproliferative Disorder at Higher Power

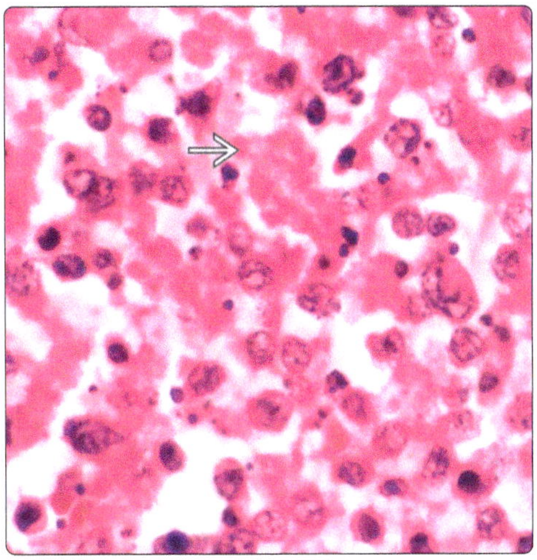

(Left) *Here is a posttransplant lymphoproliferative disorder (PTLD) with an extranodal NK-/T-cell lymphoma type. This patient developed a subcutaneous lesion after transplant. The tumor shows a nodular aggregate of malignant cells in the soft tissue →.* **(Right)** *This case of PTLD, extranodal NK-/T-cell lymphoma type shows medium-sized tumor cells with extensive necrosis → that are CD3(+), CD56(+), TIA(+), granzyme-B(+), and EBER(+).*

KEY FACTS

TERMINOLOGY

- One of the CD30(+) T-cell lymphoproliferative disorders
- Recurrent lymphoproliferative cutaneous disorder
- Disorder with self-healing lesions that regress without treatment and have atypical CD30(+) T cells in polymorphous background

CLINICAL ISSUES

- Papules or nodules at different stages of development that regress
- 20% have lymphomatoid papulosis (LyP)-associated malignant lymphoma
- Excellent prognosis

MICROSCOPIC

- Often wedge-shaped infiltrate; large atypical T cells
- Polymorphous background infiltrate
- 5 types: A, B, C, D, and E
  - Type A (mixed infiltrate)
  - Type B (mycosis fungoides-like)
  - Type C (ALCL-like)
  - Type D (cytotoxic T-cell variant)
  - Type E (angioinvasive variant)

ANCILLARY TESTS

- CD3(+), CD30(+), CD4(+), CD8(-), cytotoxic markers (+)
- t(2;5)(p23;q35) negative
- Clonal T-cell receptor gene rearrangement in 40%

TOP DIFFERENTIAL DIAGNOSES

- Primary and systemic anaplastic large cell lymphoma
  - Differentiated from LyP based on morphology and clinical course
- Reactive conditions
  - Infection and drug reaction can mimic LyP by showing clusters of atypical CD30(+) cells
- Mycosis fungoides
  - Similar to type B LyP with epidermotropism

Clinical Manifestation of LyP

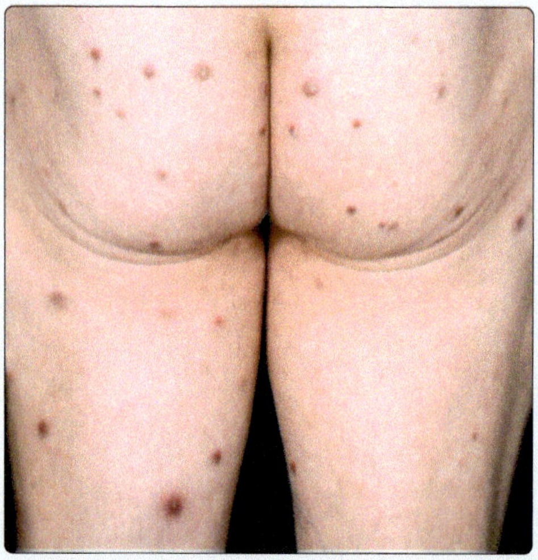

Low Magnification of LyP Type A

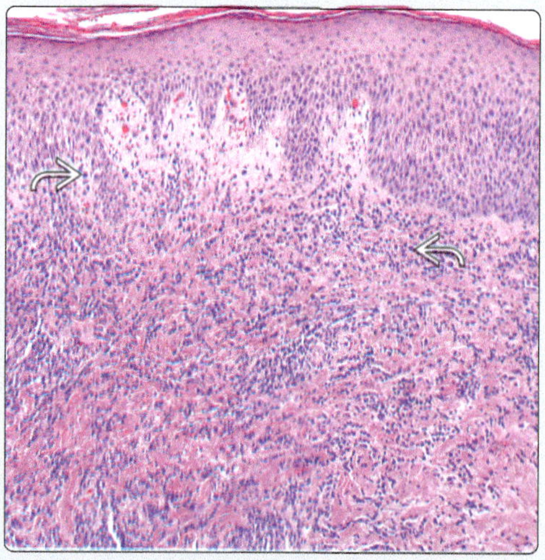

(Left) *There are papules around the buttocks and lower legs at different stages of evolution. (Courtesy R. Willemze, MD.)* **(Right)** *Epidermal acanthosis, spongiosis, and a mixed dermal infiltrate containing scattered large, hyperchromatic-staining atypical lymphocytes are shown.*

LyP Type A

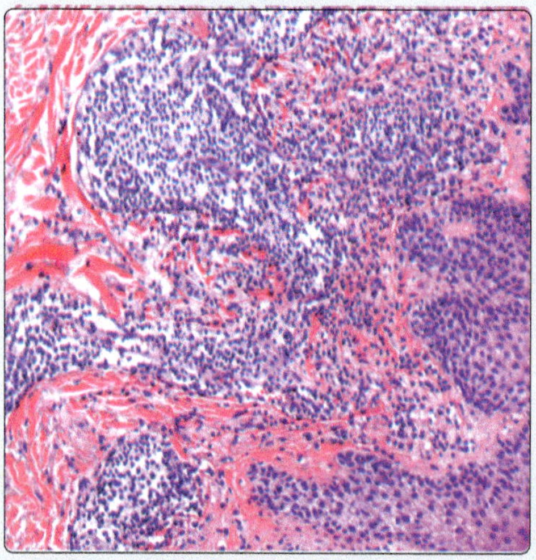

Higher Magnification of LyP Type A

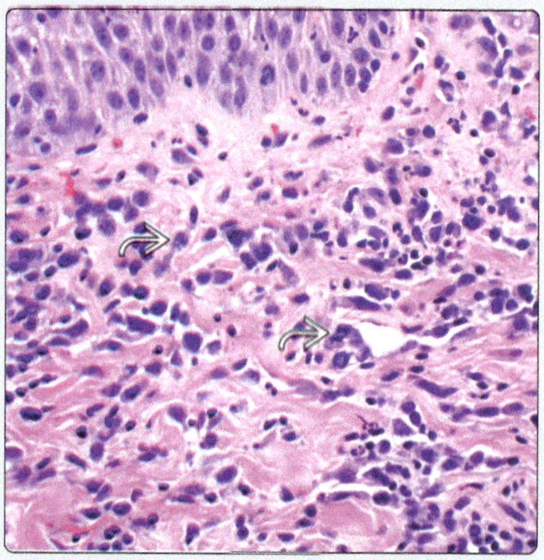

(Left) *The lesion involves the dermis and is composed of a mixed population of small- to medium-sized lymphocytes with scattered large cells. (Courtesy C. Yin, MD.)* **(Right)** *The lesion involves the dermis and is composed of a mixed population of small- to medium-sized lymphocytes with scattered large cells. Note the presence of mitotic figures.*

TERMINOLOGY

Abbreviations

- Lymphomatoid papulosis (LyP)

Definitions

- Recurrent, self-healing cutaneous lesions composed of CD30(+) atypical T cells in polymorphous inflammatory background
  - One of the CD30(+) T-cell lymphoproliferative disorders [LyP, primary cutaneous anaplastic large cell lymphoma (C-ALCL), and borderline cases]

ETIOLOGY/PATHOGENESIS

Idiopathic

- Viral infection, chronic antigenic stimulation, and immunosuppression have all been implicated as factors in some cases

CLINICAL ISSUES

Epidemiology

- Incidence
  - 0.1-0.2 cases per 100,000
- Age
  - Mostly adults, median age: 45 years, less common in children
- Sex
  - M:F = 3:1

Site

- Disease usually confined to skin
  - Common on trunk and extremities

Presentation

- Chronic, recurrent, and self-healing multiple erythematous papules or nodules
  - ± ulceration
  - Lesions at different stages of development
    - New lesions simultaneously occur at multiple anatomic sites
    - New lesions develop as old lesions regress
- May form vesicular, crusted, or hemorrhagic lesions

Natural History

- Lesions spontaneously heal with scarring
  - Individual skin lesions regress within 3-12 weeks
- Duration of disease
  - Waxing/waning clinical course; may persist for up to 40 years
- LyP-associated malignant lymphoma
  - Up to 20% of patients with LyP have another lymphoma
    - LyP may precede, proceed, or occur simultaneously with associated malignant lymphoma
    - Mycosis fungoides (MF), ALCL, Hodgkin lymphoma most common

Treatment

- Adjuvant therapy
  - No specific treatment for most patients other than follow-up to monitor changes in skin lesions
  - Sometimes low-dose methotrexate ± irradiation and psoralen ultraviolet A
  - Brentuximab vedotin has been used

Prognosis

- Excellent
  - ~ 100% 5-year survival
- 2% of associated lymphomas lead to death

MICROSCOPIC

Histologic Features

- Dermal infiltrate, often wedge-shaped or band-like, of medium- to large-sized T cells
  - Sometimes angiocentric
  - Folliculotropic if CD30(+) cells around hair follicles
- Epidermis may show ulceration, hyperkeratosis, and parakeratosis
- Variable histology with 5 subtypes (A, B, C, D, E) representing spectrum of disease
  - **Type A (mixed infiltrate)**
    - Few scattered large atypical Reed-Sternberg-like or multinucleated cells
    - Abundant reactive polymorphous inflammatory cells
  - **Type B (mycosis fungoides-like)**
    - Epidermotropism of small T cells showing cerebriform nuclei
    - Only 10% of LyP cases
    - Cannot be separated from MF by histology or immunohistochemistry
    - Type B LyP spontaneously regresses, unlike MF
  - **Type C (ALCL-like)**
    - Monotonous sheets of large atypical cells
    - Scant polymorphous background infiltrate
    - Cannot be separated from ALCL by histology or immunohistochemistry
  - **Type D (cytotoxic T-cell variant)**
    - Marked epidermotropism and CD8(+)
    - Mimics aggressive epidermotropic CD8(+) cytotoxic T-cell lymphoma
    - MUM1 focal to diffusely (+)
  - **Type E (angioinvasive variant)**
    - Clinically, rapidly progressing eschar-like ulcers
    - Angioinvasive infiltrates of medium-sized atypical lymphocytes
- Polymorphous background infiltrate
  - Histiocytes, neutrophils, eosinophils, and lymphocytes
- Biopsy may show overlapping features of type A, B, or C
- Rare histopathological variants
  - Syringotropic: Perieccrine infiltrates obliterating eccrine units
  - Granulomatous: Noncaseating granulomas
  - Follicular: ± perifollicular or intrafollicular infiltrates, cystic dilation or rupture of hair follicles, hyperplasia of follicular epithelium, follicular mucinosis and neutrophils in follicular epithelium

ANCILLARY TESTS

Immunohistochemistry

- T-cell antigens expressed: CD2(+), CD3(+), CD5(+), CD7(+)
  - ± loss of T-cell antigens (CD7 most common)

- CD30(+) necessary for diagnosis of type A and type C
  - CD30 often (-) in type B
  - ALK(-), EMA(-)
- Usually CD4(+), CD8(-), rarely CD8(+) cases (types D and E)
- Sometimes (+) for CD15, CD56 (10%), CD25, MUM1, TRAF, and Bcl-2
- Cytotoxic markers (+) (TIA1, granzyme-B, perforin)

In Situ Hybridization

- t(2;5)(p23;q35) negative

PCR

- Clonal T-cell receptor gene rearrangement
  - In ~ 40% of LyP cases
  - Identical T-cell clone in LyP lesions and LyP-associated lymphoma in same patient by sequencing studies

Genetic Testing

- No specific abnormalities

DIFFERENTIAL DIAGNOSIS

Primary and Systemic ALCL

- Also CD30(+) T-cell lymphoproliferative disorders
- Similar morphology to LyP
  - Both show proliferation of large atypical T cells
  - Both have similar immunophenotype
    - CD30 expression in LyP and ALCL
    - CD4(+) and cytotoxic markers (+)
    - ALK is (-) in LyP and cutaneous (C-ALCL), (+) in systemic ALCL
- Differentiated from LyP based on morphology and clinical course
  - ALCL usually single nodular lesion
  - Polymorphous background infiltrate not as prominent
  - t(2;5)(p23;q35) can be (+) in systemic ALCL, unlike LyP

Borderline Lesions

- Overlapping features of LyP and C-ALCL
- Unusual clinical features or discrepancy between clinical features and histology &/or immunophenotype
  - Multiple papules that do not regress
  - 1 or more nodular lesions that show mixed inflammatory infiltrate

Mycosis Fungoides

- Similar to type B LyP
  - Both LyP and MF present with epidermotropism
- Different clinical course than LyP
  - Lacks self-regressing skin lesions
  - Clinical course: Patches → plaques → tumor stage

Reactive Conditions

- Viral infections can mimic LyP
  - HSV, VZV, EBV, HPV
  - Dense infiltrate in dermis with CD30(+) T cells
  - Resolves in a few weeks
  - ± viral inclusions
  - IHC for viral antigens
  - PCR for viral DNA may be needed for definite diagnosis
- Arthropod bite reactions and dermatophyte infections can also mimic LyP
- Drug reactions can mimic LyP
  - Histology shows clusters of large CD30(+) cells in dermal T-cell infiltrate
  - History of drug use
  - Resolves after discontinuation of drug
- Pityriasis lichenoides et varioliformis acuta (PLEVA)
  - Common in children/young adults
  - Scaly erythematous/hemorrhagic lesions
  - Interface dermatitis with necrotic keratinocytes and Civatte/colloid bodies
  - CD8(+), CD30(-) (usually)
  - CD30(+) PLEVA has been described: Clinically similar to ulcerative LyP type A but no waxing or waning course typical of LyP

Classic Hodgkin Lymphoma

- Similarities to LyP
  - Hodgkin-like cells can be seen in LyP type A
  - Both tumors have polymorphous background infiltrate
  - Both are CD30(+)
- Differences from LyP
  - Rarely involves skin
  - Often CD15(+), EBER(+)
  - B-cell lymphoma, whereas LyP is T-cell proliferation
    - Classic Hodgkin lymphoma is often pax-5(+)

Primary Cutaneous Aggressive Epidermotropic CD8(+) Cytotoxic T-Cell Lymphoma

- Can be morphologically indistinguishable from cytotoxic variant of LyP (type D)
  - Both are CD8(+), CD30(+), cytoxic markers(+)
  - Worse prognosis with aggressive epidermotropic CD8(+) cytotoxic T-cell lymphoma than LyP

SELECTED REFERENCES

1. Barrett MM et al: Lymphomatoid papulosis type D: report of a case in a child and review of the literature. Pediatr Dermatol. 33(2):e52-e56, 2016
2. Bosisio FM et al: Expression of T-follicular helper markers in sequential biopsies of progressive mycosis fungoides and other primary cutaneous T-cell lymphomas. Am J Dermatopathol. 37(2):115-21, 2015
3. Duvic M et al: Results of a phase II trial of brentuximab vedotin for CD30+ cutaneous T-cell lymphoma and lymphomatoid papulosis. J Clin Oncol. 33(32):3759-65, 2015
4. Hughey LC: Practical management of CD30+ lymphoproliferative disorders. Dermatol Clin. 33(4):819-33, 2015
5. Kiavash K et al: New variant lymphomatoid papulosis type E preceding and coexisting with mycosis fungoides - a case report and review of the literature. J Cutan Pathol. ePub, 2015
6. Martires KJ et al: Characterization of primary cutaneous CD8+/CD30+ lymphoproliferative disorders. Am J Dermatopathol. 37(11):822-33, 2015
7. Newland KM et al: The efficacy of methotrexate for lymphomatoid papulosis. J Am Acad Dermatol. 72(6):1088-90, 2015
8. Ganapathi KA et al: Early lymphoid lesions: conceptual, diagnostic and clinical challenges. Haematologica. 99(9):1421-32, 2014
9. Kempf W et al: Cutaneous lymphomas: an update. Part 1: T-cell and natural killer/t-cell lymphomas and related conditions. Am J Dermatopathol. 36(2):105-23, 2014
10. Saggini A et al: A variant of lymphomatoid papulosis simulating primary cutaneous aggressive epidermotropic CD8+ cytotoxic T-cell lymphoma. Description of 9 cases. Am J Surg Pathol. 34(8):1168-75, 2010
11. de Souza A et al: Clinical, histopathologic, and immunophenotypic features of lymphomatoid papulosis with CD8 predominance in 14 pediatric patients. J Am Acad Dermatol. 61(6):993-1000, 2009
12. El Shabrawi-Caelen L et al: Lymphomatoid papulosis: reappraisal of clinicopathologic presentation and classification into subtypes A, B, and C. Arch Dermatol. 140(4):441-7, 2004
13. Kempf W et al: Fascin expression in CD30-positive cutaneous lymphoproliferative disorders. J Cutan Pathol. 29(5):295-300, 2002

H&E and CD30 Stain for LyP Type A

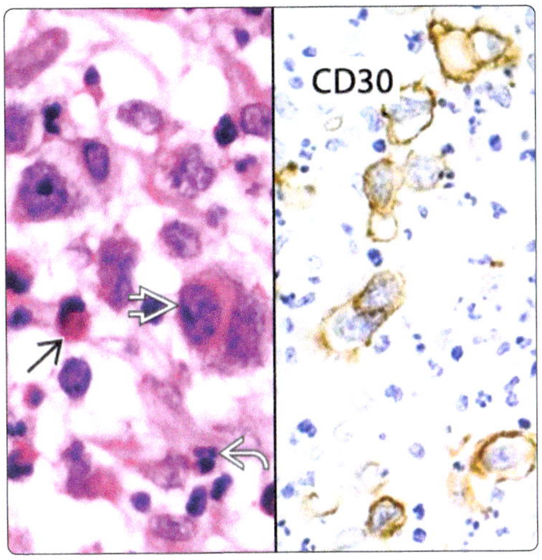

LyP Type B

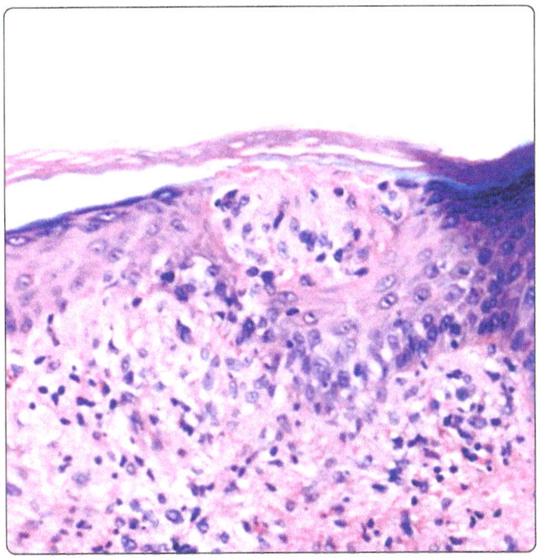

(Left) *This lymphomatoid papulosis shows a type A pattern with scattered large atypical cells and a mixed background infiltrate of eosinophils and neutrophils. The CD30 stain highlights the large atypical cells. (Courtesy M. Tomaszewski, MD.)* **(Right)** *This case of LyP has a type B pattern of infiltration with epidermotropism. There are small T cells in the epidermis with cerebriform nuclei. CD30 is negative, as expected in type B.*

LyP Type C

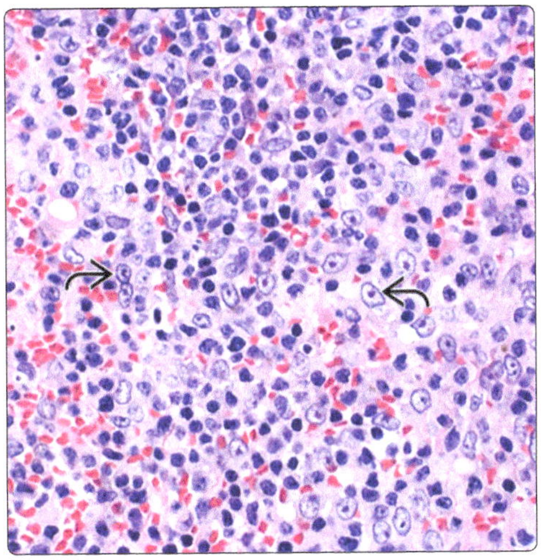

H&E and CD30 Stain for LyP Type C

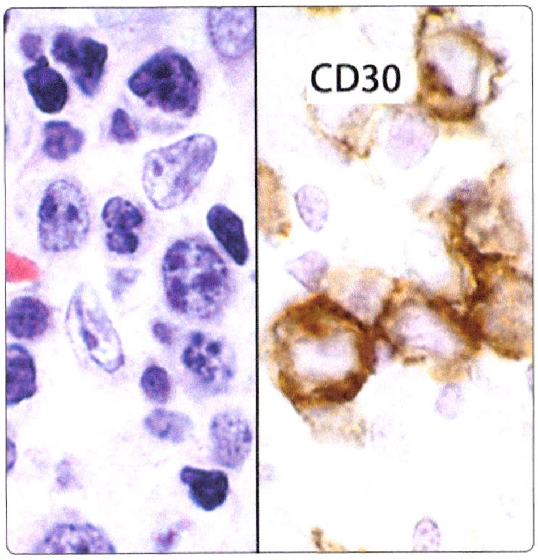

(Left) *There are sheet-like aggregates of large atypical cells with vesicular chromatin, prominent nucleoli, and pale cytoplasm, with only a sparse lymphocytic background.* **(Right)** *This high-power image of type C LyP shows that the large atypical cells express CD30 by immunohistochemical staining. The aggregates of CD30(+) T cells are similar to anaplastic large cell lymphoma. (Courtesy M. Tomaszewski, MD.)*

LyP Type D

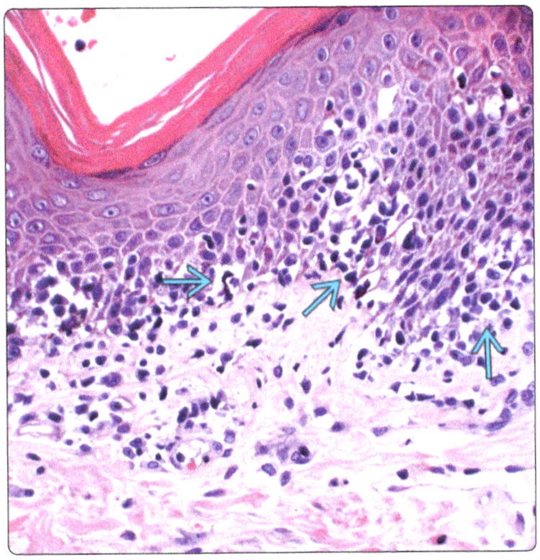

LyP Type D With Pautrier Abscess-Like Area

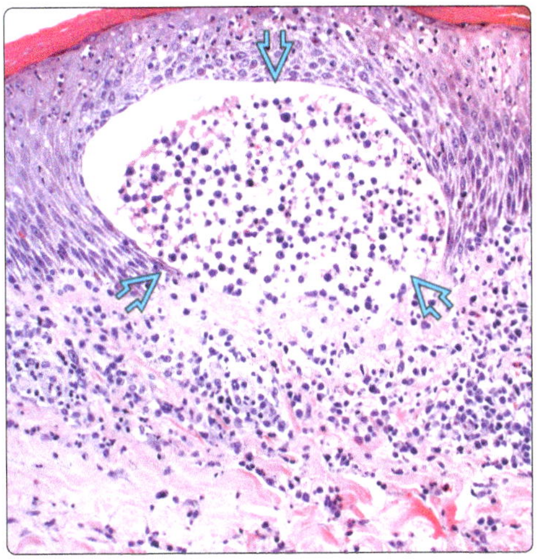

(Left) *This is an example of a type D LyP showing marked epidermotropism. The infiltrate was also CD8(+) (not shown). Given this morphology and phenotype, type D LyP mimics aggressive epidermotropic CD8(+) cytotoxic T-cell lymphoma.* **(Right)** *This is an example of a LyP type D, which is showing a large Pautrier abscess-like area. The cells in the intraepidermal abscess were CD8(+).*

CD30 Stain in LyP Type A

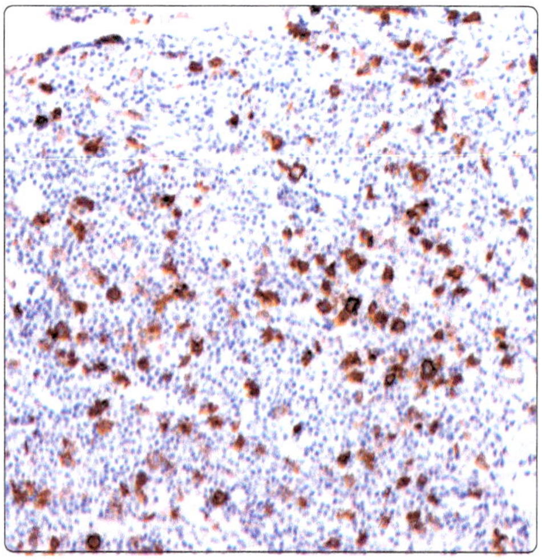

CD3 Stain in LyP

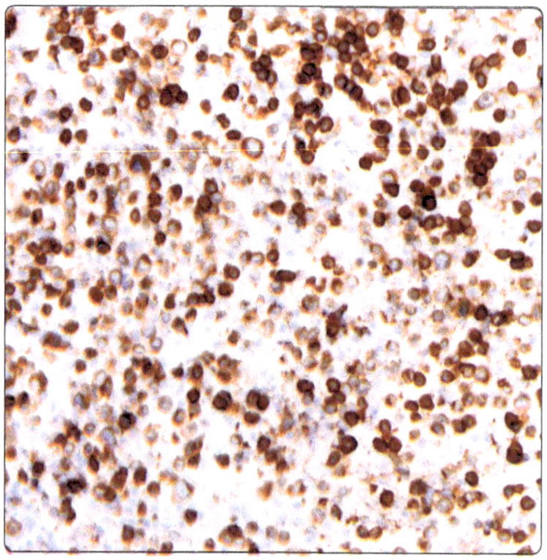

(Left) *Immunohistochemical study for CD30 in a case of LyP type A shows large atypical cells that are CD30(+), usually singly scattered, and represent a minority cell population in type A cases. (Courtesy C. Yin, MD.)* **(Right)** *CD3 is also expressed in the T-cell infiltrate, as expected in LyP. T-cell antigens, including CD2(+), CD3(+), CD5(+), and CD7(+), are immunoreactive in LyP. Sometimes there can be loss of one of the T-cell antigens, with CD7 being most common. (Courtesy C. Yin, MD.)*

CD30 Stain in LyP Type C

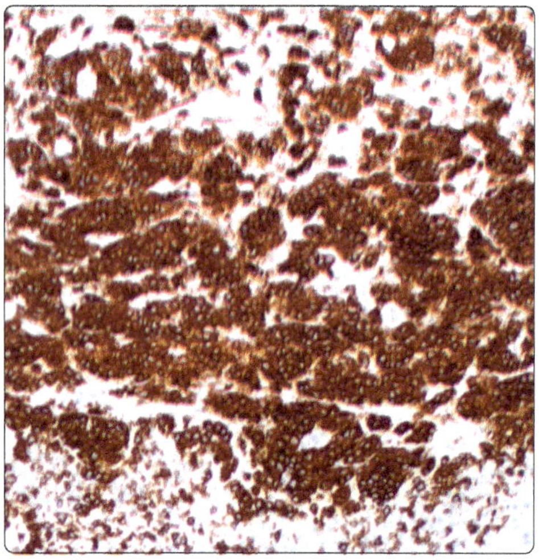

Ki-67 in LyP Type C

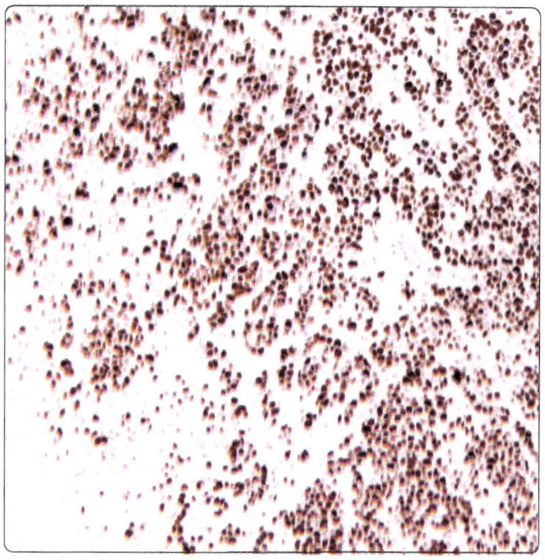

(Left) *The CD30 immunohistochemical stain is strongly and diffusely positive in the infiltrate in this case of LyP type C. CD30(+) is also seen in anaplastic large cell lymphoma and in other reactive conditions, including infections and some drug reactions. (Courtesy C. Yin, MD).* **(Right)** *Immunohistochemical study for Ki-67 in a case of LyP type C shows that lymphoid cells of LyP usually have a high proliferative rate. (Courtesy C. Yin, MD.)*

FISH for *ALK* Gene in LyP

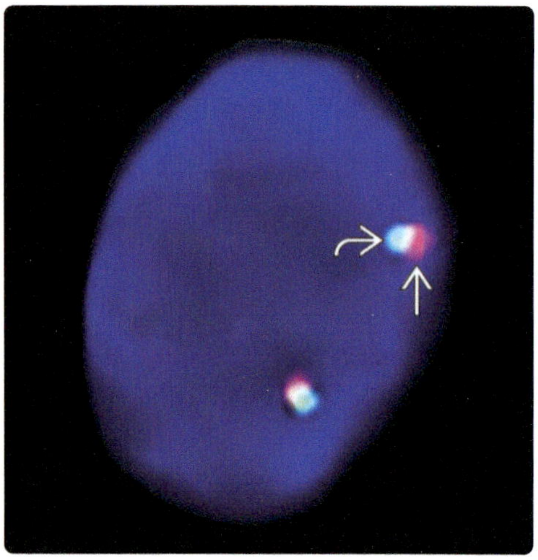

TCR-PCR of LyP

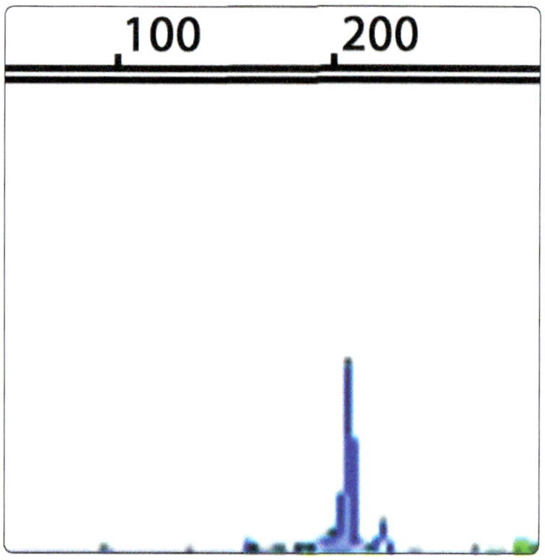

(Left) *This break-apart FISH probe for 2p23 (ALK) shows the lack of ALK rearrangement in a patient with LyP. A blue signal ➡ represents the ALK 5' region, and a pink signal ➡ represents the ALK 3' region. Two combined yellow signals indicate that ALK has not rearranged. (Courtesy N. Potter, MD and G. Nichols, MD.)* **(Right)** *The blue peak between 180 and 280 base pairs in size is suggestive of a clonal T-cell rearrangement, as is seen in 40% of cases of LyP.*

DDx of ALCL

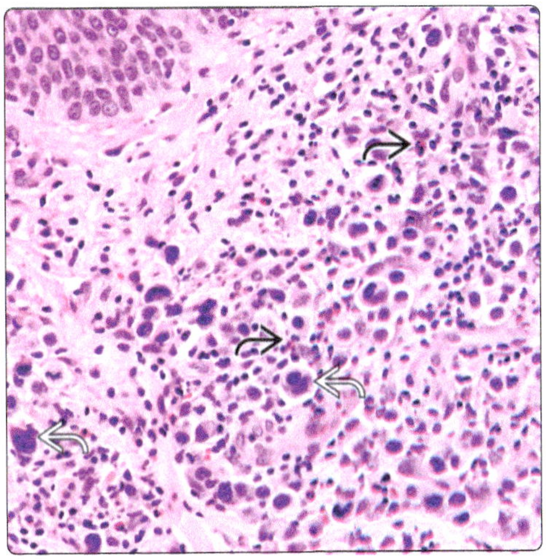

DDx of Mycosis Fungoides

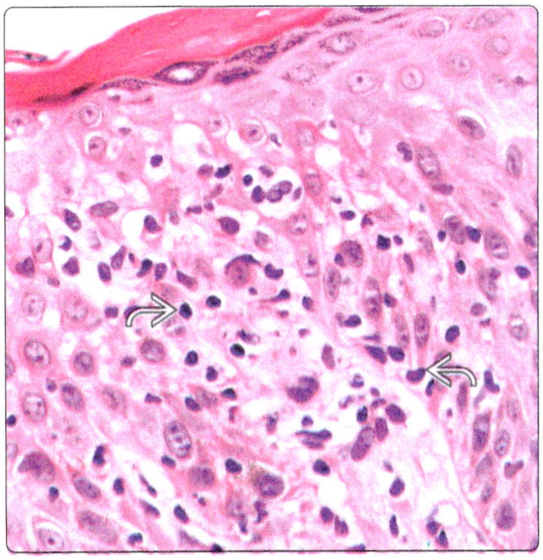

(Left) *Anaplastic large cell lymphoma shows large anaplastic cells with abundant cytoplasm and irregular multilobated nuclei, admixed with inflammatory cells including a few eosinophils. The histologic findings are essentially identical to those in LyP, and clinical findings are essential to distinguish these entities. (Courtesy C. Yin, MD.)* **(Right)** *This case of mycosis fungoides shows epidermotropism of numerous small but hyperchromatic-staining T cells in the epidermis, similar to type B LyP.*

H&E of Dermatophyte Infection

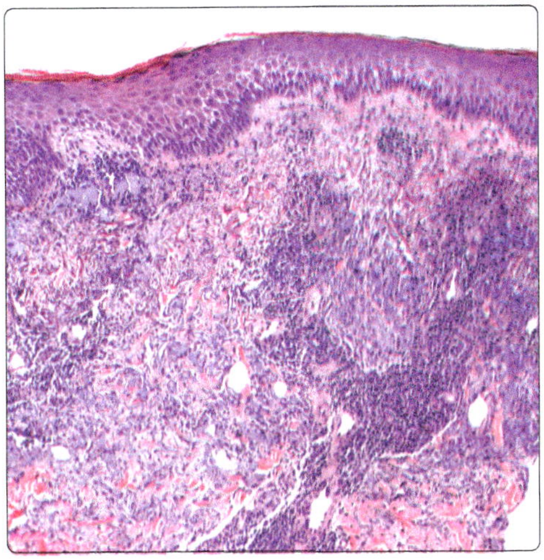

H&E of Dermatophyte Infection

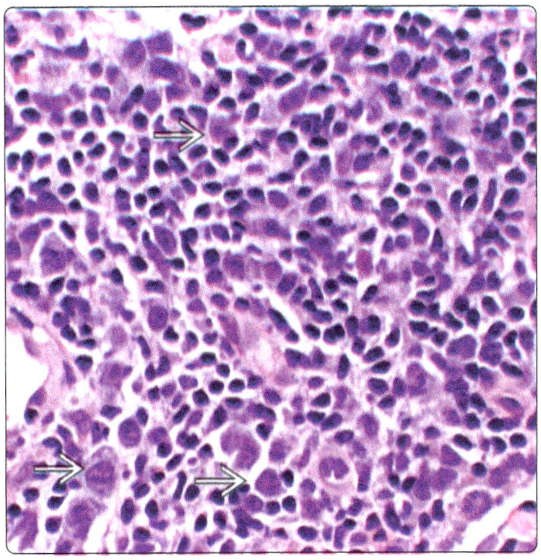

(Left) *At low power, this example of a dermatophyte infection shows a dense, atypical inflammatory infiltrate involving the entire dermis. These mononuclear cells with atypia appear similar to the atypical T cells in LyP. Many reactive conditions can mimic LyP, but the most common are infections and drug reactions.* **(Right)** *At higher power, large atypical cells in the dermis form aggregates and appear identical to those seen in LyP.*

CD30(+) Cells in Dermatophyte Infection

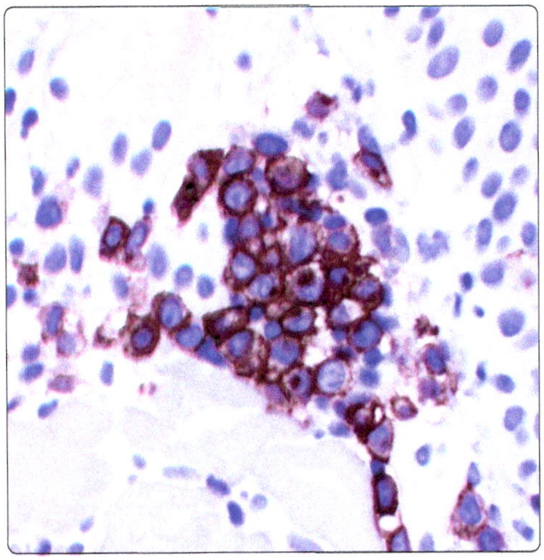

Hair Follicle in Dermatophyte Infection

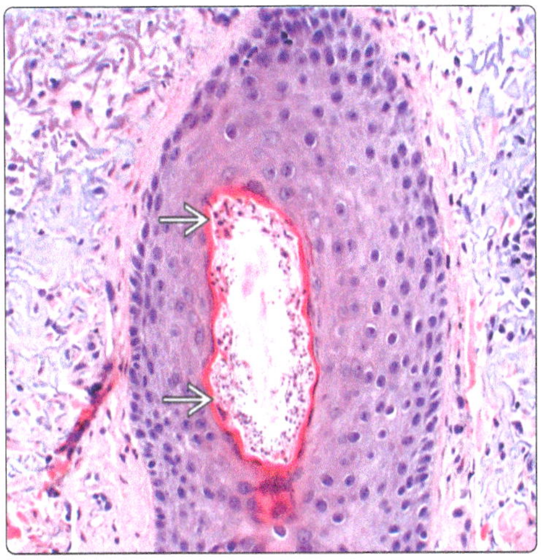

(Left) *In the same case of dermatophyte infection, high magnification of a CD30 IHC stain shows that the large atypical cells are strongly immunoreactive for CD30, just like the T cells of LyP.* **(Right)** *Also in the same case, this hair follicle contains numerous hyphal organisms, which is diagnostic for a dermatophyte infection. Infections and arthropod bite reactions can mimic LyP, especially when they show increased CD30(+) cells.*

Primary Cutaneous Anaplastic Large Cell Lymphoma

KEY FACTS

TERMINOLOGY

- One of the primary cutaneous CD30(+) T-cell lymphoproliferative disorders
  - T-cell lymphoma of atypical, usually large CD30(+) cells, without evidence of mycosis fungoides

CLINICAL ISSUES

- Solitary or localized nodules that can regress but frequently recur
- Can involve regional lymph nodes
- Treated with skin-targeted therapy for low-stage disease, chemotherapy for systemic disease
- Good prognosis, ~ 90% 10-yr survival

MICROSCOPIC

- Polymorphic background infiltrate not prominent
- Diffuse sheets of large T cells in dermis ± subcutis
- Hallmark cells with multiple nuclei (horseshoe-shaped), helpful if present

ANCILLARY TESTS

- Immunohistochemistry: CD30(+), CD15(-), CD3(+), cytotoxic markers (+), EMA(-), ALK(-), CLA(+)
- Molecular: No *ALK* gene translocations on chromosome 2
- ALK(-) ALCL shows *DUSP22* and *TP63* gene rearrangements
- Cases with *DUSP22* mutations have favorable prognosis compared to *TP63* mutations, which have more unfavorable prognosis

TOP DIFFERENTIAL DIAGNOSES

- Systemic ALCL with cutaneous involvement
  - EMA(+), ALK(+), and *ALK* gene translocations, unlike primary cutaneous anaplastic large cell lymphoma (PCALCL)
- Lymphomatoid papulosis (LyP)
  - Groups of papules that regress and recur
  - Wedge-shaped and prominent polymorphous background infiltrate
- Large cell transformation of mycosis fungoides (MF)

PCALCL on Neck

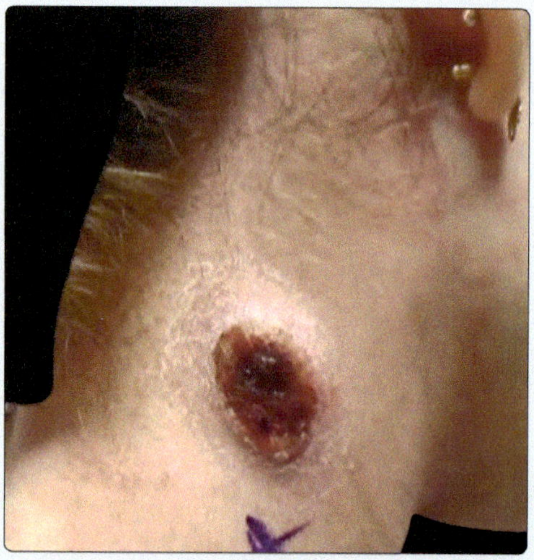

Low Magnification of PCALCL

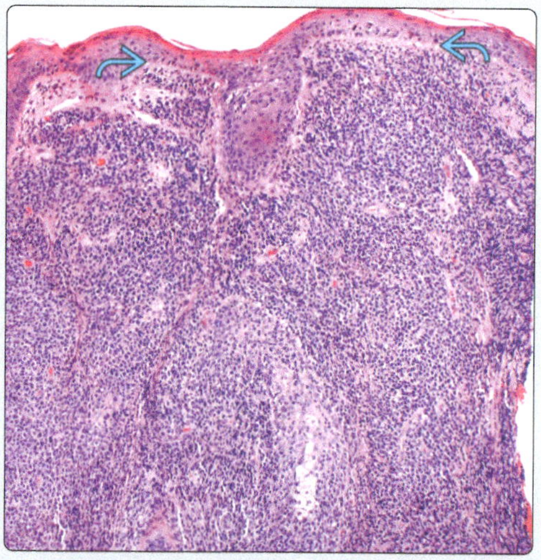

(Left) *This was a young adult female who presented with a single large, ulcerated nodular tumor on her neck.* **(Right)** *Low magnification of a primary cutaneous anaplastic large cell lymphoma (PCALCL) shows a diffuse, nodular to sheet-like dermal proliferation of large, atypical cells with hyperchromatic-staining nuclei admixed with smaller inflammatory cells. There is a grenz zone separating the infiltrate from the epidermis in this case.*

Higher Magnification of ALCL

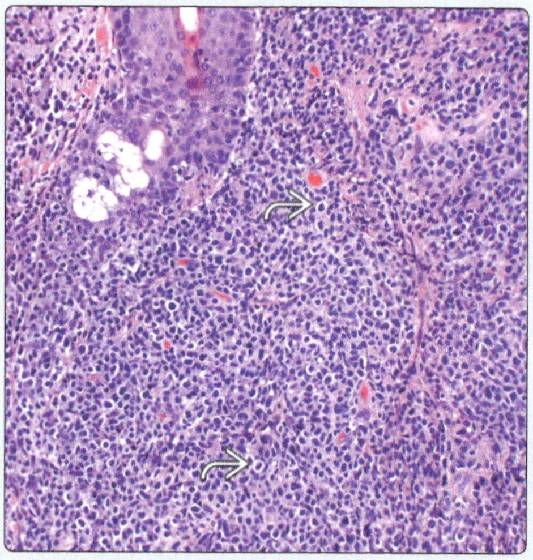

***ALK* Fluorescent In Situ Hybridization in PCALCL**

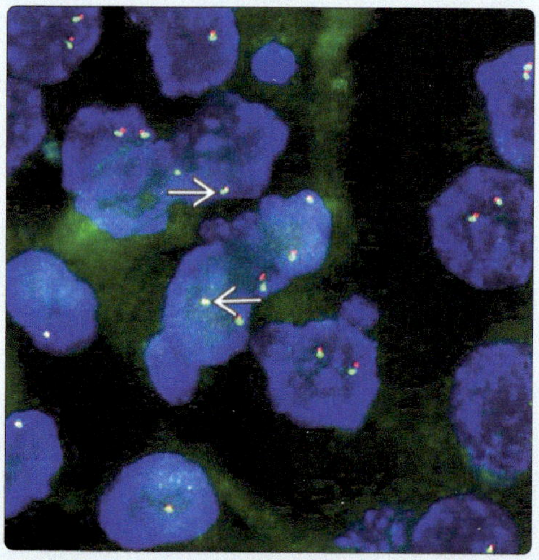

(Left) *Higher magnification shows numerous large, markedly atypical cells with amphophilic-staining cytoplasm and hyperchromatic-staining nuclei. Multiple mitotic figures are easily seen.* **(Right)** *This is a ALK FISH break-apart probe, which is showing that the signals are fused (yellow), indicating that ALK is not rearranged. ALK is rearranged in systemic ALCL, but not rearranged in PCALCL.*

TERMINOLOGY

Abbreviations

- Primary cutaneous anaplastic large cell lymphoma (PCALCL)

Synonyms

- Regressing atypical histiocytosis
- Primary cutaneous large cell T-cell lymphoma, CD30(+)

Definitions

- CD30(+) T-cell lymphoma consisting of atypical, usually large cells, without evidence of mycosis fungoides
  - One of the primary cutaneous CD30(+) T-cell lymphoproliferative disorders, including lymphomatoid papulosis (LyP) and borderline lesions

ETIOLOGY/PATHOGENESIS

Idiopathic

- Viral infection, chronic antigen stimulation, and immunosuppression may play role
- Mechanism may involve CD30/TRAF1 upregulation of NF-κB

CLINICAL ISSUES

Epidemiology

- Incidence
  - 2nd most common cutaneous T-cell lymphoma after mycosis fungoides
    - 0.1-0.2 per 100,000 people
- Age
  - Median age: 7th decade; can occur in children
- Sex
  - M:F = 2-3:1

Site

- Often trunk, face, and extremities

Presentation

- Solitary or localized nodules or papules ± ulceration
  - Growing rapidly, multifocal ~ 20%
- No clinical evidence of other cutaneous T-cell lymphoma
- No extracutaneous involvement besides regional lymph nodes
- Usually no symptoms other than mass effect
- ALK(-) ALCL is associated with breast implants

Natural History

- Partial or complete spontaneous regression (40%) but frequently recur
- Extracutaneous dissemination ~ 10%
  - Usually to regional lymph nodes

Treatment

- Solitary or localized nodules
  - Surgical excision
    - Excision is most common treatment approach
    - ~ 40% relapses
  - Radiation
    - Can be initial monotherapy or combined with surgical excision
    - ~ 40% relapses when used alone as 1st-line therapy
- Multifocal disease
  - Chemotherapy
    - CHOP or methotrexate but little evidence for their effectiveness
    - Multiagent chemotherapy for extracutaneous spread beyond regional lymph nodes

Prognosis

- Better than most T-cell lymphomas
  - ~ 90% 10-yr survival
  - Age < 60 yr and spontaneous regression are good prognostic indicators
  - Relapses confined to skin, multifocal skin lesions, or regional lymph node involvement does not yield worse prognosis

MICROSCOPIC

Histologic Features

- Diffuse sheets of large T cells in dermis ± subcutis
  - Infrequent epidermotropism ± ulceration
  - Can involve lymphatic spaces
- Tumor cells
  - Large anaplastic, pleomorphic, or immunoblastic appearance
  - Anaplastic cells with roundish shapes ± abundant cytoplasm
    - Small cell and histiocyte-rich variants are rare
  - Mitotic figures
  - Hallmark cells with multiple nuclei (horseshoe-shaped), often not seen, but helpful if present
- Polymorphic background infiltrate (eosinophils and plasma cells) uncommon, unlike LyP
  - Exceptions
    - Ulcerating ALCL has polymorphic infiltrate, fewer CD30(+) cells, and epidermal hyperplasia
    - Neutrophil-rich (pyogenic ALCL) shows clusters of neutrophils with only scattered CD30(+) cells
- Pseudoepitheliomatous hyperplasia variant
  - Likely spontaneous regression and complete resolution within a few months of initial diagnosis

ANCILLARY TESTS

Immunohistochemistry

- By definition, CD30(+) expressed by > 75% of tumor cells
- CD15(-)
- T-cell antigens express [CD2(+), CD3(+), CD5(+), CD7(+)]
  - But can show loss of T-cell antigens
- CD4(+)/CD8(-)
  - CD8(+) and CD4(-)/CD8(-) rarely
- Cytotoxic markers (+): Granzyme-B, perforin, TIA-1
- EMA(-) and ALK(-) in PCALCL
  - Usually EMA(+) and ALK(+) in systemic ALCL
  - ALK(+) skin tumor likely indicates secondary cutaneous ALCL
- Cutaneous lymphocyte antigen [CLA(+)] and HOXC5(+) in PCALCL
  - But CLA(-) in systemic ALCL
- B-cell markers (-) (CD20 and CD79)
  - Rarely pax-5(+)

Genetic Testing

- Clonal T-cell receptor gene rearrangement ~ 90%
- PCALCL does not show *ALK* gene rearrangements on chromosome 2p23
- *DUSP22 (IRF4/MUM1)* and *TP63* gene rearrangements are detected, usually in ALK(-) ALCL, but are usually not found in ALK(+) ALCL
  - Cases with *DUSP22* mutations have favorable prognosis compared to *TP63* mutations, which have more unfavorable prognosis
  - Expression of IRF4/MUM1 protein does not correlate with presence of translocation and cannot be used as surrogate marker

DIFFERENTIAL DIAGNOSIS

Systemic ALCL With Cutaneous Involvement

- Similar morphologic features and overlapping phenotype with PCALCL
- Separate disease from PCALCL, with different molecular findings and prognosis
  - Primary tumor in extracutaneous site that secondarily involves skin
  - In ALK(-) ALCL, skin may be initial manifestation; systemic involvement occurs in < 6 months
- Differences from PCALCL
  - Systemic ALCL also found in extracutaneous sites
  - Typically EMA(+) and ALK(+), unlike PCALCL
  - Translocations involving *ALK* gene
  - Less favorable prognosis [especially ALK(-) systemic ALCL]

Lymphomatoid Papulosis

- Also CD30(+) T-cell lymphoproliferative disorder but with more polymorphic background infiltrate
- Both often present with large atypical T cells
- Both have similar immunophenotype
  - CD30(+) in LyP and ALCL
  - ALK(-) in both, except for systemic ALCL
- Differentiated from ALCL based on morphology and clinical course
  - Usually more wedge-shaped infiltrate
  - Polymorphic background infiltrate is prominent
  - Groups of papules that regress without treatment and often recur
  - Better prognosis than ALCL
  - Sometimes only clinical findings can differentiate ALCL from LyP

Borderline Lesions

- Another type of primary cutaneous CD30(+) T-cell lymphoproliferative disorder
- Discrepancy between clinical features and histology/immunophenotype
  - Examples of borderline lesions
    - Case with clinical features of LyP (multiple papules/nodules), which are present with morphology more typical of ALCL (sheets of large atypical cells)
    - Case with clinical features of ALCL (solitary nonregressing lesion) with histology more like LyP (fewer atypical cells and polymorphous background infiltrate)

Large Cell Transformation of Mycosis Fungoides

- Patient with history/clinical evidence of mycosis fungoides
- Large atypical T cells with similar phenotype to ALCL
  - CD4(+), CD30(±)
- ≥ 25% large T cells in tumor
  - Can look identical to neoplastic cells in ALCL
- Often loses epidermotropism

Reactive Conditions Expressing CD30

- Viruses, arthropod bites, and drugs are most common reactive conditions that mimic ALCL
  - They can show clusters of large CD30(+) cells
  - Diagnosis may need clinical correlation or PCR for viral DNA

Classic Hodgkin Lymphoma

- Similarities to ALCL
  - Both have CD30(+) cells
  - Both have large, atypical tumor cells
  - pax-5(+) in 50% of classic Hodgkin lymphoma and rare cases of ALCL
- Differences from ALCL
  - Rare in skin
  - CD15(+)
  - EBER(+)
  - LCA(-)
  - Malignant cells not in aggregates

Diffuse Large B-Cell Lymphoma

- Similar large, atypical cells as in ALCL and can be CD30(+)
- However, strongly expresses B-cell antigens (CD19, CD20, pax-5)

SELECTED REFERENCES

1. Parrilla Castellar ER et al: ALK-negative anaplastic large cell lymphoma is a genetically heterogeneous disease with widely disparate clinical outcomes. Blood. 124(9):1473-80, 2014
2. Quintanilla-Martinez L et al: Non-mycosis fungoides cutaneous T-cell lymphomas: report of the 2011 Society for Hematopathology/European Association for Haematopathology workshop. Am J Clin Pathol. 139(4):491-514, 2013
3. Kempf W et al: EORTC, ISCL, and USCLC consensus recommendations for the treatment of primary cutaneous CD30-positive lymphoproliferative disorders: lymphomatoid papulosis and primary cutaneous anaplastic large-cell lymphoma. Blood. 118(15):4024-35, 2011
4. Feldman AL et al: PAX5-positive T-cell anaplastic large cell lymphomas associated with extra copies of the PAX5 gene locus. Mod Pathol. 23(4):593-602, 2010
5. Burg G et al: Pyogenic lymphoma of the skin: a peculiar variant of primary cutaneous neutrophil-rich CD30+ anaplastic large-cell lymphoma. Clinicopathological study of four cases and review of the literature. Br J Dermatol. 148(3):580-6, 2003
6. Bekkenk MW et al: Primary and secondary cutaneous CD30(+) lymphoproliferative disorders: a report from the Dutch Cutaneous Lymphoma Group on the long-term follow-up data of 219 patients and guidelines for diagnosis and treatment. Blood. 95(12):3653-61, 2000
7. Boulland ML et al: Primary CD30-positive cutaneous T-cell lymphomas and lymphomatoid papulosis frequently express cytotoxic proteins. Histopathology. 36(2):136-44, 2000
8. Stein H et al: CD30(+) anaplastic large cell lymphoma: a review of its histopathologic, genetic, and clinical features. Blood. 96(12):3681-95, 2000
9. Gascoyne RD et al: Prognostic significance of anaplastic lymphoma kinase (ALK) protein expression in adults with anaplastic large cell lymphoma. Blood. 93(11):3913-21, 1999

Low-Power Magnification of ALCL

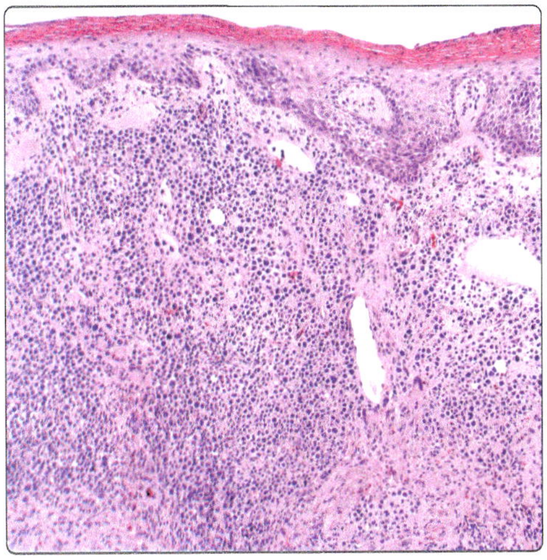

Higher Power Magnification of ALCL

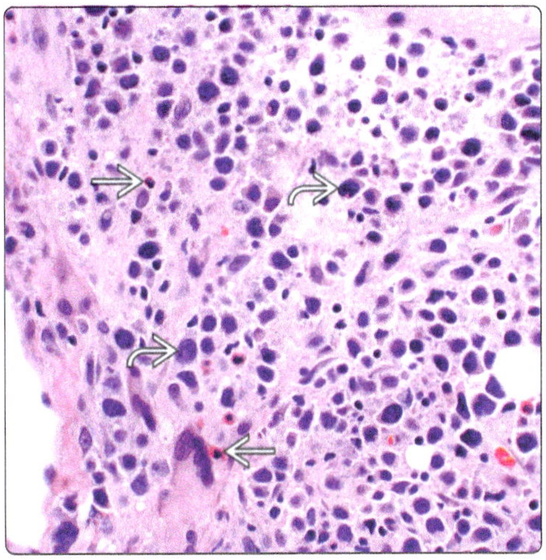

(Left) *Low-magnification histologic section from a patient with PCALCL shows a diffuse, sheet-like proliferation of numerous large atypical cells with abundant cytoplasm and hyperchromatic nuclei admixed with smaller inflammatory cells.* **(Right)** *Higher magnification of ALCL shows large atypical cells with abundant cytoplasm and irregular multilobated nuclei, admixed with a background of small inflammatory cells, including eosinophils.*

Hallmark Cells in ALCL

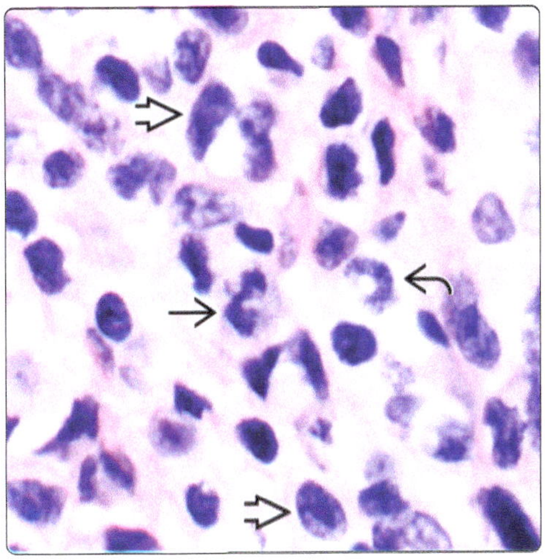

ALCL: Lymphatic Involvement and CD30(+)

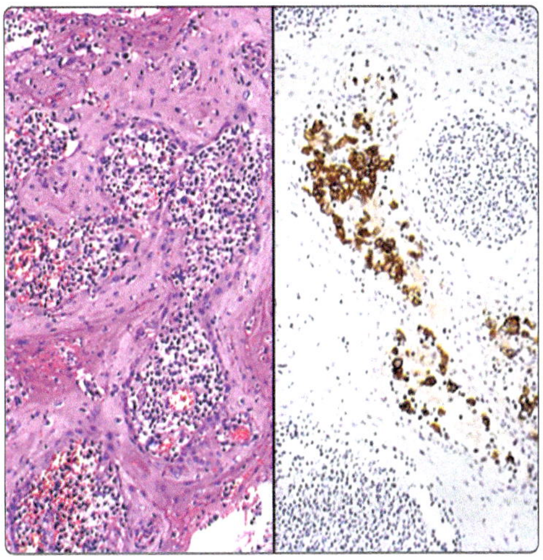

(Left) *At high power, the malignant T cells are large with dense chromatin and irregular nuclear shapes. Scattered mitotic figures are easily seen. Rare cells have the horseshoe-shaped nuclei of so-called hallmark cells. No neutrophils or eosinophils are seen.* **(Right)** *This case of ALCL is primarily involving the lymphatic spaces. The right side of the image is a CD30 immunohistochemical stain, which marks the tumor cells within the lymphatics. (Courtesy M. Tomaszewski, MD.)*

ALCL With Mucinous Stroma

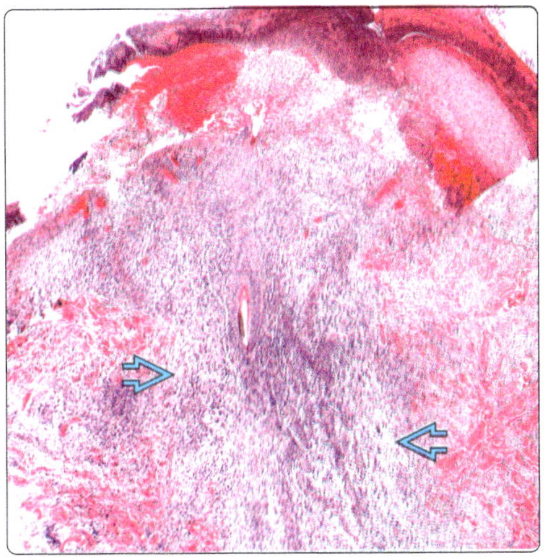

ALCL With Mucinous Stroma

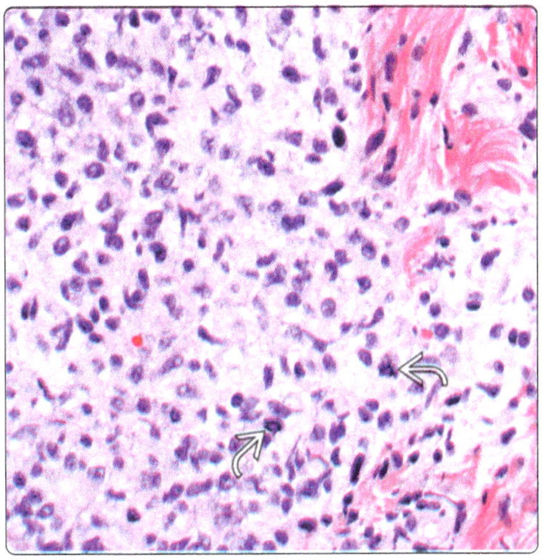

(Left) *This unusual case of ALCL showed a prominent mucinous stroma in the dermis. Note the diffuse overlying epidermal ulceration and serum crust present.* **(Right)** *High magnification of ALCL with a mucinous stroma shows a cellular nodule of markedly enlarged and atypical-appearing cells, with multiple mitoses easily identified. The cells were strongly CD30(+).*

(Left) *In this case of ALCL, on the left-sided H&E, large anaplastic-appearing malignant cells can be seen. On the right is a CD3 immunohistochemical stain that shows that the malignant cells are strongly positive for CD3, as expected in a T-cell lymphoma.* **(Right)** *This high-power image of a CD4 stain shows that the tumor cells are strongly CD4(+). CD8 (not shown) was negative. Most cases of ALCL are CD4(+)/CD8(-), and only 5% are CD4(-)/CD8(+).*

ALCL: Cytologic Features and CD3(+)

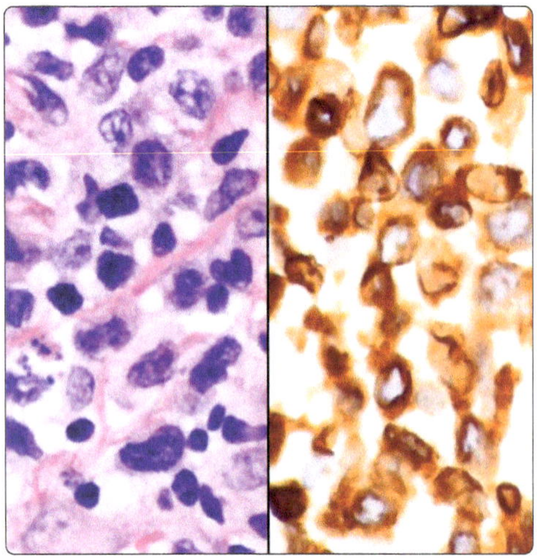

ALCL: CD4(+)

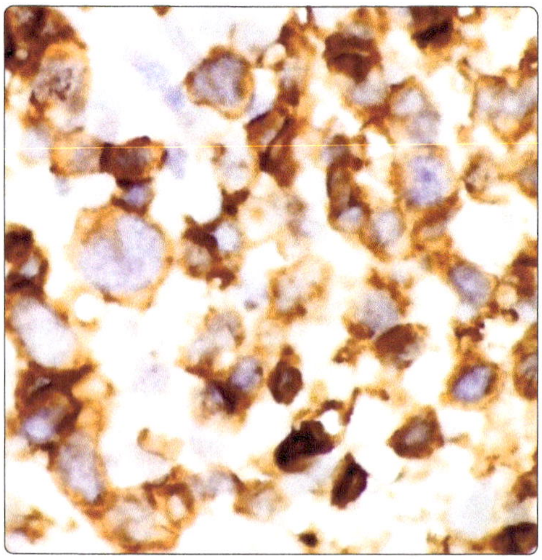

(Left) *ALK(-) immunohistochemical stain in a PCALCL is shown, which is typically ALK(-).* **(Right)** *ALK(+) immunohistochemical stain in a systemic ALCL with secondary cutaneous involvement is shown. Currently, systemic ALCL is either classified as ALK(+) or ALK(-), which are considered different diseases.*

ALK Negativity in Primary Cutaneous ALCL

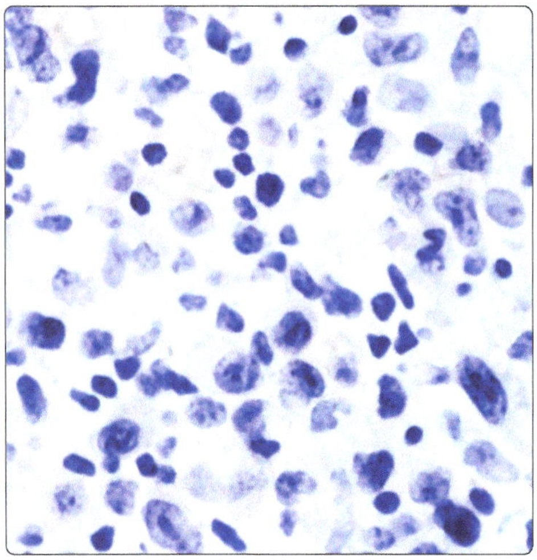

ALK Positivity In Systemic ALCL

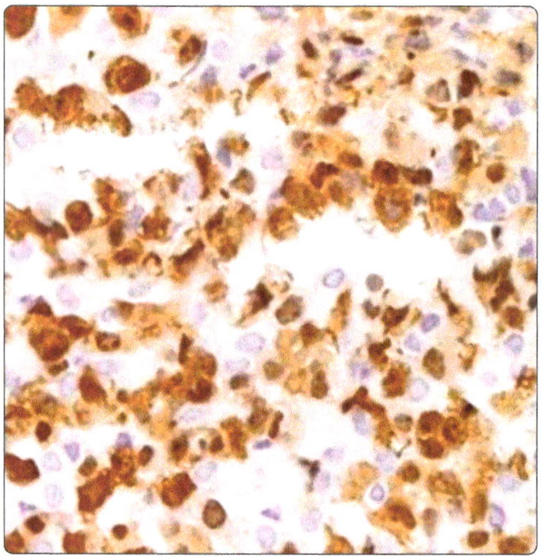

(Left) *EMA(+) immunohistochemical stain in a case of systemic ALCL with secondary involvement of skin is shown. Cases of PCALCL are typically EMA(-).* **(Right)** *This is an ALK gene break-apart probe FISH test in a case of systemic ALCL, showing ALK gene rearrangement. The yellow signal is split into a blue signal ➔, representing the 5' region of ALK and a pink signal ➔ representing the 3' region. The ALK gene is often rearranged in systemic ALCL, but not in PCALCL.*

EMA Positivity in Systemic ALCL

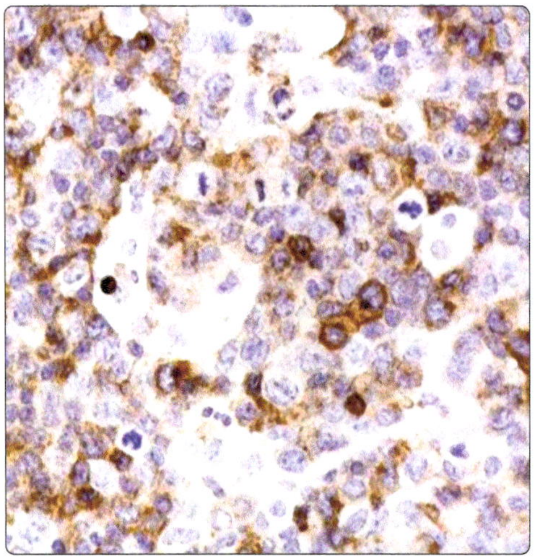

ALK Break-Apart FISH Probe

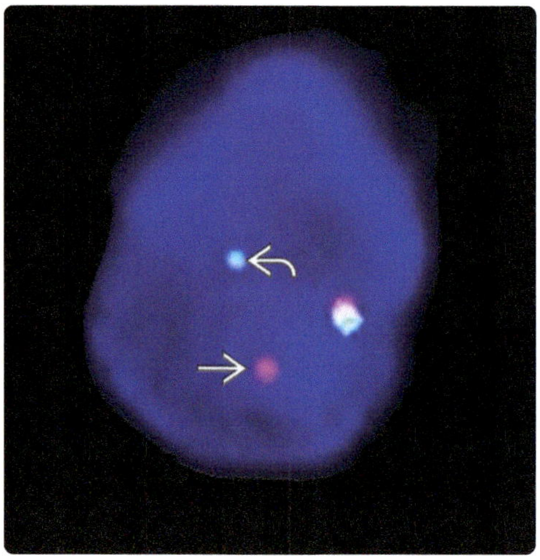

Differential Diagnosis: Lymphomatoid Papulosis

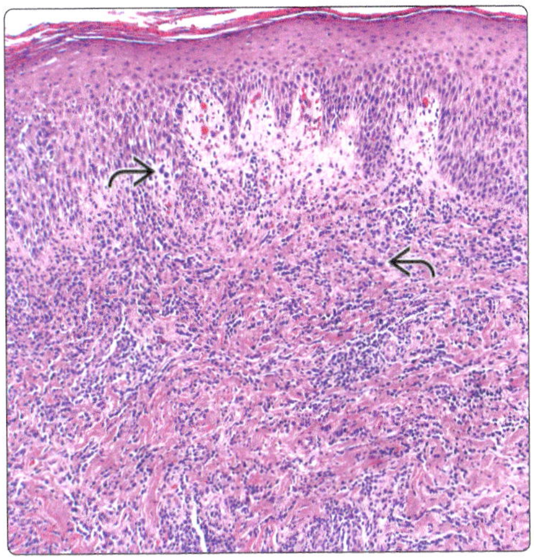

Differential Diagnosis: Lymphomatoid Papulosis

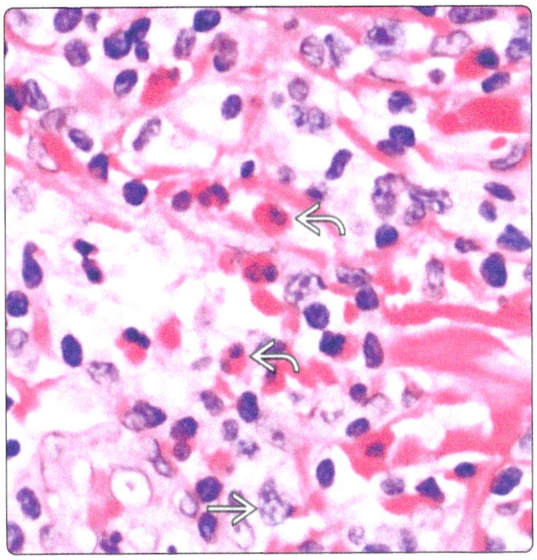

(Left) *ALCL can be difficult to distinguish from lymphomatoid papulosis (LyP), especially type C. Low magnification of LyP shows epidermal acanthosis, spongiosis, and a mixed dermal infiltrate containing scattered large, hyperchromatic-staining atypical lymphocytes ➢.* **(Right)** *This case of LyP has scattered large atypical cells ➔ as seen in ALCL but has a prominent polymorphous background infiltrate with eosinophils ➢ and histiocytes, which are not a common feature of ALCL.*

Differential Diagnosis: Systemic ALCL

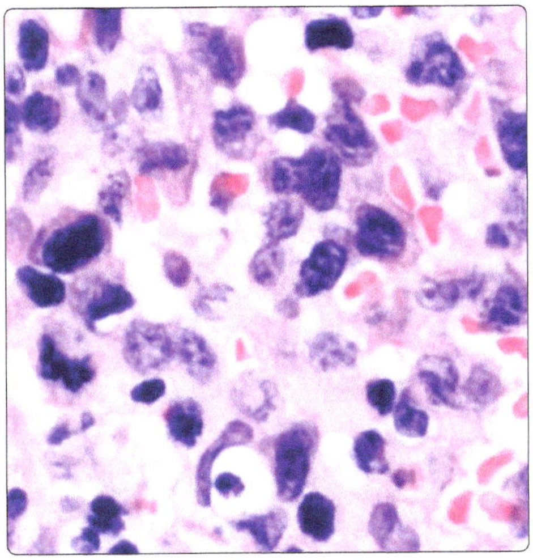

Differential Diagnosis: Primary Cutaneous Diffuse Large B-Cell Lymphoma, Leg Type

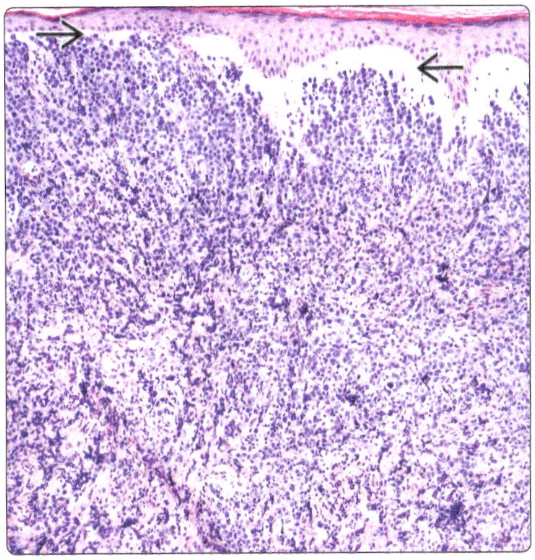

(Left) *Systemic ALCL involving the skin is shown. These are essentially indistinguishable from PCALCL without clinical history and immunohistochemistry for ALK and EMA.* **(Right)** *Primary cutaneous diffuse large B-cell lymphoma, leg type can be difficult to distinguish from ALCL without immunohistochemistry. Low magnification shows a diffuse, sheet-like infiltrate replacing the dermis with a thin grenz zone ➔ and sparing of the epidermis.*

Differential Diagnosis: Diffuse Large B-Cell Lymphoma

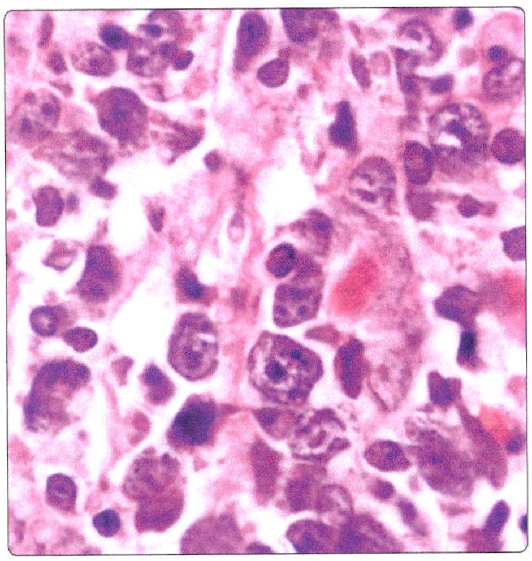

Differential Diagnosis: Diffuse Large B-Cell Lymphoma, CD20

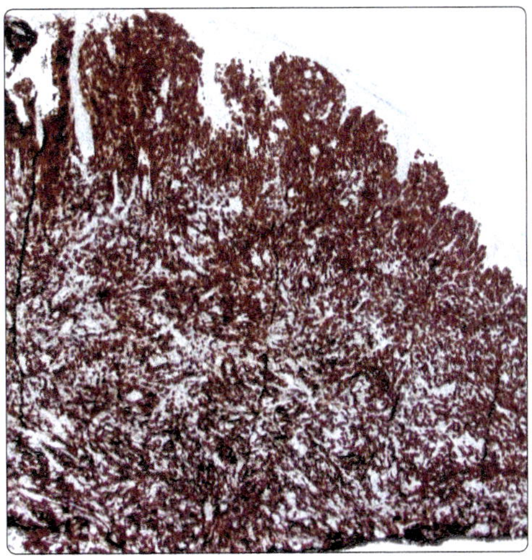

(Left) *This diffuse large B-cell lymphoma has large atypical malignant cells with morphology akin to ALCL and is CD30(+). Unlike ALCL, this case is CD20(+), CD79(+), and t(14;18)(+) by FISH.* **(Right)** *CD20 shows very strong and diffuse staining in this primary cutaneous diffuse large B-cell lymphoma, leg type. This finding excludes ALCL and is diagnostic of a B-cell lymphoma.*

Aggressive Epidermotropic CD8(+) Cytotoxic T-Cell Lymphoma

KEY FACTS

TERMINOLOGY

- Provisional diagnosis in 2008 WHO, T-cell lymphoma consisting of CD8(+) cytotoxic αβ T cells in epidermis, exhibiting aggressive clinical behavior
- Previously included in cases of peripheral T-cell lymphoma, not otherwise specified
- Often separated from other CD8(+) lymphomas based on clinical behavior

CLINICAL ISSUES

- Generalized skin lesions with ulceration and necrosis
- Aggressive clinical course
  - Often disseminated tumors, nodules, and papules
  - Rapid spread to lungs, testes, brain, and oral cavity
  - Often treated with multiagent chemotherapy
- Often spares lymph nodes
- Rare compared to other cutaneous T-cell lymphomas, such as mycosis fungoides and anaplastic large cell lymphoma

MICROSCOPIC

- Epidermotropic T-cell infiltrate
- Variably sized T cells with moderate to marked atypia
- May extend into dermis &/or subcutaneous tissue
- Ulceration, necrosis, and angioinvasion are often identified

ANCILLARY TESTS

- CD8(+), CD3(+), CD2(-/+), CD5(-), CD7(+/-), βF1(+), CD4(-), LMP1(-), CD15(-/+), CD56(+/-)
- Cytotoxic markers (+)
- Clonal for T-cell receptor gene gamma rearrangement

TOP DIFFERENTIAL DIAGNOSES

- Mycosis fungoides
  - Is rarely CD8(+), but progression to tumor stage often takes years
- Lymphomatoid papulosis
  - More benign clinical course with papules that spontaneously regress

Clinical Photograph of AECTCL

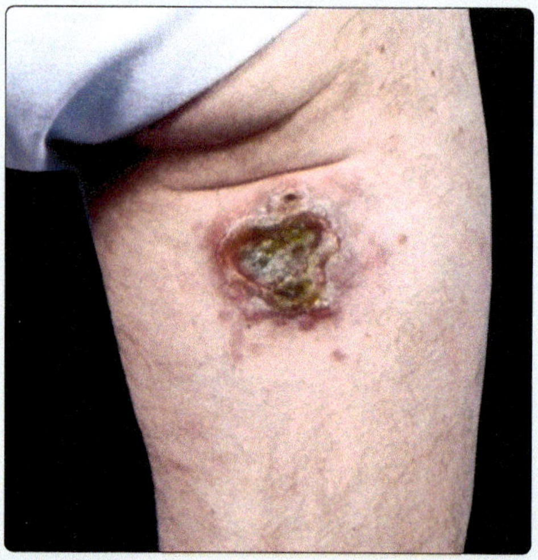

Low Magnification of AECTCL

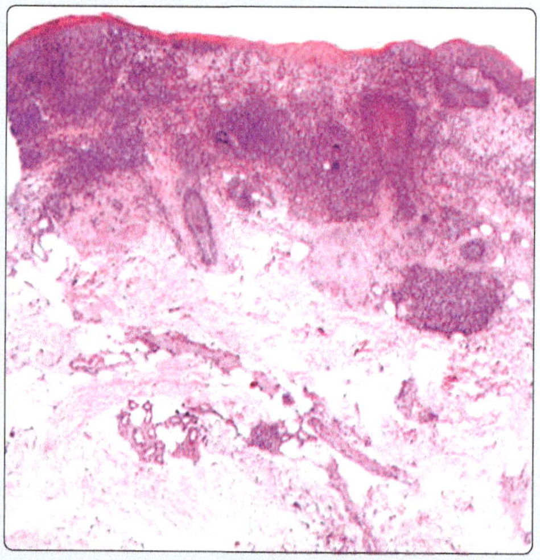

(Left) *This is a clinical photograph of a large tumor on the posterior leg of a patient with aggressive epidermotropic cytotoxic T-cell lymphoma (AECTCL). As is typical of this disease, the lesion is extensively ulcerated. (Courtesy R. Willemze, MD.)* **(Right)** *At scanning magnification of an AECTCL, there is a dense dermal lymphoid infiltrate, which also involves the epidermis. The dermal infiltrate is angiocentric, which is a common infiltration pattern in AECTCL.*

AECTCL With Epidermotropism

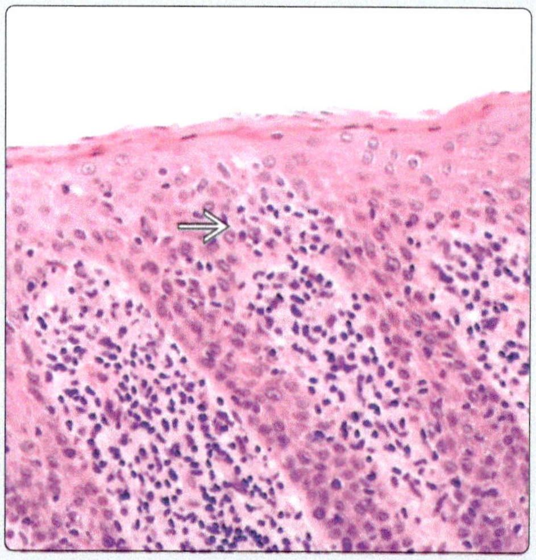

Break-Apart *ALK* FISH Probe

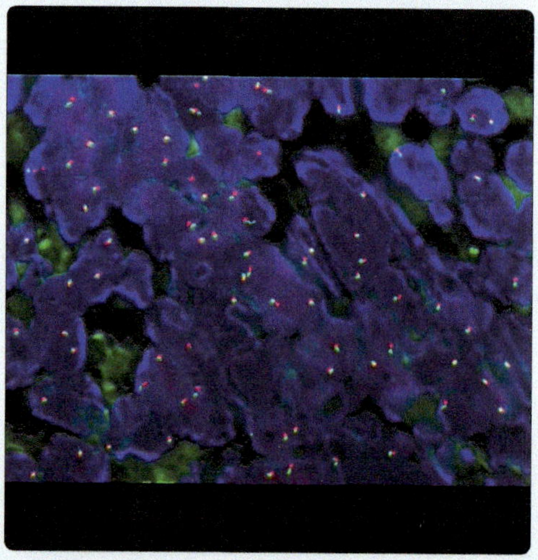

(Left) *This is a medium magnification of a case of AECTCL with considerable epidermotropism ➡. The T cells in the epidermis are medium in size with moderate atypia and coarse chromatin.* **(Right)** *This is a break-apart probe for the ALK gene by fluorescent in situ hybridization. The result is negative. No ALK gene rearrangement is seen in aggressive epidermotropic CD8(+) cytotoxic T-cell lymphoma.*

TERMINOLOGY

Abbreviations

- Aggressive epidermotropic cytotoxic T-cell lymphoma (AECTCL)

Definitions

- T-cell lymphoma consisting of CD8(+) cytotoxic αβ T cells prominently involving epidermis and exhibiting aggressive clinical behavior
  - Provisional entity in 2008 WHO Classification of Hematopoietic and Lymphoid Tissues
  - Previously included with cases of peripheral T-cell lymphoma, not otherwise specified
  - Often separated from other CD8(+) lymphomas based on clinical behavior

CLINICAL ISSUES

Epidemiology

- Incidence
  - Rare
    - < 1% of cutaneous T-cell lymphomas
- Age
  - Adults
    - Median age: 53 years
- Sex
  - M:F = 1.4:1.0

Presentation

- Skin lesions
  - Often tumors, nodules, and papules
    - Less often patches or plaques
  - Usually ulceration &/or necrosis
  - Often widespread disseminated lesions
- Rapid extracutaneous spread
  - Fairly frequent
  - Lungs, testes, brain, and oral cavity involved
  - Lymph nodes are usually spared

Treatment

- Adjuvant therapy
  - Often multiagent chemotherapy

Prognosis

- Aggressive clinical course
  - 32-month median survival
  - No difference in prognosis if tumor cells are smaller or larger
  - One study suggested that CD2(-)/CD7(+) cases have worse prognosis

MICROSCOPIC

Histologic Features

- Epidermotropism
  - Often is very prominent, with full-thickness spread and linear colonization of basal epidermis by atypical lymphocytes
- Additional epidermal changes
  - Ulceration, necrosis, or blistering common
  - Can be acanthotic or atrophic
    - Variable apoptotic keratinocytes and spongiosis
- T-cell infiltrate in dermis
  - Can involve superficial dermis &/or deeper tissues
    - Sometimes angiocentric, lichenoid, &/or adnexal
- Variable numbers of histiocytes
  - Rare eosinophils and plasma cells

Cytologic Features

- Small- to medium-sized T cells with moderate to marked atypia, coarse or blastic chromatin

ANCILLARY TESTS

Immunohistochemistry

- T-cell antigens (+) (CD3, CD2, CD7)
  - Sometimes 1 or more T-cell antigens lost
    - CD5 is most commonly lost
- Cytotoxic markers (+): Granzyme-B, perforin, and TIA1 (+)
- αβ T cells
  - βF1(+), TCR-δ-1(-)
- Cytotoxic cells
  - CD4(-), CD8(+)
- Epstein-Barr virus markers (-): (LMP1), CD15(-/+), CD56(+/-)
- High proliferative rate by MIB-1 (> 90% of tumor cells)

Genetic Testing

- Clonal for T-cell receptor gene gamma rearrangements
- Complex karyotypes seen by cytogenetics
- Loss of chr(17)p encoding *TP53* has also been reported

DIFFERENTIAL DIAGNOSIS

Mycosis Fungoides

- Vast majority of cases: CD4(+)/CD8(-), unlike AECTCL
  - Slower natural history of disease
    - Progression from patch to plaque to tumor often takes years
  - Less necrosis by morphology

Lymphomatoid Papulosis

- Similarities to AECTCL
  - Can rarely present with epidermotropism and CD8(+) T cells [type D lymphomatoid papulosis (LyP)]
  - Both CD8(+) LyP and AECTCL lack eosinophils and plasma cells
  - Both present with markedly atypical T cells with angiocentric growth pattern
- Differences from AECTCL
  - Clinical course is less aggressive for LyP
    - Presents with papules, usually nonulcerating, that often regress
    - No extracutaneous systemic involvement
  - CD30(+), which is uncommon in AECTCL

SELECTED REFERENCES

1. Kato K et al: Molecular genetic and cytogenetic analysis of a primary cutaneous CD8-positive aggressive epidermotropic cytotoxic T-cell lymphoma. Int J Hematol. 103(2):196-201, 2016
2. Martires KJ et al: Characterization of primary cutaneous CD8+/CD30+ lymphoproliferative disorders. Am J Dermatopathol. 37(11):822-33, 2015

(Left) *At medium magnification, one is more able to see the dermal infiltrate → extending into the epidermis ⇨. The T cells in the epidermis are seen singly and in small clusters, disrupting much of the epidermis.* **(Right)** *At high magnification, the epidermotropic lymphocytes show moderate atypia, with coarse chromatin and irregular nuclear contours.*

AECTCL With Epidermotropism

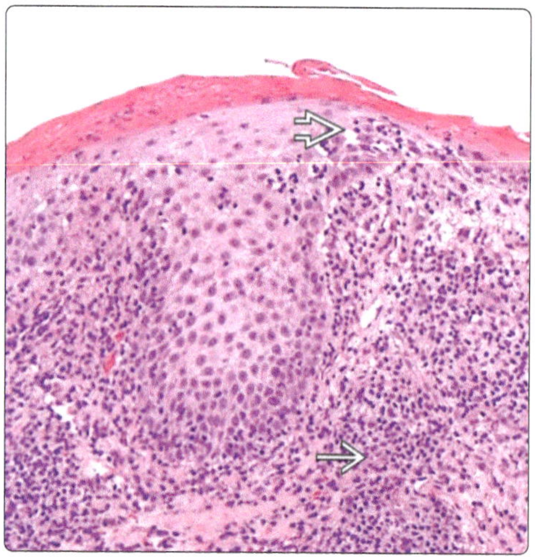

High Magnification of AECTCL

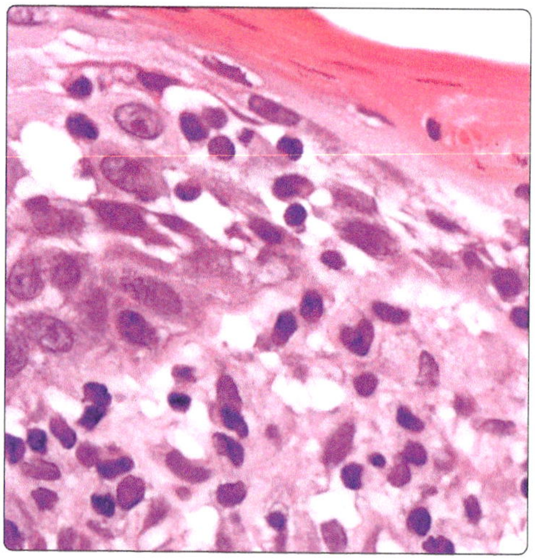

(Left) *Another case of AECTCL at high magnification demonstrates T cells that are larger in size with marked atypia ↶ and somewhat vesicular chromatin. There is a large amount of necrosis → in the background, as is often found in AECTCL. Skin ulceration was also present in some sections.* **(Right)** *CD8 shows strong cytoplasmic immunoreactivity in the malignant T cells in this case of AECTCL. The atypical CD8(+) cells are located in the dermis → and epidermis ↶.*

High Magnification of AECTCL With Necrosis

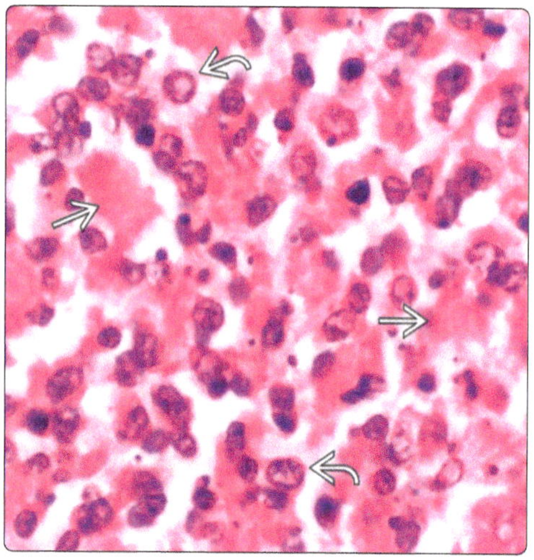

CD8 Immunohistochemistry in AECTCL

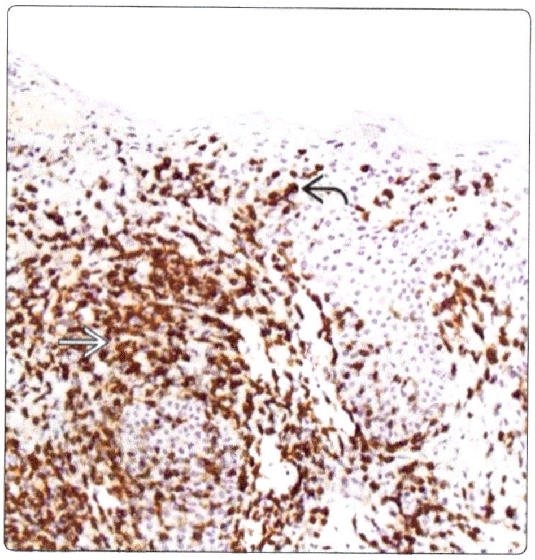

(Left) *This βF1 immunohistochemical stain strongly marks the malignant T cells in the epidermis in a case of AECTCL, indicating that these are αβ T cells. This tumor was also CD3(+), CD4(-), LMP1(-), CD15(-), and CD56(-) (not shown).* **(Right)** *This is the result of a PCR assay for the TRG gene, which shows a dominant monoclonal peak indicating T-cell receptor monoclonality.*

βF1 Immunohistochemistry

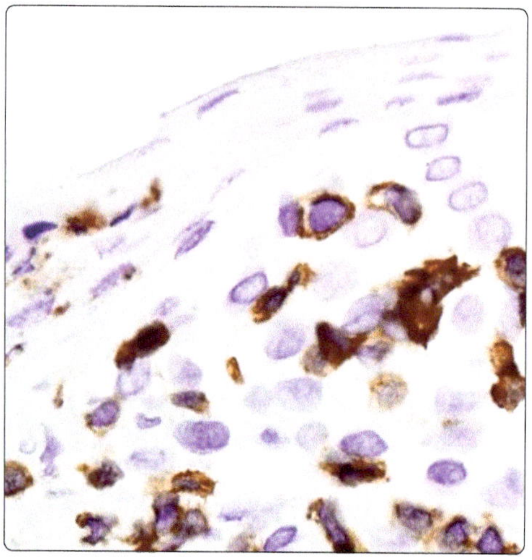

TRG Gene Rearrangement

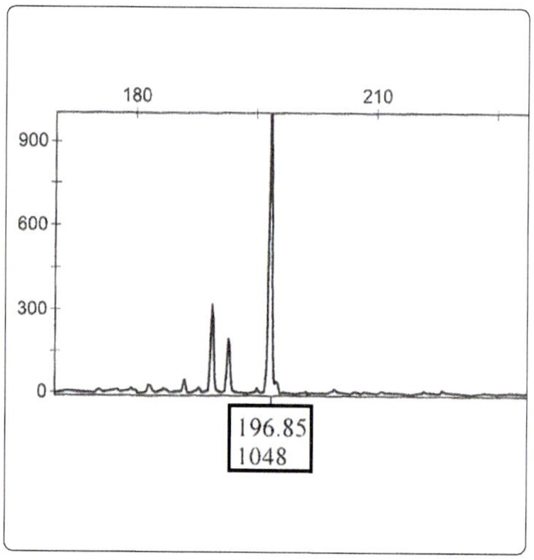

Differential Diagnosis: Mycosis Fungoides

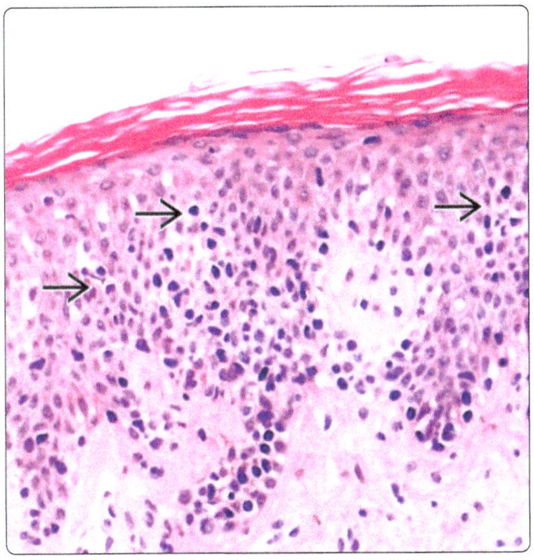

CD8 Immunohistochemical Stain in Mycosis Fungoides

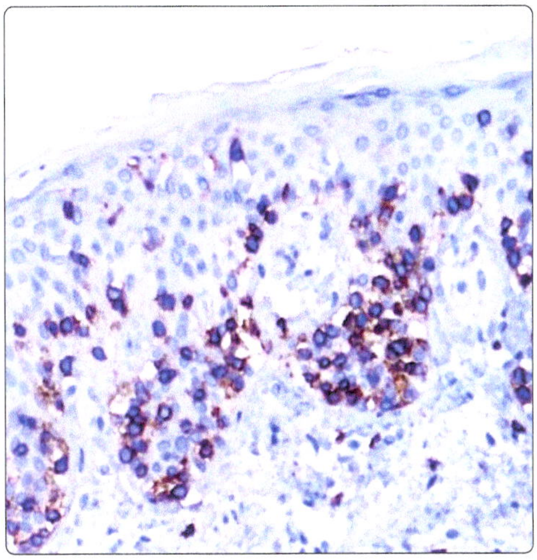

(Left) *This is a case of CD8(+) mycosis fungoides. There are malignant T cells* → *singly and scattered in the epidermis, which is a morphologic pattern identical to that seen in AECTCL.* **(Right)** *In the same case of mycosis fungoides, a CD8 IHC stain marks the T cells in the epidermis. A minority of cases of mycosis fungoides are CD4(-)/CD8(+), unlike the vast majority of AECTCL. Mycosis fungoides also lacks necrosis (which is often seen in AECTCL) and has a slower natural history of disease.*

Differential Diagnosis: Pagetoid Reticulosis

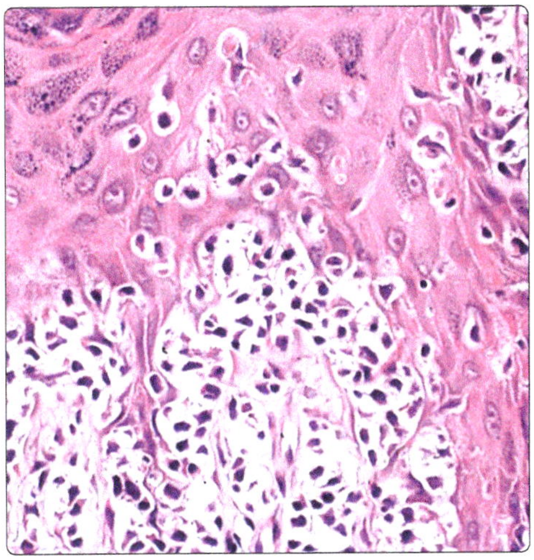

Differential Diagnosis: Lymphomatoid Papulosis, Type B

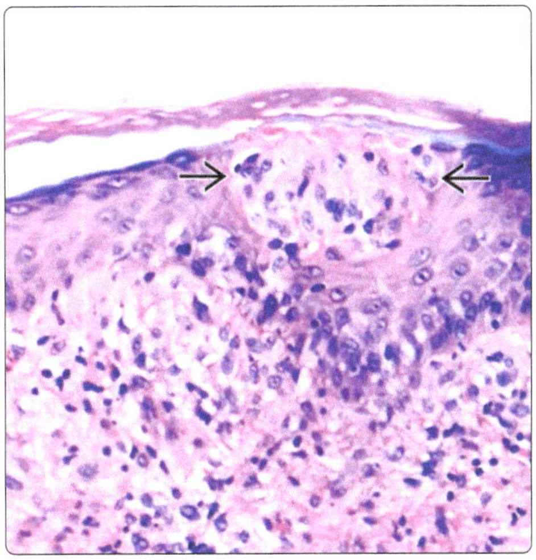

(Left) *Pagetoid reticulosis (PR) shows prominent spongiosis and haloed T cells. This extensive epidermotropism can be confused with AECTCL, but PR would be a single lesion. (Courtesy M. Tomaszewski, MD.)* **(Right)** *This case of lymphomatoid papulosis, type B shows clusters of atypical T cells* → *in the epidermis, similar to AECTCL. Both diseases present with atypical T cells, but lymphomatoid papulosis presents with self-healing, nonulcerating papules without extracutaneous involvement.*

Differential Diagnosis: Adult T-Cell Leukemia/Lymphoma

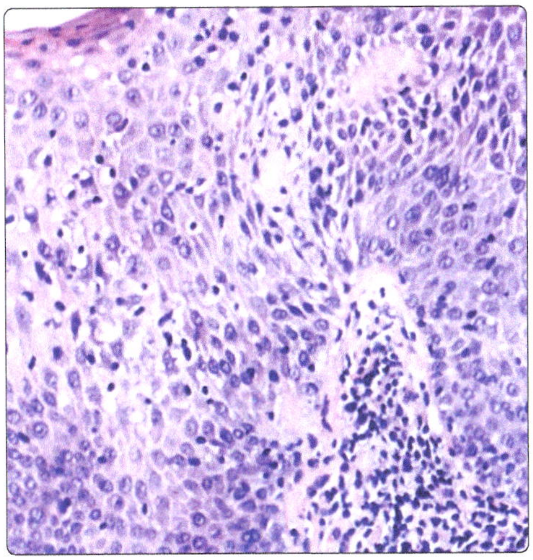

Differential Diagnosis: Spongiotic Dermatitis

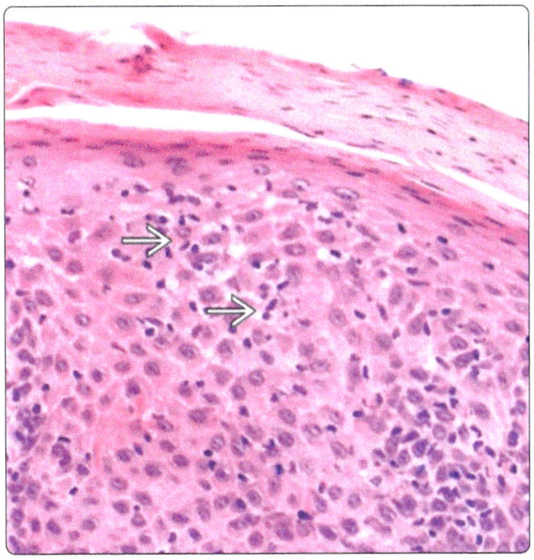

(Left) *This case of cutaneous adult T-cell leukemia/lymphoma (ATLL) is similar to AECTCL with significant epidermotropism. While both tumors show malignant epidermotropic T cells, ATLL shows CD4(+) T cells and presents in HTLV1(-) patients.* **(Right)** *In this case of a spongiotic dermatitis, there are scattered lymphocytes* → *in the spongiotic areas, mimicking epidermotropism. However, the lymphocytes are small and lack significant atypia.*

KEY FACTS

TERMINOLOGY

- T-cell lymphoma of skin with small- to medium-sized CD4(+) T cells and usually indolent clinical course
  - Provisional entity in 2008 WHO Classification of Tumors of Hematopoietic and Lymphoid Tissue
  - Lacks lesions typical of mycosis fungoides
- Cell of origin is currently thought to be follicular helper T cell

CLINICAL ISSUES

- Usually single plaque or tumor
- Good prognosis, especially if single lesion

MICROSCOPIC

- Dense dermal and subcutaneous infiltrate of small- to medium-sized pleomorphic T cells
- Sometimes focal epidermotropism
- Nodular or diffuse growth pattern
- Scattered large T cells (< 30% of total)
- Background reactive infiltrate
- Granulomatous inflammation may be present

ANCILLARY TESTS

- CD3(+), CD4(+), CD8(-), CD30(-)
- Loss of T-cell antigens
- Positive follicular helper T-cell markers (PD-1, CXCL13)
- Clonal T-cell receptor gene rearrangements
- Cytogenetics: No known abnormalities
- Epstein-Barr virus small-encoded RNA(-)

TOP DIFFERENTIAL DIAGNOSES

- Pseudolymphoma of skin
  - Very difficult to distinguish from SMPTCL
  - Both can show monoclonal T-cell receptor rearrangements
  - Both are PD-1(+)
- Mycosis fungoides
- Angioimmunoblastic T-cell lymphoma

Primary Cutaneous CD4(+) SMPTCL

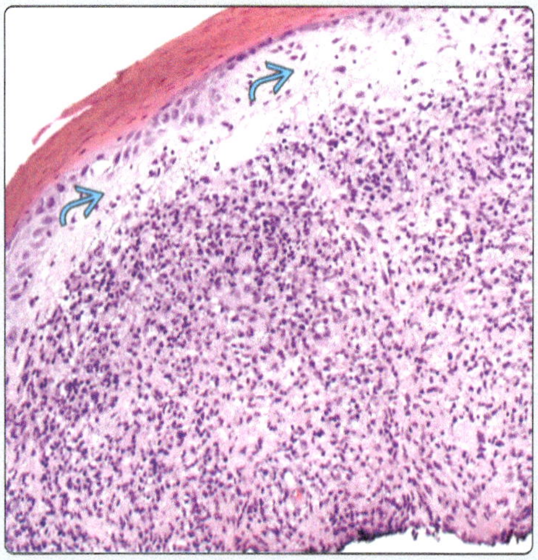

Higher Power of SMPTCL

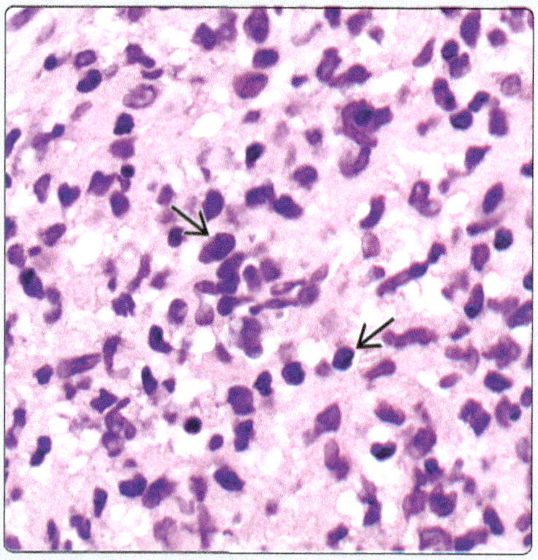

(Left) *Low-power view of a primary cutaneous CD4(+) small/medium pleomorphic T-cell lymphoma (SMPTCL) shows a dense lymphoid infiltrate filling the dermis in a diffuse pattern of infiltration. Note the sparing of the epidermis and the presence of a grenz zone* ➙. **(Right)** *At higher power magnification, the lymphocytes are small to medium in size with coarse chromatin and indistinct nucleoli. The lymphocytes show moderate atypia and pleomorphism* ➙.

High Magnification Showing Pleomorphism

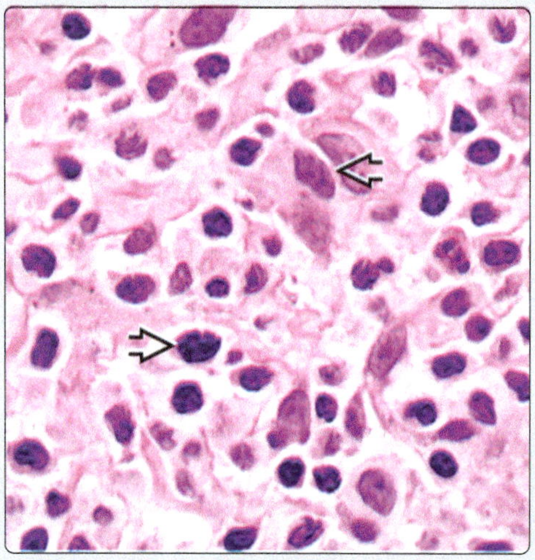

CD3 Immunostain in SMPTCL

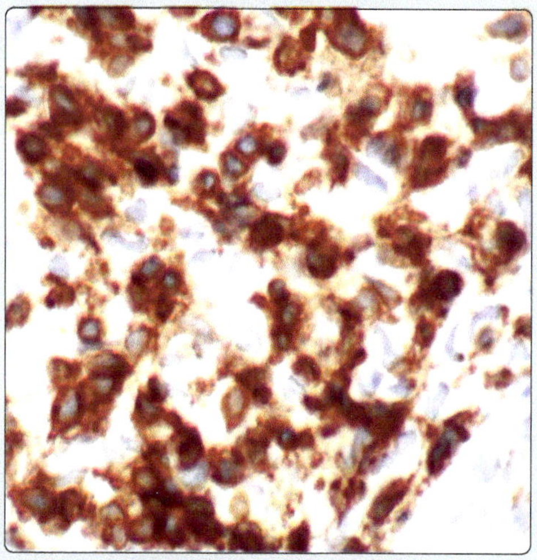

(Left) *High-power view shows there are scattered cells that are large in size* ➙ *with more significant atypia. When present, large cells should make up < 30% of the total cells.* **(Right)** *A CD3 immunohistochemical stain at high magnification shows that this case of SMPTCL is composed of a T-cell infiltrate, which is strongly and diffusely positive for CD3.*

TERMINOLOGY

Abbreviations

- Primary cutaneous CD4(+) small/medium pleomorphic T-cell lymphoma (SMPTCL)

Synonyms

- Idiopathic T-cell lymphomatoid hyperplasia/lymphoproliferative disorder

Definitions

- T-cell lymphoma/lymphoproliferative disorder of skin with small to medium-sized CD4(+) follicular helper T cells and usually indolent clinical course
  - Without typical patches/plaques of mycosis fungoides
- Provisional entity in 2008 WHO Classification of Tumors of Hematopoietic and Lymphoid Tissue
  - Nonaggressive natural history, but worrisome histologic and molecular features

ETIOLOGY/PATHOGENESIS

Postulated Normal Cell Counterpart

- Follicular helper T cell

CLINICAL ISSUES

Epidemiology

- Incidence
  - Rare
    - 2% of cutaneous T-cell lymphomas in Dutch and Austrian Cutaneous Lymphoma Group Registry
- Age
  - Median: 53 yr; range: 3-90 yr
- Sex
  - M:F = 0.5:1

Site

- Head and neck area most common
  - Upper torso often
  - Lower extremities rare

Presentation

- Single plaque or tumor
  - Less commonly > 1 tumor nodule
  - Less commonly ≥ 1 papules
  - No lesions (patches/plaques) typical of mycosis fungoides
- Usually asymptomatic
  - No lymphadenopathy
  - No systemic disease

Laboratory Tests

- No known laboratory abnormalities

Natural History

- Does not usually disseminate
  - Rarely, local recurrence is seen

Treatment

- Usually nonaggressive therapy
  - Especially if single lesion
  - Excision or local radiation therapy

Prognosis

- Mostly favorable outcome, especially if solitary lesion or localized to skin
  - Better prognosis than secondary cutaneous T-cell lymphomas
  - Better prognosis than primary cutaneous peripheral T-cell lymphoma, not otherwise specified
- Nonaggressive disease
  - Overall 5-yr survival: > 90%
- Good prognostic indicators
  - Solitary lesion
  - Disease localized to skin
- Worse prognostic indicators
  - Multiple lesions
  - Large lesions

MACROSCOPIC

General Features

- Usually single, less often multiple firm plaques and nodules

MICROSCOPIC

Histologic Features

- Dense dermal infiltrate
  - Sometimes involves subcutaneous tissue
  - Usually nonepidermotropic
    - Rarely focal epidermotropism
- Nodular or diffuse growth pattern
- Size of T cells
  - Small or medium in most cases
  - Large cells can also be seen
    - When present, should comprise < 30% of total cells
- Pleomorphic with some nuclear irregularity
- Other features
  - Background reactive infiltrate is fairly common
    - Small reactive lymphocytes, eosinophils, and histiocytes
  - ↑ reactive-appearing B cells also often present
  - Granulomatous inflammation can be seen

ANCILLARY TESTS

Immunohistochemistry

- T-cell antigens (+)
  - CD2(+), CD3(+), CD5(+), CD7(+/-)
  - May see loss of 1 or more T-cell antigens
    - CD7 > CD5, CD2
  - CD4(+), CD8(-)
- Expresses follicular helper T-cell markers
  - PD-1(+), CXCL13(+), Bcl-6(+)
- Cytotoxic markers (-)
  - TIA, GZM-B, and perforin
- CD30(-), LMP1(-)

In Situ Hybridization

- Epstein-Barr virus small-encoded RNA (EBER) (-)

PCR

- *TCR* gene rearrangement clonal
  - 60% in one series

- *IGH* immunoglobulin gene rearrangements polyclonal

Genetic Testing

- No known specific abnormalities

DIFFERENTIAL DIAGNOSIS

Atypical Reactive Lymphoid Infiltrates (Pseudolymphomas) of Skin

- Similarities to SMPTCL
  - Overlapping morphology with atypical dermal infiltrates
  - Reactive B cells and plasma cells in SMPTCL are difficult to distinguish from reactive conditions
  - PD-1(+) in both pseudolymphoma and in SMPTCL but is usually (-) in other T-cell lymphomas
- Differences from SMPTCL
  - More CD8(+) T cells
  - Lack of clonality in T-cell receptor gene rearrangement favors pseudolymphoma over SMPTCL
  - Reactive infiltrates may resolve without treatment
  - Loss of T-cell antigens favors SMPTCL
  - No one factor definitively distinguishes SMPTCL from reactive infiltrates

Mycosis Fungoides

- Similarities to SMPTCL
  - Morphology is akin to SMPTCL with infiltrate of mostly small- to medium-sized pleomorphic T cells
  - Both express T-cell markers with loss of some T-cell antigens and are CD4(+), CD8(-), CD30(-)
- Differences from SMPTCL
  - Mycosis fungoides usually presents with significant epidermotropism
  - Usually negative for follicular helper T-cell markers
    - PD-1, CXCL13, Bcl-6

Angioimmunoblastic T-Cell Lymphoma

- Similarities to SMPTCL
  - Also presents with dermal-based T-cell infiltrate
  - Also expresses follicular T-helper cell markers
    - PD-1, CXCL13, Bcl-6
- Differences from SMPTCL
  - Often presents with lymph node involvement or systemic disease
  - Morphology shows increased vasculature
  - EBER(+)
  - Worse prognosis than SMPTCL

Anaplastic Large Cell Lymphoma

- Similar histologic findings to SMPTCL
  - Atypical T-cell infiltrate in dermis
- Differences from SMPTCL
  - Often has many large atypical cells, unlike SMPTCL
    - Except small cell variant of anaplastic large cell lymphoma
  - CD30 diffusely (+)

Primary Cutaneous Peripheral T-Cell Lymphoma, Not Otherwise Specified

- Similar phenotype to SMPTCL
  - T-cell infiltrate in dermis
  - Subset expresses follicular helper T-cell markers
- Differences from SMPTCL
  - Often has > 30% large atypical cells, unlike SMPTCL
  - Worse prognosis than SMPTCL
  - Polymorphous infiltrate favors SMPTCL

Cutaneous B-Cell Lymphoma

- Including primary cutaneous marginal zone lymphoma, primary cutaneous follicle center lymphoma, and CLL
- Similar morphology to SMPTCL
  - Also presents with dermal lymphoid nodules
  - SMPTCL can have prominent B-cell component
- Differences from SMPTCL
  - B-cell markers (+)
    - CD19(+), CD20(+), CD79a(+), pax-5(+)
  - Monoclonal *IGH* immunoglobulin gene rearrangements in B-cell lymphomas
    - Polyclonal *IGH* immunoglobulin gene rearrangement in SMPTCL

Granulomatous Dermatitis

- Granulomatous inflammation can also be seen in SMPTCL but should be focal
- Atypical/pleomorphic T-cell infiltrate favors SMPTCL over granulomatous dermatitis

DIAGNOSTIC CHECKLIST

Clinically Relevant Pathologic Features

- Tissue distribution (less aggressive cases are usually solitary lesions and confined to skin)

Pathologic Interpretation Pearls

- Typical immunophenotype: CD3(+), CD4(+), CD8(-), CD30(-), EBV(-)

SELECTED REFERENCES

1. James E et al: CD4 + primary cutaneous small/medium-sized pleomorphic T-cell lymphoma: a retrospective case series and review of literature. Leuk Lymphoma. 56(4):951-7, 2015
2. Martinez F et al: Novel mutations of NFIX gene causing Marshall-Smith syndrome or Sotos-like syndrome: one gene, two phenotypes. Pediatr Res. ePub, 2015
3. Ally MS et al: Evaluation of follicular T-helper cells in primary cutaneous CD4+ small/medium pleomorphic T-cell lymphoma and dermatitis. J Cutan Pathol. 40(12):1006-13, 2013
4. Zhang L et al: Primary cutaneous CD4 positive small/medium T-cell lymphoma with high proliferation index and CD30-positive large lymphoid cells. J Cutan Pathol. 40(8):720-4, 2013
5. Cetinözman F et al: Expression of programmed death-1 in primary cutaneous CD4-positive small/medium-sized pleomorphic T-cell lymphoma, cutaneous pseudo-T-cell lymphoma, and other types of cutaneous T-cell lymphoma. Am J Surg Pathol. 36(1):109-16, 2012
6. Baum CL et al: Reappraisal of the provisional entity primary cutaneous CD4+ small/medium pleomorphic T-cell lymphoma: a series of 10 adult and pediatric patients and review of the literature. J Am Acad Dermatol. 65(4):739-48, 2011
7. Boussault P et al: Primary cutaneous CD4+ small/medium-sized pleomorphic T-cell lymphoma associated with an annular elastolytic giant cell granuloma. Br J Dermatol. 160(5):1126-8, 2009
8. Rodríguez Pinilla SM et al: Primary cutaneous CD4+ small/medium-sized pleomorphic T-cell lymphoma expresses follicular T-cell markers. Am J Surg Pathol. 33(1):81-90, 2009

SMPTCL in Superficial Dermis

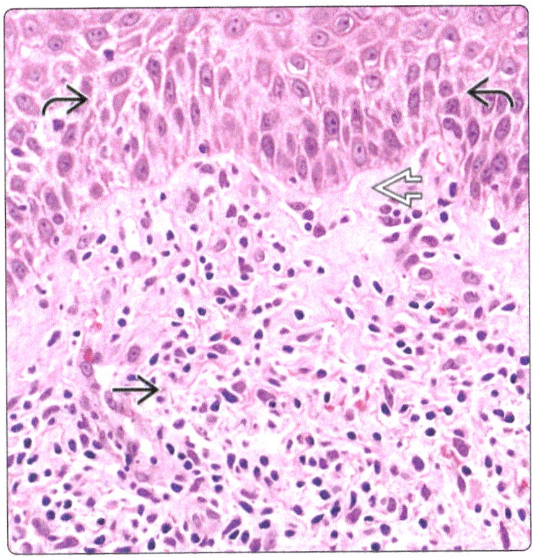

Epidermal Involvement in SMPTCL

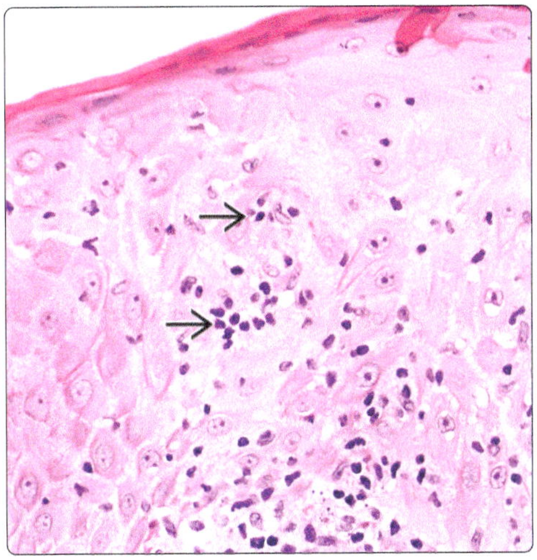

(Left) *In this case of SMPTCL, the lymphoid infiltrate is seen in the superficial dermis* → *but is separated from the epidermis* → *by a thin grenz zone* →*. In most cases, SMPTCL does not infiltrate the epidermis.* **(Right)** *Scattered small but hyperchromatic-staining T cells* → *are found in the epidermis in this case of SMPTCL. Up to 30% of cases can show focal epidermotropism.*

Higher Magnification Showing Large Cells and Small Cells

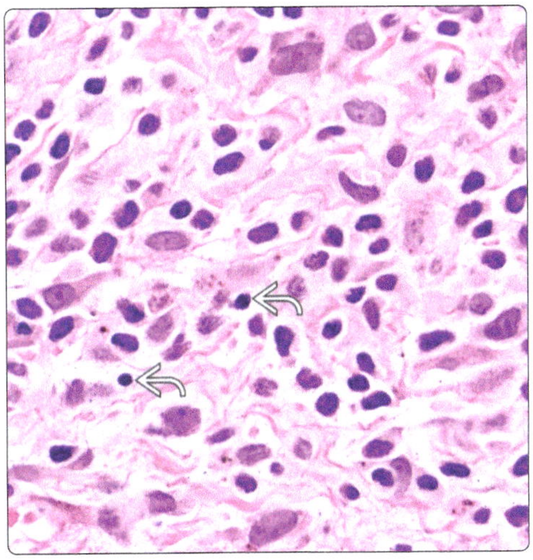

High Power of SMPTCL With Few Large Cells

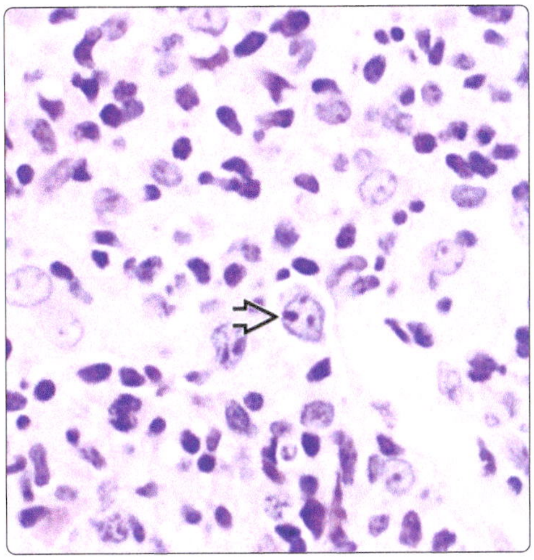

(Left) *Higher power examination of a SMPTCL shows the T cells are mostly small to medium in size and show considerable pleomorphism. Small reactive lymphocytes* → *can be used as a reference in determining the size of the tumor cells.* **(Right)** *This high-power view shows that there are scattered large cells* → *with significant atypia. When present, large cells should make up < 30% of the total cells.*

Reactive Background Reactive Infiltrate

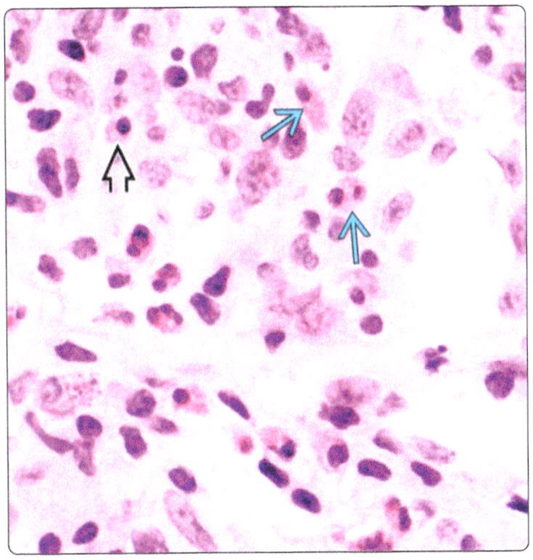

Granulomatous Inflammation

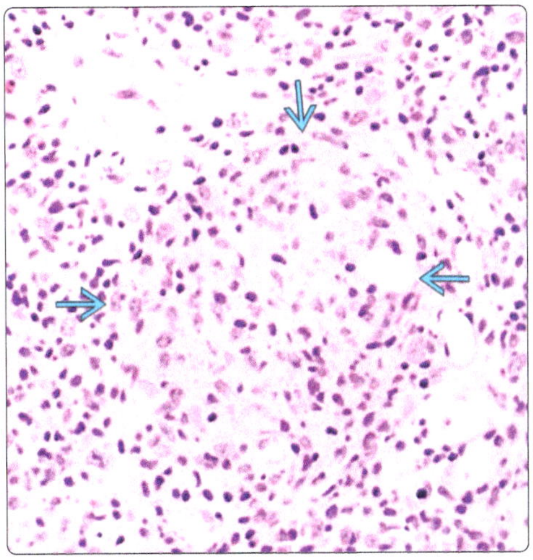

(Left) *At high power there are scattered eosinophils* → *in this case of SMPTCL. The background infiltrate can also contain neutrophils, plasma cells* →*, and histiocytes.* **(Right)** *In this same case of SMPTCL, there are focal areas with granulomatous inflammation* →*. Granulomatous inflammation is not uncommonly seen in these lesions and can be confused with a reactive process, such as an infection.*

(Left) *This CD3 immunohistochemical stain at high magnification shows that the lymphoid cells are strongly and diffusely positive for CD3.* **(Right)** *CD20 is only positive in a few scattered B cells ⮫ in this case of SMPTCL. In some cases of SMPTCL, B cells are more numerous. SMPTCL has a T-cell lineage but is often accompanied by reactive B cells.*

CD3 Immunohistochemistry in SMPTCL

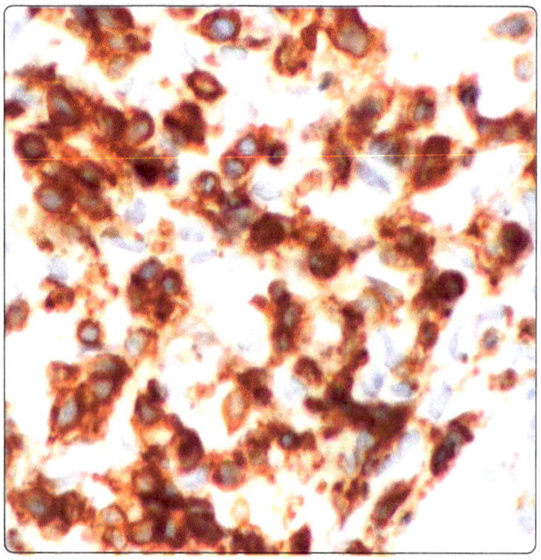

CD20 Immunohistochemistry in SMPTCL

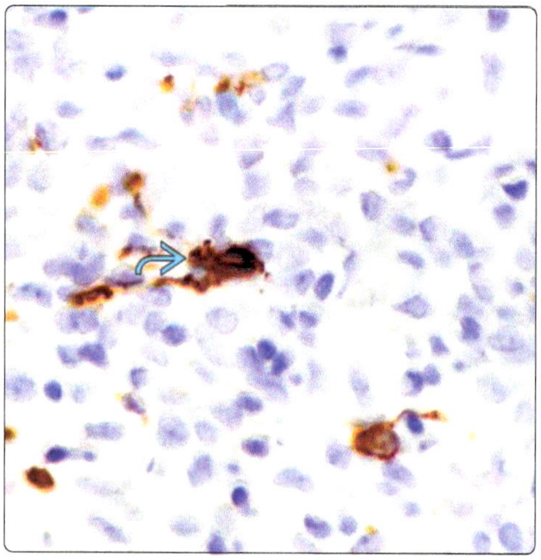

(Left) *There is strong CD4 expression in nearly all of the T cells, as is typical of this T-cell lymphoma.* **(Right)** *As compared to the previous CD4 stain, CD8 is essentially negative, with only rare cells showing a slight blush of staining ⇒. This lymphoma typically has a CD4(+), CD8(-) phenotype. Most lymphocytes are CD8(-) ⇒.*

CD4 Immunohistochemistry

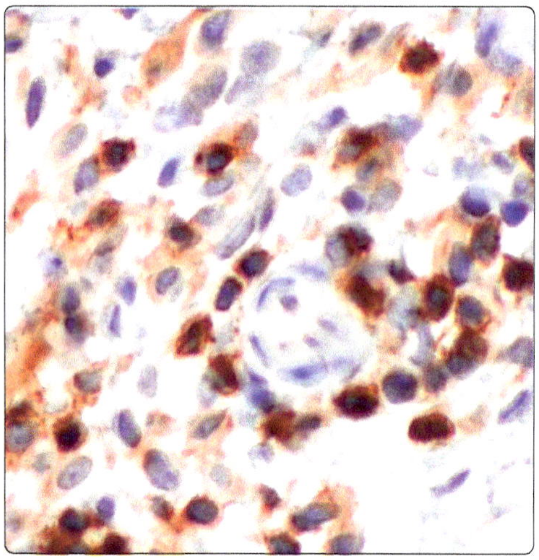

CD8 Immunohistochemistry

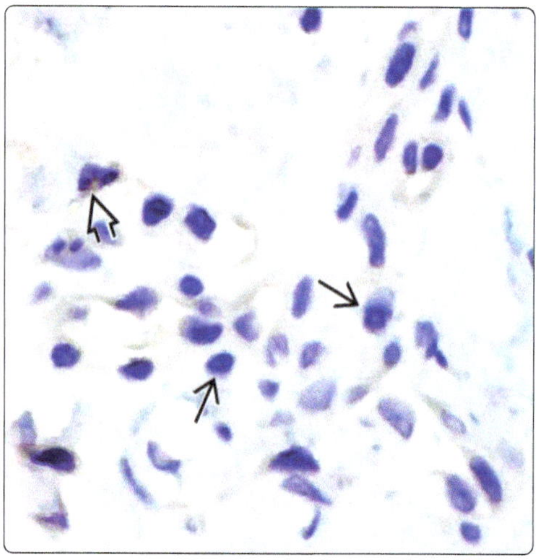

(Left) *PD-1, a marker of follicular T cells, is strongly positive in this case of SMPTCL. CXCL13 is another follicular T-cell antibody that is often expressed in SMPTCL.* **(Right)** *Medium magnification depicts loss of CD7 in most of the T cells with only rare cells ⇒ weakly expressing CD7. CD7 is the T-cell antigen most frequently lost, and CD2 is the 2nd most commonly lost.*

PD-1 Immunohistochemistry

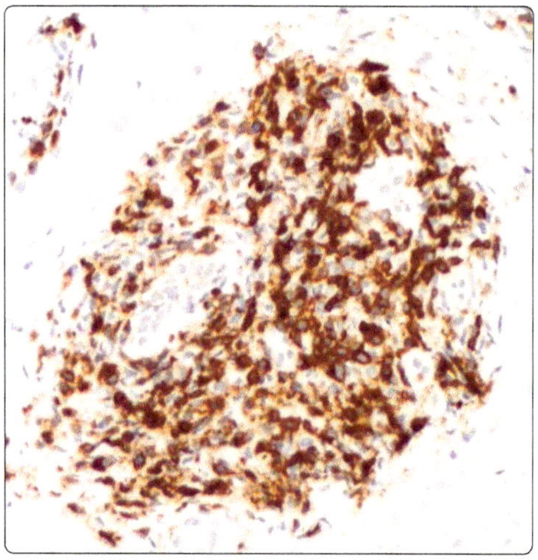

CD7 Immunohistochemistry

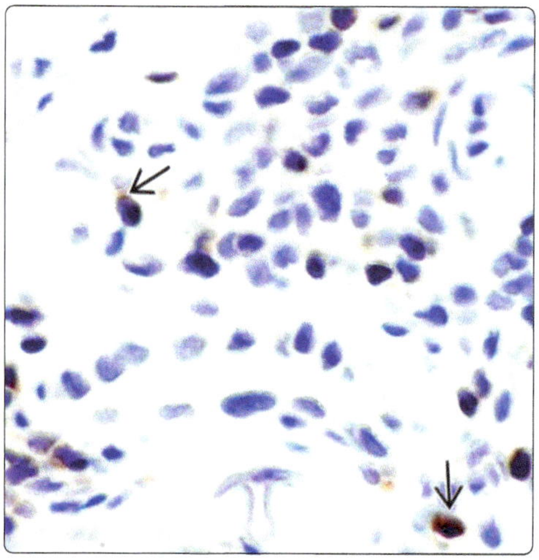

Differential Diagnosis: Reactive Lymphoid Infiltrate

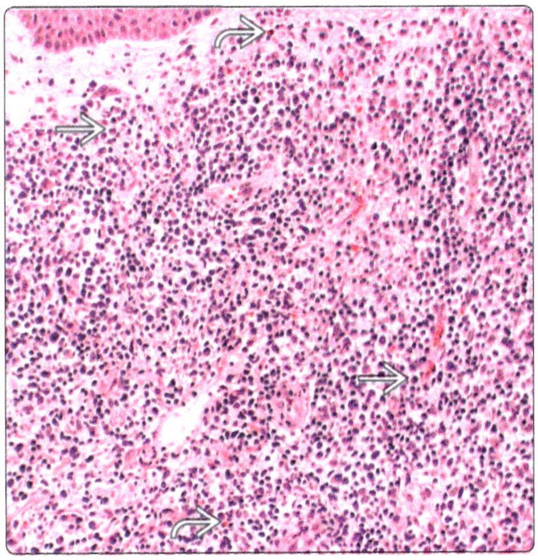

Differential Diagnosis: Mycosis Fungoides

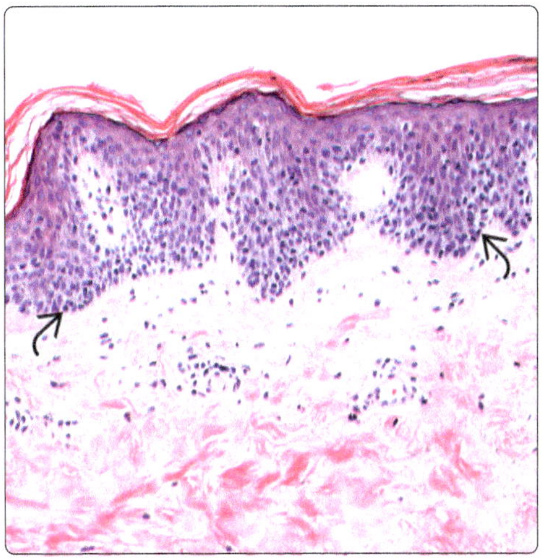

(Left) *This case of reactive lymphoid infiltrate (pseudolymphoma) developed after taking a drug. As in SMPTCL, the dermis shows a diffuse lymphoid infiltrate. However, the infiltrate contains scattered eosinophils and plasma cells and spontaneously resolved after discontinuing the medication.* **(Right)** *Mycosis fungoides (MF) has a similar immunophenotype as SMPTCL, typically composed of CD4(+), CD8(-) T cells. However, MF presents with many atypical epidermotropic cells.*

Differential Diagnosis: Primary Cutaneous Anaplastic Large-Cell Lymphoma

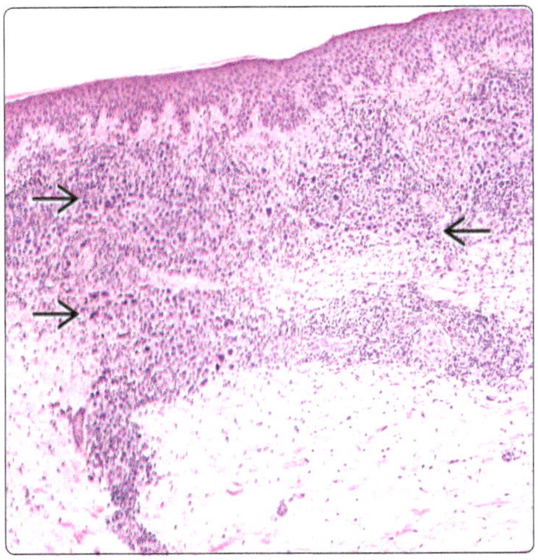

Differential Diagnosis: Peripheral T-Cell Lymphoma, Not Otherwise Specified

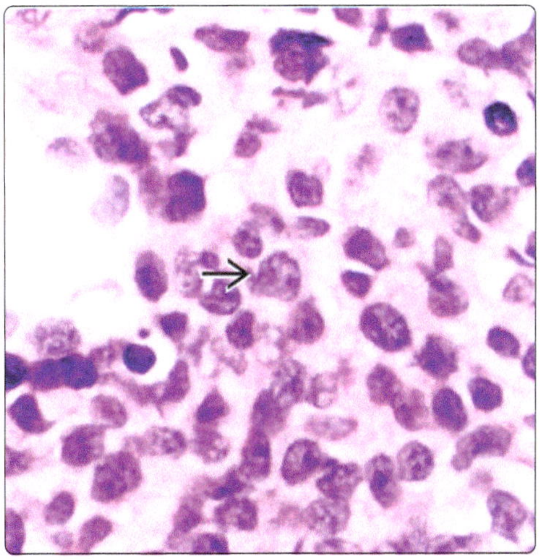

(Left) *Primary cutaneous anaplastic large-cell lymphoma (ALCL) is shown with tumor cells diffusely involving the dermis. The tumor cells are larger than expected for SMPTCL, and ALCL is not derived from follicular helper T cells. (Courtesy C. Yin, MD.)* **(Right)** *The tumor cells in PTCL-NOS are also large in size and show marked atypia. PTCL-NOS often contains tumor cells that are larger in size than SMPTCL. Less than 30% of the tumor cells in SMPTCL should be large.*

Differential Diagnosis: Primary Cutaneous Follicle Center Lymphoma

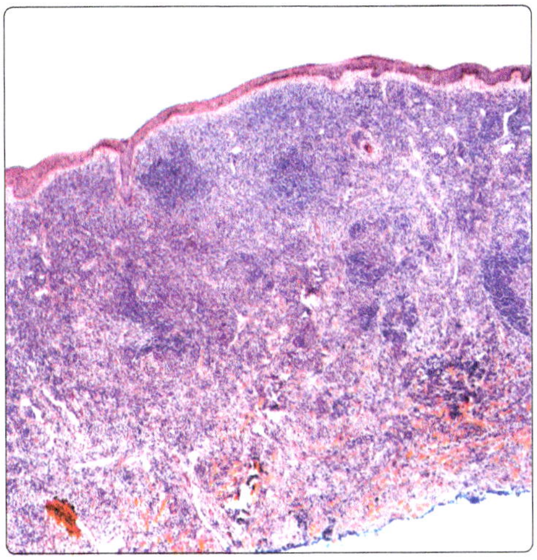

Differential Diagnosis: Chronic Lymphocytic Leukemia

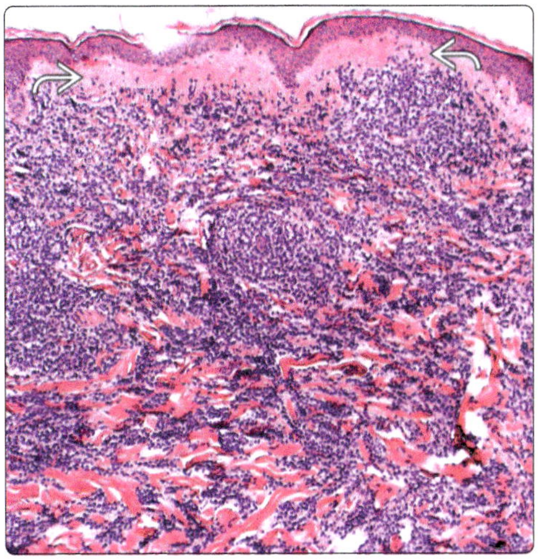

(Left) *Primary cutaneous follicle center lymphoma also presents with nodular/diffuse dermal infiltrates. However, these lymphocytes are B cells and are CD20(+), CD10(+), and show immunoglobulin heavy chain (IGH) gene rearrangements. (Courtesy R. Miranda, MD.)* **(Right)** *Chronic lymphocytic leukemia is also a dermal-based infiltrate composed of B cells, which typically involves the superficial and deep dermis. The epidermis is uninvolved and separated from the malignant B cells by a thin grenz zone.*

Cutaneous Gamma-Delta T-Cell Lymphoma

KEY FACTS

TERMINOLOGY

- T-cell lymphoma of mature γδ cells
- Separately classified from SPTCL in WHO

CLINICAL ISSUES

- Hemophagocytic syndrome in 45%
- Poor prognosis
- Treated with multiagent chemotherapy
- Stem cell transplant has been attempted with varying results

MACROSCOPIC

- Skin nodules with ulceration

MICROSCOPIC

- 3 patterns of disease: Epidermotropic, dermal, and subcutaneous
  - Malignant T cells rim around adipocytes
  - Prominent karyorrhexis/apoptosis and angioinvasion

ANCILLARY TESTS

- Immunohistochemistry: TCRδ1(+), βF1(-), CD56(+), CD4(-), CD8(-)
- EBER(-), cytotoxic markers (+)
- T-cell receptor gene rearrangement

TOP DIFFERENTIAL DIAGNOSES

- Subcutaneous panniculitis-like T-cell lymphoma
  - Panniculitis but not in dermis or epidermis; lacks ulceration; TCRδ1(-), βF1(+)
  - Much better prognosis than CGDTCL
- Peripheral T-cell lymphoma, not otherwise specified
- Lupus profundus panniculitis
  - Similar inflammation in the subcutis in panniculitic pattern
  - Lobular panniculitis, but contains plasma cells and germinal centers, unlike CGDTCL
- Mycosis fungoides/pagetoid reticulosis

CGDTCL Presenting As an Ulcerated Mass

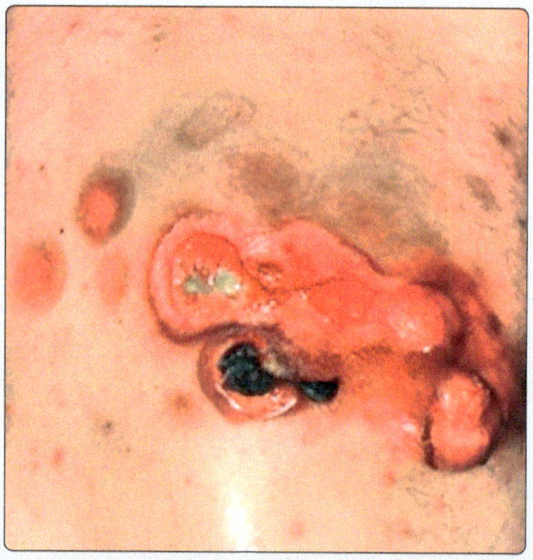

Primary CGDTCL Diffusely Involving Skin

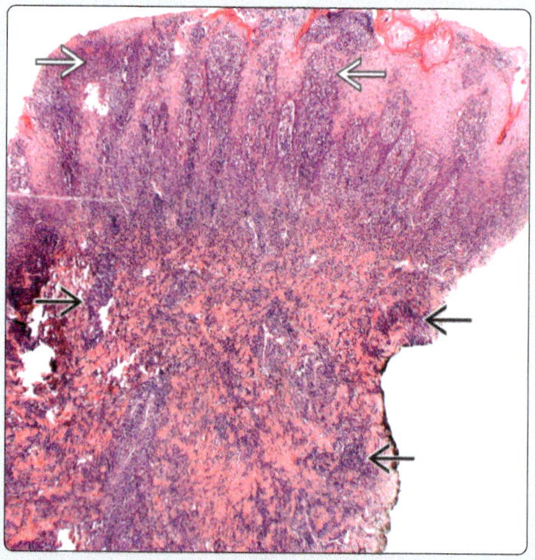

(Left) *Cutaneous γδ T-cell lymphoma (CGDTCL) shows a large raised lesion with ulcer and satellite lesions. (Courtesy C. Sander, MD.)* **(Right)** *The atypical lymphoid infiltrate diffusely involves the epidermis ➡, dermis ⇨, and also extended into the subcutaneous adipose tissue (not shown), typical of this neoplasm.*

Panniculitis With Karyorrhexis

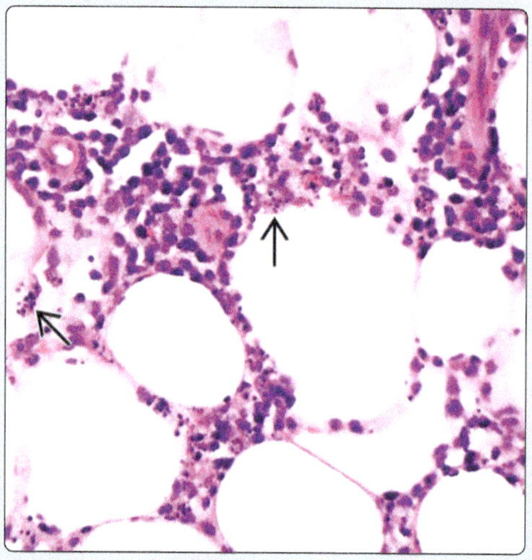

CD3 Immunohistochemical Stain in CGDTCL

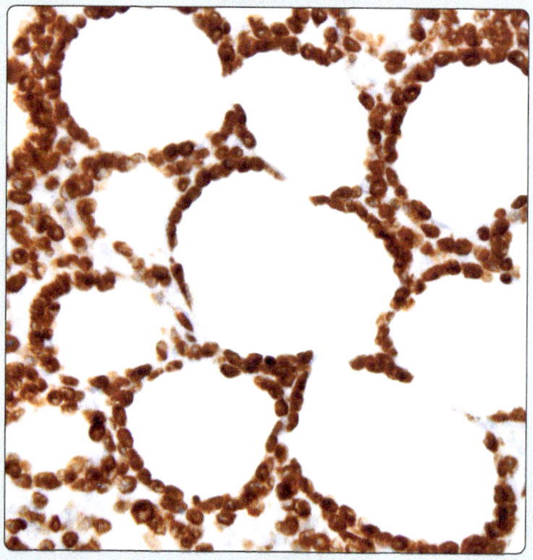

(Left) *In the same case, there is a deep infiltrate showing lobular panniculitis composed of atypical T cells rimming fat lobules with prominent apoptosis/karyorrhexis ⇨.* **(Right)** *At high power, this CD3 stain highlights the atypical T cells that are lining fat cells. This feature is common to CGDTCL and to subcutaneous panniculitis-like T-cell lymphoma. (Courtesy L. J. Medeiros, MD.)*

TERMINOLOGY

Abbreviations

- Cutaneous γδ T-cell lymphoma (CGDTCL)

Synonyms

- Subcutaneous panniculitis-like T-cell lymphoma with γδ cells

Definitions

- T-cell lymphoma arising in skin, which is composed of cytotoxic γδ T cells
  - Does not include subcutaneous panniculitis-like T-cell lymphoma composed of αβ cells

ETIOLOGY/PATHOGENESIS

Immunosuppression or Dysregulation of T Cells

- Found in many patients

Chronic Antigenic Stimulation

- Speculative but possibly involved in pathogenesis

Cell of Origin

- γδ T cells
  - Involved with mucosal and epithelial immune system function

CLINICAL ISSUES

Epidemiology

- Incidence
  - Rare tumor
    - < 1% of all cutaneous T-cell lymphomas
- Age
  - Commonly adults
- Sex
  - No gender preponderance

Site

- Mostly extremities
  - Sometimes mucosal sites, where normal γδ T cells are found
  - Metastasis common
    - Spread to lungs, liver, kidneys, oral mucosa, and brain
    - Usually not in bone marrow, lymph nodes, or spleen

Presentation

- 1 or multiple skin lesions, sometimes with ulceration
- Patches due to epidermal infiltrates
  - Plaques or nodules due to dermal infiltrates
    - ± ulcerated epidermis
- Hemophagocytic syndrome (HPS) may be present in 45% of cases
  - More often in subcutaneous lesions
    - Related to release of cytotoxic molecules
- B symptoms are frequent

Laboratory Tests

- Cytopenias and ↑ liver function tests
- HHV8, HTLV-1, and EBV serologies (-)

Treatment

- Multiagent chemotherapy ± radiotherapy
  - Aggressive therapy followed by allogeneic allogenic stem cell transplant may be promising treatment modality
  - Brentuximab vedotin can be treatment option for patients with CD30(+) CGDTCL

Prognosis

- Poor prognosis
  - 5-yr survival: ~ 11%; median survival: ~ 15 months
  - Subcutaneous disease is poor prognostic indicator
    - Better prognosis if only disease in dermis or epidermis
  - HPS is poor prognostic indicator
  - May have indolent course in children

MICROSCOPIC

Histologic Features

- May involve epidermis, dermis, &/or subcutis
  - **Epidermal**
    - Epidermotropism ranges from mild to marked
    - Can mimic mycosis fungoides or pagetoid reticulosis
  - **Dermal**
    - More dermal involvement typically present than in subcutaneous panniculitis-like T-cell lymphoma
  - **Subcutaneous**
    - Lobules mostly involved
    - Septa less frequently involved and represents secondary spilling of T cells from lobules
    - Subcutis involvement can appear identical to subcutaneous panniculitis-like T-cell lymphoma of αβ cells, including rimming of fat cells
- Malignant T cells with nuclear atypia, hyperchromasia
- Frequent necrosis/apoptosis and vascular invasion
  - Necrosis may be caused by released cytotoxic molecules
- ↑ reactive histiocytes
  - Vacuolated foamy cytoplasm from imbibed material/lipid
  - With erythrophagocytosis or cytophagocytosis

Cytologic Features

- Small to medium to large T cells with coarse, hyperchromatic-staining chromatin, sometimes vesicular nuclei, and variably prominent nucleoli

ANCILLARY TESTS

Immunohistochemistry

- T-cell antigens (CD2, CD3, CD5, CD7) (+)
  - May lose 1 or more T-cell antigens
- Most cases: CD4(-)/CD8(-)
  - Few cases: CD4(-)/CD8(+)
- TCR-δ1(+), TCR-γ1(+), βF1(-)
  - If TCRδ1 antibody is unavailable, βF1 can be used instead
    - βF1(-) may serve to assume γδ cell origin
- CD56 usually positive, unlike subcutaneous panniculitis-like T-cell lymphoma
- Cytotoxic markers (perforin, TIA1, granzyme) (+)

In Situ Hybridization

- Epstein-Barr virus small encoded receptor (EBER) (-)
  - But may be (+) in mucocutaneous γδ T-cell lymphoma

Genetic Testing

- Clonal rearrangement of *TRB* and *TRG* genes
- *IGH* not clonally rearranged
- No specific reproducible chromosomal abnormalities
  - Case report showed complex karyotype with several chromosomal translocations involving breakpoints at 9p21, 14q11.2, 14q32.1, or 16q23.1

DIFFERENTIAL DIAGNOSIS

Subcutaneous Panniculitis-Like T-Cell Lymphoma

- Previously included cases of CGDTCL until reclassification in WHO Classification of Hematopoietic and Lymphoid Tumors (2008)
- Presents with panniculitic pattern of tissue involvement similar to CGDTCL
  - Differs in morphology as subcutaneous panniculitis-like T-cell lymphoma is typically confined to subcutis
    - Does not invade dermis or epidermis in most cases
    - Epidermis is not ulcerated, contrary to CGDTCL
- Shows immunophenotype of αβ cells, not γδ cells of CGDTCL
  - BF1(+), TCRδ1(-), CD56(-), unlike CGDTCL
  - Usually CD4(-), CD8(+)
- Much better prognosis than CGDTCL
  - 5-yr survival: ~ 85%
  - Hemophagocytic syndrome less prevalent than in CGDTCL
  - Patients younger than in CGDTCL and less B symptoms
  - Often treated with systemic corticosteroids
    - Whereas CGDTCL is often treated with multiagent chemotherapy

Peripheral T-Cell Lymphoma, Not Otherwise Specified

- Similar morphology, often with dermal and subcutis involvement
- Both diseases often have pleomorphic tumor cells
- Often CD4(+) or CD8(+) cells, whereas CGDTCL is usually CD4(-)/CD8(-)
- Usually βF1(+), unlike CGDTCL, which is βF1(-)

Anaplastic Large Cell Lymphoma

- CD30(+) and CD4(+), unlike most cases of CGDTCL
- Usually in dermis and only rarely in subcutis

Mycosis Fungoides

- Atypical T cells in epidermis with lining up and clustering of cells
- CD4(+)/CD8(-) T cells; cytotoxic markers (-)
- Patch to plaque to tumor progression

Pagetoid Reticulosis

- CGDTCL with marked epidermotropism resembles pagetoid reticulosis
- Unlike CGDTCL, pagetoid reticulosis often occurs on feet
- Usually CD4(-)/CD8(+)
  - CGDTCL is usually CD4(-)/CD8(-)

Diffuse Large B-Cell Lymphoma

- Can have subcutaneous dissemination
- But will have B-cell phenotype and *IGH* gene rearrangement

Blastic Plasmacytoid Dendritic Cell Neoplasm

- Diffuse, atypical infiltrate of CD56(+) cells, like CGDTCL
  - Different phenotype than CGDTCL with cytotoxic markers (-); usually CD3(-), CD123(+), TCL1(+), CD4(+), and CD8(-)

Enteropathy-Associated T-Cell Lymphoma

- Can have subcutis dissemination
  - But will typically present with gastrointestinal mass and show features of celiac disease

Reactive Panniculitis

- **Lupus profundus panniculitis**
  - Also inflammation in subcutis in lobular panniculitis pattern
  - Can be difficult to differentiate reactive panniculitis from CGDTCL or subcutaneous panniculitis-like T-cell lymphoma
  - Features favoring lupus panniculitis over SPTCL
    - Plasma cells and germinal centers
    - Mixed inflammatory infiltrate with histiocytes, eosinophils, and neutrophils
    - Lymphocytes do not show atypia and do not rim fat cells
    - B-cell aggregates
    - Mixture of CD4(+) and CD8(+) cells
    - Vacuolar epidermal change and interstitial mucin
    - *TRB* and *TRG* rearrangements are usually not clonal, but rarely oligoclonal T-cell populations are present
    - Other clinical or lab evidence of autoimmune disease

DIAGNOSTIC CHECKLIST

Pathologic Interpretation Pearls

- Atypical lobular panniculitic γδ T-cell infiltrate with karyorrhexis and fat necrosis rimming individual fat cells
- Dermal and epidermal involvement with ulceration, unlike subcutaneous panniculitis-like T-cell lymphoma

SELECTED REFERENCES

1. Ali L et al: Gamma-delta T-cell lymphoma arising in a long-standing cutaneous plaque. J Cutan Pathol. ePub, 2015
2. Foppoli M et al: Gamma-delta t-cell lymphomas. Eur J Haematol. 94(3):206-18, 2015
3. Gibson JF et al: Hematopoietic stem cell transplantation for primary cutaneous γδ T-cell lymphoma and refractory subcutaneous panniculitis-like T-cell lymphoma. J Am Acad Dermatol. 72(6):1010-5.e5, 2015
4. Martires KJ et al: Characterization of primary cutaneous CD8+/CD30+ lymphoproliferative disorders. Am J Dermatopathol. 37(11):822-33, 2015
5. Magro CM et al: Indolent primary cutaneous γ/δ T-cell lymphoma localized to the subcutaneous panniculus and its association with atypical lymphocytic lobular panniculitis. Am J Clin Pathol. 138(1):50-6, 2012
6. Yamamoto-Sugitani M et al: Comprehensive cytogenetic study of primary cutaneous gamma-delta T-cell lymphoma by means of spectral karyotyping and genome-wide single nucleotide polymorphism array. Cancer Genet. 205(9):459-64, 2012

Epidermal Involvement in CGDTCL

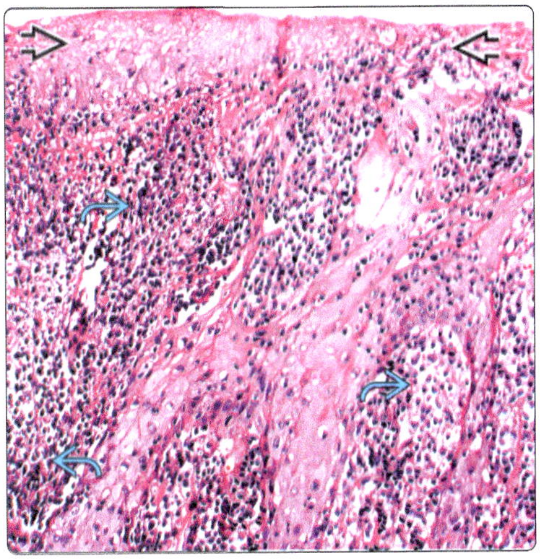

CGDTCL Mimicking Mycosis Fungoides

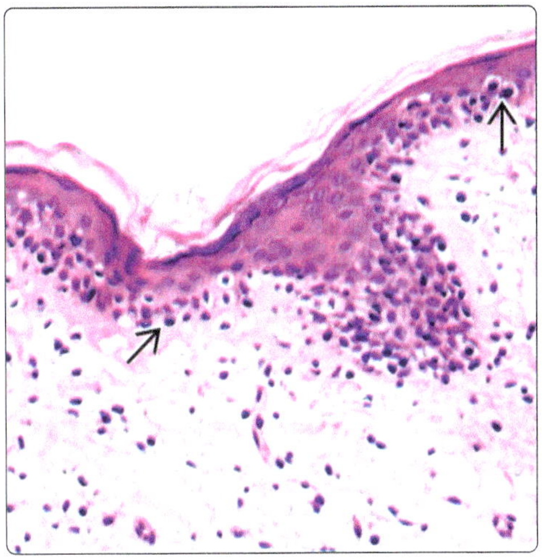

(Left) *There is ulceration of the epidermis ⇨ due to prominent infiltration by the neoplastic cells, which is commonly seen in CGDTCL. The atypical lymphoid infiltrate ↪ also diffusely involves the superficial dermis.* **(Right)** *This is an example of CGDTCL with much milder epidermal involvement. The infiltrate involves the epidermis → as small clusters and single cells with perinuclear haloes, mimicking mycosis fungoides.*

Fat Rimming in CGDTCL

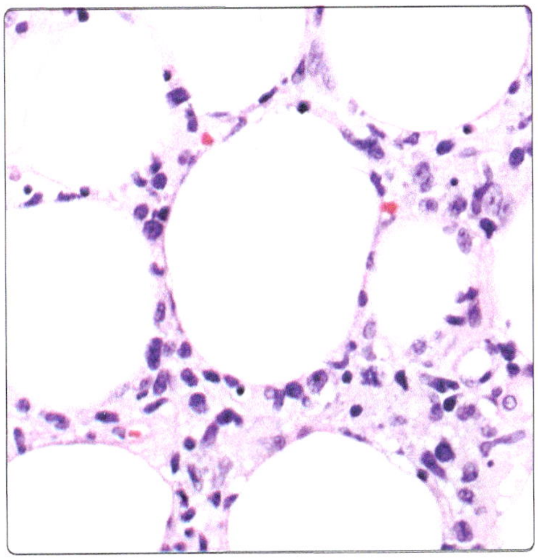

Atypical Lymphoid Cells Lining Fat Cells

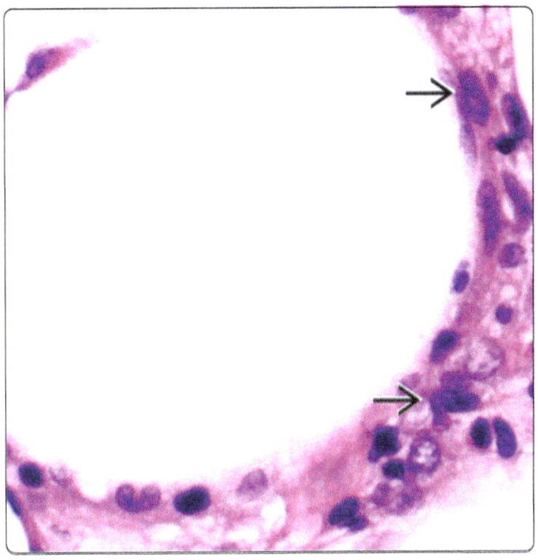

(Left) *Focusing on the subcutis, there are atypical cells that are rimming the fat, which look similar to those of subcutaneous panniculitis-like T-cell lymphoma.* **(Right)** *A higher power image of the subcutaneous tissue shows that there are atypical T cells → that line individual fat cells. These cells are more atypical than would be expected in a reactive panniculitis.*

CD3 Immunohistochemical Stain in CGDTCL

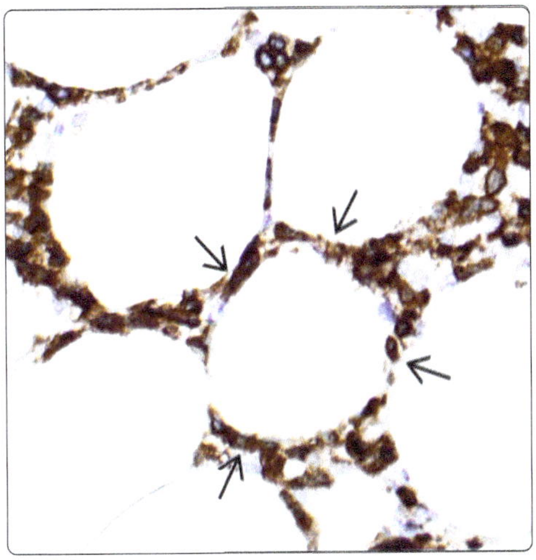

TIA1 Immunohistochemical Stain

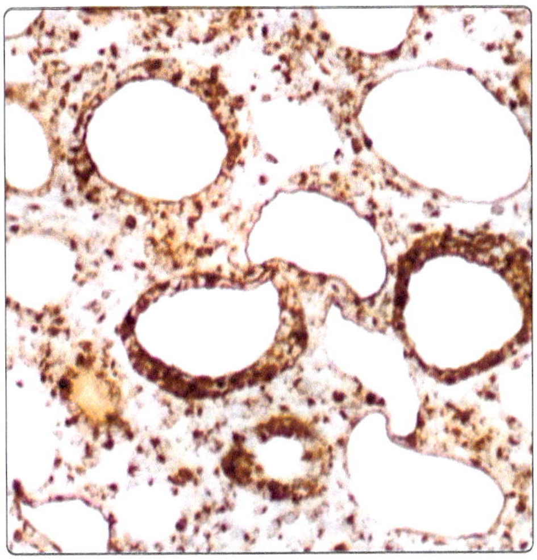

(Left) *At high power, this CD3 immunohistochemical stain highlights atypical T cells → that are lining fat cells. This feature is common to CGDTCL and to subcutaneous panniculitis-like T-cell lymphoma.* **(Right)** *This is a TIA1 immunohistochemical stain in GDTCL. Atypical neoplastic cells rimming the fat show cytotoxic granules, which strongly express TIA1. These cells were also positive for other cytotoxic markers, including granzyme-B and perforin.*

CD4 Immunohistochemical Stain

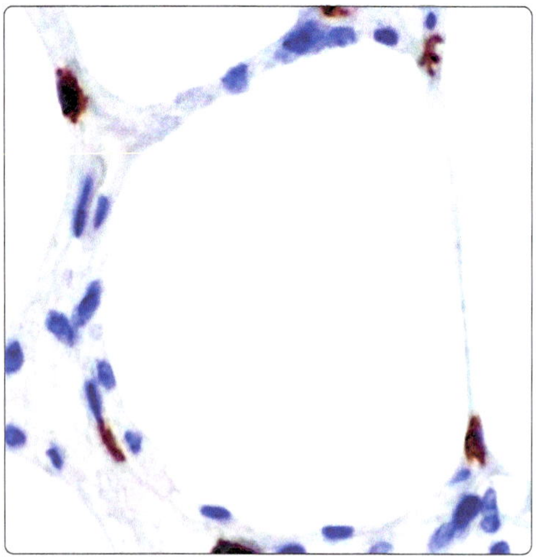

CD8 Immunohistochemical Stain

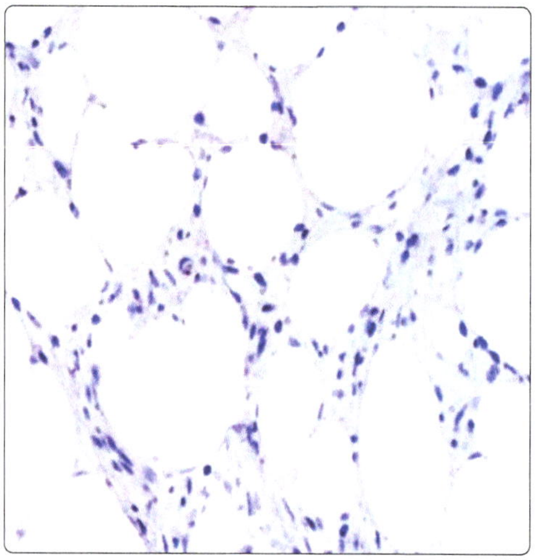

(Left) *In this example of CGDTCL, most of the malignant T cells are not immunoreactive for CD4. The few positive cells are likely histiocytes. Typically, CGDTCL are CD4(-)/CD8(-), whereas most cases of subcutaneous panniculitis-like T-cell lymphoma are CD4(-)/CD8(+).* **(Right)** *This is a CD8 immunostain in a case of CGDTCL involving the subcutis. The malignant T cells show no expression of CD8.*

CD8 Positivity in CGDTCL

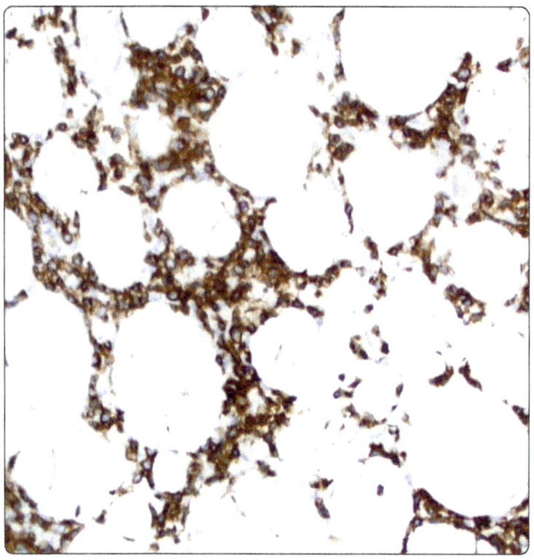

CD56 Immunohistochemical Stain

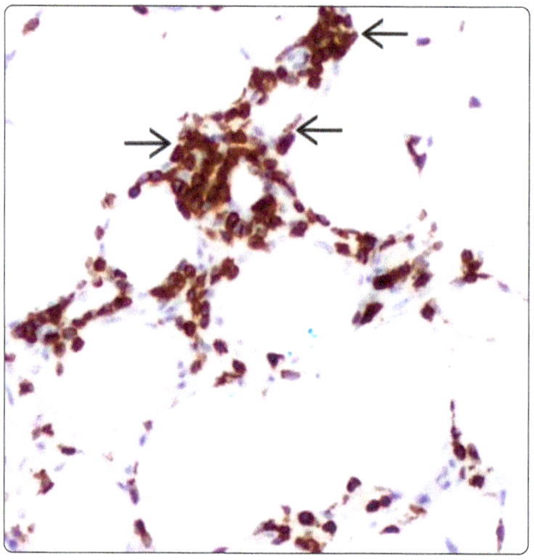

(Left) *Many of the cells of this case of CGDTCL are CD8(+). Most cases are CD8(-), but some can be focally CD8(+), and rare cases are diffusely CD8(+).* **(Right)** *This CD56 immunohistochemical stain marks the malignant T cells ⇨ in this case of CGDTCL. CD56 is differentially expressed in CGDTCL and subcutaneous panniculitis-like T-cell lymphoma, as it is usually positive in CGDTCL and negative in SPTCL.*

TCRδ-1 Immunohistochemical Stain

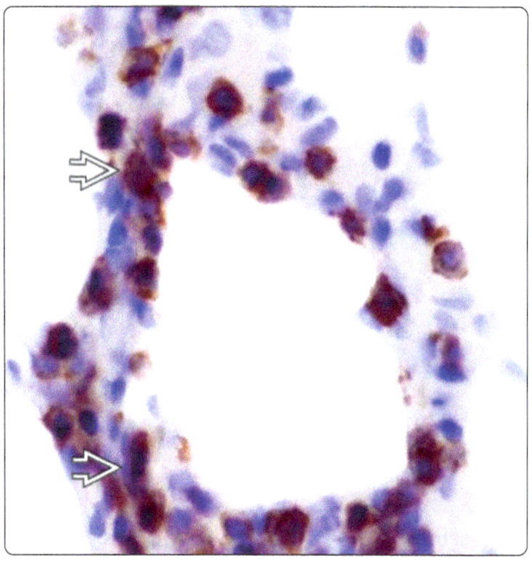

βF-1 Immunohistochemical Stain

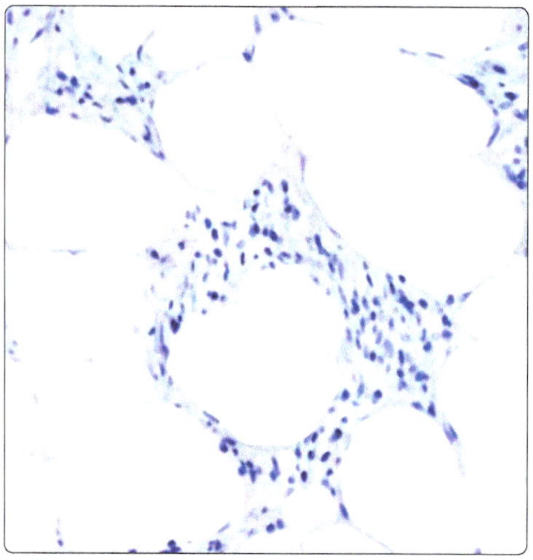

(Left) *The malignant T cells encircling adipocytes are positive for TCRδ-1 ⇨, as expected, since the tumor is composed of γδ T cells.* **(Right)** *βF1 is negative in the T cells rimming the fat. Lack of βF1 is presumptive evidence that the T cells express the γδTCR. CGDTCL is βF1(-), whereas subcutaneous panniculitis-like T-cell lymphoma is βF1(+).*

Differential Diagnosis: SPTCL

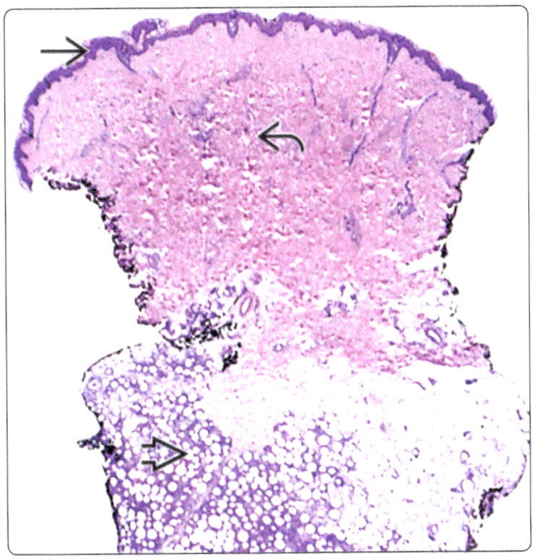

Higher Power Magnification of SPTCL

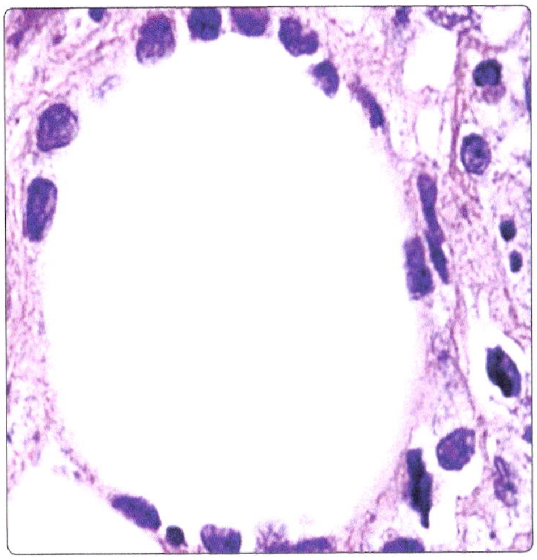

(Left) *Subcutaneous panniculitis-like T-cell lymphoma (SPTCL), which is the main differential diagnosis of subcutaneous γδ T-cell lymphoma, shows malignant T cells that are confined to the subcutis ➾, but the dermis ➢ and epidermis ➙ are not involved. (Courtesy M. Tomaszewsky, MD.)* **(Right)** *High magnification of SPTCL shows a population of atypical, hyperchromatic-staining neoplastic cells infiltrating between and around adipocytes, which appears identical to PCGDTCL.*

Differential Diagnosis: Lupus Profundus

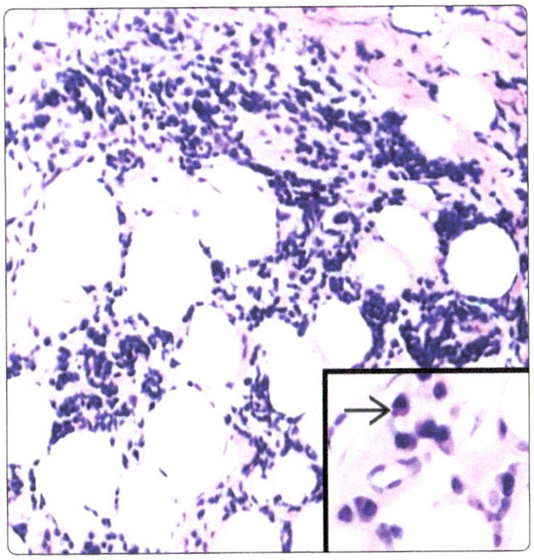

CD4/CD8 in Lupus Profundus

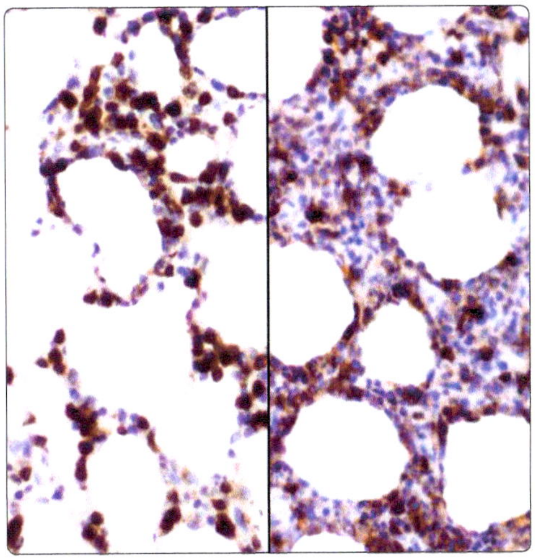

(Left) *This case of lupus profundus shows a lobular panniculitis. Scattered plasma cells are seen ➙ (lower right insert). Plasma cells and B cells are a component of lupus profundus but are not expected in CGDTCL.* **(Right)** *Lupus profundus usually has a mixture of CD4(+) & CD8(+) cells, whereas usually CGDTCL is CD4(-)/CD8(-) or CD4(-)/CD8(+). In this image of lupus profundus, the CD4 stain (left) and the CD8 stain (right) both show clusters of positive cells.*

Differential Diagnosis: Peripheral T-Cell Lymphoma, Not Otherwise Specified

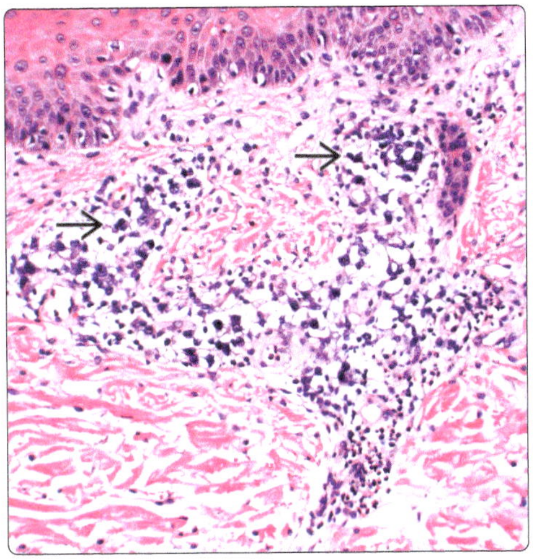

Differential Diagnosis: Pagetoid Reticulosis

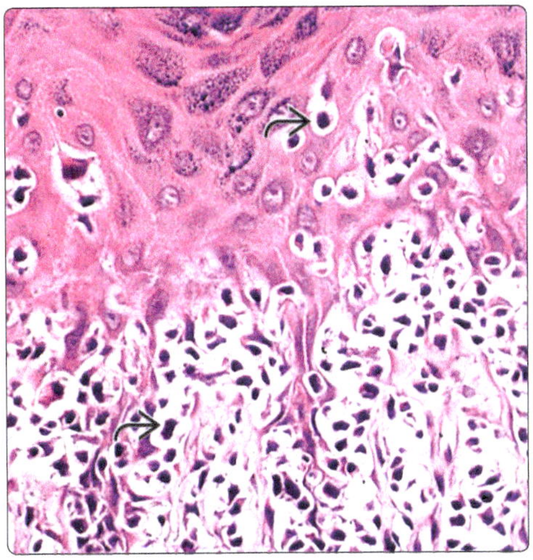

(Left) *This case of peripheral T-cell lymphoma, not otherwise specified, shows some similarities to CGDTCL with an epidermal and dermal ➙ infiltrate of atypical T cells. However, the T cells in this case are CD4(+)/βF1(+), unlike CGDTCL, which is usually CD4(-)/βF1(-).* **(Right)** *Pagetoid reticulosis can also appear similar to CGDTCL with pleomorphic cells ➢ in the epidermis. However, pagetoid reticulosis differs by having an acral distribution in most cases, and a CD4(-)/CD8(+) immunophenotype.*

Angioimmunoblastic T-Cell Lymphoma

KEY FACTS

TERMINOLOGY

- T-cell lymphoma of follicular helper T cells

CLINICAL ISSUES

- Uncommon
- Mostly adults, no gender preference
- Skin rash (50%)
- Generalized lymphadenopathy
- Autoimmune hemolytic anemia
- Polyclonal hypergammaglobulinemia
- Treatment: Chemotherapy
- Median survival: 1-2 years

MICROSCOPIC

- Skin
  - Nonspecific superficial dermal lymphocytic infiltrate with eosinophils
  - ± atypia and hyperplastic capillaries
  - May be tumor cells in skin or secondary reactive-appearing rash from cytokine production
- Lymph node: Hyperplasia of follicular dendritic cells and high endothelial venules
  - Tumor cells with clear cytoplasm, arborizing high endothelial vessels, and disrupted follicular dendritic meshworks
  - Polymorphic background inflammatory cells

ANCILLARY TESTS

- Immunophenotype
  - CD4(+) T cells, CD10(+/-), Bcl-6(+), CXCL13(+), PD1(+)
  - CD21, in disrupted follicular dendritic meshworks
- Molecular
  - EBER(+) in lymph nodes and usually EBER(-) in skin
  - Clonal *TRG* gene rearrangement
  - *RHOA* p.Gly17Val somatic mutation detected in ~ 50%

AITL at Low Magnification

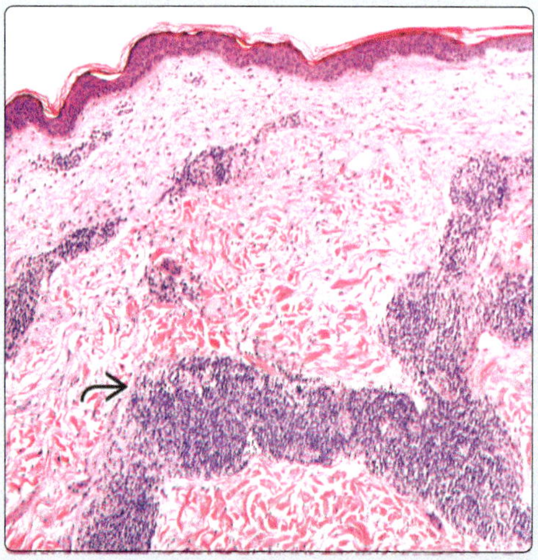

AITL at High Magnification

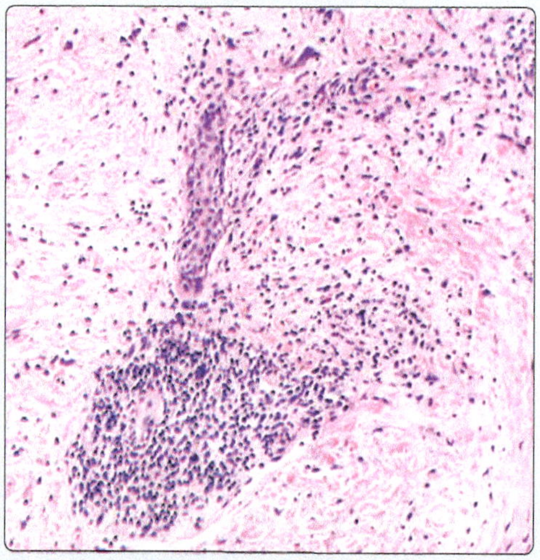

(Left) *Cutaneous involvement by angioimmunoblastic T-cell lymphoma (AITL) often shows a nonspecific dense dermal perivascular* ➔ *infiltrate at low magnification. (Courtesy S. Wang, MD.)* **(Right)** *At higher magnification, the T cells in the infiltrate only show mild atypia. In cutaneous lesions of AITL patients, the lymphocytes may or may not show significant atypia.*

PCR Test for TRG Gene Rearrangement

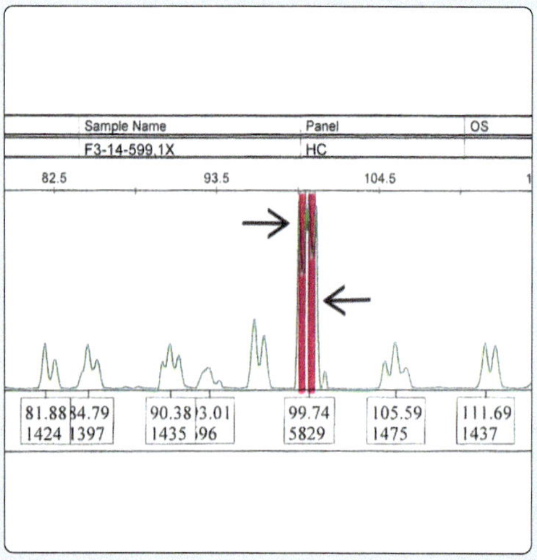

EBER In Situ Hybridization

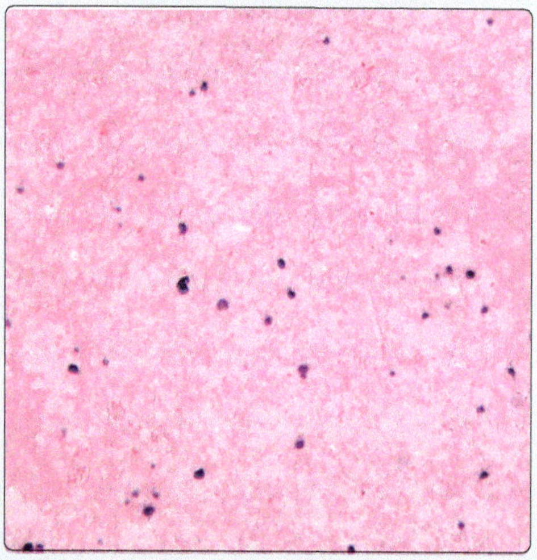

(Left) *A dominant monoclonal peak* ➔ *at position 99 is seen. This supports that this is a T-cell lymphoma. AITL can sometimes show IGH gene rearrangement. (From DP: Molecular Onc.)* **(Right)** *The test is positive in a case of AITL.*

TERMINOLOGY

Abbreviations

- Angioimmunoblastic T-cell lymphoma (AITL)

Synonyms

- Angioimmunoblastic lymphadenopathy with dysproteinemia
- Immunoblastic lymphadenopathy
- Immunodysplastic disease
- Lymphogranulomatous X

Definitions

- T-cell lymphoma of follicular helper T cells associated with
  - Systemic disease, polymorphous infiltrate, and proliferating high endothelial venules

ETIOLOGY/PATHOGENESIS

Dysfunction of Immune System

- Patients with AITL have hypergammaglobulinemia and other immune dysfunctions
  - Follicular helper T cells upregulate CXCL13 and CXCR5
  - CXCL13 promotes B-cell recruitment with B cells on high endothelial venules
  - CD21(+) follicular dendritic cells located by high endothelial venules
  - Promotes B-cell proliferation and hypergammaglobulinemia
- Cytokine dysregulation
  - Patients with AITL show abnormal cytokine dysregulation
  - Debated whether skin represents tumor or secondary reaction to cytokines

Viral Infection

- Epstein-Barr virus (EBV)
  - EBV(+) B cells are frequently seen in AITL
  - Neoplastic T cells are EBV(-)
  - Most likely secondary to patients immunocompromise
- Other viruses
  - Cytomegalovirus, herpes, and HIV also may be associated with AITL
    - PCR for human herpes virus 6B found in many AITL cases
  - Infections may be secondary to tumor

Drugs

- Implicated as causative agent in some cases (never proven)

CLINICAL ISSUES

Epidemiology

- Incidence
  - Comprises 1-2% of all non-Hodgkin lymphoma
  - 18% of all peripheral T-cell lymphomas
    - 1,000 new cases per year in USA
- Age
  - Mostly adults, middle aged to elderly
    - Rarely seen in children
  - Median age: 63
- Sex
  - M = F
- Ethnicity
  - Most common in Caucasians
  - More common in Europe than in North America

Site

- Skin
  - Frequent extranodal site
    - ~ 50% of cases have skin lesions
    - Usually secondary to systemic disease
    - Rarely, skin lesion can be 1st manifestation of disease
- Lymph node
  - Nearly all cases involve lymph nodes
- Other sites of disease
  - Often in spleen, liver, and bone marrow
    - No follicular dendritic cells in bone marrow AITL, so bone marrow AITL is CD21(-)
    - No CXCL13 in bone marrow AITL
- ~ 80-90% diagnosed with stage III or IV disease at the time of initial diagnosis

Presentation

- Skin
  - Rash, usually pruritic
    - Maculopapular eruption most common
    - Purpura, erythroderma, papulovesicular, nodules, and urticarial lesions are less common
  - Often generalized lesions
    - Frequently on trunk or extremities
  - Rash can be before, after, or same time as initial diagnosis of AITL
  - Often mimics inflammatory dermatoses
- Extracutaneous presentation
  - Generalized lymphadenopathy
  - Hepatomegaly
  - Splenomegaly
  - B symptoms
  - Arthritis/arthralgia
  - Ascites

Laboratory Tests

- Complete blood cell count
  - Anemia
    - Autoimmune hemolytic anemia
    - Cryoglobulins/cold agglutinins
    - Sometimes Coombs test (+)
  - Lymphocytes
    - Lymphopenia more often
    - Lymphocytosis less often
  - Thrombocytopenia
  - Eosinophilia
- Hypergammaglobulinemia or hypogammaglobulinemia
  - Polyclonal
  - Hypoalbuminemia
- ↑ erythrocyte sedimentation rate
- ↑ serum lactate dehydrogenase
- ↑ β-2-microglobulin
- Sometimes autoantibodies (+)
  - Rheumatoid factor
  - Antismooth muscle antibody

Natural History

- AITL-related secondary lymphomas
  - Increased risk of developing 2nd lymphoma in patients with AITL
    - Diffuse large B-cell lymphoma is most common 2nd lymphoma
    - Diffuse large B-cell lymphoma usually has EBER(+) cells

Treatment

- Adjuvant therapy
  - Combined chemotherapy
    - Treatment in most cases
  - Steroids
    - In patients who are not candidates for chemotherapy
- Autologous stem cell transplant
  - Sometimes follows treatment with chemotherapy

Prognosis

- Aggressive disease
  - Median survival: 1-2 years
- Poor prognostic indicators
  - Males
  - Anemia
  - Mediastinal lymphadenopathy

IMAGING

General Features

- Generalized lymphadenopathy
- Internal organ involvement

MICROSCOPIC

Histologic Features

- Skin
  - Usually nonspecific, variable histologic patterns
    - Often superficial dermal infiltrates with lymphocytes and eosinophils
    - Sometimes perivascular lymphocytic infiltrate
    - Sometimes sheet-like lymphocytic infiltrate
    - Lymphocytes ± atypia
    - Hyperplastic capillaries
    - Usually no epidermotropism present
  - Leukocytoclastic vasculitis is rarely seen
  - Necrotizing granulomas are occasionally present
  - May be tumor cells in skin or secondary reactive infiltrate from cytokine production
- Lymph node
  - Effaced architecture
    - Partial or complete
  - Tumor usually involves paracortical areas
    - Early disease, tumor may be only in paracortex
    - Peripheral cortical sinuses of lymph node are often patent
  - Tumor cells
    - Small to medium in size
    - Increased clear cytoplasm
  - High endothelial venules
    - ↑ vessels in tumor
    - Usually branching blood vessels
    - Follicular dendritic cells located near blood vessels
    - Periodic acid-Schiff stain highlights blood vessels
  - Follicular dendritic cell meshworks
    - Expanded and disrupted in tumor
    - Associated with high endothelial venules
  - Polymorphic background inflammatory cells
    - Often prominent
    - Eosinophils, reactive small lymphocytes, plasma cells
    - Epithelioid histiocytes give granulomatous appearance
    - B immunoblasts in paracortex
    - EBV(+) B cells
  - Lymph node follicles have variable appearance
    - Hyperplastic follicles
    - Atretic follicles (can be mistaken for Castleman lymphadenopathy)
    - No follicles

ANCILLARY TESTS

Immunohistochemistry

- Malignant T cells
  - T-cell antigens (+) (CD2, CD3, CD5, CD7)
    - Can aberrantly lose 1 or more T-cell antigens
    - Most commonly lost T-cell antigen is CD7
  - Helper T cells [usually CD4(+), CD8(-), βF1(+)]
  - Follicular helper T-cell phenotype
    - CD10(+/-), Bcl-6(+), CXCL13(+), CXCR5(+), PD1(+), SAP(+), ICOS(+)
      - ▫ In general, positivity for at least 3 of these antibodies suggest neoplasm of follicular helper T cell
    - Usually CXCL13(+) in cutaneous AITL
    - CXCR5(+): Chemokine receptor for CXCL13; CXCL13-CXCR5 axis plays role in formation of germinal centers in secondary lymphoid organs
    - Often CD10(-) in cutaneous AITL
- Follicular dendritic cell meshworks
  - CD21, CD23, CD35, and clusterin positive
- ↑ reactive B cells
  - Express B-cell markers (CD19, CD20, pax-5, CD79a)

Flow Cytometry

- Loss of 1 or more T-cell antigens
  - Most commonly lost T-cell antigen is CD7
- CD10 coexpressed on subset of T cells

In Situ Hybridization

- EBV small-encoded RNA (EBER)
  - 80-90% of lymph nodes (+)
    - Usually negative in skin lesions

PCR

- Clonal *TRB* and *TRG* gene rearrangement in 87% of lymph nodes with AITL
  - Some skin infiltrates show clonal T-cell receptor gene rearrangement
    - Identical clones can be seen in skin and lymph node
- Clonal *IGH* gene rearrangement in 25% of lymph nodes with AITL

Genetic Testing

- *RHOA* p.Gly17Val somatic mutation
  - Detected in ~ 50%
  - *RHOA* is GTPase protein of RAS family
  - Mutation also detected in small percentage of peripheral T-cell lymphoma, not otherwise specified cases and in some NK-/T-cell lymphomas
- Cytogenetic findings
  - Trisomy of chromosomes 3, 5, 21 reported
  - Loss of 6q and gain of X reported, 1p alterations
- Potentially frequent mutations in epigenetic regulators (TET2, DNMT3A, IDH2)

DIFFERENTIAL DIAGNOSIS

Cutaneous Infiltrates With Reactive T Cells

- Variety of entities can show nonspecific perivascular T-cell infiltrates in skin
  - Differential diagnosis includes
    - Infections
    - Drug reactions
    - Lymphocytic vasculitis
    - Granulomatous disease if granulomatous inflammation is seen
  - T cells have minimal atypia and are often CD8(+)
  - Usually no clonal *TRG* gene rearrangements
  - No increase in CD21(+) follicular dendritic cells
  - T cells will not coexpress CD10 and will be EBER(-)
  - Clinical history is helpful in making diagnosis

Anaplastic Large Cell Lymphoma

- Common in skin (primary cutaneous anaplastic large cell lymphoma)
- CD30(+); ALK/EMA(-)
- EBER(-)

Peripheral T-Cell Lymphoma, Not Otherwise Specified

- Similarities to AITL
  - Both are malignant T-cell lymphomas, expressing T-cell antigens
  - Some peripheral T-cell lymphoma, not otherwise specified have follicular T-cell profile, similar to AITL in gene expression arrays
  - Sometimes increased high endothelial venules
- Differences from AITL
  - No increased follicular dendritic cells or high endothelial venules
  - EBER(-)

Primary Cutaneous CD4(+) Small/Medium T-Cell Lymphoma

- Solitary lesion, usually head and neck or upper trunk
- Follicular helper T-cell markers (+) (i.e., PD1) like AITL
- Lacks hypergammaglobulinemia and lymphadenopathy that is seen in AITL

T Cell/Histiocyte-Rich Large B-Cell Lymphoma

- Similarities to AITL
  - Both tumors have more T cells than B cells
- Differences from AITL
  - Large atypical B cells and small reactive-appearing T cells in TCRLBCL
    - Often large atypical T cells and small B cells in AITL
  - Clonal *IGH* gene rearrangement
  - No increased follicular dendritic cells
  - EBER(-)

EBV(+) Diffuse Large B-Cell Lymphoma of Elderly

- Both are EBV(+) malignant tumors
- Differences from AITL
  - Usually polyclonal *TRG* gene rearrangement and clonal *IGH* gene rearrangement
  - No increased follicular dendritic cells
  - EBV(+) in sheets of large B cells and far fewer in number in AITL
  - No aberrant T-cell antigens

DIAGNOSTIC CHECKLIST

Clinically Relevant Pathologic Features

- Hypergammaglobulinemia and autoimmune hemolytic anemia

Pathologic Interpretation Pearls

- T-cell lymphoma with arborizing high endothelial venules and increased background inflammatory cells
- CD3(+), CD10(+), CXCL13(+)

SELECTED REFERENCES

1. Ondrejka SL et al: Angioimmunoblastic T-cell lymphomas with the RHOA p.Gly17Val mutation have classic clinical and pathologic features. Am J Surg Pathol. 40(3):335-41, 2016
2. Chiba S et al: G17V RHOA: Genetic evidence of GTP-unbound RHOA playing a role in tumorigenesis in T cells. Small GTPases. 6(2):100-3, 2015
3. Odejide O et al: A targeted mutational landscape of angioimmunoblastic T-cell lymphoma. Blood. 123(9):1293-6, 2014
4. Couronné L et al: TET2 and DNMT3A mutations in human T-cell lymphoma. N Engl J Med. 366(1):95-6, 2012
5. Dorfman DM et al: CD200 (OX-2 membrane glycoprotein) is expressed by follicular T helper cells and in angioimmunoblastic T-cell lymphoma. Am J Surg Pathol. 35(1):76-83, 2011
6. Hatanaka K et al: Methotrexate-associated lymphoproliferative disorders mimicking angioimmunoblastic T-cell lymphoma. Pathol Res Pract. 206(1):9-13, 2010
7. Smithberger ES et al: Primary cutaneous angioimmunoblastic T-cell lymphoma histologically mimicking an inflammatory dermatosis. J Drugs Dermatol. 9(7):851-5, 2010
8. Rodriguez-Justo M et al: Angioimmunoblastic T-cell lymphoma with hyperplastic germinal centres: a neoplasia with origin in the outer zone of the germinal centre? Clinicopathological and immunohistochemical study of 10 cases with follicular T-cell markers. Mod Pathol. 22(6):753-61, 2009
9. Yoon GS et al: Angioimmunoblastic T cell lymphomas: frequent cutaneous skin lesions and absence of human herpes viruses. Ann Dermatol. 21(1):1-5, 2009
10. Ortonne N et al: Characterization of CXCL13+ neoplastic t cells in cutaneous lesions of angioimmunoblastic T-cell lymphoma (AITL). Am J Surg Pathol. 31(7):1068-76, 2007
11. Jayaraman AG et al: Cutaneous involvement by angioimmunoblastic T-cell lymphoma: a unique histologic presentation, mimicking an infectious etiology. J Cutan Pathol. 33 Suppl 2:6-11, 2006
12. Brown HA et al: Cutaneous involvement by angioimmunoblastic T-cell lymphoma with remarkable heterogeneous Epstein-Barr virus expression. J Cutan Pathol. 28(8):432-8, 2001

(Left) *Low-power magnification of a skin biopsy from a patient with AITL who had a maculopapular rash shows a nonspecific, mostly perivascular* → *lymphocytic infiltrate.* **(Right)** *In contrast, this AITL skin lesion shows diffuse, large sheets of malignant lymphocytes* ↪. *This sheet-like distribution pattern is less common.*

AITL at Low Magnification

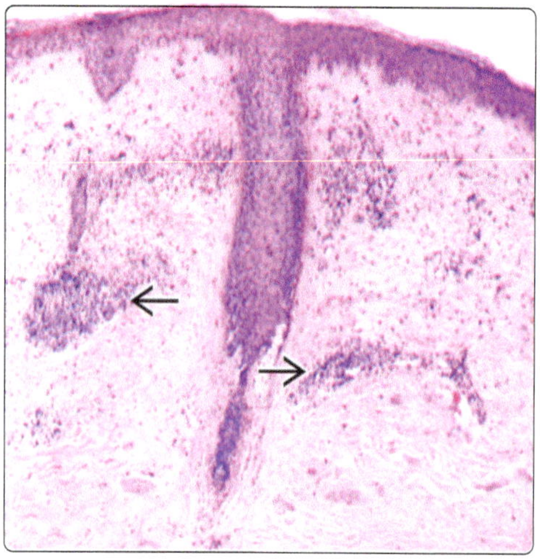

AITL at Low Magnification

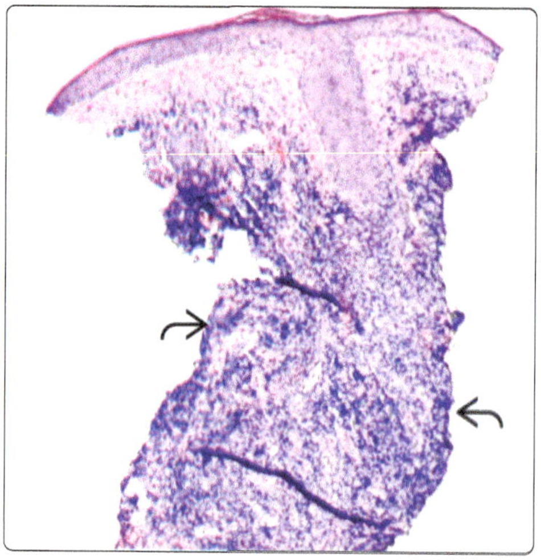

(Left) *In another case of cutaneous AITL, the infiltrate is confined to the dermis* →, *and the epidermis* ➡ *is uninvolved. Most skin lesions in patients with AITL do not show epidermotropism.* **(Right)** *The stain shows strongly positive staining of the dermal T cells. CD20 only marks rare scattered B cells (not shown).*

Epidermis vs. Dermis in AITL

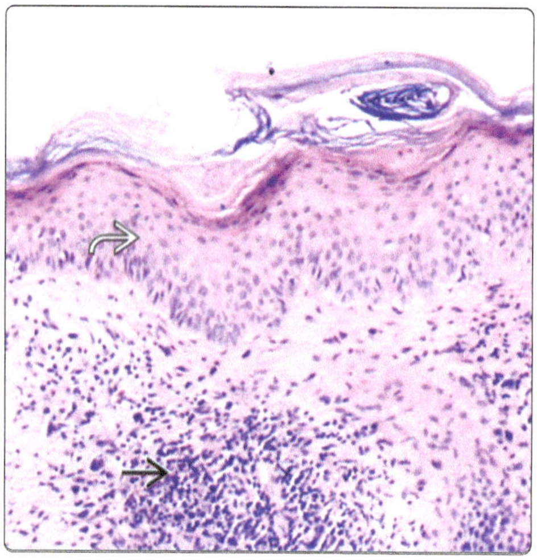

CD3 Immunohistochemistry in AITL

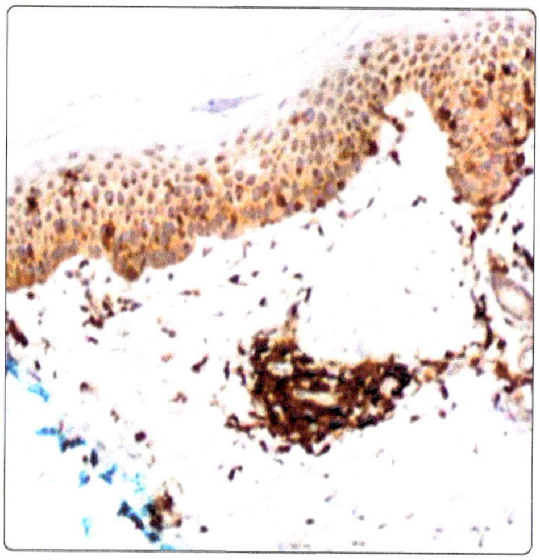

(Left) *The stain shows strong cytoplasmic expression in cutaneous AITL. The T cells are positive for CD4 but negative for CD8 (not shown).* **(Right)** *CXCL13 is typically positive in cutaneous AITL. This CXCL13 immunostain shows that the T cells are strongly immunoreactive. Cutaneous lesions in patients with AITL are often positive for CXCL13 but may be negative for CD10 (not shown).*

CD4 Immunohistochemistry in AITL

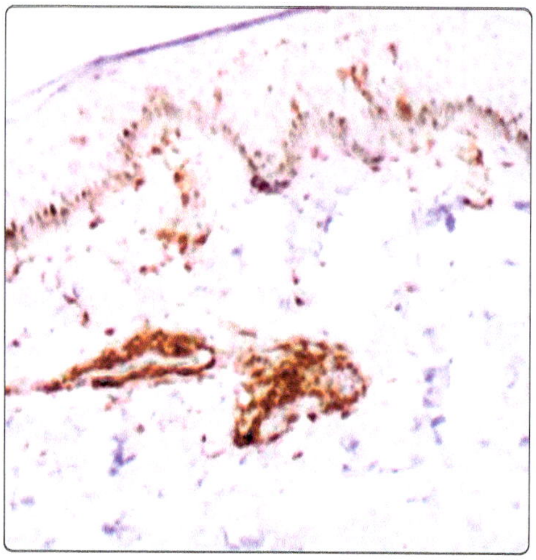

CXCL13 Immunohistochemistry in AITL

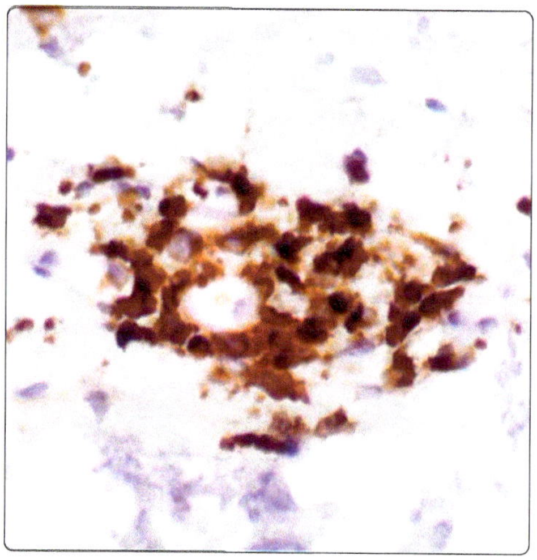

AITL in Lymph Node

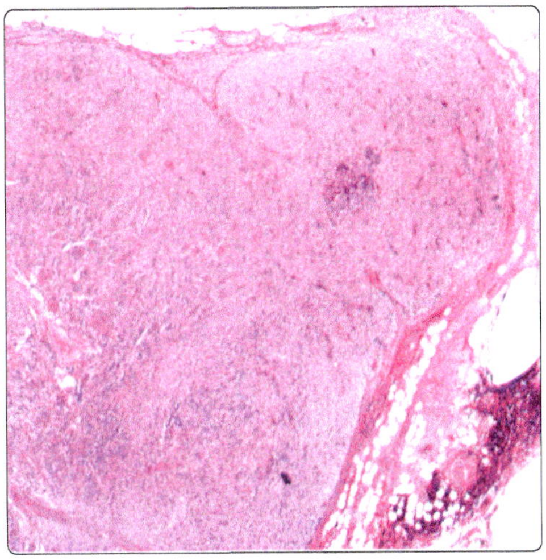

AITL in Lymph Node

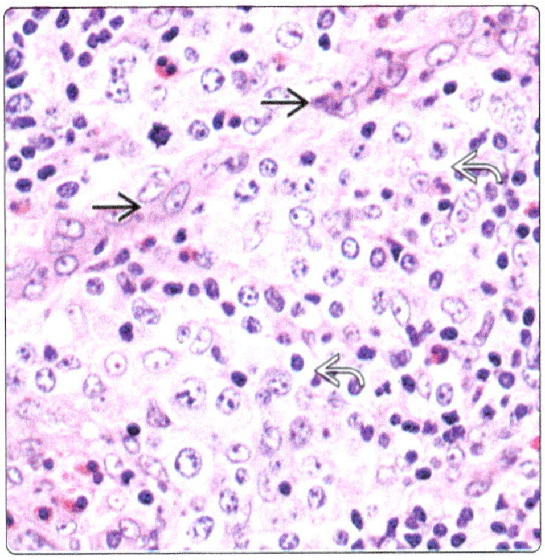

(Left) *This lymph node is involved with AITL. At low power, the architecture is effaced by the tumor. Sometimes residual follicles, open subcapsular sinuses, and a paracortical tumor distribution are seen.* **(Right)** *At high-power magnification, there are increased high endothelial venules ➔ surrounded by neoplastic cells with clear-staining cytoplasm ➔.*

Inflammatory Cells in AITL

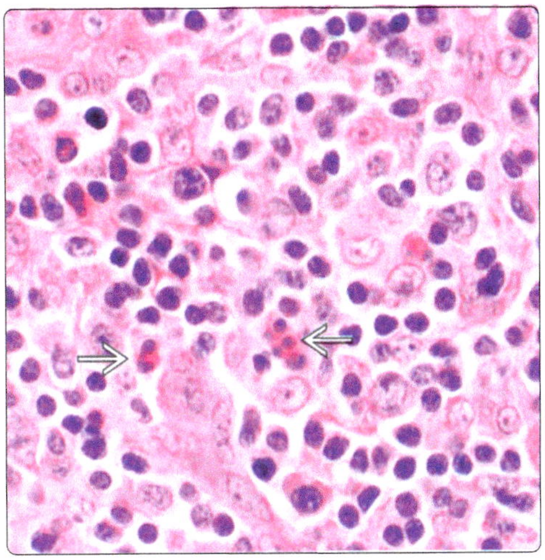

Bone Marrow With AITL

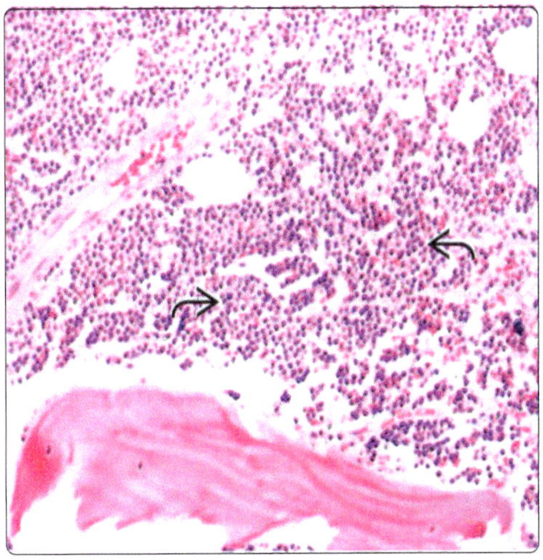

(Left) *In AITL, the tumor cells are often accompanied by a mixed inflammatory infiltrate. In this image, there are scattered eosinophils ➔.* **(Right)** *Bone marrow involvement in AITL often presents as a nodular infiltrate, either paratrabecular or nonparatrabecular. In the bone marrow, collections of tumor cells ➔, as well as small lymphocytes, eosinophils, and histiocytes, are present.*

DLBCL in Association With AITL

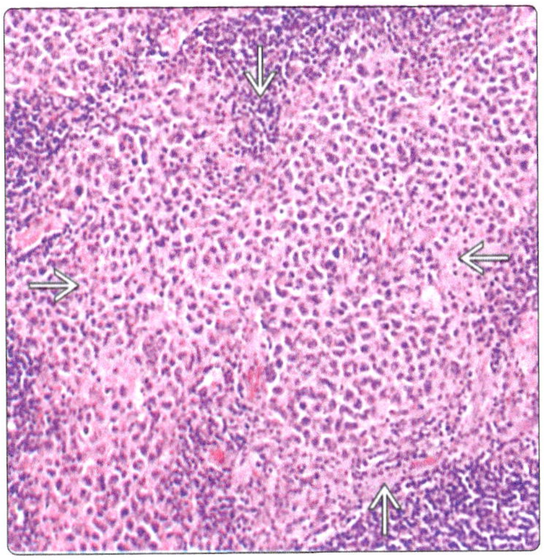

CD20 Immunohistochemistry in DLBCL

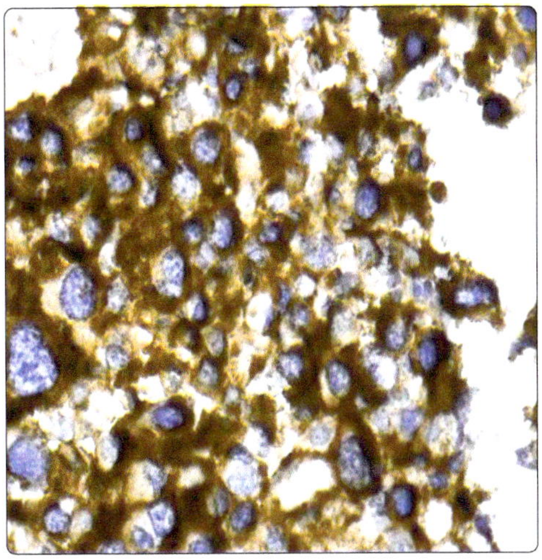

(Left) *Histologic examination shows diffuse large B-cell lymphoma (DLBCL) in a patient with AITL. Patients with AITL can also develop B-cell lymphomas, which are thought to arise from B-cell immunoblasts in the AITL. In this image, the lymph node shows a nodular collection of large, atypical B cells ➔.* **(Right)** *In this case of DLBCL in a patient with AITL, CD20 strongly highlights the large, atypical B cells of the DLBCL.*

(Left) *High magnification of a lymph node involved by AITL shows that there are arborizing high endothelial venules → amidst medium-sized neoplastic clear cells ↪.* **(Right)** *PD1 is strongly positive in this case of AITL. PD1 is 1 of the antigens found in follicular helper T cells that is expressed in AITL. (Courtesy S. Wang, MD.)*

AITL in Lymph Node

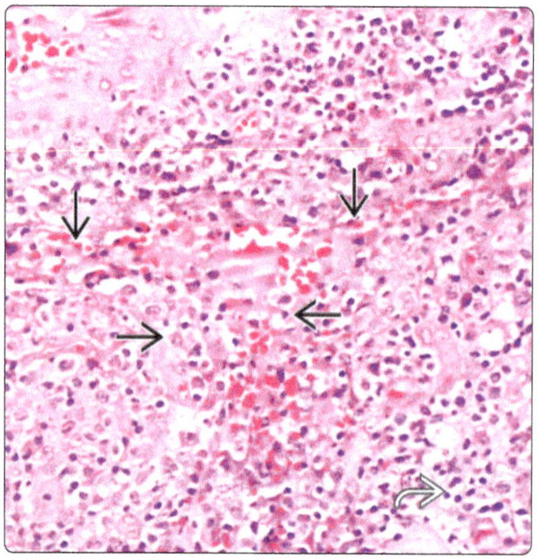

PD1 Immunohistochemistry in AITL

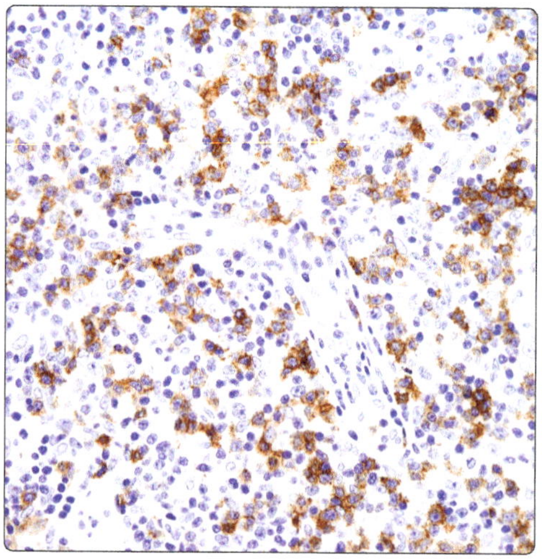

(Left) *At high magnification, this CD3 immunostain is positive in the tumor cells of AITL. AITL often expresses multiple T-cell antigens but may aberrantly lose more T-cell markers.* **(Right)** *This CD10 immunostain is coexpressed on the same T cells as in the previous CD3 image. Positive CD10 and CD3 cells are commonly seen in AITL.*

CD3 Immunohistochemistry in AITL

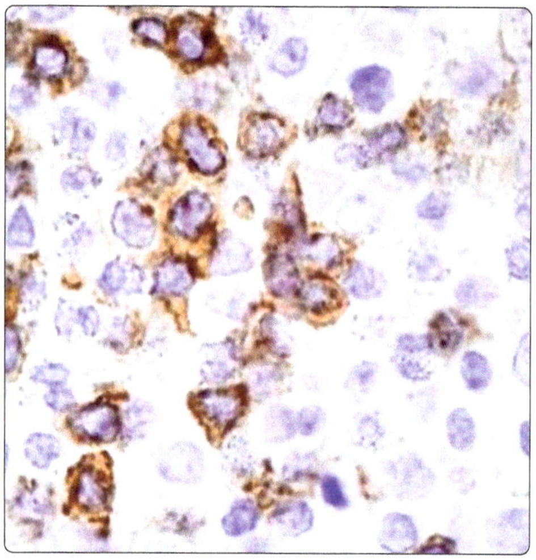

CD10 Immunohistochemistry in AITL

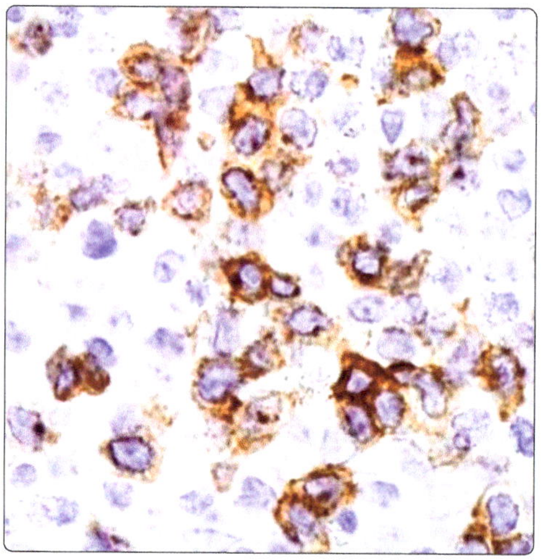

(Left) *This EBER stain by in situ hybridization is positive → in scattered cells in this case of AITL. Approximately 80-90% of lymph nodes with AITL show positive EBER cells, but skin lesions are often negative.* **(Right)** *This CD21 stain marks the follicular dendritic cells →, which surround blood vessels in AITL ↪. Lymph nodes with AITL typically show expanded and disrupted follicular dendritic cells.*

EBER In Situ Hybridization in AITL

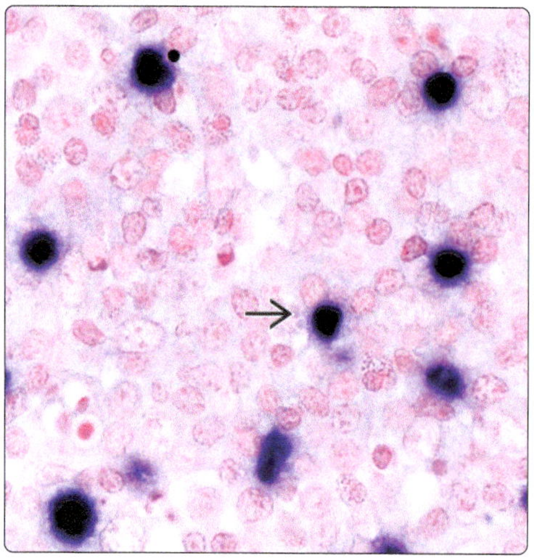

CD21 Immunohistochemistry in AITL

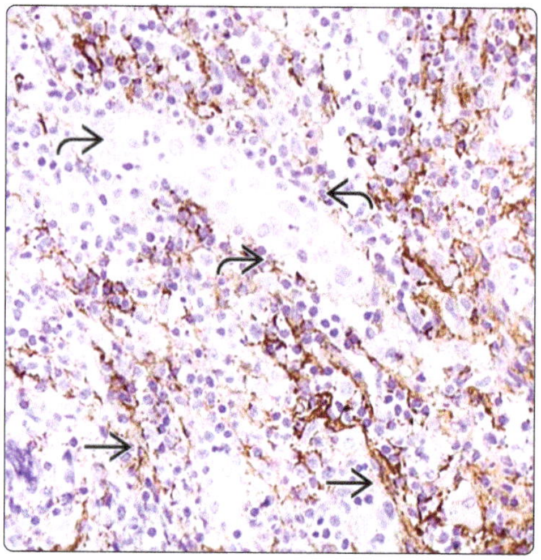

DDx: Drug Reaction

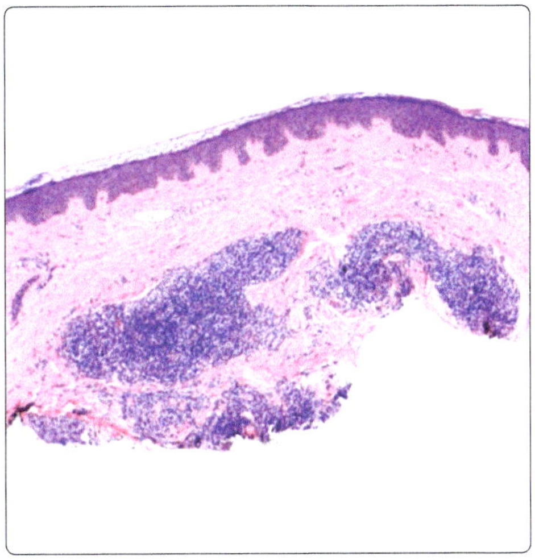

DDx: Small Medium Pleomorphic T-Cell Lymphoma

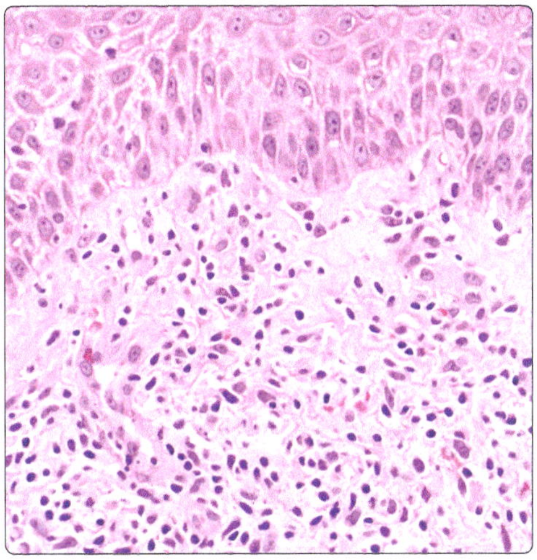

(Left) *In this drug reaction from a patient on chlorambucil, there is a prominent angiocentric T-cell infiltrate. Angiocentric dermal infiltrates are also commonly seen in AITL. To differentiate between these diagnoses, an appropriate clinical history is required.* **(Right)** *This primary cutaneous small medium pleomorphic CD4(+) T-cell lymphoma (SMPTCL) has a superficial perivascular T-cell infiltrate like AITL. However, in SMPTCL, the T cells are negative for CD10 and EBER.*

DDx: Peripheral T-Cell Lymphoma, Not Otherwise Specified

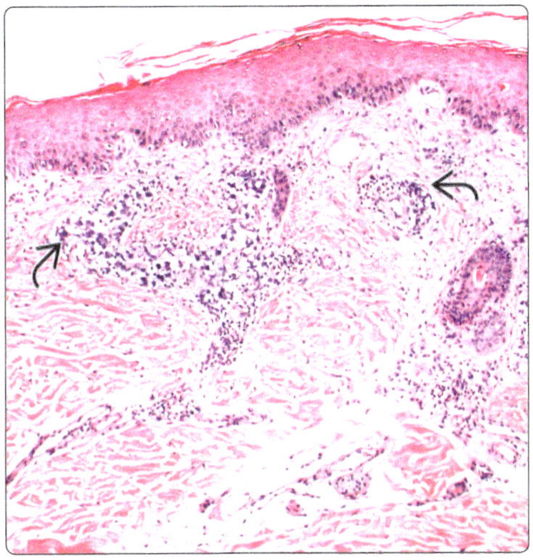

DDx: Hodgkin Lymphoma

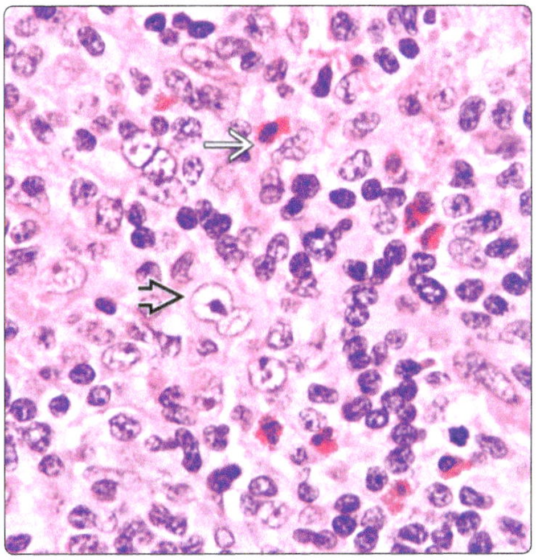

(Left) *Peripheral T-cell lymphoma, not otherwise specified (PTCL-NOS) shows an atypical T-cell infiltrate* ⇨ *surrounding the superficial blood vessels and adnexal structures. PTCL-NOS is often in the differential diagnosis of AITL.* **(Right)** *Hodgkin lymphoma (HL) can look like AITL with large atypical cells* ⇨ *and mixed inflammation* ➔*, but the large atypical cells in HL are CD45(-), CD30(+), and CD15(+). (Courtesy S. Wang, MD.)*

DDx: T-Cell/Histiocyte-Rich Large B-Cell Lymphoma

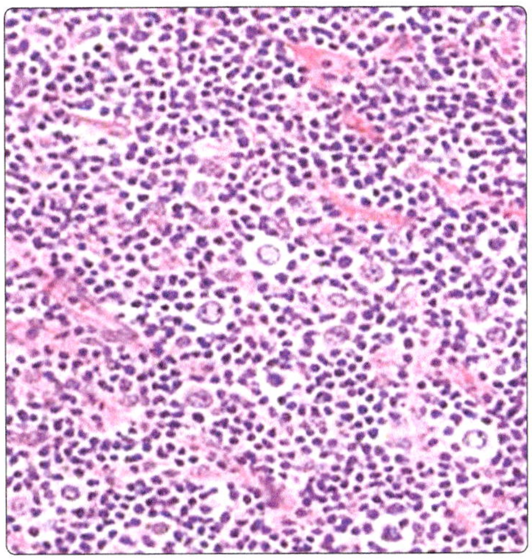

DDx: CD20 Immunohistochemistry in TCRLBCL

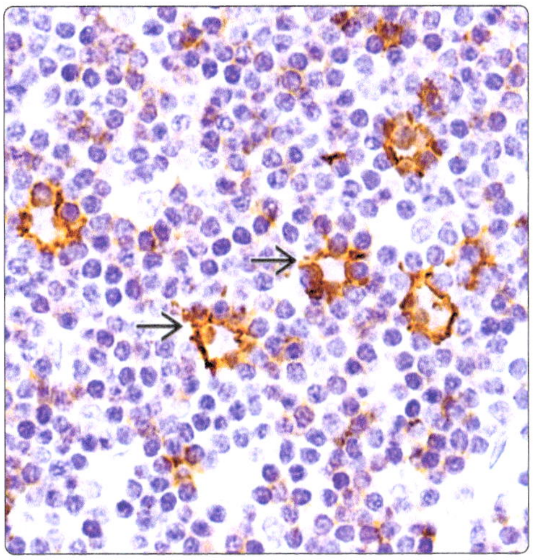

(Left) *T-cell/histiocyte-rich large B-cell lymphoma (TCRLBCL) can look similar to AITL. In this case of TCRLBCL, there are scattered large neoplastic cells in a background of small lymphocytes and histiocytes.* **(Right)** *CD20 highlights the large neoplastic B cells* ⇨ *in TCRLBCL. In AITL, the atypical cells would be negative for CD20 and positive for CD3. The large B cells are usually negative for EBV, unlike many cases of AITL.*

Systemic T-Cell and NK-Cell Lymphomas Involving Skin

KEY FACTS

TERMINOLOGY

- Systemic T-cell or NK-cell lymphoma that has spread to skin
- Morphology of primary and secondary skin lymphomas are similar

ETIOLOGY/PATHOGENESIS

- Epstein-Barr virus infection in some lymphomas

CLINICAL ISSUES

- Often multiple lesions, less often single lesion
- Most commonly in adults
- Usually much worse prognosis than primary cutaneous lymphoma
- Frequently aggressive chemotherapy, contrary to many primary cutaneous T-cell lymphomas, which are treated with more conservative therapy

MICROSCOPIC

- Variably sized T cells with increased clear cytoplasm, often with eosinophils
- Immunohistochemistry and flow cytometry typically show loss of at least 1 T-cell antigen
- *TCR-β* and *TCR-γ* gene rearrangement

TOP DIFFERENTIAL DIAGNOSES

- Peripheral T-cell lymphoma, unspecified, includes any T-cell lymphomas that do not fit into better defined subtype of T-cell lymphoma
- Systemic ALK(+) anaplastic large cell lymphoma: Often large atypical tumor cells in dermis, sometimes hallmark cells with multiple (horseshoe-shaped nuclei)
- Angioimmunoblastic T-cell lymphoma presents as superficial perivascular T-cell infiltrates with increased reactive inflammatory cells and high endothelial venules

Systemic Anaplastic Large Cell Lymphoma Involving Skin

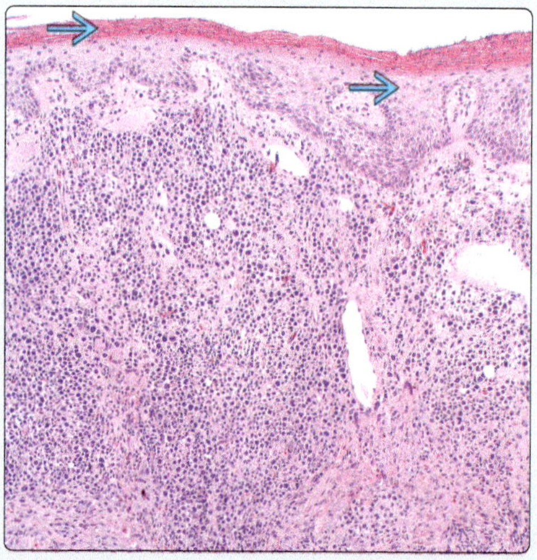

Systemic Anaplastic Large Cell Lymphoma Involving Skin

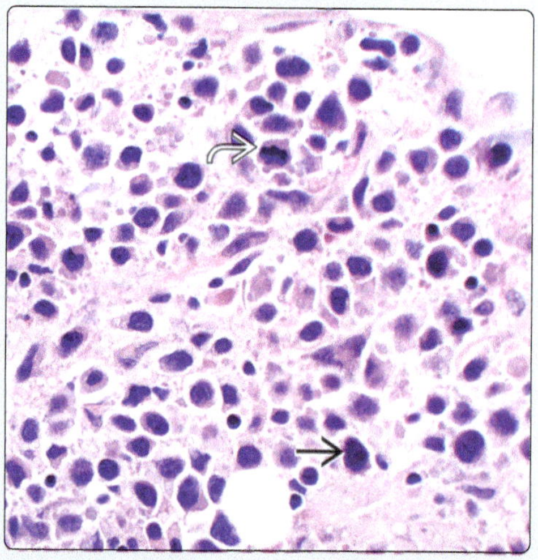

(Left) *At low magnification, the lymphoid infiltrate diffusely fills the superficial and deep dermis. The epidermis is not involved.* **(Right)** *At higher power, the tumor cells in systemic anaplastic large cell lymphoma (ALCL) are large and pleomorphic appearing with irregular nuclear contours, vesicular chromatin, and indistinct nucleoli. Mitotic figures are seen.*

PCR of T-Cell Receptor Gamma

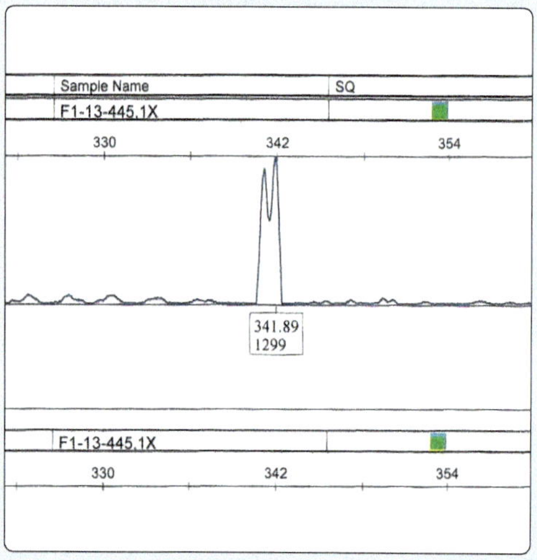

In Situ Hybridization for EBER

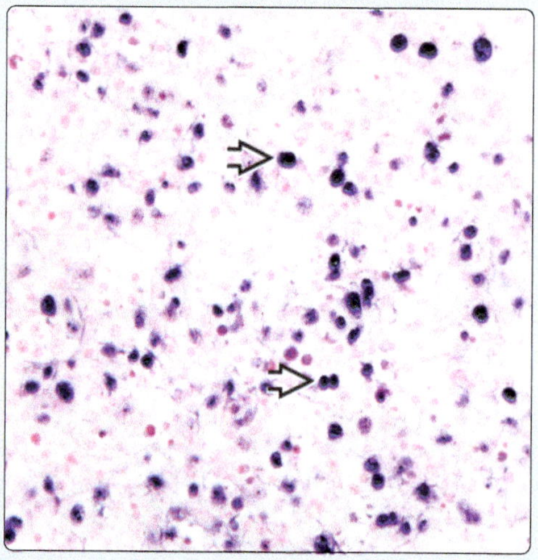

(Left) *A dominant monoclonal peak was seen on PCR testing for T-cell receptor gamma at position 341, which indicates that this is a monoclonal T-cell process. T-cell monoclonality is typically seen in all of the systemic T-cell lymphomas and is tested for either TRB or TRG.* **(Right)** *In situ hybridization for EBER is often useful in separating out some kinds of systemic T-cell lymphomas from others. Angioimmunoblastic T-cell lymphoma and peripheral T-cell lymphoma (PTCL), NOS can both be EBER(+), but ALCL is always EBER(-).*

TERMINOLOGY

Abbreviations

- Systemic T-cell lymphoma involving skin

Synonyms

- Secondary cutaneous T-cell lymphoma

Definitions

- T-cell or NK-cell lymphoma that has spread to skin as secondary site of disease
  - Lymphoma originates systemically but involves skin
  - Morphology of primary and secondary skin lymphomas are similar
    - Clinical behavior and treatment of each is divergent

ETIOLOGY/PATHOGENESIS

Depends on Type of NK-/T-Cell Lymphoma

- Can be therapy related
- Epstein-Barr virus infection in some lymphomas
  - Including angioimmunoblastic T-cell lymphoma (AITL) and extranodal NK-/T-cell lymphoma, nasal type

CLINICAL ISSUES

Epidemiology

- Incidence
  - Secondary cutaneous lymphomas make up 50% of all cutaneous lymphomas, excluding mycosis fungoides
  - Secondary T-cell lymphoma in skin is less common than systemic B-cell lymphoma in skin
  - Types of systemic T-cell and NK-cell lymphomas commonly associated with secondary cutaneous involvement
    - Peripheral T-cell lymphoma, not otherwise specified (PTCL, NOS) (20-30% with cutaneous lesions)
    - AITL (~ 50% with cutaneous lesions)
    - Extranodal NK-/T-cell lymphoma, nasal type (8-20% with cutaneous lesions)
    - Anaplastic large cell lymphoma (ALCL)
- Age
  - Any age but mostly adults
    - Systemic ALCL displays bimodal distribution that includes children, whereas primary cutaneous ALCL is primarily found in adults
- Sex
  - Occurs in both males and females

Presentation

- Often multiple lesions, less often single lesions
  - Usually tumors or nodules
  - Any cutaneous site, no site of predilection
  - Skin involvement may present at time of initial diagnosis or develop later

Treatment

- Usually adjuvant therapy
  - Frequently aggressive chemotherapy, contrary to many primary cutaneous T-cell lymphomas, which are treated with more conservative therapy

Prognosis

- Depends on type of T-cell lymphoma but usually poor prognosis
  - Higher stage than primary cutaneous lymphoma
  - Usually much worse prognosis than primary cutaneous lymphoma
- ALK(-) ALCL has worse prognosis than primary cutaneous ALCL or systemic ALK(+) ALCL

MICROSCOPIC

Histologic Features

- Morphology and immunophenotype sometimes identical to systemic disease
- **PTCL, NOS**
  - All T-cell lymphomas that do not fit into better defined subtype of T-cell lymphoma
    - Other types of T-cell lymphoma must 1st be excluded
  - Wide variety of morphologic appearances
  - Usually atypical nodular or diffuse dermal T-cell infiltrate sparing epidermis, which may extend to subcutis
    - Medium to large T cells, often with markedly pleomorphic nuclei
    - Sometimes immunoblastic T cells or Reed-Sternberg-like T cells
  - Background reactive infiltrate, including small lymphocytes, plasma cells, and eosinophils
  - Variable degrees of vascular proliferation
  - Can be confused with infection, granuloma annulare, lupus or dermatomyositis, panniculitis, and vasculitis
  - Variants include lymphoepithelioid (Lennert lymphoma), follicular, and T zone
- **Systemic ALK(+) ALCL**
  - 30% involve skin
  - Often large atypical tumor cells in dermis, sometimes hallmark cells with multiple (horseshoe-shaped) nuclei
  - Usually no epidermotropism
  - Can involve lymphatic spaces
- **Systemic ALK(-) ALCL**
  - Same histology as systemic ALK(+) ALCL but considered different disease from primary cutaneous ALCL
  - Strong and uniform expression of CD30 but lacking ALK expression
  - Poorer prognosis than ALK(+) ALCL
  - Can be bcl-2(+) unlike ALK(+) ALCL
- **AITL**
  - Superficial perivascular infiltrates with lymphocytes, eosinophils, often plasma cells and histiocytes
  - Less often, may show more sheet-like, destructive dermal T-cell infiltrates
  - Increased numbers of high endothelial venules
  - Hyperplasia of follicular dendritic cells
- **Extranodal NK-/T-cell lymphoma, nasal type**
  - Cytotoxic lymphocytes with prominent cytoplasmic azurophilic granules
    - Tumor cells are angiocentric and angiodestructive
  - Dense dermal infiltrate
    - ~ 30% of cases show rare foci of epidermotropism
  - Perivascular/periadnexal
  - Medium/large irregular cells, sometimes with blastic chromatin

- Coagulative necrosis in most cases

Cytologic Features

- Depend on subtype of systemic T-cell or NK-cell lymphoma

ANCILLARY TESTS

Immunohistochemistry

- **PTCL, NOS**
  - Expresses some T-cell antigens but may lack 1 or more T-cell antigens
  - Usually CD4(+)/CD8(-)
    - Rarely CD8(+)/CD4(-), CD4(+)/CD8(+), or CD4(-)/CD8(-)
  - CD30 (+/-), CXCL13(-), PD-1(-), CD10(-), Bcl-6(-)
  - Usually cytotoxic antigens (-)
  - EBER is only rarely positive
- **Systemic ALK(+) ALCL**
  - CD30(+), usually CD4(+)
  - ALK and EMA (+) by IHC, whereas primary cutaneous ALCL is almost always ALK and EMA (-)
    - ALK(+) in skin lymphoma should warrant clinical evaluation for extracutaneous ALCL
    - Lack of ALK in skin lymphoma is not definite evidence for primary cutaneous ALCL, however
  - Clusterin expression may be seen in noncutaneous ALCL (not confirmed in later studies)
  - Cutaneous lymphocyte antigen and HOXC5(-) in systemic ALCL but HOXC5(+) in primary cutaneous ALCL
- AITL
  - T-cell antigen (+) (CD2, CD3, CD5, CD7)
    - Can lose 1 or more T-cell antigens
    - CD7 most commonly lost
  - Helper T cells
    - Usually CD4(+)/CD8(-)/TCR-βF1(+)
  - Follicular helper T-cell phenotype
    - CD10(-/+), Bcl-6(+), CXCL13(+), CCR5(+), SAP(+), ICOS(+), PD-1(+)
    - Often CD10(-) in cutaneous AITL
    - Usually CXCL13(+) in cutaneous AITL
  - Follicular dendritic T-cell meshworks
    - Usually CD21, CD23, CD35, and clusterin (+)
  - ↑ reactive B cells
    - Express B-cell markers (CD20, CD79, pax-5)
  - Often EBER(+) in lymph nodes but EBER(-) in skin
- **Extranodal NK-/T-cell lymphoma, nasal type**
  - T-cell antigens (+) (CD2, CD3, CD7)
  - CD56(+)
  - Cytotoxic markers (+): TIA1, granzyme B, granzyme M, perforin
  - EBER(+) and LMP(+)
  - CXCL13, OCT2, and IRF4 more common in NK-cell origin; PD-1 more common in T-cell origin

Molecular Tests

- *TCR* gene rearrangements are seen in all T-cell lymphomas
- Systemic ALCL
  - Translocations involving *ALK* are common t(2;5), unlike primary cutaneous ALCL
  - Subsets of ALK(-) ALCL
    - *DUSP22* translocation: Survival rate similar to ALK(+) ALCL
    - *TP63* translocation: Rare, aggressive progression
- *IRF4* translocations are found in primary cutaneous ALCL but not in systemic ALCL or lymphomatoid papulosis
- G17V *RHOA* mutation may be driving molecular event for AITL and can be seen in some PTCL, NOS
  - Frequent mutations in *TET2*, *IDH2*, *DNMT3A*, and *RHOA* genes in AITL

DIFFERENTIAL DIAGNOSIS

Primary Cutaneous T-Cell Lymphomas

- May show overlapping features
- Often have to prove there is no extracutaneous lymphoma by clinical and imaging studies

B-Cell Lymphomas

- Express B-cell antigens and show *IGH* gene rearrangement

DIAGNOSTIC CHECKLIST

Pathologic Interpretation Pearls

- SCTLs have higher stage and worse prognosis than most primary cutaneous T-cell lymphomas
- SCTLs are treated more aggressively with chemotherapy than most primary cutaneous T-cell lymphomas

SELECTED REFERENCES

1. Hapgood G et al: The biology and management of systemic anaplastic large cell lymphoma. Blood. 126(1):17-25, 2015
2. Inghirami G et al: Peripheral T-cell and NK cell lymphoproliferative disorders: cell of origin, clinical and pathological implications. Immunol Rev. 263(1):124-59, 2015
3. Lee WJ et al: Secondary cutaneous lymphoma: comparative clinical features and survival outcome analysis of 106 cases according to lymphoma cell lineage. Br J Dermatol. 173(1):134-45, 2015
4. Kinney MC et al: Anaplastic large cell lymphoma: twenty-five years of discovery. Arch Pathol Lab Med. 135(1):19-43, 2011
5. Pan ST et al: Cutaneous peripheral T-cell lymphoma of cytotoxic phenotype mimicking extranodal NK/T-cell lymphoma. Am J Dermatopathol. 33(2):e17-20, 2011
6. Sánchez-Schmidt JM et al: Primary cutaneous CD30+ anaplastic large-cell lymphomas show a heterogeneous genomic profile: an oligonucleotide arrayCGH approach. J Invest Dermatol. 131(1):269-71, 2011
7. Wada DA et al: Specificity of IRF4 translocations for primary cutaneous anaplastic large cell lymphoma: a multicenter study of 204 skin biopsies. Mod Pathol. 24(4):596-605, 2011
8. Berti E et al: Cutaneous extranodal NK/T-cell lymphoma: a clinicopathologic study of 5 patients with array-based comparative genomic hybridization. Blood. 116(2):165-70, 2010
9. Liao JB et al: Clinicopathologic analysis of cutaneous lymphoma in taiwan: a high frequency of extranodal natural killer/t-cell lymphoma, nasal type, with an extremely poor prognosis. Arch Pathol Lab Med. 134(7):996-1002, 2010
10. Park S et al: Primary cutaneous Epstein-Barr virus-associated T-cell lymphoproliferative disorder-2 cases with unusual, prolonged clinical course. Am J Dermatopathol. 32(8):832-6, 2010
11. Querfeld C et al: Primary cutaneous and systemic anaplastic large cell lymphoma: clinicopathologic aspects and therapeutic options. Oncology (Williston Park). 24(7):574-87, 2010
12. Choi YL et al: Extranodal NK/T-cell lymphoma with cutaneous involvement: 'nasal' vs. 'nasal-type' subgroups--a retrospective study of 18 patients. Br J Dermatol. 160(2):333-7, 2009
13. Feldman AL et al: Recurrent translocations involving the IRF4 oncogene locus in peripheral T-cell lymphomas. Leukemia. 23(3):574-80, 2009
14. Schwartz EJ et al: Immunohistochemical characterization of nasal-type extranodal NK/T-cell lymphoma using a tissue microarray: an analysis of 84 cases. Am J Clin Pathol. 130(3):343-51, 2008

Systemic PTCL, NOS Involving Skin

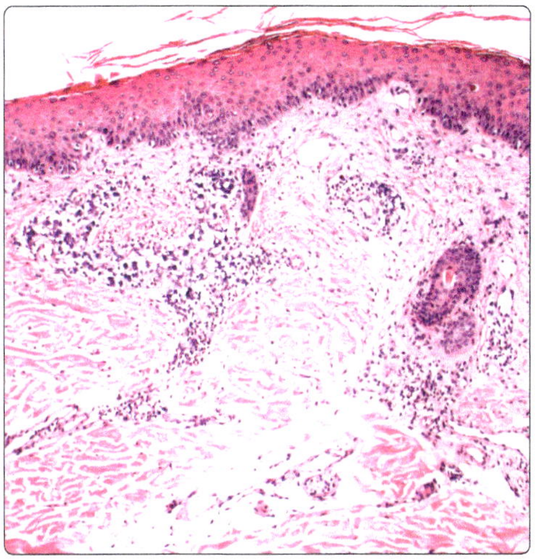

Systemic PTCL, NOS Involving Skin

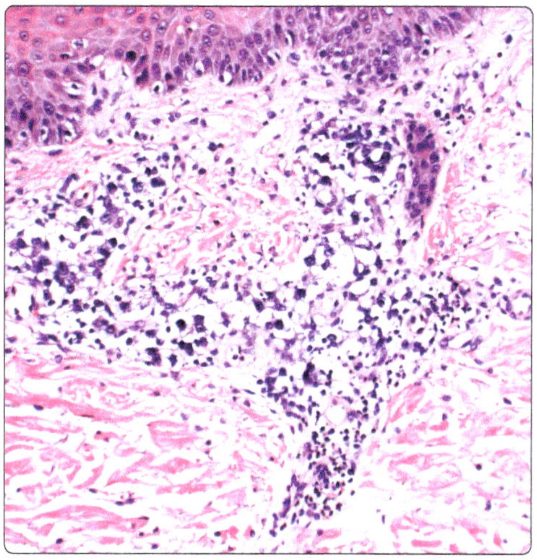

(Left) *Several years ago, the patient was diagnosed with PTCL of the cervical and inguinal lymph nodes and now presents with multiple tumor nodules on his thigh, which was diagnosed as PTCL, NOS.* **(Right)** *This PTCL, NOS presents as a superficial and deep, mostly perivascular lymphoid infiltrate.*

Systemic PTCL, NOS Involving Skin

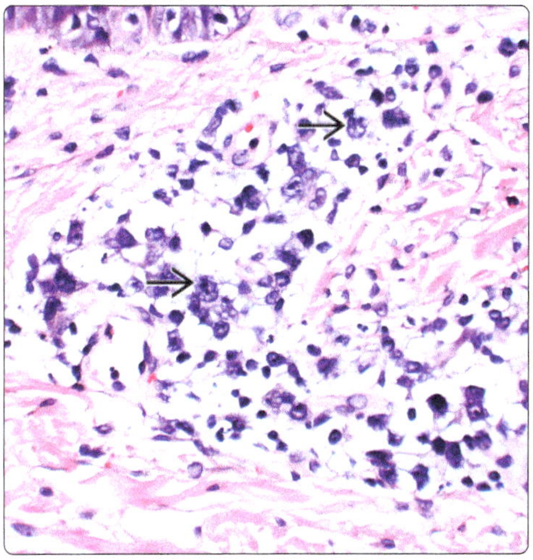

PTCL, NOS With CD3

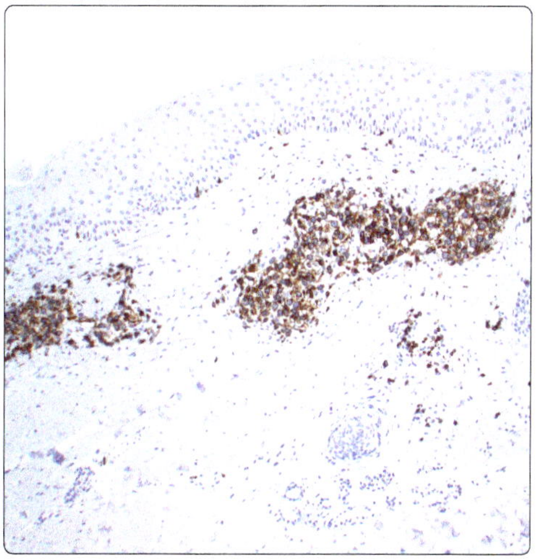

(Left) *On high magnification, the malignant T cells in PTCL, NOS range from medium to large in size. Some of the larger cells have coarse chromatin and enlarged nucleoli ⇒.* **(Right)** *CD3 immunohistochemical stain is strongly positive in this PTCL, NOS. PCR also showed TCR gamma gene rearrangement.*

PTCL, NOS With CD4

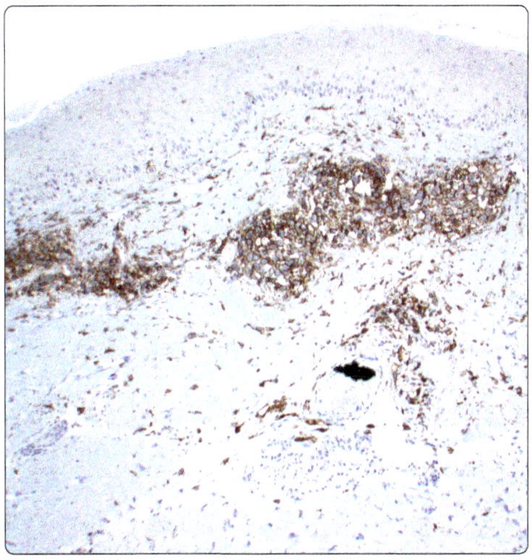

PTCL, NOS With CD30

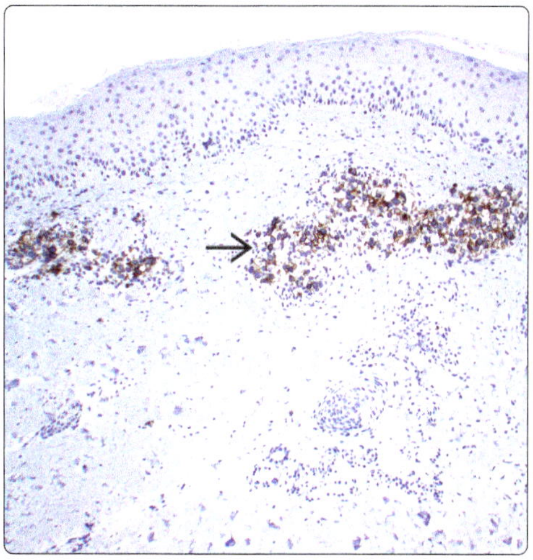

(Left) *CD4 immunohistochemical stain shows that the same CD3(+) T cells also strongly express CD4. CD8 (not shown) was negative.* **(Right)** *CD30 marker was positive ⇒ in this PTCL, NOS, even though it was negative in the original lymph node biopsies. Gain of CD30 expression can be seen in many cases and does not indicate that this is ALCL. No ALK translocations were identified in the lymph nodes or skin biopsies.*

Systemic Anaplastic Large Cell Lymphoma Involving Skin

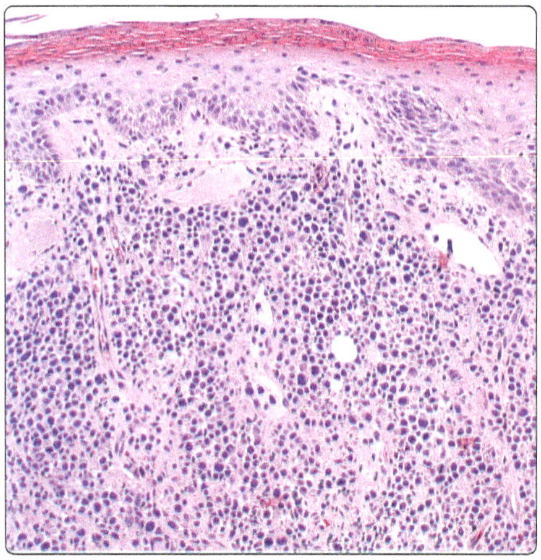

Anaplastic Large Cell Lymphoma Involving Lymphatic Spaces

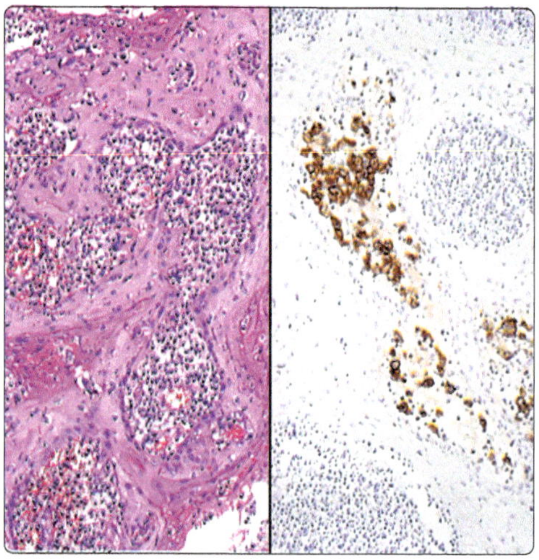

(Left) *Two years ago, the patient had been diagnosed with ALCL in the lymph nodes. There is a diffuse dermal lymphoid infiltrate of large, markedly atypical cells.* **(Right)** *The image on the right is a CD30 immunohistochemical stain, which marks the tumor cells with a lymphatic distribution. (Courtesy M. Tomaszewski, MD.)*

Anaplastic Large Cell Lymphoma, CD4(+)

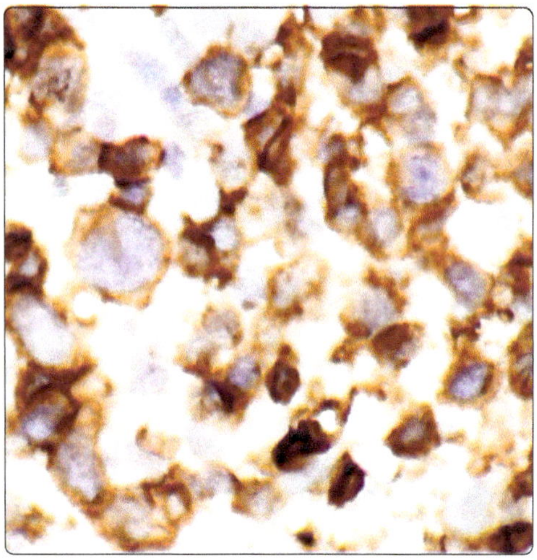

Anaplastic Large Cell Lymphoma, EMA(+)

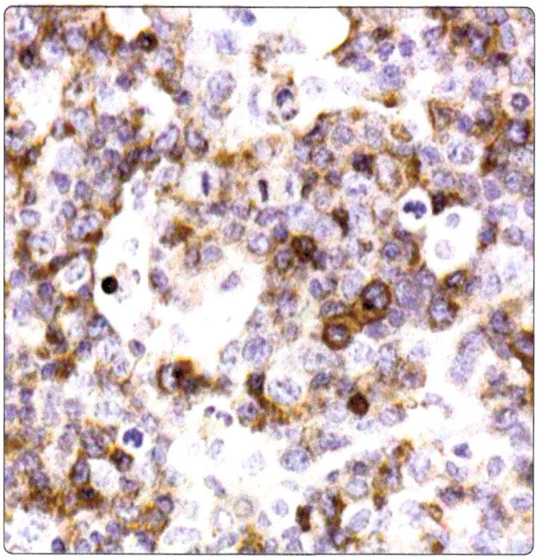

(Left) *This high-power image of a CD4 IHC stain shows that the tumor cells are strongly CD4(+). CD8 (not shown) was negative. Most cases of ALCL are CD4(+)/CD8(-), and only 5% are CD4(-)/CD8(+).* **(Right)** *This is an EMA(+) stain in a case of systemic ALCL with secondary involvement of the skin. Systemic cases are often EMA(+), whereas primary cutaneous ALCL is usually EMA(-).*

Systemic ALK(+) Anaplastic Large Cell Lymphoma Involving Skin

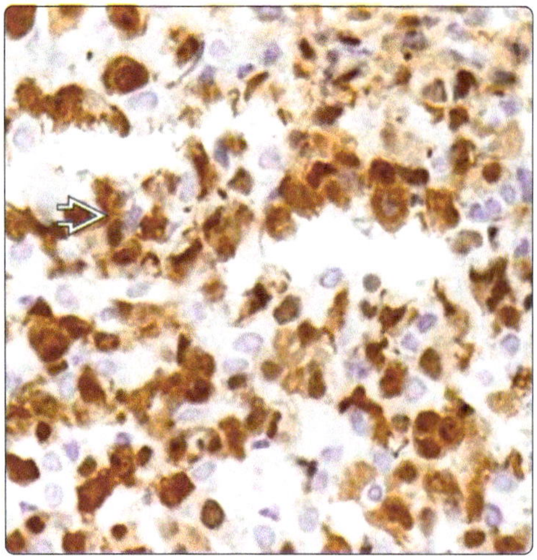

Translocation of ALK in Anaplastic Large Cell Lymphoma

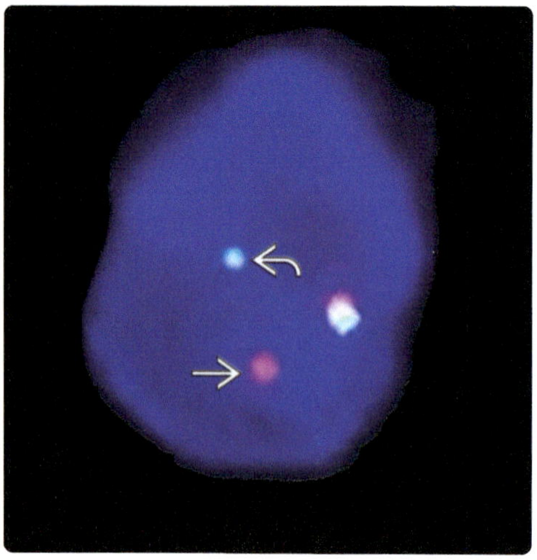

(Left) *This systemic ALCL with secondary cutaneous involvement strongly expresses ALK by immunostaining ⇨. Currently, systemic ALCL is either classified as ALK(+) or ALK(-), and these are considered different diseases.* **(Right)** *This is a break-apart probe FISH test for 2p23 (ALK). The blue signal ↶ represents the 5' region of ALK, and the pink signal → represents the 3' region of ALK. ALK rearrangements are usually seen in systemic ALCL but not primary cutaneous ALCL.*

Systemic Angioimmunoblastic T-Cell Lymphoma Involving Skin

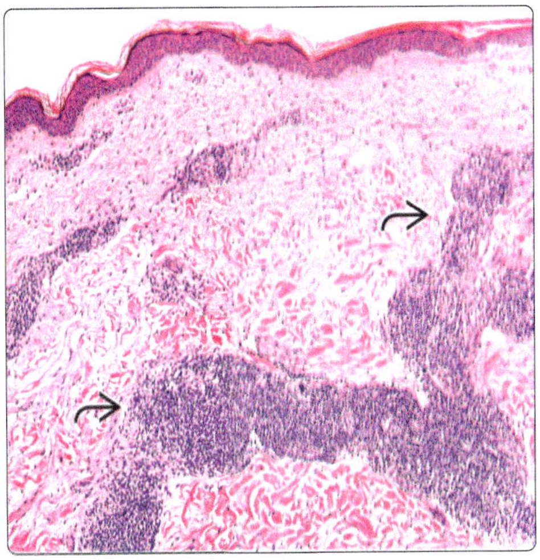

Systemic Angioimmunoblastic T-Cell Lymphoma Involving Skin

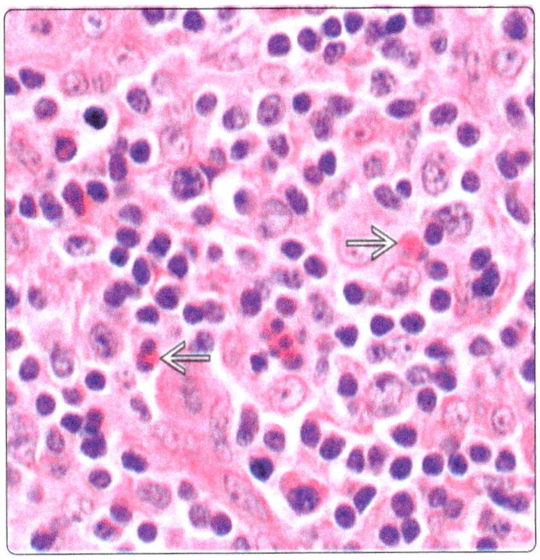

(Left) *Cutaneous involvement by angioimmunoblastic T-cell lymphoma (AITL) often shows a nonspecific dense dermal perivascular* ➡ *infiltrate at low magnification. (Courtesy S. Wang, MD.)* **(Right)** *In AITL, the tumor cells are often accompanied by a mixed inflammatory infiltrate. In this image, there are scattered eosinophils present* ➡.

Systemic Angioimmunoblastic T-Cell Lymphoma Involving Skin

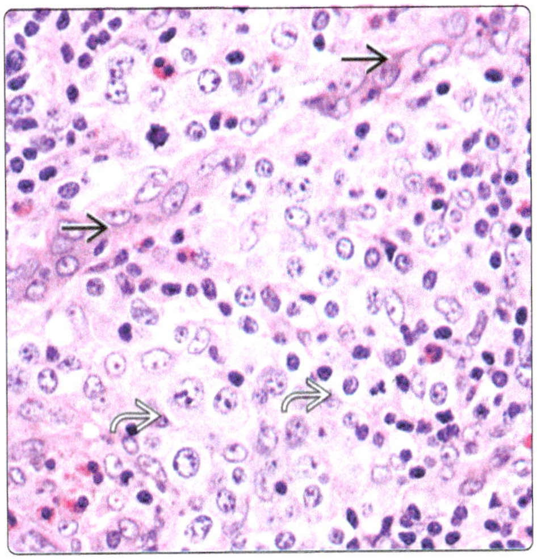

Angioimmunoblastic T-Cell Lymphoma, CD3(+)

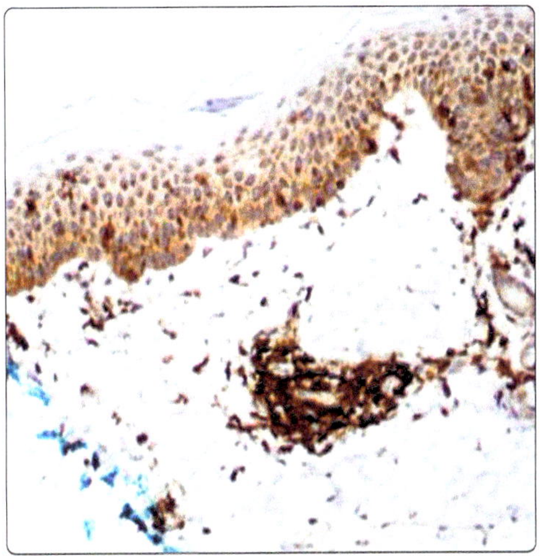

(Left) *At higher power, there are increased high endothelial venules* ➡ *surrounded by neoplastic cells with clear cytoplasm* ➡. **(Right)** *In this CD3 immunohistochemical stain, CD3 is strongly positive in the dermal T cells. CD20 only marked rare scattered B cells (not shown).*

Angioimmunoblastic T-Cell Lymphoma, CD4(+)

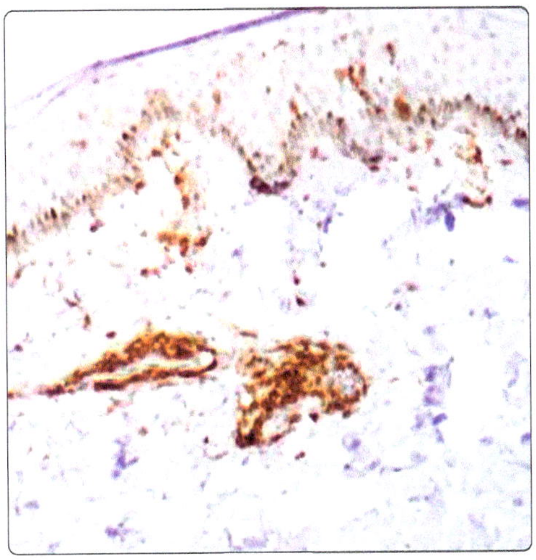

Angioimmunoblastic T-Cell Lymphoma, CXCL13(+)

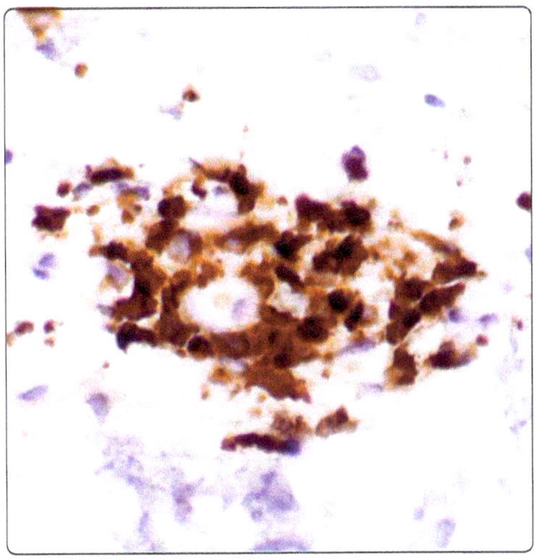

(Left) *This is a CD4(+) immunohistochemical stain showing strong cytoplasmic expression in cutaneous AITL. The T cells are CD4(+) but CD8(-) (not shown).* **(Right)** *CXCL13 is positive in cutaneous AITL. The T cells are strongly immunoreactive for CXCL13. Cutaneous lesions in patients with AITL are often CXCL13(+) but are often CD10(-) (not shown).*

Leukemia Cutis

KEY FACTS

TERMINOLOGY

- Clinically identifiable cutaneous lesions secondary to cutaneous infiltration by neoplastic leukocytes (myeloid or lymphoid)

CLINICAL ISSUES

- Presentation may precede [aleukemic leukemia cutis (LC)], coincide, or manifest as recurrence of leukemia
- Acute monocytic, myelomonocytic, and T-cell leukemias show highest incidence of LC
  - Occurs in 10-15% of patients with AML
  - Occurs in 20-70% of mature T-cell leukemias
  - Occurs in up to 25% of CLL/SLL cases
- Frequency higher among children than adults

MICROSCOPIC

- Perivascular, periadnexal, diffuse, and nodular infiltrates can be seen
- Stromal fibrosis often present
- Large cells with oval to convoluted nuclei, immature finely dispersed chromatin, occasional nucleoli (myeloid LC)
- Intermediate-sized round nuclei, immature dispersed chromatin, inconspicuous nucleoli, scant cytoplasm (LBL)

ANCILLARY TESTS

- Flow cytometry evaluation of suspected lesions can be helpful

TOP DIFFERENTIAL DIAGNOSES

- Inflammatory dermatoses
- Mature B-cell lymphomas
- Mature T-cell lymphomas
- Blastic plasmacytoid dendritic cell neoplasm

DIAGNOSTIC CHECKLIST

- Diagnosis requires careful histologic and immunohistochemical examination
- Correlation with clinical data, bone marrow, and peripheral blood findings also necessary

Clinical Presentation of Myeloid Sarcoma

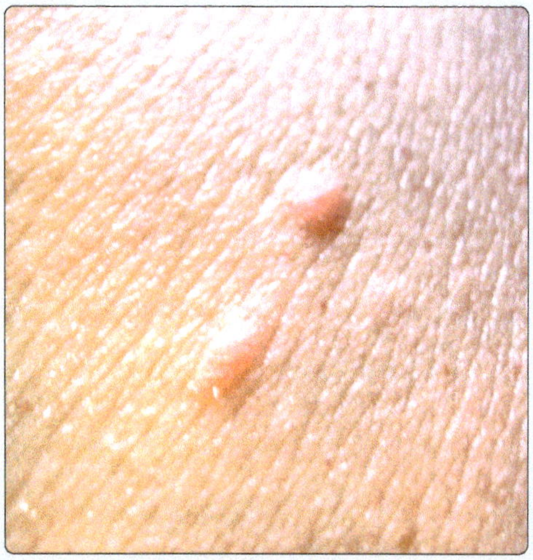

Clinical Presentation of Acute Myeloid Leukemia/Myeloid Sarcoma

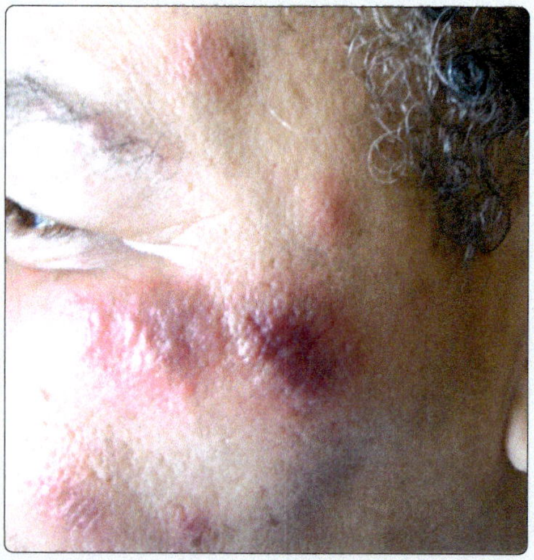

(Left) *Clinical image shows 2 small papules in a patient with acute myeloid leukemia (AML). Histologic examination confirmed leukemic infiltrates consistent with myeloid sarcoma (MS). (Courtesy V. Tonkovic-Capin, MD.)* **(Right)** *Clinical photograph shows an adult male with a known history of AML who later presented with multiple violaceous plaques on the left side of the face. Histologic examination revealed findings of MS consistent with recurrent AML. (Courtesy M. Jackson, MD.)*

Leukemia Cutis at Low Magnification

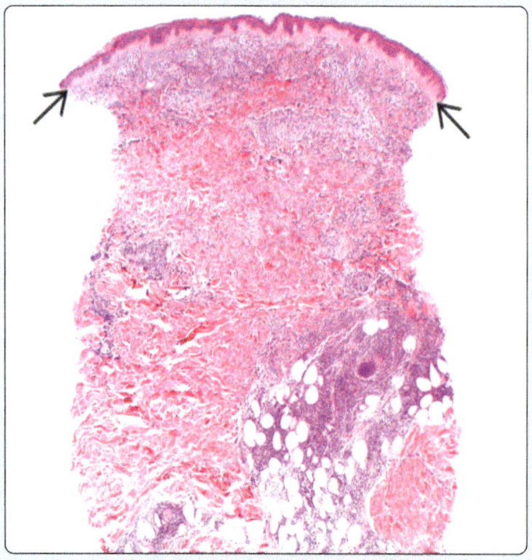

Higher Magnification of Myeloid Sarcoma

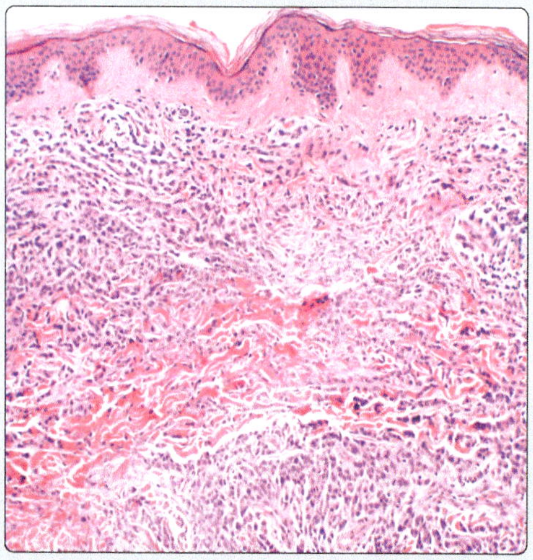

(Left) *A punch biopsy shows leukemic infiltrates in the superficial and deep dermis, extending into the subcutaneous adipose tissue. Sparing of the epidermis with a thin grenz zone ⇒ is noted.* **(Right)** *Diffuse dermal cellular infiltrates composed of large pleomorphic cells with sparing of the epidermis are shown in this example of cutaneous MS. This finding represents the initial manifestation of recurrent AML.*

TERMINOLOGY

Abbreviations

- Leukemia cutis (LC)

Synonyms

- Myeloid sarcoma (MS), granulocytic sarcoma, extramedullary myeloid cell tumor, chloroma
  - When composed of myeloid cells
- Monoblastic sarcoma
  - When composed of monocytic precursors

Definitions

- Clinically identifiable cutaneous lesions secondary to cutaneous infiltration by neoplastic leukocytes (myeloid or lymphoid)

ETIOLOGY/PATHOGENESIS

Mechanisms of Skin Homing

- Underlying process has not been defined
  - May involve coexpression of CLA and its interaction with specific chemokines
- Predilection for sites with cutaneous inflammation (e.g., tumors, Sweet syndrome, psoriasis)

CLINICAL ISSUES

Epidemiology

- Incidence
  - Acute monocytic, myelomonocytic, and T-cell leukemias show highest incidence of LC
  - LC can be observed in all forms of acute myeloid leukemia (AML)
  - Occurs in 10-15% of patients with AML
    - Varies widely with AML subtype
    - Up to 50% of patients with acute myelomonocytic and monocytic types
  - Is seen in up to 25% of chronic lymphocytic leukemia/small lymphocytic lymphoma (CLL/SLL) cases
  - Occurs in 20-70% of mature T-cell leukemias
    - 40-70% of adult T-cell leukemia/lymphoma (ATLL)
    - 25-30% of T-cell prolymphocytic leukemia (T-PLL)
  - Unusual in patients with precursor B- or T-cell lymphoblastic leukemia/lymphomas (LBL) and plasma cell leukemia
  - Occurs in 25-30% of infants with congenital leukemia
- Age
  - Frequency higher among children than adults

Site

- Most commonly involves extremities (legs > arms)
- Back, chest, scalp, and face may also be involved
- Preferential involvement at sites of previous or concomitant inflammation
  - Sweet syndrome, herpes zoster, insect bites, psoriasis

Presentation

- Presentation may precede (aleukemic LC), coincide with, or manifest as recurrence of acute leukemia
  - Most cases present after diagnosis of systemic leukemia
  - < 10% present prior to blood or bone marrow involvement (aleukemic LC or primary extramedullary leukemia)
- Single or multiple skin lesions
  - Violaceous, red-brown, or hemorrhagic papules, nodules, and plaques of varying sizes
  - Erythematous papules and nodules most commonly reported
  - Blueberry muffin appearance
    - Firm blue, red, or purple nodules in generalized distribution
    - Term historically used to describe cutaneous involvement in children with congenital leukemia
- Oral petechiae
- Thickening of gums
  - Oral lesions more common in adults
- Other sites of extramedullary involvement are frequent (e.g., meninges)

Laboratory Tests

- Lactate dehydrogenase and β2-microglobulin
  - Higher levels reported in patients with LC
- Serology for HTLV-1 in cases of ATLL

Treatment

- Options, risks, complications
  - Managed by treating underlying leukemia
    - Systemic chemotherapy
    - Bone marrow transplantation
  - Local therapy (e.g., radiation)

Prognosis

- Poor prognosis
  - Generally manifestation of disease progression
- LC in context of congenital myelogenous leukemia is exception
  - Not associated with worse prognosis
  - Spontaneous regression of LC without treatment has been observed
- Prognosis in CLL patients is good
  - Exception of blastic transformation (Richter syndrome)

MICROSCOPIC

General Histologic Features

- Low-power patterns of involvement
  - Perivascular &/or periadnexal
  - Dense, diffuse, and nodular
  - Subtle superficial interstitial infiltrate (rare)
- Stromal fibrosis often seen
- Lineage determination unreliable by histology alone

Myeloid and Monoblastic Sarcoma

- Perivascular, periadnexal, diffuse, and nodular infiltrates can be seen
- Epidermotropism is very rare
- Myeloid blasts and granulocytic precursors predominate
  - Large cells with oval to convoluted nuclei, immature finely dispersed chromatin, occasional nucleoli
  - Nuclei may appear more cleaved/convoluted and cytoplasm more abundant with monocytic differentiation

- Mitotic figures and apoptotic cells

Precursor B- or T-Cell Lymphoblastic Leukemia/Lymphomas

- Deep-seated infiltrates
  - Perivascular &/or diffuse
- Cells typically appear monomorphous
  - Intermediate-sized round nuclei, immature dispersed chromatin, inconspicuous nucleoli, scant cytoplasm
- Cytomorphologic features of B- and T-LBL are nearly identical
- Lack epidermotropism
- Frequent mitotic figures and apoptotic bodies
  - Starry-sky pattern may be present
- Stromal fibrosis

Mature B-Cell Lymphoproliferative Neoplasms

- Most commonly, CLL/SLL
  - Patterns of involvement
    - Perivascular and periadnexal
    - Nodular and diffuse
    - Band-like
    - Pseudoproliferation centers may be visible in large lesions
  - Monotonous population of small lymphoid cells
    - Round nuclei
    - Mature heterogeneous chromatin
  - Lesions may occur at sites previously involved by inflammatory &/or infectious agents or epithelial malignancies

Mature T-Cell Lymphoproliferative Neoplasms

- **ATLL**
  - Superficial band-like infiltrate with prominent epidermotropism and Pautrier-like microabscesses
  - Often resembles mycosis fungoides (MF)
  - Perivascular infiltrates ± angioinvasion
  - Heterogeneous infiltrates
    - Small, intermediate, large, and pleomorphic T cells
- **T-PLL**
  - Perivascular &/or periadnexal infiltrate
  - Focal epidermotropism
  - Stromal edema
  - Heterogeneous cytomorphology
    - Typically larger than normal lymphocytes
    - Round to irregular nuclei
    - ± prominent nucleoli
- **Sézary syndrome (SS)**
  - Patterns can be indistinguishable from MF
  - Upper and middermal infiltrates are most common
  - Perivascular &/or interstitial dermal infiltrates
  - Epidermotropism often present but may be focal
    - May be absent in significant proportion of cases
    - Lack of epidermotropism does not exclude diagnosis
  - Cytomorphology
    - Small to medium-sized cells
    - Often have irregular, twisted nuclear contours
    - Larger perivascular lymphocytes more common in SS

ANCILLARY TESTS

Flow Cytometry

- Evaluation of suspected lesions can be useful
- Aberrant antigen expression patterns helpful in defining but not always specific to neoplasia

PCR

- T- and B-cell clonality studies
  - May be helpful
  - False-positive results can occur in reactive infiltrates
  - Tests should be interpreted with caution
    - Always interpret in context of clinicopathologic findings
  - Monoclonal rearrangements for B-cell receptor gene
    - Present in majority of B-LBL, CLL
  - Monoclonally rearranged T-cell receptor genes
    - Present in majority of T-LBL

Genetic Testing

- Molecular abnormalities reflect those of respective leukemia type
- **MS**
  - FISH probes to evaluate for specific recurrent cytogenetic abnormalities are available in some specialized labs
    - Can be performed on paraffin-embedded tissue
    - May aid in classification of aleukemic MS
  - Chromosome 8 abnormalities
    - Common in AML patients with LC (30-40%)
- Molecular genetic studies in other subtypes of LC are limited

DIFFERENTIAL DIAGNOSIS

Inflammatory Dermatoses

- Requires careful histologic and immunohistochemical examination
  - Immature B- or T-cell phenotype (TdT, CD1a, CD34) excludes inflammatory disorder
- Flow cytometry can be helpful
  - Neoplastic processes more likely to show antigen loss &/or aberrant antigen expression patterns
  - Additional tissue held for possible flow cytometry studies can be valuable
- Distinction by B- and T-cell clonality studies can be problematic
- Clinicopathologic correlation is essential

Mature B-Cell Lymphomas

- Extranodal B-cell lymphomas may involve skin as primary site
- Nodal B-cell lymphomas may involve skin as secondary site
- Express multiple B-cell antigens
  - CD19, CD20, CD79a, pax-5, MUM1
  - May express CD10, Bcl-2, and Bcl-6 (follicular lymphomas)
- Lack TdT, CD34, MPO, lysozyme

Mature T-Cell Lymphomas

- Extranodal T-cell lymphomas may involve skin as primary site

Immunohistochemical Patterns of Leukemia Cutis

Diagnostic Type	Positive	Variable	Negative	Comments
Myeloid (granulocytic) sarcoma	CD34, CD43, CD117, MPO, lysozyme	CD4, CD45	CD68(PG-M1), CD10	MPO and lysozyme are often most helpful in demonstrating myeloid lineage
Myeloid (monoblastic) sarcoma	CD4, CD43, CD68(PG-M1), lysozyme	CD10, CD45, MPO, CD117	CD34	MPO and lysozyme are often most helpful in demonstrating myeloid lineage
Precursor B-ALL	CD10, CD19, CD34, CD43, CD79a, TdT	CD20, CD45		
Precursor T-ALL	CD1a, CD2, CD3, CD5, CD10, CD99, TdT	CD4, CD8		Surface CD3 may be absent; CD99 is nonspecific; combination of CD3 with TdT &/or CD1a considered most specific
Chronic lymphocytic leukemia/small lymphocytic lymphoma	CD5, CD19, CD20(dim), CD23, CD43, CD45, CD79a, pax-5			
Adult T-cell leukemia/lymphoma	CD2, CD3, CD4, CD5, CD25	CD7	CD1a, TdT, TIA1, granzyme-B	Diminished or loss of CD7 is common
T-cell prolymphocytic leukemia	CD3, CD4, CD45RO, TCL1		CD1a, CD34, TdT	CD4 and CD8 coexpressed in 25% of cases
Sézary syndrome	CD3, CD4, CD25, CD45RO			Loss of diminished CD7 and CD26 are common; rare cases may express CD8; larger cells may express CD30

- Nodal T-cell lymphomas may involve skin as secondary site
- May show bone marrow involvement but lack peripheral blood involvement
- Express mature T-cell antigens without TdT or CD1a

Blastic Plasmacytoid Dendritic Cell Neoplasm

- Usually presents with solitary or multiple skin lesions
- 10-20% associated with or develop into AML
- Resembles MS
- Expresses CD4, CD43, CD45RA, CD56, and plasmacytoid dendritic cell antigens (CD123, CD303, TCL1)
  - CD7 and CD33 expression is relatively common
  - Lysozyme (-) and MPO(-)
- CD4 and CD56 alone cannot be used to differentiate from MS
  - MS commonly expresses CD4, and rarely expresses CD56

Langerhans Cell Histiocytosis

- Langerhans cells have abundant eosinophilic cytoplasm and coffee bean-shaped nuclei with nuclear grooves
- Frequently accompanied by numerous eosinophils
- Complete phenotypic analysis should be performed
  - Expresses CD1a and S100

Histiocytic Sarcoma

- Substantial overlap between monocytic sarcoma and histiocytic sarcoma
- Composed of frankly atypical and pleomorphic-appearing histiocytes by morphology and IHC
- By definition, no evidence of blood or bone marrow involvement

Poorly Differentiated Carcinoma

- Often presents with large aggregates of atypical tumor cells in dermis
- Glandular differentiation (±)
- History of carcinoma may be known
- Should show expression of at least some cytokeratins; often p63 and CK5/6 (+) in primary cutaneous tumors

Merkel Cell Carcinoma

- Histomorphologic features may overlap
- Expresses cytokeratins, CK20 (perinuclear dot-like pattern), and neuroendocrine markers, including chromogranin and synaptophysin
- Lacks expression of lymphoid and myeloid markers

DIAGNOSTIC CHECKLIST

Pathologic Interpretation Pearls

- Diagnosis requires careful histologic and immunohistochemical examination
- Correlation with clinical data, bone marrow, and peripheral blood findings also necessary
- Aleukemic LC is frequently misdiagnosed as atypical lymphoid infiltrate or lymphoma
  - Immunophenotyping is essential to make distinction

SELECTED REFERENCES

1. Cruz Manzano M et al: Rosacea-like leukemia cutis: A Case Report. Am J Dermatopathol. ePub, 2016
2. Tran C et al: Chilblain-like leukaemia cutis. BMJ Case Rep. 2016, 2016
3. Wong SM et al: Rare skin manifestations successfully treated with primary B-cell chronic lymphocytic leukemia treatment. J Cutan Pathol. ePub, 2016
4. Campuzano-García AE et al: Leukemia cutis in a patient with pre-B-cell acute lymphoblastic leukemia. JAAD Case Rep. 1(6):364-7, 2015
5. Cho-Vega JH et al: Leukemia cutis. Am J Clin Pathol. 129(1):130-42, 2008
6. Barzilai A et al: Aleukemic monocytic leukemia cutis. Cutis. 69(4):301-4, 2002
7. Ratnam KV et al: Leukemia cutis. Dermatol Clin. 12(2):419-31, 1994

(Left) *High-power view highlights the cytomorphologic detail of the leukemic blasts in this case of cutaneous MS. Note the variably pleomorphic large nuclei with dispersed fine chromatin and inconspicuous nucleoli. Occasional mitotic figures are noted* ➲. **(Right)** *IHC stain for lysozyme highlights numerous leukemic blasts in a patient with previously diagnosed and treated AML. The findings are consistent with recurrent AML.*

High Magnification of Myeloid Sarcoma

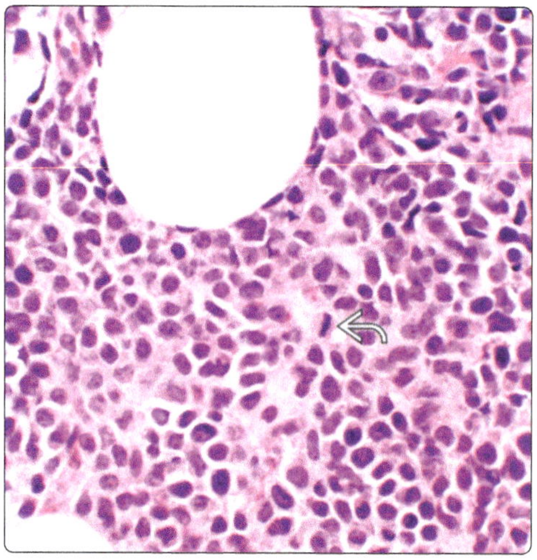

Lysozyme Immunohistochemical Stain in AML

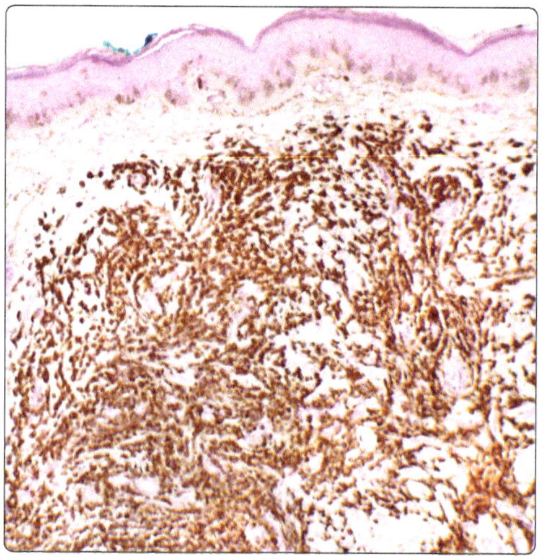

(Left) *IHC staining with CD68 at high-power magnification highlights numerous leukemic blasts with monocytic differentiation in a patient with previously diagnosed and treated AML.* **(Right)** *IHC staining with CD34 highlights the vascular structures* ⇨ *but is negative in the leukemic blasts. Leukemic blasts with monocytic differentiation are frequently negative for CD34; however, this finding alone should does not exclude the diagnosis of MS.*

CD68 Immunohistochemical Stain in AML

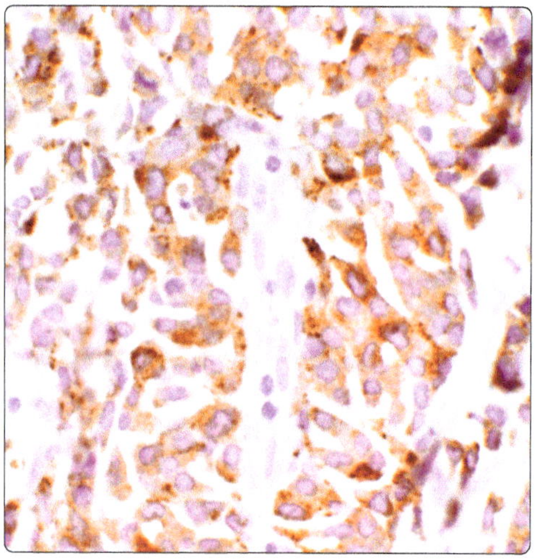

CD34 Immunohistochemical Stain in AML

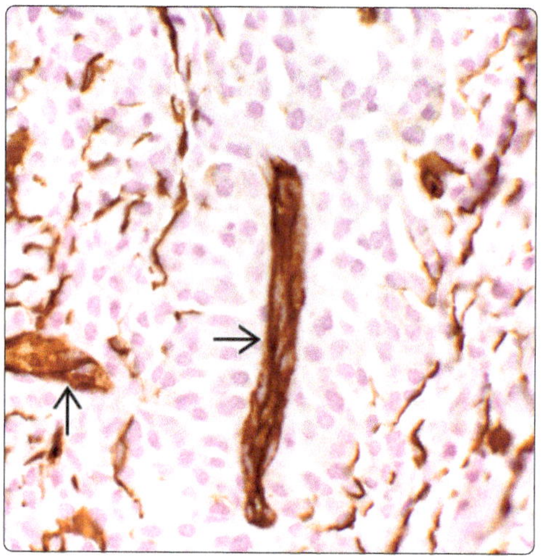

(Left) *This is a case of B-LBL involving the skin. In this field, the lymphoblasts fill the dermis and surround blood vessels. The monomorphic cytomorphology is more typical of B- and T-cell LBL. (Courtesy C. Bueso-Ramos, MD, PhD.)* **(Right)** *IHC for TdT shows positive nuclear staining, consistent with B-LBL. This pattern of staining is also observed in T-LBL. Additional B- and T-cell lineage markers are necessary to determine the lineage of the tumor. (Courtesy C. Bueso-Ramos, MD, PhD.)*

B-Cell Lymphoblastic Leukemia/Lymphomas Leukemia Cutis

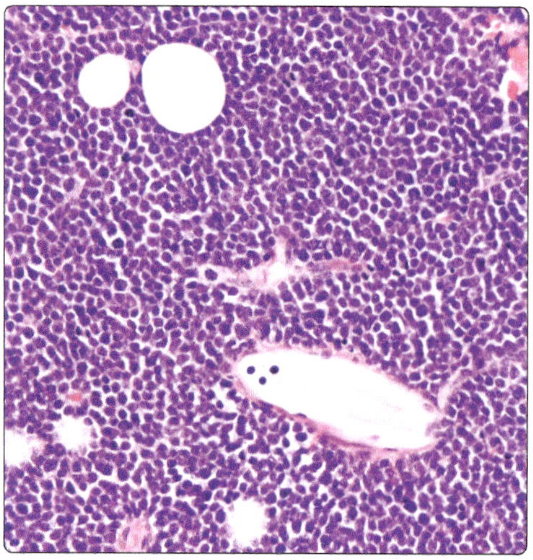

TdT Immunohistochemical Stain in B-LBL

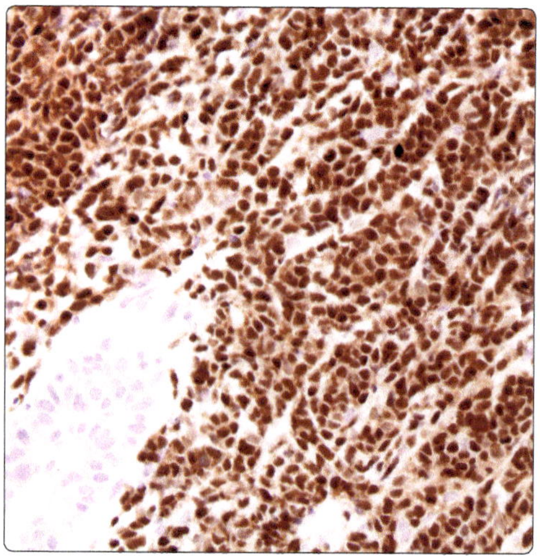

Histologic Features of Chronic Lymphocytic Leukemia/Small Lymphocytic Lymphoma

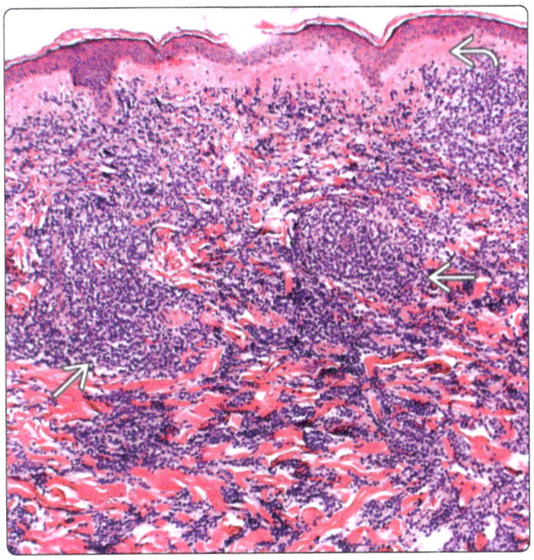

CD20 Immunohistochemical Stain in CLL

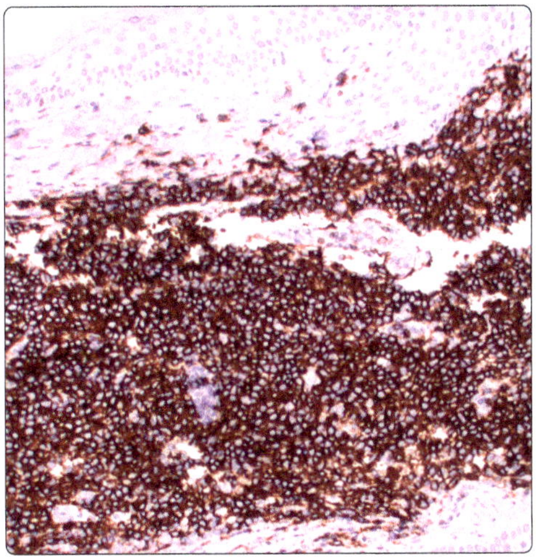

(Left) *Skin with involvement by CLL/SLL is shown. The lymphoid cells ➡ are in the superficial and deep dermis and show a dense, sheet-like growth pattern. The epidermis is uninvolved and separated from the malignant B-cell infiltrate by a thin grenz zone ↪. No germinal centers are present.* **(Right)** *The lymphoid infiltrate shows strong CD20 reactivity in a patient with CLL/SLL. The strong and diffuse reactivity is consistent with a mature B-cell lymphoma, although CD20 can also be aberrantly expressed in some B-LBLs.*

Differential Diagnosis: Blastic Plasmacytoid Dendritic Cell Neoplasm

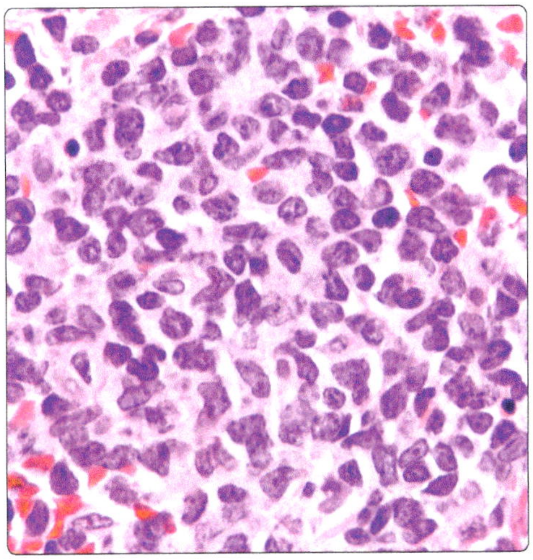

Differential Diagnosis: Diffuse Large B-Cell Lymphoma

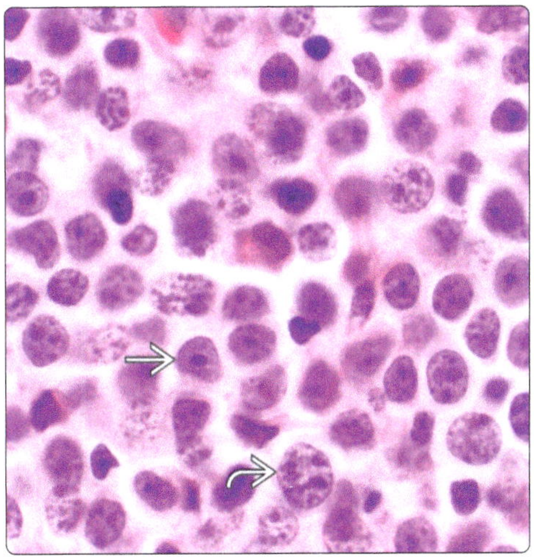

(Left) *This case of BPDCN shows cells with prominent pleomorphism and blastic-appearing chromatin, cytologic features that suggest a differential of MS with monocytic differentiation. However, stains for CD56, TCL1, and CD123 can help make this distinction.* **(Right)** *A mixture of both centroblasts ↪ and immunoblasts ➡ are seen in this diffuse large B-cell lymphoma. A mature B-cell phenotype with negative MPO and lysozyme makes the distinction from leukemia cutis.*

Differential Diagnosis: Primary Cutaneous Follicle Center Lymphoma

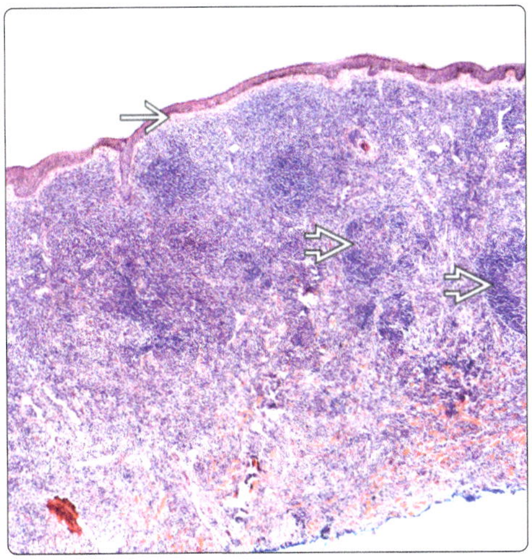

Differential Diagnosis: Primary Cutaneous Marginal Zone Lymphoma

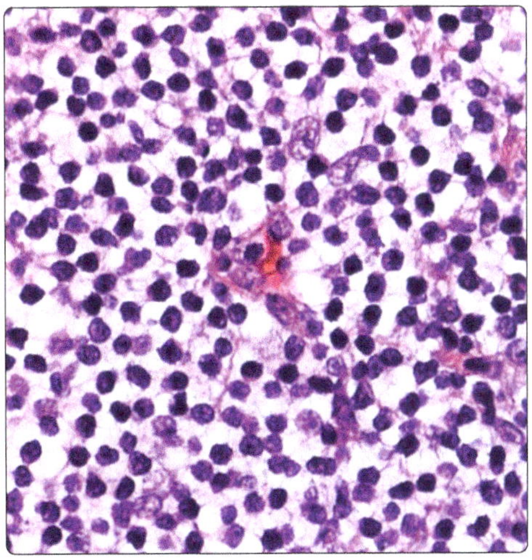

(Left) *Primary cutaneous follicle center lymphoma displays a dense lymphocytic infiltrate in the dermis, sparing the subepidermal layer (grenz zone ➡). The neoplasm contains ill-defined follicles ⇨. (Courtesy R. Miranda, MD.)* **(Right)** *In many cases of primary cutaneous marginal zone lymphoma, the tumor cells have a monocytoid appearance. In this image, the monocytoid cells have increased amounts of clear cytoplasm.*

KEY FACTS

TERMINOLOGY

- Tumor of plasmacytoid dendritic cells, initially involves skin and disseminates
- Categorized within acute myeloid leukemia and related neoplasms in 2008 WHO classification

CLINICAL ISSUES

- Initial presentation as asymptomatic cutaneous lesion without disseminated symptoms
- Natural history is clinically aggressive with involvement of bone marrow and blood
- Gender/sex
  - Middle age to elderly, male predominance
- Multiple skin lesions
  - Usually eventually disseminated disease
- Prognosis and therapy
  - No established standard therapy
  - Therapy similar to acute leukemia may be effective
  - Poor response to lymphoma chemotherapy

MICROSCOPIC

- Diffuse dermal infiltrate, spares epidermis, of medium-sized cells with blastic chromatin

ANCILLARY TESTS

- Immunohistochemistry: CD123(+), CD4(+), CD56(+), TCL1(+), TdT(+) (sometimes)
- Molecular tests
  - All *IGH* gene rearrangement studies are nonclonal
  - Most T-cell receptor gene rearrangement studies are nonclonal
  - EBV-encoded small nuclear RNA (EBER) (-)

TOP DIFFERENTIAL DIAGNOSES

- Leukemia cutis
- Extranodal NK-/T-cell lymphoma, nasal type
- Peripheral T-cell lymphoma, not otherwise specified
- Metastatic malignant melanoma
- Poorly differentiated carcinoma

Clinical Photograph

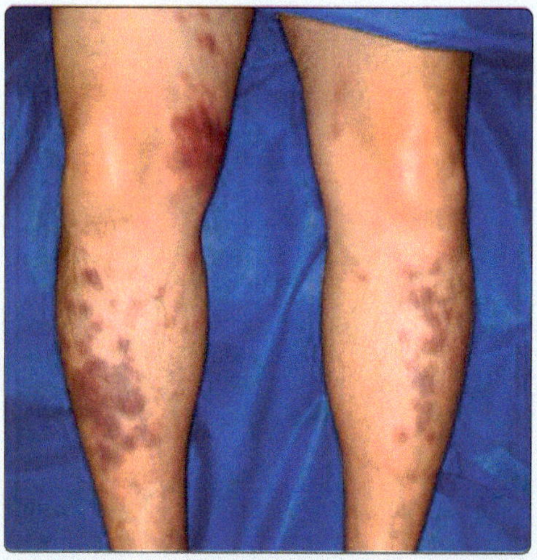

BPDCN With Diffuse Dermal Involvement

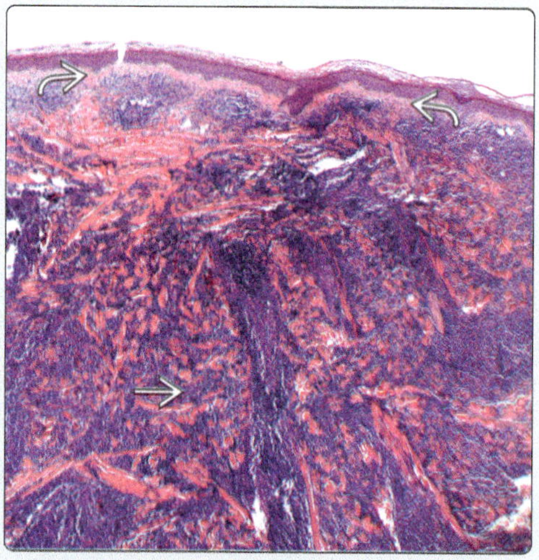

(Left) *This patient rapidly developed generalized, indurated, purplish-red, well-defined papules and coalescent plaques over his legs, which were diagnosed as blastic plasmacytoid dendritic cell neoplasm (BPDCN). (Courtesy J. Alonso, MD.)* **(Right)** *This cutaneous BPDCN shows diffuse dermal replacement by a proliferation of small blue tumor cells with an infiltrative pattern, dissecting between collagen bundles ➡. The epidermis is spared, with a grenz zone ↷.*

BPDCN at High Magnification

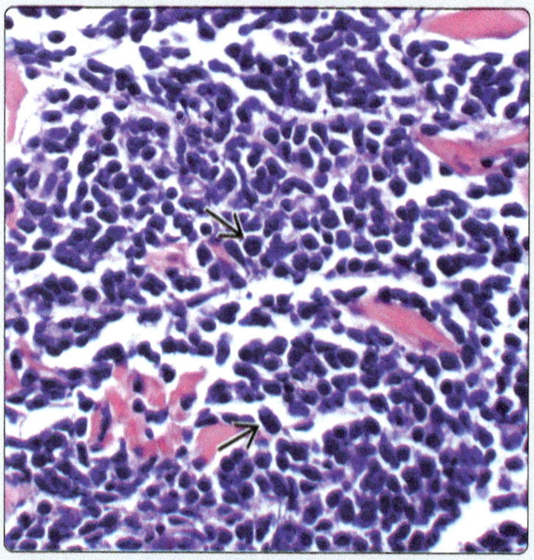

CD123 Immunohistochemical Stain in BPDCN

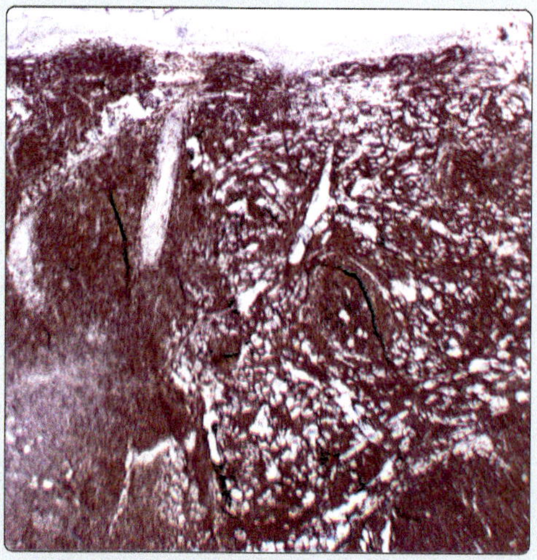

(Left) *At high magnification, the tumor cells have dense, homogeneous, blast-like chromatin ⇨. Nucleoli are not identifiable in this field.* **(Right)** *This cutaneous BPDCN shows very strong and diffuse staining with CD123, which is considered a relatively specific marker for this tumor.*

TERMINOLOGY

Abbreviations

- Blastic plasmacytoid dendritic cell neoplasm (BPDCN)

Synonyms

- CD4(+)/CD56(+) hematodermic neoplasm
- Blastic NK-cell lymphoma

Definitions

- Aggressive tumor of precursor plasmacytoid dendritic cells, which usually involves skin; frequently culminates in leukemia
  - Categorized within acute myeloid leukemia and related neoplasms in 2008 WHO classification, even though it is tumor of plasmacytoid dendritic cells

ETIOLOGY/PATHOGENESIS

Plasmacytoid Dendritic Cells

- Plasmacytoid dendritic cells (PDCs) are found in T-cell areas of hematopoietic tissue
  - Found in lymph node, bone marrow, blood, and spleen (subcapsular)
    - Enter lymph node and mucosa in response to immune activation
- Functions of plasmacytoid dendritic cells
  - Interferon-γ production and IL-3α expression
  - Dendritic cell differentiation following exposure to IL3 and CD40
- Immunophenotype of plasmacytoid dendritic cells
  - CD4, CD123, BDCA-2, CLA, TCL1, HLA-DR, CD43, CD68 (+)
  - CD56, TdT, TIA1, perforin (-)
- Diseases with ↑ plasmacytoid dendritic cells
  - Castleman lymphadenopathy
  - Kikuchi-Fujimoto disease
  - Classic Hodgkin lymphoma
  - Chronic granulomatous inflammation
  - Psoriasis
  - Lupus erythematosus
  - Chronic myelomonocytic leukemia

Etiology

- Undetermined, but some cases associated with myelodysplasia

CLINICAL ISSUES

Epidemiology

- Incidence
  - Rare
    - 0.4% of all hematopoietic neoplasms
    - < 1% of cutaneous lymphomas
- Age
  - Usually middle age to elderly
    - Can occur in children
  - Median: 65 yr
    - Range: 8-96 yr
- Sex
  - M:F = 3.3:1.0
- Ethnicity
  - No association

Site

- Often presents in > 1 anatomic site
- Skin
  - Usually 1st manifestation of disease
  - Eventually skin involvement in nearly all patients
  - 50% confined to skin at initial staging
- Bone marrow and peripheral blood
  - Occurs with progression of disease
  - 60-90% of cases
  - There are rare leukemia variants without skin involvement that are recognized with intensive immunophenotyping
  - Can be subtle infiltrates in bone marrow
- Regional lymph nodes involved in ~ 50%
- Other organs that have been reported to be involved by BPDCN
  - Liver, spleen, tonsils, nasopharynx, conjunctiva, kidneys, central nervous system

Presentation

- Generalized, localized, or solitary cutaneous lesions
  - Macules, plaques, &/or tumors
    - Sometimes erythema &/or purpura
- Lymphadenopathy and rarely B symptoms

Laboratory Tests

- Cytopenias
  - Thrombocytopenia most common
- Monocytosis is sometimes present

Natural History

- Relapse and metastasis in most cases
  - Soft tissue and CNS frequently at relapse but rare at diagnosis
- Leukemia
  - Often relapses as leukemia
    - 10-20% of cases develop into acute myeloid leukemia
    - Often myelomonocytic leukemia
  - Presents more like leukemia than lymphoma

Treatment

- Multiagent chemotherapy
  - Non-Hodgkin lymphoma chemotherapy (R-CHOP) has short-term remission rates of only 40%
  - More aggressive regiments, such as hyper CVAD, has better response
  - 90% of cases relapse after chemotherapy
- Hematopoietic stem cell transplantation
  - Intrathecal chemotherapy followed by allogeneic bone marrow transplantation sometimes performed
- Anti-CD33 antibody might be treatment possibility in cases that express CD33

Prognosis

- Poor
  - Median survival ~ 13 months
    - Less aggressive in children with median survival of 3 yr
    - Often favorable initial response to chemotherapy but eventual relapse

MACROSCOPIC

General Features

- Nodules, tumors, or plaques of skin, which may have ulceration

MICROSCOPIC

Histologic Features

- Skin
  - Dermal infiltrate
    - Typically extends into subcutaneous tissue
    - Spares epidermis, with grenz zone
  - Growth pattern
    - Diffuse, if extensive involvement
    - Perivascular and periadnexal
  - Increased mitotic figures
  - Extravasated erythrocytes
  - Scattered reactive T cells amidst tumor cells
- Lymph node
  - Effacement of lymph node architecture
    - Often interfollicular and medullary involvement by tumor
    - Sometimes tumor in sinuses
- Bone marrow
  - Aggregates of tumor cells or scattered tumor cells
    - Often interstitial distribution
  - Residual bone marrow often shows dysplasia
- Peripheral blood
  - Circulating tumor cells may resemble myeloid, monocytoid, or lymphoid blasts

Cytologic Features

- Morphology of blasts
  - Fine blastic chromatin, resembling lymphoblast or myeloblast
  - Medium-/large-sized cells with 1 or more small nucleoli and sparse cytoplasm
    - Sometimes tumor cells have more atypia and coarse chromatin

ANCILLARY TESTS

Immunohistochemistry

- Plasmacytoid dendritic cell antibodies
  - CD123(+), BDCA-2/CD303(+)
    - These are 2 most specific markers
  - CD4(+)
    - May be weakly (+)
  - CD56(+)
    - May be weakly (+)
    - Rarely CD56 is (-) and does not exclude diagnosis
  - TCL1(+)
    - Also (+) in some lymphomas, but (-) in AML
    - Can differentiate BPDCN from AML
- Other antibodies
  - CD68(+)
    - 50% of cases with cytoplasmic dot positivity
  - MxA(+), marker for interferon-γ
  - CD45RA(+/-), CD43(+) CLA(+), Bcl-6(+/-)
- Immunohistochemical markers (-)
  - Blast markers (-)
    - CD34(-), CD117(-)
    - TdT(+) in 1/2 of cases but usually in only fraction of tumor cells
  - Most myeloid markers (-)
    - CD13(-), CD15(-), lysozyme(-), CD163(-), myeloperoxidase (-)
    - But CD33 and CD43 can be (+)
  - Most B-cell markers (-)
    - CD19(-), CD20(-), CD79a(-)
    - pax-5 and MUM1 can be (+)
  - Most T-cell markers (-)
    - CD3(-), CD5(-)
    - CD2, CD45RA, and CD7 can rarely be (+)

In Situ Hybridization

- EBV-encoded small nuclear RNA (EBER) (-)

PCR

- *IGH* gene rearrangement studies are polyclonal
- Most T-cell receptor gene rearrangement studies are polyclonal

Genetic Testing

- Complex chromosomal abnormalities (2/3 of cases)
  - 6 major cytogenetic abnormalities identified: 5q, 12p, 13q, 6q, 15q, 9
  - Genomic imbalances predominate mostly losses
  - Deletion of 5q appears to be most common chromosomal aberration
- No single cytogenetic abnormality is considered specific for BPDCN
- Molecular alterations
  - *NRAS* and *ATM* are most common mutated genes
  - *CDKN1B, RB1, KRAS, IDH2,* and *KIT* have less frequent point mutations
  - *TP53* and *PTEN* mutations are rare
  - *CDKN2A* (~ 27%) and *RB1* (~ 9%) deletions
  - *TET2* mutations in absence of other mutations commonly observed in AML
  - Aberrant activation of the NF-kB pathway

DIFFERENTIAL DIAGNOSIS

Acute Myeloid Leukemia/Myeloid Sarcoma

- Tumor cells of BPDCN have immature features of myeloid blasts
- Both acute myeloid leukemia (AML) and BPDCN may express CD56, CD4, CD33, CD123, TdT
  - CD123(+) but weak in AML
- Presence of Auer Rods and cytoplasmic granules indicative of AML
- Multiple myeloid markers favor acute myeloid leukemia
  - i.e., MPO, CD13, and CD33
  - MPO(+) and lysozyme(+) in AML but BPDCN (-)
- Multiple plasmacytoid dendritic cell markers favors BPDCN over acute myeloid leukemia
  - i.e., CD123, BDCA-2
  - CD123 is only weakly (+) in AML
  - TCL1 can be (+) in BPDCN but is (-) in AML

Immunophenotype of Blastic Plasmacytoid Dendritic Cell Neoplasm

CD4	CD56	CD123	TCL	TdT	MPO	CD3
Positive	Positive	Positive	Positive	Sometimes positive	Negative	Negative

Chronic Myelomonocytic Leukemia

- May have nodules of plasmacytoid dendritic cells in bone marrow
- PDCs have round nuclei with fine chromatin, eosinophilic cytoplasm, and distinct cytoplasmic borders
- CD123(+)

Precursor T-Cell Acute Lymphoblastic Leukemia/Lymphoma

- Similarities to BPDCN
  - Tumor cells with blastic chromatin, similar to BPDCN
  - May express CD56 ± CD4
  - Both are often TdT(+)
- Differences from BPDCN
  - Multiple B-cell antigens or T-cell antigens favor B-cell acute lymphoblastic leukemia or T-acute lymphoblastic leukemia (T-ALL), respectively
  - TdT is usually strongly (+) in all tumor cells in ALL
  - Younger age of patients in ALL
  - Often mediastinal mass in T-ALL
  - Clonal T-cell receptor gene rearrangements
  - CD10(+) in ALL
    - CD1a can be (+), CD123 and BDCA2 usually (-)

Extranodal NK-/T-Cell Lymphoma, Nasal Type

- May express CD56 ± CD4
  - Prominent necrosis, angioinvasion, CD2(+), EBER(+), and cytotoxic markers (+)
  - CD123(-) and TCL1(-)
  - T-cell receptor gamma rearrangements clonal
  - Tumor cells usually do not have blast-like chromatin

Peripheral T-Cell Lymphoma, Not Otherwise Specified

- May express CD56 ± CD4
- Differences from BPDCN
  - T-cell lymphomas express more T-cell antigens than just CD43 and CD4
  - Clonal T-cell receptor gene rearrangement common in T-cell lymphoma

Mature B-Cell Lymphomas

- Differences from BPDCN
  - B-cell lymphomas express multiple B-cell antigens
    - CD20, CD19, pax-5, CD79a, MUM1
    - B-cell lymphomas are often CD10 and Bcl-6 (+)
  - Molecular findings
    - B-cell lymphomas have clonal *IGH* gene rearrangements
    - t(14;18) in diffuse large B-cell lymphoma
    - t(8;14) and other *MYC* translocations in Burkitt lymphoma

Precursor B-Cell Lymphoblastic Leukemia/Lymphoma

- Blastic cells look similar to BPDCN
- TdT often more uniformly (+)
- Multiple B-cell antigens (+)
- *IGH* gene rearrangements

Metastatic Melanoma

- Similarities to BPDCN
  - Often presents with nodular aggregates of tumor cells in dermis
  - Tumor cells are large, atypical, and may show diffuse, sheet-like pattern
- Differences from BPDCN
  - Melanin may be seen microscopically
  - Expresses melanoma markers by immunohistochemistry
    - S100, MART-1/Melan-A, HMB-45, tyrosinase, SOX10

Metastatic Poorly Differentiated Carcinoma

- Similarities to BPDCN
  - Can present with large aggregates of tumor cells in dermis
  - Tumor cells are large, atypical, and may not form glands
- Differences from BPDCN
  - Any glandular differentiation favors carcinoma
  - History of carcinoma
  - Typically express at least some cytokeratins, dependent on type of tumor

DIAGNOSTIC CHECKLIST

Clinically Relevant Pathologic Features

- Skin lesions
  - Usually macules, nodules, or plaques
  - Often disseminated
- Can be associated with myelodysplasia or leukemia

Pathologic Interpretation Pearls

- Atypical round to oval tumor cells with blast-like chromatin
- Needs extensive immunophenotyping
  - CD123(+), CD4(+), CD56(+), TCL1(+), TdT(+), MPO(-)

SELECTED REFERENCES

1. Facchetti F et al: Neoplasms derived from plasmacytoid dendritic cells. Mod Pathol. Feb;29(2):98-111, 2016
2. Kim JH et al: Blastic plasmacytoid dendritic cell neoplasm: analysis of clinicopathological feature and treatment outcome of seven cases. Ann Dermatol. 27(6):727-37, 2015
3. Nguyen CM et al: Blastic plasmacytoid dendritic cell neoplasm in the pediatric population: a case series and review of the literature. Am J Dermatopathol. 37(12):924-8, 2015
4. Riaz W et al: Blastic plasmacytoid dendritic cell neoplasm: update on molecular biology, diagnosis, and therapy. Cancer Control. 21(4):279-89, 2014
5. Shi Y et al: Blastic plasmacytoid dendritic cell neoplasm: a clinicopathologic review. Arch Pathol Lab Med. 138(4):564-9, 2014

(Left) *BPDCN shows the dermis replaced by a diffuse proliferation of tumor cells with an infiltrative pattern, dissecting between collagen bundles* ➡*. The epidermis is spared, with a grenz zone* ⮫*. (Courtesy L. J. Medeiros, MD.)* **(Right)** *Higher magnification of BPDCN shows the superficial dermis replaced by the neoplasm. The epidermis is uninvolved, and a distinct grenz zone* ➡ *can be appreciated. (Courtesy L. J. Medeiros, MD.)*

BPDCN With Diffuse Dermal Infiltration

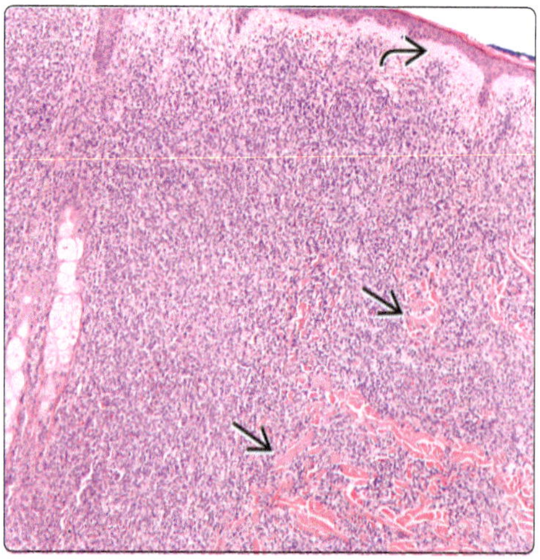

Higher Magnification of BPDCN

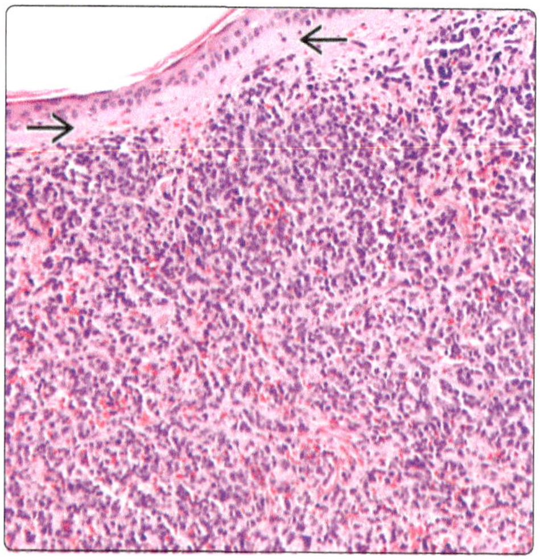

(Left) *Immunohistochemical stain for CD303 (BDCA-2) is strongly positive in this cutaneous BPDCN. This marker and CD123 are typically considered the most specific markers for this tumor.* **(Right)** *Deep involvement in BPDCN shows the tumor cells extending into the deep subcutaneous fat. Tumor is seen infiltrating around individual fat cells* ➡*.*

Positive Immunohistochemistry for CD303

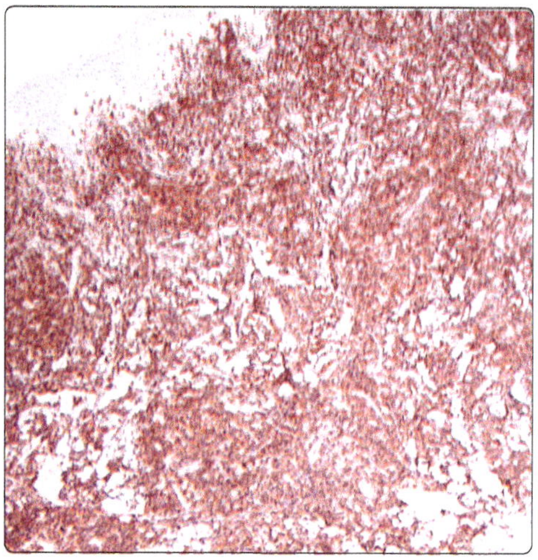

Subcutis Involvement by BPDCN

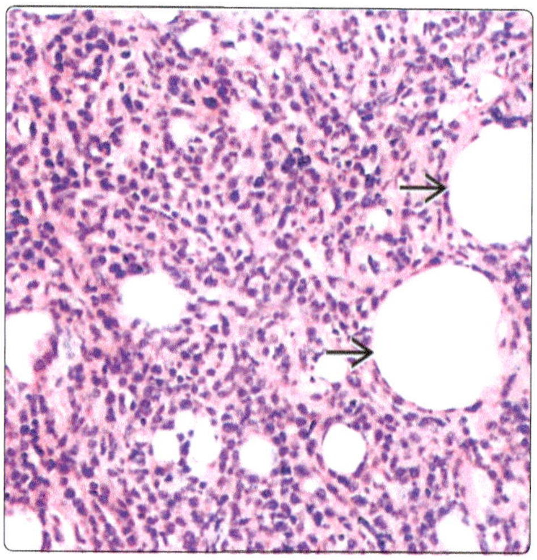

(Left) *At high magnification, the tumor cells have a fine, homogeneous, blast-like chromatin pattern* ➡*. One or more small nucleoli can be seen in some of the cells. This is the classic morphology of the tumor cells in BPDCN.* **(Right)** *High magnification of another case of BPDCN shows that the neoplastic cells are small to intermediate in size. These cytologic features suggest a differential diagnosis with lymphoblastic lymphoma and small cell T-cell lymphomas.*

Fragile Blast-Like Chromatin in BPDCN

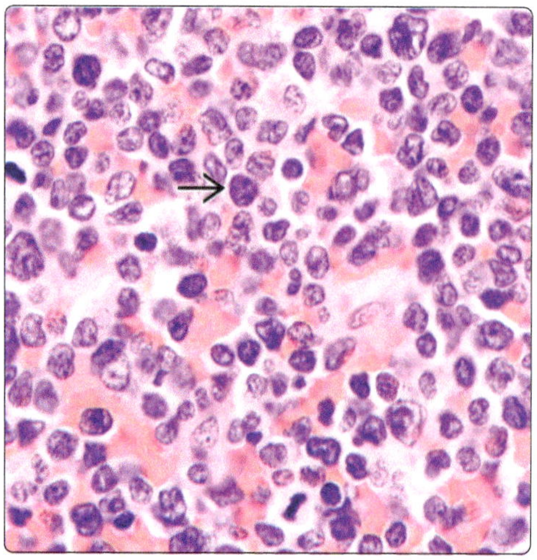

Smaller Cell Size in BPDCN

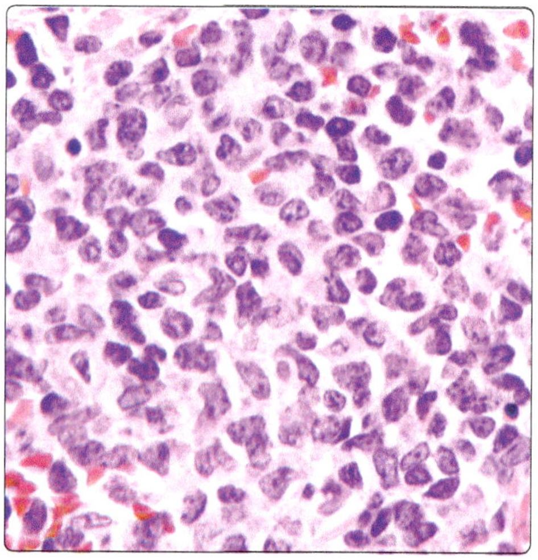

CD4 Immunohistochemical Stain in BPDCN

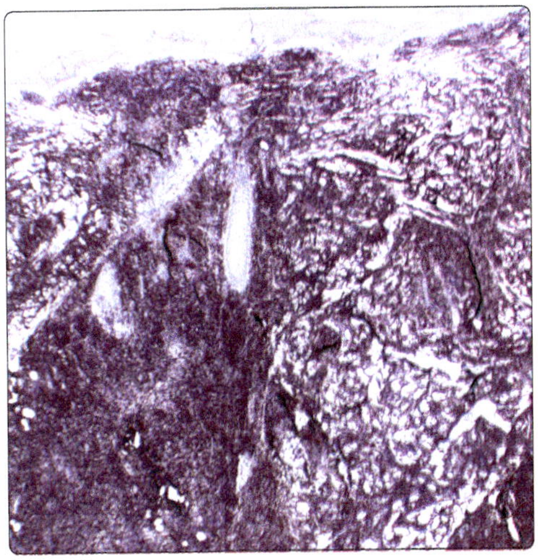

TCL1 Immunohistochemical Stain in BPDCN

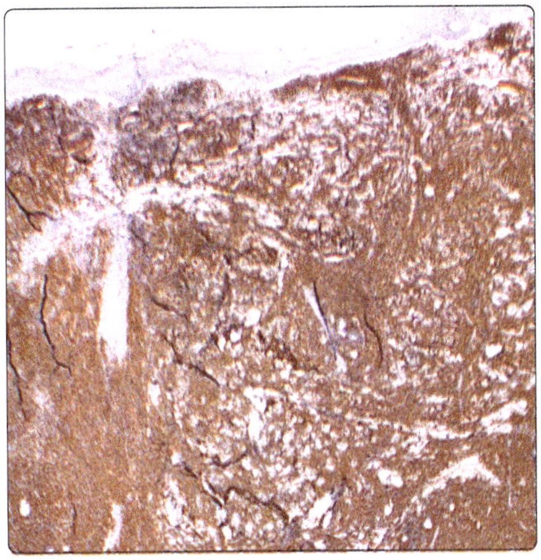

(Left) *This CD4 immunostain is diffusely strongly positive as would be expected in a case of BODCB.* **(Right)** *TCL1 is another marker often expressed by these tumors, although it is not specific for BPDCN.*

CD56 Immunohistochemical Stain in BPDCN

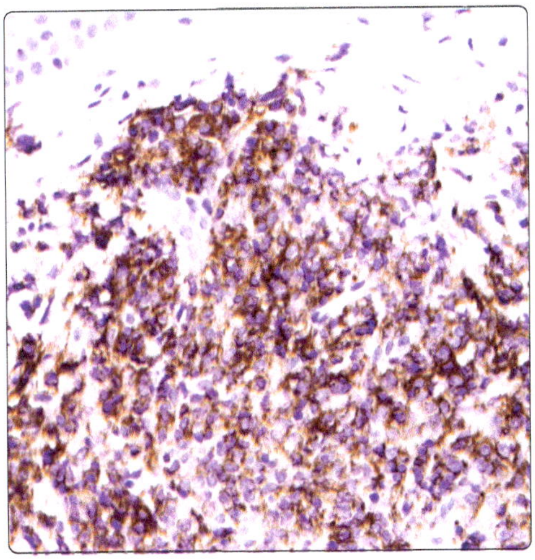

CD123 Immunohistochemical Stain in BPDCN

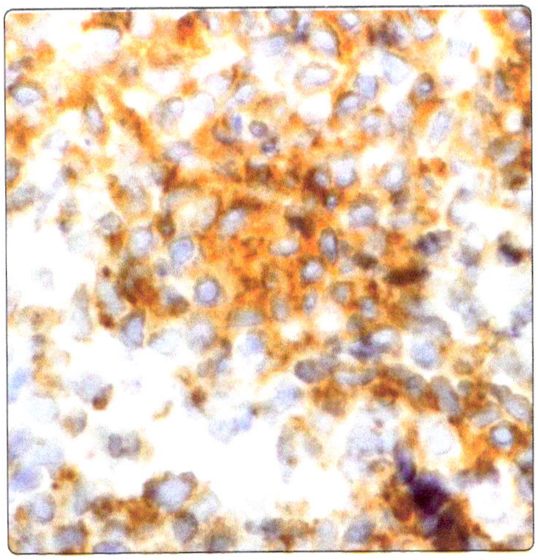

(Left) *High magnification of BPDCN involving the dermis shows the neoplastic cells strongly CD56(+). (Courtesy L. J. Medeiros, MD.)* **(Right)** *BPDCN is typically positive with CD123, since CD123 is a marker of plasmacytic dendritic cells. BDCA-2 and MXA are other plasmacytic dendritic cell markers that are often positive in BPDCN.*

Negative PCR For *IGH* Gene Rearrangement

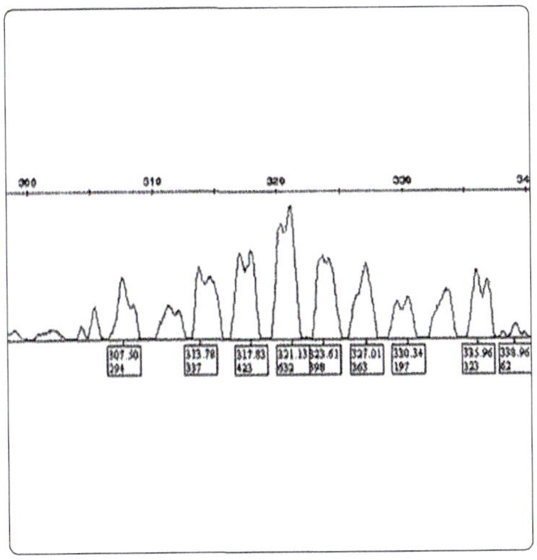

Negative PCR For *TRG* Gene Rearrangement

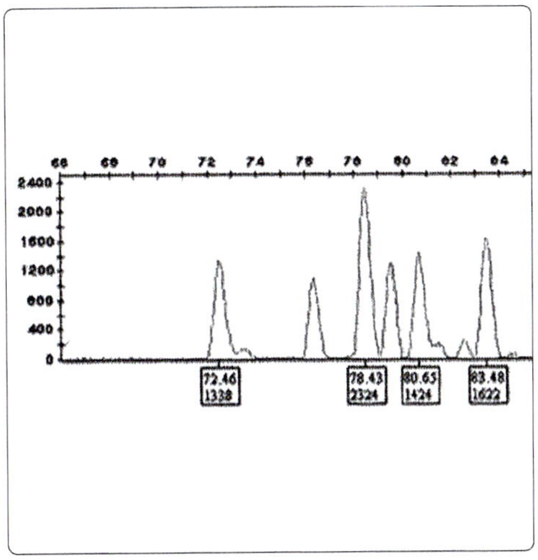

(Left) *This is an example of PCR for immunoglobulin gene rearrangements (IGH). No dominant monoclonal peak is observed, and there is a bell-shaped curve signal distribution. IGH gene rearrangements should not be detected in BPDCN.* **(Right)** *This is an example of PCR for T-cell receptor gamma gene rearrangements (TRG). No dominant monoclonal peak is observed in the assay. Like IGH, TRG gene rearrangements should not be detected in BPDCN.*

Lymph Node Involvement by BPDCN

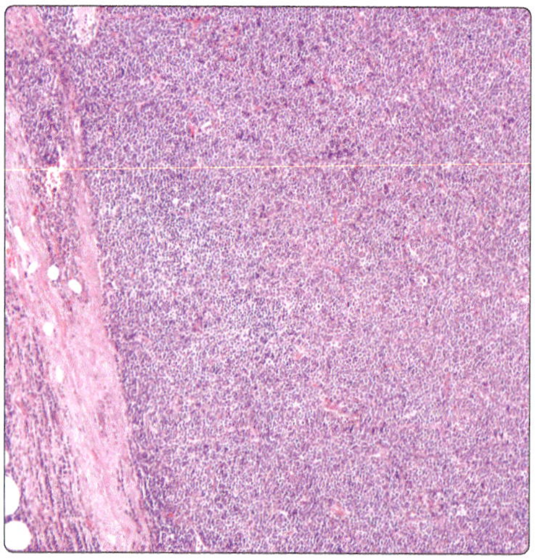

Higher Power of Lymph Node Involvement by BPDCN

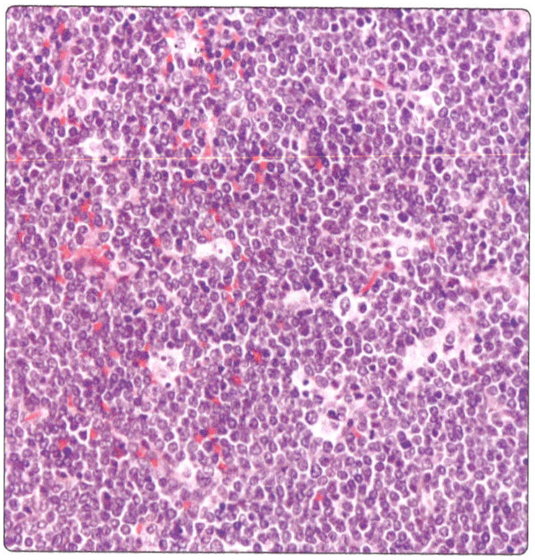

(Left) *In this case of BPDCN involving a lymph node, the neoplasm completely replaces the lymph node and has a diffuse pattern. (Courtesy L. J. Medeiros, MD.)* **(Right)** *At higher magnification, the tumor cells are small and have immature chromatin resembling, in part, lymphoblasts. (Courtesy L. J. Medeiros, MD.)*

CD4 Immunohistochemical Stain in BPDCN

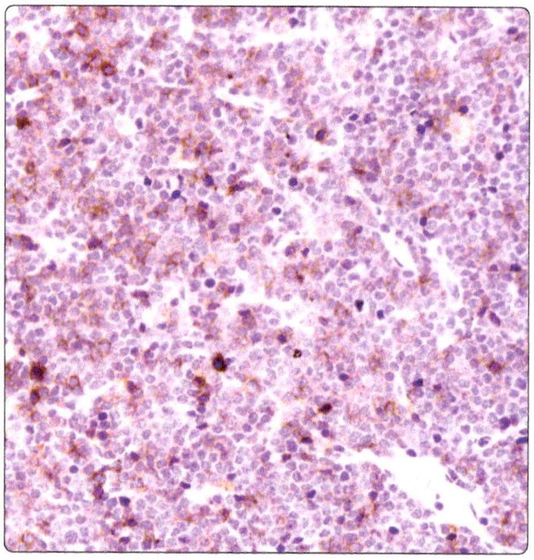

CD56 Immunohistochemical Stain in BPDCN

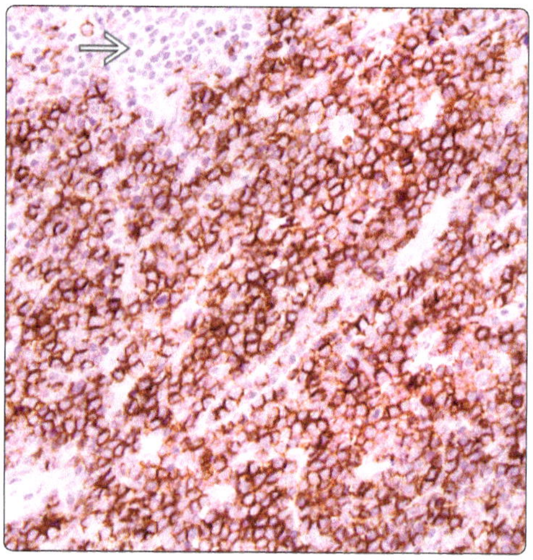

(Left) *The neoplastic cells in this LN case of BPDCN express CD4 with dim intensity and a cytoplasmic staining pattern. (Courtesy L. J. Medeiros, MD.)* **(Right)** *The neoplastic cells are CD56(+). A residual follicle ➔ is CD56(-). (Courtesy L. J. Medeiros, MD.)*

TCL1 Immunohistochemical Stain in BPDCN

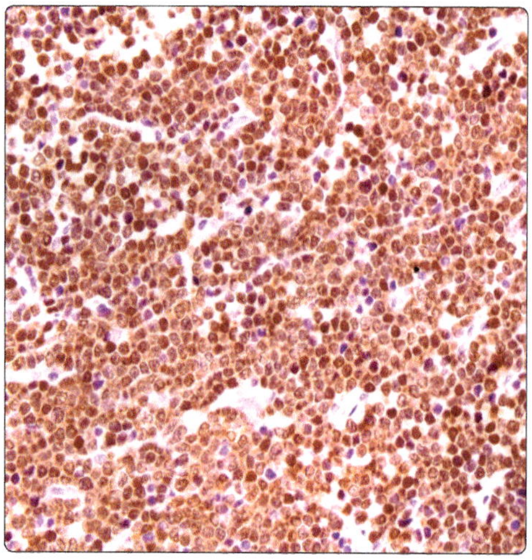

CD123 Immunohistochemical Stain in BPDCN

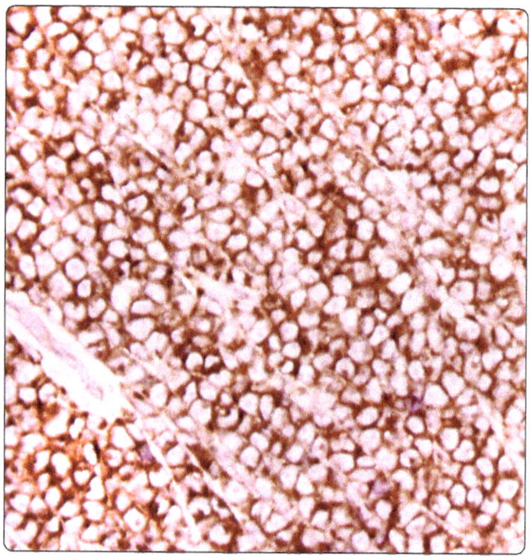

(Left) *The neoplastic cells are strongly TCL1(+) with a nuclear pattern of expression. TCL1 expression is present in these neoplasms and helpful in the differential diagnosis. (Courtesy L. J. Medeiros, MD.)* **(Right)** *The neoplastic cells are strongly CD123(+). Expression of CD123 is characteristic of this neoplasm and very helpful in the differential diagnosis. (Courtesy L. J. Medeiros, MD.)*

Differential Diagnosis: Leukemia Cutis

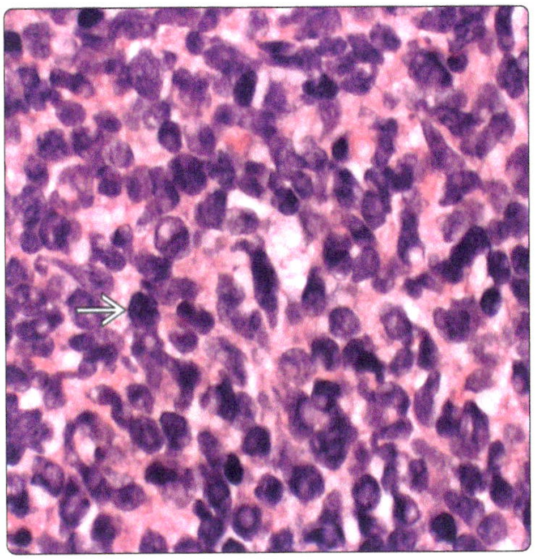

MPO Immunohistochemical Stain in Leukemia Cutis

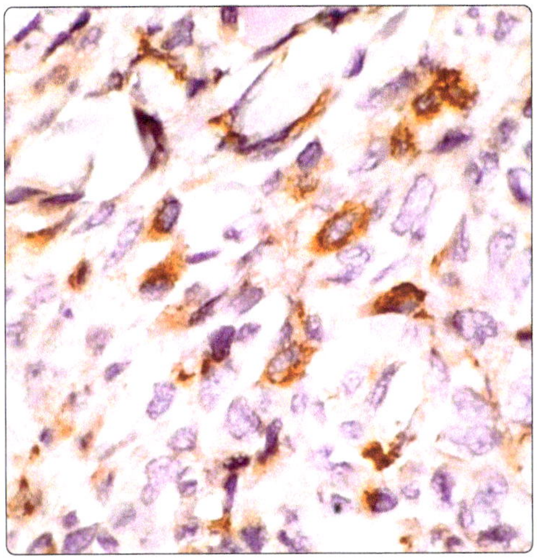

(Left) *Leukemia cutis must be excluded in all cases of BPDCN. In this case of leukemia cutis, the infiltrate filled the dermis. At high power, the tumor cells are large* → *with fine blastic chromatin.* **(Right)** *In this MPO stain of leukemia cutis, the tumor cells are myeloperoxidase (+). The tumor cells were also CD15(+), CD68(+), and CD4(+), showing monocytic differentiation.*

Differential Diagnosis: Diffuse Large B-Cell Lymphoma

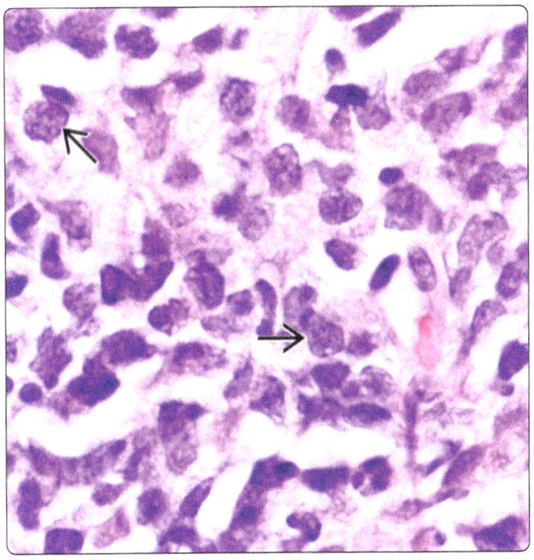

Differential Diagnosis: Anaplastic Large Cell Lymphoma

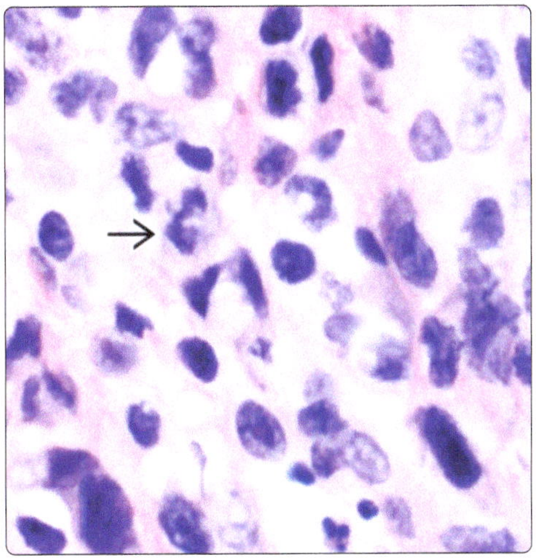

(Left) *Diffuse large B-cell lymphoma is in the differential diagnosis of BPDCN. This case shows a diffuse dermal infiltrate with large malignant cells with coarse chromatin* ⇨*. This case had a different immunophenotype from BPDCN, expressing pax-5 and CD20 and was positive for t(14;18).* **(Right)** *This case of anaplastic large cell lymphoma has a similar morphology to BPDCN with a diffuse dermal infiltrate of large malignant cells* ⇨ *but a different phenotype [CD30(+), ALK(+/-)].*

Differential Diagnosis: Melanoma

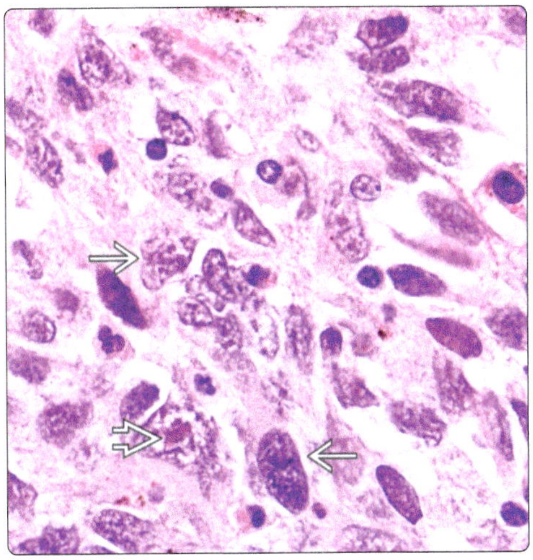

Differential Diagnosis: Small Cell Carcinoma

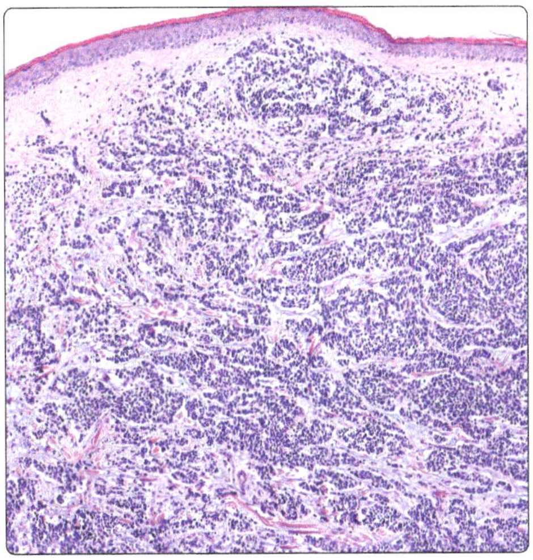

(Left) *Melanoma can also be mistaken for BPDCN. In this case of melanoma, the tumor cells show more atypia* → *and prominent nucleoli* → *and are typically S100(+), HMB-45(+), MART-1/Melan-A(+), and tyrosinase (+).* **(Right)** *Metastatic small cell carcinoma of the lung shows a diffuse, infiltrative pattern in the dermis, with sparing of the epidermis and separation from it by a grenz zone. However, the tumor cells are typically strongly CK7(+) and TTF-1(+).*

KEY FACTS

TERMINOLOGY

- Formation of blood cells (erythroid cells, myeloid cells, megakaryocytes) outside bone marrow
- Most common in liver and spleen; rare in skin
- Hematopoiesis occurs in skin in early embryonic life

ETIOLOGY/PATHOGENESIS

- Associated with viral infections, hematopoietic disorders, and neoplasms
- Also entities that lack bone marrow hematopoiesis

CLINICAL ISSUES

- Depends on aggressiveness of patient's underlying disorder
- Usually, underlying disorder is treated rather than extramedullary hematopoiesis (EMH)
- Erythema, single lesions, plaques, ulcers, or bullae

MICROSCOPIC

- Dermis with myeloid cells, erythroid cells, and megakaryocytes at all stages of maturation
- 1, 2, or all 3 hematopoietic cell lines may be identified with predominant type depending on associated condition
- Dysplasia is not seen in reactive EMH
- Dysplasia is often identified in extramedullary hematopoiesis associated with myeloid neoplasm
- Peripheral blood can often show leukoerythroblastosis, especially if patient has primary myelofibrosis

ANCILLARY TESTS

- Myeloid cells positive for CD33, CD13, CD43, and CD15
- Erythroid cells positive for hemoglobin A
- Megakaryocytes express factor VIII and CD61
- Leder stain is positive in myeloid cells

TOP DIFFERENTIAL DIAGNOSES

- Leukemia cutis
- Chronic myeloproliferative neoplasms

(Left) *This is a skin biopsy specimen with extramedullary hematopoiesis (EMH), as evidenced by the large megakaryocyte* →. **(Right)** *This cutaneous lesion contains small clusters of nucleated red blood cells* ↪, *which were positive for a hemoglobin A immunostain (not shown).*

EMH With Megakaryocyte

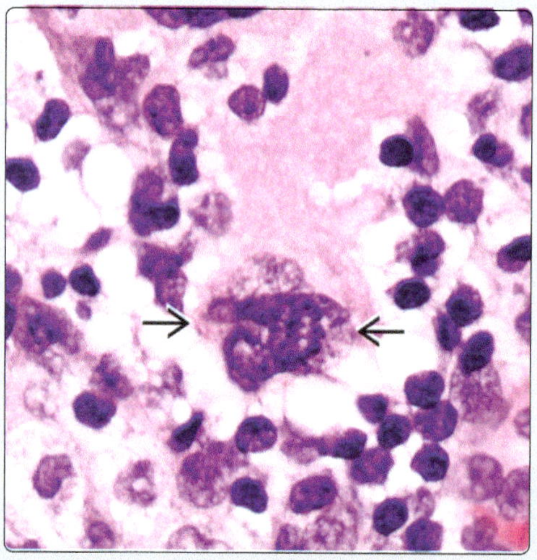

EMH With Erythroid Cells

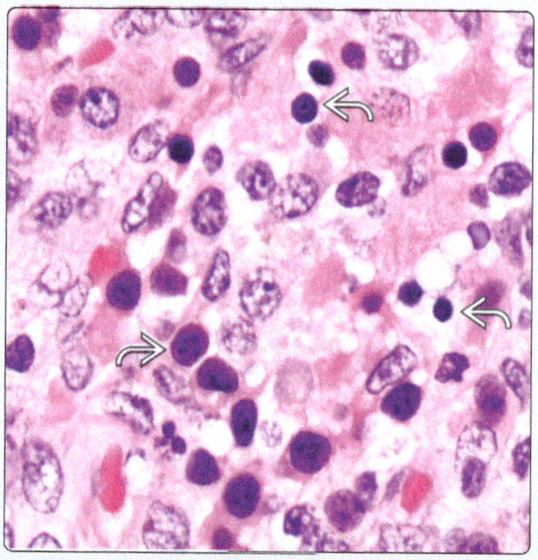

(Left) *This is a factor VIII immunostain in EMH of the skin. The megakaryocytes are positive for factor VIII. Other megakaryocyte markers include CD61, CD34, and LMP.* **(Right)** *This is a hemoglobin A immunostain in a skin biopsy specimen with EMH; the stain is highlighting erythroid cells.*

Factor VIII Immunohistochemistry

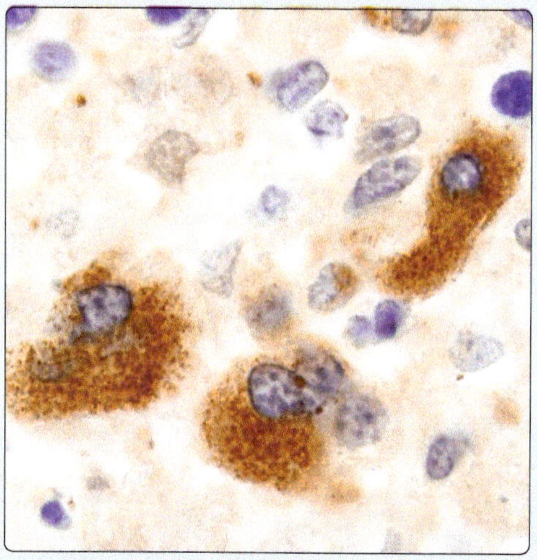

Hemoglobin A Immunohistochemistry

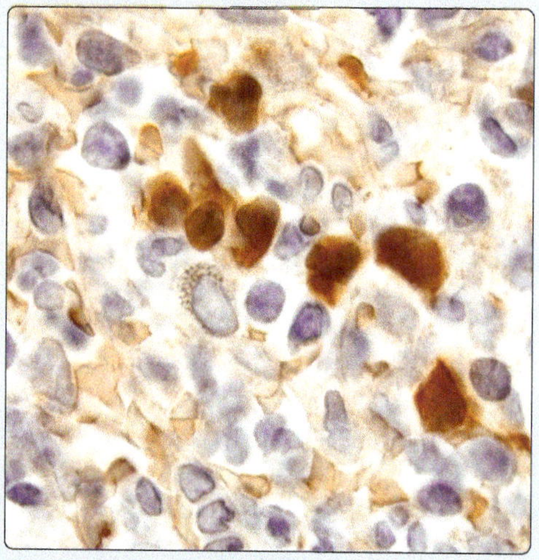

TERMINOLOGY

Abbreviations

- Extramedullary hematopoiesis (EMH)

Definitions

- Formation of blood cells (including nucleated red blood cells, lymphocytes, and megakaryocytes) outside of bone marrow
  - Occurs most commonly in liver and spleen
    - Also found in other organs, including lymph nodes, kidney, adrenal, gastrointestinal tract, lung, breast, central nervous system
  - Hematopoiesis occurs in skin early in embryonic life

ETIOLOGY/PATHOGENESIS

Viral Infection

- Has been reported in skin in neonates with intrauterine viral infections including
  - Cytomegalovirus
  - Coxsackievirus
  - Rubella

Hematopoietic Disorders

- In neonates, EMH occurs in congenital hematologic disorders including
  - Hemolytic disease of newborn
  - Twin transfusion syndrome
- In adults, EMH is seen with hematopoietic disorders
  - All myeloproliferative neoplasms are associated with EMH
    - Primary myelofibrosis is most common, especially in patients who have had splenectomy
    - Essential thrombocythemia, polycythemia vera, and chronic myelogenous leukemia have also been reported

Neoplasms

- Can also develop in variety of tumors
  - Pilomatrixomas can rarely show EMH

CLINICAL ISSUES

Presentation

- Variable and depends on associated disease
  - Erythema, single lesions, plaques, ulcers, or bullae
  - EMH can develop in surgical wounds
  - Blueberry muffin appearance is multiple violaceous papulonodular lesions in neonates with EMH
- Patients with EMH in spleen develop splenomegaly

Treatment

- Usually, underlying disorder is treated rather than EMH

Prognosis

- Depends on aggressiveness of patient's underlying disorder

MICROSCOPIC

Histologic Features

- Occurs in superficial and deep dermis
- Polymorphic infiltrate with myeloid cells, erythroid cells, and megakaryocytes
  - Cells are at all stages of maturation; thus, can present with myelocytes, promyelocytes, bands, and neutrophils
  - Megakaryocytes are often most easily seen elements
- Often perivascular distribution
- Can cause fibrosis in skin, liver, and spleen
- Peripheral blood can often show leukoerythroblastosis, especially if patient has primary myelofibrosis
- In liver, EMH occurs in sinusoids

ANCILLARY TESTS

Immunohistochemistry

- Myeloid cells can be highlighted by myeloperoxidase, CD33, CD13, CD43, MAC387, and CD15
- Erythroid cells are immunoreactive with hemoglobin A and glycophorin
- Megakaryocytes express factor VIII, CD61, CD34, and LMP
- CD45RB is positive in all myeloid cells, erythroid cells, and megakaryocytes

Special Stains

- Leder stain is positive in myeloid cells

DIFFERENTIAL DIAGNOSIS

Leukemia Cutis

- Early myeloid cells of EMH can rarely be mistaken for acute myeloid leukemia
- Early erythroid cells could be confused with acute erythroid leukemia
- Blast cell markers, such as CD34 and CD117, are usually positive

Chronic Myeloproliferative Neoplasms

- Similarly can present with proliferations of myeloid cells, erythroid cells, &/or megakaryocytes

SELECTED REFERENCES

1. LeBlanc RE et al: JAK2-positive cutaneous myelofibrosis presenting as sclerosing extramedullary hematopoietic tumors on the scalp: case presentation and review of the literature. J Cutan Pathol. Nov;42(11):858-62, 2015
2. Sheikh U et al: Extramedullary hematopoiesis: cytomorphologic, histologic, and radiologic findings in sixteen cases. Acta Cytol. 59(2):144-8, 2015
3. Rajiah P et al: Extramedullary hematopoiesis in unusual locations in hematologically compromised and noncompromised patients. Skeletal Radiol. 40(7):947-53, 2011
4. Smith J et al: Extramedullary haematopoiesis secondary to hereditary spherocytosis. Br J Haematol. 154(5):543, 2011
5. Miyata T et al: Cutaneous extramedullary hematopoiesis in a patient with idiopathic myelofibrosis. J Dermatol. 35(7):456-61, 2008
6. Haniffa MA et al: Cutaneous extramedullary hemopoiesis in chronic myeloproliferative and myelodysplastic disorders. J Am Acad Dermatol. 55(2 Suppl):S28-31, 2006
7. Fernández Aceñero MJ et al: Extramedullary hematopoiesis in an adult. J Am Acad Dermatol. 48(5 Suppl):S62-3, 2003
8. Revenga F et al: Cutaneous extramedullary hematopoiesis. Int J Dermatol. 39(12):957-8, 2000
9. Patel BM et al: Cutaneous extramedullary hematopoiesis. J Am Acad Dermatol. 32(5 Pt 1):805-7, 1995
10. Mizoguchi M et al: Cutaneous extramedullary hematopoiesis in myelofibrosis. J Am Acad Dermatol. 22(2 Pt 2):351-5, 1990
11. Schofield JK et al: Cutaneous extramedullary hematopoiesis with a preponderance of atypical megakaryocytes in myelofibrosis. J Am Acad Dermatol. 22(2 Pt 2):334-7, 1990
12. Hocking WG et al: Cutaneous extramedullary hematopoiesis following splenectomy for idiopathic myelofibrosis. Am J Med. 76(5):956-8, 1984
13. Kuo T: Cutaneous extramedullary hematopoiesis presenting as leg ulcers. J Am Acad Dermatol. 4(5):592-6, 1981

KEY FACTS

TERMINOLOGY

- Heterogeneous group of clonal neoplastic proliferations of mast cells in ≥ 1 organ system
  - Cutaneous mastocytosis: Confined to skin
  - Systemic mastocytosis: Involvement of at least 1 organ ± skin lesions

ETIOLOGY/PATHOGENESIS

- Frequently associated with somatic activating point mutations within *KIT* protooncogene
  - Most common mutation: D816V in exon 17 encoding tyrosine kinase domain
  - Provides relative resistance to prototypical tyrosine kinase inhibitor imatinib
- About 30% of SM cases associated with *TET2* mutations

CLINICAL ISSUES

- 2/3 of cases occur in children
- Prognosis depends on disease category
  - Pediatric-onset CM has favorable outcome
- ~ 80% of patients with mastocytosis have evidence of skin involvement

MICROSCOPIC

- Multifocal compact or diffuse compact mast cell infiltrates
- Diffuse interstitial infiltration pattern
- Cytology varies, but abnormal features are almost always detected, including spindling and hypogranularity
- Frequent bi- or multilobated nuclei usually indicate aggressive disease

ANCILLARY TESTS

- Neoplastic mast cells may express aberrant CD2 &/or CD25

TOP DIFFERENTIAL DIAGNOSES

- Reactive mast cell hyperplasia
- Cutaneous lymphoma
- Myeloid and lymphoid neoplasms with eosinophilia

(Left) *This mastocytoma of the skin was present at birth on the right neck of this newborn. Mastocytomas of the skin occur almost exclusively in infants. (Courtesy S. Vanderhooft, MD.)* **(Right)** *Low-power microscopic image of a mastocytoma of the skin in an infant shows a dense infiltrate of mast cells with epidermal sparing that showed round nuclei with abundant basophilic-staining cytoplasm at high power.*

Clinical Photograph of Mastocytoma of Skin

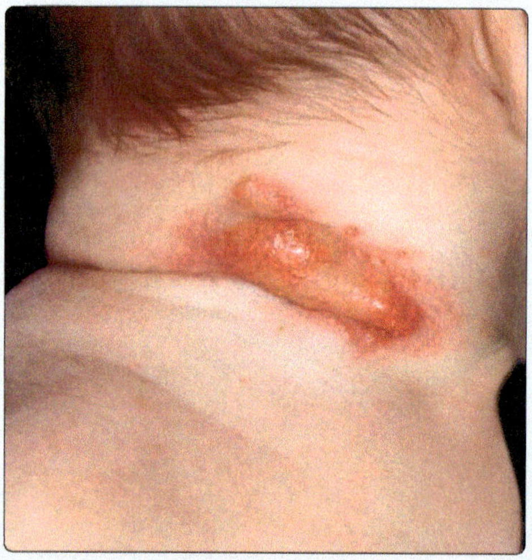

Mastocytoma of Skin

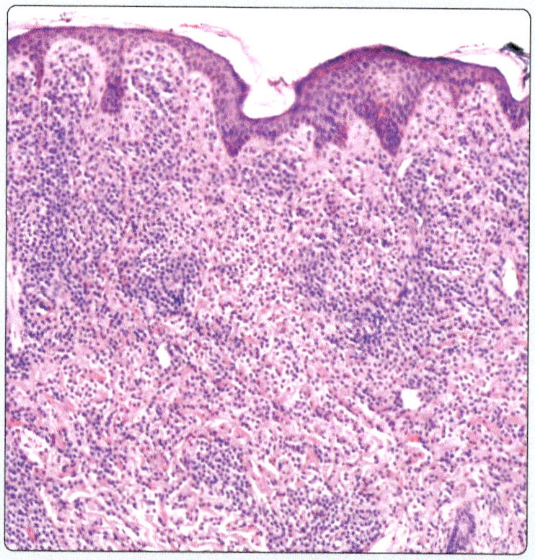

(Left) *Telangiectasia macularis eruptiva perstans (TMEP) is characterized by a relatively subtle, predominantly perivascular infiltrate of mast cells, which can be easily missed at low magnification. At higher magnification, increased numbers of oval to spindled perivascular mast cells with granular cytoplasm can be seen* ⮳. **(Right)** *CD117 strongly highlights the increased numbers of perivascular spindle-shaped mast cells in TMEP.*

Cutaneous Mastocytosis: TMEP Variant

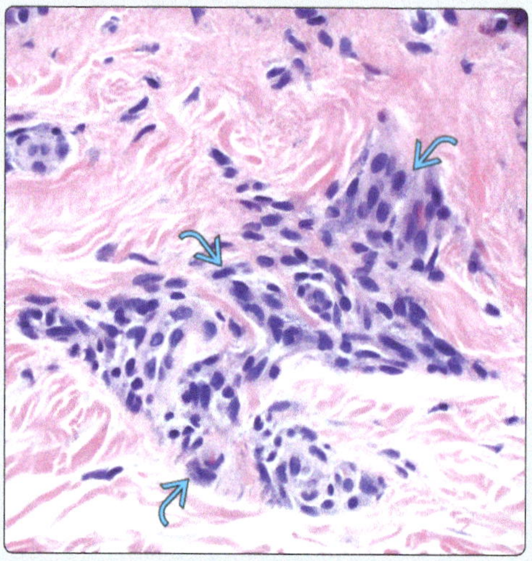

CD117 (KIT) Immunohistochemistry in TMEP

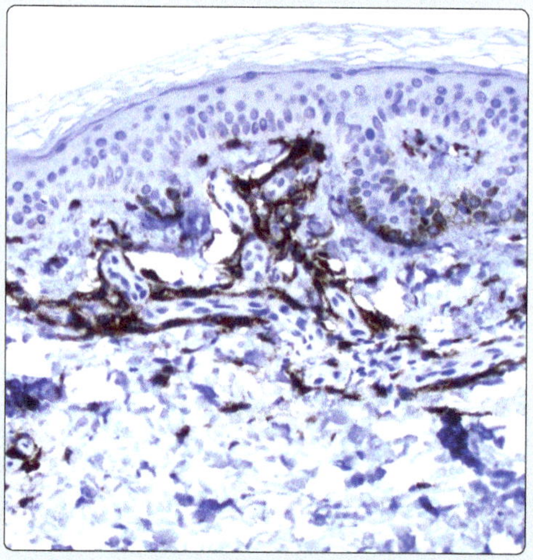

TERMINOLOGY

Abbreviations

- Cutaneous mastocytosis (CM)
- Systemic mastocytosis (SM)

Synonyms

- Mast cell disease

Definitions

- Heterogeneous group of clonal, neoplastic mast cell proliferations that accumulate in 1 or more organ systems
- Subtypes based mainly on distribution of disease and clinical manifestations
  - **CM**: Mast cell infiltrates confined to skin
    - Urticaria pigmentosa (UP)/maculopapular cutaneous mastocytosis (MPCM)
    - Telangiectasia macularis eruptiva perstans (TMEP)
    - Diffuse cutaneous mastocytosis
    - Mastocytoma of skin
  - **SM**: Involvement of at least 1 extracutaneous organ ± skin lesions
    - Indolent systemic mastocytosis (ISM)
    - Systemic mastocytosis with associated clonal hematological non-mast cell lineage disease (SM-AHNMD)
    - Aggressive systemic mastocytosis (ASM)
    - Mast cell leukemia (MCL)
    - Mast cell sarcoma (MCS)
    - Extracutaneous mastocytoma

ETIOLOGY/PATHOGENESIS

Molecular Background

- Frequently associated with somatic activating point mutations within *KIT* protooncogene
  - Encodes tyrosine kinase receptor for stem cell factor (SCF)
  - Various mutations result in ligand-independent activation of KIT tyrosine kinase
    - Constitutively activated KIT leads to clonal proliferation of mast cells
  - Most common mutation: D816V in exon 17 encoding tyrosine kinase domain
    - Identified in ≥ 95% of adults with SM when sensitive methods are used
    - Present in 35% of pediatric CM cases
    - Provides relative resistance to prototypical tyrosine kinase inhibitor imatinib
- Pediatric CM historically regarded as reactive condition with transient dysregulation of local growth factors
- Rare familial cases with germline mutations of *KIT* have been reported
- In patients with SM-AHNMD, additional genetic defects are detected depending on type of associated clonal hematological non-mast cell lineage disease (AHNMD)
- ~ 30% of SM cases associated with *TET2* mutations
  - *TET2* acts as putative tumor suppressor gene
  - 50% of those cases also carry *KIT* D816V mutation

CLINICAL ISSUES

Epidemiology

- Incidence
  - Very rare
    - Lack exact numbers with regard to frequency
    - Calculated incidence of 5-10 new cases per million population per year in various studies
  - CM
    - UP: Most common CM variant
    - Mastocytoma of skin (10-15% of pediatric CM cases)
    - Diffuse CM (rare)
  - SM
    - ISM: Most common SM variant (46% of SM cases)
    - SM-AHNMD (40% of SM cases)
    - ASM (12% of SM cases)
    - MCL, MCS, and extracutaneous mastocytoma are extremely rare
- Age
  - Occurs at any age
    - 2/3 occur in children in 1st 2 years of life
  - CM most common in children, less frequent in adults
  - SM generally diagnosed after 2nd decade of life, rare in pediatric population
- Sex
  - CM: Slight male predominance
  - SM: M:F = 1:1-1:3

Site

- ~ 80% of patients with mastocytosis have evidence of skin involvement
- CM: Mast cell infiltrates confined to skin
- SM: Involvement of at least 1 extracutaneous organ ± skin lesions
  - Bone marrow (BM) almost always involved
  - Skin lesions occur in ≥ 50% of cases, more often in those with indolent disease
  - Spleen, lymph nodes, liver, and gastrointestinal tract mucosa
  - Rarely peripheral blood (PB) shows leukemia
  - Any tissue may be affected

Presentation

- **CM**
  - Includes 3 distinct clinicohistopathologic entities
  - Characterized by 2 main groups of symptoms
  - Skin lesions due to mast cell infiltrate and release of mediators (flushing, blistering, pruritus)
    - Lesions can urticate when stroked (Darier sign) in 1/2 of cases
  - Systemic symptoms due to release of mast cell mediators (histamine most significant)
    - Headache
    - GI manifestations including acid reflux disease, peptic ulcer disease, and diarrhea
    - Respiratory symptoms including shortness of breath and asthma exacerbations
    - Cardiovascular symptoms including tachycardia, hypotension, syncope, or rarely, even shock
- **UP/MPCM**

- Widespread distribution of tan macules and occasionally nodules or plaques
- Most lesions show intraepidermal accumulation of melanin pigment
- Sparing of palms, soles, face, and scalp
- In children, typically involving head and lateral face
- Special forms
  - TMEP: Brown macules and erythema with telangiectasias on trunk and extremities, usually in adults, higher incidence of associated systemic mastocytosis
  - Plaque form: Nonpigmented, plaque-forming lesions in young children
  - Nodular form: Brown nodules
  - Blistering variant (bullous mastocytosis): Exaggeration of urticaria due to chymase cleaving dermal-epidermal junction
- **Diffuse CM**
  - Diffusely thickened skin with orange peel appearance and yellow-red discoloration
  - In more severe variant, blistering may precede mast cell infiltration
    - Differential diagnosis with congenital bullous diseases
  - More likely associated with severe systemic symptoms (higher concentrations of mast cells)
    - GI manifestations (including severe diarrhea), hypotension, or even shock
- **Mastocytoma of skin**
  - Single indurated red-brown macule, papule, plaque, or tumor measuring ≤ 4 cm in diameter
    - Multiple mastocytomas in different locations have been reported
  - Almost exclusively in infants
  - Slight predilection for trunk, but also occurs on extremities, head, and neck
- **SM**
  - Includes 6 distinct clinicohistopathologic entities
  - Symptoms grouped into few categories
  - Constitutional symptoms
    - Fatigue, weight loss, fever, diaphoresis
  - Skin manifestations
    - Pruritus, urticaria, dermographism
  - Mediator-related systemic events (due to release of histamine, eicosanoids, proteases, and heparin)
    - Same as CM systemic symptoms
  - Musculoskeletal complaints
    - Bone pain, osteopenia/osteoporosis, fractures, arthralgias, myalgias
  - Symptoms related to organ impairment due to mast cell infiltrates (absent in indolent but present in aggressive variants)
    - Splenomegaly (often minimal)
    - Lymphadenopathy and hepatomegaly (less frequent)
  - Hematological abnormalities
    - Anemia, leukocytosis, eosinophilia (frequent), neutropenia, and thrombocytopenia
    - BM failure only in aggressive or leukemic variants
    - Significant numbers of circulating mast cells are suggestive of MCL
    - 30-40% of SM has AHNMD diagnosed before, simultaneously with, or after SM diagnosis
    - Any defined myeloid or lymphoid malignancy possible, myeloid predominates chronic myelomonocytic leukemia most common

Laboratory Tests

- Serum total tryptase
  - Persistently elevated (> 20 ng/mL suggestive of SM, used as minor criterion for diagnosis)
    - Criterion not valid in SM-AHNMD
  - Normal to slightly elevated in patients with CM
    - Usually reserved for adult work-up of CM
- Histamine
  - May be very elevated in diffuse CM but are rarely part of routine work-up for CM

Treatment

- CM
  - Alleviate symptoms with antihistamines and topical steroids
  - Prevent episodes by avoiding mast cell degranulators
    - Physical stimuli (temperature changes, rubbing/friction, intense physical exertion)
    - Foods (spicy foods, citrus fruits, cheese, alcohol)
    - Medications (antibiotics, aspirin, lidocaine, etc.)
  - Educate and reassure families
- SM
  - Currently no cure
  - PKC412 tyrosine kinase inhibitor may be effective in treating SM with mutated *KIT*
- ASM, MCL, and MCS
  - Candidates for cytoreductive therapies

Prognosis

- Depends on disease category
- Pediatric-onset CM has favorable outcome
  - Majority of cases have improvement of symptoms over time
    - Complete regression by adolescence in > 50%
    - Very low likelihood of progressive disease
  - Transformation to SM rare, but more likely in diffuse CM than UP
- In adults, cutaneous lesions generally do not regress and are often associated with SM (usually ISM)
- SM
  - Usually normal life expectancy
  - Patients with aggressive variants may survive only a few months
  - SM-AHNMD depends on associated hematological disorder
  - Predictors of poorer prognosis for SM
    - Late onset of symptoms, absence of CM, thrombocytopenia, elevated LDH, anemia, BM hypercellularity, abnormal myeloid maturation patterns, PB smear abnormalities, elevated alkaline phosphatase, and hepatosplenomegaly
    - Percentage and morphology of mast cells in BM smears is independent predictor of survival

MICROSCOPIC

General Microscopic Features

- Normal mast cells in tissue sections (H&E)

- Loosely scattered
- Round to oval nuclei with clumped chromatin and inconspicuous nucleoli
- Low nuclear:cytoplasmic ratio with numerous basophilic cytoplasmic granules

- Neoplastic mast cells
  - Cytology varies, but abnormal features (including spindling and hypogranularity) are almost always detected
    - More pronounced in high-grade lesions; occurrence of metachromatic blast cells is usual feature of mast cell leukemia
    - Frequent bi- or multilobated nuclei ("promastocytes") usually indicates aggressive mast cell proliferation
    - Mitotic figures in mast cells do occur, but are infrequent even in aggressive or leukemic variants
  - Pattern of infiltrate may vary depending on tissue
  - Perivascular collections of mast cells seen in TMEP
  - Multifocal compact or diffuse compact mast cell infiltrates
    - Highly compatible with diagnosis
    - Additional immunohistochemical and molecular studies are still recommended
  - Diffuse interstitial infiltration pattern
    - Loosely scattered mast cells in absence of compact aggregates
    - Also observed in reactive mast cell hyperplasia and myelomastocytic leukemia
    - Additional immunohistochemical and molecular studies are necessary to establish diagnosis

Microscopic Features of CM

- UP
  - Aggregates of round to spindle-shaped mast cells in papillary and reticular dermis
  - Often in perivascular (especially in TMEP) and periadnexal location
  - Mast cells are fewer in adults than in children
- Diffuse CM
  - Band-like infiltrate of mast cells in papillary and upper reticular dermis
- Mastocytoma of skin
  - Dense sheets of mature-appearing, highly metachromatic mast cells in papillary and reticular dermis
  - May extend into subcutaneous tissues
  - Abundant cytoplasm
  - No cytologic atypia (distinguishes it from extremely rare MCS of skin)
  - Highest concentration of mast cells compared with other types of CM

Microscopic Features of SM

- Bone marrow: 4 types of infiltrates
  - Multifocal, sharply demarcated compact infiltrates of mast cells
    - Paratrabecular, perivascular, &/or parafollicular in location
    - "Mixed infiltrates" composed of mast cells, intermingled with lymphocytes, eosinophils, histiocytes, and fibroblasts
  - Monomorphic infiltrate with spindle-shaped mast cells that abut or stream along bony trabeculae
    - Significant reticulin fibrosis and thickening of adjacent bone are frequent
  - Diffuse replacement of BM by compact mast cell infiltrates
    - Resembles sheets of fibroblasts
  - Compact infiltrates composed exclusively of round hypergranular mast cells (rare)
    - Tryptase positive round cell infiltration of BM (TROCI-BM)
  - Careful examination of BM not involved by mastocytosis is crucial
    - Unremarkable: ISM with skin and BM involvement or isolated BM mastocytosis
    - Extremely hypercellular due to proliferation of cells of non-mast cell lineages (reactive or coexisting hematopoietic neoplasm)
  - Reactive, nonclonal mast cell hyperplasia may accompany variety of hematological disorders (lymphoplasmacytic lymphoma and hairy cell leukemia)
- Lymph node
  - Focal or diffuse infiltrates, often paracortical
  - Hyperplasia of germinal centers, angioneogenesis, tissue eosinophilia, plasmacytosis, and reticulin/collagen fibrosis may be present
- Spleen
  - Red &/or white pulp may be involved
  - Eosinophilia and fibrosis are frequent
- Liver
  - Small granulomatoid foci of mast cells within periportal tracts and loosely scattered mast cells within sinusoids
- GI tract mucosa
  - Involvement frequently suspected clinically
  - Various patterns may be seen

Diagnostic Criteria

- CM
  - Skin lesions show typical clinical features of UP/MPCM, diffuse CM, or solitary mastocytoma
  - Mast cells in multifocal or diffuse pattern
  - Lack features/criteria of SM
- SM
  - Major criterion and 1 minor criterion or at least 3 minor criteria are present

ANCILLARY TESTS

Immunohistochemistry

- Normal mast cells express CD9, CD33, CD45, CD68, and CD117 (KIT)
  - Tryptase expressed in virtually all mast cells irrespective of stage of maturation or neoplastic state
  - Chymase expressed in subpopulation of mast cells
    - Highly specific but less sensitive for atypical and immature mast cells than CD117
- Neoplastic mast cells have similar antigen profile to normal mast cells
  - In contrast, coexpress CD2 &/or CD25
    - Distinguish from CD2(+) T cells

Diagnostic Criteria for Systemic Mastocytosis*

Major Criterion**	Minor Criteria**
Multifocal, compact, dense mast cell infiltrates (≥ 15 mast cells in aggregates) in bone marrow or tissue sections	> 25% of mast cells show atypical, spindled, or immature morphologies in smears or tissue sections
	D816V KIT mutation present
	Mast cells show aberrant expression of CD2 &/or CD25
	Total serum tryptase level > 20 ng/mL***

**Adapted from WHO 2008 classification. **Diagnosis of SM made when major and 1 minor criterion or ≥ 3 minor criteria are present. ***Parameter not valid if associated clonal hematological non-mast cell lineage disease is present.*

Classification of Mastocytosis*

Categories	Comments
Cutaneous mastocytosis	Lacks features/criteria of SM
Systemic mastocytosis	1 major and 1 minor or ≥ 3 minor criterion are present
Mast cell leukemia	≥ 20% mast cells in bone marrow; usually ≥ 10% mast cells in peripheral blood
Mast cell sarcoma	High-grade cytology; unifocal lesion; destructive; no evidence for SM
Extracutaneous mastocytoma	Low-grade cytology; unifocal lesion; nondestructive; no evidence for SM
Indolent systemic mastocytosis	Low mast cell burden; skin lesions typical
Aggressive systemic mastocytosis	≥ 1 of the following: Bone marrow dysfunction, hepatomegaly with liver function impairment, ascites, portal hypertension, skeletal involvement, splenomegaly, malabsorption, and weight loss
Systemic mastocytosis with associated clonal hematological non-mast cell lineage disease	Meets SM criteria and meets WHO criteria for a clonal hematopoietic non-mast cell lineage disorder (i.e., MDS, MPN, AML, lymphoma)

**Adapted from WHO 2008 classification.*

  - CD25 expression may be inconsistent or even undetectable in well-differentiated SM or subgroup of MCL

DIFFERENTIAL DIAGNOSIS

Reactive Mast Cell Hyperplasia

- Lacks compact mast cell infiltrates, no atypical cytology, and no aberrant antigen expression
- May be seen in BM following toxic or inflammatory exposures

Congenital Bullous Diseases

- Blistering variants of UP and diffuse CM can clinically resemble bullous diseases
- No significant mast cell infiltrate on skin biopsy

Cutaneous Lymphoma

- Mast cells only mildly increased, if any
- Evaluate with appropriate IHC panel

Myelomastocytic Leukemia

- Advanced myeloid neoplasm with elevated numbers of immature atypical mast cells
- Criteria for SM not met

Myeloid and Lymphoid Neoplasms With Eosinophilia

- Exclude *FIP1L1-PDGFRA* rearrangement in cases with PB and BM eosinophilia
- Serum tryptase and BM mast cells may be increased but typically less than SM
- Mast cells do not form large compact aggregates as in SM

Child Abuse

- CM can clinically resemble multiple bruises

SELECTED REFERENCES

1. Hermans MA et al: Systemic mastocytosis: a cohort study on clinical characteristics of 136 patients in a large tertiary centre. Eur J Intern Med. ePub, 2016
2. Pieri L et al: Clinical presentation and management practice of systemic mastocytosis. A survey on 460 Italian patients. Am J Hematol. ePub, 2016
3. Severino M et al: Telangiectasia macularis eruptiva perstans (TMEP): a form of cutaneous mastocytosis with potential systemic involvement. J Am Acad Dermatol. ePub, 2016
4. Bodemer C et al: Pediatric mastocytosis is a clonal disease associated with D816V and other activating c-KIT mutations. J Invest Dermatol. 130(3):804-15, 2010
5. Klco JM et al: Molecular pathology of myeloproliferative neoplasms. Am J Clin Pathol. 133(4):602-15, 2010
6. Parker RI: Pediatric mast cell disease: what's the big (hematologic) deal? Pediatr Blood Cancer. 53(4):527-8, 2009
7. Uzzaman A et al: Pediatric-onset mastocytosis: a long term clinical follow-up and correlation with bone marrow histopathology. Pediatr Blood Cancer. 53(4):629-34, 2009
8. Briley LD et al: Cutaneous mastocytosis: a review focusing on the pediatric population. Clin Pediatr (Phila). 47(8):757-61, 2008
9. Metcalfe DD: Mast cells and mastocytosis. Blood. 112(4):946-56, 2008

Clinical Image of Cutaneous Mastocytosis

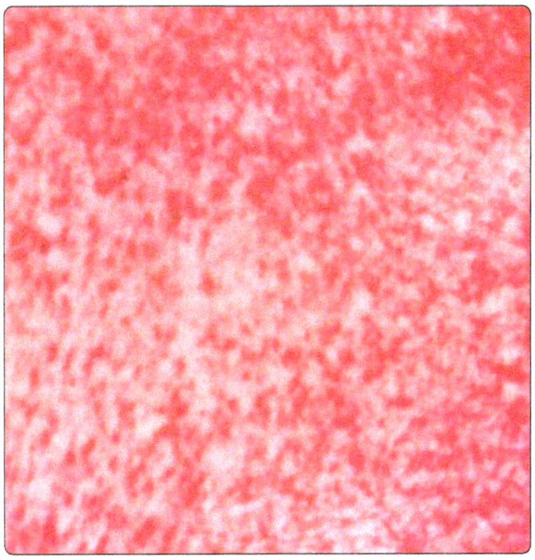

Clinical Image of Cutaneous Mastocytosis

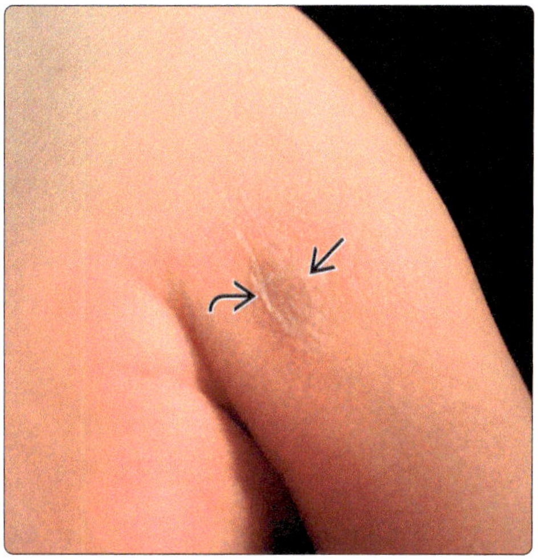

(Left) *Clinical image of maculopapular cutaneous mastocytosis shows macular and maculopapular brown skin lesions. The pigmentation is usually caused by an intraepidermal accumulation of melanin. (Courtesy C. Bueso-Ramos, MD, PhD.)* **(Right)** *Brownish-red plaque → on the thumb of a 5-year-old boy shows a positive Darier sign where a linear wheal ↷ has formed at the site of a scratch by the wooden end of a cotton swab. (Courtesy J. Hall, MD.)*

Cutaneous Mastocytosis Shows Dermal Infiltrate

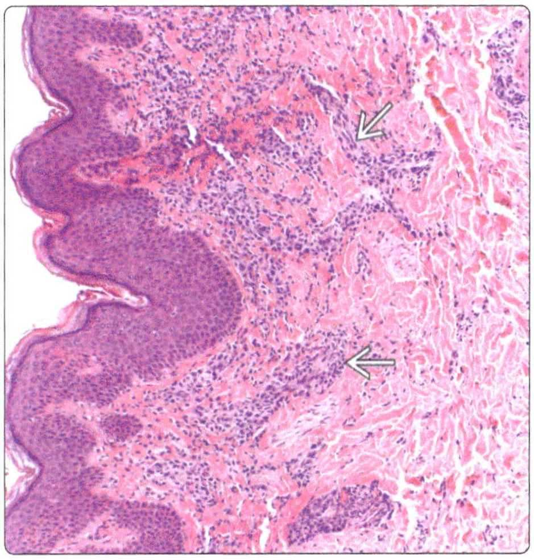

Cutaneous Mastocytosis at Higher Magnification

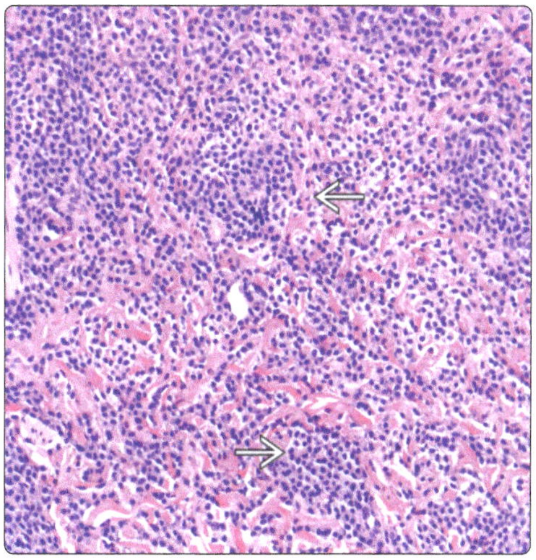

(Left) *Cutaneous mastocytosis at intermediate magnification shows the dermal mast cell infiltrate →. The mast cells show variable cytologic features, with some showing spindled nuclei and other areas showing more round nuclei, and abundant basophilic cytoplasm.* **(Right)** *Cutaneous mastocytosis at higher power highlights the dermal mast cell infiltrate →. The mast cells show variable cytologic features including both spindled and round nuclei. All contain abundant basophilic cytoplasm.*

Cutaneous Mastocytosis at Higher Magnification

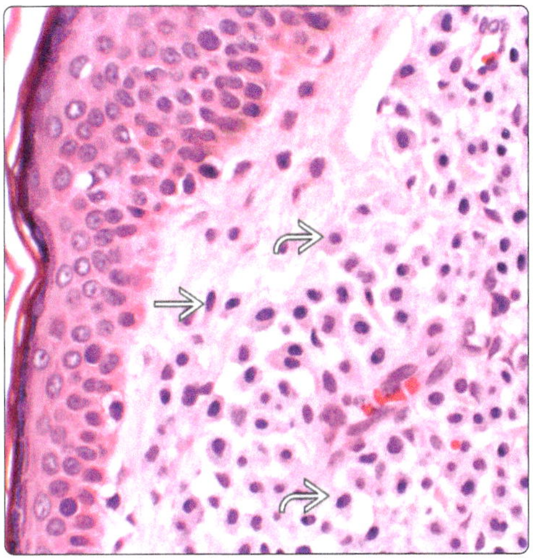

Mastocytoma: High Magnification Showing Cytologic Details

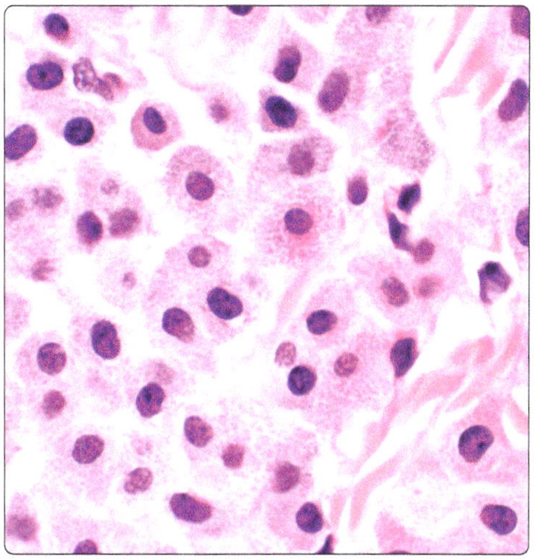

(Left) *High magnification of cutaneous mastocytosis displays a dense dermal mast cell infiltrate. This infiltrate in an adult should prompt staging to exclude systemic mastocytosis (SM). Note the variable cytologic features, which include both spindled → and round to oval nuclei ↷.* **(Right)** *High-power view of mastocytoma highlights the cytologic features, which include enlarged round to oval nuclei with abundant basophilic granular cytoplasm.*

Systemic Mastocytosis in Bone Marrow Aspirate

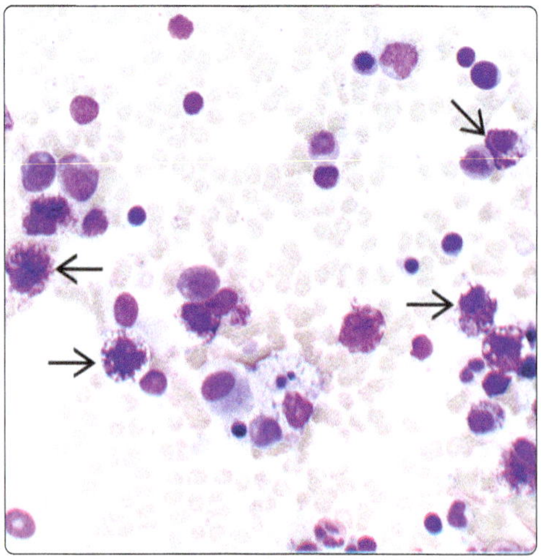

Systemic Mastocytosis in Bone Marrow

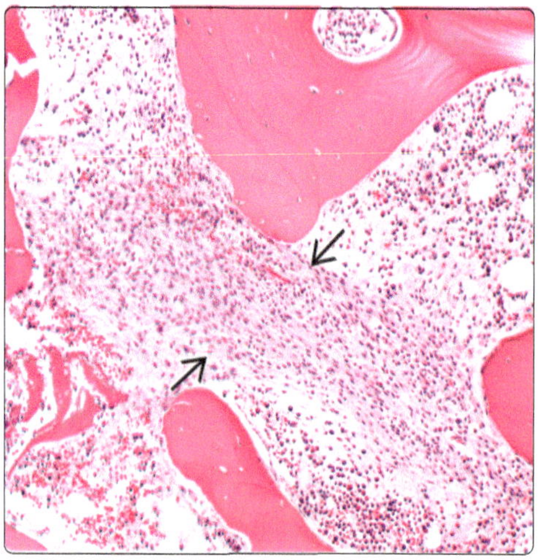

(Left) *Bone marrow aspirate in a patient with SM shows many mast cells ➡. Mast cells were readily identified away from the spicules, whereas in many patients with a clinical suspicion of SM, careful inspection of the spicules for mast cells is required.* **(Right)** *Core biopsy from a patient with SM shows a cohesive aggregate of atypical mast cells ➡. This finding meets both major (> 15 mast cells in aggregate) and minor (> 25% are of spindle-shaped) criteria for SM.*

Systemic Mastocytosis at High Magnification

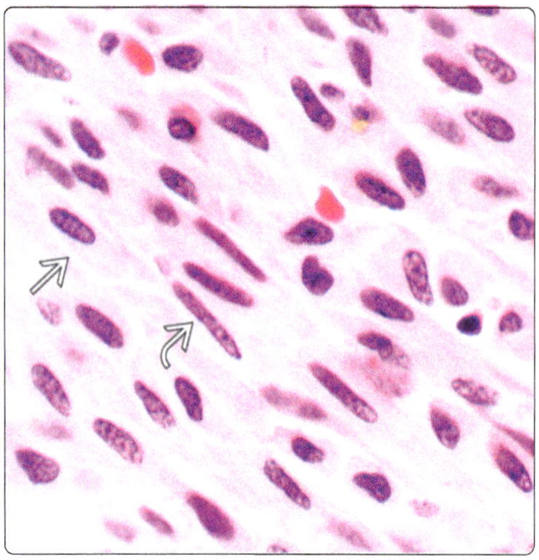

Systemic Mastocytosis: Mast Cell Tryptase

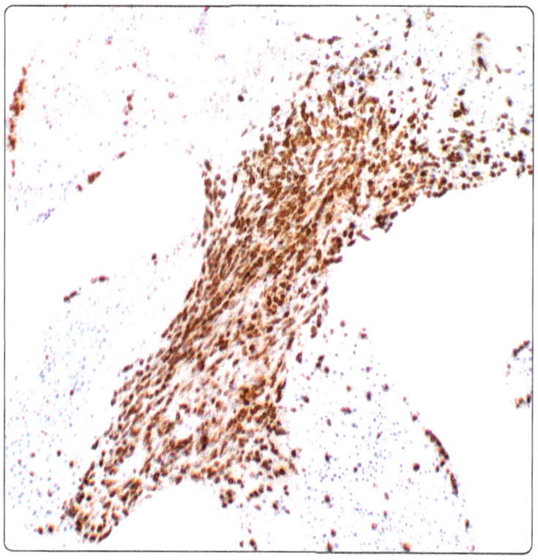

(Left) *Atypical mast cells forming a cohesive aggregate in a bone marrow core biopsy are shown at high power. Note the spindle-shaped nuclei ➡ and the prominent cell borders ➡ that are typical of mast cell infiltrates.* **(Right)** *Mast cell tryptase shows positive cytoplasmic reactivity in the mast cells that are forming an atypical cohesive aggregate in this core biopsy specimen. The findings are consistent with a diagnosis of SM.*

Extracutaneous Mastocytoma: CD2 Stain

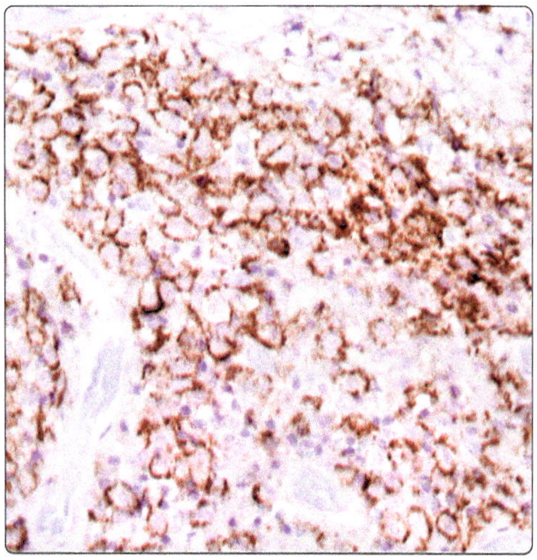

Systemic Mastocytosis: CD25 Stain

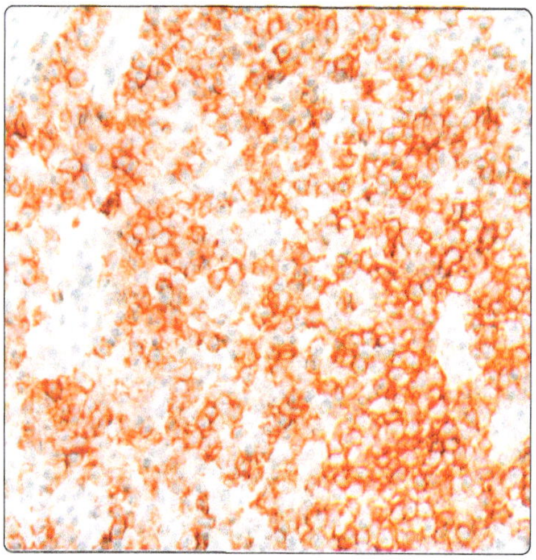

(Left) *An extracutaneous mastocytoma involving soft tissue of the shoulder is shown. Immunohistochemistry for CD2 highlights the mast cells. CD2 expression by mast cells is aberrant and supports mast cell neoplasia. (Courtesy C. Bueso-Ramos, MD, PhD.)* **(Right)** *IHC for CD25 shows a compact cluster of mast cells in this bone marrow biopsy specimen. Reactivity of mast cells with CD25 fulfills a minor diagnostic criterion for the diagnosis of SM. (Courtesy C. Bueso-Ramos, MD, PhD.)*

Mast Cell Leukemia in Peripheral Blood Smear

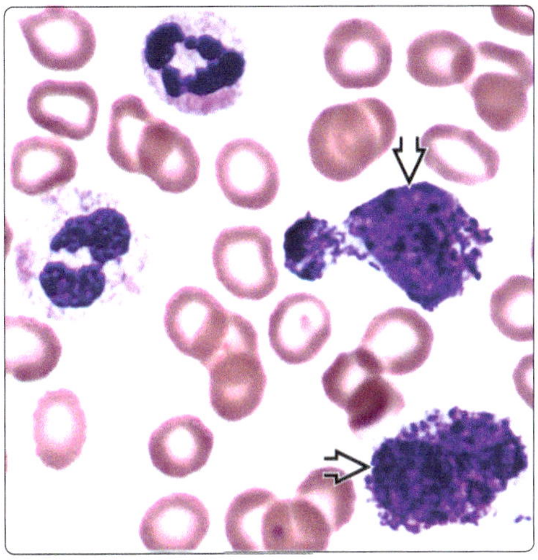

Mast Cell Leukemia in Bone Marrow

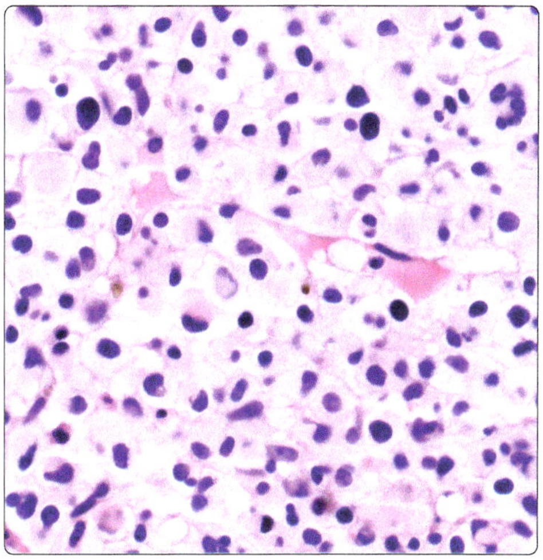

(Left) *Two circulating, well-granulated mast cells are seen in this smear from a patient with mast cell leukemia (MCL). "Leukemic" MCL typically shows > 10% circulating mast cells. (Courtesy K. Reichard, MD.)* **(Right)** *MCL is an aggressive form of mastocytosis and often a differential diagnostic consideration. In contrast to SM, the mast cells are more often round rather than spindled and account for ≥ 20% of BM aspirate nucleated cells. (Courtesy K. Reichard, MD.)*

Systemic Mastocytosis With AHNMD

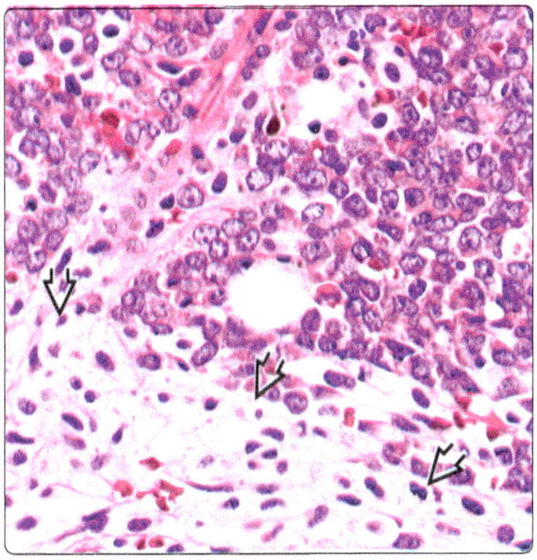

Systemic Mastocytosis in Spleen

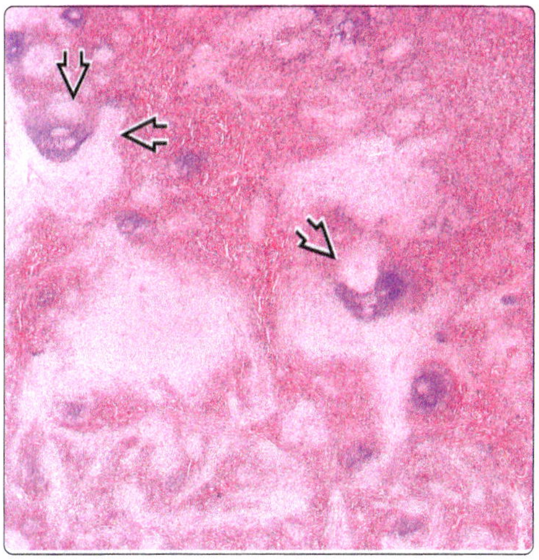

(Left) *Bone marrow shows a mast cell cluster adjacent to acute myeloid leukemia (AML) with t(8;21)(q22;q22), consistent with associated clonal hematological non-mast cell lineage disease. (Courtesy K. Reichard, MD.)* **(Right)** *Spleen in a patient with SM is shown. Note perifollicular pale mast cell aggregates. Characteristically patchy fibrosis is associated with and can obscure mast cells. (Courtesy C. Bueso-Ramos, MD, PhD.)*

Myelomastocytic Leukemia

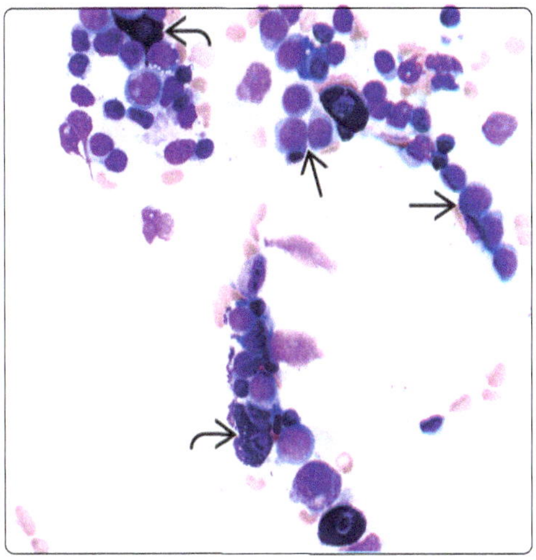

Mast Cell Hyperplasia: CD117 Stain

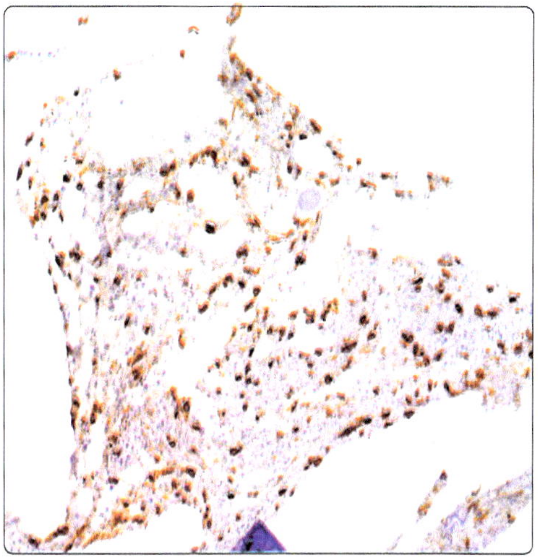

(Left) *Myelomastocytic leukemia is an exceedingly rare diagnosis. Myeloid blasts are a key component of the diagnosis along with neoplastic mast cells. (Courtesy K. Reichard, MD.)* **(Right)** *Mast cells are highlighted by a CD117 stain. Mast cell hyperplasia may occur after potent myeloablative chemotherapy or other massive toxic insult. In contrast to SM, the mast cells do not form compact aggregates. (Courtesy K. Reichard, MD.)*

PART II
SECTION 1
Benign Melanocytic Tumors (Nevi)

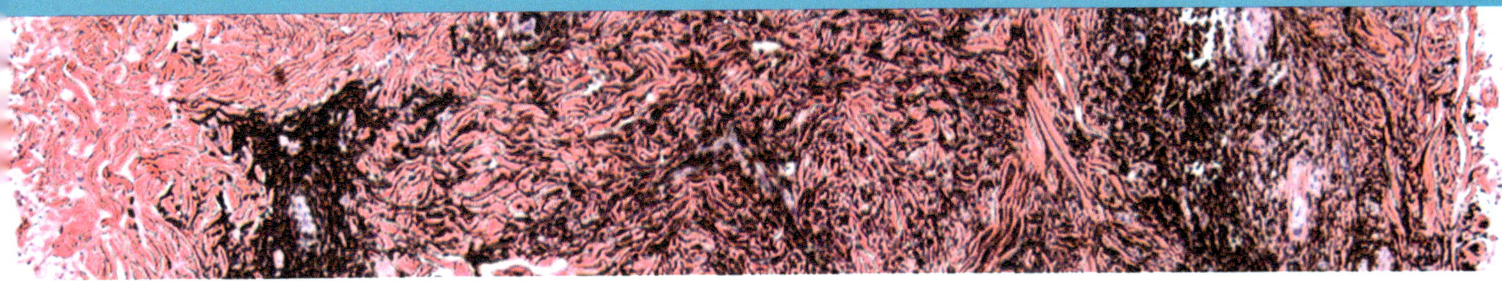

Congenital Melanocytic Nevi

KEY FACTS

CLINICAL ISSUES

- Present at birth, by definition
- However, some congenital melanocytic nevi may be tardive and not readily noticeable at birth
- Categorized by size
  - < 1.5 cm = small
  - > 1.5 cm to < 20 cm = medium
  - > 20 cm = large
- Risks, particularly for large congenital melanocytic nevus
  - ~ 5% risk of developing cutaneous melanoma
  - Neurocutaneous melanosis

MICROSCOPIC

- Melanocytes usually extend into lower reticular dermis and sometimes subcutaneous tissue
- Infiltration of
  - Arrector pili muscle
  - Adnexal structures
  - Nerves
- Clustering around blood vessels
- Cells become smaller and more dispersed with depth
- Nodular proliferations (more common in large nevi)
  - Based in dermis, no epidermal involvement or necrosis

TOP DIFFERENTIAL DIAGNOSES

- Acquired melanocytic nevi: Not present at birth
  - Usually limited to upper 1/2 of reticular dermis)
- Atypical (dysplastic/Clark) melanocytic nevi: Not present at birth
  - Junctional component shows cytologic atypia, bridging, and lateral extension beyond intradermal cells, which are often limited to upper 1/2 of reticular dermis
- Malignant melanoma arising in congenital nevus
  - In differential diagnosis of dermal nodular proliferation, very rare if age is < 1 yr
  - Well-demarcated, highly cellular nodules of atypical epithelioid to spindled cells with cytologic atypia; nuclear pleomorphism and necrosis often present

Congenital Melanocytic Nevus

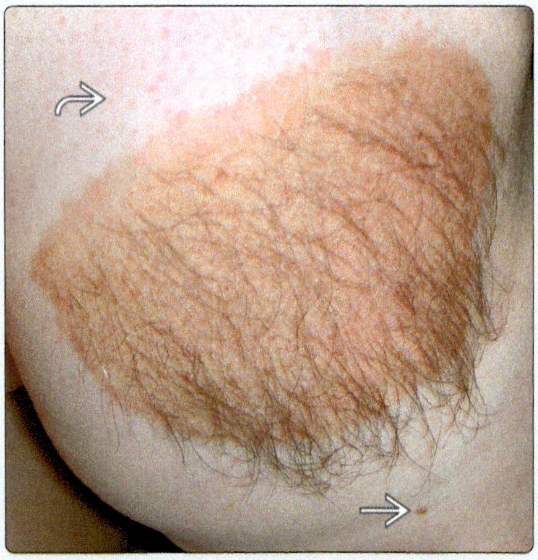

Compound, Predominantly Intradermal Congenital Nevus

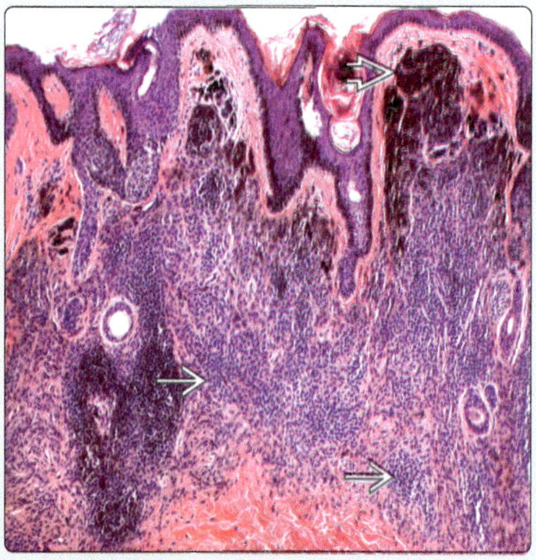

***(Left)** This light tan, medium-sized congenital melanocytic nevus, which measured 10 x 8 cm, has coarse terminal hairs within it. The patient also has keratosis pilaris and an acquired melanocytic nevus. **(Right)** This congenital compound nevus has nests of larger, more heavily pigmented superficial cells progressing to smaller, less pigmented cells deeper in the dermis, consistent with maturation with dermal descent.*

Congenital Intradermal Nevus

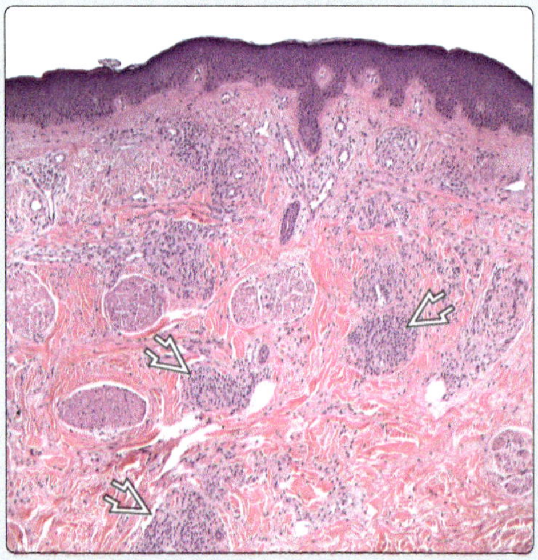

Congenital Junctional Nevus

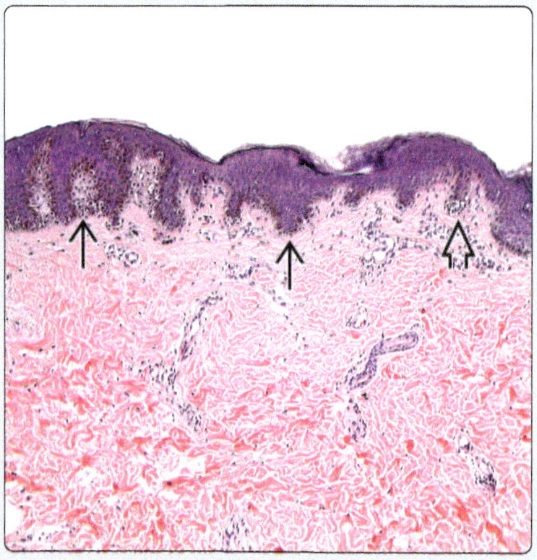

***(Left)** This congenital intradermal melanocytic nevus extends deeply throughout the dermis, with clustering of melanocytes around vessels and adnexa. **(Right)** Some congenital nevi, especially if small, may be purely junctional, with scattered nests and single melanocytes at the tips and sides of rete, mimicking an acquired junctional melanocytic nevus.*

TERMINOLOGY

Synonyms

- Giant/bathing suit/garment-type melanocytic nevus

CLINICAL ISSUES

Epidemiology

- Incidence
  - 1% of newborns
- Age
  - Present at birth, by definition
  - However, some congenital melanocytic nevi may be tardive
    - Not readily noticeable at birth; usually become more obvious with age (generally by age 2)

Presentation

- Categorized by size
  - Small
    - < 1.5-cm diameter
    - Round to oval, symmetric
    - Color is variation of brown; may be speckled
    - Surface may be pebbled &/or hairy
  - Medium
    - > 1.5-cm, < 20-cm diameter
    - Round to oval, symmetric; color is brown to black, may be speckled
    - Surface may be pebbled &/or hairy
  - Large
    - > 20-cm diameter
    - Often involves back; dark color, brown to black
    - Surface thickened with increased hair; may make it difficult to follow these lesions for changes over time
    - Satellite nevi often present
    - Underlying soft tissue hypertrophy may be present
    - Proliferative nodules, usually < 5 mm in diameter, may develop with time

Treatment

- Sometimes completely excised (if possible) for cosmetic purposes or to reduce risk of melanoma
- Nodules developing within congenital melanocytic nevi
  - At the least: Should be biopsied and followed clinically
  - May be judicious to conservatively excise and follow clinically

Prognosis

- Risk of developing cutaneous malignant melanoma in congenital melanocytic nevi
  - Risk highest for large subtype, estimated at ~ 5%; median age: ~ 5 years (average age: ~ 13 years)
  - Risk quite low (to possibly none) in small to medium subtypes
- Patients with large congenital melanocytic nevi on head/neck/trunk
  - At risk for neurocutaneous melanosis, also with risk for primary central nervous system melanoma

MICROSCOPIC

Histologic Features

- May be heterogeneous within 1 lesion
- Epidermis may be normal or hyperplastic
  - Lentiginous array of melanocytes may be seen
  - Focal pagetoid scatter may be present
- Small congenital melanocytic nevi may be junctional only
- Most nevi extend into lower reticular dermis and sometimes subcutaneous tissue
- Dermal involvement
  - Occasionally periadnexal or perivascular predominant in small nevi
  - Generally diffuse and interstitial
  - Rows of single melanocytes between collagen bundles
  - Infiltration of arrector pili muscle, adnexal structures, and nerves, with clustering around vessels
  - Cells become smaller with depth and less dense (maturation)
- Nodular proliferations (more common in large nevi)
  - Variable morphology of melanocytes (spindled, epithelioid, round)
  - Nodule not well demarcated from (blends into) surrounding nevus
  - Lack of epidermal involvement and necrosis
  - Mitoses may be prominent
  - Cytologic atypia usually not prominent
- Large lesions may contain bone, cartilage, fat, vascular proliferation

Cytologic Features

- Melanocytes, particularly junctional, may show slightly enlarged nuclei with small nucleoli

DIFFERENTIAL DIAGNOSIS

Acquired Melanocytic Nevi

- History (not present at birth) may be key
- Generally do not extend as deeply as congenital nevi (i.e., limited to upper 1/2 of reticular dermis)
- Dermal involvement with only periadnexal/perivascular clusters of melanocytes seen more commonly in congenital nevi

Atypical (Dysplastic/Clark) Melanocytic Nevi

- History (not present at birth) may be key
- Junctional component shows cytologic atypia, bridging, and lateral extension beyond intradermal cells
- Generally limited to upper 1/2 of reticular dermis

Melanoma Arising in a Congenital Nevus

- In differential diagnosis of dermal nodular proliferation
- Very rare if age is < 1 yr
- Well-demarcated, highly cellular nodules of atypical epithelioid to spindled cells with cytologic atypia
- Nuclear pleomorphism and necrosis often present

SELECTED REFERENCES

1. Magaña M et al: Congenital melanocytic nevus: two clinicopathological forms. Am J Dermatopathol. 37(1):31-7, 2015
2. Shah KN: The risk of melanoma and neurocutaneous melanosis associated with congenital melanocytic nevi. Semin Cutan Med Surg. 29(3):159-64, 2010

Common Acquired Melanocytic Nevi

KEY FACTS

TERMINOLOGY

- Benign melanocytic nevus, junctional melanocytic nevus, compound melanocytic nevus, intradermal melanocytic nevus, common melanocytic nevus

ETIOLOGY/PATHOGENESIS

- Believed by some to arise from intraepidermal melanocytes

CLINICAL ISSUES

- Not present at birth
- Majority develop in adolescence
- Increase with age up to 3rd decade

MICROSCOPIC

- Flat surface to slightly raised to polypoid
- Epidermis varies (e.g., thin or seborrheic keratosis-like)
- Well circumscribed
- Generally symmetrical from side to side
- Melanocytes arranged in regular clusters/nests, particularly at junction
- Mitoses generally absent
- Melanin pigment often limited to junctional or superficial dermal nests
- Dermal maturation: Type A nevus cells superficially, type B and C nevus cells in dermis
  - Type A nevus cells: Epithelioid
  - Type B nevus cells: Lymphocytoid
  - Type C nevus cells: Spindled, neuroid

TOP DIFFERENTIAL DIAGNOSES

- Atypical/dysplastic nevus
- Congenital melanocytic nevus
- DDx of junctional lentiginous melanocytic nevus
  - Lentigo
- DDx of intradermal nevus (especially neurotized)
  - Neurofibroma

Acquired Junctional Nevus

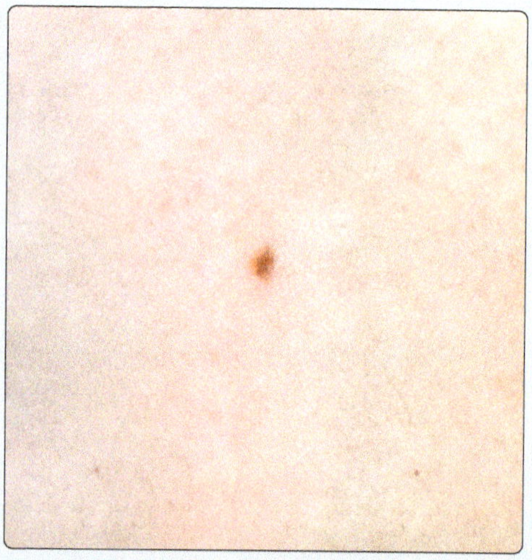

Junctional Nevus With Pigment Incontinence

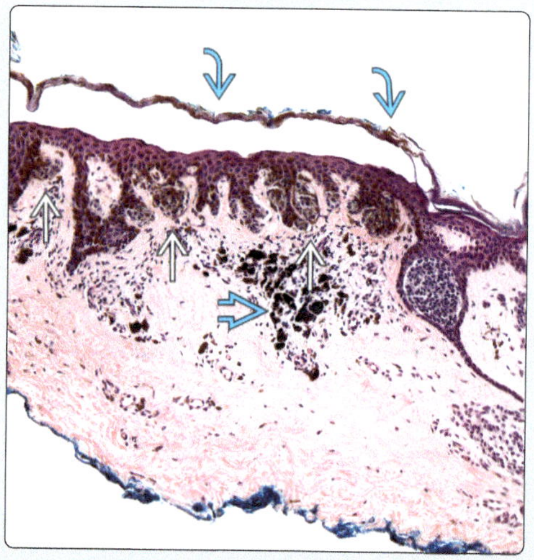

(Left) *This clinical photo shows a nevus as an oval macule with even, light brown pigmentation. There is overall symmetry with a smooth border; the size was measured to be 2 x 1 mm.* **(Right)** *This junctional melanocytic nevus shows nests at the tips of rete ridges. The presence of pigmented parakeratosis and pigment incontinence likely corresponds to a dark color clinically.*

Junctional Nevus at Higher Magnification

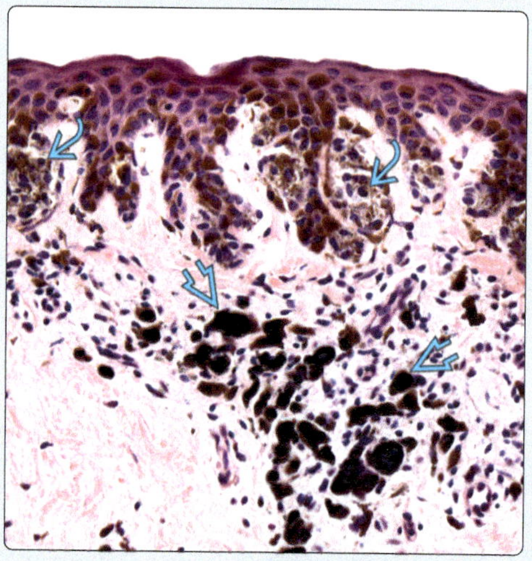

Compound Nevus With Congenital Features

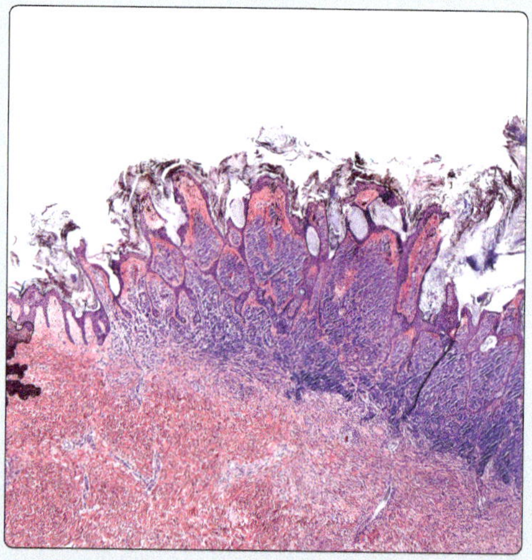

(Left) *Higher magnification of the same junctional nevus shows nests of regular size with > 3-5 melanocytes. Note the small, hyperchromatic-staining nuclei. The nuclei of dermal melanophages are usually not detectable due to heavy cytoplasmic melanin.* **(Right)** *This compound melanocytic nevus shows overlying epidermal hyperplasia. This configuration has been labeled by some authors as "Unna nevus" or "keratotic melanocytic nevus."*

TERMINOLOGY

Synonyms

- Junctional melanocytic nevus, compound melanocytic nevus, intradermal melanocytic nevus, common mole, common melanocytic nevus, nevocellular nevus

ETIOLOGY/PATHOGENESIS

Exact Etiology Unknown

- Believed by some to arise from intraepidermal melanocytes
- Others have suggested that melanocytic nevi arise from nerves or pluripotential cells

Tumor vs. Hamartoma

- Still debated
- Evidence for tumor
  - Studies showing that some nevi are clonal
  - Growth advantage of nevus cells over epidermal, dendritic melanocytes in cell culture
  - Similar expression of different markers by nevi and malignant melanoma
  - Presence of mutations in *BRAF* oncogene in majority of nevi (> 80%)
- Evidence for hamartoma
  - Other proliferative elements: Epidermal, follicular, sebaceous and connective tissue
  - Studies showing that some nevi are polyclonal

CLINICAL ISSUES

Epidemiology

- Incidence
  - Number of acquired nevi
    - Increases with age up to 3rd decade
    - May be related to familial predisposition
    - Sun exposure in childhood also linked to development of nevi
    - More common in lighter skinned individuals
- Age
  - Not present at birth
  - Majority develop in adolescence
  - Density of nevi generally decreases after 4th decade

Presentation

- Junctional lesions
  - Flat to minimally raised macule/very thin papule
  - Generally < 6 mm, but may be larger
  - Color often variation of brown
- Compound lesions
  - Slightly raised papule
  - Variable color (brown, flesh-colored, pink)
  - May contain hair
- Intradermal lesions
  - Papule, may be pedunculated
  - Variable color (brown, skin-colored, pink)
  - May contain hair

Natural History

- Abtropfung hypothesis of Unna
  - Melanocytes are initially junctional
  - With chronologic time (aging), melanocytes drop off into dermis, creating compound melanocytic lesions
  - With more time, junctional melanocytes may have all dropped off, creating intradermal melanocytic lesions
  - Intradermal melanocytic lesions may eventually shed or become acrochordons
    - Degenerative changes include balloon cell change and fatty change
- Alternative hypothesis
  - Nevi begin in dermis
- Not all melanocytic nevi display progressive changes; some arrest at given stage indefinitely
- Melanocytic nevi can undergo clinical and histopathologic changes during pregnancy, as well as after various forms of surgical and nonsurgical trauma

Prognosis

- Benign; very low risk of transformation to melanoma

MICROSCOPIC

Histologic Features

- Flat surface to slightly raised to polypoid
- Well circumscribed
- Melanocytes arranged in nests at tip of retes, particularly at junction of epidermis and dermis and superficial dermis
- Nest defined as cluster of at least 3 (some authors) or 5 (other authors) melanocytes
- Generally symmetrical from side to side
- Orderly arrangement of nests at junction and in superficial dermis
- Regular nest size
- Cell and nest size sometimes enlarged in younger patients
- Junctional component, when present
  - Often ends peripherally with nests
  - Nests centered at tips and sometimes sides of rete
  - Variable numbers of single, rounded melanocytes present in basal layer (may predominate in junctional lentiginous melanocytic nevus)
  - Pagetoid spread unusual (may be seen in nevi of special sites and irritated/traumatized nevi), look for parakeratosis
- Intradermal component, when present, matures with increasing dermal depth
  - Melanocytes near base are smaller in diameter (type B, lymphocytoid) than those in superficial dermis (type A, epithelioid), i.e., maturation
    - Superficial dermis: Type A cells: Epithelioid with pink to finely pigmented cytoplasm and oval to round nuclei, sometimes with small nucleoli; multinucleate cells (with clustered nuclei or wreath-like arrangement of nuclei) may also be seen
    - Toward base of lesion: Type B cells: Lymphocyte-like with round, blue nuclei and little cytoplasm
    - Base of lesion may be composed of type C cells: Spindled and neural in appearance (these cells predominate in neurotized nevus)
- Mitoses generally absent
- Melanin pigment often limited to junctional or superficial dermal nests
- Specific patterns that may be present
  - Pseudovascular pattern

- Melanocytes line empty spaces, giving appearance of vessels
- Degenerative pattern
  - a.k.a., fatty change or lipomatous differentiation
  - Lipocytes are interspersed among melanocytes
  - Degeneration may also manifest with balloon cells or sebocyte-like cells; these have prominent, vacuolated cytoplasm
- Additional findings that may be seen include
  - Dermal ossification
    - Termed "nevus of Nanta"
  - Epidermal spongiosis
    - Termed Meyerson nevus
  - Epidermal hyperplasia that resembles seborrheic keratosis
    - Term keratotic melanocytic nevus proposed by some
  - Stromal desmoplasia
    - Termed desmoplastic (sclerotic) melanocytic nevus
  - Bizarre cells with enlarged nuclei in dermis with generally absent mitoses
    - Termed ancient melanocytic nevus

Cytologic Features

- Type A nevus cells
  - Epithelioid
    - Pink to light blue cytoplasm
    - Oval, pale nucleus
    - May see intranuclear pseudoinclusion: Lighter staining around area within nucleus
- Type B nevus cells
  - Lymphocytoid
    - Little cytoplasm
    - Round, blue nucleus
    - May see intranuclear pseudoinclusion: Lighter staining round area within nucleus
- Type C nevus cells
  - Spindle-shaped with pink cytoplasm (can appear neural)
- Multinucleate cells
  - Arrangement of nuclei
    - Wreath-like (Touton giant cell-like)
    - Clumped (mulberry-type)

DIFFERENTIAL DIAGNOSIS

Atypical (Dysplastic or Clark) Nevus

- In compound lesions, junctional component extends beyond dermal component (shoulder phenomenon)
- Bridging of nests across rete ridges
- Nest size variable and irregular
- Single melanocytes often seen between nests
- May be asymmetric side to side
- Papillary dermal fibrosis (lamellar and concentric)
- Perivascular lymphocytes
- Dermal component, if present, shows maturation
- Deep mitoses absent
- Cytologically, melanocytes may show enlarged nuclei with nucleoli and increased cytoplasm; cytoplasm may be finely pigmented (smoky)

Congenital Melanocytic Nevus

- History (present at birth) may be key
- Often deeper than acquired melanocytic nevi
- Melanocytes
  - May involve and track down arrector pili muscle
  - May cluster around vessels/adnexal structures
  - Often splay singly through collagen toward base

Combined Nevus

- Banal or "ordinary" junctional, compound, or intradermal melanocytic nevus
- Additionally, 2nd type of nevus (most commonly blue nevus but may also be deep-penetrating or Spitz nevus type) present

Lentigo (Simplex or Solar)

- In differential diagnosis of junctional lentiginous melanocytic nevus
- Increased number of single melanocytes in basal layer of epidermis may be seen in some cases
- Nests of melanocytes absent

Neurofibroma

- In differential of intradermal nevus with extensive neurotization
- Fragmented collagen, so-called shredded carrots appearance, darker than stroma
- Short, spindled cells with tapered nuclei in light pink stroma
- Lacks nests/clusters of melanocytic cells

Nevoid Melanoma

- May be in differential of ancient melanocytic nevus
- Presence of cytologic atypia, pleomorphism, and mitotic activity; lack of maturation
- Mitoses and inflammation uncommonly present in ancient melanocytic nevus

Desmoplastic Melanoma

- In differential of desmoplastic (sclerotic) melanocytic nevus
- Overlying changes of melanoma in situ often present
- Atypical spindled cells with hyperchromatic-staining nuclei infiltrate dermis
- Perivascular and interstitial lymphocytes often present

SELECTED REFERENCES

1. Sardana K et al: Optimal management of common acquired melanocytic nevi (moles): current perspectives. Clin Cosmet Investig Dermatol. 7:89-103, 2014
2. Wilford CE et al: Atypical histopathologic features in a melanocytic nevus after cryotherapy and pregnancy. J Cutan Pathol. 41(10):802-5, 2014
3. Karram S et al: Predictors of BRAF mutation in melanocytic nevi: analysis across regions with different UV radiation exposure. Am J Dermatopathol. 35(4):412-8, 2013
4. Yeh I et al: Clonal BRAF mutations in melanocytic nevi and initiating role of BRAF in melanocytic neoplasia. J Natl Cancer Inst. 105(12):917-9, 2013
5. Kerl H et al: Ancient melanocytic nevus: a simulator of malignant melanoma. Am J Dermatopathol. 33(2):127-30, 2011
6. Barnhill RL et al: State of the art, nomenclature, and points of consensus and controversy concerning benign melanocytic lesions: outcome of an international workshop. Adv Anat Pathol. 17(2):73-90, 2010
7. Tokuda Y et al: Histogenesis of congenital and acquired melanocytic nevi based on histological study of lesion size and thickness. J Dermatol. 37(12):1011-8, 2010
8. Takata M et al: Genetic alterations in melanocytic tumors. J Dermatol Sci. 43(1):1-10, 2006

Compound Nevus With Congenital Features

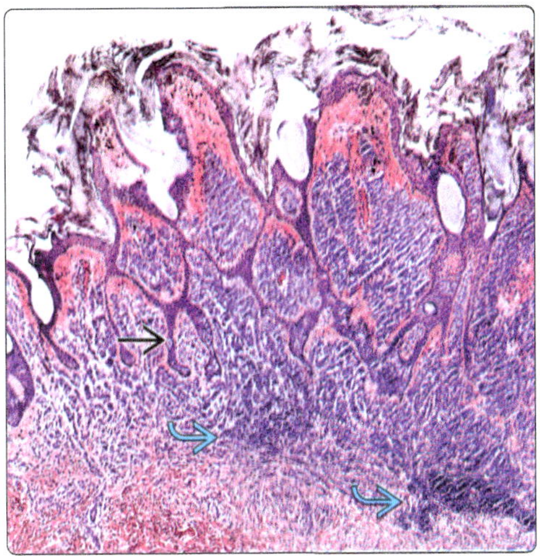

Intradermal Nevus With Congenital Features

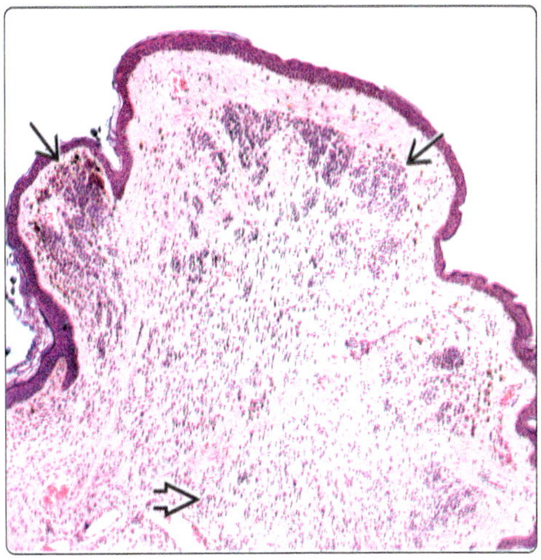

(Left) *There are a few intraepidermal nests. The dermal melanocytes mature with increasing dermal depth. In this maturation process, the nevus cells become smaller to resemble lymphocytes, i.e., type B or lymphocytoid melanocytes.* **(Right)** *This polypoid intradermal melanocytic nevus shows dermal melanocytes with a congenital pattern and maturation. There are nested, larger melanocytes near the surface, and smaller, more oval to spindle-shaped melanocytes toward the base.*

Intradermal Nevus With Congenital Features

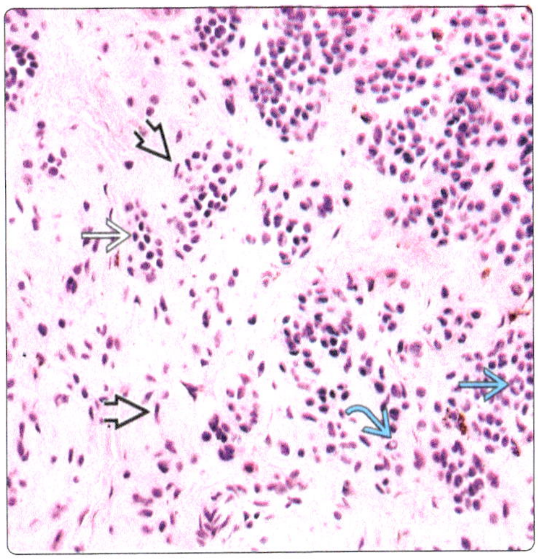

Maturation in Dermal Component

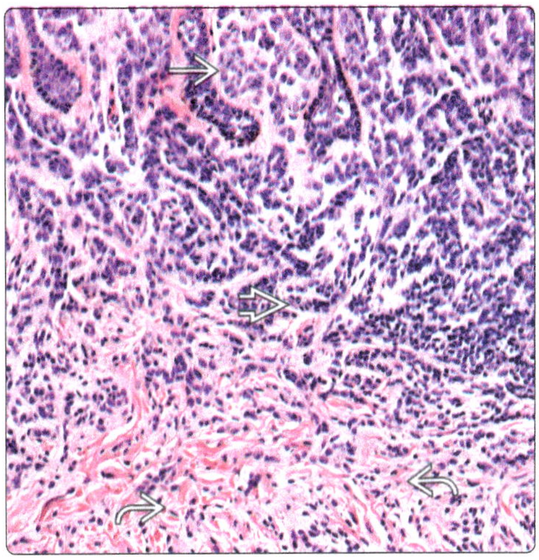

(Left) *Type B (lymphocytoid) and type C (spindled) cells are shown. Note the focal pseudonuclear inclusions and rare multinucleate cells.* **(Right)** *In another example of proper maturation, the dermal component matures from superficial nested type A (epithelioid) to type B (small, lymphocytoid) to type C (spindled/neuroid) cells at the base.*

Balloon Cell Nevus

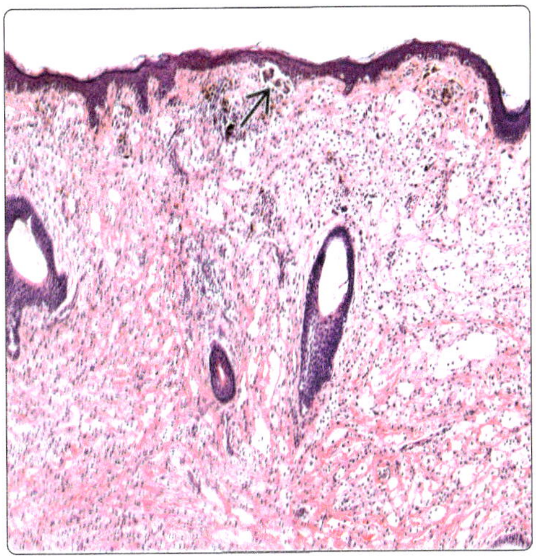

Balloon Cell Nevus at High Magnification

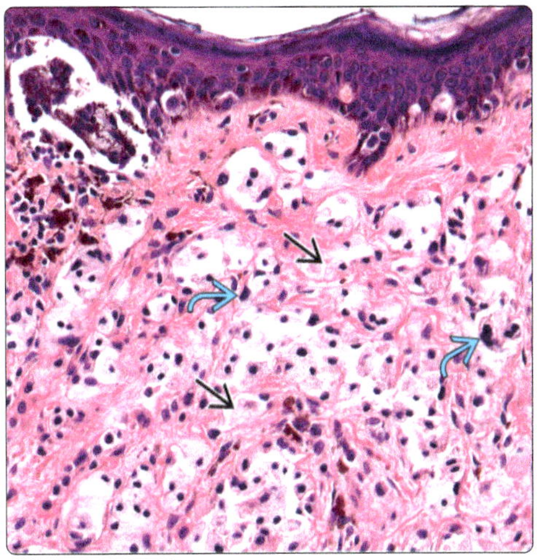

(Left) *This is a compound balloon cell nevus. The balloon (or sebocyte-like) cells are a degenerative phenomenon. There are a few remaining junctional nests of pigmented melanocytes present.* **(Right)** *Higher magnification shows that the balloon cells (sebocyte-like cells) have foamy/vacuolated cytoplasm and pyknotic, hyperchromatic nuclei. Note the lack of nuclear pleomorphism or mitotic figures.*

KEY FACTS

TERMINOLOGY

- Blue nevus (BN)
- Dendritic BN, common BN, sclerotic BN
- Benign melanocytic tumor composed of spindle-shaped and dendritic melanocytes and melanophages
- Heterogeneous group of acquired and congenital melanocytic tumors

CLINICAL ISSUES

- Occur in any age; wide range of locations
- Well-demarcated, slightly raised papules (< 1 cm in diameter)
- Color ranges from blue to gray to blue-black to black
- Excellent prognosis; no significant malignant potential

MICROSCOPIC

- Well-demarcated, wedge-shaped dermal melanocytic tumor with variable amount of collagenosis
- Hypocellular lesions, but can grow in short fascicles with overlying grenz zone
- Dermal sclerosis with variable amount of collagen in tumor stroma
- Heavy to sometimes light mixture of melanophages
- Variants include melanotic BN, sclerotic BN, and agminated BN (multiple adjacent similar satellite lesions)
- **Cytologic features**
  - Variable amount of granular melanin in cytoplasm and within dendritic processes
  - Minimal nuclear atypia and pleomorphism
  - Mitotic figures are rare to absent
- May present as 1 component in combined nevi

TOP DIFFERENTIAL DIAGNOSES

- Desmoplastic Spitz nevus
- Desmoplastic acquired melanocytic nevus
- Desmoplastic melanoma
- Dermatofibroma

Clinical Photograph of Blue Nevus on Forehead

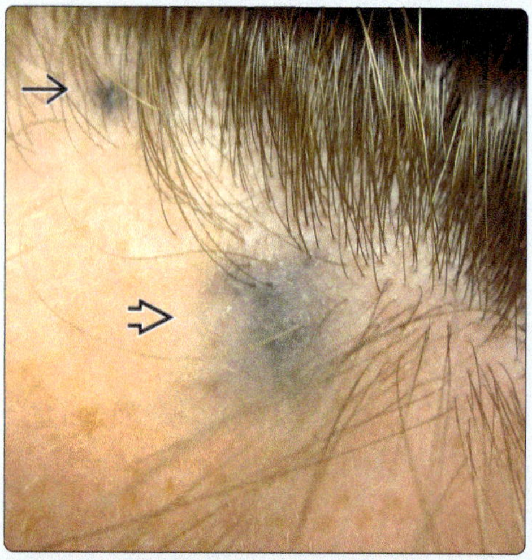

Blue Nevus Dermoscopy

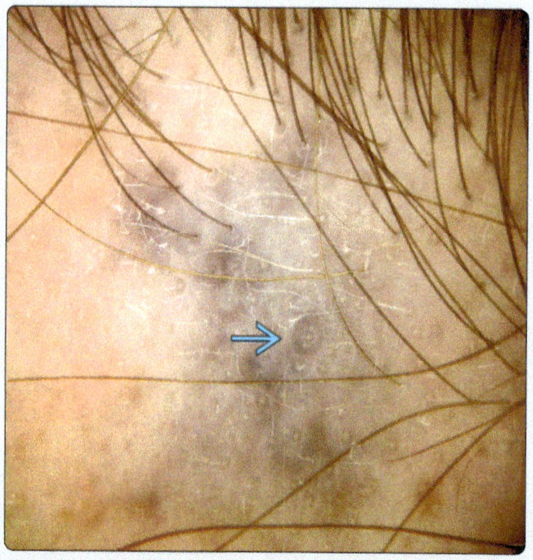

(Left) *Clinically, blue nevus (BN) can appear as a blue to gray patch or macule, resembling a bruise or graphite tattoo. There are 2 such lesions seen on the hairline of this individual; a small macule ➔ and an adjacent larger patch ⇨. (Courtesy J. Finch MD.)* **(Right)** *BN under dermoscopy shows an intact, evenly pigmented reticular pattern. It shows a jagged outline with perifollicular accentuation ➔. It is evenly pigmented. (Courtesy J. Finch MD.)*

Scanning Magnification of Blue Nevus

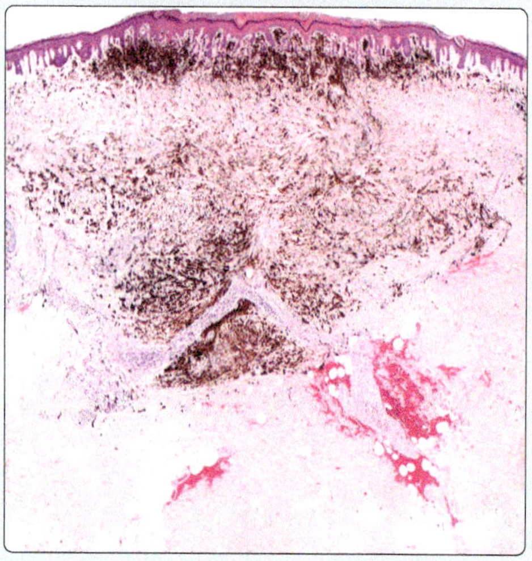

High Magnification of Blue Nevus

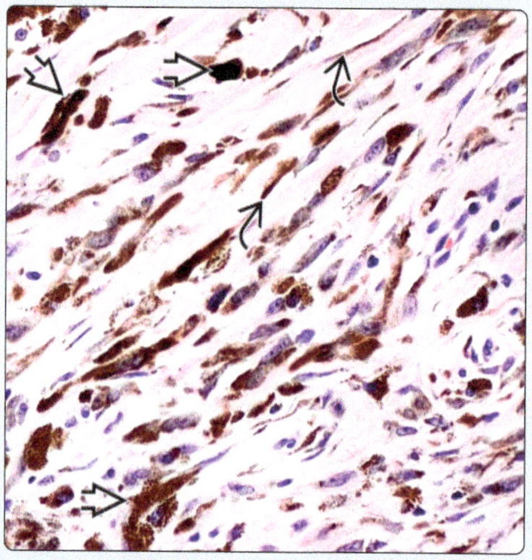

(Left) *Scanning magnification of a BN shows a symmetrical, wedge-shaped, and evenly pigmented melanocytic tumor present throughout the dermis. This is heavily melanized.* **(Right)** *High-power magnification of a conventional BN shows 2 cell types: Spindled to dendritic melanocytes ⇨, which possess long dendritic processes, and melanophages. These cells have abundant, heavily pigmented cytoplasm, often masking the nuclei ⇨.*

TERMINOLOGY

Abbreviations

- Blue nevus (BN)

Synonyms

- Dendritic BN, common BN, sclerotic BN

Definitions

- Heterogeneous group of acquired and congenital melanocytic tumors
- Composed predominantly of spindled to dendritic-shaped melanocytes
- Varying degrees of cellularity, melanin pigment, and dermal sclerosis

ETIOLOGY/PATHOGENESIS

Developmental Anomaly

- May represent aberrant melanocytic precursor migration in development

CLINICAL ISSUES

Epidemiology

- Incidence
  - Very common
  - Predilection for females
- Age
  - Principally in children
  - However, can occur later in life at any age

Site

- Most occur in skin, commonly on extremities and face
  - Backs of hands and feet, buttocks, face, and scalp
- Other documented extracutaneous anatomic sites include
  - Subungual region, orbit, conjunctiva, oral cavity

Presentation

- Well-demarcated, slightly raised papule or nodule (< 1 cm in diameter)
- Range in color from blue to gray to blue-black to black
- Sclerosing variants appear hypopigmented

Treatment

- Surgical approaches
  - Simple excision

Prognosis

- Excellent; no significant malignant potential

MICROSCOPIC

Histologic Features

- Hypocellular lesions, but can grow in short fascicles with overlying grenz zone
- Dermal sclerosis with variable amount of collagen in tumor stroma
- Ill-defined dermal or submucosal proliferation of 2 cell types
  - Elongated melanocytes with spindled and fine dendritic processes
  - Melanophages with coarse cytoplasmic melanin pigment
- Variants
  - Amelanotic BN (lack of significant pigmentation)
  - Sclerotic BN (prominent stromal sclerosis)
  - Agminated BN (multiple adjacent similar satellite lesions)
  - May present as 1 component in combined nevi

Cytologic Features

- Melanocytes
  - Bipolar, spindled-shaped
  - Elongated dendritic processes
  - Variable amount of granular melanin in cytoplasm and within dendritic processes
  - Minimal nuclear atypia
  - Mitotic figures are almost always absent
- Melanophages
  - Round, ample cytoplasm
  - Abundant, coarse cytoplasmic melanin pigment
  - Nuclei difficult to see due to heavy melanin pigment

DIFFERENTIAL DIAGNOSIS

DDx of Sclerosing (Desmoplastic) Blue Nevus

- Desmoplastic Spitz nevus
- Desmoplastic acquired melanocytic nevus
- Desmoplastic melanoma
  - Immunostains for HMB-45 and MART-1/Melan-A are usually negative in desmoplastic melanoma but positive in BN
- Dermatofibroma
  - Mixture of spindled and histiocytic-appearing cells with vacuolated cytoplasm
  - Overlying epidermal hyperplasia with basilar hyperpigmentation
  - Pigmented cells can be present, but contain hemosiderin [Fe(+)], not melanin

DDx of Amelanotic Blue Nevus

- Dermatofibroma
  - Mixture of spindled and histiocytic-appearing cells with vacuolated cytoplasm
  - Overlying epidermal hyperplasia with basilar hyperpigmentation

DIAGNOSTIC CHECKLIST

Clinically Relevant Pathologic Features

- Slate-gray to blue round papule/macule

Pathologic Interpretation Pearls

- Typically heavily pigmented, should see ill-defined dermal spindle cell to dendritic proliferation associated with sclerotic collagen
- Under high-power magnification, search for dendritic processes originating from elongated cells

SELECTED REFERENCES

1. Zembowicz A et al: Blue nevi and variants: an update. Arch Pathol Lab Med. 135(3):327-36, 2011
2. Murali R et al: Blue nevi and related lesions: a review highlighting atypical and newly described variants, distinguishing features and diagnostic pitfalls. Adv Anat Pathol. 16(6):365-82, 2009
3. Massi G et al: Histological diagnosis of nevi and melanoma. Darmstadt, Germany: Steinkopff Verlag, 2004

(Left) *Dermoscopic image shows an evenly pigmented patch with a well-defined rim. (Courtesy J. Finch, MD.)* **(Right)** *This black to blue papule on the left chin of an elderly woman shows a darkly and evenly pigmented papule ⇨, which has sharply defined edges. This is in contrast to a lightly pigmented macule of solar lentigo →. (Courtesy J. Finch, MD.)*

Dermoscopy of Blue Nevus

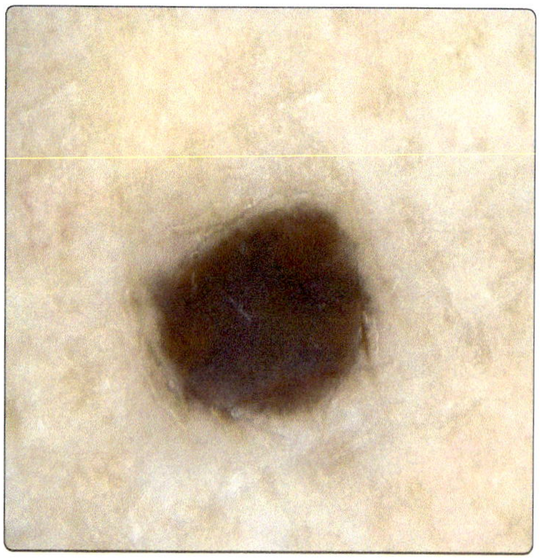

Clinical Image of Blue Nevus

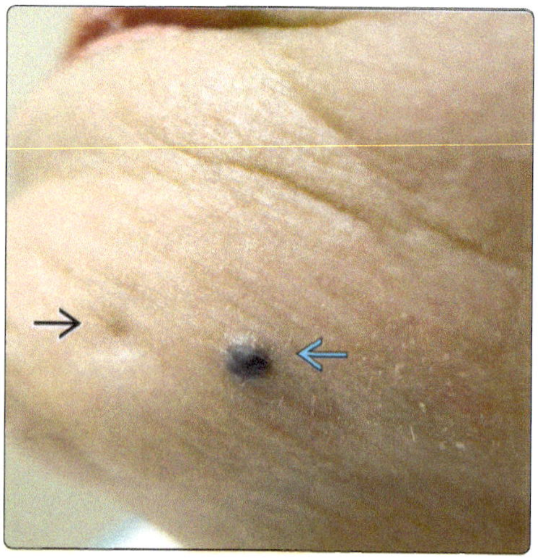

(Left) *Combined nevus has a similar clinical appearance ➡ to conventional BN but histologically is composed of more than 1 population of melanocytes. (Courtesy J. Finch, MD.)* **(Right)** *Under low-power examination, there are 2 distinct areas of heavy ⇧ and light → pigmentation. The lesional cells intimately involve the adnexa, which are intact. In this example of combined intradermal and BN, the type B intradermal nevus cells ↪ are seen in the superficial dermis.*

Clinical Image of Combined Nevus

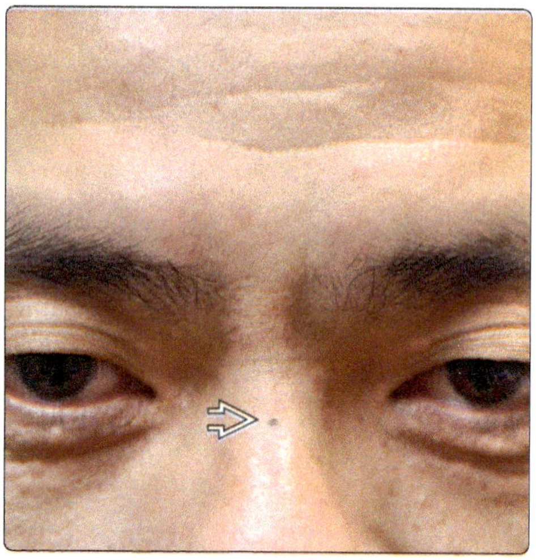

Combined Nevus at Low Magnification

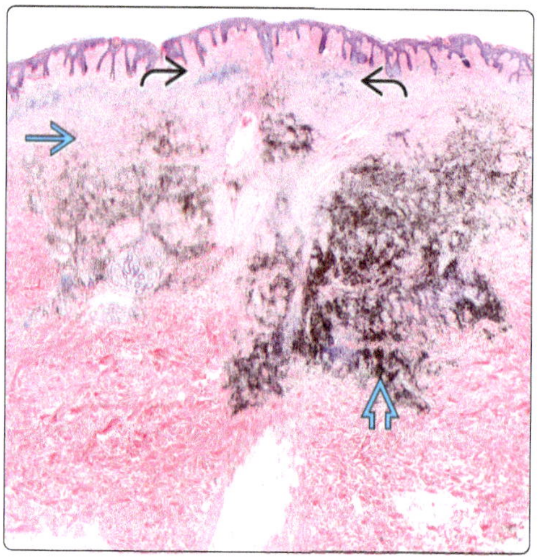

(Left) *Medium-power examination shows dendritic spindle cells wrapping around collagen bundles ↪, mimicking a dermatofibroma. The melanocytic proliferation is deeply penetrating to reticular collage, resembling a deep penetrating nevus. The neurovascular bundles ⇨ and the adnexa → are intact.* **(Right)** *There are lightly melanized spindle cells with delicate dendritic processes ↪ and some melanophages ⇨ under higher magnification. Note the trapped collagen bundles ⇨.*

Combined Nevus at Intermediate Magnification

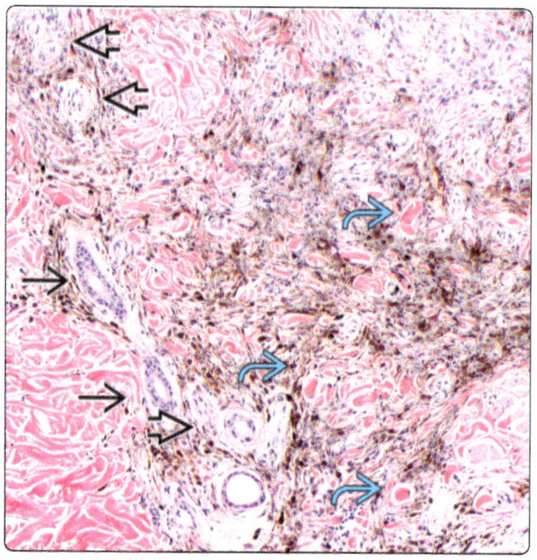

Combined Nevus at High Magnification

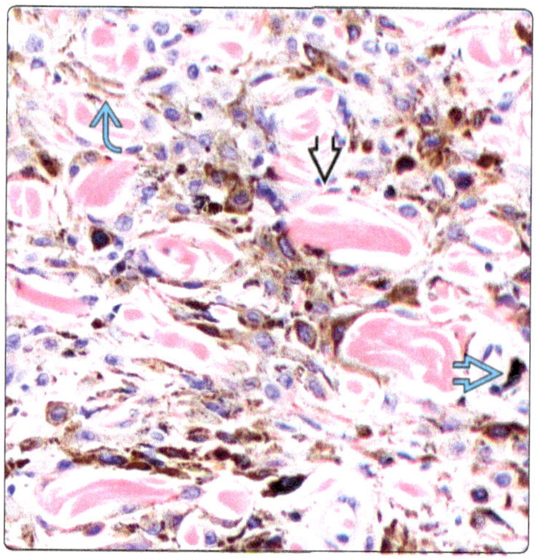

Sclerotic Blue Nevus

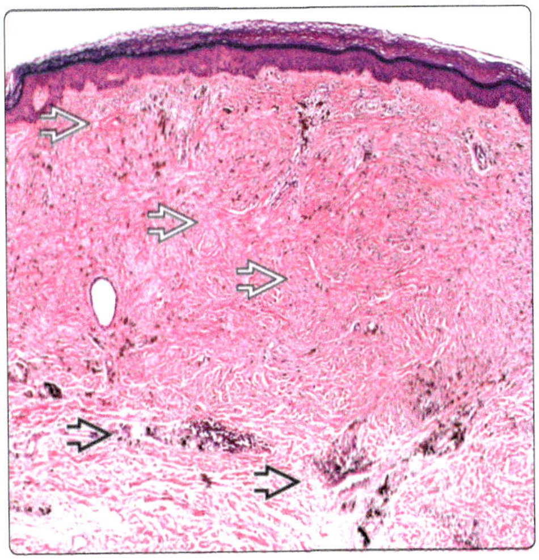

High Magnification of Sclerotic Blue Nevus

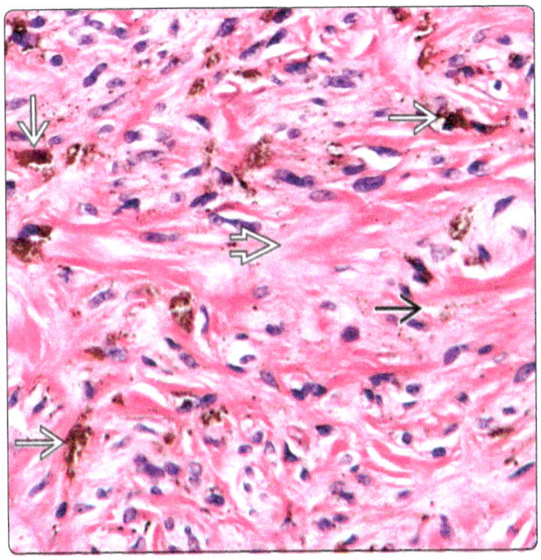

(Left) *This is an example of a BN showing pronounced hyalinizing collagenosis in the stroma, typical of a sclerotic variant. Note the decreased number of melanocytes and increased dense collagenous stroma. Melanophages are evident at the base of the lesion.* **(Right)** *High-power magnification of a BN demonstrates prominent sclerotic collagen in the tumor stroma and scattered melanophages. The delicate dendritic processes are evident.*

High Magnification of Blue Nevus

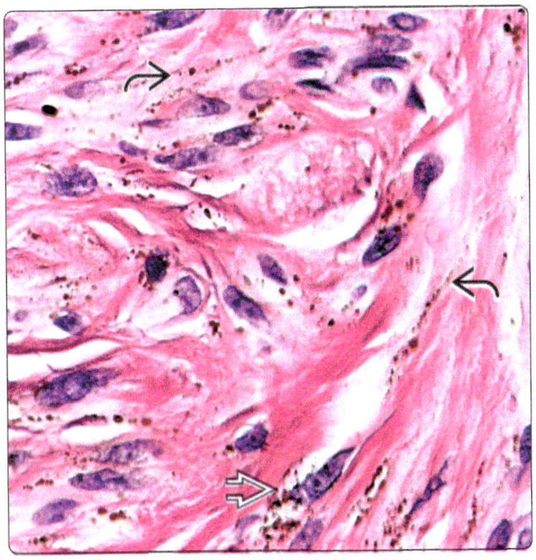

Low Magnification of Blue Nevus

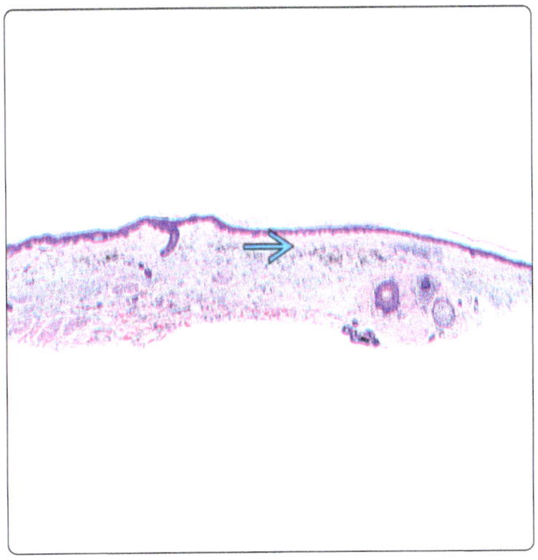

(Left) *High-power magnification shows numerous melanocytes with very fine dendritic processes and fine granular melanin pigment in their cytoplasm.* **(Right)** *Biopsy of a small patch shows a few pigmented cells admixed with mostly solar elastosis under low-power examination. This can be an expected feature in the chronically sun-exposed skin, where the clinical concern may be rule out lentigo maligna.*

Blue Nevus With Small Spindled Cells

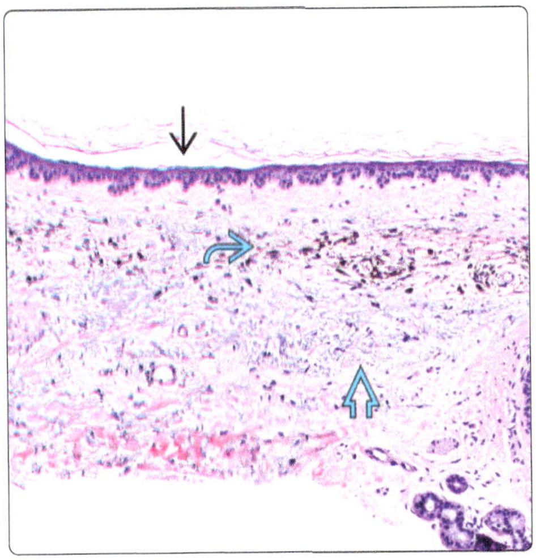

High Magnification of Blue Nevus

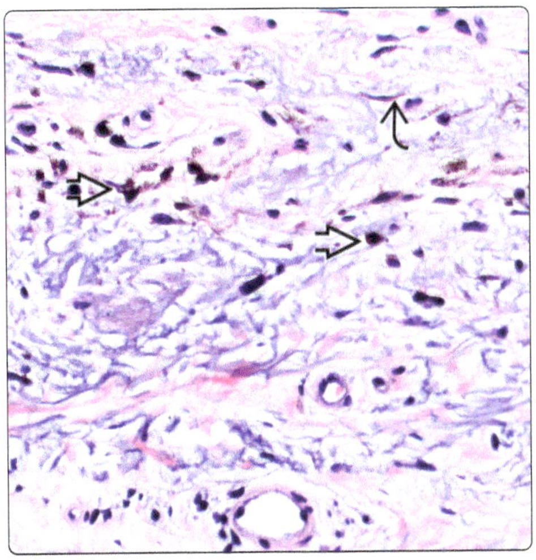

(Left) *Thin spindle cells are admixed with elastic fibers. Note the absence of any junctional melanocytes. In a chronically sun-exposed skin biopsy, examine the epidermis for subtle melanocytic proliferation. This is especially important, if the epidermis shows atrophic changes.* **(Right)** *The identification of dendritic processes emanating from pigmented spindle cells is highly characteristic of BN. Numerous melanophages are also seen.*

Cellular Blue Nevi

KEY FACTS

TERMINOLOGY

- Cellular variant of blue nevus

CLINICAL ISSUES

- Occurs in children and young adults
- Female predominance
- Heavily pigmented black/blue nodule or plaque; tends to occur on buttocks and sacrococcygeal region
- Local recurrences if incompletely excised; very low incidence of transformation into melanoma

MICROSCOPIC

- Dumbbell-shaped architecture at low magnification; often extends deeply
- Superficial and peripheral desmoplasia with conventional blue nevus cells and melanophages are often conspicuous
- Oval and spindle-shaped cells with bland cytology
- Lack of mitoses or necrosis
- **Cytologic features**
  - Ovoid, clear cells are abundant
  - Clear cells show small, round to oval monomorphous nuclei; eosinophilic or clear cytoplasm
  - Heavily pigmented spindled and dendritic cells alternate with clear cells

TOP DIFFERENTIAL DIAGNOSES

- Atypical cellular blue nevus
- Melanoma arising in or mimicking cellular blue nevus (malignant blue nevus)
- Desmoplastic melanoma

DIAGNOSTIC CHECKLIST

- Clinical features
  - Heavily pigmented black or blue nodule or plaque
- Pathologic features
  - Should not show multiple mitoses or necrosis (both of which favor malignancy)

(Left) *Gray to dark blue tumor on the scalp of a middle-aged woman shows central ulceration related to trauma. (Courtesy J. Finch, MD.)* **(Right)** *Dermoscopy of the same lesion shows a uniformly gray nodule. (Courtesy J. Finch, MD.)*

Clinical Image of a CBN

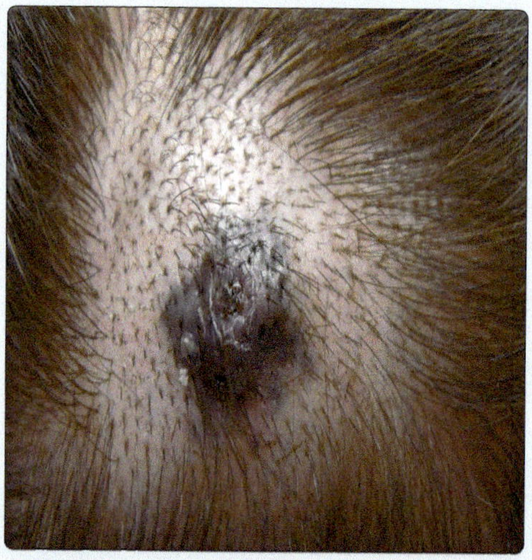

Dermatoscopic Image of a CBN

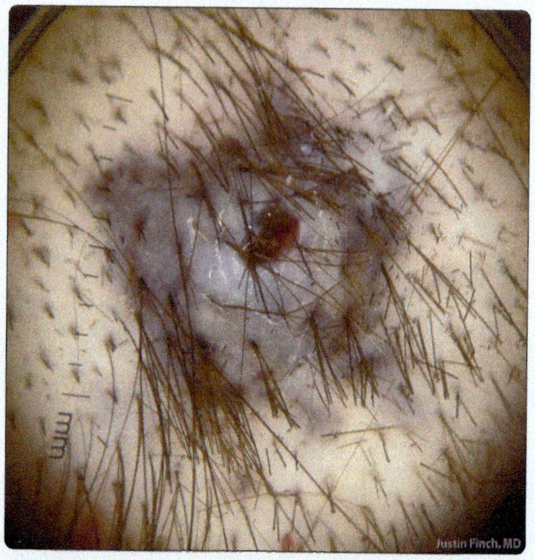

(Left) *At this low power, a conventional blue nevus (CBN) showing nodular growth with deep pushing border is identified.* **(Right)** *The lesion is heavily pigmented and shows small nests/nodules, of oval to spindle-shaped melanocytes.*

CBN at Scanning Magnification

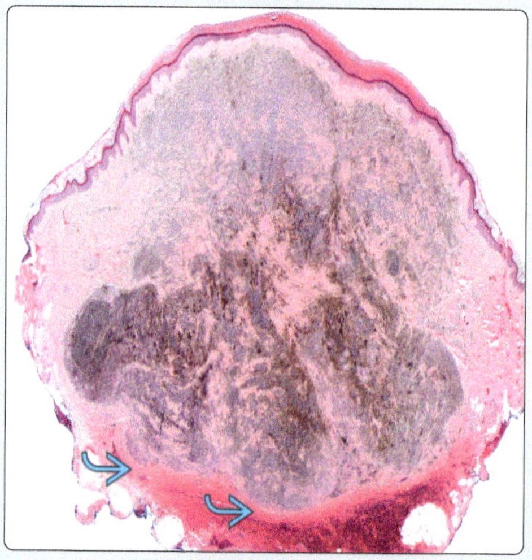

CBN at Low Magnification Showing Base of Lesion

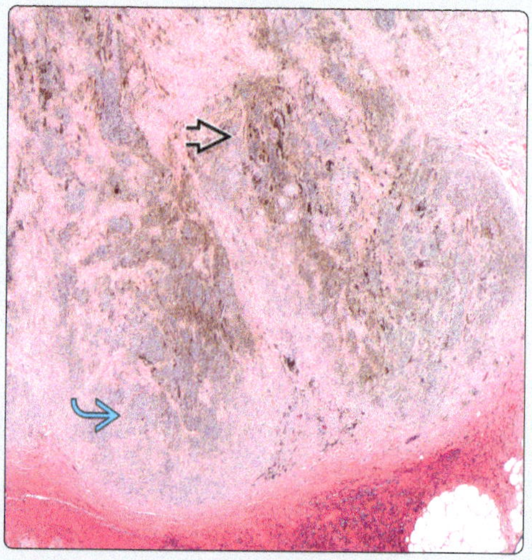

TERMINOLOGY

Abbreviations

- Cellular blue nevus (CBN)

Definitions

- Uncommon cellular variant of blue nevus

CLINICAL ISSUES

Epidemiology

- Age
  - Occurs in childhood and young adult life; mean: 33 years
- Sex
  - Female predominance (F:M ~ 2:1)
- Ethnicity
  - All affected

Site

- Mostly occurs on sacrococcygeal regions and buttock but may also be located on scalp, neck, face, hands, and extremities (especially dorsal foot)

Presentation

- Heavily pigmented, slow-growing, black or blue nodule or plaque typically ranging 1-2 cm and sometimes up to 6 cm in diameter
- Ulceration may be seen in lesions appearing in area with growth restriction, such as dorsal foot
- Rarely can be with satellitosis, characterized clinically by development of macules around a central papule or nodule, and may thus mimic melanoma

Treatment

- Surgical approaches
  - Simple excision

Prognosis

- Benign but may rarely recur
- Regional lymph node involvement and benign metastases to regional lymph nodes with CBN are rare, but well documented
  - Resulting lymphadenopathy is prone to misdiagnosis as metastatic malignant melanoma
- Has rare potential for malignant transformation, and affected patients have poor clinical outcome

MICROSCOPIC

Histologic Features

- Architecture consists of central mass with adjacent ramifications
  - These have dumbbell or peninsula-like shape occupying place of effaced hair follicles, deeply extending into subcutis
- In addition, superficial and peripheral desmoplasia are often conspicuous
- Lesion is much more cellular in center, with ovoid and spindled pale cells in large nests, lobules, or fascicles
- Collagen bundles between cells are thickened
- Exhibits classic features of common blue nevus in areas, i.e., dendritic, heavily pigmented melanocytes with numerous densely pigmented melanophages
- Margins are usually pushing
- Epidermis is usually unremarkable unless has junctional component, as seen in combined nevi

Cytologic Features

- Can be biphasic
  - Plump spindled cells with pale cytoplasm, round to oval vesicular nuclei and small, inconspicuous nucleoli
  - Elongated bipolar or dendritic melanocytes containing melanin, resembling common blue nevus
- Heavily pigmented spindled and dendritic cells alternate with clear cells
- Usually no, or only mild, atypia and nuclear pleomorphism
- Necrosis and mitotic index (i.e., > 2-3% are typically absent)

ANCILLARY TESTS

Immunohistochemistry

- MIB-1 labeling index can be helpful and should be < 2-3% according to one study
- p16 expression maybe lost in atypical CBN or those with malignant potential

DIFFERENTIAL DIAGNOSIS

Atypical Cellular Blue Nevus

- CBN that exhibits atypia insufficient for diagnosis of malignancy
- Cytologic atypia can be focal or diffuse
- No necrosis, and mitotic rate of < 2 per mm^2

Melanoma Arising in or Mimicking Cellular Blue Nevus (Malignant Blue Nevus)

- Malignant cytology in areas, often with benign blue nevus component
  - Atypia with hyperchromatic nuclei and obvious nucleoli in majority of cells
- Sarcoma-like solid sheets of atypical spindle cells
- Large sheets or nodules of atypical cells with oval or epithelioid shape
- Prominent mitoses (increased numbers, often atypical) and cellular necrosis

Desmoplastic Melanoma

- Lymphocytic infiltrate often prominent
- Desmoplastic melanoma often is achromic, in contrast to CBN, which has many melanophages
- Desmoplastic melanoma typically only positive for S100 and SOX10; CBN show diffuse HMB-45 and MART-1/Melan-A staining as well

DIAGNOSTIC CHECKLIST

Clinically Relevant Pathologic Features

- Heavily pigmented black or blue nodule or plaque ranging from 1-2 cm in diameter (even up to 6 cm)

Pathologic Interpretation Pearls

- Should not exhibit multiple mitoses or necrosis (both of which favor malignancy)

SELECTED REFERENCES

1. Yaman B et al: Atypia and differential diagnosis in cellular blue nevi: clinicopathological study of 21 cases. Turk Patoloji Derg. 31(2):89-94, 2015

CBN Showing Well-Nested Pattern

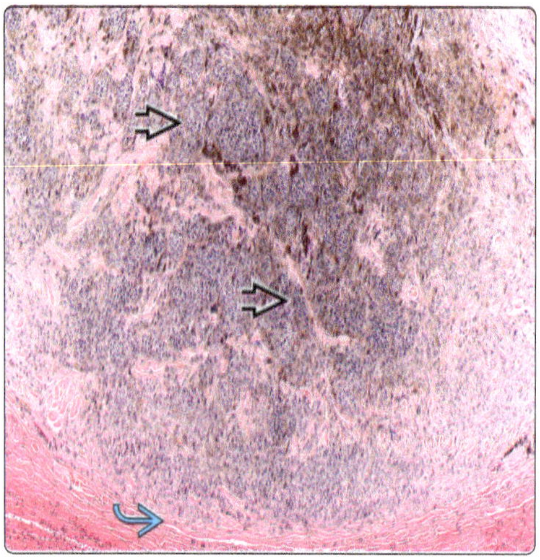

CBN at High Magnification

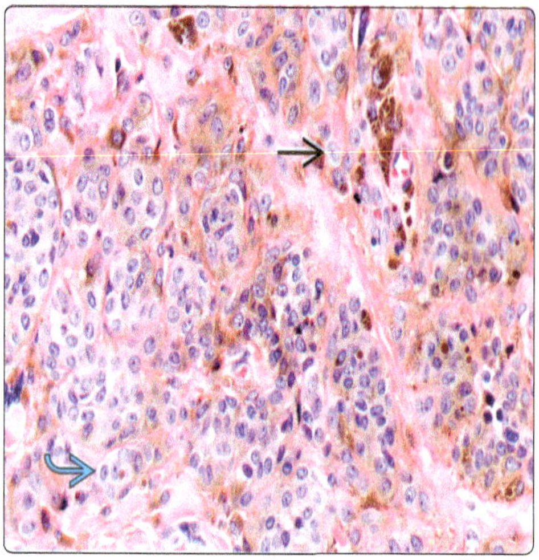

(Left) *The same lesion at a higher magnification shows a well-nested pattern, some coalescing into nodules with a smooth pushing border.* **(Right)** *The cytology shows round to oval nuclei with smooth nuclear membranes. The chromatin is evenly dispersed and small nucleoli are identified.*

CBN at Scanning Magnification

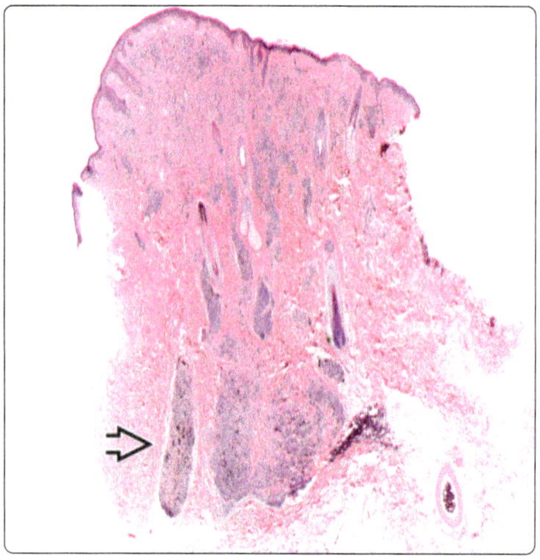

CBN, Deep Component of Lesion

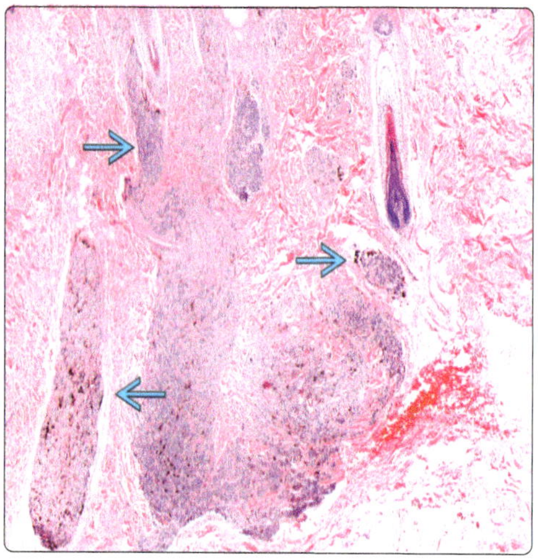

(Left) *Another lesion at scanning magnification shows deep extension of pigmented, smooth fascicles into the subcutaneous adipose tissue.* **(Right)** *Multiple well-defined fascicles are identified. Note the well-circumscribed borders of the nests and fascicles.*

CBN, Well-Nested Deep Component

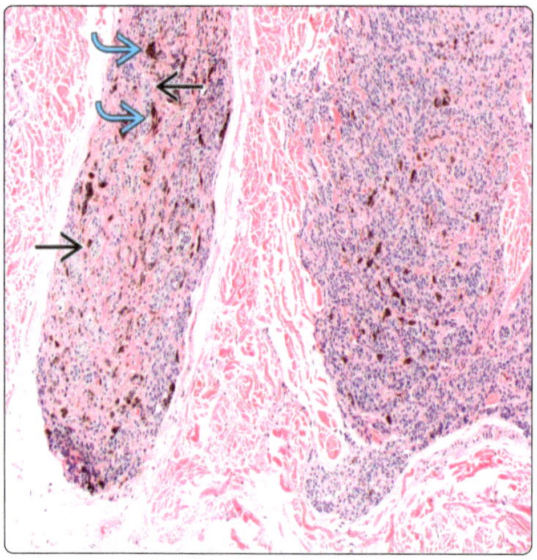

CBN at High Magnification

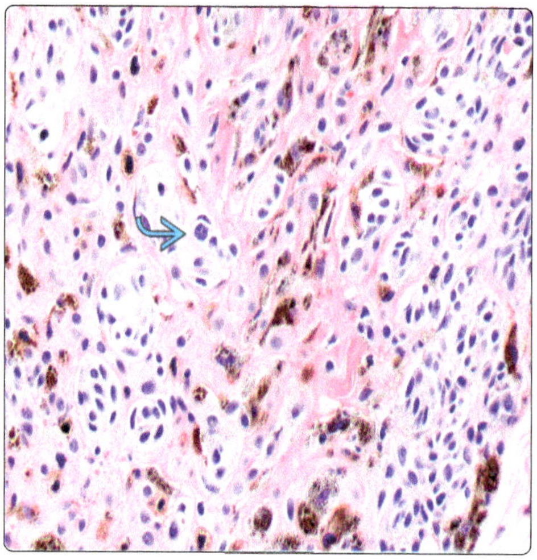

(Left) *The fascicles of small nested melanocytes with gray cytoplasm are surrounded by melanophages.* **(Right)** *Cytology shows round to oval nuclei with smooth nuclear membrane and evenly dispersed chromatin. The nucleoli are inconspicuous. No mitoses were identified.*

CBN in Lymph Node at Low Magnification

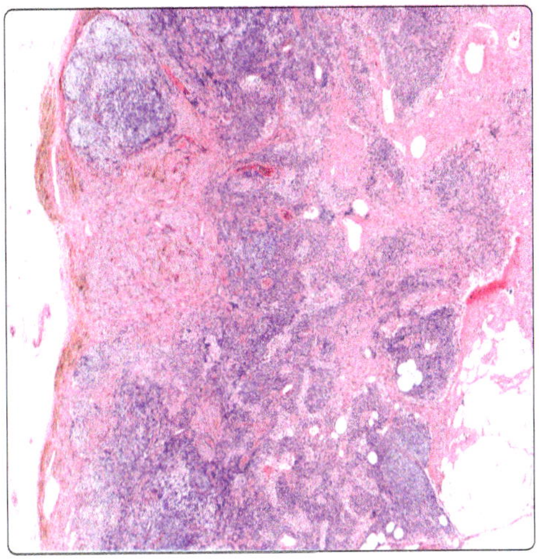

CBN in Lymph Node at Intermediate Magnification

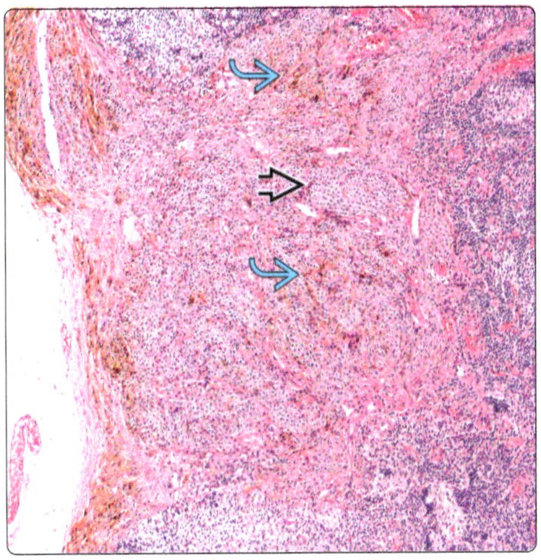

(Left) *This rare case of a CBN in a 34-year-old man was discovered as a black lymph node during herniorrhaphy.* **(Right)** *Small round nests ⮕ surrounded by melanophages ⮕ are identified. This resembles a cutaneous CBN.*

CBN in Lymph Node at High Magnification

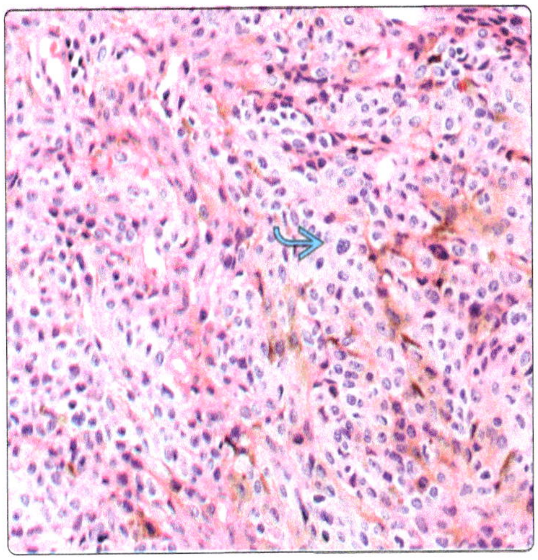

CBN at Scanning Power

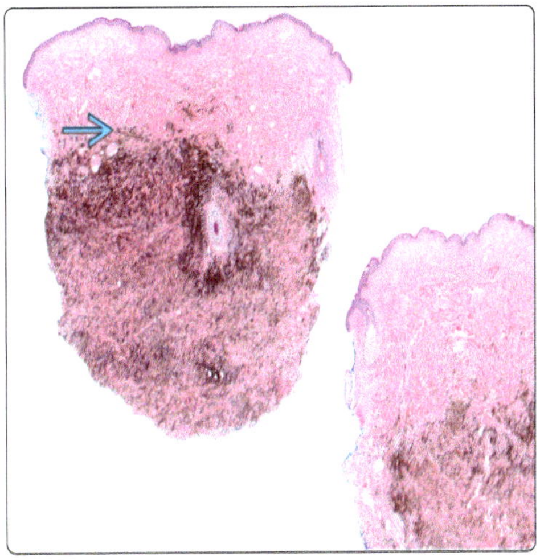

(Left) *Cytology shows small round to oval nuclei with even chromatin and inconspicuous nucleoli ⮕. No mitoses were identified.* **(Right)** *A 25-year-old Indian man presented with a 1.5-cm black plaque. This lesion is deep seated, starting from the mid dermis ⮕, without distinctive nodules, extending to the deep edge of the punch biopsy.*

CBN at Intermediate Power

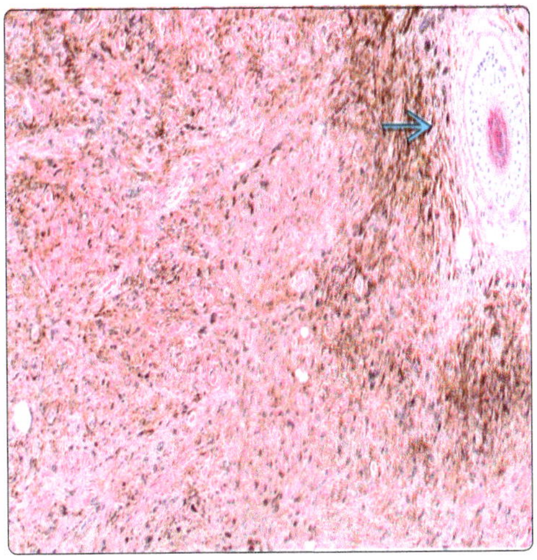

CBN at High Power Showing Spindled to Dendritic Cells

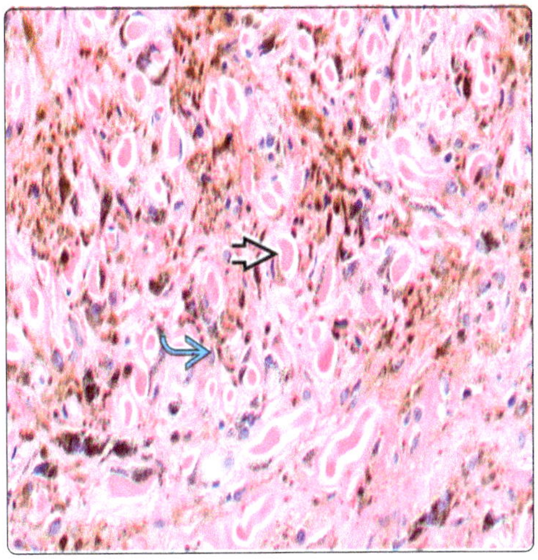

(Left) *The adnexa are well-preserved ⮕, a sign of benignity.* **(Right)** *The lesion is heavily melanized and most of the cells are spindled with dendritic processes ⮕. Collagen trapping ⮕ is identified, resembling a dermatofibroma.*

Combined Nevi

KEY FACTS

TERMINOLOGY

- Presence of 2 or more distinct populations of melanocytes
or
- Presence of 2 or more types of melanocytic nevi

CLINICAL ISSUES

- Generally in young adults
- Size usually < 6 mm
- Pigment of lesion often very dark brown to black or blue-black
- Site
  - May be more common on head and neck

MICROSCOPIC

- Lesion overall orderly, symmetric, and well circumscribed
- Most commonly: Compound/intradermal melanocytic nevus plus blue nevus
- Others types of combined nevi include compound or intradermal nevus plus pigmented spindle or spitzoid cells

TOP DIFFERENTIAL DIAGNOSES

- Blue nevus (common and cellular types)
  - Composed of dendritic to spindled melanocytes and melanophages
  - Cellular often shows deep extension into dermis/subcutaneous
- Deep penetrating nevus
  - Wedge-shaped architecture
  - Often deep extension into dermis/subcutaneous
  - Junctional nests may be present
  - Dermal component composed of epithelioid/spindled melanocytes in nests bordered by melanophages
  - Occasionally, bulbous/pushing margin is present
- Congenital melanocytic nevus: Present at birth
  - May extend deep into dermis or subcutaneous tissue
  - May infiltrate arrector pili, adnexal structures, nerves
  - Maturation with depth

Combined Nevus With Conventional and Blue Nevus Components

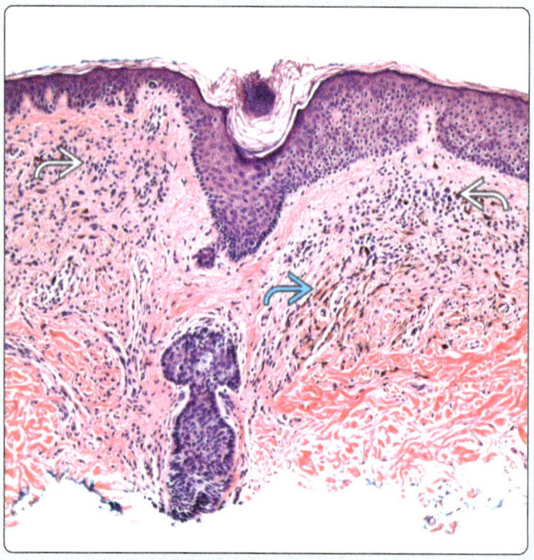

Combined Nevus: Conventional and Spitz

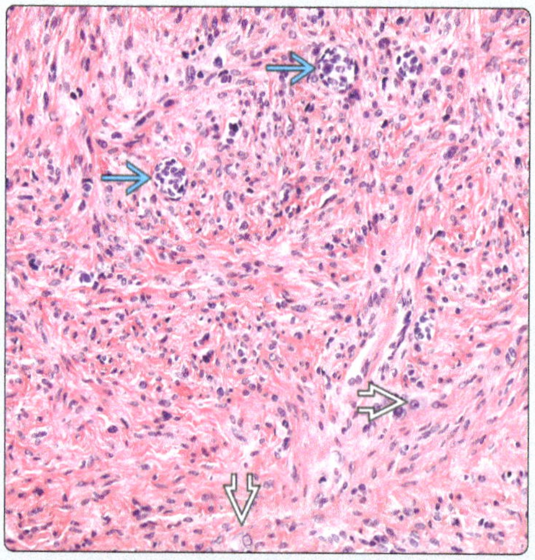

(Left) *This is an example of a combined nevus of the most common type (i.e., composed of a conventional compound melanocytic nevus ➡ and a blue nevus ↪). The lesion is symmetric and bland appearing.* **(Right)** *This combined nevus has conventional nevomelanocytes → (small cells with oval to round nuclei, some in round nests) as well as larger cells with eosinophilic cytoplasm and larger nuclei (spitzoid cells ⇨).*

Differential Diagnosis: Spitz Nevus, Desmoplastic Type

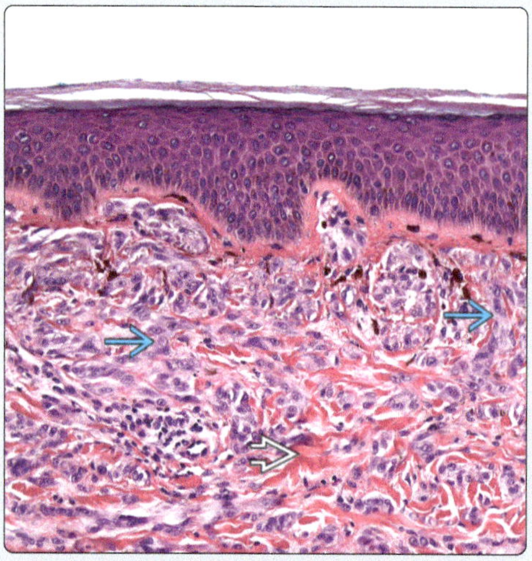

Differential Diagnosis: Deep Penetrating Nevus

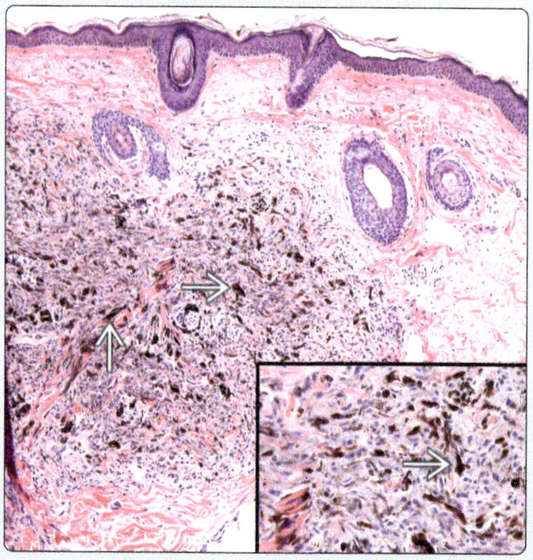

(Left) *The differential diagnosis of a combined nevus may include other less common nevi, such as a desmoplastic Spitz nevus. The cells are large with eosinophilic cytoplasm →. There are interspersed melanophages and a sclerotic stroma ⇨.* **(Right)** *The differential diagnosis of a combined nevus can also include a deep penetrating nevus, shown here, with a nodular collection of finely pigmented spindled to epithelioid cells in fascicles with many interspersed melanophages ⇨.*

TERMINOLOGY

Synonyms

- Melanocytic nevus with phenotypic heterogeneity, clonal nevus, nevus with focal epithelioid component, combined Spitz nevus, inverted type A nevus

Definitions

- Presence of 2 or more distinct populations of melanocytes (i.e., type A melanocytic nevus cells and spindled or dendritic cells) **or**
- Presence of 2 or more types of melanocytic nevi (i.e., intradermal melanocytic and blue or Spitz)

CLINICAL ISSUES

Presentation

- Generally in young adults
- Any site but may be more common on head and neck
- Pigment often very dark brown to black or blue/black
- Lesion may have small focus of blue to blue/black color in background of lighter pigment
- Size usually < 6 mm

Prognosis

- No significant malignant potential

MICROSCOPIC

Histologic Features

- All combined nevi
  - Lesion overall symmetric, well-circumscribed, orderly arrangement of melanocytes
- Most common type of combined nevus
  - Intradermal or compound melanocytic nevus plus blue nevus
    - Blue nevus component: Variable composition of dendritic melanocytes, melanophages, and fibrosis; may extend deeply &/or have plexiform configuration
- Another type of combined nevus: Compound or intradermal melanocytic plus pigmented spindle cells or spitzoid/epithelioid cells
  - Pigmented spindle cells in nests/fascicles **or**
  - Spitzoid/epithelioid cells in nests/fascicles
    - Large cells with round to oval nuclei, often with melanin pigment

Cytologic Features

- Most common type of combined nevus
  - Intradermal melanocytes
    - Type A: Round cells with pink cytoplasm, round nuclei, small nucleoli may be visible (epithelioid)
    - Type B: Resemble lymphocytes with round, blue nuclei and little cytoplasm
    - Mulberry-type giant cells: Molded, tightly packed nuclei with little cytoplasm
    - Giant cells with wreath-like arrangement of nuclei at periphery of cells
  - Blue nevus-type melanocytes
    - Melanocytes with dendritic processes and cytoplasmic melanin

DIFFERENTIAL DIAGNOSIS

DDx of Combined Nevus (Compound or Intradermal Melanocytic Plus Blue Nevus)

- Blue nevus (common)
- Compound blue nevus: Rare lesion
  - Junctional component composed of nonnested dendritic melanocytes
- Congenital melanocytic nevus
  - Lacks dendritic and spindle-shaped melanocytes
- Cellular blue nevus
  - Lacks junctional component
  - Melanophages, pigmented dendritic melanocytes, and cellular nests or lobules of spindled melanocytes (often with little melanin pigment)
  - May have bulbous/pushing margin into subcutaneous fat
- Deep penetrating nevus
  - Wedge-shaped architecture
  - Often deep extension into dermis/subcutaneous
  - Junctional nests may be present
  - Dermal component composed of pigmented spindled melanocytes in nests bordered by melanophages
  - Nests/fascicles of cells may be centered around adnexal/neurovascular structures in dermis
  - Occasionally, bulbous/pushing margin is present

DDx of Combined Compound or Intradermal Melanocytic Plus Spitzoid/Epithelioid Nevus

- Spitz nevus
  - Lacks conventional nevus component
  - Composed of variable proportions of spindled and epithelioid-shaped cells
- Melanoma arising in dermis of melanocytic nevus
  - Large expansile nests/sheets of atypical cells (pleomorphic, enlarged, hyperchromatic)
  - Mitoses (atypical &/or deep) often common

DIAGNOSTIC CHECKLIST

Pathologic Interpretation Pearls

- Combined nevi
  - Either combination of 2 or more types of melanocytic nevi **or** combination of 2 or more melanocytic cell types in 1 lesion

SELECTED REFERENCES

1. Heng YK et al: Congenital combined melanocytic nevus of the scalp with associated alopecia areata. Am J Dermatopathol. 35(4):486-8, 2013
2. Baran JL et al: Combined melanocytic nevi: histologic variants and melanoma mimics. Am J Surg Pathol. 35(10):1540-8, 2011
3. Barnhill RL et al: State of the art, nomenclature, and points of consensus and controversy concerning benign melanocytic lesions: outcome of an international workshop. Adv Anat Pathol. 17(2):73-90, 2010
4. de Giorgi V et al: Dermoscopic features of combined melanocytic nevi. J Cutan Pathol. 31(9):600-4, 2004
5. Scolyer RA et al: Combined naevus: a benign lesion frequently misdiagnosed both clinically and pathologically as melanoma. Pathology. 36(5):419-27, 2004
6. Kamino H et al: Compound blue nevus: a variant of blue nevus with an additional junctional dendritic component. A clinical, histopathologic, and immunohistochemical study of six cases. Arch Dermatol. 126(10):1330-3, 1990
7. Gartmann H et al: [Combined occurrence of blue nevus and nevus cell nevus in one and the same tumor ('combined nevus').] Z Hautkr. 52(7):389-98, 1977

Halo Nevi

KEY FACTS

TERMINOLOGY

- Nevus with clinically depigmented halo surrounding pigmented area

ETIOLOGY/PATHOGENESIS

- Thought to be reaction to melanocytic antigens

CLINICAL ISSUES

- Usually young patients (children and young adults)
- May be associated with melanoma, typically at another site, in older patients

MICROSCOPIC

- Nevus associated with dense inflammatory infiltrate
- Infiltrate typically shows lichenoid pattern in dermis
- Nests predominate in early lesions, single cells later
  - May be absent in late stage (regressed) lesions
- Melanocytic markers may be useful to confirm presence of melanocytes
- Spitzoid features may be present in some cases (halo Spitz nevi)
- Reactive atypia may be seen
- Dermal component should show evidence of maturation with descent
- Mitoses should be rare to absent

ANCILLARY TESTS

- Melanocytic markers may be useful to confirm presence of melanocytes
  - S100, SOX10, Melan-A, HMB-45, p16

TOP DIFFERENTIAL DIAGNOSES

- Melanoma
  - Can show associated inflammatory infiltrate but usually milder than halo nevi
  - Lack of symmetry and circumscription
  - Pagetoid scatter and dermal mitoses may be present
- Myerson nevus (eczematous nevus)

Clinical Photograph of Halo Nevi

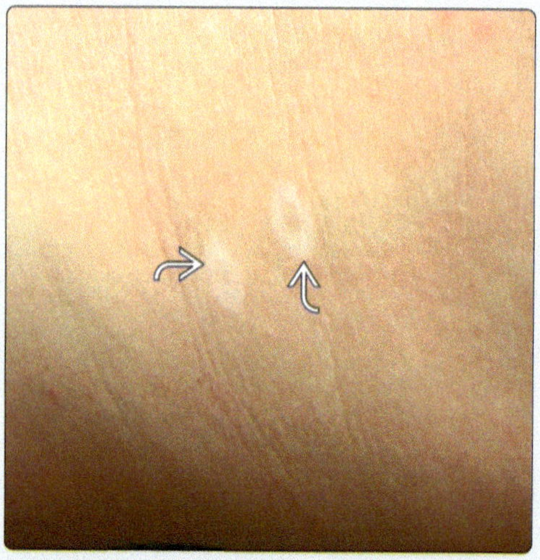

Halo Nevus Showing Dense, Band-Like Inflammatory Infiltrate

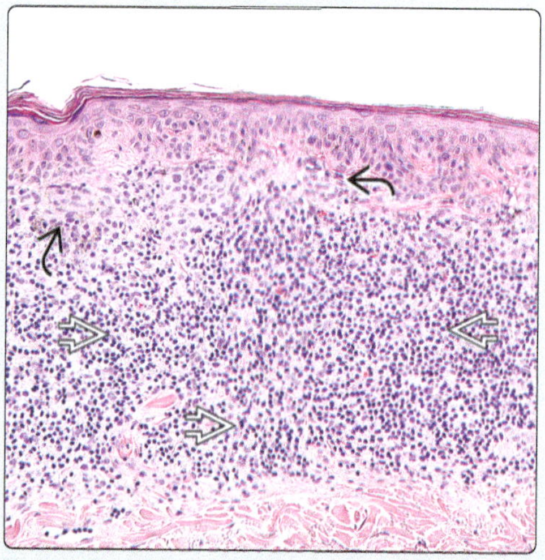

(Left) *Two halo nevi seen on the back of a young adult are oval, well demarcated, and depigmented (skin colored or paler). With time, the white area may replace the nevus entirely ➡.* **(Right)** *Halo nevus is characterized by a dense, band-like lymphohistiocytic infiltrate in the dermis ➡. Several junctional and superficial nests of melanocytes ➡ can be appreciated upon close inspection.*

Halo Nevus at Higher Magnification

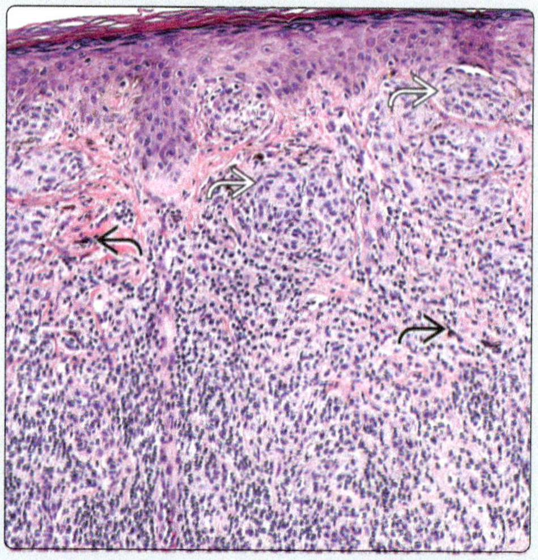

Melan-A Immunohistochemistry in Halo Nevus

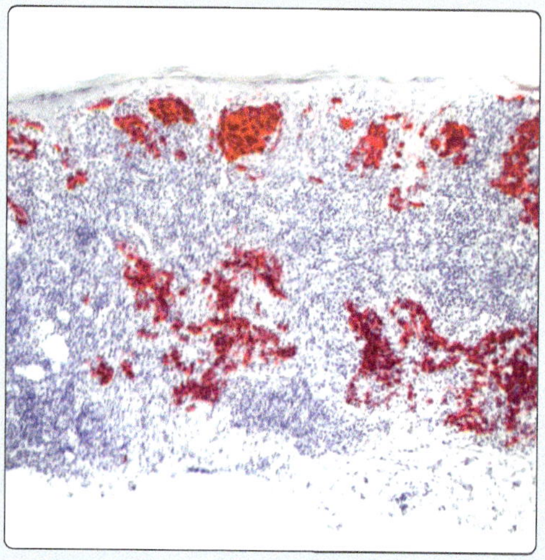

(Left) *Higher magnification shows a dense lymphohistiocytic infiltrate with scattered melanophages ➡. The melanocytes are mildly enlarged and atypical appearing ➡ but show no mitotic activity.* **(Right)** *Melan-A immunohistochemistry in a halo nevus strongly highlights the residual junctional and dermal cells. S100 and Melan-A are usually diffusely positive, whereas HMB-45 usually only highlights the junctional cells (which can be useful in the differential with melanoma).*

TERMINOLOGY

Synonyms

- Sutton nevus
- Nevus depigmentosa centrifugum

Definitions

- Nevus with clinically depigmented halo surrounding pigmented area
- Dense inflammatory infiltrate typically present
  - Histologically heavily inflamed nevi that lack clinical halo may be said to show halo reaction/phenomenon, but they are not true halo nevi

ETIOLOGY/PATHOGENESIS

Inflammatory Process

- Thought to be reaction to melanocytic antigens
- Infiltrate includes numerous T cells, including cytotoxic CD8(+) cells that may induce melanocyte apoptosis

CLINICAL ISSUES

Epidemiology

- Age
  - Usually young patients (children and young adults)
  - Patients over 40 years old uncommon
    - Should raise concern for possibility of melanoma at another site

Site

- Most common on back but may occur at any site

Presentation

- Pigmented lesion
  - Depigmented halo surrounds lesion
  - Central lesion eventually loses pigmentation
- Often multiple

Natural History

- Progressively loses pigmentation over several months
  - Central nevus
    - Initially pigmented; may show erythema before regressing

Treatment

- Surgical approaches
  - Complete conservative excision is curative

Prognosis

- Excellent
- May be associated with melanoma, typically at another site, in older patients

MICROSCOPIC

Histologic Features

- Compound nevus associated with dense inflammatory infiltrate
- Infiltrate typically shows lichenoid (band-like) pattern in dermis
  - Composed mostly of lymphocytes with scattered histiocytes and melanophages
  - Rarely, clinically typical-appearing halo nevi can lack significant inflammation
- Nevus may be of any type but usually conventional compound nevus
  - Junctional and dermal nests are surrounded by dense inflammatory infiltrate
  - Nests predominate in early lesions, single cells in later lesions
    - May be completely absent in late-stage lesions
  - Dermal component should show evidence of maturation with descent
  - Reactive atypia may be present but should be low grade (mild/moderate)
    - Severe atypia should raise suspicion for melanoma
  - Mitoses should be rare to absent
    - May be difficult to determine if mitosis is in inflammatory or stromal cell vs. melanocyte
  - Spitzoid features may be present in some cases (halo Spitz nevi)
- Epidermis shows loss of pigmentation and normal melanocytes at periphery of lesion

ANCILLARY TESTS

Immunohistochemistry

- Melanocytic markers may be useful to confirm presence of melanocytes if not obvious on histologic sections
  - S100, SOX10, MART-1/Melan-A, HMB-45, and tyrosinase
    - HMB-45 often positive in junctional cells but negative in dermal component (may be useful in favoring nevus over melanoma)
    - Staining for p16 can also be useful: Often strong in nevi, weak to negative in melanoma

DIFFERENTIAL DIAGNOSIS

Melanoma

- May be heavily inflamed in some cases
  - But usually shows more patchy infiltrate than halo nevi
- Shows greater degree of cytologic and architectural atypia
- Pagetoid scatter also usually present
- Lack of maturation (if invasive)
- Lack of symmetry and circumscription
- Dermal mitotic figures, loss of p16, and elevated Ki-67 proliferative rate often seen

Myerson Nevus (Eczematous Nevus)

- Eczematous (spongiotic) reaction involving nevus
- May show eczematous halo clinically
- Milder inflammation with eosinophils usually present

SELECTED REFERENCES

1. Weyant GW et al: Halo nevus: review of the literature and clinicopathologic findings. Int J Dermatol. 54(10):e433-5, 2015
2. Martín JM et al: Spontaneous regression of multiple melanocytic nevi after melanoma: report of 3 cases. Am J Dermatopathol. 36(11):e183-8, 2014
3. Ohtsuka T: Multiple Sutton nevi: Hypomelanocytic halo development around 28 melanocytic nevi. J Dermatol. 36(6):355-7, 2009
4. Moretti S et al: Fibrosis in regressing melanoma versus nonfibrosis in halo nevus upon melanocyte disappearance: could it be related to a different cytokine microenvironment? J Cutan Pathol. 34(4):301-8, 2007
5. Frank SB et al: The halo nevus. Arch Dermatol. 89:367-73, 1964

KEY FACTS

TERMINOLOGY

- Melanocytic nevi of special sites
- Benign melanocytic nevus with unusual histological features that can mimic dysplastic nevus or melanoma
- Unusual histopathology is attributed to anatomic location and not neoplastic features

CLINICAL ISSUES

- Special site designation, anatomic locations include flexural skin or skin folds, acral, genital, and scalp

MACROSCOPIC

- Light to dark brown papule or plaque with areas of pigmentary change
- Dermoscopy can show prominent pigment net, sometimes with bizarre lines, and large globules

MICROSCOPIC

- Asymmetry and poor peripheral circumscription
- Large junctional nests of melanocytes located at tips, sides, and between rete ridges
- Involvement of skin adnexa
- Focal poorly nested, lentiginous proliferation of melanocytes along dermoepidermal junction

TOP DIFFERENTIAL DIAGNOSES

- Atypical (dysplastic) nevus
- Melanoma
- Nevoid melanoma

DIAGNOSTIC CHECKLIST

- If focally traumatized (presence of parakeratosis), there may be upward migration of isolated melanocytes
- This finding should not be used in isolation; may lead to overdiagnosis
- If mitotic figure is identified, step-leveled sections should be examined for additional mitoses

Displaced Junctional Nests in Breast Nevus

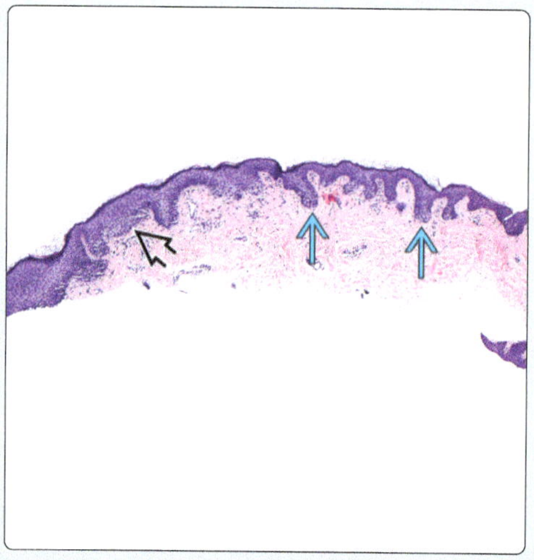

Papillary Dermal Fibroplasia in Breast Nevus

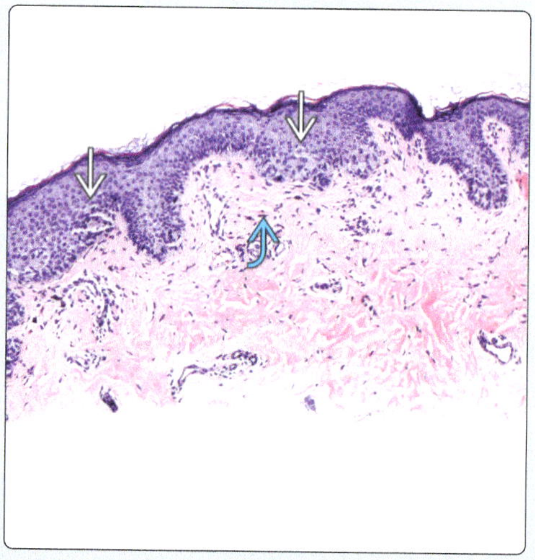

(Left) *At this low power, a junctional melanocytic proliferation is evident on the breast of a 25-year-old woman. Most nests ➡ appear at the tips of rete ridges. However, there are apparently displaced nests on the left side of the lesion ➡.* **(Right)** *These nests ➡ appear to be overlying papillary dermal fibroplasia ➡ and are not laterally displaced or fused as seen in atypical/dysplastic nevi.*

High Magnification: Banal Cytology

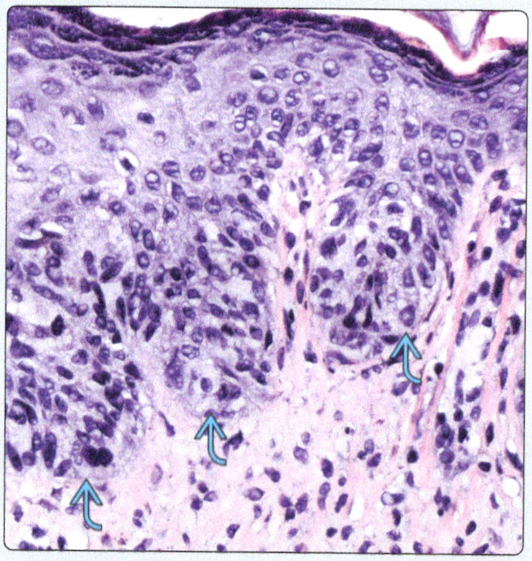

High Magnification: Lack of Cytological Atypia

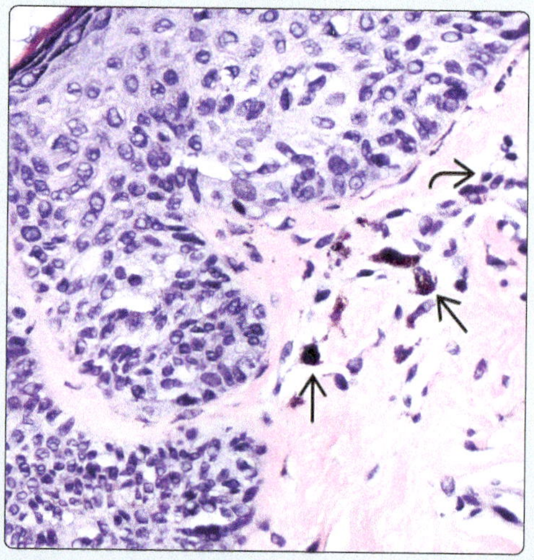

(Left) *Higher power examination exhibits no macronucleoli, vesicular nuclei, or hyperchromasia. Note how the nests ➡ blend in with epidermal keratinocytes.* **(Right)** *Another focus of the same lesion shows nested melanocytes devoid of cytological atypia. Note the melanin incontinence ➡ and sparse lymphohistiocytic inflammation ➡ in the superficial dermis.*

TERMINOLOGY

Synonyms

- Melanocytic nevi of special sites

Definitions

- Benign melanocytic nevi with unusual histological features that can mimic dysplastic nevi or melanoma
  - Unusual histopathologic findings are attributed to anatomic location and not neoplastic features
  - Architectural &/or cytological abnormalities do not correlate with aggressive clinical behavior

CLINICAL ISSUES

Presentation

- Special site designation includes the following anatomic locations
  - Acral
  - Genital
  - Scalp
  - In and around ear
  - Breast and milk line
  - Flexural skin (skin folds at axillae, antecubital and popliteal fossae, and umbilicus)

Treatment

- Surgical approaches
  - Shave or simple excision

Prognosis

- Excellent

MACROSCOPIC

General Features

- Light to dark brown papule or plaque with areas of pigmentary change
- Dermoscopy can show prominent pigment network, sometimes with bizarre lines, and large globules

MICROSCOPIC

Histologic Features

- Asymmetry and poor peripheral circumscription
- Large junctional nests of melanocytes located at tips, sides, and between rete ridges
  - Some nests are randomly scattered along dermoepidermal junction, resembling atypical/dysplastic nevi
  - Nests show variation in shape with frequent bizarre forms
  - Dyscohesion of tumor cells within nests
- Involvement of skin adnexa
- Focal poorly nested, lentiginous proliferation of melanocytes along dermoepidermal junction
- Focal upward migration of isolated melanocytes in central part of lesion, especially if traumatized
- Dermal melanocytic component is cytologically bland
  - Matures properly with increasing dermal depth
  - Occasional mitotic activity can be seen
  - Cell are set in fibroplasia or may be focally inflamed

Cytologic Features

- Mild atypia characterized by hyperchromatic nuclei and inconspicuous nucleoli
  - Occasionally severe but focal cytological atypia may be present
- Pale cytoplasm with dusty melanin

DIFFERENTIAL DIAGNOSIS

Atypical (Dysplastic) Nevus

- Architectural atypia
  - Junctional nests extend beyond intradermal component
  - Lateral displacement of nests in rete ridges
- Cytological atypia characterized by melanized cytoplasm, pleomorphic and hyperchromatic-staining nuclei

Melanoma

- Often shows marked and diffuse pagetoid scatter
  - Or lentiginous, confluent growth pattern (lentigo maligna type)
- Marked cytological atypia
  - Slightly cherry-red macronucleoli
    - Or if hyperchromatic, nucleoli are inapparent
  - Irregular and thickened nuclear membrane
  - Pleomorphic nuclei

Nevoid Melanoma

- Deceptively benign-appearing, hypercellular melanocytic proliferation
- Cytologically, nuclei can be bland
- Mid to deep dermal mitoses

DIAGNOSTIC CHECKLIST

Pathologic Interpretation Pearls

- Asymmetry and poor peripheral circumscription
- Large junctional nests of melanocytes located at tips, sides, and between rete ridges
- Dermal melanocytic component is cytologically bland
- If focally traumatized (presence of parakeratosis), there may be upward migration of isolated melanocytes
  - This finding should not be used in isolation; may lead to overdiagnosis
- If mitotic figure is identified, step-leveled sections should be examined for additional mitoses
- Scalp lesions of adolescents can have more strikingly worrisome features
  - Large, bizarrely shaped nests
  - Scattered disorderly nests along dermoepidermal junction with follicular involvement

SELECTED REFERENCES

1. Arps DP et al: Atypical umbilical naevi: histopathological analysis of 20 cases. Histopathology. 66(3):363-9, 2015
2. Fisher KR et al: Histologic features of scalp melanocytic nevi. J Am Acad Dermatol. 68(3):466-72, 2013
3. Hofmann-Wellenhof R: Special criteria for special locations 2: scalp, mucosal, and milk line. Dermatol Clin. 31(4):625-36, ix, 2013
4. Cheung WL et al: Dermatopathology updates on melanocytic lesions. Dermatol Clin. 30(4):617-22, vi, 2012
5. Mason AR et al: Nevi of special sites. Clin Lab Med. 31(2):229-42, 2011

(Left) *This vulvar nevus of a middle-aged woman shows a heavily melanized, fairly symmetrical-appearing, compound melanocytic nevus. Note that it starts* → *and ends* → *with small nests.* **(Right)** *The nests are at the tips of rete* →*, some of which are more melanized* → *than others. There is a focally band-like lymphohistiocytic infiltrate* → *in the papillary dermis.*

Vulvar Compound Nevus

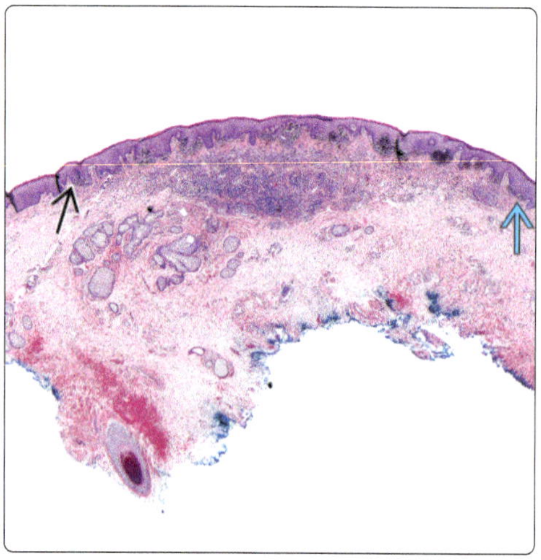

Vulvar Compound Nevus With Focal Lichenoid Infiltrate

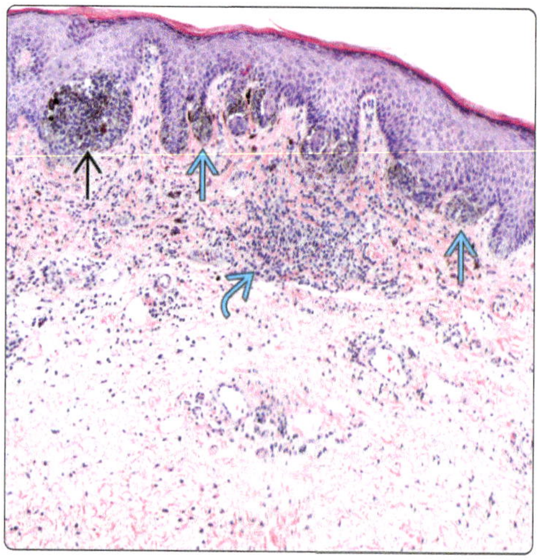

(Left) *Another edge of the same lesion shows well-nested junctional growth* →*. Papillary dermal fibroplasia* → *hugs the nests, mimicking an atypical/dysplastic nevus.* **(Right)** *High magnification of a vulvar nevus shows that the nuclei are not enlarged, irregular in shape, or hyperchromatic-staining. The nucleoli are inconspicuous to small.*

Papillary Dermal Fibroplasia

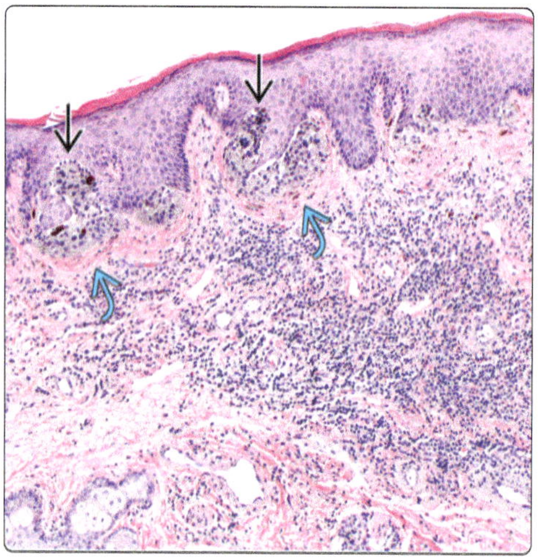

High Magnification: Lack of Cytological Atypia

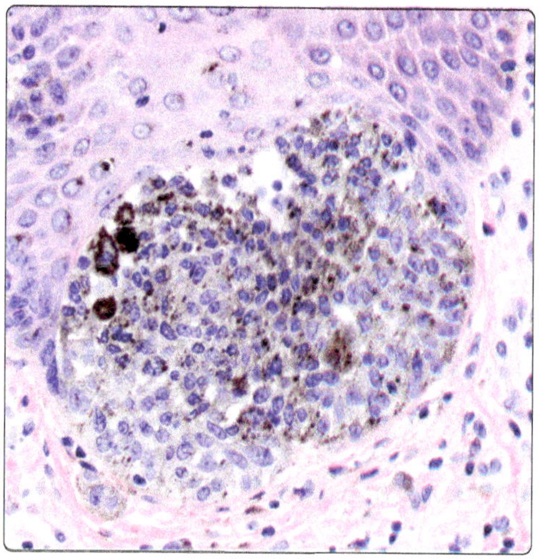

(Left) *High magnification of another area shows that the nuclear membranes are smooth, not thickened* →*.* **(Right)** *This partial biopsy of a clinically atypical-appearing pigmented lesion shows a hypermelanotic, hypercellular melanocytic proliferation. It may appear atypical; however, the dermal cells become smaller (mature)* → *with increasing dermal depth, and some disperse* →*.*

High Magnification: Banal Cytology

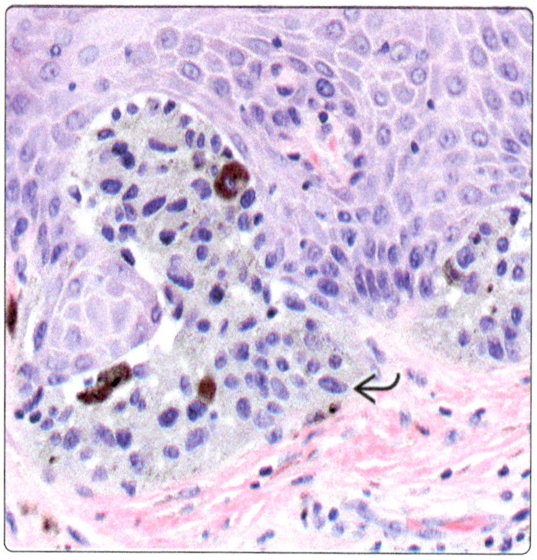

Vulvar Atypical Compound Nevus

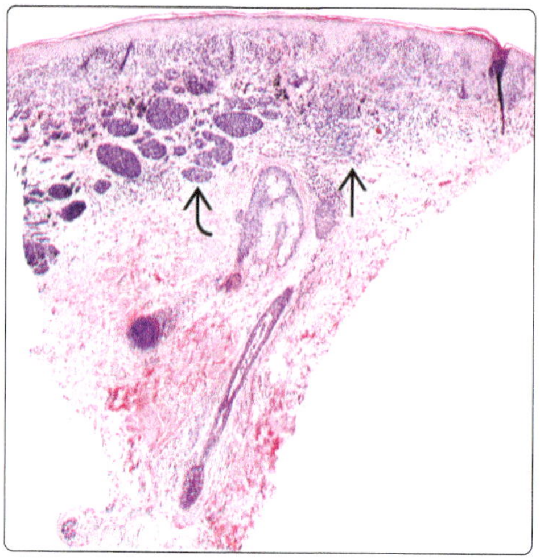

Lack of Pagetoid Upward Scatter in Vulvar Atypical Compound Nevus

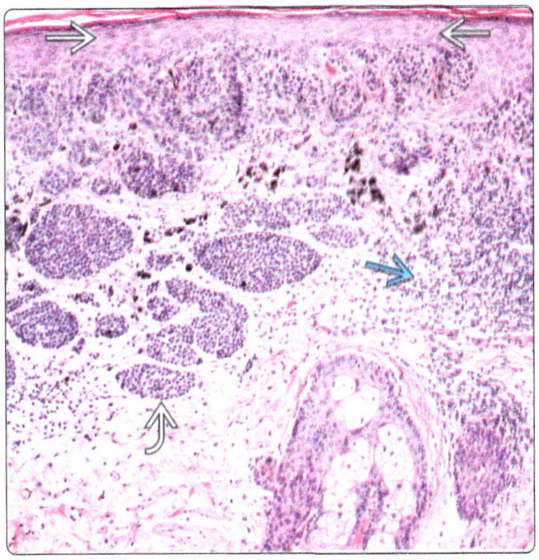

Hypercellular Focus Devoid of Cytological Atypia

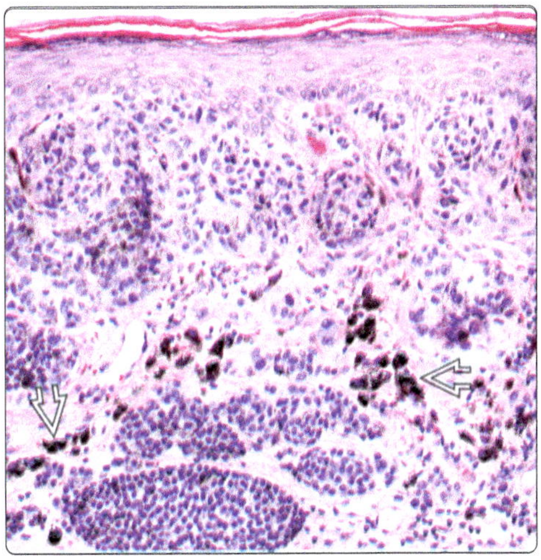

(Left) *Note the lack of significant pagetoid scatter ➡ and maturation of dermal nests ➡ with descent. The lesion is accompanied by patchy to focally lichenoid infiltrate ➡.* **(Right)** *The same area is shown under higher magnification. Although they are quite hypercellular, the junctional and dermal cells lack significant cytological atypia. Scattered melanophages are also present in the papillary dermis ➡.*

Higher Magnification: Large Dermal Cells

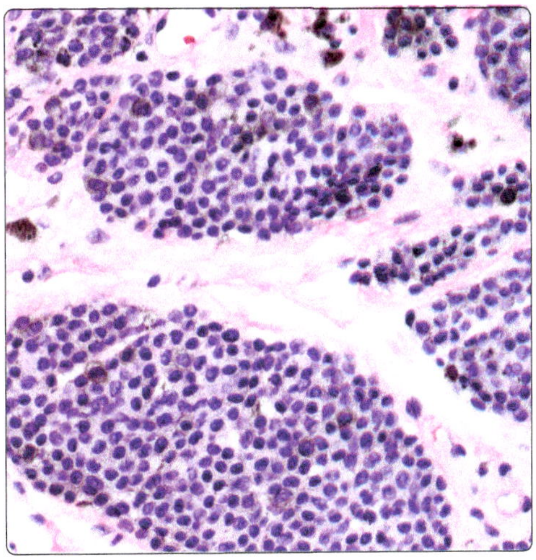

Lack of Cytological Atypia in Vulvar Atypical Compound Nevus

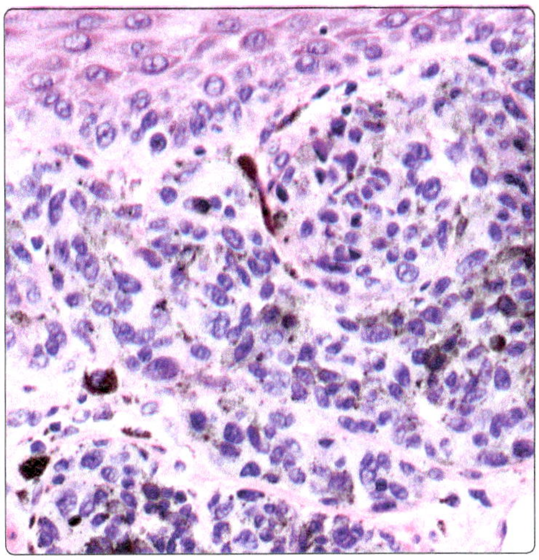

(Left) *Although the cells are crowded and show mild nuclear hyperchromasia in the large dermal nests, they are devoid of mitoses and mature with increasing dermal depth. The nuclei are small and uniform with inconspicuous nucleoli, which are reassuring features.* **(Right)** *The nuclei have small to inconspicuous nucleoli and smooth nuclear membrane. No marked nuclear atypia or pleomorphism is identified.*

Ki-67 Immunohistochemistry in Vulvar Nevus

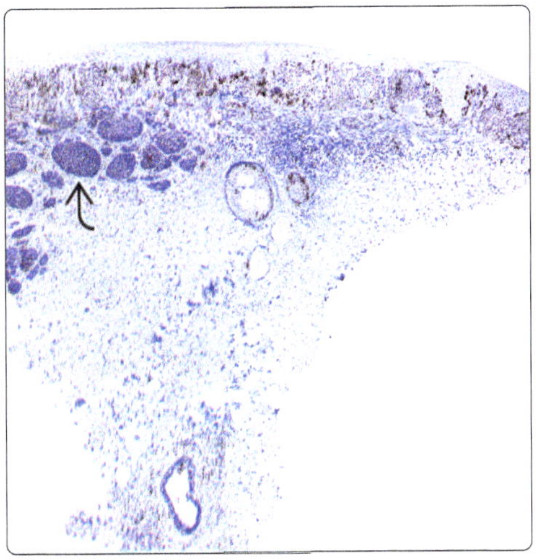

Ki-67 Immunohistochemistry at Higher Magnification

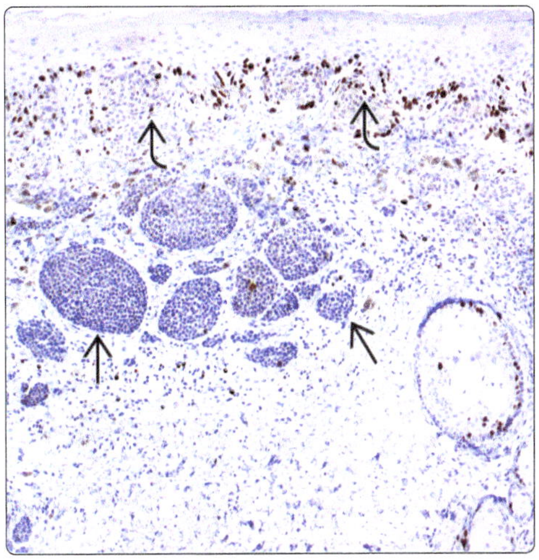

(Left) *Although there were no mitoses identified, a low proliferative in the dermal component ➡ can be confirmed by Ki-67 immunostaining, providing reassurance of benignancy.* **(Right)** *Only the junctional melanocytes have a mildly elevated (~ 10%) labeling index for Ki-67 ➡. The dermal nests are virtually negative ➡.*

Inverted Type A (Clonal) Nevi

KEY FACTS

TERMINOLOGY

- Inverted type A nevus (ITAN)
- Benign melanocytic nevus with inverted maturation of dermal melanocytes
- Clonal nevus (superficial)
- Deep-penetrating nevus (deep seated)

CLINICAL ISSUES

- Usually thin brown papule with eccentric small focus of dark pigmentation within less pigmented macule
- Shave or simple excision is usually curative
- Recent color change in otherwise benign preexisting nevus

IMAGING

- Dermoscopy shows regular and uniform brown globules with eccentric small blue-grey blotch

MICROSCOPIC

- Collection of nests with distinctively epithelioid morphology, type A nevus cells, at or near bottom of lesion
- Surrounded by numerous melanophages
- Nuclei of type A cells are round-to-plum/oval in shape with finely melanized cytoplasm
- Mitoses absent or rare

ANCILLARY TESTS

- Examine additional deeper histological sections looking for mitoses
- Bleached sections can be helpful in examining cytological details in case of heavily pigmented lesion
- Ki-67 can be helpful in detecting high labeling index (>15%) if mitoses are not found

DIAGNOSTIC CHECKLIST

- Look very carefully for mitoses by examining multiple step-leveled histologic sections

ITAN Clinical

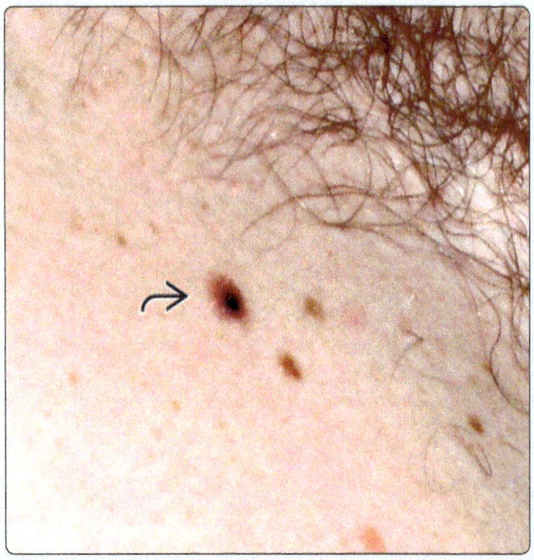

ITAN at Scanning Magnification

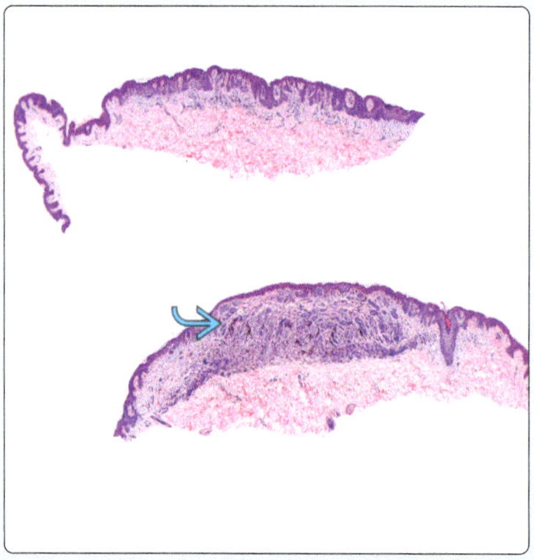

(Left) *Clinically, an inverted type A nevus (ITAN) is* → *compared to other pigmented papules. ITAN has an eccentrically placed dark papule upon an evenly pigmented flat area. The lesional borders are sharp in contrast to dysplastic nevus. (Courtesy R. McClintok, MD.)* **(Right)** *At scanning magnification, the nevus resembles an ordinary nevus with admixed melanophages* →.

ITAN at Low Magnification

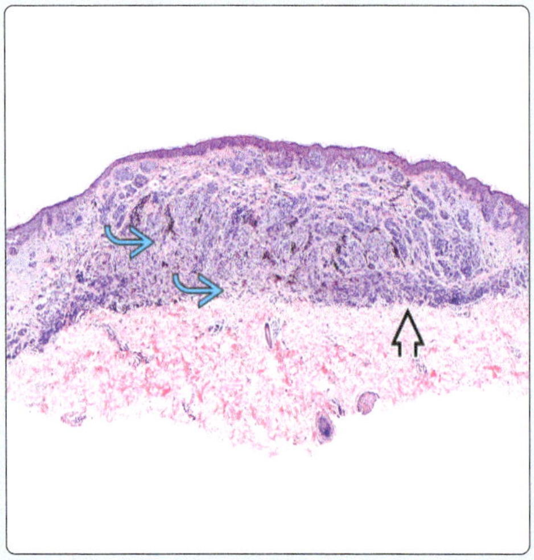

ITAN at Intermediate Magnification Showing Maturation

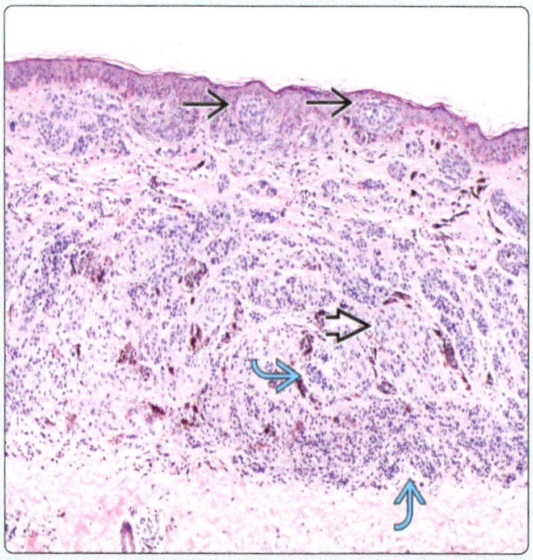

(Left) *At low power, the more epithelioid nests are identified in the middermis toward the bottom of the lesion* →. *There is also a 2nd population of type B cells* →, *resembling lymphocytes at this power.* **(Right)** *Under medium-power magnification, the type A nevus nests* → *are contrasted to the type B cells* →. *There is also a junctional component* →.

TERMINOLOGY

Abbreviations

- Inverted type A nevus (ITAN)

Synonyms

- Clonal nevus (superficial)
- Deep penetrating nevus (deep seated)

Definitions

- Benign melanocytic nevus with inverted maturation of dermal melanocytes

CLINICAL ISSUES

Presentation

- Recent color change in otherwise benign preexisting nevus
- Usually thin brown papule with eccentric small focus of dark pigmentation within less pigmented macule

Treatment

- Surgical approaches
  - Shave or simple excision is usually curative

Prognosis

- Excellent, no reported local recurrence or metastasis

IMAGING

General Features

- Dermoscopy shows regular and uniform brown globules with eccentric small blue-grey blotch

MICROSCOPIC

Histologic Features

- Collection of nests with distinctively epithelioid morphology, type A nevus cells
  - Cells located at or near bottom of lesion
  - Type A nevus cells are typically present in superficial dermis
    - Location deep in reticular dermis gives its name, "inverted type A"
- May have variants or admixed with cell types
  - Purely type A (epithelioid nevus cells)
  - Type B (lymphoid nevus cells)
  - Type C (spindled nevus cells)
  - Dendritic blue cells
- Surrounded by numerous melanophages

Cytologic Features

- Nuclei of type A cells are round-to-plum/oval in shape with finely melanized cytoplasm
- Even chromatin with inconspicuous nucleoli
- Nuclear membrane is smooth
- Mitoses are absent to extremely rare

ANCILLARY TESTS

Histochemistry

- Examine additional deeper histological sections looking for mitoses
- Bleached sections can be helpful in examining the cytological details in case of heavily pigmented lesion

Immunohistochemistry

- KI-67 can be helpful in detecting high labeling index (>15%) if mitoses are not found

DIFFERENTIAL DIAGNOSIS

Clonal Nevus

- Has considerable histological and cytological overlap with ITAN; some authors believe they are synonymous
- In clonal nevi, epithelioid (type A) cells are typically situated in superficial dermis
  - In ITAN, these cells are located deep in reticular dermis

Deep Penetrating Nevus

- Symmetrical, wedge-shaped nodule with broad base typically extends deep into subcutaneous adipose tissue
- Lacks characteristic type A nevus cells

Combined Nevus

- Usually contains type B melanocytes with other cell types like spindled, bipolar cells with dendritic processes, resembling blue nevus

DIAGNOSTIC CHECKLIST

Clinically Relevant Pathologic Features

- Epithelioid type A nevus cells with gray, finely melanized cytoplasm
- Lack of mitoses by deeper sections &/or low mitotic index are reassuring

Pathologic Interpretation Pearls

- Look very carefully for mitoses by examining multiple step-leveled histologic sections
- Do not rely on cytological maturation (reduction of nuclear size) with increasing dermal depth
  - Inverted nature by definition is atypical but does not warrant malignant diagnosis

SELECTED REFERENCES

1. Balagula Y et al: Dermoscopy of a clonal (inverted type A) nevus in a child. J Am Acad Dermatol. 71(5):e187-9, 2014
2. Baran JL et al: Combined melanocytic nevi: histologic variants and melanoma mimics. Am J Surg Pathol. 35(10):1540-8, 2011
3. High WA et al: Is melanocytic nevus with focal atypical epithelioid components (clonal nevus) a superficial variant of deep penetrating nevus? J Am Acad Dermatol. 55(3):460-6, 2006
4. Huynh PM et al: The clinical appearance of clonal nevi (inverted type A nevi). Int J Dermatol. 43(12):882-5, 2004
5. Scolyer RA et al: Combined naevus: a benign lesion frequently misdiagnosed both clinically and pathologically as melanoma. Pathology. 36(5):419-27, 2004
6. Ball NJ et al: Melanocytic nevi with focal atypical epithelioid cell components: a review of seventy-three cases. J Am Acad Dermatol. 30(5 Pt 1):724-9, 1994
7. Pulitzer DR et al: Histologic classification of the combined nevus. Analysis of the variable expression of melanocytic nevi. Am J Surg Pathol. 15(12):1111-22, 1991

(Left) *The same lesion is shown at high magnification. The gray, lightly melanized cytoplasm with banal nuclei are characteristic.* **(Right)** *Another example shows a mixture of lightly stained area (type A) contrasted with the darkly stained areas at scanning magnification. Melanophages are evident even at this magnification.*

ITAN at High Magnification Showing Melanized Cytoplasm

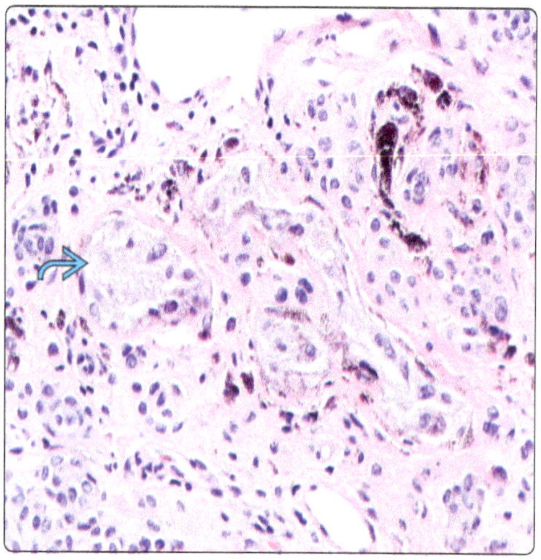

ITAN at Scanning Magnification

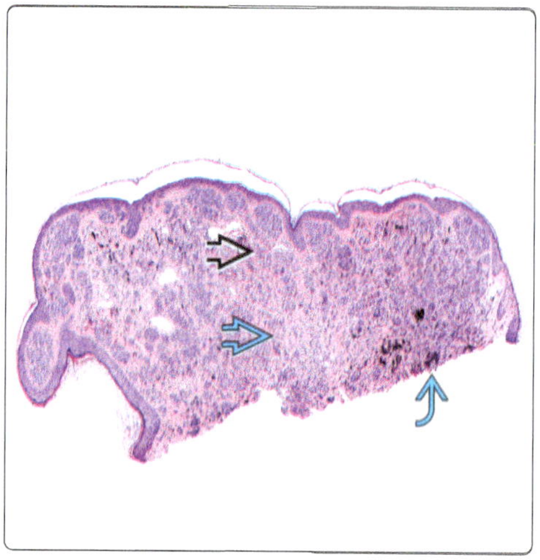

(Left) *Under medium-power magnification, the type A nests stand out in contrast to the surrounding type B nests.* **(Right)** *The type A cells have a banal cytology with finely melanized cytoplasm. The nuclear membranes are smooth and chromatin is evenly distributed. There is no significant nuclear pleomorphism. Mitoses are lacking in the deep aspect of the lesion. Some nucleoli are barely conspicuous.*

ITAN at Intermediate Magnification

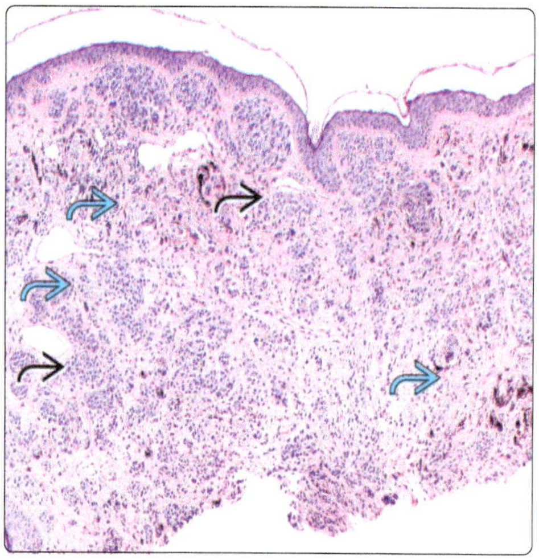

ITAN-Banal Cytology at High Magnification

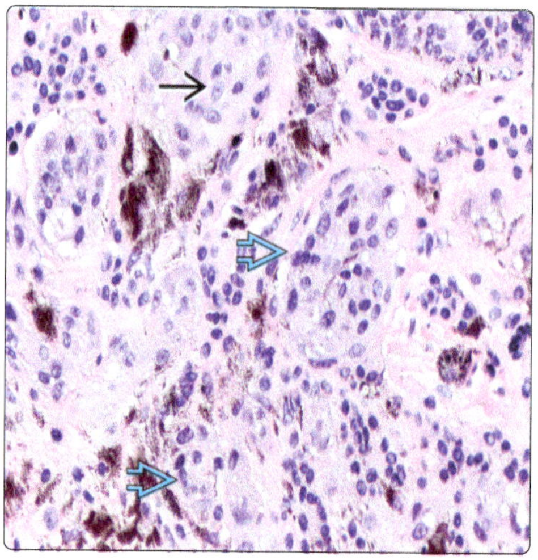

(Left) *This example is wedge-shaped and symmetrical. The unusual feature at this magnification is the lack of maturation with increasing dermal depth.* **(Right)** *The nests do mature with increasing dermal depth but extend deep into the reticular dermis, resembling a deep penetrating nevus.*

ITAN: Example Mimicking Deep Penetrating Nevus

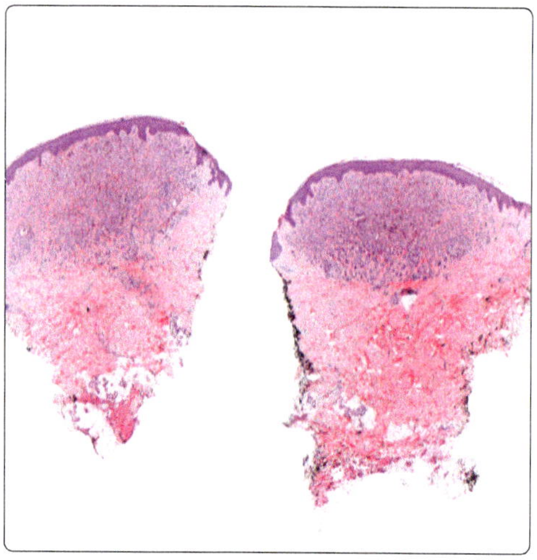

ITAN Resembling Deep Penetrating Nevus

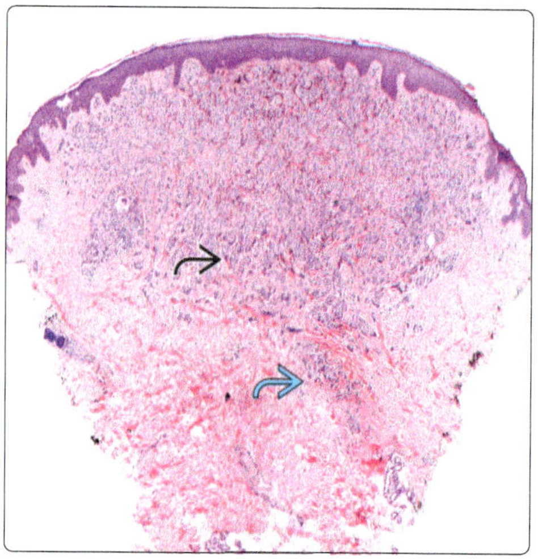

ITAN at Intermediate Magnification

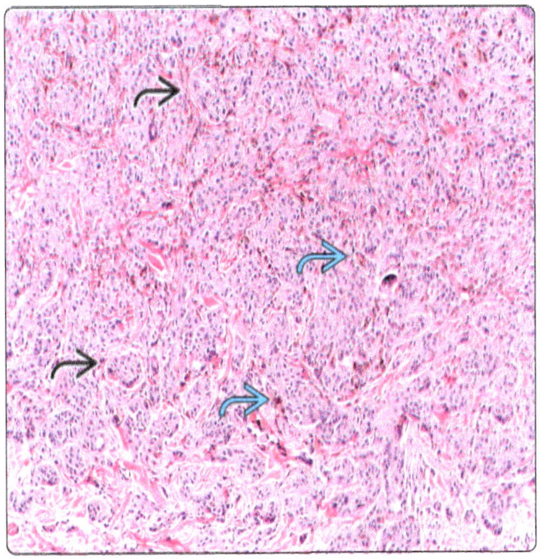

ITAN at High Power Showing Cytologic Features

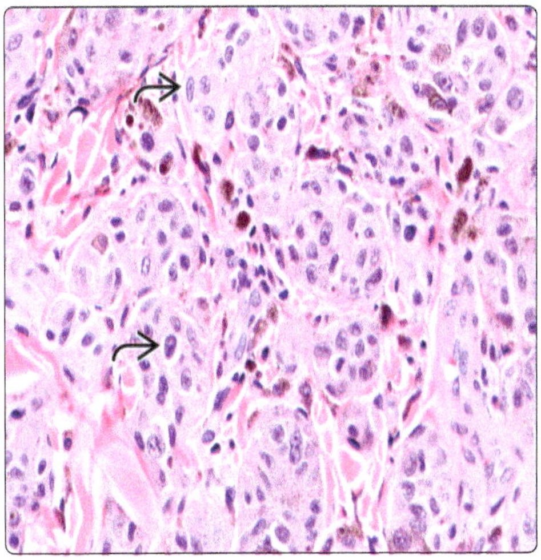

(Left) *This example has a predominately epithelioid morphology. It is well nested, and the nests are surrounded by numerous melanophages.* **(Right)** *Under high-power magnification, the nests have a round outline. The nuclei are vesicular with conspicuous nucleoli. No mitoses are found under high magnification.*

Another ITAN at Low Magnification

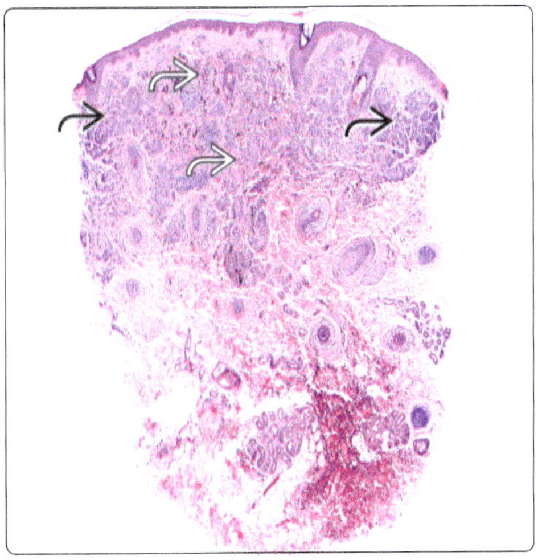

ITAN at Intermediate Power

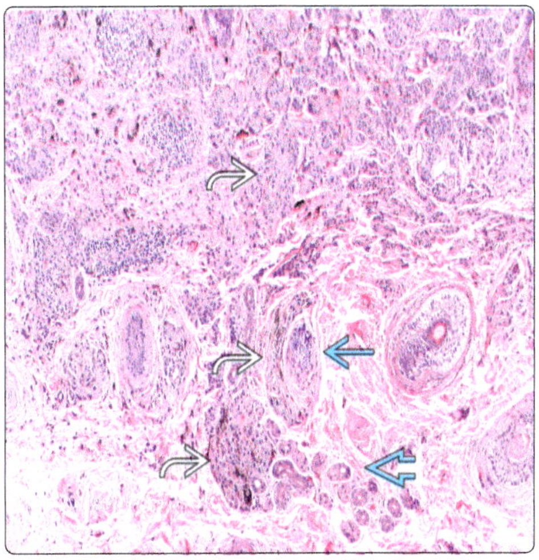

(Left) *This punch biopsy of facial skin shows 2 populations of nests: (1) Darker, closer to the periphery and (2) Lighter, more central.* **(Right)** *The gray, lightly melanized nests extend deep into the reticular dermis and wrap around the hair follicle and eccrine apparatus.*

ITAN at High Power Showing Cytologic Features

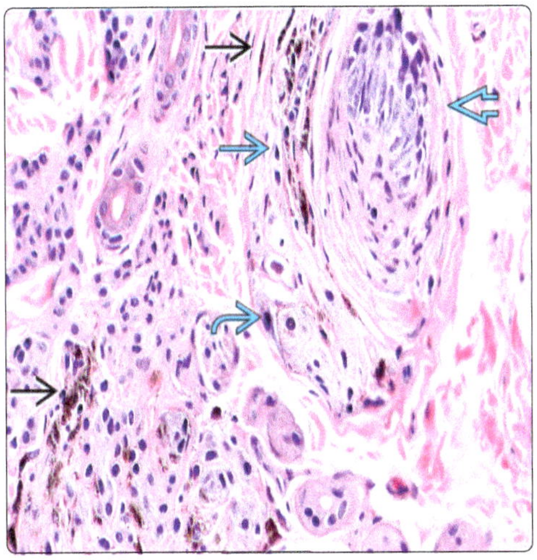

ITAN Plaque-Like Example at Low Power

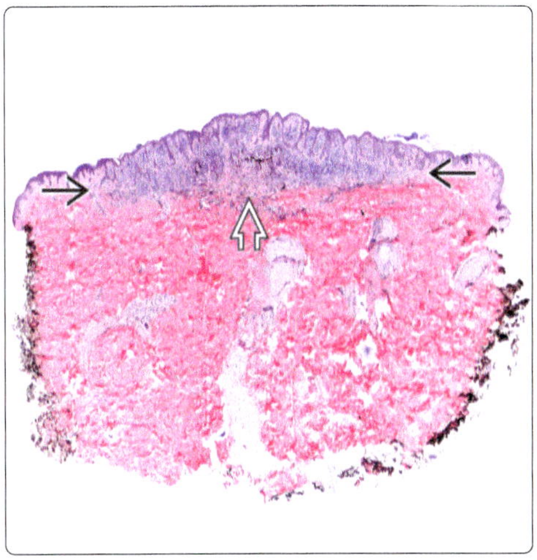

(Left) *The small, hyperchromatic nuclei and somewhat smudged chromatin are reassuring benign features. Adnexa (hair follicle in this case) are preserved. Numerous melanophages are evident.* **(Right)** *This example on back skin shows a plaque-like intradermal growth, resembling a congenital melanocytic nevus. The tumor fills the papillary dermis and is centrally pale.*

KEY FACTS

TERMINOLOGY

- Plexiform spindle cell nevus
- Benign, uncommon variant of melanocytic nevus (blue nevus)
- Frequent participant in combined nevus, where it is associated with ordinary nevus
- Characterized by wedge-shaped or plexiform growth pattern

ETIOLOGY/PATHOGENESIS

- Often associated with 2nd nevoid subtype, thereby overlapping with combined nevus

CLINICAL ISSUES

- Patients between 10-30 years
- Head (face) and neck, back (upper trunk), and proximal extremities
- Irregular dark brown to black papule or nodule measuring 0.2-1.0 cm in diameter
- Deep penetrating nevus-like atypical borderline tumors can be associated with regional lymph node metastasis

MICROSCOPIC

- Wedge-shaped (inverted triangle) outline, extending to deep dermis and subcutaneous adipose tissue
- Extending deep involving (wrapping around) blood vessels, nerves, and adnexa (plexiform pattern)
- Cells have epithelioid to round to fusiform nuclei
- Normal-appearing mitotic figures are few and present in only small minority of lesions

TOP DIFFERENTIAL DIAGNOSES

- Malignant melanoma
- Cellular blue nevus
- Combine nevus with features of common blue
- Spitz nevus
- Inverted type-A nevus
- Plexiform spindle cell nevus

DPN Showing Wedge-Shaped Infiltrate

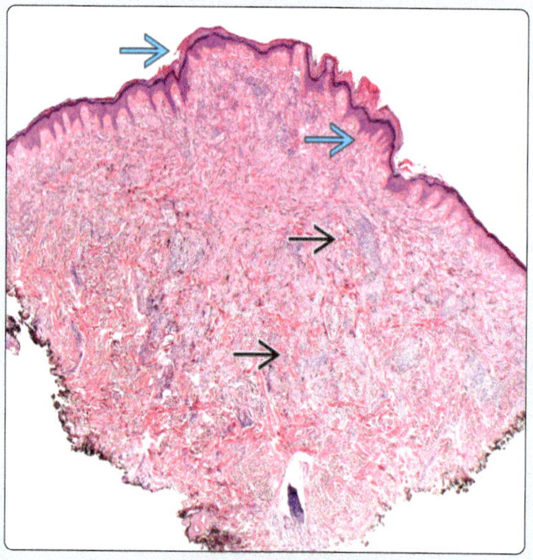

DPN: Inflamed With Melanophages

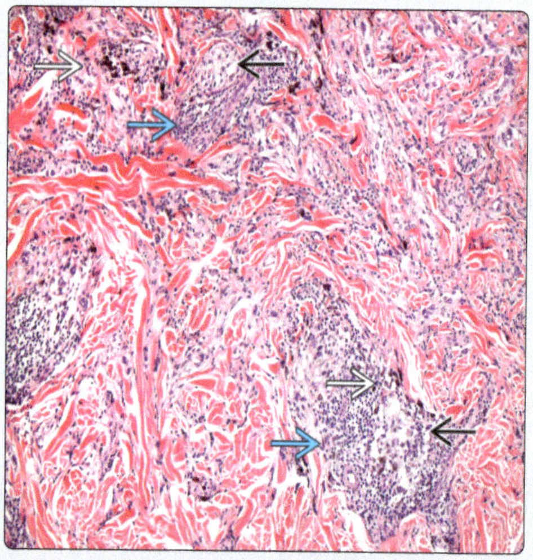

(Left) *This is a subtle case of deep penetrating nevus (DPN) on low-power examination. There are, however, dermally located subtle nests and fascicles of melanocytes* → *. There is no junctional* → *component.* **(Right)** *There is a lymphocytic infiltrate* → *that surrounds the lightly melanized fascicles and nests of melanocytes* → *. Note the melanophages* → *located deep in the reticular dermis.*

Melanocytes Intervening Between Collagen Bundles

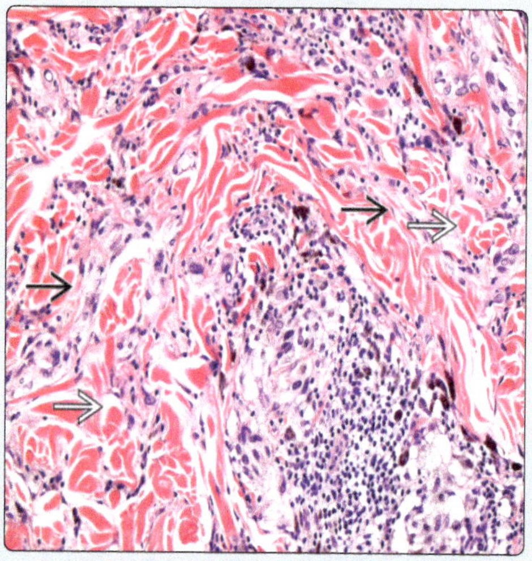

Mild Cytological Atypia in DPN

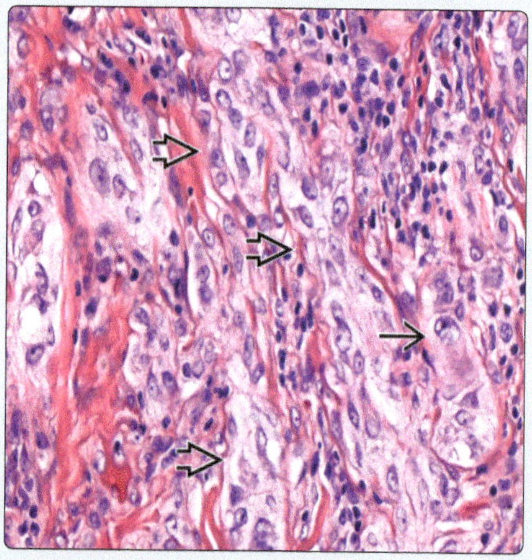

(Left) *This power shows cords and smaller fascicles of melanocytes* → *that intervene between collagen bundles. This feature may be more prominent in plexiform spindle cell tumors. It can resemble a dermatofibroma as the melanocytes "trap" collagen bundles* → *.* **(Right)** *High-power examination shows mild, focal nuclear pleomorphism and prominent nucleoli* → *. The remainder of nuclei are fusiform with smooth nuclear membranes and conspicuous nucleoli* → *. No mitoses were found in this example.*

TERMINOLOGY

Abbreviations

- Deep penetrating nevus (DPN)

Synonyms

- Plexiform spindle cell nevus

Definitions

- Benign, uncommon variant of melanocytic nevus (likely blue nevus variant)
  - Characterized by wedge-shaped or plexiform growth pattern

ETIOLOGY/PATHOGENESIS

Histological Variance

- Often associated with 2nd nevoid subtype, thereby overlapping with combined nevus

CLINICAL ISSUES

Epidemiology

- Patients between 10-30 years

Site

- Head (face) and neck, back (upper trunk), and proximal extremities

Presentation

- Irregular dark brown to black papule or nodule measuring 0.2-1.0 cm in diameter
- May show variegation in color, including shades of brown, blue, and black
  - Can create initial clinical concern for malignant melanoma (29% of cases)

Natural History

- Lesions without cytological atypia and low mitotic activity show no local recurrences and no distant metastases
- DPN-like borderline tumors can be associated with regional lymph node metastasis
  - May exhibit potential for melanoma progression despite normal cytogenetic profile

Treatment

- Surgical approaches
  - When devoid of atypia, it is treated by simple excision
  - Patients with DPN-like borderline tumors should be aggressively managed

Prognosis

- Patients with typical plexiform spindle cell melanocytic tumors do well
- Patients with DPN-like borderline tumors may show lymph node involvement (33%)
  - Can rarely recur or metastasize

MICROSCOPIC

Histologic Features

- Wedge-shaped (inverted triangle) outline, extending to deep dermis and subcutaneous adipose tissue
- Extending deep involving (wrapping around) blood vessels, nerves, and adnexa (plexiform pattern)
- Heavily pigmented macrophages are sparse to abundant

Cytologic Features

- Pale to lightly melanized cytoplasm
- Cells have epithelioid to round to fusiform nuclei
- Cytological atypia (e.g., nuclear hyperchromasia or pleomorphism) is rare
- Normal-appearing mitotic figures are few and present in only small minority of lesions

ANCILLARY TESTS

Immunohistochemistry

- PCNA or other markers of cell cycle, e.g., Ki-67
  - Like other melanocytic nevi, DPN shows low proliferation index in melanocytes, i.e., 5%

Comparative Genomic Hybridization

- DPN-like borderline tumors may deceptively show normal cytogenetics by comparative genomic hybridization (cGH) and FISH

DIFFERENTIAL DIAGNOSIS

Malignant Melanoma

- Atypical junctional melanocytic component
- Nonrandom cytological atypia of dermal melanocytes

Cellular Blue Nevus

- Nests and fascicles of poorly pigmented melanocytes with ovoid nuclei
  - Inconspicuous nucleoli and clear cytoplasm

Combined Nevus With Features of Common Blue

- Pigmented, spindled-shaped (with dendrites), and small epithelioid (type B) melanocytes

Spitz Nevus

- Raining down pattern of epithelioid and spindled melanocytes

Inverted Type A Nevus

- Distinct epithelioid cells deep within lesion (reticular dermis)

Plexiform Spindle Cell Nevus (Likely DPN Variant)

- Predominately spindled cells spread between collagen fibers

DIAGNOSTIC CHECKLIST

Pathologic Interpretation Pearls

- Acquire deeper histological sections looking for mitoses

SELECTED REFERENCES

1. Hung T et al: The plexiform spindle cell nevus nevi and atypical variants: report of 128 cases. Hum Pathol. 45(12):2369-78, 2014
2. Magro CM et al: Deep penetrating nevus-like borderline tumors: a unique subset of ambiguous melanocytic tumors with malignant potential and normal cytogenetics. Eur J Dermatol. 24(5):594-602, 2014
3. High WA et al: Is melanocytic nevus with focal atypical epithelioid components (clonal nevus) a superficial variant of deep penetrating nevus? J Am Acad Dermatol. 55(3):460-6, 2006

(Left) *This example shows heavy pigmentation throughout the lesion and the dermis. The outline is wedge-shaped and resembles an imaginary, inverted triangle. Note the deep extension into the reticular dermis, giving the 1st impression of a DPN.* **(Right)** *Higher power examination reveals a hypercellular area, resembling a cellular blue nevus. The melanocytic cytoplasm ranges from being lightly to heavily melanized. Note the fascicular growth rather than the nested pattern.*

Heavily Melanized DPN With Wedge-Shaped Outline

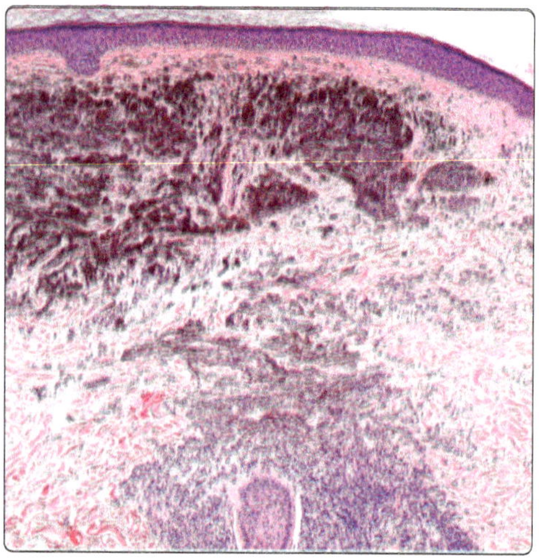

Small Epithelioid Cytology in DPN

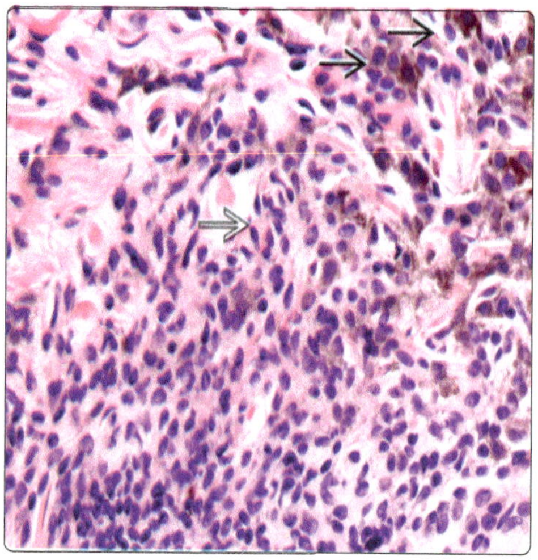

(Left) *In this field, the melanocytes respect the follicular adventitia. The cells abut the adventitia but do not invade it. These cells can also involve neurovascular bundles. However, there is no necrosis or loss of adnexa.* **(Right)** *Among the numerous heavily melanized, epithelioid melanocytes, there are rare fusiform to spindled nevus cells. The dendritic processes are evident. This may be why some consider this nevus a variant of blue nevus.*

DPN Cells Respecting Adventitia

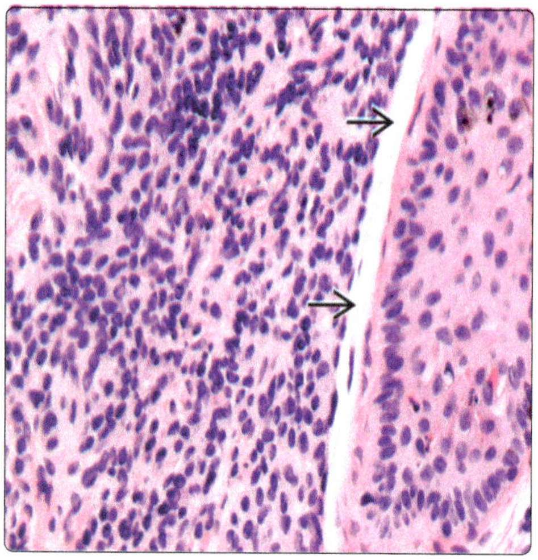

Rare Spindled Cells in DPN

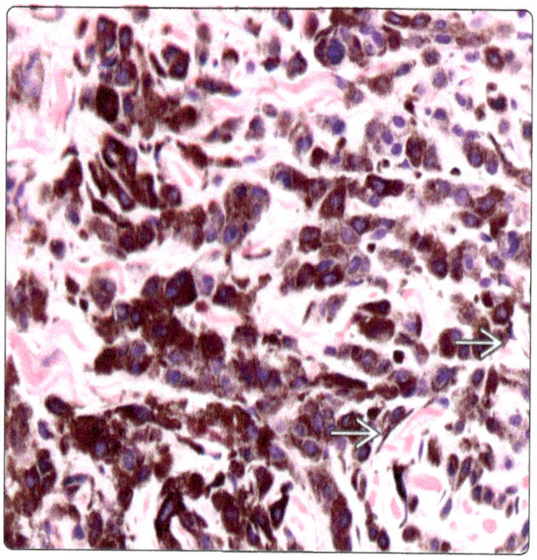

(Left) *This lesion also shows a heavily melanized, wedge-shaped tumor that penetrates down to Clark anatomic level IV, mimicking a DPN. However, this lesion has 2 cell types: Small epithelioid type B and the spindled melanocytes with dendrites.* **(Right)** *This field shows the deep extension of short, spindled melanocytes that wrap around the eccrine ducts, nerve bundles, and blood vessels. Note the collagen trapping by spindled melanocytes in the deeper areas. Also note the type B nevomelanocytes.*

Differential Diagnosis: Combined Nevus

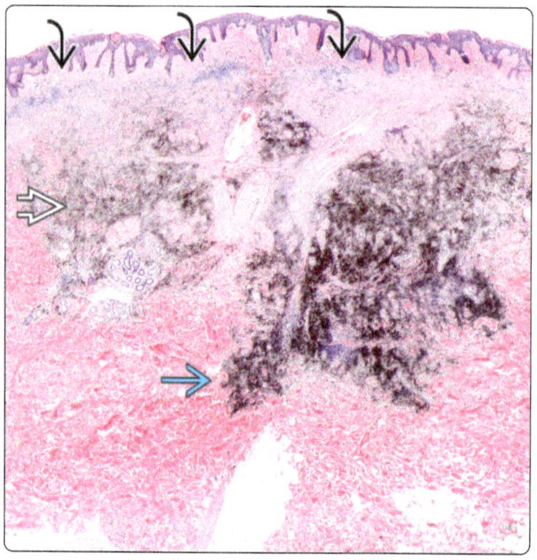

Combined Nevus Involving Neurovascular Bundles and Adnexa

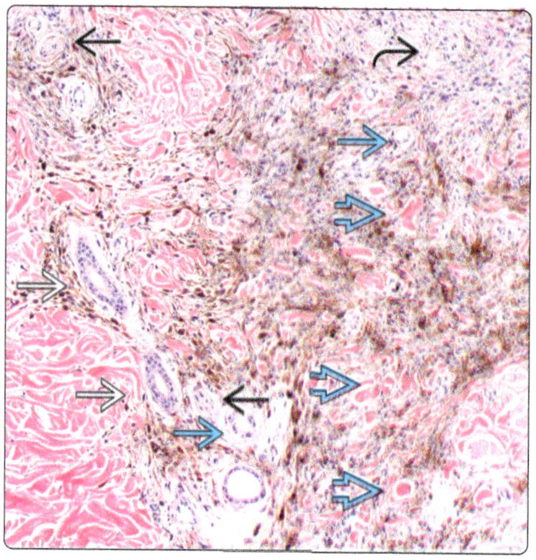

Combined Nevus Showing Benign Cytology

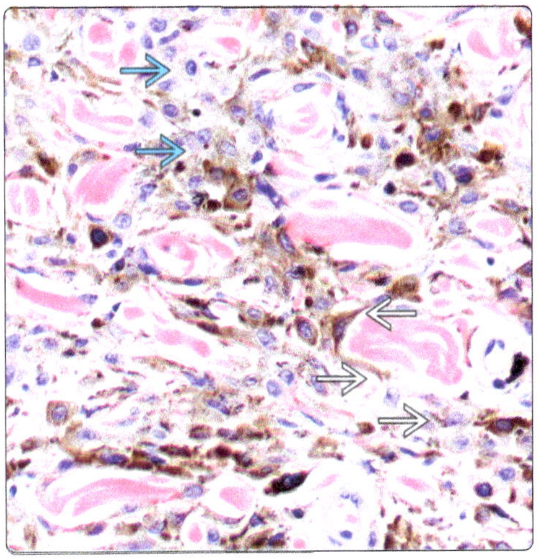

Differential Diagnosis: Cellular Blue Nevus

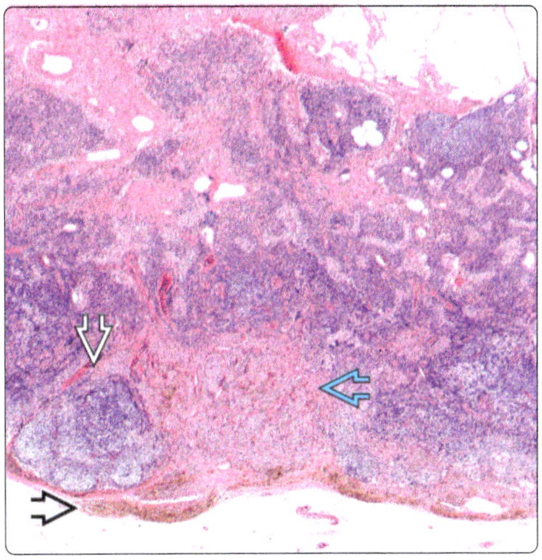

(Left) *The cytopathology is benign to mildly atypical: Slight nuclear pleomorphism and conspicuous nucleoli ➡. Also found are spindled melanocytes with delicate dendrocytes ➡. Note the absence of melanocytic nests or fascicles.* **(Right)** *Cellular blue nevus can resemble a DPN by virtue of its deep involvement of subcutaneous adipose tissue. However, a dumbbell appearance ➡, small epithelioid ➡, and spindled melanocytes with melanophages ➡ are evident here.*

Differential Diagnosis: Cellular Blue Nevus

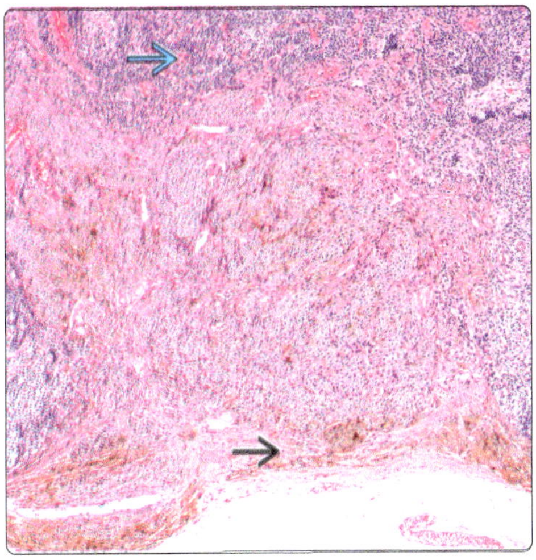

Differential Diagnosis: Cellular Blue Nevus at High Magnification

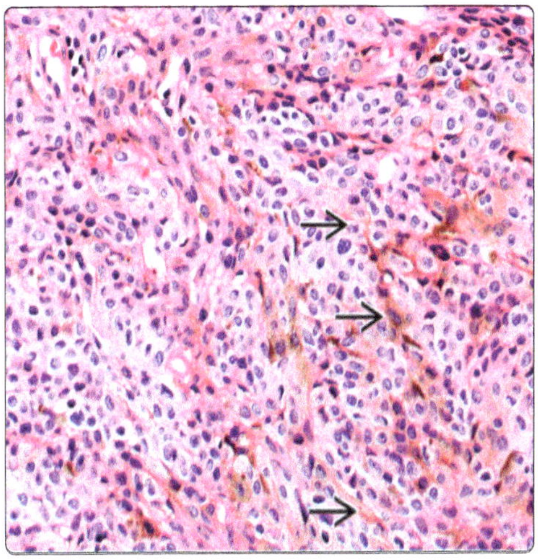

(Left) *In this medium-power magnification, a focus of clear cell melanocytes with pale cytoplasm is apparent. The focus is surrounded by a sparse lymphoid infiltrate above ➡ and a zone of spindled melanocytes admixed with melanophages below ➡.* **(Right)** *A higher magnification shows that the nevus cells have pale cytoplasm with uniform round to oval vesicular nuclei and conspicuous nucleoli. There are intervening pigmented spindled cells ➡.*

Differential Diagnosis: Inverted Type A Nevus

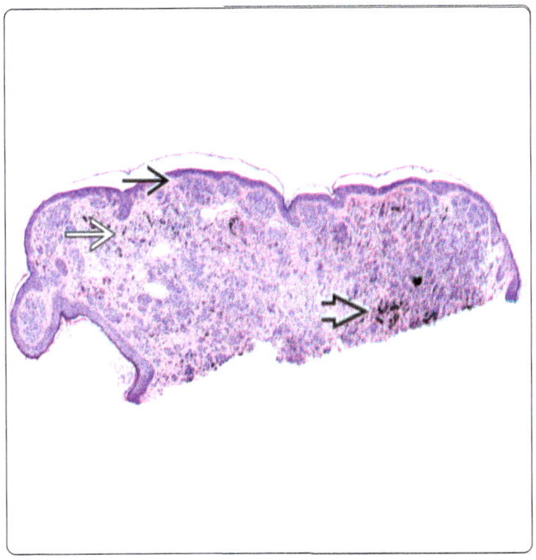

Differential Diagnosis: Inverted Type A Nevus at High Power

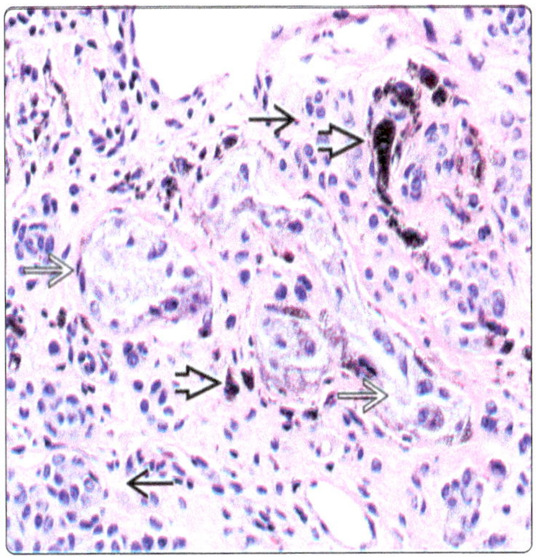

(Left) *Inverted type A nevi can have a deep extension into the reticular dermis, not appreciated in this superficial shave biopsy. Note the type B ➡ and type A ➡ areas admixed with melanophages ➡. The type A areas appear to be more pale with less hyperchromatic nuclei.* **(Right)** *Under higher magnification, the type B (or lymphoid) ➡ and type A (epithelioid) ➡ melanocytes become evident. These areas are admixed with melanophages ➡. The type A areas appear to be more pale with less hyperchromatic nuclei.*

Conjunctival Melanocytic Nevi

KEY FACTS

TERMINOLOGY

- Conjunctival melanocytic nevus
- Primary acquired melanosis (PAM)
- Acquired or congenital conjunctival nevi
- Most common tumors of conjunctiva, accounting for up to 53% of all conjunctival neoplasms

CLINICAL ISSUES

- Most common in young Caucasians, with mean age at presentation of ~ 32 years
- Most commonly arise in bulbar conjunctiva, caruncle, or plica semilunaris
- Circumscribed flat to slightly raised macules or papules
- Juvenile conjunctival nevus rapidly grow and can look clinically concerning, leading to biopsies
- PAM is acquired, usually unilateral, flat, pigmented lesion

MICROSCOPIC

- Junctional: Nested but sometimes also lentiginous proliferations of type A or type B cells confined to epithelium
- Compound: Intraepithelial components shows type A, or less commonly, type B melanocytes
- Subepithelial (counterpart of intradermal nevus): Have predominantly type B or C melanocytes in substantia propria without intraepithelial component
- Juvenile conjunctival nevus exhibit confluent growth pattern in junctional component
- Paradoxical "reverse" maturation in subepithelium seen in juvenile conjunctival nevus
- PAM without atypia (similar to solar lentigo &/or jentigo in skin)

ANCILLARY TESTS

- Melanocytes should express usual melanocytic markers, MART-1/Melan-A, HMB-45, and S100

Conjunctival Nevus With Prominent Epithelial Cysts

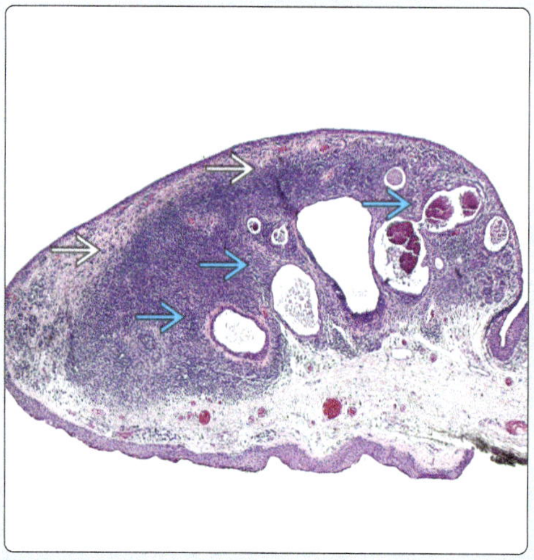

Epithelial Cysts With Sulfur Granules

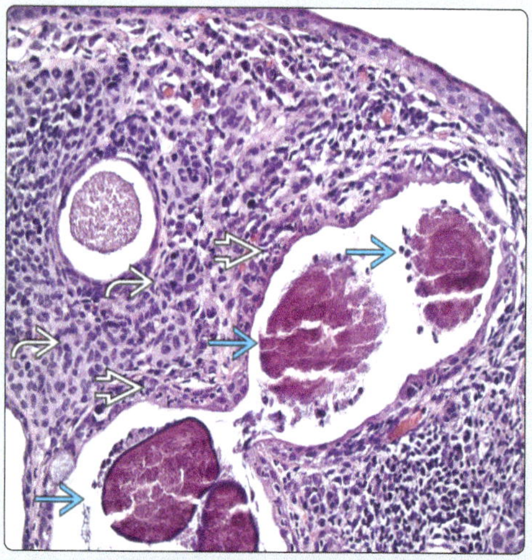

(Left) *Conjunctival melanocytic nevi (50%) can exhibit numerous epithelial-lined cysts located within the lesion, as seen here under scanning magnification. This is a useful finding, supporting benignancy. Note the lymphohistiocytic infiltrate hugging the lesion.* **(Right)** *Higher power magnification shows the cysts to contain sulfur granules and invoke a neutrophilic response. The nested nevomelanocytes, surrounding the infected cysts, are devoid any cytological atypia.*

Juvenile Conjunctival Nevus

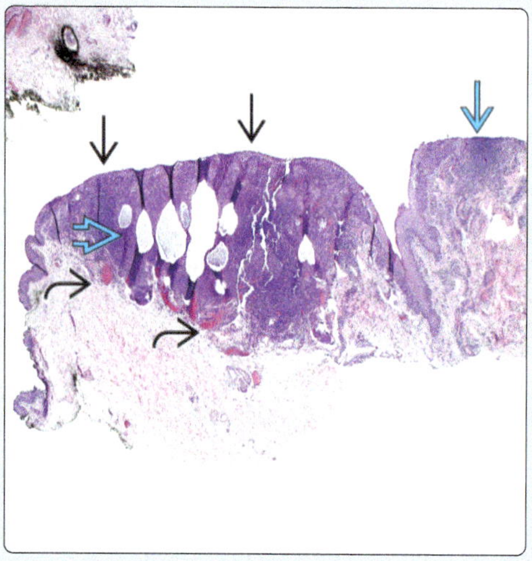

Confluent Growth Pattern and Reverse Maturation

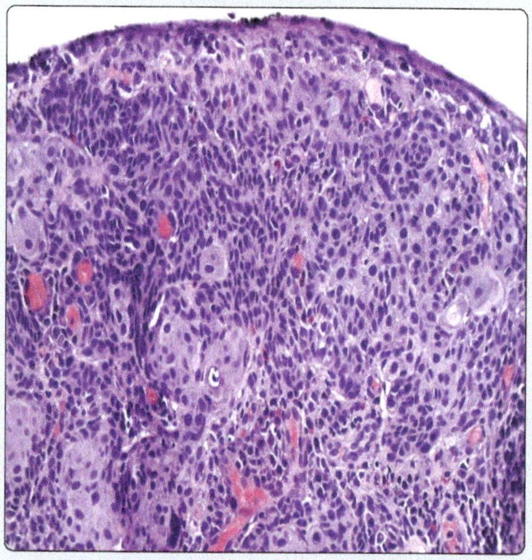

(Left) *At this scanning magnification, a hypercellular proliferation appears to occupy the subepithelium underneath the conjunctival epithelium. There is intralesional cystic degeneration. There is a focus of intense lymphohistiocytic infiltrate commonly seen in these lesions.* **(Right)** *A higher magnification is shown from the same lesion. The subepithelial component does not appear to decrease in the nuclear:cytoplasmic ratio. This paradoxical maturation is an expected feature.*

TERMINOLOGY

Synonyms

- Acquired or congenital conjunctival nevi
- Primary acquired melanosis (PAM)
  - Not secondary melanosis due to inflammation or systemic disease

Definitions

- Most common tumors of conjunctiva, accounting for up to 53% of all conjunctival neoplasms

CLINICAL ISSUES

Epidemiology

- Most common in young Caucasians, with mean age at presentation of ~ 32 years
- Juvenile conjunctival nevus occurs in children and adolescents
- PAM occurs in middle-aged or elderly Caucasians

Site

- Most commonly arise in bulbar conjunctiva, caruncle, or plica semilunaris
- PAM occurs on bulbar conjunctiva

Presentation

- Circumscribed flat to slightly raised macules or papules
- Juvenile conjunctival nevi rapidly grow and can look clinically concerning, leading to biopsies
- PAM is acquired, usually unilateral, flat, pigmented lesion

Natural History

- Malignant melanoma can develop in less than 1% of conjunctival nevi

Treatment

- Surgical approaches
  - Conjunctival nevi do not require treatment if clinically stable

Prognosis

- Conjunctival nevi have excellent prognosis
- PAM without atypia can recur in about 11% cases, but it does not progress to melanoma

MICROSCOPIC

Histologic Features

- Anatomic classification (similar to skin)
  - Junctional: Nested but sometimes also lentiginous proliferations of type A or type B cells confined to epithelium
  - Compound: Intraepithelial components shows type A, or less commonly, type B melanocytes
    - Similar to those in skin, melanocytes become smaller (nuclear:cytoplasmic ratio decreased) with increasing dermal depth
    - Formation of intralesional epithelial cysts lined by conjunctival epithelium and goblet cells (found in 50% of cases)
  - Subepithelial (counterpart of intradermal nevus): Have predominantly type B or C melanocytes in substantia propria without intraepithelial component
- Juvenile conjunctival nevus
  - Confluent growth pattern in junctional component
  - Paradoxical "reverse" maturation in subepithelium
    - i.e., nuclear and cytoplasmic size of melanocytes forming subepithelial component is greater than that of junctional component
  - Prominent inflammatory infiltrate
    - May obscure architecture of nevus
    - Misleading impression of cytologic atypia
- PAM without atypia (similar to solar lentigo &/or jentigo in skin)
  - Basal keratinocytic hyperpigmentation ± melanocytic hyperplasia
  - No melanocytic hyperplasia
    - If present, it is mildly cellular and limited to basal layer

Cytologic Features

- Melanocytic cell-shaped cytology (similar to skin)
  - Nests of oval cells (type A): Vesicular chromatin and conspicuous nucleoli
  - Sheets of oval to cuboidal cells (type B): Hyperchromatic and smooth nuclear membrane
  - Spindle-like cells in subepithelium (type C): Vesicular to hyperchromatic chromatin

Histologic Variants (Similar to Skin)

- Include combined nevus, inverted type A nevus, balloon cell nevus, Spitz nevus, pigmented spindle cell nevus, and blue nevus

ANCILLARY TESTS

Immunohistochemistry

- Melanocytes should express usual melanocytic markers, MART-1/Melan-A, HMB-45, and S100

Genetic Testing

- One study suggests that FISH may be helpful in better classifying atypical conjunctival melanocytic proliferations from nevi

DIFFERENTIAL DIAGNOSIS

Primary Acquired Melanosis With Atypia

- Melanocytic hyperplasia with atypia

DIAGNOSTIC CHECKLIST

Clinically Relevant Pathologic Features

- Acquire clinical information such as age and race

Pathologic Interpretation Pearls

- Be cautious with conjunctival nevi with prominent lentiginous growth pattern that are partially sampled

SELECTED REFERENCES

1. Zembowicz A et al: Melanocytic lesions of the conjunctiva. Arch Pathol Lab Med. 134(12):1785-92, 2010

(**Left**) *This lesion shows a prominent banal junctional component with adjacent inflammatory infiltrate. Also seen is a focus with limited pagetoid scatter. This finding, in isolation, should not be overinterpreted as these lesions may often show tangential sectioning of the epithelium.* (**Right**) *A higher magnification of the same field in the lesion shows a robust junctional component that extends into the subepithelium. There are no subepithelial nests. The presence of apical clefting suggests benignancy.*

Junctional Component With Limited Pagetoid Scatter in Conjunctival Nevus

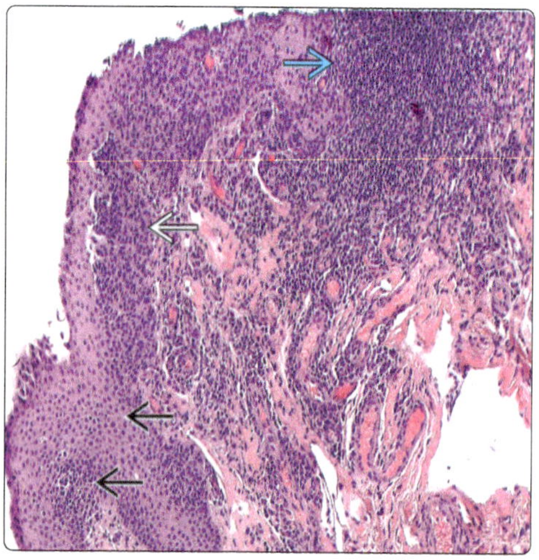

High Magnification of Junctional Component

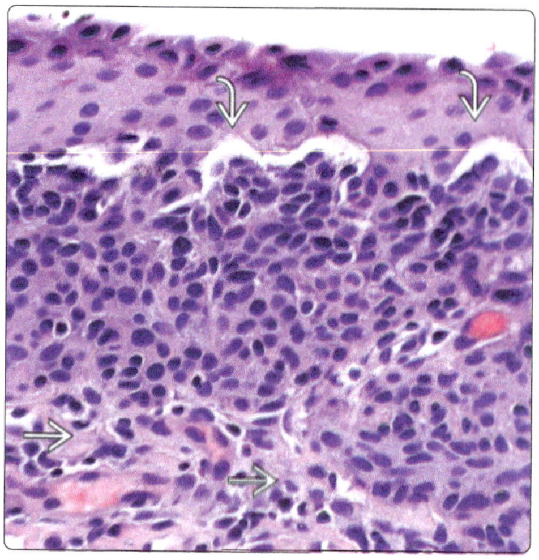

(**Left**) *This field of junctional component shows focal upward ascent of banal melanocytes, which should not be over diagnosed as malignant. Moreover, there are banal junctional nests throughout the conjunctiva (nonkeratinizing epithelium).* (**Right**) *This field (same lesion) reveals a junctional melanocytic component and epithelial induction, which appears more eosinophilic. There are epithelial microcysts and goblet cells.*

Conjunctival Nevus With Limited Pagetoid Scatter

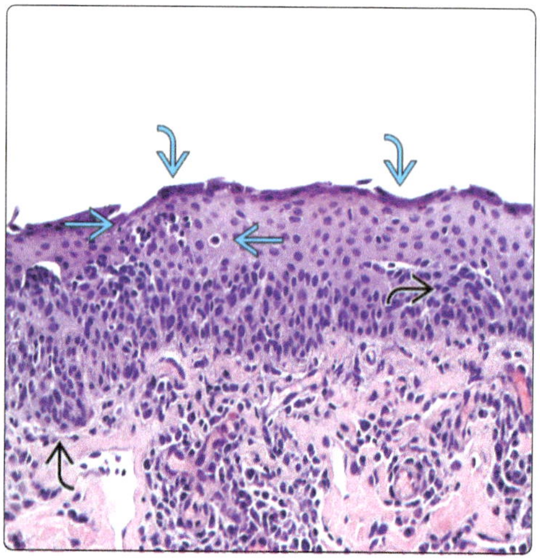

Associated Epithelial Cysts and Goblet Cells

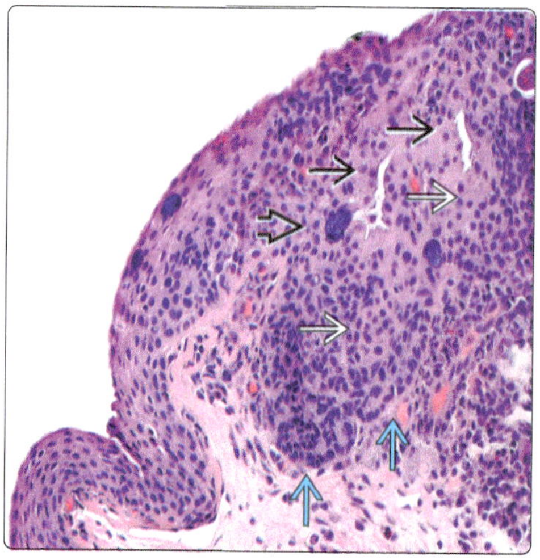

(**Left**) *Note the banal cytology of type B cells located in the junctional component, with evenly distributed chromatin. These melanocytes appear to "blend in" with the keratinocytes. Epithelial microcysts and goblet cells are shown at a higher power magnification.* (**Right**) *High-power examination of the junctional component melanocytes shows smooth nuclear membranes & ample eosinophilic cytoplasm. Melanocytic cytoplasmic membrane is indistinct, blending in with the keratinocytes.*

Blended Appearance of Melanocytes and Keratinocytes

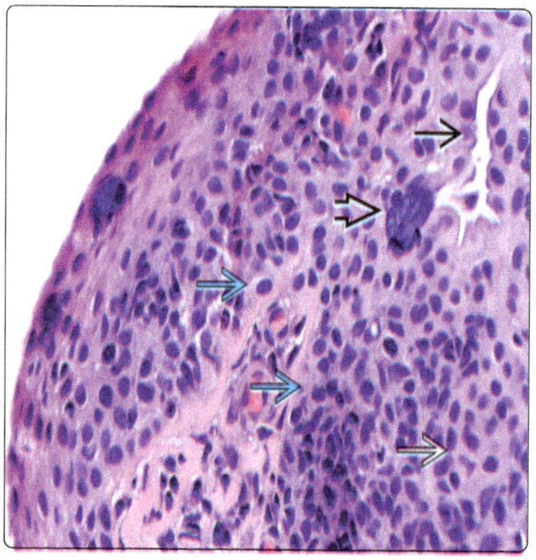

High Magnification Showing Benign Cytopathology

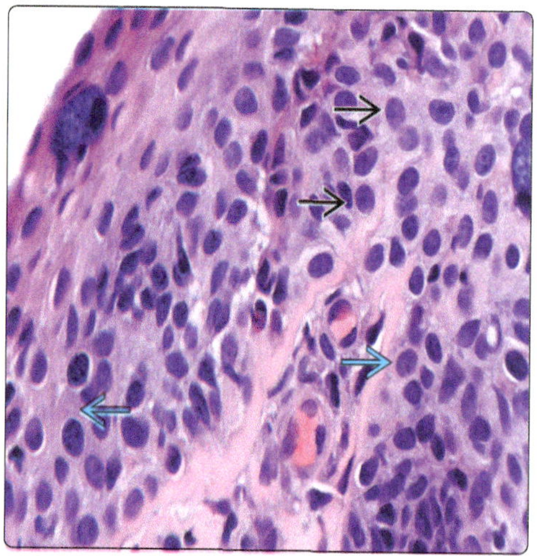

Conjunctival Nevus With Goblet Cells and Epithelial Cysts

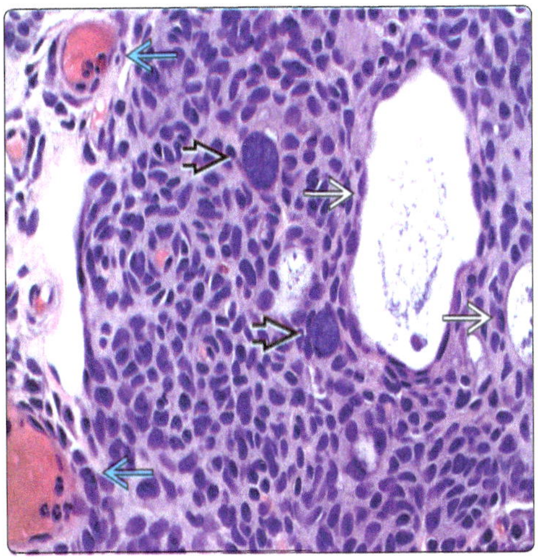

High Magnification Showing Benign Cytopathology

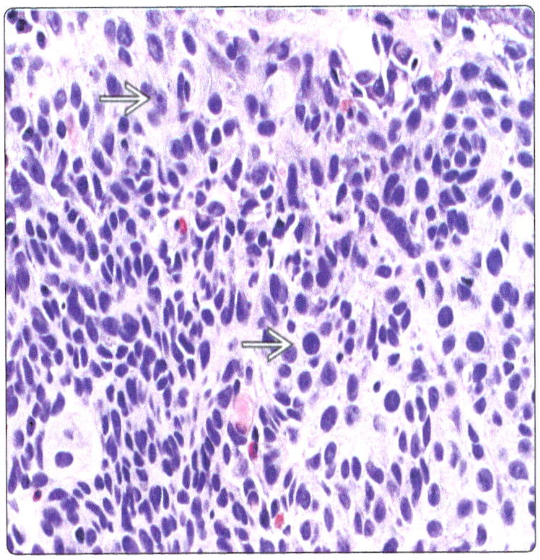

(Left) *The presence of goblet cells and epithelial-lined cysts are reassuring features. They support evidence of benignancy. Note the smooth nuclear membrane outline and hyperchromasia. Capillary-sized blood vessels are noted.* **(Right)** *High-power magnification shows evenly distributed chromatin and conspicuous nucleoli in most of the cells in this field. There are no mitoses, apoptosis, or necrosis.*

Heavily Pigmented Conjunctival Nevus

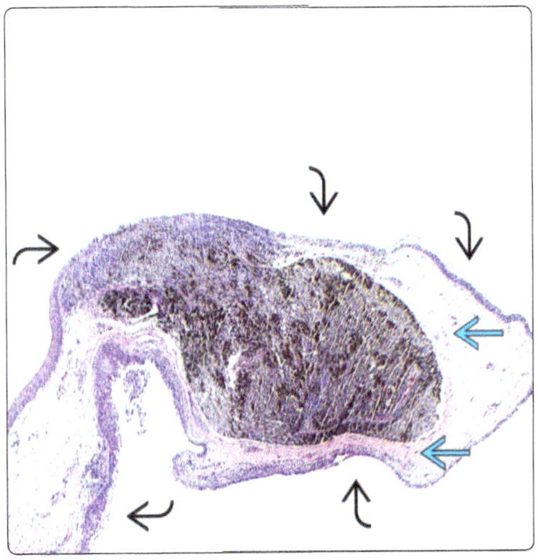

Combined Juvenile Conjunctival and Inverted Type A Nevus

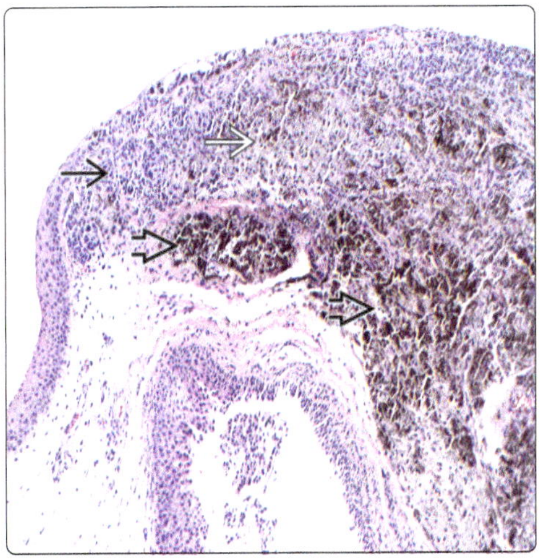

(Left) *The scanning magnification of this lesion shows a heavily pigmented pedunculated nodule within the subepithelium. The biopsy shows an intact, continuous conjunctival covering all around the nodule.* **(Right)** *A medium-power examination shows pale and darker cellular areas. This field is admixed with a significant number of melanophages.*

Combined Type B and Type A Nevomelanocytes

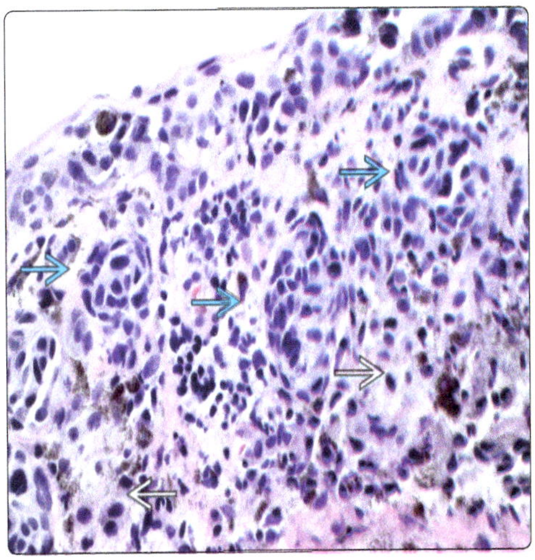

Banal Cytopathology of Type A Melanocytes

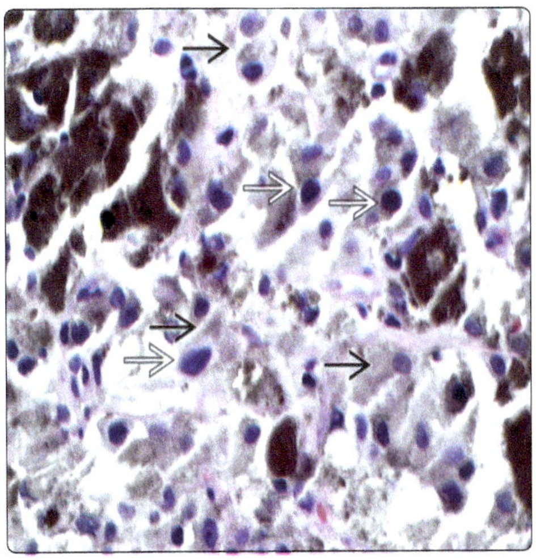

(Left) *This field (same lesion) shows the combined presence of both type B "lymphoid" nevus cells and type A epithelioid nevomelanocytes. This feature is analogous to a cutaneous inverted type A nevus with a combined type B component.* **(Right)** *Ample, epithelioid cytoplasm that is lightly melanized gives a blue-gray to pink quality. The nuclei are oval to round with even chromatin and inconspicuous nucleoli.*

Dermal Melanocytoses (Nevus of Ota and Ito, Mongolian Spot)

KEY FACTS

CLINICAL ISSUES

- Nevus of Ota and Ito and Mongolian spot
  - Often evident at birth
  - Occasionally manifest later in life
  - Different clinical course
    - Generally stable over time (nevus of Ota and Ito)
    - Resolution with time (Mongolian spot)
  - Blue to gray macule/patch
- Nevus of Ota
  - Near/involving eye
- Nevus of Ito
  - Shoulder area
- Mongolian spot
  - Generally on back

MICROSCOPIC

- Dendritic melanocytes in dermis
- Dermis generally otherwise normal (without sclerosis)

TOP DIFFERENTIAL DIAGNOSES

- Blue nevus
  - Clinically, confluent macule or patch of blue pigmentation, generally not present at birth
  - Histologically dendritic/spindled melanocytes in dermis with variable numbers of melanophages
- Hori nevus
  - Acquired in adulthood, female predominance
  - More common in Asian populations
  - Involves malar cheeks, generally bilateral
  - Often composed of numerous brown macules that may become gray over time
- Becker nevus
  - Clinically tan to brown patch on shoulder/upper back area; may show hypertrichosis within lesion
  - Histologically: Basal layer melanin pigment, smooth muscle bundles in dermis, ± hypertrichosis
- Child abuse

Mongolian Spot in Sacral Region

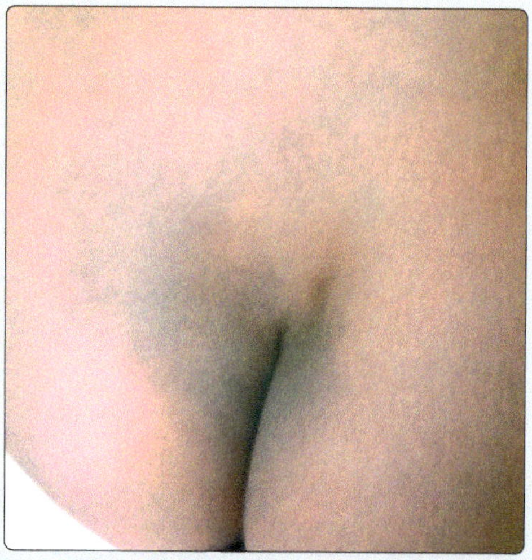

Mongolian Spot on Arm

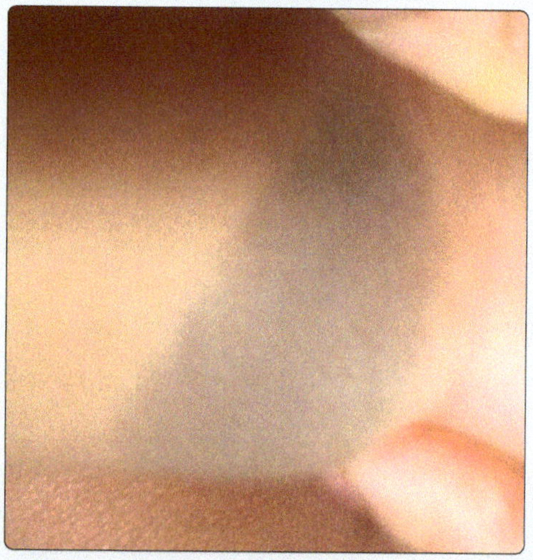

(Left) *This is the classic location for a Mongolian spot, over the sacral area. There may also be patches in other areas of the back.* **(Right)** *This is an aberrant Mongolian spot located on the arm. It was present at birth. These lesions overlap with blue nevi and do not always resolve.*

Mongolian Spot at Low Magnification

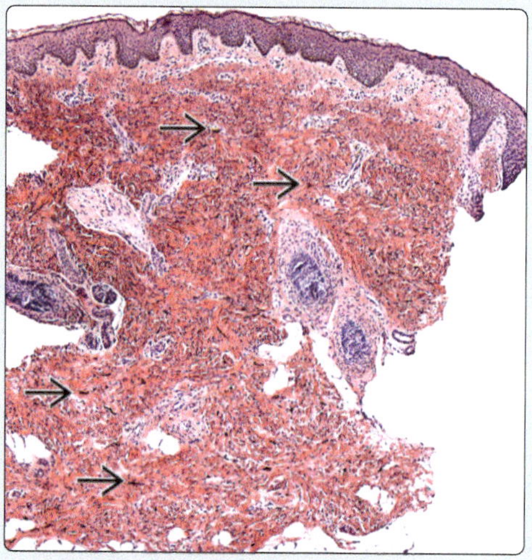

Mongolian Spot at High Magnification

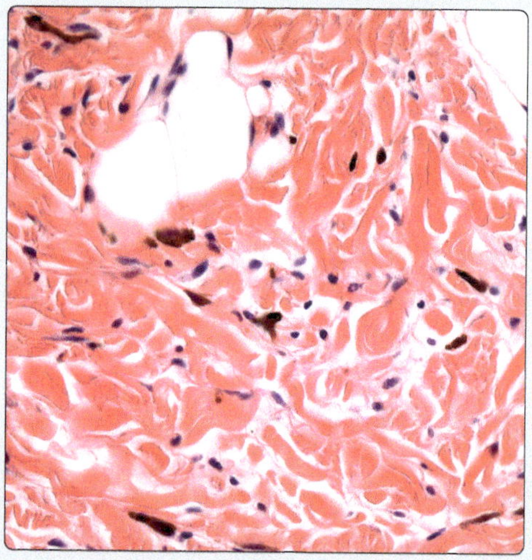

(Left) *This low-magnification view of a Mongolian spot shows a normal epidermis and pigmented cells* ➡ *scattered through the dermis.* **(Right)** *This high-magnification view of a Mongolian spot shows dendritic melanocytes with cytoplasmic melanin pigment in the deep dermis.*

CLINICAL ISSUES

Epidemiology

- Age
  - Often evident at birth but occasionally manifest later
- Ethnicity
  - More common in Asians

Site

- Nevus of Ota
  - Located near/involving eye (conjunctiva)
    - In distribution of trigeminal nerve (ophthalmic/maxillary)
- Nevus of Ito
  - Located on shoulder/deltoid area
- Mongolian spot
  - Located most commonly on back, especially lumbosacral
  - Rarely, in so-called aberrant form, may involve extremities
    - When located in areas other than back, overlaps with blue nevi

Presentation

- Nevus of Ota/Ito
  - Often unilateral
  - Color often blue to gray
  - Variably sized mottled patch
- Mongolian spot
  - Generally 1 or more patches of blue to gray
  - Evident at birth
  - May be associated with nevus flammeus (capillary malformation), nevus spilus, &/or nevus anemicus (so-called phacomatosis pigmentovascularis)

Natural History

- Nevus of Ota and Ito generally stable over time
- Mongolian spots generally fade by age 5
  - Aberrant Mongolian spots may not fade

Treatment

- Benign, no treatment necessary
- Laser may be used if treatment is desired for cosmetic purposes

Prognosis

- Very rarely, malignancy has been reported to develop within nevus of Ota and Ito
- Rarely, nevus of Ota associated with deafness
- Rarely, extensive Mongolian spots associated with inheritable storage disease

MICROSCOPIC

Histologic Features

- Nevus of Ota and Ito and Mongolian spot show similar histologic features
  - Dendritic melanocytes in dermis, may cluster around adnexal structures/vessels/nerves
    - Nevus of Ota/Ito: Melanocytes may be sparse to more numerous, usually in upper dermis
    - Mongolian spot: Melanocytes may be sparse, usually in deeper dermis, often arranged parallel to epidermis
  - Dermis generally otherwise normal (without sclerosis)
  - Melanophages generally absent

Cytologic Features

- Melanocytes
  - Not atypical, dendritic, melanin pigment in cytoplasm

DIFFERENTIAL DIAGNOSIS

Nevus of Ota

- Blue nevus
  - Clinically, confluent macule or patch of blue pigmentation, generally not present at birth
  - Histologically dendritic/spindled melanocytes in dermis with variable numbers of melanophages
- Hori nevus
  - Clinically
    - Acquired in adulthood, female predominance
    - More common in Asian populations
    - Involves malar cheeks, generally bilateral
    - Often composed of numerous brown macules that may become gray over time
- Sun nevus
  - Clinically acquired in adulthood, unilateral hyperpigmented macules in malar area
  - Histologically similar to nevus of Ota or Ito

Nevus of Ito

- Becker nevus
  - Clinically tan to brown patch on shoulder/upper back area; may show hypertrichosis within lesion
  - Histologically
    - Basal layer may show increased melanin pigment
    - Increased smooth muscle bundles in dermis
    - Hair follicles may be increased in number
- Macular amyloid
  - Clinically on shoulder/upper back area with rippled pattern of hyperpigmentation
  - Histologically
    - Deposits of amyloid in papillary dermis, ± pigment incontinence, no melanocytes

Mongolian Spot

- Child abuse
  - In contrast to bruising from child abuse, Mongolian spots present at birth, shows uniform blue-gray color
- Patch-like blue nevus
  - Aberrant Mongolian spot may be indistinguishable clinically from patch-like blue nevus
  - Histologically similar, although patch-like blue nevus is more cellular

SELECTED REFERENCES

1. Tse JY et al: Melanoma arising in a nevus of Ito: Novel genetic mutations and a review of the literature on cutaneous malignant transformation of dermal melanocytoses. J Cutan Pathol. Jan;43(1):57-63, 2015
2. Park JM et al: Acquired bilateral nevus of Ota-like macules (Hori nevus): etiologic and therapeutic considerations. J Am Acad Dermatol. 61(1):88-93, 2009

KEY FACTS

TERMINOLOGY

- Paraganglioma-like dermal melanocytic tumor (PLDMT)
- Rare dermal-based, low-grade melanocytic tumor with histologic similarities to paraganglioma

CLINICAL ISSUES

- Very rare tumors
- Typically occur in young adults, more often in females
- Usually occur on extremities
- Complete excision should be recommended

MICROSCOPIC

- Nodular dermal-based melanocytic tumor
- Relatively well-circumscribed, unencapsulated, and symmetric appearing
- Typically composed of packets of oval to spindle-shaped cells surrounded by thin fibrous septa
- Uniform nuclei, small nucleoli, clear cytoplasm
- Mitotic activity may be present but is usually low

ANCILLARY TESTS

- Positive for S100; MART-1/Melan-A, and HMB-45 (variable)

TOP DIFFERENTIAL DIAGNOSES

- Clear cell/balloon cell melanoma
  - Pagetoid spread and lentiginous hyperplasia in junctional component
  - Dermal component shows greater cytologic atypia and mitotic activity than PLDMT
- Clear cell sarcoma
  - Occurs on extremities, usually in young adults
  - Typically based in deep subcutis but may invade dermis
  - t(12;22), *EWSR1/ATF1* fusion
- Primary dermal melanoma
  - Rare variant of melanoma located in dermis &/or subcutaneous tissues
  - Large, well-circumscribed nodule, which mimics metastatic melanoma in most cases
- Perivascular epithelioid cell tumor

PLDMT at Low Magnification

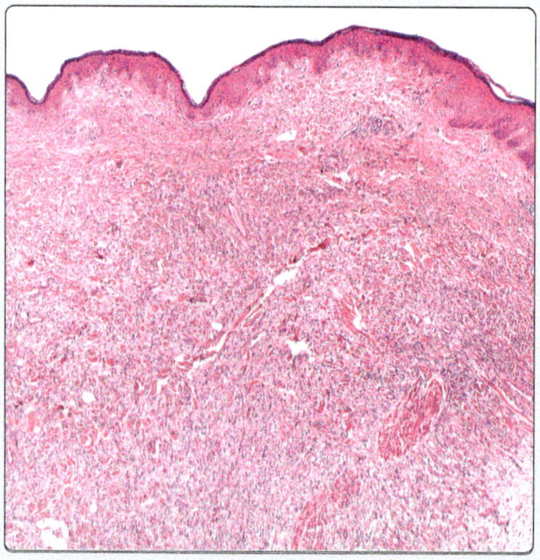

PLDMT at High Magnification Showing Nests of Clear Cells

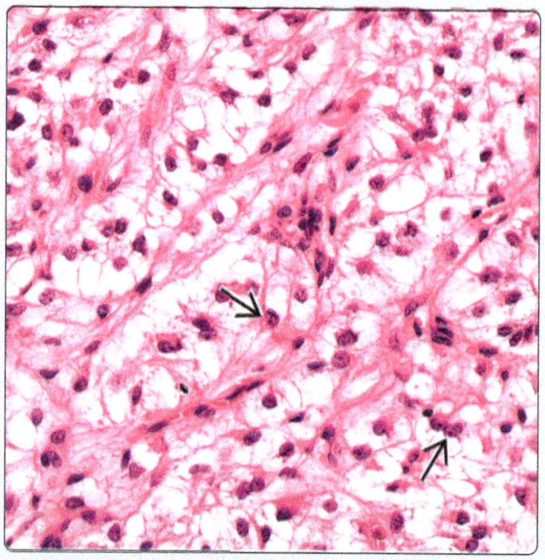

(Left) *Histologic sections show a diffuse proliferation of clear cells located in the dermis. Paraganglioma-like dermal melanocytic tumor (PLDMT) is often a well-circumscribed, but unencapsulated, dermal-based tumor that can extend into the subcutis.* **(Right)** *High magnification shows that the tumor is composed of closely packed nests of cells with clear or granular cytoplasm and round to oval nuclei with small nucleoli* ⇨.

Immunohistochemical Staining for S100

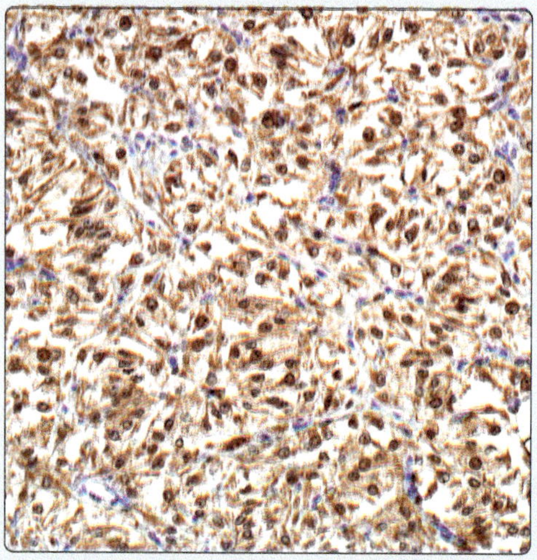

Immunohistochemical Staining for HMB-45

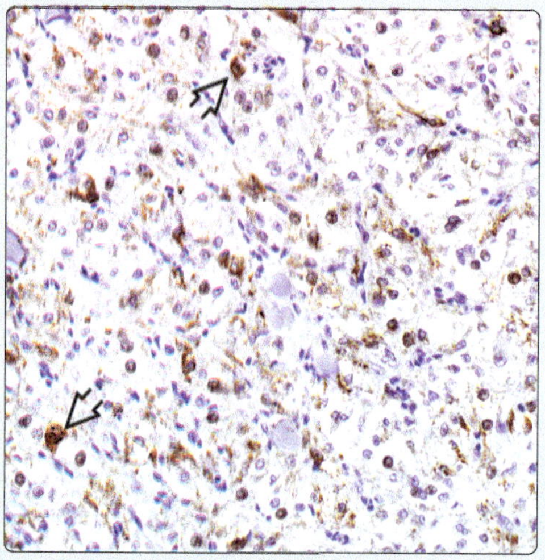

(Left) *Immunostaining for S100 shows diffuse nuclear and cytoplasmic positivity. This helps in the distinction from perivascular epithelioid cell tumor, which is usually negative or only very focally positive for S100 (but positive for other melanocytic markers, including HMB-45 and MART-1/Melan-A).* **(Right)** *The lesional cells also show scattered cytoplasmic positivity for HMB-45* ⇨.

TERMINOLOGY

Abbreviations

- Paraganglioma-like dermal melanocytic tumor (PLDMT)

Definitions

- Dermal-based, low-grade melanocytic tumor with histologic similarities to paraganglioma

CLINICAL ISSUES

Epidemiology

- Incidence
  - Very rare tumors; only 12 cases reported to date
- Age
  - Typically occur in young adults
    - Range: 18-53 years
    - Mean: 35 years
- Sex
  - M < F

Site

- Usually occur on extremities
  - Mostly lower limb
    - Thigh, knee, lower leg

Presentation

- Dermal-based mass lesion
  - Clinically amelanotic in most cases

Treatment

- Surgical approaches
  - Complete excision should be recommended, given uncertain biologic potential of these tumors

Prognosis

- Local recurrences rare
- No metastases reported to date

MACROSCOPIC

General Features

- Circumscribed dermal-based nodule

MICROSCOPIC

Histologic Features

- Nodular dermal-based melanocytic tumor
  - Relatively well-circumscribed, nonencapsulated, and symmetric-appearing tumor
    - Focal infiltrative features at edges of tumor may be seen in some cases
- Typically composed of well-formed packets of bland, pale to clear-staining, oval-shaped cells, mimicking paraganglioma
  - Nests are surrounded by thin fibrous septa
  - Cells show moderate amounts of clear cytoplasm
  - Only focal, fine cytoplasmic melanin pigment may be found in some cases
- Mitotic activity may be present but is usually low (1-4/10 HPF)

Cytologic Features

- Uniform, oval to spindle-shaped nuclei
- Small nucleoli
- Abundant clear cytoplasm
- No high-grade cytologic atypia described

ANCILLARY TESTS

Immunohistochemistry

- Positive for S100, variably so for MART-1/Melan-A and HMB-45

Genetic Testing

- *EWSR1* (EWS)/*ATF1* gene rearrangement (seen in clear cell sarcoma) absent

DIFFERENTIAL DIAGNOSIS

Clear Cell/Balloon Cell Melanoma

- Atypical proliferation of large, clear-staining melanocytes, often with overlying in situ component
- Pagetoid spread and lentiginous hyperplasia in junctional component
- Dermal component shows greater cytologic atypia and mitotic activity than PLDMT

Clear Cell Sarcoma of Soft Parts

- Young adults, often on lower extremity
- Typically based in deep subcutis but may invade dermis
- Immunohistochemistry similar to that of PLDMT
  - Multiple melanocytic markers typically expressed
- Characterized by t(12;22), *EWSR1/ATF1* fusion

Perivascular Epithelioid Cell Tumor

- Rare tumors composed of nests and sheets of bland-appearing clear cells
- HMB-45 and MART-1/Melan-A (+), usually only weakly/focally positive for S100
- SMA(+) and variably so for desmin and CK (unlike in PLDMT)

Primary Dermal Melanoma

- Very rare variant of melanoma located in dermis &/or subcutaneous tissues
- Well-circumscribed, large, cellular nodule, which mimics metastatic melanoma in most cases
- Cytologic atypia, mitotic activity, sometimes necrosis
- S100, MART-1/Melan-A, and HMB-45 (+)
- Lacks t(12;22), *EWSR1/ATF1* fusion

DIAGNOSTIC CHECKLIST

Clinically Relevant Pathologic Features

- Mitotic rate may be important if higher than usual

Pathologic Interpretation Pearls

- Dermal melanocytes in small nests in fibrous septa

SELECTED REFERENCES

1. Thyvalappil A et al: Paraganglioma-like dermal melanocytic tumor. Indian J Dermatol. 60(1):80-1, 2015
2. Zinovkin DA et al: Paraganglioma-like dermal melanocytic tumor: a rare skin lesion. Exp Oncol. 37(2):156-7, 2015
3. Cimpean AM et al: Paraganglioma-like dermal melanocytic tumor: a case report with particular features. Int J Clin Exp Pathol. 3(2):222-5, 2009
4. Walsh SN et al: PEComas: a review with emphasis on cutaneous lesions. Semin Diagn Pathol. 26(3):123-30, 2009

Atypical (Dysplastic) Melanocytic Nevi

KEY FACTS

TERMINOLOGY

- Dysplastic nevi, Clark nevi
- Pigmented lesions with clinical, architectural, and cytologic atypia, characterized into familial and sporadic atypical nevi

CLINICAL ISSUES

- Adolescents to young and old adults
- Any location may be involved (especially those with familial type)
- Typically > 6 mm in diameter (range: 8-10 mm)
- Variegate pigmentation with irregular borders
- Central papule with peripheral macular flare or fuzzy appearance

MICROSCOPIC

- Presence of shouldering phenomenon in compound nevi
- Lentiginous proliferation of melanocytes that fuse adjacent rete ridges via proliferation of single cells and nests
- Lamellar and concentric fibroplasia
- Range of cytologic atypia
  - Enlarged cells with abundant, dusky cytoplasm
  - Nuclear pleomorphism (mild to severe)
  - Small to prominent nucleoli

TOP DIFFERENTIAL DIAGNOSES

- Common acquired nevus
  - May show some shouldering but no melanocytic atypia
- Congenital melanocytic nevus
  - Often have greater intradermal than junctional component
  - Band-like distribution of intradermal nevus cells extending down adnexal structures
- Malignant melanoma
  - Lack of symmetry and circumscription
  - Lack of maturation with increasing dermal depth
  - Often show mitoses and marked nuclear atypia, with irregular chromatin and large nucleoli

Clinical Photograph: Dysplastic Nevus

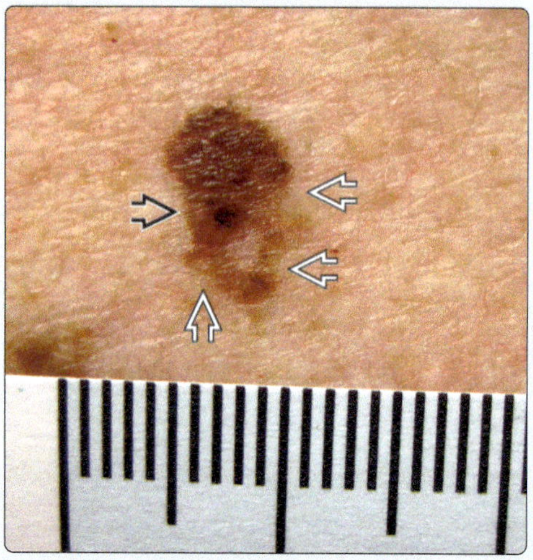

Dermoscopy of Same Lesion

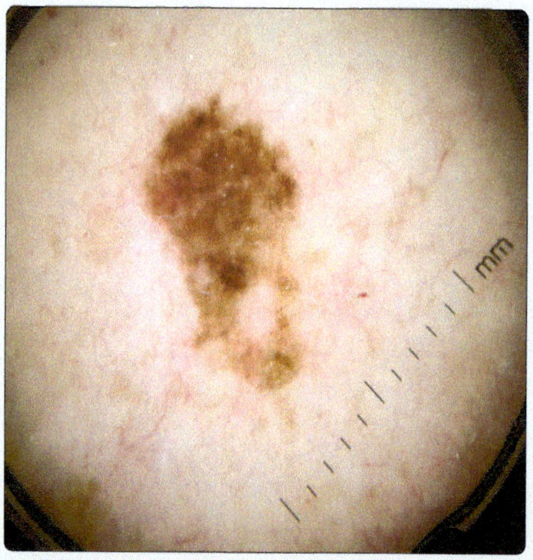

(Left) *A 0.9-cm, 2-color compound dysplastic nevus shows a dark papule ➡ and less pigmented advancing macule ➡. (Courtesy J. Finch, MD.)* **(Right)** *There is an interruption in the reticular pigmentation network. (Courtesy J. Finch, MD.)*

Clinical Photograph: Dysplastic Nevus

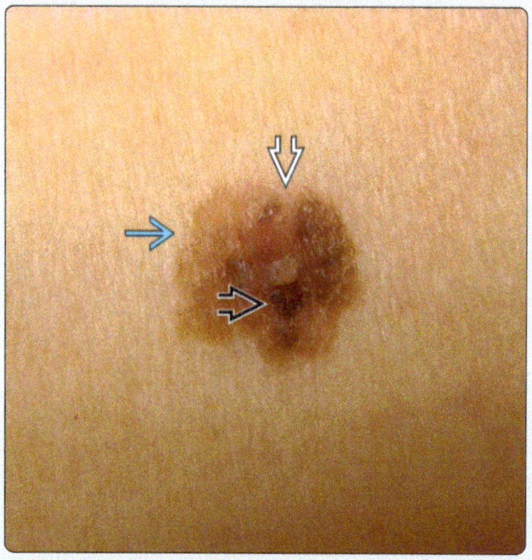

Dermoscopy of Same Lesion

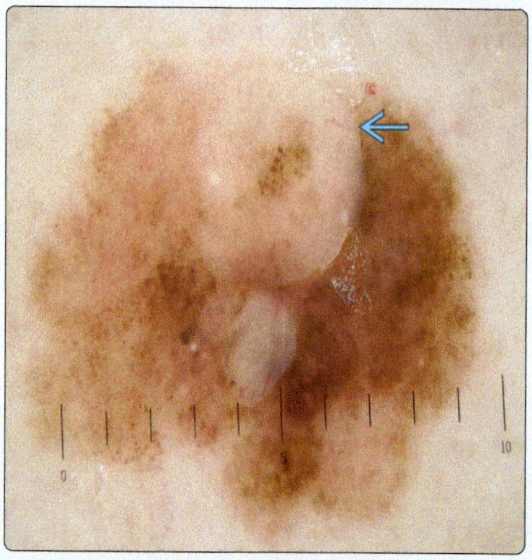

(Left) *Another large (1.1 cm) compound dysplastic nevus shows darkly ➡ and lightly ➡ melanized papules. The advancing edge has a smudged border ➡. (Courtesy J. Finch, MD.)* **(Right)** *The disrupted pigmentary network is characteristic. Prominent blood vessels ➡ are evident in vivo and microscopically. (Courtesy J. Finch, MD.)*

TERMINOLOGY

Abbreviations

- Atypical melanocytic nevi (AMN)

Synonyms

- Dysplastic nevi, Clark nevi

Definitions

- Pigmented lesions with clinical, architectural, and cytologic atypia
  - May be separated into familial and sporadic atypical/dysplastic nevi
- Likely clinical markers for overall increased risk of developing melanoma
- Variant of melanocytic nevi, which may represent precursor lesions for melanoma (controversial)
- Controversial entity, as some believe it represents only another type of nevus
  - There are overlapping clinicopathological features that exist between AMN and common acquired melanocytic nevi

CLINICAL ISSUES

Epidemiology

- Age
  - Adolescents to young and old adults

Site

- Any location may be involved (especially those with familial type)
  - Trunk, trunk extremities (lower legs in women), buttocks, and external genitalia
  - Including face, scalp, doubly covered areas (breasts in women, bathing trunk area in men and women)
  - Be wary of partially biopsied "atypical" lesions on face of elderly or chronically sun-exposed skin
    - Some cases may mimic early evolving melanoma, lentigo maligna type

Presentation

- Central papule, typically 8-10 mm
- Irregular borders and variegate pigmentation
- Peripheral macular flare
- Fuzzy border

Treatment

- Surgical approaches
  - Excision with 5-mm clinical margins for severely atypical nevi
    - Most agree that margin-positive severely dysplastic nevi should be removed with surgical margin
  - Simple excision for moderately AMN
    - Reexcision of mildly and mildly/moderately atypical nevi may not be necessary
    - Rarely results in clinically significant change in diagnosis

Prognosis

- Once adequately excised, should have very low risk of local recurrence and little, if any, risk of melanoma

MICROSCOPIC

Histologic Features

- Junctional or compound nevus with architectural disorder and asymmetry (major criteria)
  - Extension of peripheral nests beyond dermal component (shoulder phenomenon) in compound nevi
    - Typically 3 rete ridges beyond center of lesion
  - Lentiginous proliferation of melanocytes that fuse (bridge across) adjacent rete ridges
    - Fusion occurs via proliferation of single cells and nests
  - Pagetoid scatter may be focally present but usually limited to center of lesion
  - Lateral displacement of nests (in contrast to usual tips of rete location)
  - Dermal nevus cells get smaller and more spindled from superficial to lower dermis (maturation with dermal depth)
- Subepidermal lamellar (stacked) fibroplasia parallel to epidermis (minor criteria)
- Circumferential fibroplasia surrounding nests (minor criteria)
- Vascular proliferation in reticular dermis (minor criteria)
- Chronic inflammation with melanin incontinence (melanophages in papillary dermis) (minor criteria)

Cytologic Features

- Ample brown-gray cytoplasm (major criteria)
- Nuclear pleomorphism (greater in more moderate and severe-grade lesions) (major criteria)
- Nuclear diameter larger than spinous layer epidermal keratinocyte, especially in moderately to severely atypical lesions
- Densely hyperchromatic chromatin pattern
- Nucleolar prominence (greater in higher grade lesions)

ANCILLARY TESTS

PCR

- Expression of specific microRNAs is dysregulated in AMN compared to melanoma

Genetic Testing

- Genetics of AMN remain understudied; however, there is documented relationship between AMN and familial melanoma
  - 30-40% of these families harbor mutation in *CDKN2A* locus, which encodes p16 and ARF tumor suppressor proteins
    - p16 mutation-carriers were more likely to have ≥ 2 clinically atypical nevi
- One study found *BRAF* wild-type melanoma in situ arising in *BRAF* V600E mutant dysplastic nevus

DIFFERENTIAL DIAGNOSIS

Common Acquired Nevus

- May exhibit some shouldering of junctional component
- May show lamellar fibroplasia
  - Especially lesions on back
- Lacks nuclear atypia, pleomorphism, and gray cytoplasm

Grading Criteria for Cytologic Atypia in Atypical Melanocytic Nevi

Features	Mildly Dysplastic	Moderately Dysplastic	Severely Dysplastic
Nuclear size	Same as a keratinocyte	1.5-2.0x keratinocyte	> 2x keratinocyte
Chromatin	Hyperchromatic	Hyperchromatic to vesicular	Vesicular
Nucleolus	Absent	Usually absent	Prominent
Dusky cytoplasm	Little	Little to abundant	Usually abundant

Atypia is determined subjectively by comparing the nuclear features of atypical melanocytic nevi to those of midlayer epidermal keratinocytes. Modified from Weinstock MA et al: Reliability of the histopathologic diagnosis of melanocytic dysplasia. The Dysplastic Nevus Panel. Arch Dermatol. 133(8):953-8, 1997; McKee PH et al: Diagnostic Atlas of Melanocytic Pathology. Philadelphia: Elsevier, 2009.

Congenital Melanocytic Nevus

- Often have greater intradermal than junctional component
- Band-like distribution of intradermal nevus cells, which surround adnexal structures
  - Nevus cells extend around neurovascular bundles
  - Splaying of collagen bundles
- May show neurotization and pseudovascular spaces, especially in larger lesions
- Lacks nuclear pleomorphism and gray cytoplasm

Malignant Melanoma

- Lack of symmetry and circumscription
- Shows significant cytologic atypia
  - Often marked nuclear atypia, with irregular chromatin and large nucleoli
- Lack of maturation with increasing dermal depth
- Mitoses often present; may be atypical or deep dermal
- Shows consumption of epidermis

DIAGNOSTIC CHECKLIST

Clinically Relevant Pathologic Features

- Large pigmented macule with shades of tan and brown, with irregular and fuzzy borders
- Presence of AMN is important risk factor for developing cutaneous melanoma

Pathologic Interpretation Pearls

- Symmetric lesion with shoulder phenomenon and cytological atypia
- Fusion of retes can be useful clue
- Look for lateral expansion of retes via melanocytic proliferation
- Lacks consumption of epidermis

SELECTED REFERENCES

1. Tan JM et al: BRAF wild-type melanoma in situ arising in a BRAF V600E mutant dysplastic nevus. JAMA Dermatol. 151(4):417-21, 2015
2. Babapoor S et al: A novel miR-451a isomiR, associated with amelanotypic phenotype, acts as a tumor suppressor in melanoma by retarding cell migration and invasion. PLoS One. 9(9):e107502, 2014
3. Strazzula L et al: The utility of re-excising mildly and moderately dysplastic nevi: A retrospective analysis. J Am Acad Dermatol. 71(6):1071-6, 2014
4. Kozubek J et al: In-depth characterization of microRNA transcriptome in melanoma. PLoS One. 8(9):e72699, 2013
5. Duffy K et al: The dysplastic nevus: from historical perspective to management in the modern era: part I. Historical, histologic, and clinical aspects. J Am Acad Dermatol. 67(1):1.e1-16; quiz 17-8, 2012
6. Duffy K et al: The dysplastic nevus: from historical perspective to management in the modern era: part II. Molecular aspects and clinical management. J Am Acad Dermatol. 67(1):19.e1-12; quiz 31-2, 2012
7. Brenn T: Atypical genital nevus. Arch Pathol Lab Med. 135(3):317-20, 2011
8. Sommer LL et al: Persistent melanocytic nevi: a review and analysis of 205 cases. J Cutan Pathol. 38(6):503-7, 2011
9. Zembowicz A et al: Nevus/melanocytoma/melanoma: an emerging paradigm for classification of melanocytic neoplasms? Arch Pathol Lab Med. 135(3):300-6, 2011
10. McKee PH et al: Diagnostic Atlas of Melanocytic Pathology. Philadelphia: Elsevier, 2009
11. Crowson AN et al: The Melanocytic Proliferations: A Comprehensive Textbook of Pigmented Lesions. New York: Wiley-Liss, 2001
12. Elder DE: Dysplastic naevi: an update. Histopathology. 56(1):112-20, 2010
13. Walters RF et al: Consumption of the epidermis: a criterion in the differential diagnosis of melanoma and dysplastic nevi that is associated with increasing breslow depth and ulceration. Am J Dermatopathol. 29(6):527-33, 2007
14. Liu L et al: Mutation of the CDKN2A 5' UTR creates an aberrant initiation codon and predisposes to melanoma. Nat Genet. 21(1):128-32, 1999
15. Pollock PM et al: Haplotype analysis of two recurrent CDKN2A mutations in 10 melanoma families: evidence for common founders and independent mutations. Hum Mutat. 11(6):424-31, 1998
16. Weinstock MA et al: Reliability of the histopathologic diagnosis of melanocytic dysplasia. The Dysplastic Nevus Panel. Arch Dermatol. 133(8):953-8, 1997
17. Elder DE et al: The early and intermediate precursor lesions of tumor progression in the melanocytic system: common acquired nevi and atypical (dysplastic) nevi. Semin Diagn Pathol. 10(1):18-35, 1993
18. Roth ME et al: The histopathology of dysplastic nevi. Continued controversy. Am J Dermatopathol. 13(1):38-51, 1991
19. Barnhill RL et al: Correlation of histologic architectural and cytoplasmic features with nuclear atypia in atypical (dysplastic) nevomelanocytic nevi. Hum Pathol. 21(1):51-8, 1990
20. White WL: Re: A. R. Rhodes, M. C. Mihm, and M. A. Weinstock. Dysplastic Melanocytic Nevi: a Reproducible Histologic Definition Emphasizing Cellular Morphology. Mod Pathol 2:306, 1989. Mod Pathol. 3(1):99, 1990
21. Elder DE et al: The dysplastic nevus syndrome: our definition. Am J Dermatopathol. 4(5):455-60, 1982
22. Clark WH Jr et al: Origin of familial malignant melanomas from heritable melanocytic lesions. 'The B-K mole syndrome'. Arch Dermatol. 114(5):732-8, 1978
23. Lynch HT et al: Familial atypical multiple mole-melanoma syndrome. J Med Genet. 15(5):352-6, 1978

Clinical Photograph: Atypical Compound Nevus

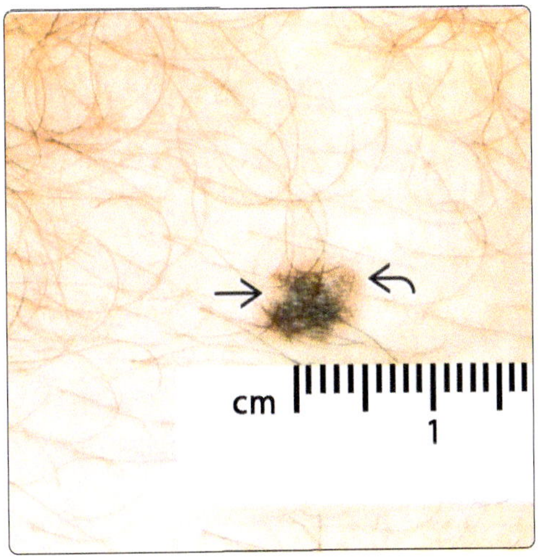

Compound Dysplastic Melanocytic Nevus

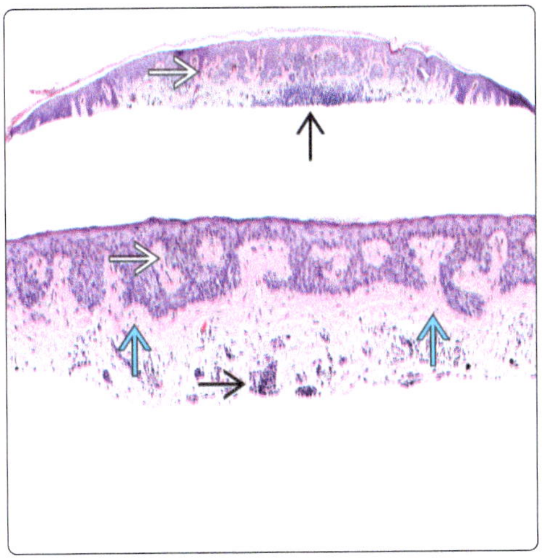

(Left) *Clinical photograph of an atypical compound nevus shows a pigmented lesion with somewhat irregular borders. Note the central papular area surrounded by a macular periphery. (Courtesy P. Duray, MD.)* **(Right)** *There are junctional nests, laterally placed, and a dermal component that matures with increasing dermal depth. Note lamellar fibroplasia that hugs the rete ridges.*

Lichenoid Inflammatory Infiltrate

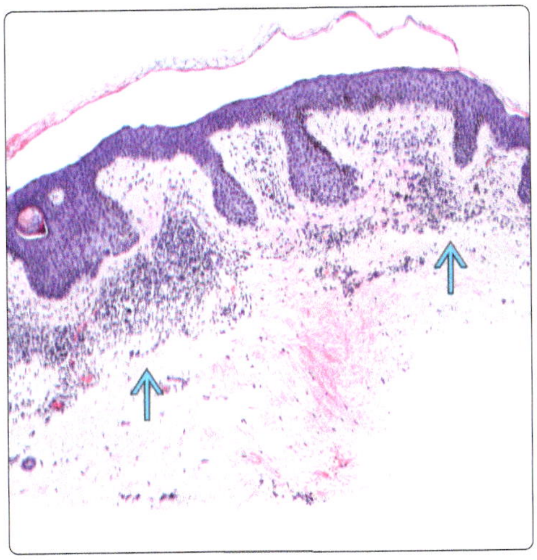

Lateral Displacement of Junctional Nests

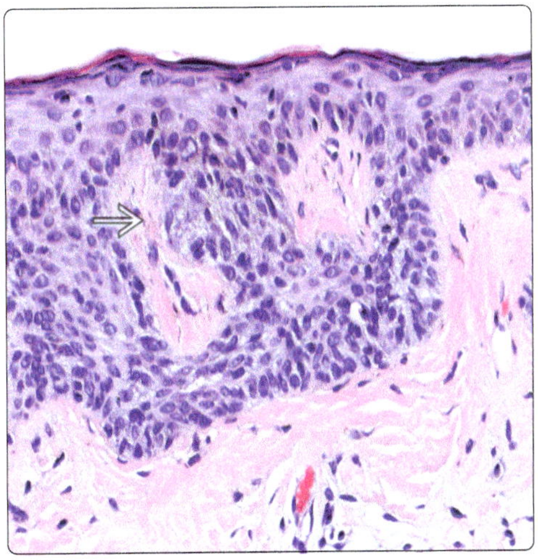

(Left) *Dysplastic nevi can often display a band-like inflammatory infiltrate, composed of lymphocytes and histiocytes, hugging the dermal fibroplasia.* **(Right)** *Lateral displacement of nests is a typical finding in dysplastic melanocytic nevi. Cytologically, the nuclei are small, and oval with slight pleomorphism. No nucleoli are evident. The cytoplasm is light gray.*

Dysplastic Nevus on Facial Skin

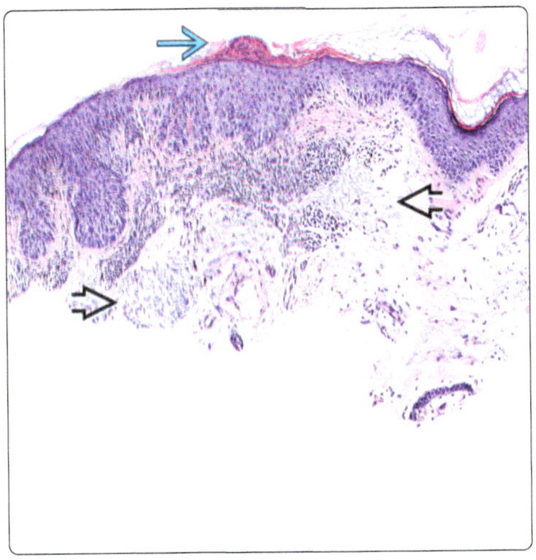

Dermal Component

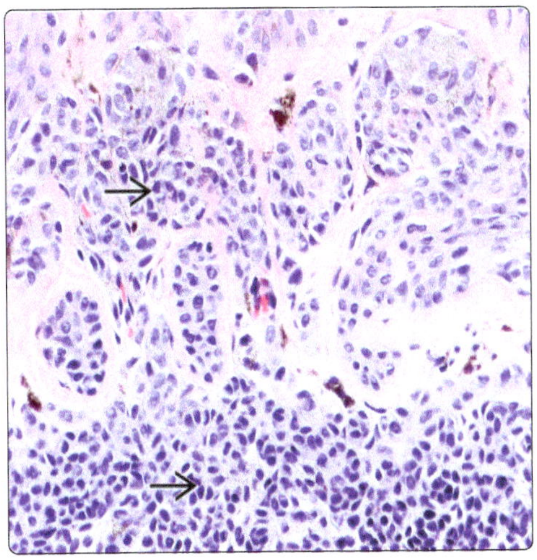

(Left) *These lesions can be challenging, especially in the older individual with evident solar elastosis. Note the mound of parakeratosis that denotes prior trauma at this site.* **(Right)** *The dermal cells do become smaller with increasing dermal depth.*

(Left) *Limited pagetoid upward scatter ➡ can be expected. This finding can be concerning for melanoma in situ; however, the finding of parakeratosis can partially explain the pagetoid scatter. SOX10 (or MITF) immunostaining can be helpful.* **(Right)** *Some dysplastic nevi, especially those in young to middle-aged women on the extremities, can display some features associated with Spitz nevi. The dermal nests → mature with increasing dermal depth.*

Pagetoid Upward Scatter

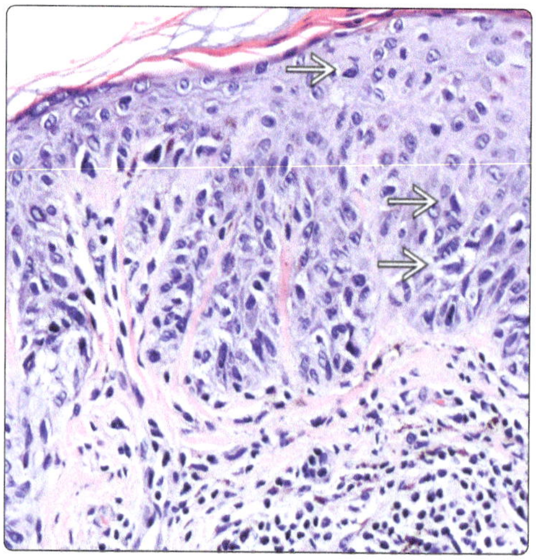

Dysplastic Nevus With Spitz Features

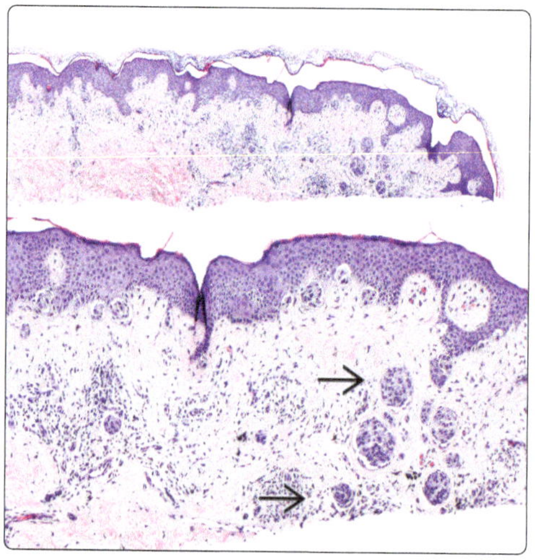

(Left) *The cells have epithelioid cytology with dysplastic gray or light brown cytoplasm ⇨. Note the apical clefts ➡ seen in Spitz nevi.* **(Right)** *Inflammatory regression in dysplastic nevi can be concerning. The lichenoid infiltrate is patchy, heavy, and nodular ⇨ in some areas and mild in others ➡.*

Dysplastic Nevus With Spitz Cytology

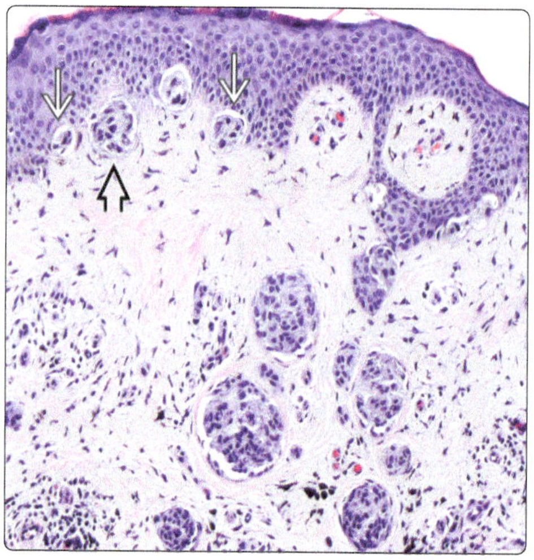

Dysplastic Nevus With Inflammatory Regression

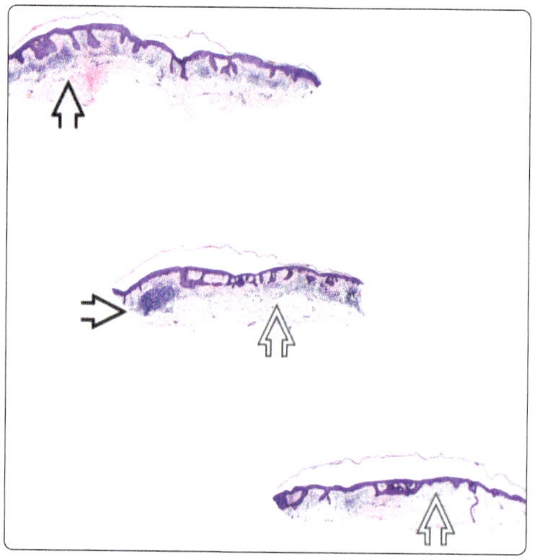

(Left) *There is an interruption ➡ in the junctional melanocytic proliferation. Some nests remain →. The lichenoid inflammation can hide the dermal nests ⇨. Note the vertically oriented blood vessels ➡.* **(Right)** *Gray cytoplasm and small, hyperchromatic nuclei are evident ⇨. Note the dermal nests →, melanin incontinence ⇨, and blood vessels ➡ in the inflammatory infiltrate.*

Inflammatory Regression

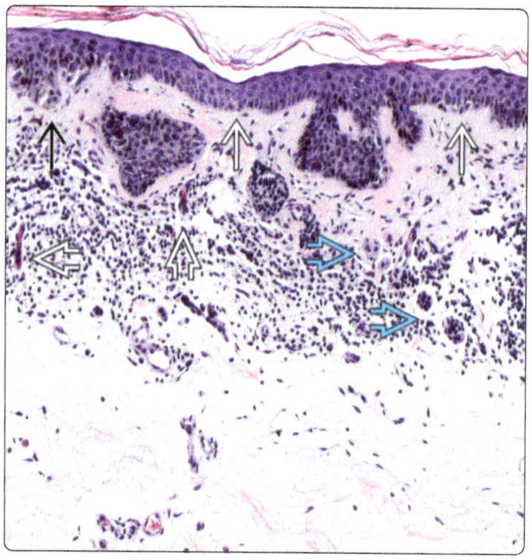

Cytology of Regression

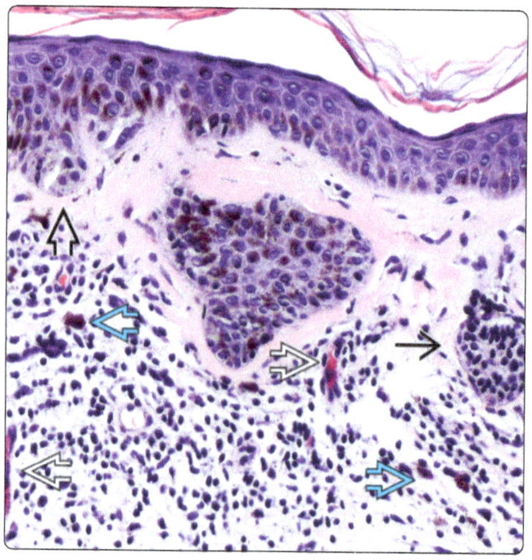

Differential Diagnosis: Melanoma In Situ

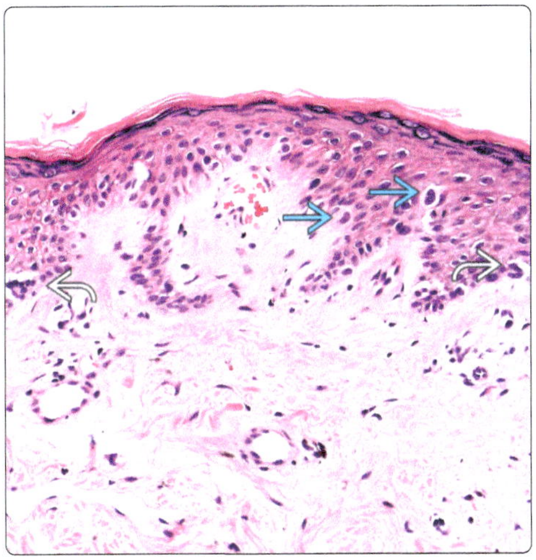

Differential Diagnosis: Melanoma In Situ

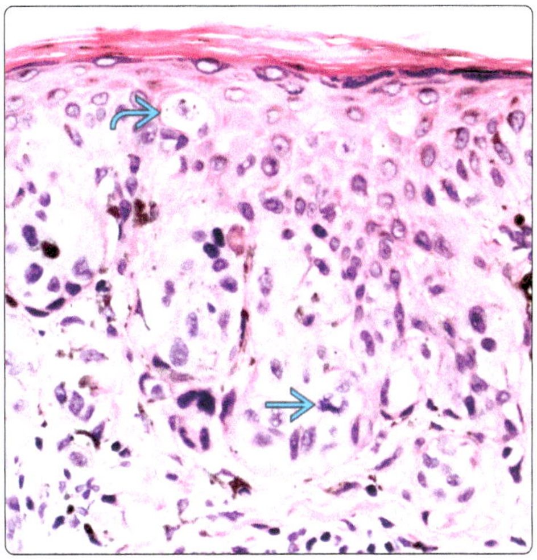

(Left) *Melanoma in situ, lentigo maligna type, shows a proliferation of single, atypical lentiginous and multinucleated melanocytic cells along the dermal-epidermal junction.* **(Right)** *Melanoma in situ, superficial spreading type, shows a prominent atypical intraepidermal proliferation of large, epithelioid-shaped melanocytes with pagetoid spread and junctional mitotic figures.*

Mildly Atypical Junctional Nevus

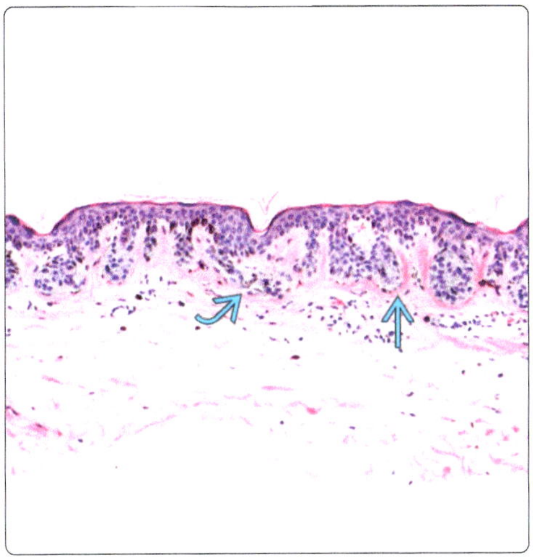

Mildly Atypical Compound Nevus

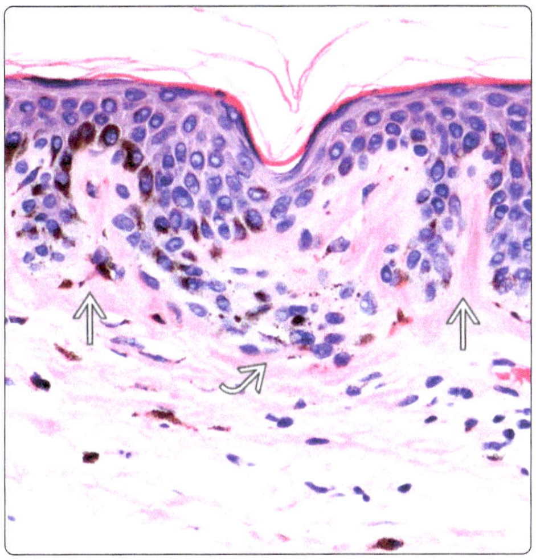

(Left) *Low-power magnification of a mildly atypical junctional nevus shows a fusion of rete ridges and concentric fibroplasia that surrounds the nests of junctional melanocytes.* **(Right)** *High-power magnification shows the junctional melanocytic proliferation fusing 2 adjacent rete ridges. The concentric fibroplasia prominently hugs the junctional atypical melanocytic nevi.*

Severely Atypical Junctional Nevus

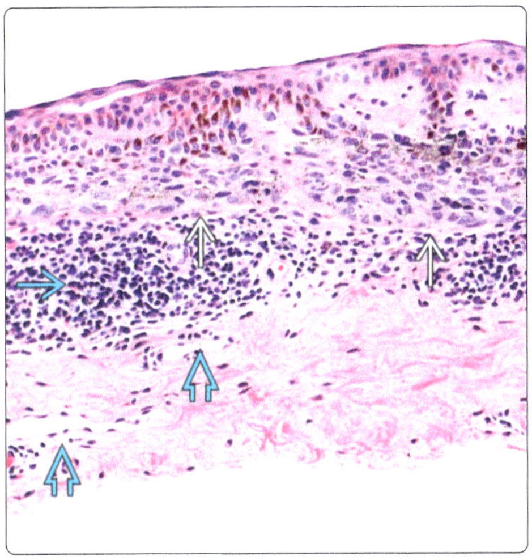

Severely Atypical Junctional Nevus

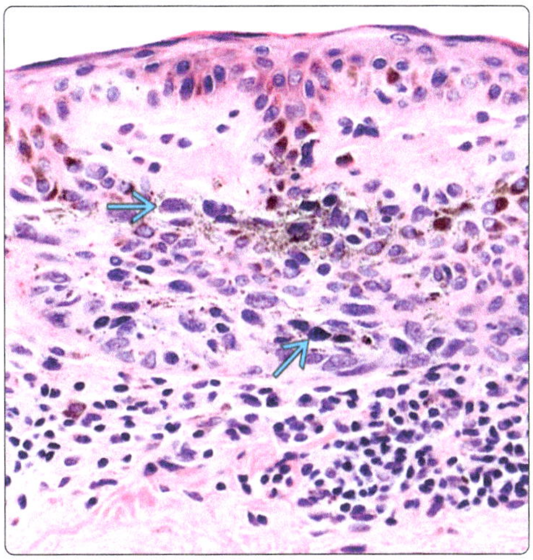

(Left) *This severely atypical nevus exhibits a junctional proliferation of atypical melanocytes, which fuse the rete ridges together. A chronic inflammatory infiltrate and a few slightly dilated blood vessels are noted in the dermis.* **(Right)** *High-power magnification of a severely atypical nevus shows atypical melanocytes with gray or brown pigmented cytoplasm and pleomorphic, hyperchromatic-staining nuclei.*

Spitz (Spindle and Epithelioid Cell) Nevi

KEY FACTS

CLINICAL ISSUES

- Benign melanocytic tumor
- Most common in children and young adults
- Common sites: Face, trunk, extremities
- Pink or flesh-colored, dome-shaped dermal papule or nodule

MICROSCOPIC

- Junctional, compound, and dermal forms
- Symmetric, well circumscribed in most cases
- Varying proportions of spindled and epithelioid melanocytes
  - Spindle cells much more common
  - Epithelioid cells usually dispersed individually throughout lesion
- Melanocytes "mature" by becoming smaller from superficial to deep
- Kamino bodies: Eosinophilic globules at dermal-epidermal junction
- Artifactual clefting of papillary dermal nests from overlying epidermis often present
- Can show atypical features (atypical Spitz nevus/tumor)
  - Pleomorphic cells with large, irregular nuclei and prominent eosinophilic nucleoli
  - Increased mitoses may be seen
- **Variants: Halo Spitz nevus, desmoplastic Spitz nevus**

TOP DIFFERENTIAL DIAGNOSES

- Spitzoid melanoma; findings suspicious for melanoma include
  - Patients usually > 10 years old
  - Lesions usually > 1 cm
  - Ulceration and increased mitoses often present
  - Asymmetry and poor circumscription
  - Subcutaneous involvement
- Pigmented spindle cell nevus of Reed (usually leg of young adult female)
- Conventional melanocytic nevi

Clinical Photograph of Spitz Nevus

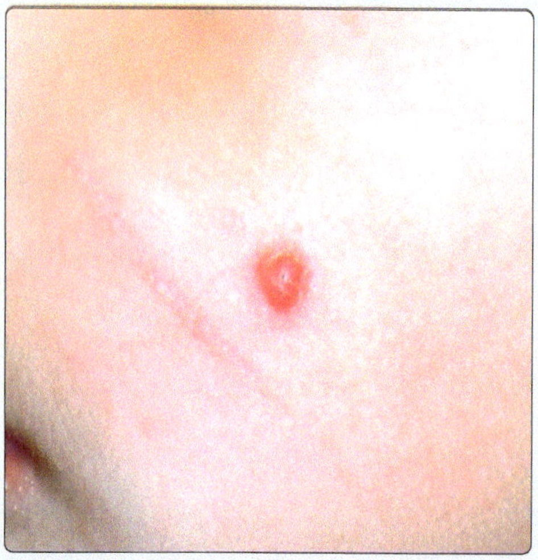

Classic Spitz Nevus

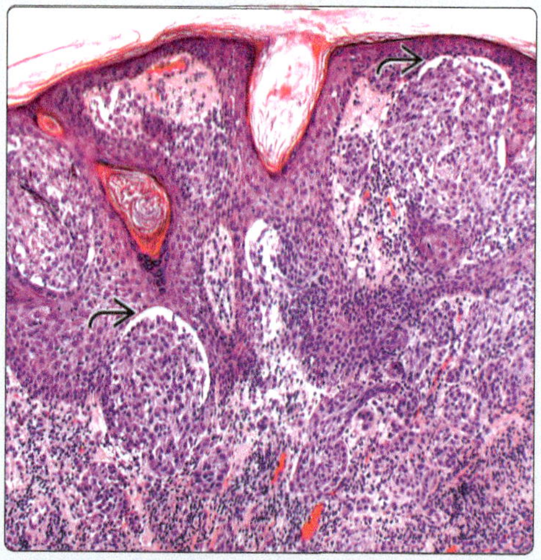

(Left) *A small, symmetric pink papule, typical of a Spitz nevus, is shown on the face of a child. (Courtesy R. J. Antaya, MD.)* **(Right)** *Histologic examination of a classic Spitz nevus shows nests of spindled and epithelioid-shaped melanocytes at the dermal-epidermal junction and in the dermis. Note the clefting artifact overlying several of the nests ➔.*

Spitz Nevus at High Magnification

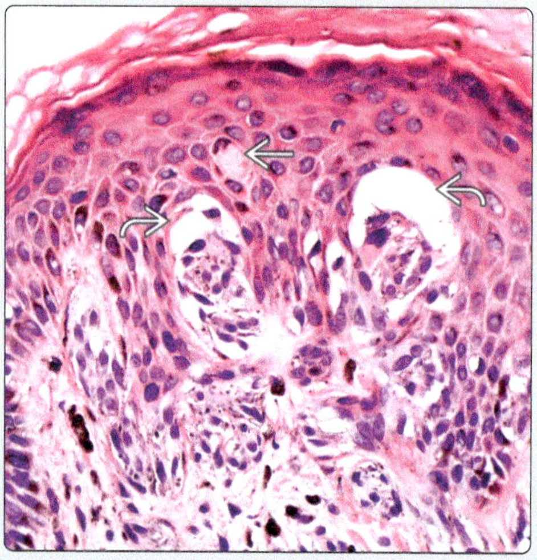

Kamino Body in Spitz Nevus

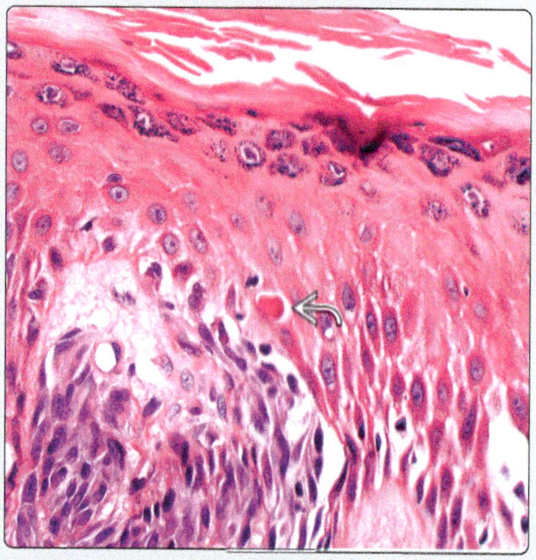

(Left) *High-power examination of a Spitz nevus shows small nests of epithelioid to spindled melanocytes with overlying artifactual clefting ➔ and an eosinophilic Kamino body ➔.* **(Right)** *High-power examination of this case shows a small, densely eosinophilic-staining Kamino body ➔, which is an eosinophilic globule found at the dermal-epidermal junction. These are typical of Spitz nevi but are not seen in most cases.*

TERMINOLOGY

Synonyms

- Spindle and epithelioid cell nevus
- Benign juvenile melanoma (outdated term)

CLINICAL ISSUES

Site

- Trunk
- Head and neck
- Extremities, especially thigh

Presentation

- Most common in children and young adults
  - May occur at all ages
- Solitary
  - Can be clustered or disseminated

Treatment

- Complete conservative excision

Prognosis

- Benign tumors; only very rare malignant transformation
- Low recurrence rate, even after incomplete excision

MACROSCOPIC

General Features

- Dome-shaped dermal nodule
- Pink or flesh colored

Size

- Usually < 1 cm

MICROSCOPIC

Histologic Features

- Junctional, compound, and dermal forms
  - Most common type is compound with prominent dermal component
- Symmetric, well-circumscribed proliferation
  - Usually no lateral extension of junctional nests beyond dermal component
- Varying proportions of spindled and epithelioid melanocytes
  - Spindle cells more common in most cases
  - Epithelioid cells usually dispersed individually throughout lesion
- Spindle cells are arranged in fascicles perpendicular to epidermis
- Small clusters of melanocytes can be seen in epidermis
  - Can see pagetoid spread of few single melanocytes
- Artifactual clefting of junctional nests from overlying epidermis
- Kamino bodies
  - Eosinophilic globules at dermal-epidermal junction
  - PAS(+) and trichrome (+)
- Melanocytes show "maturation" as they become smaller from superficial to deep
  - Important clue for differentiating from melanoma
- Other common features
  - Vascular and sometimes edematous stroma
  - Pseudoepitheliomatous hyperplasia often seen
- **Halo Spitz nevus**
  - Nevus with depigmented rim
  - Heavy lymphocytic infiltrate with sparing of adjacent basal melanocytes
  - Often seen in combined Spitz and melanocytic nevus
- **Desmoplastic Spitz nevus**
  - Tend to occur in young adults on extremities
  - Usually dermal-based lesions
  - Dense, hyalinized collagenous stroma
- **Atypical Spitz nevus/tumor**
  - Some cases show features overlapping between typical Spitz nevus and spitzoid melanoma
  - Atypical features include
    - Large, irregular nuclei with prominent eosinophilic nucleoli
    - Increased numbers of (typical) mitoses
    - Marked cellular pleomorphism

DIFFERENTIAL DIAGNOSIS

Spitzoid Melanoma

- Asymmetry and poor circumscription at low magnification
- No maturation of melanocytes with dermal descent
- Cells typically show more coarse chromatin, anaplastic nuclear features
- Deep &/or atypical mitoses
- Findings that should raise suspicions for melanoma include
  - Patient > 10 years of age
  - Lesion > 1 cm
  - Ulceration present
  - Subcutaneous involvement

Pigmented Spindle Cell Nevus of Reed

- Typically considered variant of Spitz nevus
- Usually occur in young adult women on extremities (especially thighs)
- Predominantly junctional proliferation, with only small superficial dermal component in most cases
- Cells show prominent pigmentation, unlike most Spitz nevi

Conventional Melanocytic Nevi

- Conventional nevi are composed of small, round to epithelioid-appearing cells
- Lack streaming together (or raining down) of cells
- Kamino bodies and characteristic clefting around junctional nests are not present

SELECTED REFERENCES

1. Lallas A et al: Atypical Spitz tumours and sentinel lymph node biopsy: a systematic review. Lancet Oncol. 15(4):e178-83, 2014
2. Kerner M et al: Spitz nevi: a bridge between dermoscopic morphology and histopathology. Dermatol Clin. 31(2):327-35, 2013
3. Al Dhaybi R et al: p16 expression: a marker of differentiation between childhood malignant melanomas and Spitz nevi. J Am Acad Dermatol. 65(2):357-63, 2011
4. George E et al: Immunohistochemical evaluation of p16INK4A, E-cadherin, and cyclin D1 expression in melanoma and Spitz tumors. Am J Clin Pathol. 133(3):370-9, 2010
5. Requena C et al: Spitz nevus: a clinicopathological study of 349 cases. Am J Dermatopathol. 31(2):107-16, 2009
6. Allen AC et al: Histogenesis and clinicopathologic correlation of nevi and malignant melanomas; current status. AMA Arch Derm Syphilol. 69(2):150-71, 1954

PART II

SECTION 2

Malignant Tumors (Melanomas and Related Lesions)

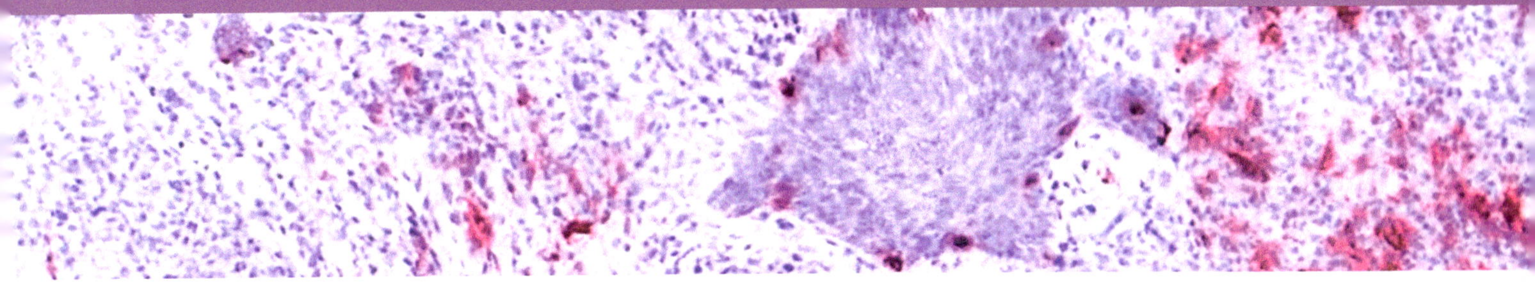

Melanoma In Situ

Invasive Melanoma

Melanoma In Situ, Lentigo Maligna Type

KEY FACTS

TERMINOLOGY

- Melanoma in situ, lentigo maligna type (MIS-LMT)
- Hutchinson melanotic freckle

CLINICAL ISSUES

- Most common on face (in women) and on scalp, neck, and ears (in men)
- Nonpalpable broad, slowly evolving pigmented patch
- Strikingly variegated colors with irregular borders

CYTOPATHOLOGY

- Small, angulated nuclei
- Nuclear hyperchromasia
- Scant cytoplasm, typically without melanin granules

MICROSCOPIC

- Ill-defined lentiginous proliferation of atypical melanocytes along dermal-epidermal junction replacing basal keratinocytes
- Epidermal atrophy accompanied by cytological atypia
- Typically limited pagetoid upward scatter of melanocytes
- Ill-defined peripheral borders (trailing off of single cells)

TOP DIFFERENTIAL DIAGNOSES

- Invasive lentigo maligna melanoma
- Actinic (solar) melanocytic hyperplasia
- Atypical (dysplastic) nevus
- Reed (pigmented spindle cell) nevus

DIAGNOSTIC CHECKLIST

- Clinical
  - Slowly evolving large pigmented patch on chronically sun-exposed areas
- Pathological
  - Epidermal atrophy and effaced rete ridges, in background of solar elastosis
  - Melanocytes at the dermal-epidermal junction are cytologically atypical

Melanoma In Situ, Lentigo Maligna on Cheek

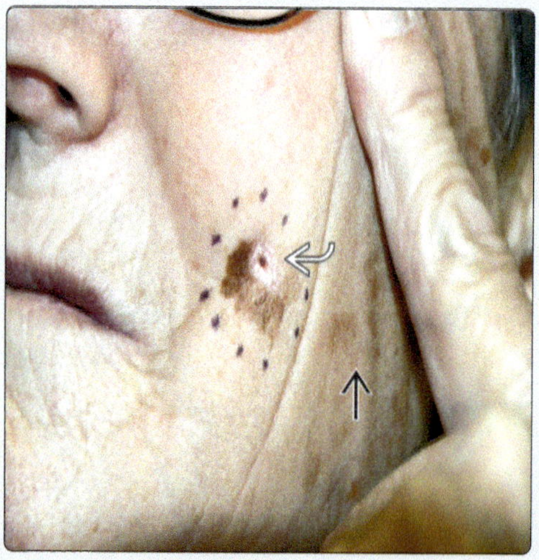

MIS-LMT on Cheek

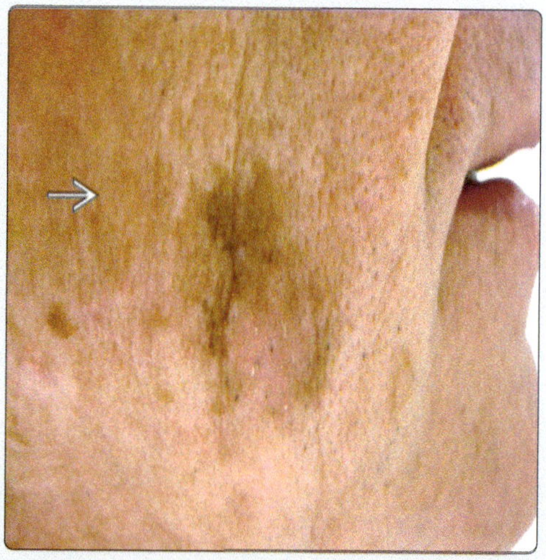

(Left) *Multicolor pigmented patch on the facial cheek of an elderly woman shows evidence of regression. Such lesions should be biopsied. Note the posterior lightly pigmented patches. (Courtesy J. Finch, MD.)* **(Right)** *Another 2-toned pigmented patch on a chronically sun-exposed cheek is ill defined. Due to the unclear borders, more than 1 biopsy may be needed to determine its extent. (Courtesy J. Finch, MD.)*

MIS-LMT on Temple

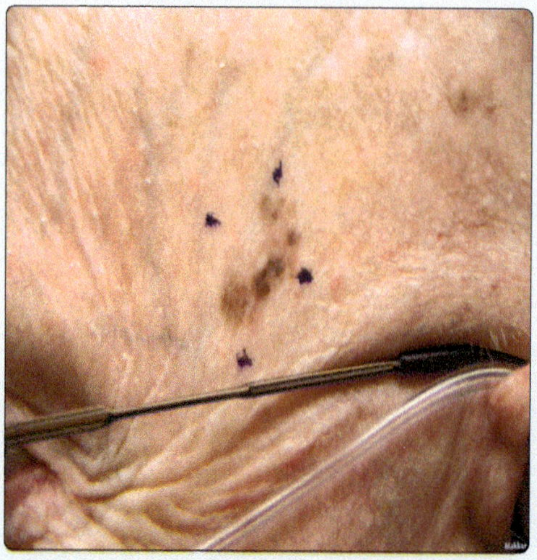

Clinical Photograph of MIS-LMT

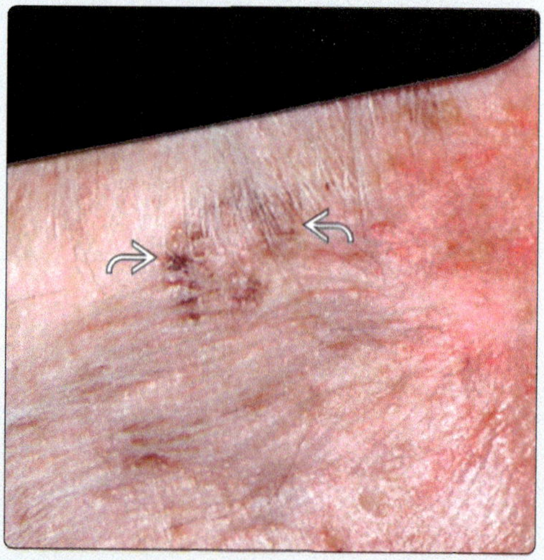

(Left) *Multicolor irregular patch on a chronically sun-exposed temple warrants a biopsy. (Courtesy J. Finch, MD.)* **(Right)** *Clinical photograph of a lentigo maligna type of melanoma in situ shows an irregularly shaped and unevenly pigmented patch on the scalp of an elderly patient.*

TERMINOLOGY

Abbreviations

- Melanoma in situ, lentigo maligna type (MIS-LMT)

Synonyms

- Hutchinson melanotic freckle

Definitions

- Slowly evolving, indolent melanoma subtype that usually presents on head and neck (sun-exposed regions) in older patients

ETIOLOGY/PATHOGENESIS

Environmental Exposure

- Long-term exposure to ultraviolet irradiation

CLINICAL ISSUES

Epidemiology

- Incidence
  - Very common subtype of melanoma in situ: ~ 5% overall lifetime risk
- Age
  - Older adults, usually > 72 years
- Sex
  - Slight female predominance

Site

- Most common on face (in women) and on scalp, neck, and ears (in men)

Presentation

- Nonpalpable, broad lesion (size > 1 cm), can sometimes cover large portion of affected area
- Strikingly variegated colors of tan, brown, dark brown, black admixed with gray or blue-black

Treatment

- Surgical approaches
  - Excision with clear margins (usually 5-mm clinical margins recommended)

Prognosis

- Surgical margins of at least 5 mm give cure rates of 90-95%
- Low incidence of associated invasive melanoma

MICROSCOPIC

Histologic Features

- Lentiginous proliferation of atypical melanocytes along dermal-epidermal junction replacing basal keratinocytes
  - Mostly single cells, but irregular nests may also be present
- Typically limited pagetoid upward scatter of melanocytes
- Ill-defined peripheral borders (trailing off of single cells)
- Extension of atypical melanocytes along adnexal structures
- Epidermal atrophy and effacement of rete ridges
- Marked solar elastosis

Cytologic Features

- Nuclei are small, hyperchromatic, and often angulated (may resemble lymphocytes)
- Scanty cytoplasm, typically without melanin granules

ANCILLARY TESTS

Immunohistochemistry

- SOX10 and MITF can be very useful to highlight ill-defined junctional melanocytic hyperplasia
  - May be particularly important in setting of chronically sun-exposed skin (better than Mart-1/MelanA)

Genetic Testing

- Frequently increased copy number of *CCND1* (cyclin-D1) and lower rates of *BRAF* mutations compared to intermittently sun-exposed skin

DIFFERENTIAL DIAGNOSIS

Invasive Lentigo Maligna Melanoma

- Typically microinvasive spindle cell/desmoplastic type, and dermal component can be difficult to identify
- Multiple deeper level sections (and, in more difficult cases, immunohistochemistry) should be used to exclude invasion

Actinic (Solar) Melanocytic Hyperplasia

- Seen in heavily sun-damaged skin
- Consists of scattered single atypical cells along dermal-epidermal junction
- Not nested or confluent; does not involve adnexal epithelium
  - SOX10 and MITF does not typically reveal lentiginous overgrowth of junctional melanocytes

Atypical (Dysplastic) Nevus

- Severely atypical junctional nevi can be difficult to distinguish from MIS-LMT
  - Especially on small, partial biopsies
- Features such as symmetry, circumscription, and lack of confluence favor nevus
  - Complete excision may be necessary to evaluate these features

Reed (Pigmented Spindle Cell) Nevus

- Hyperplastic (not atrophic) epidermis, lateral margins are sharply defined (no trailing off of single cells)
- Cells may be atypical but are typically monomorphous (not pleomorphic, as in MIS-LMT)

DIAGNOSTIC CHECKLIST

Clinically Relevant Pathologic Features

- Large pigmented patch, slowly evolving indolent melanoma subtype on chronically sun-exposed regions

Pathologic Interpretation Pearls

- Epidermal atrophy and effaced rete ridges, in background of solar elastosis
- Trace dermal-epidermal junction using medium to high magnification to look for cytological atypia

SELECTED REFERENCES

1. Curtin JA et al: Distinct sets of genetic alterations in melanoma. N Engl J Med. 353(20):2135-47, 2005
2. Crowson AN et al: The precursors of malignant melanoma. Recent Results Cancer Res. 160:75-84, 2002

(Left) *Scanning power view shows that there are dense inflammatory aggregates in the papillary dermis.* **(Right)** *There are ill-defined, poorly nested, and intraepidermal areas of melanocytic hyperplasia overlying the inflammatory infiltrate identified on higher magnification.*

Shave Biopsy of MIS-LMT in Chronically Sun-Exposed Skin

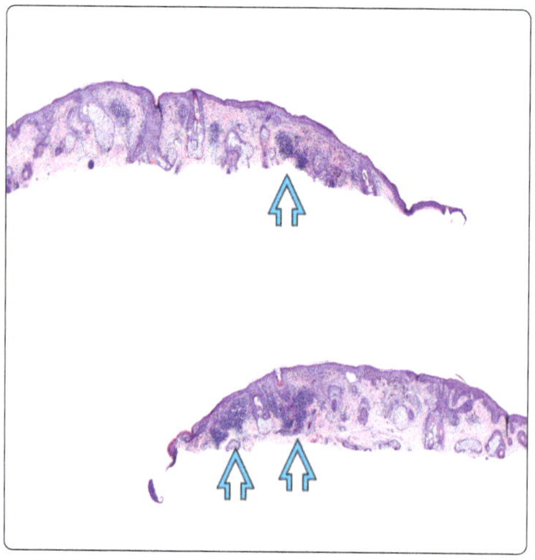

MIS-LMT

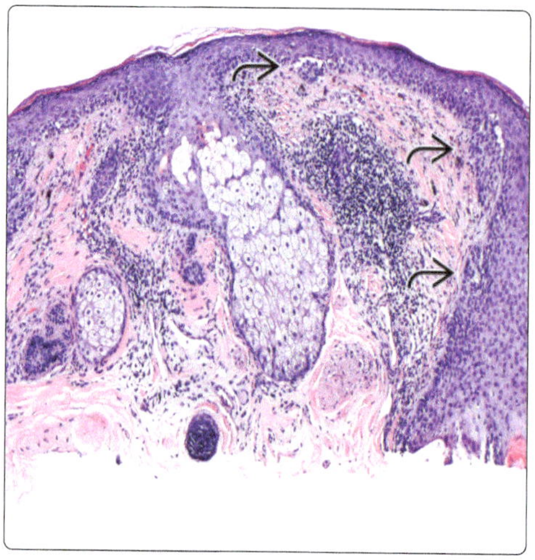

(Left) *Ill-defined melanocytic nests extend down hair follicular epithelium. The papillary dermis reveals fibrosis, lymphohistiocytic infiltrate, and melanin incontinence.* **(Right)** *Poorly defined melanocytic hyperplasia involves both the interfollicular and follicular epithelium.*

Adnexal Extension in MIS-LMT

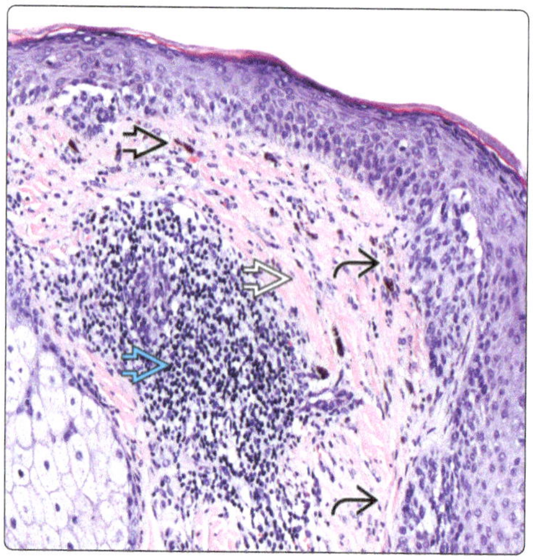

Interfollicular and Follicular Involvement in MIS-LMT

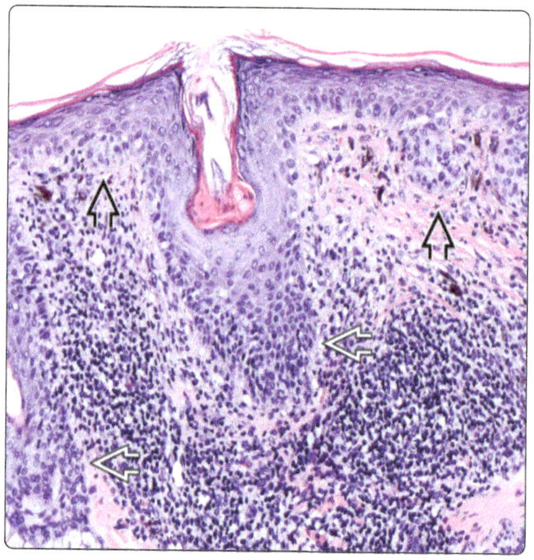

(Left) *The combination of patchy lymphohistiocytic infiltrate, papillary dermal fibrosis, and solar elastosis should raise concern for early changes of lentigo maligna.* **(Right)** *A closer examination shows atypical intraepidermal melanocytic hyperplasia. Note dermal fibrosis and vertically oriented blood vessels related to regression.*

Ill-Defined Melanocytic Hyperplasia in MIS-LMT

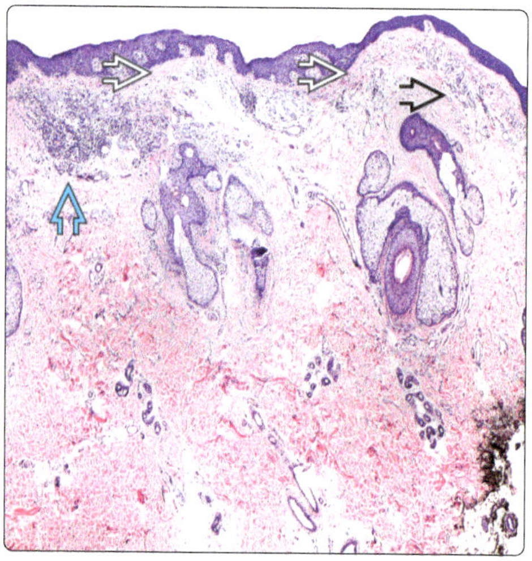

Higher Magnification of MIS-LMT

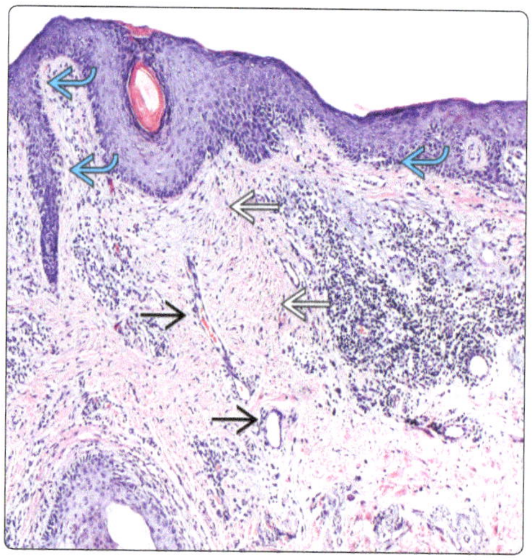

Absent Pagetoid Upward Migration of Melanocytes in MIS-LMT

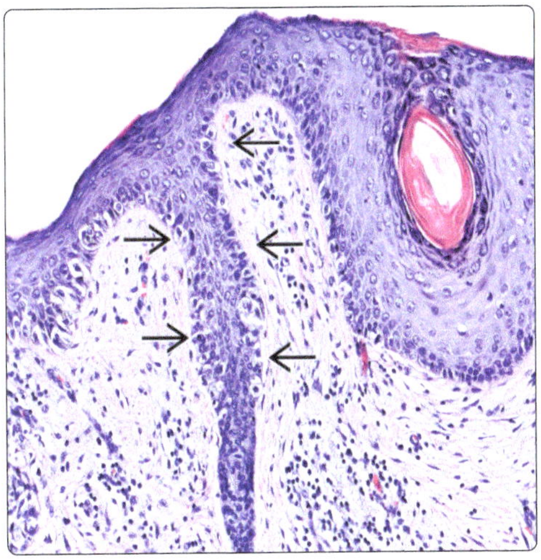

MIS-LMT at Low Magnification

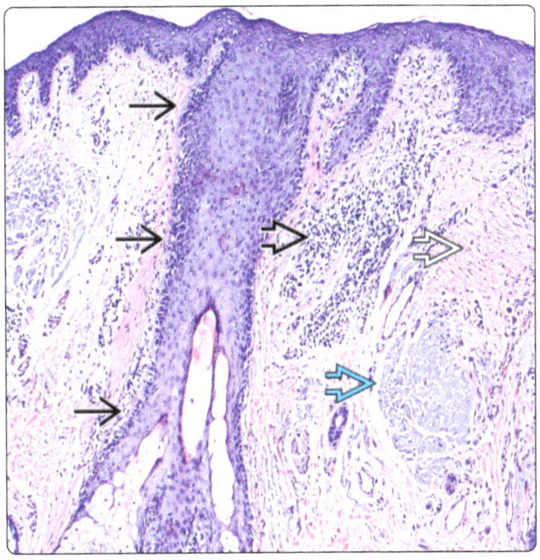

(Left) *The atypical melanocytes grow in a lentiginous manner* → *without upward migration through the layers of epidermis. The nuclei are small, angulated, and without nucleoli.* **(Right)** *Solar elastosis* →, *patchy inflammatory infiltrate* →, *dermal fibrosis* →, *and lentiginous junctional melanocytic hyperplasia* → *are hallmarks of lentigo maligna.*

Lack of Dermal Invasion in MIS-LMT

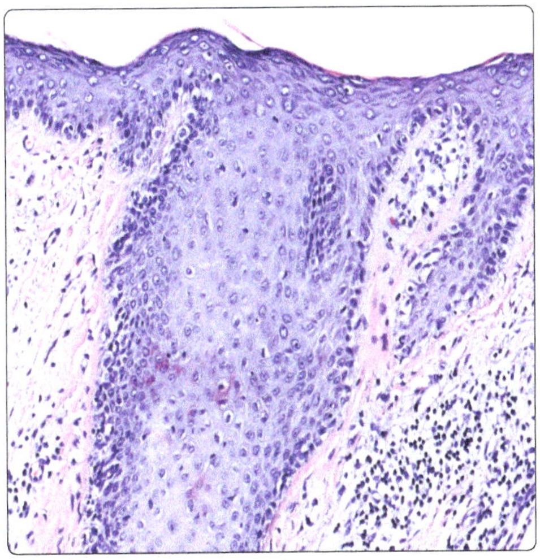

MART-1 Overstaining in Junctional Melanocytes and Keratinocytes in MIS-LMT

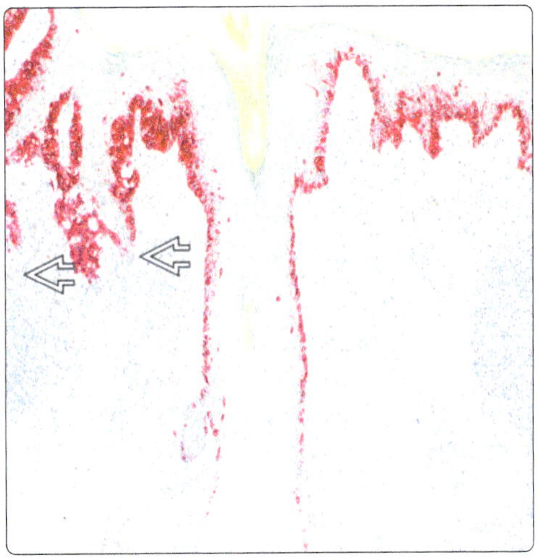

(Left) *Lentiginous, junctional melanocytic hyperplasia can be very extensive, corresponding to the clinical appearance of an ill-defined patch. There are no invasive dermal melanocytes.* **(Right)** *IHC for MART-1 exaggerates the numbers of intraepidermal melanocytes but confirms lack of early dermal invasion* →.

SOX10 Does Not Overstain Junctional Melanocytes in MIS-LMT

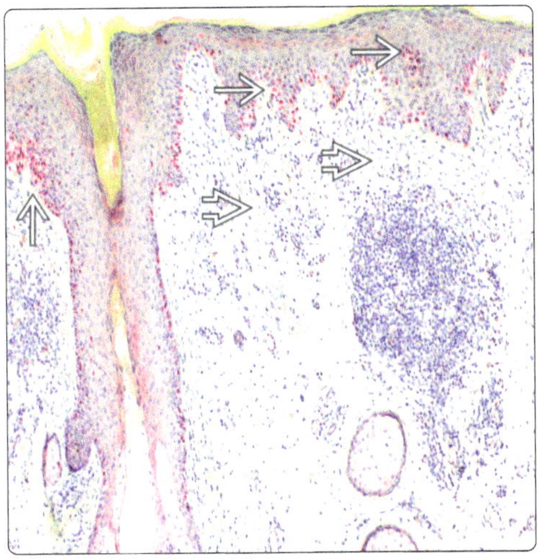

Higher Power of Nuclear Staining by SOX10

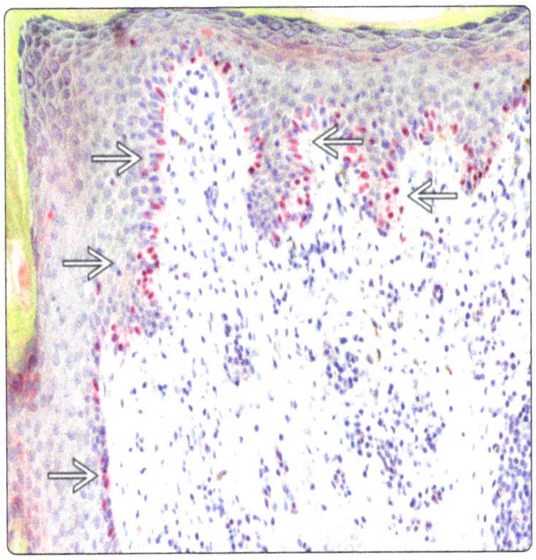

(Left) *SOX10 IHC specifically highlights the nuclei of junctional melanocytes* → *using the red protocol. It also confirms lack of dermal invasion* →. **(Right)** *Higher magnification shows lentiginous, junctional melanocytic hyperplasia is highlighted by red nuclei* →.

(Left) *The junctional proliferation of melanocytes appear hypercellular even at the scanning magnification especially on the facial cheek of an elderly. There is a deep scar from another procedure at this site.* **(Right)** *The lentiginous growth along the dermal-epidermal junction and lack of nesting are typical of melanoma in situ, lentigo maligna (MIS-LM) type.*

MIS-LMT

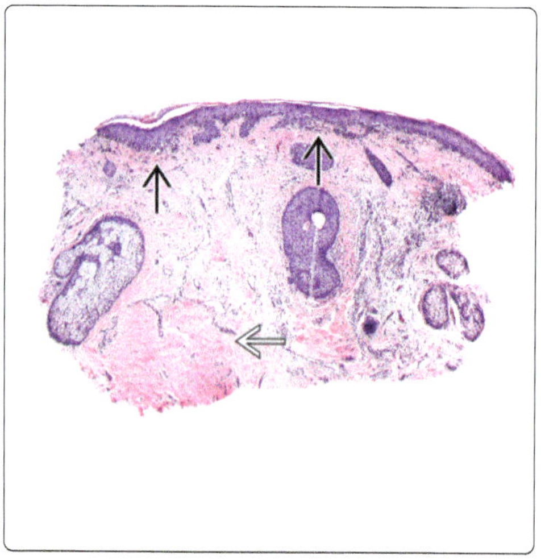

Lentiginous Proliferation of Atypical Melanocytes in MIS-LMT

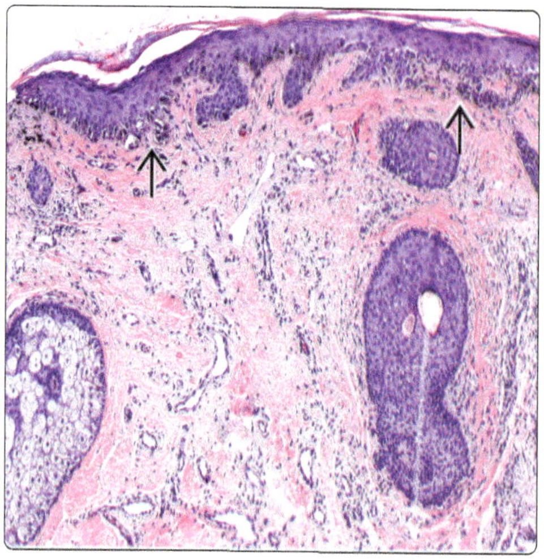

(Left) *Atypical melanocytes involve the follicular epithelium. There is dermal fibrosis with melanin incontinence.* **(Right)** *There are some scattering of atypical melanocytes in the epidermis seen in MIS-LM; however, they do not reach the granular cell layer. Adnexal involvement by melanoma cells is depicted.*

Higher Magnification Showing Adnexal Involvement

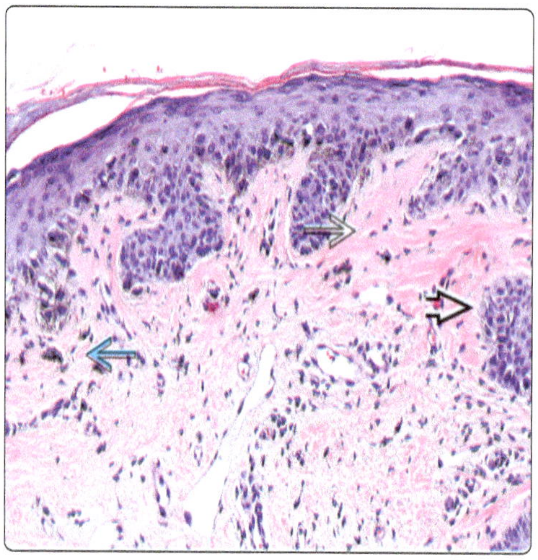

SOX10 Highlights Limited Upward Scatter of Atypical Melanocytes

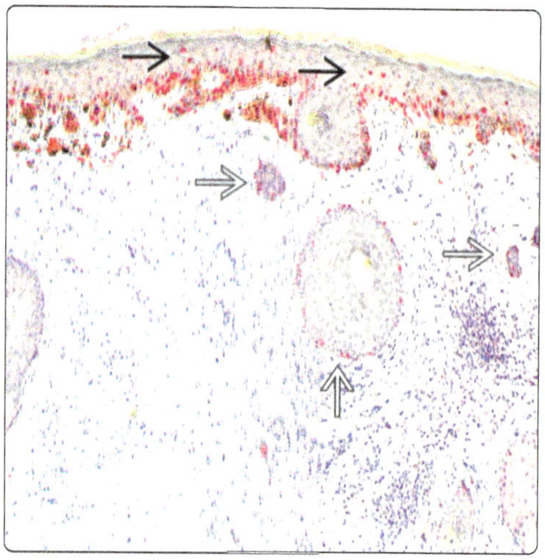

(Left) *Scanning magnification shows another MIS-LM type as a broad, inflamed intraepidermal melanocytic proliferation.* **(Right)** *High magnification of MIS-LMT shows almost complete replacement of the basal layer by atypical cells. Focal pagetoid upward scatter is also noted in this case.*

MIS-LMT at Low Magnification

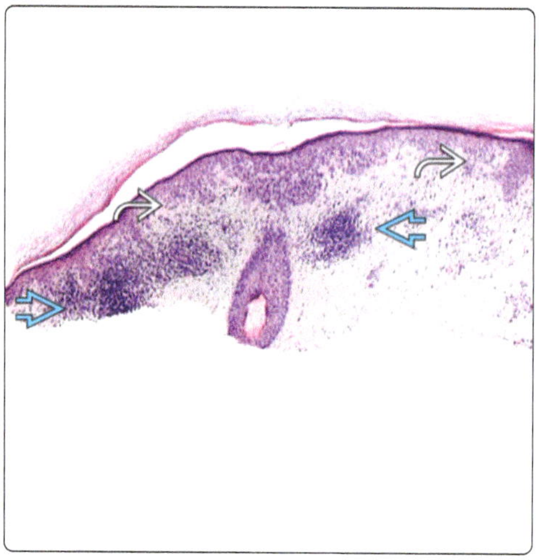

MIS-LMT With Limited Pagetoid Spread

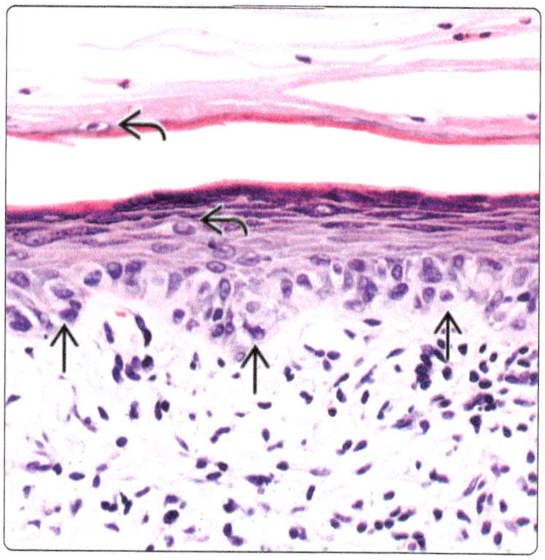

Shave Biopsies of MIS-LMT

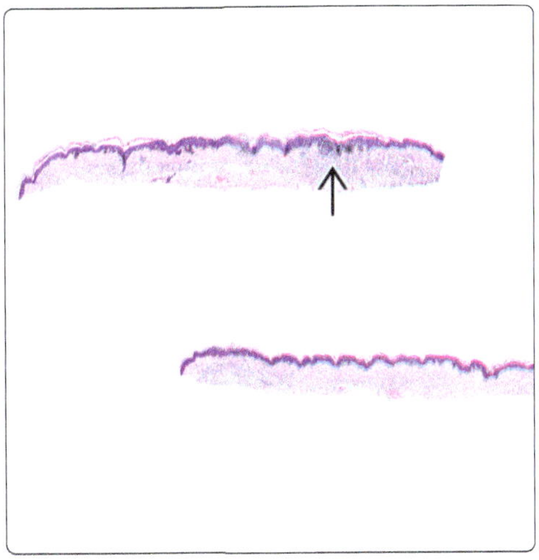

Early MIS-LMT and Solar Lentigo

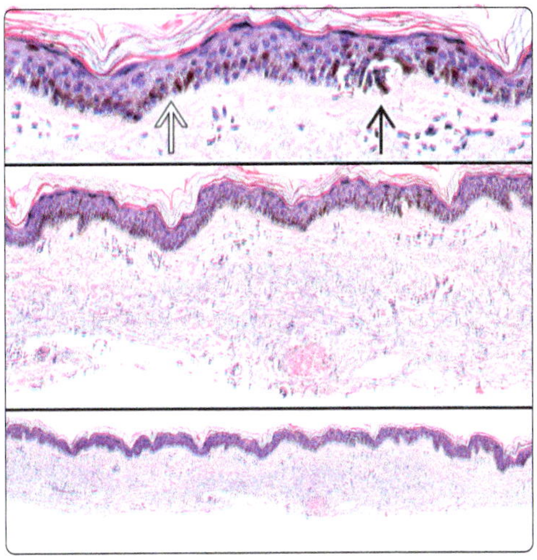

(Left) *Some lesions are very broad and are almost entirely shaved. Two such pieces are shown here. Focal pigmented proliferation* → *is identified even on scanning magnification.* **(Right)** *Early lentiginous proliferations of atypical melanocytes* → *are difficult to diagnose with certainty, especially if complicated by changes of solar lentigo. Hyperpigmentation is identified in the basilar keratinocytes* ➡. *The same field is shown in high (top), medium (middle), and low power (bottom).*

Early MIS-LMT

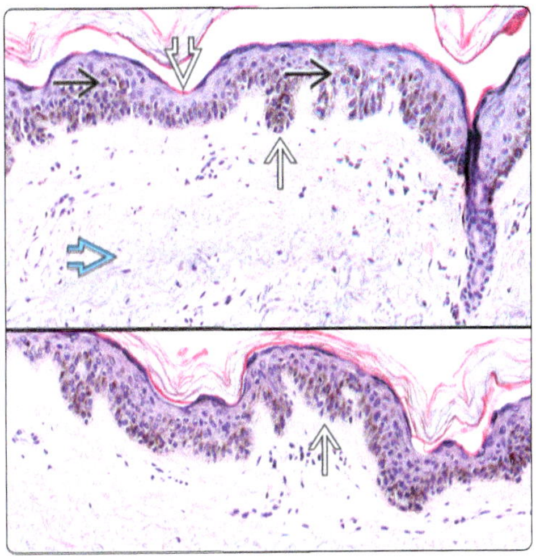

MITF Aids in Identification of Epidermal Melanocytes

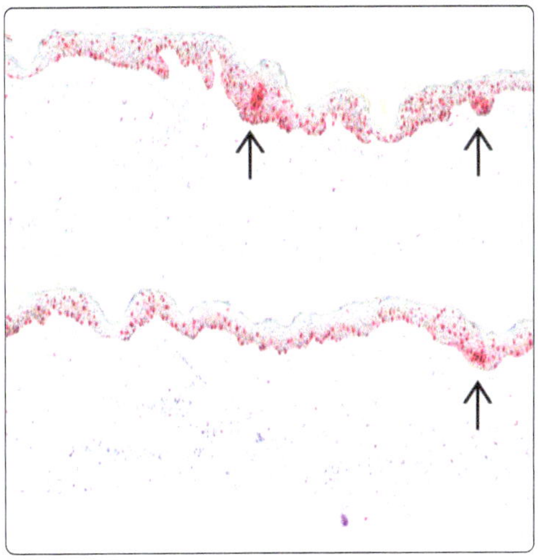

(Left) *Atypical intraepidermal melanocytes* → *are seen associated with hyperpigmented keratinocytes* ➡. *Note the epidermal atrophy* ➡ *and solar elastosis* ⇨. **(Right)** *MITF highlights the nuclei of poorly nested, lentiginous melanocytes* →.

SOX10 IHC in Early MIS-LMT

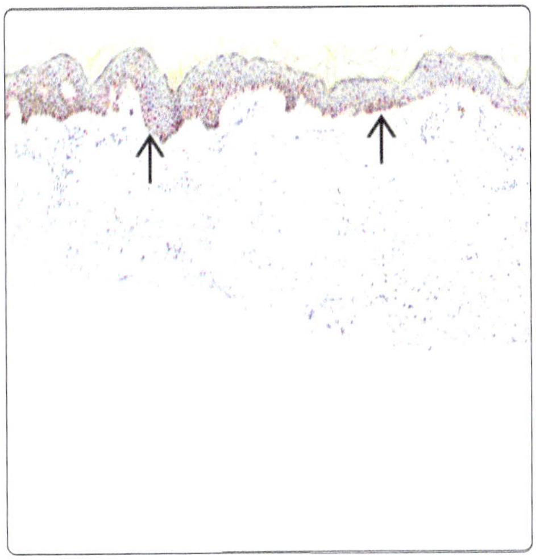

MART Overstains Epidermis in MIS-LMT

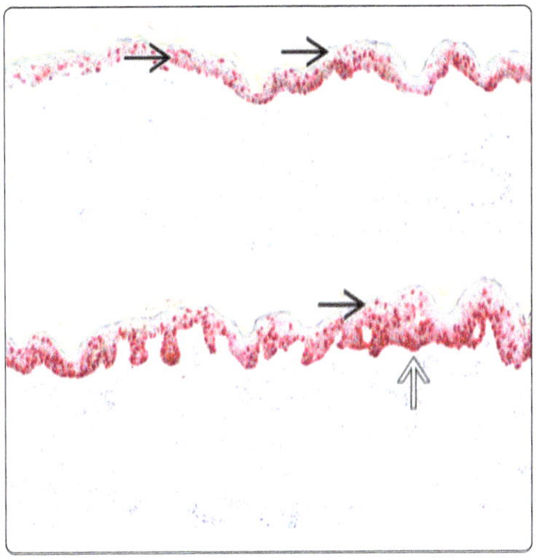

(Left) *SOX10 identifies the hard-to-find melanocytes (nuclei)* → *in early lesions of MIS-LMT.* **(Right)** *In the sun-damaged epidermis, MART IHC can exaggerate the melanocytic hyperplasia. It can highlight melanocytes* → *and basilar keratinocytes* ➡.

KEY FACTS

TERMINOLOGY

- Melanoma in situ composed mostly of irregular nests spreading along dermal-epidermal junction
- Melanoma in situ, superficial spreading type (MFS-SST)

CLINICAL ISSUES

- Most common variant of melanoma in situ
- Broad pigmented macule, variegated colors, irregular borders
- Sites vary: Often back (in men), legs (in women)
- Excellent prognosis

MICROSCOPIC

- Asymmetric, poorly circumscribed lesion with lateral expansion of large nests of atypical melanocytes
- Spread of atypical single cells and nests along junction (radial growth phase)
- Abundant pagetoid scatter of atypical melanocytes into spinous layer, often at periphery of lesion
- Large cells with ample cytoplasm
- Nuclear hyperchromasia and pleomorphism

TOP DIFFERENTIAL DIAGNOSES

- Severely atypical (dysplastic) junctional nevus
- Traumatized melanocytic nevus
- Melanocytic nevus of special site
- Reed (pigmented spindle cell) nevus
- Mammary and extramammary Paget disease

DIAGNOSTIC CHECKLIST

- Clinical: Large macule with variegated colors and irregular borders
- Pathologic: Large, irregular junctional nests, and lateral expansion of atypical melanocytes, often with abundant pagetoid spread

Pigmented Patch With Irregular Border and Lichenification

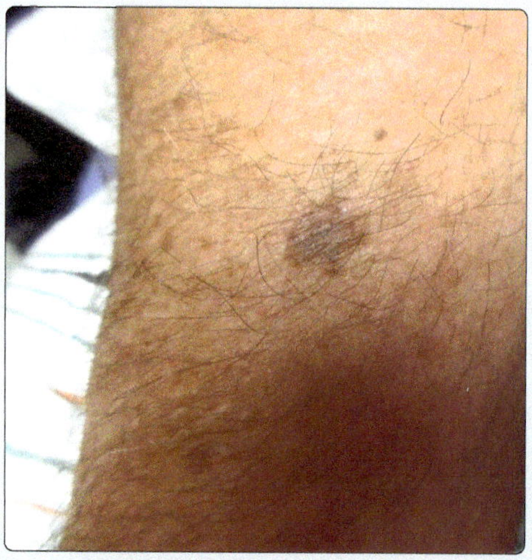

2-Tone Patch With Irregular Borders

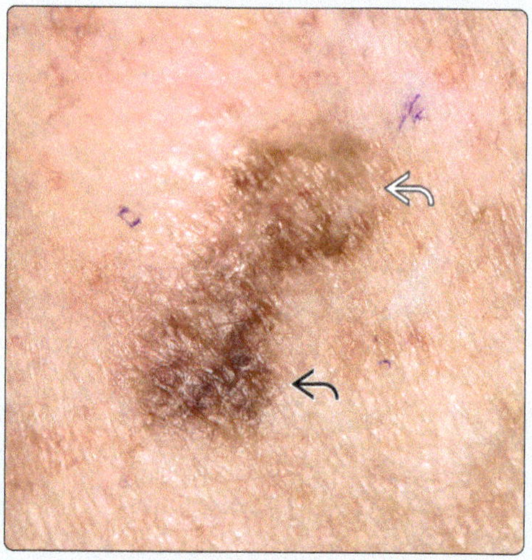

(Left) *This patch may resemble a lichenified keratosis. However, a shove biopsy showed a definitive melanoma in situ, superficial spreading type (MIS-SST). The lesional borders are distinct but irregular. (Courtesy J. Finch, MD.)* **(Right)** *The areas of hypo- ➔ and hyperpigmentation ➔ are concerning for melanoma. The depigmented area is concerning for regression. (Courtesy J. Finch, MD.)*

Radial Nesting in MIS-SST

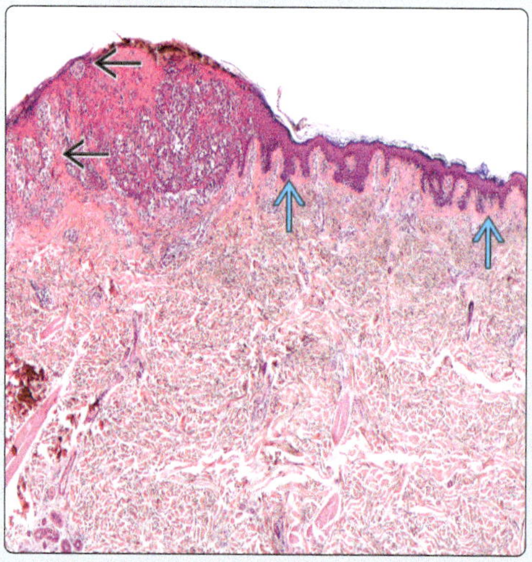

MIS-SST at Higher Magnification

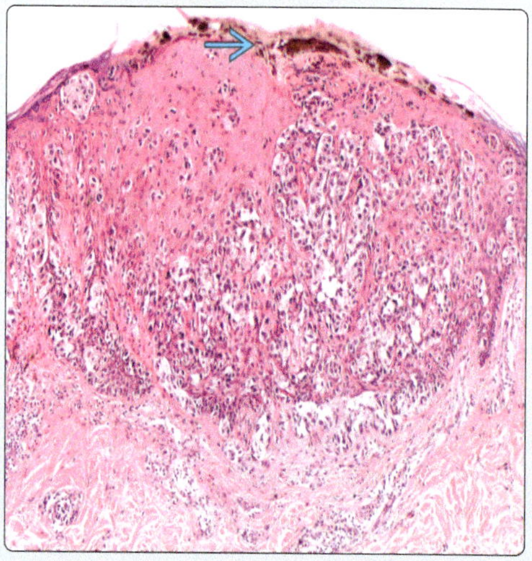

(Left) *The scanning magnification shows a papular growth in this atypical melanocytic lesion. Radial nesting of melanocytes ➔ at the edge is the defining feature of MIS-SST. There is an accompanying lentiginous melanocytic proliferation ➔.* **(Right)** *There is an extensive pagetoid scatter of melanocytes. Note the pigmented parakeratosis ➔ containing melanocytes.*

TERMINOLOGY

Abbreviations

- Melanoma in situ, superficial spreading type (MIS-SST)

Synonyms

- Superficial spreading melanoma in situ

Definitions

- Earliest stage of melanoma limited to epidermis, showing spread along dermoepidermal junction (radial growth phase)

CLINICAL ISSUES

Epidemiology

- Incidence
  - Most common variant of melanoma
- Age
  - Generally adults
- Sex
  - Males and females, different site predilections
- Ethnicity
  - Typically light-colored persons (especially red hair and skin type I/II)

Site

- Varies according to gender, on back (in men) and on legs (in women)
  - Intermittently sun-exposed areas (as opposed to chronically sun-exposed areas in lentigo maligna type of melanoma in situ)

Presentation

- Large dark brown macule (average size: 2.5 cm)
- Variegated color with shades of tan, brown, black, blue-black, red (due to inflammation or vascular ectasia), gray and white (zones of regression)
- Irregular borders

Treatment

- Surgical approaches
  - Complete excision with 5-mm clear margins is standard treatment

Prognosis

- Excellent prognosis
- Almost all patients are cured with adequate excision
- 100% survival at 5 and 10 years has been reported

MICROSCOPIC

Histologic Features

- Asymmetric, poorly circumscribed lesion with lateral expansion of large nests of atypical melanocytes
  - Irregular distribution of nests, which can be confluent with indented borders
- Increased numbers of single atypical melanocytes involving both rete ridges and suprapapillary plates
- Typically abundant pagetoid spread of atypical melanocytes located in spinous layer
  - Pagetoid spread at periphery of lesion (as opposed to only central focal spread in atypical and irritated nevi)
- Large artifactual clefts between nests and epidermis above
- No dermal invasion, but dense irregularly distributed inflammatory dermal infiltrate

Cytologic Features

- Large cells with ample cytoplasm
- Nuclear hyperchromasia and pleomorphism
  - Large eosinophilic or purple nucleoli often seen
- Mitotic figures often present

ANCILLARY TESTS

Immunohistochemistry

- Expression of p16 often lost (but positive in most melanocytic nevi)
- Ki-67 often shows elevated nuclear proliferative rate (> 10-15%)

DIFFERENTIAL DIAGNOSIS

Atypical (Dysplastic) Junctional Melanocytic Nevus

- Should show symmetry and circumscription at low magnification
  - Can be difficult to assess on partial biopsy
- Typically shows less pagetoid upward scatter of melanocytes
  - If present, should be in center of lesion

Irritated/Traumatized Melanocytic Nevi and Nevi Located on Special Sites

- In cases of suspected trauma, search for parakeratosis &/or serum above focus of pagetoid spread
- Recognize clinical setting and anatomic site

Reed (Pigmented Spindle Cell) Nevus

- Hyperplastic (not atrophic) epidermis, lateral margins are sharply defined (no trailing off of single cells)
- Composed mostly of spindle-shaped cells, which may be atypical but are often monomorphous (not pleomorphic as in MIS-SST)

DIAGNOSTIC CHECKLIST

Clinically Relevant Pathologic Features

- Large macule with variegated colors and irregular borders

Pathologic Interpretation Pearls

- Large junctional lesion with lateral expansion of atypical melanocytes, often with abundant pagetoid spread

SELECTED REFERENCES

1. Bhatt VR et al: Clinicopathologic characteristics and management trends of cutaneous invasive and in situ melanoma in older patients: a retrospective analysis of the National Cancer Data Base. Ther Adv Med Oncol. 7(1):4-11, 2015
2. Kutzner H et al: Histological and genetic evidence for a variant of superficial spreading melanoma composed predominantly of large nests. Mod Pathol. 25(6):838-45, 2012
3. Duncan LM: The classification of cutaneous melanoma. Hematol Oncol Clin North Am. 23(3):501-13, ix, 2009
4. Massi G et al: Histological Diagnosis of Nevi and Melanoma. 1st ed. Darmstadt: Steinkopff Verlag, 2004
5. Crowson et al: The Melanocytic Proliferations: A Comprehensive Textbook of Pigmented Lesions. 1st ed. New York: Wiley-Liss, 2001
6. Lopansri S et al: Clinical and pathological correlation of malignant melanoma. J Cutan Pathol. 6(3):180-94, 1979

(Left) *A shave biopsy of this lesion showed MIS. Note that there are areas of hyperpigmentation in an unevenly toned pigmented patch. (Courtesy J. Finch, MD.)* **(Right)** *The disrupted pigmentary network pattern is identified. Note the increase in blood vasculature. The hyperpigmented foci are evident. (Courtesy J. Finch, MD.)*

Irregularly Pigmented Patch

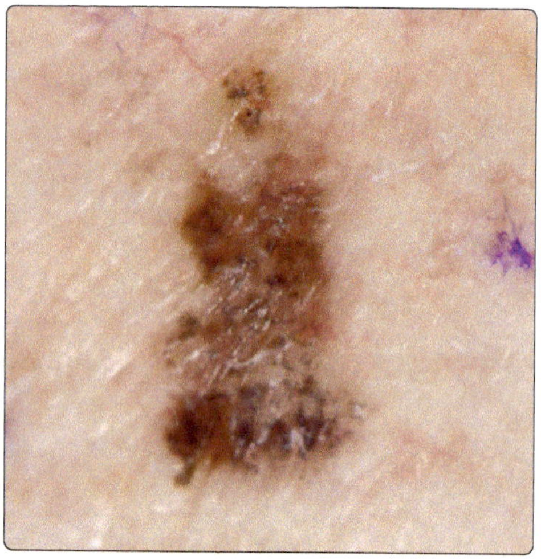

Dermoscopy of Same Lesion

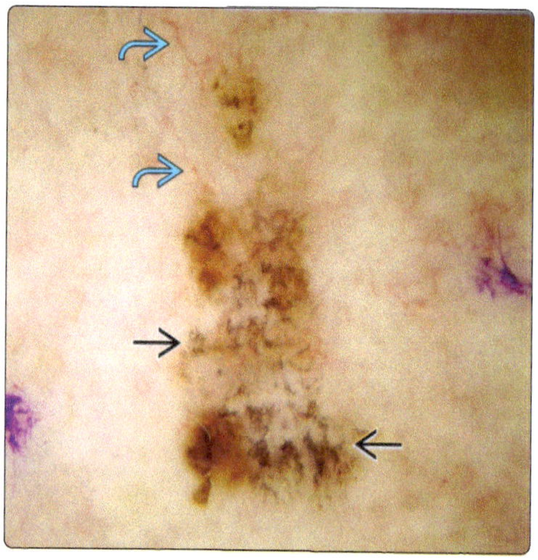

(Left) *The melanocytes appear in single and nested patterns. They are found in all layers of the epidermis.* **(Right)** *The intraepidermal melanocytes have oval to round nuclei, open chromatin, and more than 1 conspicuous nucleolus per cell. A mitotic figure is seen.*

Nesting and Scattering in MIS-SST

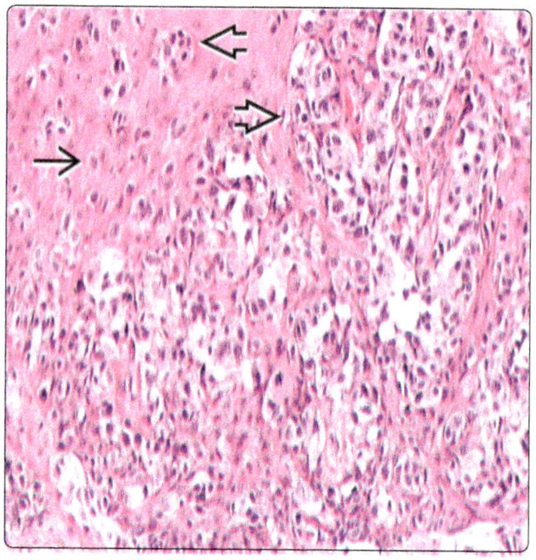

High Magnification Showing Melanoma Cytology

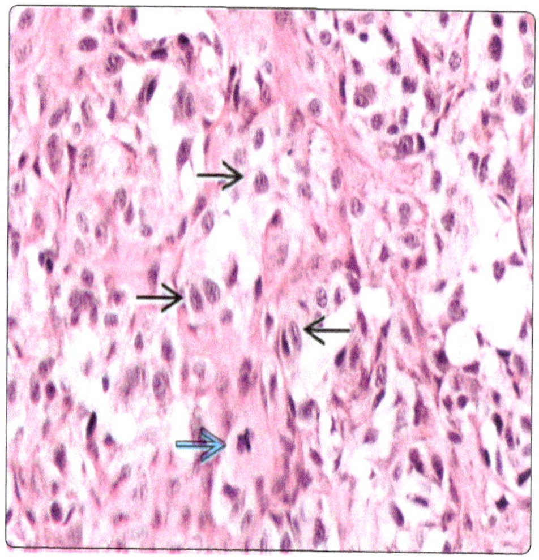

(Left) *Low magnification of a MIS-SST shows an atypical intraepidermal melanocytic proliferation in all layers of the epidermis and irregular nests of atypical cells along the dermal-epidermal junction.* **(Right)** *Higher power magnification reveals multifocal pagetoid scatter of atypical, epithelioid-shaped melanocytes throughout all layers of the epidermis.*

Low Magnification of MIS-SST

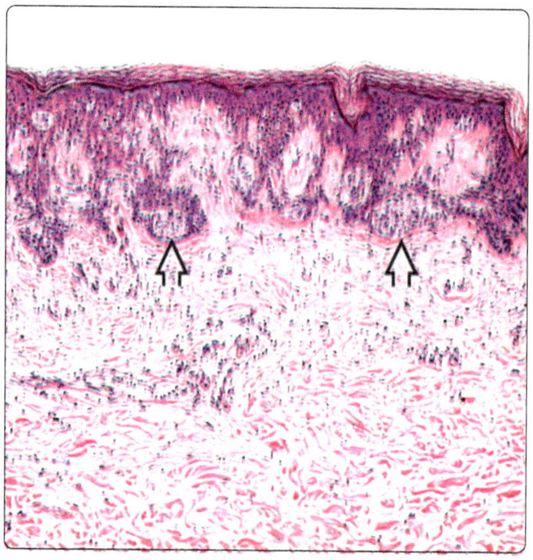

Multifocal Pagetoid Scatter of Melanocytes in MIS-SST

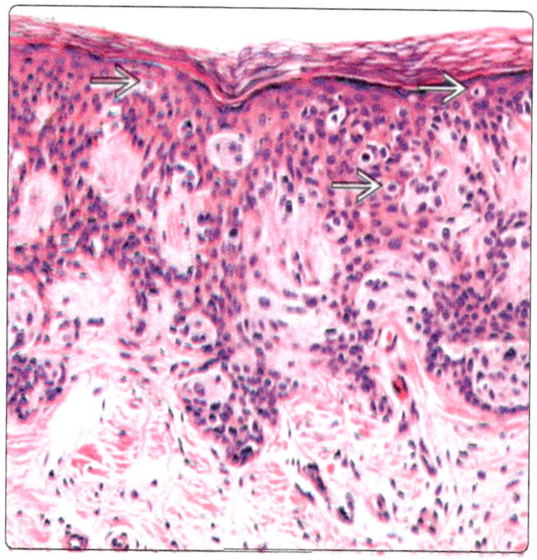

MIS-SST With Atypical Junctional Mitosis

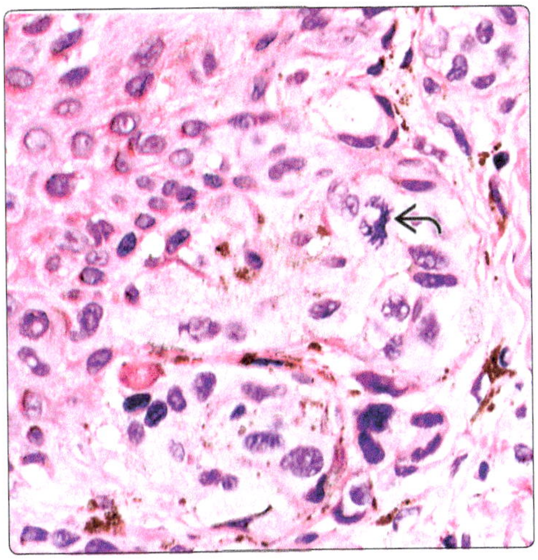

MIS-SST in Sun-Exposed Skin

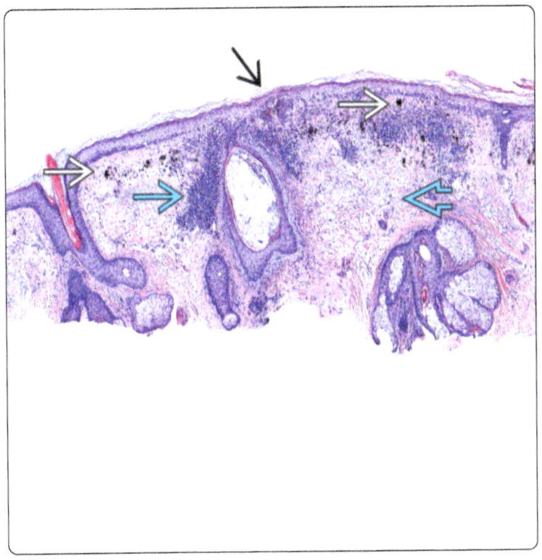

(Left) *High magnification of another case of MIS-SST shows nests of enlarged, atypical cells. Note the atypical (crab-like) mitosis.* **(Right)** *Even at this scanning magnification, patchy inflammation and irregular pigmentation are concerning. There is an overlying atypical junctional and poorly nested melanocytic hyperplasia. The dermis shows marked solar elastosis.*

Poorly Nested Radial Growth in MIS-SST

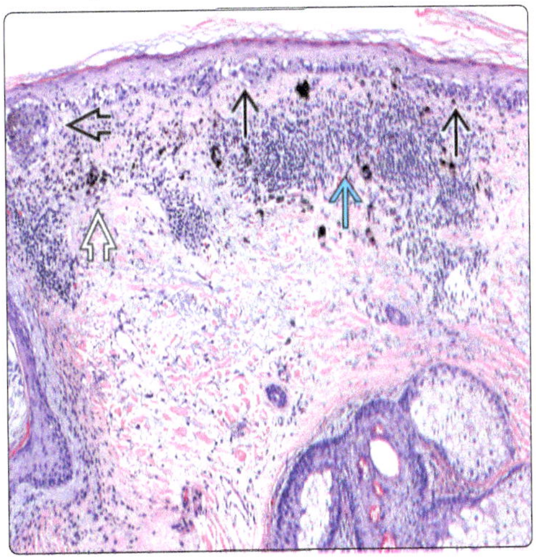

Consumption of Epidermis in MIS-SST

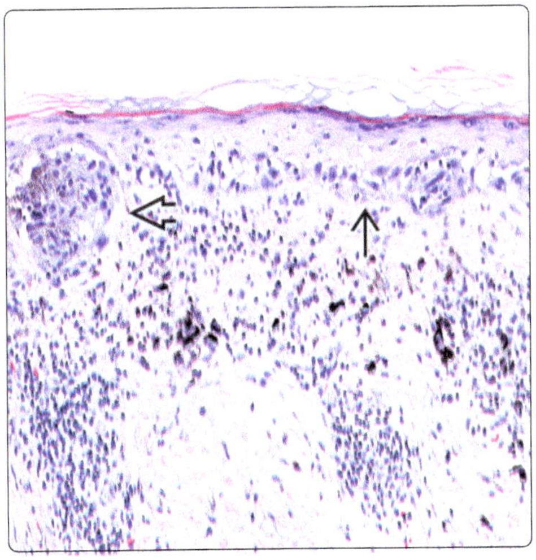

(Left) *This example shows poorly nested and lentiginous growth patterns. Note the lichenoid inflammatory infiltrate with melanin incontinence. Deep dermal solar elastosis is evident.* **(Right)** *Both nested and lentiginous patterns are identified, and are confirmed under a higher magnification. The lentiginous melanocytes are "consuming" the epidermis, a feature of melanoma.*

Lentiginous Pattern in MIS-SST

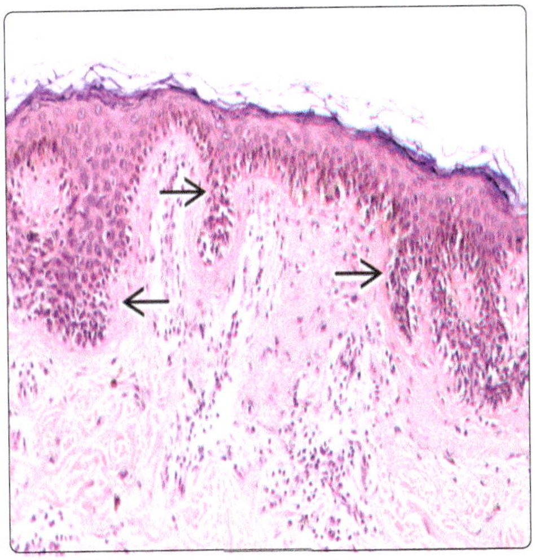

Lentiginous Growth of Melanocytes in MIS-SST

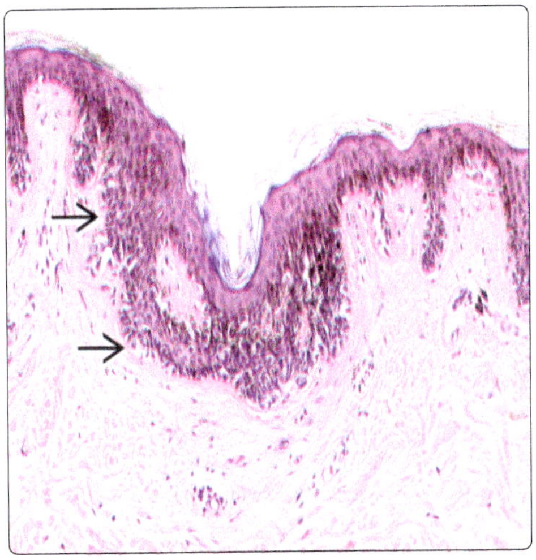

(Left) *In some lesions, a focal lentiginous growth can be seen in an otherwise mostly nested pattern. This lentiginous pattern is concerning for melanoma even though there is no extensive pagetoid upward scatter of melanocytes.* **(Right)** *Another example shows a lentiginous growth pattern of melanocytes. This is consistent with melanoma in situ, despite the lack of pagetoid upward scatter.*

KEY FACTS

TERMINOLOGY

- Melanoma in situ, not otherwise specified (MIS, NOS)
- Cases that cannot be clearly categorized as either lentigo maligna, acral lentiginous, or superficial spreading type of melanoma in situ

CLINICAL ISSUES

- Uncommon tumors
- Typically occur in elderly patients
- Usually located on sun-exposed areas, especially cheeks, upper trunk, and arms
- Borders of lesions are irregular, asymmetric, and often notched
- Lesions are dark, broad macules ~ 0.8 cm in diameter
- Complete excision with 5.0-mm clear margins
- Mohs surgery may also be effective but is controversial

MICROSCOPIC

- Asymmetric, poorly circumscribed atypical junctional melanocytic proliferation
- Single atypical melanocytes with lentiginous spread and pagetoid upward scatter
- Peripheral trailing off of single atypical cells
- Spitzoid features may be present in some cases
  - Cells are markedly enlarged and atypical to bizarre-appearing

TOP DIFFERENTIAL DIAGNOSES

- Melanoma in situ, superficial spreading type
- Melanoma in situ, lentigo maligna type
- Atypical (dysplastic) junctional melanocytic nevus
- Irritated/traumatized nevi and nevi of special sites
- Reed (pigmented spindle cell) nevus

Clinical Photograph of MIS, NOS

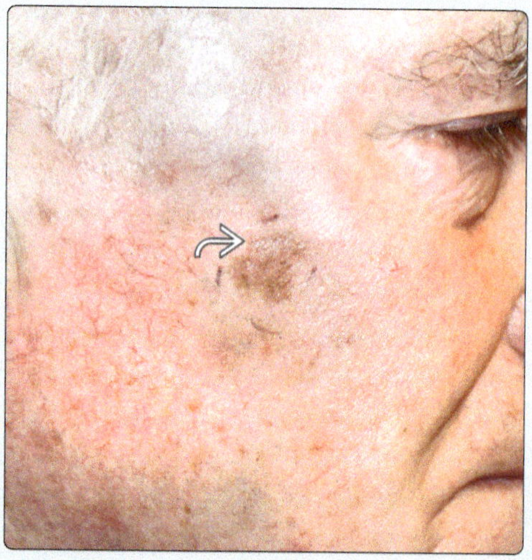

Irregular Patch on Sun-Exposed Skin

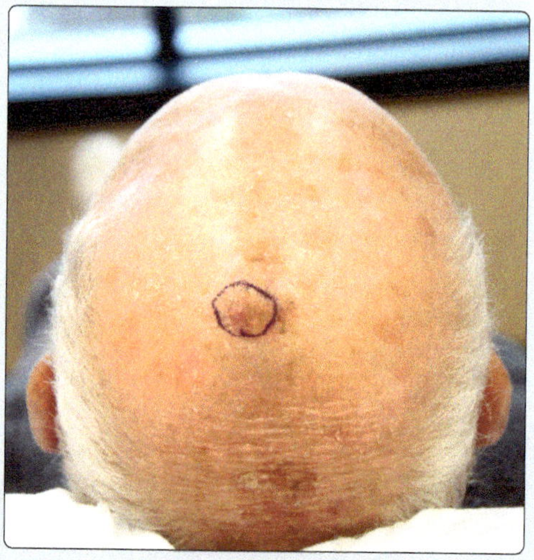

(Left) *This lightly pigmented patch on chronically sun-exposed skin has irregular borders. It appears to be ill-defined, and a biopsy is needed to rule in melanoma. The biopsy proved a melanoma in situ (MIS). The lesion is evenly pigmented; however, there are less pigmented foci ➡, suggestive of early regression.* **(Right)** *There is a growing pigmented patch (circled) in a background of sun damage, lentigines, and actinic keratoses. The ill-defined patch should raise concern and be biopsied. (Courtesy J. Finch, MD.)*

MIS Showing Hypercellular Junctional Growth

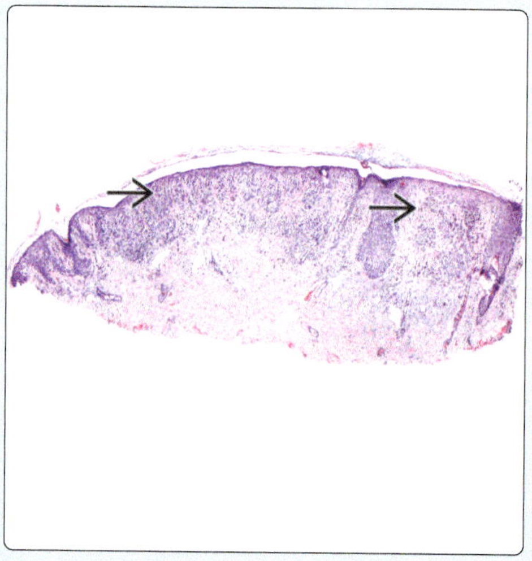

MIS Showing Upward Scatter of Melanocytes

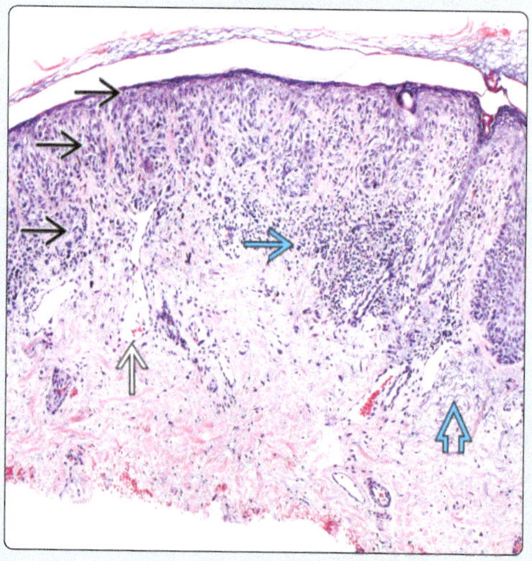

(Left) *Under scanning magnification, there is an overgrowth of intraepidermal melanocytes ➡. This configuration should raise concern for MIS, even at scanning magnification.* **(Right)** *There is migration of melanocytes throughout all the epidermal layers ➡. A patchy lymphocytic infiltrate ➡, telangiectasia ➡, and solar elastosis ➡ are noted. Note how the melanocytes outnumber the keratinocytes.*

TERMINOLOGY

Abbreviations

- Melanoma in situ, not otherwise specified (MIS, NOS)

Definitions

- Cases that cannot be clearly categorized as either lentigo maligna, acral lentiginous, or superficial spreading type of melanoma in situ

CLINICAL ISSUES

Epidemiology

- Incidence
  - Uncommon tumors
- Age
  - Typically occur in elderly patients

Site

- Usually located on sun-exposed areas, especially cheeks, upper trunk, and arms

Presentation

- Borders of lesions are irregular, asymmetric, and often notched
- Lesions are dark, broad macules ~ 0.8 cm in diameter
- Mottled pigmentation

Treatment

- Surgical approaches
  - Complete excision with 5.0-mm clear margins
  - Mohs surgery may also be effective, but is controversial

Prognosis

- Excellent: Little recurrence potential with adequate surgical margins

MICROSCOPIC

Histologic Features

- Melanocytic proliferation typically characterized by both lentiginous junctional spread (similar to lentigo maligna) and irregular nesting and pagetoid spread (similar to superficial spreading type of MIS)
- Asymmetric, poorly circumscribed junctional melanocytic lesion
  - Peripheral trailing off of single atypical cells
  - Melanocytes extend laterally beyond last nests
- Spitzoid features may be present in some cases
  - Cells are markedly enlarged and atypical to bizarre-appearing
  - Composed of mixture of spindled and epithelioid-shaped cells
  - Markedly atypical junctional spitzoid lesions in adults are much more likely to represent MIS than atypical Spitz nevus
- Dermis may show dense but irregularly distributed inflammatory dermal infiltrate

Cytologic Features

- Nuclear atypia and pleomorphism
  - Large eosinophilic or purple nucleoli
- Mitotic figures often present

ANCILLARY TESTS

Immunohistochemistry

- HMB-45, SOX10, and MITF can be used to confirm diagnosis of MIS
  - Can also identify superficially invasive cells

DIFFERENTIAL DIAGNOSIS

Melanoma In Situ, Superficial Spreading Type

- Proliferation of predominantly nested and pagetoid melanocytes
- Broad, asymmetric junctional spread of irregularly shaped and sized nests

Melanoma In Situ, Lentigo Maligna Type

- Proliferation of predominantly single lentiginous cells along dermal-epidermal junction
- Less nesting and pagetoid scatter than MIS-NOS and MIS, superficial spreading type

Atypical (Dysplastic) Junctional Melanocytic Nevus

- Should show symmetry and circumscription at low magnification
  - Can be difficult, if not impossible, to assess on partial biopsy
- Typically shows less atypia and pagetoid upward scatter of melanocytes
  - If present, should be focal in center of lesion

Irritated/Traumatized Junctional Nevi and Nevi of Special Sites

- Search for parakeratosis &/or serum above foci of pagetoid spread
- Important to recognize clinical setting and anatomic site

Reed (Pigmented Spindle Cell) Nevus

- Usually occurs on extremities in young adults, more common in females
- Hyperplastic epidermis, lateral margins are sharply defined
- Composed mostly of spindle-shaped cells, which may be atypical, but are often monomorphous
  - Cells typically heavily pigmented, and numerous melanophages present in dermis

DIAGNOSTIC CHECKLIST

Pathologic Interpretation Pearls

- Single atypical melanocytes as well as irregular nesting and areas of limited pagetoid scatter

SELECTED REFERENCES

1. Danga ME et al: Melan-A positive dermal cells in malignant melanoma in situ. J Cutan Pathol. 42(6):388-93, 2015
2. King R: Lentiginous melanoma. Arch Pathol Lab Med. 135(3):337-41, 2011
3. Erickson C et al: Treatment options in melanoma in situ: topical and radiation therapy, excision and Mohs surgery. Int J Dermatol. 49(5):482-91, 2010
4. Gerami P et al: Superficial melanocytic neoplasms with pagetoid melanocytosis: a study of interobserver concordance and correlation with FISH. Am J Surg Pathol. 34(6):816-21, 2010
5. Ramos-Herberth FI, Karamchandani J, Kim J, et al: SOX10 immunostaining distinguishes desmoplastic melanoma from excision scar. J Cutan Pathol 2010;37(9):944-952.

(Left) *Note the upward (pagetoid) scatter of melanocytes without significant epidermal atrophy. Nearly the entire epidermis is filled with highly atypical melanocytes, which outnumber the keratinocytes.* **(Right)** *In MIS, NOS, features of both lentigo maligna and superficial spreading melanoma can be seen. Note the junctional growth of melanocytes and their extension along the follicular epithelium. Focally radial growth or a nested pattern can also be seen.*

MIS, NOS Showing Pagetoid Scatter of Melanocytes

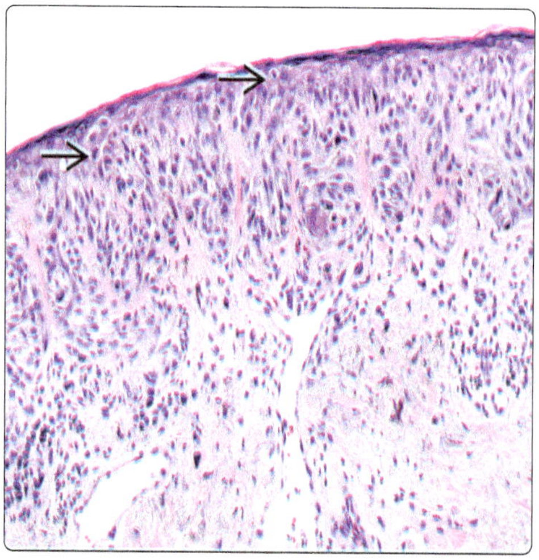

Poorly Nested, Junctional Growth in MIS, NOS

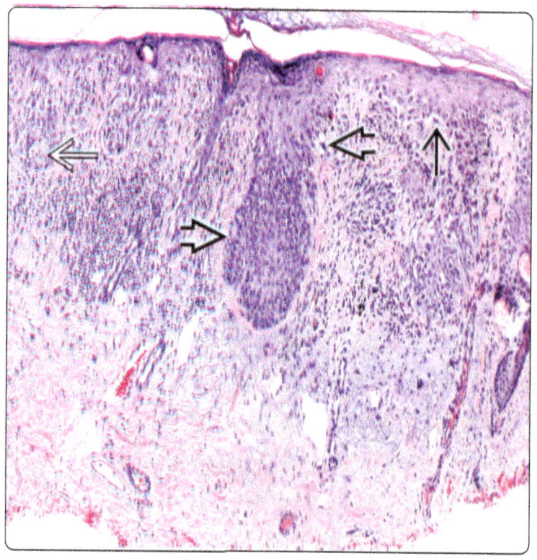

(Left) *Shown at higher magnification, there are atypical melanocytes that extend down the follicular epithelium. The dermis also appears hypercellular, concerning for microinvasion. However, there is a point of connection to the epidermis, excluding an invasive focus.* **(Right)** *Focal large, bizarre-appearing spitzoid cells are present along the junction. There are foci of pagetoid scatter of atypical melanocytes. Note the lymphoid infiltrate in the papillary dermis and nodular elastosis.*

Involvement of Follicular Epithelium in MIS, NOS

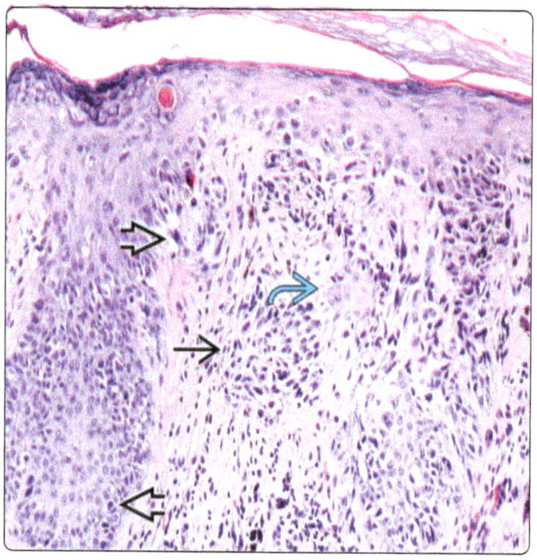

Nested and Pagetoid Scatter of Melanocytes in MIS, NOS

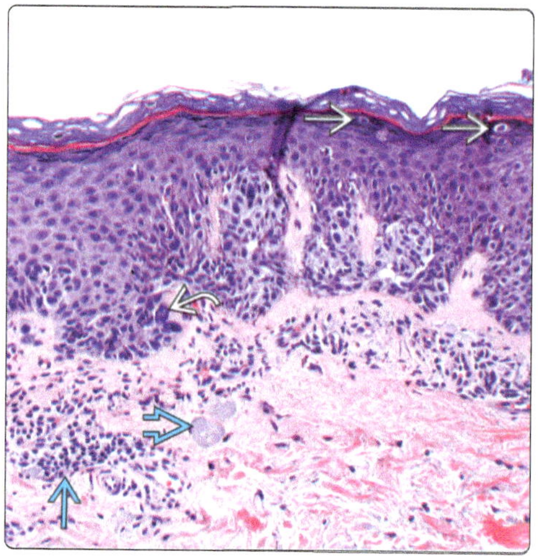

(Left) *This image shows a lentiginous junctional growth pattern of melanocytes that are poorly nested. There is also pagetoid upward scatter. The dermis shows a patchy inflammatory infiltrate and melanin incontinence.* **(Right)** *Higher power magnification shows a predominantly lentiginous proliferation of atypical cells along the dermal-epidermal junction. The nests are bridging by joining across the rete ridges. Limited pagetoid upward scatter is also seen.*

Lentiginous Growth and Pagetoid Scatter in MIS, NOS

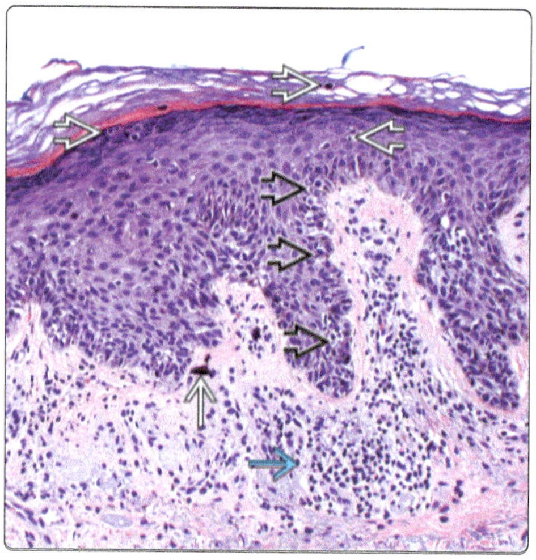

Mostly Lentiginous Growth in MIS, NOS

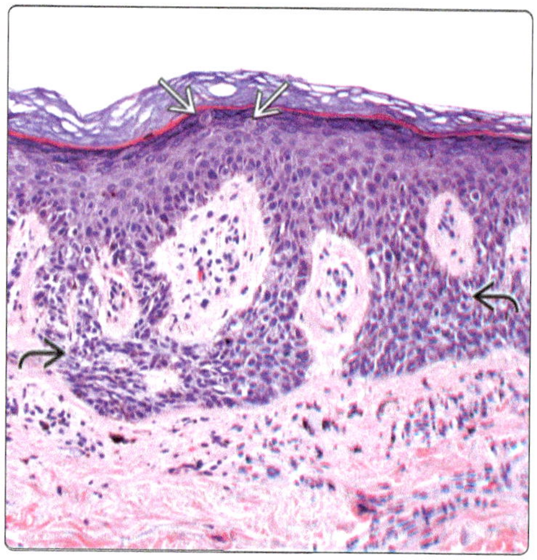

Broad, Atypical Melanocytic Proliferation

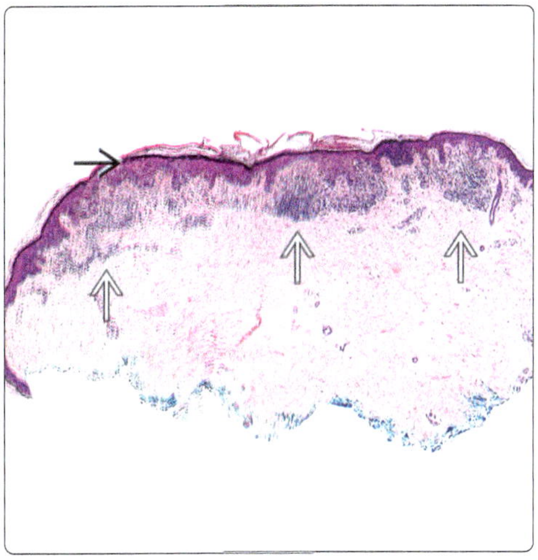

Hypercellular Epidermis in MIS, NOS

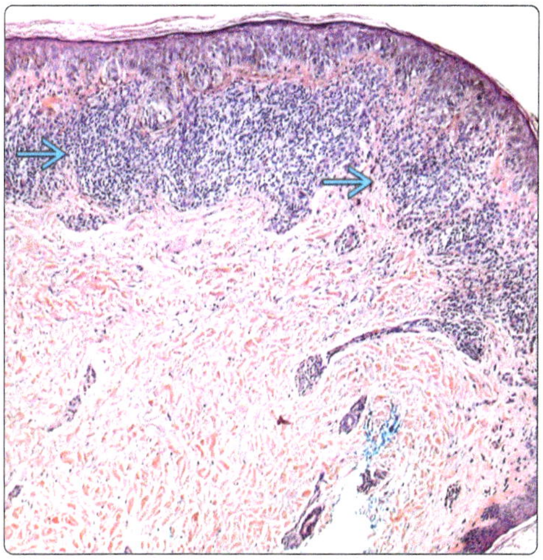

(Left) *Scanning magnification of a MIS shows a broad intraepidermal melanocytic proliferation* ➙*. The lesion is associated with a brisk lymphocytic host response in the dermis* ➙*.* **(Right)** *Low-power magnification of the same case shows spindled and epithelioid atypical intraepidermal melanocytes. The configuration is somewhat vertical, resembling a Spitz nevus. The papillary dermis is filled with a band-like inflammatory infiltrate* ➙*, obliterating the junctional component.*

Focal Pagetoid Scatter in MIS, NOS

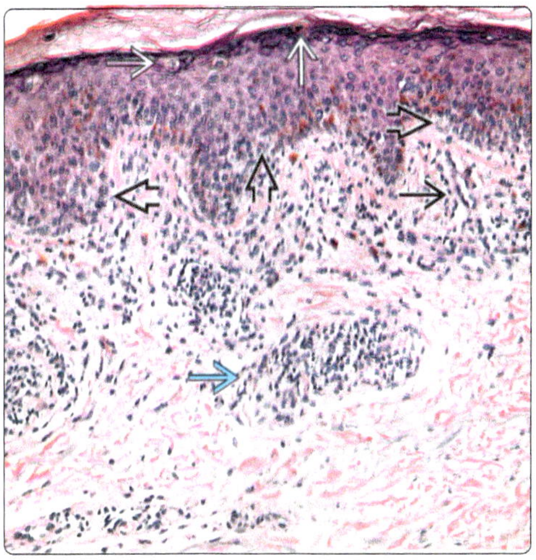

Incomplete Nesting Pattern in MIS, NOS

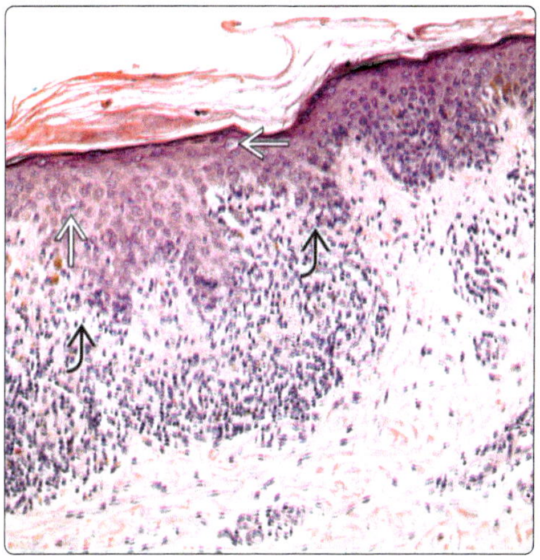

(Left) *High-power view shows limited and focal pagetoid upward scatter* ➙*. There is a lack of peripheral nesting, but there is lentiginous growth of melanocytes* ➙*. These findings are sufficient for the diagnosis of MIS. Note the vertically oriented blood vessels* ➙ *and patchy inflammation* ➙*.* **(Right)** *This field shows incomplete nesting of melanocytes* ➙*. There is only focal pagetoid upward scatter* ➙*. The papillary dermis shows a relatively dense lymphocytic infiltrate (below the melanocytic proliferation).*

Spindled and Epithelioid Cytology in MIS, NOS

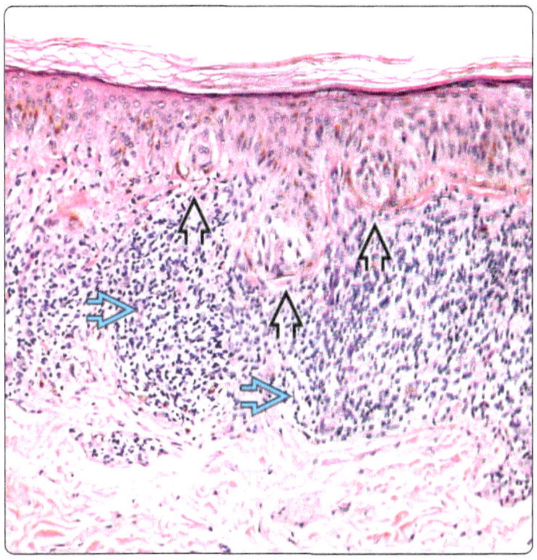

Overlapping Features: Junctional and Lentiginous Growth Patterns

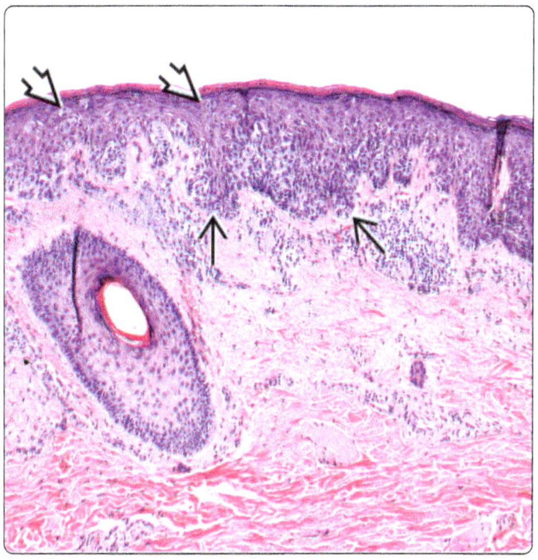

(Left) *This field shows vertically oriented spindled and epithelioid atypical melanocytes* ➙ *in a poorly nested configuration, resembling a spitzoid MIS. The dermis shows a brisk lymphocytic host response* ➙*.* **(Right)** *MIS is shown with overlapping features of lentigo maligna and superficial spreading types. There is relatively prominent pagetoid scatter* ➙ *and irregular nesting, as well as a proliferation of atypical lentiginous cells* ➙ *along the junction.*

(Left) *Higher magnification shows numerous atypical single lentiginous cells* ⇒ *and a few irregular nests* ⇒ *along the junction. There is marked globular solar elastosis* ⇒. **(Right)** *Melanoma in situ, not otherwise specified shows numerous atypical lentiginous cells* ⇒ *along the junction (similar to lentigo maligna), but there is also focal pagetoid scatter* ⇒ *and irregular nesting* ⇒ *(similar to MIS, superficial spreading type).*

Higher Magnification of MIS, NOS Showing Some Nesting

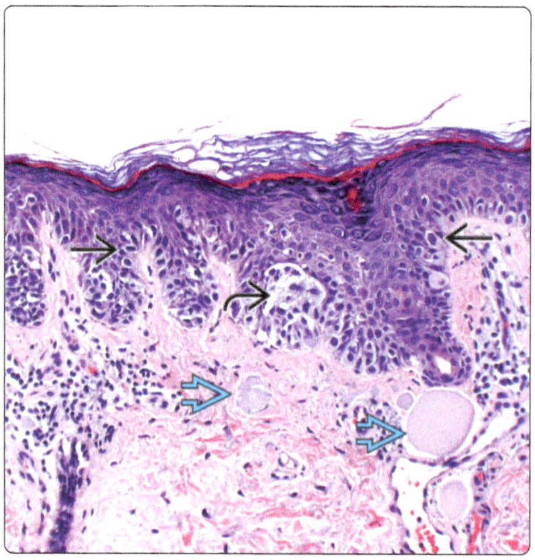

Mostly Lentiginous Growth in MIS, NOS

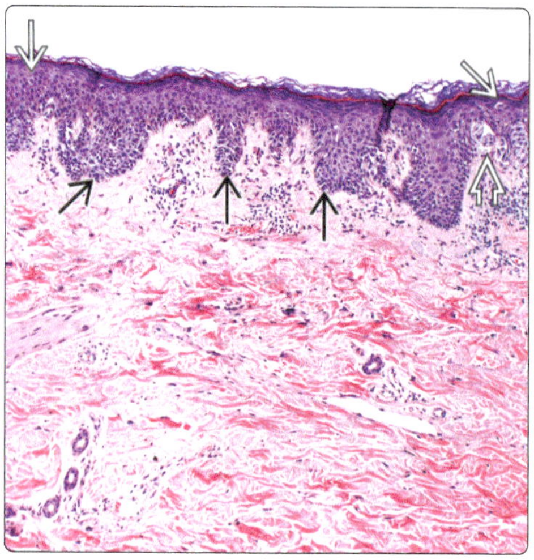

(Left) *There is marked, thick solar elastosis* ⇒ *extending deep beyond the papillary to reticular dermis. The overlying melanocytes are well nested with retraction artifact* ⇒. *There is melanin incontinence in the papillary dermis* ⇒. **(Right)** *This example resembles a verruca vulgaris with dense overlying hyperkeratosis and parakeratosis* ⇒. *However, the epidermis is hypercellular without distinct nesting. Careful examination of the epidermis is warranted to search for melanocytic hyperplasia.*

MIS, NOS: Well-Nested Pattern Example

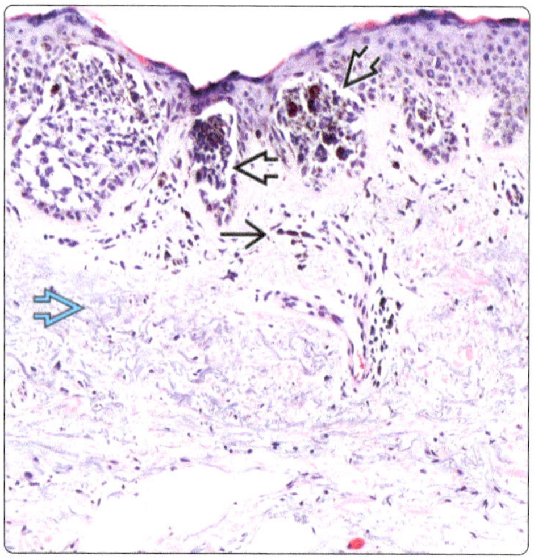

Hyperkeratotic Example of MIS, NOS

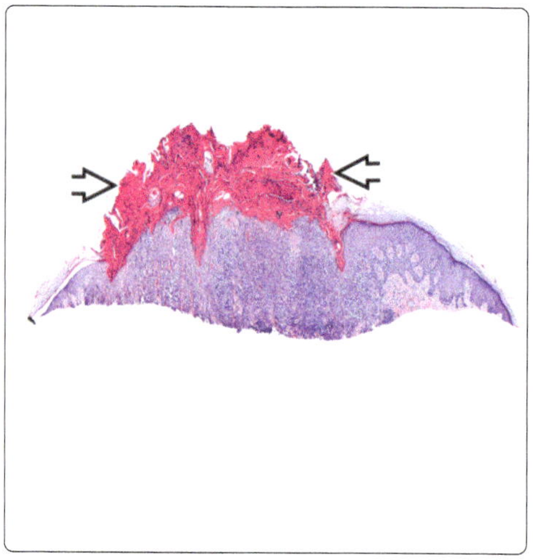

(Left) *The epidermis is hypercellular* ⇒, *resembling a squamous cell carcinoma in situ arising in a wart. However, even at this power, there are no keratin pearls or eosinophilia that are seen in squamous cell carcinoma.* **(Right)** *There are melanocytes in all the layers of the epidermis* ⇒. *There is only focal, irregular nesting seen in this field. Atypical melanocytes are found in the stratum corneum* ⇒ *via transepidermal elimination.*

Hypercellular Epidermis in MIS, NOS

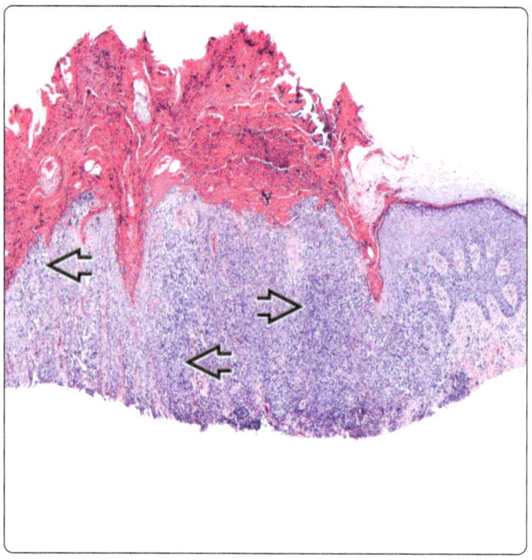

Extensive Pagetoid Scatter in MIS, NOS

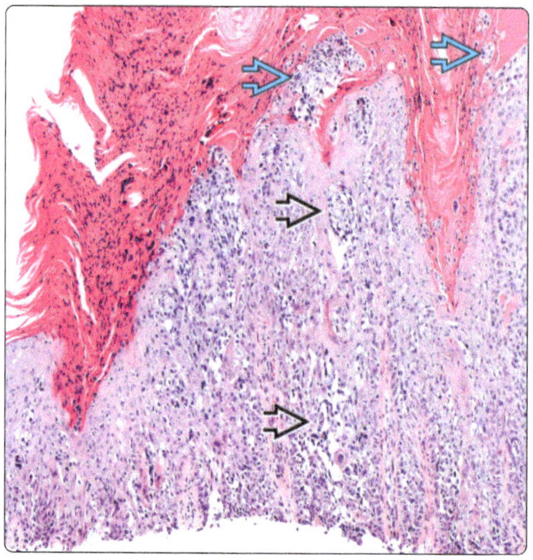

MIS-NOS at Low Magnification

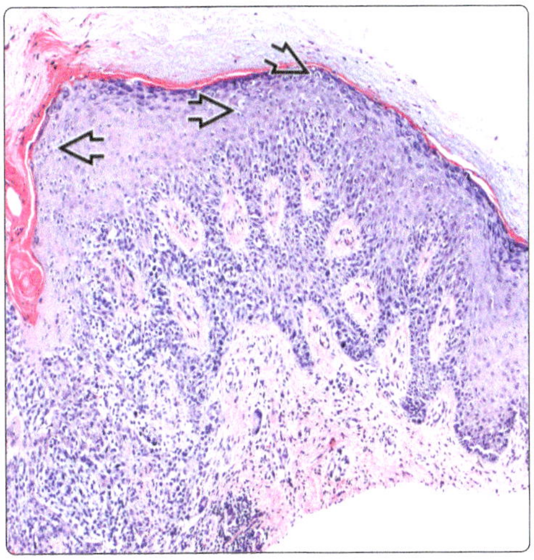

Upward Scatter of Melanocytes in MIS, NOS

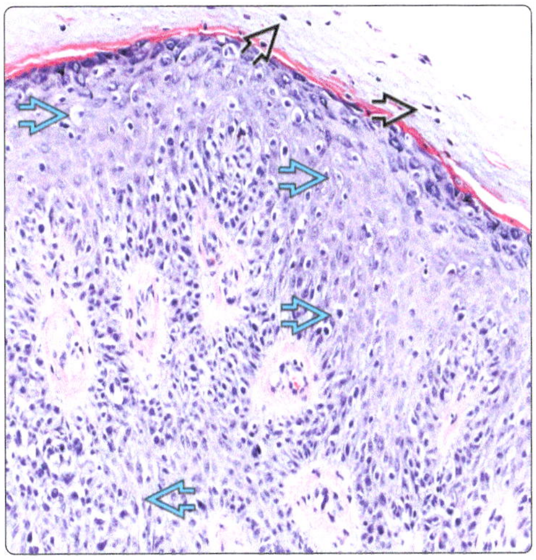

(Left) *This field bears a closer resemblance to MIS. There is extensive upward scatter of melanocytes* ⇨*. There are melanocytes in all the layers of epidermal keratinocytes; however, no definitive nesting is observed.* **(Right)** *There are melanocytes in all the layers of epidermis* ⇨*, even in the stratum corneum* ⇨*. Note the associated keratinocytic hyperplasia, which may mask the melanocytic proliferation.*

SOX10 Immunostaining in MIS, NOS

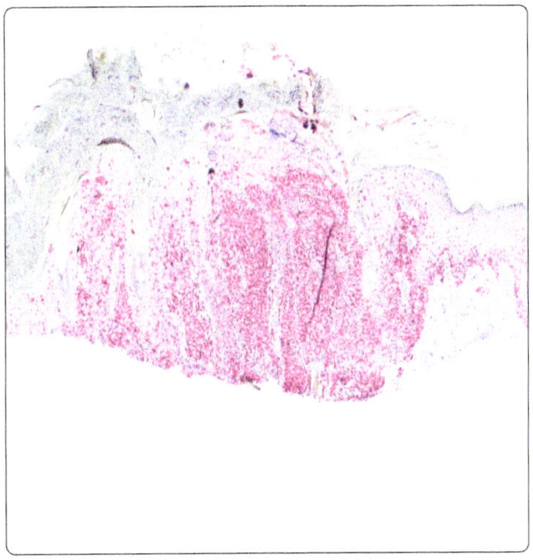

SOX10 Showing Extensive Pagetoid Scatter and Focal Microinvasion

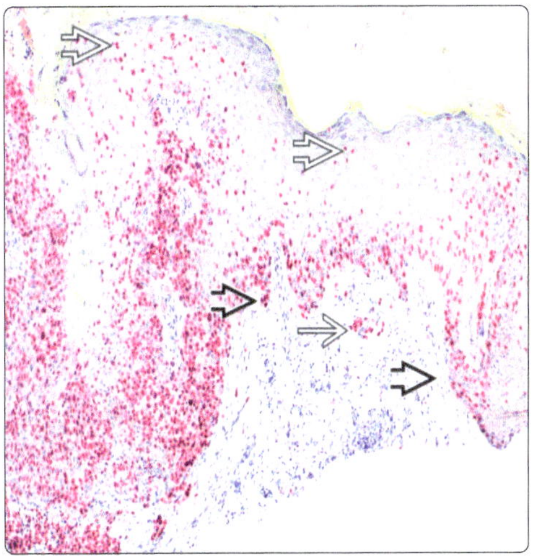

(Left) *Immunostaining for SOX10 highlights all of the intraepidermal melanocytes, helpful in confirming the melanocytic differentiation. The extent of melanocytic hyperplasia may be rather surprising, compared to the histologic findings.* **(Right)** *The junctional* ⇨ *and pagetoid* ➡ *melanocytes are highlighted. There are a few cells* ➡ *invading the papillary dermis. SOX10 is more helpful than MITF, especially in looking for dermal invasion.*

MITF Immunostaining in MIS, NOS

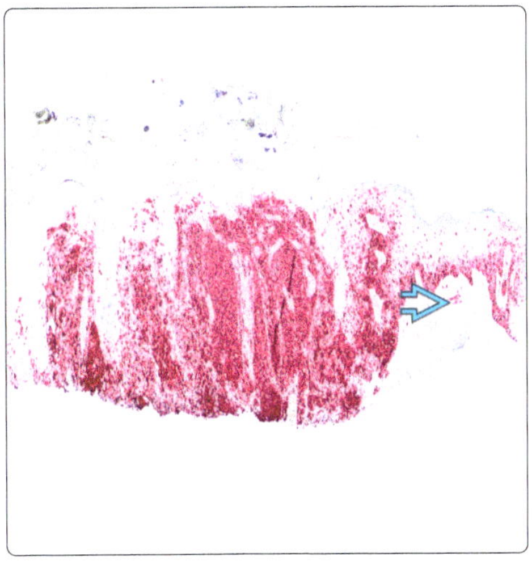

Extensive Pagetoid Scatter in MIS, NOS by MITF

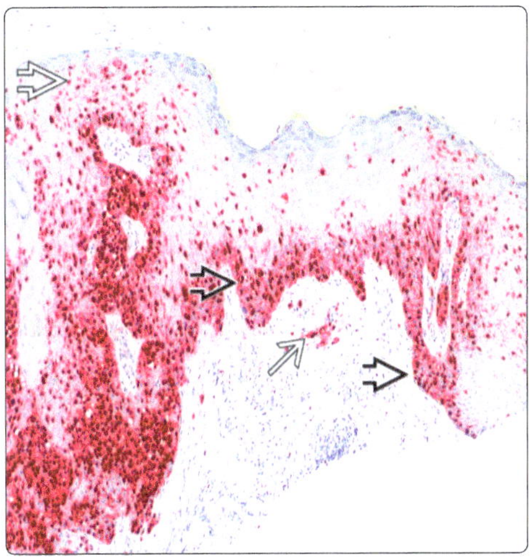

(Left) *Similarly, the immunostaining for MITF highlights all of the intraepidermal melanocytes. Even at this power, the focal dermal invasion* ⇨ *is evident. However, MITF can falsely highlight dermal histiocytes or multinucleated giant cells, especially in scars.* **(Right)** *The junctional* ⇨ *and pagetoid* ➡ *melanocytes are highlighted. There are a few cells* ➡ *invading the papillary dermis. MITF typically has a cytoplasmic blush, but the most intense staining is found in the nuclei of the melanocytes.*

KEY FACTS

TERMINOLOGY

- Histologically diverse group of melanocytic tumors
- Malignant cutaneous melanocytic neoplasm arising in children

ETIOLOGY/PATHOGENESIS

- Classified according to mode of occurrence and histology

CLINICAL ISSUES

- Knowledge of clinical dimensions is of maximum importance
  - Ensure viewing of entire lesion before making benign diagnosis
  - Can be difficult, especially in cases of giant congenital melanocytic nevus (CMN)
- Accounts for 1-3% of all childhood malignancies
- Slight female predominance
- 50% arise in association with preexisting lesion
- 50% arise de novo

MICROSCOPIC

- Lack of circumscription
  - One of most powerful criteria for diagnosing melanoma
- Consumption of overlying epidermis
- Pagetoid spread of melanocytes
- Lack of maturation with increasing dermal depth
- Deep dermal mitoses
- Pigment present deep in lesion
- Absence of Kamino bodies
- Melanomas arising in giant CMN
- Inflammatory infiltrate can be helpful, especially if asymmetrical
- High nuclear:cytoplasmic ratio
- Prominent nucleoli, often appear cherry red

ANCILLARY TESTS

- FISH assays targeting most common chromosomal aberrations can be helpful
- Spitz nevi tend to demonstrate isolated gains of 11p

Nodular Melanoma

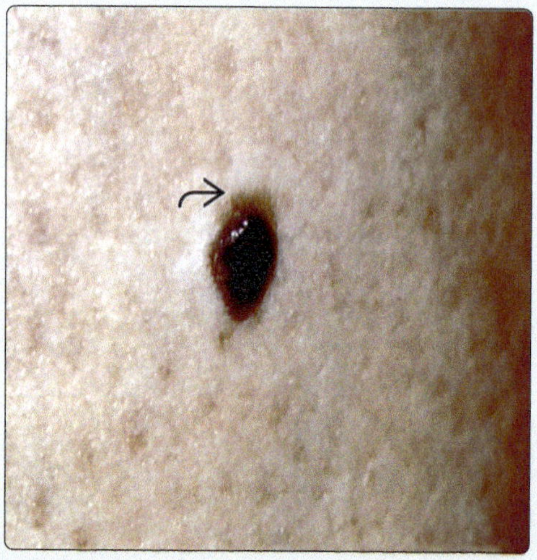

Nodular Melanoma Mimicking Nevus

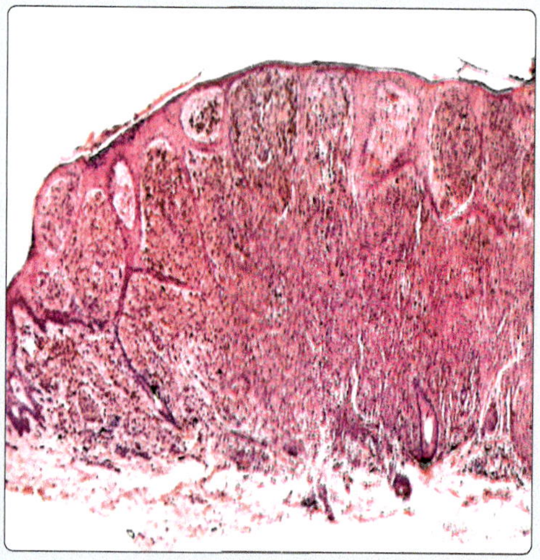

(Left) *This nodular melanoma presents as a dark brown asymmetric nodule with leakage of melanin around the edge of the lesion.* **(Right)** *A nevoid melanoma arising in a 4-year-old child is shown. The lesion is centrally hypercellular and does not appear to properly mature with increasing dermal depth. There were deep atypical melanocytes and mitoses present on high power.*

Multiple Mitotic Figures

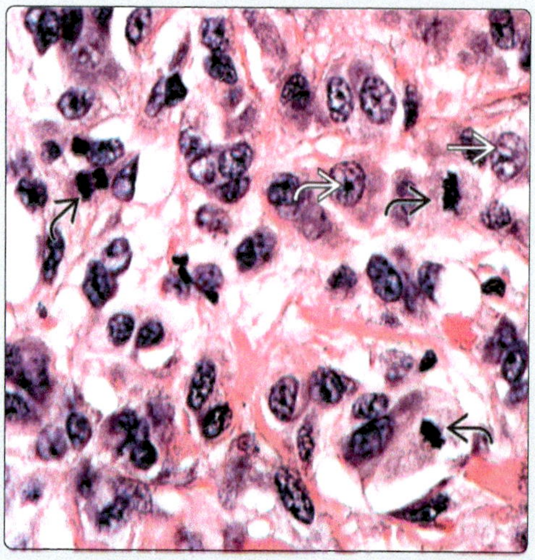

Ulcerated Melanoma

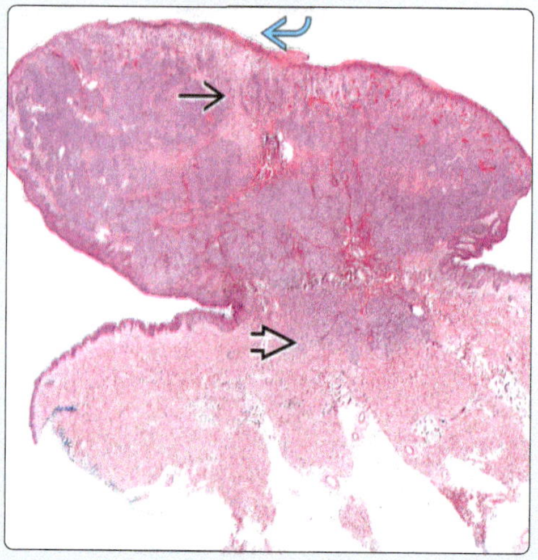

(Left) *High magnification of a melanoma arising in a 4-year-old child shows an area with prominent cytologic atypia and multiple mitotic figures. The melanoma cells have large nuclei with open chromatin and macronucleoli.* **(Right)** *At scanning magnification, this ulcerated polypoid, pedunculated melanocytic proliferation appears malignant even in a child. Note failure to mature with increasing dermal depth from the ulcer bed to the lower end of reticular dermis.*

TERMINOLOGY

Abbreviations

- Malignant melanoma (MM)

Synonyms

- Melanoma of childhood

Definitions

- Histologically diverse group of melanocytic tumors
- Malignant cutaneous melanocytic neoplasm arising in children

ETIOLOGY/PATHOGENESIS

Classification of Pediatric Melanoma

- Classified according to mode of occurrence and histology
  - Transformation from giant congenital melanocytic nevus (CMN)
  - In association with congenital predisposing conditions
  - Development from preexisting nevus
  - Transplacental melanoma

CLINICAL ISSUES

Epidemiology

- Incidence
  - Accounts for 1-3% of all childhood malignancies
  - Accounts for < 0.5% of all melanomas
  - 7x more frequent in 2nd decade than 1st decade of life
  - On rise in children and teenagers
- Age
  - Prepubescent melanoma
    - Congenital and infantile melanomas are rare
    - Develops transplacentally, de novo, or within CMN, especially giant congenital nevi
  - Postpubescent melanoma
    - > 14 years
    - Clinical features and prognosis tend to resemble adult counterparts
- Sex
  - Slight female predominance

Site

- Can occur anywhere on skin
  - Rarely mucous membranes and meninges

Presentation

- 50% arise in association with preexisting lesion
  - 30% arise within giant CMN (> 20 cm)
    - 50-70% before puberty
    - Tend to arise within dermis
    - Worse prognosis
  - 20% in association with other cutaneous nevi
    - Small to medium-sized CMNs
    - Acquired melanocytic nevi
    - More likely to occur after puberty
- 50% arise de novo
- May arise within neurocutaneous melanosis
  - Rare but carries high risk of malignant transformation in children
  - Median age: 3 years
  - Up to 2/3 of patients may develop primary intracranial melanomas
- Signs and symptoms may include
  - Rapid increase in size of lesion, hemorrhage, ulceration, change in color, loss of previously regular borders, pruritus, lymphadenopathy
- Important clinical signs ("ABCD" criteria)
  - **A**symmetry
  - **B**order irregularity
  - **C**olor/pigmentation irregularities
  - **D**iameter of 6 mm or greater
- **Risk factors**
  - Fair skin
  - Giant CMN (bathing trunk nevus)
    - Risk correlates with size, depth, and number of nevomelanocytes
    - Occurs in 1 in 20,000 newborns
    - ≥ 20 cm in largest diameter
    - Up to 5-7% risk of malignant transformation
  - Dysplastic nevus syndrome
  - Numerous acquired melanocytic nevi
    - Independent risk factor
  - Sporadic atypical nevi
    - Independent risk factor
  - Xeroderma pigmentosum
  - Albinism
  - Immunosuppression
  - Family history of melanoma (familial melanoma)
    - Occur at younger age
    - Often multifocal
    - Germline mutations of *CDKN2A* tumor suppressor gene

Treatment

- Options, risks, complications
  - Surgical resection with standard margins
    - Treatment of choice for primary disease
    - Potentially curative
    - May also include sentinel lymph node biopsy or regional lymphadenectomy
    - Both NCCN and AAD publish online guidelines for surgical margins
  - Chemotherapy of minimal benefit
  - Experimental immunotherapy of unproven benefit
  - Treatment protocols based on adult population

Prognosis

- Most important prognostic factors
  - Depth of invasion
    - Most accurately measured by Breslow thickness
    - Clark level is of questionable significance
  - Stage at diagnosis
    - Stage IV 5-year survival rate (34%)
    - Stage I-II 5-year survival rate (90%)
- Other poor prognostic indicators
  - Previous nonmelanocytic malignancies, nodular type, fusiform cytology, vertical growth phase
  - High dermal mitotic activity, ulceration, vascular invasion, age > 10 years, and presence of metastases at diagnosis
  - Presence of ulceration upstages tumor (e.g., T2a to T2b)

- Overall 5-year survival ~ 79%
- Survival characteristics similar to adult population

MACROSCOPIC

Size

- Usually > 7 mm

MICROSCOPIC

Histologic Features

- May or may not have ulceration
- Consumption of overlying epidermis
  - Especially helpful in resolving Spitz nevus vs. spitzoid melanoma differential diagnosis
  - Defined as thinning of epidermis with attenuation of basal and suprabasal layers
    - Rete ridges are lost in areas of direct contact with neoplastic melanocytes
- Asymmetry
  - One of most powerful histologic criteria
  - Nests showing
    - Variability in size and shape
    - Haphazard interval and array
  - Haphazard arrangement of solitary epidermal melanocytes
- Poor circumscription
  - Lesion does not start or end in nests
  - Difficult to discern where lesion begins and ends
  - Single melanocytes predominate at edge of lesion
- Pagetoid spread of melanocytes
  - Ascent of single melanocytes above dermoepidermal junction
  - Can also be present in Spitz nevi (sometimes full nests) and acral nevi
  - Should not be at periphery of Spitz or acral nevi
- Lack of maturation with increasing dermal depth
  - Deeper melanocytes as large as superficial ones
- Deep dermal mitoses
- Pigment present deep in lesion
- Atypical melanocytes
  - Atypical features not always present
  - May have marked nuclear pleomorphism
  - Melanocytes may be small and spindled or epithelioid
- Confluence of melanocytes
- Absence of Kamino bodies
- Melanomas arising in giant CMN
  - When arising in type 1 CMN, usually arises at dermal-epidermal junction
  - When arising in type 2 CMN, usually arises in dermal component
- Inflammatory infiltrate can be helpful, especially if asymmetrical
  - Often seen surrounding invasive component

Cytologic Features

- High nuclear:cytoplasmic ratio
- Prominent nucleoli, often appear cherry red
- Marked nuclear pleomorphism
- Hyperchromasia
- Dusty melanin

Histologic Subtypes

- **Superficial spreading melanoma**
  - Most common subtype
  - Found on nonsun-exposed skin
  - Characteristic radial (lateral) growth phase
  - Asymmetrical proliferation of atypical epithelioid-appearing melanocytes
    - Cells often have abundant cytoplasm, fine melanin pigmentation, pleomorphic vesicular nuclei, prominent cherry-red nucleoli, and scattered mitotic figures
  - Pagetoid spread of single melanocytes common
  - Epidermal acanthosis with effacement of rete ridges
  - FISH and comparative genomic hybridization (CGH) studies less sensitive
- **Acral lentiginous melanoma**
  - Found on palms and soles
  - More common in Asian and black populations
  - Acanthosis and elongation of epidermal ridges infiltrated by atypical melanocytes
    - Often pleomorphism, hyperchromasia, conspicuous nucleoli, and mitoses
    - Fixation retraction artifact
  - Scattered foci of junctional nests
  - Lichenoid chronic inflammatory infiltrate
  - Includes subungual melanomas
    - Most often affect large toe
  - FISH and CGH studies more sensitive
- **Nodular melanoma**
  - Large nodules of oval to round epithelioid melanocytes
  - May be symmetrical in all directions
  - Lacks intraepidermal melanocytic proliferation
  - FISH and CGH studies more sensitive
- **Spindle cell melanoma**
  - Spindled cytology
  - S100 and SOX10 only reliable immunostains
    - Often HMB-45 and MART-1/Melan-A (-)
- Other rare melanoma variants
  - Spitzoid, amelanotic, balloon cell, pedunculated, nevoid, small cell, and myxoid

ANCILLARY TESTS

Immunohistochemistry

- S100(+); considered most sensitive marker
- HMB-45 and MART-1/Melan-A (+); more specific but less sensitive than S100
- Usually MITF, SOX10, KBA62, and tyrosinase (+)

In Situ Hybridization

- FISH assays targeting most common chromosomal aberrations can be helpful
  - Probes vary from institution to institution, but 6p25, 6q23, Cep6, and 11q13 are often used

Array Comparative Genomic Hybridization

- Can be very helpful adjunctive test, especially for most difficult cases
- Most benign nevi show no chromosomal aberrations
- Spitz nevi tend to demonstrate isolated gains of 11p
- > 96% of MMs demonstrate chromosomal aberrations

- Most common are gains of chromosome 1q, 6p, 7p, 7q, 8q, 17q, and 20q or losses of 6q, 9p, 9q, 10q, 10p, and 11q
- Benign proliferations in CMNs can show chromosomal aberrations
  - These differ from aberrations found in melanomas arising in CMNs, which are similar to melanomas arising de novo

DIFFERENTIAL DIAGNOSIS

Spitz Nevus

- Preferentially involves head and neck of children
- Usually < 1 cm in diameter
- Characterized by large spindled &/or epithelioid cells
- Features that support diagnosis of Spitz nevus
  - Symmetry, maturation with depth, wedge-shaped silhouette
  - Melanocytic nests clutched by rete ridges or showing pagetoid spread
  - Clefts around nests
  - Kamino bodies
    - Dull, pink globules often situated above tips of dermal papillae
    - No published case reports of well-formed Kamino bodies in melanoma proven by metastatic spread

Melanocytic Nevus

- Symmetrical and well-circumscribed nests of melanocytes
- Typically lacks cytologic atypia and pagetoid spread
  - Pagetoid spread can be seen in middle of Spitz, acral, and irritated/traumatized nevi
- Melanocytes mature with depth
- Lacks deep mitoses
- Usually lacks lymphocytes
  - Exceptions include irritated nevi, Spitz nevi, halo nevi, and dysplastic nevi

Atypical (Dysplastic) Nevus

- Pigmented papules, macules, and plaques
- Clinical features may resemble melanoma
- Diagnostic features
  - Lateral dislocation of nests
  - Shouldering of nests
    - Nests extend at least 3 rete ridges beyond dermal component (architectural atypia)
  - Melanocytes display hyperchromatic, pleomorphic nuclei (cytological atypia)

Benign Proliferative Nodule in Giant Congenital Melanocytic Nevi

- Area of higher cell density and nuclear enlargement with higher mitotic activity in CMN
- Can also be hamartoma arising in giant CMN
  - Nonmelanocytic cells, such as smooth muscle, nerve, or sebaceous cells, normally also present
- Typically become softer in time, stop growing, and subsequently become smaller or regress completely

STAGING

AJCC

- Staging does not differ from that for adults
- **Breslow thickness**
  - Measurement in mm from top of granular layer to deepest point of invasion
  - Extension along adnexal structures is not measured
  - Considered most important prognostic indicator and more accurate than Clark levels
- Ulceration and mitotic figures may increase stage and result in T1 tumors
  - Presence will change stage from T1a to T1b
    - Sentinel lymph node examination may be performed

REPORTING

Misdiagnosis

- Commonly occurs
- Up to 40% of pediatric melanomas initially misdiagnosed as benign
- Up to 60% of patients < 20 years experience delay in treatment

Points of Diagnostic Confusion

- Similar histologic presentations as Spitz nevi
- Atypia in proliferative nodules of giant CMN

Uncertainty

- Is not uncommon in these difficult lesions and challenging patient population
- Consultation encouraged of any markedly atypical/highly suspicious lesion
  - Expert review of cases often needed and improves patient care
- Often only true measure of malignancy in pediatric population is death or distant metastasis

SELECTED REFERENCES

1. Gerami P et al: Histomorphologic assessment and interobserver diagnostic reproducibility of atypical spitzoid melanocytic neoplasms with long-term follow-up. Am J Surg Pathol. 38(7):934-40, 2014
2. Bangash HK et al: What's new in prognostication of melanoma in the dermatopathology laboratory? Clin Dermatol. 31(3):317-23, 2013
3. Kozubek J et al: In-depth characterization of microRNA transcriptome in melanoma. PLoS One. 8(9):e72699, 2013
4. Dadras SS: Molecular diagnostics in melanoma: current status and perspectives. Arch Pathol Lab Med. 135(7):860-9, 2011
5. Berk DR et al: Melanoma and melanocytic tumors of uncertain malignant potential in children, adolescents and young adults-the Stanford experience 1995-2008. Pediatr Dermatol. 27(3):244-54, 2010
6. Ducharme EE et al: Pediatric malignant melanoma: an update on epidemiology, detection, and prevention. Cutis. 84(4):192-8, 2009
7. Jen M et al: Childhood melanoma. Clin Dermatol. 27(6):529-36, 2009
8. Ma Z et al: Profiling and discovery of novel miRNAs from formalin-fixed, paraffin-embedded melanoma and nodal specimens. J Mol Diagn. 11(5):420-9, 2009
9. Downard CD et al: Melanoma in children and adolescents. Surg Oncol. 16(3):215-20, 2007
10. Krengel S et al: Melanoma risk in congenital melanocytic naevi: a systematic review. Br J Dermatol. 155(1):1-8, 2006
11. Ferrari A et al: Does melanoma behave differently in younger children than in adults? A retrospective study of 33 cases of childhood melanoma from a single institution. Pediatrics. 115(3):649-54, 2005
12. Hantschke M et al: Consumption of the epidermis: a diagnostic criterion for the differential diagnosis of melanoma and Spitz nevus. Am J Surg Pathol. 28(12):1621-5, 2004
13. Saenz NC et al: Childhood melanoma survival. Cancer. 85(3):750-4, 1999

Melanoma With Nodular Growth Pattern

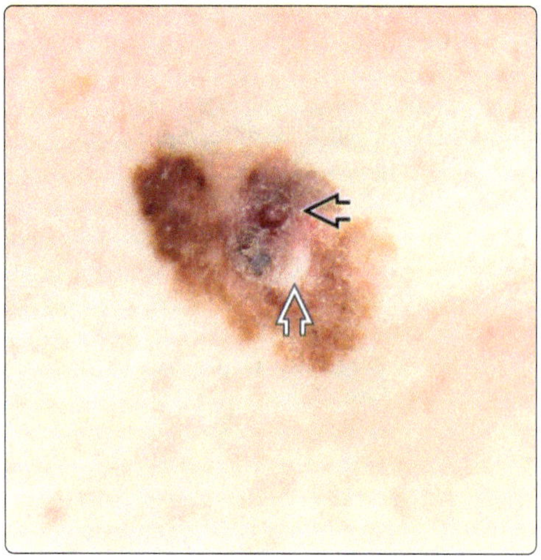

Melanoma With Pagetoid Spread of Melanocytes

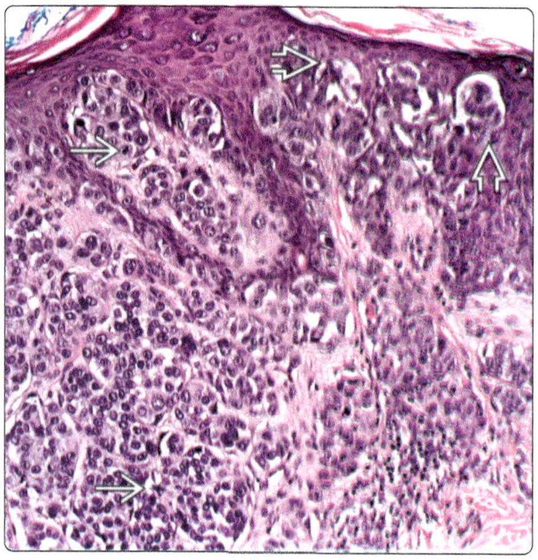

(Left) *Clinical photograph shows a large melanoma with variegated color, jagged border, and irregular surface, all of which are concerning clinical signs. Note the papular growth within the patch and central scar (regression).* **(Right)** *This image shows melanoma from the back of a 16-year-old girl. The lesion is composed of atypical epithelioid cells with several mitotic figures, and there are atypical cells advancing up through the epidermis (pagetoid spread). (Courtesy C. Cockerell, MD.)*

Melanoma on Face of Child

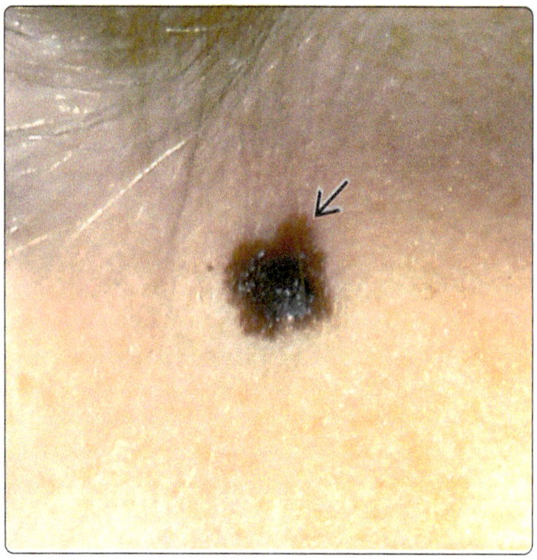

Pagetoid Spread in Melanoma, Superficial Spreading Type

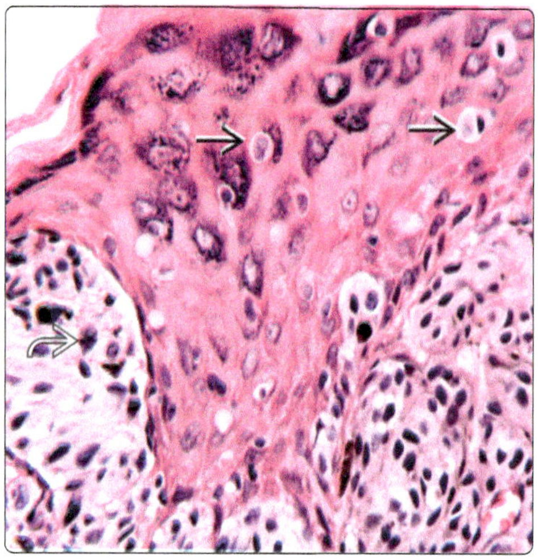

(Left) *This preauricular, superficial spreading melanoma is larger than 6 mm in diameter with an irregular border, asymmetry, and pseudopod of different color on the superior edge.* **(Right)** *Superficial spreading melanoma shows prominent pagetoid spread and obvious atypia with nuclear hyperchromasia, pleomorphism, and cytologic atypia. An atypical mitosis is also present.*

Nodular Melanoma, Evenly Pigmented

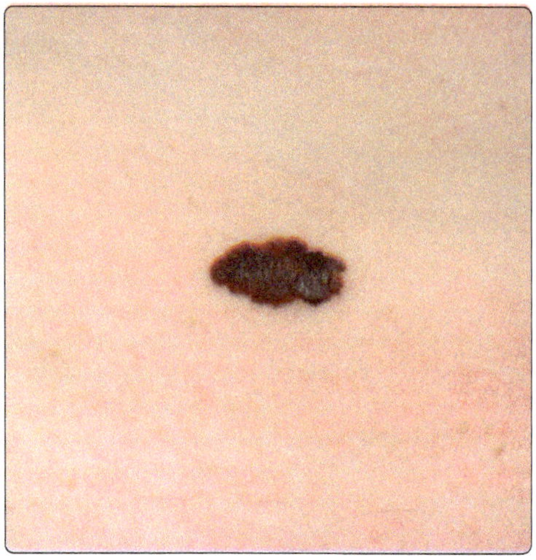

Melanoma With Lack of Maturation With Increasing Dermal Depth

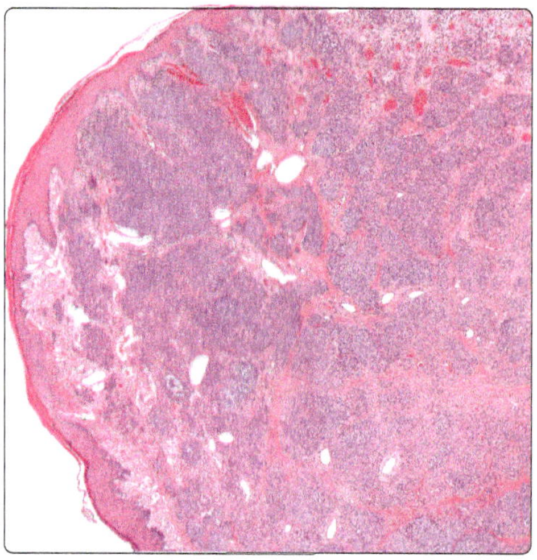

(Left) *This lesion appears deceptively benign by mimicking a seborrheic keratosis. Note the asymmetry and irregular borders. (Courtesy J. Wu, MD.)* **(Right)** *In nodular melanoma, these are usually sharply circumscribed edges containing nests of oval to round, atypical, epithelioid melanocytes growing throughout the dermis. Lack of maturation (uniform cells throughout) and large irregular nests are other helpful features. (Courtesy G. Fraga, MD.)*

Asymmetric, Atypical Melanocytic Neoplasm, Extending Into Subcutaneous Adipose Tissue

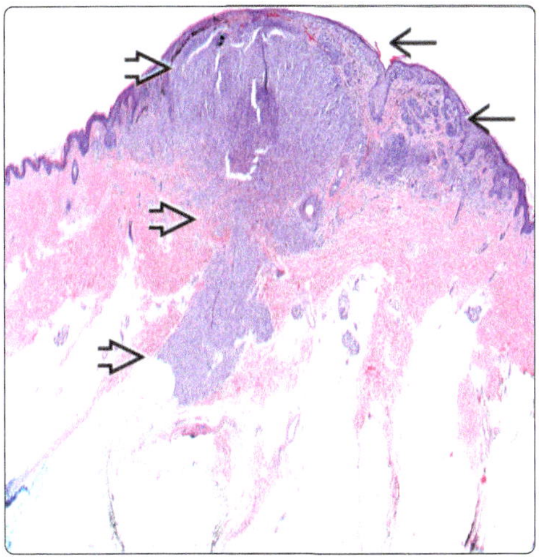

Extensive Pagetoid Scatter

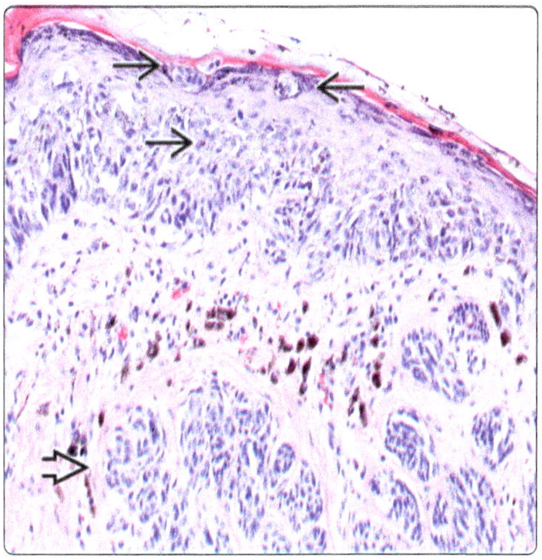

(Left) *This lesion from the trunk of an 11-year-old child mimics a deep penetrating nevus to the left ⇨ and a compound proliferation to the right →. This type of asymmetry at scanning magnification is an atypical feature.* **(Right)** *The same lesion at the right corner is shown at a higher magnification to reveal an extensive pagetoid upward scatter of melanocytes →. Note the dermal component underneath ⇨, which fails to mature with increasing dermal depth. The cytology is epithelioid and spindled.*

Deep Extension Into Subcutis

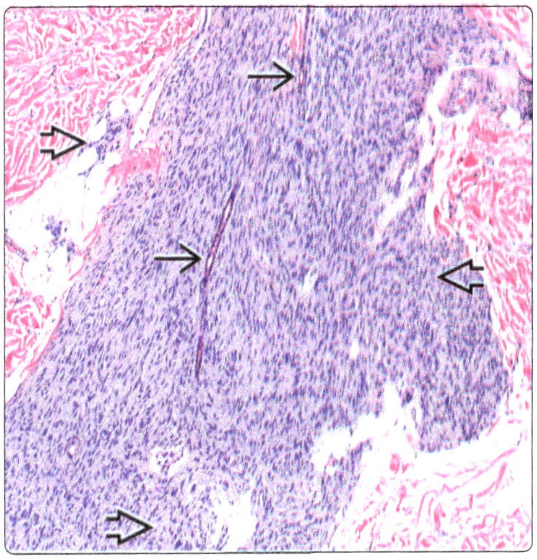

Spindled, Sheet-Like Growth Pattern

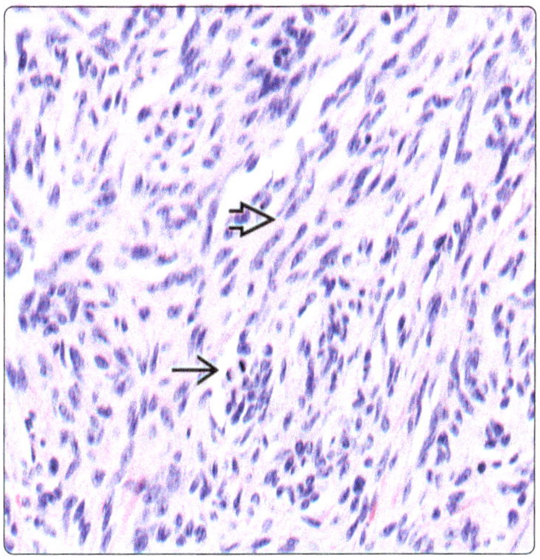

(Left) *A sheet-like melanocytic proliferation ⇨ extends into the subcutaneous adipose tissue. There is no maturation with increasing dermal depth. The eccrine ducts → are left intact.* **(Right)** *Pseudosarcomatous appearance ⇨ is displayed of the sheet-like growth. Note that the cytoplasmic borders are indistinct, showing a syncytial pattern. A mitotic figure → is identified.*

Mitotic Figure, Deep Within Lesion

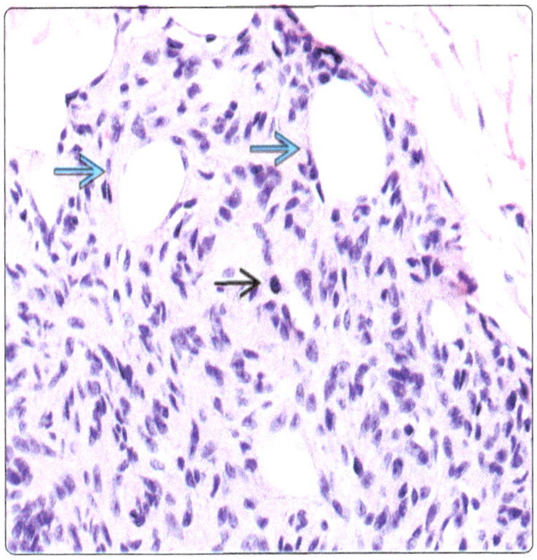

High Proliferation Index by Ki-67 IHC

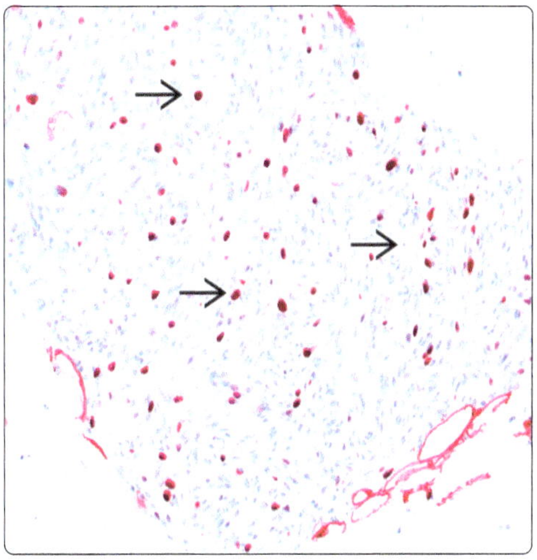

(Left) *Another normal-appearing mitotic figure → is identified deep within the neoplasm. Adipose tissue ⇨ is surrounded by the tumor. The nuclei are plump, spindled with vesicular nuclei and prominent nucleoli.* **(Right)** *Ki-67 or MIB-1 (red nuclei) → can be helpful in demonstrating the labeling index of proliferation. It is defined by the percentage of positive cells, indicative of cycling cells. The labeling index > 15% can be a feature of malignancy, confirming the deeply situated mitotic figures found by histology.*

(Left) *This nodular lesion appeared on the thigh of a 5-year-old child. Although somewhat symmetrical, it does not appear to mature with increasing dermal depth. The tumor cells extend to the deep inked tissue margin.* **(Right)** *Under medium-power magnification, there is no pagetoid spread in the epidermis. However, the lesion is focally inflamed. There are sheets of epithelioid cells, a concerning feature.*

Highly Atypical Spitz Melanocytic Tumor

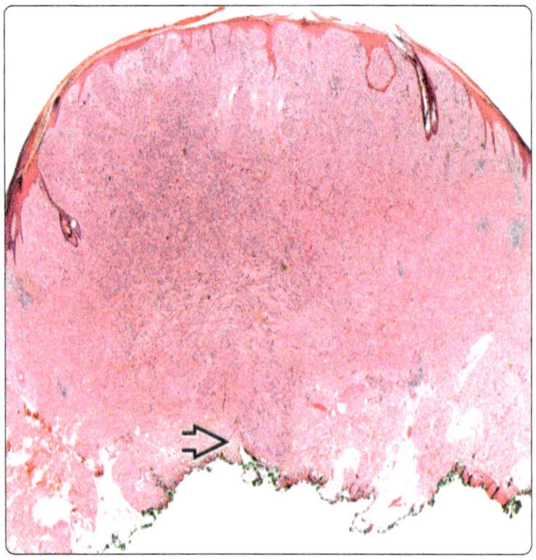

Atypical Spitz Tumor

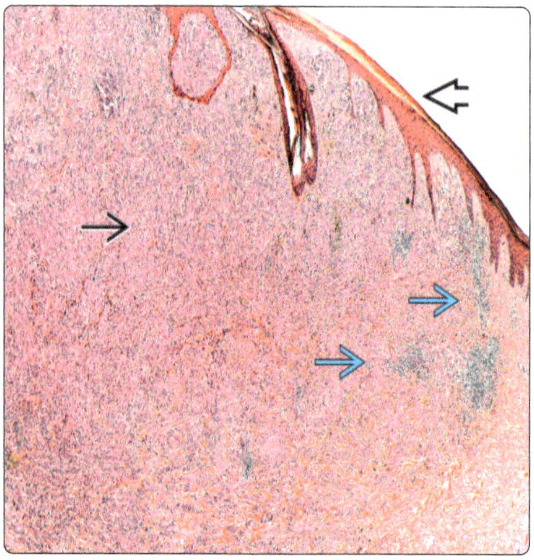

(Left) *At high-power magnification, the large epithelioid cells are destroying the remaining portion of pilar muscle.* **(Right)** *At the advancing front of the same lesion, there is perineural invasion. Although there is no significant mitotic activity, loss of cellular maturation combined with perineural invasion are highly suspicious for malignancy.*

Consumption of Pilar Muscle

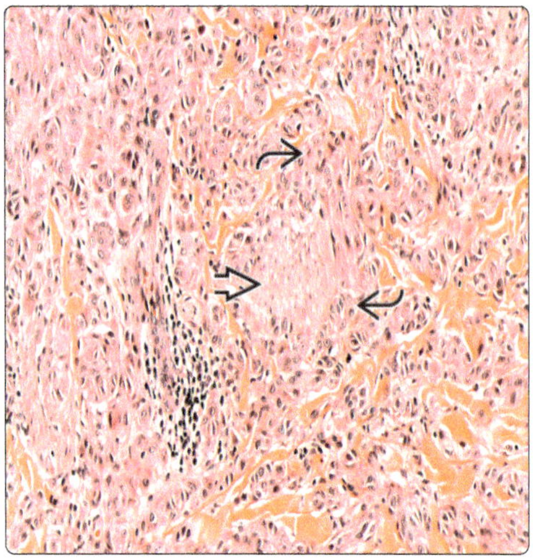

Perineural Invasion

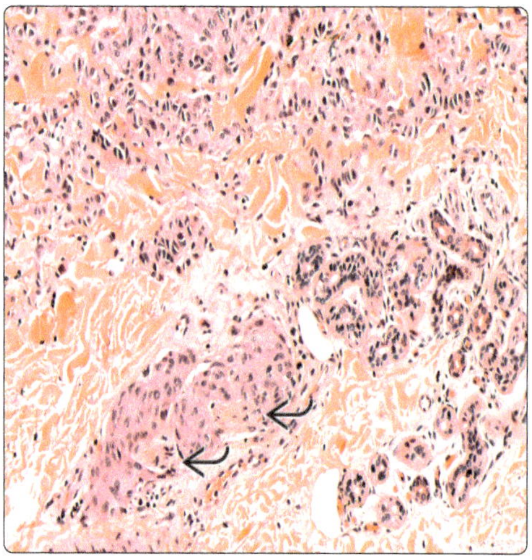

(Left) *This is a scanning magnification of a calf lesion excised from a 3-year-old child. Note the asymmetric proliferation to the right to be contrasted from more basophilic nodules and nests to the left. Note the focal melanin incontinence and extension into the subcutis.* **(Right)** *Higher power magnification of the right area shows large epithelioid nests with vesicular nuclei and prominent nucleoli. There is no maturation with increasing dermal depth. The mitotic index was 9/mm².*

Asymmetric Nodular Neoplasm

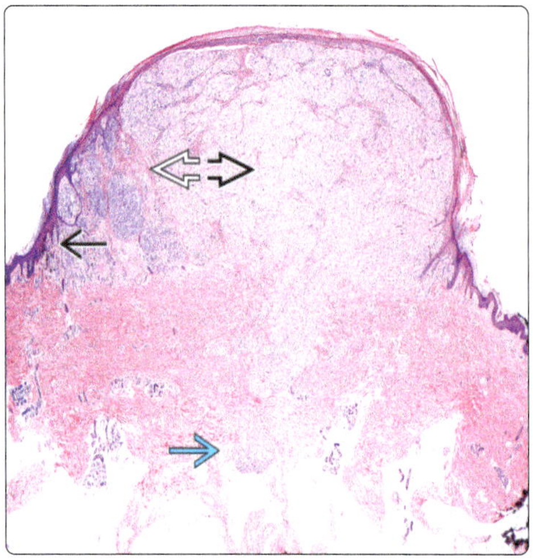

Lack of Maturation and Mitoses

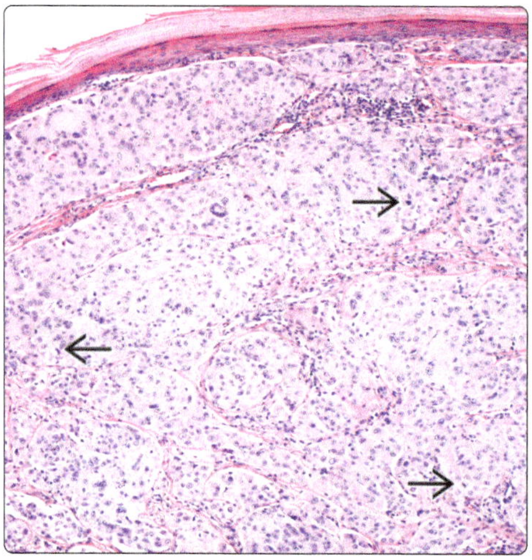

MicroRNA In Situ Hybridization for miR-211 (Red Nuclei)

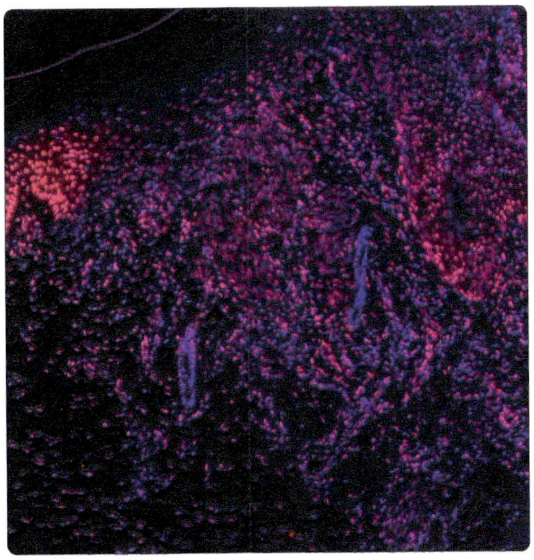

MicroRNA In Situ Hybridization for miR-211

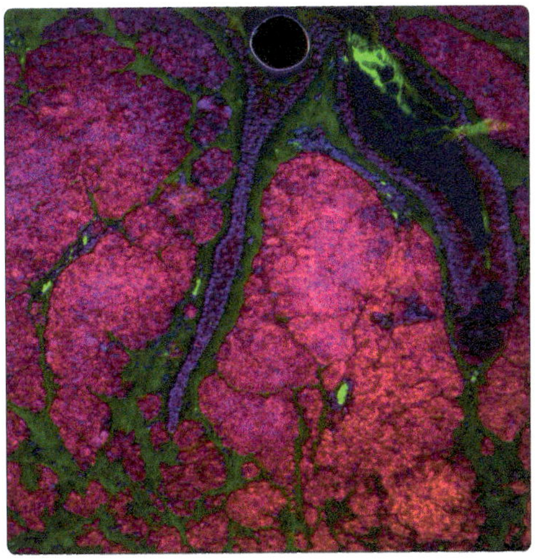

(Left) *In-depth characterization of miRNA transcriptome studies have shown that melanocytic nevi express miR-211, which is lost in melanoma. The previous lesion in a 3 year old highly expressed miR-211, suggesting a benign outcome. After 5 years of follow-up, the child remains metastasis-free, and PET scans have been negative.* **(Right)** *A melanocytic nevus expresses high levels of miR-211 (red). The expression is diffuse and uniform. The green channel shows formalin-induced fluorescence in the reticular collagen.*

Giant Congenital Melanocytic Nevus

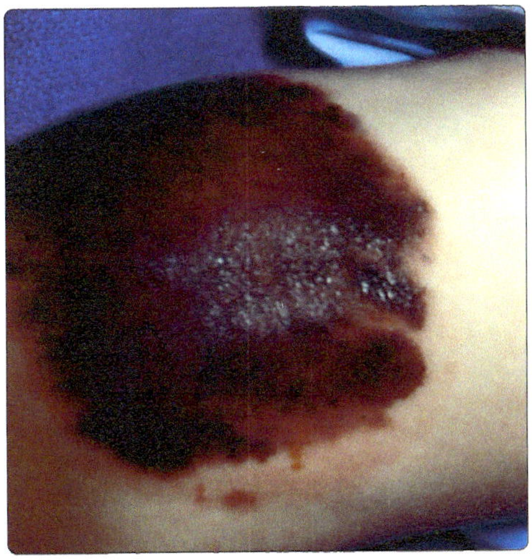

Melanoma Arising in Giant Congenital Melanocytic Nevus

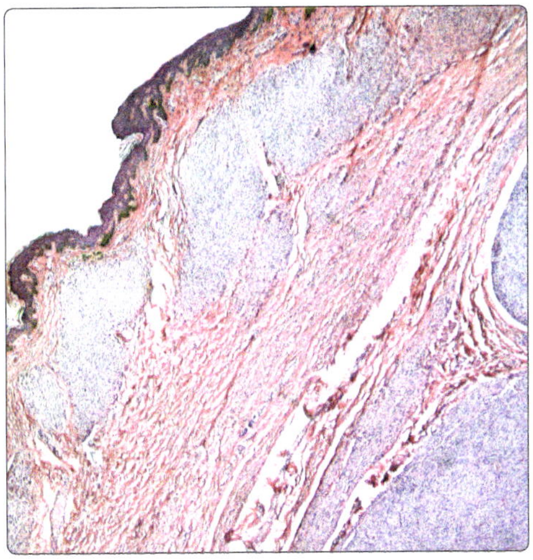

(Left) *This is a giant congenital pigmented nevus on the lower back of a newborn. Unfortunately, a melanoma developed in this lesion that was ultimately fatal.* **(Right)** *Note the large dermal nests showing sheets or nodular proliferation in the background of a congenital nevus. This cellular nodule shows a high number of cells per unit area, a high mitotic index.*

Large Nodules and Sheeting of Melanocytes

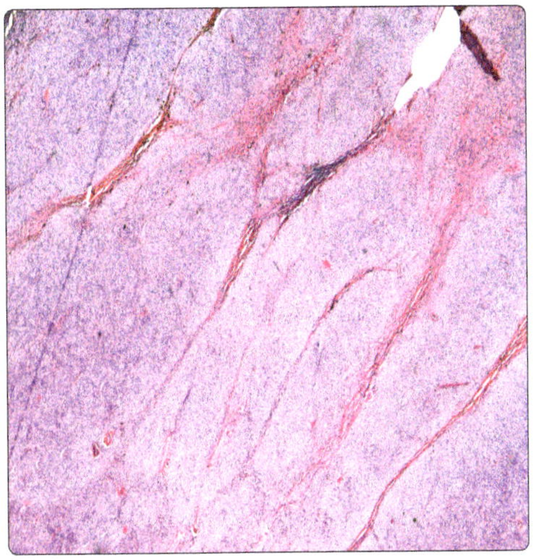

DDx: Compound Melanocytic Nevus

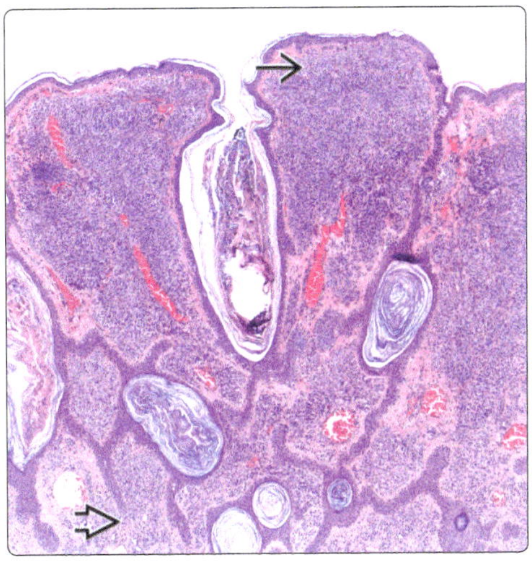

(Left) *One should examine the excision specimen of giant congenital nevi for areas of nodular proliferation, which may be indicative of malignant transformation.* **(Right)** *This is a compound nevus for comparison. Note how the lesion is symmetric and the melanocytes seem to "mature" as you move down the lesion from epidermis ➡ to the bottom of the lesion ⇨. (Courtesy UCSF Department of Dermatopathology.)*

Atypical/Borderline and Malignant Spitz Tumors

KEY FACTS

TERMINOLOGY

- Atypical Spitz tumor (AST)
- Spitz tumor of borderline/uncertain malignant potential
- Spitzoid melanoma

ETIOLOGY/PATHOGENESIS

- Typically occur in young patients without any known risk factors for melanoma

CLINICAL ISSUES

- Very rare tumors
- Mostly young patients; range: 2-30 years
- Prognosis difficult to predict
  - Most patients have good prognosis, with only minority of cases progressing to systemic disease or death

MICROSCOPIC

- **Severely atypical/borderline Spitz tumor**
  - Typically, large and deep cellular compound melanocytic tumors
  - May appear symmetric and well circumscribed at low power
  - Cells show severe cytologic atypia with nuclear hyperchromasia, enlarged nucleoli, irregular chromatin, and abundant amphophilic or dense eosinophilic cytoplasm
  - Mitotic figures often present, increased compared to conventional Spitz nevi
- **Spitzoid melanoma**
  - Also large and deep tumors
  - Frank atypia and pleomorphism present
  - Junctional component often shows irregular nesting, confluence, and prominent pagetoid upward scatter
  - Multiple mitotic figures usually present
  - Often atypical &/or deep

Clinical Photograph of Atypical Spitz Tumor

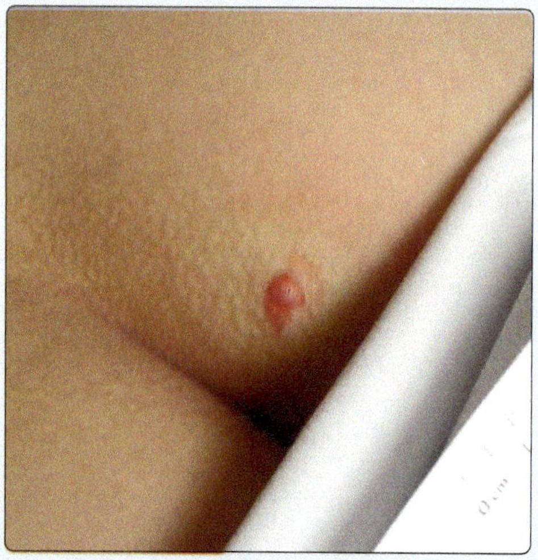

Severely Atypical Spitz Tumor

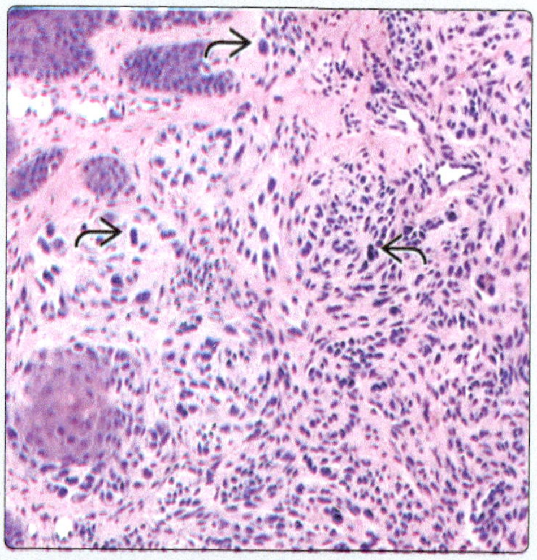

(Left) *This is an atypical compound Spitz tumor on the buttock of a 16-year-old patient. Despite the clinically banal appearance, there was severe cytologic atypia and multiple dermal mitotic figures identified, histologically.* **(Right)** *This severely atypical compound Spitz tumor shows a predominantly intradermal population of atypical spindled cells with nuclear enlargement, hyperchromasia, and focally prominent nucleoli.*

Spitzoid Melanoma

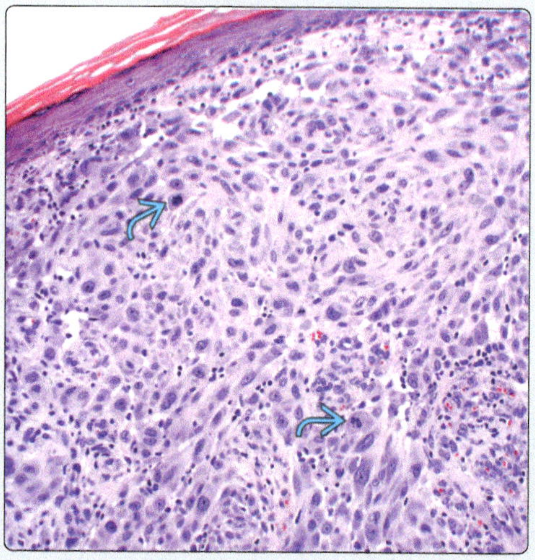

HMB-45 Immunohistochemistry in Spitzoid Melanoma

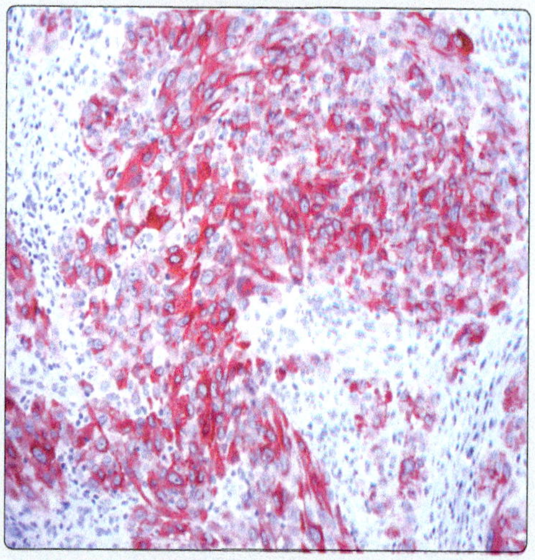

(Left) *This is an example of spitzoid melanoma in a young adult. The dermal cells are markedly enlarged, atypical, and pleomorphic appearing. In addition, there are multiple mitotic figures in this field.* **(Right)** *This spitzoid melanoma shows strong HMB-45 staining in the dermis. Although not always positive, strong dermal HMB-45 expression in an atypical melanocytic proliferation should raise suspicion for melanoma.*

TERMINOLOGY

Abbreviations

- Atypical Spitz tumor (AST)

Definitions

- Atypical/borderline Spitz tumor: Severely atypical melanocytic proliferation with features intermediate between Spitz nevus and spitzoid melanoma
- Malignant Spitz tumor: Malignant melanocytic proliferation with spitzoid features

ETIOLOGY/PATHOGENESIS

Unknown

- Typically occur in young patients without any known risk factors for melanoma

Possible Genetic Role

- Suggested by chromosome 11p amplification in minority of Spitz nevi
- Complex chromosomal alterations typically seen in melanoma

CLINICAL ISSUES

Epidemiology

- Incidence
  - Very rare tumors
- Age
  - Mostly young patients; range: 2-30 years
  - Malignant tumors more common in postpuberty

Presentation

- Dermal papule or nodule

Treatment

- Surgical approaches
  - Complete and wider excision is standard therapy
    - Typically ≥ 5-mm clinical margins for atypical/borderline tumors
    - Spitzoid melanomas should be treated with same margins as invasive melanomas of same Breslow depth
  - Sentinel lymph node biopsy remains controversial

Prognosis

- Difficult to predict
  - Most patients have relatively good prognosis, with only minority of cases progressing to metastasis and death

MICROSCOPIC

Histologic Features

- **Severely atypical/borderline Spitz tumor**
  - Typically, large and deep cellular compound tumor
  - May appear symmetric and well circumscribed
  - Composed of nests, fascicles, and often sheet-like collections of melanocytes
  - Junctional component is variable
    - May show irregular nesting, confluence, and areas of pagetoid upward scatter
  - Dermal melanocytes often do not show maturation with dermal descent (unlike most typical Spitz nevi)
  - Severe cytologic atypia with nuclear hyperchromasia, enlarged nucleoli, irregular chromatin, and abundant amphophilic or dense eosinophilic cytoplasm
  - Mitotic figures often present, increased compared to conventional Spitz nevi
    - Few deep &/or atypical mitoses may be seen
- **Spitzoid melanoma**
  - Also large and deep tumors
  - Frank atypia and pleomorphism present
  - Junctional component often shows irregular nesting, confluence, and prominent pagetoid upward scatter
  - Multiple mitotic figures usually present
    - More numerous than in AST
    - Often deep &/or atypical
  - Lymphovascular invasion may be present

ANCILLARY TESTS

Genetic Testing

- FISH: Typically negative in AST, positive in melanoma
- CGH: Complex alterations usually seen in melanoma

DIFFERENTIAL DIAGNOSIS

Spitz Nevus

- Typically smaller, more well-circumscribed and symmetric-appearing proliferation
- Lack of marked cytologic atypia and pleomorphism
- Mitotic figures may be present but are typically superficial and nonatypical appearing

Conventional Melanoma

- Less likely to be considered in differential diagnosis
- Usually shows mostly epithelioid cells, rather than mixture of spindled and epithelioid cells in AST
- Spindle cell-predominant lesions can be seen in lentigo maligna melanoma, acral lentiginous melanoma
- Lacks clefting artifact, epidermal hyperplasia, and Kamino bodies

DIAGNOSTIC CHECKLIST

Pathologic Interpretation Pearls

- Large lesion composed of nests, fascicles, and often sheet-like collections of atypical spindled and epithelioid melanocytes
- Mitotic figures often present, increased in numbers, and may be atypical (especially in spitzoid melanomas)

SELECTED REFERENCES

1. Dika E et al: Spitzoid tumors in children and adults: a comparative clinical, pathological, and cytogenetic analysis. Melanoma Res. 25(4):295-301, 2015
2. Moscarella E et al: Clinical and dermoscopic features of atypical Spitz tumors: a multicenter, retrospective, case-control study. J Am Acad Dermatol. 73(5):777-84, 2015
3. Cerroni L et al: Melanocytic tumors of uncertain malignant potential: results of a tutorial held at the XXIX Symposium of the International Society of Dermatopathology in Graz, October 2008. Am J Surg Pathol. 34(3):314-26, 2010
4. Ludgate MW et al: The atypical Spitz tumor of uncertain biologic potential: a series of 67 patients from a single institution. Cancer. 115(3):631-41, 2009
5. Murali R et al: Sentinel lymph node biopsy in histologically ambiguous melanocytic tumors with spitzoid features (so-called atypical spitzoid tumors). Ann Surg Oncol. 15(1):302-9, 2008

(Left) *This is an example of an atypical desmoplastic Spitz tumor, which shows a predominantly dermal distribution and associated dense stromal sclerosis. Even at this low magnification, scattered enlarged, pleomorphic, and hyperchromatic-staining nuclei are evident.* **(Right)** *High magnification of atypical desmoplastic Spitz tumor shows several enlarged, bizarre-appearing nuclei with multiple nucleoli.*

Atypical Desmoplastic Spitz Tumor

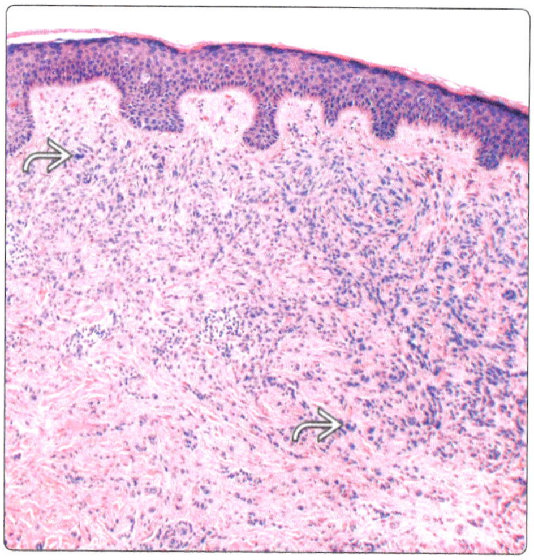

Atypical Desmoplastic Spitz Tumor at High Magnification

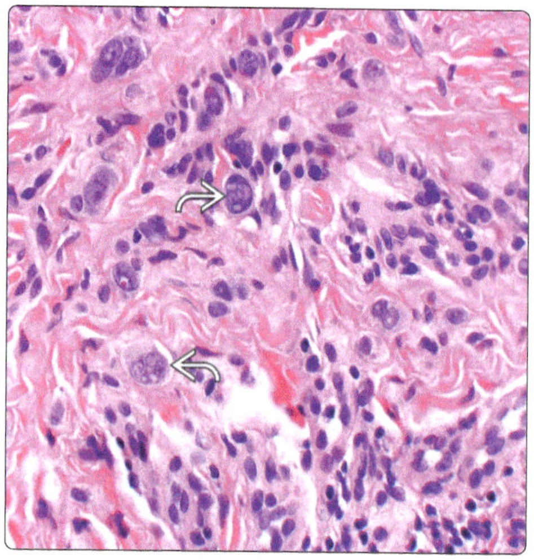

(Left) *This is an example of a severely atypical compound Spitz tumor, with the intradermal component composed mostly of atypical epithelioid cells with cytoplasmic pigmentation (which is unusual in conventional Spitz nevi). Note the presence of several mitotic figures.* **(Right)** *Higher magnification of a severely atypical Spitz tumor shows the intradermal component composed of atypical epithelioid cells with cytoplasmic pigmentation. Note the presence of mitotic figures.*

Severely Atypical Spitz Tumor

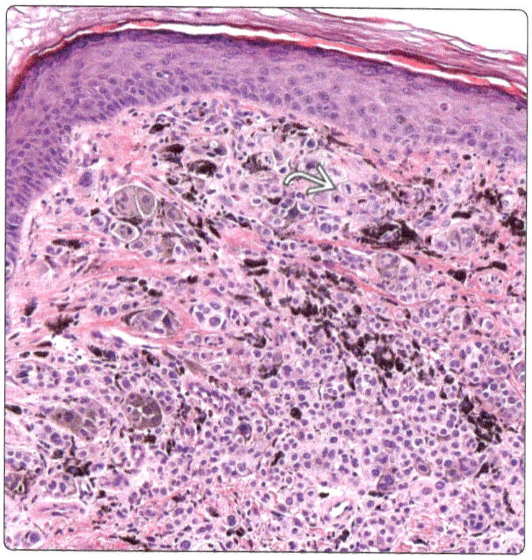

Severely Atypical Spitz Tumor at Higher Magnification

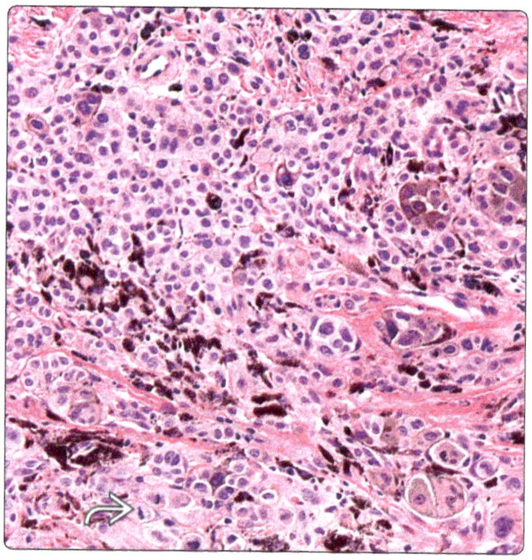

(Left) *This severely atypical Spitz tumor shows partial loss of p16 expression, with only scattered cells staining. Although most nevi show p16 staining, and most melanomas lose expression, this marker may or may not be useful, as not all melanoma cases are negative.* **(Right)** *Ki-67 often shows an elevated proliferative rate in atypical and malignant Spitz tumors. This case shows scattered enlarged dermal nuclei staining, although the overall rate is relatively low.*

Immunohistochemistry for p16 in Atypical Spitz Tumor

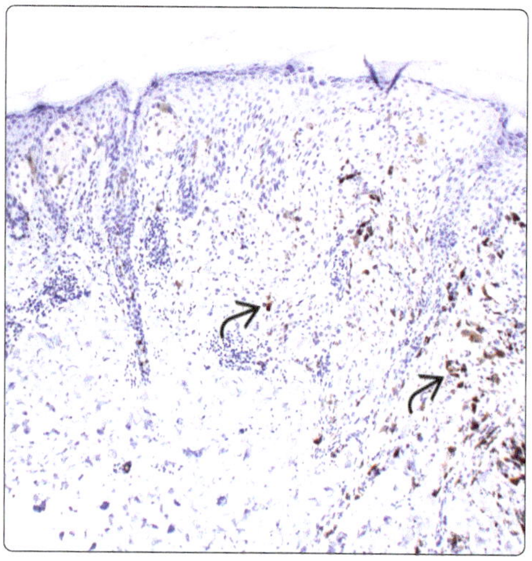

Ki-67 Immunohistochemistry in Atypical Spitz Tumor

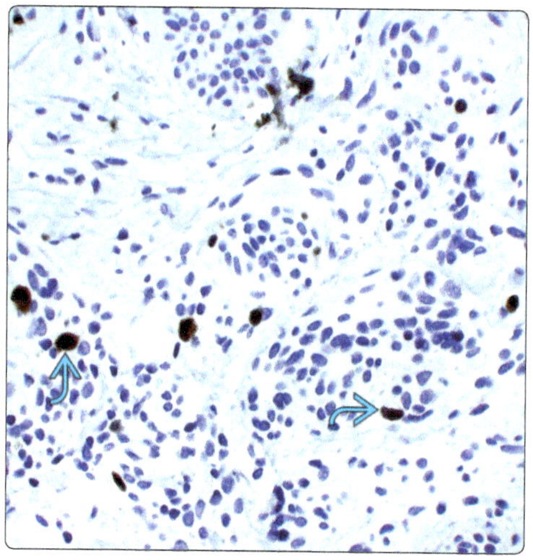

Spitzoid Melanoma With Atypical Mitosis

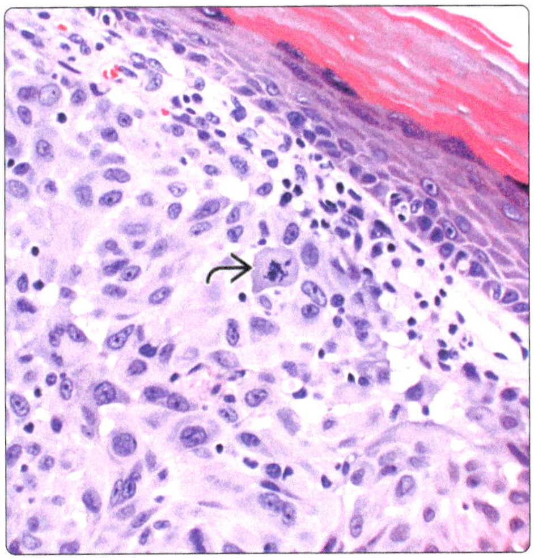

Melan-A Stain Highlights Superficial Lymphatic Invasion

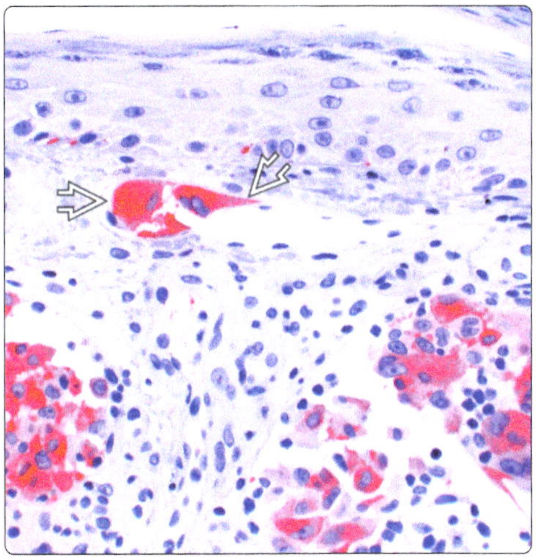

(Left) *This is a high-magnification view of a spitzoid melanoma involving the dermis that shows severe cytologic atypia, marked pleomorphism, and an atypical mitotic figure .* **(Right)** *A Melan-A stain highlights a focus of superficial lymphatic invasion in the same case of spitzoid melanoma.*

Pagetoid Spread in Spitzoid Melanoma

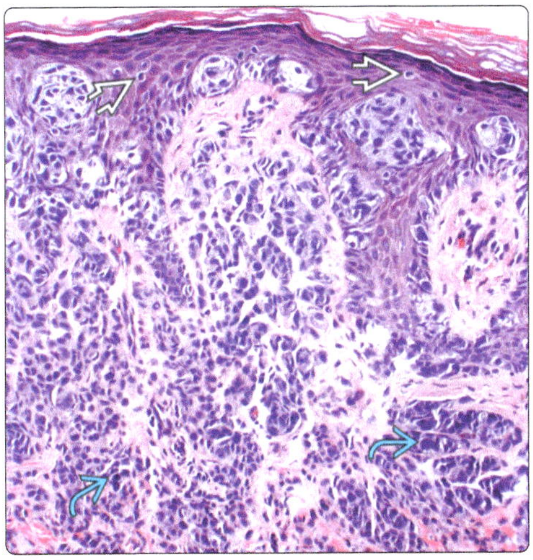

HMB-45 Stain in Spitzoid Melanoma

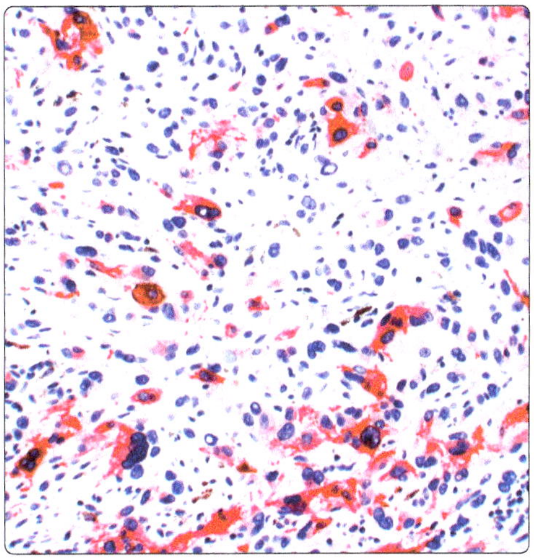

(Left) *This is another example of a spitzoid melanoma in a young adult patient. Multifocal pagetoid spread is identified . In addition, many atypical, hyperchromatic-staining nuclei are seen in the dermal component.* **(Right)** *HMB-45 in a spitzoid melanoma shows strong cytoplasmic staining of many of the enlarged, atypical-appearing epithelioid and spindled cells in the dermis.*

Spitzoid Melanoma Arising in Nevus

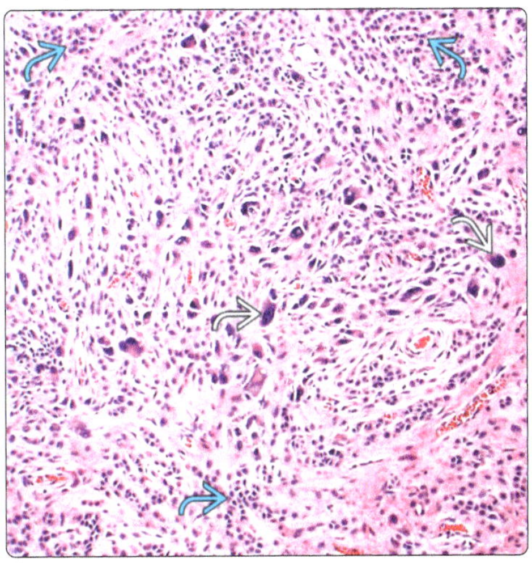

Loss of p16 in Spitzoid Melanoma

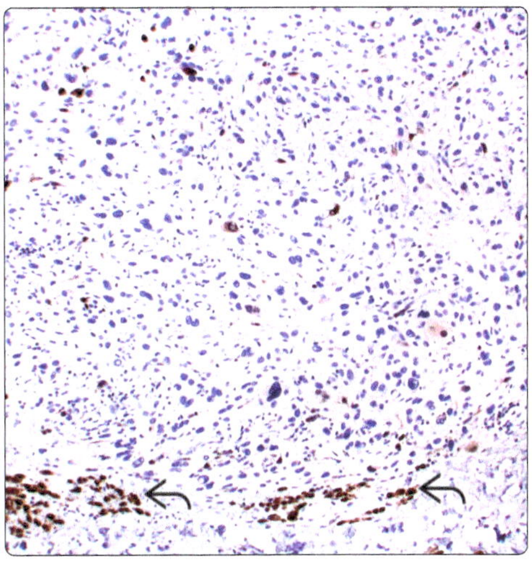

(Left) *This is a rare case of a spitzoid melanoma arising in a large congenital nevus in a child. Note the markedly atypical and bizarre-appearing spitzoid cells , surrounded by small, bland-appearing conventional nevus cells .* **(Right)** *Immunohistochemistry for p16 shows loss of expression in most of the cells in this case of spitzoid melanoma arising in a large congenital nevus. The surrounding benign nevus cells show strong nuclear and cytoplasmic staining .*

KEY FACTS

TERMINOLOGY

- Indolent melanoma subtype that typically evolves slowly
- a.k.a. invasive melanoma, lentigo maligna type

CLINICAL ISSUES

- Usually occurs on head and neck (sun-exposed regions) of elderly patients
- Broad patch with irregular, mottled pigmentation and irregular borders
- Slowly evolving, indolent but invasive type melanoma
- Surgical margins of at least 5 mm give cure rates of 90-95%

MICROSCOPIC

- Confluence of atypical melanocytes replacing basilar keratinocytes forming cleft
- Epidermal atrophy and loss of rete ridges
- Tumor cells extend along adnexal structures
- Invasion of dermis by atypical cells, usually in nests &/or fascicles
- Dermal component often shows spindle cell &/or desmoplastic melanoma features

ANCILLARY TESTS

- Positive for melanocytic immunohistochemical markers, especially SOX10 and S100
- Can be helpful in identifying focal microinvasion

TOP DIFFERENTIAL DIAGNOSES

- Reed (pigmented spindle cell) nevus
- Dysplastic compound melanocytic nevus
- Invasive melanoma, superficial spreading type

DIAGNOSTIC CHECKLIST

- Look for epidermal atrophy
- Confluent nesting along junction
- Adnexal extension
- Dermal invasion, often composed of spindled cells
  - May be difficult to identify, especially if desmoplastic type or heavily inflamed

Papular Growth in Pigmented Patch

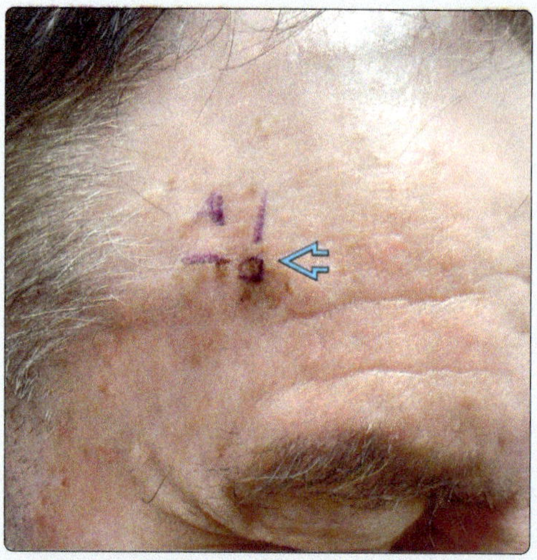

Darkly Pigmented Papule on Elderly Earlobe

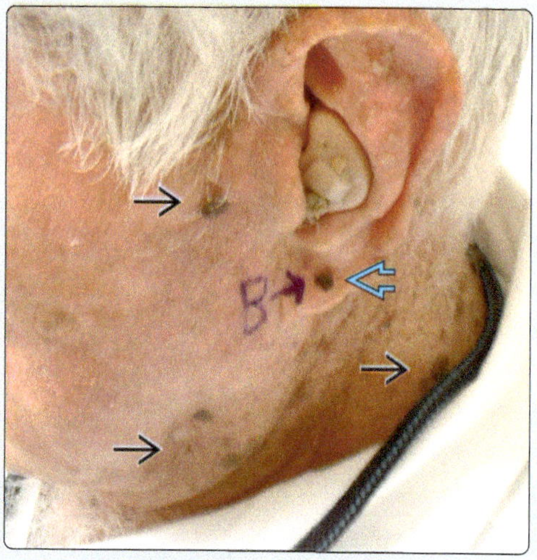

(Left) *The marked area ⊡, prior to biopsy, shows a papular growth in an ill-defined pigmented patch. This raises concern for a microinvasive melanoma. (Courtesy J. Finch, MD.)* **(Right)** *The marked lesion is concerning for melanoma ⊡. This lesion stands out among the many seborrheic keratoses ⊡ on the left face and neck. (Courtesy J. Finch, MD.)*

Atypical Pigmented Lesion With Inflammatory Regression of LMM

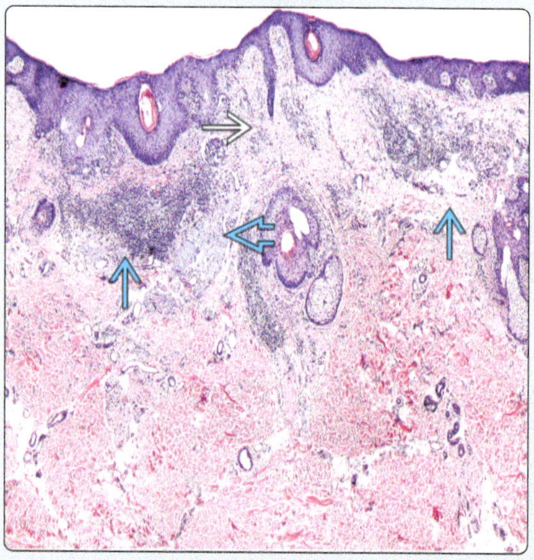

Microinvasive Nest of LMM

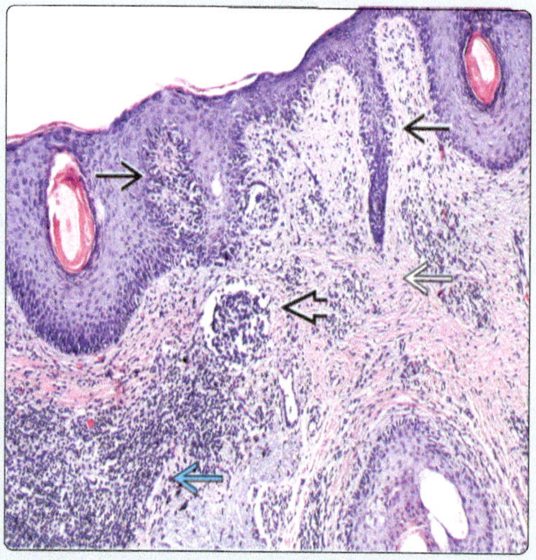

(Left) *This broad, atypical melanocytic proliferation displays fibrosis ⊡ and patchy, inflammatory infiltrate ⊡, consistent with inflammatory regression. Even the solar elastosis ⊡ is interrupted in the area of fibrosis.* **(Right)** *Above the lentiginous atypical, melanocytic proliferation ⊡, there is a prominent invasive nest ⊡ in the papillary dermis. Note the fibrosis (interrupted solar elastosis) ⊡ and inflammation ⊡.*

TERMINOLOGY

Abbreviations

- Lentigo maligna melanoma (LMM)

Synonyms

- Invasive melanoma, lentigo maligna type
- Hutchinson freckle (clinical term, which typically refers to melanoma in situ, lentigo maligna type)

Definitions

- Indolent melanoma subtype that evolves slowly and usually presents on head and neck (sun-exposed regions) in older patients

CLINICAL ISSUES

Epidemiology

- Age
  - Older patients, typically > 60 years old

Site

- Usually on head and neck (sun-exposed regions)

Presentation

- Broad patch with nodule, may grow 5-10 cm or larger
- Variegated colors
- Irregular borders

Natural History

- Slowly evolving, indolent but invasive type melanoma

Treatment

- Surgical approaches
  - Complete excision; margins depend on depth of invasion
  - Mohs surgery if poorly defined margins; recurrence rates of < 1%
- Drugs
  - Imiquimod cream is controversial but has shown promise for subset of patients
    - Long-term follow-up and several posttreatment biopsies are encouraged, even with lack of clinical recurrence

Prognosis

- Surgical margins of at least 5 mm give cure rates of 90-95%

MICROSCOPIC

Histologic Features

- Severely atypical compound melanocytic proliferation with junctional lentiginous component (typical of lentigo maligna)
  - Confluence of melanocytes replacing basilar keratinocytes, often forming cleft
  - Numerous solitary units and small nests of atypical cells along basilar layer
  - Extension of atypical melanocytes along adnexal structures
  - Epidermal atrophy and effacement of rete ridges
- Predominantly lymphocytic dermal infiltrate may obscure junctional component
- Invasion of dermis by atypical cells, usually in nests &/or fascicles
  - Dermal component often shows spindle cell &/or desmoplastic melanoma features
  - Often deeply invasive with no evidence of maturation
- Solar elastosis present, typically severe

Cytologic Features

- Cells are angulated and may be spindled
- Scant cytoplasm with only few, if any, melanin granules
- Nuclei are hyperchromatic and pleomorphic-appearing

ANCILLARY TESTS

Immunohistochemistry

- Positive for melanocytic immunohistochemical markers, especially SOX10 and S100
  - Can be helpful in identifying focal microinvasion

DIFFERENTIAL DIAGNOSIS

Reed (Pigmented Spindle Cell) Nevus

- Hyperplastic epidermis, symmetry, and well-defined peripheral margins
- Tumor cells are spindle-shaped and may show atypia but are usually monomorphous

Dysplastic Compound Melanocytic Nevus

- Less cytological atypia
- No basal confluence of nevus cells or adnexal extension
- Dermal component matures with increasing depth

Invasive Melanoma, Superficial Spreading Type

- Junctional component shows greater nesting and pagetoid spread compared to lentigo maligna
- Dermal component often nested and composed mostly of epithelioid-shaped cells
  - Not composed of oval to spindled cells of LMM
- Not associated with spindle cell/desmoplastic melanoma

DIAGNOSTIC CHECKLIST

Pathologic Interpretation Pearls

- Look for epidermal atrophy
- Confluent nesting along junction, especially in chronically sun-exposed skin
- Adnexal extension
- Dermal invasion, often composed of spindled cells
  - May be difficult to identify, especially if desmoplastic type or heavily inflamed

SELECTED REFERENCES

1. Van Meurs T et al: Treatment of lentigo maligna with imiquimod cream: a long-term follow-up study of 10 patients. Dermatol Surg. 36(6):853-8, 2010
2. Raziano RM et al: Staged margin control techniques for surgical excision of lentigo maligna. G Ital Dermatol Venereol. 144(3):259-70, 2009
3. van Meurs T et al: Recurrence of lentigo maligna after initial complete response to treatment with 5% imiquimod cream. Dermatol Surg. 33(5):623-6; discussion 626-7, 2007
4. Tannous ZS et al: Progression to invasive melanoma from malignant melanoma in situ, lentigo maligna type. Hum Pathol. 31(6):705-8, 2000
5. Flotte TJ et al: Lentigo maligna and malignant melanoma in situ, lentigo maligna type. Hum Pathol. 30(5):533-6, 1999

(Left) *Clinical photograph of lentigo maligna melanoma (LMM) on the nose of an elderly patient shows irregular pigmentation. Both in situ and invasive melanoma were present on biopsy. (Courtesy P. Hsu, MD.)* **(Right)** *The close-up of another irregularly pigmented patch on chronically sun-exposed skin showed invasive melanoma, lentigo maligna type. White streaks and surrounding depigmented areas are clinically suggestive of regression. (Courtesy J. Finch, MD.)*

LMM, Invasive and In Situ

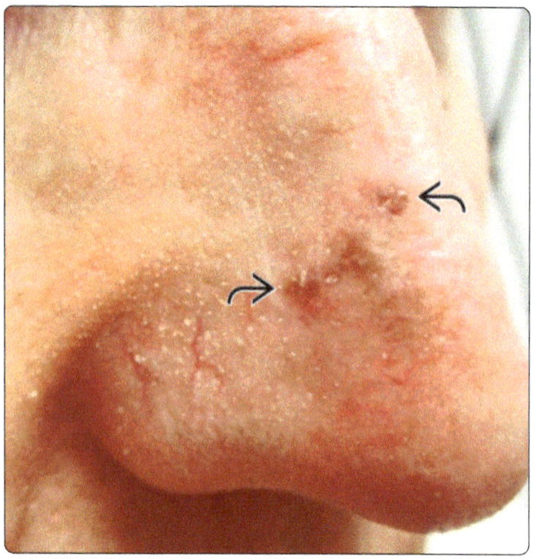

LMM With Regression

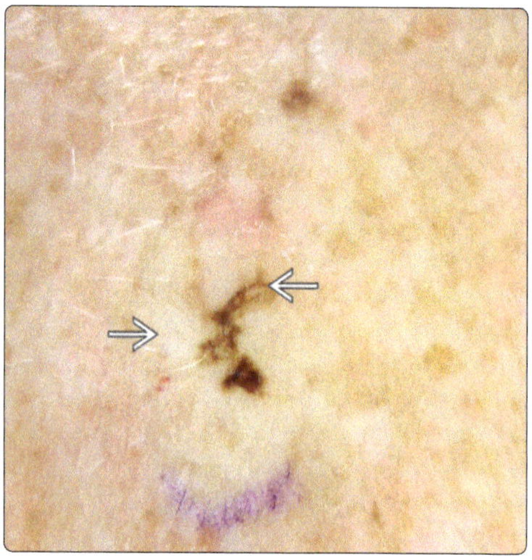

(Left) *Although the melanocytic nest is very close the epidermis, it appears to be completely separated from it. There are intervening fibroblasts.* **(Right)** *The nuclei are small with open chromatin and conspicuous nucleoli. Although the banal cytology may raise the differential of an intradermal melanocytic nevus, the cytology resembles that of the junctional melanocytes.*

LMM, Close Proximity to Epidermis

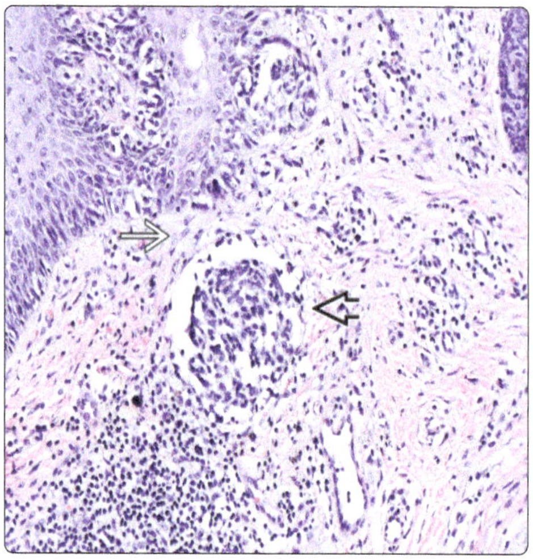

LMM at Higher Magnification Showing Small Cells, Banal Cytology

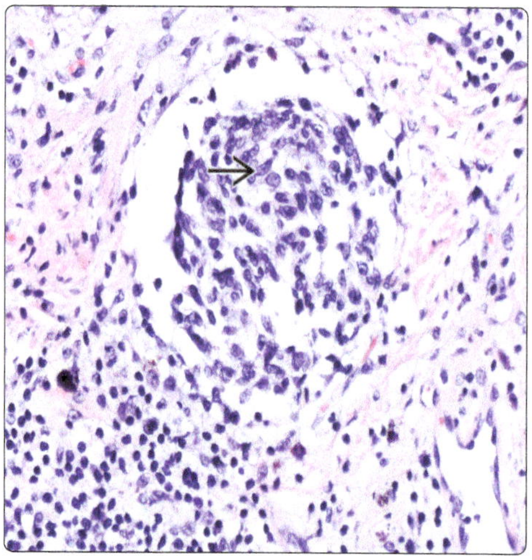

(Left) *This papular lesion appears suspicious for melanoma since it is a new pigmented lesion on chronically sun-exposed skin in an elderly patient. This is confirmed by solar elastosis being pushed down by the melanocytic growth.* **(Right)** *The presence of fibrosis with patchy, lymphohistiocytic infiltrate, melanin incontinence, and disrupted melanocytic proliferation are defining features of inflammatory regression.*

Solar Elastosis Pushed Down

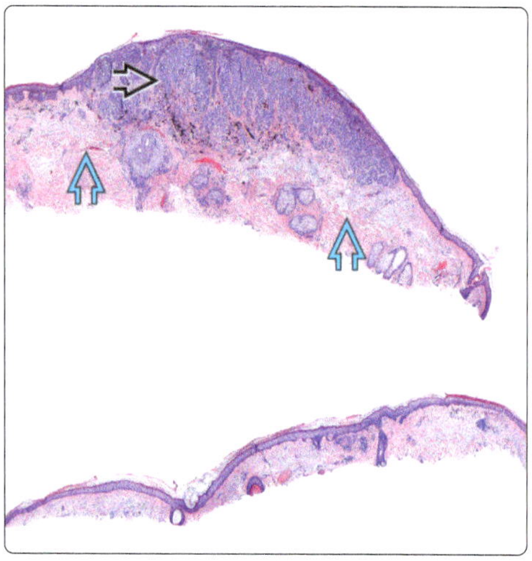

Inflammatory Regression

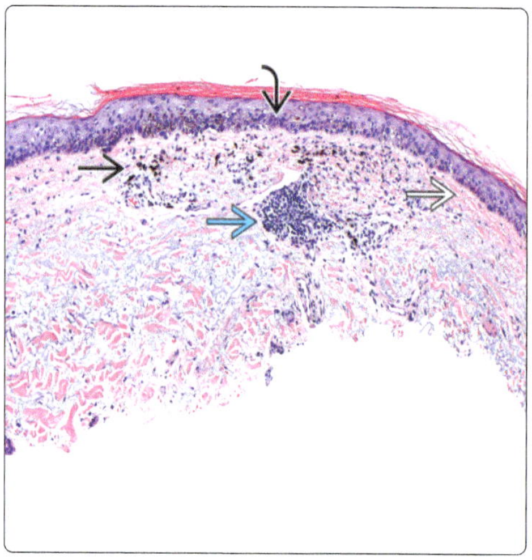

Invasive Melanoma, Lentigo Maligna Type

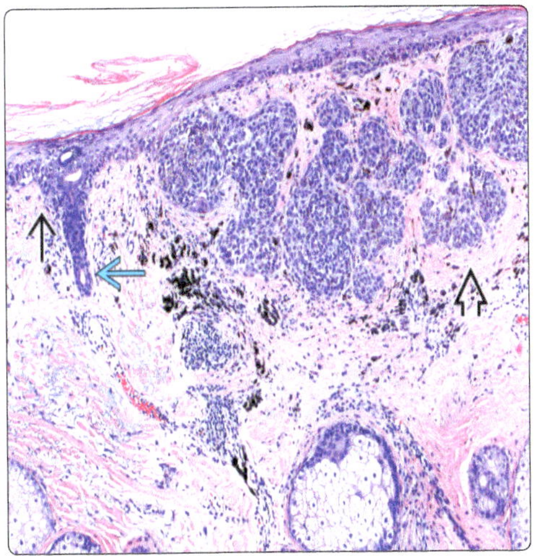

Small Cell Cytology in LMM

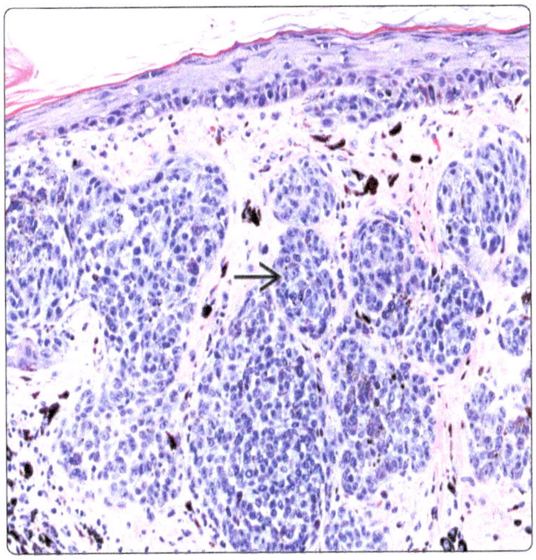

(Left) *The invasive dermal component is evident and indicates vertical growth phase . The adjacent junctional melanocytes track down an acrosyringium entering the epidermis and other adnexal structures (not shown in this field).* **(Right)** *The cytology is that of small epithelioid cells with round to oval nuclei. There are prominent nucleoli throughout the nests.*

Microinvasive LMM, Obscured by Inflammation

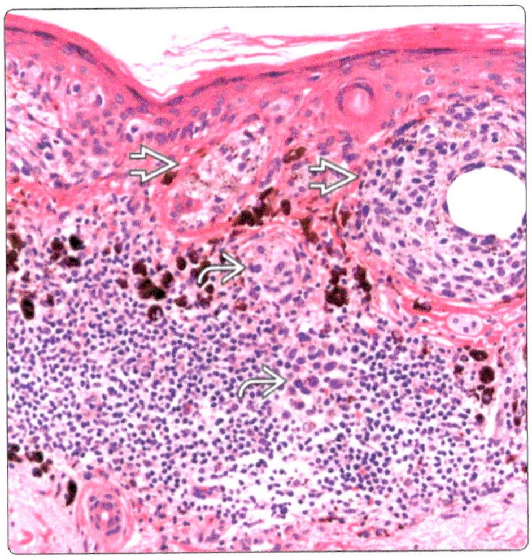

Lentiginous Growth Without Nesting and Small Invasive Melanoma

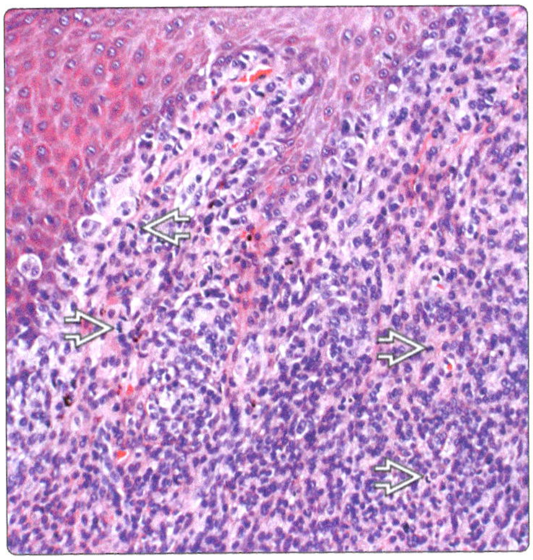

(Left) *LMM shows epidermal atrophy, consumed rete ridges, and an atypical junctional melanocytic lesion . The papillary dermis is obscured by a dense lymphocytic infiltrate, but focal invasion is present .* **(Right)** *High-power examination reveals the invasive melanoma with numerous mitoses in the superficial dermis. Again, the small melanoma cytology is evident. It is critical that these cells are examined carefully and not dismissed as "lymphocytes."*

Small, Spindle Cell Cytology in LMM

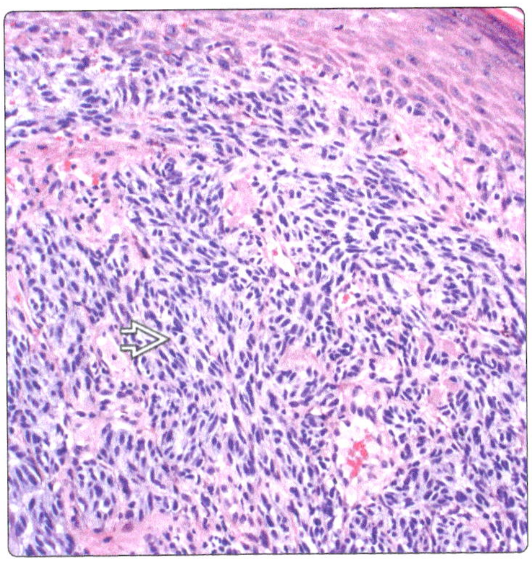

Dermal Invasion Confirmed

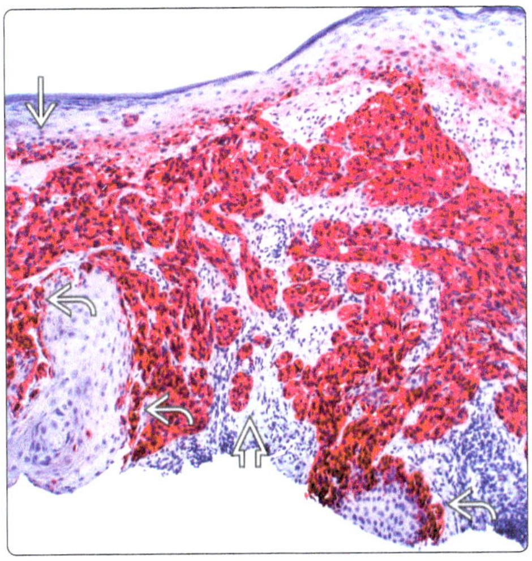

(Left) *This lesion shows a dermally invasive focus of melanoma cells growing in sheets. The cells are again small but spindled in shape. A mitosis is identified.* **(Right)** *HMB-45 immunohistochemistry shows strong and diffuse staining of the in situ and dermally invasive melanoma cells, consistent with invasive melanoma. Note the florid involvement of the adnexal structures .*

KEY FACTS

TERMINOLOGY

- Malignant melanoma, superficial spreading type (MM-SST)
- Most common variant of invasive melanoma

CLINICAL ISSUES

- Varies according to gender; occurs most often on back (in men) and on legs (in women)
- Broad macule with variegated colors
- Irregular borders
- Presence of papule/nodule may represent invasive component

MICROSCOPIC

- Proliferation of single atypical melanocytes involving both rete ridges and suprapapillary plates
- Abundant pagetoid spread of atypical melanocytes located in spinous layer
- Broad invasive front in which invasive dermal cells appear similar to overlying melanoma in situ (radial growth phase)
- Highly atypical melanocytes form confluent nests or nodule in dermis
- Lack of maturation of dermal component
- Dense but irregularly distributed inflammatory dermal infiltrate (mostly lymphocytes)
- Asymmetrical distribution of melanin pigment
- Enlarged, atypical epithelioid cells
- Nuclear pleomorphism, prominent nucleoli, and dermal mitoses

ANCILLARY TESTS

- MM-SST tends to show *BRAF*-activated mutations

TOP DIFFERENTIAL DIAGNOSES

- Severely dysplastic compound melanocytic nevus
  - Typically appears symmetric and well circumscribed at low magnification
  - Lack of dermal mitoses; presence of dermal maturation
- Atypical Reed nevus

Clinical Photograph of MM-SST

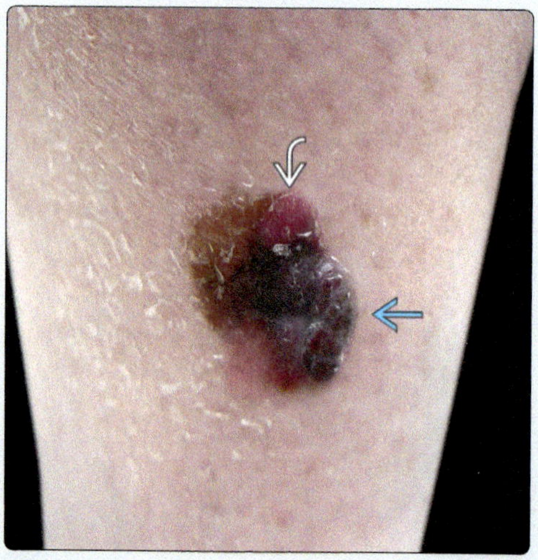

Clinical Photograph of MM-SST, With Regression

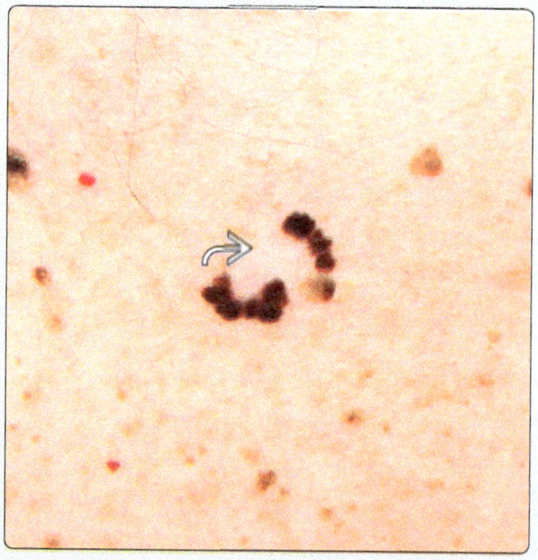

(Left) *Large, growing patch with variegated colors proved to be a melanoma, superficial spreading type (MM-SST) on histological examination. Note the patch at the edge represents the horizontal growth, and the plaque represents the invasive component. (Courtesy J. Finch, MD.)* **(Right)** *Clinical photograph of a MM-SST shows darkly pigmented areas surrounding a central area of regression. (Courtesy J. Wu, MD.)*

Low Magnification of MM-SST

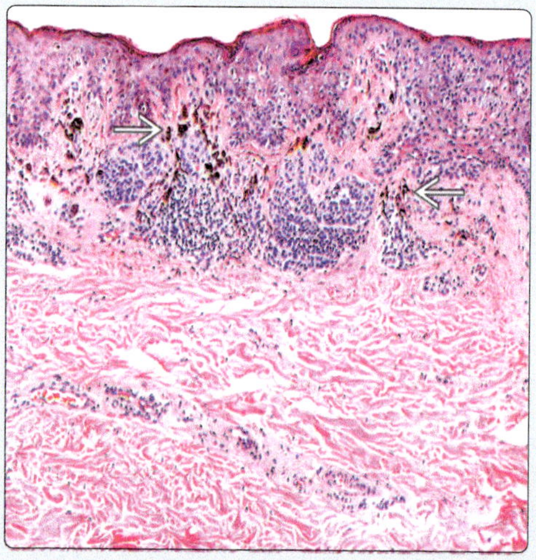

High Magnification of MM-SST

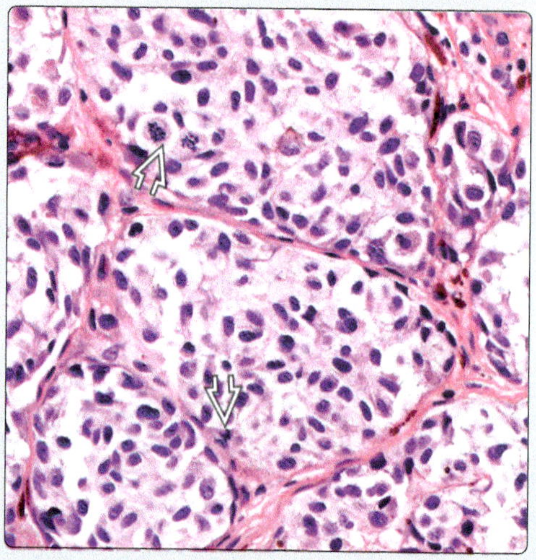

(Left) *Low-power magnification of a MM-SST shows a highly atypical compound melanocytic proliferation with mild dermal inflammation with scattered melanophages.* **(Right)** *The dermal component is composed of highly atypical cells, which fail to mature from the superficial to deeper dermis. Multiple mitoses are easily found.*

TERMINOLOGY

Abbreviations

- Malignant melanoma, superficial spreading type (MM-SST)

Definitions

- Most common variant of invasive melanoma
- Characterized histologically by pagetoid upward spread and lateral expansion of large dermal nests of atypical melanocytes

CLINICAL ISSUES

Epidemiology

- Incidence
  - 6th most common cancer in USA with increasing incidence
- Sex
  - Both men and women; more common overall in men
- Ethnicity
  - Typically persons with red hair and skin type I/II; can occur in other ethnicities

Site

- Varies according to gender; on back (in men) and on legs (in women)

Presentation

- Large dark brown macule (average size: 2.5 cm)
- Variegated color with shades of tan, brown, black, blue-black, red (inflammation or vascular ectasia), gray, and white; irregular borders

Treatment

- Surgical approaches
  - Complete excision with clear margins

Prognosis

- Varies according to Breslow depth, ulceration, and mitotic index

MACROSCOPIC

Size

- Typically > 1 cm in diameter

MICROSCOPIC

Histologic Features

- Lateral expansion of large nests of atypical melanocytes in both epidermis and dermis, i.e., radial growth phase
  - Proliferation of single atypical melanocytes involving both rete ridges and suprapapillary plates
  - Abundant pagetoid spread of atypical melanocytes located in spinous layer
  - Irregular distribution of nests, which can be confluent with indented borders
  - Large artifactual clefts between nests and epidermis above
  - Highly atypical melanocytes form confluent nests or nodule in dermis
  - Nuclear:cytoplasmic ratio does not change with increasing dermal depth, i.e., dermal melanocytes fail to mature with increasing depth in dermis
- Dense but irregularly distributed inflammatory dermal infiltrate (mostly lymphocytes)
- Asymmetrical distribution of melanin pigment in dermis

Cytologic Features

- Enlarged, atypical epithelioid cells
- Nuclear pleomorphism
- Large eosinophilic or purple nucleoli
- Presence of mitoses in dermal component

ANCILLARY TESTS

Genetic Testing

- MM-SST tends to show *BRAF*-activated mutations
- Melanomas with *BRAF* mutations show distinct morphological features
  - Increased upward migration
  - Nested formation of intraepidermal melanocytes
  - Larger, rounder (epithelioid), and more pigmented tumor cells

DIFFERENTIAL DIAGNOSIS

Severely Atypical (Dysplastic) Compound Melanocytic Nevus

- Typically appears symmetric and well circumscribed at low magnification
  - May need excisional specimen to adequately evaluate these features
- Less cytological atypia and mitotic activity than melanoma
  - Dermal mitoses highly suspicious for melanoma
- Less pagetoid spread
- Dermal component should mature with increasing dermal depth

Atypical Reed Nevus

- Hyperplastic epidermis, lateral margins are sharply defined (no trailing off of single cells)
- Composed mostly of spindle-shaped cells, which may be atypical, but are often monomorphous (not pleomorphic as in MM-SST)
- Kamino bodies may be present

Metastatic Melanoma (With Epidermotropism)

- Dermal component that is much larger than intraepidermal component
- Uniform cytologic atypia in dermal component
- Lymphatic invasion typically present (may need levels &/or immunohistochemistry, i.e., D2-40/podoplanin or CD31 to identify)

SELECTED REFERENCES

1. Foth M et al: Prognostic and predictive biomarkers in melanoma: an update. Expert Rev Mol Diagn. Feb;16(2):223-37, 2015
2. Reichrath J et al: Ultraviolet damage, DNA repair and vitamin D in nonmelanoma skin cancer and in malignant melanoma: an update. Adv Exp Med Biol. 810:208-33, 2014
3. Pacheco I et al: Towards new therapeutic approaches for malignant melanoma. Expert Rev Mol Med. 13:e33, 2011
4. Piris A et al: AJCC melanoma staging update: impact on dermatopathology practice and patient management. J Cutan Pathol. 38(5):394-400, 2011
5. Balch CM et al: Multivariate analysis of prognostic factors among 2,313 patients with stage III melanoma: comparison of nodal micrometastases versus macrometastases. J Clin Oncol. 28(14):2452-9, 2010

(Left) *Another clinical example of superficially invasive MM-SST with focal regression* ➡ *is shown. (Courtesy J. Finch, MD.)* **(Right)** *Scanning view of this ulcerated MM-SST shows a deeply invasive component* ➡ *associated with a dense dermal lymphocytic infiltrate.*

Clinical Photograph of MM-SST, With Regression

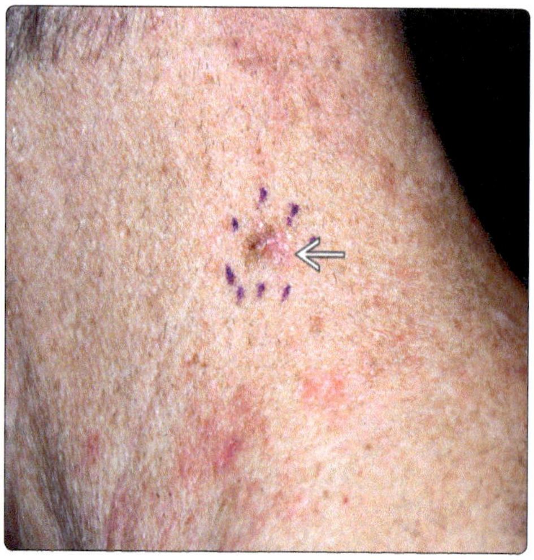

MM-SST at Scanning Magnification With Ulceration

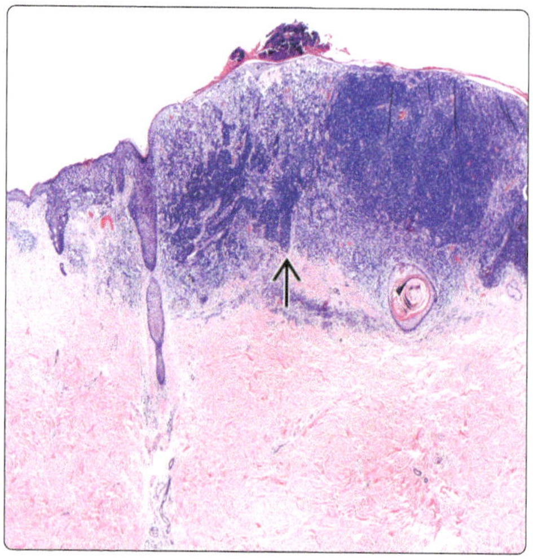

(Left) *Low-power view of the same case shows pagetoid upward scatter within the epidermis and the nested pattern of growth at the edge* ➡*, the defining feature of MM-SST.* **(Right)** *Fibrosis and vertically oriented blood vessels* ➡ *with lymphohistiocytic infiltrate* ➡ *and interrupted junctional component* ➡ *define regression. The peripheral nests* ➡ *define radial growth. Note the in situ cells with extensive pagetoid scatter* ➡ *involving the follicular and interfollicular epidermis.*

MM-SST at Low Magnification

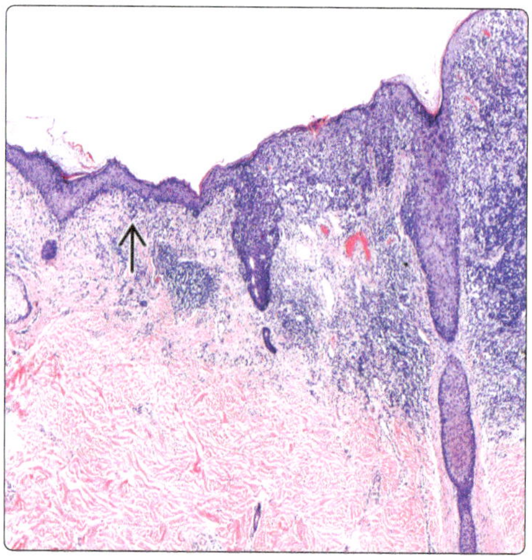

MM-SST at Intermediate Magnification

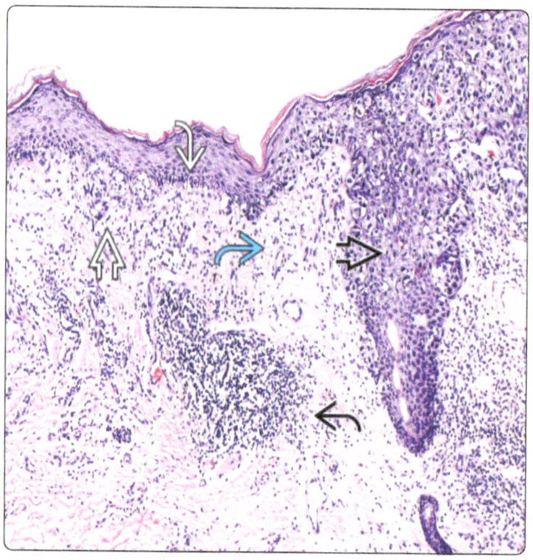

(Left) *On closer examination, there is nuclear pleomorphism among the large oval to round nuclei. There is hyperchromasia* ➡ *and prominent nucleoli* ➡*. There is no maturation with increasing dermal depth.* **(Right)** *HMB-45 often shows strong and diffuse staining in the invasive dermal component, a finding which can be useful in the differential diagnosis with an atypical nevus (which is typically weak/negative for HMB-45 in the dermis).*

MM-SST at High Magnification

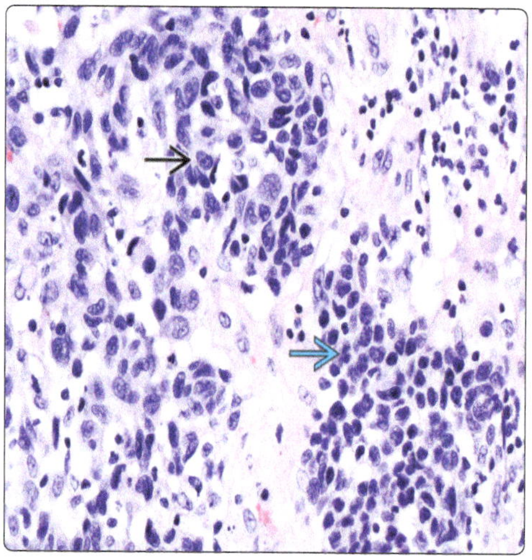

HMB-45 Immunohistochemistry in MM-SST

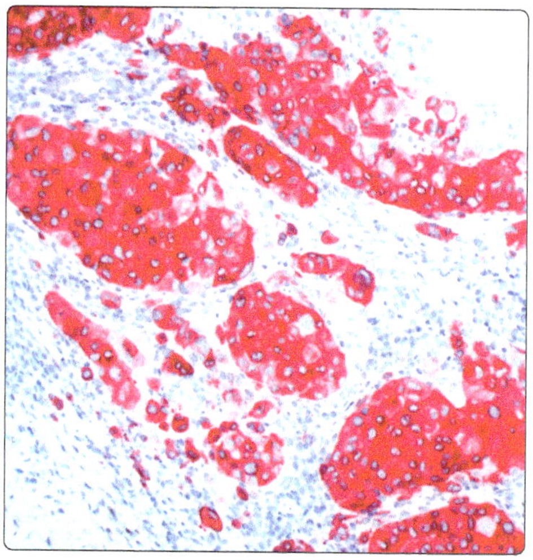

Clinical Photograph of MM-SST

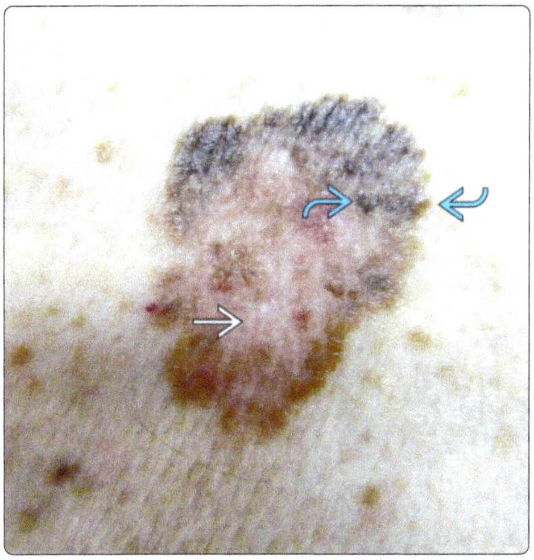

MM-SST at Low Magnification

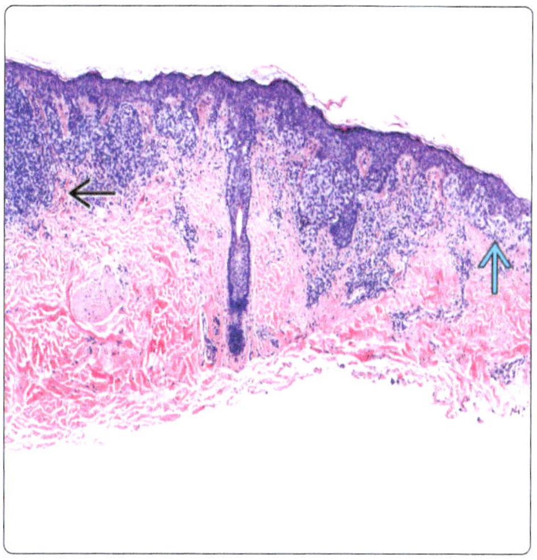

(Left) *Another clinical example shows an enlarging patch with papules →. The white areas in the center represent regression →. (Courtesy J. Finch, MD.)* **(Right)** *Low-power view shows the junctional → and invasive → components with the broad, junctional component extending well beyond the invasive component.*

MM-SST, In Situ Component

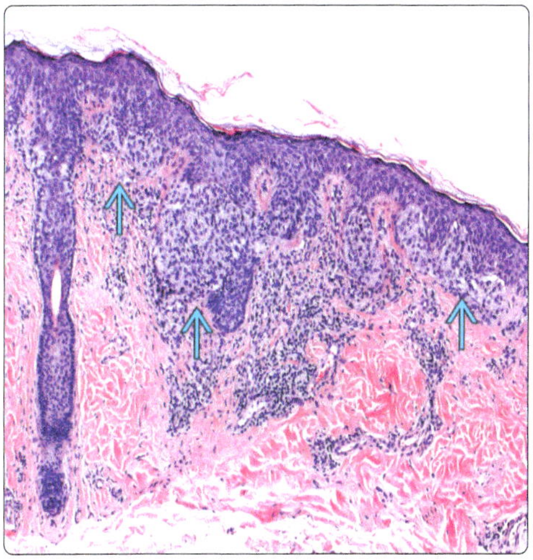

MM-SST, High Magnification With Dermal Infiltrate

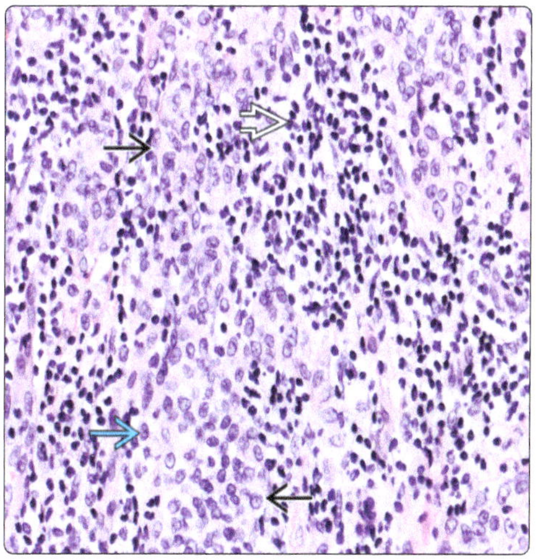

(Left) *The junctional nests → in horizontal growth phase are the defining feature in superficial spreading type of melanoma.* **(Right)** *This focus shows poorly formed nests with small oval nuclei. Although there are inconspicuous to small nucleoli →, the nuclei fail to become smaller with increasing dermal depth →. Note the clusters and patches of tumor infiltrating lymphocytes →.*

MM-SST, Lack of Maturation

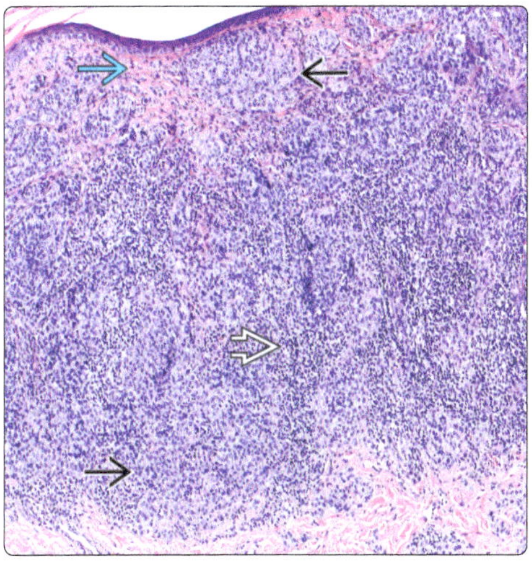

MM-SST, Invasive Component

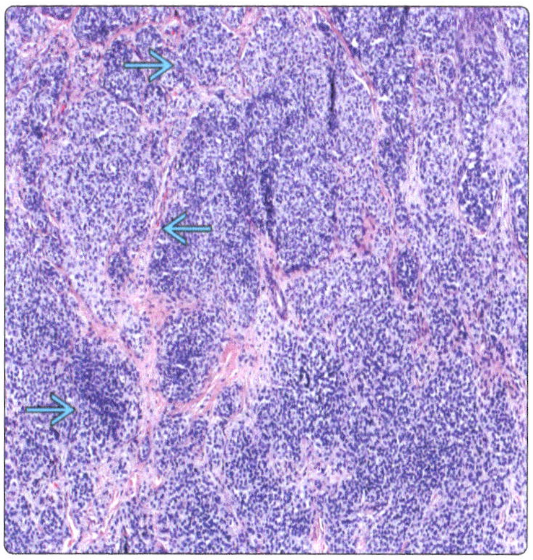

(Left) *The rete ridges are wiped out →, and there is no maturation → in the dermis. The invasive component is infiltrated by numerous small lymphocytes →.* **(Right)** *The invasive component fails to mature with increasing dermal depth; that is, the nuclei → remain the same size.*

(Left) *Another example of MM-SST shows a dome-shaped, predominantly dermal-based tumor, raising the possibility of an epidermotropic melanoma metastasis. Two distinct cell populations are noted: Large, pale cells superficially and small, hyperchromatic cells at the deeper aspect (preexisting nevus).* **(Right)** *The presence of irregularly scattered intraepidermal nests with scalloped borders define the radial growth phase. The dermal cells fail to mature with increasing depth.*

MM-SST at Low Magnification

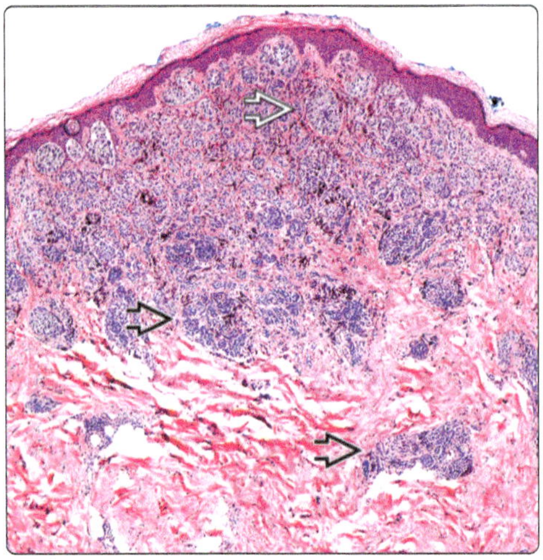

MM-SST at Higher Magnification

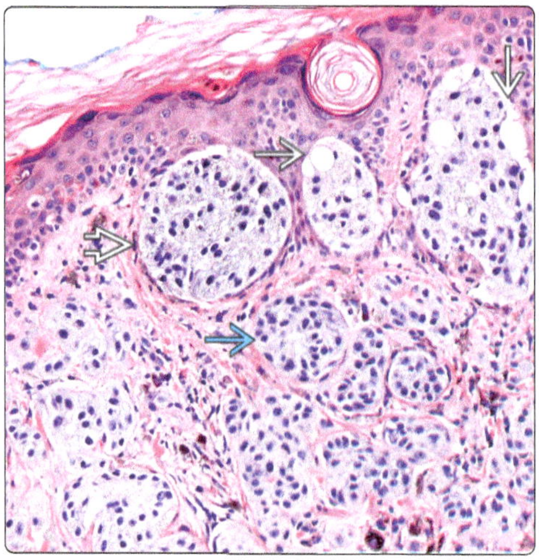

(Left) *High-power magnification shows atypical cells with ample gray-melanized cytoplasm with nuclear hyperchromasia and pleomorphism. Melanophages are noted in this case.* **(Right)** *Immunohistochemistry for p16 can be useful in some cases, as it is often weak to negative in invasive melanomas, but expressed in atypical nevi. This case shows patchy, mostly weak cytoplasmic staining.*

High Magnification of Dermal Nests in MM-SST

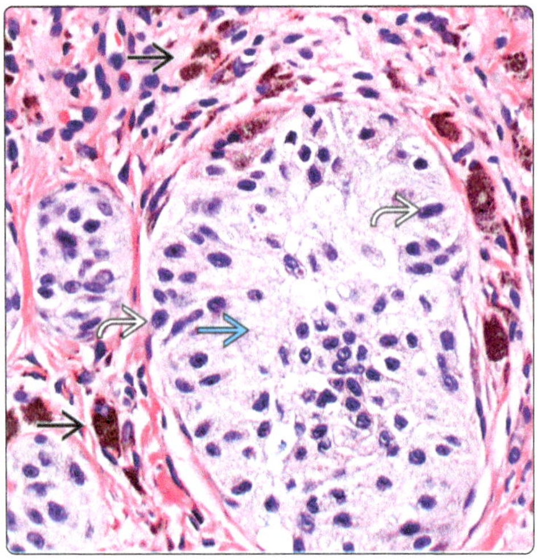

Immunohistochemistry for p16 in MM-SST

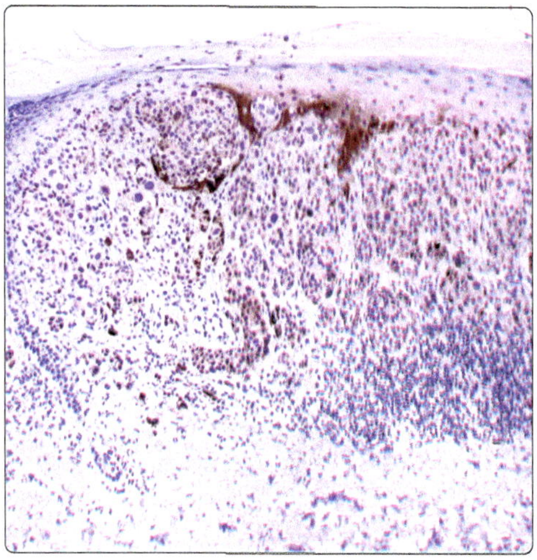

(Left) *Low-power examination shows melanoma in situ with pagetoid spread, superficial spreading type, overlying the invasive melanoma. This case was complicated by a preexisting intradermal melanocytic nevus.* **(Right)** *High-power magnification shows the dermal component, which demonstrates prominent cytologic atypia and 2 adjacent mitoses.*

Invasive MM-SST, With Associated Nevus

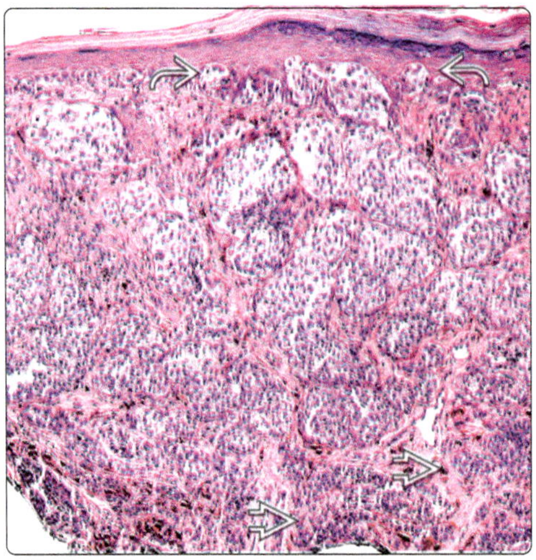

High Magnification of MM-SST

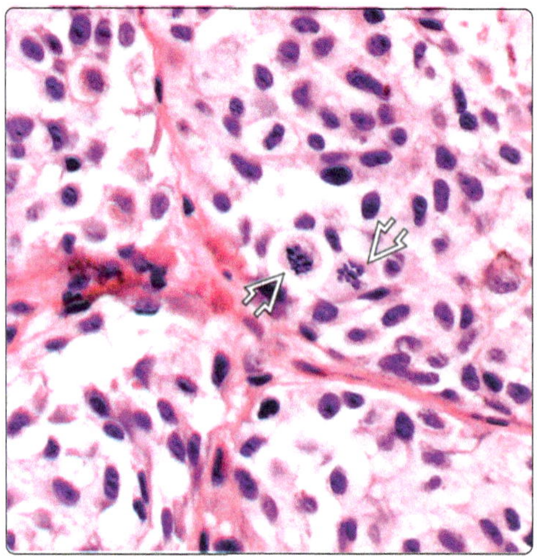

Differential Diagnosis: Atypical Recurrent Nevus With Dermal Scar

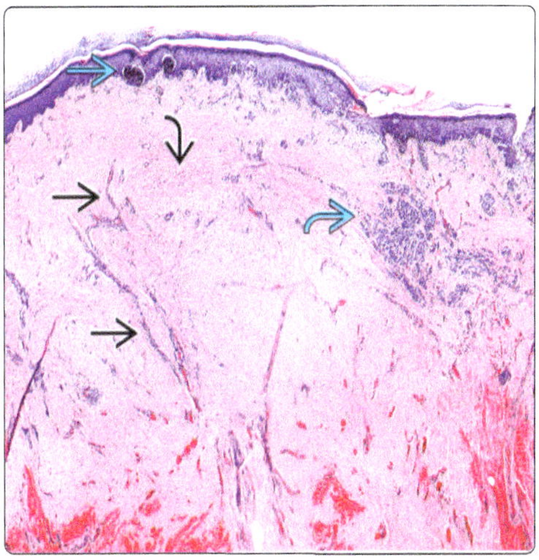

Differential Diagnosis: Atypical Recurrent Nevus With Dermal Scar

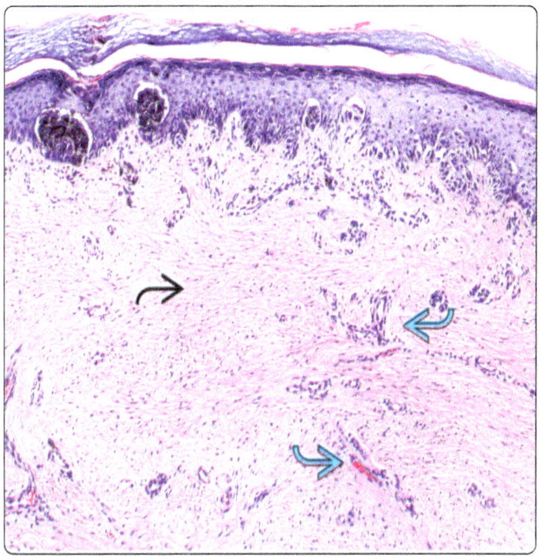

(Left) *In recurrent nevus, the junctional nests → are overlying a dermal scar →. The scar is defined by dermal fibrosis and vertically oriented prominent blood vessels →. The dermal component → matures with increasing dermal depth.* **(Right)** *The junctional component is well nested. Note the prominent dermal blood vessels → in the fibrotic area →.*

Differential Diagnosis: Recurrent Nevus

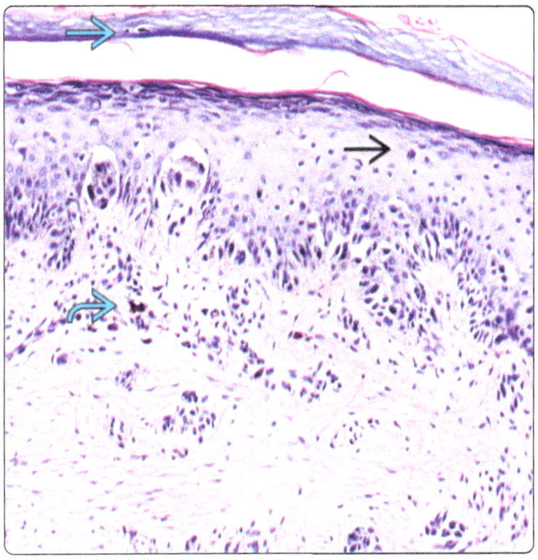

Differential Diagnosis: Atypical Recurrent Nevus at High Magnification

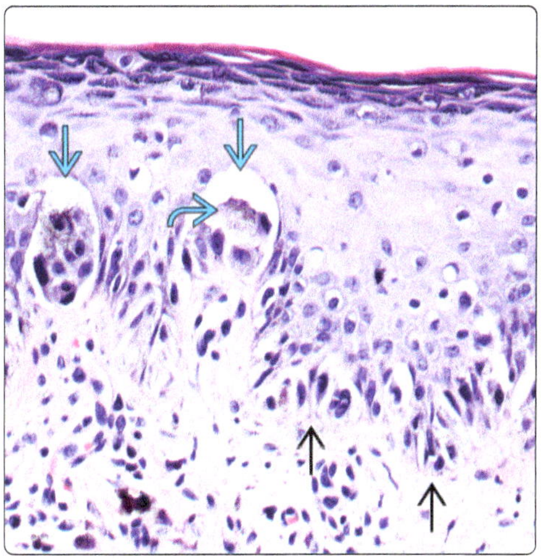

(Left) *Limited pagetoid scatter → may be evident. Melanin deposition in the dermis → &/or stratum corneum → are consistent with prior trauma (i.e., previous biopsy) in recurrent nevi.* **(Right)** *In this recurrent nevus, the junctional nests show apical clefts → (often considered a benign finding), not dyscohesion. The cytoplasm is heavily melanized →. The nuclei are round to oval and hyperchromatic →.*

Differential Diagnosis: Atypical Pigmented Spindle Cell Nevus

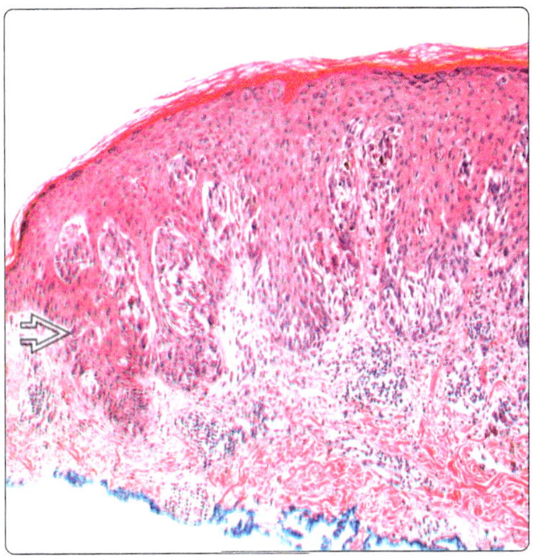

Differential Diagnosis: Atypical Pigmented Spindle Cell Nevus

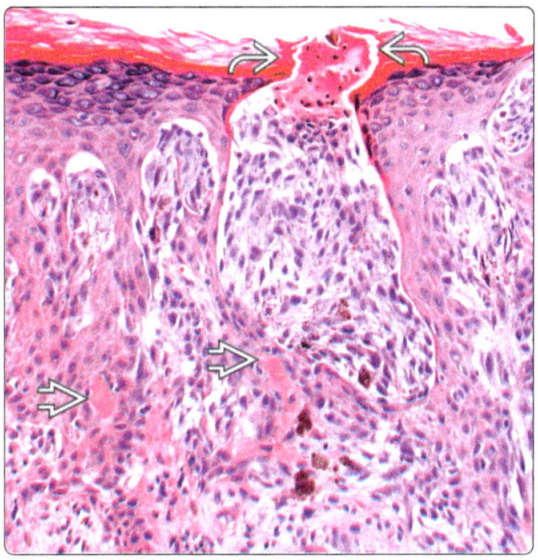

(Left) *Atypical pigmented spindle cell nevus (of Reed) shows a predominantly junctional proliferation of atypical spindle-shaped cells in irregular nests. Note the sharp lateral circumscription → as opposed to the trailing off of cells seen in MM-SST.* **(Right)** *High magnification of the center of an atypical Reed nevus shows pagetoid spread eroding through the granular layer →, but the cells are more uniform and spindled compared to MM-SST. Note the presence of Kamino bodies →.*

Melanoma, Nodular Type

KEY FACTS

TERMINOLOGY

- Nodular, predominantly dermal-invasive melanoma
- Invasive melanoma that histologically lacks radial growth phase
- Radial growth phase is defined by prominent junctional component

CLINICAL ISSUES

- Elevated, firm, rapidly growing nodule
- 2nd most common subtype of invasive melanoma (after superficial spreading type)
- Median age of onset: 49 years
- May grow very quickly
- Lead to poor prognosis in most cases

MICROSCOPIC

- Junctional component is small, and nodule may be separated from epidermis
- Areas of nodular/sheet-like growth pattern
- Epithelioid cell morphology with vesicular nuclei, prominent nucleoli
- Pleomorphic nuclei with hyperchromasia
- Mitoses often numerous, present deep in dermal component
- Preferential growth in dermis, rather than epidermis
- At border of lesion, confluent nests of abnormal melanocytes may be seen

TOP DIFFERENTIAL DIAGNOSES

- Superficial spreading type of invasive melanoma
- Spitz nevus
- Metastatic melanoma (with epidermotropism)

DIAGNOSTIC CHECKLIST

- Nodular, predominantly dermal-based lesion
- Prominent vertical growth phase with sheeting growth pattern

Crusted Scalp Tumor

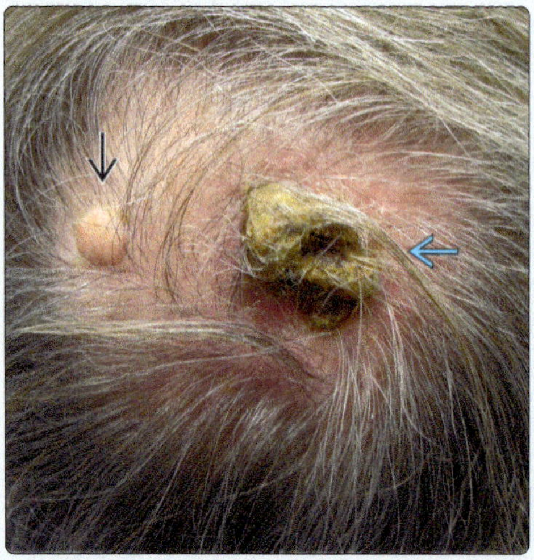

MM-NT

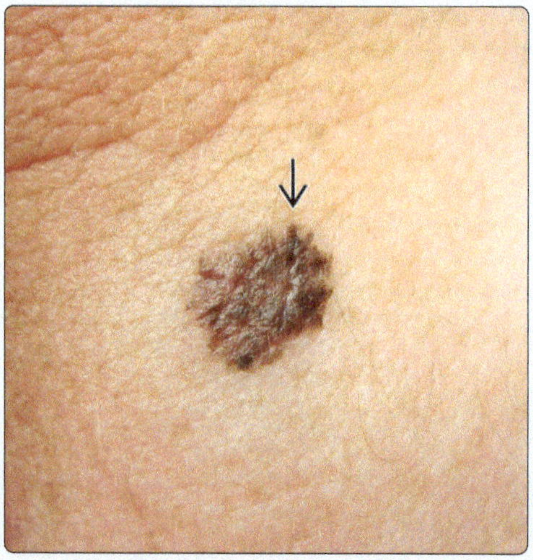

(Left) *The tumor → is crusted on the scalp of this elderly man. The skin-colored nodule on the left → is benign, either a neurofibroma or a neurotized intradermal nevus. (Courtesy J. Finch, MD.)* **(Right)** *This lesion was located on the posterior neck of a middle-aged man. Although it has a stuck-on appearance, it has uneven, jagged edges →. The biopsy showed melanoma, nodular type (MM-NT). (Courtesy J. Finch, MD.)*

MM-NT With Collarette Formation

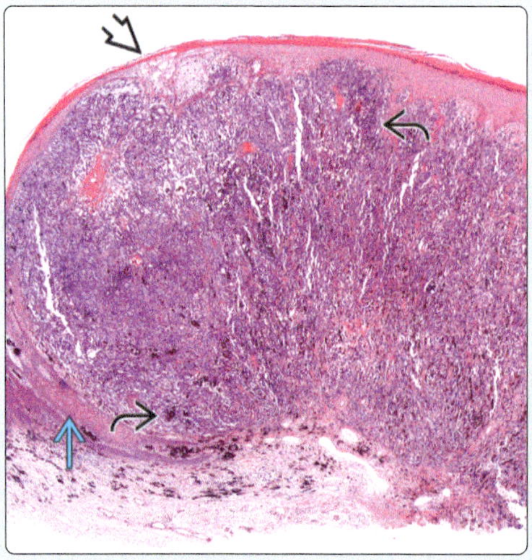

MM-NT at Higher Magnification

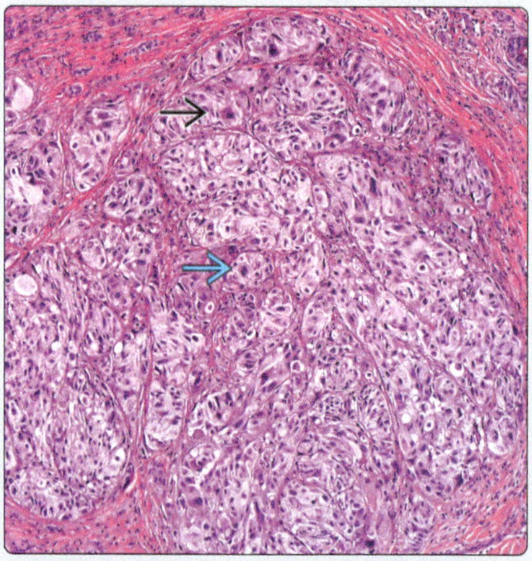

(Left) *Low-power examination of a melanoma, nodular type shows a large, expansile dermal nodule with irregular pigmentation → and areas of epidermal thinning and necrosis → (but no complete ulceration in this section). There is collarette formation → and no radial growth phase.* **(Right)** *There is proliferation of melanoma cells in nests and nodules. There is significant nuclear pleomorphism and hyperchromasia →. Mitotic figures → are easily found.*

TERMINOLOGY

Abbreviations

- Melanoma, nodular type (MM-NT)

Definitions

- Invasive melanoma that histologically lacks radial growth phase

CLINICAL ISSUES

Epidemiology

- Incidence
  - 2nd most common subtype of invasive melanoma (after superficial spreading type)
- Age
  - Median age of onset: 49 years

Site

- Typically on backs of males and legs of females

Presentation

- Raised, firm, dome-shaped mass of varied color
  - May be black, reddish, partially pigmented, or even achromatic
  - May have unequal color distribution or be homogeneous in color
  - Dominant color is black, with brown being 2nd most common color

Natural History

- May grow very quickly
  - Are commonly relatively new-onset lesions that lack radial growth phase
- More commonly are deeply invasive than other types of melanoma

Prognosis

- Depends on depth of invasion (Breslow depth), ulceration, and mitotic index
- Lymphatic invasion and lymph node metastasis are significant poor prognostic indicators
  - Median survival with metastasis: 4.4 months

MICROSCOPIC

Histologic Features

- Preferential growth in dermis, rather than epidermis
- Junctional component is tiny or absent, except at borders of lesion
  - Nodule may be separated from epidermis by thin rim of collagen
- At border of lesion, confluent nests of abnormal melanocytes may be seen
- Within lesion, nests have varying amounts of pigmentation
  - Some lesions may even appear to completely lack pigment
  - However, small granules of melanin will be often found histologically
    - If needed, melanin stain can be used
- Smaller nodules, sheets of melanocytes, or closely apposed nests are usually found
- May find focal to sheet-like areas of necrosis

Cytologic Features

- Epithelioid cell morphology with vesicular nuclei
- Pleomorphic nuclei with hyperchromasia
- Prominent, cherry-red macronucleoli
- Mitoses present deep in dermal component

ANCILLARY TESTS

Immunohistochemistry

- Same immunohistochemical markers as superficial spreading type

DIFFERENTIAL DIAGNOSIS

Superficial Spreading Type of Invasive Melanoma

- Shows broader atypical junctional component
  - Often extends laterally well beyond dermal component
- Dermal component often broader than that in MM-NT
  - Composed mostly of irregular nests (less nodular/sheet-like areas)

Spitz Nevus

- Younger patients (children to young adults)
- Symmetrical, well-circumscribed architecture at low magnification
- Composed of mixture of spindled and epithelioid cells in most cases
- Hyperkeratotic epidermis (not irregular thinning), often with clefting around nests
- Kamino bodies
- Mitoses usually superficial and nonatypical

Metastatic Melanoma (With Epidermotropism)

- Dermal component that is much larger than intraepidermal one
- Uniform atypical cytology in dermal component
- Lymphatic invasion almost always present
  - May need step-leveled sections or immunohistochemistry, i.e., D2-40/podoplanin

DIAGNOSTIC CHECKLIST

Clinically Relevant Pathologic Features

- Depth of invasion
- Ulceration
- Mitotic rate

Pathologic Interpretation Pearls

- Nodular, predominantly dermal-based lesion
- Prominent vertical growth phase with sheeting growth pattern

SELECTED REFERENCES

1. Cicchiello M et al: An assessment of clinical pathways and missed opportunities for the diagnosis of nodular melanoma versus superficial spreading melanoma. Australas J Dermatol. May;57(2):97-101, 2015
2. Pacheco I et al: Towards new therapeutic approaches for malignant melanoma. Expert Rev Mol Med. 13:e33, 2011
3. Erkurt MA et al: Nodular melanoma presenting with rapid progression and widespread metastases: a case report. J Med Case Reports. 3:50, 2009
4. Segura S et al: In vivo microscopic features of nodular melanomas: dermoscopy, confocal microscopy, and histopathologic correlates. Arch Dermatol. 144(10):1311-20, 2008
5. Warycha MA et al: Changes in the presentation of nodular and superficial spreading melanomas over 35 years. Cancer. 113(12):3341-8, 2008

(Left) *Scanning magnification shows lack of radial growth phase and epidermal collarette formation. There is uneven pigmentation and an inflammatory infiltrate that hugs the tumor pushing front.* **(Right)** *The same nodular melanoma is shown under medium-power magnification. There is epidermal consumption but no in situ component or junctional nesting is identified.*

Small MM-NT

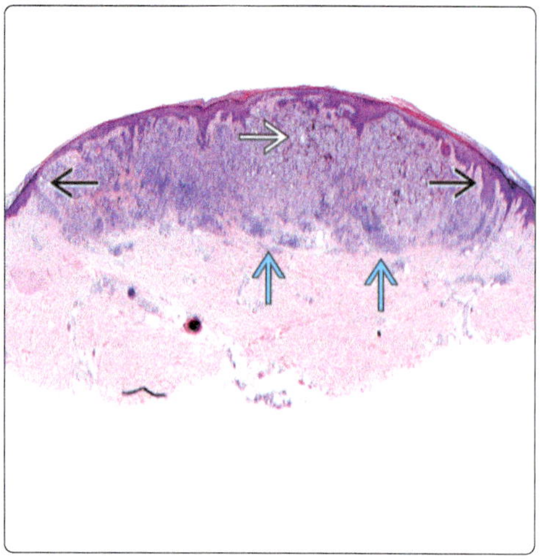

Lack of Radial Growth Phase in MM-NT

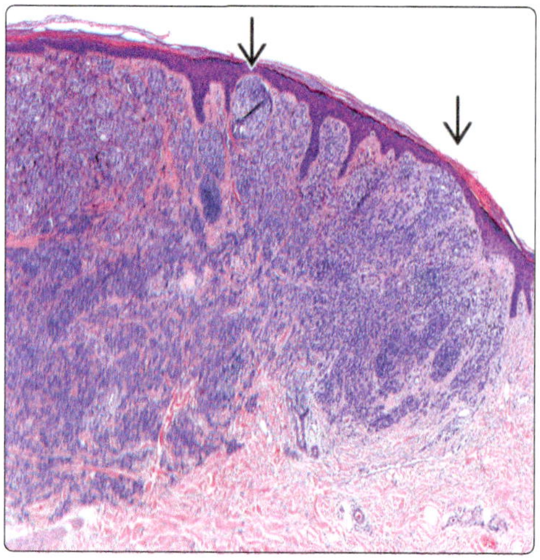

(Left) *This field shows 2 distinct cell populations. One is large and epithelioid; the other smaller, "nevoid" cells. There is focal lymphocytic [typically CD8(+) killer T cells].* **(Right)** *Another nodular melanoma shows an epidermal collarette and lack of a radial growth phase. This lesion is ulcerated and showed numerous mitotic figures on higher power examination.*

2-Cell Population in MM-NT

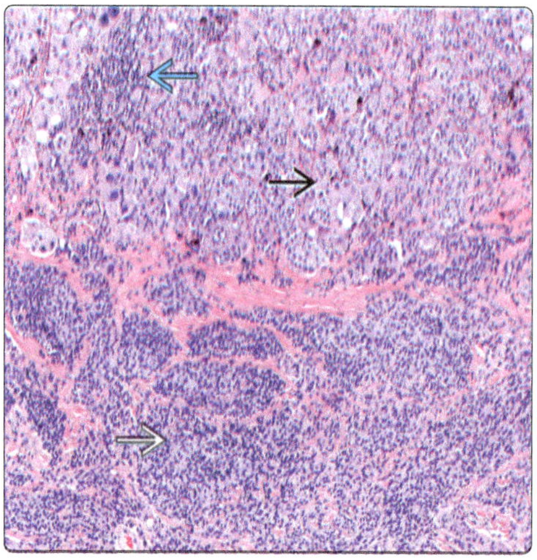

Collarette Formation in MM-NT

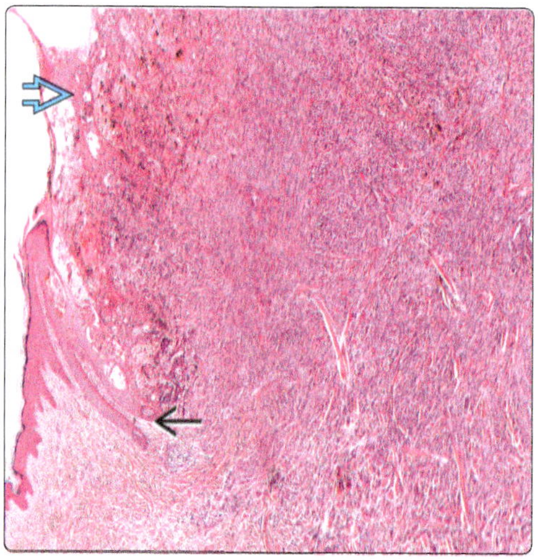

(Left) *This exophytic, nodular growth is unevenly pigmented. It lacks maturation with increasing dermal depth even at this scanning magnification. Epidermal collarette formation is evident.* **(Right)** *Although the lesion is nodular with an epidermal collarette, there is clearly a focus of radial growth phase, as seen by nested, lentiginous growth of melanoma cells.*

Papulonodular Growth in MM-NT

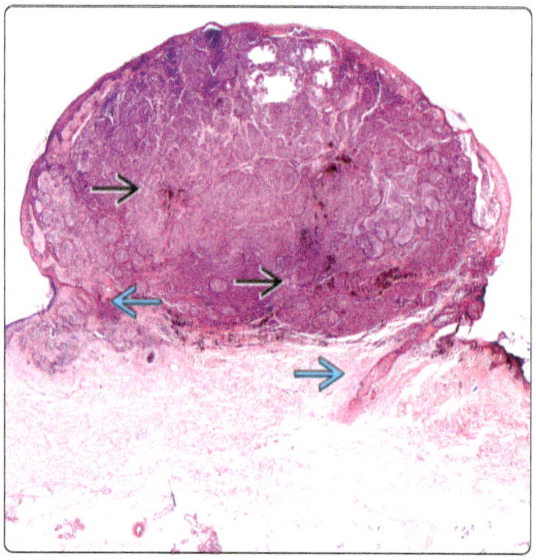

Radial Growth Phase in MM-NT

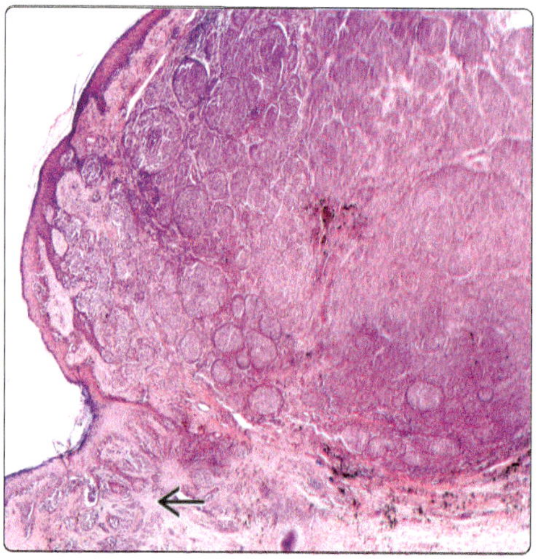

No Radial Growth Phase in MM-NT

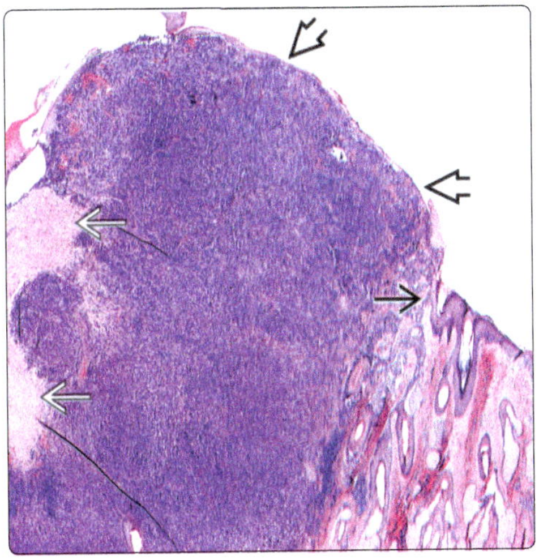

Inflamed Junctional Activity in MM-NT

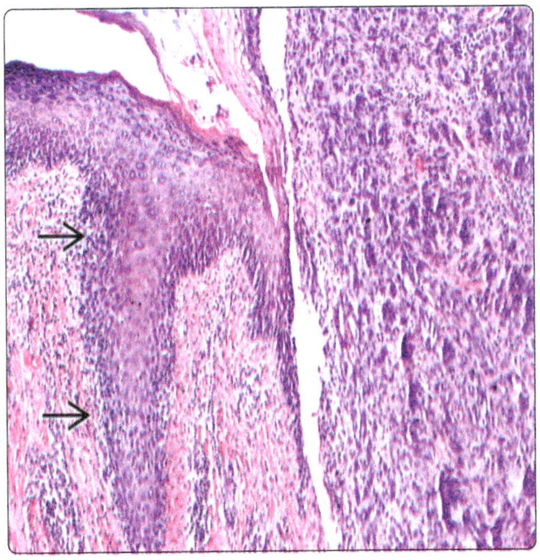

(Left) *Scanning magnification of a nodular melanoma shows a large nodule with broad areas of overlying ulceration ⇨ and large areas of necrosis ➡. There is no radial growth phase in the periphery →.* **(Right)** *Medium-power magnification shows a lack of radial growth phase. There is no nesting or melanoma in situ component. The lymphocytic exocytosis mimics a junctional component →.*

High Magnification Showing Melanoma Cytology in MM-NT

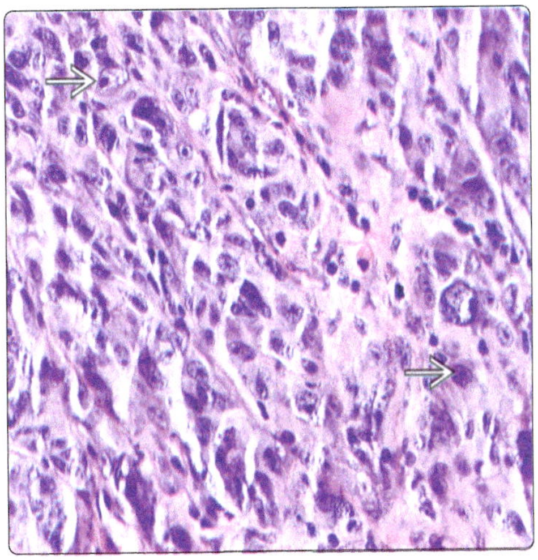

Ulcerated MM-NT at Low Magnification

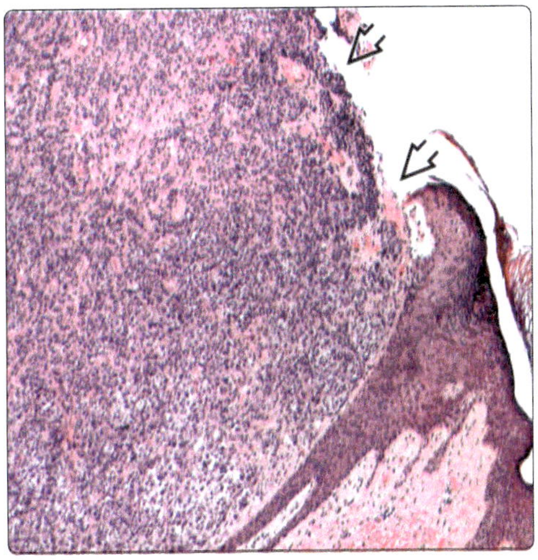

(Left) *High-power magnification shows sheets of melanoma cells with bizarre cytology (pleomorphic nuclei, thick and irregular nuclear membranes, and prominent nucleoli ➡).* **(Right)** *Low-power examination of a nodular malignant melanoma shows a large, expansile dermal nodule with significant epidermal thinning and full-thickness ulceration ⇨. The dermis exhibits a nodular to sheet-like cellular tumor.*

MM-NT With Sheet-Like Growth at High Magnification

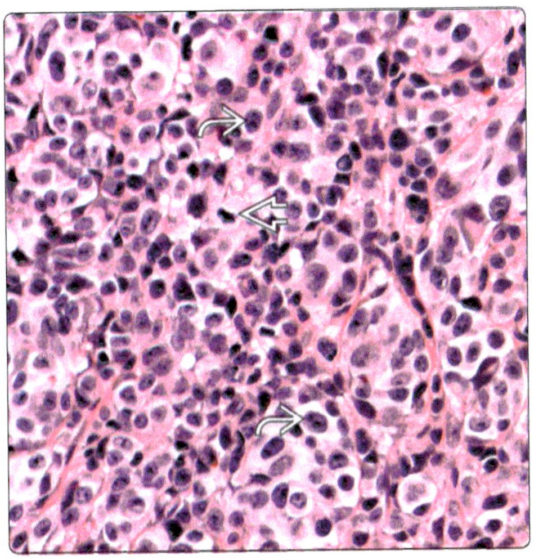

Vascular Invasion in MM-NT

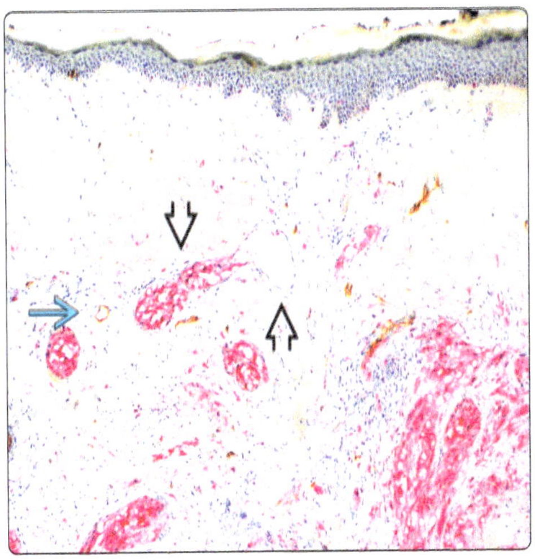

(Left) *High magnification shows a sheet-like growth pattern. The cells are markedly atypical and usually epithelioid-shaped, with vesicular nuclei and prominent nucleoli ➦. A mitotic figure is present ➡ in this field.* **(Right)** *S100 (red)/podoplanin (brown) double immunostains show vascular invasion. It is defined by the presence of tumor in podoplanin (-) vessels ⇨. The adjacent lymphatics → are free of tumor thrombi.*

KEY FACTS

TERMINOLOGY

- Invasive melanoma that often resembles inflamed scar
- Desmoplastic melanoma (DM)

CLINICAL ISSUES

- Firm, skin-colored, tan or pink plaque or nodule
- Presents in sun-damaged skin of elderly adults

MICROSCOPIC

- Ill-defined spindle cell neoplasm with highly infiltrative pattern of growth
- Overlying epidermis may show melanoma in situ (usually lentigo maligna type)
- Discrete dermal lymphoid aggregates admixed with abundant collagen
- Severe solar elastosis
- Pure and combined (more cellular) subtypes

ANCILLARY TESTS

- Usually immunostains for S100 and SOX10 (+)

TOP DIFFERENTIAL DIAGNOSES

- Dermal scar
- Desmoplastic nevus
- Spindle cell squamous cell carcinoma
  - HMWCKs(+), p63; S100(-)
- Atypical fibroxanthoma
  - S100(-); CD10/CD68/CD99 (+)
- Dermatofibroma: FXIIIA/CD10 (+); S100(-)
- Dermatofibrosarcoma protuberans: CD34(+); S100(-)
- Neural tumors
  - S100/SOX10 (+); CD34(+) (not in DM)
- Leiomyosarcoma
  - Actin/desmin (+), S100(-)

(Left) *Desmoplastic melanoma (DM) may resemble an inflamed scar on a low-power examination. However, aggregates of lymphoid cells and prominent solar elastosis are usually identified and are helpful findings.* **(Right)** *Unlike a scar, DM under high-magnification examination shows hyperchromatic-staining atypical spindle cells surrounded by abundant collagen bundles.*

Scar-Like Appearance in DM

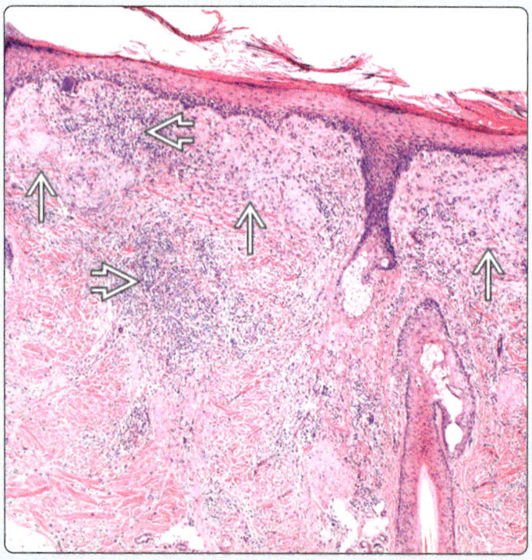

Cytological Atypia in DM

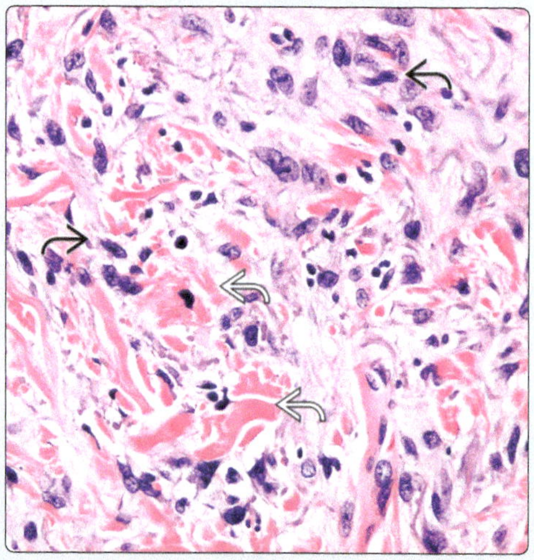

(Left) *This punch biopsy shows hyperkeratosis overlying an expanded dermis, mimicking an inflamed scar. There are discrete lymphoid aggregates throughout the dermis that should raise suspicion for DM.* **(Right)** *The presence of scar-like dermis and multiple lymphoid aggregates should be followed up by SOX10 (or S100) immunohistochemistry to confirm DM as in this case. The nuclei of tumor cells are strongly positive.*

Dermal Lymphoid Aggregates in DM

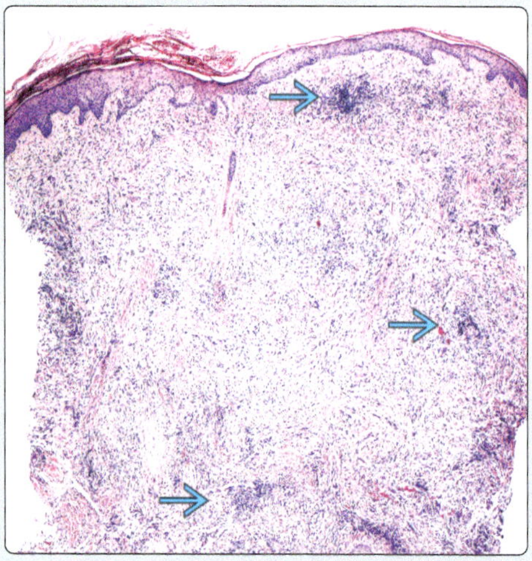

SOX10 Immunohistochemistry in DM

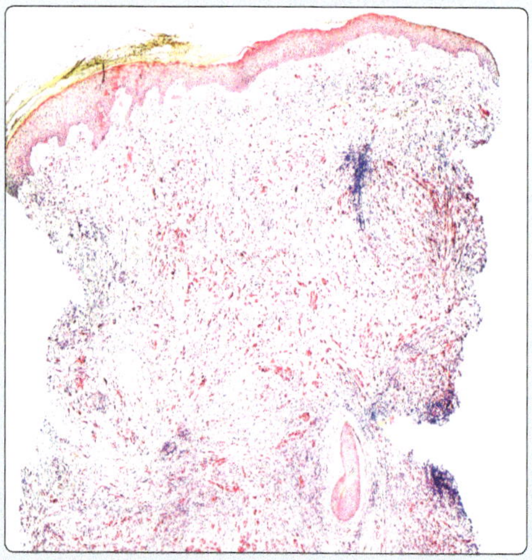

TERMINOLOGY

Abbreviations

- Desmoplastic melanoma (DM)

Synonyms

- Desmoplastic/neurotropic melanoma

Definitions

- Form of invasive melanoma composed of spindle cells associated with dense stromal collagen
  - Resembles scar

CLINICAL ISSUES

Epidemiology

- Age
  - Presents in sun-damaged skin of elderly adults

Presentation

- Firm, skin-colored, tan or pink plaque or nodule
- Sometimes depressed

Treatment

- Surgical approaches
  - It is important to resect DMs with clear surgical margins
  - There is increasing evidence that sentinel lymph node biopsy may not be indicated for "pure" variants

Prognosis

- Tumor thickness (Breslow depth)
- Clark level (IV vs. V)
- Histological subtype: Pure (longer disease-free survival) vs. combined
  - Pure subtype is defined as > 90% scar-like areas
  - Combined subtype is defined as densely cellular spindle cell collections
    - Lacks significant scar-like areas (> 10%)
- Tumor mitotic rate

MICROSCOPIC

Histologic Features

- Ill-defined spindle cell neoplasm with highly infiltrative pattern of growth
- Overlying epidermis may show melanoma in situ (usually lentigo maligna type)
- Stromal collagen on scanning magnification resembles scar
- Spindle cells are arranged in fascicles and merge with scar-like areas
- Cellular density and cytologic atypia can vary based on histologic subtype
- Discrete dermal lymphoid aggregates
- Solar elastosis

Cytologic Features

- Pure subtype shows
  - Spindle cells with often deceptively mild cytological atypia
  - Nuclear hyperchromasia
  - Irregular nuclear contours
  - Minimal nuclear pleomorphism
  - Inconspicuous mitotic activity
- Combined subtype shows
  - Greater cellularity and plump, elongated cells
  - Vesicular nuclei and prominent nucleoli

ANCILLARY TESTS

Immunohistochemistry

- Typically strongly S100(+)
- Often SOX10 and KBA62 (+)

DIFFERENTIAL DIAGNOSIS

Fresh or Old Scar

- Dense collagen bundles, usually oriented parallel to epidermis
- Verticalized blood vessels

Desmoplastic Nevi

- Desmoplastic Spitz nevus
  - Occurs in young adults, not elderly
  - Often shows scattered epithelioid cells
- Desmoplastic intradermal nevus

Spindle Cell Squamous Cell Carcinoma

- Spindle cell and desmoplastic squamous cell carcinoma can histologically mimic DM
- HMWCKs(+), p63; S100(-)

Atypical Fibroxanthoma

- Also occurs in heavily sun-damaged skin of elderly
- Usually more cellular proliferation of frankly atypical, enlarged pleomorphic cells
- Lacks stromal desmoplasia in most cases
- S100(-); CD10/CD68/CD99 (+)

Fibrohistiocytic Tumors

- Dermatofibroma
  - Collagen entrapment and overlying epidermal hyperplasia
  - Lacks significant cytologic atypia
  - Usually CD10/CD68/FXIIIA (+); S100(-)
- Dermatofibrosarcoma protuberans
  - Bland cellular spindle cell proliferation with storiforming
  - CD34(+); S100(-)

Neural Tumors

- Neurofibroma
  - Lacks significant cytologic atypia or lymphoid aggregates
  - S100/SOX10 (+); CD34(+) (not in DM)
- Superficial malignant peripheral nerve sheath tumor
  - Rare, but shows similar immunohistochemical profile as DM [S100(+), SOX10(+/-)]

Leiomyosarcoma

- Fascicles of eosinophilic-staining cells
  - Actin/desmin (+), S100(-)

SELECTED REFERENCES

1. Busam KJ: Desmoplastic melanoma. Clin Lab Med. 31(2):321-30, 2011
2. Ramos-Herberth FI et al: SOX10 immunostaining distinguishes desmoplastic melanoma from excision scar. J Cutan Pathol. 37(9):944-52, 2010

Desmoplastic Melanoma

(Left) *Aggregates of lymphoid infiltrate and solar elastosis are readily found in the superficial aspect of most cases of DM. These features are clues to suggest the diagnosis.* **(Right)** *Poorly nested, lentiginous growth of atypical melanocytes in the epidermis and follicular epithelium is consistent with an in situ component, lentigo maligna. This finding is helpful in confirming the diagnosis.*

Superficial Aspect of DM

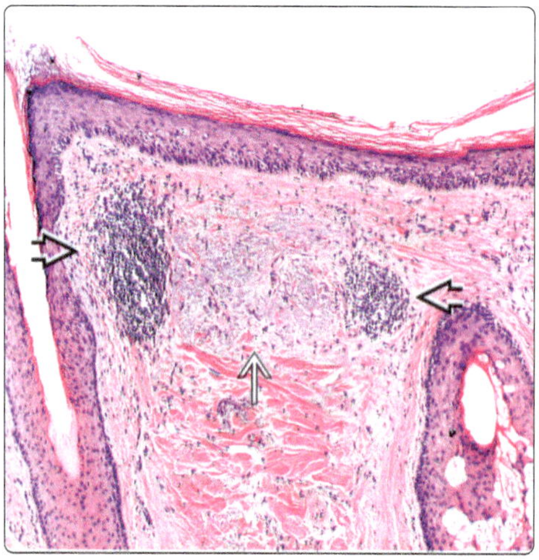

Lentigo Maligna Associated With DM

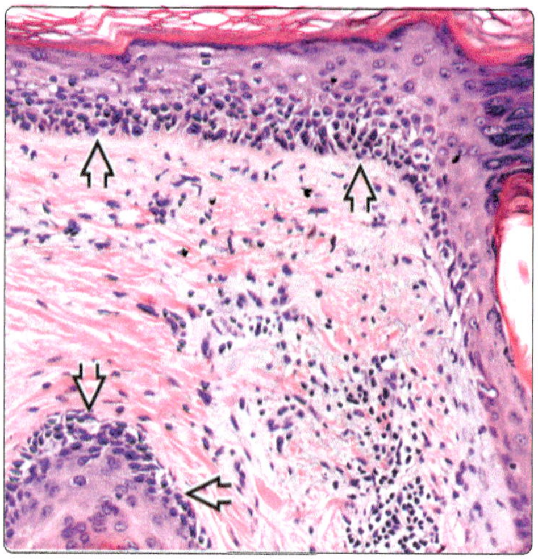

(Left) *An example of DM arising in very severely solar-damaged skin, with a relatively dense chronic inflammatory infiltrate in the dermis is shown. Note the small focus of overlying melanoma in situ.* **(Right)** *This DM shows a very dense lymphoid infiltrate at the deep aspect of the tumor. There is adjacent stromal desmoplasia with scattered atypical, hyperchromatic-staining spindle cells [which were strongly S100(+), not shown].*

Marked Solar Elastosis in DM

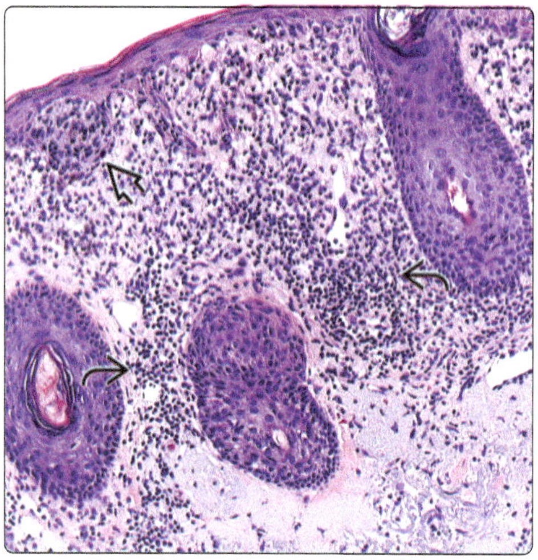

Dense Lymphoid Infiltrate in DM

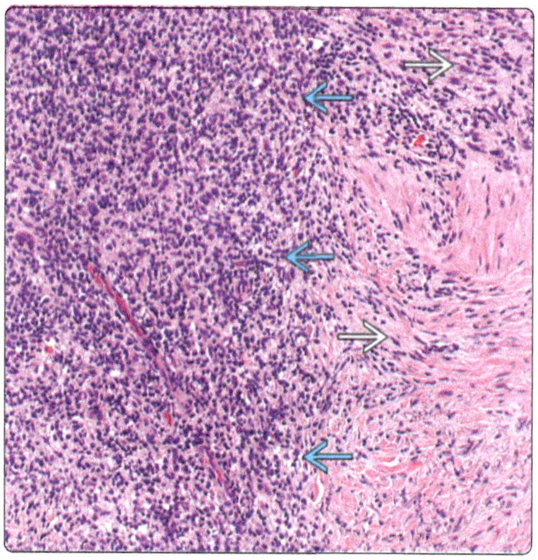

(Left) *An area of DM shows stromal sclerosis with hyalinized balls of collagen resembling those seen in dermatofibromas. However, note the presence of atypical, hyperchromatic nuclei and adjacent lymphoid aggregates.* **(Right)** *Mitotic figures may be seen in DM, but they are usually sparse. Additional sections may be needed to search for mitotic activity.*

DM Mimicking Dermatofibroma

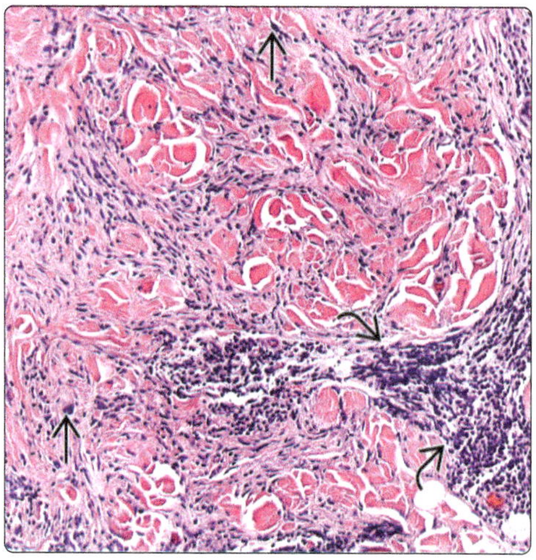

Cytology of DM at High Magnification

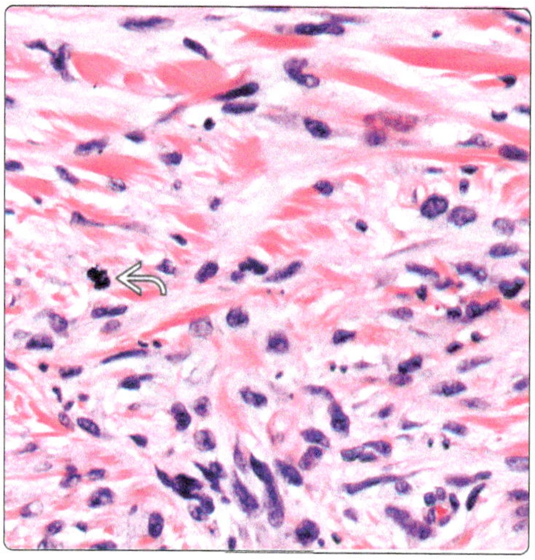

S100 Immunohistochemistry in DM

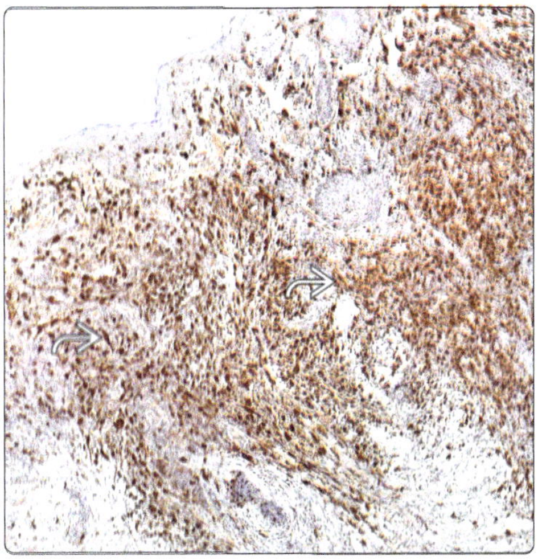

Melan-A Immunohistochemistry in DM

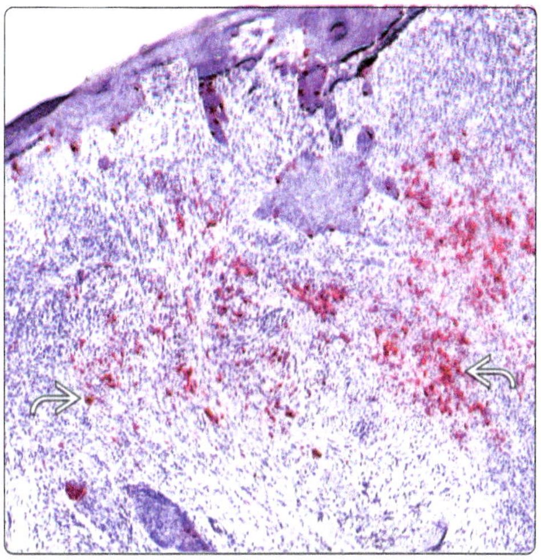

(Left) *S100 immunohistochemistry shows strong and diffuse nuclear and cytoplasmic staining of the dermal spindle cell population in DM. In this example, there was no in situ component.* **(Right)** *Melan-A stain shows patchy staining of a portion of tumor cells. Although most often negative in DM, markers such as MART-1/Melan-A, HMB-45, and tyrosinase, can occasionally be positive (reportedly in up to 20-25% of cases).*

Differential Diagnosis: Desmoplastic Nevus

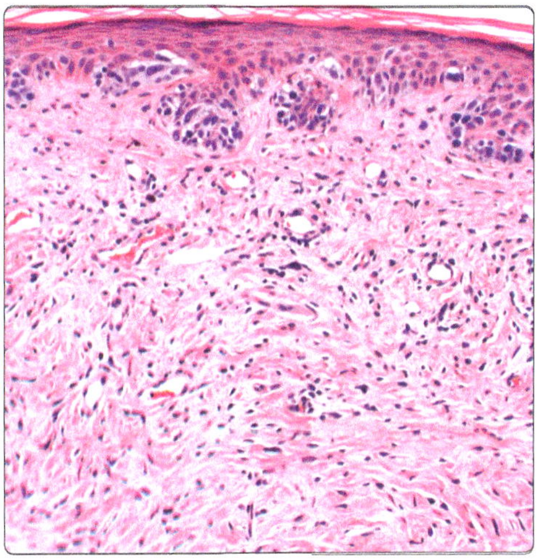

Differential Diagnosis: Desmoplastic Spitz Nevus

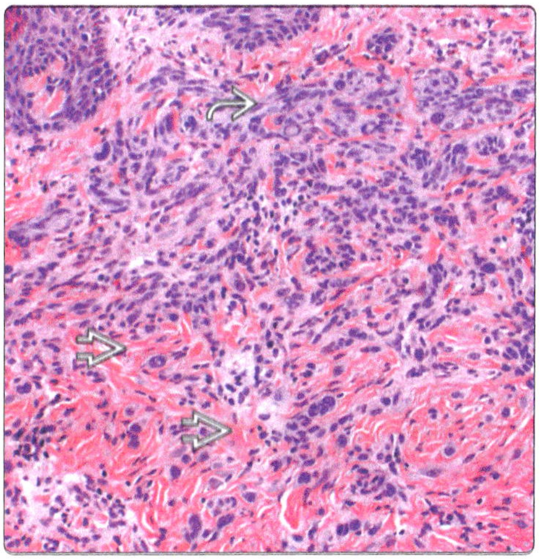

(Left) *Atypical combined nevus with a desmoplastic nevus component in the dermis is shown. The junctional component is moderately atypical, but the dermal cells are small and bland-appearing. Note the lack of severe solar elastosis and lymphoid aggregates typical of desmoplastic melanoma.* **(Right)** *Desmoplastic Spitz nevus shows spindled and epithelioid cells arrayed in irregular nests, short fascicles, and cords in a dense, hyalinized-appearing stroma. These tumors typically occur in young adults.*

Differential Diagnosis: Atypical Dermatofibroma/Fibrous Histiocytoma

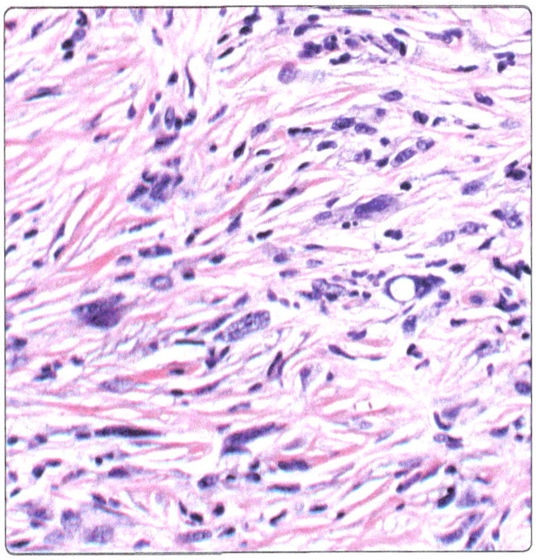

Differential Diagnosis: Dermatofibrosarcoma Protuberans

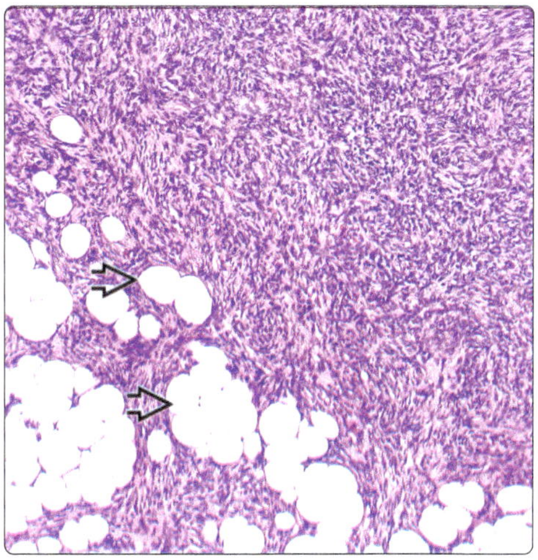

(Left) *Atypical dermatofibroma shows a proliferation of enlarged and pleomorphic spindle-shaped and histiocytoid cells, which are larger than those typically seen in DM. In addition, the cells are S100(-) and CD10/CD68/FXIIIA (+).* **(Right)** *H&E shows deep dermal and subcutaneous involvement by a cellular spindle cell tumor with honeycombing adipose tissue entrapment. These tumors are more cellular than DM, lack the stromal desmoplasia, and are S100(-)/CD34(+).*

KEY FACTS

TERMINOLOGY

- Uncommon variant of conventional melanoma that looks deceptively benign

CLINICAL ISSUES

- Melanoma is not suspected clinically

MICROSCOPIC

- Dome-shaped or verrucous
- Exhibits pseudomaturation
- Increased mitotic activity or proliferation index
- Imparts nevoid appearance on initial examination
- Cells mimic type A nevus cells
- Can also mimic lymphocytes

ANCILLARY TESTS

- Immunostaining for Ki-67 (MIB-1) to determine proliferation index (> 5-10% supports diagnosis)

TOP DIFFERENTIAL DIAGNOSES

- Atypical melanocytic nevus
- Congenital melanocytic nevus
- Combined melanocytic nevus

DIAGNOSTIC CHECKLIST

- Finding 1 dermal mitotic figure alone usually does not justify diagnosis of melanoma, especially if superficial; however, it indicates need to look for other clues to support diagnosis of melanoma
- Nevoid melanoma is classic diagnostic trap
- Diagnosis is not infrequently made retrospectively after appearance of metastases
- Look for sheet-like growth pattern in dermis
- Beware of hypercellular areas in dermis
- Search for lack of cellular dispersion at bottom of lesion
- Examine for mitoses, especially multiple, deep, or atypical forms

Small, Nevoid Appearance

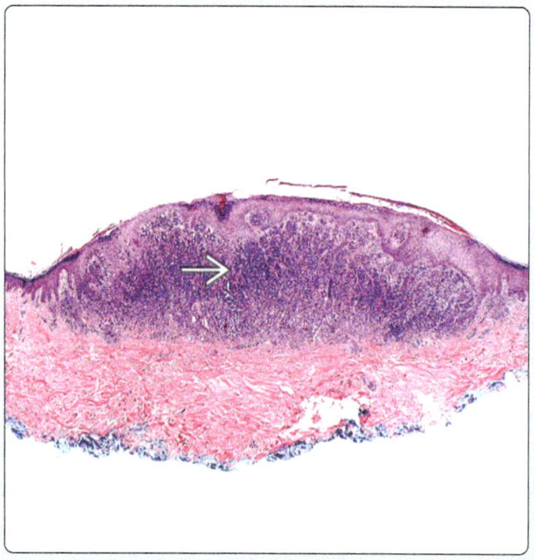

Numerous Mitotic Figures

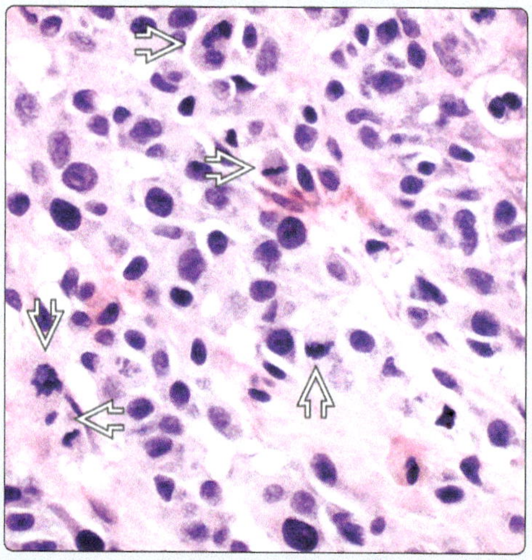

(Left) *Nevoid melanoma is deceptively symmetrical, mimicking an intradermal nevus on low-power examination. The only clue is hypercellularity (blue appearance) ➡ and lack of maturation, which should invoke a closer scrutiny.* **(Right)** *On high-power examination, numerous mitotic figures ➡ are easily found in this nevoid melanoma. This finding is usually surprising given the small size and symmetry on low-power examination.*

Deceptive Symmetry

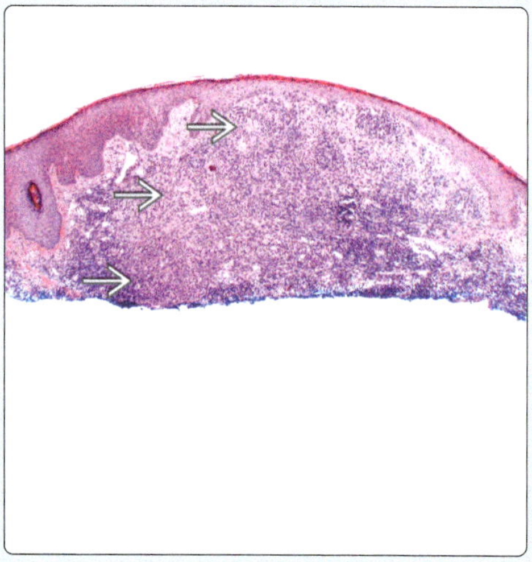

Lack of Maturation

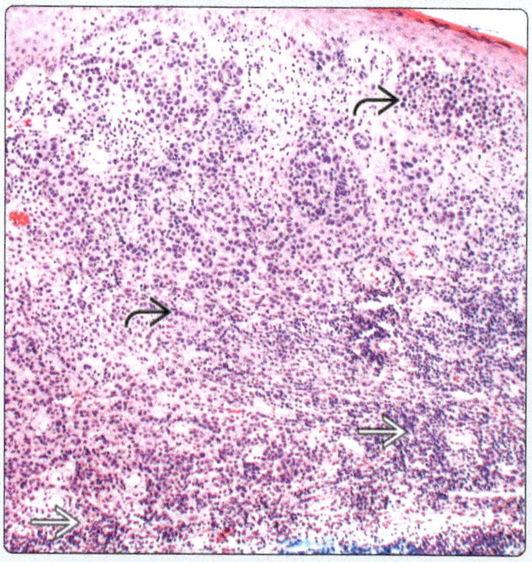

(Left) *Low-power examination shows a deceptively symmetrical-appearing compound, predominantly intradermal proliferation, mimicking a nevus. There is lack of maturation with increasing dermal depth ➡ and central hypercellularity.* **(Right)** *Higher magnification shows that the cells are hyperchromatic staining ⇨ and do not show definite evidence of maturation with dermal descent. Note also the relatively dense surrounding lymphoid infiltrate ➡. There is an atypical component focally seen.*

TERMINOLOGY

Synonyms

- Some cases have been described as "minimal deviation melanoma," but this term is very controversial and should be avoided

Definitions

- Uncommon variant of melanoma that shows histological features mimicking a nevus

ETIOLOGY/PATHOGENESIS

Environmental Exposure

- Likely solar/UV radiation related, similar to most types of melanoma

CLINICAL ISSUES

Presentation

- Occurs in wide age range
- Can be ubiquitous, but occurs more frequently on back and extremities
- Dome-shaped papule or nodule or verrucous lesion
- Often not recognized clinically as melanoma
  - Can resemble nevus or basal cell carcinoma

Treatment

- Surgical approaches
  - Complete excision with clear margins
  - Sentinel lymph node biopsy often performed for staging, especially if lesion is thicker than 1.0 mm or
    - Level IV
    - Ulcerated
    - Exhibits dermal mitotic figures

Prognosis

- Similar to conventional melanoma
- Determined by AJCC staging, especially depth of invasion (Breslow depth), ulceration, and mitotic activity

MICROSCOPIC

Histologic Features

- At scanning magnification, there are 2 variants
  - Verrucous or papillated
    - Mimics polypoid intradermal melanocytic nevus
  - Flat or dome-shaped
    - Mimics ordinary intradermal or compound melanocytic nevus
- Imparts nevoid appearance on initial examination
  - Cells mimic type A nevus cells
  - Can also mimic lymphocytes
- Tightly packed, it forms sheets of relatively banal-appearing nevoid cells
  - Hypercellular
  - Sheets, not nests, are often present
- Slightly asymmetric
- Predominantly intradermal
- May exhibit pseudomaturation with increasing dermal depth
  - At low-power examination, it may appear that intradermal cells mature
  - However, atypia and mitotic figures should be identified at high magnification

Cytologic Features

- Abundant eosinophilic cytoplasm
- Round to oval vesicular nuclei
- Prominent nucleoli seen at high magnification
- Nuclear pleomorphism, best appreciated at high magnification
- Mitotic activity present, often deep within lesion
- Atypical mitotic figures may be seen

DIFFERENTIAL DIAGNOSIS

Atypical Melanocytic Nevus

- Usually compound lesion with shouldering
- No sheeting
- Lack of prominent nucleoli and mitotic activity

Congenital Melanocytic Nevus

- Band-like proliferation of cells surrounding adnexal structures
- Matures properly with increasing dermal depth

Combined Melanocytic Nevus

- May show mixture of type A nevus cells with other cell types
  - Type B or C nevus cells
- Matures properly with increasing dermal depth

DIAGNOSTIC CHECKLIST

Clinically Relevant Pathologic Features

- Finding 1 dermal mitotic figure alone usually does not justify diagnosis of melanoma, especially if superficial in non-sundamaged skin; however, it indicates need to look for other clues to support diagnosis of melanoma
- Nevoid melanoma is classic diagnostic trap
  - Diagnosis is not infrequently made retrospectively after appearance of metastases

Pathologic Interpretation Pearls

- Look for sheet-like growth pattern in dermis
- Beware of hypercellular areas in dermis
- Search for lack of cellular dispersion at bottom of lesion
- Examine for mitoses, especially multiple, deep, or atypical forms

SELECTED REFERENCES

1. Diwan AH et al: Nevoid melanoma. Clin Lab Med. 31(2):243-53, 2011
2. Massi G et al: Histological Diagnosis of Nevi and Melanoma. New York: Springer-Verlag, 2004
3. Zembowicz A et al: Morphological analysis of nevoid melanoma: a study of 20 cases with a review of the literature. Am J Dermatopathol. 23(3):167-75, 2001
4. McNutt NS: "Triggered trap": nevoid malignant melanoma. Semin Diagn Pathol. 15(3):203-9, 1998
5. McNutt NS et al: Nevoid malignant melanoma: morphologic patterns and immunohistochemical reactivity. J Cutan Pathol. 22(6):502-17, 1995
6. Wong TY et al: Nevoid melanoma: a clinicopathological study of seven cases of malignant melanoma mimicking spindle and epithelioid cell nevus and verrucous dermal nevus. Hum Pathol. 26(2):171-9, 1995
7. Blessing K et al: Verrucous naevoid and keratotic malignant melanoma: a clinico-pathological study of 20 cases. Histopathology. 23(5):453-8, 1993
8. Muhlbauer JE et al: Minimal deviation melanoma: a histologic variant of cutaneous malignant melanoma in its vertical growth phase. J Invest Dermatol. 80 Suppl:63s-65s, 1983

Symmetrical, Dome-Shaped Papule in Nevoid Malignant Melanoma

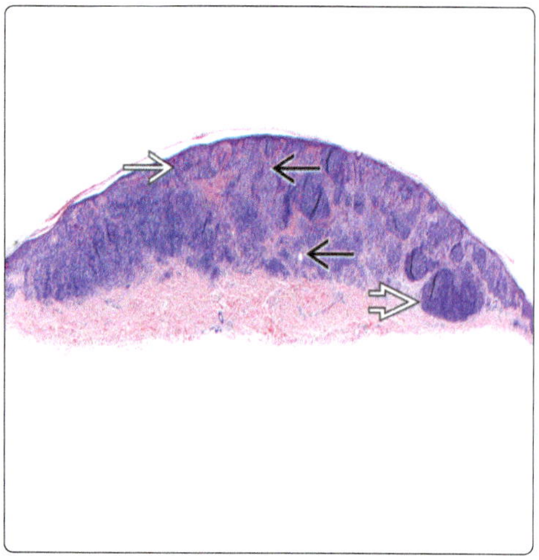

Lack of Maturation in Nevoid Malignant Melanoma

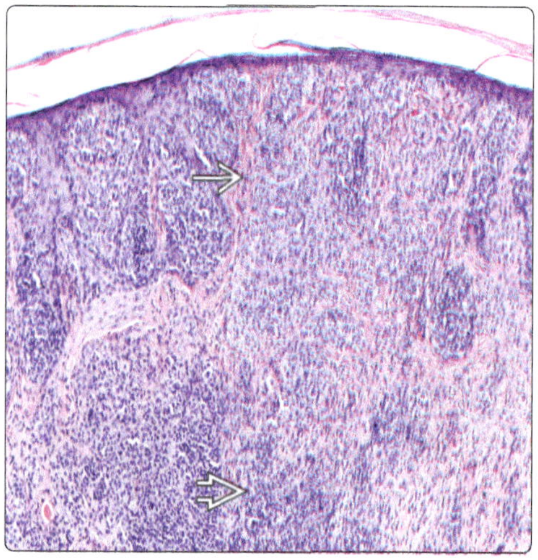

(Left) *Another case of nevoid melanoma is depicted. There is a junctional component and nodular growth on the right side of the lesion. There is lack of maturation with increasing dermal depth.* **(Right)** *Lack of maturation is defined as failure of nevus cells to get smaller as one moves from the top to the bottom of the lesion. In addition, there is nuclear hyperchromasia that remains.*

Mitotic Figure in Nevoid Malignant Melanoma

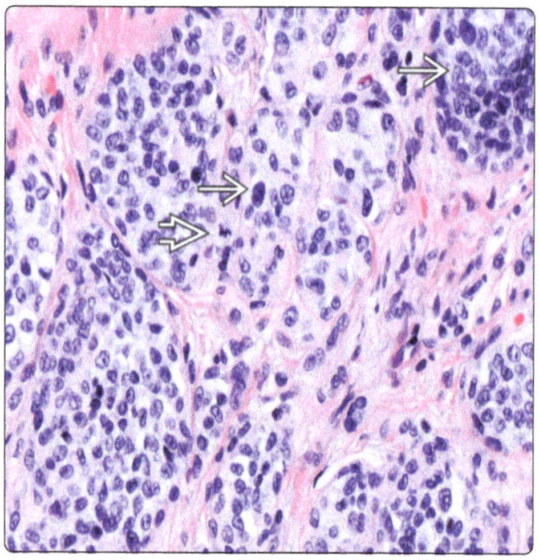

Dermal Mitosis in Nevoid Melanoma

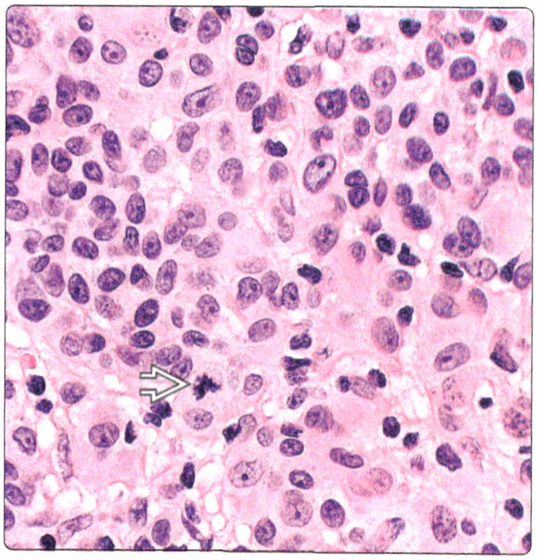

(Left) *Although there is a perception of symmetry and small size, an intradermal mitotic figure can be found, an ominous sign of nevoid melanoma. Moreover, there is focal nuclear pleomorphism.* **(Right)** *High magnification shows large cells with eosinophilic cytoplasm, and a mitotic figure is seen deep in the lesion. Although junctional mitoses can be seen, intradermal mitosis (even 1) with lack of maturation should raise concern for nevoid melanoma.*

Deceptively Small Nevoid Malignant Melanoma Example

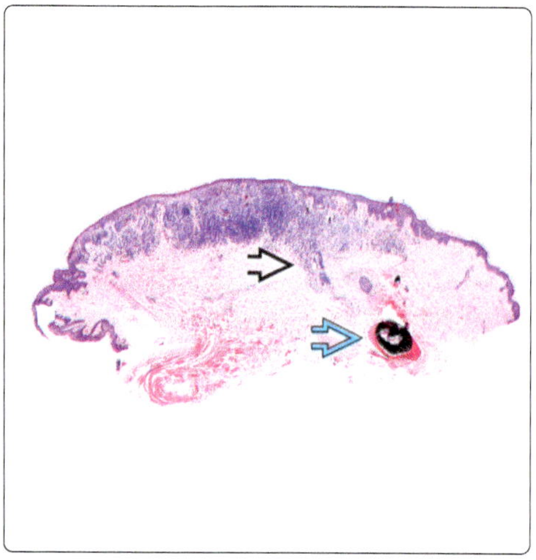

Lack of Maturation in Nevoid Malignant Melanoma

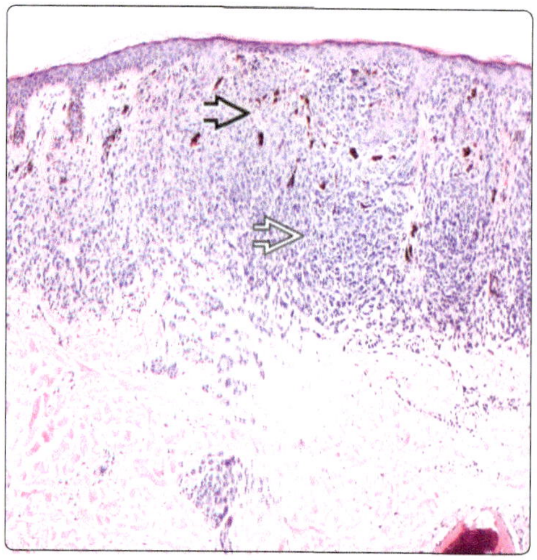

(Left) *Another nevoid melanoma shows a symmetrical, small melanocytic tumor with some congenital features (condensation of melanocytes around adnexa). There is an incidental osteoma cutis.* **(Right)** *A medium-power examination of the previous lesion shows hyperchromasia and dysmaturation with increasing dermal depth. There is marked uneven, melanin incontinence throughout the dermis.*

Nuclear Hyperchromasia & Pleomorphism in Nevoid Malignant Melanoma

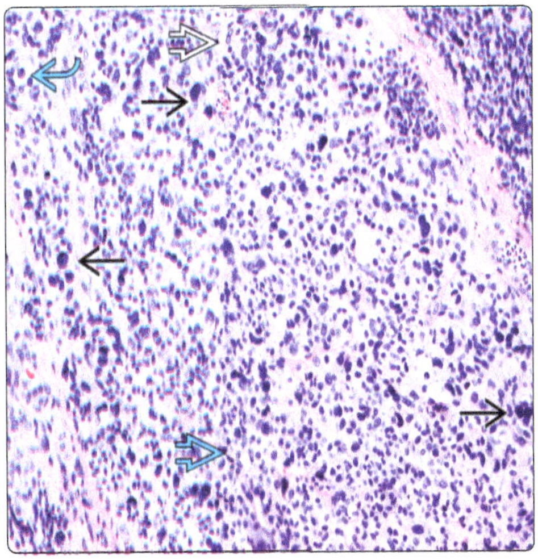

Nevoid Malignant Melanoma Presenting as Ulcerated Papule

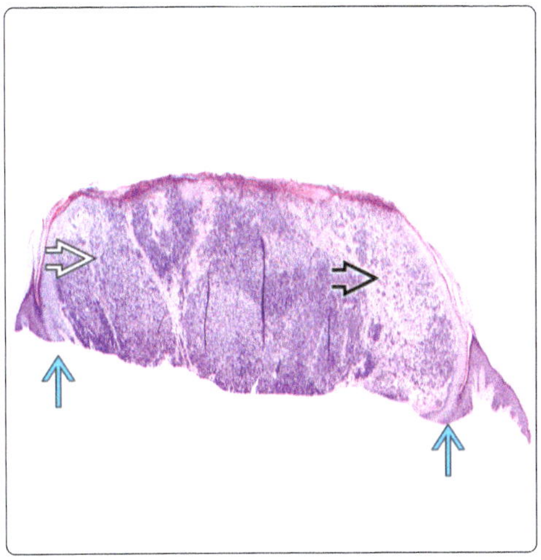

(Left) *Examining the lesion from top to bottom reveals dysmaturation with increasing dermal depth. Moreover, there is a significant nuclear pleomorphism. Also found are apoptotic bodies, but no sheet-like necrosis is found. There were mitotic figures in other fields (not shown).* **(Right)** *This lesion is somewhat asymmetrical, where it is nodular on the left and more nested on the right side of the lesion. Note the collarette formation and lack of radial growth phase.*

Nevoid Malignant Melanoma With Prominent Dysmaturation

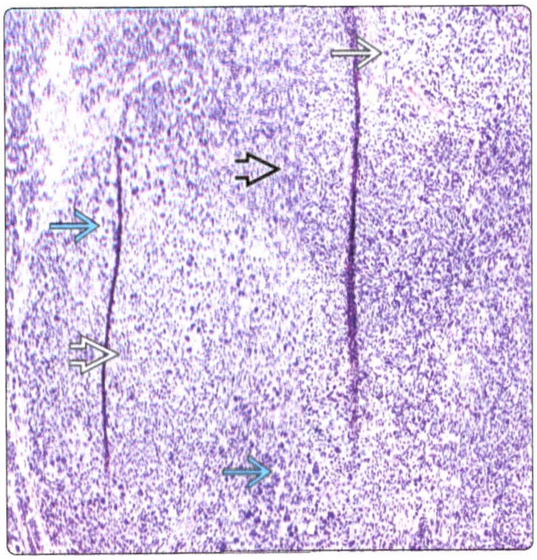

Hypercellular Area

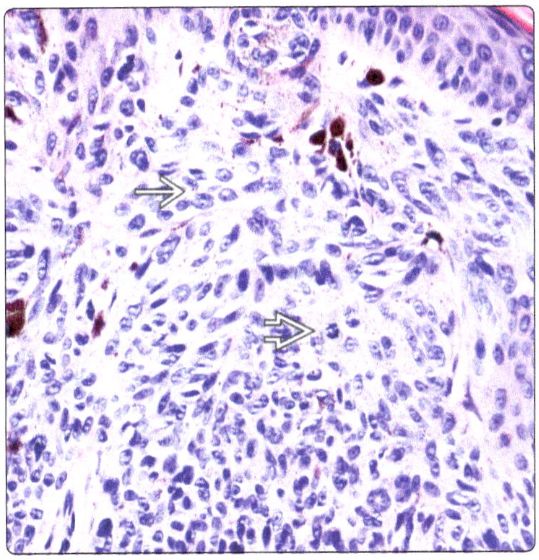

(Left) *There is significant dysmaturation with increasing dermal depth. Note the vaguely pale nodular growth on the lower left and upper right. The area in between appears more hyperchromatic. Within the pale nodule, there is marked nuclear pleomorphism.* **(Right)** *The hypercellular areas need to be closely examined for the presence of mitotic figure(s). There is a short, spindled to epithelioid morphology with open chromatin and conspicuous nucleoli.*

Ki-67 Immunohistochemistry in Nevoid Malignant Melanoma

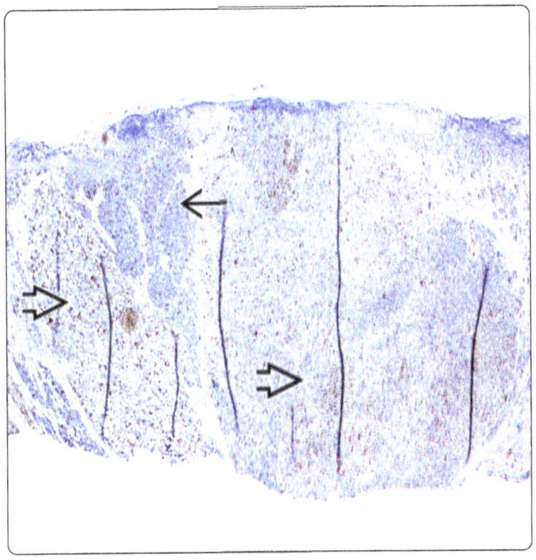

High Labeling Index in Nevoid Malignant Melanoma

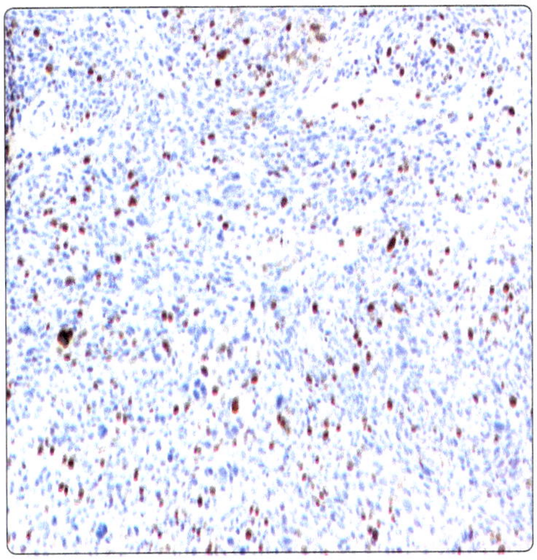

(Left) *Ki-67 immunohistochemistry can be helpful in lesions where mitotic figures are not readily identified. This lesion shows a surprisingly high mitotic index, even at this low-power examination. Note there are proliferation hot spots compared to others.* **(Right)** *Labeling index is defined as the percentage of positive tumor nuclei out of the total tumor nuclei. Typically, an index higher than 10-15% is considered worrisome for melanoma.*

Acral Lentiginous Melanoma

KEY FACTS

TERMINOLOGY

- Acral melanoma that grows in lentiginous pattern
- Acral lentiginous melanoma (ALM)

CLINICAL ISSUES

- < 5% of all malignant melanomas
- Most often on sole of foot or subungual region
- Most frequently reported symptoms are change in size, bleeding, change in color, and becoming raised or nodular
- Relatively uncommon in Caucasians, but most common subtype of melanomas in Asians and Africans

MICROSCOPIC

- Lentiginous proliferation of atypical melanocytes with rare pagetoid scatter
- ALM in situ may present with very few atypical melanocytes
- Nesting at dermal-epidermal junction
  - Rare to absent in early lesions, prominent and confluent in late lesions
  - Nests are irregular in size and shape, randomly alternate with single melanocytes
- Cells show elongated, ovoid hyperchromatic nuclei with little cytoplasm
- Elongated, ovoid shape with little cytoplasm

TOP DIFFERENTIAL DIAGNOSES

- Acral melanocytic nevus
- Spindle cell melanoma
- Clinical differential
  - Subungual hematoma caused by trauma (talon noir)
  - Tinea nigra (darkly pigmented macule with irregular borders)

DIAGNOSTIC CHECKLIST

- Early lesions are difficult to diagnose
- Very few neoplastic melanocytes may be present
- Exercise caution when evaluating partially sampled lesions

Acral Melanoma Presenting as Unevenly Pigmented Plaque

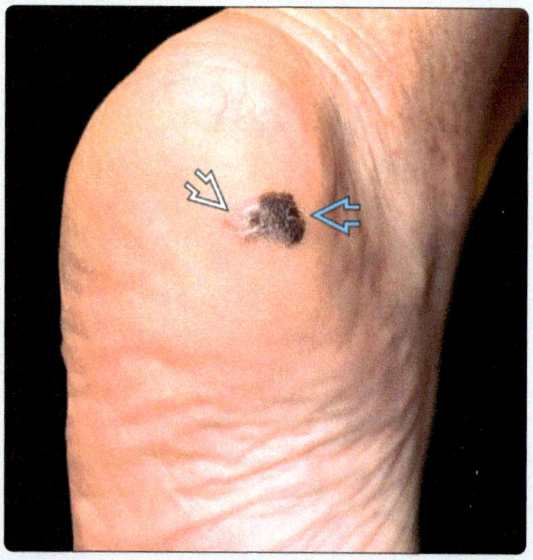

Early Lentiginous Growth in ALM

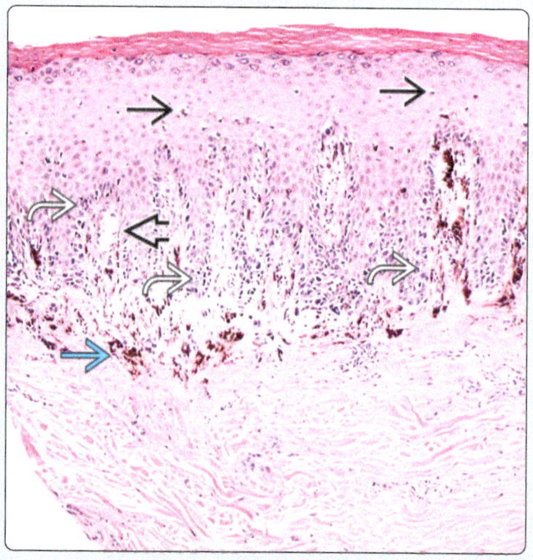

(Left) *The heel of this patient shows a dark brown plaque with early depigmentation and an erythematous rim. The lesion has a sharp border on the medial aspect. (Courtesy J. Finch, MD.)* **(Right)** *Lentiginous growth of atypical melanocytes is seen in this early in situ lesion. Only rare upward scatter of atypical melanocytes is identified. A Meissner corpuscle is seen in the dermis. There is marked uneven melanin incontinence.*

Poorly Nested Pattern in ALM

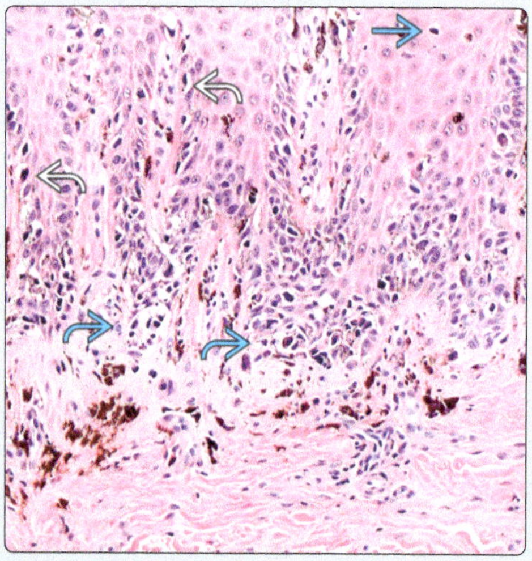

Angulated, Hyperchromatic Nuclei in ALM at High Magnification

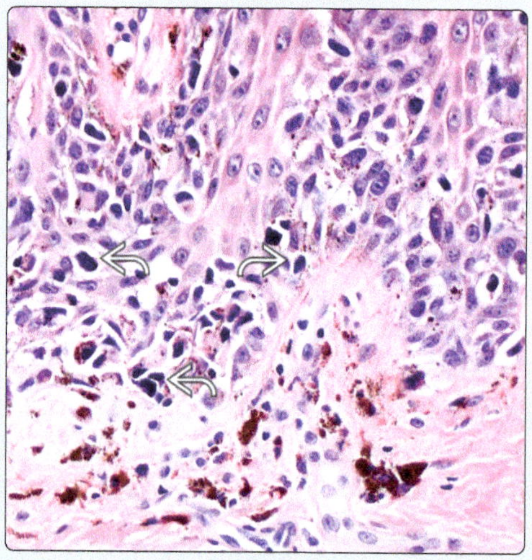

(Left) *There is a lentiginous growth and poorly nested growth pattern identified at the dermal-epidermal junction. There is only limited pagetoid upward scatter, unlike cutaneous melanoma. The finding of lentiginous growth with cytological atypia is sufficient for the diagnosis of melanoma in situ, acrolentiginous type.* **(Right)** *Higher magnification of same lesion shows angulated, hyperchromatic nuclei with scant amounts of cytoplasm. Note the melanocytic hyperplasia has replaced most of the basal keratinocytes.*

TERMINOLOGY

Abbreviations

- Acral lentiginous melanoma (ALM)

Definitions

- Form of cutaneous melanoma that microscopically grows in lentiginous array and occurs on acral sites
  - Palms and soles
  - Digits and subungual regions

CLINICAL ISSUES

Presentation

- < 5% of all malignant melanomas
- More common on sole of foot or in subungual region of big toe or thumb
- Most frequently reported symptoms are change in size, bleeding, change in color, and becoming raised or nodular
  - May remain flat or present as large, pigmented macule
  - Lesion becomes darker and more irregular as it progresses
  - Invasive areas may be associated with hyperkeratotic plaques, papules, nodules, and even ulceration
  - Spreads rapidly
- Average age at diagnosis: 60-70 years
- Relatively uncommon in Caucasians, but most common subtype of melanomas in Asians and Africans

Treatment

- Surgical approaches
  - Wide surgical excision and amputation give comparable survival rates
  - In many cases of subungual melanomas, amputation is preferred due to relative lack of soft tissue between tumor and bone beneath nail

Prognosis

- Compared to other cutaneous melanomas, disease-specific survival rates are lower
  - 5-year melanoma-specific survival rates: 80.3%
  - 10-year melanoma-specific survival rates: 67.5%
- Compared to other melanomas matched for Breslow thickness, prognosis is same

MACROSCOPIC

Dermoscopic Exam

- Shows parallel ridge pattern, where globules may be seen symmetrically along both sides of furrows

Areas of Regression

- Appear as gray-white coloration
- Become extensive in larger, invasive lesions

Epiluminescent Examination

- Differentiates benign from malignant
  - Benign lesions display pigmentation following depressions between dermatoglyphic ridges
  - Melanomas display pigmentation overlying dermatoglyphic ridges

MICROSCOPIC

Histologic Features

- Growth pattern of atypical melanocytes
  - Early lesions
    - Lentiginous array
    - Scattered among basal layer keratinocytes
  - Late lesions
    - Lentiginous array is no longer present
    - Confluent at dermal-epidermal junction
    - Invasion of atypical cells into dermis
- Nesting at dermal-epidermal junction
  - Early lesions
    - Absent to poorly formed
  - Late lesions
    - Prominent and confluent
    - Nests are irregular in size and shape, and they randomly alternate with single melanocytes
- ALM in situ may present with very few atypical melanocytes before progressing to invasive ALM
- Inflammatory response in superficial dermis
  - Lichenoid pattern with areas of subepidermal clefts
  - Leukocytes typically found in dermis except early lesions

Cytologic Features

- Elongated, ovoid shape with little cytoplasm
- Nuclei are
  - Hyperchromatic
  - Vertically oriented
  - Angulated
- Little nucleolar detail
- Pagetoid cells may appear epithelioid
- Invasive cells appear spindled

DIFFERENTIAL DIAGNOSIS

Acral Melanocytic Nevus

- Need to examine entire lesion, especially periphery, to differentiate acral melanocytic nevus from early lesion of ALM

Spindle Cell Melanoma

- Dermal component of ALM is frequently spindle-shaped
- Lacks overlying melanoma in situ with characteristic features of ALM in situ

Clinical Differential

- Tinea nigra (darkly pigmented macule with irregular borders)
- Subungual hematoma caused by trauma (talon noir)

DIAGNOSTIC CHECKLIST

Pathologic Interpretation Pearls

- Early lesions are difficult to diagnose
  - Very few neoplastic melanocytes may be present
- Exercise caution when evaluating partially sampled lesions

SELECTED REFERENCES

1. Wu XC et al: Racial and ethnic variations in incidence and survival of cutaneous melanoma in the United States, 1999-2006. J Am Acad Dermatol. 65(5 Suppl 1):S26-37, 2011

(Left) *The 1st toe exhibits melanoma of the nail matrix in an elderly woman. Note the uneven pigmentation and rough surface* → *of the nail plate. The proximal fold is darkly pigmented* →. **(Right)** *This lesion is located at the medial aspect of the 2nd toe in a young man. Such ulcerated appearance, rapid nodular growth, and acral site may clinically mimic a pyogenic granuloma or a traumatic event. Such lesions, especially in young individuals, should be biopsied to exclude an acral melanoma.*

Clinical Photograph of Subungual ALM

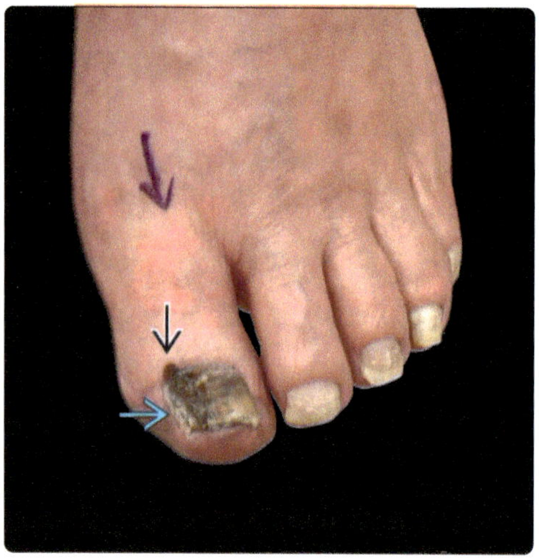

Ulcerated ALM on Toe

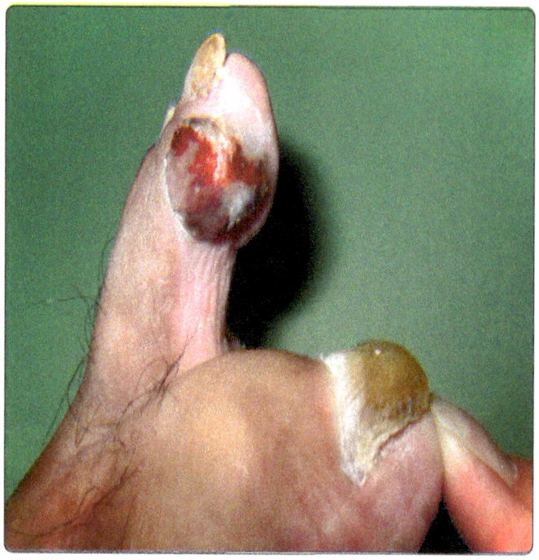

(Left) *Another acral melanoma presents as a darkly, unevenly pigmented patch. Note the darker, hyperkeratotic center* → *with a brown peripheral rim* →. *The border of the peripheral rim is jagged.* **(Right)** *This punch biopsy shows an asymmetrical melanocytic proliferation by virtue of pagetoid upward scatter* → *in one area and dermal invasion in another* →. *There is uneven pigmentation* → *deep within the lesion. Note an artificial area of subepidermal clefting* →.

Clinical Photograph of ALM on Plantar Surface

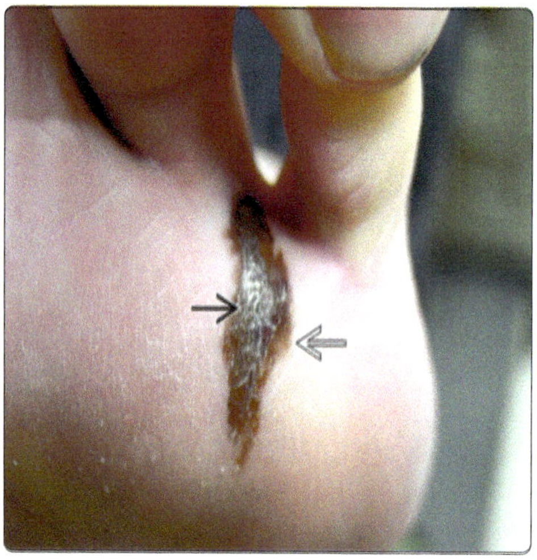

Asymmetrical, Compound ALM at Low Magnification

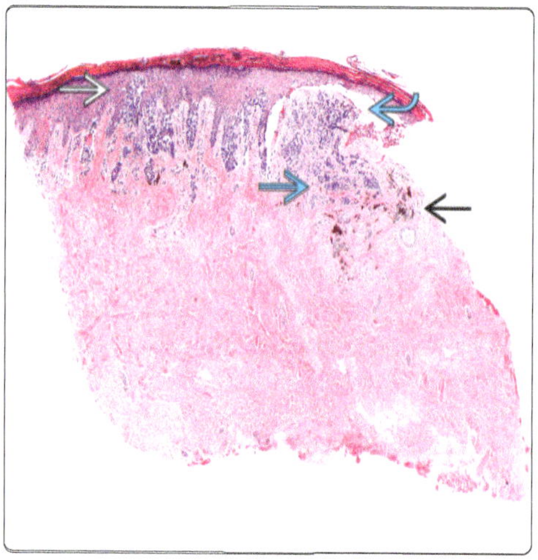

(Left) *There is significant pagetoid upward scatter of melanoma cells* → *throughout all the layers of the acral epidermis. Transepidermal elimination of melanin, seen as pigmented parakeratosis* →, *was also found. Dermal invasion* → *is evident.* **(Right)** *The dermal melanoma cells are cytologically identical to the lentiginous cells by virtue of angulated, polygonal nuclei* →. *The chromatin is open, and nucleoli are conspicuous* →.

Marked Pagetoid Spread and Pigmented Parakeratosis in ALM

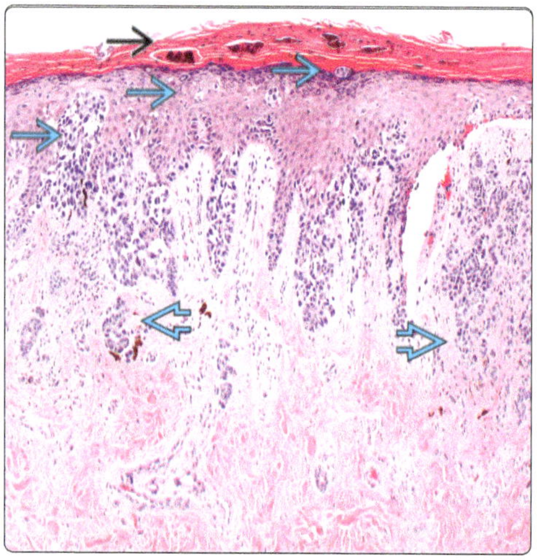

Cytology of Dermal Invasion in ALM at High Magnification

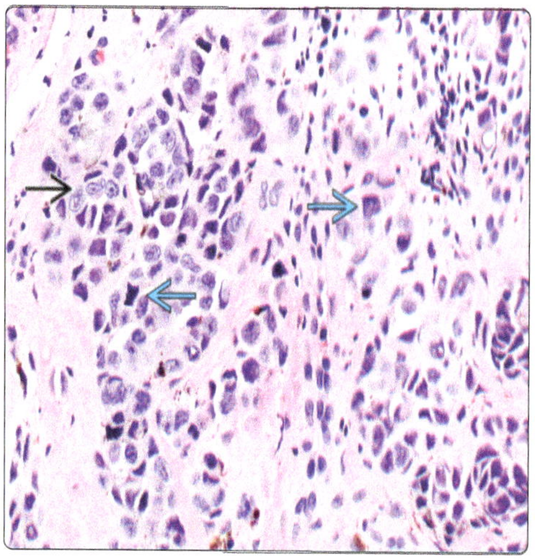

ALM at Low Magnification Showing Nodular Growth

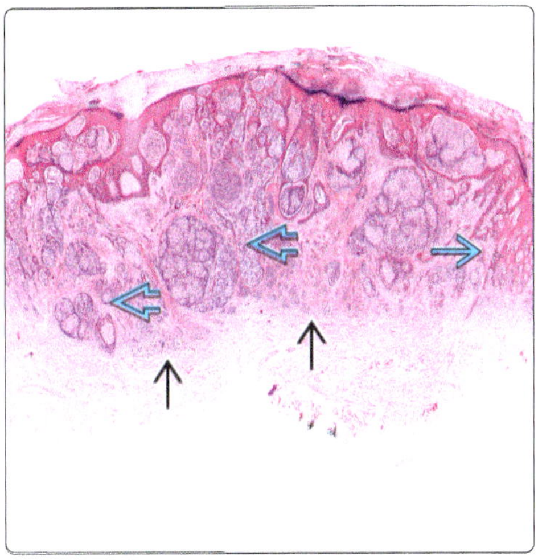

Pagetoid Upward Scatter at Higher Magnification

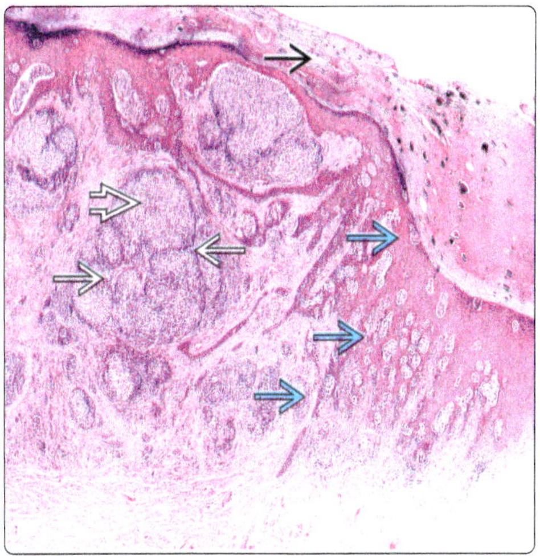

(Left) This acral melanoma is readily diagnosed as it shows significant pagetoid upward scatter ➡ at one edge and an invasive nodular growth ⇨ in the dermis. There are small nests at the advancing edge ➡. (Right) There is a prominent pagetoid upward scatter of melanoma cells ➡ throughout all the layers of the acral epidermis. There are even melanoma cells ➡ in the thick stratum corneum. The dermal component is nodular ⇨ with fibrous septa ⇨.

High Magnification of ALM Showing Fascicular Growth

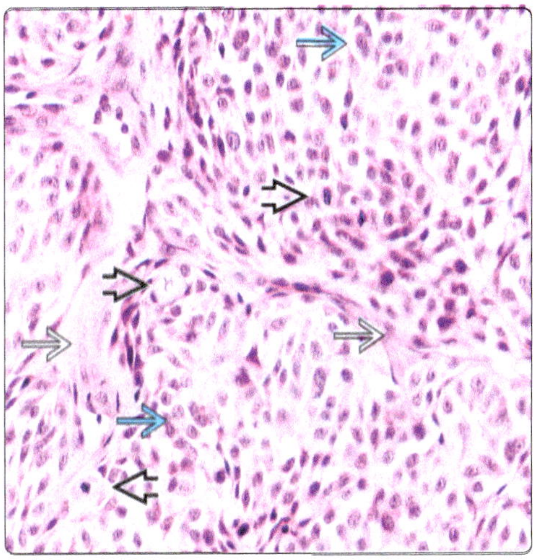

Differential Diagnosis: Acral Melanocytic Nevus

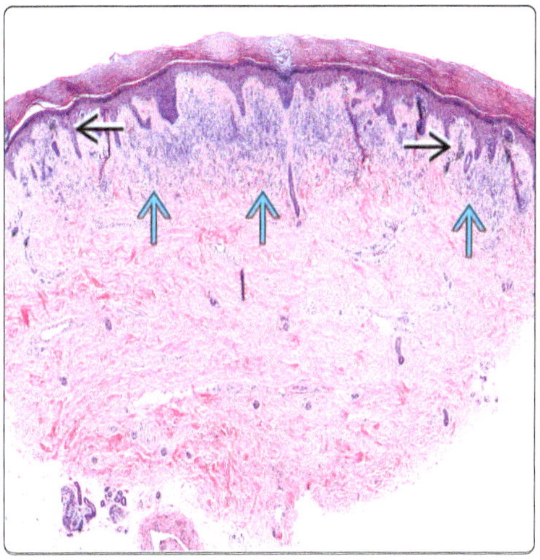

(Left) The dermal nodules, separated by fibrotic trabeculum ⇨, show a vaguely fascicular growth composed of short spindle cells with open chromatin and prominent nucleoli ➡. Mitotic figures ⇨ are evident. (Right) This punch biopsy shows the complete profile of a compound melanocytic nevus, acral type, facilitating its diagnosis. There is a symmetrical intradermal component ➡ with even pigmentation ➡.

Focal Junctional Component in Acral Melanocytic Nevus

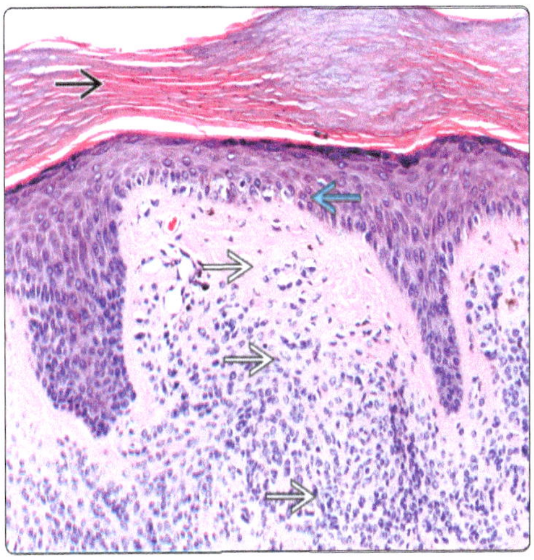

Differential Diagnosis: Acral Junctional Melanocytic Nevus

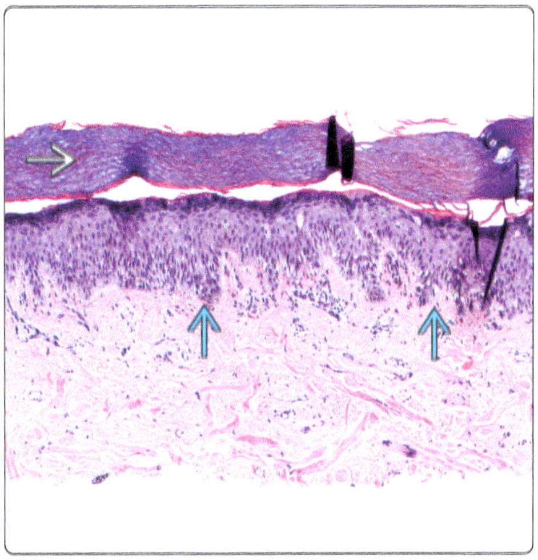

(Left) There is light pigmentation ➡ in the stratum corneum. The junctional component is focally lentiginous ➡ but lacks cytological atypia. The dermal component matures properly with increasing depth ⇨. (Right) There is a thick stratum corneum ⇨ compatible with the acral location. There is a contiguous lentiginous proliferation of melanocytes ➡ without cytological atypia. Periphery of lesion could be visualized in the biopsy, showing a well-circumscribed melanocytic nevus (not shown).

KEY FACTS

TERMINOLOGY

- Malignant neural crest-derived neoplasm with melanocytic differentiation

CLINICAL ISSUES

- Extremely rare, accounting for < 1% of all melanomas
  - Represent < 0.5% of all oral malignancies
- Mean in 6th-7th decades
- M > F (2.5-3:1)
- Hard palate and maxillary alveolus are most common sites of involvement (~ 80%)
- Cervical lymph node metastases reported in > 50% of cases at presentation
- Asymmetric, painless, pigmented lesion with irregular borders
- Radical surgical excision
- Overall, poor prognosis (median: 2 years)

IMAGING

- Oral cavity mass with high T1 signal on MR

MICROSCOPIC

- In situ component with pagetoid spread of single or multiple melanoma cells in superficial epithelium
- Epithelioid or spindle-shaped morphology of melanocytes containing fine melanin granules
  - 15% of oral melanomas have little to no melanin
- 1/3 of cases have bone/cartilage invasion

ANCILLARY TESTS

- **Positive**: S100, SOX10, HMB-45; tyrosinase, melan-A, MITF

TOP DIFFERENTIAL DIAGNOSES

- Spindle cell squamous cell carcinoma, metastatic melanoma, pleomorphic sarcoma

Palatal MM With Satellite Lesions

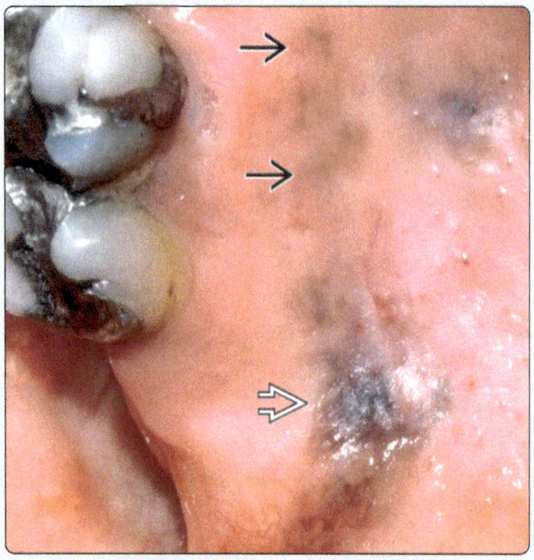

Epithelioid Melanocytes in Nodular MM

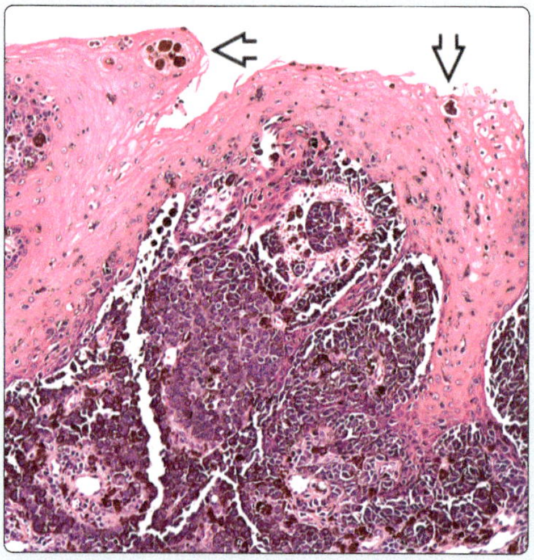

(Left) *Primary mucosal melanoma (MM) of the hard palate presents as a diffuse, patchy area of heavy pigmentation with irregular borders ⇒. Satellite lesions are noted away from the main area of pigmentation →.* **(Right)** *Nodular melanoma of the hard palate shows epithelioid malignant melanocytes, some with melanin pigment, expanded into the lamina propria. Individual melanocytes ⇒ are seen in the upper layers of the mucosa (pagetoid spread).*

Pseudoepitheliomatous Hyperplasia in MM

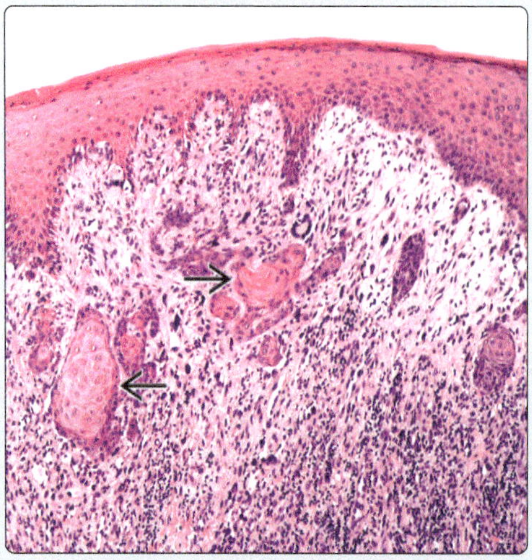

HMB-45 Highlights Melanocytes in MM

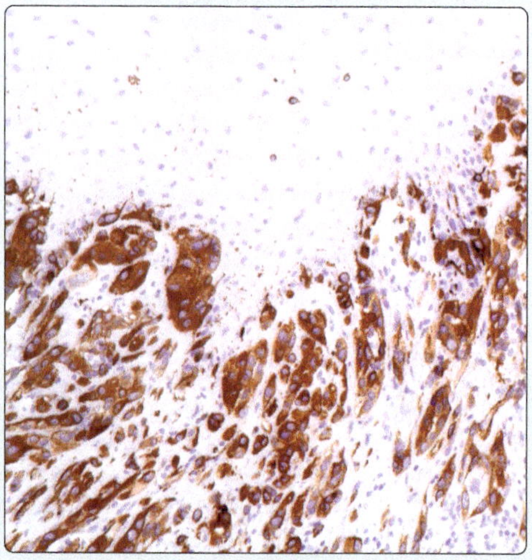

(Left) *There is a concurrent pseudoepitheliomatous hyperplasia → present in association with an atypical melanocytic proliferation. An inflammatory infiltrate is also present. The melanoma may be obscured or missed due to this process.* **(Right)** *HMB-45 immunohistochemistry highlights the melanocytes present both in the basal layer as well as in the submucosa. This is one of the more specific markers for melanoma. It is important to know that staining can be patchy or focal.*

TERMINOLOGY

Definitions

- Malignant neural crest-derived neoplasm with melanocytic differentiation in oral cavity
  - Atypical melanocytes at epithelial-connective tissue interface with upward migration or connective tissue invasion

ETIOLOGY/PATHOGENESIS

Etiology

- Unknown: Not related to preexisting mucosal nevi or physiologic pigmentation
- Increased frequency of *KIT* (c-KIT, CD117) mutations in mucosal melanomas have been reported
  - Mutation not often detected in cutaneous melanomas
- BRAF mutations **not** detected in mucosal melanoma, but seen in cutaneous melanomas

CLINICAL ISSUES

Epidemiology

- Incidence
  - Extremely rare, accounting for < 1% of all melanomas
    - 0.02/100,000 population/year in USA
  - Represent ~ 40% of all head and neck mucosal melanomas
  - Represent < 0.5% of all oral malignancies
  - Unlike cutaneous melanoma, oral melanoma incidence has been stable
- Age
  - Mean: 6th-7th decades; rare in pediatric patients
- Sex
  - M > F (2.5-3:1)
- Ethnicity
  - More common in Japan and western Africa

Site

- Hard palate and maxillary alveolus are most common sites of involvement (~ 80%)
- Remaining 20% include
  - Mandibular gingivae
  - Buccal mucosa
  - Floor of mouth and tongue

Presentation

- Most arise de novo, although 1/3 are preceded by pigmented lesion for few months or years
  - Melanosis reported before development of melanoma
- Asymmetric, painless, pigmented lesion
  - Irregular borders or outlines
  - Black, purple, red, gray
    - 15% of oral melanomas are amelanotic
  - Macular, with nodular areas
- Many patients present at advanced stage with pain, ulceration, loose teeth
- Cervical lymph nodes metastases reported in up to 50% of cases at presentation
  - Lymph node metastases increase when tumor thickness > 5 mm
- Distant metastases seen in ~ 50% of patients at presentation

Treatment

- Surgical approaches
  - Radical surgical excision
    - Clear margins not always possible due to adjacent vital structures, resulting in local control rates of < 50%
  - Some institutions recommend regional lymph node dissection, even in clinically negative neck
- Adjuvant therapy
  - No clear cut evidence that chemotherapy or immunotherapy for oral melanoma provides any survival benefits
    - Generally used for palliative purposes
  - Not recommended as single modality treatment
- Radiation
  - May provide prolonged palliation but does not appear to provide any survival benefits

Prognosis

- Overall, poor prognosis
  - Median survival: 2 years
  - 5-year survival: 5-10%
- High rates of metastases to liver, brain, and lung
- Worse prognosis suggested by
  - Thickness > 5 mm
  - Vascular invasion
  - Necrosis
  - Significant pleomorphism
  - Older age
  - High stage

IMAGING

MR Findings

- Best imaging study is multiplanar MR
- Oral cavity mass with high T1 signal on MR
  - Melanotic melanomas show increased signal due to melanin, free radicals, metal ions, and hemorrhage, giving high or intermediate T1 signal

MACROSCOPIC

General Features

- Brown to black pigmented lesion with irregular borders
- Flat macule extends laterally (radial growth phase); nodular lesion (vertical growth phase)
  - Some oral melanomas lack radial growth phase
- Satellite lesions of melanoma are common

Sections to Be Submitted

- Bone &/or cartilage for staging

Size

- Range: Up to 4 cm generally

MICROSCOPIC

Histologic Features

- Radial growth phase similar to junctional lentiginous melanoma

Immunohistochemistry

Antibody	Reactivity	Staining Pattern	Comment
S100	Positive	Nuclear & cytoplasmic	Diffuse and strong
SOX10	Positive	Nuclear	Diffuse and strong
HMB-45	Positive	Cytoplasmic	Most tumor cells positive
Tyrosinase	Positive	Cytoplasmic	Variably reactive in most cases
Melan-A103	Positive	Cytoplasmic	Variably reactive in most cases
MITF	Positive	Nuclear	Positive in most cases
CD117	Positive	Cytoplasmic	Isolated tumor cells positive
NSE	Positive	Cytoplasmic	Variably present in many cases
Desmin	Negative		
CD45RB	Negative		
CK-PAN	Negative		

- Pagetoid spread (in situ): Single or multiple melanoma cells within epithelium
- Atypical melanocytes in basal layer spreading laterally
- Invasion of melanoma cells into lamina propria
- Prominent dendritic processes may be seen
- May have pseudoepitheliomatous hyperplasia

- Nodular growth phase
  - Epithelioid or spindle-shaped morphology to melanocytes containing fine melanin granules
    - 15% of oral melanomas have little to no melanin
  - 1/3 of cases have bone/cartilage invasion
  - Vascular and perineural invasion not readily noted
  - Mitoses tend to be infrequent but are increased in invasive tumors
  - Pleomorphic cells with atypical mitoses
    - Polygonal, spindled, epithelioid, small cell
    - Intranuclear cytoplasmic inclusions, prominent nucleoli
  - Squamous surface ulceration or atrophy is common
  - Pseudoepitheliomatous hyperplasia adjacent to tumor may be seen

ANCILLARY TESTS

Histochemistry

- Melanin can be highlighted with Fontana-Masson or Schmorl stains

Immunohistochemistry

- **Positive**: S100, SOX10, HMB-45, tyrosinase, Melan-A, MITF, vimentin
- **Negative**: Pan-cytokeratin, myogenic markers, epithelial membrane antigen

Genetic Testing

- *NRAS* and *KIT* mutations have been identified in mucosal melanomas
  - May be useful for targeted therapies

DIFFERENTIAL DIAGNOSIS

Spindle Cell Squamous Cell Carcinoma

- Should be considered when there is no pigmentation
- Junctional origin frequently present
- High-grade tumors, significant pleomorphism, increased mitoses
- **Positive**: Up to 70% epithelial markers, p63, p40; **negative**: Melanoma markers

Pleomorphic Sarcoma

- High-grade spindled cell tumor, lacking surface origin or involvement
- By definition, lacks melanomocytic and epithelial markers

Metastatic Melanoma

- Extremely rare, with very few reported cases
- Most common: Tongue, buccal mucosa, lip
- Clinical history required
- *BRAF* or *KIT* useful in selected cases, but not IHC

Clinical Differential Diagnosis

- May be clinically worrisome for mucosal melanoma, but can be easily separated by histologic examination
  - **Oral nevi**: Intraoral nevi usually single and quite small
  - **Melanoacanthoma**: Rapid growth of this benign lesion usually dictates biopsy to rule out melanoma
  - **Physiologic pigmentation**: Generally diffuse
  - **Smoker's melanosis**
  - **Amalgam tattoo**
  - **Medication-related pigmentation**: Chloroquine and minocycline can cause oral pigmentation
  - **Systemic diseases**: Addison disease, Peutz-Jeghers syndrome, Laugier-Hunziker syndrome

SELECTED REFERENCES

1. López F et al: Update on primary head and neck mucosal melanoma. Head Neck. Jan;38(1):147-55, 2014
2. Prasad ML et al: Prognostic significance of regulators of cell cycle and apoptosis, p16(INK4a), p53, and bcl-2 in primary mucosal melanomas of the head and neck. Head Neck Pathol. 6(2):184-90, 2012
3. Shuman AG et al: Mucosal melanoma of the head and neck: predictors of prognosis. Arch Otolaryngol Head Neck Surg. 137(4):331-7, 2011
4. Moreno MA et al: Management of mucosal melanomas of the head and neck: did we make any progress? Curr Opin Otolaryngol Head Neck Surg. 18(2):101-6, 2010
5. Bachar G et al: Mucosal melanomas of the head and neck: experience of the Princess Margaret Hospital. Head Neck. 30(10):1325-31, 2008
6. Beadling C et al: KIT gene mutations and copy number in melanoma subtypes. Clin Cancer Res. 14(21):6821-8, 2008

PET Scan of Palatal Melanoma

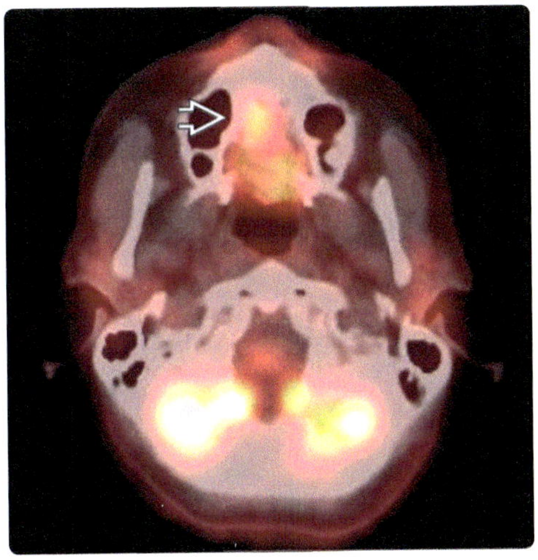

Palatal MM

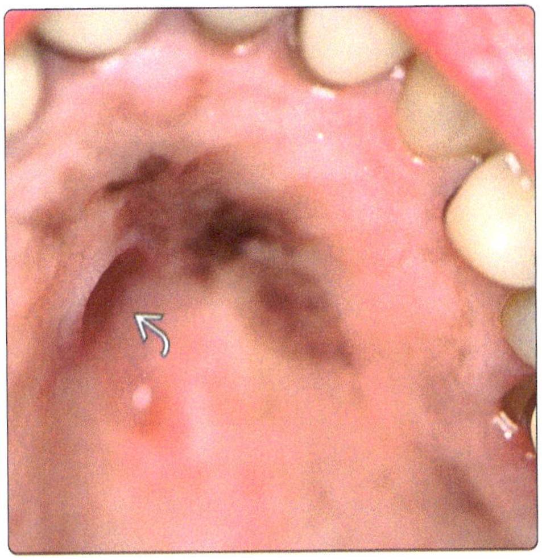

(Left) *This PET scan of a palatal melanoma shows FDG uptake ➡ in the region corresponding to the pigmentation seen clinically. Although this patient had no cervical metastases, up to 75% of oral melanomas have metastases at presentation.* **(Right)** *Image shows a 65-year-old woman with newly diagnosed palatal mucosal melanoma status post punch biopsy ➡. The hard palate and maxillary alveolus account for 80% of reported cases. Most cases are pigmented, although 15% of oral melanomas are amelanotic.*

Recurrent MM

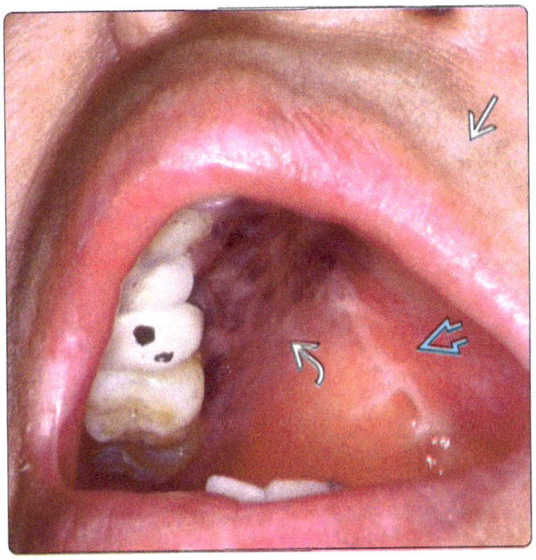

Lentiginous Junctional Growth Pattern in MM

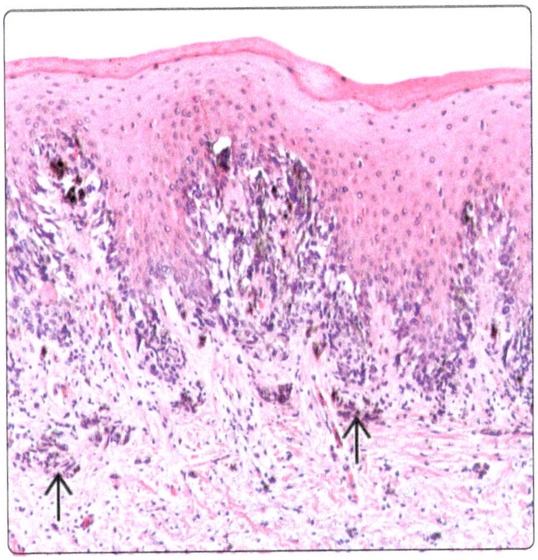

(Left) *This patient had a hemimaxillectomy for palatal mucosal melanoma. The surgical scar is evident ➡ as is lack of teeth in this area resulting in lip asymmetry ➡. The recurrence presents as numerous satellite lesions on the contralateral palate ➡.* **(Right)** *The majority of the proliferation in this melanoma is noted at the epithelial-stromal junction. However, isolated nests of atypical melanocytes ➡ are noted within the superficial region of the stroma. Inflammatory cells are inconspicuous.*

Lentiginous Junctional Pattern in MM

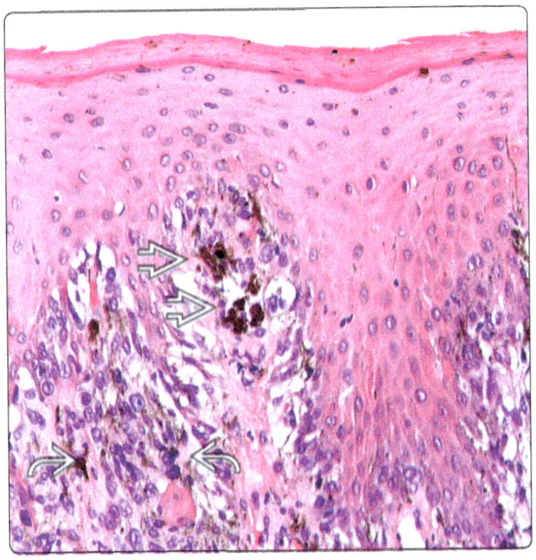

Strong, Diffuse S100 Staining in MM

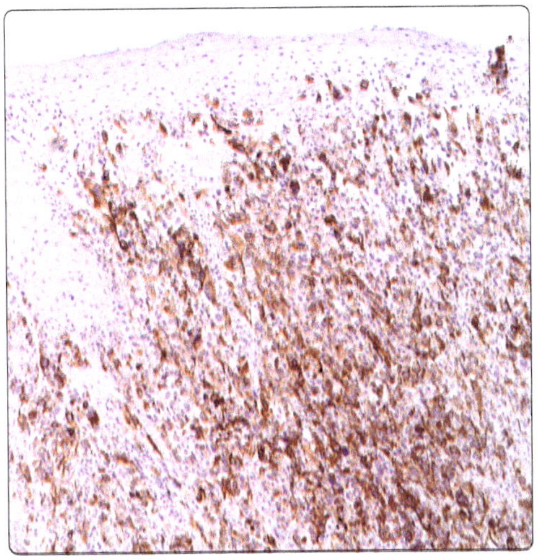

(Left) *High-power histology shows junctional lentiginous melanoma of the hard palate with numerous atypical melanocytes present in the basal epithelium ➡ with invasion into the superficial submucosa ➡.* **(Right)** *S100 shows very strong and diffuse nuclear and cytoplasmic reactivity in the neoplastic cells as they expand from the surface epithelium into the stroma. Depth of invasion is difficult to assess for oral melanoma.*

KEY FACTS

TERMINOLOGY

- Mucosal malignant melanoma
- Vulvar melanoma, vaginal melanoma, penile melanoma

ETIOLOGY/PATHOGENESIS

- *KIT* mutations and *NRAS* mutations are most frequent
  - Opportunity for targeted therapy

CLINICAL ISSUES

- Rare lesions: Comprise only 2% or less of melanomas
- Vulva (most frequent site in females)
- Glans penis (most common site in males)
- Macular to nodular to polypoid lesions
- Usually pigmented brown to black
  - Foci of regression appear red, gray, or white
  - Amelanotic lesions may occur

MICROSCOPIC

- Different histological variants may affect genital area
  - Lentiginous type
  - Superficial spreading type
  - Nodular invasive type
  - Desmoplastic/neurotropic melanoma
- Melanoma in situ typically is broad, poorly circumscribed, asymmetric lesion
- Invasive melanoma shows lack of maturation with descent, dermal mitoses

TOP DIFFERENTIAL DIAGNOSES

- Atypical genital nevi
  - Younger patients
  - Architectural and cytologic atypia
  - Focal pagetoid spread
  - Maturation with descent (deep mitoses are absent)
- Nevi associated with lichen sclerosus
  - Show features reminiscent of recurrent nevus phenomenon

Melanoma Affecting Glans Penis

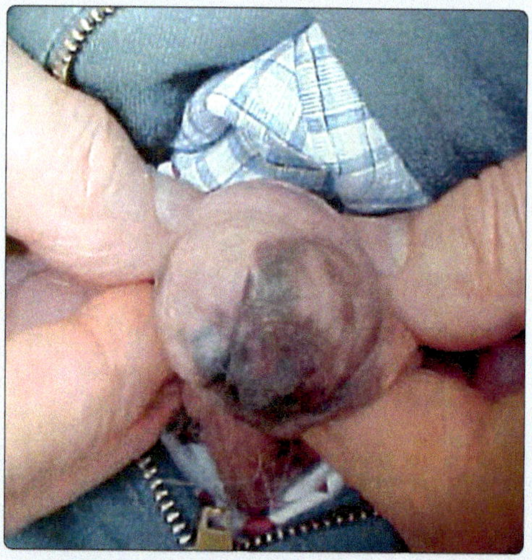

Lentiginous Melanoma In Situ Component

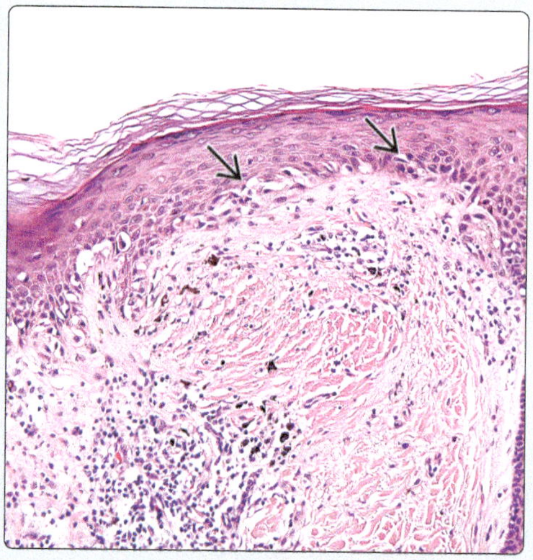

(Left) *Clinical photograph shows a mucosal melanoma on the glans penis of an elderly patient. Histologic examination showed a deeply invasive nodular type melanoma with foci of regression.* **(Right)** *Mucosal melanoma in situ of the vulva shows a lentiginous → and confluent pattern of growth without significant pagetoid spread (similar to lentigo maligna).*

Mucosal Melanoma With Pseudoglandular Structures

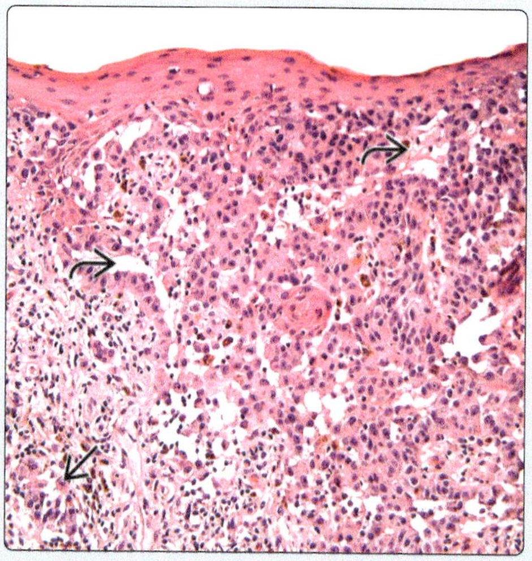

Nodular Melanoma of Vulva

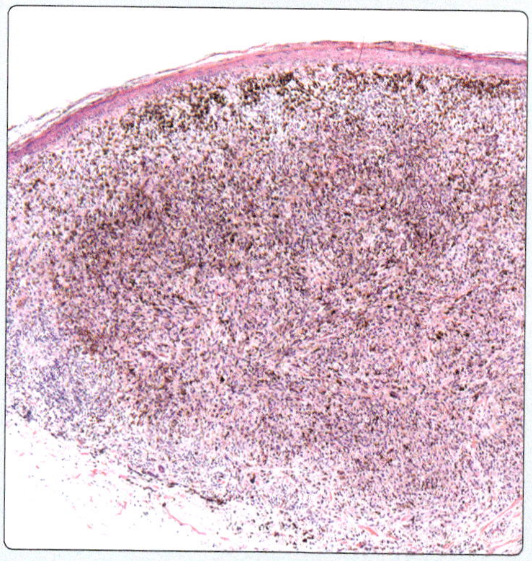

(Left) *This invasive mucosal melanoma shows dyscohesive growth of epithelioid melanocytes mimicking glandular structures ↪ seen in Paget disease. Note the focal invasive component →.* **(Right)** *This is a nodular invasive melanoma of the labia majora with prominent, diffuse pigmentation. Deep lesions such as this tend to have a bad prognosis.*

TERMINOLOGY

Abbreviations

- Mucosal malignant melanoma (MMM)

Synonyms

- Vulvar melanoma, vaginal melanoma, penile melanoma

Definitions

- In situ or invasive melanoma on genitalia

ETIOLOGY/PATHOGENESIS

Unknown in Most Cases

- Spectrum of somatic mutations in MMM differs from malignant melanoma (MM) arising on sun-exposed skin and are more similar to those seen in acral MM
  - *KIT* mutations (~ 30% of cases)
  - *NRAS* mutations (~ 20% of cases)
  - *BRAF* mutations are almost always absent
  - High frequency of gene amplifications throughout genome
- 6% are associated with nevi
- Family history and genetic susceptibility

CLINICAL ISSUES

Epidemiology

- Incidence
  - Rare
    - ~ 2% of all melanomas in females
    - Even less frequent in males
- Age
  - Most in 6th to 7th decades

Site

- Females
  - Vulva, vagina, and cervix
    - Labia majora and clitoris (most frequent sites)
- Males
  - Penis and scrotum
    - Glans (most frequent site)

Presentation

- Flat to nodular to polypoid lesions
- Irregular to well-defined borders
- Usually pigmented, brown or black
  - 27% of vulvar MM may be amelanotic
    - Such lesions mimic squamous cell carcinoma or Paget disease
- Areas of regression may appear red, gray, or white

Treatment

- Surgical approaches
  - Surgical excision (complete excision of early lesions associated with best outcome)
  - Sentinel node biopsy for staging purposes
- Adjuvant therapy
  - Chemotherapy or immunotherapy (no definitive evidence of improved survival)
  - Molecularly targeted therapy (under investigation)

Prognosis

- Tumor thickness is most important parameter
- MMM has poorer prognosis compared to cutaneous melanoma
- Published 5-year survival for mucosal melanoma varies between 17-55%
  - Vulva melanoma has been found to have better prognosis than vaginal and penile in recent publication

MACROSCOPIC

General Features

- Few millimeters to several centimeters papular to nodular lesion

MICROSCOPIC

Histologic Features

- Different histological variants may affect genital areas
  - Lentiginous (similar to lentigo maligna and acral lentiginous melanoma)
  - Superficial spreading type
  - Nodular type
  - Desmoplastic/neurotropic melanoma
- Neoplastic cells vary in morphology
  - Epithelioid, spindled, or nevoid
- Melanoma in situ
  - Confined to epidermis
  - Lack of symmetry and circumscription
  - Pagetoid spread may be absent/minimal to prominent
- Invasive
  - Superficial or deep invasion
  - Lack of maturation with descent
  - Mitoses may be present (including deep and atypical)
- Variable amount of melanin pigment
- Ulceration &/or regression may be present

DIFFERENTIAL DIAGNOSIS

Atypical Genital Nevi

- Typically occur in younger patients
- Show maturation with descent (deep mitoses are absent)
- May show pagetoid spread, but usually focal

Genital Nevi Arising in Lichen Sclerosus et Atrophicus

- Show features similar to recurrent nevi
- Maturation (deep mitoses are absent)

DIAGNOSTIC CHECKLIST

Pathologic Interpretation Pearls

- Deep mitosis is a feature of MM and not genital nevi

SELECTED REFERENCES

1. Sanchez A et al: Primary genitourinary melanoma: epidemiology and disease-specific survival in a large population-based cohort. Urol Oncol. 34(4):166.e7-166.e14, 2016
2. Carvajal RD et al: Phase II study of nilotinib in melanoma harboring KIT alterations following progression to prior KIT inhibition. Clin Cancer Res. 21(10):2289-96, 2015
3. Bastian BC: The molecular pathology of melanoma: an integrated taxonomy of melanocytic neoplasia. Annu Rev Pathol. 9:239-71, 2014

KEY FACTS

CLINICAL ISSUES

- Wide age range, usually in 5th-8th decades
- Anterior nasal septum > maxillary sinus
- Wide local excision is treatment of choice, followed by adjuvant radiation
- 5-year disease-free survival < 20%

MACROSCOPIC

- Most are polypoid, with surface ulceration/erosion common
- Range: Up to 6 cm; mean: 2-3 cm

MICROSCOPIC

- Protean histology, mimic of many other primary tumor types
- Junctional activity and epithelial migration (pagetoid spread) help to confirm primary tumor
- Many patterns of growth
  - Peritheliomatous: Distinctive and unique for sinonasal melanoma
- Variety of cell types can be seen
  - Undifferentiated, epithelioid, polygonal, small cell, plasmacytoid, rhabdoid, giant cell
- Prominent, irregular, brightly eosinophilic, enlarged nucleoli
- Intranuclear cytoplasmic inclusions usually present
- Melanin-containing tumor cells can be seen

ANCILLARY TESTS

- **Positive**: S100, SOX10, HMB-45, Melan-A, tyrosinase, vimentin

TOP DIFFERENTIAL DIAGNOSES

- Olfactory neuroblastoma
- Sinonasal undifferentiated carcinoma
- Rhabdomyosarcoma
- Meningioma
- Leiomyosarcoma, biphenotypic sinonasal sarcoma

Cartilage Destruction by Melanoma

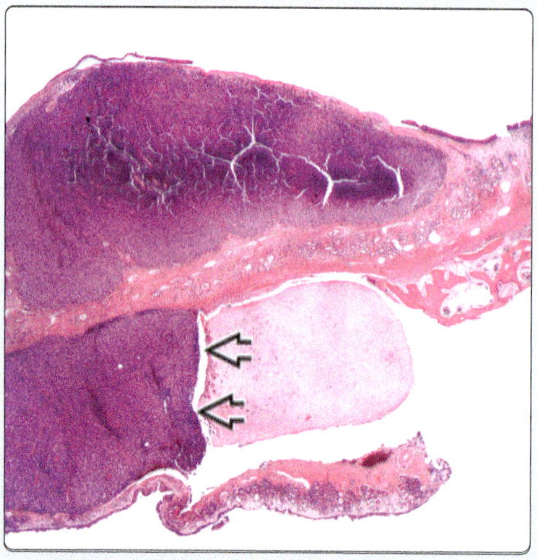

Junctional Melanoma Confirms Primary Melanoma

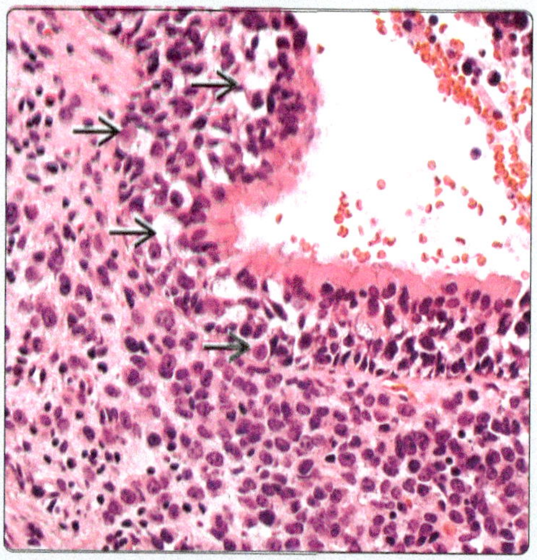

(Left) *The nasal septum cartilage ➡ is being destroyed by the infiltrative neoplasm. The tumor forms a thick, sheet-like distribution. No pattern of growth can be seen at this magnification, although ulceration is present.* **(Right)** *Neoplastic, atypical junctional melanocytes are noted within the respiratory epithelium, arranged in pagetoid spread ➡. The tumor cells are also present within the stroma. This change helps to confirm a primary tumor.*

Spindled Cells in STMMM

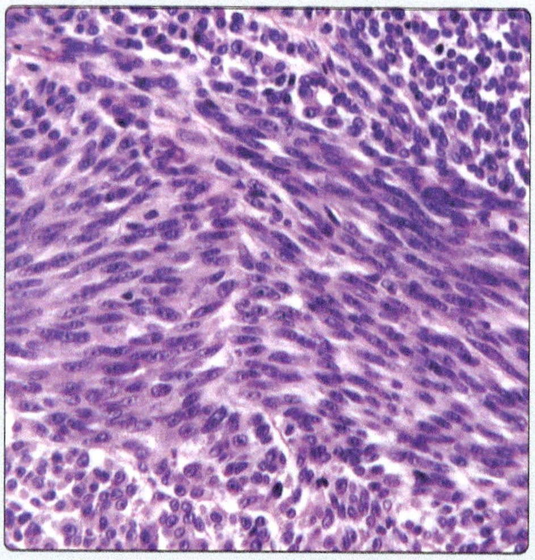

Pigmented STMMM

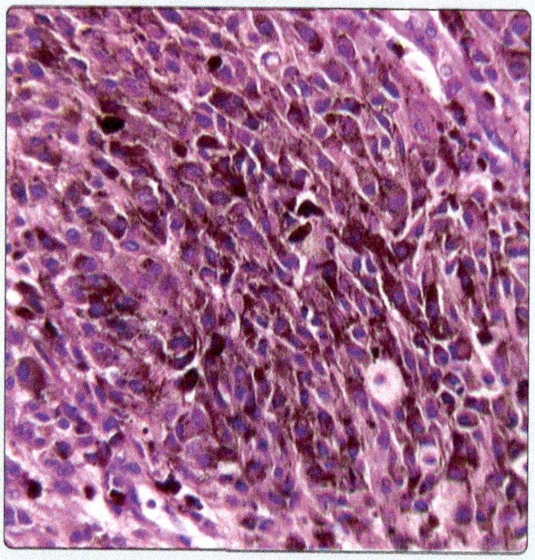

(Left) *The neoplastic cells are arranged in a short fascicular architecture, comprised of spindled cells. Nucleoli are quite prominent.* **(Right)** *Hematoxylin and eosin shows a spindled to polygonal population of highly atypical, pigmented neoplastic cells. These changes are characteristic for a pigmented melanoma. The pigment must be within the atypical cells (rather than histiocytes) to qualify as a pigmented melanoma.*

TERMINOLOGY

Definitions

- Neural crest-derived neoplasms originating from melanocytes and demonstrating melanocytic differentiation

ETIOLOGY/PATHOGENESIS

Environmental Exposure

- Formalin, possibly radiation, &/or UV exposure

CLINICAL ISSUES

Epidemiology

- Incidence
  - Rare
    - Represents < 1% of all melanomas
    - < 5% of all sinonasal tract neoplasms
    - 15-20% of all skin melanomas occur in head and neck
    - Sinonasal tract and nasopharynx mucosal malignant melanoma (STMMM) represent < 4% of all head and neck melanomas
- Age
  - Wide range, usually in 5th-8th decades
- Sex
  - Equal gender distribution
- Ethnicity
  - Increased incidence in Japanese patients

Site

- ~ 15-20% of melanomas arise in head and neck
  - 80% are cutaneous in origin
  - Ocular origin account for majority of remaining malignant mucosal melanoma (MMM)
  - Sinonasal tract is next most common site
- Anterior nasal septum > maxillary sinus

Presentation

- Nasal obstruction
- Epistaxis or nasal discharge
  - Melanorrhea: Black-flecked (melanin) discharge
- Polyp
- Pain is uncommon

Treatment

- Options, risks, complications
  - Metastatic melanoma to sinonasal tract can develop but is vanishingly rare
  - Breslow thickness and Clark level are not used in sinonasal tract
- Surgical approaches
  - Wide local excision is treatment of choice
- Radiation
  - Adjuvant postoperative radiation therapy may improve locoregional control but does not affect survival

Prognosis

- Poor overall
- 5-year survival: 17-47%
  - 5-year disease-free survival: < 20%
- Recurrences are common
- Poor prognosis associated with
  - Obstruction as presenting symptom; nasopharynx or mixed site of involvement; tumor ≥ 3 cm; undifferentiated histology; high mitotic count; recurrence; stage of tumor
- Tyrosine kinase inhibitors may work when protooncogene *KIT* mutations are detected

IMAGING

Radiographic Findings

- Usually identifies extent of tumor and bone invasion
- PET tends to show posterior nasal cavity and sinus tumors better than anterior nasal tumors
- Locoregional and metastatic disease can be detected

MACROSCOPIC

General Features

- Most are polypoid
- White to gray, brown, or black
- Surface ulceration/erosion is common

Size

- Range: Up to 6 cm; mean: 2-3 cm

MICROSCOPIC

Histologic Features

- Protean histology, mimic of many other primary tumor types
- Junctional activity and epidermal migration (pagetoid spread) help to confirm primary tumor
- Surface ulceration is common, obscuring in situ component
- Bone or soft tissue invasion is common
- Many patterns of growth
  - Peritheliomatous: Distinctive and unique for STMMM
  - Epithelioid, solid, organoid, sheets, nests, papillary structures
  - Fascicles and interlacing bundles, storiform, hemangiopericytoma-like
  - Meningothelial
- Variety of cell types can be seen
  - Undifferentiated
  - Epithelioid, polygonal
  - Small cell, plasmacytoid, rhabdoid, giant cell
- Vesicular nuclei, although sometimes hyperchromatic
- Prominent, irregular, brightly eosinophilic, enlarged nucleoli
- Intranuclear cytoplasmic inclusions usually present
- Melanin-containing tumor cells can be seen
- Tumor cell necrosis is common
- Mitotic figures, including atypical forms, usually easily found and increased in numbers
- Inflammation may be present but not of consequence
- Desmoplastic type fibrosis can be seen but is not common
- Perineural invasion, when present, is poor prognostic indicator
- Tumor depth of invasion (Clark) impossible to accurately assess
- Tumor thickness (Breslow) not meaningful in sinonasal tract

Lymphatic/Vascular Invasion

- Usually present but difficult to assess

Margins

- Difficult to assess, as samples are frequently fragmented and removed piecemeal

ANCILLARY TESTS

Histochemistry

- Fontana-Masson: Melanin bleach confirms melanin in cytoplasm

Immunohistochemistry

- **Positive**: S100, HMB-45, Melan-A, SOX10, microphthalmia transcription factor (MIFT), tyrosinase, vimentin
- p16 expression is lost in most MMM (74%) but is **not** correlated with worse prognosis

Genetic Testing

- Comparative genomic hybridization (CGH) shows chromosome arm 1q is gained in nearly all tumors studied
- Gains of 6p (93%) and 8q (57%) are also identified
- Protooncogene KIT can be assessed in metastatic mucosal melanomas, therapeutic target for tyrosine kinase inhibitors
    - *BRAF* is **not** usually assessed in setting of MMM (< 10% harbor mutations)

Electron Microscopy

- Premelanosomes and melanosomes confirm melanocytic origin

DIFFERENTIAL DIAGNOSIS

Olfactory Neuroblastoma

- Lobular architecture
- Fibrillary matrix material associated with rosettes and pseudorosettes
- **Positive**: CD56, chromogranin, synaptophysin, and sustentacular S100

Sinonasal Undifferentiated Carcinoma

- Small cells with high nuclear:cytoplasmic ratio
- Necrosis, destructive growth, and vascular invasion
- **Positive**: Strong, diffuse keratin; **negative**: Melanoma markers

Rhabdomyosarcoma

- Tends to develop in younger patients (although not alveolar type)
- Nests, alveolar patterns are similar
- Strap and rhabdoid patterns are helpful
- Cross striations can confirm diagnosis
- **Positive**: Desmin, MYOD1, myogenin, SMA, MSA, CD56

Meningioma

- Usually secondary in sinonasal tract from intracranial primary
- Meningothelial pattern, spindled cells with intranuclear cytoplasmic inclusions
- **Positive**: EMA, CK7 (prepsammomatous); **negative**: SOX10, S100 (usually)

Leiomyosarcoma

- Fascicular architecture, frequently associated with necrosis and high mitotic index
- Perinuclear vacuoles and cigar-shaped nuclei are rare in melanoma
- **Positive**: Muscle markers; **negative**: Melanoma markers

Biphenotypic Sinonasal Sarcoma

- Poorly circumscribed, invasive, cellular spindle cell tumor with epithelial inclusions and low mitoses
- **Positive**: S100, SMA, MSA; **negative**: SOX10, HMB-45, Melan-A, tyrosinase

Plasma Cell Myeloma (Plasmacytoma)

- Hematologic neoplasm giving sheet-like pattern of plasmacytoid cells
- Hof zone, paranuclear clearing, and rounded nuclei with clock face-like chromatin distribution
- **Positive**: CD138, CD79a, κ or λ, and other hematologic markers
- Lymphoma is uncommonly in the differential diagnosis

Melanotic Neuroectodermal Tumor of Infancy

- Tumor of neonatal period, affecting gnathic bones
- Biphasic tumor with small and large cells, with pigment easily identified

Metastatic Melanoma

- While theoretic consideration, junctional/pagetoid spread helps to exclude this possibility
- Clinical and radiographic examinations are only way to make definitive distinction

Mesenchymal Chondrosarcoma

- Small, undifferentiated cell appearance, but if enough sections are taken, cartilaginous features can be seen
- **Positive**: S100 (chondrocytic tumors are positive); **negative**: HMB-45, tyrosinase, Melan-A

SELECTED REFERENCES

1. Lazarev S et al: Mucosal Melanoma of the Head and Neck: A Systematic Review of the Literature. Int J Radiat Oncol Biol Phys. 90(5):1108-1118, 2014
2. López F et al: Update on primary head and neck mucosal melanoma. Head Neck. Jan;38(1):147-55, 2014
3. Jangard M et al: Primary sinonasal malignant melanoma: a nationwide study of the Swedish population, 1960-2000. Rhinology. 51(1):22-30, 2013
4. Keller DS et al: Outcomes in patients with mucosal melanomas. J Surg Oncol. 108(8):516-20, 2013
5. Koivunen P et al: Accuracy of the current TNM classification in predicting survival in patients with sinonasal mucosal melanoma. Laryngoscope. 122(8):1734-8, 2012
6. Vandenhende C et al: Sinonasal mucosal melanoma: retrospective survival study of 25 patients. J Laryngol Otol. 126(2):147-51, 2012
7. Clifton N et al: Malignant melanoma of nasal cavity and paranasal sinuses: report of 24 patients and literature review. J Laryngol Otol. 125(5):479-85, 2011
8. Wenig BM: Undifferentiated malignant neoplasms of the sinonasal tract. Arch Pathol Lab Med. 133(5):699-712, 2009
9. Dauer EH et al: Sinonasal melanoma: a clinicopathologic review of 61 cases. Otolaryngol Head Neck Surg. 138(3):347-52, 2008
10. Prasad ML et al: Clinicopathologic differences in malignant melanoma arising in oral squamous and sinonasal respiratory mucosa of the upper aerodigestive tract. Arch Pathol Lab Med. 127(8):997-1002, 2003
11. Thompson LD et al: Sinonasal tract and nasopharyngeal melanomas: a clinicopathologic study of 115 cases with a proposed staging system. Am J Surg Pathol. 27(5):594-611, 2003

Immunohistochemistry

Antibody	Reactivity	Staining Pattern	Comment
S100	Positive	Nuclear & cytoplasmic	Diffuse and strong stain usually; identified in ~ 90% of cases
HMB-45	Positive	Cytoplasmic	Variably reactive in most cases (~ 75%)
SOX10	Positive	Nuclear	Strong and diffuse in nearly all tumor cells
Tyrosinase	Positive	Cytoplasmic	Variably reactive in most cases (~ 75%)
Melan-A103	Positive	Cytoplasmic	Variably reactive in majority of cases (~ 66%)
MITF	Positive	Nuclear	Positive in majority of cases (~ 55%)
NSE	Positive	Cytoplasmic	Positive in < 50% of tumor cells, often focal
CD117	Positive	Cytoplasmic	Positive in ~ 33% of cases
CD99	Positive	Cytoplasmic	Positive in ~ 25% of cases
Vimentin	Positive	Cytoplasmic	All tumor cells
CD56	Positive	Cell membrane & cytoplasm	~ 7% of cases
Synaptophysin	Positive	Cytoplasmic	Nonspecific in ~ 10% of cases
EMA	Positive	Cytoplasmic	< 5% of tumor cells
Chromogranin-A	Negative		
CD45RB	Negative		
CK-PAN	Negative		
GFAP	Negative		
Actin-HHF-35	Negative		
Actin-sm	Negative		
Desmin	Negative		
MYOD1	Negative		

Mucosal Melanoma of Head and Neck

Classification	Description
Primary Tumor (T)	
T3	Mucosal disease only
T4a	Moderately advanced disease (deep soft tissue, cartilage, bone, skin)
T4b	Very advanced disease [brain, dura, skull base, lower cranial nerves (IX, X, XI, XII), masticator space, carotid artery, prevertebral space]
Regional Lymph Nodes (N)	
NX	Regional lymph nodes cannot be assessed
N0	No lymph node metastasis
N1	Regional lymph node metastases
Distant Metastasis (M)	
M0	No distant metastases
M1	Distant metastasis
Prognostic Groups	
III	T3 N0 M0
IVA	T4a N0 M0
	T3-T4a N1 M0
IVB	T4b, any N M0
IVC	Any T, any N, M1

AJCC Staging, 7th edition.

(Left) *This coronal view of the nasal cavity and sinuses demonstrates a large, polypoid mass ➡ arising from and destroying the cartilage of the septum. These findings are nonspecific for melanoma.* **(Right)** *Isolated junctional neoplastic cells ➡ are noted in this malignant mucosal melanoma (MMM). The neoplastic cells in the stroma show pleomorphism and a plasmacytoid appearance, identical to the junctional cells. Pigment is easily identified.*

Computed Tomography of STMMM

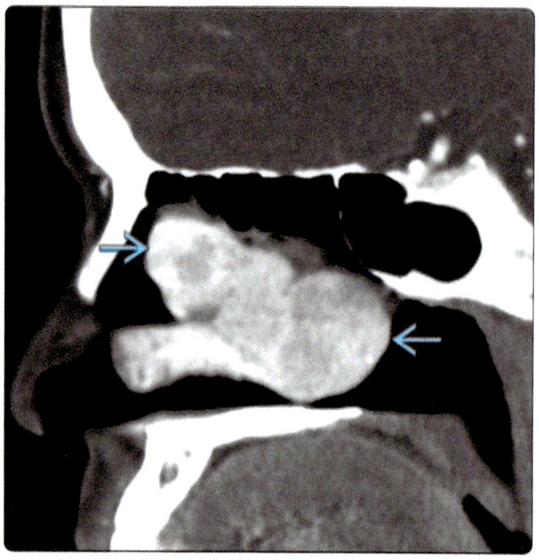

Junctional or Pagetoid Spread in STMMM

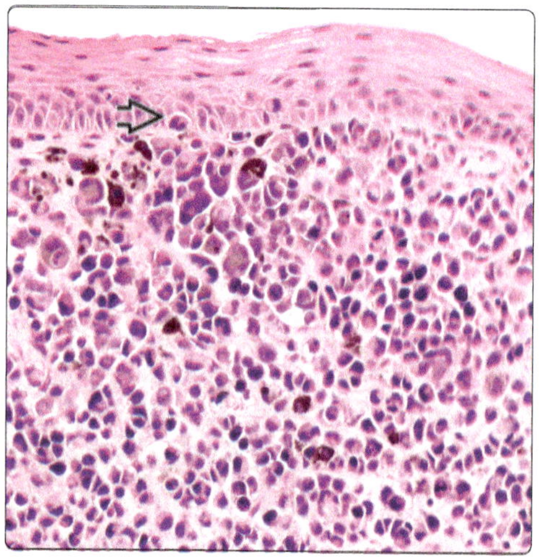

(Left) *This peritheliomatous or perivascular ➡ distribution of the neoplastic cells is quite characteristic for melanoma. It is thought to represent viable tumor cells remaining around vessels. This pattern can be seen in other tumors, but not to the same frequency as it is in melanoma.* **(Right)** *MMM can be arranged in a number of different architectures, with a fascicular architecture seen here. The spindle cells are arranged in short, intersecting fascicles. The cells are somewhat syncytial in appearance.*

Peritheliomatous Pattern in STMMM

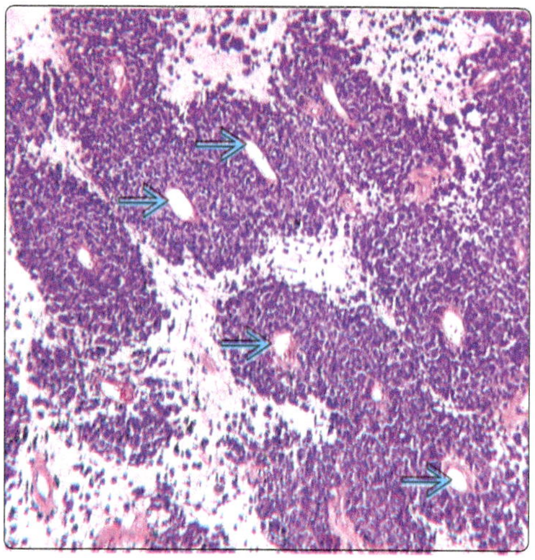

Fascicular Architecture in STMMM

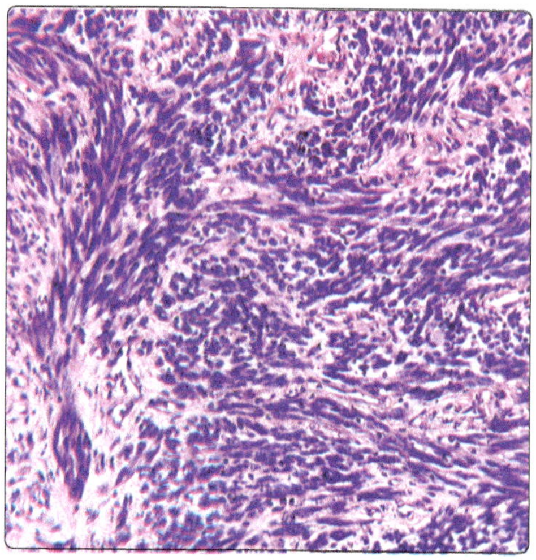

(Left) *There is a whorled, meningothelial pattern to this melanoma. This pattern can mimic a meningioma. S100 can be positive in both lesions, although SOX10 and HMB-45 are negative in meningioma. Note the mitosis ➡.* **(Right)** *It is not uncommon to have an undifferentiated or small round blue cell appearance to MMM. There is a slightly plasmacytoid appearance to the cells. Note the very prominent nucleoli. Pigment is absent.*

Meningothelial Pattern in STMMM

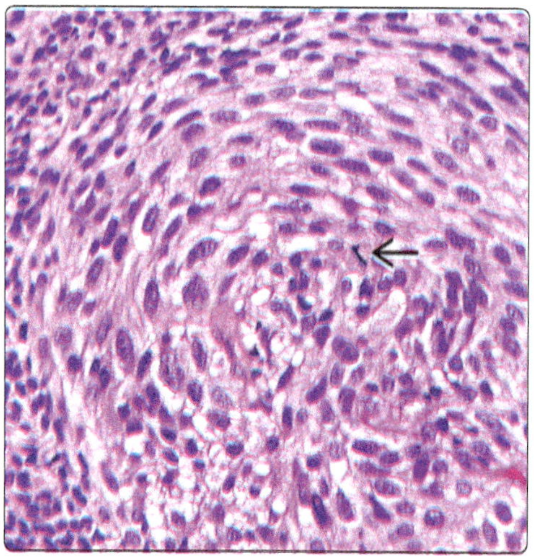

Undifferentiated Cytology Pattern in STMMM

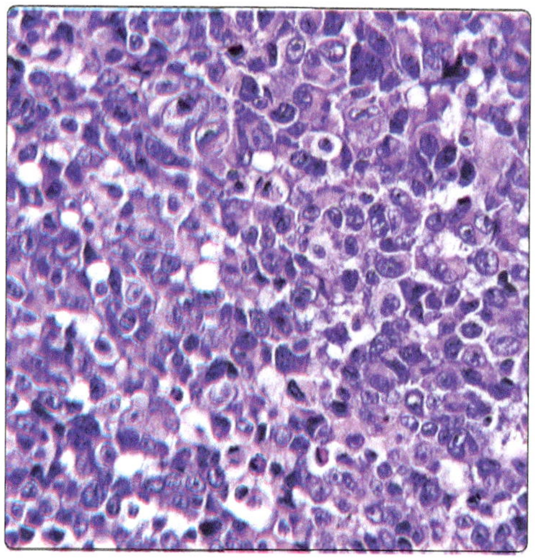

STMMM With Plasmacytoid Cytology

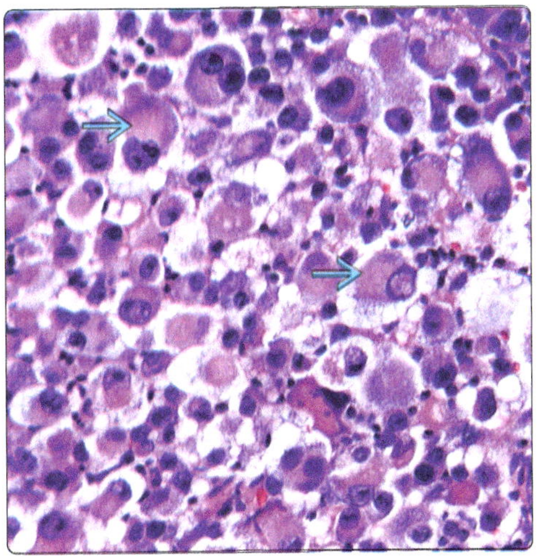

STMMM With Rhabdoid Cytology

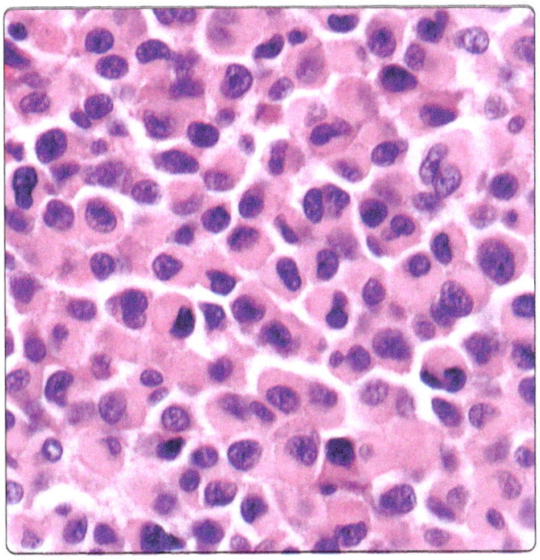

(Left) *This tumor shows a very pronounced plasmacytoid appearance, including a Hof zone adjacent to the nucleus ➡. There are intranuclear cytoplasmic inclusions as well as binucleation in this MMM.* **(Right)** *A rhabdoid appearance with darkly opacified, eosinophilic cytoplasm is the dominant pattern in this MMM. Nucleoli are not as enlarged. Mitotic figures, necrosis, and pigment are not appreciated.*

STMMM With Solid Sheet of Undifferentiated Cells

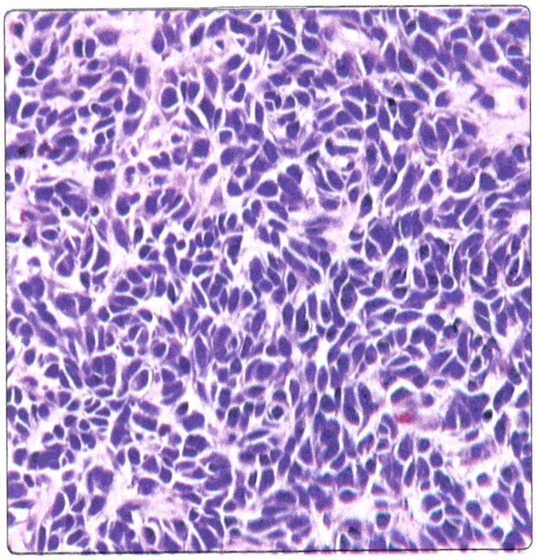

Pleomorphic Cells With Intranuclear Cytoplasmic Inclusions in STMMM

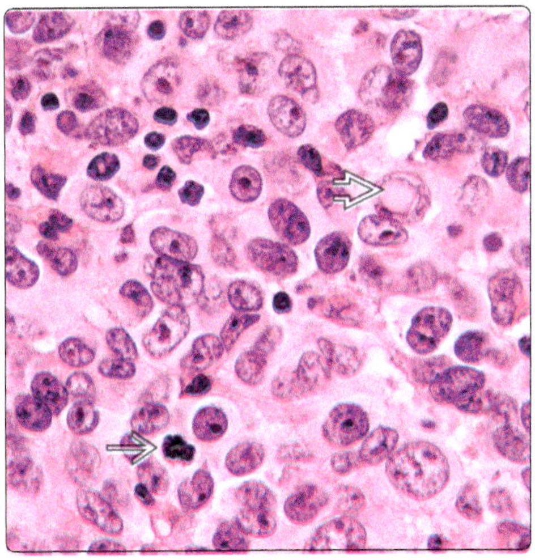

(Left) *There is a sheet-like pattern of undifferentiated neoplastic cells in this melanoma. There is a high nuclear:cytoplasmic ratio, but other characteristic histologic features are absent. Immunohistochemistry is most helpful in this setting.* **(Right)** *Pleomorphic polygonal cells comprise this melanoma. There is remarkable variability between cells. Prominent, eosinophilic nucleoli are noted, along with intranuclear cytoplasmic inclusions ➡. Mitotic figures are also noted ➡.*

STMMM With S100-Positive Reaction

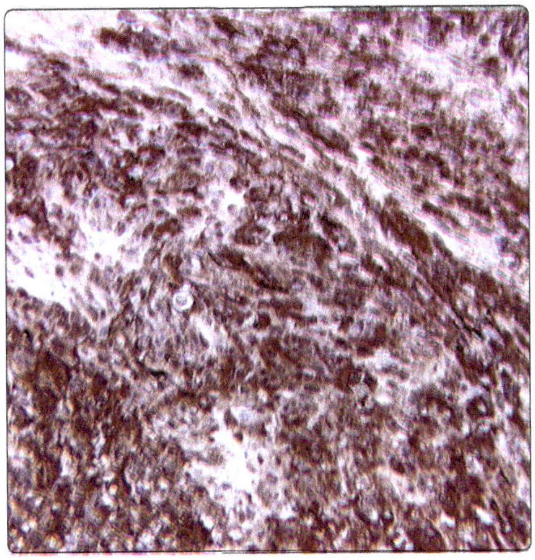

STMMM With Tyrosinase Positive Cells

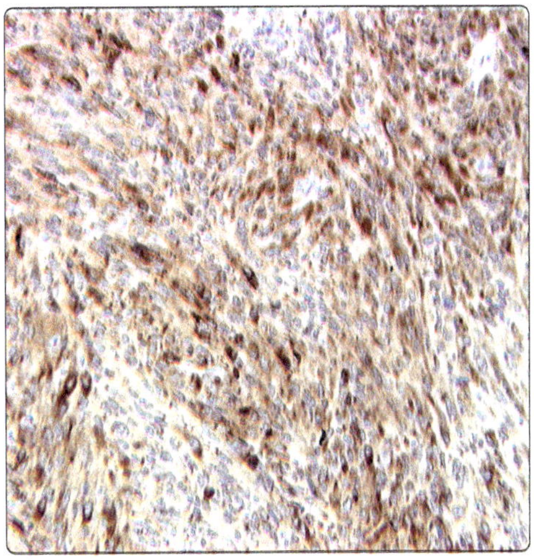

(Left) *Positive S100 is immunoreactive in this spindled cell melanoma. There is both cytoplasmic and nuclear reactivity with this marker that highlights nearly all of the cells.* **(Right)** *The neoplastic cells show a strong and diffuse cytoplasmic reaction with tyrosinase in this spindled cell melanoma. An atypical spindled tumor has a broad differential in this location, with IHC helping to reach a definitive diagnosis.*

KEY FACTS

TERMINOLOGY

- Malignant proliferation of conjunctival melanocytes that commonly arises in setting of primary acquired melanosis (PAM) with atypia

CLINICAL ISSUES

- Rare; accounts for only 2-3% of ocular cancers
- More common in older individuals (mean age at presentation: 50-60 years)
- Exceedingly rare in children younger than 15 years of age (only 28 reported cases)
- Bulbar conjunctiva close to limbus is most common location
- Majority of cases (53-75%) arise in setting of PAM with atypia
- Avoiding manipulation of tumor during surgery reduces local recurrence rate and lymphatic spread
- All should be completely excised with 2- to 3-mm tumor-free margins
- Sentinel lymph node biopsy is recommended for high-risk tumors
- Conjunctival melanoma arising in association with PAM has higher risk of local recurrence

MICROSCOPIC

- Conjunctival cysts are extremely rare
- Intraepithelial component showing pagetoid growth
- Radial extension of intraepithelial component
- Lack of maturation toward base of lesion
- Invasion of sclera or cornea, especially if through Bowman membrane or into conjunctival stroma
- Significant cytological atypia: Large nuclear size and prominent nucleoli
- Mitotic activity

TOP DIFFERENTIAL DIAGNOSES

- Conjunctival nevus
- Juvenile conjunctival nevus

(Left) *Clinical image shows an expansile pigmented patch ⇨ at the limbus ⇨ and adjacent to the iris ➡. Bulbar conjunctiva close to the limbus is the most common location for primary acquired melanosis (PAM).* **(Right)** *Scanning magnification of this conjunctival shave biopsy shows a lentiginous basilar proliferation ⇨ that stands out even at the this power. The radial extension appears to be extensive.*

Conjunctival Melanoma Presenting as Pigmented Patch

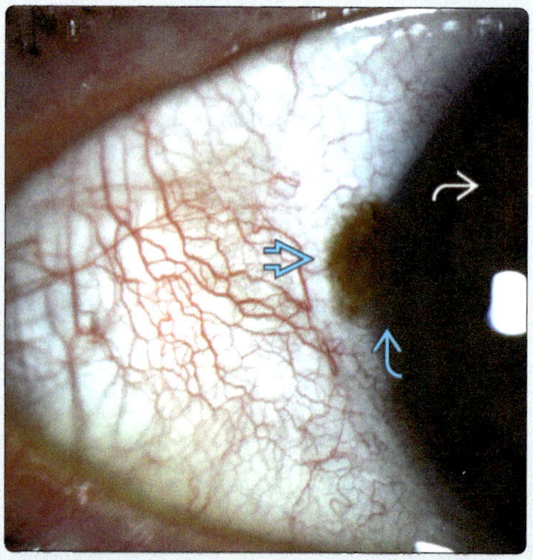

Scanning Magnification of PAM With Atypia

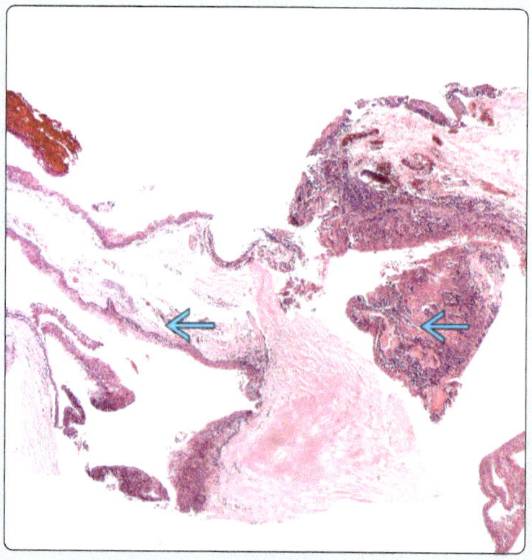

(Left) *Higher magnification of the same case confirms that atypical melanocytes ⇨ have replaced the basilar keratinocytes in the conjunctiva. There is some pagetoid upward scatter of melanocytes →.* **(Right)** *High-power magnification shows poorly nested proliferation of atypical melanocytes in the same lesion of PAM with atypia. The upward scatter →, nuclear hyperchromasia ⇨, and nuclear pleomorphism resembles cutaneous melanoma in situ.*

Higher Magnification of PAM With Atypia

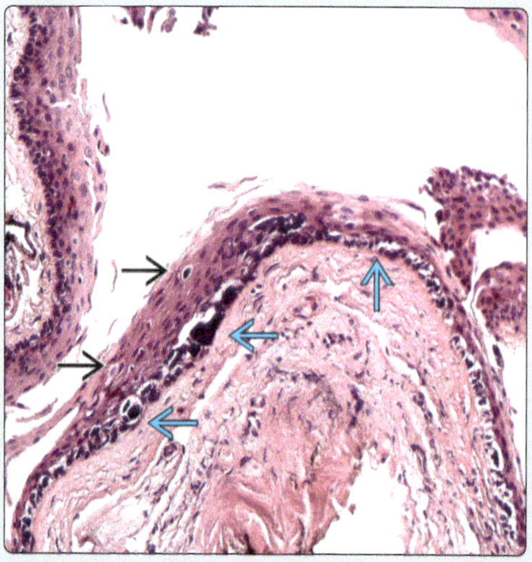

Higher Magnification Shows Nuclear Hyperchromasia and Pleomorphism

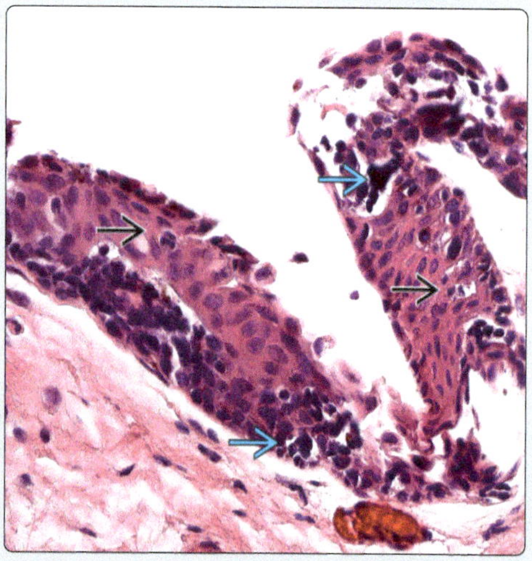

TERMINOLOGY

Synonyms

- Conjunctival malignant melanoma

Definitions

- Malignant proliferation of conjunctival melanocytes commonly associated with primary acquired melanosis (PAM) with atypia

CLINICAL ISSUES

Epidemiology

- Incidence
  - Rare; accounts for only 2-3% of ocular cancers
- Age
  - More common in older individuals (mean age at presentation: 50-60 years)
  - Exceedingly rare in children younger than 15 years of age (only 28 reported cases)

Presentation

- Bulbar conjunctiva close to limbus is most common location

Natural History

- Majority of cases (53-75%) arise in setting of PAM with atypia
- Remainder (18-30%) arise de novo
- Minority of cases (5%) are associated with preexisting melanocytic nevus

Treatment

- Options, risks, complications
  - Avoiding manipulation of tumor during surgery reduces local recurrence rate and lymphatic spread
- Surgical approaches
  - All should be completely excised with 2- to 3-mm tumor-free margins
  - Sentinel lymph node biopsy recommended for high-risk tumors
- Adjuvant therapy
  - Risk of recurrence is reduced with adjuvant cryotherapy, irradiation, or topical chemotherapy

Prognosis

- Conjunctival melanoma arising in association with PAM has higher risk of local recurrence
- 10-year survival rate: 70-86%
- After 10 years, 50% of tumors will recur locally and about 25% will metastasize
- Adverse clinical prognostic indicators include
  - Nonbulbar (fornix, palpebral) location
  - Involvement of lymphatics-rich caruncle
  - Invasion of skin, into eye or brain

Suspicious Clinical Features

- Extension into cornea and attachment to sclera
- Lack of mobility in relation to sclera

MICROSCOPIC

Histologic Features

- Conjunctival cysts are extremely rare
- Intraepithelial component showing pagetoid growth
- Radial extension of intraepithelial component beyond lateral edge of subepithelial component
- Lack of maturation toward base of lesion
- Invasion of sclera or cornea, especially if through Bowman membrane or into conjunctival stroma
- Patchy or band-like inflammation at base of lesion

Cytologic Features

- Conjunctival melanoma can be composed of 1 or combination of 4 different cell types
  - Small polyhedral cells
  - Epithelioid cells
  - Balloon cells
  - Spindle cells
    - Purely spindle cell melanomas have been found to be less aggressive
- Significant cytological atypia: Large nuclear size and prominent nucleoli
- Mitotic activity

ANCILLARY TESTS

Immunohistochemistry

- Melanocytes should express usual melanocytic markers, including MART-1/Melan-A, HMB-45, and S100

Genetic Testing

- FISH may be helpful in better classifying atypical conjunctival melanocytic proliferations from nevi

DIFFERENTIAL DIAGNOSIS

Conjunctival Nevus

- Lesion composed of small polyhedral cells can also be seen in conjunctival nevus

Juvenile Conjunctival Nevus

- Radial extension of intraepithelial component can also be seen during rapid growth phase of juvenile conjunctival nevi
- Paradoxical "reverse" maturation where subepithelial cells are larger than intraepithelial ones
- Patchy or band-like inflammation at base of lesion

DIAGNOSTIC CHECKLIST

Clinically Relevant Pathologic Features

- Acquire additional clinical information like age and race

Pathologic Interpretation Pearls

- Look for invasion of sclera or cornea if represented in specimen

SELECTED REFERENCES

1. Zembowicz A et al: Melanocytic lesions of the conjunctiva. Arch Pathol Lab Med. 134(12):1785-92, 2010
2. Shields JA et al: Primary acquired melanosis of the conjunctiva: experience with 311 eyes. Trans Am Ophthalmol Soc. 105:61-71; discussion 71-2, 2007
3. Sugiura M et al: Low-risk and high-risk histologic features in conjunctival primary acquired melanosis with atypia: Clinicopathologic analysis of 29 cases. Am J Surg Pathol. 31(2):185-92, 2007

PAM With Atypia: Lentiginous Proliferation of Melanocytes

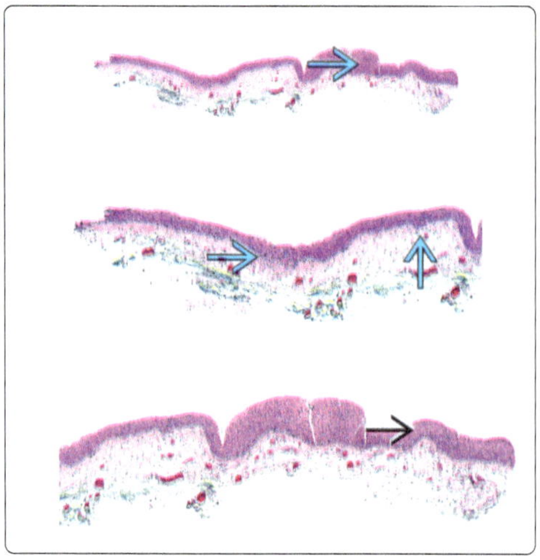

PAM With Atypia Resembles Cutaneous Melanoma In Situ

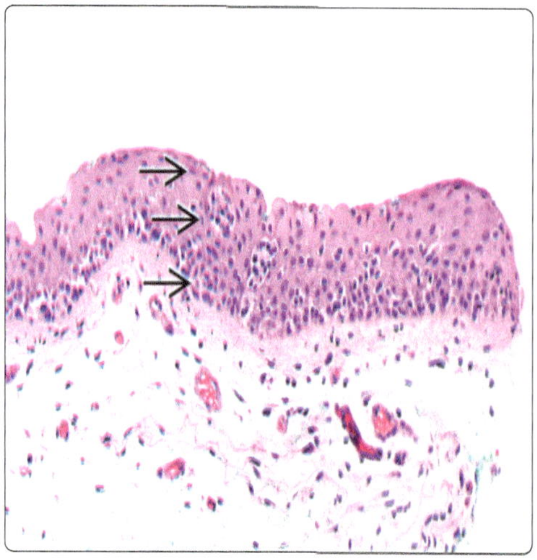

(Left) *Composite shows a conjunctival shave biopsy at scanning magnification, where basilar hyperchromatic cells → can be identified in the conjunctiva. The bottom piece (shown at 40x) reveals pagetoid scatter of melanocytes → in the conjunctiva.* **(Right)** *Medium-power magnification demonstrates scatter of atypical melanocytes → throughout all the layers of this thin conjunctiva. This is sufficient for the diagnosis of PAM with atypia.*

PAM With Atypia at Higher Magnification

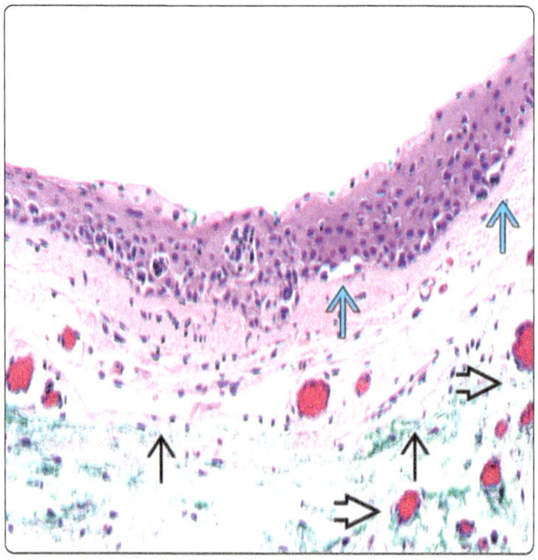

Nuclear Hyperchromasia and Pleomorphism at High Magnification

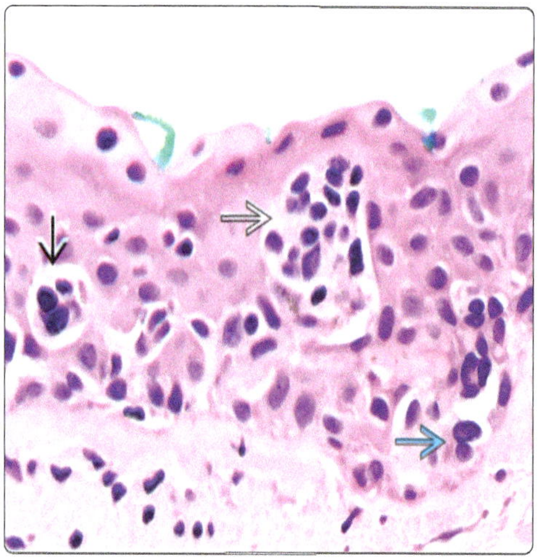

(Left) *Note the junctional proliferation of atypical melanocytes producing a clefting artifact → at the basal layer. There are no subepithelial melanocytes, i.e., devoid of invasion. There are dilated lymphatics → and capillary-size blood vessels → in the subepithelium.* **(Right)** *Same focus at high power shows intraepithelial melanocytes with significant nuclear hyperchromasia → and pleomorphism →; some exhibit prominent nucleoli →, which are more difficult to appreciate with hyperchromasia.*

Conjunctival Melanoma Resembling Inverted Type-A Nevus

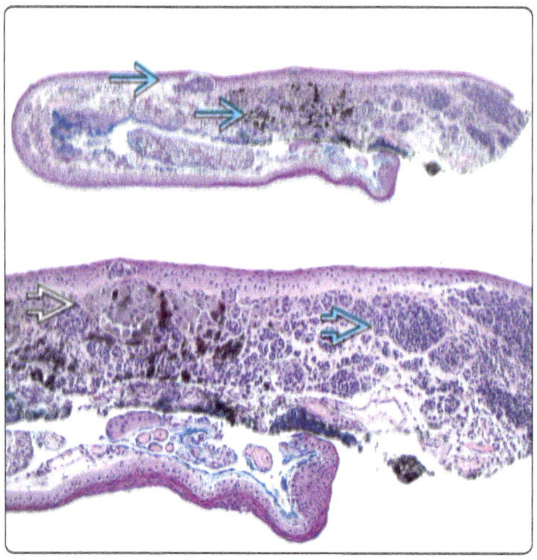

Large Intraepithelial Nest in Conjunctival Melanoma

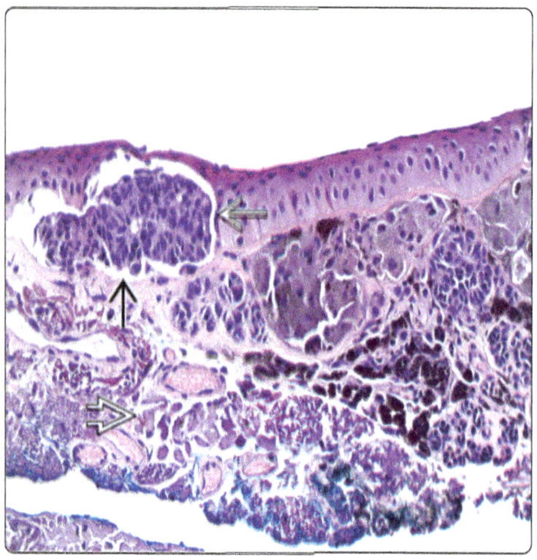

(Left) *Composite figure shows a deeply melanized compound melanocytic proliferation → in a shave biopsy of conjunctiva (top). Higher magnification (bottom) shows 2 cell populations in the subepithelium. One is epithelioid and heavily melanized (type A) →, and the other has small "lymphoid" appearance (type B) →.* **(Right)** *This field shows a large intraepithelial nest → with epithelial consumption producing a retraction artifact →. Marked solar elastosis → is identified.*

Epithelial Consumption and Malignant Cytopathology in Conjunctival Melanoma

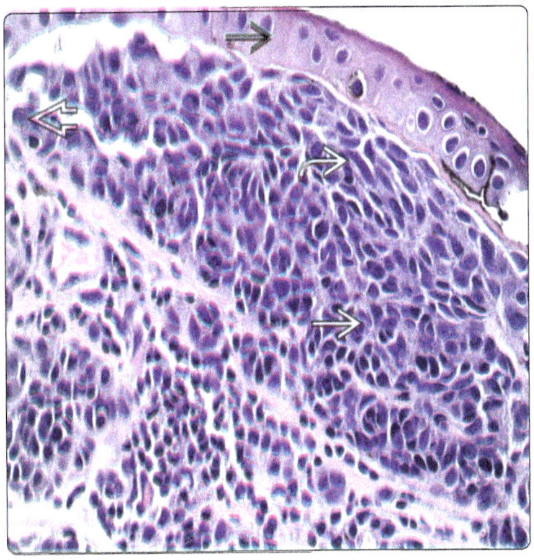

2 Cellular Populations in Conjunctival Melanoma

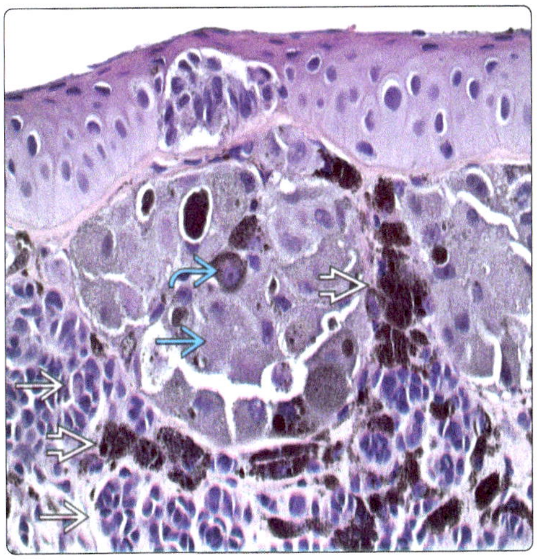

(Left) *This field shows only 2-3 layers of conjunctival keratinocytes remain as the large melanoma nest has consumed the rest of it. The nest is composed of oval to short spindle cells with nuclear hyperchromasia and pleomorphism. There are prominent nucleoli.* **(Right)** *There are large epithelioid cells with ample gray-brown cytoplasm and macronucleoli. In addition, there are smaller, basaloid cells with nuclear hyperchromasia and pleomorphism. Melanophages are found.*

Another Example of Conjunctival Melanoma

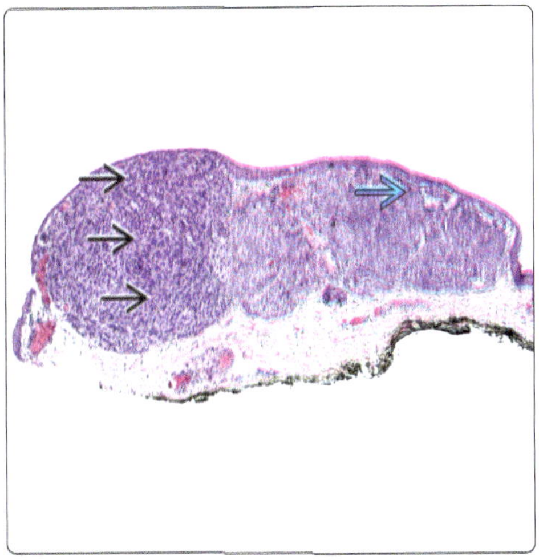

Malignant Cytopathology in Conjunctival Melanoma

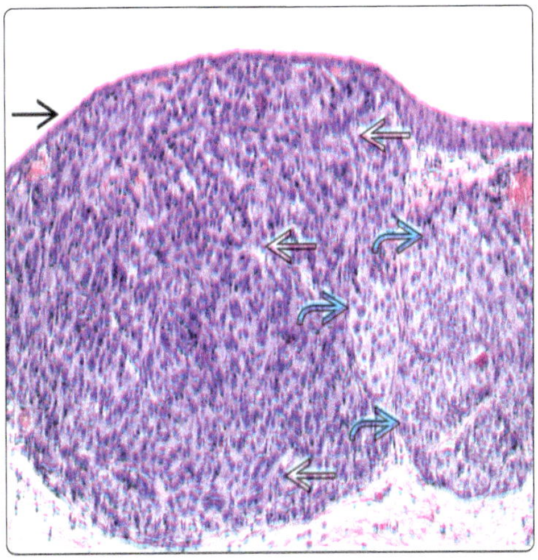

(Left) *Scanning magnification shows a papule that is compound but predominantly subepithelial. There are small intraepithelial nests with retraction artifact. The lesion is mainly situated in the lamina propria without any evidence of maturation with increasing depth.* **(Right)** *The subepithelial nodular growth is consuming conjunctiva; a thin single layer remains. There are large epithelioid cells with macronucleoli adjacent to smaller, basaloid cells.*

Conjunctival Melanoma at Low Magnification

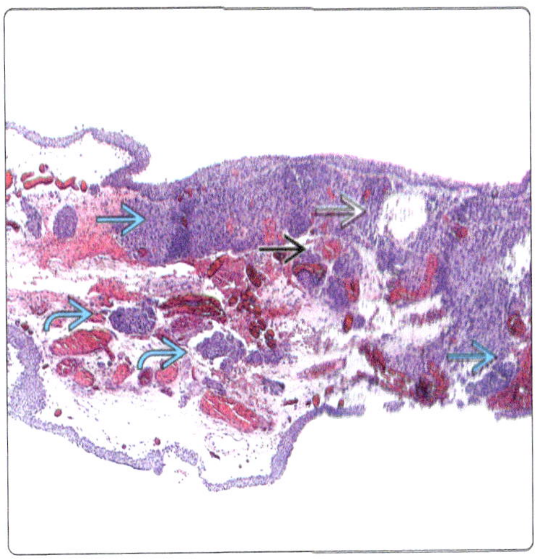

Perineural Invasion and Malignant Cytopathology in Conjunctival Melanoma

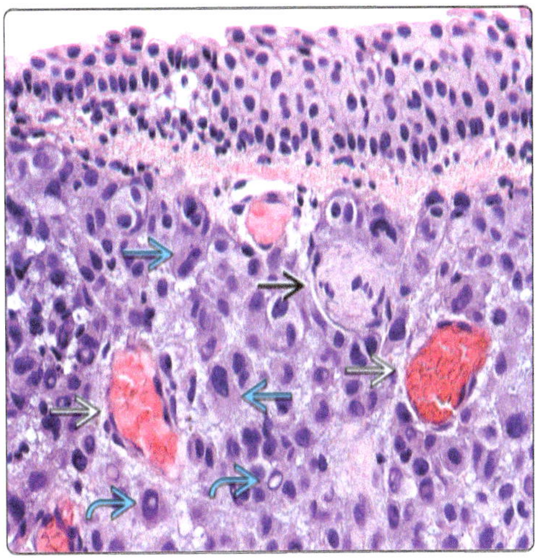

(Left) *Scanning magnification of this lesion shows a predominantly subepithelial melanoma composed of nodules and tumor nests. Note the angiogenic blood vessels and dilated lymphatics.* **(Right)** *There are large epithelioid cells with ample eosinophilic cytoplasm and nuclear pseudoinclusions. There are prominent angiogenic capillaries intimately associated with the melanoma cells. Perineural invasion is also identified.*

Malignant Cellular Blue Nevus (Melanoma Arising in Cellular Blue Nevus)

KEY FACTS

TERMINOLOGY

- Malignant cellular blue nevus
- Dermal-based melanocytic neoplasm with associated cellular blue nevus or features simulating cellular blue nevus

ETIOLOGY/PATHOGENESIS

- May be associated with solar damage
- Mutations in *GNAQ* and *GNA11* have been reported

CLINICAL ISSUES

- Very rare tumor
- Usually occurs in adults; more common in males
- May appear blue, bluish-gray, or bluish-black clinically
- Complete and wider surgical excision is necessary for local removal

MICROSCOPIC

- Cellular, dermal-based, nodular melanocytic tumor
- Often asymmetric, appears poorly circumscribed
- Cytologic atypia is usually very marked
- Mitotic figures present, often atypical
- May show areas of necrosis
- Areas of benign cellular blue nevus may be present

TOP DIFFERENTIAL DIAGNOSES

- Cellular blue nevus
    - Symmetric and well circumscribed
    - Often shows dumbbell-like appearance at low power
    - Cells lack prominent cytologic atypia, mitotic activity, and necrosis
- Atypical cellular blue nevus
    - Shows overlapping features with cellular blue nevus, but with increased cytologic atypia
    - May have some mitoses, but not numerous or atypical
- Metastatic melanoma
    - Usually mostly epithelioid-appearing melanocytes, fewer spindled cells, and no dendritic cells

(Left) *This was a very large and deep cellular lesion in an older adult patient. Note the central focus of necrosis surrounded by cellular nodules of hyperchromatic-appearing cells.* **(Right)** *This malignant blue nevus shows densely cellular areas of atypical spindled melanocytes forming fascicular (sarcoma-like) arrangements.*

Malignant Cellular Blue Nevus With Necrosis

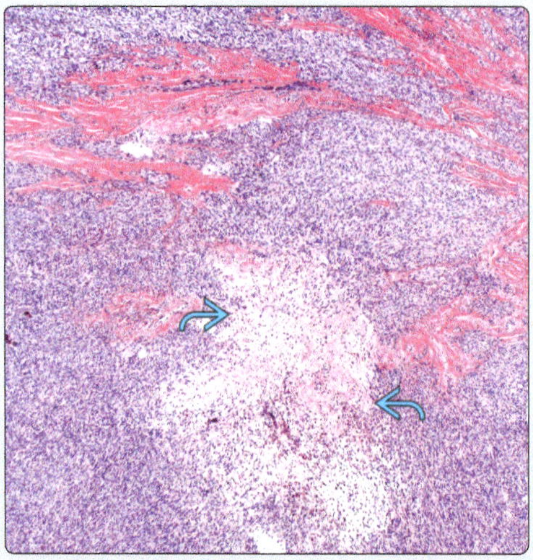

Densely Cellular Fascicles of Spindle Cells in Malignant Cellular Blue Nevus

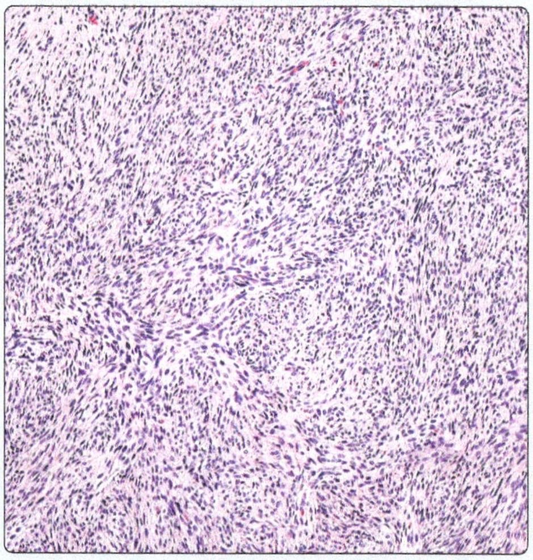

(Left) *High magnification of a heavily pigmented malignant cellular blue nevus (MCBN) demonstrates significant nuclear atypia with prominent nucleoli and a mitotic figure in this case.* **(Right)** *Ki-67 immunostaining shows increased nuclear positivity in this malignant cellular blue nevus, with scattered enlarged, atypical-appearing nuclei staining.*

High Magnification of Heavily Pigmented Malignant Cellular Blue Nevus

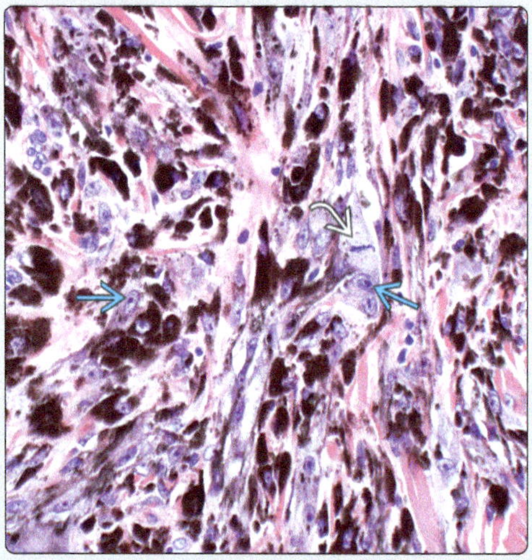

Ki-67 Immunostaining in Malignant Cellular Blue Nevus

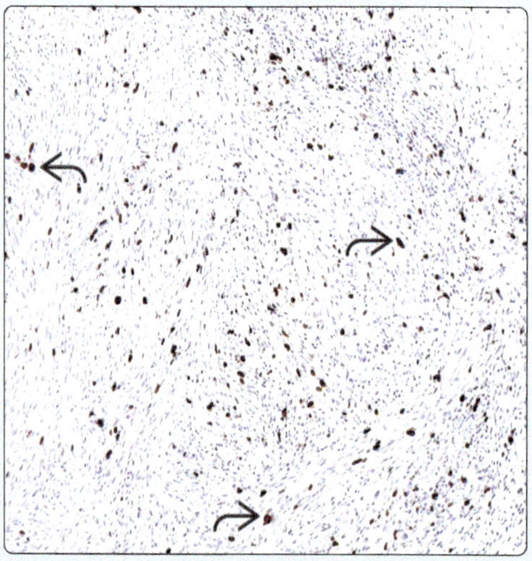

TERMINOLOGY

Abbreviations

- Malignant cellular blue nevus (MCBN)

Synonyms

- Melanoma arising in cellular blue nevus
- Melanoma mimicking cellular blue nevus

Definitions

- Malignant dermal-based melanocytic neoplasm with associated cellular blue nevus or features simulating cellular blue nevus

ETIOLOGY/PATHOGENESIS

Environmental Exposure

- May be related to solar damage

Genetics

- Multiple chromosomal abnormalities reported in some cases
- Mutations in *GNAQ* and *GNA11* have been reported
- Loss of nuclear BAP1 expression also recently identified

CLINICAL ISSUES

Epidemiology

- Incidence
    - Very rare tumor
- Age
    - Usually occurs in adults

Presentation

- Dermal mass/nodular lesion
    - May appear blue, bluish-gray, or bluish-black

Treatment

- Surgical approaches
    - Complete and wider surgical excision is necessary for local removal

Prognosis

- Controversial
    - Originally thought to be very aggressive, but recent reports may indicate lower malignant potential

MICROSCOPIC

Histologic Features

- Cellular, dermal-based, nodular melanocytic tumor
    - Proliferation of atypical spindle-shaped cells in fascicles and lobules
    - Often asymmetric, appears poorly circumscribed at low magnification
    - May extend into subcutis
    - Cytologic atypia is usually very marked
    - Mitotic figures present
        - Often atypical, and may be > 2/HPF
    - May show areas of necrosis
- Typically lacks epidermal involvement
- Areas of benign cellular blue nevus may be present
    - Some authorities require presence of associated nevus, but this is controversial

Cytologic Features

- Spindle-shaped cells with hyperchromatic-staining nuclei

ANCILLARY TESTS

Immunohistochemistry

- Elevated proliferative activity can be shown by Ki-67 and PCNA
- p16 often shows loss of expression (positive in cellular blue nevi)

DIFFERENTIAL DIAGNOSIS

Cellular Blue Nevus

- Dermal-based cellular melanocytic proliferation
    - Often symmetric and well circumscribed at low magnification
- Lobules and fascicles of oval to spindle-shaped cells
- Often shows dumbbell-like appearance at low-power examination
- Peripheral areas often show conventional blue nevus-like pattern with hypocellular areas of melanocytes associated with dermal fibrosis and melanophages
- Cells lack prominent cytologic atypia, mitotic activity, and necrosis
    - Few mitotic figures can be present, especially in cellular areas

Atypical Cellular Blue Nevus

- Shows overlapping features with cellular blue nevus but with increased atypia
- Lobules and fascicles of atypical oval to spindled cells
- May show some asymmetry and infiltrative features
- Scattered mitotic figures may be present, but they are not numerous or atypical-appearing as in MCBN
- Necrosis should be lacking

Metastatic Melanoma

- Lacks junctional component, similar to malignant blue nevus but also shows
    - More epithelioid-appearing melanocytes, fewer spindled cells (most cases), and no dendritic cells
    - Fewer melanophages (unless regressing) and less surrounding dermal fibrosis
    - No associated benign blue nevus component
- Clinical history and complete examination may be necessary for distinction in some cases

SELECTED REFERENCES

1. Hung T et al: Cellular blue nevomelanocytic lesions: analysis of clinical, histological, and outcome data in 37 cases. Am J Dermatopathol. ePub, 2016
2. Chang LM et al: p16 expression is lost in severely atypical cellular blue nevi and melanoma compared to conventional, mildly, and moderately atypical cellular blue nevi. ISRN Dermatol. 2014:348417, 2014
3. Loghavi S et al: Melanoma arising in association with blue nevus: a clinical and pathologic study of 24 cases and comprehensive review of the literature. Mod Pathol. 27(11):1468-78, 2014
4. Martin RC et al: So-called "malignant blue nevus": a clinicopathologic study of 23 patients. Cancer. 115(13):2949-55, 2009
5. Barnhill RL et al: Atypical cellular blue nevi (cellular blue nevi with atypical features): lack of consensus for diagnosis and distinction from cellular blue nevi and malignant melanoma ("malignant blue nevus"). Am J Surg Pathol. 32(1):36-44, 2008

Malignant Cellular Blue Nevus at Scanning Magnification

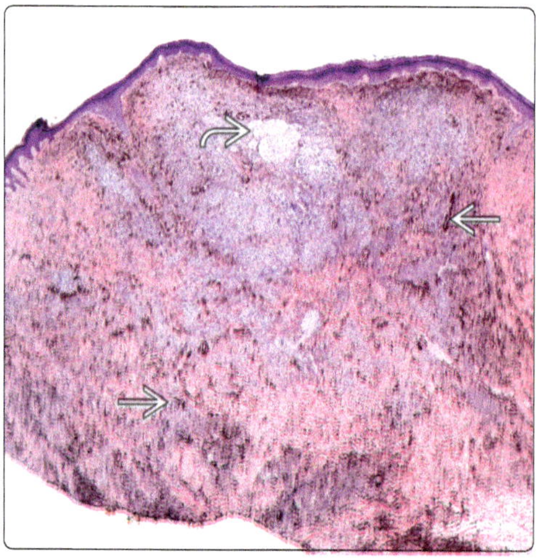

Higher Magnification of Malignant Cellular Blue Nevus Showing Mitoses

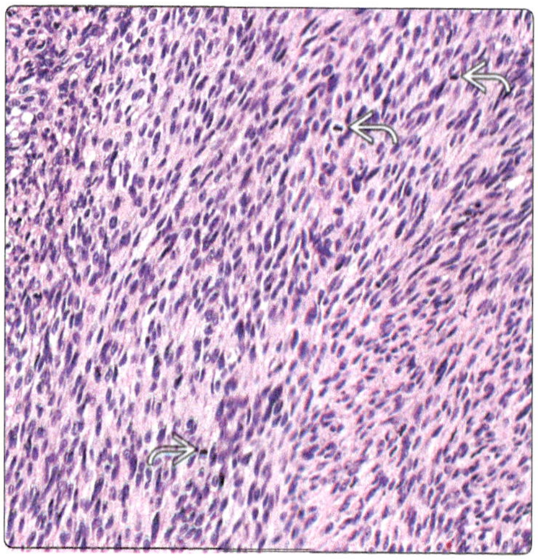

(Left) *Malignant blue nevus at low magnification appears similar to a cellular blue nevus, with lobules of pale-staining cells surrounded by darker-staining pigmented spindle cells and melanophages. However, there was significant atypia and atypical mitoses identified on high magnification.* **(Right)** *Higher magnification of a malignant cellular blue nevus shows a densely cellular area composed of fascicles of hyperchromatic-staining cells with multiple mitotic figures.*

Focus of Necrosis in Malignant Cellular Blue Nevus

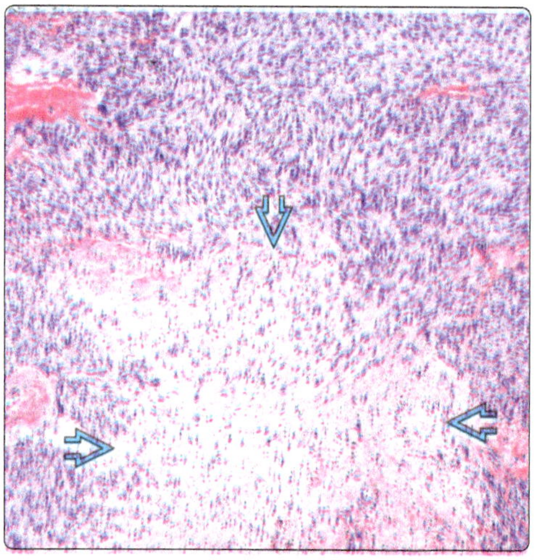

Ki-67 Immunohistochemistry in Malignant Cellular Blue Nevus

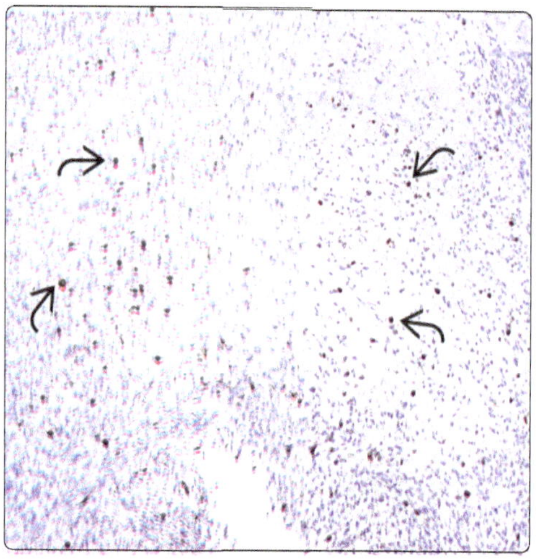

(Left) *This field shows a deep focus of necrosis in an MCBN surrounded by atypical oval to spindled cells with nuclear hyperchromasia.* **(Right)** *Ki-67 in the same case shows increased numbers of melanocytic nuclei staining around the area of necrosis, consistent with a malignant tumor.*

Heavily Pigmented Malignant Cellular Blue Nevus

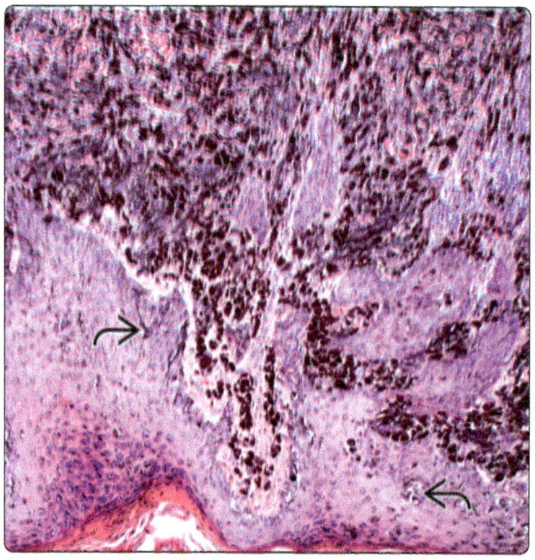

Higher Magnification of Heavily Pigmented Malignant Cellular Blue Nevus

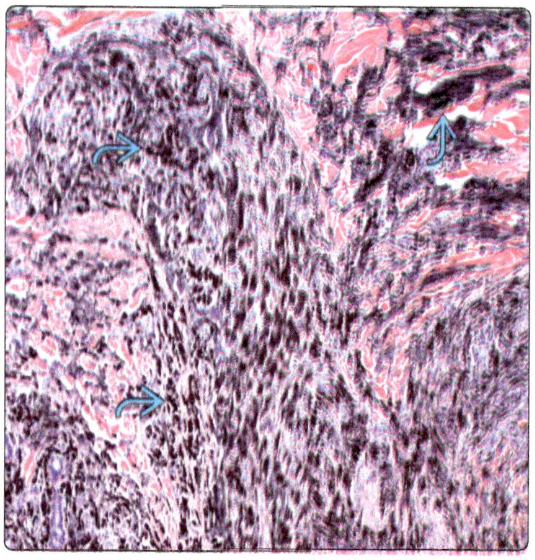

(Left) *This is another example of MCBN showing a proliferation of heavily pigmented cells in the superficial dermis. Note the presence of an atypical junctional lentiginous and pagetoid component, which is lacking in benign cellular blue nevi.* **(Right)** *Higher magnification of the dermal component shows fascicles of heavily pigmented cells surrounded by stromal fibrosis and numerous melanophages, findings often seen in blue nevi and deep penetrating nevi.*

Malignant Cellular Blue Nevus With Densely Cellular Fascicles

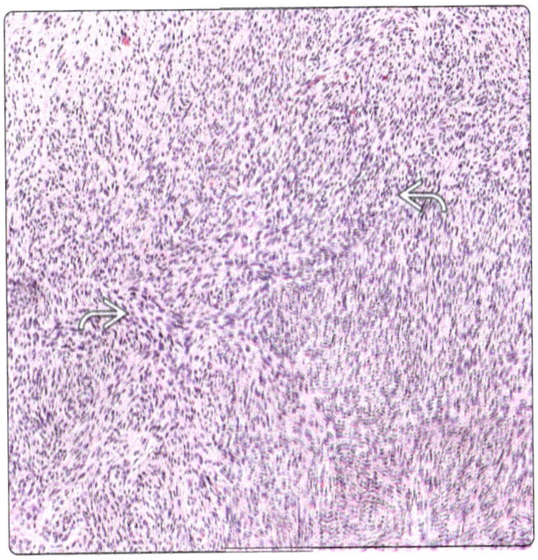

Malignant Cellular Blue Nevus With Prominent Pigmentation

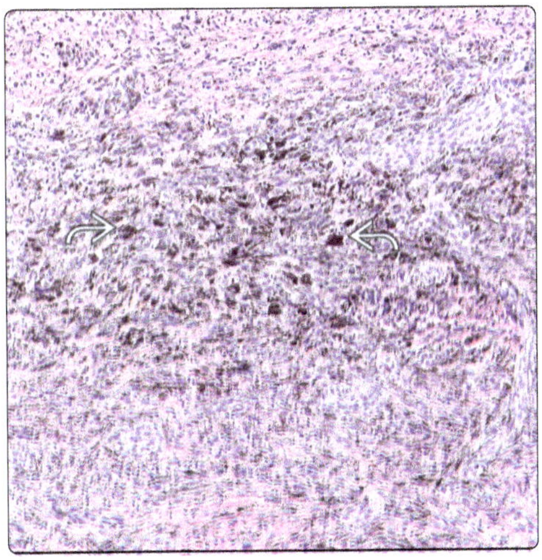

(Left) *Low magnification of another malignant cellular blue nevus shows densely cellular collections of hyperchromatic-staining cells forming irregular fascicles.* **(Right)** *This example shows more heavily pigmented oval to spindled melanocytes and scattered associated melanophages.*

Differential Diagnosis: Cellular Blue Nevus

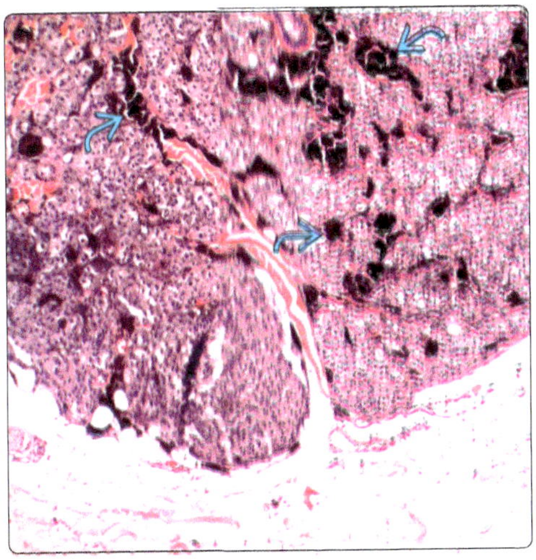

Differential Diagnosis: Cellular Blue Nevus

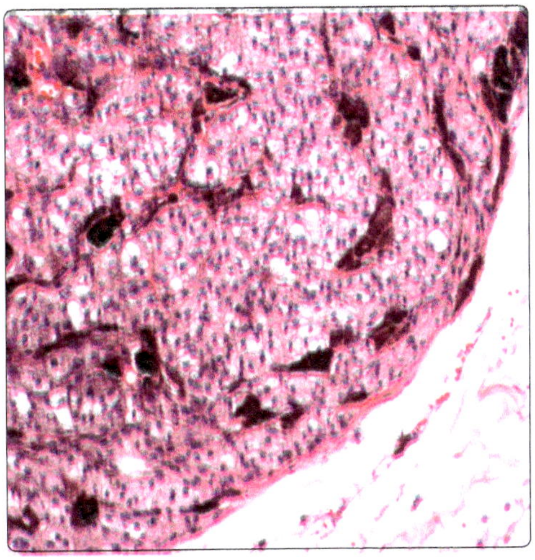

(Left) *Cellular blue nevus is composed of well-circumscribed lobules of pale- to clear-staining melanocytes associated with numerous melanophages. They show no evidence of high-grade atypia or atypical mitotic figures.* **(Right)** *Higher magnification of cellular blue nevus shows well-circumscribed lobules of pale- to clear-staining melanocytes associated with numerous melanophages. Note the lack of high-grade atypia or mitotic figures.*

Differential Diagnosis: Deep Penetrating Nevus

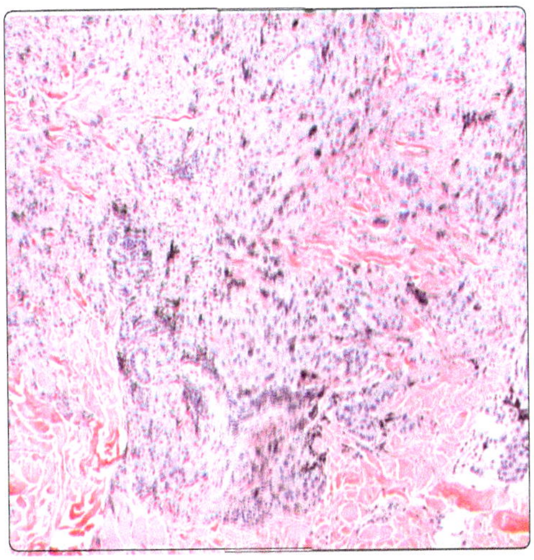

Immunohistochemistry for p16 in DPN

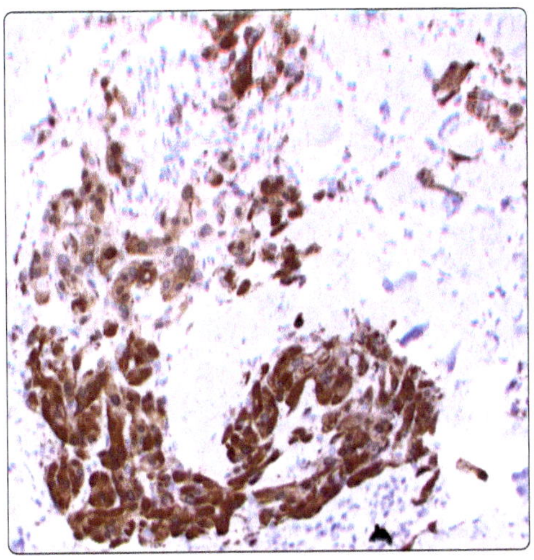

(Left) *Deep penetrating nevus (DPN) is often considered a subtype of cellular blue nevus but is composed of smaller nests and fascicles of oval to spindled-shaped melanocytes. In addition, the lesion often shows more of a wedge-shaped distribution at low magnification.* **(Right)** *DPN, like most benign melanocytic tumors, typically shows diffuse p16 expression. Loss of p16 is often seen in melanoma, including MCBN.*

Pigmented Epithelioid Melanocytoma ("Animal-Type Melanoma")

KEY FACTS

TERMINOLOGY

- Heavily pigmented, deeply invasive melanocytic proliferation with low-grade malignant potential
- Very controversial entity, not universally accepted (especially inclusion of some epithelioid blue nevi in this category)

CLINICAL ISSUES

- Heavily pigmented, dome-shaped nodule
- Occur sporadically or in association with Carney complex
- Low-grade malignant potential
- Complete excision necessary
- Extremities, trunk, and head and neck are most commonly affected sites
- Heavily pigmented, dome-shaped, or verrucous nodule ≥ 1.0 cm in diameter

MICROSCOPIC

- Deep dermal tumor with frequent involvement of subcutis
- More cellular in center and shows infiltrative growth pattern at periphery
- Composed of 3 principal cell types
    - Medium-sized epithelioid cells, large epithelioid cells, and spindled cells
- Spindled blue nevus-like cells
- Large epithelioid cells
- Does not exhibit brisk dermal mitotic activity

ANCILLARY TESTS

- Loss of expression for protein kinase A regulatory subunit 1-α

TOP DIFFERENTIAL DIAGNOSES

- Malignant blue nevus
- Atypical cellular blue nevus
- Cellular blue nevus
- Common blue nevus

Extensive Pigmentation in PEM

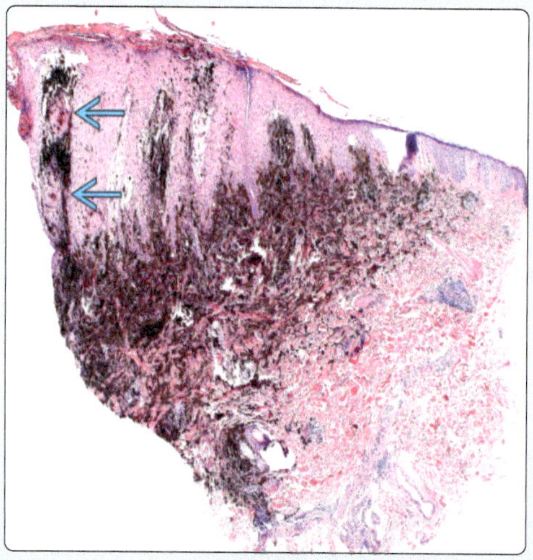

Intraepidermal Melanophages in PEM

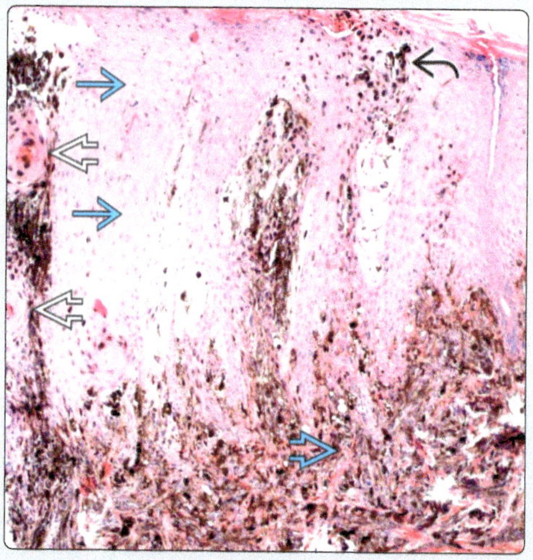

(Left) *A punch biopsy from an 11-year-old girl, right posterior auricular, shows a heavily pigmented compound melanocytic tumor with overlying epidermal hyperplasia and squamous proliferation →. Typically, pigmented epithelioid melanocytoma (PEM) is over pigmented out of proportion to the tumor.* **(Right)** *Among the epidermal psoriasiform hyperplasia →, there lies intraepidermal melanophages →. The squamous eddies → are reactive and not neoplastic. Large epithelioid dermal cells are evident →.*

High Magnification of Large Epithelioid Cytology

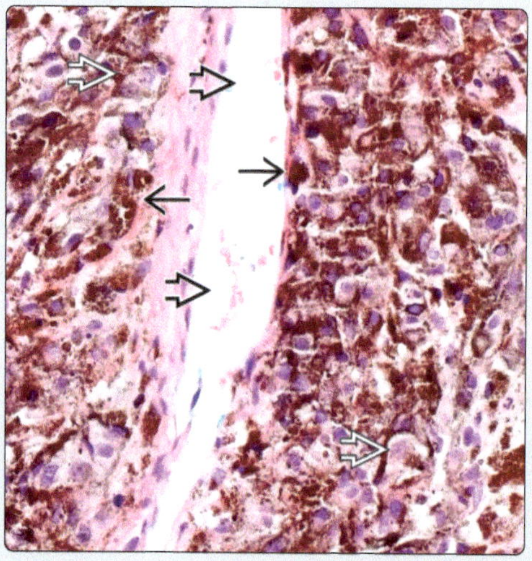

Nodal Metastasis in PEM

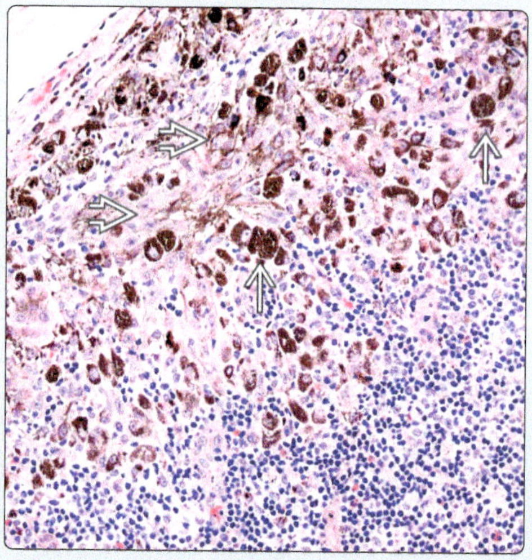

(Left) *High magnification shows large epithelioid cells → with open chromatin and cherry-red macronucleoli. The melanophages are packed with chunky clusters of melanin →, masking the nuclei. The tumor cells condense around the blood vessels and lymphatics but do not invade vascular spaces →.* **(Right)** *A sentinel lymph node biopsy from the 11-year-old girl diagnosed with PEM shows melanophages → and large epithelioid tumor cells →, seen in multiple foci throughout the lymph node.*

TERMINOLOGY

Abbreviations

- Pigmented epithelioid melanocytoma (PEM)

Synonyms

- Older terms, not recommended
  - Animal-type melanoma

Definitions

- Heavily pigmented, deeply invasive melanocytic proliferation with low-grade malignant potential
- Very controversial entity, not universally accepted (especially inclusion of some epithelioid blue nevi in this category)

ETIOLOGY/PATHOGENESIS

Genetic Syndrome

- May occur sporadically or in association with Carney complex

CLINICAL ISSUES

Site

- Extremities, trunk, and head and neck are most commonly affected sites

Presentation

- Heavily pigmented, dome-shaped, or verrucous nodule ≥ 1.0 cm in diameter
- Often of long duration

Treatment

- Surgical approaches
  - Complete excision necessary
  - Most experts recommend sentinel lymph node biopsy
  - Systemic therapy may not be indicated, given lower malignant potential of PEM

Prognosis

- Has capacity to metastasize to lymph nodes but with less frequent systemic spread
- Short-term follow-up suggests better prognosis for PEM than for conventional metastatic melanoma

MICROSCOPIC

Histologic Features

- Extends into deep reticular tissue and subcutaneous fat along adnexal structures or neurovascular bundles
- More cellular in center and shows infiltrative growth pattern at periphery
- Abuts epidermis and often associated with epidermal hyperplasia
  - However, some are separated from epidermis by grenz zone of uninvolved papillary dermis
- Composed of 3 principal cell types (listed from most to least abundant)
  - Medium-sized epithelioid cells with exorbitant intracellular coarse melanin
    - Unclear if these cells are all melanocytic in nature, as some have features of tumor-infiltrating macrophages
  - Spindled blue nevus-like cells
    - Found singly or in small groups penetrating among surrounding stromal collagen bundles
  - Large epithelioid cells
    - May be multinucleated
- Does not exhibit brisk dermal mitotic activity
- Rarely exhibits necrosis

Cytologic Features

- Depends on cell type
  - Medium-sized epithelioid cells have heavily pigmented cytoplasm obscuring nuclei
    - Oval and regular nuclei contain multiple small eosinophilic nucleoli
  - Spindled blue nevus-like cells have vesicular nuclei with amphophilic cytoplasm
  - Large epithelioid cells have large vesicular nuclei with prominent macronucleoli and abundant cytoplasm
    - Melanin granules at periphery of cytoplasm, giving cells fried egg appearance

ANCILLARY TESTS

Immunohistochemistry

- Loss of expression for protein kinase A regulatory subunit 1-α

DIFFERENTIAL DIAGNOSIS

Malignant Blue Nevus

- Melanoma arising in or mimicking blue nevus
  - Has blue nevus (blue nevus-like) component
  - Dermal mitoses and tumor necrosis are common

Atypical Cellular Blue Nevus

- Usually shows areas of cellular blue nevus
- Tumor necrosis and ulceration are rare
- Atypical mitoses not observed

Cellular Blue Nevus

- Shows dumbbell-shaped cellular dermal lobules of bland-appearing melanocytes
- Often shows surrounding areas of more conventional blue nevus

Common Blue Nevus

- Does not show pigmented epithelioid cells of PEM
- Dermal sclerosis, common in blue nevus, is rarely seen in PEM

DIAGNOSTIC CHECKLIST

Pathologic Interpretation Pearls

- Finding fried egg cells can be helpful
- Melanin-bleached sections are helpful in evaluation of cytological details

SELECTED REFERENCES

1. Dadras SS et al: Transplantable malignant melanoma in LT.B6 congenic mice resembling pigmented epithelioid melanocytoma in humans. J Invest Dermatol. 134(6):1772-5, 2014

(Left) *This is an excisional biopsy of a black tumor on the back. At scanning magnification, the dermal expansion, by heavily melanized tumor cells, resembles a blue nevus or malignant blue nevus. The extent of melanization seems out of proportion. No geographic areas of necrosis are identified.* **(Right)** *The lesion is deeply invasive into the reticular collagen (Clark level IV) but has a smooth, noninfiltrative border. There is an area of eosinophilic collagen but no definitive necrosis was identified.*

PEM: Heavily Pigmented Dermal Neoplasm

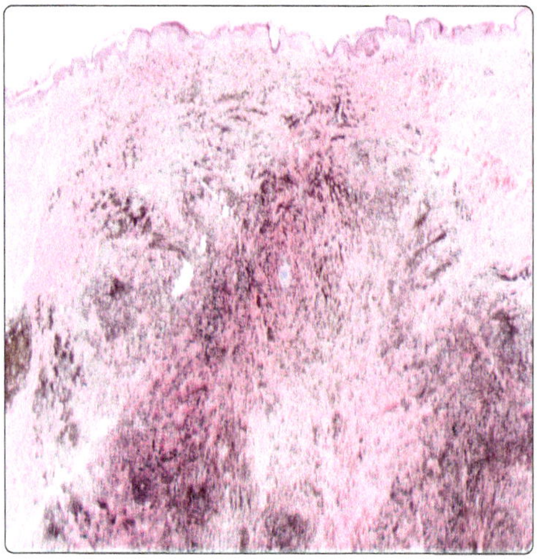

PEM: Deeply Invasive but With Smooth Border

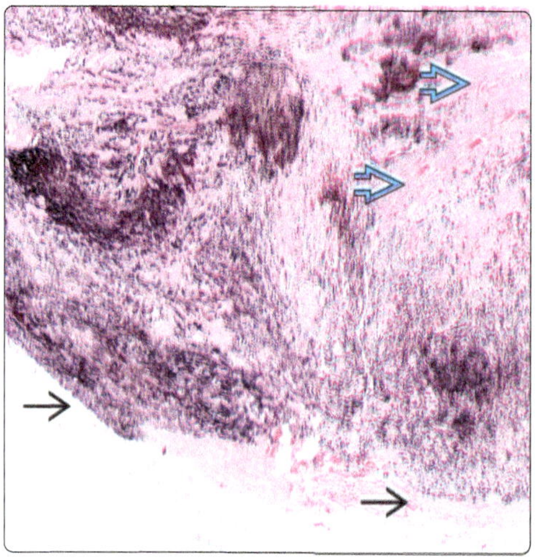

(Left) *There are large epithelioid cells with dendritic processes, similar to blue nevus. However, this lesion is very large and the pigmentation is out of proportion. The large cells are less melanized compared to the melanophages.* **(Right)** *As grey horses that naturally develop PEM, so can an experimental mouse model. The dermis is overwhelmed by a heavily pigmented melanocytic tumor, replacing the adnexa. A distinct nodule is evident with adjacent areas of melanophages.*

Large Epithelioid Cells in PEM

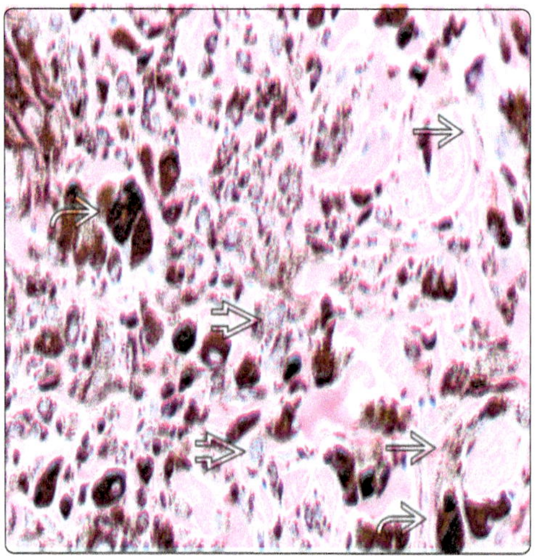

LT.B6 Congenic Mouse Tumor Mimicking PEM

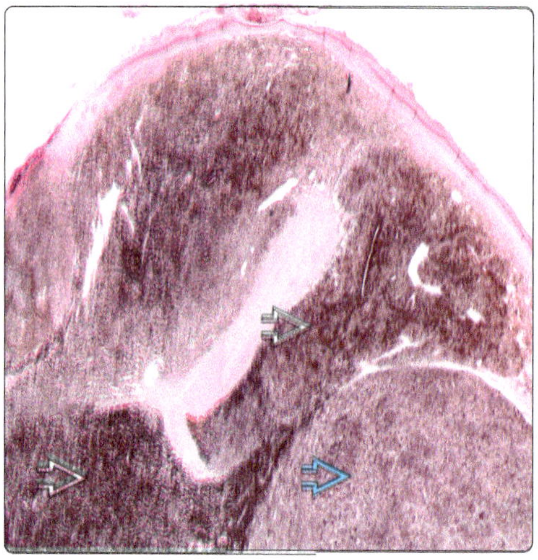

(Left) *The nodule is deeply invasive into the reticular dermis, but the pushing border is smooth and well defined. Similar to the human counterpart, there is no necrosis.* **(Right)** *There are numerous large epithelioid cells that are less pigmented than the adjacent melanophages. The epithelioid cells have open chromatin with prominent nucleoli. A dendritic meshwork is evident.*

Smooth Tumor Border in Mouse Tumor

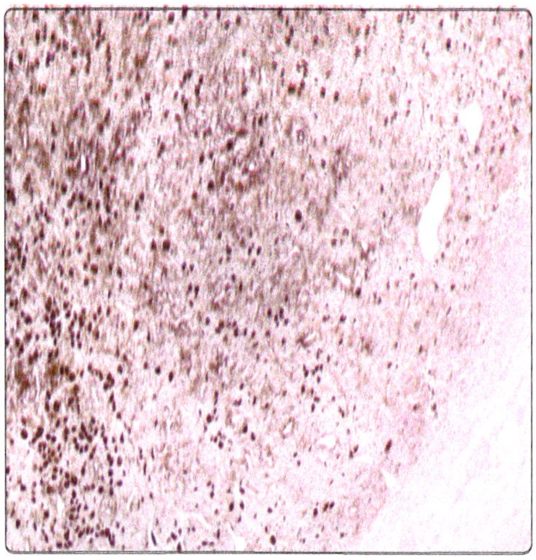

Large Epithelioid Cytology in Mouse Tumor

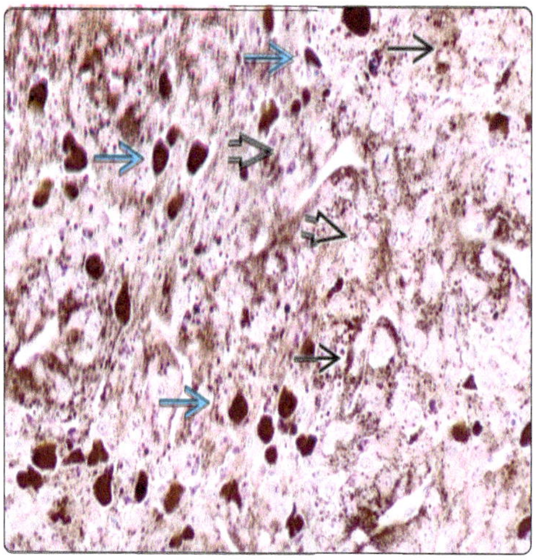

Differential Diagnosis: Malignant Cellular Blue Nevus

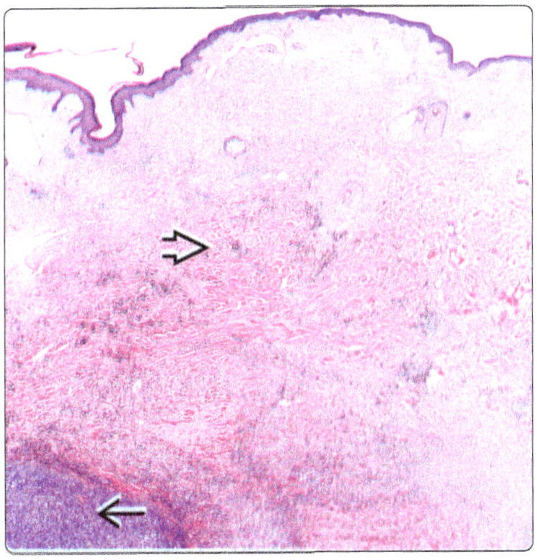

Dermal Tumor Nodule and Adjacent Necrosis in Malignant Cellular Blue Nevus

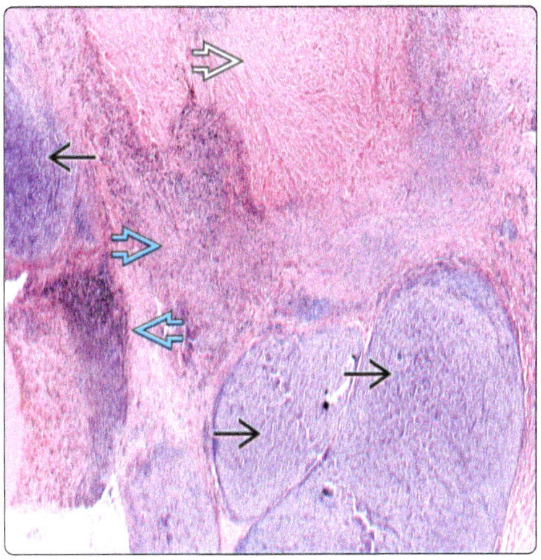

(Left) *A deeply invasive, pigmented neoplasm is depicted here, expanding the reticular dermis. A blue nevus-like area → is evident in the superficial aspect of the lesion. The tumor is not over pigmented. An amelanotic blue nodule → is identified.* **(Right)** *Deep in the lesion, there are amelanotic blue tumor nodules → adjacent to large areas of necrosis →. Zones of melanophages → are evident at the rim of necrosis.*

Malignant Cellular Blue Nevus at Higher Magnification

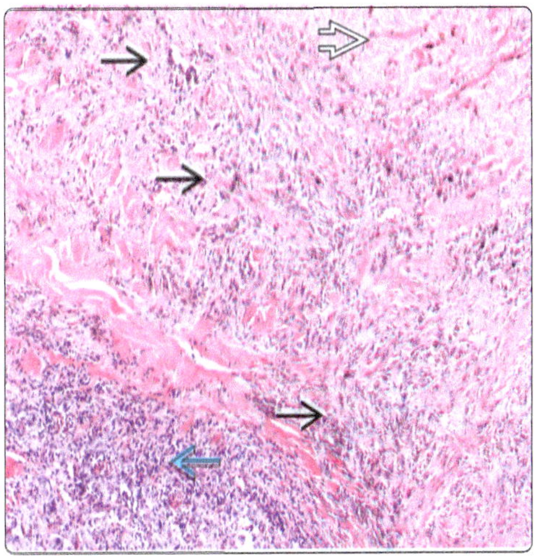

Small Blue Epithelioid Cytology in Malignant Cellular Blue Nevus

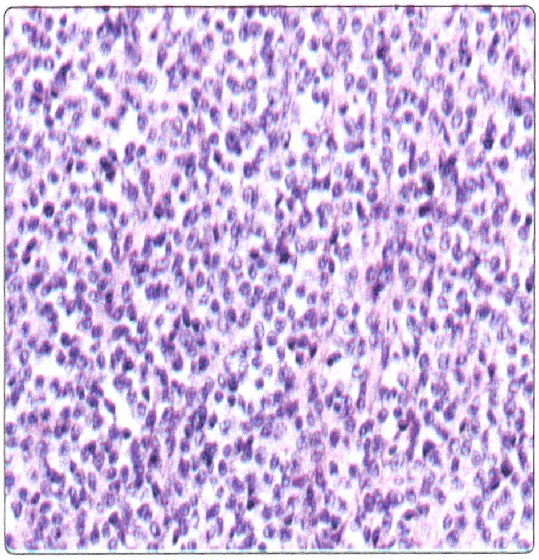

(Left) *A zone of necrosis → with a rim of melanophages → and lymphohistiocytic infiltrate → is identified.* **(Right)** *A high-power examination of the depigmented nodules shows a composition of tightly packed small blue lymphoid-like epithelioid cells in this malignant blue nevus. Surprisingly, no brisk mitotic activity is identified in this area.*

Differential Diagnosis: Cellular Blue Nevus

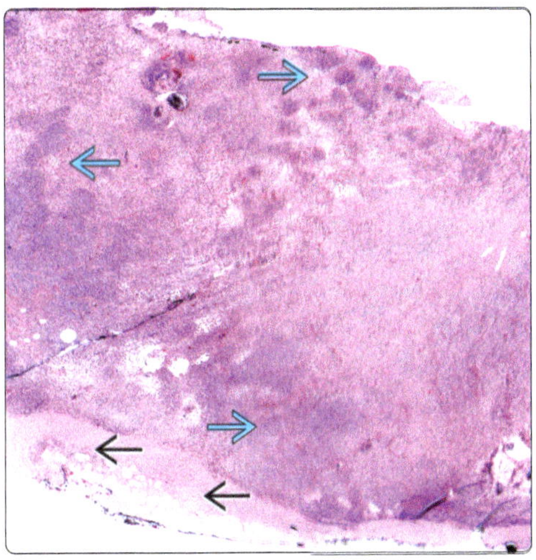

Lack of Cytological Atypia in Cellular Blue Nevus

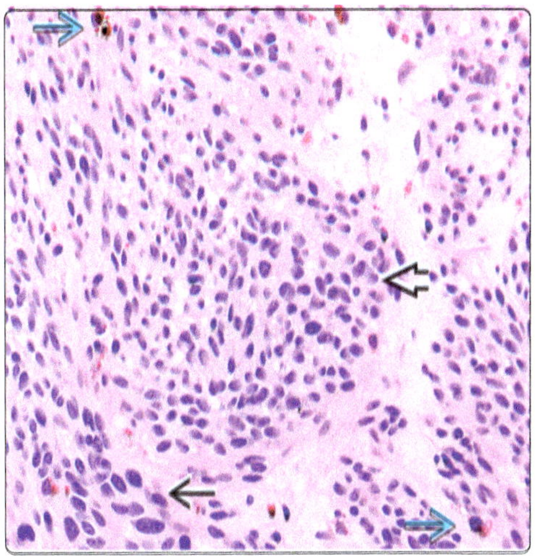

(Left) *This excisional biopsy shows a hypercellular, deep-seated melanocytic tumor that extends deeply into subcutaneous adipose tissue →. There are areas of vague nodularity →. Lack of melanin pigmentation is noted and is in contrast to pigmented epithelioid melanocytoma.* **(Right)** *A closer examination of a nodule shows fusiform → to epithelioid nuclei →. The chromatin is evenly dispersed with conspicuous nucleoli. The nuclear membrane is smooth and no mitoses are found. Only focal melanin → is evident.*

KEY FACTS

TERMINOLOGY

- Primary dermal melanoma (PDM)
- Primary cutaneous melanoma arising in dermis or subcutis, mimicking metastatic melanoma (MM)
- By definition, lacks any evidence of epidermal involvement, ulceration, or regression

CLINICAL ISSUES

- Often clinically suspected to be cyst or epithelial tumor
- Extremely rare tumors
- Typically occur in older adults
- Presents as dermal mass in sun-damaged skin
- Complete and wider excision necessary
- Complete clinical and imaging studies required in order to exclude possibility of MM

MICROSCOPIC

- Nodular, well-circumscribed, dermal &/or subcutaneous based
- By definition, no overlying epidermal involvement, ulceration, or evidence of regression can be present
- Composed of highly atypical melanocytes
- Variable mixture of cell types: Typically epithelioid but may be spindle-shaped, rhabdoid, or pleomorphic
- Mitoses are often easily identified; necrosis may be present

TOP DIFFERENTIAL DIAGNOSES

- Metastatic melanoma
  - Should be history of previous or concurrent melanoma
  - Well-circumscribed dermal &/or subcutaneous nodular mass, features very similar to PDM
- Primary nodular melanoma
  - Overlying junctional component &/or ulceration should be present
- Spitzoid melanoma
  - Occur in younger patients
  - Typically shows mixture of spindled and epithelioid-shaped cells, similar to Spitz nevi

Clinical Photograph of PDM on Scalp

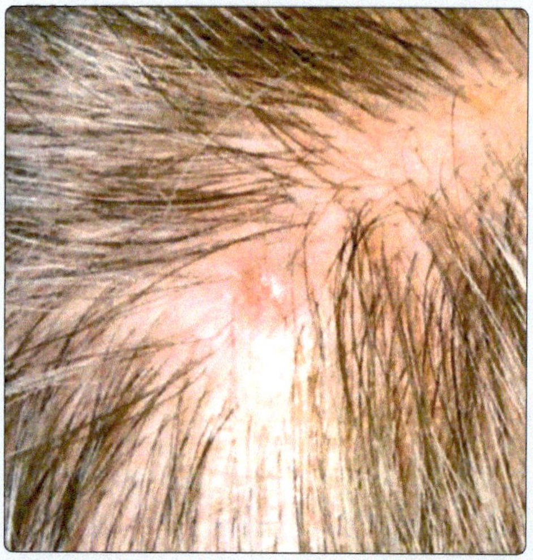

PDM at Scanning Magnification

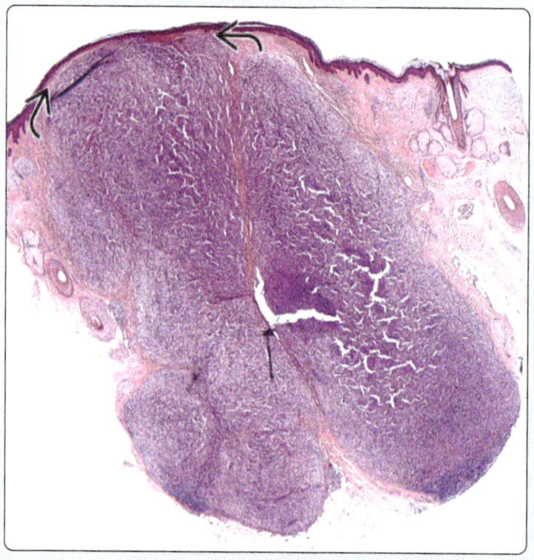

(Left) *Clinical photograph shows a nodular-appearing, flesh-colored lesion on the scalp of a patient. Most cases of primary dermal melanoma (PDM) are not pigmented and are often thought to be a cyst or epithelial tumor clinically. (Courtesy S. Swetter, MD.)* **(Right)** *Low magnification of a PDM shows a well-circumscribed, dermal-based nodule, mimicking metastatic melanoma. Note the grenz zone ➜ separating the tumor from the overlying epidermis.*

High Magnification of PDM

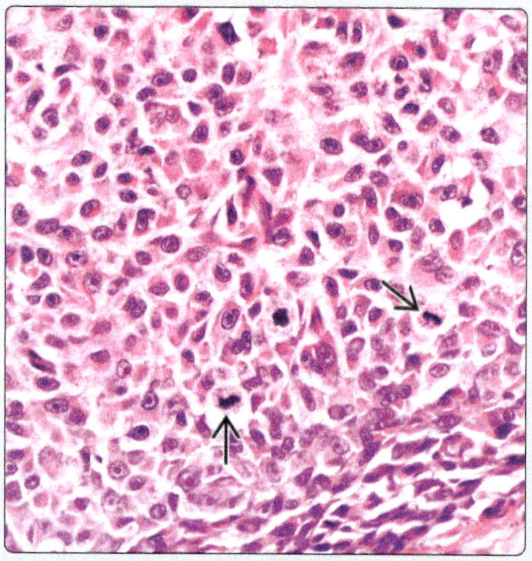

PDM With Focal Pigmentation

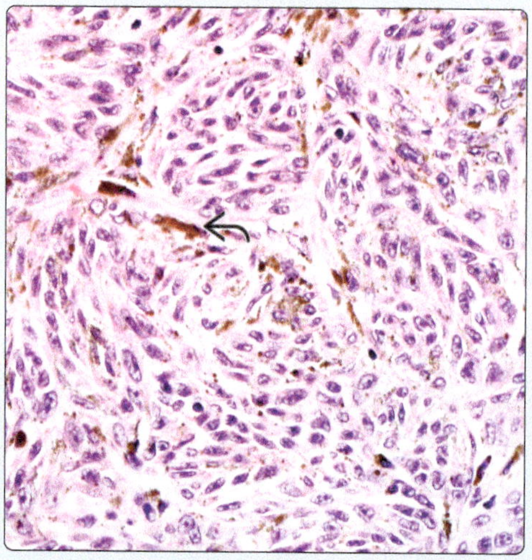

(Left) *High magnification of PDM typically shows marked cytologic atypia and multiple mitotic figures ➜.* **(Right)** *Most cases of PDM are amelanotic, although a few are pigmented. This case was composed of oval- to spindle-shaped cells with scattered cytoplasmic pigmentation and melanophages ➜.*

TERMINOLOGY

Abbreviations

- Primary dermal melanoma (PDM)

Synonyms

- Dermal &/or subcutaneous melanoma

Definitions

- Primary melanoma arising in dermis or subcutis, typically mimicking metastatic melanoma (MM)
- Clinically, lack of prior or concurrent melanoma by history and imaging studies
- Histologically, lack of any evidence of epidermal involvement, ulceration, or regression

ETIOLOGY/PATHOGENESIS

Unknown

- Typically arises in sun-damaged skin of elderly, thus may be related to solar damage

CLINICAL ISSUES

Epidemiology

- Incidence
  - Extremely rare (estimated incidence: < 0.1% of all melanoma cases)
- Age
  - Typically occur in older adults (mean age: 70 years)

Presentation

- Dermal mass in sun-damaged skin
  - Often clinically suspected to be cyst or epithelial tumor
- Amelanotic in most cases

Treatment

- Surgical approaches
  - Complete and wider excision necessary (margins typical for invasive melanoma)
  - Typically, sentinel lymph node biopsy will also be performed for staging purposes

Prognosis

- Relatively good, especially compared to MM of unknown origin and similar depth primary nodular melanomas

Clinical Work-Up

- Complete clinical and imaging studies necessary in order to exclude possibility of MM

MACROSCOPIC

General Features

- Large, solid to cystic, dermal-based nodule
- Typically not pigmented

MICROSCOPIC

Histologic Features

- Atypical nodular dermal-based melanocytic tumor
  - Typically well-circumscribed, unencapsulated deep dermal &/or subcutaneous mass
  - By definition, no overlying epidermal involvement, ulceration, or evidence of regression can be present
    - Multiple sections should be examined to exclude these features
  - Variable mixture of cell types: Typically epithelioid but may be spindle-shaped, rhabdoid, or pleomorphic appearing
  - Mitoses are often easily identified
  - Necrosis may be present

Cytologic Features

- Cytologic atypia prominent, with enlarged nuclei and prominent nucleoli

ANCILLARY TESTS

Immunohistochemistry

- Strongly positive for melanocytic markers by immunohistochemistry (IHC), including S100, MART-1/Melan-A, and HMB-45 in most cases
- Lower levels of p53, Ki-67, cyclin-D1, and D2-40 (lymphovascular spaces) compared to MM and nodular-type melanomas

DIFFERENTIAL DIAGNOSIS

Metastatic Melanoma

- Ideally, there should be history of previous or concurrent melanoma
  - If no history, complete clinical examination and imaging studies should be performed
- Well-circumscribed dermal &/or subcutaneous nodular mass, features very similar to PDM
- Epidermal involvement may rarely be seen (epidermotropic metastasis)
- IHC typically shows higher levels of Ki-67, cyclin-D1, p53, and D2-40 compared to PDM

Primary Nodular Melanoma

- Predominantly dermal-based, nodular lesion with deep invasion
- By definition, at least focal overlying epidermal involvement &/or ulceration
- IHC may show higher levels of Ki-67, cyclin-D1, p53, and D2-40 compared to PDM

Spitzoid Melanoma

- Can be dermal-based in some cases but most are compound tumors
- Typically show mixture of spindled and epithelioid-shaped cells, similar to Spitz nevi
- More often occur in adolescents and young adults

SELECTED REFERENCES

1. Doepker MP et al: Dermal melanoma: a report on prognosis, outcomes, and the utility of sentinel lymph node biopsy. J Surg Oncol. 113(1):98-102, 2016
2. Sidiropoulos M et al: Primary dermal melanoma: a unique subtype of melanoma to be distinguished from cutaneous metastatic melanoma: a clinical, histologic, and gene expression-profiling study. J Am Acad Dermatol. 71(6):1083-92, 2014
3. Cassarino DS et al: Primary dermal melanoma: distinct immunohistochemical findings and clinical outcome compared with nodular and metastatic melanoma. Arch Dermatol. 144(1):49-56, 2008
4. Swetter SM et al: Primary dermal melanoma: a distinct subtype of melanoma. Arch Dermatol. 140(1):99-103, 2004

KEY FACTS

TERMINOLOGY

- Rare variants of melanoma, including chondroid, osseous, myxoid, rhabdoid, and balloon cell melanoma

ETIOLOGY/PATHOGENESIS

- Related to UV exposure in most cases

CLINICAL ISSUES

- Very rare tumors

MICROSCOPIC

- Most variants often show areas of more conventional-appearing melanoma &/or overlying melanoma in situ
- **Balloon cell/clear cell melanoma**
  - Composed of enlarged cells with abundant clear to vacuolated-appearing cytoplasm
- **Chondroid melanoma**
  - Malignant epithelioid cells associated with prominent myxochondroid-appearing matrix
- **Osteoid melanoma**
  - Malignant epithelioid cells associated with prominent osteoid-appearing material
- **Myxoid melanoma**
  - Atypical epithelioid cells scattered in prominent myxoid matrix
- **Small cell melanoma**
  - Nests and sheets of small, hyperchromatic-staining cells with scant cytoplasm (high nuclear:cytoplasmic ratio)
- **Rhabdoid melanoma**
  - Proliferation of markedly enlarged and atypical-appearing melanocytes with abundant eosinophilic-staining cytoplasm

TOP DIFFERENTIAL DIAGNOSES

- Nevi
- Chondroma or other tumors with cartilaginous differentiation
- Osteoma or other tumors with osseous differentiation
- Benign cutaneous myxoid proliferations

Balloon Cell Melanoma

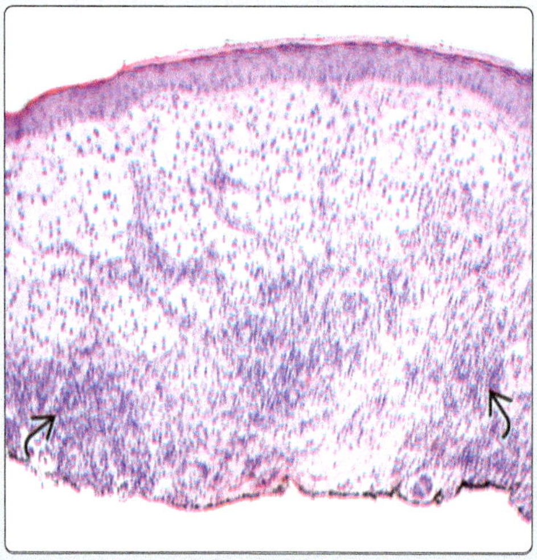

Myxoid Melanoma

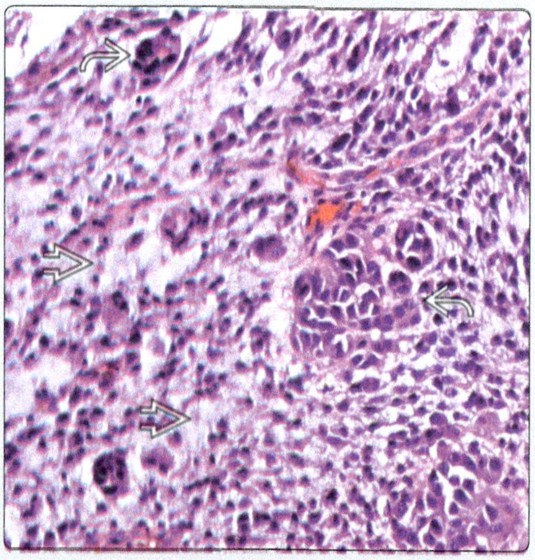

(Left) *Balloon cell melanoma is composed of nests of large, pale- to clear-staining cells with abundant vacuolated cytoplasm (mimicking sebocytes). Note the associated lymphocytic infiltrate ➔.* **(Right)** *High magnification of myxoid melanoma shows many single tumor cells and small nests ➔ floating in a prominent mucinous stroma ➔.*

Spindle Cell/Pleomorphic Melanoma

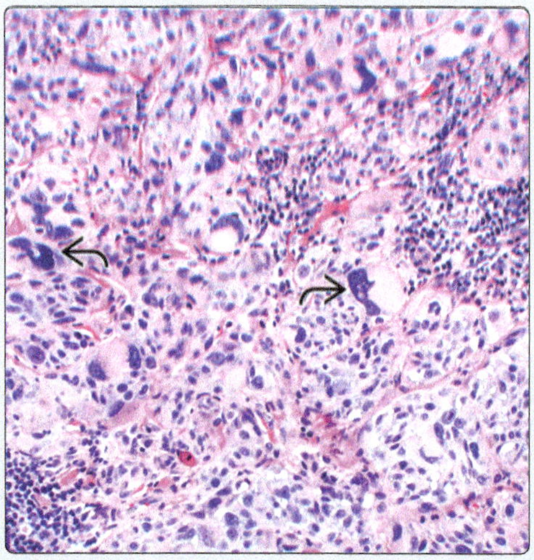

S100 Immunohistochemical Stain in Spindle Cell/Pleomorphic Melanoma

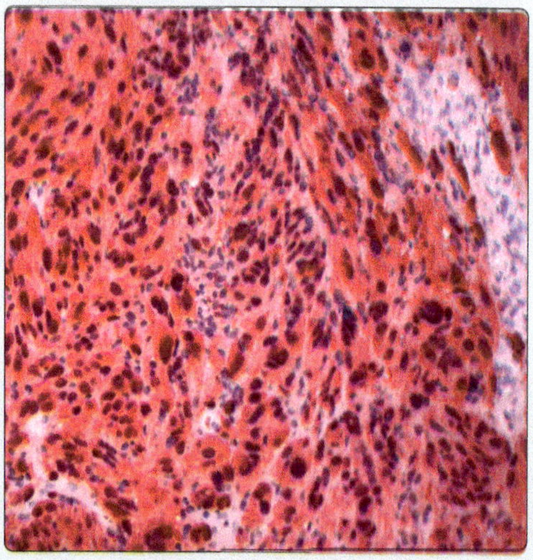

(Left) *This is a case of spindle cell/pleomorphic melanoma, which can mimic spindle cell carcinoma, atypical fibroxanthoma, and pleomorphic sarcoma (as well as other sarcomas). Note the frankly pleomorphic, bizarre-appearing tumor giant cells ➔.* **(Right)** *S100 (red chromogen) shows strong and diffuse staining in this case of spindle cell/pleomorphic melanoma, essentially excluding the other tumors in the differential diagnosis.*

TERMINOLOGY

Definitions

- Rare variants of melanoma, including clear cell/balloon cell, chondroid, osteoid, myxoid, and rhabdoid melanoma

ETIOLOGY/PATHOGENESIS

Environmental Exposure

- Related to UV exposure in most cases

CLINICAL ISSUES

Site

- Sun-damaged skin, typically head and neck region, upper trunk, forearms

Presentation

- Usually present as papule or nodule with irregular, asymmetric borders

Treatment

- Surgical approaches
  - Complete and wide excision, with clinical margins based on Breslow depth

Prognosis

- Depends on typical melanoma prognostic features, such as Breslow depth, ulceration, mitotic count, and presence of perineural or angiolymphatic invasion

MICROSCOPIC

Histologic Features

- Depends on histologic variant
- Most cases often show areas of conventional-appearing melanoma &/or overlying melanoma in situ
- **Clear cell/balloon cell melanoma**
  - Enlarged cells with abundant clear- to vacuolated-appearing cytoplasm
  - May appear deceptively bland in some cases
- **Chondroid melanoma**
  - Malignant epithelioid cells associated with myxochondroid-appearing matrix
  - Often shows areas of overlying melanoma in situ or more conventional melanoma with nesting
- **Osteoid melanoma**
  - Malignant epithelioid cells associated with prominent osteoid-appearing material
- **Myxoid melanoma**
  - Atypical epithelioid to spindle-shaped cells scattered in prominent myxoid matrix
- **Small cell melanoma**
  - Nests and sheets of small, hyperchromatic-staining cells with scant cytoplasm (high nuclear:cytoplasmic ratio)
  - Mimics basal cell carcinoma, Merkel cell carcinoma, or other neuroendocrine carcinomas
- **Rhabdoid melanoma**
  - Proliferation of enlarged and atypical-appearing cells with abundant eosinophilic cytoplasm
  - Peripheral displacement of nucleus by cytoplasmic material (intermediate filaments)
- **Signet ring cell melanoma**
  - Atypical epithelioid cells with pale- to clear-staining cytoplasm
  - Peripheral displacement of nucleus

Cytologic Features

- Cells are usually enlarged and atypical appearing with hyperchromatic nuclei, prominent nucleoli

ANCILLARY TESTS

Immunohistochemistry

- Most are typically positive for melanocytic markers, including S100, MART-1/Melan-A, HMB-45, tyrosinase, and SOX10

DIFFERENTIAL DIAGNOSIS

Nevi

- Compound nevi may show balloon cell features, rarely osteoid or chondroid material
- Nevus cells lack significant cytologic atypia, pleomorphism, or mitotic activity

DDx of Chondroid Melanoma

- Chondroma or other tumors with cartilaginous differentiation
  - Benign chondrocytes in myxocollagenous stroma
  - Lacks evidence of melanocytic differentiation by IHC

DDx of Osteoid Melanoma

- Osteoma or other tumors with osseous differentiation
  - Benign osteoclasts and mature-appearing bone
  - IHC(-) for melanocytic differentiation

DDx of Myxoid Melanoma

- Benign cutaneous myxoid proliferations
  - Bland-appearing, spindle-shaped fibroblasts or myofibroblasts in myoid stroma
  - Often prominent vascularity (e.g., myxoma, angiomyxoma)
- Malignant cutaneous myxoid proliferations
  - Myxofibrosarcoma: Atypical spindle-shaped cells in myxoid stroma with prominent chicken-wire pattern of vessels
  - Myxoid liposarcoma (extremely rare in skin): Also shows chicken-wire vascularity

SELECTED REFERENCES

1. Inskip M et al: Pigmented primary cutaneous balloon cell melanoma demonstrating balloon cells in the dermoepidermal junction: a brief case report with dermatoscopy and histopathology. Int J Dermatol. 55(2):e110-2, 2016
2. Joana Devesa P et al: Cartilaginous melanoma: case report and review of the literature. An Bras Dermatol. 88(3):403-7, 2013
3. Gharpuray-Pandit D et al: Rhabdomyoblastic differentiation in malignant melanoma in adults: report of 2 cases. Int J Surg Pathol. 15(1):20-5, 2007
4. Inoue T et al: Metastatic myxoid melanoma with partial regression of the primary lesion. J Cutan Pathol. 34(6):508-12, 2007
5. Rütten A et al: Primary cutaneous signet-ring cell melanoma: a clinico-pathologic and immunohistochemical study of two cases. Am J Dermatopathol. 25(5):418-22, 2003
6. Blessing K et al: Small cell malignant melanoma: a variant of naevoid melanoma. Clinicopathological features and histological differential diagnosis. J Clin Pathol. 53(8):591-5, 2000
7. Lucas DR et al: Osteogenic melanoma. a rare variant of malignant melanoma. Am J Surg Pathol. 17(4):400-9, 1993

Clear Cell Melanoma

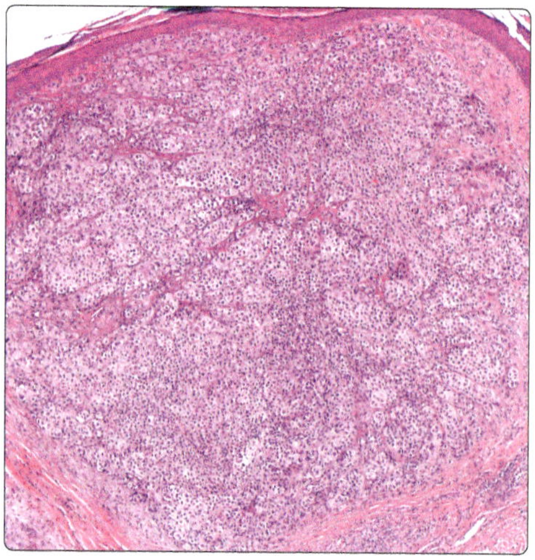

Clear Cell Melanoma at High Magnification

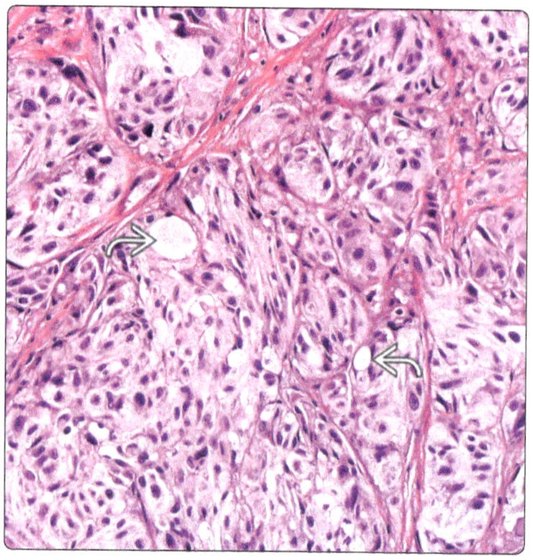

(Left) *Clear cell melanoma shows a dense, nodular to sheet-like dermal proliferation of pale-staining cells. These tumors can mimic clear cell sarcoma, but the superficial location would be highly unusual.* **(Right)** *High magnification of clear cell melanoma shows atypical cells with abundant pale- to clear-staining cytoplasm and cytoplasmic vacuoles ➡. The nests are surrounded by fibrous bands, mimicking clear cell sarcoma.*

Small Cell Melanoma

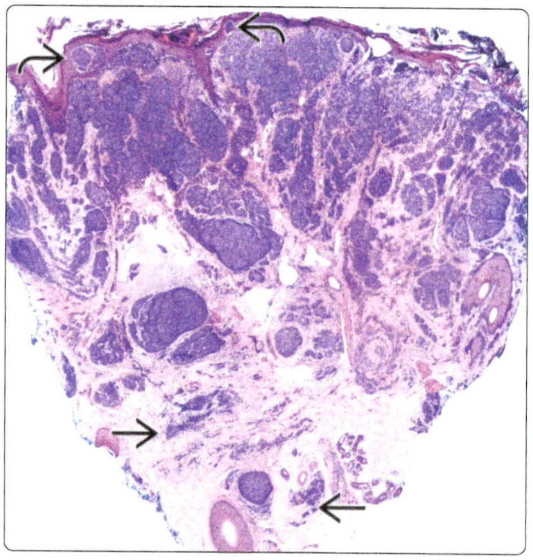

Small Cell Melanoma at Higher Magnification

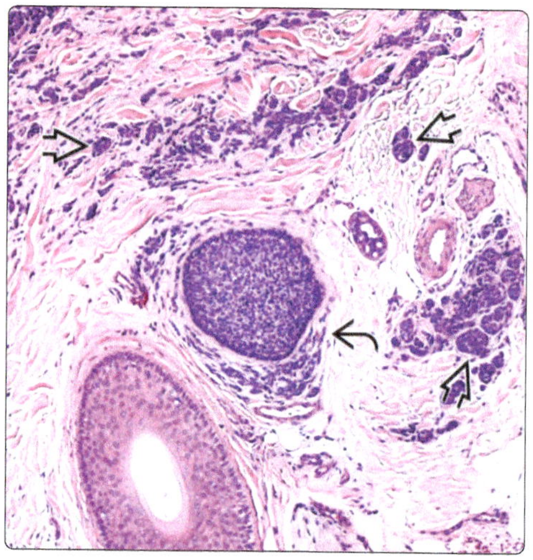

(Left) *Small cell melanoma shows a diffusely invasive tumor extending into the deep dermis ➡. These cases can be mistaken for basal cell carcinoma or Merkel cell carcinoma at low magnification. However, an overlying melanoma in situ component ➡ is present, providing a clue to the diagnosis, which can be confirmed by IHC.* **(Right)** *Higher magnification shows infiltrating nests ➡, cords, and single small blue cells extending into the deep dermis and surrounding adnexal structures ➡.*

Plasmacytoid Melanoma

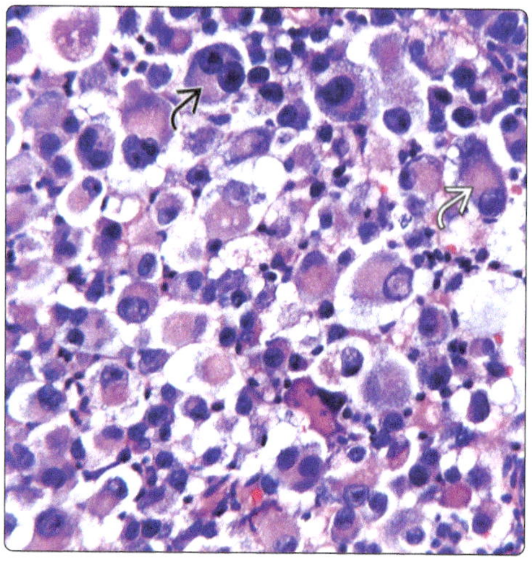

Rhabdoid Melanoma

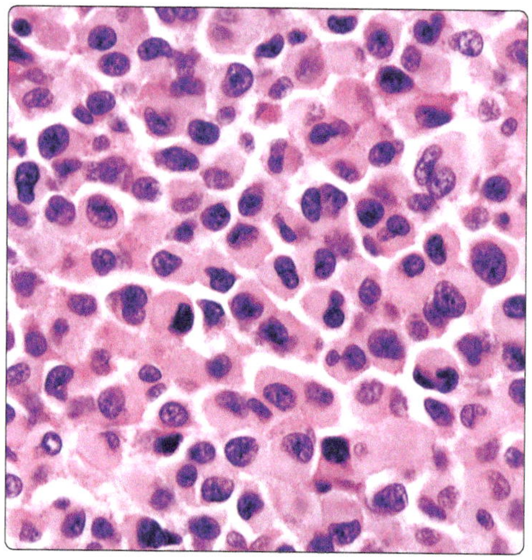

(Left) *Plasmacytoid and rhabdoid-appearing melanoma shows cells with peripherally displaced nuclei and eosinophilic- to pale-staining cytoplasm, focally mimicking the perinuclear hof ➡ of plasma cells. A few binucleated, Reed-Sternberg-like cells are also present ➡.* **(Right)** *Rhabdoid melanoma shows a population of rhabdoid-appearing cells with peripherally displaced nuclei and prominent eosinophilic-staining cytoplasm.*

Myxoid Melanoma With Scattered Nests

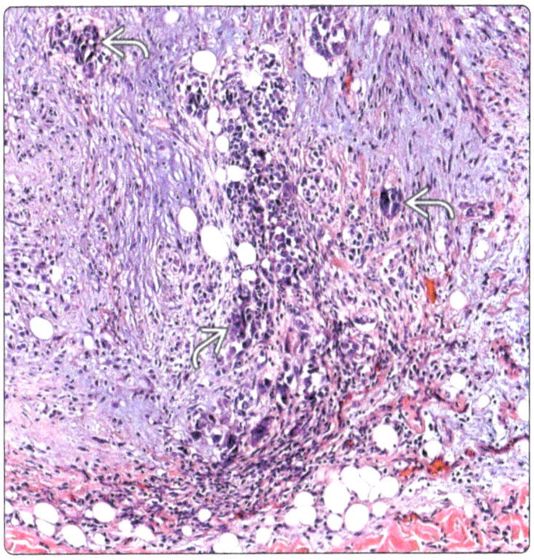

Myxoid Melanoma With Prominent Spindle Cells

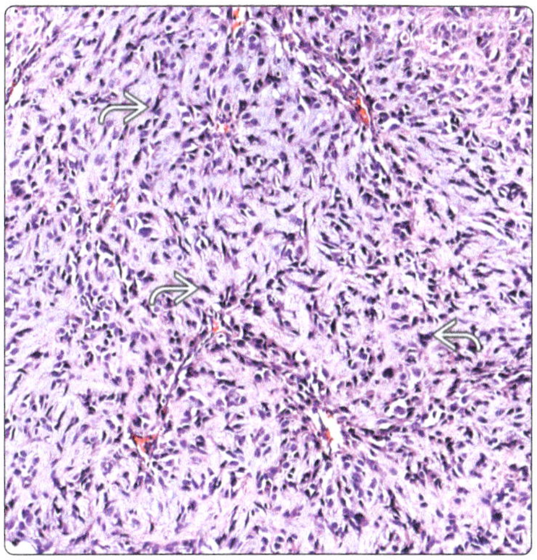

(Left) *Myxoid melanoma at low magnification shows a deeply invasive tumor associated with a very prominent mucinous stroma. However, scattered irregular nests* ➦ *of atypical tumor cells can be identified.* **(Right)** *Myxoid melanoma in another area shows a proliferation of markedly atypical-appearing, hyperchromatic-staining, oval- to spindle-shaped cells* ➦*. These findings mimic a myxoid sarcoma, such as a high-grade myxofibrosarcoma.*

Osteoid Melanoma

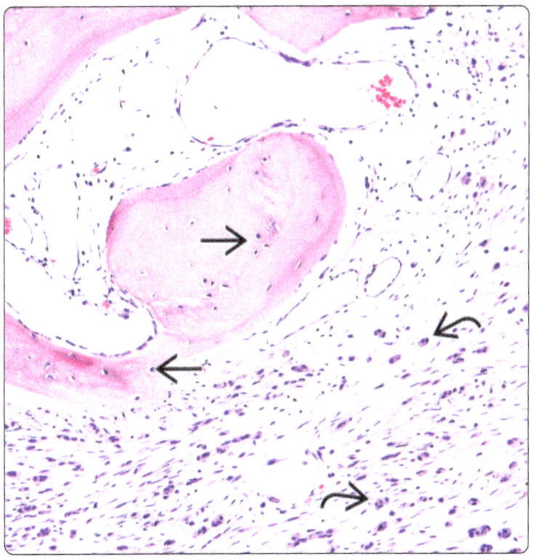

Osseous Melanoma at High Magnification

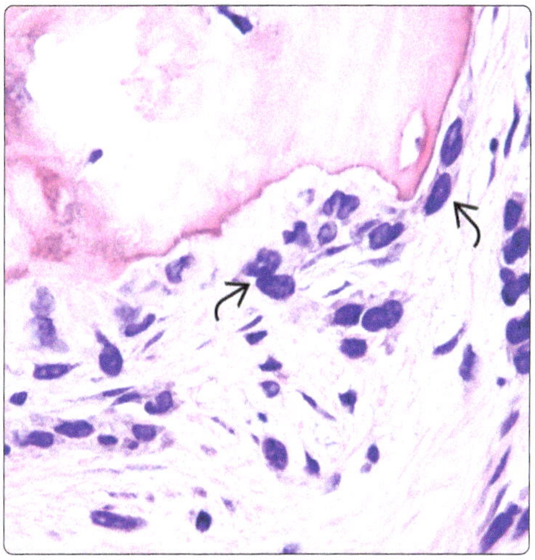

(Left) *Osteoid melanoma shows a focus of ossification with atypical-appearing, oval- to spindle-shaped cells with perinuclear halos* ➡ *embedded in a dense osseous matrix. Note the mixed spindled and epithelioid cell population with focal nests* ➦ *in the surrounding stroma.* **(Right)** *High magnification shows atypical oval to spindled cells* ➦ *with nuclear hyperchromasia adjacent to a focus of ossification.*

Spindle Cell/Pleomorphic Melanoma

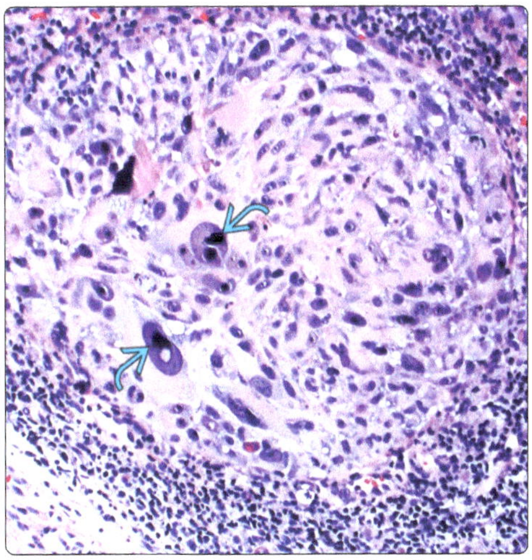

HMB-45 in Spindle Cell/Pleomorphic Melanoma

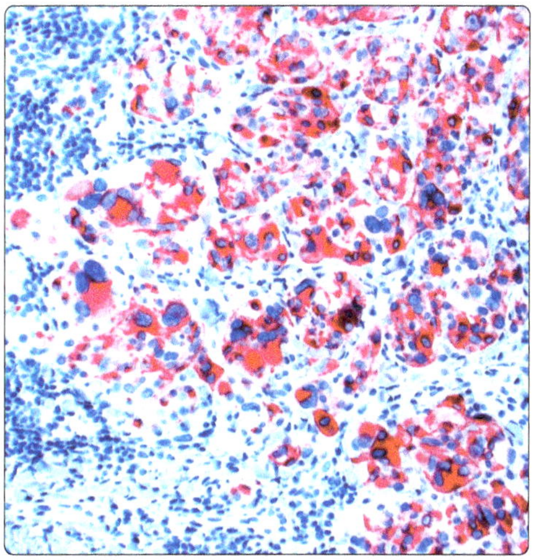

(Left) *This example of spindle cell/pleomorphic melanoma shows markedly atypical and bizarre-appearing tumor cells, many of which have macronucleoli* ➦*.* **(Right)** *HMB-45 (red chromogen) shows strong and diffuse cytoplasmic staining in this case of spindle cell/pleomorphic melanoma.*

TERMINOLOGY

Abbreviations

- Primary tumor (pT), regional lymph nodes (pN), distant metastasis (pM)

Definitions

- **pTX**: Primary tumor cannot be assessed (i.e., partial biopsy or completely regressed melanoma)
- **pT0**: No evidence of primary tumor
- **pTis**: Melanoma in situ (no evidence of invasion)
- **pT1**: Melanoma 1.0 mm or less in thickness
  - pT1a: Melanoma ≤ 1.0 mm, no ulceration, no mitoses
  - pT1b: Melanoma ≤ 1.0 mm, with ulceration &/or mitoses (≥ 1/mm²)
- **pT2**: Melanoma > 1.0 - 2.0 mm in thickness
  - pT2a: Melanoma > 1.0 - 2.0 mm, no ulceration
  - pT2a: Melanoma > 1.0 - 2.0 mm, with ulceration
- **pT3**: Melanoma greater than 2.0-4.0 mm in thickness
  - pT3a: Melanoma > 2.0 - 4.0 mm, no ulceration
  - pT3a: Melanoma > 2.0 - 4.0 mm, with ulceration
- **pT4**: Melanoma greater than 4.0 in thickness
  - pT4a: Melanoma > 4.0 mm, no ulceration
  - pT4a: Melanoma > 4.0 mm, with ulceration
- **pNX**: Regional lymph nodes cannot be assessed
- **pN0**: No regional lymph node metastasis
- **pN1**: Metastasis to 1 regional lymph node
  - pN1a: Clinically occult metastasis (micrometastasis)
  - pN1b: Clinically apparent metastasis (macrometastasis)
- **pN2**: Metastasis in 2-3 regional lymph nodes or intralymphatic regional metastasis without nodal involvement
  - pN2a: Clinically occult metastasis (micrometastasis)
  - pN2b: Clinically apparent metastasis (macrometastasis)
  - pN2c: Satellite or in-transit metastasis without nodal metastases
- **pN3**: Metastasis in 4 or more regional lymph nodes, or matted lymph nodes, or in-transit or satellite metastases with positive regional nodes
- **pM1** (required only if there is confirmed metastasis)
  - pM1a: Metastasis to skin, subcutaneous tissue, or distant lymph node(s)
  - pM1b: Metastasis to lung
  - pM1c: Metastasis to all other visceral sites or distant metastasis associated with elevated serum LDH levels

SELECTED REFERENCES

1. Boland GM et al: Principles of melanoma staging. Cancer Treat Res. 167:131-48, 2016
2. Caldarella A et al: How staging of thin melanoma is changed after the introduction of TNM 7th edition: a population-based analysis. J Cancer Res Clin Oncol. 142(1):73-6, 2016
3. Egger ME et al: Prognostic factors in melanoma patients with tumor-negative sentinel lymph nodes. Surgery. 159(5):1412-21, 2016
4. Gonzalez AB et al: Status of the regional nodal basin remains highly prognostic in melanoma patients with in-transit disease. J Am Coll Surg. ePub, 2016
5. Hafström A et al: Sentinel lymph node biopsy staging for cutaneous malignant melanoma of the head and neck. Acta Otolaryngol. 136(3):312-8, 2016
6. Mahar AL et al: Critical assessment of clinical prognostic tools in melanoma. Ann Surg Oncol. ePub, 2016
7. Bartlett EK et al: Current staging and prognostic factors in melanoma. Surg Oncol Clin N Am. 24(2):215-27, 2015
8. Cheng Y et al: Stage-specific prognostic biomarkers in melanoma. Oncotarget. 6(6):4180-9, 2015
9. Gyorki DE et al: Sentinel lymph node biopsy in T4 melanoma: an important risk-stratification tool. Ann Surg Oncol. ePub, 2015
10. Hieken TJ et al: The effect of the AJCC 7th edition change in T1 melanoma substaging on national utilization and outcomes of sentinel lymph node biopsy for thin melanoma. Melanoma Res. 25(2):157-63, 2015
11. Kyrgidis A et al: Sentinel lymph node biopsy followed by lymph node dissection for localised primary cutaneous melanoma. Cochrane Database Syst Rev. 5:CD010307, 2015
12. Larson AR et al: Impact of the 2009 AJCC staging guidelines for melanoma on the number of mitotic figures reported by dermatopathologists at one institution. J Cutan Pathol. 42(8):536-41, 2015
13. McGregor JM et al: Sentinel node biopsy in cutaneous melanoma: time for consensus to better inform patient choice. Br J Dermatol. 172(3):552-4, 2015
14. Ramos M et al: Completeness of T, N, M and stage grouping for all cancers in the Mallorca Cancer Registry. BMC Cancer. 15:847, 2015
15. Zoras O et al: Uncertainties in the management of melanoma nodal metastasis. Eur J Surg Oncol. 41(7):811-3, 2015
16. Chu VH et al: Impact of the 2009 (7th edition) AJCC melanoma staging system in the classification of thin cutaneous melanomas. Biomed Res Int. 2013:898719, 2013
17. Edge SB, et al: AJCC Cancer Staging Manual. 7th Ed. New York, NY: Springer. 325-344, 2010

Melanoma In Situ (Tis)

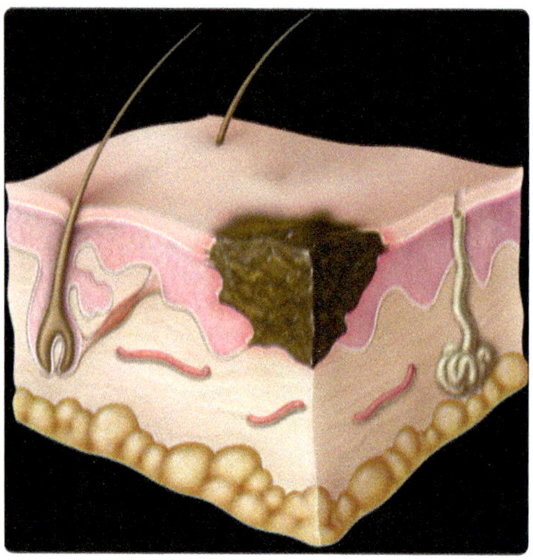

Metastatic Melanoma on PET/CT Scan

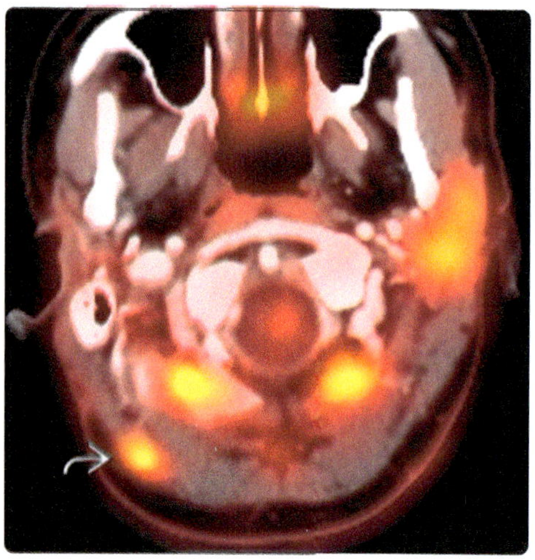

(Left) *Tis melanoma is a melanoma in situ with no evidence of dermal invasion.* **(Right)** *Axial fused PET/CT in a patient with melanoma shows intense FDG activity ➯ in a lesion in the right posterior neck musculature, consistent with metastatic disease (M1a).*

T1a Invasive Melanoma

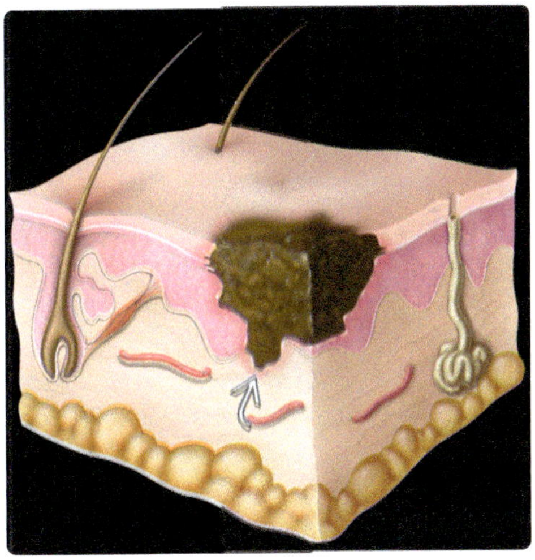

T1b Invasive Melanoma

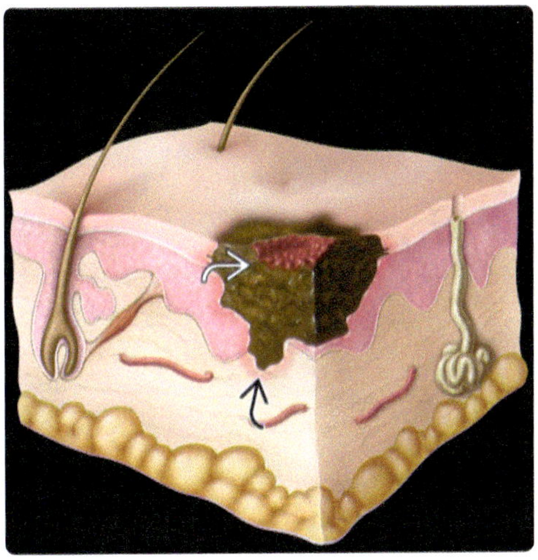

(Left) *T1a invasive melanoma shows a tumor with superficial invasion ≤ 1.0 mm in thickness, without ulceration or evidence of dermal mitotic activity.* **(Right)** *T1b invasive melanoma shows a tumor invasive ≤ 1.0 mm in thickness, with ulceration &/or evidence of dermal mitotic activity (≥ 1/mm²). T1b tumors are clinically more aggressive and have a higher incidence of metastasis than T1a tumors.*

T2a Invasive Melanoma

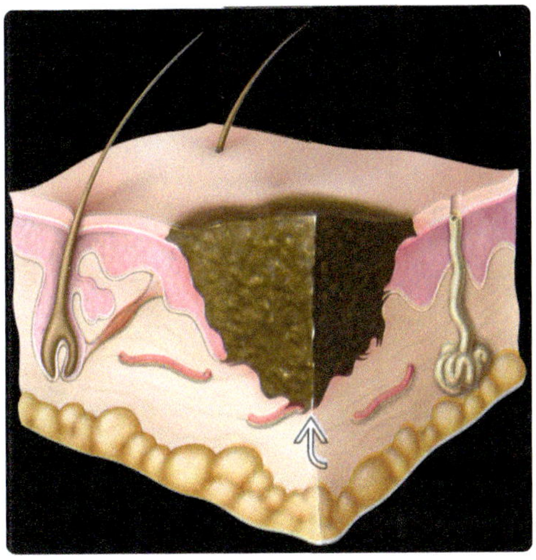

T2b Invasive Melanoma

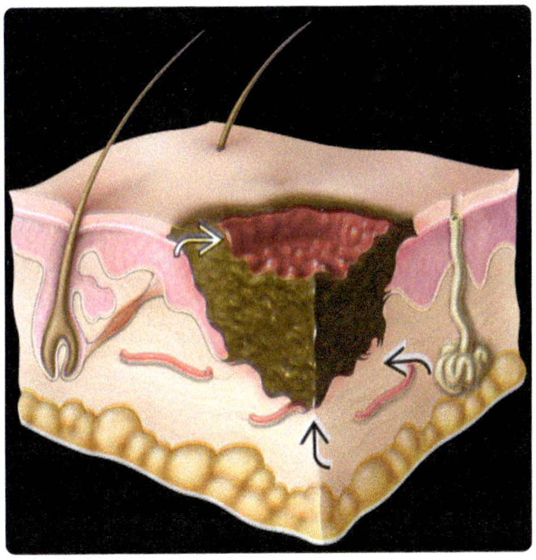

(Left) *T2a melanoma invades to > 1.0 mm in thickness, but is ≤ 2.0 mm in depth, and lacks evidence of ulceration.* **(Right)** *T2b melanoma invades to > 1.0 mm in thickness, but is ≤ 2.0 mm in depth, and shows evidence of ulceration. Ulceration is one of the worst prognostic findings.*

T3a Invasive Melanoma

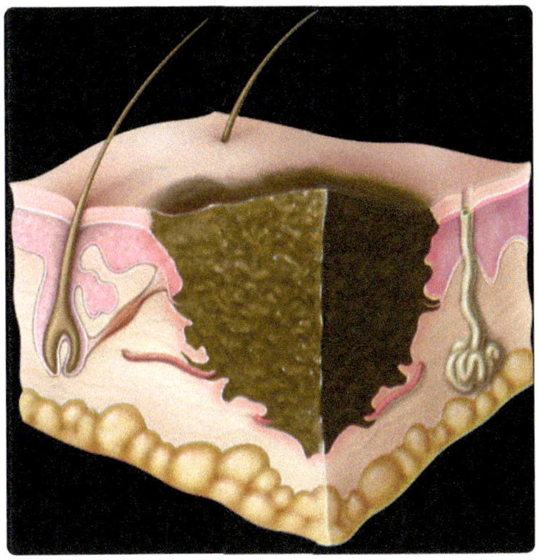

T3b Invasive Melanoma

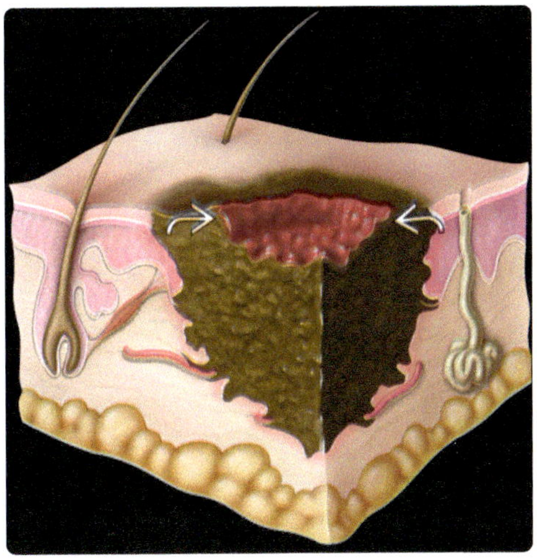

(Left) *T3a melanoma invades to > 2.0 mm in thickness, but is ≤ 4.0 mm in depth, and lacks evidence of ulceration.* **(Right)** *T3b melanoma invades to > 2.0 mm in thickness, but is ≤ 4.0 mm in depth, and shows evidence of ulceration.*

INDEX

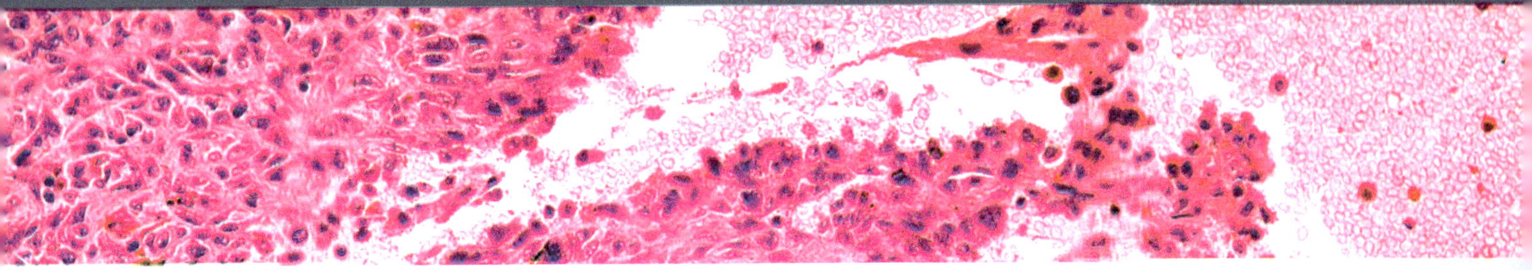

A

INDEX

INDEX

C

INDEX

INDEX

INDEX

D

F

INDEX

INDEX

I

M

INDEX

INDEX

INDEX

O

P

INDEX

INDEX

R

S

U

V

W

X

Z